CURRENT PEDIATRIC DIAGNOSIS & TREATMENT

5TH EDITION

current
PEDIATRIC
DIAGNOSIS
& TREATMENT

By

C. HENRY KEMPE, MD
Professor of Pediatrics and Microbiology
University of Colorado School of Medicine
Denver

HENRY K. SILVER, MD
Professor of Pediatrics
University of Colorado School of Medicine
Denver

DONOUGH O'BRIEN, MD, FRCP
Professor of Pediatrics
University of Colorado School of Medicine
Denver

And Associate Authors

Lange Medical Publications
LOS ALTOS, CALIFORNIA 94022

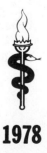

1978

A Concise Medical Library for Practitioner and Student

Current Pediatric Diagnosis & Treatment, 5th ed. $17.00

Current Medical Diagnosis & Treatment 1978 (annual revision). Edited by M.A. Krupp and M.J. Chatton. 1098 pp.   1978

Current Surgical Diagnosis & Treatment, 3rd ed. Edited by J.E. Dunphy and L.W. Way. 1139 pp, *illus.*   1977

Current Obstetric & Gynecologic Diagnosis & Treatment. Edited by R.C. Benson. 911 pp, *illus.*   1976

Review of Physiological Chemistry, 16th ed. H.A. Harper, V.W. Rodwell, and P.A. Mayes. 681 pp, *illus.*   1977

Review of Medical Physiology, 8th ed. W.F. Ganong. 599 pp, *illus.*   1977

Review of Medical Microbiology, 12th ed. E. Jawetz, J.L. Melnick, and E.A. Adelberg. 542 pp, *illus.*   1976

Review of Medical Pharmacology, 5th ed. F.H. Meyers, E. Jawetz, and A. Goldfien. 740 pp, *illus.*   1976

Basic & Clinical Immunology. Edited by H.H. Fudenberg, D.P. Stites, J.L. Caldwell, and J.V. Wells. 653 pp, *illus.*   1976

Basic Histology, 2nd ed. L.C. Junqueira, J. Carneiro, and A.N. Contopoulos. 453 pp, *illus.*   1977

Clinical Cardiology. M. Sokolow and M.B. McIlroy. 659 pp, *illus.*   1977

General Urology, 8th ed. D.R. Smith. 492 pp, *illus.*   1975

General Ophthalmology, 8th ed. D. Vaughan and T. Asbury. 379 pp, *illus.*   1977

Correlative Neuroanatomy & Functional Neurology, 16th ed. J.G. Chusid. 448 pp, *illus.*   1976

Principles of Clinical Electrocardiography, 9th ed. M.J. Goldman. 412 pp, *illus.*   1976

The Nervous System. W.F. Ganong. 226 pp, *illus.*   1977

Handbook of Obstetrics & Gynecology, 6th ed. R.C. Benson. 772 pp, *illus.*   1977

Physician's Handbook, 18th ed. M.A. Krupp, N.J. Sweet, E. Jawetz, E.G. Biglieri, and R.L. Roe. 754 pp, *illus.*   1976

Handbook of Pediatrics, 12th ed. H.K. Silver, C.H. Kempe, and H.B. Bruyn. 723 pp, *illus.*   1977

Handbook of Poisoning: Diagnosis & Treatment, 9th ed. R.H. Dreisbach. 559 pp.   1977

To

Robert J. Glaser, MD

in recognition of his contribution to the growth of the
Department of Pediatrics of the University of Colorado School of Medicine
and in gratitude for his support and encouragement during his years
as Dean of the School of Medicine (1957–1963).

Table of Contents

Preface

The Fifth Edition of this book introduces many changes made necessary by changing concepts or shifts of emphasis in the diagnosis and treatment of pediatric disorders. The chapters on the respiratory tract and mediastinum, orthopedics, developmental problems of childhood, and neoplastic diseases have been completely rewritten, and several new names have been added to the list of contributors. All of the contributors are or have been members of the pediatrics department faculty at University of Colorado Medical Center.

In spite of the many changes, we continue to take aim at the objectives of the First Edition, published in 1970: to be useful without being encyclopedic; to emphasize what is more common and more important, but to include also what is uncommon though still important; to pass on to the student and younger pediatrician the practical bedside tips that are his due from foregoing generations of pediatricians who often worked with little else, but to emphasize also the modern aspects of sophisticated procedure; and to balance our desire to leave nothing pertinent unsaid against the necessity of getting the book done and of a size and at a price with which everyone can be satisfied. Our attempt, as always, is to present the basic principles of diagnosis and treatment along with sufficient detail to cover actual management of a patient in clinical practice, plus important current references to which the reader can turn for more detailed study as the need arises.

We have been most pleased by the acceptance this book has achieved over a wide spectrum of users, including medical students and practitioners, nursing students and nurses, pediatric nurse practitioners, and other health workers.

Translations have been completed in Spanish, Polish, and Serbo-Croatian and will soon be available in Italian and French.

The authors wish to stress that the popular *Handbook of Pediatrics* (Silver, Kempe, & Bruyn) continues to be revised and reissued on alternate years. That book is now in its Twelfth Edition and serves an entirely different purpose.

C. Henry Kempe, MD
Henry K. Silver, MD
Donough O'Brien, MD, FRCP

Denver
March, 1978

Authors

Charles S. August, MD
Disorders of Immune Mechanisms
Associate Professor of Pediatrics, University of Pennsylvania School of Medicine.

Frederick C. Battaglia, MD
The Newborn Infant
Professor and Chairman, Department of Pediatrics, University of Colorado Medical Center.

John G. Brooks, MD
Respiratory Tract & Mediastinum
Assistant Professor of Pediatrics, University of Colorado Medical Center.

John D. Burrington, MD
Emergencies & Accidents
Professor, Department of Surgery, and Chief, Section of Pediatric Surgery, Pritzker School of Medicine, The University of Chicago.

H. Peter Chase, MD
Normal Childhood Nutrition & Its Disorders
Associate Professor of Pediatrics, University of Colorado Medical Center.

Henry E. Cooper, Jr., MD
Adolescence
Associate Professor of Pediatrics and Director of Adolescent Clinic, University of Colorado Medical Center.

Ernest K. Cotton, MD
Respiratory Tract & Mediastinum
Professor of Pediatrics, University of Colorado Medical Center.

Burris R. Duncan, MD
Ambulatory Pediatrics
Associate Professor of Pediatrics, University of Colorado Medical Center.

Robert E. Eilert, MD
Orthopedics
Assistant Clinical Professor of Orthopedic Surgery, University of Colorado Medical Center; Chairman, Department of Orthopedics, The Children's Hospital, Denver.

Jerry J. Eller, MD
Infections: Bacterial & Spirochetal
Associate Professor of Pediatrics and Microbiology and Head, Section of Pediatric Infectious Diseases, The University of Texas Health Science Center, San Antonio.

Philip P. Ellis, MD
Eye
Professor of Surgery and Head, Division of Ophthalmology, University of Colorado Medical Center.

William K. Frankenburg, MD
Development
Associate Professor of Pediatrics, University of Colorado Medical Center.

Vincent A. Fulginiti, MD
Immunization; Infections: Viral & Rickettsial; Infections: Mycotic
Professor and Head, Department of Pediatrics, University of Arizona College of Medicine, Tucson.

John H. Githens, MD
Hematologic Disorders
Professor of Pediatrics, University of Colorado Medical Center.

Stephen I. Goodman, MD
Genetic & Chromosomal Disorders, Including Inborn Errors of Metabolism
Associate Professor of Pediatrics, University of Colorado Medical Center.

Ronald W. Gotlin, MD
Endocrine Disorders; Diagnostic & Therapeutic Procedures
Associate Professor of Pediatrics, University of Colorado Medical Center.

Keith B. Hammond, MS, FIMLT
Interpretation of Biochemical Values
Senior Instructor of Pediatrics and Director, Pediatric Microchemistry Laboratories, University of Colorado Medical Center.

William Hathaway, MD
Hematologic Disorders
Professor of Pediatrics, University of Colorado Medical Center.

Roger Hollister, MD
Immune Complex Diseases
Assistant Professor of Pediatrics, University of Colorado Medical Center; Senior Staff Physician, Department of Pediatrics, National Jewish Hospital and Research Center, Denver.

Charlene P. Holt, MD
Neoplastic Diseases
Mountain States Tumor Institute, Boise, Idaho.

Olof H. Jacobson, DDS
Teeth
Clinical Associate Professor of Dentistry, University of Colorado, School of Dentistry; Chief of Dental Service, The Children's Hospital, Denver.

T. Jacob John, MBBS, MRCP, DCH
Infections: Parasitic
Professor of Microbiology and Chief, Enterovirus Laboratory, Christian Medical College and Hospital, Vellore, Tamil Nadu, India.

Richard B. Johnston, Jr., MD
Disorders of Immune Mechanisms
Professor of Pediatrics, University of Colorado Medical Center; Director, Department of Pediatrics, National Jewish Hospital and Research Center, Denver.

C. Henry Kempe, MD
Fever of Undetermined Origin; Anti-infective Chemotherapeutic Agents & Antibiotic Drugs
Professor of Pediatrics and Microbiology, University of Colorado Medical Center.

Ruth S. Kempe, MD
Personality Development
Assistant Professor in Psychiatry and Pediatrics, University of Colorado Medical Center.

Anthony J. Kisley, MD
Psychosocial Aspects of Pediatrics & Psychiatric Disorders
Assistant Clinical Professor of Psychiatry, University of Colorado Medical Center.

Georgeanna J. Klingensmith, MD
Endocrine Disorders
Assistant Professor of Pediatrics, University of Colorado Medical Center; Chief, Department of Endocrinology and Metabolism, The Children's Hospital, Denver.

Lula O. Lubchenco, MD
Infant Feeding
Professor of Pediatrics and Co-Director, Newborn Service Division of Perinatal Medicine, University of Colorado Medical Center.

Gary M. Lum, MD
Kidney & Urinary Tract
Assistant Professor of Pediatrics and Medicine (Nephrology) and Director of Pediatric Dialysis, University of Colorado Medical Center.

Harold P. Martin, MD
Developmental Problems of Childhood
Associate Professor of Pediatrics, John F. Kennedy Child Development Center, University of Colorado Medical Center.

Rawle M. McIntosh, MD
Kidney & Urinary Tract
Professor of Pediatrics, University of Colorado Medical Center.

Ida Nakashima, MD
Adolescence
Assistant Director, Adolescent Clinic, University of Colorado Medical Center.

Gerhard Nellhaus, MD
Neurologic & Muscular Disorders
Associate Clinical Professor of Pediatrics and Neurology, University of Colorado Medical Center.

James J. Nora, MD
Cardiovascular Diseases
Professor of Pediatrics and Director of Pediatric Cardiology, University of Colorado Medical Center.

Donough O'Brien, MD, FRCP
Normal Childhood Nutrition & Its Disorders; Kidney & Urinary Tract; Immune Complex Diseases; Diabetes Mellitus; Genetic & Chromosomal Disorders, Including Inborn Errors of Metabolism; Fluid & Electrolyte Therapy; Interpretation of Biochemical Values
Professor of Pediatrics, University of Colorado Medical Center.

William H. Parry, MD
Respiratory Tract & Mediastinum
Assistant Clinical Professor of Pediatrics, University of Colorado Medical Center.

David S. Pearlman, MD
Allergic Disorders
Associate Clinical Professor of Pediatrics, University of Colorado Medical Center; Attending Allergist, Division of Pediatric Clinical Immunology, National Jewish Hospital and Research Center, Denver.

Robert G. Peterson, MD, PhD
Drug Therapy
Assistant Professor of Pediatrics and Pharmacology, University of Colorado Medical Center.

LTC Richard O. Proctor, MD, MPH&TM, FAAP
Infections: Parasitic
Clinical Associate Professor of Pediatrics, The University of Texas Health Science Center, San Antonio.

Dane G. Prugh, MD
Psychosocial Aspects of Pediatrics & Psychiatric Disorders
Professor of Psychiatry and Pediatrics, University of Colorado Medical Center.

Arthur Robinson, MD
Genetic & Chromosomal Disorders, Including Inborn Errors of Metabolism
Professor and Chairman, Department of Biophysics and Genetics, University of Colorado Medical Center; Chief of Professional Services, National Jewish Hospital and Research Center, Denver.

Claude C. Roy, MD
Gastrointestinal Tract; Liver & Pancreas
Professor of Pediatrics, Hospital Ste. Justine, University of Montreal.

Barry H. Rumack, MD
Poisoning; Drug Therapy
Assistant Professor of Pediatrics and Medicine, University of Colorado Medical Center; Director, Rocky Mountain Poison Center, Denver General Hospital.

Barton D. Schmitt, MD
Ambulatory Pediatrics; Ear, Nose, & Throat; Battered Child Syndrome
Associate Professor of Pediatrics, University of Colorado Medical Center.

Henry K. Silver, MD
History & Physical Examination; Growth & Development; Endocrine Disorders; Diagnostic & Therapeutic Procedures; Drug Therapy
Professor of Pediatrics, University of Colorado Medical Center.

Arnold Silverman, MD
Gastrointestinal Tract; Liver & Pancreas
Associate Professor of Pediatrics, University of Colorado Medical Center; Director of Pediatrics, Denver General Hospital.

James K. Todd, MD
Urinary Tract Infections
Assistant Professor of Pediatrics, University of Colorado Medical Center.

David G. Tubergen, MD
Neoplastic Diseases
Associate Professor of Pediatrics, University of Colorado Medical Center; Director, Pediatric Oncology, The Children's Hospital, Denver.

William L. Weston, MD
Skin
Assistant Professor of Medicine (Dermatology) and Pediatrics, University of Colorado Medical Center.

Robert R. Wolfe, MD
Cardiovascular Diseases
Assistant Professor of Pediatrics, University of Colorado Medical Center.

Anne S. Yeager, MD
Anti-infective Chemotherapeutic Agents & Antibiotic Drugs
Assistant Professor of Pediatric Infectious Diseases, Stanford University Medical Center.

1...

History & Physical Examination

Henry K. Silver, MD

HISTORY

General Considerations in Taking the History

For many pediatric problems, the history is the most important single factor in making a proper assessment.

A. Interpretation of History: The presenting complaint as given by the informant may be a minor part of the problem. One should be prepared to go on, if necessary, to a more productive phase of the interview, which may have little or no apparent relationship to the complaint as originally presented.

B. Source of History: The history should be obtained from the mother or from whoever is responsible for the care of the child. Much valuable information can be obtained also from the child.

C. Direction of Questioning: Allow the informant to present the problem as she sees it; then fill in with necessary past and family history and other pertinent information. The record should also include whatever may be disclosed concerning the parents' temperaments, attitudes, and methods of rearing children.

Questions should not be prying, especially about subjects likely to be associated with feelings of guilt or shame; however, the informant should be allowed to volunteer information of this nature when she is prepared to do so.

D. Recorded History: The history should be a detailed, clear, and chronologic record of significant information. It should include the parents' interpretation of the present difficulty and should indicate the results they expect from consultation.

E. Psychotherapeutic Effects: In many cases the interview and history-taking is the first stage in the psychotherapeutic management of the patient and the parents.

HISTORY OUTLINE: GENERAL

The following outline should be modified and adapted as appropriate for the age and sex of the child and the reason for the visit to the physician:

Name, address, home phone number, sex, date and place of birth, race, religion, nationality, referred by, father's and mother's names, father's and mother's occupations, business telephone numbers.

Date: _____ Hospital or case number: _____

Previous entries: Dates, diagnoses, therapy, other data.

Summary of correspondence or other information from physicians, schools, etc.

Presenting Complaint (PC)

Patient's or parent's own brief account of the complaint and its duration.

Present Illness (PI) (or Interval History)

When was the patient last entirely well?

How and when did the disturbance start?

Health immediately before the illness.

Progress of disease; order and date of onset of new symptoms.

Specific symptoms and physical signs that may have developed.

Pertinent negative data obtained by direct questioning.

Aggravating and alleviating factors.

Significant medical attention and medications given and over what period.

In acute infections, statement of type and degree of exposure and interval since exposure.

For the well child, determine factors of significance and general condition since last visit.

Examiner's opinion about the reliability of the informant.

Previous Health

A. Antenatal: Health of mother during pregnancy. Medical supervision, diet, infections such as rubella, etc, other illnesses, vomiting, preeclampsia-eclampsia, other complications; Rh typing and serology, pelvimetry, medications, x-ray procedure.

B. Natal: Duration of pregnancy, birth weight, kind and duration of labor, type of delivery, sedation and anesthesia (if known), state of infant at birth, resuscitation required, onset of respiration, first cry.

C. Neonatal: Apgar score; color, cyanosis, pallor, jaundice, cry, twitchings, excessive mucus, paralysis, convulsions, fever, hemorrhage, congenital abnormalities, birth injury. Difficulty in sucking, rashes, excessive weight loss, feeding difficulties.

Development

(1) First raised head, rolled over, sat alone, pulled up, walked with help, walked alone, talked (meaningful words; sentences).

(2) Urinary continence during night; during day.

(3) Control of feces.

(4) Comparison of development with that of siblings and parents.

(5) Any period of failure to grow or unusual growth.

(6) School grade, quality of work.

Nutrition

A. Breast or Formula: Type, duration, major formula changes, time of weaning, difficulties.

B. Vitamin Supplements: Type, when started, amount, duration.

C. "Solid" Foods: When introduced, how taken, types.

D. Appetite: Food likes and dislikes, idiosyncrasies or allergies, reaction of child to eating.

Illnesses

A. Infections: Age, types, number, severity.

B. Contagious Diseases: Age, complications following measles, rubella, chickenpox, mumps, pertussis, diphtheria, scarlet fever.

C. Others.

Immunization & Tests

Indicate type, number, reactions, age of child.

A. Inoculations: Diphtheria, tetanus, pertussis, measles, poliomyelitis, typhoid, mumps, others.

B. Oral Immunizations: Poliomyelitis.

C. Percutaneous Vaccination: Smallpox. ("Take" or not? Scar?)

D. Recall immunizations ("boosters").

E. Serum Injections: Passive immunizations.

F. Tests: Tuberculin, Schick, serology, others.

Operations

Type, age, complications; reasons for operations; apparent response of child.

Accidents & Injuries

Nature, severity, sequelae.

Family History

(1) Father and mother (age and condition of health). What sort of people do the parents characterize themselves as being?

(2) Marital relationships. Little information should be sought at first interview; most information will be obtained indirectly.

(3) Siblings. Age, condition of health, significant previous illnesses and problems.

(4) Stillbirths, miscarriages, abortions; age at death and cause of death of immediate members of family.

(5) Tuberculosis, allergy, blood dyscrasias, mental or nervous diseases, diabetes, cardiovascular diseases, kidney disease, rheumatic fever, neoplastic diseases, congenital abnormalities, cancer, convulsive disorders, others.

(6) Health of contacts.

Personality History

A. Relations With Other Children: Independent or clinging to mother; negativistic, shy, submissive; separation from parents; hobbies; easy or difficult to get along with. How does child relate to others? Physical deformities affecting personality.

B. School Progress: Class, grades, nursery school, special aptitudes, reaction to school.

Social History

A. Family: Income; home (size, number of rooms, living conditions, sleeping facilities), type of neighborhood, access to playground. Localities in which patient has lived. Who cares for patient if mother works?

B. School: Public or private, overcrowded, type of students.

C. Insurance: Blue Cross, Blue Shield, or other health insurance?

Habits

A. Eating: Appetite, food dislikes, how fed, attitudes of child and parents to eating.

B. Sleeping: Hours, disturbances, snoring, restlessness, dreaming, nightmares.

C. Exercise and play.

D. Urinary, bowel.

E. Disturbances: Excessive bedwetting, masturbation, thumbsucking, nailbiting, breath-holding, temper tantrums, tics, nervousness, undue thirst, others. Similar disturbances among members of family.

System Review

A. Ears, Nose, and Throat: Frequent colds, sore throat, sneezing, stuffy nose, discharge, postnasal drip, mouth breathing, snoring, otitis, hearing, adenitis.

B. Teeth: Age of eruption of deciduous and permanent; number at 1 year; comparison with siblings.

C. Cardiorespiratory: Frequency and nature of disturbances. Dyspnea, chest pain, cough, sputum, wheeze, expectoration, cyanosis, edema, syncope, tachycardia.

D. Gastrointestinal: Vomiting, diarrhea, constipation, type of stools, abdominal pain or discomfort, jaundice.

E. Genitourinary: Enuresis, dysuria, frequency, polyuria, pyuria, hematuria, character of stream, vaginal discharge, menstrual history, bladder control, abnormalities of penis or testes.

F. Neuromuscular: Headache, nervousness, dizziness, tingling, convulsions, habit spasms, ataxia, muscle or joint pains, postural deformities, exercise tolerance, gait.

G. Endocrine: Disturbances of growth, excessive fluid intake, polyphagia, goiter, thyroid disease.

H. Special senses.

I. General: Unusual weight gain or loss, fatigue, skin color or texture, other abnormalities of skin, temperature sensitivity, mentality. Pattern of growth (record previous heights and weights on appropriate graphs). Time and pattern of pubescence.

The Health Record

Every patient should have a comprehensive medical and health record containing all pertinent information. The parents should be given a summary of this record (including data regarding illnesses, operations, idiosyncrasies, sensitivities, heights, weights, special medications, and immunizations).

PHYSICAL EXAMINATION

Every child should receive a complete systematic examination at regular intervals. One should not restrict the examination to those portions of the body considered to be involved on the basis of the presenting complaint.

Approaching the Child

Adequate time should be spent in allowing the child and the examiner to become acquainted. The child should be treated as an individual whose feelings and sensibilities are well developed, and the examiner's conduct should be appropriate to the age of the child. A friendly manner, quiet voice, and a slow and easy approach will help to facilitate the examination. If the examiner is not able to establish a friendly relationship but feels that it is important to proceed with the examination, it should be done in an orderly, systematic manner in the hope that the child will then accept the inevitable.

The examiner's hands should be washed in warm water before examining the child and the hands should be warm.

Observation of Patient

Although the very young child may not be able to speak, one still may receive much information by being observant and receptive. The total evaluation of the child should include impressions obtained from the time the child first enters, ie, it should not be based solely on the period during which the patient is on the examining table. In general, more information is obtained by careful inspection than from any of the other methods of examination.

Holding for Examination

A. Before Age 6 Months: The examining table is usually well tolerated.

B. Age 6 Months to 3–4 Years: Most of the examination may be performed while the child is held in the mother's lap or over her shoulder. Certain parts of the examination can sometimes be done more easily with the child in the prone position or held against the mother so that the child does not see the examiner.

Removal of Clothing

Clothes should be removed gradually to prevent chilling and to avoid the development of resistance in a shy child. In order to save time and to avoid creating unpleasant associations with the doctor in the child's mind, undressing the child and taking the temperature are best performed by the mother. The physician should respect the marked degree of modesty that may be exhibited by some children.

Sequence of Examination

In most cases it is best to begin the examination of the young child with an area that is least likely to be associated with pain or discomfort. The ears and throat should usually be examined last. The examiner should develop a regular sequence of examination that can be adapted as required by special circumstances.

Painful Procedures

Before performing a disagreeable, painful, or upsetting examination, the examiner should tell the child (1) what is likely to happen and how the child can assist, (2) that the examination is necessary, and (3) that it will be performed as rapidly and as painlessly as possible.

GENERAL PHYSICAL EXAMINATION
(See also Chapter 2.)

Temperature, pulse rate, and respiratory rate (TPR); blood pressure, weight, and height. The weight should be recorded at each visit; the height should be determined at monthly intervals during the first year, at 3-month intervals in the second year, and twice a year thereafter. The height, weight, and head circumference of the child should be compared with standard charts and the approximate percentiles recorded. Multiple measurements at intervals are of much greater value than single ones since they give information regarding the pattern of growth that cannot be determined by single measurements.

Rectal Temperatures

During the first years of life the temperature should be taken by rectum (except for routine temperatures of the premature infant, where axillary temperatures are sufficiently accurate). The child should be laid face down across the mother's lap and held firmly with her left forearm placed flat across the child's back; with the left thumb and index finger, she can separate the buttocks and insert the lubricated thermometer with the right hand.

Rectal temperature may be 1° F higher than oral temperature. A rectal temperature up to 37.8° C (100° F) may be considered normal in a child.

Apprehension and activity may elevate the temperature.

General Appearance

Does the child appear well or ill? Degree of prostration; degree of cooperation; state of comfort, nutrition, and consciousness; abnormalities; gait, posture, and coordination; estimate of intelligence; reaction to parents, physician, and examination; nature of cry and degree of activity; facies and facial expression.

Skin

Color (cyanosis, jaundice, pallor, erythema), texture, eruptions, hydration; edema, hemorrhagic manifestations, scars, dilated vessels and direction of blood flow, hemangiomas, café-au-lait areas and nevi, mongolian (blue-black) spots, pigmentation, turgor, elasticity, and subcutaneous nodules. Striae and wrinkling may indicate rapid weight gain or loss. Sensitivity, hair distribution and character, and desquamation.

Practical notes:

(1) Loss of turgor, especially of the calf muscles and skin over the abdomen, is evidence of dehydration.

(2) The soles and palms are often bluish and cold in early infancy; this is of no significance.

(3) The degree of anemia cannot be determined reliably by inspection, since pallor (even in the newborn) may be normal and not due to anemia.

(4) To demonstrate pitting edema in a child it may be necessary to exert prolonged pressure.

(5) A few small pigmented nevi are commonly found, particularly in older children.

(6) Spider nevi occur in about one-sixth of children under 5 years of age and almost half of older children.

(7) "Mongolian spots" (large, flat black or blue-black areas) are frequently present over the lower back and buttocks; they have no pathologic significance.

(8) Cyanosis will not be evident unless at least 5 gm of reduced hemoglobin are present; therefore, it develops less easily in an anemic child.

(9) Carotenemic pigmentation is usually most prominent over the palms and soles and around the nose, and spares the conjunctiva.

Lymph Nodes

Location, size, sensitivity, mobility, consistency. One should routinely attempt to palpate suboccipital, preauricular, anterior cervical, posterior cervical, submaxillary, sublingual, axillary, epitrochlear, and inguinal lymph nodes.

Practical notes:

(1) Enlargement of the lymph nodes occurs much more readily in children than in adults.

(2) Small inguinal lymph nodes are palpable in almost all healthy young children. Small, mobile, nontender shotty nodes are commonly found as residua of previous infection.

Head

Size, shape, circumference, asymmetry, cephalhematoma, bosses, craniotabes, control, molding, bruit, fontanel (size, tension, number, abnormally late or early closure), sutures, dilated veins, scalp, hair (texture, distribution, parasites), face, transillumination.

Practical notes:

(1) The head is measured at its greatest circumference; this is usually at the midforehead anteriorly and around to the most prominent portion of the occiput posteriorly. The ratio of head circumference to circumference of the chest or abdomen is usually of little value.

(2) Fontanel tension is best determined with the quiet child in the sitting position.

(3) Slight pulsations over the anterior fontanel may occur in normal infants.

(4) Although bruits may be heard over the temporal areas in normal children, the possibility of an existing abnormality should not be overlooked.

(5) Craniotabes may be found in the normal newborn infant (especially the premature) and for the first 2–4 months.

(6) A positive Macewen's sign ("cracked pot" sound when skull is percussed with one finger) may be present normally as long as the fontanel is open.

(7) Transillumination of the skull can be performed by means of a flashlight with a sponge rubber collar so that it forms a tight fit when held against the head.

Face

Symmetry, paralysis, distance between nose and mouth, depth of nasolabial folds, bridge of nose, distribution of hair, size of mandible, swellings, hypertelorism, Chvostek's sign, tenderness over sinuses.

Eyes

Photophobia, visual acuity, muscular control, nystagmus, mongolian slant, Brushfield spots, epicanthic folds, lacrimation, discharge, lids, exophthalmos or enophthalmos, conjunctiva; pupillary size, shape, and reaction to light and accommodation; media (corneal opacities, cataracts), fundi, visual fields (in older children).

Practical notes:

(1) The newborn infant usually will open his or her eyes if placed prone, supported with one hand on the abdomen, and lifted over the examiner's head.

(2) Not infrequently, one pupil is normally larger than the other. This sometimes occurs only in bright or in subdued light.

(3) Examination of the fundi should be part of every complete physical examination, regardless of the age of the child; dilatation of pupils may be necessary for adequate visualization.

(4) A mild degree of strabismus may be present during the first 6 months of life but should be considered abnormal after that time.

(5) To test for strabismus in the very young or uncooperative child, note where a distant source of

light is reflected from the surface of the eyes; the reflection should be present on corresponding portions of the 2 eyes.

(6) Small areas of capillary dilatation are commonly seen on the eyelids of normal newborn infants.

(7) Most infants produce visible tears during the first few days of life.

Nose

Exterior, shape, mucosa, patency, discharge, bleeding, pressure over sinuses, flaring of nostrils, septum.

Mouth

Lips (thinness, downturning, fissures, color, cleft), teeth (number, position, caries, mottling, discoloration, notching, malocclusion or malalignment), mucosa (color, redness of Stensen's duct, enanthems, Bohn's nodules, Epstein's pearls), gums, palate, tongue, uvula, mouth breathing, geographic tongue (usually normal).

Practical note: If the tongue can be extended as far as the alveolar ridge, there will be no interference with nursing or speaking.

Throat

Tonsils (size, inflammation, exudate, crypts, inflammation of the anterior pillars), mucosa, hypertrophic lymphoid tissue, postnasal drip, epiglottis, voice (hoarseness, stridor, grunting, type of cry, speech).

Practical notes:

(1) Before examining a child's throat it is advisable to examine the mouth first. Permit the child to handle the tongue blade, nasal speculum, and flashlight in order to overcome fear of the instruments. Then ask the child to stick out his or her tongue and say "Ah," louder and louder. In some cases this may allow an adequate examination. In others, a cooperative child may be asked to "pant like a puppy"; during this time, the tongue blade is applied firmly to the rear of the tongue. Gagging need not be elicited in order to obtain a satisfactory examination. In still other cases, it may be expedient to examine one side of the tongue at a time, pushing the base of the tongue to one side and then to the other. This may be less unpleasant and is less apt to cause gagging.

(2) Young children may have to be restrained to obtain an adequate examination of the throat. Eliciting a gag reflex may be necessary if the oral pharynx is to be adequately seen.

(3) The small child's head may be restrained satisfactorily by having the mother place her hands at the level of the child's elbows while the arms are held firmly against the sides of the child's head.

(4) If the child can sit up, the mother is asked to hold the child erect in her lap with his or her back against her chest. She then holds the child's left hand in her left hand and the child's right hand in her right hand and places them against the child's groin or lower thighs to prevent the child from slipping down from her lap. If the throat is to be examined in natural light,

the mother faces the light. If artificial light and a head mirror are used, the mother sits with her back to the light. In either case, the physician uses one hand to hold the head in position and the other to manipulate the tongue blade.

(5) Young children seldom complain of sore throat even in the presence of significant infection of the pharynx and tonsils.

Ears

Pinnas (position, size), canals, tympanic membranes (landmarks, mobility, perforation, inflammation, discharge), mastoid tenderness and swelling, hearing.

Practical notes:

(1) A test for hearing is an important part of the physical examination of every infant.

(2) Examine the ears of all sick children.

(3) Before actually examining the ears, it is often helpful to place the speculum just within the canal, remove it and place it lightly in the other ear, remove it again, and proceed in this way from one ear to the other, gradually going farther and farther, until a satisfactory examination is completed.

(4) In examining the ears, as large a speculum as possible should be used and should be inserted no farther than necessary, both to avoid discomfort and to avoid pushing wax in front of the speculum so that it obscures the field. The otoscope should be held balanced in the hand by holding the handle at the end nearest the speculum. One finger should rest against the head to prevent injury resulting from sudden movement by the child.

(5) The child may be restrained most easily while lying on the abdomen.

(6) Low-set ears are present in a number of congenital syndromes, including several that are associated with mental retardation. The ears may be considered low-set if they are below a line drawn from the lateral angle of the eye to the external occipital protuberance.

(7) Congenital anomalies of the urinary tract are frequently associated with abnormalities of the pinnas.

(8) To examine the ears of an infant, it is usually necessary to pull the auricle backward and downward; in the older child, the external ear is pulled backward and upward.

Neck

Position (torticollis, opisthotonos, inability to support head, mobility), swelling, thyroid (size, contour, bruit, isthmus, nodules, tenderness), lymph nodes, veins, position of trachea, sternocleidomastoid (swelling, shortening), webbing, edema, auscultation, movement, tonic neck reflex.

Practical note: In the older child, the size and shape of the thyroid gland may be more clearly defined if the gland is palpated from behind.

Thorax

Shape and symmetry, veins, retractions and pulsations, beading, Harrison's groove, flaring of ribs, pigeon breast, funnel shape, size and position of nipples, breasts, length of sternum, intercostal and substernal retraction, asymmetry, scapulas, clavicles.

Practical note: At puberty, in normal children, one breast usually begins to develop before the other. In both sexes, tenderness of the breasts is relatively common. Gynecomastia is not uncommon in boys.

Lungs

Type of breathing, dyspnea, prolongation of expiration, cough, expansion, fremitus, flatness or dullness to percussion, resonance, breath and voice sounds, rales, wheezing.

Practical notes:

(1) Breath sounds in infants and children normally are more intense and more bronchial, and expiration is more prolonged, than in adults.

(2) Most of the young child's respiratory movement is produced by abdominal movement; there is very little intercostal motion.

(3) If one places the stethoscope over the mouth and subtracts the sounds heard by this route from the sounds heard through the chest wall, the difference usually represents the amount produced intrathoracically.

Heart

Location and intensity of apex beat, precordial bulging, pulsation of vessels, thrills, size, shape, auscultation (rate, rhythm, force, quality of sounds—compare with pulse as to rate and rhythm; friction rub—variation with pressure), murmurs (location, position in cycle, intensity, pitch, effect of change of position, transmission, effect of exercise).

Practical notes:

(1) Many children normally have sinus arrhythmia. The child should be asked to take a deep breath to determine its effect on the rhythm.

(2) Extrasystoles are not uncommon in childhood.

(3) The heart should be examined with the child erect, recumbent, and turned to the left.

Abdomen

Size and contour, visible peristalsis, respiratory movements, veins (distention, direction of flow), umbilicus, hernia, musculature, tenderness and rigidity, tympany, shifting dullness, tenderness, rebound tenderness, pulsation, palpable organs or masses (size, shape, position, mobility), fluid wave, reflexes, femoral pulsations, bowel sounds.

Practical notes:

(1) The abdomen may be examined while the child is lying prone in the mother's lap or held over her shoulder, or seated on the examining table with the back to the doctor. These positions may be particularly helpful where tenderness, rigidity, or a mass must be palpated. In the infant the examination may be aided by having the child suck at a "sugar tip" or nurse at a bottle.

(2) Light palpation, especially for the spleen, often will give more information than deep.

(3) Umbilical hernias are common during the first 2 years of life. They usually disappear spontaneously.

Male Genitalia

Circumcision, meatal opening, hypospadias, phimosis, adherent foreskin, size of testes, cryptorchidism, scrotum, hydrocele, hernia, pubertal changes.

Practical notes:

(1) In examining a suspected case of cryptorchidism, palpation for the testicles should be done before the child has fully undressed or become chilled or had the cremasteric reflex stimulated. In some cases, examination while the child is in a hot bath may be helpful. The boy should also be examined while sitting in a chair holding his knees with his heels on the seat; the increased intra-abdominal pressure may push the testes into the scrotum.

(2) To examine for cryptorchidism, start above the inguinal canal and work downward to prevent pushing the testes up into the canal or abdomen.

(3) In the obese boy, the penis may be so obscured by fat as to appear abnormally small. If this fat is pushed back, a penis of normal size is usually found.

Female Genitalia

Vagina (imperforate, discharge, adhesions), hypertrophy of clitoris, pubertal changes.

Practical note: Digital or speculum examination is rarely done until after puberty.

Rectum & Anus

Irritation, fissures, prolapse, imperforate anus. The rectal examination should be performed with the little finger (inserted slowly). Note muscle tone, character of stool, masses, tenderness, sensation. Examine stool on glove finger (gross, microscopic, culture, guaiac) as indicated.

Extremities

A. General: Deformity, hemiatrophy, bowlegs (common in infancy), knock-knees (common after age 2), paralysis, edema, coldness, posture, gait, stance, asymmetry.

B. Joints: Swelling, redness, pain, limitation, tenderness, motion, rheumatic nodules, carrying angle of elbows, tibial torsion.

C. Hands and Feet: Extra digits, clubbing, simian lines, curvature of little finger, deformity of nails, splinter hemorrhages, flat feet (feet commonly appear flat during first 2 years), abnormalities of feet, dermatoglyphics, width of thumbs and big toes, syndactyly, length of various segments, dimpling of dorsa, temperature.

D. Peripheral Vessels: Presence, absence, or diminution of arterial pulses.

Spine & Back

Posture, curvatures, rigidity, webbed neck, spina bifida, pilonidal dimple or cyst, tufts of hair, mobility, mongolian spot; tenderness over spine, pelvis, or kidneys.

Neurologic Examination (After Vazuka.)

A. Cerebral Function: General behavior, level of consciousness, intelligence, emotional status, memory, orientation, illusions, hallucinations, cortical sensory interpretation, cortical motor integration, ability to understand and communicate, auditory-verbal and visual-verbal comprehension, recognition of visual object, speech, ability to write, performance of skilled motor acts.

B. Cranial Nerves:

1. I (olfactory)—Identify odors; disorders of smell.

2. II (optic)—Distant and near visual acuity, visual fields, ophthalmoscopic examination, retina.

3. III (oculomotor), IV (trochlear), and VI (abducens)—Ocular movements, strabismus, ptosis, dilatation of pupil, nystagmus, pupillary accommodation, and pupillary light reflexes.

4. V (trigeminal)—Sensation of face, corneal reflex, masseter and temporal muscles, maxillary reflex (jaw jerk).

5. VII (facial)—Wrinkle forehead, frown, smile, raise eyebrows, asymmetry of face, strength of eyelid muscles, taste on anterior portion of tongue.

6. VIII (acoustic)—

a. Cochlear portion—Hearing, lateralization, air and bone conduction, tinnitus.

b. Vestibular—Caloric tests.

7. IX (glossopharyngeal), X (vagus)—Pharyngeal gag reflex, ability to swallow and speak clearly; sensation of mucosa of pharynx, soft palate, and tonsils; movement of pharynx, larynx, and soft palate; autonomic functions.

8. XI (accessory)—Strength of trapezius and sternocleidomastoid muscles.

9. XII (hypoglossal)—Protrusion of tongue, tremor, strength of tongue.

C. Cerebellar Function: Finger to nose; finger to examiner's finger; rapidly alternating pronation and supination of hands; ability to run heel down other shin and to make a requested motion with foot; ability to stand with eyes closed; walk; heel to toe walk; tremor; ataxia; posture; arm swing when walking; nystagmus; abnormalities of muscle tone or speech.

D. Motor System: Muscle size, consistency, and tone; muscle contours and outlines; muscle strength; myotonic contraction; slow relaxation; symmetry of posture; fasciculations; tremor; resistance to passive movement; involuntary movement.

E. Reflexes:

1. Deep reflexes— Biceps, brachioradialis, triceps, patellar, Achilles; rapidity and strength of contraction and relaxation.

2. Superficial reflexes—Abdominals, cremasteric, plantar, gluteal.

3. Pathologic reflexes—Babinski, Chaddock, Oppenheim, Gordon.

● ● ●

General References

Barness LA: *Manual of Pediatric Physical Diagnosis,* 4th ed. Year Book, 1972.

Frankenburg W & others: *Denver Developmental Screening Test Reference Manual,* revised 1975 ed. LADOCA Project & Publishing Foundation, 1975.

Judge RD, Zuidema GD (editors): *Physical Diagnosis: A Physiologic Approach to the Clinical Examination,* 2nd ed. Little, Brown, 1968.

Morgan WL, Engel GL: *The Clinical Approach to the Patient.* Saunders, 1969.

Richmond JB, Green M: *Pediatric Diagnosis,* 2nd ed. Saunders, 1962.

2...
Growth & Development*

Henry K. Silver, MD

Body measurements and developmental landmarks provide the best and most practical means of evaluating the health of the individual child because physical growth and developmental sequence follow a relatively smooth and clearly defined pattern. Growth and development generally progress along expected lines only when the functions of the individual are successfully integrated into a working whole. Failure of the individual to conform to the expected human pattern is completely nonspecific in etiologic terms, since it may equally well result from malnutrition, genetic deficiency, psychologic maladaptation, protracted illness, or a number of other causes. The physician, alerted by disturbances in growth, needs to seek out the specific causes.

Physical or psychologic growth and development generally have a smooth pattern of progression, but some deviation from this pattern is to be expected. The variation between racial groups can be great because of unfavorable factors in some cultures. The reference data given here apply to the USA and other Western countries. The reference "norms" are derived from the measurement of many individuals and may not be entirely applicable to an individual child.

There is no demonstrated advantage for the relatively large child over the relatively small child, although children falling outside the fifth and 95th percentiles are more likely to contract particular diseases or be prone to contract them. Gradual and relatively minor change over a period of months or years from one percentile level within the group to another need not be considered as evidence of disease, but marked deviations should be regarded with suspicion. The physician must constantly bear in mind that integration of function occurs within the individual and that disruption of the child's own pattern of growth and development is of greater significance than a deviation from the total population of any one set of measurements.

A knowledge of growth and development is of practical importance in relation to the sick child. Diseases tend to have more impact and to lead to greater permanent impairment when they occur during periods of rapid growth and development than when they occur during intervals of slower growth. For example,

*See also Index and other pertinent chapters.

loss of growth in the long bones of one leg over a period of several months due to osteomyelitis or prolonged casting in the preadolescent child is of lesser ultimate significance to the alignment of his spine than it would be if he had been at the peak of his adolescent growth.

Development and growth are continuous dynamic processes occurring from conception to maturity, and they take place in an orderly sequence which is approximately the same for all individuals. At any particular age, however, wide variations are to be found among normal children which reflect the active response of the growing individual to numberless hereditary and environmental factors.

GROWTH

The body as a whole and its various tissues and organs have characteristic growth patterns which are essentially the same in all individuals (Fig 2–1). *Development* signifies maturation of organs and systems, acquisition of skills, ability to adapt more readily to stress, and ability to assume maximum responsibility and to achieve freedom in creative expression. *Growth* refers to a change in size resulting from the multiplication of cells or the enlargement of existing ones.

Rate of growth is generally more important than actual size, and height and weight data must be considered in relation to the variability within a certain age. For more accurate comparisons, data should be recorded both as absolute figures and as percentiles for a particular age.

A number of extrinsic and intrinsic factors influence the rate of total growth and growth of various organ systems. Some of the more important extrinsic factors are nutritional status, climate, season, illness, and activity.

Serial measurements of growth are the best indicators of health. Pertinent measurements should be plotted to determine the pattern of growth and to compare them with normal standards. Graphs designating percentile distribution are particularly useful.

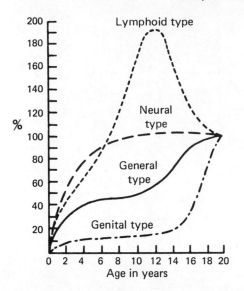

Figure 2–1. Graph showing major types of postnatal growth of various parts and organs of the body. *Lymphoid type:* Thymus, lymph nodes, intestinal lymphoid masses. *Neural type:* Brain and its parts, dura, spinal cord, optic apparatus, many head dimensions. *General type:* Body as a whole, external dimensions (with exception of head and neck), respiratory and digestive organs, kidneys, aorta and pulmonary trunks, spleen, musculature as a whole, skeleton as a whole, blood volume. *Genital type:* Testis, ovary, epididymis, uterine tube, prostate, prostatic urethra, seminal vesicles. (From RE Scammon. Redrawn and reproduced, with permission, from Holt, McIntosh, & Barnett: *Pediatrics,* 13th ed, Appleton-Century-Crofts, 1962, as redrawn from Harris & others: *Measurement of Man.* University of Minnesota Press, 1930.)

Fetal Growth (See Fig 2–2; Tables 2–1 and 2–2.)

A. Placental Transport:

1. Substances that pass through the placenta by simple diffusion are oxygen, carbon dioxide, water, and urea. Some that diffuse are present in lower concentration in the fetus (thyroxine, cholesterol, bilirubin, insulin, progesterone, estrogen), whereas still others are transported actively across the placenta and appear in the fetal blood in higher concentration than in maternal blood (amino acids, glucose, glycerol, fatty acids, minerals).

2. Phosphorus, iodine, and iron are relatively more concentrated on the fetal side of the placenta. Total calcium is present in higher concentration in the blood of the fetus than in the maternal blood, but ionizable calcium is present in equal concentrations in both.

3. Water-soluble vitamins are found in higher concentrations in fetal blood, but fat-soluble vitamins are present in lower concentrations in the fetus.

4. Lipids cross the placenta poorly.

5. The placenta acts as a barrier against thyroid-stimulating hormone, growth hormone, nucleic acids, neutral fats, and many bacteria and viruses.

6. The placenta produces estrogens, progestins, and gonadotropins.

B. Etiology of Fetal Abnormalities: Dietary deficiencies, infections, and numerous other factors in the pregnant woman may cause no manifest symptoms in her while producing significant abnormalities in the offspring; the pregnant woman may fare better than her offspring. Major malformations are present in 1–3.6% of newborn and stillborn infants; minor anomalies have been noted in as many as 15% of newborns.

C. Metabolic Factors:

1. The main source of energy for the growing fetus is carbohydrate.

2. Oxygen saturation in the fetus is lower than that found after birth.

Length and Height (See Figs 2–2 to 2–4, 2–7 to 2–10, and 2–14; Tables 2–1, 2–3, and 2–4.)

A. In Utero:

1. Maximal growth in length occurs during the sixth and seventh months of pregnancy.

2. During fetal life the rate of growth is extremely rapid. During the early months the fetal rate of gain in length is greater than the rate of gain in weight when expressed as percentage of value at birth. By the eighth month the fetus has achieved 80% of his birth length and only 50% of his birth weight. After the second fetal month the greatest relative increase in length is due to an increase in the growth of the extremities.

B. Neonatal:

1. Firstborn infants are usually smaller than later-born infants.

2. At birth, boys are slightly bigger than girls in both height and weight.

3. At birth, the ratio of the lower to the upper segment of the body (as measured from the pubis) is approximately 1:1.7. Subsequently, the legs grow more rapidly than the trunk (Fig 2–5).

C. Childhood: (Figs 2–3, 2–4; Table 2–3.) Height increases at a slowly declining rate until the onset of puberty, when a great spurt in growth occurs. Changes in height are slower in responding to factors that are detrimental to growth than are changes in weight.

1. Birth length is doubled by approximately age 4 and tripled by age 13.

2. The average child grows approximately 20 inches (50.8 cm) in the 9 months prior to birth, 10 inches (25.4 cm) in the first year of life, 5 inches (12.7 cm) in the second, 3–4 inches (7.6–10.2 cm) in the third, and approximately 2–3 inches (5.1–7.6 cm) per year until the growth spurt of puberty appears.

3. At 2 years of age, the midpoint in height is the umbilicus, whereas at adulthood the midpoint is slightly below the symphysis pubica.

4. At *3* years of age, the average child is *3* feet (91.4 cm) tall, and at *4* years, *40* inches (101.6 cm) tall. At *3.5* years the average child weighs *35* pounds (15.9 kg).

5. The legs and feet grow more rapidly than the trunk during childhood. During the first 2–3 years, the feet are flat, and there is an inward bowing of the legs from the knees to the ankles. The feet are often inter-

Table 2–1. Fetal and newborn dimensions and weights of the body and its organs.*

Age (Fetal) in Weeks†	Crown-heel (cm)	Crown-rump (cm)	Head Circ. (cm)	Body Wt (gm)	Adrenal (gm)	Brain (gm)	Heart (gm)	Kidney (gm)	Liver (gm)	Lungs (gm)	Pancreas (gm)	Pituitary (gm)	Spleen (gm)	Thymus (gm)	Thyroid (gm)
Prenatal and Newborn															
12	9.0	7.5	7.4	18.6	.087	2.32	.098	.163	.097	.69	.013		.006	.010	.026
16	16.7	12.8	12.6	100	.417	14.4	.662	.962	5.94	3.23	.095	.011	.086	.122	.133
20	24.2	17.7	17.6	310	1.07	43.0	2.08	2.77	16.8	8.18	.314	.024	.410	.553	.352
24	31.1	21.9	22.3	670	2.02	91.0	4.47	5.69	34.5	15.2	.695	.040	1.16	1.53	.684
28	37.1	25.5	26.3	1150	3.16	153	7.70	9.43	57.4	23.7	1.22	.058	2.43	3.14	1.08
30	39.8	27.1	28.1	1400	3.78	189	9.78	11.5	70.3	28.2	1.53	.067	3.26	4.18	1.33
32	42.4	28.5	29.9	1700	4.44	228	11.6	13.8	84.3	33.0	1.88	.076	4.25	5.41	1.54
34	44.8	29.9	31.5	2000	5.11	268	13.7	16.2	100.0	37.8	2.24	.085	5.36	6.77	1.78
36	47.0	31.2	33.1	2450	5.77	309	15.9	18.6	113.0	42.7	2.61	.094	6.55	8.22	2.01
38	49.1	32.4	34.4	2900	6.45	352	18.2	21.0	129.0	47.5	3.01	.103	7.86	9.82	2.26
40	51.0	33.5	35.7	3150	7.10	394	20.6	23.5	143.5	52.5	3.40	.111	9.22	11.5	2.50
Age (Years)						**Postnatal**									
1					4	875	43	62	350	160		0.15	30	23	
5					5	1250	90	110	575	305		0.23	55	28	
10					6	1325	145	150	825	450		0.33	77	31	
15					8	1340	245	220	1275	675		0.48	125	27	
						Adult‡									
Male					6	1375	300	320	1600	1000			165	14	
Female					6	1280	250	280	1500	750			150	14	

*Adapted from Edith Boyd.
†Time from first day of last menstrual period.
‡Adapted from several sources.

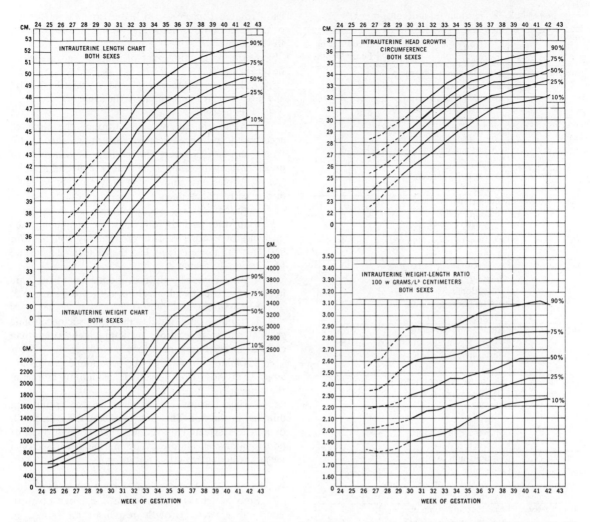

Figure 2—2. Colorado intrauterine growth charts. (Reproduced, with permission, from Lubchenco LO & others: Pediatrics 37:403, 1966.) These values are lower than those reported by others.

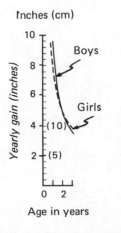

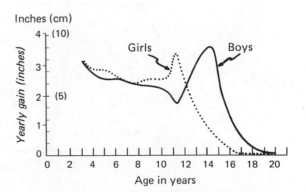

Figure 2—3. Growth rate from birth to age 3 (both sexes).

Figure 2—4. Growth rate from age 3–20 (both sexes).

Table 2—2. Human fetal development.*

		Fetal Age in Lunar Months
Integument	Three-layered epidermis	3
	Body hair begins	4
	Skin glands form, sweat and sebaceous	4
Mouth	Lip fusion complete	2
	Palate fused completely	3
	Enamel and dentin depositing	5
	Primordia of permanent teeth	6—8
Gastrointestinal	Bile secreted	3
	Rectum patent	3
	Pancreatic islands appear	3
	Fixation of duodenum and colon	4
Respiratory	Definitive shape of lungs	3
	Maxillary sinuses developing	4
	Elastic fibers appear in lung	4
Urogenital	Kidney able to secrete	2½
	Vagina regains lumen	5
	Testes descend into scrotum	7—9
Vascular	Definitive shape of heart	1½
	Heart becomes 4-chambered	3½
	Blood formation in marrow begins	3
	Spleen acquires typical structure	7
Nervous	Commissures of brain complete	5
	Myelinization of cord begins	5
	Typical layers of cortex	6
Special senses	Nasal septum complete	3
	Retinal layers complete, light-perceptive	7
	Vascular tunic of lens pronounced	7
	Eyelids open	7—8

*Reproduced, with permission, from Arey LB: *Developmental Anatomy: A Textbook and Laboratory Manual of Embryology,* 5th ed. Saunders, 1947.

nally rotated ("pigeon-toed") due to internal torsion of the tibia or varus deformity of the medial aspect of the forefoot.

6. During the first year of life, boys grow slightly faster than girls.

7. Between the ages of 1 and 9 years, both boys and girls grow at approximately the same rate.

D. Pubescence:

1. Although children pass through the phase of accelerated growth associated with pubescence at different chronologic ages, the pattern or sequence of pubescent growth tends to be similar in all children.

2. Adolescents undergoing early puberty are taller during early pubescence but have an earlier cessation of growth than adolescents undergoing late puberty.

3. In the period following the menarche, the median growth for girls is approximately 3 inches (7.6 cm), but the range is from less than 1 inch (2.5 cm) up to 7 inches (17.8 cm).

4. Boys whose height is at the median at age 2 are likely to be twice as tall as adults as they were at age 2.

E. Environmental Factors:

1. Children of middle and low socioeconomic groups in this generation are appreciably taller than children in previous generations.

2. Children from high socioeconomic groups are larger than those from lower socioeconomic groups in the same area.

3. Height gains are maximal in the spring and minimal in the fall. The growth of well nourished children is less affected by seasons than is the growth of poorly nourished children. The mechanism in seasonal factors affecting growth is not known.

Weight (See Figs 2—2, 2—6 to 2—10; Table 2—4.)

Body weight is probably the best index of nutrition and growth. Growth responses are noted in changes in weight before they are noted in other aspects of growth. The greatest weight gain occurs in the fall, the least gain in the spring. Obese children are usually taller and exhibit an advanced bone age.

A. Neonatal:

1. The average infant weighs approximately 7 lb 5 oz (3333 gm) at birth.

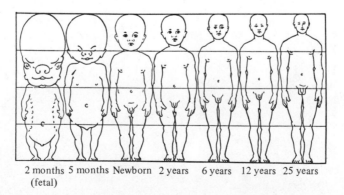

2 months   5 months   Newborn   2 years   6 years   12 years   25 years
(fetal)

Figure 2—5. Relative proportions of head, trunk, and extremities at different ages. (From Stratz, modified by Robbins & others: *Growth.* Yale Univ Press, 1928.)

2. Within the first few days of life, the newborn loses up to 10% of his birth weight. This loss is attributable to loss of meconium, urine, and physiologic edema, and less intake. By 10 days of age, the newborn has generally regained his birth weight.

B. Childhood: (Fig 2—6.)

1. The increment in weight is approximately 1 oz (30 gm)/day during the early months of life.

2. Between the ages of 3 and 12 months, the weight of the child in pounds is equal to his age in months plus 11.

3. Birth weight is doubled between the fourth and fifth months of age, tripled by the end of the first year, and quadrupled by the end of the second year. Between the ages of 2 and 9 years, the annual increment in weight averages about 5 lb per year.

4. At 7 years, the average child weighs 7 times his birth weight.

C. Adolescence: During adolescence, the most rapid gain in weight usually occurs in the year before menarche.

Head & Skull (See Figs 2—5, 2—11, and 2—12.)

Measurements of the head serve as an estimate of brain growth. Growth of the skull as determined by increasing head circumference is a much more accurate index of brain growth than is the presence or size of the fontanel.

A. In Utero: During pregnancy, the cranium increases in size much more rapidly than the rest of the body.

B. Newborn: At birth, the head is approximately three-fourths of its total mature size whereas the rest of the body is only one-fourth its adult size.

C. Childhood:

1. The brain grows very rapidly during infancy and then grows relatively less. At birth, the head makes up one-fourth of the infant's length; by 25 years of age, the head measures only one-eighth of the body length.

2. Cranial sutures do not ossify completely until early adulthood.

3. While the *averages* of head and chest circumference in the first 4 years of life are approximately equal, during this period the head circumference may normally be from 5 cm larger to 7 cm smaller than the chest.

D. Fontanels:

1. Six fontanels (anterior, posterior, 2 sphenoid, and 2 mastoid) are usually present at birth.

2. The anterior fontanel normally closes between 10 and 14 months of age but may be closed by 3 months or remain open until 18 months.

3. The posterior fontanel usually closes by 2 months but in some children may not be palpable even at birth.

E. Other:

1. The pineal gland may be visualized roentgenographically in 10% of children beyond the tenth year and in 80% of adults of advanced age.

2. The eustachian tube is shorter and more horizontal at birth than later.

Table 2—3. Approximate percentage of mature height achieved at each age.

Age in Years	Boys			Girls		
	Average	Accelerated	Retarded	Average	Accelerated	Retarded
Birth	29			31		
1	42	45	40	45	48	42
2	50	51	47	53	55	50
3	54	56	52	57	60	55
4	58	60	56	62	65	60
5	62	64	60	66	69	64
6	65	68	64	69	73	68
7	69	71	67	74	76	72
8	72	74	70	78	80	75
9	75	77	73	81	84	78
10	78	80	76	84	88	81
11	81	83	80	88	93	85
12	84	87	82	93	97	88
13	87	91	85	97	98	91
14	92	96	88	98	99	95
15	96	98	92	99	99	98
16	98	99	96	99	99	99
16½					100	
17	99	100	98	100		99
17½		100				
18	100		99			100
18½	100					
19			100			
20			100			

Table 2—4. Percentiles for weight and height: Birth to 5 years and 5—18 years.*

Percentiles (Boys)						Percentiles (Girls)				
3	10	50	90	97		3	10	50	90	97
					Birth					
5.8	6.3	7.5	9.1	10.1	Weight in pounds	5.8	6.2	7.4	8.6	9.4
2.63	2.86	3.4	4.13	4.58	Weight in kg	2.63	2.81	3.36	3.9	4.26
18.2	18.9	19.9	21.0	21.5	Length in inches	18.5	18.8	19.8	20.4	21.1
46.3	48.1	50.6	53.3	54.6	Length in cm	47.1	47.8	50.2	51.9	53.6
					3 Months					
10.6	11.1	12.6	14.5	16.4	Weight in pounds	9.8	10.7	12.4	14.0	14.9
4.81	5.03	5.72	6.58	7.44	Weight in kg	4.45	4.85	5.62	6.35	6.76
22.4	22.8	23.8	24.7	25.1	Length in inches	22.0	22.4	23.4	24.3	24.8
56.8	57.8	60.4	62.8	63.7	Length in cm	55.8	56.9	59.5	61.7	63.1
					6 Months					
14.0	14.8	16.7	19.2	20.8	Weight in pounds	12.7	14.1	16.0	18.6	20.0
6.35	6.71	7.58	8.71	9.43	Weight in kg	5.76	6.4	7.26	8.44	9.07
24.8	25.2	26.1	27.3	27.7	Length in inches	24.0	24.6	25.7	26.7	27.1
63.0	63.9	66.4	69.3	70.4	Length in cm	61.1	62.5	65.2	67.8	68.8
					9 Months					
16.6	17.8	20.0	22.9	24.4	Weight in pounds	15.1	16.6	19.2	22.4	24.2
7.53	8.07	9.07	10.39	11.07	Weight in kg	6.85	7.53	8.71	10.16	10.98
26.6	27.0	28.0	29.2	29.9	Length in inches	25.7	26.4	27.6	28.7	29.2
67.7	68.6	71.2	74.2	75.9	Length in cm	65.4	67.0	70.1	72.9	74.1
					12 Months					
18.5	19.6	22.2	25.4	27.3	Weight in pounds	16.8	18.4	21.5	24.8	27.1
8.39	8.89	10.07	11.52	12.38	Weight in kg	7.62	8.35	9.75	11.25	12.29
28.1	28.5	29.6	30.7	31.6	Length in inches	27.1	27.8	29.2	30.3	31.0
71.3	72.4	75.2	78.1	80.3	Length in cm	68.9	70.6	74.2	77.1	78.8
					15 Months					
19.8	21.0	23.7	27.2	29.4	Weight in pounds	18.1	19.8	23.0	26.6	29.0
8.98	9.53	10.75	12.34	13.33	Weight in kg	8.21	8.98	10.43	12.07	13.15
29.3	29.8	30.9	32.1	33.1	Length in inches	28.3	29.0	30.5	31.8	32.6
74.4	75.6	78.5	81.5	84.2	Length in cm	71.9	73.7	77.6	80.8	82.8
					18 Months					
21.1	22.3	25.2	29.0	31.5	Weight in pounds	19.4	21.2	24.5	28.3	30.9
9.57	10.12	11.43	13.15	14.29	Weight in kg	8.8	9.62	11.11	12.84	14.02
30.5	31.0	32.2	33.5	34.7	Length in inches	29.5	30.2	31.8	33.3	34.1
77.5	78.8	81.8	85.0	88.2	Length in cm	74.9	76.8	80.9	84.5	86.7
					2 Years					
23.3	24.7	27.7	31.9	34.9	Weight in pounds	21.6	23.5	27.1	31.7	34.4
10.57	11.2	12.56	14.47	15.83	Weight in kg	9.8	10.66	12.29	14.38	15.6
32.6	33.1	34.4	35.9	37.2	Length in inches	31.5	32.3	34.1	35.8	36.7
82.7	84.2	87.5	91.1	94.6	Length in cm	80.1	82.0	86.6	91.0	93.3
					2½ Years					
25.2	26.6	30.0	34.5	37.0	Weight in pounds	23.6	25.5	29.6	34.6	38.2
11.43	12.07	13.61	15.65	16.78	Weight in kg	10.7	11.57	13.43	15.69	17.33
34.2	34.8	36.3	37.9	39.2	Length in inches	33.3	34.0	36.0	37.9	38.9
86.9	88.5	92.1	96.2	99.5	Length in cm	84.5	86.3	91.4	96.4	98.7
					3 Years					
27.0	28.7	32.2	36.8	39.2	Weight in pounds	25.6	27.6	31.8	37.4	41.8
12.25	13.02	14.61	16.69	17.78	Weight in kg	11.61	12.52	14.42	16.96	18.96
35.7	36.3	37.9	39.6	40.5	Length in inches	34.8	35.6	37.7	39.8	40.7
90.6	92.3	96.2	100.5	102.8	Length in cm	88.4	90.5	95.7	101.1	103.5
					4 Years					
30.1	32.1	36.4	41.4	44.3	Weight in pounds	29.2	31.2	36.2	43.5	48.2
13.65	14.56	16.51	18.78	20.09	Weight in kg	13.25	14.15	16.42	19.73	21.86
38.4	39.1	40.7	42.7	43.5	Length in inches	37.5	38.4	40.6	43.1	44.2
97.5	99.3	103.4	108.5	110.4	Length in cm	95.2	97.6	103.2	109.6	112.3
					5 Years					
33.6	35.5	40.5	46.7	50.4	Weight in pounds	32.1	34.8	40.5	49.2	52.8
15.24	16.1	18.37	21.18	22.86	Weight in kg	14.56	15.79	18.37	22.32	23.95
40.2	40.8	42.8	45.2	46.1	Length in inches	39.4	40.5	42.9	45.4	46.8
102.0	103.7	108.7	114.7	117.1	Length in cm	100.0	103.0	109.1	115.4	118.8

*The figures for the group from 0—5 years are from Studies of Child Health & Development, Department of Maternal & Child Health, Harvard School of Public Health; those for the group from 5—18 years are from studies by and are reproduced by courtesy of Howard V. Meredith, Iowa Child Welfare Research Station, The State University of Iowa. The figures for 5 years are given twice; their variations are due to the different populations of children used for each group.

Table 2—4 (cont'd). Percentiles for weight and height: Birth to 5 years and 5—18 years.

	Percentiles (Boys)					Percentiles (Girls)				
3	10	50	90	97		3	10	50	90	97
					5 Years					
34.5	36.6	42.8	49.7	53.2	Weight in pounds	33.7	36.1	41.4	48.2	51.8
15.65	16.6	19.41	22.54	24.13	Weight in kg	15.29	16.37	18.78	21.86	23.5
40.2	41.5	43.8	45.9	47.0	Height in inches	40.4	41.3	43.2	45.4	46.5
102.1	105.3	111.3	116.7	119.5	Height in cm	102.6	105.0	109.7	115.4	118.0
					6 Years					
38.5	40.9	48.3	56.4	61.1	Weight in pounds	37.2	39.6	46.5	54.2	58.7
17.46	18.55	21.91	25.58	27.71	Weight in kg	16.87	17.96	21.09	24.58	26.63
42.7	43.8	46.3	48.6	49.7	Height in inches	42.5	43.5	45.6	48.1	49.4
108.5	111.2	117.5	123.5	126.2	Height in cm	108.0	110.6	115.9	122.3	125.4
					7 Years					
43.0	45.8	54.1	64.4	69.9	Weight in pounds	41.3	44.5	52.2	61.2	67.3
19.5	20.77	24.54	29.21	31.71	Weight in kg	18.73	20.19	23.68	27.76	30.53
44.9	46.0	48.9	51.4	52.5	Height in inches	44.9	46.0	48.1	50.7	51.9
114.0	116.9	124.1	130.5	133.4	Height in cm	114.0	116.8	122.3	128.9	131.7
					8 Years					
48.0	51.2	60.1	73.0	79.4	Weight in pounds	45.3	48.6	58.1	69.9	78.9
21.77	23.22	27.26	33.11	36.02	Weight in kg	20.55	22.04	26.35	31.71	35.79
47.1	48.5	51.2	54.0	55.2	Height in inches	46.9	48.1	50.4	53.0	54.1
119.6	123.1	130.0	137.3	140.2	Height in cm	119.1	122.1	128.0	134.6	137.4
					9 Years					
52.5	56.3	66.0	81.0	89.8	Weight in pounds	49.1	52.6	63.8	79.1	89.9
23.81	25.54	29.94	36.74	40.73	Weight in kg	22.27	23.86	28.94	35.88	40.78
48.9	50.5	53.3	56.1	57.2	Height in inches	48.7	50.0	52.3	55.3	56.5
124.2	128.3	135.5	142.6	145.3	Height in cm	123.6	127.0	132.9	140.4	143.4
					10 Years					
56.8	61.1	71.9	89.9	100.0	Weight in pounds	53.2	57.1	70.3	89.7	101.9
25.76	27.71	32.61	40.78	45.36	Weight in kg	24.13	25.9	31.89	40.69	46.22
50.7	52.3	55.2	58.1	59.2	Height in inches	50.3	51.8	54.6	57.5	58.8
128.7	132.8	140.3	147.5	150.3	Height in cm	127.7	131.7	138.6	146.0	149.3
					11 Years					
61.8	66.3	77.6	99.3	111.7	Weight in pounds	57.9	62.6	78.8	100.4	112.9
28.03	30.07	35.2	45.04	50.67	Weight in kg	26.26	28.4	35.74	45.54	51.21
52.5	54.0	56.8	59.8	60.8	Height in inches	52.1	53.9	57.0	60.4	62.0
133.4	137.3	144.2	151.8	154.4	Height in cm	132.3	137.0	144.7	153.4	157.4
					12 Years					
67.2	72.0	84.4	109.6	124.2	Weight in pounds	63.6	69.5	87.6	111.5	127.7
30.48	32.66	38.28	49.71	56.34	Weight in kg	28.85	31.52	39.74	50.58	57.92
54.4	56.1	58.9	62.2	63.7	Height in inches	54.3	56.1	59.8	63.2	64.8
138.1	142.4	149.6	157.9	161.9	Height in cm	137.8	142.6	151.9	160.6	164.6
					13 Years					
72.0	77.1	93.0	123.2	138.0	Weight in pounds	72.2	79.9	99.1	124.5	142.3
32.66	34.97	42.18	55.88	62.6	Weight in kg	32.75	36.24	44.95	56.47	64.55
56.0	57.7	61.0	65.1	66.7	Height in inches	56.6	58.7	61.8	64.9	66.3
142.2	146.6	155.0	165.3	169.5	Height in cm	143.7	149.1	157.1	164.8	168.4
					14 Years					
79.8	87.2	107.6	136.9	150.6	Weight in pounds	83.1	91.0	108.4	133.3	150.8
36.2	39.55	48.81	62.1	68.31	Weight in kg	37.69	41.28	49.17	60.46	68.4
57.6	59.9	64.0	67.9	69.7	Height in inches	58.3	60.2	62.8	65.7	67.2
146.4	152.1	162.7	172.4	177.1	Height in cm	148.2	153.0	159.6	167.0	170.7
					15 Years					
91.3	99.4	120.1	147.8	161.6	Weight in pounds	89.0	97.4	113.5	138.1	155.2
41.41	45.09	54.48	67.04	73.3	Weight in kg	40.37	44.18	51.48	62.64	70.4
59.7	62.1	66.1	69.6	71.6	Height in inches	59.1	61.1	63.4	66.2	67.6
151.7	157.8	167.8	176.7	181.8	Height in cm	150.2	155.2	161.1	168.1	171.6

Table 2—4 (cont'd). Percentiles for weight and height: Birth to 5 years and 5—18 years.

Percentiles (Boys)						Percentiles (Girls)				
3	10	50	90	97		3	10	50	90	97
					16 Years					
103.4	111.0	129.7	157.3	170.5	Weight in pounds	91.8	100.9	117.0	141.1	157.7
46.9	50.35	58.83	71.35	77.34	Weight in kg	41.64	45.77	53.07	64.0	71.53
61.6	64.1	67.8	70.7	73.1	Height in inches	59.4	61.5	63.9	66.5	67.7
156.5	162.8	171.6	179.7	185.6	Height in cm	150.8	156.1	162.2	169.0	172.0
					17 Years					
110.5	117.5	136.2	164.6	175.6	Weight in pounds	93.9	102.8	119.1	143.3	159.5
50.12	53.3	61.78	74.66	79.65	Weight in kg	42.59	46.63	54.02	65.0	72.35
62.6	65.2	68.4	71.5	73.5	Height in inches	59.4	61.5	64.0	66.7	67.8
159.0	165.5	173.7	181.6	186.6	Height in cm	151.0	156.3	162.5	169.4	172.2
					18 Years					
113.0	120.0	139.0	169.0	179.0	Weight in pounds	94.5	103.5	119.9	144.5	160.7
51.26	54.43	63.05	76.66	81.19	Weight in kg	42.87	46.95	54.39	65.54	72.89
62.8	65.5	68.7	71.8	73.9	Height in inches	59.4	61.5	64.0	66.7	67.8
159.6	166.3	174.5	182.4	187.6	Height in cm	151.0	156.3	162.5	169.4	172.2

Nervous System

The CNS makes up one-fourth of the total body weight in the second fetal month, one-tenth at birth, one-twentieth at age 5, and only one-fiftieth of the total weight at full maturity.

A. Myelinization:

1. Myelinization begins by the fourth fetal month and is evident first in the ventral and dorsal spinal routes. The cerebral cortex and thalamus are the last to be myelinated. Myelinization in the cord proceeds in a cephalocaudal direction. At birth, all the cranial nerves, with the exception of the optic and olfactory, are myelinated. At that time, the autonomic nervous system is mature, and some of the segmented spinal nerves are mature, fully myelinated, and functional.

2. The brain stem, those tracts going to the cortex, and some of the finer configurations of the cortex of the brain as well as the nerve tracts connecting the cortex with lower centers are immature and probably incompletely myelinated. Minimal cortical function is present; function is primarily on a subcortical level.

3. Efferent fibers to the voluntary muscles begin to become myelinated soon after birth.

4. Myelinization of the spinal cord, brain stem, and cortex may not be completed for at least 2 years.

B. Reflexes:

1. The cough reflex, Moro reflex, Chvostek's sign, the walking reflex, the patellar reflex, and the grasping reflex are present at birth.

2. The Babinski reflex is seldom elicited in the newborn infant but appears somewhat later and may persist for a year or more.

3. The abdominal and cremasteric reflexes usually cannot be elicited in the neonatal period, nor can the Achilles tendon reflex nor the tonic neck reflex, which is quite inconstant in the newborn but is usually present in the normal 1-month-old infant.

4. By 6 months, superficial reflexes are present.

C. Blood-Brain Barrier: The blood-brain barrier appears to be more permeable during early infancy than later.

The Respiratory System

A. In Utero:

1. Respiratory movements take place in utero; an exchange of amniotic fluid in the alveoli occurs.

2. The first patterns of respiratory movements become manifest at about the 20th week of pregnancy.

3. The fetus and the newborn can withstand anoxia more effectively than can adults.

B. Newborn:

1. The onset of respiration in the newborn infant is probably dependent on a number of factors, including stimulation of the tactile and thermal receptors on the skin, as well as hypoxia.

2. Respiration in infants is largely diaphragmatic during the first years of life.

C. Childhood:

1. The respiratory rate decreases steadily during childhood, averaging approximately 30/minute during

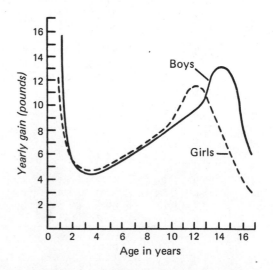

Figure 2—6. Yearly gain in weight. (Redrawn and reproduced, with permission, from Barnett: *Pediatrics,* 14th ed. Appleton-Century-Crofts, 1968.)

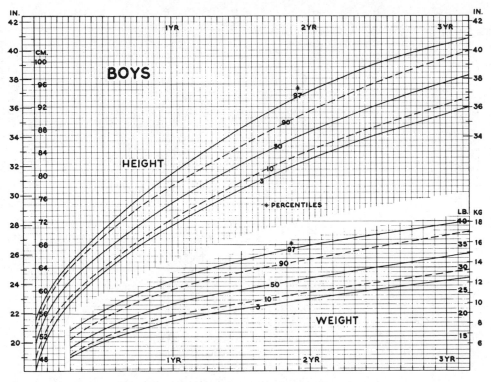

Figure 2—7. Height and weight for boys, age 1–3 years. (Harvard School of Public Health data.)

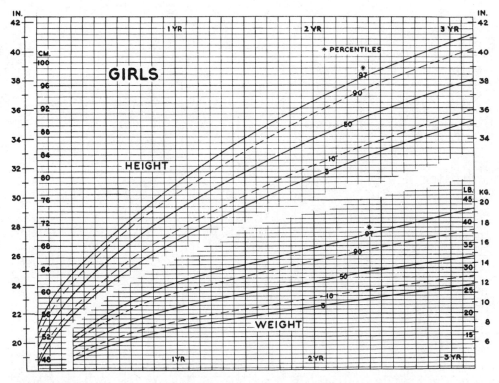

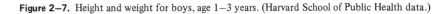

Figure 2—8. Height and weight for girls, age 1–3 years. (Harvard School of Public Health data.)

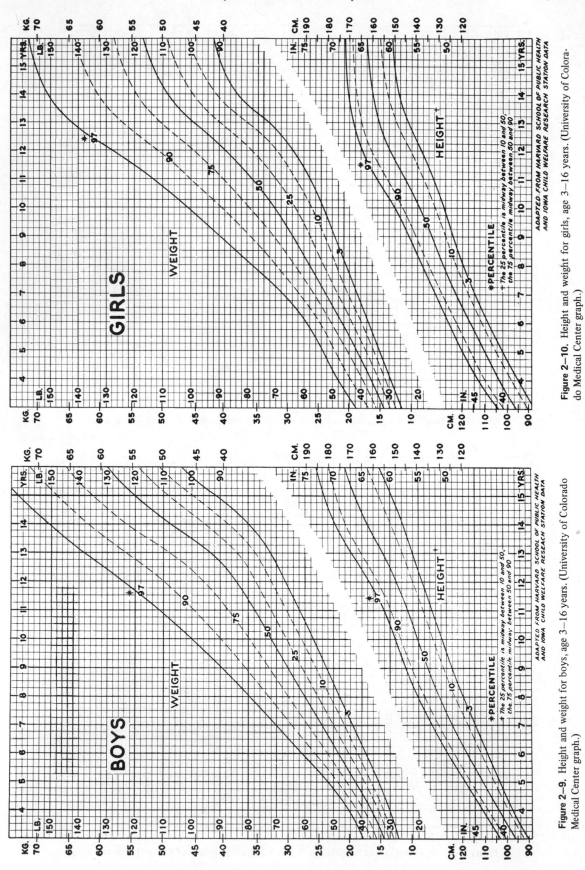

Figure 2–10. Height and weight for girls, age 3–16 years. (University of Colorado Medical Center graph.)

Figure 2–9. Height and weight for boys, age 3–16 years. (University of Colorado Medical Center graph.)

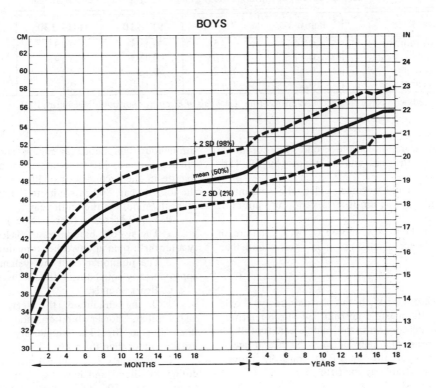

Figure 2—11. Head circumference for boys, birth to 18 years. (Nellhaus: Pediatrics 41:106, 1968.)

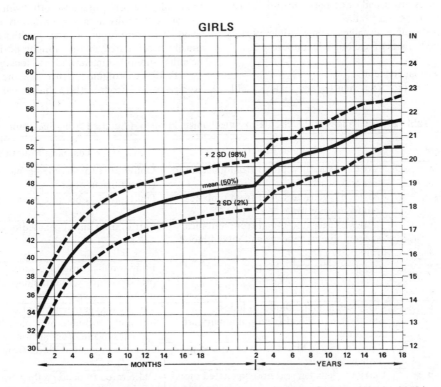

Figure 2—12. Head circumference for girls, birth to 18 years. (Nellhaus: Pediatrics 41:106, 1968.)

Table 2—5. Upper limits of the normal P—R interval in children.*

Pulse Rate	Below 70	71—90	91—110	110—130	Above 130
Birth—18 months	0.16	0.15	0.145	0.135	0.125
18 months—6 years	0.17	0.165	0.155	0.145	0.135
6—13 years	0.18	0.17	0.16	0.15	0.14
13—17 years	0.19	0.18	0.17	0.16	0.15

*Reproduced, with permission, from Ashman & Hull: *Essentials of Electrocardiography.* Macmillan, 1941.

the first year, 25/minute in the second year, 20/minute during the eighth year, and 18/minute by the 15th year.

2. As the child becomes older, the amount of oxygen in the expired air decreases and the amount of CO_2 increases.

D. Adult: Men expel more CO_2 with each breath and have a larger alkali reserve in their blood than women.

Sinuses

A. Newborn: At birth, the mastoid process is only a single cell—the mastoid antrum—and has a relatively wide communication with the middle ear. Its cellular structure appears gradually between birth and age 3. Pneumatization of the tip of the mastoid process becomes demonstrable by the fifth year.

B. Childhood:

1. Maxillary and ethmoid sinuses are present at birth but are usually not aerated and usually cannot be seen by x-ray examination for at least 6 months. The sphenoid sinuses are usually not pneumatized (or visible) until after the third year.

2. Frontal sinuses usually become visible by x-ray between 3 and 9 years of age but seldom before 5.

The Cardiovascular System

A. Heart Rate: The heart rate falls steadily throughout childhood, averaging about 150 beats/minute in utero, 130 beats/minute at birth, 105 beats/minute in the second year of life, 90 beats/minute in the fourth year, 80 beats/minute in the sixth year, and 70 beats/minute in the tenth year.

B. Blood Pressure: (Table 18—5.)

1. The systolic blood pressure is lower immediately after birth than at any other time during life.

2. The pulmonary and the systemic pressures are approximately equal during the first weeks of life.

C. Heart Sounds:

1. During childhood, the heart sounds have a higher pitch, shorter duration, and greater intensity than later in life. The pulmonary second sound is usually louder than the aortic.

2. Innocent ("functional") murmurs are common during childhood and have been reported to occur in approximately 50% of children at some time during childhood, with a peak incidence between the ages of 6 and 9.

3. Less than 10% of murmurs present at birth are the result of a congenital lesion that will persist.

4. A "venous hum" is commonly noted in childhood. It is continuous, located in the parasternal area, usually accentuated in the upright position, and may be either sub- or supraclavicular in location.

D. Heart Volume: Heart volume decreases an average of 25% from birth to the second day as a result

Table 2—6. Changes in the circulatory mechanism at birth. (Adapted from Scammon.)

Structure	Prenatal Function	Postnatal Function
Umbilical vein	Carries oxygenated blood from placenta to liver and heart.	Obliterated to become ligamentum teres (round ligament of liver).
Ductus venosus	Carries oxygenated blood from umbilical vein to inferior vena cava.	Obliterated to become ligamentum venosum.
Inferior vena cava	Carries oxygenated blood from umbilical vein and ductus venosus and mixed blood from body and liver.	Carries only unoxygenated blood from body.
Foramen ovale	Connects right and left atria.	Functional closure by 3 months, although probe patency without symptoms may be retained by some adults.
Pulmonary arteries	Carry some mixed blood to lungs.	Carry unoxygenated blood to lungs.
Ductus arteriosus	Shunts mixed blood from pulmonary artery to aorta.	Generally occluded by 4 months and becomes ligamentum arteriosum.
Aorta	Receives mixed blood from heart and pulmonary arteries.	Carries oxygenated blood from left ventricle.
Umbilical arteries	Carry oxygenated and unoxygenated blood to the placenta.	Obliterated to become the vesical ligaments on the anterior abdominal wall.

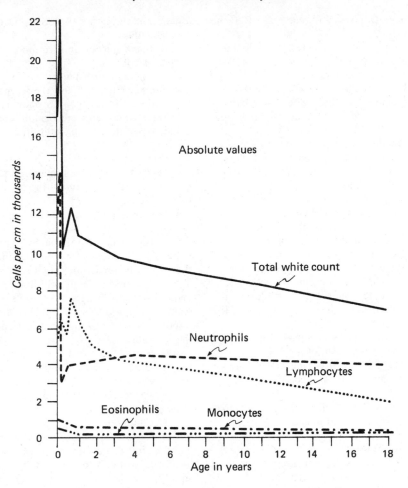

Figure 2—13. Life patterns of leukocytes. (Redrawn and reproduced from: *Dynamics of Development: Euthenic Pediatrics.* by D Whipple. Copyright 1966 by McGraw-Hill. Used with permission of McGraw-Hill Book Company.)

of both the fluid shift from the vascular compartment and a decreasing flow of blood through the ductus arteriosus.

E. Blood Volume: The total blood volume ranges from 80—110 ml/kg in the newborn infant; averages 115 ml/kg in the premature infant during the first several weeks of life; and is 75—100 ml/kg in the older infant and child and 70—85 ml/kg in the adult.

F. Electrocardiography: (Table 2—5.) During the first months of life there is a tendency to right axis deviation on the ECG.

G. Anatomic Changes Occurring at Birth: (Table 2—6.) The ductus arteriosus and the foramen ovale close functionally soon after birth; anatomic obliteration of the ductus is complete by the fourth month of postnatal life, whereas anatomic closure of the foramen ovale does not occur until toward the end of the first year.

H. Other:

1. In early childhood, the axis of the heart is more nearly transverse than in later life.

2. Sinus arrhythmia is a normal phenomenon during childhood.

The Blood (See Table 38—3 and Fig 2—13.)

A. In Utero: The first blood-forming centers in the fetus are found in connective tissue (mesenchyme). This later shifts to the liver (most active), spleen, and mesonephros, and finally to the bone marrow. At birth, production of formed elements in the blood occurs primarily in the bone marrow. The liver and spleen retain the ability to make blood cells until early childhood at times of pathologic stress such as excessive hemorrhage.

B. Newborn:

1. If the umbilical cord is not clamped for 2—3 minutes after delivery of the infant, 75—135 ml of blood will be transferred from the placenta to the infant. Late clamping will produce a red blood cell count which is approximately 1 million/cu mm higher, a hemoglobin level approximately 2.5 gm/100 ml higher, and a hematocrit 7% higher than if early clamping were carried out.

2. Nucleated red cells and immature lymphocytes may be present in the newborn but disappear within the first week of life.

3. At birth, 5% of all red blood cells may be

reticulocytes; they drop to less than 1% after the second week.

4. Up to 5% of nucleated red blood cells (as a percentage of the total number of nucleated cells) may be present normally for several days after birth.

5. Normally, the number of leukocytes and erythrocytes and the amount of hemoglobin is relatively greater immediately after birth than at any other time in life.

C. Fetal Hemoglobin: Fetal hemoglobin accounts for 80% of total hemoglobin at birth (cord blood), 75% of the total at 2 weeks of age, 55% at 5 weeks, and falls to 5% by 20 weeks of life.

D. White Cells: (Fig 2–13.)

1. The leukocyte count is high at birth, rises slightly during the first 48 hours after birth, falls for the next 2 or 3 weeks, and then rises again. In some children, it reaches its highest level in life sometime before the seventh month; the leukocyte count then falls gradually throughout the remainder of childhood.

2. The lymphocyte count is highest during the first year of life and then falls progressively during the remainder of childhood.

3. The eosinophil count is higher during early infancy than at any other time of life.

4. The basophil count remains essentially unchanged during childhood; at puberty, it falls to adult levels.

E. Sedimentation Rate: Children have an elevated sedimentation rate as contrasted to adults.

The Gastrointestinal Tract

A. Newborn: Gas may be visualized roentgenographically almost immediately after birth in the stomach, within 2 hours in the ileum, and, on the average, in 3 or 4 hours in the rectum.

B. Enzymes:

1. There is a deficiency of the starch-splitting enzyme amylase during early infancy; this prevents optimal handling of long chain polysaccharides. Amylase is present in significant amounts in the pancreatic juice by 3 months of age.

2. Lipase activity is low throughout early childhood. In contrast, trypsin activity is adequate from birth except in the premature infant, in whom low levels are often found.

C. Ketone Bodies: Ketone bodies are not formed as readily by the liver of the young infant as by the older child; acetone is seldom found in the urine at any time during the first 6 months of life.

D. Gastric Acidity: Gastric juice acidity is low during infancy and rises during childhood, with a marked increase during adolescence. Acidity is greater in boys than in girls.

E. Transit Time: Food passes through the stomach more rapidly in the infant than in the older child. Protein digestion is less complete in the stomach of the infant than in the older child.

F. Stomach Capacity: The capacity of the stomach is approximately 30–90 ml at birth, 90–150 ml at 1 month, 210–360 ml at 1 year, approximately 500 ml at 2 years, and averages 750–900 ml in later childhood.

G. Other:

1. Some spitting-up is common in early infancy in almost all children.

2. The abdomen tends to be prominent in infants and toddlers. In the infant, the ascending and descending portions of the colon are short compared with the transverse colon, and the sigmoid extends higher into the abdomen than during later life.

The Urinary System

A. In Utero: The kidney functions during fetal life and contributes some urine to the amniotic fluid, but the fetal kidney probably does not participate in the regulation of electrolyte balance.

B. Newborn:

1. In the kidney of the full-term infant at birth there is a full quota of nephrons, but this may not be the case in the premature infant.

2. The first urine usually has a specific gravity of about 1.015. During the first weeks of life, the urine is scanty and quite dilute (probably as a result of poor response to antidiuretic hormone and immaturity of the renal tubules).

3. During the neonatal period, there is a low clearance of sodium, chloride, and urea, resulting in a hypotonic urine as compared to plasma.

4. The percentage of uric acid is higher in the urine of the neonate than later.

C. Childhood:

1. Renal immaturity probably exists for several months after birth; during the second year of life, the histologic structure of the kidney reaches its mature structure.

2. Glucose and albumin may normally be present in the urine.

D. Urine Volume: The average infant secretes 15–50 ml of urine per 24 hours during the first 2 days of life, 50–300 ml/day during the next week, 250–400 ml/day during the next 2 months, and 400–500 ml/day by the latter half of the first year. There is subsequently a gradual increase in urinary output; 700–1000 ml are secreted during ages 5–8 and 700–1500 ml between the ages of 8 and 14.

E. Glomerular Filtration: Glomerular filtration rate is low during the first 9 months of life, as are urea clearance, renal plasma flow, and maximal tubular excretory capacity also.

F. Creatine and Creatinine:

1. Creatine is excreted in large amounts by the infant and to a lesser degree by children to the time of puberty; the male adult excretes almost no creatine, whereas female adults excrete very little.

2. Creatinine output increases throughout the growing period, the quantity being directly related to the amount of body musculature.

Fat, Muscle, & Body Water

A. Fat: The body contains equal amounts of fat and protein at or shortly before birth; subsequently, the amount of fat exceeds the amount of protein.

1. Fat is first laid down about the sixth month of pregnancy.

2. The fat of the fetus and newborn infant has a higher degree of saturation, a higher melting point, and contains more palmitic but less stearic and oleic acids than the fat of the older child or adult.

3. There is a gradual decrease in the body stores of fat from the middle of the first year to the age of 6 or 7 years; girls tend to retain more fat than boys, but the differences are slight during childhood. Fat begins to reaccumulate from age 6–7 up to puberty. At that time, the amount of fat decreases in the male but continues to increase in the female.

B. Muscle:

1. At birth, muscle constitutes a smaller portion (20–25%) of the total body weight as compared to that in the adult.

2. During the second trimester of pregnancy, skeletal musculature forms about one-sixth of the body weight; at birth, one-fifth to one-fourth; in early adolescence, one-third; and in early maturity, approximately two-fifths. The gain in musculature during childhood equals the growth of all other organs, systems, and tissues combined.

C. Body Water:

1. The water content of the body is approximately 95% by weight in early fetal life; 65–75% at birth; and 55–60% at maturity.

2. The infant ingests and excretes approximately 20% of his total body fluid daily, whereas the adult has a water exchange of only 5% of his total body fluid. For the infant, this represents nearly 50% of his extracellular fluid volume; for the adult, 14% of extracellular fluid volume.

Temperature, BMR, & Steroids (See Table 2–7.)

A. Body Temperature: Body temperature during childhood is on the average 37.3° C (99.1° F) in the first year, 37.5° C (99.4° F) in the fourth year, 37° C (98.6° F) in the fifth year, and 36.7° C (98° F) in the 12th year. During childhood, there is no appreciable

Table 2–7. Average body temperatures in well children under basal conditions.*

Age	Temperature and Standard Deviation	
	F	C
3 months	99.4 (0.8)	37.4 (0.4)
6 months	99.5 (0.6)	37.5 (0.3)
1 year	99.7 (0.5)	37.6 (0.2)
3 years	99.0 (0.5)	37.2 (0.2)
5 years	98.6 (0.5)	37.0 (0.2)
7 years	98.3 (0.5)	36.8 (0.2)
9 years	98.1 (0.5)	36.7 (0.2)
11 years	98.0 (0.5)	36.7 (0.2)
13 years	97.8 (0.5)	36.5 (0.2)

*From *Growth and Development of Children*, by Ernest H. Watson, MD. Copyright © 1967. Year Book Medical Publishers, Inc. Used by permission.

difference in the body temperature of boys and girls, but after adolescence women tend to have a higher temperature than men.

B. Basal Metabolic Rate (BMR):

1. Fetal metabolism is lower than that of the newborn.

2. The BMR is highest in the young infant and falls continuously throughout life.

3. Boys and girls have comparable basal metabolic rates, but the rate is higher in men than in women.

C. Steroids:

1. Plasma levels of 17-ketosteroids at birth and for a few days thereafter are 2–5 times higher than in the adult; urinary excretion is higher in the neonatal period than later in infancy.

2. The plasma levels and the urinary excretion of 17-hydroxycorticosteroids are decreased in the newborn infant when compared with the mother's levels (which are elevated, particularly during vaginal delivery). Plasma levels remain low for the first 1–2 weeks after birth, gradually rising to adult levels.

Organs of Special Sense

A. Tactile Sensation:

1. At birth the newborn infant has mature sensory receptors for pressure, pain, and temperature from the entire body surface, from the mouth, and from the external genitalia; the infant also has mature pain receptors in the viscera and proprioceptive receptors in muscles, joints, and tendons.

2. A response to touch is first elicited in the region of the face, particularly the lips.

B. Taste: The ability to taste is present in the newborn infant, and the 4 basic tastes can be distinguished at this time.

C. Smell: The human infant is born with fully mature receptors for olfaction; the infant may have a stronger sense of smell than the older individual, but this is difficult to test.

D. Hearing:

1. Normal infants can hear almost immediately after birth, but because of a lack of myelinization of cortical auditory pathways they respond to sounds at a subcortical level. Voluntary muscular action in response to sound is present in the average infant by 2 months of age.

2. Although the hearing mechanism in the ear is anatomically mature soon after birth, full maturity of total auditory function may not be present for 5–7 years.

3. The infant can localize a direction of sound by the middle of the first year.

E. Vision: (Table 2–8.) The visual system is relatively immature at birth. The eyeball is less spherical the cornea is larger, the anterior chamber is more shallow, and the lens more spherical than in the older individual. Because of a lack of myelinization of cerebral neural pathways, the striated muscles which move the eyeballs are not under voluntary control.

1. Anatomic considerations–

a. The macula begins to differentiate during the

first month of life, is well organized by 4 months, and is histologically mature by 8 months.

b. Final development of the macula is reached at about 6 years of age.

c. Tears can be produced during the early weeks of life.

d. The newborn infant is hyperopic; the eyeball grows rapidly for the first 8 years of life, becoming even more hyperopic as a result of changes in the

Table 2—8. Chronology of ophthalmic development.

Age	Level of Development
Birth	Awareness of light and dark. The infant closes his eyelids in bright light.
Neonatal	Rudimentary fixation on near objects (3—30 inches).
2 weeks	Transitory fixation, usually monocular at a distance of roughly 3 feet.
4 weeks	Follows large conspicuously moving objects.
6 weeks	Moving objects evoke binocular fixation briefly.
8 weeks	Follows moving objects with jerky eye movements. Convergence is beginning to appear.
12 weeks	Visual following now a combination of head and eye movements. Convergence is improving. Enjoys light objects and bright colors.
16 weeks	Inspects own hands. Fixates immediately on a 1-inch cube brought within 1—2 feet of eye. Vision 20/300—20/200 (6/100—6/70).
20 weeks	Accommodative convergence reflexes all organizing. Visually pursues lost rattle. Shows interest in stimuli more than 3 feet away.
24 weeks	Retrieves a dropped 1-inch cube. Can maintain voluntary fixation of stationary object even in the presence of competing moving stimulus. Hand-eye coordination is appearing.
26 weeks	Will fixate on a string.
28 weeks	Binocular fixation clearly established.
36 weeks	Depth perception is dawning.
40 weeks	Marked interest in tiny objects. Tilts head backward to gaze up. Vision 20/200 (6/70).
52 weeks	Fusion beginning to appear. Discriminates simple geometric forms, squares and circles. Vision 20/180 (6/60).
12—18 months	Looks at pictures with interest.
18 months	Convergence well established. Localization in distance crude—runs into objects which he sees.
2 years	Accommodation well developed. Vision 20/40 (6/12).
3 years	Convergence smooth. Fusion improving. Vision 20/30 (6/9).
4 years	Vision 20/20 (6/6).

cornea and lens. The eyeball reaches its adult size at about age 8 and then tends to become comparatively myopic. Thus, hyperopia is to be expected in the preschool and early school years.

e. Some children may have brief episodes of transient strabismus during the first few months of life. These usually clear spontaneously. Irrespective of age, strabismus that is present for prolonged periods needs ophthalmologic consultation and evaluation as soon as recognized. Mature adult function of the eye muscles is usually reached by the end of the first year.

2. Functional considerations—

a. At birth there is an awareness of light and dark, and an infant is capable of rudimentary fixation on near objects.

b. The newborn is capable of peripheral vision, but other visual functions are deficient.

c. Pupillary response is present in late fetal life.

d. The ability to fixate well is usually present by 2—3 months of age.

e. Perception of bright colors is probably present at 3—5 months of age.

f. Depth perception develops at about 9 months of age but does not reach a mature level until age 6.

g. Convergence begins to appear at approximately 8 weeks of age. At 4 months, vision is 20/300—20/200 (6/100—6/70). By 7 months of age, binocular fixation is clearly established. Depth perception becomes apparent at 9 months. At 10 months, vision is 20/200 (6/70). At 1 year, fusion is beginning to appear, and at 18 months convergence is well established. At 2 years, accommodation is well developed; vision is 20/40 (6/12). By 3 years fusion is appearing and vision is 20/30 (6/9). Vision becomes 20/20 (6/6) at age 4.

h. Fusion of images probably occurs by the sixth year of life.

Immune Mechanisms (See Chapter 15.)

A. In Utero:

1. Antibodies of low molecular weight—7S immunoglobulin G (IgG)—may appear in higher concentration in fetal than in maternal blood. Antibodies of high molecular weight—19S immunoglobulin M (IgM)—are usually found in low concentration in the fetus.

2. The placenta permits the transfer of 7S IgG molecules to the fetus but selectively withholds the IgM and IgA. Transfer of gamma globulin from mother to fetus takes place principally in the last trimester of pregnancy; blood levels of gamma globulin are higher in the full-term infant than in the premature.

3. Immunoglobulins are normally not synthesized in utero. Macroglobulins (19S IgM) may be synthesized in response to antigenic stimulation.

B. Newborn and Infancy:

1. During the first months of postnatal life, the infant has passive immunity to certain diseases to which the mother was immune, but such immunity is generally limited to those whose antibodies are carried in the 7S IgG fraction. Maternal immunity carried solely in macroglobulins is not passed on.

2. In the newborn period, the blood contains a

Table 2—9. Time of appearance of sexual characteristics in American girls.*

Pelvis	Female contour assumed and fat deposition begins	8—10 years
Breasts	First hypertrophy or budding	9—11 years
	Further enlargement and pigmentation of nipples	12—13 years
	Histologic maturity	16—18 years
Vagina	Secretion begins and glycogen content of epithelium increases with change in cell type	11—14 years
Pubic hair	Initial appearance	10—12 years
	Abundant and curly	11—15 years
Axillary hair	Initial appearance	12—14 years
Acne	Varies considerably	12—16 years

*From *Growth and Development of Children*, by Ernest H. Watson, MD. Copyright © 1967. Year Book Medical Publishers, Inc. Used by permission.

Table 2—10. Time of appearance of sexual characteristics in American boys.*

Breasts	Some hypertrophy, often assuming a firm nodularity	12—14 years
	Disappearance of hypertrophy	14—17 years
Testes and penis	Increase in size begins	10—12 years
	Rapid growth	12—15 years
Pubic hair	Initial appearance	12—14 years
	Abundant and curly	13—16 years
Axillary hair	Initial appearance	13—16 years
Facial and body	Initial appearance	15—17 years
Acne	Varies considerably	14—18 years
Mature sperm	Average range	14—16 years

*From *Growth and Development of Children*, by Ernest H. Watson, MD. Copyright © 1967. Year Book Medical Publishers, Inc. Used by permission.

relatively high level of passively transmitted 7S IgG and an absence or marked deficiency of 7S and 19S IgM. The 7S IgG which was passively transferred from the mother gradually disappears from the infant's circulation. The lowest level of gamma globulin is reached about the 15th to 80th days.

3. The newborn can manufacture antibody (macroglobulins) as early as the end of the first week of life. By the end of the first year, the child can produce 19S IgM as effectively as the adult. However, the newborn is unable to synthesize 7S IgG.

C. Childhood: In the normal adult, the presence of 19S IgM is followed within a period of 1—2 weeks by the appearance of 7S IgG, but in the infant relatively little 7S IgG appears subsequent to 19S IgM formation.

Adolescent Changes (See Tables 2—9 and 2—10.)

A. Both Sexes:

1. The adolescent growth spurt in both sexes is probably due to the production of androgens.

2. Girls mature earlier than boys.

3. Children destined to mature sexually at an early age tend to be tall and have an advanced bone age; late-maturing children are short and show epiphyseal retardation.

4. Sexual maturation is more closely correlated with bone maturation than with chronologic age.

B. Girls: (Table 2—9.)

1. The vaginal mucosa is converted from columnar to squamous type shortly before menarche. This is associated with an increased glycogen content of the mucosa and a lowering of the pH.

2. The maximal yearly increase in height occurs during the year before menarche in most girls.

3. Climate apparently has little effect on sexual development. Nigerian girls and Eskimo girls have their menarche at approximately the same age.

4. If environmental and nutritional factors are similar, girls of different races tend to have their menarche at the same approximate age.

5. During the first 1—2 years following menarche, the menstrual periods of most girls are anovulatory.

6. The first several menses are often irregular, and the interval between periods may be longer or shorter than is characteristic of later life.

7. Girls with early menarche have a more accelerated growth curve than girls with late menarche, but the duration of their growth is shorter.

8. Girls who mature late are taller (on the average) when final stature is attained.

C. Boys: (Table 2—10.) Some degree of breast hypertrophy (gynecomastia) is relatively common in boys at puberty.

"Bone Age" (Epiphyseal Development)
(See Table 2—11 and Fig 2—14.)

The ideal method of evaluating bone age would be based upon x-rays of all of the bones. However, this is not practical due to limitations of time, cost, and danger of excessive radiation. At all ages, the most useful areas to evaluate are the wrists and hands; prior to the age of 2 years, x-rays of the feet and knees are also valuable.

The time of appearance and union of various epiphyseal centers follows a specific sequential pattern during both intra- and extrauterine life.

At birth, the average full-term infant has 5 ossification centers demonstrable by x-ray: the distal end of the femur, the proximal end of the tibia, the calcaneus, the talus, and the cuboid.

The clavicle is the first bone to calcify in utero, calcification beginning during the fifth fetal week.

Epiphyseal development of girls is consistently ahead of that of boys throughout childhood.

Table 2—11. Time of appearance of epiphyseal ossification centers.*

Hand and Wrist

Age (Year//Month†) Percentile (Boys)			Epiphyseal Centers	Age (Year//Month†) Percentile (Girls)		
5	50‡	95		5	50‡	95
Birth	0//2.5	0//4	Capitate	< term§	0//2.25	0//4
Birth	0//3.5	0//6	Hamate	< term§	0//2.5	0//5
0//8	1//0	2//0	Distal radius	0//6	0//10	1//6
1//0	1//6	2//0	Proximal third carpal	0//9	0//11	1//3
1//0	1//6	2//0	Proximal second and fourth carpal	0//9	0//11	1//6
1//3	1//6	2//3	Second metacarpal	0//9	0//11	1//6
1//0	1//6	2//3	Distal first carpal	0//9	1//0	1//6
1//3	1//9	2//6	Third metacarpal	0//9	1//0	1//6
1//6	2//0	2//6	Fourth metacarpal	1//0	1//3	1//9
1//6	2//0	2//6	Proximal fifth carpal	1//0	1//3	2//0
1//6	2//0	2//6	Middle third and fourth carpal	1//0	1//3	2//0
1//6	2//3	3//0	Fifth metacarpal	1//0	1//6	2//0
1//6	2//3	3//0	Middle second carpal	1//0	1//6	2//0
1//0	2//3	4//6	Triquetrum	1//0	1//6	3//0
2//0	2//3	3//0	First metacarpal	1//6	1//6	2//6
2//6	3//0	3//6	Proximal first carpal**	1//3	1//9	2//6
2//6	3//6	5//0	Middle fifth carpal**	1//6	2//0	3//3
1//6	4//0	5//6	Lunate**	2//6	3//0	4//0
3//6	5//3	6//6	Greater multangular**	2//6	4//0	5//6
3//6	5//3	6//6	Lesser multangular**	2//6	4//0	5//6
4//0	5//3	7//0	Navicular**	3//0	4//0	6//6
6//0	7//0	8//0	Distal ulna	5//0	5//6	7//0
10//0	11//0	13//0	Pisiform	7//6	8//0	10//6

Extremities
(Excluding Hand and Wrist)

< term§	< term§	2 weeks	Distal femur	< term§	< term§	1 week
< term§	< term§	2 weeks	Proximal tibia	< term§	< term§	1 week
< term§	2 weeks	6 weeks	Tarsal cuboid	< term§	1 week	2 weeks
Birth	3 weeks	0//2	Head of humerus	Birth	2 weeks	0//1
0//3	0//4	0//9	Distal tibia	0//2	0//3	0//8
0//4	0//5	0//10	Head of femur	0//3	0//4	0//8
0//5	0//7	1//6	Capitellum of humerus	0//3	0//5	1//0
0//7	1//0	2//0	Greater tuberosity of humerus	0//4	0//8	1//6
0//8	1//0	2//0	Distal fibula	0//8	0//9	1//6
2//6	3//6	4//6	Greater trochanter of femur	2//0	2//6	4//0
3//0	4//0	5//6	Proximal fibula	2//0	2//6	4//6
3//6	5//0	7//6	Proximal radius	3//0	4//0	6//0
4//6	6//0	8//0	Medial epicondyle of humerus	3//0	3//6	6//0
7//6	10//0	12//0	Trochlea of humerus	6//0	8//0	10//0
8//0	10//6	12//0	Proximal ulna	6//6	8//0	9//6
10//0	12//0	13//0	Lateral epicondyle of humerus	8//0	9//6	11//0

*Adapted from Marian Maresh. Compiled from data obtained from the Harvard Growth Study, Fels Institute, Brush Foundation, and the University of Colorado Child Research Council.
†Eg, 1//3 = 1 year 3 months.
‡50th percentile and mean are approximately the same in most studies.
§< term = before term.
**Centers which are most variable in time and order of appearance.

Table 2–12. Dental growth and development.

Primary or Deciduous Teeth

	Calcification		Eruption*		Shedding	
	Begins At	Complete At	Maxillary	Mandibular	Maxillary	Mandibular
Central incisors	4th fetal month	18–24 months	6–10 months (2)	5–8 months (1)	7–8 years	6–7 years
Lateral incisors	5th fetal month	18–24 months	8–12 months (3)	7–10 months (2)	8–9 years	7–8 years
Cuspids	6th fetal month	30–39 months	16–20 months (6)	16–20 months (6a)	11–12 years	9–11 years
First molars	5th fetal month	24–30 months	11–18 months (5)	11–18 months (3)	9–11 years	10–12 years
Second molars	6th fetal month	36 months	20–30 months (7)	20–30 months (7a)	9–12 years	11–13 years

Secondary or Permanent Teeth

	Calcification			Eruption*	
	Begins At		Complete At	Maxillary	Mandibular
Central incisors		3–4 months	9–10 years	7–8 years (3)	6–7 years (2)
Lateral incisors	Maxilla	10–12 months	10–11 years	8–9 years (5)	7–8 years (4)
	Mandible	3–4 months			
Cuspids		4–5 months	12–15 years	11–12 years (11)	9–11 years (6)
First premolars		18–24 months	12–13 years	10–11 years (7)	10–12 years (8)
Second premolars		24–30 months	12–14 years	10–12 years (9)	11–13 years (10)
First molars		Birth	9–10 years	5½–7 years (1)	5½–7 years (1a)
Second molars		30–36 months	14–16 years	12–14 years (12)	12–13 years (12a)
Third molars	Maxilla	7–9 years	18–25 years	17–30 years (13)	17–30 years (13a)
	Mandible	8–10 years			

*Figures in parentheses indicate order of eruption. Many otherwise normal infants do not conform strictly to the stated schedule.

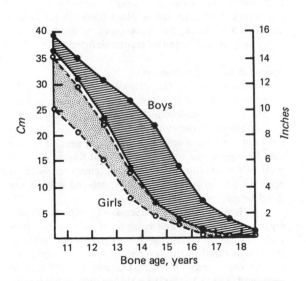

Figure 2–14. Growth expectancy at bone ages indicated. (Redrawn and reproduced, with permission, from Holt, McIntosh, & Barnett: *Pediatrics,* 13th ed. Appleton-Century-Crofts, 1962, as redrawn from Harris & others: *Measurement of Man.* Univ of Minnesota Press, 1930.)

DEVELOPMENT*
(See Table 2–15; Figs 2–15 and 2–16.)

The physician is as responsible for the preservation of health as for the treatment of disease. In order to carry out the former and to identify developmental deviations which may require further assessment, persons responsible for child care must understand the dynamic process involved in what we call development. Development applies to the maturation of organs and systems as well as the acquisition of skills and the ability to adapt to new situations.

Progress of Development
Development is a continuous process that starts with conception and follows an orderly sequential course until death. Children sit before they stand, say single words before they speak phrases and sentences, and draw circles before they can draw squares.

*William K. Frankenburg, MD.

Development does not proceed at a constant rate but in bursts of rapid progress interrupted by resting plateaus.

The developmental process takes place in a cephalocaudal direction: control of the head precedes control of the arms, and both precede control of the legs.

Development in the extremities progresses in a proximo-distal direction: control of the arms and legs occurs before control of the wrists and fingers and the feet and toes.

Development proceeds from the massive to the specific. Initially, a young infant seeing a toy moves his entire body; at a later age, he reaches with one hand to grasp it. When an infant learns to say "milk," he may use the word to mean, "Bring me a glass of milk" or "Take the milk"—or the word milk may be used to signify any other drink. Eventually, the word is used to denote what we mean by milk and is combined with other words to form sentences.

Factors Influencing Development

There are "critical periods" of development. At these times, interference with the normal course of development may result in permanent developmental deficits. Just as rubella during the first trimester of pregnancy may result in congenital anomalies, so may untreated cretinism, phenylketonuria, galactosemia, or malnutrition during the first few months after birth result in permanent developmental deficits. On the other hand, rubella, uncontrolled phenylketonuria, hypothyroidism, galactosemia, or malnutrition occurring later in life are usually not associated with permanent significant developmental deficits. Similarly, emotional and psychologic deprivation early in life may produce permanent deficits in personality development.

The pattern of normal development may be influenced by a number of factors, including genetic determinants of rates of development. In certain families, a number of individuals may have a delay in language development. Genetic factors may also determine the intactness of enzyme systems, ie, they may be responsible for inborn errors of metabolism.

Environmental factors may, in turn, influence the genetic alternatives. For example, the infant genetically destined to develop cretinism, with its resultant brain damage, may be protected if exogenous thyroid is given. Failure to be appropriately stimulated at critical periods may result in neurologic deficits. Thus, persons deprived of light and auditory stimulation for a prolonged period of time may temporarily develop hallucinations and EEG changes. Environmental influences can either inhibit or enhance the child's motivation and curiosity, and may contain models from which the child learns.

Practice has only a slight influence on normal development; maturation usually plays a much greater role in determining the rate of development.

DEVELOPMENT OF MOTOR SKILLS

The newborn infant can perform a number of motor movements, but these are mainly reflex in character.

Motor development involving the hands tends to proceed along a definite sequential course. First the child looks from his hand to the object. Next, he attempts to grasp objects with 2 hands. Then he learns to grasp with the palm of the hand, first using the ulnar side of the hand and later the radial side. Eventually, he grasps objects with the thumb and index finger.

DEVELOPMENT OF SPEECH & LANGUAGE

The normal development of speech and language requires exposure to language, normal structures of the organs of speech, and the following abilities: hearing in the normal speech frequencies (between 250–4000 cycles/second); comprehending what is heard; recalling what has been heard before; formulating a response; and controlling the muscles of speech. On the average, infants manifest speech and language development as shown in Table 2–13.

Normal Variations in Speech & Language Development

A normal 2-year-old child may have a vocabulary varying from a few words to well over 2000 words. First children tend to speak earlier than subsequent children; twins later than singletons. In some studies, girls developed language earlier than boys. Early development of language is often found in intellectually gifted children, but slow onset of speech is not necessarily an indication of mental deficiency.

Speech & Language Disorders

Though speech and language problems can be detected within the first few years of life, they usually do not come to professional attention until school age.

A. Delayed Development of Speech: If a child does not produce words by 2½ years of age, his speech may be considered to be retarded, but this may not be particularly significant if normal comprehension is present. The principal causes of delayed speech are listed below.

1. Hearing loss or hypoacusis—The effect of hearing loss upon speech and language development varies with the age at which the loss began (more severe in the younger child), the severity of loss, the configuration of the threshold audiogram, and the efficacy of treatment. (See Chapter 11.) Hypoacusis is frequently associated with incorrect articulation of **b**, **f**, and **u**. The sounds of **d**, **y**, and **w** are frequently substituted for **g**, **l**, and **r**, respectively. The child with a high-frequency hearing loss may react normally to the

Table 2–13. Normal speech and language development.

Age	Speech	Language
1 month	Throaty sounds	
2 months	Vowel sounds ("eh"), coos	
2½ months	Squeals	
3 months	Babbles, initial vowels	
4 months	Guttural sounds ("ah," "goo")	
7 months	Imitates speech sounds	
10 months		"Dada" or "Mama" nonspecifically.
12 months		One word other than Mama or Dada.
13 months		Three words.
15–18 months	Jargon (language of his own)	Six words.
21–24 months		Two- to 3-word phrases.
2 years	Vowels uttered correctly	Approximately 270 words; uses pronouns.
3 years	Some degree of hesitancy and uncertainty common	Approximately 900 words; intelligible 4-word phrases.
4 years		Approximately 1540 words; intelligible 5-word phrases or sentences.
6 years		Approximately 2560 words; intelligible 6- or 7-word sentences.
7–8 years	Adult proficiency	

spoken voice or to sounds of low frequency, clapping of hands, or banging of doors. Hypoacusis, therefore, should only be ruled out by means of a complete audiologic evaluation.

2. Central nervous system dysfunction—The most common type of CNS dysfunction associated with delayed speech development is mental retardation. Neurologic impairments anywhere in the complex speech mechanism may be manifested in delayed speech and language development. Any child with delayed speech development should be evaluated intellectually in terms of his nonverbal as well as his verbal adaptive skills.

3. Maternal deprivation—Children reared without adequate mothering may have delayed speech development. Though other aspects of the child's development may also be delayed, the delay in language is frequently the most prominent. Historically, these children may show a lack of parent-child interaction—diminished affect, decreased motivation, failure to demonstrate stranger anxiety, inability to communicate nonverbally, and a history of an insatiable appetite.

4. Infantile autism—One of the most common manifestations of autism is a delay in speech (see above), probably because of a primary problem in relating to people.

5. Elective mutism—In this condition, children do not talk to certain persons but speak freely at home or elsewhere. Frequently such children are shy. Birth of a sibling may cause a child to stop talking or to talk less and to regress in his development in other ways.

6. Socially disadvantaged background—Since language is learned from other people, deprived environments may fail to provide suitable reinforcement and a sufficient variety of environmental experiences to bring about verbal facility. Children from the lower socioeco-

nomic classes may demonstrate significant deficits in vocabulary, use of adjectives and adverbs, ability to construct complex sentences, and a general delay in development of articulation. Their speech and language are similar to normal speech and language of nondisadvantaged children of a younger age.

7. Familial delay—Occasionally, a delay in speech development (possibly due to delayed myelinization) affects several members of a family. The child usually comprehends normally. The delay in speech seldom persists beyond 3 years of age.

8. Histidinemia—In this rare familial aminoaciduria, delayed speech development may occur with mental retardation.

9. Twins—Twins are often late talkers.

10. Bilingualism—Monolingual children are more advanced than bilingual children in language expression but show no differences in the rate of development of language comprehension.

B. Voice Defects (Dysphonia): The loss or impairment of tone and volume is due to excessive loudness and pitch. Though it is generally a functional process, it may evolve into an organic condition with the production of vocal nodules. It may also be due to structural defects (eg, papilloma of the larynx).

C. Articulation Disorders: Articulation errors may be due to omissions, distortions, substitutions, or a combination of these.

1. Causes of articulation disorders—

a. Physiologic and anatomic causes—Defects in the cerebrum and cranial nerves which innervate the muscles of the lips, tongue, and palate may produce articulation defects. Inadequate velopharyngeal closure may also cause articulation disorders, since normal articulation involves movement of the velum between the pendant position to closure against the posterior

Table 2—14. Evaluation of articulation disorders.*

	Age in Years						
	2½–3	3–3½	4–4½	4½–5	5–5½	5½–6	6 and older
Normal number of sounds articulated correctly	7 or more	15 or more	16 or more	18 or more	22 or more	24 or more	25 or more
Normal intelligibility	Understandable half the time or more	Easy to understand					

*Adapted from Drumwright A & others: The Denver articulation screening exam. J Speech Hear Disord 38:3, 1973.

pharyngeal wall. Inappropriate closure removes the nasality from nasal consonants. Inadequate closure results in resonant properties such as "talking through the nose." Causes of inadequate closure are a cleft palate, a submucous cleft, and velar paresis or disproportion between the soft palate and the posterior pharynx. Since the adenoids sometimes form part of the posterior surface against which the soft palate closes, removal of the adenoids may produce inadequate closure. Children with inadequate closure sometimes present with a history of fluids coming out of the nose during drinking. Failure of fusion of upper lip and hypoplasia of the mandible are other causes of articulation disorders.

b. Environmental factors—Since a child replicates the speech heard in his home, articulation errors may be due to racial, cultural, and regional differences or to imitation of articulation errors of the parents. The later a child starts to learn a second language, the more likely he will be to have difficulty in articulating the new language.

2. Evaluation of articulation disorders—The Denver Articulation Screening Exam* is a useful, simple, accurate instrument for determining if a child's articulation is appropriate for his age. The test is designed to detect articulation problems in children age 2½–6 years. To administer the test, one determines the child's ability to correctly articulate each of the 30 italicized sounds found in the following 22 words.

1. *t*able	9. *th*umb	16. wago*n*
2. shi*rt*	10. too*th*brush	17. *g*u*m*
3. *d*oor	11. *s*ock	18. *h*ouse
4. tru*n*k	12. vac*uu*m	19. *p*encil
5. *j*umping	13. *y*arn	20. *f*ish
6. zi*pp*er	14. *m*o*th*er	21. *l*eaf
7. *gr*apes	15. *tw*inkle	22. *c*arr*o*t
8. *fl*ag		

The child's articulation is also evaluated for general intelligibility as he puts words together in sentences or phrases (Table 2–14). An abnormal response either in the articulation of single words or in

*Amelia F. Drumwright, University of Colorado Medical Center, 1971.

general intelligibility should be a cause for a diagnostic evaluation by a speech pathologist.

The evaluation should also include a complete neurologic assessment; evaluation of general development or intelligence; assessment of social maturity with a scale such as the Vineland Social Maturity Scale; physical examination of the oropharyngeal cavity; lateral head x-rays during speech production to determine the degree of velopharyngeal closure; and a complete audiologic examination.

D. Dysrhythmia: Three to 4% of children manifest a lack of normal language fluency. In general, lack of fluency is due to interference in the normal control of the respiratory mechanism during speech. Dysrhythmias may be in the form of undue prolongation of word sounds, arrest of speech—mainly at the beginning of a sentence (hesitation)—or repetition of syllables at the beginning of phrases or sentences. Young children between ages 2½–4 years normally manifest breaks in the rhythm of speech, with repetitions being most common.

E. Cluttering: Cluttering is a rapid nervous speech marked by omission of sounds or syllables. The child who clutters may repeat syllables or short words and be unaware of his speech disturbance. Cluttering is due to a dissociation between thinking and speaking. Thus, a child may "get lost" in the middle of a sentence. Individual sounds may be articulated correctly, but the articulation breaks down when the child speaks in longer sentences. Some children who clutter also manifest dysrhythmic handwriting. There is often a family history of cluttering. Occasionally, cluttering may lead to stuttering.

F. Stuttering: Stuttering is a disturbance of rhythm and fluency of speech by an intermittent blocking, convulsive repetition, or prolongation of sounds, syllables, words, or phrases. It is probably caused by many factors. Both organic and psychogenic factors are considered to play a role. Fifty percent of people who stutter begin to do so before age 5, and most begin to stutter before age 11. Between ages 2 and 5, stuttering is usually transient or benign. Stuttering is 2–4 times more frequent in boys. Stuttering causes considerable anxiety in parents, who may then call the child's attention to it in an attempt to make him stop. This, in turn, makes the child more anxious and self-conscious and aggravates the problem. The child may avoid words which are difficult for him to enunciate, and he may avoid speaking at all. Facial and body movements may be associated with stuttering.

Since one of the factors precipitating or aggravating stuttering is anxiety, it is important to determine the circumstances which led to it. If the stuttering persists or if it has its onset after 11 years of age, the child should be referred to an experienced speech pathologist.

Drumwright A: *Denver Articulation Screening Exam.* University of Colorado Medical Center, 1971.
De Hirsch K: Stuttering and cluttering: Developmental aspects of dysrhythmic speech. J Special Education 2:143, 1969.
Morris HL & others: An articulation test for assessing competency of velopharyngeal closure. J Speech Hear Disord 1:48, 1961.
Raph JB: Language and speech deficits in culturally disadvantaged children: Implications for the speech clinician. J Speech Hear Disord 32:203, 1967.

DEVELOPMENTAL SCREENING*
(See Fig 2–15.)

There is general agreement that the physician who gives routine pediatric care should have some knowledge of child development and be able to identify abnormal developmental delays.

The Denver Developmental (Frankenburg-Dodds) Screening Test (DDST) is a device for detecting developmental delays in infancy and the preschool years. The test is administered with ease and speed and lends itself to serial evaluations on the same test sheet.

Test Materials
Skein of red wool, box of raisins, rattle with a narrow handle, small aspirin bottle, bell, tennis ball, test form, pencil, 8 one-inch cubical counting blocks.

General Administration Instructions
The mother should be told that this is a developmental screening device to obtain an estimate of the child's level of development and that it is not expected that the child be able to perform each of the test items. This test relies on observations of what the child can do and on reports by a parent who knows the child. Direct observation should be used whenever possible. Since the test requires active participation by the child, every effort should be made to put the child at ease. The younger child may be tested while sitting on the mother's lap. This should be done in such a way that he can comfortably reach the test materials on the table. The test should be administered before any frightening or painful procedures. A child will often withdraw if the examiner rushes demands upon the child. One may start by laying out 1 or 2 test materials

*Adapted from Frankenburg WK, Goldstein A, Camp B: The revised Denver Developmental Screening Test: Its accuracy as a screening instrument. J Pediatr 79:988, 1971.

in front of the child while asking the mother whether he performs some of the personal-social items. It is best to administer the first few test items well below the child's age level in order to assure an initial successful experience. To avoid distractions, it is best to remove all test materials from the table except those required for the test being administered.

Steps in Administering the Test
(1) Draw a vertical line on the examination sheet through the 4 sectors (gross motor, fine motor adaptive, language, and personal-social) to represent the child's chronologic age. Place the date of the examination at the top of the age line. For premature children, subtract the months premature from the chronologic age.

(2) The items to be administered are those through which the child's chronologic age line passes unless there are obvious deviations. In each sector one should establish the area where the child passes all of the items and the point at which he fails all of the items.

(3) In the event that a child refuses to do some of the items requested by the examiner, it is suggested that the parent administer the item, provided she does so in the prescribed manner.

(4) If a child passes an item, a large letter "P" is written on the bar at the 50% passing point. "F" designates a failure, and "R" designates a refusal.

(5) Failure to perform an item passed by 90% of children of the same age should be considered significant, although not necessarily abnormal.

(6) Note date and pertinent observations of parent and child behavior (how child feels at time of the evaluation, relation to the examiner, attention span, verbal behavior, self-confidence, etc).

(7) Ask the parent if the child's performance was typical of his performance at other times.

(8) To retest the child on the same form, use a different color pencil for the scoring and age line.

(9) Instructions for administering footnoted items are given below.

Interpretations
The test items are placed into 4 categories: gross motor, fine motor adaptive, language, and personal-social. Each of the test items is designated by a bar which is so located under the age scale as to indicate clearly the ages at which 25%, 50%, 75%, and 90% of the standardization population could perform the particular test item. The left end of the bar designates

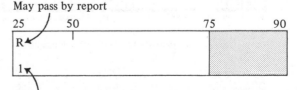

Footnote # (To be filled in from list on p 35.)

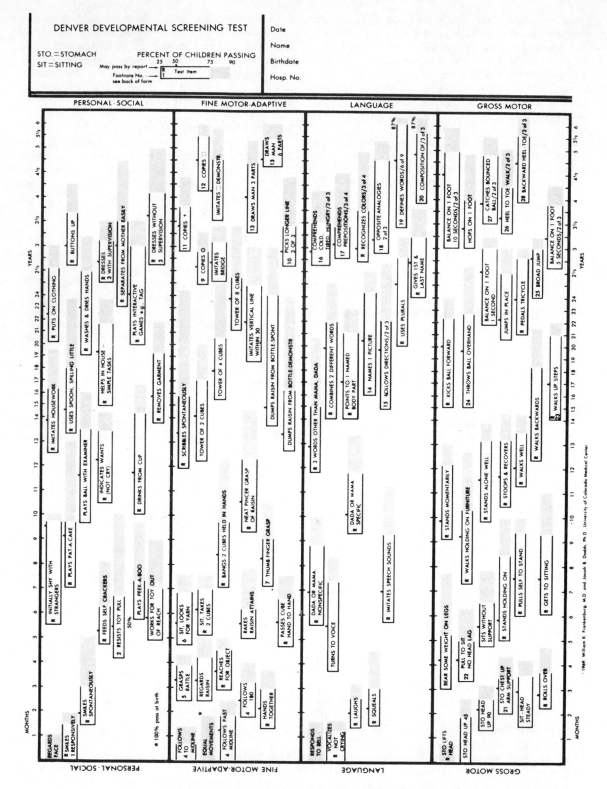

Figure 2–15. Denver Developmental Screening Test. (See p 35 for footnoted items.)

Table 2—15. Developmental charts for ages 3—15 years.*

Ages 3—4 Years

Activities to be observed:
Climbs stairs with alternating feet.
Begins to button and unbutton.
"What do you like to do that's fun?" (Answers using plurals, personal pronoun, and verbs.)
Responds to command to place toy *in, on,* or *under* table.
Draws a circle when asked to draw a man (girl, boy).
Knows his sex. ("Are you a boy or a girl?")
Gives full name.
Copies a circle already drawn. ("Can you make one like this?")

Activities related by parent:
Feeds self at mealtime.
Takes off shoes and jacket.

Ages 4—5 Years

Activities to be observed:
Runs and turns without losing balance.
May stand on one leg for at least 10 seconds.
Buttons clothes and laces shoes. (Does not tie.)
Counts to 4 by rote.
"Give me 2 sticks." (Able to do so from pile of 4 tongue depressors.)
Draws a man. (Head, 2 appendages, and possibly 2 eyes. No torso yet.)
"You know the days of the week. What day comes after Tuesday?"
Gives appropriate answers to: "What must you do if you are sleepy? Hungry? Cold?"
Copies + in imitation.

Activities related by parent:
Self care at toilet. (May need help with wiping.)
Plays outside for at least 30 minutes.
Dresses self except for tying.

Ages 5—6 Years

Activities to be observed:
Can catch ball.
Skips smoothly.
Copies a + already drawn.
Tells his age.
Concept of 10 (eg, counts 10 tongue depressors). May recite to higher number by rote.
Knows his right and left hand.
Draws recognizable man with at least 8 details.
Can describe favorite television program in some detail.

Activities related by parent:
Does simple chores at home. (Taking out garbage, drying silverware, etc.)
Goes to school unattended or meets school bus.
Good motor ability but little awareness of dangers.

Ages 6—7 Years

Activities to be observed:
Copies a △.
Defines words by use. ("What is an orange?" "To eat.")
Knows if morning or afternoon.
Draws a man with 12 details.
Reads several one-syllable printed words. (My, dog, see, boy.)
Uses pencil for printing name.

Ages 7—8 Years

Activities to be observed:
Counts by 2s and 5s.
Ties shoes.
Copies a ◇.
Knows what day of the week it is. (Not date or year.)
Reads paragraph #1 Durrell:

Reading:
Muff is a little yellow kitten. She drinks milk. She sleeps on a chair. She does not like to get wet.

Corresponding arithmetic:

7	6	6	8
+ 4	+ 7	− 4	− 3

No evidence of sound substitution in speech (eg, *fr* for *thr*).
Adds and subtracts one-digit numbers.
Draws a man with 16 details.

Ages 8—9 Years

Activities to be observed:
Defines words better than by use. ("What is an orange?" "A fruit.")
Can give an appropriate answer to the following: "What is the thing for you to do if . . .
    —you've broken something that belongs to someone else?"
    —a playmate hits you without meaning to do so?"
Reads paragraph #2 Durrell:

Reading:
A little black dog ran away from home. He played with two big dogs. They ran away from him. It began to rain. He went under a tree. He wanted to go home, but he did not know the way. He saw a boy he knew. The boy took him home.

Corresponding arithmetic:

	45		
67	16	14	84
+ 4	+ 27	− 8	− 36

Is learning borrowing and carrying processes in addition and subtraction.

*Modified from Leavitt SR, Goodman H, Harvin D: Pediatrics 31:499, 1963.

[cont'd]

Table 2–15 (cont'd). Developmental charts for ages 3–15 years.

Ages 9–10 Years

Activities to be observed:

Knows the month, day, and year.

Names the months in order. (Fifteen seconds, one error.)

Makes a sentence with these 3 words in it: (One of 2. Can use words orally in proper context.)

1. work . . . . money . . . . men
2. boy . . . . river . . . . ball

Reads paragraph #3 Durrell:

Reading:

Six boys put up a tent by the side of river. They took things to eat with them. When the sun went down, they went into the tent to sleep. In the night, a cow came and began to eat grass around the tent. The boys were afraid. They thought it was a bear.

Corresponding arithmetic:

$$\begin{array}{ccc} 5204 & 23 & 837 \\ -\,530 & \times\,3 & \times\,7 \end{array}$$

Should comprehend and answer question: "What was the cow doing?"

Learning simple multiplication.

Ages 10–12 Years

Activities to be observed:

Should read and comprehend paragraph #5 Durrell:

Reading:

In 1807, Robert Fulton took the first long trip in a steamboat. He went one hundred and fifty miles up the Hudson River. The boat went five miles an hour. This was faster than a steamboat had ever gone before. Crowds gathered on both banks of the river to see this new kind of boat. They were afraid that its noise and splashing would drive away all the fish.

Corresponding arithmetic:

$$\begin{array}{ccc} 420 \\ \times\,29 & 9\overline{)72} & 31\overline{)62} \end{array}$$

Answer: "What river was the trip made on?"

Ask to write the sentence: "The fishermen did not like the boat."

Should do multiplication and simple division.

Ages 12–15 Years

Activities to be observed:

Reads paragraph #7 Durrell:

Reading:

Golf originated in Holland as a game played on ice. The game in its present form first appeared in Scotland. It became unusually popular and kings found it so enjoyable that it was known as "the royal game." James IV, however, thought that people neglected their work to indulge in this fascinating sport so that it was forbidden in 1457. James relented when he found how attractive the game was, and it immediately regained its former popularity. Golf spread gradually to other countries, being introduced in America in 1890. It has grown in favor until there is hardly a town that does not boast of a private or public course.

Corresponding arithmetic:

$$536\overline{)4762} \qquad \begin{array}{c} \frac{1}{3} \\ +\,\frac{1}{3} \end{array} \qquad \begin{array}{c} 7\frac{1}{6} \\ -\,\frac{3}{4} \end{array}$$

Reduce fractions to lowest forms.

Ask to write sentence: "Golf originated in Holland as a game played on ice."

Answers questions:

"Why was golf forbidden by James IV?"

"Why did he change his mind?"

Does long division, adds and subtracts fractions.

---

the age at which 25% of the standardization population could perform the item; the point shown at the top of the bar, 50%; the left end of the shaded area, 75%; and the right end of the bar the age at which 90% of the standardization population could perform the item.

Failure to perform an item passed by 90% of children of the same age should be considered significant. Such a failure may be emphasized by coloring the right end of the bar of the failed item. Several failures in one sector are considered to be developmental delays. These delays may be due to:

(1) The unwillingness of the child to use his ability:

(a) Due to temporary phenomena, such as fatigue, illness, hospitalization, separation from the parent, fear, etc.

(b) General unwillingness to do most things that are asked of him; such a condition may be just as detrimental as an inability to perform.

(2) An inability to perform the item due to:

(a) General retardation.

(b) Pathologic factors such as deafness or neurologic impairment.

(c) Familial pattern of slow development in one or more areas.

If unexplained developmental delays are noted and are a valid reflection of a child's abilities, he should be rescreened a month later. If the delays persist, he should be further evaluated with more detailed diagnostic studies.

Caution: The DDST is not an intelligence test. It is intended as a screening instrument for use in clinical practice to note whether the development of a particular child is within the normal range.

Directions for Footnoted Items

(1) Try to get child to smile by smiling or by talking or waving to him. Do not touch him.

(2) When child is playing with toy, pull it away from him. Pass if he resists.

(3) Child does not have to be able to tie shoes or button in the back.

(4) Move yarn slowly in an arc from one side to the other, about 6 inches above child's face. Pass if eyes follow 90° to midline. (Past midline, 180°.)

(5) Pass if child grasps rattle when it is touched to the backs or tips of fingers.

(6) Pass if child continues to look where yarn disappeared or tries to see where it went. Yarn should be dropped quickly from sight from tester's hand without arm movement.

(7) Pass if child picks up raisin with any part of thumb and a finger.

(8) Pass if child picks up raisin with the ends of thumb and index finger using an overhand approach.

(9) Copy. Pass any enclosed form. Do not name form. Do not demonstrate.

(10) "Which line is *longer*?" (Not *bigger*.) Turn paper upside down and repeat. (Pass 3 of 3 or 5 of 6.)

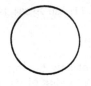

(11) Copy. Pass any crossing lines. Do not name form. Do not demonstrate.

(12) Have child copy first. If he fails, demonstrate. Do not name form.

(13) When scoring symmetrical forms, each pair (2 arms, 2 legs, etc) counts as one part.

(14) Point to picture and have child name it. (No credit is given for sounds only.)

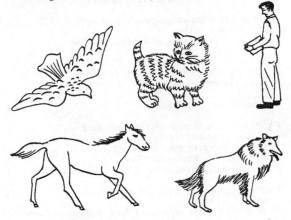

(15) Tell child to, "Give block to Mommie." "Put block on table." "Put block on floor." Pass 2 of 3.

(16) Ask child, "What do you do when you are cold?" "Hungry?" "Tired?" Pass 2 of 3.

(17) Tell child to, "Put block on table." ". . . under table." ". . . in front of chair." ". . . behind chair." Pass 3 of 4. (Do not help child by pointing or by moving head or eyes.)

(18) Ask child, "If fire is hot, ice is —." "Mother is a woman, Dad is a —." "A horse is big, a mouse is —." Pass 2 of 3.

(19) Ask child, "What is a ball?" ". . . a lake?" ". . . a desk?" ". . . a house?" ". . . a banana?" ". . . a curtain?" ". . . a ceiling?" ". . . a hedge?" ". . . a pavement?" Pass if defined in terms of use, shape, what it is made of, or general category (eg, banana is *fruit*, not just *yellow*). Pass 6 of 9.

(20) Ask child, "What is a spoon made of?" ". . . a shoe made of?" ". . . a door made of?" (No other objects may be substituted.) Pass 3 of 3.

(21) When placed on stomach, child lifts chest off table with support of forearms and/or hands.

(22) When child is on back, grasp his hands and pull him to sitting position. Pass if head does not hang back.

(23) Child may use wall or rail only, not a person. May not crawl.

(24) Child must throw ball overhand 3 feet to within arm's reach of tester.

(25) Child must perform standing broad jump over width of test sheet (8½ inches).

(26) Tell child to walk forward, heel within 1 inch of toe.

(27) Bounce ball to child, who should stand 3 feet away from tester. Child must catch ball with hands, not arms, in 2 out of 3 tries.

(28) Tell child to walk backward, toe within 1 inch of heel. Tester may demonstrate. Child must walk 4 consecutive steps in 2 out of 3 tries.

Date and behavioral observations: (How child feels at time of test, relation to tester, attention span, verbal behavior, self-confidence, etc.)

Smile: In response to an adult or to his voice . . . .

Vocalize: Utters sounds spontaneously or on . . . .
    stimulation
Head control: No head lag when pulled to sitting   . . . .
    position from supine
Hand control: Grasps toy with one or both hands   . . . .
    when toy is dangled in midline above his chest
Roll over: From back to abdomen . . . .

Sit alone: For several moments . . . .

Crawl: By rolling over and over, pushing along . . . .
    on stomach or back, or any other means
Prehension: Brings together thumb and   . . . .
    forefinger to pick up small objects
Pull up: To standing position . . . .

Walk with support: By holding to playpen, ...
    furniture, or an adult
Stand alone: Without any support, for several moments . . . .

Walk alone: Several steps . . . .

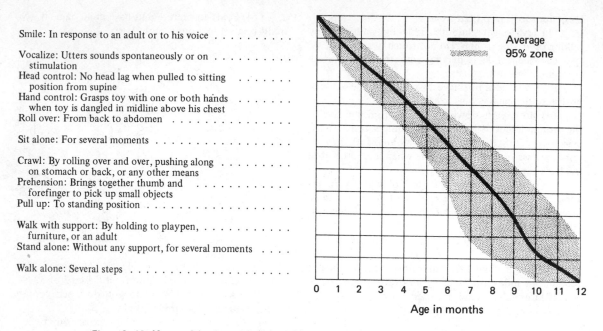

Figure 2—16. Norms of development. (Adapted from Aldrich & Norval: J Pediatr 29:304, 1946.)

PERSONALITY DEVELOPMENT*

Personality development is a dynamic process, and no summary can give a complete picture of what takes place. The goal of the individual, both as a child and as an adult, is to be able to work, to play, to master personal problems, and to love and be loved in a manner that is creative, socially acceptable, and personally gratifying.

The development of personality is a complicated process involving all aspects of the individual and his environment. The process varies from one child to another, but on the whole all children pass through various phases of development of which details differ but of which the broad general outlines are essentially the same.

Each of these successive stages of development is characterized by definite problems which the child must solve if he is to proceed with confidence to the next. The highest degree of functional harmony will be achieved when the problems of each stage are met and solved at an orderly rate and in a normal sequence. On the other hand, it is well to remember that the successive personality gains which the child makes are not rigidly established once and for all but may be reinforced or threatened throughout the life of the individual. Even in adulthood a reasonably healthy personality may be achieved in spite of previous misfortunes and defects in the developmental sequence.

In considering psychologic development it is important to remember that it takes place within a

*Ruth S. Kempe, MD

cultural milieu. Not only the form of large social institutions but the framework of family life, the attitudes of parents, and their practices in child-rearing will be conditioned by the culture of the period.

Psychologic development in childhood may be roughly divided into 5 stages: infancy (birth to 18 months), early childhood (18 months to 5 years), later childhood (5–12 years), early adolescence (12–16 years), and late adolescence (16 years to maturity).

Infancy

Perhaps the most striking features of the first year are the great physical development which takes place and the infant's growing awareness of himself as an entity separate from his environment.

Much of the psychologic development of the first year is interrelated with physical development, ie, dependent upon the maturation of the body to the extent that the child can discriminate self and nonself. Knowledge of the environment comes with increasing sharpening of the senses (from indiscriminate mouthing to coordinated eye-hand movements). Beginning of mastery over the environment comes with increasingly adept coordination, the development of locomotion, and the beginnings of speech. The realization of himself as an individual in relation to an environment including other individuals is the basis upon which interpersonal relationships are founded.

The newborn infant is at first aware only of his bodily needs—ie, the presence or absence of discomfort (cold, wet, etc). The pleasure of relief from discomfort gradually becomes associated with mothering and later (when perception is sufficient for recognition) with the mother. The child derives a feeling of security when his needs are satisfied and from contact with the mother. The feeding situation provides the first opportunity for development of this feeling of security, and it is therefore important for the physician to ensure that this is a happy event.

The development of the first emotional relationship, then, comes through this close contact with the mother. It no longer will be just a meeting of the infant's physical needs but a sustained physical contact and emotional interaction with one person. Prolonged absence of this relationship, if no satisfactory substitute is provided, is damaging to the personality. If permanent, it leads to restriction of personality development, even to pseudoretardation in all areas. Such behavior may also occur in a home situation, but it is more striking and more common in infants who remain for long periods of time in the hospital or in other institutions where the nursing personnel is inadequate (either in number or ability) to give sufficient personalized and kindly attention to each child. If the infant is deprived of the security and affection necessary to produce a sense of trust, he may respond with listlessness, immobility, unresponsiveness, indifferent appetite, an appearance of unhappiness, and insomnia. In other cases the continued deprivation of consistent care in infancy may not become apparent until later life, when the individual may feel that he has no reason to trust people; this may result in his feeling no sense of responsibility toward his fellow men.

No particular technics are necessary to develop a baby's feeling of security. The infant is not easily discouraged by an inexperienced mother's mistakes; rather the child seems to respond to the warmth of her feeling and her eagerness to keep trying. The feeling of security derived from satisfactory relationships during the first year is probably the most important single element in the personality. It makes it possible for the child to accept restrictions without fearing that each restriction implies total loss of love.

Toward the end of the first year, other personal relationships also are developing, particularly with the father, who is now recognized as comparable in importance with the mother. Relationships perhaps are also forming with siblings.

Early Childhood

In early childhood the child's horizon continues to widen. Increased body control makes possible the development of many physical skills. The very important development of speech permits extension of the social environment and increasing ability to understand and perfect social relationships.

Perhaps the central problem of early childhood is still, however, the development of control over the instinctive drives, particularly as they arise in relationship to the parents. The acceptance of limitations on the need for bodily love (the realization that complete infantile dependency is not permitted or desirable) and the control of aggressive feelings are prime examples. This control of primitive feelings is largely accomplished through the psychologic process of "identification" with the parents—the desire in the child to be like the parents and to emulate them. With this desire comes the beginnings of conscience, the child's incorporation into his own personality of the moral values of the parents.

The child now begins to have a feeling of autonomy—of self-direction and initiative. The child 18 months to 2½ years of age is actively learning to exercise the power of "yes" and "no." The difficulty the 2-year-old has in making up his mind between the 2 often leads to parental misunderstanding; he may say "no" when he really means "yes," as if he were compelled to exercise this new "will" even against his better judgment.

At this period, parental "discipline" becomes very important. Discipline is an educative means by which the parent teaches the child how to become a self-respecting, likeable, and socially responsible adult. Disciplinary measures have value chiefly as they serve this educative function; if used as an end in themselves, to establish the "authority" of the parent irrespective of the issues at hand, they usually lead only to warfare (open or surreptitious) between parent and child.

The goal is to allow the child to develop the feeling that he is a responsible human being, while at the same time he learns that he is able to use the help and guidance of others in important matters. The favorable result is self-control without loss of self-esteem. As adults, we should allow a child increasingly wide latitude in undergoing experiences which permit him to make the choices he is ready and able to make, and yet we must also teach him to accept restrictions when necessary.

Firmness and consistency in the parent are necessary, for the child must be protected against the potential anarchy of his poorly developed judgment. Perhaps the most constructive rule a parent can follow is to decide which kinds of conformity are really important and then to clearly and consistently require obedience in these areas. Then "discipline" will have the positive goal of making the child socially compatible without making him feel guilty about his basic drives or stifling his need for some expression of independence.

Later Childhood

In this period, the child achieves a rapid intellectual growth and actively begins to establish himself as a member of society. Psychiatrists call this the latency period, because the force of the primitive drives has been fairly successfully controlled, expressed in a socially acceptable way, or repressed. The energy derived from the instinctive drives of which society does not permit direct expression is diverted into the great drive for knowledge—a process of "sublimation." At no time in life does the individual learn more avidly and quickly. Reading and writing (the intellectual skills) and a vast body of information are quickly assimilated. The preoccupation with fantasy gradually subsides, and the child wants to be engaged in real tasks he can carry through to completion. Even in play activities, the emphasis is on developing mental and bodily skills through interest in sports and games.

Late childhood is also a period of conformity to the group. The environment enlarges to include the school and, particularly, other children. Much of the emotional satisfaction previously derived from the parents is now derived from the child's relationships with his peers. His desire to become a member of this larger group of his equals tends to make the qualities of cooperation and obedience to the will of the group (elements of democracy) important. It also paves the way for questioning of the parental values where these differ from those of the group: a direct impact of broader cultural values upon the environment of the home.

Early Adolescence

After the comparative calm of late childhood, early adolescence is a period of upheaval. With the great changes in body size and configuration comes a new confusion about the physical self (the "body image"). Sexual maturation brings with it a resurgence of the strong instinctual drives which have been successfully repressed for several years. In our culture, in contrast to some primitive cultures, the sexual drive is not permitted direct expression in adolescence in spite of physical readiness.

The calm emotional adjustment is disrupted. Again the child has to learn to control strong feelings: love, hate, and aggression. Again the relationship to the parents is disturbed. The former docile acceptance of them as most important, most powerful, is replaced by rebellion. Yet as strongly as the adolescent rebels and insists on independence from his parents, just as strongly does he feel again the old dependence which, although not openly admitted, is revealed in his unwillingness to accept personal responsibility and his tendency to rely on parental care.

Again his position as an individual must be realigned, not in relation to the family circle but in relation to society. Adolescents are constantly preoccupied with how they appear in the eyes of others as compared with their own conceptions of themselves. They find comfort in conformity with their own age group, and fads in clothing and manners reach a peak in early adolescence.

Perhaps most helpful to parents is the ability to "ride" with each swing in adolescent behavior and not assume that each change accurately presages the personality of the future adult. Adolescents are inexperienced in their new roles as potential adults, and their behavior tends to be erratic and extreme. Calm and stability provided by the parents can do much to keep them in equilibrium.

Late Adolescence

By the 16th year most children have again reached comparative equilibrium. Body growth has slowed somewhat, and the adolescent has had time to adapt to his new physique. He has acquired comparative mastery over his biologic drives to the extent that they can now be channeled into more constructive patterns, the beginning of heterosexual social activity, which eventually leads to the choice of a marital partner.

The relationship to the parents is now more mature. With the discovery that responsible independence is neither frightening nor overwhelming but a position possible to maintain, the adolescent can cease to rebel and can accept his parents' help in planning constructively for his adulthood.

Again learning is rapid, particularly for the intelligent youth, who can absorb much more than a junior high school education.

Active preparation for adulthood characterizes late adolescence in our culture, although, as in more primitive cultures, some adolescents will have already taken on the responsibilities of job and marriage. Biologically, this is certainly feasible; it is the complexity and competition of our modern culture which so greatly prolong the emergence into full adulthood.

• • •

General References

Frankenburg WK, Camp W: *Pediatric Screening Tests.* Thomas, 1975.

McCammon RW: *Human Growth and Development.* Thomas, 1970.

Watson EH, Lowrey GH: *Growth and Development of Children,* 5th ed. Year Book, 1967.

Whipple DV: *Dynamics of Development: Euthenic Pediatrics.* McGraw-Hill, 1966.

3...
The Newborn Infant

Frederick C. Battaglia, MD

The care of the newborn infant is part of "perinatal medicine," which encompasses the fields of obstetrics and neonatology and involves a close working relationship between obstetricians and pediatricians in caring for the mother, the fetus, and the newborn infant.

During the past few years, services within neonatology have been divided into 3 levels of infant care (low-risk, level 1; intermediate care, level 2; and intensive care, level 3) and 2 levels of obstetric services (a "regular" or low-risk service and a high-risk service).

The low-risk level 1 nurseries are usually for full-term infants and often function as "rooming-in" units. All personnel working in this nursery pay special attention to encouraging and developing good parental skills, initiate screening tests for various metabolic problems such as phenylketonuria and hypothyroidism, and are alert for signs of congenital infections, particularly group B streptococcal infections, which attack newborn infants regardless of their gestational age or size. Level 1 units should have excellent neonatal treatment facilities where newborn infants who are ill can be cared for briefly and their condition stabilized in preparation for possible transport to level 2 or level 3 units.

Level 2 nurseries care for most sick newborn infants, including most preterm infants of about 32 weeks' gestational age or more whose weight is 1300–1500 gm or more. Most infants with intrauterine growth retardation or infants of diabetic mothers can be cared for in these units. These nurseries rarely attempt to treat infants requiring arterial catheterization, respiratory care, or intubation, but they do care for infants requiring intravenous infusions or management of infections or a variety of metabolic problems. In general, infants are discharged from this unit directly to the parents without transport to a level 1 unit.

Level 3 nurseries care for sick infants regardless of their size, gestational age, or severity of illness. In general, these nurseries treat infants for a relatively short period of time during the acute phase of a critical illness. Once the condition of the infants has improved sufficiently, they are discharged to the nearest level 2 nursery, which is often much closer to their homes.

Past Obstetric History

The past history of the infant is important regardless of the severity of the current illness. To a considerable extent, the past history of an infant is actually the obstetric history of the mother. Maternal age, interval between pregnancies, and previous therapeutic or spontaneous abortions, particularly in the early teens, are factors that have profound effects on neonatal outcome. Birth weight and gestational age of other infants born to the parents should be plotted as in Fig 3–1 to enable the physician to recognize any striking change in pregnancy outcome or the continuation of a consistent pattern of intrauterine growth characteristic of previous pregnancies. Maternal weight gain or loss during pregnancy, dietary fads, and possible drug ingestion should be noted, as well as the family history and a review of any current maternal illnesses such as toxemia, asthma, etc.

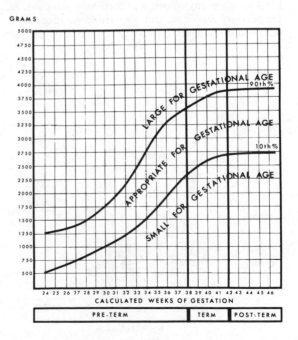

Figure 3–1. Classification of newborn infants by birth weight and gestational age. (University of Colorado Medical Center. Reproduced, with permission, from Battaglia FC, Lubchenco LO: J Pediat 71:160, 1967.)

39

INTRAUTERINE GROWTH RATE

The intrauterine growth rate of an infant is affected by many factors, including the mother's general health, the health of the fetus, and the condition of the placenta. During the intrauterine period, virtually any organ system disease can affect the growth rate of the child, sometimes temporarily and in other instances permanently. The weight of the infant may reflect the total genetic and environmental status. Thus, maternal toxemia may lead to small-for-gestational age (SGA) infants; the longer the toxemia has been present during the pregnancy, the more striking the degree of growth retardation. Similarly, congenital rubella infection usually produces some degree of growth retardation (see Fig 3–2).

It is important to have some means of recognizing marked deviations in intrauterine growth rate as soon after birth as possible. Many different birth weight-gestational age growth curves are available and are useful for initial screening purposes. One classification of newborn infants based upon birth weight and gestational age is presented in Fig 3–1. Fig 3–2 shows some of the conditions affecting the fetus and producing deviations from normal intrauterine growth rate.

Birth Weight

In the past, prematurity was defined as a birth weight of less than 2500 gm. Today, the age and the birth weight of an infant are recognized as separate and equally important factors. Birth weight is important because many physiologic and metabolic processes, eg, temperature regulation and the need for environmental temperature support, are a function of size and are relatively independent of the infant's gestational age. Thus, relative surface area increases as weight decreases. For practical purposes, many physicians distinguish a category of "very-low-birth-weight" (VLBW) infants. These are infants with birth weights of less than 1000 gm, whose problems of metabolism, thermal regulation, water and electrolyte balance, etc are exceedingly complex regardless of their gestational age.

Gestational Age

Determination of gestational age must be based on the maternal history correlated with certain findings during the pregnancy, eg, rate of change of uterine height above the symphysis and the time when fetal heart sounds and movement were first noted.

Many additional tests can help to determine gestational age during pregnancy. These include serial ultrasound examinations to determine biparietal diameter and its rate of growth, amniotic fluid examination for creatinine concentration, and assessment of lecithin/sphingomyelin ratios. Correct determination of gestational age is especially important when elective termination of pregnancy is considered.

After delivery, a clinical estimation of gestational age should be based on physical characteristics and the neurologic examination, which change predictably with increasing gestational age.

Length & Head Size

Most newborns who present with intrauterine growth retardation in weight show relatively less deviation from normal in length and head circumference. Length and head growth appear to be protected to some extent under circumstances of intrauterine undernutrition. However, in severe and prolonged intrauterine undernutrition, such as occurs in the discordant twin, all body proportions may be affected.

Weight-Length Ratio

The weight-length ratio (Fig 2–2) aids in identifying fetal growth abnormalities. It increases with fetal age, ie, the baby becomes heavier for his length as he approaches full term. In intrauterine growth retardation, the weight-length ratio decreases since the rate of growth in weight is affected more than length. The ratio is calculated using the following formula:

$$\frac{100 \times \text{Weight in gm}}{(\text{Length in cm})^3}$$

Battaglia FC, Lubchenco LO: A practical classification of newborn infants by weight and gestational age. J Pediatr 71:159, 1967.

Davies PA, Tizard JPM: Very low birth weight and subsequent neurological defect. Dev Med Child Neurol 17:3, 1975.

Jones MD, Battaglia FC: Intrauterine growth retardation. Am J Obstet Gynecol 127:540, 1977.

Lowry GH: *Growth and Development of Children*, 6th ed. Year Book, 1973.

Lubchenco LO & others: Intrauterine growth in length and head circumference as estimated from live births at gestational ages from 26 to 42 weeks. Pediatrics 37:403, 1966.

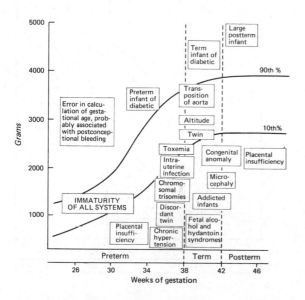

Figure 3–2. Conditions associated with intrauterine growth related to birth weight and gestational age classification. (Reproduced, with permission, from: Nutricia Symposium. HE Stenfert Korese, NV. Leiden, Holland, 1968.)

PHYSICAL EXAMINATION

The physical examination of the newborn should be appropriate for the age of the infant. Four separate time periods are identified in the term infant, and in each of these periods specific information and problems are being sought. The first examination is immediately after birth, usually in the delivery room, and is aimed at both identifying life-threatening abnormalities which require immediate attention and at evaluating the infant's ability to adjust to extrauterine life. A thorough or "complete" examination is not appropriate at this time. The second time interval is the "transition" period, which may last 1–4 hours. In this second evaluation, the infant is observed but not disturbed unless problems arise. He is weighed, measured, and classified by birth weight and gestational age. Specific problems which are likely to occur, as indicated by these parameters, may be investigated. The complete examination, or third evaluation, is ideally performed after 12–24 hours and should be thorough. The fourth evaluation is done at the time of hospital discharge. The discharge examination may be brief and is performed in the presence of the mother so that she and the examiner may assess the infant's condition and discuss the findings.

Considerable effort is currently being expended to find ways to evaluate the infant with the least disturbance to the mother-child interaction and with the least disruption of an environment conducive to the development of good parenting patterns.

THE INFANT IMMEDIATELY AFTER BIRTH

Evaluations

A. Apgar Score: Immediate evaluation of the newborn at 1 and 5 minutes after birth is a valuable routine procedure (Table 3–1). The newborn in the best condition (Apgar score 8–10) is vigorous, pink, and crying. A moderately depressed baby (Apgar score 5–7) appears cyanotic, with slow and irregular respirations but has good muscle tone and reflexes. The severely depressed infant (Apgar score 4 or less) is limp, pale or blue, apneic, and has a slow heart rate. The 5-minute Apgar score is the more useful indicator of neonatal and long-term prognosis.

One should be cautious, however, in attempting to interpret low Apgar scores in very-low-birth-weight infants. Partly because of their marked immaturity, which militates against normal muscle tone, and partly because of their very small size, which predisposes to more severe shock, very-low-birth-weight infants often have low Apgar scores unassociated with subsequent increased morbidity or mortality rates.

B. Chest: Auscultation of the lungs may reveal sticky rales with the first few breaths. In the healthy infant, air exchange is good almost immediately. Respiratory rate ranges from 30–60 for the first few minutes and may be irregular. The heart rate may be variable but should remain above 100/minute and stabilize between 120–160/minute.

Positive pressure resuscitation is rarely required when the heart rate is consistently above 100/minute. Resuscitation and the various stages of physiologic support supplied during resuscitation are discussed later in this chapter.

C. Temperature: The maintenance of body temperature is always important but especially so in the very-low-birth-weight infant and in the infant severely depressed as a result of perinatal asphyxia. The temperature of a newborn infant cannot be maintained within the thermal neutral zone without detailed attention to all aspects of care. At birth, the infant's skin must always be toweled dry of amniotic fluid because evaporative heat losses are enormous, and no radiant heat will support body temperature if the skin is wet. A radiant heater, preferably in combination with a mattress warmer, should be used to supplement a warm environment if the infant remains nude immediately after birth (Fig 3–3).

Body temperature will fall precipitously in a cool environment unless adequate precautions are taken. As the fall in body temperature occurs, the infant becomes cyanotic—first in the hands and feet, then in the face, and finally over the entire body—and may develop grunting respirations and retractions.

A change in the distribution of cardiac output occurs in infants who are allowed to become hypothermic. This altered state causes metabolic acidosis,

Table 3–1. Infant evaluation at birth (Apgar score).* One minute and 5 minutes after complete birth of infant (disregarding cord and placenta), the following objective signs should be observed and recorded.

Points	0	1	2
1. Heart rate	Absent	Slow (<100)	>100
2. Respiratory effort	Absent	Slow, irregular	Good, crying
3. Muscle tone	Limp	Some flexion of extremities	Active motion
4. Response to catheter in nostril (tested after oropharynx is clear)	No response	Grimace	Cough or sneeze
5. Color	Blue or pale	Body pink; extremities blue	Completely pink

*Reproduced, with permission, from Apgar V: JAMA 168:1985, 1958.

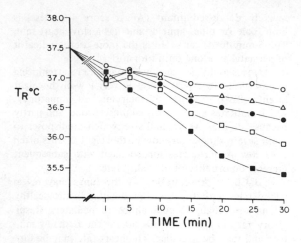

Figure 3–3. Mean deep body temperatures (T_R) of each group during the first 30 minutes of life. T_R is on the ordinate and minutes postdelivery on the abscissa. ■ wet infants in room air; □ dry infants in room air; ● wet infants under the radiant heater; △ dry infants wrapped in a blanket; ○ dry infants under the radiant heater. (Reproduced, with permission, from Dahm LS, James LS: Newborn temperature and calculated heat loss in the delivery room. Pediatrics 49:504, 1972.)

gradually increasing hypoxia, and other clinical findings associated with these abnormalities.

D. Skin: Cyanosis of the peripheral portions of the extremities is common for a short time after birth. The presence of generalized cyanosis, pallor, petechiae, ecchymoses, or plethora requires further investigation. The amount of vernix should be noted and related to clinical estimation of gestational age. Jaundice at birth is a grave finding and requires immediate evaluation.

Pallor in the newborn infant may indicate possible acute hemorrhage that is draining into the maternal circulation. It may be caused by a tear in a placental vessel. Ecchymoses of the skin, particularly in preterm babies following breech vaginal deliveries, may be a manifestation of extensive hemorrhage into the deep muscles of the back or buttocks, which may be severe enough to cause shock. In all cases of suspected hemorrhage, prompt expansion of blood volume should be achieved by means of placental blood, albumin, Plasmanate, or some other appropriate colloid solution. Blood volume expansion should always be achieved in doubtful cases because there are no conditions occurring in the newborn infant at delivery that are likely to be confused with acute blood loss in which volume expansion would be harmful.

E. Abdomen: The abdomen should be soft and somewhat scaphoid immediately after birth. As the bowel fills with air, the abdomen becomes more full. Abdominal organs are easily palpated during this early period. A marked and persistent scaphoid abdomen suggests diaphragmatic hernia with some abdominal contents within the chest. A distended abdomen suggests such problems as organomegaly, ascites, and bowel obstruction.

F. General Appearance: The infant's sex, size, and

development in relation to gestational age, and the presence of malformations or odd facies or body appearance should be noted. Any asymmetric movements may suggest an injury to the cervical or the brachial plexus. In such cases, movement of the chest wall should be carefully observed for any suggestion of a phrenic nerve injury producing asymmetric respiration. The examination for potential birth injuries should be very carefully carried out in all infants who are large for gestational age.

Fetal Adnexa

A. Amniotic Fluid: The color, appearance, and the estimated volume of amniotic fluid should be noted. Normal amniotic fluid at term is a light straw color. Bright red fresh blood or chocolate-colored old blood pigments may be present.

In normal pregnancy, amniotic fluid volume increases until approximately the 35th week of gestation and then decreases at a rate of approximately 100 ml per week. At term the volume is about 700 ml. Polyhydramnios is present if the amniotic fluid volume is 3 times the normal value or is greater than 2000 ml. Polyhydramnios occurs in association with those congenital anomalies that prevent normal fetal swallowing or absorption of amniotic fluid. These abnormalities include (1) major CNS anomalies such as anencephaly and (2) gastrointestinal tract obstruction, including tracheo-esophageal fistula and duodenal or jejunal stenosis. Oligohydramnios occurs in association with "prune belly" syndrome, renal agenesis, or urinary obstruction, all of which are lesions that reduce fetal urine production and thereby affect a major source of amniotic fluid. When the fluid is meconium-stained, the obstetrician and pediatrician should observe special precautions (see p 62).

B. Umbilical Cord:

1. Gross appearance—The cord of term infants with small placentas is likely to be thin and stained yellow. Meconium staining of the cord indicates prior fetal distress. The cord is usually inserted concentrically on the placenta. When the insertion is velamentous, arising away from the placental margin and supported only by the amnion, there is increased risk of fetal hemorrhage during delivery. Velamentous insertions of the cord occur more frequently with multiple births.

2. Length—A very short cord is uncommon but can result in abruptio placentae or rupture of the cord. A very long cord (75 cm or more) may loop around the body and neck, resulting in a relatively short cord during delivery. Occasionally a nuchal cord is the cause of fetal distress.

3. Single umbilical artery—The vessels of the umbilical cord are best observed in a freshly cut section at birth. Normally, 2 arteries and one vein are present. A single artery is present in approximately 1% of births. The incidence rises to 5–6% in twins. The twin with a single umbilical artery is often smaller than the twin with 2 arteries. A single umbilical artery is considered a congenital vascular malformation. Associated congenital abnormalities, especially of the cardiovascular, gastrointestinal, or urinary systems, may be present, although the incidence of associated anomalies is not high enough to justify special diagnostic tests in the absence of any specific clinical signs.

4. Prolapsed cord—Prolapsed umbilical cord with compression during labor causes acute fetal distress. This is an obstetric emergency, and prompt treatment is necessary if the life and welfare of the baby are to be preserved. Perinatal mortality with prolapsed umbilical cord is about 35%.

C. Placenta: Placental weight and the infant's birth weight are directly related. Placental weight establishes an upper limit to the infant's size which may or may not be attained depending upon other in utero conditions. A small placenta is invariably associated with a small infant. However, large placentas, particularly if they are abnormal (eg, as a result of hydrops fetalis or congenital infections), may occur with infants who are not large. The small placenta with multiple small infarcts is characteristic of the woman with chronic hypertensive vascular disease and is associated with infants who are small for gestational age. Examination of the placenta is particularly helpful in multiple pregnancies. An arteriovenous anastomosis between placentas can be recognized by the injection of a dye or of milk into the placental vessels of one fetus; if one chorion is present, the twins must be monozygotic or identical. When 2 chorions and 2 amnions are present, the twins can be either monozygotic or dyzygotic.

THE INFANT DURING THE
FIRST FEW HOURS AFTER BIRTH

During the first few hours after birth, the normal baby progresses through a fairly predictable sequence of events recovering from the stress of delivery and adaptation to extrauterine life. The baby neither requires nor easily tolerates the handling involved with a complete physical examination. However, a considerable portion of the physical examination and evaluation of the newborn can be based on careful observation of the infant. This is especially important during the birth recovery period in order to identify early—but without excessive handling—the infant who is at increased risk of developing problems. Observation of abnormal findings such as hypotension, pallor, cyanosis, plethora, jaundice, birth injury, respiratory distress, abdominal distention, hyperactivity, abnormal birth recovery period, or discrepant clinical estimation of gestational age requires early, more detailed evaluation. The nurses caring for the infant play a vital role in observing and evaluating the infant during this period. (See p 46 for description of the complete physical examination, and p 52 for routine care of the newborn during this period.)

Birth Recovery Period

Desmond has described the physical findings associated with the postnatal adjustment in normal infants.

A. First Stage: For 30–60 minutes after delivery, the infant is active, with eyes open and alert and muscle tone increased. The heart and respiratory rates are rapid, and transient rales may be heard. Bowel sounds are absent. The infant may drool or vomit mucus. Respirations may be accompanied by flaring of the alae nasi, and costal retractions.

B. Second Stage: Between about 30 minutes and 2 hours, there is a decrease in heart and respiratory rates; motor activity declines; and the infant falls asleep.

C. Third Stage: After about 2 hours, the infant arouses. He again shows an increase in heart rate, vasomotor instability, and irregular respirations with rest periods. Oral mucus is present. Bowel sounds appear, and meconium is passed. The infant gradually stabilizes and may give a loud cry of hunger.

Recognition of an abnormal birth recovery period may be an important clue to underlying disease. Significant deviation from the basic sequence of events may result from a variety of influences. The preterm infant's response is prolonged. Infants with low Apgar scores show an initial delay in the first stage but may then recover rapidly. Drugs administered to the mother, birth trauma, and disease in the newborn may alter the birth recovery events.

Clinical Estimation of Gestational Age

The onset of the mother's last menstrual period is the basic information from which the period of gestation is calculated. During pregnancy, observations of increasing fundal height, onset of fetal movement, detection of fetal heart beat, and certain laboratory tests aid in determining the degree of fetal maturity.

It is possible to estimate the gestational age of the infant by examination after birth since fetal physical characteristics and neurologic development progress in a predictable fashion with increasing gestational age. Table 3–2 itemizes the clinical criteria used in determining gestational age and outlines the physical and neurologic findings observed in the infant born at various gestational ages.

There are 2 charts presented in Table 3–2 for estimating gestational age. The first, designed for use during the first hours after birth, includes the physical characteristics plus 3 items related to muscle tone. The second chart is a neurologic examination based on items indicating normal neurologic development. The examination for gestational age during the first hours requires very little manipulation of the infant yet gives adequate data for assessing gestational age at the time it is most needed. The later neurologic examination will help confirm gestational age when discrepancies exist between the age obtained from menstrual history and age derived from the clinical findings. It is also used when individual items vary considerably.

Intrauterine growth retardation due to undernutrition—rather than due to fetal malformation—alters the physical characteristics associated with gestational age in the following ways:

Table 3–2. Clinical estimation of gestational age. An approximation based on published data. Adapted from Lubchenco LO: P Clin North America 17:125, 1970.

Examination First Hours

WEEKS GESTATION

PHYSICAL FINDINGS		Descriptions (left → right, weeks 20 → 48)
Vernix		Appears (≈21) · Covers body, thick layer (≈24–28) · On back, scalp, in creases (≈38) · Scant, in creases (≈40–41) · No vernix (≈42+)
Breast tissue and areola		Areola and nipple barely visible, no palpable breast tissue (≈23) · Areola raised (≈35) · 3–5 mm nodule (≈36–37) · 5–6 mm (≈38–39) · 7–10 mm (≈40–41) · ?12 mm (≈44)
Ear	Form	Flat, shapeless (≈24) · Beginning incurving superior (≈33–34) · Incurving upper 2/3 pinnae (≈36–37) · Well-defined incurving to lobe (≈40)
	Cartilage	Pinna soft, stays folded (≈23) · Cartilage scant, returns slowly from folding (≈32–33) · Thin cartilage, springs back from folding (≈38–39) · Pinna firm, remains erect from head (≈42)
Sole creases		Smooth soles without creases (≈23) · 1–2 anterior creases (≈33) · 2–3 anterior creases (≈35–36) · Creases anterior 2/3 sole (≈37) · Creases involving heel (≈39–40) · Deeper creases over entire sole (≈42)
Skin	Thickness & appearance	Thin, translucent skin, plethoric, venules over abdomen, edema (≈22) · Smooth, thicker, no edema (≈33–34) · Pink (≈37) · Few vessels (≈39) · Some desquamation pale pink (≈40) · Thick, pale, desquamation over entire body (≈43)
	Nail plates	Appear (≈23) · Nails to finger tips (≈33) · Nails extend well beyond finger tips (≈44)
Hair		Appears on head (≈25) · Eye brows and lashes (≈27) · Fine, woolly, bunches out from head (≈29) · Silky, single strands, lays flat (≈38)
Lanugo		Appears (≈21) · Covers entire body (≈24) · Vanishes from face (≈33) · Present on shoulders (≈38) · No lanugo (≈42)
Genitalia	Testes	Testes palpable in inguinal canal (≈30) · In upper scrotum (≈37) · In lower scrotum (≈41)
	Scrotum	Few rugae (≈30) · Rugae, anterior portion (≈38) · Rugae cover (≈40) · Pendulous (≈42)
	Labia & clitoris	Prominent clitoris, labia majora small, widely separated (≈31) · Labia majora larger, nearly cover clitoris (≈36) · Labia minora and clitoris covered (≈41)
Skull firmness		Bones are soft (≈24) · Soft to 1″ from anterior fontanelle (≈29) · Spongy at edges of fontanelle, center firm (≈35) · Bones hard, sutures easily displaced (≈38) · Bones hard, cannot be displaced (≈43)
Posture	Resting	Hypotonic, lateral decubitus (≈22) · Hypotonic (≈26) · Beginning flexion, thigh (≈30) · Stronger hip flexion (≈32) · Frog-like (≈35) · Flexion, all limbs (≈36) · Hypertonic (≈39) · Very hypertonic (≈42)
Recoil - leg		No recoil (≈21) · Partial recoil (≈32) · Prompt recoil (≈39)
Arm		No recoil (≈21) · Begin flexion, no recoil (≈34) · Prompt recoil, may be inhibited (≈37) · Prompt recoil after 30″ inhibition (≈43)

Week scale: 20 21 22 23 24 25 26 27 28 29 30 31 32 33 34 35 36 37 38 39 40 41 42 43 44 45 46 47 48

Confirmatory Neurologic Examination To Be Done After 24 Hours

Weeks Gestation

	Physical Findings	20–48 (text entries by gestational week)
Tone	Heel to ear	No resistance (20–26); Some resistance (30–32); Impossible (35–)
	Scarf sign	No resistance (20–26); Elbow passes midline (32–33); Elbow at midline (36–38); Elbow does not reach midline (43–)
	Neck flexors (head lag)	Absent (20–28); Head in plane of body (38–40); Holds head (43–)
	Neck extensors	Head begins to right itself from flexed position (34–35); Good righting cannot hold it (36); Holds head few seconds (39); Keeps head in line with trunk >40″ (41); Turns head from side to side (45–)
	Body extensors	Straightening of legs (33); Straightening of trunk (37); Straightening of head and trunk together (44–)
	Vertical positions	When held under arms, body slips through hands (26–28); Arms hold baby, legs extended? (34); Legs flexed, good support with arms (38–)
	Horizontal positions	Hypotonic, arms and legs straight (26–30); Arms and legs flexed (37); Head and back even, flexed extremities (39–40); Head above back (44–)
Flexion angles	Popliteal	No resistance (20–); 150° (29); 110° (33); 100° (35); 90° (39); 80° (41)
	Ankle	45° (32); 20° (37); 0 (41)
	Wrist (square window)	90° (29); 60° (33); 45° (36); 30° (39); 0 (41)
Reflexes	Sucking	Weak, not synchronized with swallowing (26–); Stronger, synchronized (33); Perfect (35); Perfect, hand to mouth (39); Perfect (43)
	Rooting	Long latency period slow, imperfect (27–); Hand to mouth (31); Brisk, complete, durable (36); Complete (43)
	Grasp	Finger grasp is good, strength is poor (26–); Stronger (33); Stronger (38); Can lift baby off bed, involves arms (40); Hands open (45)
	Moro	Barely apparent (22–); Weak, not elicited every time (26); Stronger (33); Complete with arm extension, open fingers, cry (35); Arm adduction added (41); ?Begins to lose Moro (45)
	Crossed extension	Flexion and extension in a random, purposeless pattern (26–); Extension, no adduction (32); Extension, adduction (34); Still incomplete (36); Complete with arm extension, open fingers, cry (38); Extension, adduction, fanning of toes (39); Complete (43)
	Automatic walk	Minimal (31); Begins tiptoeing, good support on sole (32); Fast tiptoeing (36); Heel-toe progression, whole sole of foot (40); A pre-term who has reached 40 weeks walks on toes (43); ?Begins to lose automatic walk (47)
	Pupillary reflex	Absent (20–); Appears (30); Present (32)
	Glabellar tap	Absent (20–); Appears (33); Present (35)
	Tonic neck reflex	Absent (20–); Appears (29); Present (32)
	Neck-righting	Absent (20–); Appears (34); Present after 37 weeks (38–)

A pre-term who has reached 40 weeks still has a 40° angle

(1) Diminished growth or absence of breast tissue.

(2) Loss of vernix and desquamation of the skin prior to term.

(3) Meconium staining of the skin and nails due to fetal distress with bowel evacuation.

(4) Weight is affected first, followed by decreased growth in length and, in severe undernutrition, head circumference.

(5) Neurologic examination is least affected and is usually appropriate for the actual gestational age.

COMPLETE NEWBORN PHYSICAL EXAMINATION

A complete physical examination should be done on each newborn within 24 hours after delivery. However, it should be delayed until the baby has stabilized following birth because of the infant's limited tolerance to handling during the birth recovery period (see p 41). Careful observation for abnormal findings during this time by the physician and nursing staff will identify those infants who require earlier, more detailed examination and evaluation.

A rigid sequence for doing various parts of the newborn physical examination is not necessary. It may not be possible to complete the entire examination at one time, in which case the balance can (and must) be finished later. The goal is to provide a complete record of the newborn which will contain essential information for reference as the infant grows and if later problems develop. Take advantage of quiet periods to perform portions of the examination which require it. The baby can usually be quieted sufficiently by using a pacifier or by having him held by the examiner or the mother.

There are distinct advantages in having the mother present and assisting the examination: (1) Her participation with the examiner in this intimate evaluation of her baby can enhance the development of the normal mother-baby relationship. (2) Her response and involvement with the baby can be observed, allowing early identification of problems in mothering that may exist. (3) She can be reassured immediately about minor variations in normal findings. (4) The meaning and plan for evaluation of significant abnormal findings can be discussed, allowing early involvement with the sick baby.

When abnormal findings are observed, they must be documented and a plan for evaluation developed. In caring for the newborn, it is crucial that abnormal findings be reevaluated at frequent intervals. Changes in physical findings such as heart murmurs can occur rapidly.

The basic approach to the newborn physical examination is modified somewhat from that described in Chapter 1 because of the special problems the newborn often presents:

(1) **Observation**: Observation is particularly im-portant in the newborn examination. A major portion of the information gathered will be obtained by patient, careful observation of the infant prior to his being disturbed and during various stages of activity. The usual order is to observe the infant generally and then to concentrate on specific areas for more detailed observation.

(2) **Auscultation**: Listen to the heart, lungs, abdomen, and head when the baby is quiet. Be alert for any asymmetry in breath sounds.

(3) **Palpation and manipulative procedures**: These must be timed in order to obtain reliable information but without disturbing the infant to such a degree that valid observations cannot be made. Adequate palpation of the abdomen and portions of the neurologic examination must be done with the infant quiet; examination of the mouth, throat, and ears can be done adequately even in an actively crying infant.

General Appearance & Evaluation

A. Vital Signs and Physical Measurements: These may be obtained from the nurse's record or during the course of the examination. It is usually not possible to make these observations first, since the baby will become fussy. Length, weight, and head circumference are measured and plotted on the intrauterine growth charts related to gestational age. Blood pressure may be determined by the flush or Doppler method (see p 325).

B. Appearance: The general appearance, maturity, nutritional status, presence of abnormal facies or body deformities, and state of well-being are noted. Before the baby is disturbed, observe the resting position (which frequently reflects the position assumed in utero), quality of respirations, color, and character of sleep pattern. While the baby is being undressed, observe his response to handling and general muscle tone. The usual quieting response upon being picked up and held may be demonstrated after undressing.

Specific Observations

A. Skin:

1. Color and appearance—The skin becomes erythematous for a few hours after birth, then fades to its normal appearance. The presence of *jaundice* and age at onset of jaundice should always be noted. *Peripheral cyanosis* (acrocyanosis) is commonly present, particularly when extremities are cool. *Generalized cyanosis* is an important observation requiring immediate evaluation.

Pallor may be due to acute blood loss at the time of delivery or to gastrointestinal bleeding from a variety of causes or may be iatrogenic, particularly in the preterm infant who has had multiple samples of blood drawn for blood chemistry and blood gas measurements. Even so-called "microchemistries" can lead to appreciable blood loss in infants weighing less than 1200 gm. The amount of blood withdrawn each time and the total taken for sampling should be recorded. Plethora suggests polycythemia, which may lead to hyperviscosity syndrome. It occurs frequently in infants of diabetic mothers, small-for-gestational-age babies, and twins who have received a twin-twin transfusion. *Vernix caseosa,* a whitish, greasy material, normally covers the body of the fetus, decreasing in amount as term approaches. It is usually present in body creases of term infants but may be completely absent on a postterm infant. *Dry skin,* with cracking and peeling of the superficial layers, is common in infants who are postterm or have had intrauterine growth retardation. Normal skin is present underneath. *Edema* may be generalized (usually indicating serious renal, cardiac, or other systemic disease) or localized (dorsum of extremities in Turner's disease, eyelids with acute conjunctivitis). *Meconium staining* of the umbilical cord, vernix, nails, and skin suggests prior fetal distress. The *preterm infant's skin* is more translucent and may be covered with fine lanugo hair.

2. Skin lesions—Many lesions are present on the skin of normal newborns and must be differentiated from significant skin disease. *Mongolian spots*—bluishblack areas of pigmentation over the back and buttocks—are seen with more frequency in dark-skinned races. *Capillary hemangiomas* are common over the occiput, eyelids, forehead, nares, and lips. These lesions tend to decrease in size and intensity as the child grows. A few *petechiae* are seen over the presenting part. Numerous or fresh petechiae should suggest thrombocytopenia. *Milia* are the small, yellowish-white papular areas over the nose and face. *Erythema toxicum* is characterized by an evanescent rash with lesions in different stages—erythematous macules, papules, or small vesicles containing eosinophils—that spread to a variable extent over the skin, more commonly on the trunk. It occurs with decreasing frequency in preterm infants.

Staphylococcal or streptococcal infection of the skin in preterm babies may resemble erythema toxicum, a diagnosis that should always be made with caution in preterm infants.

B. Head: Note size, shape, symmetry, and general appearance of the head. *Molding* of the presenting part due to pressures during labor and delivery causes transient deformation of the head. *Head circumference* measurement may be affected by molding. *Caput succedaneum* is an area of edema over the presenting part which extends across suture lines. This differentiates it from a *cephalhematoma,* bleeding into the subperiosteal space on the surface of a skull bone (most commonly the parietal), which is circumscribed by the borders of the individual skull bone. The quantity of blood loss draining into a cephalhematoma can be significant in contributing to anemia appearing soon after birth and in causing early hyperbilirubinemia. Normally, the size of the *anterior fontanel* varies from 1–4 cm in any direction; it is smaller when the sutures are overriding. It is soft, pulsates with the baby's pulse, and becomes slightly depressed when the baby is upright and quiet. The *posterior fontanel* barely admits a finger. A *third fontanel,* a bony defect along the sagittal suture in the parietal bones, may be present. The sutures may feel open to a variable degree or may be

overriding. These findings are usually of no clinical importance. *Craniosynostosis* presents as a ridge along one or more sutures and is associated with increasing cranial deformity.

Increased intracranial pressure in the newborn is associated with increasing head circumference and a full anterior fontanel. *Skull fractures* resulting from birth trauma may be linear or depressed but are rarely associated with the common cephalhematoma.

Transillumination—the degree of light transmitted through the head—should be done in any baby suspected of having neurologic disease. The procedure is done in a completely dark room after the examiner's eyes have become dark-adapted. The circle of light extending beyond the flange of the transillumination flashlight should be no more than 1.5 cm in term or up to 2 cm in preterm infants. Excessive light transmission occurs when diminished brain tissue is present, such as that observed with collection of subdural fluid, hydrocephalus, or brain atrophy.

Computerized tomography (CT scans) in preterm infants may reveal moderately advanced hydrocephalus in the absence of the classical signs of a bulging or full fontanel and increased transillumination. Even if other physical signs of hydrocephalus are not present, a CT scan should be obtained whenever the head circumference increases rapidly, particularly in preterm infants prone to episodes of intracranial hemorrhage.

C. Face: The general appearance and symmetry of the face are observed. *Odd facies* are often associated with specific syndromes and should alert the examiner to search for other abnormalities. Localized swelling, ecchymoses, or asymmetry may result from birth pressure or the use of forceps during delivery. *Facial nerve palsy* is observed when the baby cries; the unaffected side of the mouth moves normally, giving a distorted facial grimace. When injury is more extensive, the eyelid will remain partially open on the affected side. Facial edema can be marked following a face presentation and can be severe enough to cause airway obstruction. A moderate restriction of water intake for 24—48 hours is in order for infants with facial edema because they are prone to dilutional hyponatremia.

D. Eyes: The eyes of each newborn should be examined carefully at least once during his nursery stay—preferably before silver nitrate prophylaxis is given, since periorbital edema and conjunctivitis may make examination difficult following the procedure. This is particularly important when eye disease or head trauma is suspected. An ophthalmologist should be readily available for consultation, since loss of vision may result from delay in proper diagnosis and treatment.

Eye examination should include evaluation of the periorbital structures, nerve function, anterior orbital structures, and light reflex. If indicated, an ophthalmoscopic examination through dilated pupils may be done after examination has ruled out the presence of glaucoma or anterior chamber hemorrhage. Phenylephrine (10%), tropicamide (0.5%), or homatropine (5%) may be used—1 drop in each eye, repeated once in 15 minutes if needed. (Do not use atropine because of the danger of systemic toxicity.)

The eyes are usually open and alert for the first 30 minutes and then tend to be closed during sleep for the next few hours. The baby will open his eyes when awake, especially when picked up. He will look toward a light and may focus briefly on the examiner's face. The size, shape, and position of the eyes and the presence of epicanthal folds are noted. Eyelid swelling and some conjunctival discharge are frequent after instillation of silver nitrate, but the possibility of infection must always be considered. *Eyelid movement* is observed. Occasional *uncoordinated eye movements* are common, but persistent irregular movements (nystagmus, eye deviation) are abnormal. *Acute dacryocystitis* associated with swelling and redness along the course of the lacrimal duct may become apparent in the newborn period. Corneal or lens *opacities* and *pupil size* can be observed with an ordinary flashlight. *Iris* abnormalities, such as Brushfield spots and colobomas, are noted. *Anterior chamber hemorrhage* may occur following eye trauma during birth but may not be apparent for several hours. A fluid level of blood will form when the baby is upright. *Congenital glaucoma* must be recognized early to preserve vision. The cornea is large (> 11 mm) and is often cloudy as a result of edema. Photophobia is common. Enlargement of the entire eye is a late finding.

Chorioretinitis may occur as a result of congenital toxoplasmosis, cytomegalic inclusion disease, or herpesvirus hominis infection. Small *retinal hemorrhages* are commonly observed in normal newborns, but more extensive hemorrhage is indicative of trauma or bleeding disorder. *Tumors* are rare in the newborn; retinoblastoma must be considered if the light reflection is grayish-yellow or absent or if strabismus or a dilated pupil is noted. Orbital hemangiomas may displace the eye in the orbit.

E. Nose: The shape and size of the nose are noted. Deformities may be due to in utero pressure, but many congenital syndromes are associated with abnormal nose configuration. Nasal discharge, noisy breathing, or complete obstruction to breathing may be present, suggesting choanal atresia or other nasal abnormality. When nasal obstruction is present, the infant may become cyanotic or apneic, since about one-third of term infants are obligatory nasal breathers. Nasal obstruction from mucous discharge can occur in those infants born with an upper respiratory tract infection acquired as a viral infection in utero. Flaring of the alae nasi occurs with increased respiratory effort.

F. Ears: Malformed or malpositioned (low-set or rotated) ears are often associated with other congenital abnormalities, especially of the urinary tract. The amount of cartilage in the pinnas is related to maturity. The *tympanic membranes* may be visualized with careful examination. Fluid may be present behind the drum for the first few hours.

Otitis media occurs fairly frequently in the neonatal period, particularly in preterm infants, in those with deformities of the palate, or in those who have been intubated for long periods of time (particularly with nasotracheal intubations). A careful examination of the eardrums should be made whenever sepsis or other infection is suspected.

Congenital deafness may be detected by standardized hearing screening tests in the newborn period (see p 250).

G. Mouth: Observe the lips and mucous membranes for pallor and cyanosis. The membranes should be moist in a normally hydrated infant. *Epithelial pearls* or retention cysts are noted on the gum margins and at the junction of the soft and hard palates. *Natal teeth* may be present—usually soft incisors—and may need to be removed in order to avoid the risk of aspiration. *High-arched palate* may be present as an isolated finding or may be associated with abnormal facies. *Cleft lip and palate* should be noted. Most newborns have relatively small *mandibles* that cause no problem. When the mandibles are very small, as in Pierre Robin syndrome, difficulty in breathing may occur when the tongue blocks the airway as it falls back against the pharynx. In the prone position, the baby usually has less respiratory difficulty. Some *drooling* of mucus is common in the first few hours after birth; excessive drooling occurs with esophageal atresia. The *tonsils* and *adenoids* are quite small in newborns.

H. Neck: Position, symmetry, range of motion, and muscle tone are noted. *Webbing* of the neck suggests Turner's syndrome. Enlargement of the *thyroid* may occur in the newborn and must be evaluated. *Sinus tracts* may be seen as remnants of branchial clefts. *Torticollis* due to shortening or spasm of one sternocleidomastoid muscle may occur when there is hemorrhage or fibrosis in the body of the muscle. A persistent *tonic neck reflex*, assumed spontaneously and maintained by the infant, may be caused by brain damage. A very *short neck* may be associated with cervical vertebral abnormalities.

I. Vocalization: Note character of the *cry*. A high-pitched cry suggests brain damage. A hoarse cry results from inflammation or edema of the larynx or vocal cord paralysis. A whining "cat's cry" occurs with the syndrome of partial deletion of the short arm of chromosome 5. A weak cry may be a general sign occurring in a sick infant. A delay in vocalizing the cry after the baby appears to be crying is noted in congenital hypothyroidism.

Expiratory grunting occurs with respiratory distress due to many causes—notably the respiratory distress syndrome. *Inspiratory stridor* is associated with partial obstruction of the upper airway during inspiration such as occurs with the soft, collapsible tracheal structures of congenital stridor.

J. Thorax: Note shape, symmetry, position, and development of the thorax, nipples, and breast tissue. Determine the respiratory rate and the character of the respirations.

Absent *clavicles* permit unusual anterior movement of the shoulders. Fracture of the clavicle is detected by tenderness and crepitus at the fracture site and limited movements of that arm. After a few days, callus is formed and the deformity can be easily visualized and felt. *"Fullness" of the thorax* due to increased anteroposterior diameter occurs with overexpansion of the lungs. Note asymmetry in expansion of the 2 sides or retractions during inspiration in the subcostal, intercostal, xiphoid, and suprasternal areas. These signs indicate pulmonary disease or airway obstruction.

K. Lungs: Auscultation of newborn lungs reveals bronchovesicular or bronchial breath sounds. Fine rales may be present during the first few hours. When there is a pneumothorax or pneumomediastinum, the breath sounds and heart sounds may be distant and the percussion sound may be hyperresonant. Decreased air entry and expiratory grunting are noted in respiratory distress syndrome. A chest x-ray must be obtained when abnormal lung findings are suspected because of the limited usefulness of physical findings alone in evaluation of respiratory disease.

L. Heart and Vascular System: Physical examination of the heart and vascular system and the physiologic changes of the perinatal period which affect these physical findings are described in Chapter 13.

M. Abdomen: The abdomen will appear slightly scaphoid at birth but will become more protuberant as the bowel fills with air. The abdominal organs are most easily palpated soon after birth, before the bowel becomes distended. A markedly scaphoid abdomen associated with respiratory distress suggests the presence of a diaphragmatic hernia. These are generally on the left side. An *omphalocele* may be present at birth; sometimes it may be small and may be included in the cord clamp if not recognized. *Umbilical hernias* are common and usually cause no difficulty. *Absence of abdominal musculature* or "prune belly" syndrome may occur in association with severe urinary tract abnormalities.

Abdominal distention may occur with intestinal obstruction or paralytic ileus in an infant with peritonitis or generalized sepsis. Palpation of the abdomen for organs or masses should be done with a light touch. The spleen tip is felt from the patient's right side and is sometimes 2—3 cm below the left costal margin. The liver usually is palpable 1—2 cm below the right costal margin. The lower poles of both kidneys should be felt. Abdominal muscle rigidity and apparent abdominal tenderness should be evaluated.

The outline of a distended *bladder* may be seen above the symphysis and may be felt as a ballottable mass in the lower abdomen. Contraction of bladder muscles with voiding often occurs with palpation.

Superficial veins may appear prominent over the abdominal wall with or without pathologic conditions.

The *umbilical cord* begins drying within hours after birth, becomes loose from the underlying skin by 4—5 days, and falls off by 7—10 days. Occasionally, a granulating stump remains which heals faster if treated with silver nitrate cauterization.

N. Genitalia: Male and female genitalia show findings characteristic of gestational age (Table 3—2). In most term male infants, the scrotum is pendulous, with rugae completely covering the sac. The testes have completely descended. The size of the scrotum and the penis varies widely in individual normal infants. The foreskin is adherent to the glans.

In females, the labia majora at term completely cover the labia minora and clitoris. A hymenal ring may be visible as a protruding tab of tissue. During the first few days after birth, a white mucous discharge that may contain blood issues from the vagina. Occasionally, a thin septum produced by fusion of the labia minora covers the vagina. The fusion is easily disrupted with a blunt probe.

O. Anus and Rectum: Observe anatomy and muscle tone of the anus. *Patency* should be checked if meconium has not been passed; use a soft catheter or little finger—not a rectal thermometer or other rigid object. *Irritation* or *fissures* may occur after the immediate newborn period. A firm *meconium plug* may be present.

"Meconium plug" syndrome may occur in the newborn with hard meconium producing total intestinal obstruction. These infants generally appear well despite marked abdominal distention. Once the plug is passed, the distention is rapidly relieved and does not recur.

P. Extremities and Back: The arms and legs should be relatively symmetrical in anatomy and function. Obvious *major abnormalities* of the extremities include absence of a bone, clubfoot, fusion or webbing of digits, or missing parts. *Hip dislocation* is suspected when there is limitation of abduction of the hips or when a click can be felt when the femur is pressed downward and then abducted. The legs may be unequal in length, and extra skin folds in the affected thigh are seen. *Palsies* involving the extremities are recognized when there are limited movements of the extremities, especially if only one is involved. *Fractures* may present with the same findings; in addition, swelling and crepitation are felt. Note the size and shape of the hands and feet. Deformities are frequent with *chromosomal abnormalities*.

The back is observed for curvature, spinal defects such as meningomyelocele, and dimples or defects overlying the lower lumbar spine.

Q. Neurologic Examination: The neurologic behavior of the newborn has become more clearly understood in recent years. Certain test items and observations on muscle tone are useful in assessing gestational age since normal neurologic development follows a predictable course (Table 3—2).

Other items, described below, are those traditionally associated with abnormal CNS function (Prechtl & Beintema), and still others (Brazelton) attempt to test higher centers of CNS function. The authors referred to stress the importance of testing the infant during specific awake-asleep states. A guide to the items applicable in each of the neurologic examinations is detailed in Table 3—3.

1. Traditional neurologic examination—Head circumference, sutures, fontanels, presence of cephalhematoma have been described, and evidence of jaundice, plethora, cyanosis, and sepsis are included in a neurologic examination because of the potential association with CNS pathology (eg, kernicterus, meningitis, alteration of CNS circulation and oxygen supply). Facial palsies and ocular disorders have been described.

Some observations are made while the infant is completely undisturbed; some involve minimal handling; and some can only be made by observing responses to specific stimuli. The infant should not be too hungry or too sleepy. Because a prolonged examination may exhaust the infant or cause irritability, the examination may have to be done in parts.

a. General observations—Paucity of *spontaneous movements* may be as important as abnormal movements. Discordant movements of one limb or of one side, hyperactivity, opisthotonos, athetoid movements, and movements ranging from tremors or jerks to frank

convulsions may be seen in the infant with CNS damage. Brief seizures may present as momentary cessation of movements in a crying infant. Continuous chewing or sucking movements, protrusion of the tongue, and frequent yawning are other abnormal movements.

Resting position is observed without disturbing the infant. *Asymmetry* of the skull, face, jaw, or extremities may result from intrauterine pressures. The infant may be passively "folded" into the position of comfort assumed in utero.

b. Muscle tone—Test recoil of the extremities. Extend the legs and then release; both legs return promptly to the flexed position in the term infant. Extend arms alongside the body; upon release, there is prompt flexion at the elbows in the term infant. The amount of flexion and extension around joints is further tested

---

Table 3–3. The neurologic examinations of the newborn. The first is evaluation of normal neurologic development; the second is the classical neurologic examination for CNS disease; and the third extends the evaluation to include function of higher CNS centers and to elucidate individual behavior.

(1) NORMAL NEUROLOGIC DEVELOPMENT (Estimate of gestational age) (From Dargassies & others.)	(2) ABNORMAL CNS FUNCTION (From Prechtl & Beintema.)		(3) FUNCTION OF HIGHER CNS CENTERS & BEHAVIOR (From Brazelton.)
Muscle tone	**Muscle tone**		**Response decrements**
Resting posture	Resting posture and recoil		Visual
Recoil of extremities	Opisthotonos vs frog position		Auditory
Horizontal suspension	Hypertonic vs hypotonic		Tactile
Vertical suspension	Flopping hand and foot		**Orientation:** visual
Heel to ear	Unequal tone		Inanimate
Popliteal angle	Pull to sit		Animate
Scarf sign	Spontaneous movements		**Orientation:** auditory
Neck extensors } pull to sit	Lack of or excessive		Inanimate
Neck flexors	Fisting		Animate
Body extensors	Tremors → seizures		**General behavior (tone, irritability,**
Standing	Passive movement		**spontaneous motor behavior,**
Reflexes	**Reflexes**		**maturity)**
Suckling	Moro	Hand grasp	Level of consciousness
Rooting	Knee jerk	Plantar grasp	Initial state
Grasp	Ankle clonus	Tonic neck	Predominant state
Crossed extension	Biceps	Crawling	Alertness
Automatic walk	Suck and root	Babinski	Lability of state
Moro	**Eyes**		Rapidity of build-up
Tonic neck	Strabismus, nystagmus		**Specific behavior**
Neck righting	Abnormal movements		Cuddliness
Pupillary	Setting sun		Consolability
Glabellar tap	Doll's eyes		Hand-to-mouth
Babinski	Corneal reflex		Self-quieting
Magnet	Ophthalmologic examination		Smiles
Flexion angles	**Face**		Lability of state
Ankle	Expression		Lability of skin color
Wrist (square window)	Facial palsies		Rapidity of build-up
	Cry		**Reflexes**
	High-pitched		Defensive movements
	Skull		
	Sutures		
	Fontanels		
	Cephalhematoma		
	Other		
	Jaundice	Abdominal	
	Plethora	distention	
	Cyanosis	Skin turgor	

at the neck, trunk, shoulders, elbows, wrists, hips, knees, and ankles.

Another means of testing for tone is by flopping the hand and foot. As the wrist is moved sharply back and forth, the hand flops for a brief period and then the infant resists the movement and holds the hand or wrist firm. Normal term infants show approximately as much flopping as resistance to this maneuver.

A general impression of hypotonia or hypertonia can be gained from this testing. The *hypertonic* baby is usually jittery and startles easily; his fists are tightly closed, the arms in tight flexion, and the legs stiffly extended. The *hypotonic* or *lethargic* infant is "floppy" and has little head control. The extremities fall to the bed loosely when picked up and released. Recoil of arms and legs to the flexed position after being extended helps determine tone as well as gestational age.

c. Rooting reflex—The rooting reflex occurs so early in gestation that its absence in a viable baby should cause concern. However, the rooting reflex is strongest when the infant is hungry and may disappear after feeding. The reflex is elicited in 4 areas: at both corners of the mouth and on the upper and lower lips at the midline. The mouth opens or the head turns toward the side of the stimulus.

d. Sucking reflex—The sucking reflex can be obtained by placing a finger in the baby's mouth and noting the vigor of the movements and the amount of suction produced. A hypertonic or irritable infant makes biting rather than sucking movements.

e. Traction response: Head flexion and extension—The infant's hands and wrists are grasped and he is pulled gently to a sitting position. In the term infant, there is at first a head lag and then active flexion of the neck muscles so that the head and chest are in line when the infant reaches the vertical position. He maintains his head in the upright position for a few seconds, and the head then falls forward. He then will raise his head again, either spontaneously or following a slight stimulus such as stroking the upper lip.

f. Grasp reflex—

(1) **Fingers**—Stimulate the palm with a finger, and the infant will close his fingers on it. The grasp should be sufficiently strong in the term infant so that he can be lifted from the table by holding onto the examiner's finger.

(2) **Toes**—Pressing the ball of the foot elicits a definite and prompt toe flexion.

g. Biceps, triceps, knee, and ankle tendon reflexes—These are best elicited with the finger rather than a percussion hammer. The infant must be relaxed.

h. Ankle clonus—Normally present in the newborn; sustained clonus is abnormal.

i. Incurvation of the trunk—The infant is lifted up and held over the hand in a prone position. The amount of flexion of the head and body is noted for an additional estimate of tone. The incurvation reflex is obtained by stroking or applying intermittent pressure with the finger parallel to the spine, first on one side and then the other, watching for a movement of the pelvis to the stimulated side.

j. Righting reaction—When the infant is lifted from the table vertically, he will usually flex his legs. If the soles of the feet then touch the table, he will respond with the righting reflex, ie, first his legs will extend, then the trunk, and the head.

k. Placing—The baby is held vertically with his back against the examiner and one leg held out of the way. The other leg is moved forward so that the dorsum of the foot touches the edge of the examining table. The baby will flex the knee and bring his foot up as though he were trying to step onto the table.

l. Automatic walking—Following the preceding tests, the ability to perform automatic walking movements is evaluated. The baby is inclined forward to begin automatic walking. When the sole of one foot touches the table, he tends to right himself with that leg and the other foot flexes. As the next foot touches the table, the reverse action occurs. Term infants will walk on the entire sole of the foot, whereas preterm infants often walk on their toes.

m. Moro (startle) reflex—When eliciting the Moro response, observe the arms, hands, and cry. The arms show abduction at the shoulder and extension of the elbow, followed by adduction of the arms in most infants. The hands show a prominent spreading or extension of the fingers. Any abnormality in the movements should be noted, such as jerkiness or tremor, slow response, or asymmetric response. A cry follows the startle and should be vigorous. The nature of the cry is important—absent, weak, high-pitched, or excessive.

The Moro reflex may be elicited in several ways:

(1) Holding the baby's hands, lift his body and neck (but not his head) off the examining table and quickly let go.

(2) Holding the infant with one hand supporting his head and the other supporting his body, allow the head to drop a few centimeters rather suddenly.

(3) Holding the infant in both hands, lower both hands rapidly a few centimeters so that he experiences a sensation of falling.

(4) If the baby is quiet in the bassinet, lift the head of the bassinet a few centimeters and let it drop.

2. The Brazelton examination—This behavioral assessment of the newborn is presented as a research tool with an elaborate scoring system and, when it is used as such, observer reliability must be established. However, items in the examination lend themselves to routine application. The examination includes items from the Prechtl-Beintema examination (Table 3–3).

The various tests and observations are all done in relation to specific states. The infant should pass through all 6 states during the examination.

During the testing, observations on lability of state, skin color, rapidity of build-up, self-quieting activity, startle responses, irritability, and spontaneous movements are noted and recorded.

a. Response decrements—Visual (flashlight), auditory (rattle and bell), and tactile (pinprick) stimuli are presented repetitively to the infant in states 1, 2, or 3. The response to each is noted and the time of the decrement noted.

b. Orientation (state 4)—The infant's ability to orient to and attend to visual stimuli, both animate and inanimate, is tested, and his orientation to auditory stimuli is noted. Again, animate and inanimate sounds are presented.

c. Behavior—Cuddliness is defined as molding of the body of the infant to the examiner and can be elicited in the arms or by placing the infant over the shoulder. Consolability is scored on the number of ways necessary to quiet the infant, ranging from the examiner's face, voice, hand on belly, to holding, rocking, and finally a pacifier. Self-quieting activity is observed when the infant has reached state 6. He may not be able to quiet himself at all, or he may be quiet for brief periods. He may have the capacity to quiet himself for sustained periods. Associated with self-quieting is hand-to-mouth facility, which may range from brief swipes to thumbsucking.

d. Defensive movements—In this part of the examination, the observer tests the infant's ability to remove a cloth placed over his face.

THE DISCHARGE EXAMINATION

Since the complete examination has already been performed, only supplemental observations need be made at discharge. The infant should be examined at the mother's bedside, and she should be given ample opportunity to raise questions. The physician should check the late appearance of medical problems such as jaundice, infection, skin rashes, etc and be aware of maternal behavior which may affect care of the infant. Plans for medical follow-up are made at this time.

Amiel-Tison C: Neurological evaluation of the maturity of newborn infants. Arch Dis Child 43:89, 1968.

Brazelton TB: Assessment of the infant at risk. Clin Obstet Gynecol 16:361, 1973.

Brazelton TB: *Neonatal Behavioral Assessment Scale.* Spastics International Medical Publications. Heinemann, 1973.

Dubowitz LMS & others: Clinical assessment of gestational age in the newborn infant. J Pediatr 77:1, 1970.

Froehlich LA, Fujikura T: What prognosis with single umbilical artery? Pediatrics 52:6, 1973.

Malan AF, Higgs SC: Gestational age assessment in infants of very low birthweight. Arch Dis Child 50:322, 1975.

Nicolopoulos D & others: Estimation of gestational age in the neonate: A comparison of clinical methods. Am J Dis Child 130:477, 1976.

Smith DW: *Recognizable Patterns of Human Malformation.* Saunders, 1970.

Solomon LM, Esterly NB: *Neonatal Dermatology.* Saunders, 1973.

THE NORMAL NEWBORN

CARE OF THE NORMAL NEWBORN

Immediately After Delivery

The normal term newborn infant is cared for in a level 1 unit that is preferably organized as a rooming-in unit and that aims to treat pregnancy and delivery not as parts of a disease process but as a normal and happy event in family life. However, adequate objective observation of the infant is necessary in order to recognize the development of any problems requiring medical assistance. A common problem in the term newborn infant is mild respiratory depression resulting from anesthesia given to the mother. Frequently the only therapy necessary is a short period of assisted ventilation with a bag and mask at the time of delivery.

Certain routines must be performed after delivery to make certain that the infant is adapting smoothly to extrauterine life and that there are no immediate life-threatening problems.

A. Nasopharyngeal Suction: Gentle suctioning with a bulb syringe is done during or immediately after delivery to remove mucus or blood and to clear the airway of obstructive debris.

B. Positioning: The infant should be positioned so that secretions do not pool in the pharynx, where they may be aspirated.

C. Apgar Scoring: Determined at 1 and 5 minutes (Table 3–1).

D. Physical Examination: See pp 41 ff.

E. Maintain Body Temperature: Every effort should be made to prevent a fall in body temperature. This is especially important in cool, air-conditioned delivery rooms. Evaporative heat loss from wet skin and radiant heat loss into the cool environment can be excessive unless special precautions are taken. The baby should be wiped dry, wrapped in a warm blanket, and placed in a warm environment until he is stabilized and able to maintain his temperature well.

F. Stomach Tube: Passing an orogastric tube should *not* be routine. Stimulation of the posterior pharynx and esophagus may cause bradycardia and apnea. Therefore, if the procedure is required, it should be done in the nursery after the baby has stabilized. An exception is a delivery complicated by polyhydramnios, when it is important to rule out the possibility of a tracheo-esophageal fistula by passing a soft rubber catheter into the stomach.

G. Umbilical Cord, Membranes, and Placenta: Examine after each delivery for abnormalities.

H. Eye Prophylaxis: Routine eye prophylaxis against gonorrheal infection must be done as defined by local health codes. One percent silver nitrate is instilled carefully into each eye so that the conjunctival surface is adequately bathed in the solution. Single dose vials are preferred. The eyes are not irrigated with water or saline.

I. Identification: Done before the baby is removed from the delivery area.

J. Cord Blood Collection: At least 10–20 ml of clotted cord blood in 2 tubes should be collected. One tube is used for blood typing, Coombs testing, serologic examination, and other tests that may be needed soon. The other tube should go to the nursery with the infant and be kept in a refrigerator, where it will be available if other tests are required as the baby is further evaluated. This second tube should be retained until the baby is discharged or for 7 days, or should go with the baby if he is transferred to another nursery for care.

K. Mother-Baby Relationship: Important aspects of developing mother-baby relationships optimally occur in the delivery area (see p 56).

L. Transfer to Nursery: If the nursery is adjacent to the delivery area, the baby may be carried, adequately protected from chilling. It may be easier to transport him in an incubator. Specially designed transport incubators are available for use when the nursery is far removed from the delivery area by time or distance. In addition to heat, these special incubators provide for visibility, easy access to the infant, and oxygen administration.

In the Transitional Nursery Area

An area or room in the nursery should be designated for admission of newborns from the delivery room for careful observation during the birth recovery period. All newborns should be admitted to this area except sick babies or those at high risk who are admitted directly to the special care nursery. All babies are potentially at risk, and most of those who will become sick during their nursery stay can be identified in the first few hours after birth by careful observation and evaluation. The nursery staff play a vital role during this time in evaluating the infant and identifying those who require special attention.

A. Data Compilation and the Medical Record: Record the expected due date and verify calculated gestational age. Determine and record birth weight, length, and head circumference. The medical record should be designed to relate to problems that the baby presents as well as to record the data required for the infant's care and for evaluation of the nursery service activities.

B. Classification: Determine the baby's newborn classification based on birth weight and gestational age (Fig 3–1), identifying all those that are outside the low-risk, term, appropriate-for-gestational-age group.

C. Prognosis: Make an estimate of the mortality risk based on birth weight and gestational age. In general, infants with a 10% or greater chance of dying, based on these criteria, should be placed in a special care nursery. Other factors that may contribute to the risk of a particular newborn must also be considered in determining the level of care that he should receive. Examples of these additional factors include maternal hypertension, drug therapy, diabetes, Rh sensitization, bleeding, infection, and previous neonatal death.

D. Examination: The appropriate examination at this time includes a review of the maternal and immediate perinatal history, noting whether fetal monitoring was done and, if so, whether results were normal; clinical estimation of gestational age; evaluation of pulmonary and cardiac status, including routine blood pressure measurement; and notation of factors that may influence the baby's course (see pp 43 ff). A careful review of potential drug exposure must be made.

E. Birth Recovery Period: Observe for sequence of events related to birth recovery and note deviations from normal pattern (see p 43).

Observe for presence of abnormal symptoms or signs which may suggest developing problems. Findings that are unimpressive by themselves may acquire significance if observed and recorded objectively. A check list of significant observations can be an important part of the nurse's notes (Table 3–4).

F. Temperature Control: After delivery and until the baby has stabilized, his body temperature may be labile. This is especially true when rooms are cool and the baby is not swaddled. Cooling should be avoided, since it will delay the normal cardiovascular adjustments required of the infant after birth. Radiant heat devices designed for use with newborns are ideal for this purpose in the transitional nursery area.

G. Vitamin K: Administer phytonadione, 1 mg IM, to every newborn routinely as part of the admission procedure to the nursery.

H. First Urine and Stool: Time must be noted. If these events have not occurred prior to transfer to the general care nursery, a special note must be made.

I. Care and Feeding: After the baby has stabilized and his condition is good, he will awaken and act hungry. At this time he may be bathed, dressed, and given his first feeding. This may be at 2–10 hours of age. These events should be well tolerated in a normal baby and confirm that he is at low risk.

J. Physician Responsibility: The physician responsible for the care of the newborn reviews the history and neonatal course and performs a complete physical examination after the baby is stable, preferably before 24 hours of age. The mother may be present at the time of this examination. If any significant abnormalities have been identified before the physician's expected visit, he is notified of the abnormality immediately so that he may evaluate the problem earlier.

Continued Care in the Level 1 Nursery

Although a registered nurse will supervise the area, the bulk of the day-to-day care in a level 1 nursery may be given by personnel at lower professional levels who are trained in the care of newborns. The emphasis is on well baby care, enhancing successful mother-baby relationships, feeding, and teaching care technics. However, the staff must be continually alert for any significant evidence of illness that may require evaluation.

A. Admission: The staff should review the baby's history and immediate postnatal events in order to be aware of any problems.

Table 3—4. Check list of significant observations in newborns.

DATE						
TIME						

ACTIVITY	✓	ACTIVE				
	+	Activity decreased				
	+	Tires easily				
	+	Lethargic				
	+	Floppy				
	+	Irritable				
	+	Pacifier required				
	+	Frantic				
	+	Swaddled				
	+	Tremors				
	+	Twitching				
	+	Rigid				
	+	Opisthotonos				
	+	Moro poor or absent				

APPEARANCE	✓	COLOR STABLE				
	+	Pallor				
	+	Plethora				
	+	Mottled				
	+	Harlequin syndrome				
	+	Jaundice				
	+	Dusky				
	+	Cyanosis: Generalized				
	+	Circumoral				
	+	Circumocular				
	+	Extremities				
	+	Tearing				
	+	Eye discharge				

FEEDINGS (GASTROINTESTINAL)	✓	HUNGRY				
	✓	DEMANDING				
	✓	SUCKS WELL				
	+	Sucks poorly				
	✓	GAVAGED WELL				
	✓	Gavaged well/slowly				
	+	Gavaged poorly				
	+	Gavage resisted				
	+	Mucus on tube				
	+	Mucus, other				
	+	Drooled				
	+	Gagged				
	+	Regurgitated				
	+	Abdomen distended				
	cm	Abdomen, circumference				
	+	Hiccup				
	+	Sore buttocks				

DATE						
TIME						

RESPIRATIONS	✓	CRY GOOD				
	+	Cry high-pitched				
	+	Cry weak				
	+	Sneezes				
	+	Stuffy nose				
	+	Yawning				
	+	Hoarseness				
	+	Stridor				
	✓	RESPIRATIONS: REGULAR				
	+	Shallow				
	+	Labored				
	+	Deep				
	+	Irregular				
	+	See-saw				
	+	Periodic breathing				
	+	Rest periods: < 10 sec				
	+	10–30 sec				
	+	Apnea > 30 sec				
	+	Alae nasi dilated				
	+	Cough				
	+	Grunting				
	+	Retraction				

SKIN	✓	SKIN NORMAL				
	+	Dry and peeling				
	+	Irritated				
	+	Petechiae (area)				
	+	Ecchymosis (area)				
	+	Bleeding (area)				
	+	Dehydrated				
	+	Edema				
	+	Pustular rash				
	+	Erythema toxicum				
	+	Other rash (specify)				
	+	Abscess (area)				
	+	Sclerema				
	+	Umbilical redness				
	+	Umbilical oozing				

DIRECTIONS: This record is completed by the nurse, indicating presence of findings (✓), severity (+, ++, +++), timing (ac, pc), etc. This check list is used instead of routine nursing notes. Capitalized items indicate normal findings. Each column signifies a period of observations. Significant additional data are recorded in the Progress Notes. A 24-hour summary of nursing observations is given to the physician at morning rounds. These observations and the physician's findings provide the necessary data base on which a decision is made concerning illness. (Adapted from Lubchenco LO: P Clin North America 8:471, 1961.)

B. Duration of Stay: Following an uncomplicated perinatal course, mother and baby may stay in the hospital only 2–5 days (up to 7 days following cesarean section). The short hospitalization permits the mother and baby to have an earlier "rooming in" experience in their own home. If there is an understanding adult helper in the home, freeing the mother to care for the baby, the benefits of this early adjustment can be great. However, early discharge is accompanied by definite risk of delay in detecting problems: breast feeding is not established; the severity of "physiologic" jaundice cannot be evaluated; and subtle symptoms of illness may not be recognized before discharge.

C. Adapting Nursery Activity to Needs of Mother and Child: The life situation of the mother and the family is important in their acceptance of the newborn baby. Favorable conditions exist when the mother is married, the child is wanted at this time, there is some financial security, and the parents themselves are emotionally mature. Even when these favorable factors are operative, however, there may be adverse factors which interfere with satisfactory adjustment. Problems in pregnancy, a difficult delivery, birth of an abnormal or premature infant, and development of maternal or infant illness are a few such factors. The nursery staff should understand the needs of the mother and child and show their willingness to meet these needs. The following suggestions will help (see also Mother-Baby Relationship, below): (1) Become acquainted with the mother and father—before delivery if possible. (2) Show an interest in the total family unit. (3) Visit the mother daily while she is in the hospital and be attentive to her expressed anxieties. (4) Institute flexible schedules of feeding, especially for mothers who are breast feeding. (5) Institute flexible schedules for the amount of time the baby and mother spend together. (6) Examine the infant in the mother's presence. Above all, it is important that *both* physicians and nurses respect the diversity of life styles and approaches to parenting. The health care team should *assist* the parents and infant, not *dictate* any particular approach to the family. Parents should not be made to feel guilty if they do not choose to use rooming-in nursery arrangements, natural childbirth, or breast feeding. Criticism is often implied when parents do not choose the same approach to childbirth and infant care that the health care team would, despite the fact that different approaches to parenting and family life are equally compatible with development of a healthy child.

D. Rooming-In: The optimal family-centered program is the rooming-in situation with mother and baby together in the room under the supervision of an understanding and helpful nurse, with unrestricted visiting by the father. The mother can get instruction in caring for the baby as she watches her baby being examined, and her questions about the significance of findings can be answered as they arise. Continued help and encouragement from well trained nurses for the mother who is breast feeding are very helpful. Rooming-in may be continuous in a separate unit or modi-fied, using existing postpartum and nursery facilities. Close cooperation between obstetric and pediatric medical and nursing personnel is essential.

1. Continuous rooming-in—A separate unit with separate nursing staff is arranged so that the mothers may have the babies with them as much as they desire. A nursery room located in the unit is available for babies at other times. The nursing staff cares for mothers and babies and plays an effective role in teaching—encouraging successful breast feeding when that method is desired, as well as being alert to problems in mother-baby relationships. Mothers or babies who present particular care problems will benefit from continuous rooming-in.

2. Modified rooming-in—It is feasible to adapt the routine schedule of activities in the postpartum and nursery units to allow the babies to remain with their mothers for variable periods, depending on the mother's individual desires and needs. Feeding on demand, modification of visiting rules and patient activities, and a helpful, interested attitude on the part of the staff will ensure a successful program of modified rooming-in.

E. Screening for Disease: Since nearly all babies in the USA are born in hospitals, an excellent opportunity exists to screen mother and baby for disease that has not become manifest during their stay in the hospital. Some of these tests can be routine, and some are required by law:

1. Blood type and direct Coombs test to identify potential blood group incompatibilities.

2. Serologic test for syphilis.

3. Elevated serum phenylalanine and other amino acids.

4. TSH or T_4 measurements.

5. Other tests may be done when indicated—screening for hearing, IgM, sex chromatin, galactosemia, G6PD deficiency, etc.

F. Preparation for Discharge:

1. Perform a physical examination—preferably with the mother in attendance—and discuss the care of the cord, circumcision, genitalia, etc as the baby is examined.

2. Make sure the mother has mastered and understood the reasons for procedures for caring for the baby. Give her ample opportunity to discuss questions she may have.

Now that infants are being discharged from the nursery earlier and parents are assuming more of the routine care of the newborn at home, it is important to explain to parents the need to observe the infant for jaundice. They should be prepared to bring the infant to their physician as soon as significant signs are noted. It is not unusual for infants discharged early from nurseries to have jaundice that goes unrecognized until bilirubin levels exceed 15–20 mg/100 ml.

3. Give feeding instructions and a written formula. Careful attention to preparation of the formula is essential, since improperly prepared formula is dangerous to the infant.

4. Vitamin and iron supplementation may be re-

quired. Most proprietary infant formulas contain adequate vitamins. If breast milk or whole or evaporated cow's milk formulas are used, supplementation with vitamins A, C, and D is recommended.

5. Give an appointment to the physician's office or clinic in 2–3 weeks for well baby care or specific problem follow-up.

6. Make sure the mother knows whom to call if she has questions or if problems develop.

7. Check identification of baby and of person accepting responsibility for the infant at time of discharge.

Frankenburg WK, Camp BW: *Pediatric Screening Tests.* Thomas, 1975.

Jackson E: Family centered maternity care. In: *Problems of Infancy and Early Childhood.* Josiah Macy Jr Foundation Conference, 1950.

Klaus MH, Kennell JH: Mothers separated from their newborn infants. Pediatr Clin North Am 17:1015, 1970.

Lubchenco LO & others: Neonatal mortality rate: Relationship to birth weight and gestational age. J Pediatr 81:814, 1972.

MOTHER-BABY RELATIONSHIP

Mothers' feelings for their newborn infants may vary over a range extending from strong feelings of love and protection to complete rejection. Many factors that affect a woman's capacity for mothering are ingrained, ie, dependent on her genetic endowment, her relationship with her own parents, and cultural practices. Other factors include her marital status, financial situation, and attitudes about the pregnancy. Obstetric and nursery routines and attitudes of hospital personnel also affect the mother's ability to relate to her child. The separation of mother and baby at birth and during much of the postnatal period is probably the most arbitrary and potentially harmful of current postnatal practices.

Development of Maternal Attachment to the Infant

The mother's emotional attachment to the baby begins early in pregnancy. If the fetus or newborn dies, she will go through a process of mourning, even following an early abortion. During the early months she may be preoccupied with the certainty of the diagnosis of pregnancy. Fetal movements are the first concrete evidence that she is truly going to have a baby. These movements are usually pleasant and associated with considerable fantasy. At this time, the parents often decide on a choice of names for the baby.

Behavior After Birth

The mother's initial thoughts at the moment of birth are usually, "Is my baby all right?" and, "Is it a boy or a girl?" The answer may provoke profound expressions of joy or, at times, withdrawal and tears. When the mother is given the opportunity in the delivery room to hold her infant, she will regard him with tenderness, tending to concentrate on his eyes. Klaus and Kennel have observed a pattern of examination and touching that the mother follows when the nude infant is presented to her at about 1 hour of age. She usually begins with fingertip touching of the extremities and proceeds to palm contact of the trunk within a few minutes. There is noticeable attention paid to the infant's eyes.

Both the mother and the infant may go through a stage of wakefulness during the first hour after birth. The baby is wide-eyed, alert, and responsive. The mother's wakefulness may persist until she has held her infant and fed him. It is as though the birth process is not finished until she has cared for her child. Following this period of wakefulness, both the mother and the infant fall into a deep sleep lasting several hours.

Implication for Hospital Care of Mother and Infant

If these observations give some insight into the needs of the mother and baby, then the routines of delivery and nursery care must be reoriented. Prolonged separation of mother and baby and rigidity of schedules and routine activities in the postnatal areas may be playing a significant negative role in development of normal mother-baby relationships.

Guidelines to Provide Optimal Mother-Baby Relationships

(1) The mother's comfort and access to her baby are of prime importance.

(2) The physician responsible for the baby's care should talk with parents—preferably together—at least once a day, and more frequently if the baby is ill. It is important to explore their understanding of the disease and its causes and to assess their reaction to the fact of their baby's illness.

(3) If the baby is ill, the mother should be prepared for the baby's appearance and for the equipment used in the special care nursery before she goes to visit her infant. An informed individual must be with her to answer questions and give support while she is there. Physical contact with the baby should be allowed whenever possible.

(4) The physician and nurse should not overburden the mother with details or concerns of care and prognosis during the early period. Optimism about prognosis is essential whenever possible. The mother is developing an important relationship with the infant during this time which should not be interrupted by needless anxieties.

The Sick Baby

Occasionally an infant has a grave illness or serious congenital anomaly requiring immediate management. If the difficulty has been anticipated, the problems will have been prepared for prior to delivery. If the occurrence is unexpected, the following guidelines will be helpful:

(1) A prompt survey of the seriousness of the condition and decisions about immediate treatment are

urgently required. Additional help or immediate transfer to the nursery may be required.

(2) The mother will sense the seriousness of the situation if she is awake at the delivery. An absent cry and increased activity around the baby cannot be disguised. A word to the mother that indicates there is a problem and that the baby's welfare is being considered first is vital. Some indication of the type of trouble should be given, eg, "He has a defect of his spine," or "He has difficulty breathing."

(3) If the baby is likely to die or must be removed from the room immediately, she should be told these facts and be assured that someone will return soon to report what is happening.

(4) Should the mother see a sick or deformed infant? Yes, for many reasons. Even a glimpse of the infant will prevent a grossly exaggerated imaginary picture from forming in the mother's mind. If possible, the mother should be allowed to see and touch her infant in order to complete the perinatal experience. If the appearance of the infant is gruesome, she will require preparation for later reunion plus added support and understanding. If the infant dies, it is especially important that she see the infant so that she will be able to accomplish the mourning process. These comments also apply when a stillbirth has occurred.

(5) No emotionally charged comments should be made to the parents. Decisions involving long-term outcome and disposition should be postponed.

(6) The parents will go through a period of shock and disappointment, often associated with feelings of guilt, and will require understanding and emotional support from the physician during the succeeding days and weeks.

Genetic Counseling

The likelihood of genetic defects reappearing in future pregnancies need not be considered or discussed immediately after the birth of an abnormal child. At some point in the following weeks, the perceptive physician will recognize the parents' need for additional information and will offer genetic counseling. Sufficient information is available about most defects to allow satisfactory assessment of the chance of recurrence of an abnormality. Interested and informed concern by the physician will aid the parents in arriving at realistic plans for future pregnancies.

Relinquishing an Infant

Although pregnancy in the unmarried does not carry the same social stigma as in the past, there is still much misunderstanding about emotional aspects of the adoption process in such cases. Relinquishment of the baby should be presented as an acceptable alternative to pregnant women carrying an unwanted child. They should be aware of the current favorable adoption statistics showing that infants will almost certainly be placed in appropriate homes. Another popular belief is that "The mother does not want to see or hear about the child"; that "She does not want to become attached to it"; or that "She might change her mind."

However, since the mother already has related to the fetus early in pregnancy, special feelings cannot be avoided when she relinquishes the infant for adoption. If she can see and touch the baby, the experience of pregnancy and delivery can be completed rather than forever shrouded in uncertainty, denial, and fantasy because the mother can work through her feelings more easily. Predelivery counseling is desirable, including informed discussion of expected emotional reactions after delivery. The process of delivery and immediate handling by the mother may be the same as for the mother who is keeping her baby.

The *earliest possible* placement of the infant in a permanent adoptive home is best for the new parents and for the baby.

Klaus MH & others: Maternal attachment: The importance of the first postpartum days. N Engl J Med 286:460, 1972.
Milunsky A (editor): *The Prevention of Mental Retardation and Genetic Disease.* Saunders, 1975.

FEEDING OF THE NEWBORN*

Feeding schedules in newborn nurseries have tended to be fairly rigid, primarily for the convenience of the staff. The result has been that some babies are awake and hungry for long periods and others must be awakened to be fed, and neither is optimal from the baby's point of view. "Demand feeding"—allowing the baby to eat when he is awake and hungry—usually leads to optimal intake and eventual establishment of a "schedule" which will be both satisfying to the baby and reasonable for the family. Initiating demand feeding in the nursery is entirely feasible and most easily done with a modified or continuous rooming-in program where the mother can respond to the baby's needs with ease.

What, When, & How Much to Feed?

The first water feeding should be offered as the birth recovery period is ending and the baby appears hungry; this may be as early as 3–6 hours of age in many normal term infants. The baby should appear actively hungry and should have normal bowel sounds and no abdominal distention. When these conditions are met, the exact composition of the first feeding is of relatively little importance.

The first feeding may be sterile water or 5% glucose in water. One water feeding is usually sufficient, although in occasional cases several may be required to make certain that feedings are well tolerated. Full-strength milk formula (approximately 20 kcal/oz) or breast feedings can then be given. Diluted or concentrated formulas do not appear to have any special advantages. Most commercially available modified cow's milk formulas are satisfactory during the hospital stay.

---

*Infant feeding as such is discussed in Chapter 4.

Prepackaged units are recommended for use in the nursery since they provide a maximum of convenience and safety.

The initial feeding may consist of a few swallows or several ounces. As feedings are established, the baby should be allowed to regulate the volume and frequency of feedings so long as his fluid and caloric requirements are met. By the third day he should receive a minimum of 100 ml/kg/day and will soon thereafter start taking about 120 kcal and 180 ml/kg/day or more, allowing for hunger satisfaction and optimal growth.

Methods of Feeding

A. Bottle Feeding: Most commercial bottles and nipples are satisfactory. If the nipple hole needs to be enlarged, this can easily be done with a hot needle. For premature or debilitated babies, a soft nipple with easy flow (cross-cut hole) is required.

B. Breast Feeding: (See also Chapter 4.) When a mother wants to nurse her infant, success or failure is related to the amount of factual information given her and to the emotional support of physician and nurses. The staff can share the role of listening, giving factual data, and encouraging the mother to continue nursing long enough to overcome occasional problems she may have in establishing lactation. Having a nurse present when the mother first attempts to feed, providing explanation of physiologic processes, and making her physically comfortable will assure success.

A variable amount of breast engorgement occurs on about the third day after delivery. The engorgement may interfere with nursing because the infant is unable to grasp the nipple. A nipple shield may be used to reduce the areolar engorgement and to draw out the nipple. The infant may then nurse directly from the breast. Prolonged use of the shield interferes with complete emptying of the breasts. Nipple soreness is minimized if the nursing time is kept to approximately 5 minutes during the prelactation period until milk flow is established. Only a bland ointment should be used on the nipples.

1. Variations of hunger—The mother should be forewarned that her infant will seem to become more hungry about the fourth or fifth day and will want to nurse more frequently. This behavior lasts only 1–2 days. The baby will then return to a less frequent feeding schedule.

2. Nursing premature and sick infants—The mother who wishes to nurse premature, sick, or debilitated infants may be successful if given some additional suggestions. She must empty her breasts several times a day with a mechanical pump or by manual expression to maintain lactation until her infant is able to nurse from the breast. The supply will increase in a few days after the infant begins to nurse. If the baby does not empty the breast, milk production can be increased if she pumps the breast after feedings. She may have insufficient milk for a few days, and a supplement immediately following feeding will be necessary until supply increases.

C. Gavage Feeding: Intermittent gavage feeding should be used when the baby has a weak sucking and swallowing reflex or tires easily. Gavage feeding can be done safely with minimal handling. However, in a sick infant with danger of abdominal distention, regurgitation, and aspiration, gavage feeding has the same risk as nipple feeding.

Indwelling orogastric tubes have been used for long-term feedings of small premature infants. A small polyethylene (rather than rubber) catheter must be used to minimize local irritation. The location of the end of the tube must be checked before each feeding to be sure it has remained in the stomach.

Some centers handling newborn infants prefer nasogastric tubes although these have 2 disadvantages: They tend to obstruct breathing, particularly in preterm babies who are obligate nasal breathers, and, since they constitute a foreign body in the nasopharynx, they can predispose to otitis media and blockage of the eustachian tube. Occasionally, a preterm baby of less than 32 weeks' gestation may tolerate gastric feedings of any kind poorly. These infants can be fed successfully using oroduodenal tubes. It was once thought that such tubes would have to be placed in the jejunum to avoid potential interference with biliary drainage. However, oroduodenal tubes are easily passed and seem to carry far less risk than nasojejunal tubes, which have had a fairly high rate of complications, including perforations of the small bowel.

D. Gastrostomy: This procedure can be done easily and relatively safely in infants in the rare instances when it is indicated. It should be done by an experienced surgeon with careful attention to special problems of the newborn. The main indications are in surgical conditions such as tracheo-esophageal fistula, chest surgery, and some bowel surgery to aid in the pre- and postoperative care.

E. Intravenous Fluids: Intravenous fluids are always required in preterm babies, in very-low-birth-weight infants, and in any critically ill infant. The fluids are given primarily to ensure adequate hydration and electrolyte intake. A multivitamin preparation should be added to provide water-soluble vitamins, since infants are born with poor reserves of these vitamins. Water and electrolyte intake must be adjusted to the needs of each infant, based on a record of intake and output which should be reviewed at least every 12 hours. The amount administered should maintain normal plasma sodium concentrations, a urine osmolarity between 150 and 250 mOsm/kg of water, and a urine flow rate between 1 and 3 ml/kg/hour. In general, the amount of water administered in the form of 10% glucose should be in the range of 80–150 ml/kg/day, and sodium intake should be between 1.5–3 mEq/kg/day. The higher figures apply to the smaller preterm infants. Potassium, 2 mEq/kg/day, should be added to the intravenous fluids. If metabolic acidosis is not present, the sodium is given as sodium bicarbonate and the potassium as potassium chloride. If metabolic acidosis is present, both sodium and potassium salts are given as the salts of metabolizable anions.

F. Parenteral Alimentation: The recent development of effective methods to provide adequate nutrition by the vascular route represents a major advance in meeting nutritional needs in those rare instances where babies cannot take sufficient feedings orally for a prolonged period. Several specific solutions have been devised which consist of water, glucose, amino acids, electrolytes, and vitamins. The solution is usually delivered through a central venous catheter. Newborns likely to benefit from this technic are primarily those babies with gastrointestinal abnormalities which do not allow adequate oral feedings or have associated severe malabsorption.

G. Special Considerations:

1. Termination of intravenous feedings—Intravenous fluids are discontinued gradually to avoid reactive hypoglycemia and to provide supplemental fluids until oral intake is satisfactory. When several oral feedings have been retained, the infusion may be discontinued.

2. Feeding preterm infants—Even in small preterm infants, early feedings are preferred over a period of prolonged starvation and dehydration. For babies who are very small or sick, intravenous feeding of 10% glucose in water with maintenance electrolytes will fill this need until oral or gavage feedings can be started safely. Babies who are well and will tolerate oral feedings may be fed by nipple or gavage. Nipple or gavage feedings should begin with sterile water or 5% glucose in water. Formula at standard dilution (20 kcal/oz) is started as soon as water feedings are tolerated. Small infants begin at 2–5 ml/feeding at 2- to 3-hour intervals, gradually increasing to the desired 24-hour volume as tolerated (120 kcal and 180 ml/kg or more). Larger infants begin at 5–15 ml/feeding at 3-hour intervals. With gavage feedings, gastric emptying can be checked by aspirating the stomach before feedings until a regular feeding pattern occurs. Replace aspirated fluid and add milk to the volume desired for that feeding.

Nipple feedings can be substituted for gavage feedings gradually when the baby shows increased activity before feeding and begins sucking on the gavage tube. Transition is made slowly, as babies will tire easily with nipple feedings. Demand feeding of prematures is desirable. Intake will vary, and each baby will tend to establish his own pattern. Feeding is satisfactory when optimal weight gain occurs.

3. Discharge formula—A variety of formulas are available for feeding after the baby goes home. Anticipate the confusion that may occur about how to make up the particular formula the baby is given. Clear instructions for preparation of the baby's formula must be given in written form for the mother's reference.

No prepared formula may be considered ideal to replace mother's milk. However, the standard milk preparations available provide satisfactory nutrition. Proprietary formulas usually come in 3 forms: concentrated liquid, requiring dilution with equal parts of water; ready-to-feed, requiring no dilution; and powdered, diluted one scoop (provided in can) to 2 oz of water. An evaporated milk formula for use during the first weeks consists of 13 oz of evaporated milk, 19 oz of water, and 1½ oz of corn syrup; this provides about 21 kcal/oz.

Applebaum RM: The modern management of successful breast feeding. Pediatrics 17:203, 1970.

Catz C, Giacoia GP: Drugs and breast milk. Pediatr Clin North Am 19:151, 1972.

Davidson M: Formula feeding of normal term and low birth weight infants. Pediatr Clin North Am 17:913, 1970.

Quinby GE Jr & others: Parenteral nutrition in the neonate. Clin Perinatol 2:59, 1975.

Raiha NCR & others: Milk protein quantity and quality in low birthweight infants. Pediatrics 57:659, 1976.

Sinclair JC & others: Supportive management of the sick neonate: Parenteral calories, water, electrolytes. Pediatr Clin North Am 17:793, 1970.

SPECIAL CARE OF THE HIGH-RISK INFANT

GENERAL CONCEPTS & PROCEDURES

Each hospital service that delivers babies must be able to respond to the urgent needs of the newborn who is acutely ill at birth or develops an acute problem during his newborn stay. In many cases the danger can be anticipated and appropriate arrangements made for care of the high-risk infant by having needed personnel and equipment available or by transferring the baby to a special care nursery as soon as the need is recognized. Ideally, when the baby's problem is identified during pregnancy, he should be delivered at the hospital where special care can be provided. The special care nursery provides specially trained physicians and nurses, related medical subspecialty support (pediatric surgery, birth defects, neurology, etc), service support (x-ray, laboratory), and equipment and facilities geared to the special needs and care of sick newborn infants.

Transport to Special Care Nursery

Referral guidelines should be constantly in force in order to expedite transfer when the need arises. The special care nursery may be in another hospital, perhaps some distance away. Telephone consultation about the infant's problem and management facilitates the transfer and allows the staff to be prepared to provide for his specific needs. Adequate clinical information, a consent for treatment at the referral nursery, a tube of clotted mother's blood, and the tube of cord blood should accompany the infant. The mother's blood may be required to evaluate jaundice or serve for cross-match if a transfusion is required.

Stabilization of the sick newborn prior to transport minimizes his risk during transport. Temperature maintenance requires special attention. Check for hypoglycemia and treat with intravenous glucose; 10% glucose water at 3—4 ml/kg/hour is recommended during transport. Hypoventilation must be recognized and methods of supporting ventilation instituted prior to transport. Evaluation of acid-base status should be made and treatment instituted by means of assisted ventilation or bicarbonate therapy (or both if indicated). Under no conditions should more than 3 mEq $NaHCO_3$/kg be given. Hypotension may be detected; a mean blood pressure of less than 40 mm Hg should be treated by means of blood volume expanders. Chest x-ray (anteroposterior and cross-table lateral) and hematocrit are usually indicated.

Certain problems require special attention related to transport, as illustrated by these examples. Any enclosed pocket of air will expand if the baby is transported to a higher altitude. Therefore, pneumothorax, diaphragmatic hernia, and bowel obstruction usually need tube and suction decompression prior to transport. The blind upper pouch of esophageal atresia needs constant suction to avoid overflow aspiration of saliva. A large omphalocele presents a special problem of temperature control because of the large evaporative surface. This should be covered with gauze packs moistened with warm (37° C [98.6° F]) saline solution and enclosed with plastic wrap during transport in order to prevent evaporative heat loss.

Care of Sick Newborn

A careful review of the history, physical examination, and prior treatment is essential. Diagnostic procedures should be done on clear indication and may have to be spaced, depending on how well the baby tolerates handling. Procedures should be done in the nursery whenever possible and should include portable x-rays, exchange transfusions, and minor surgery. If the infant must be removed from the nursery, one of the nursery staff should accompany him, taking along resuscitation and other needed emergency equipment.

Procedures used in the care of sick newborns are described in the following section and in Chapter 34. Management of specific problems is described in the following portion of this chapter and in appropriate sections throughout the book. Adequate space, trained personnel, and safe equipment must be provided. Careful medical records must be kept: history, physical examination, progress notes, problem list and plan for management, nursing observations, data recording and graphing of selected data to clarify clinical course, and documentation of orders and procedures.

Drugs

Information about the pharmacology of many drugs used in the newborn period is meager. Newer drugs may not have been adequately studied to determine dosage and safety for young infants. Many unfortunate complications of drug therapy in newborns have occurred. Therefore, use only those drugs whose safety has been documented by adequate pharmacologic study or long clinical observation. Except when very

specific indications leave no choice, avoid newer drugs when familiar drugs will give adequate effect.

Drug administration to newborns presents some special problems. Dosage is small, and proper calculation of dose and measuring of drug must be assured. Mixing certain drugs must be avoided, eg, penicillin and kanamycin, sodium bicarbonate and calcium salts.

Convalescent Care

The baby may receive intermediate and convalescent care in the special care area or he may be transferred to the general care nursery or back to the referring hospital. Frequent observation and evaluation of the infant's progress should be done. Routine recording of certain data aids in identifying infants with developing problems: Record weight daily or twice weekly; length and head circumference weekly; hematocrit and acid-base status weekly. The mother should be encouraged to participate in the baby's care to the greatest extent possible.

Discharge

Each infant's course is reviewed for short- and long-term problems that might be anticipated. The problem list is updated and plans for follow-up care are made. Screening tests are done. Clear feeding and care instructions are given to the mother.

Battaglia FC & others: Water and electrolyte balance. Chapter 13 in: *Perinatal Medicine: Review and Comments.* Vol 2. Mosby, 1978.

Cunningham MD, Smith FR: Stabilization and transport of severely ill infants. Pediatr Clin North Am 20:359, 1973.

Kuhns LR, Poznanski AK: Endotracheal tube position in the infant. J Pediatr 78:991, 1971.

Segal S (editor): *Transport of High-Risk Newborn Infants.* Canadian Pediatric Society, 1972.

Tronick E & others: Regional obstetric anesthesia and newborn behavior: Effect over the first ten days of life. Pediatrics 58:94, 1976.

PERINATAL RESUSCITATION

It is no longer adequate to begin resuscitation of the newborn after delivery; instead, the entire sequence of decisions made by obstetricians, pediatricians, and family physicians throughout the course of labor and delivery must be seen as significantly affecting the condition of the infant at birth. Parturition and the many endocrine and cardiovascular changes it induces in the mother and infant begin sometime before uterine contractions actually start. However, attention focuses most closely on the time of labor, when synchronous cervical dilatation and uterine contractions lead to delivery of the infant. Labor constitutes a stress that is perfectly normal and well tolerated by the full-term, healthy infant delivered after an uncomplicated pregnancy. However, the stress of labor and delivery may cause marked fetal distress in pregnancies having one or more complications, eg, intra-uterine growth retardation. Frequently, the small-for-gestational age infant shows no evidence of fetal distress until labor and delivery, at which time there is a high incidence of fetal distress.

For this reason, it is important to emphasize pre-planning for delivery by the entire health care team. The preplan not only considers the optimal time and mode of delivery (ie, vaginal versus cesarean section) that would minimize fetal and maternal complications but also considers what level of care will be required by the mother and infant. The latter evaluation determines which hospital in the community will be used for delivery. Increasing emphasis is being placed on determining the best setting for delivery before the birth takes place so that the parents can be informed that delivery is anticipated, for example, at a level 3 perinatal center. This contrasts with the past practice of delivery at any community hospital followed by transport of a critically ill infant to some referral nursery.

Table 3−5 shows the various stages of resuscitation of the fetus or newborn infant, beginning with decisions made while the infant is in the birth canal and continuing with traditional resuscitation of the infant following delivery. Effective preplanning based on multiple assessments of gestational age and maturity can virtually eliminate the complication of elective delivery of a preterm baby who subsequently develops iatrogenic hyaline membrane disease.

Intrapartum Resuscitation

Intrapartum resuscitation is based on knowledge of the changes in uterine and umbilical flow that occur during parturition and during the stress of uterine contractions. Certainly in high-risk pregnancies the obstetrician must continuously assess the condition of the fetus through measurements of maternal blood pressure, maternal acid-base status and oxygenation of the mother, intrauterine pressure recordings, instantaneous fetal heart rate recordings, and occasional scalp pH measurements. Therapy to support the maternal circulation and uterine blood flow rest on basic physiologic principles. The uterine vascular bed is a unique part of the vascular system because at the end of pregnancy it functions as a maximally dilated bed, ie, the arterioles are for the most part fully dilated.

Table 3−5. Perinatal resuscitation.

Intrapartum
  Provide oxygen therapy.
  Position mother on her side.
  Support circulation; avoid any hypotension.
At delivery
  Collect placental blood.
  Suction nasopharynx prior to delivery of thorax
    for meconium-stained amniotic fluid.
Traditional postnatal resuscitation
  See Fig 3−4.

Thus, they cannot accommodate any fall in maternal arterial blood pressure with further vasodilatation. This contrasts strikingly with vascular beds in most other organs of the body, which can respond to maternal hypotension by vasodilatation and maintenance of blood flow to that organ. Thus, any fall in maternal blood pressure is reflected in a fall in uterine blood flow and potential uterine and fetal hypoxia. This physiologic relationship accounts for attempts to avoid maternal hypotension by infusing isotonic salt solutions or colloid into the mother or by placing the mother on her side to avoid pressure from the gravid uterus upon the inferior vena cava, which would reduce return of blood to the right side of the heart.

The second physiologic principle is that oxygen tension in the most highly oxygenated blood of the fetus, ie, the umbilical venous blood, tends to equilibrate with uterine *venous* P_{O_2}, not with maternal arterial P_{O_2}.

When oxygen in high concentration is given to the mother, her arterial P_{O_2} rises to very high levels, but the P_{O_2} in the uterine vein does not and increases to a much smaller extent. This increase in uterine vein P_{O_2} leads to a small but very important increase in umbilical venous P_{O_2}. Since the oxygen affinity of fetal blood is greater than that of adult blood and since the human fetus functions on the steep part of its oxygen dissociation curve, the small change in oxygen tension effects a very large change in oxygen content in the umbilical venous blood. This is why oxygen therapy is used when there is any evidence of fetal distress. The fact that oxygen tension in fetal blood increases when oxygen is given to the mother has been documented in several clinical studies by fetal scalp P_{O_2} measurements. Careful medical management during labor and delivery is important not only in what it actively provides for the mother and fetus but also in what it avoids, eg, potentially depressant drugs, complications of obstetric anesthesia, and maternal hyponatremia, which will be reflected in hyponatremia in the newborn.

Obstetric Management at Delivery

Because unexpected complications at delivery can develop in the form of prolapse of the umbilical cord, unexpected dystocia of a head or shoulder, etc, it is important−particularly at medical centers where a choice can be made−that the most experienced obstetrician be available for the delivery of high-risk infants. Two useful procedures in the pediatric management of the newborn are the following: First, it is useful if the obstetrician draws 20 ml of placental blood from the umbilical cord after delivery of the newborn. This is obtained with a 20 gauge needle and 20 ml syringe under sterile conditions. The needle is moistened with heparin at a 1:1000 dilution. The dead space of the needle and syringe will contain sufficient heparin to heparinize 20 ml blood to a concentration of 4 units/ml. This blood is then readily available for use if the infant is hypotensive or requires blood volume expansion. If the blood is not needed, it can then be discarded or can be used for certain blood chemistry studies. One of the few clinically useful measurements that can be made on umbilical cord blood is a measurement of sodium concentration whenever the possibility of dilutional hyponatremia in the mother and infant is suspected.

A second procedure is performed whenever meconium-stained amniotic fluid is noticed at delivery. The obstetrician should deliver the head of the infant and then suction the nasopharynx, using a catheter and a DeLee trap before the shoulders are delivered and the thorax expands. This simple procedure has markedly reduced the incidence of severe meconium aspiration pneumonitis.

Resuscitation of the Newborn Infant

The flow chart presented in Fig 3—4 diagrams the resuscitation procedures for newborn infants according to the severity of the neonatal depression shown at delivery. A few general comments apply to all infants. A senior pediatrician skilled in the mechanics of resuscitation and in the evaluation of depressed infants of any weight or gestational age should be present for the delivery of every high-risk infant. In multiple pregnancies, there should always be one physician present for each infant. The knowledge of the attending physi-

cian should encompass far more than skills in airway management; an emphasis on the technic and practice of skillful intubation may overshadow a physician's inability to recognize clinical signs of impending shock or other problems in low-birth-weight infants. Ideally, a staff nurse from the neonatal intensive care unit should be present at the delivery of a high-risk infant. This enables the high-risk obstetrics nurse to concentrate exclusively upon the care of the mother. In addition, nurses from intensive care units are familiar with all the equipment and procedures required for support of the circulation and other procedures in high-risk infants. At medical centers with residency training programs, the physician and nursing staff should be supplemented by pediatric house staff members who assist in resuscitation for both training and service purposes.

The basic approach to resuscitation should center on adequate oxygenation and temperature support of the infant. It should ensure that these needs are met promptly and should de-emphasize pharmacologic management. The mechanics of resuscitation are far more important than the use of any pharmacologic agents, including sodium bicarbonate. All newborn infants, even the low-risk, full-term newborn infant, require adequate temperature support at delivery. In

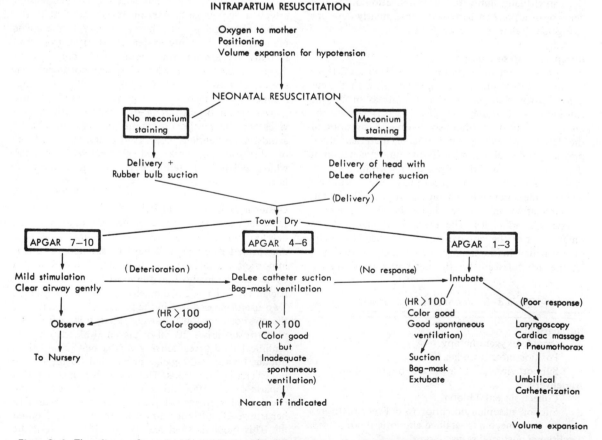

Figure 3—4. Flow diagram for perinatal resuscitation. (Modified and reproduced, with permission, from Lemons JA, Battaglia FC: Resuscitation of the newborn. Pages 811—814 in: *Current Therapy 1977.* Conn HF [editor] . Saunders, 1977.)

addition, every delivery suite should have adequate lighting and a gentle suction source for aspiration of the oro- or nasopharynx. Temperature support of the infant requires that a radiant heat source be provided and that the infant's skin be toweled dry to prevent the enormous evaporative heat losses that would otherwise occur.

A comment is in order about resuscitation of the very-low-birth-weight infant. Such infants may have depressed (<3) initial Apgar scores at 1 minute, even though their subsequent course is uncomplicated and the umbilical venous and arterial pH and base excess were normal at delivery. These observations suggest that the Apgar score may provide an inadequate assessment of the condition of the very immature infant. The obvious important implication of this observation is that the physician may interpret a low Apgar score as an indication of a poor prognosis and may therefore hesitate to provide prompt and effective resuscitation to the very-low-birth-weight baby. *The decision to withhold prompt and effective resuscitative measures should never be made on the basis of the low Apgar score in the very immature infant.* If prompt intervention and the establishment of adequate ventilation are carried out in small newborn infants, further steps are rarely required. Of 94 infants at Colorado General Hospital whose birth weights were less than 1500 gm, only one infant required additional resuscitative steps despite the fact that half the infants had initial 1-minute Apgar scores of less than 4. The routine use of alkali therapy and various cardiac stimulants in the delivery room should be vigorously discouraged. Temperature support of the very-low-birth-weight infant requires more than a radiant heater and drying of the skin; a gentle heat source should be placed below the infant. It may be either a circulating warm water pad or one of several chemical thermogenic heating pads. The latter are useful in transporting the very-low-birth-weight infant to the nursery because the infant can be transported on the pad and yet still be wrapped in a silver swaddler or some similar insulation material.

When volume expansion is required in very-low-birth-weight infants, placental blood, albumin infusions at 5–10 gm/100 ml, or Plasmanate is preferred. In the rare cases in which sodium bicarbonate may be required for resuscitation, it should always be diluted to an isotonic solution and should generally be given in the same solution used to administer albumin.

OXYGEN THERAPY

The development of retrolental fibroplasia is directly related to increased arterial oxygen tensions. Therefore, careful monitoring of arterial P_{O_2} is required to avoid this complication and yet provide adequate oxygenation.

A second organ injured by administration of oxygen in high concentrations is the lung. Prolonged exposure to high ambient oxygen concentrations will produce fatal bronchopulmonary dysplasia. Since this condition is caused by exposure of the surface of the respiratory tract to high concentrations rather than by a high arterial P_{O_2}, it may to some extent be unavoidable in those infants with severe hyaline membrane disease who require high oxygen concentrations in inspired air to ensure acceptable arterial oxygen tension. Positive pressure ventilation with high oxygen concentrations increases the risk of pulmonary damage. Bronchopulmonary dysplasia has occurred less frequently when negative pressure respirators were used or when infants did not require high peak inspiratory and peak expiratory pressure for effective ventilation.

Supplemental oxygen administration is needed for infants whose arterial oxygen tensions fall below 50–60 mm Hg. Cyanosis does not provide an accurate indication of arterial oxygen levels and cannot be used as a guide for continued oxygen therapy. The use of equipment to maintain an ambient oxygen concentration at less than 40% is not recommended because arterial P_{O_2} levels exceeding 100 mm Hg may occur at this concentration and a limit of 40% may be insufficient for an infant with respiratory distress.

The oxygen should be warmed (31–34° C) and humidified and delivered through the incubator air intake system or by use of a head box or plastic hood.

Guidelines for Oxygen Therapy

(1) Maintain arterial oxygen between 50–80 mm Hg, not to exceed 100 mm Hg.

(2) Measure and record inspiratory oxygen concentration at infant's nose accurately and frequently; also each time blood gases are drawn.

(3) Arterial oxygen tension determinations may be done from the descending aorta or the temporal, brachial, or radial arteries. Values from blood obtained from a warmed heel are less reliable and may be used only when a more reliable source is not available.

(4) If blood gas measurements are not available, oxygen supplementation may be administered in concentrations just high enough to relieve cyanosis. However, because of the special risk of retrolental fibroplasia and other toxic effects of oxygen administration, the infant should be transferred for care where these measurements are available.

(5) Infants who have received oxygen therapy should have a careful eye examination for evidence of retrolental fibroplasia prior to discharge.

Committee on Fetus and Newborn: Oxygen therapy in the newborn infant. Pediatrics 47:1086, 1971.

Hull D: Lung expansion and ventilation during resuscitation of the asphyxiated newborn. J Pediatr 75:47, 1969.

Kuhns LR, Poznanski AK: Endotracheal tube position in the infant. J Pediatr 78:991, 1971.

Lemons JA, Battaglia FC: Resuscitation of the newborn. Pages 811–814 in: *Current Therapy 1977.* Conn HF (editor). Saunders, 1977.

Stern L: The use and misuse of oxygen in the newborn infant. Pediatr Clin North Am 20:447, 1973.

Turberville DF, Bowen FW, Killam AP: Intracranial hemorrhage in kittens: Hypernatremia versus hypoxia. J Pediatr 89:294, 1976.

PHOTOTHERAPY

Light energy enhances the degradation of unconjugated bilirubin in the skin to colorless by-products which are apparently nontoxic. Full-spectrum fluorescent bulbs are preferred to blue lights so that the baby can be observed under normal light. Otherwise, observation of skin color for pallor, cyanosis, or other conditions is virtually impossible. Certain important routines must be followed whenever phototherapy is used:

(1) Phototherapy should be used only when significant unconjugated (indirect) hyperbilirubinemia is present; its use with elevated conjugated (direct) bilirubin levels is contraindicated ("bronze baby syndrome").

(2) The etiologic basis for jaundice must always be sought.

(3) Bilirubin levels must be determined serially while the infant is receiving phototherapy; skin jaundice is not a reliable indicator of serum bilirubin levels.

(4) The indication for exchange transfusion and other methods of management of neonatal jaundice are not changed by phototherapy.

(5) Phototherapy should be administered in alternating light and dark cycles. The optimal cycle is not known, although most centers prefer a repeating cycle of 6 hours of phototherapy followed by 2 hours without therapy.

(6) The eyes should be protected from intense light by appropriate patching. The patch must be applied carefully and should be removed at regular intervals to examine the eyes; conjunctivitis and corneal abrasion are the main hazards.

(7) The use of phototherapy or an open radiant heater (or both) produces considerable evaporative water losses in infants. It is customary to increase free water intake during phototherapy by about 25% and to follow urine flow rates and specific gravities carefully in order to readjust fluid intake as required. An increase in the evaporative water loss may be associated with an increase in caloric requirements. This may constitute an additional nutritional problem in certain instances in which nutrition has been inadequate for other reasons. Phototherapy also increases gastrointestinal transit time and may interfere with the absorption of drugs administered orally.

(8) Electrical and mechanical safety of the phototherapy unit must be assured.

Lucey JF: Neonatal jaundice and phototherapy. Pediatr Clin North Am 19:829, 1972.

OTHER PROCEDURES

Umbilical artery and vein catheterization, cutdowns, monitors, respirators and other ventilatory assistance devices, radiant heaters, and other procedures and equipment are used extensively in the care of sick newborns. These procedures are described in other sections of this book (Chapters 12 and 34).

Kitterman JA & others: Catheterization of umbilical vessels in newborn infants. Pediatr Clin North Am 17:895, 1970.

THE PRETERM INFANT

Babies born prematurely make up the major portion of newborns who are at increased risk. (For definitions and classification, see the early sections of this chapter.) Gestational age and birth weight correlate well with mortality risk.

Physiologic Handicaps Due to Prematurity

The increased risk due to prematurity is largely due to the functional and anatomic immaturity of various organs. Some of the more important examples are as follows:

(1) Weak sucking, swallowing, gag, and cough reflexes, leading to difficulty in feeding and danger of aspiration.

(2) Pulmonary immaturity and a pliable thorax, leading to hypoventilation and hypoxia with respiratory and metabolic acidosis.

(3) Decreased ability to maintain body temperature.

(4) Limited ability to excrete solutes in urine.

(5) Increased susceptibility to infection.

(6) Limited iron stores and rapid growth, leading to later anemia.

(7) Tendency to develop rickets due to rapid growth with diminished intake of calcium and vitamin D.

(8) Nutritional disturbances secondary to feeding difficulties and diminished absorption of fat and fat-soluble vitamins.

(9) Immaturity of some metabolic processes, which influences the metabolism of certain nutrients and drugs as well as maintenance of normal homeostasis.

Care of the Preterm Infant

A. Delivery Room: See Perinatal Resuscitation on p 60 for resuscitation procedures for preterm infants.

B. Care in Nursery: Babies born at 36–38 weeks' gestation may need only general nursery care, stabilizing uneventfully after birth and going home with the mother. The more premature infant will require special care in either a level 2 or level 3 nursery.

Incubator Care

Recently, there has been a tendency to care for small, preterm, or growth-retarded infants under open radiant heaters instead of in incubators because it is more convenient for nurses and doctors to examine infants and adjust tubes and equipment. However, easy accessibility introduces the risk of infection from contact with hospital personnel, whereas incubator care tends to remind the staff of the need for scrupulous hand washing and other isolation procedures. Another disadvantage of the open radiant heater is the increased evaporative water losses and increased caloric requirements that may occur, particularly in very-low-birthweight infants; occasionally, very-low-birth-weight infants may require more than 175 ml/kg/day of free water intake to prevent hypertonicity secondary to dehydration. Thus, incubator care still has some advantages over open radiant heaters. The incubators should be set to maintain skin temperature at 36–37° C (96.8–98.6° F). This generally requires an air temperature of 32–36° C (89.6–96.8° F). The larger and more mature the infant, the lower the incubator temperature required to achieve a thermal neutral zone with minimal oxygen consumption.

Satisfactory incubators may be either servocontrolled or manually controlled. The use of manually controlled incubators for temperature regulation encourages observation of the infant's thermal stability and increases the chances that elevations of body temperature will be noted more readily. Humidification of the incubator environment by the addition of water is no longer routine because the inspired air, supplemented with oxygen, has often already been warmed and humidified and because there is concern that the high humidity within the incubator may encourage the growth of hydrophilic organisms (eg, pseudomonas) on the inner surfaces, thus predisposing to infections with these organisms.

Transfer From an Incubator to Bassinet

When the premature infant who is swaddled is able to maintain his body temperature without added environmental heat, he is placed in an open bassinet. This usually may be done when the infant reaches 1800–2000 gm. His body temperature should be monitored to be sure he continues to maintain a normal temperature. This step represents one more reduction in the level of support the infant requires.

Feeding

See pp 57 ff.

Growth of Preterm Infant

In order to monitor the growth, hydration, and nutrition of preterm infants, standard postnatal growth curves can be used and further data added. Each day the infant's daily weight, the total water intake (in ml/kg/day), and the total caloric intake (kcal/kg/day) are plotted on the same graph (Fig 3–5). For purposes of plotting calories and hydration, the weight in grams along the ordinate can be used as units of caloric and water intake.

Examination

Evaluation and diagnostic procedures are done gently and carefully. The baby may not tolerate excessive handling well, so that the examination should be tempered by a practical consideration of the baby's condition. Careful observation will provide much information, diminishing the amount of handling needed for the physical examination. Whenever possible, procedures should be done without removing the baby from the incubator and should be done within the nursery environment.

Supplements

A. **Vitamins:** For infants receiving adequate

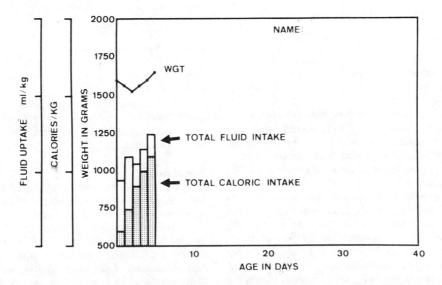

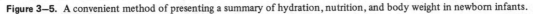

Figure 3–5. A convenient method of presenting a summary of hydration, nutrition, and body weight in newborn infants.

amounts of milk, vitamins A, C, and D are given as supplements if they are not present in adequate amounts in the formula being used. Phytonadione (vitamin K_1, AquaMephyton), 1 mg IM, is given on admission to the nursery.

When infants receive only intravenous or intra-arterial fluids during the first few days of life, a water-soluble multivitamin preparation should be added to the fluids to ensure adequate intake of water-soluble vitamins.

B. Iron: Infants with birth weight less than 1800 gm need supplemental iron, since their iron stores at birth are limited and there is rapid growth with an increase in red cell mass during the first year of life. Oral iron supplementation is begun after the first week of life in these infants.

Discharge

Discharge from the hospital usually occurs when the infant weighs 2000–2500 gm and is eating well and coexistent medical problems have resolved or are sufficiently improved. In the nursery, the parents are encouraged to visit the baby frequently and help care for and feed their child. A social worker or visiting nurse may be very helpful in aiding the mother to care for the baby and in helping to solve the special problems related to prolonged mother-infant separation, disease, or handicaps.

Follow-Up Care

Long-term follow-up care is especially important for babies discharged from level 2 or level 3 nurseries because of the high incidence of significant handicaps occurring later: cerebral palsy, deafness, learning and perceptual problems, and mental retardation. Early recognition of these handicaps and appropriate treatment when indicated will improve outcome.

MULTIPLE BIRTHS

Twinning occurs in about one out of 90 pregnancies. The incidence of twins increases with the mother's age and parity. There is a familial tendency toward dizygotic twinning.

Dizygotic twinning occurs with increased frequency following the use of drugs, eg, clomiphene, which induce ovulation and which may be used in the treatment of infertility. Twins may develop from a single ovum (monozygotic, identical) or from 2 ova (dizygotic, fraternal).

About one-third of twins are of the single ovum type. About one-third of identical twins have a double placenta, amnion, and chorion. However, if the partition between the twins consists of 2 layers of transparent amnion without an intervening chorion, a diagnosis of monozygotic twinning can be made with certainty. Similarly, if the twins are of opposite sexes the diagnosis of dizygotic twins is made with certainty. It

is important to determine if the twins are monozygotic or dizygotic, since the information may be crucial later in life if questions of organ transplantation occur. Certain complications such as twin-twin transfusion syndrome occur more frequently with single chorion placentation.

Intrauterine Growth

The fetal growth pattern in multiple pregnancy differs from that of a single fetus. Intrauterine growth retardation occurs at a given total weight of all fetuses regardless of the number. Thus, intrauterine growth retardation appears in each fetus later in gestation in triplets than for quadruplets and still later in twins. In addition, the greater the number of fetuses, the earlier in pregnancy labor will occur, ie, triplets tend to be delivered earlier than twins. Thus, infants in multiple pregnancies are more likely to be affected by problems of preterm delivery and intrauterine growth retardation than are singletons. Discordant twins whose birth weights differ markedly (by at least 20% or more) often are found in association with twin-twin transfusion syndrome and are more common when there is a single chorion, as in monozygotic twins. The larger, plethoric twin tends to be much more ill than the anemic, smaller one when twin-twin transfusion syndrome occurs, perhaps because hypervolemia and hyperviscosity may contribute to the symptoms in the larger twin.

Complications of Multiple Births

(1) Preterm delivery: Pregnancy is usually several weeks shorter with twins.

(2) Polyhydramnios: Ten times more common.

(3) Preeclampsia and eclampsia: Three times more common.

(4) Placenta previa: More frequent, presumably from increased placental mass.

(5) Abruptio placentae: May occur with second twin placenta due to reduction in size of uterus following delivery of the first twin.

(6) Presentation: Breech and other abnormal presentations are more frequent.

(7) Duration of labor: Usually not much longer, though uterine contractions after delivery may be poor, with subsequent bleeding.

(8) Prolapse of the cord: Seven times more frequent than in single deliveries because of abnormal presentations and rupture of the second twin's membranes when unengaged.

Prognosis

The morbidity and mortality risks in multiple births are greater than with single births. More second-born twins die than firstborn twins.

Follow-up studies of twins for later growth and development are conflicting, with some studies supporting a continued discrepancy in size of the 2 twins into adulthood and other studies being unable to demonstrate persistent differences in developmental size from those recorded in single births.

Benirschke K: Multiple birth: Signal for scrutiny. Hosp Pract 1:25, 1966.

Fujikura T, Froehlich LA: Mental and motor development in monozygotic co-twins with dissimilar birth weights. Pediatrics 53:884, 1974.

Wilson RS: Twins: Measure of birth size at different gestational ages. Ann Hum Biol 1:57, 1975.

SPECIFIC DISEASES OF THE NEWBORN

RESPIRATORY DISEASES

1. APNEA

Apnea is defined as cessation of respiration for 30 seconds or longer and is accompanied by cyanosis and bradycardia. It must be distinguished from *periodic breathing* (see below), in which the apnea is brief (usually less than 10 seconds) and is not accompanied by cyanosis or bradycardia.

Apnea may be a sign of serious significance in the newborn. Apnea can occur at any time during the neonatal period, particularly in very immature infants. Generally, the appearance of severe apneic episodes in a previously well preterm baby signals the onset of some other serious illness (eg, meningitis, sepsis, intracranial hemorrhage, etc), but in some instances apnea apparently unassociated with any metabolic problem or illnesses may occur. Virtually any serious illness may precipitate apneic episodes. For this reason, apneic attacks require a thorough evaluation of the infant's condition, with particular attention directed to any infection or CNS disorder as a possible cause of the attacks. Severe apneic attacks in a previously well infant may be an indication for an EEG study. An infant may have seizures that have not been clinically recognized as the basis for the apneic episodes. Apneic episodes in infants with neonatal seizures will often stop when seizures are controlled and successfully treated with anticonvulsants. If apneic episodes are frequent, an oral loading dose of theophylline, 5 mg/kg, can be given. A blood level reading should be obtained 2 hours after administration of the loading dose, at which time the drug level is likely to be at its peak. A maintenance dose is adjusted on the basis of blood level readings but is generally in the range of 1–2 mg/kg every 12 hours, given orally.

Aranda JV & others: Pharmacokinetic aspects of theophylline in premature newborns. N Engl J Med 295:413, 1976.

Daily WJR, Klaus M, Meyer HBP: Apnea in premature infants: Monitoring, incidence, heart rate changes and an effect of environmental temperature. Pediatrics 43:510, 1969.

Gupta JM, Tizard JPM: The sequence of events in neonatal apnea. Lancet 2:55, 1967.

2. PERIODIC BREATHING

In the small premature infant, a form of Cheyne-Stokes respiration has been described. It characteristically consists of a rhythm of 8–12 respiratory cycles followed by a pause or apneic period of approximately 10 seconds. Periodic breathing is so frequent in premature infants that it scarcely causes concern, and the phrase "rest periods" is often used to describe the breathing pattern. The infant with periodic breathing does not become cyanotic; in fact, studies have shown that he is better ventilated than the premature infant with regular respirations.

Periodic breathing is related to altitude as well as to prematurity, since instances of periodic breathing occur in full-term infants in Denver (1 mile above sea level).

Periodic breathing tends to occur after the first few days of life. This finding is not associated with significant changes in heart rate and has no prognostic significance.

3. RESPIRATORY DISTRESS

It is generally useful to divide pulmonary disorders of the newborn into 3 categories based upon physical and radiologic findings.

(1) Hyaline membrane disease with marked hypoexpansion and reduced lung volume and involving all lung fields: An inspiratory chest x-ray has the appearance of an expiratory film. On physical examination the findings are consistent with decreased lung volume and include marked intercostal retraction, suprasternal retraction, and grunting. Air entry is uniformly poor throughout all lung fields.

(2) Disorders with increased or normal pulmonary expansion, hilar infiltrates, rales, and rhonchi: This group includes congenital bacterial pneumonias (generally caused by group B streptococci), "wet lung" syndrome, transient tachypnea of the newborn, and hyperviscosity syndrome. Wheezing may be present. The chest x-ray shows a slightly enlarged heart and streaky infiltrates radiating from the hilus of the lung following the general pattern of the lymphatic and venous drainage of the lung. The peripheral lung fields are clear. Although some of the diseases in this category are quickly diagnosed (eg, hyperviscosity syndrome with the help of a hematocrit determination), congenital bacterial pneumonias and "wet lung" syndrome cannot be easily diagnosed. For this reason, infants in whom a tentative diagnosis of "wet lung" syndrome has been made should be treated with antibiotics until bacterial infection is clearly ruled out.

(3) Disorders with normal lung expansion, relatively clear lung fields, and marked hypoxemia: The condition most commonly associated with these findings is transient persistence of the fetal circulation.

Any congenital heart lesion with inadequate pulmonary blood flow will also have these findings. Occasionally, "shock lung" following a severe hypoxic and hypotensive episode will also have these signs. More commonly, however, shock lung has a clinical spectrum comparable to that of "wet lung" syndrome. Transient persistence of the fetal circulation may cause marked arterial hypoxemia with clear lung fields.

Treatment

A. Hyaline Membrane Disease: Treatment includes early administration of continuous positive airway pressure, careful monitoring of inspiratory oxygen concentration, and appropriate supportive care of temperature, hydration, and nutrition. If CO_2 retention is marked or if oxygenation is inadequate, respirator support should be used.

Continuous positive airway pressure is normally begun at pressures of 4–6 cm water. The concentration of inspired oxygen is adjusted to maintain an arterial P_{O_2} greater than 50 mm Hg. If positive pressure ventilation is required, lower pressures can be used to achieve adequate oxygenation if inspiratory-expiratory ratios of 1.0 or greater are used. Peak inspiratory pressures greater than 24–26 cm water are rarely required.

General supportive care is crucial in avoiding iatrogenic complications or other problems. Hypothermia should be avoided since this will increase the infant's oxygen requirements. An infusion of 10% glucose with appropriate sodium intake provided as $NaHCO_3$ should be given because infants with hyaline membrane disease almost invariably demonstrate combined respiratory and metabolic acidosis. The quantities of water and sodium required will vary depending upon the size and maturity of the infant; general guidelines have been given above. Frequently, infants severely ill with hyaline membrane disease may require circulatory support with intravenous infusion of colloid or red blood cells. However, expansion of circulating blood or plasma volume should not be confused with expansion of extracellular volume caused by the increased administration of sodium and water. Expansion of extracellular volume should be avoided.

B. Treatment of Conditions in ¶ (2): In general, infants with diseases in this category will not require respiratory support and can be managed satisfactorily in level 2 nursery units. In the presence of congestion or "wet lung" syndrome, restriction of water and sodium intake during the first 2 days of life is useful. Occasionally, "benign continuous positive airway pressure" (ie, CPAP not requiring intubation) will also improve oxygenation and avoids the use of excessively high concentrations of inspired oxygen. Since diseases in this category cannot be distinguished early in their courses from congenital bacterial pneumonia, particularly group B streptococcal pneumonia, infants with these diseases should be given antibiotics and cultures should be performed until congenital bacterial pneumonia has been ruled out. Hyperviscosity syndrome can be treated simply by a small exchange transfusion

with plasma sufficient to lower the central hematocrit to less than 65.

C. Treatment of Conditions in ¶ (3): In many cases of transient persistence of the fetal circulation, CO_2 retention is not marked and respirator care is not required. Therapy consists of frequent adjustments of inspired oxygen concentration. During the first 24–48 hours, pulmonary vascular resistance may increase or decrease at frequent intervals. For this reason, inspired oxygen concentration must be readjusted often. Otherwise there is the risk of alternating periods of hypoxia and hyperoxia, with the possibility of retrolental fibroplasia. When transient persistence of the fetal circulation is very severe, tolazoline (Priscoline) in a dose of 1–2 mg/kg IV may be safely used to vasodilate the pulmonary vascular bed. It should be emphasized that tolazoline is a general alpha-adrenergic blocking agent and has histamine-like activity. As such it will cause vasodilatation in other vascular beds besides that of the lung. Severe and irreversible shock may occur if colloid in the form of plasma or whole blood is not given at the time of tolazoline administration. Mean arterial blood pressure should be carefully monitored during and following tolazoline therapy.

Brumley GW: The critically ill child. 16. Respiratory distress syndrome of the newborn. Pediatrics 47:758, 1971.

Capitanio MA, Kirkpatrick JA Jr: Roentgen examination in the evaluation of the newborn infant with respiratory distress. J Pediatr 75:896, 1969.

Gregory GA: Respiratory care of newborn infants. Pediatr Clin North Am 19:311, 1972.

Knelson JH & others: Physiologic significance of grunting respirations. Pediatrics 44:393, 1969.

Krouskop RW, Brown EG, Sweet AY: The early use of continuous positive airway pressure in the treatment of idiopathic respiratory distress syndrome. J Pediatr 87:263, 1975.

Krouss AN, Klain DB, Auld PAM: Chronic pulmonary insufficiency of prematurity. Pediatrics 55:55, 1975.

Sundell H & others: Studies on infants with type II respiratory distress syndrome. J Pediatr 78:754, 1971.

HEART DISEASE

See Chapter 13 for discussions of physiologic changes in circulation in the perinatal period and specific congenital and acquired heart diseases. Treatment of heart failure in the newborn is discussed on p 334.

Signs & Symptoms of Heart Failure in the Newborn

Heart failure in the newborn infant may be difficult to recognize because the signs and symptoms are not the same as in older infants. The infant in early failure will show only an increased heart and respiratory rate and perhaps irritability. Auscultation of the lungs rarely reveals evidence of pulmonary edema. X-ray examination may show the heart to be enlarged, but in newborn infants minimal cardiac enlargement is difficult to determine, particularly if there is a large thymus shadow. Assessing heart size by physical examination is even more difficult.

Increasing liver size is an important finding. An enlarged or enlarging liver, in the absence of other disease, is good evidence of heart failure. Liver size should be followed as a means of evaluating the effectiveness of treatment.

Peripheral edema is frequent in preterm babies but rarely as a sign of heart failure. When it does occur as a result of heart failure, it is a late and ominous sign. In general, peripheral edema reflects excessive sodium and water intake rather than heart failure. Echocardiography, a new and powerful noninvasive tool requiring little manipulation of the infant, enables physicians to safely perform serial examinations of critically ill infants. It has been useful in assessing the strength of myocardial contractions, facilitating the early diagnosis of various congenital anomalies of the heart, and providing an estimate of left atrial size through measurements of left atrial-aortic route diameters (LA:AO ratios). The latter measurement is particularly useful in monitoring the progress of preterm babies with a patent ductus arteriosus.

Treatment of acute heart failure of whatever cause consists of restricting water intake to the amount of evaporative losses and eliminating sodium intake. If water restriction is coupled with complete sodium restriction, hyponatremia will not result even if potent diuretics are used. This regimen can be instituted along with a single dose of furosemide and digitalization of the infant. After 12–24 hours, water and sodium intake may then be increased, with the degree of water and sodium administered depending upon the clinical course of the infant.

JAUNDICE IN THE NEWBORN

Jaundice is the most frequent clinical problem in the neonatal period. The age at onset, the degree of jaundice, and the condition of the baby are important observations in determining the cause and significance of jaundice.

When red blood cells break down, the iron and protein are stored and reused. However, the porphyrin ring must be detoxified and excreted from the body. It is reduced to bilirubin (unconjugated, indirect) in the reticuloendothelial cells and is then transported to the liver via the blood, bound to albumin. In the liver, the bilirubin is conjugated mainly to bilirubin diglucuronide (conjugated, direct) and excreted through the biliary ducts to the gut. In the intestine it would normally be converted to urobilinogen by bacterial action, effectively removing it from consideration. However, since the newborn intestine is sterile, this step does not take place. Conjugated bilirubin excreted in the bile can be hydrolyzed back to bilirubin, which then may be reabsorbed if the bowel content is not evacuated.

The degree of jaundice that develops will depend upon the rate of red cell breakdown (bilirubin load), the rate of conjugation, the rate of excretion, and the amount of bilirubin reabsorbed from the intestine. In normal term infants, red blood cells have an average life span of about 100 days; therefore 1% of the cells is removed from the circulation every day. The average capacity of the liver to conjugate bilirubin in the first few days of life approximately equals the bilirubin load, since about half of infants will show laboratory evidence of a significant rise in bilirubin levels and about one-third show clinical jaundice. Jaundice tends to occur first in the head and neck. As the unconjugated bilirubin concentration increases, more of the body appears jaundiced; jaundice involving most of the body surfaces including the palms and soles occurs only with markedly elevated bilirubin concentration. Early feedings and glycerin suppositories have been shown to minimize the degree of jaundice in the newborn period, presumably by enhancing early evacuation of meconium from the gut and eliminating the bilirubin present in the intestine.

In contrast, any problems leading to gastrointestinal obstruction in the newborn infant tend to be associated with an increased incidence of jaundice.

Bilirubin levels should be determined periodically on all jaundiced infants because of the special danger of kernicterus in the newborn (see p 86).

Etiology of Jaundice in the Newborn

A. **Increased Rate of Hemolysis:** (All patients in this category have an increased unconjugated bilirubin concentration and an increased reticulocyte count.)

　1. Patients with positive Coombs test (this category includes all patients with isoimmunization, including ABO incompatibility, Rh incompatibility, etc).

　2. Patients with negative Coombs test.

　　a. Abnormal red cell shapes, including spherocytosis, elliptocytosis, pyknocytosis, stomatocytosis.

　　b. Red cell enzyme abnormalities: glucose-6-phosphate dehydrogenase deficiency, pyruvate kinase deficiency.

B. **Decreased Rate of Conjugation:** Unconjugated bilirubin elevated, reticulocyte count normal.

　1. Immaturity of bilirubin conjugation ("physiologic jaundice").

　2. Congenital familial nonhemolytic jaundice (inborn errors of metabolism affecting glucuronyl transferase system and bilirubin transport).

　3. Breast milk jaundice?

C. **Abnormalities of Liver Function:** Conjugated and unconjugated bilirubin elevated, Coombs test negative, reticulocyte count normal.

　1. Hepatitis—Viral, parasitic, bacterial, toxic.

　2. Metabolic abnormalities—

　　a. Galactosemia.

　　b. Glycogen storage diseases.

c. Infant of diabetic mother.

d. Cystic fibrosis.

3. Biliary atresia.

4. Choledochal cyst.

5. Obstruction at ampulla of Vater (annular pancreas).

6. Sepsis.

1. ISOIMMUNIZATION DUE TO ABO BLOOD GROUP INCOMPATIBILITY

ABO blood group incompatibility is the most common form of isoimmunization but a less severe clinical problem than Rh-D incompatibility, which is second in frequency.

Management of Pregnancy

Anti-A and anti-B antibodies are not demonstrated by antibody screening tests since O cells are used. Since ABO incompatibility imposes only a slight risk on the fetus, there is ample time to evaluate the infant after delivery at term. Amniotic fluid bilirubin determination is not helpful in management of these pregnancies.

Diagnosis

There is no satisfactory way to predict which infants with ABO incompatibility will develop significant hyperbilirubinemia. However, the presence of a potential problem can be anticipated by comparing the blood groups of the mother and baby (which is the reason for recommending routine blood typing on cord blood of all babies). Blood group combinations that represent incompatibility are as follows:

Mother	Infant
O	A or B
A	B or AB
B	A or AB
AB	No incompatibility

Hemoglobin levels are normal or nearly so. Mild reticulocytosis may be present. Spherocytes are commonly found on the smear of peripheral blood.

Physical examination is usually normal except for jaundice, which may develop in the first 48 hours. More severe involvement occasionally occurs, usually with B–O incompatibility.

Coombs testing can be done whenever potential incompatibility exists. The direct Coombs test is usually positive if done carefully. The indirect Coombs test will be positive in the presence of antibody if type-specific cells are used, although a strongly positive reaction is uncommon. If in doubt about the sensitivity of a Coombs test, it is best to assume that sensitization is present whenever maternal-infant major blood group incompatibility exists. Serial bilirubin levels are then obtained in those infants who become jaundiced.

Note: Babies who may have both ABO and Rh isoimmunization (eg, mother is type O Rh-negative; baby type A Rh-positive) will often be protected from Rh sensitization. However, such a baby with a positive direct Coombs test should have indirect Coombs testing for both antibodies.

Management

Give supportive care and phototherapy as described for Rh sensitization (see below). Exchange transfusion should be used to keep bilirubin levels below 20 mg/100 ml. Cord values or early rates of bilirubin rise are not indications for transfusion in ABO sensitization, since these do not predict eventual bilirubin levels.

2. ISOIMMUNIZATION DUE TO Rh & SIMILAR RED CELL ANTIGENS

Isoimmunization due to Rh antigens (D, E, C^W c, or e), Kell (Kk), Duffy (Fy), Lutheran (Lu), and Kidd (Jk) factors may have a similar clinical picture. The involved red cell antigen is always absent from the mother's red cells; therefore, if fetal red cells containing the antigen cross the placenta, the mother will produce antibodies to the "foreign" antigen. The IgG antibodies cross the placenta and enter the fetal circulation. When antibody forms a complex with fetal red cell antigen, the cells will be removed from the circulation at an increased rate, leading to anemia and increased bilirubin load.

Diagnosis

A. Maternal Past History: History of affected infant or unexplained jaundice, anemia, or fetal death.

B. Current Pregnancy: Blood type and antibody screening should be done on all pregnant women as early as possible. Antibody screening is an easy and inexpensive means of demonstrating the presence or absence of red cell antibody. If antibody is absent in an Rh-negative woman early in pregnancy, it should be repeated frequently throughout the second and third trimesters. Significant sensitization to blood groups other than D is unlikely to occur when no antibody exists in the initial screening. When antibody screening is positive, the specific antibody should be identified and an indirect Coombs titer determined to establish the degree of sensitization.

C. Amniocentesis and Amniotic Fluid Analysis: Amniotic fluid analysis should be done early on all pregnant women with significant elevated Rh antibody titers to determine if the fetus is affected and to evaluate the severity of the disease. A clinical estimate of severity of disease in the fetus is then made, using the prediction graph based on clinical experience with that method (Fig 3–6 and Table 3–6).

D. Infant at Birth: Blood type on cord blood compared with mother's blood type will indicate

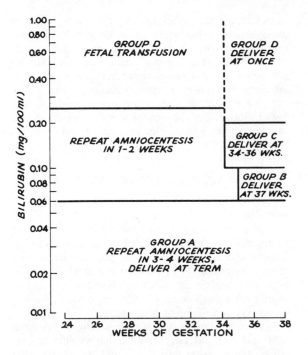

Figure 3—6. Prediction graph; management of Rh-sensitized pregnancies based on serial amniotic fluid bilirubin concentrations. Location of dashed line dividing management of group D patients is determined by relative risks of premature delivery and intrauterine transfusion. Because of absorbance characteristics of bilirubin, the concentration of bilirubin in mg/100 ml approximates delta optical density (Δ OD) of Liley (eg, 0.100 mg/100 ml bilirubin approximates a Δ OD of 0.100). (Redrawn and reproduced, with permission, from Brazie JV & others: An improved, rapid procedure for the determination of amniotic fluid bilirubin and its use in predicting the course of Rh-sensitized pregnancies. Am J Obstet Gynecol 104:80, 1969.)

Table 3—6. Patient groups in Rh-D isoimmunization.

Group A: Fetus mildly affected or unaffected. Repeat amniocentesis in 3—4 weeks. Deliver at or near term. Newborn in good condition. If affected, there is time after delivery to evaluate infant.

Group B: Moderate disease; fetus at risk of developing hydrops if pregnancy continues beyond 37 weeks. Repeat amniocentesis in 1—2 weeks. Deliver at 37 weeks. Newborn may be more severely affected. Anticipate immediate evaluation and need for treatment.

Group C: More severe disease; fetus at risk of developing hydrops if pregnancy continues to 37 weeks. Risk of premature delivery less than risk of intrauterine transfusion. Repeat amniocentesis in 1—2 weeks. Deliver at 34—36 weeks. Newborn more severely affected and premature. Anticipate immediate evaluation and need for treatment.

Group D: Severely affected fetus; hydrops likely prior to 34 weeks. Risk of intrauterine transfusion less than risk of very premature delivery. Intrauterine transfusions indicated. Deliver at 34 weeks or later, if possible. Newborn condition variable, depending on the efficiency of the fetal transfusion and the degree of prematurity. Anticipate immediate evaluation and need for treatment.

In severely affected infants, one or more intrauterine transfusions may be required for fetal survival. In a moderately ill infant, it may be safer to allow the pregnancy to reach 34 weeks' or more gestation and then deliver a somewhat anemic preterm baby.

It is important to evaluate the severity of the disease because this is a deciding factor in determining when exchange transfusions are required.

B. Newborn at Delivery:

(1) The first indication for a postnatal exchange transfusion of packed red blood cells immediately after birth is to correct anemia and reduce plasma volume, thus helping to alleviate high output failure. In such cases, the first exchange transfusion may be done essentially on cardiovascular indications, and the volume should be relatively small, just enough to increase hemoglobin concentration and reduce plasma volume. This indication for exchange transfusion may exist whether or not intrauterine transfusions have already been performed. The presence of cardiovascular indications for immediate exchange transfusion implies severe disease. An infant with severe disease often requires both paracentesis to reduce the volume of ascitic fluid and positive pressure ventilation on a respirator to ensure adequate oxygenation.

(2) A second indication for an immediate exchange transfusion is severe sensitization in an infant who is not hydropic. In this case, an exchange trans-

potential blood group incompatibility. Direct Coombs test done on cord blood will be positive if the baby's cells are coated with antibody. This is diagnostic of isoimmunization. A positive indirect Coombs test indicates the presence of antibody in the baby's serum but does not confirm the presence of blood group incompatibility.

Prevention of Rh-D Isoimmunization

The passive administration of human $Rh_0(D)$ immune globulin (RhoGAM) to the Rh-negative, unsensitized mother has proved successful in preventing sensitization when she has delivered an Rh-positive infant.

After delivery, the Rh-negative woman must receive RhoGAM within 72 hours if it is indicated. This is also true after delivery of a stillborn infant or after abortion.

Management

A. During Pregnancy: Fig 3—6 and Table 3—6 summarize the management of an affected pregnancy related to estimated severity of disease in the fetus.

fusion is done to remove affected red cells, since it is far more efficient to remove potential bilirubin while it is still packaged in red blood cells as hemoglobin rather than when it is free bilirubin distributed in fat depots throughout the body. Sensitization as an indication for exchange transfusion depends on whether or not intrauterine transfusions have been done. When several intrauterine transfusions have been performed, the infant's circulating red blood cells at birth may be virtually all donor red cells. In such a case, an early exchange to remove affected infant cells would be useless. The Kleihauer technic should be employed on umbilical cord blood in order to determine what percentage of circulating red cells are fetal cells.

(3) The third indication for exchange transfusion is to remove the bilirubin that has already formed. This indication for exchange transfusion may develop at any time whether or not intrauterine transfusions have been performed.

Exchange transfusions involve replacement of approximately twice the infant's blood volume. To estimate the volume of donor blood required, the infant's blood volume is usually calculated as constituting 8–10% of body weight. Type O Rh-negative blood may be used, particularly when plans must be made before delivery for an exchange transfusion immediately after birth. ABO type-specific blood may be used if the baby's ABO type is known. Donor blood should always be cross-matched with maternal serum. Fresh heparinized blood may be used safely for exchange transfusion but has little advantage over citrate-phosphate-dextrose (CPD) blood. The latter represents less of an acid load than acid-citrate-dextrose (ACD) blood. It has been widely used, since, unlike heparinized blood, it can be stored for some time. It is not necessary to buffer either ACD or CPD blood before use. Attempts to minimize the pH change prior to exchange transfusion are not only unnecessary but may be dangerous and lead to an increased risk of cardiac arrhythmias when blood with high pH but very low calcium activity is infused close to the heart. Metabolic complications associated with erythroblastosis fetalis include the following: (1) Severe hypoglycemia secondary to pancreatic islet cell hyperplasia and occurring most frequently following an exchange transfusion using blood that has a high glucose concentration (eg, CPD blood). The glucose concentration in the infant is sustained during the transfusion but falls rapidly following the procedure. (2) Cardiac arrhythmia associated with delayed return of normal calcium activity when CPD or ACD blood is used for an exchange transfusion. The fall in calcium activity is not necessarily associated with a fall in total calcium concentration in the plasma. The risk of cardiac arrhythmias is compounded if calcium activity falls when other factors affecting function may also be changing (temperature of the solution, glucose concentration in the blood, etc). For this reason, all solutions infused into the inferior vena cava should be warmed to body temperature or administered very slowly to avoid any sudden change in temperature within the heart. Be-

cause of all the other problems requiring medical management immediately after birth, these infants should be delivered at hospitals that can provide optimal obstetric and neonatal care. The infants should not be delivered at one hospital and transferred to an intensive care nursery at another hospital.

All infants with erythroblastosis should be followed closely, particularly for signs of severe anemia that may develop later in the neonatal period.

3. OTHER CAUSES OF JAUNDICE

Infection

Jaundice secondary to bacterial infection is most commonly due to organisms (*Escherichia coli,* staphylococci, and streptococci) which produce hemolyzing toxins, increasing the rate of red cell breakdown. The bilirubin is mainly unconjugated. Jaundice may appear shortly after birth or later in the first week, depending on severity and timing of the infection.

Jaundice due to agents such as viruses (cytomegalic inclusion disease, hepatitis, herpes simplex, rubella, etc), parasites (toxoplasmosis), and *Treponema pallidum* is associated with elevations of both conjugated and unconjugated bilirubin as a result of liver cell injury and obstruction of biliary canaliculi.

Abnormal Red Cell Metabolism

Two inborn errors of metabolism in the red cells may result in an increased rate of hemolysis: glucose-6-phosphate dehydrogenase (G6PD) deficiency and pyruvate kinase deficiency. The first is a very common enzyme defect but usually becomes evident only after coincident exposure of the mother or baby to substances such as naphthalene or primaquine. Hereditary spherocytosis may present with a hemolytic crisis in the newborn period, causing jaundice and anemia. Synthetic vitamin K preparations are oxidants and thus will cause increased hemolysis of red blood cells if administered in excessive amounts to patients with G6PD deficiency.

Extravascular Hemorrhage

Bleeding within the body, as in cephalhematoma, extensive purpura, or CNS hemorrhage, may result in elevated levels of unconjugated bilirubin because of the increased load of hemoglobin which is broken down to bilirubin. Recent studies have stressed the tendency to underestimate the degree of bleeding into muscle and soft tissues of preterm babies who have suffered from apparently superficial bruising. In some preterm babies delivered after difficult breech extractions, the bleeding into muscles of the back and buttocks may be extensive enough to cause irreversible shock and total muscle necrosis in the newborn period.

Immaturity of Glucuronyl Transferase Enzyme System ("Physiologic Jaundice")

"Physiologic jaundice" is a catchall term referring

to the condition occurring in all newborn infants who have jaundice but who have not been shown to have any specific disease leading to increased hemolysis or decreased liver function. It is a diagnosis made by exclusion of other more serious diseases.

The onset of jaundice occurs on the late second or third day in an otherwise well baby and reaches its peak at 5–7 days. The cause is apparently a delay in maturation of the glucuronyl transferase enzyme to conjugate bilirubin, although other factors may be operative as well. Clinical jaundice is evident in about one-third of full-term infants. Serum unconjugated bilirubin is increased, but other laboratory findings are normal. Bilirubin levels rarely exceed 12 mg/100 ml in full-term infants or 15 mg/100 ml in premature infants.

Treatment consists of adequate hydration and caloric intake. Occasionally, phototherapy is required; rarely, exchange transfusions are needed. The prognosis is excellent.

Metabolic Defects in the Liver

Galactosemia and glycogen storage disease may cause jaundice in the newborn. In galactosemia, symptoms (which may include hypoglycemia) begin after milk feedings are established. Mild jaundice usually has its onset after the third day and persists into the second week of life.

Obstruction of Biliary Ducts

Bile duct obstruction is manifested principally by an elevation in the level of conjugated bilirubin, but a significant degree of unconjugated bilirubinemia secondary to liver cell injury will also be present. Jaundice may begin on the third day, as with physiologic jaundice, but will persist and become increasingly intense as the conjugated bilirubin levels rise. With persistent jaundice of this type, the skin takes on a greenish-yellow hue.

Prolonged & Persistent Jaundice in the Newborn

Most causes of jaundice in the newborn are transient. When jaundice persists into the second week of life, one of the following conditions may be considered:

(1) In small premature infants, jaundice will persist longer due to the delayed maturation of the glucuronyl transferase enzyme system.

(2) Liver disease or anomaly: If there are persistent and increasing levels of conjugated and unconjugated bilirubin, the diagnostic work-up is urgent because irreversible cirrhosis may develop in the presence of a surgically correctable lesion. Therefore, intrahepatic biliary atresia and neonatal hepatitis must be differentiated from extrahepatic atresia, choledochal cysts, or other correctable abnormality. Liver function tests, needle biopsy, and the clinical course may help, but open biopsy and operative cholangiogram are usually necessary to identify the cause of the jaundice.

(3) Choledochal cysts cause obstruction by intermittent filling of the cyst with bile, which causes tor-

sion of the duct. The jaundice is usually intermittent and variable and is often associated with a palpable mass in the upper right quadrant of the abdomen.

Freda VJ: Hemolytic disease of the newborn. Chapter 19 in: *Textbook of Obstetrics and Gynecology,* 3rd ed. Danforth DN (editor). Harper & Row, 1977.

INFECTIONS IN THE NEWBORN

GENERALIZED BACTERIAL SEPSIS

The fetus and newborn are unusually susceptible to generalized, sometimes overwhelming infection. The symptoms may be deceptively mild until the infection is far-advanced, making early recognition and treatment more difficult. Immunoglobulin G (IgG) is transferred from the mother to the fetus, providing passive protection against some organisms. Antibodies to gram-negative organisms are contained in the IgM fraction, which is not transferred to the fetus—one reason why *Escherichia coli* is the most common etiologic agent in bacterial infection in the newborn period. Other gram-negative organisms, staphylococci, streptococci, pneumococci, and other less common organisms also cause disease. Many of these bacteria produce hemolysins which increase the rate of hemolysis of red blood cells, resulting in hyperbilirubinemia. Other toxins may be produced which cause systemic and cellular injury. Bacteria that are usually considered nonpathogenic in older children may cause clinical disease in the newborn. Infection is frequently generalized, being manifest as septicemia. Blood cultures are frequently positive.

Clinical Findings

A. History: A negative maternal or neonatal history does not exclude the possibility of congenital infection. The mother may have had active infection during pregnancy which is transmitted directly to the fetus.

Amnionitis is frequently associated with neonatal sepsis. If any of the clinical signs of amnionitis are present in the mother (eg, fever, uterine tenderness), appropriate cultures should be obtained and antibiotic therapy administered. Premature rupture of the membranes is less ominous if it is unassociated with other clinical signs of infection.

B. Signs: The infant may show jaundice and lethargy; poor feeding with delayed gastric emptying, regurgitation, and the danger of aspiration; and symptoms resulting from localization of infection in a particular organ.

C. Laboratory Findings: Cultures of blood and rectal and cord base swabs should be done whenever infection is suspected and before antimicrobial therapy is started. Carefully obtained cord blood for culture can be very helpful in determining the causative organism in a baby who develops sepsis. The white blood cell and differential counts are useful in the early diagnosis of bacterial infection; elevation of the band count occurs early in the illness. Extremely low granulocyte counts, particularly in the first 24 hours of life, are an ominous sign and should always be regarded as indicating overwhelming bacterial infection until proved otherwise.

Treatment

A. General Measures: Early diagnosis, supportive care, and specific antimicrobial therapy are the ingredients of effective management of bacterial infections in the newborn period. Frequent reevaluation is essential. The following categories based on information obtained from the history, physical examination, and careful evaluation of the clinical course will help direct management in an individual case.

1. Suspected sepsis—If infection is being considered in the differential diagnosis, obtain cultures and other diagnostic studies and observe carefully. Preterm babies or infants who are ill from other causes must be treated immediately because one cannot wait for serial observations for a more definitive diagnosis and because these infants are less able to cope with the additional stress of infection.

2. Probable sepsis—If a presumptive diagnosis of infection is made—based on clinical findings or because the baby is seriously ill and infection may be present—obtain cultures and other diagnostic studies and treat with antibiotics. Observe carefully. If the diagnosis proves incorrect, antibiotics may be stopped.

3. Proved sepsis—If cultures or other diagnostic studies have demonstrated a significant pathogen or definite clinical confirmation of infection, treat with antibiotics after cultures have been obtained.

B. Antimicrobial Therapy: When a definite etiologic diagnosis has not been established, the antibiotics chosen should cover both gram-negative and gram-positive bacteria; should be bactericidal rather than bacteriostatic; and should be safe when given in proper dosage for the newborn. Ampicillin and kanamycin fit these criteria well in most cases. Gentamicin may replace kanamycin in the presence of resistant $E coli$ or pseudomonas. Other antibiotics should be given only on specific indications. Gentamicin should be used with caution in the very-low-birth-weight infant, since it may produce ototoxicity; the half-life in the very-low-birth-weight infant is unknown. Therapy usually should be continued for 2–3 days beyond the time when the infection appears to have cleared and the baby is well. Continued observation is required to make certain the infection does not recur. Negative blood cultures obtained after antibiotics are discontinued confirm the adequacy of treatment.

McCracken GH Jr: Pharmacologic basis for antimicrobial therapy in newborn infants. Clin Perinatol 2:139, 1975.

Sever JL: *Infectious Agents and Fetal Disease.* McGraw-Hill, 1970.

Symposium on intrauterine infections. Birth Defects 4:1, 1968.

SPECIFIC BACTERIAL INFECTIONS

1. EPIDEMIC DIARRHEA OF THE NEWBORN

Acute diarrhea in infants may be associated with certain types of pathogenic *Escherichia coli* and klebsiella. When it occurs in the nursery, it is potentially quite virulent and communicable. Constant surveillance, quick recognition and treatment, and active measures to avoid epidemic spread are required.

Clinical Findings

Because of the virulence of diarrhea and the rapidity of spread among infants in a nursery, emphasis must be placed on early recognition and identification of the etiologic agent. The spread to other infants is chiefly via hand contamination; therefore, hand washing and stool care are the chief measures of control of the epidemic.

A. Symptoms and Signs: Infection with pathogenic gram-negative organisms may be asymptomatic or may cause mild to very severe diarrhea. Pathogenic strains should be suspected particularly when diarrhea occurs in epidemics in infant nurseries. Examination shows dehydration and electrolyte alterations appropriate to the severity of the diarrhea. The diarrhea is often bloody. The amount of fluid lost in the stools is frequently underestimated. Careful physical examination and frequent weighing are most helpful in determining the degree of dehydration.

B. Laboratory Findings: Over the past few years it has become clear that traditional methods of serotyping or phage-typing gram-negative organisms cannot identify those strains that are virulent for the gastrointestinal tract. Thus, these methods of identification have little clinical value. Several different bioassays have been used to point out some characteristic of bacterial virulence, ie, some assays identify those strains producing heat-labile enterotoxin; others identify strains causing increased tissue invasiveness. However, none of these technics are widely available, and they must still be regarded as tools for clinical research rather than as established clinical diagnostic procedures. In the future, these technics should clarify much of the confusion about the nature of epidemic diarrhea of the newborn and necrotizing enterocolitis.

Differential Diagnosis

Other causes of diarrhea include salmonellae, shigellae, and staphylococci. Viruses probably cause diarrhea in the newborn but have been infrequently isolated. Often no etiologic agent can be demonstrated.

Treatment

Fluid and electrolyte losses must be replaced promptly by the intravenous route, followed by oral maintenance of electrolytes and calories. Treatment of shock with blood volume expanders may be needed.

Give neomycin orally and specific antibiotic therapy systemically depending upon the organisms isolated and their antibiotic sensitivities.

Prognosis

Not all patients will have organisms eliminated from the bowel, although they will become asymptomatic. These infants should be followed closely for recurrence of diarrhea.

Echeverria PD, Chang CP, Smith D: Enterotoxigenicity and invasive capacity of enteropathogenic serotypes of *Escherichia coli.* J Pediatr 89:8, 1976.
Nelson JD: Duration of neomycin therapy for enteropathogenic *Escherichia coli* diarrhea disease: A comparative study of 113 cases. Pediatrics 48:248, 1971.

2. PNEUMONIA

Pneumonia may be present at birth or may be acquired after delivery. Two organisms are associated with overwhelming pneumonia at birth or soon thereafter: group B streptococci and *Listeria monocytogenes.* Infection with group B streptococci is far more common in the USA; the latter is apparently more common in some areas of Europe. Both can cause fulminant sepsis and pneumonia leading to death in a few hours. Infants colonized with group B streptococci during passage through the birth canal should be treated with penicillin until the organisms are eradicated. In addition, several congenital viral infections may present with pneumonia at birth.

As stated earlier in the chapter, when a tentative diagnosis of "wet lung" syndrome is made, infants should be treated with antibiotics until congenital bacterial pneumonia can be excluded as a cause of symptoms.

3. MENINGITIS

Since meningitis results from blood-borne organisms, its presence should be suspected in any infant with septicemia. Whenever a diagnosis of meningitis is suspected, a lumbar puncture should be done before antibiotic therapy is started.

Irritability in an infant with symptoms of sepsis is a strong reason to suspect meningitis. Localizing physical findings may include a bulging anterior fontanel, meningeal irritation with opisthotonos, and convulsions. Serial head circumference measurements are essential. Newborn infants may respond to CNS infection with little if any localizing findings. *E coli* is a common cause.

General supportive care should include intravenous fluids to avoid vomiting and aspiration of stomach contents. Give specific therapy with antibiotics effective against both gram-positive and gram-negative organisms until the etiologic agent is identified. The drugs should be administered at the highest dosage level safe for newborn infants. Treatment is continued until lumbar punctures show completely normal spinal fluid and negative cultures.

The infant should be observed closely for evidence of recurrence of infection. If infection recurs, an anatomic abnormality of the skull, spinal cord, or vertebral column may be present which allows seeding of organisms to take place—eg, a dermal sinus, fibrin deposits in the base of the brain from the original meningitis, or subdural collections of fluid and small abscesses which have not cleared completely. Localized or generalized brain damage or evidence of developing hydrocephalus should be anticipated.

Greensher J & others: Lumbar puncture in the neonate: A simplified technique. J Pediatr 78:1034, 1971.
Overall JC: Neonatal bacterial meningitis. J Pediatr 76:499, 1970.

4. OSTEOMYELITIS

Osteomyelitis is quite rare and is almost always secondary to septicemia in the newborn infant; in rare cases it may be secondary to organisms introduced when a femoral puncture or bone marrow examination is performed. The most common organisms are staphylococci, streptococci, and *E coli.*

Physical examination will reveal localization of the infection to a bone or joint. There will be tenderness, swelling, redness of the area, and limitation of movement of the extremity involved. The diagnosis is confirmed by aspiration of joint or subperiosteal material for smear and culture. X-ray changes (which may not be present for 1–2 weeks) include periosteal elevation and calcification.

Specific antibiotic therapy should be aimed at the organism most likely to cause the disease. Treatment should be continued until the child is completely well, evidence of local inflammation has completely subsided, and x-rays show that healing is well under way. Follow-up examination and x-rays should be done to make certain that there is no recurrence.

5. PYELONEPHRITIS

Pyelonephritis in newborns is usually secondary to septicemia rather than contamination via the lower urinary tract. Abnormal fistulous connections between the bowel and the urinary tract, patent urachus, vesicovaginal fistula, or other structural anomaly of the urinary tract associated with obstruction will predispose to urinary tract infection.

Newborn infants with symptoms of infection may have a focus of infection in the urinary tract. This is especially true if the baby is suspected of having a urinary tract anomaly.

A specimen taken by means of suprapubic aspiration is desirable for examination and culture. Colony counts above 10,000 organisms/ml of urine in a clean, freshly voided specimen, or any colonies in a suprapubic tap, should be considered evidence of infection. For reasons which are not clearly understood, pyelonephritis in the newborn infant is often associated with jaundice. Other diagnostic procedures such as intravenous urography or cystography may be needed to demonstrate congenital anomalies or obstruction of the urinary tract.

Antibiotics should be continued until the urine is normal and cultures negative. Underlying urinary tract pathology may require specific treatment. A baby with documented urinary tract infection must be followed for a long time with repeated urine cultures to be sure that infection does not recur after therapy is discontinued. Underlying urinary tract anomalies and obstruction make recurrence or continued chronic infection more likely.

6. OMPHALITIS

A normal umbilical cord stump will mummify and separate at the skin level. Saprophytic organisms occasionally cause a small amount of purulent material to form at the base of the cord. Other organisms may colonize and cause infection, especially *E coli,* streptococci, and staphylococci.

Omphalitis is a potential danger when umbilical vessels are catheterized for administration of intravenous fluids or exchange transfusion. Strict aseptic technic and immediate removal of catheters at the first sign of any complication are important. The risk of omphalitis is greater with umbilical vein catheterization than with umbilical artery catheterization; however, the risk of hemorrhage is much greater with arterial catheters.

Redness and edema of the skin around the umbilicus indicate cellulitis. Serosanguineous or purulent discharge indicates progress of the infection. Systemic reaction occurs as infection becomes more severe. Culture of skin around the cord base and blood cultures should be done.

Appropriate antibiotics for gram-positive and gram-negative organisms are given until the cause is specifically identified, and they are continued until all evidence of disease has disappeared and blood cultures are negative.

Local therapeutic measures should also be used and include drying the base of the cord thoroughly with absolute ethanol swabs and swabbing the area with one of the surgical soaps containing an organic iodide.

Since staphylococcal epidemics in nurseries often begin with an outbreak of several apparently minor infections of the skin in infants, even relatively minor infections should receive aggressive treatment and should stimulate a review of hand washing technics among nursery personnel.

The extent of infection into omphalic vessels determines the prognosis. Septic thrombophlebitis can lead to hepatic abscess, generalized septicemia, and portal vein thrombosis.

7. SKIN INFECTIONS

The skin is exposed first to all of the organisms in the birth canal and then to staphylococci upon contact with nursery personnel and the family. The mere presence of staphylococci on the skin does not indicate pathogenicity, nor does it mean that clinical infection will follow. It is important to watch for evidence of skin infection in babies or their families during their nursery stay and after they have left the nursery. If clinical infection occurs, careful evaluation of nursery babies and personnel must be made to determine which strain of staphylococcus caused the infection and how prevalent it is.

Treatment of both babies and personnel may be necessary to rid a nursery of a prevailing virulent organism.

Colonization by organisms other than staphylococci—usually *E coli* or candida—may take place in a newborn infant who is debilitated, has received antibiotic therapy, or has been so well isolated that staphylococcal colonization has not taken place.

Clinical Findings

A. Symptoms and Signs: Infection is manifested by skin pustules with an erythematous base. These may rupture, releasing purulent exudate, and become encrusted. The degree of involvement of the skin may be variable, from a few lesions to extensive coalescing lesions spread over most of the body. *Cellulitis* due to streptococci (less often staphylococci) may spread rapidly. *Ritter's disease* is a grave form of cellulitis caused by staphylococci in which invasion of the skin is extremely rapid, with sloughing of the superficial layers, leaving extensive denuded, weeping areas.

Localized infections may occur around the circumcision site or umbilicus. Breast abscess may occur.

B. Laboratory Findings: Appropriate local cultures and blood cultures should be done. Specific phage typing of staphylococci may be necessary to determine the prevalence of a pathogenic strain in an epidemic.

Treatment

Systemic antibiotic therapy should always be used for infections that cause more than the most superficial lesions. When the infection is definitely localized and superficial, it may be treated by repeated cleansing with a soap containing an organic iodide preparation.

Melish ME, Glasgow LA: Staphylococcal scalded skin syndrome: The expanded clinical syndrome. J Pediatr 78:958, 1971.

8. GROUP B STREPTOCOCCUS SEPSIS

As mentioned earlier, group B streptococcus recently has been identified as a significant cause of sepsis in the newborn. It is acquired before or during delivery from the maternal birth canal. The mother is usually asymptomatic, but culture of the cervix is positive. It may cause generalized septicemia and pneumonia at birth or shortly thereafter, or may present as meningitis a few days or weeks later. Identification of group B streptococcus-positive women before delivery is important, since adequate treatment may remove the danger of infection in the infant.

Franciosi RA & others: Group B streptococcal neonatal and infant infections. J Pediatr 82:707, 1973.
Howard JB, McCracken GH: The spectrum of group B streptococcal infections in infancy. Am J Dis Child 128:815, 1974.

VIRAL INFECTIONS

Neonatal viral infections are likely to be generalized, to cause signs and symptoms of multiple organ involvement, and to have a progressive course resulting in multiple permanent sequelae or death. They are usually acquired before or during delivery. These infections must be considered in the differential diagnosis of severely ill newborns. Although they involve multiple organs, they frequently have individual characteristics which permit a diagnosis in the newborn period. Specific etiologic diagnosis will require viral cultures and serial serum antibody titers.

1. CYTOMEGALIC INCLUSION DISEASE

Congenital cytomegalovirus infection usually follows an apparently normal pregnancy and delivery, although the mother may have an infectious mononucleosis-type illness. The clinical course varies from severely affected infants with fulminating sepsis through intermediate stages with varying degrees of CNS involvement to apparently normal infants. In the severe form, the infant is acutely ill at birth with signs of multiple organ involvement. He tends to be small for gestational age and have a disproportionately small head circumference. CNS signs include symptoms of meningoencephalitis and later development of muscle weakness or spasticity. Chorioretinitis has been observed. Mental retardation accompanies the severe form.

In the intermediate form, the newborn shows few signs early. Neonatal jaundice and petechiae are common. After a month or more, feeding difficulties, irritability, muscle weakness, and spasticity may develop.

Cases of congenital cytomegalovirus infection have been documented in which no clinical evidence of disease existed and no late sequelae were reported.

IgM in cord blood is usually elevated. CSF is abnormal—with elevated protein and white cell count—and epithelial cells in the urine show inclusion bodies. Cytomegalovirus may be cultured from the urine, saliva, and CSF. Skull x-rays may show calcification. A rising or persistent cytomegalovirus antibody titer in the infant confirms the diagnosis.

Treatment is supportive, and the prognosis for full recovery in clinically evident cases is poor.

Burnbaum G & others: Cytomegalovirus infections in the newborn. J Pediatr 75:789, 1969.
Monif GRG & others: The correlation of maternal cytomegalovirus infection during varying stages in gestation with neonatal involvement. J Pediatr 80:17, 1972.

2. RUBELLA

Congenital rubella infection occurs as a result of rubella infection in the mother during pregnancy. The earlier in pregnancy the disease occurs, the more severely affected the fetus is likely to be—particularly during the first trimester. Infection may involve the placenta or fetus (or both) and may persist throughout pregnancy and for a variable period after delivery. A newborn with congenital rubella, therefore, must be considered contagious to those taking care of him—particularly any personnel who are pregnant. Evidence is inconclusive that gamma globulin administered to the mother at the time of exposure or during clinical rubella protects the fetus.

The incidence of major anomalies—some of which may not be apparent immediately at birth—has been estimated to range from 20% to 60% depending on the time of infection in utero. Therefore, it is essential that the clinical diagnosis of rubella in a pregnant woman be confirmed by culture and by hemagglutination inhibition antibody titer of paired sera drawn 10 days apart. Vaccination with attenuated live rubella virus is now possible to prevent the disease.

Rubella should be considered in a baby with thrombocytopenia with petechiae or purpura, hepatitis, microcephaly, congenital heart disease (patent ductus arteriosus is the most common lesion), low birth weight for gestational age, cataracts, hepatosplenomegaly, myocarditis, and interstitial pneumonia. X-rays show characteristic longitudinal radiolucent areas in the distal metaphyses of long bones. Cultures of the baby's nasopharynx, throat secretions, and stool are usually positive, often for several weeks after delivery. Antibody titers, liver function tests, and long bone x-rays are needed. Thrombocytopenia, sometimes only transient, is a consistent finding.

No specific treatment is available. The prognosis is variable, depending on the degree of involvement of various organs. The highest incidence of severe involvement occurs with infection soon after conception. Despite microcephaly, these children do not show evidence of mental retardation in later life.

Kibrick S, Loria RM: Rubella and cytomegalovirus: Current concepts of congenital and acquired infection. Pediatr Clin North Am 21:513, 1974.

Macfarlane DW & others: Intrauterine rubella, head size and intellect. Pediatrics 55:797, 1975.

3. HERPESVIRUS HOMINIS

Congenital or neonatal infection with herpesvirus hominis is now commonly recognized. Infant infection is usually secondary to genital infection in the mother, primarily with type 2 herpesvirus hominis. The spectrum of infection in the baby may extend from subclinical, with apparent recovery, to generalized multiple organ involvement and death. Skin vesicles are common and are sometimes present at birth. CNS, eye, and generalized visceral involvement occurs frequently. Later handicaps are common in survivors, particularly when the CNS is affected.

The diagnosis is made by virus culture from maternal and infant lesions and by demonstrating inclusion bodies and positive fluorescent antibodies in cytologic preparations of cells from the margins of skin lesions. A rising antibody titer in the baby is confirmatory.

Treatment is supportive. Idoxuridine has been given with variable results. Isolation technics should be instituted to minimize spread to personnel or other susceptible infants.

Prevention may be attempted by cesarean delivery when maternal genital lesions are present, thus avoiding fetal contact with the lesions during delivery, though this is not always effective. This should be done while membranes are intact to minimize the chance of ascending infection.

Nahmias AJ & others: Infection of the newborn with *Herpesvirus hominis*. Adv Pediatr 17:185, 1970.

4. OTHER VIRAL INFECTIONS

Echoviruses, coxsackieviruses, myxoviruses, and a variety of other viruses may cause congenital infection. They should be considered when meningoencephalitis, pneumonia, myocarditis, hepatitis, cataracts, or other unexplained disease is present.

Varicella may occur in a fetus or newborn if the mother develops the disease during her pregnancy. The baby will develop clinical disease—usually typical skin vesicles—after the usual incubation period of 2–3 weeks. The clinical course is usually modified in the infant, presumably by passive antibodies from the mother. The disease is contagious while active lesions are present.

INFECTIONS DUE TO OTHER CAUSES

1. TOXOPLASMOSIS

Toxoplasmosis is caused by the parasite *Toxoplasma gondii.* The clinical features of congenital toxoplasmosis closely resemble those of cytomegalic inclusion disease with a similar spectrum of degree of involvement. More severe clinical disease is associated with intrauterine growth retardation, microcephaly or hydrocephaly, microphthalmia, chorioretinitis, calcifications in skull x-rays, thrombocytopenia, and jaundice.

Diagnosis is confirmed by antibody titers which rise or persist in the baby. IgM in cord blood is usually elevated. The organism may be cultured, but this must be done only under special conditions because of the danger of laboratory infection.

Many infants affected at birth die during the neonatal period. Those who survive are usually handicapped, with mental retardation, convulsions, neuromuscular disease, poor vision, and microcephaly or hydrocephaly.

2. CONGENITAL SYPHILIS: See Chapter 26.

GASTROINTESTINAL DISEASES IN THE NEWBORN
(See also Chapter 16.)

TRACHEO-ESOPHAGEAL FISTULA & ESOPHAGEAL ATRESIA

Determination of abnormal anatomy is usually made on clinical grounds (Fig 3–7). X-ray demonstra-

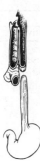
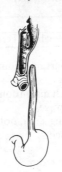

Type A
Symptoms and Signs:

Excessive mucus, aspiration
of saliva.
Scaphoid abdomen.
No gas in bowel on x-ray.
Cannot pass catheter into
stomach.
Gradually increasing respira-
tory distress.
Polyhydramnios.

Type B
Symptoms and Signs:

Polyhydramnios.
Coughing, choking, and
pneumonia from birth.
Scaphoid abdomen.
No gas in bowel on x-ray.

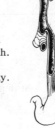

Type C
Symptoms and Signs:

Most common (80% of
cases).
Excessive mucus.
Gradually increasing respira-
tory distress.
Polyhydramnios frequent
but not severe.
Gas in bowel on x-ray.

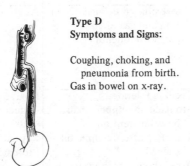
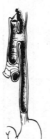

Type D
Symptoms and Signs:

Coughing, choking, and
pneumonia from birth.
Gas in bowel on x-ray.

Type E
Symptoms and Signs:

Difficult to diagnose.
Coughing or cyanosis with
feeding.
Chronic aspiration pneu-
monia.

Figure 3—7. Types of tracheo-esophageal fistula and clinical findings.

tion of the upper pouch should be done by instilling no more than 1–2 ml of contrast medium if a plain film with a radiopaque catheter in place is not adequate.

When fistula is present alone, the diagnosis may be difficult to confirm. Careful evaluation must be done in any baby who has respiratory symptoms, particularly coughing, choking, and cyanosis associated with feeding. The differential diagnosis includes pharyngeal muscle weakness, vascular rings, and esophageal diverticula.

Treatment varies depending upon the type of lesion and the degree of abnormality present. Frequent or continuous gentle suctioning of the upper pouch and pharynx will minimize tracheal aspiration of saliva. Generally, gastrostomy is performed early and the fistula ligated at that time. If the ends of the esophagus are too far apart for a direct anastomosis, the upper pouch is exteriorized. After a sufficient period of growth, during which time the infant is fed through the gastrostomy, a primary repair of the esophagus is made.

When the lungs are clear enough to permit surgery, the fistula is closed and, if the 2 ends of the esophagus are close enough, primary anastomosis may be done. However, if this cannot be done easily, closing the fistula and exteriorizing the upper pouch onto the neck is a satisfactory interim measure until final repair is done later.

Careful attention to fluid, electrolyte, and caloric requirements, as well as infection, is important during preparation for surgery and in the postoperative period. Associated congenital anomalies, particularly cardiac and other gastrointestinal abnormalities, may coexist. Evaluation for these should be made prior to surgery.

INTESTINAL OBSTRUCTION

A newborn infant with abdominal distention and vomiting must be suspected of having intestinal obstruction. Fig 3–8 lists the symptoms at various levels of obstruction.

The level of intestinal obstruction can usually be determined and the decision whether or not to undertake surgery can usually be made by careful review of the history and physical examination. A plain film of the abdomen is frequently all that is needed to confirm the clinical impression.

Additional work-up should be done only when needed to clarify the diagnosis or to aid in planning surgery. Unnecessary studies put the baby through needless procedures and delay definitive treatment. The baby may tolerate surgery better soon after birth than he will later. Needless delay must be avoided when vascular supply to the bowel may be compromised. Again, careful attention to the baby's needs in preparation for surgery and during the postoperative period is important.

Surgery may consist of definitive repair of the abnormality or may be palliative, ie, decompression of the bowel followed later by repair of the primary lesion.

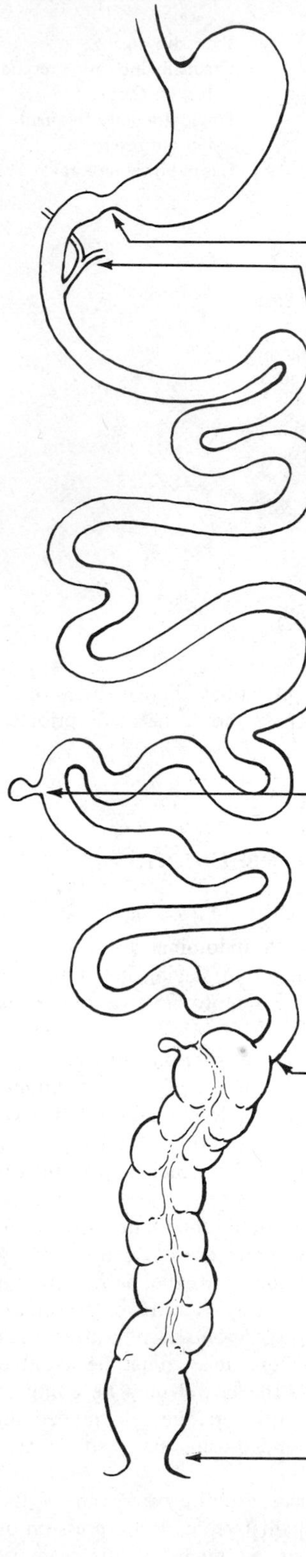

Region of Obstruction	Level	Signs and Symptoms	
		Newborn Period	**Pregnancy and Delivery**
Stomach Pylorus	A	Early part of feeding tolerated. Stomach distention with gastric waves. Vomiting soon, not bile-stained. X-ray shows gas to level of obstruction.	Polyhydramnios present. Usually over 30 ml stomach content at delivery.
Proximal duodenum Ampulla of Vater	B	Above plus additional distention and gas-filled first part of duodenum.	As above.
Distal duodenum & jejunum Meckel's diverticulum	C	Feeding tolerated. Stomach and upper small bowel distention. Vomiting after feeding, bile-stained. X-ray shows gas in upper small bowel.	Degree of polyhydramnios decreases as lesion descends gastrointestinal tract. Stomach contents at birth bile-stained.
Ileum Ileocecal valve	D	Several feedings tolerated. Gradually increasing distention. Less stomach distention. Vomiting after several feedings, bile-stained.	No polyhydramnios. No increased stomach contents at birth.
Colon	E	More feedings tolerated. More gradual, generalized abdominal distention. Vomiting later, gradually increasing in amount, bile-stained.	As above.
Rectum & anus	F	Above symptoms and signs still more delayed. Physical examination confirms diagnosis.	As above.

Figure 3–8. Sites of intestinal obstruction and clinical findings.

Lesions Causing Intestinal Obstruction (Fig 3—8)

A. Atresia and Stenosis: (Levels A, B, C, D, E.) Intestine is narrowed below the level of obstruction.

B. Meconium Ileus: (Level D.) A common presenting clinical picture of cystic fibrosis in the newborn. Small bowel obstruction with very palpable doughy loops of gut. Meconium contains protein. Sweat chloride test may be abnormal.

C. Hypertrophic Pyloric Stenosis: (Level A.) Symptoms begin after 2—3 weeks. Gradually increasing vomiting after feedings, not bile-stained, associated with gastric distention and peristaltic waves. May occur in premature infant while still in the nursery.

D. Meconium Plug: (Levels D, E.) Usually cured by diagnostic barium enema. Check bowel movement carefully during or following barium enema for evidence of typical meconium plug followed by normal meconium.

E. Malrotation With or Without Midgut Volvulus: (Levels C, D.) Urgent because of vascular insufficiency if associated with volvulus.

F. Volvulus: (Levels C, D.) Urgent because of vascular insufficiency.

G. Congenital Peritoneal Bands: (Levels C, D.) May occur alone or in association with malrotation.

H. Incarcerated Hernia, Internal or External: (Levels A, C, D.) Always check the inguinal area when bowel obstruction is present. Acquired intra-abdominal hernia follows surgery or adhesions, or may occur through the diaphragm.

I. Annular Pancreas: (Levels B, C.) X-ray may show abnormality.

J. Duplication and Enteric Cysts: (Levels A, B, C, D, E.) Anywhere along gut; may have associated anomalies (hemivertebrae, neurologic).

K. Intussusception: (Level D.) Usually lower small bowel, crampy, intermittent symptoms, blood in stool which may have a currant jelly appearance. Careful barium enema may reduce the intussusception. If not, surgery is required.

L. Peritoneal Adhesions: (Levels C, D.) Follows bowel perforation, peritonitis, or abdominal surgery.

M. Aganglionosis (Hirschsprung's Disease): (Levels D, E.) Often presents as lower bowel obstruction in newborn. Barium enema with a small amount of barium may demonstrate typical constricted lesion. Rectal biopsy is diagnostic.

N. Paralytic Ileus: (Secondary to sepsis, respiratory distress syndrome, CNS damage, etc.) Generalized distention, decreased bowel sounds, associated with other serious disease.

O. Anal and Lower Rectal Stenosis or Atresia: (Level F.) Can be recognized by careful examination of the perineum at the initial physical examination. The abnormal anatomy may consist of stenosis of the anal opening, an imperforate membrane covering the anal opening, an unformed anus and terminal rectum, or atresia of the rectum. Fistulas may exist between the terminal rectum and the perineum or vagina or urinary tract. Their presence should be carefully searched for in each case because of the complications, particularly contamination and infection of the urinary tract.

Capitanio MA, Kirkpatrick JA: Roentgenographic evaluation of intestinal obstruction in the newborn infant. Pediatr Clin North Am 17:983, 1970.

OTHER ABDOMINAL SURGICAL CONDITIONS

Appendicitis & Meckel's Diverticulum

These disorders may occur in the newborn period and always present difficult diagnostic problems. The infant will show general symptoms of illness and may have abdominal distention, decreased bowel sounds, and constipation. Fever and leukocytosis may not be present. Careful examination of the abdomen will usually show localizing findings of peritonitis. The appendix is often ruptured at the time of diagnosis. Meckel's diverticulum may present with sudden gastrointestinal bleeding.

Omphalocele

Omphalocele will be present at birth and requires early surgical consultation. Care is needed to keep the sac from rupturing before surgery.

Ruptured Abdominal Viscera

A ruptured abdominal viscus will present with peritonitis and pneumoperitoneum if the stomach or bowel is perforated. Rupture of a solid viscus presents with hemoperitoneum, anemia, and shock.

Pneumoperitoneum

Pneumoperitoneum may occur spontaneously, particularly in very immature infants. The rupture is often in the large bowel along the hepatic flexure. In contrast to the findings of necrotizing enterocolitis, the bowel is entirely normal except for the perforation. Depending on when the perforation occurs, postoperative complications may be minimal, since the bowel contents are often sterile.

Pneumoperitoneum may also result from dissection by air along the mediastinum and through the diaphragm next to the esophagus, with rupture into the peritoneal cavity. This complication develops in infants receiving positive pressure ventilation with the respirator set at relatively high pressures. With positive pressure ventilation, air may accumulate rapidly in the peritoneal cavity, and continuous drainage of air from the peritoneum may be required to allow adequate movement of the diaphragm. Although the accompanying pneumomediastinum or pneumothorax is generally obvious, it occasionally may be inapparent.

HEMATOLOGIC DISORDERS

BLEEDING DISORDERS

The most common causes of bleeding in the newborn are vascular accidents, clotting deficiencies (vitamin K-dependent factors being the most common), thrombocytopenia, and disseminated intravascular coagulation.

Hemorrhagic Disease of the Newborn (Hypoprothrombinemia)

Vitamin K-dependent clotting factors (factors II, VII, IX, X) are normal at birth but decrease within 2–3 days. In vitamin K-deficient babies, these levels may be very low, resulting in prolonged bleeding times. Bleeding may occur into the skin or gastrointestinal tract, at the site of injection or circumcision, or at internal sites. Small amounts of vitamin K are sufficient to correct the clotting factor defects unless liver function is immature in a very sick or premature infant. All newborns should receive 1 mg of vitamin K IM on admission to the nursery.

Blood in Vomitus or Stool

Swallowing maternal blood during delivery is not uncommon. If enough has been ingested, the baby may vomit bright red or dark blood or may pass stool containing dark or bright red, fresh-appearing blood. Clinical evidence of acute blood loss is lacking, but a transient rise in BUN may occur. Blood of maternal origin may be differentiated from infant blood by testing for fetal hemoglobin, which is resistant to alkali denaturation: a small amount of red bloody stool or vomitus is mixed with 5–10 ml of water and centrifuged. To 5 parts of pink supernatant, add 1 part 0.25 N sodium hydroxide. If fetal hemoglobin is present, the solution stays pink; if adult hemoglobin is present, it becomes brown.

Gastrointestinal bleeding in the newborn may be due to trauma, peptic ulcer, duplication of bowel, Meckel's diverticulum, intussusception, volvulus, hemangioma or telangiectasis of the bowel, polyp, rectal prolapse, anal fissure (a common cause of a small amount of blood in the stool in infants), infection (salmonellae, shigellae), systemic bleeding disorders (particularly hemorrhagic disease of the newborn), and tumors.

If blood is of maternal origin, no treatment is needed. If bleeding is of fetal origin, treat as for acute blood loss with blood transfusions and supportive care and then proceed with diagnosis and treatment of the underlying disease. The most common intrinsic cause of bloody vomitus is a gastric ulcer, which seldom causes massive bleeding and perforation. The bleeding generally can be managed with frequent oral milk feedings alone. If blood loss has been significant but transfusion is not necessary, iron supplementation may be required during the first few months.

ANEMIA

Acute blood loss before or during delivery can occur into the maternal circulation, the amniotic sac, into a twin fetus in the twin-twin transfusion syndrome, or into the vagina. Acute blood loss after delivery may be external (gastrointestinal, circumcision site, umbilical stump) or internal (fracture site, cephalhematoma, CNS or pulmonary hemorrhage, soft tissue hematoma, injured internal organ). Anemia may be secondary to hemolysis (isoimmunization, acquired hemolytic disease, red cell metabolic abnormalities) or to congenital aplastic or hypoplastic anemia.

The degree of bleeding, which may occur at many sites during delivery (including muscle and skin), is frequently underestimated. In general, whenever there is serious doubt about the extent of bleeding in the fetus, the infant's blood volume should be expanded with plasma expanders or whole blood.

If severe anemia is chronic or due to acute hemolysis, transfusion may have to be done with sedimented red cells, using small volume exchange transfusions to avoid overloading the vascular space.

POLYCYTHEMIA

Unusually high hematocrits are seen in newborn infants infrequently in some pediatric services and in as many as 5% of all births in others. Polycythemia results in increased blood viscosity, particularly when the hematocrit exceeds 70%. A peripheral hematocrit of 70% is an indication for performing a venous hematocrit. If the venous hematocrit is greater than 65%, hyperviscosity is invariably present. The cause of polycythemia is not always apparent. Known causes include fetofetal transfusions in twins, leaving one twin anemic and the other plethoric. It is often seen in small-for-gestational-age infants but frequently occurs in the infant of the diabetic mother as well.

Hyperviscosity decreases effective perfusion of the capillary beds of the microcirculation and increases the work load of the heart. Clinical manifestations include an enlarged heart, pulmonary perihilar infiltrates, tachypnea, oxygen dependency, priapism, and CNS signs ranging from increased jitteriness to overt seizures.

Treatment is indicated for symptomatic infants. Long-term neurologic sequelae have been reported in a high percentage of children who were symptomatic during the neonatal period.

Treatment consists of administering a small isovolumetric exchange transfusion using plasma or isotonic 5% albumin solution as the donor fluid. Phlebotomy should not be done for several reasons, partly because it reduces the hematocrit slowly and partly because reduction in circulating blood volume may cause additional undesirable problems.

Hathaway WE: Coagulation problems in the newborn. Pediatr Clin North Am 17:929, 1970.

Humbert JR & others: Polycythemia in small for gestational age infants. J Pediatr 75:812, 1969.

Kontras SB: Polycythemia and hyperviscosity syndromes in infants and children. Pediatr Clin North Am 19:919, 1972.

Wirth FH, Goldberg KE, Lubchenco LO: Neonatal hyperviscosity: Incidence and effect of partial plasma exchange transfusion. Pediatr Res 9:373, 1975.

METABOLIC DISORDERS

HYPOGLYCEMIA

The umbilical cord blood glucose concentration is slightly lower than that of the mother. During the hours after delivery, the blood glucose concentration of the infant decreases (rarely below 30–40 mg/100 ml), and by 6–12 hours of age it stabilizes between 50–80 mg/100 ml. Blood glucose levels below 30 mg/100 ml are considered abnormal.

Hypoglycemia is frequent in 2 extremes of altered intrauterine nutrition: the infant of the diabetic mother, who is well nourished, with abundant glycogen and fat stores; and the infant with intrauterine growth retardation, who is undernourished, with minimal glycogen and fat deposits. (These conditions are discussed separately below.) In addition, hypoglycemia is associated with Beckwith's syndrome, erythroblastosis fetalis, islet cell tumor, leucine sensitivity, glycogen storage disease, and galactosemia. Hypoglycemia may occur in any sick infant and is frequent after birth asphyxia.

The manifestations of hypoglycemia in the newborn may be mild and nonspecific: lethargy, poor feeding, regurgitation, apnea, and twitching. As symptoms become more severe, the baby will develop pallor, sweating, cool extremities, and prolonged apnea and convulsions.

Blood glucose concentration should be measured frequently during the first few days of life in all infants at risk of hypoglycemia, particularly small-for-gestational age infants, infants with erythroblastosis, those born of diabetic mothers, and those with asphyxia at birth.

Infants of Diabetic Mothers

Infants of diabetic mothers have special problems because they are large for gestational age. Even in pregnant women whose diabetes has been under good control, the blood glucose concentration will vary more in a 24-hour period than in normal women. In addition, other compounds in the blood, such as free fatty acids and insulin, are present in abnormal amounts. Such findings contribute to the birth of large-for-gestational age infants to mothers whose diabetes would appear to be relatively mild. Excessive size in the infant is associated with an increased incidence of birth trauma, particularly following vaginal delivery. In a vertex delivery, the injuries occur generally to the head and neck and include stretching or tearing of the cervical or brachial plexus, leading to peripheral nerve injuries (eg, Erb's palsy or phrenic nerve paralysis). The latter condition may cause tachypnea as well as a need for an increased concentration of oxygen in inspired air in the infant immediately after birth. However, this need is unassociated with hyaline membrane disease.

Infants of diabetic mothers also have problems related to the diabetes in the mother. These problems include hypocalcemia, hypoglycemia, and hypercoagulability with hyperviscosity leading to complications such as renal vein thrombosis, hyperbilirubinemia, respiratory distress, cardiomyopathy, and an increased incidence of congenital anomalies.

Two forms of respiratory distress can occur in infants of diabetic mothers: (1) Hyaline membrane disease occurs in higher frequency in these infants than in infants of comparable gestational age. (2) "Wet lung" syndrome may develop during the first few days of life in infants of diabetic mothers. This pulmonary problem may be related to cardiomyopathy, with cardiomegaly, evidence of pulmonary congestion, and abnormal ventricular septal findings appearing on echocardiography. The cardiac findings tend to resolve slowly over the first 3–5 days of life.

Infants With Intrauterine Growth Retardation

Infants with intrauterine growth retardation (small-for-gestational-age infants) can be born after normal uncomplicated pregnancies, but such infants usually are found in association with a maternal problem such as chronic vascular disease, toxemia, congenital infection, chronic ingestion of alcohol, ingestion of phenytoin, heroin, or morphine, or multiple pregnancies.

Chromosomal trisomies in the fetus may also account for small size or intrauterine growth retardation.

Regardless of the cause of intrauterine growth retardation, these infants tend to be at increased risk of fetal distress during labor and delivery and should be attended by an obstetrician, a pediatrician, and nurses specially trained in high-risk perinatal medicine. Birth asphyxia is the biggest danger facing these infants; if it can be avoided by good obstetric and neonatal care, the other problems of small-for-gestational-age infants (eg, hypoglycemia, hyperviscosity syndrome) are generally easier to manage.

If birth asphyxia occurs, other complications may follow (eg, hypocalcemia and renal injury leading to oliguria or anuria and meconium aspiration pneumonitis producing respiratory distress).

Small-for-gestational-age infants should receive 100 ml/kg/day of 10% glucose infusion to maintain blood glucose concentrations greater than 40 mg/100 ml. Dextrostix or some other means of measuring blood glucose concentrations should be used. Some infants will develop hypoglycemia in spite of this therapy, in which case the glucose concentrations or the flow rate of the infusion should be increased proportionately. In rare instances, small-for-gestational-age infants may develop marked hyperglycemia and a transient diabetes mellitus–like syndrome. Insulin therapy is rarely required and seldom need be given past the first week of life. The small-for-gestational-age infant with hypoglycemia and a very high hematocrit (capillary hematocrit greater than 75) is likely to show the most severe clinical signs of hypoglycemia, presumably reflecting a reduction in cerebral plasma flow. These infants should have a small exchange transfusion with plasma to reduce the hematocrit and to correct the hypoglycemia.

Fluge G: Neurological findings at follow-up in neonatal hypoglycemia. Acta Paediatr Scand 64:629, 1975.

Lubchenco LO, Bard H: Incidence of hypoglycemia in newborn infants classified by birth weight and gestational age. Pediatrics 47:831, 1971.

Pagliara AS & others: Hypoglycemia in infancy and childhood. (2 parts.) J Pediatr 82:365, 558, 1973.

HYPOCALCEMIA

The fetal plasma during fetal life has a higher total calcium concentration and a higher calcium activity than during neonatal or adult life. In general, hypocalcemia in the newborn infant may be defined as a plasma concentration less than about 3.5 mEq/liter (7 mg/100 ml). Within the range of 3.2–4 mEq/liter, infants vary considerably in clinical hypocalcemic signs. Infants are generally symptomatic at levels below 3.2 mEq/liter. Hypocalcemia is most likely to occur at 2 times: shortly after birth and toward the end of the second or third week of life. Hypocalcemia occurring shortly after birth has been associated with infants of diabetic mothers, sepsis of the newborn, perinatal asphyxia, and maternal hyperparathyroidism.

Clinical Findings

A. Symptoms and Signs: The infant may be twitchy, tremulous, or have frank convulsions, although many babies with low serum calcium levels are without apparent symptoms. Hypocalcemia rarely causes life-threatening symptoms in the immediate newborn period but later may cause severe tetany of the newborn.

B. "Tetany of the Newborn": This disorder occurs in the third or fourth week of life, almost exclusively in infants fed evaporated milk formulas. Cow's milk formulas contain high concentrations of phosphates, which are not cleared adequately by the kidney. This leads to elevation of serum phosphorus with a secondary lowering of the serum calcium and clinical tetany. It is not known why only a small number of babies are at risk.

Treatment

A. Oral Calcium: Oral administration of calcium lactate or gluconate is the preferred method of treatment. Calcium can either be given as a diluted solution or added to formula feedings several times a day in a dose of 0.5–1 gm/kg/day.

In "tetany of the newborn" it is advisable to lower the solute and phosphorus loads as well as to provide extra calcium. This can be done by using one of the commercially available low-solute formulas.

B. Intravenous Calcium: Intravenous administration of calcium solutions may occasionally be necessary. The infusion must be given slowly, diluted with an equal amount of glucose in water. The heart rate is monitored carefully during the infusion and immediately afterward; cardiac slowing and arrest can occur as a result of rapid administration of calcium salts. The response to intravenous calcium is usually only transient. (*Note:* Calcium salts cannot be added to intravenous solutions that contain $NaHCO_3$, since they will precipitate as calcium carbonate.)

Clark PCN: Hypocalcemic and hypomagnesemic convulsions. J Pediatr 70:806, 1970.

Shaw JCL: Evidence for defective skeletal mineralization in low-birthweight infants: Absorption of calcium and fat. Pediatrics 57:16, 1976.

Tsang RC & others: Hypocalcemia in infants of diabetic mothers. J Pediatr 80:384, 1972.

LATE METABOLIC ACIDOSIS

Late metabolic acidosis may occur in preterm infants during the first weeks of life. Early findings consist of a diminished rate of weight gain in spite of adequate intake associated with a falling serum total CO_2 content and a relatively alkaline urine for the degree of metabolic acidosis present. This disease is usually transient and responds to treatment with the addition of 3 mEq of $NaHCO_3$/kg/day to formula feedings.

Kildeberg P: Disturbances of hydrogen ion balance occurring in premature infants. 2. Late metabolic acidosis. Acta Paediatr Scand 53:517, 1964.

• • •

INFANTS OF NARCOTIC ADDICTS

Withdrawal symptoms occur in about two-thirds of infants born to mothers who are addicted to heroin, methadone, or related drugs. Symptoms consist primarily of increased tremors, irritability and hyperactivity, hypertonicity, sweating, yawning, sneezing, excessive hunger and salivation, nasal stuffiness, and regurgitation. More severely affected babies may have vomiting, diarrhea, respiratory distress, and convulsions. This clinical picture of increased activity—often frantic behavior—is typical enough to suggest the diagnosis even though a history of drug abuse had not been elicited prior to delivery. Infants may be small for gestational age. Confirmation can be obtained by doing a screening test for drug excretory products on the urine of mother or baby.

Treatment

Observe carefully for onset and progression of symptoms. Give no specific treatment until symptoms develop.

With onset of significant irritability, tremors, and hyperactivity, sedation is required. Phenobarbital, 8–12 mg/kg/day in divided doses every 4–6 hours, is recommended because of its safety and predictability of effect. The dose may need to be increased cautiously to provide adequate control of symptoms, but respiratory depression must be avoided. Phenobarbital blood levels should be obtained in infants treated near the limits of the therapeutic range, since phenobarbital plasma clearances in newborn infants vary considerably from one infant to another. Continue dose until withdrawal symptoms subside—a few days or several weeks—and then gradually decrease the dose. In addition to sedation, swaddling the baby and using a pacifier may help control the excessive activity, allowing the baby to rest between feedings.

Prognosis

The prognosis is good for the health of the baby. Careful evaluation of the family unit must be made in each case. The baby may be cared for by the mother, but continued interest and long-term support by the health team and the mother's active involvement with a drug treatment program are essential. Otherwise, arrangements for care of the infant by temporary placement must be considered.

Neumann LL, Cohen SN: The neonatal narcotic withdrawal syndrome: A therapeutic challenge. Clin Perinatol 2:99, 1975.

Rothstein P, Gould JB: Born with a habit: Infants of drug-addicted mothers. Pediatr Clin North Am 21:307, 1974.

RETROLENTAL FIBROPLASIA

Retrolental fibroplasia (RLF) may affect the eyes of some preterm infants who have received oxygen therapy. Other factors may also play a role in the pathogenesis of RLF, since it is seen occasionally in preterm babies who have been closely monitored during oxygen therapy. The retinal vessels become dilated and tortuous. As the severity increases, vessels proliferate into the vitreous, fibrosis occurs, and the retina becomes elevated. Permanent damage will vary in degree from none to complete detachment of the retina and blindness. Glaucoma may occur later in more severe cases. Early mild stages are reversible. Prevention consists of avoiding elevated oxygen tensions in arterial blood (greater than 90 mm Hg). Unlike bronchopulmonary dysplasia, retrolental fibroplasia is not produced by high oxygen concentrations in the ambient air but rather by high oxygen tensions in the arterial blood. Each newborn who has received oxygen administration should have a careful ophthalmoscopic examination before discharge from the nursery. (See also Oxygen Therapy, p 273.)

BRAIN & NEUROLOGIC DISEASE

Brain damage in newborn full-term infants is usually due to physical trauma at birth or to perinatal asphyxia; congenital anomalies and infections of the CNS are the next most common causes. Most of the brain damage due to trauma or asphyxia is preventable, primarily through improved obstetric care and, secondarily, through improved neonatal care immediately following delivery.

1. PROLONGED & SEVERE HYPOXIA

Intrauterine hypoxia causes brief tachycardia in the fetus and increased fetal movement, followed by depression and bradycardia. Meconium may be passed into the amniotic fluid and subsequently aspirated. At delivery, the infant is hypotonic, cyanotic, and pale, and makes little or no respiratory effort. The Apgar score is less than 3.

Hypoxia causes a redistribution of cardiac output, with the brain and the heart receiving increased blood flow while the lung and certain other organs have markedly decreased blood flow even with relatively moderate degrees of hypoxia. If hypoxia is severe, other organs such as the skin, muscle, and gastrointestinal tract also have reduced blood flow and become underperfused with blood of low oxygen content. This state leads to an increasingly severe metabolic acidosis. Active resuscitation is indicated, and prolonged assisted ventilation may be necessary. After a variable period, the infant may make spontaneous respiratory efforts and gradually establish spontaneous respirations. A high-pitched, irritable cry, absent or poor Moro reflex, diminished or absent deep tendon reflexes, decreased muscle tone, and retinal hemorrhages are common.

By the second day of life, reflexes become hyperactive and muscle tone increases, sometimes asymmetrically. There may be less spontaneous activity and a weak sucking reflex. Spasticity associated with mental and physical retardation, including slow head growth, may be expected. However, some babies recover without any demonstrable handicap.

2. HEMORRHAGE DUE TO TRAUMA

Trauma that may result in subarachnoid, intraventricular, or cerebral hemorrhage is usually associated with a history of difficult delivery, often precipitous or breech. The baby may appear well after birth, but within a few hours develops clinical findings of irritability, increased muscle tone, high-pitched cry, respiratory distress, decreased or absent Moro and sucking reflexes, increased or asymmetric muscle tone, twitching, retinal hemorrhages, and dilated pupils. Convulsions may occur. Anemia and shock will occur if bleeding has been of sufficient volume. If bleeding is mild and does not recur, symptoms will begin to improve. The degree of permanent neurologic damage will depend on the extent and location of the injury.

3. CONGENITAL ANOMALY

Microcephaly, hydrocephaly, hydranencephaly, and other congenital abnormalities can be identified in the newborn period.

Lesions that involve an open neural tube defect with communication between the CSF and amniotic fluid can be diagnosed prenatally by assay of the α-fetoprotein in the amniotic fluid.

4. TREATMENT OF THE BRAIN-DAMAGED NEWBORN

The infant who has sustained an injury to the CNS requires special care and observation. Specific therapeutic measures should be instituted for the treatment of hydrocephalus and subdural hematoma. Good supportive care can reduce the risk of additional injury from hemorrhage, hypoglycemia, hypocalcemia, or aspiration pneumonia. A precise prognosis is often not possible in the first days of life and should be made with caution. Periodic reassessment and reevaluation throughout infancy are often needed. This should be explained to the parents. Parents need to know *and believe* that the physician and the rest of the health care team will continue to provide support, advice, and assistance after the infant leaves the nursery. Parents should be helped to relate well to the child. If the parents feel sure of the continued interest and support of the medical staff, they will be more ready to accept a rather indefinite prognosis and more willing to wait until the extent of damage is fully known.

5. CONVULSIONS

Seizures occurring at the time of delivery or very shortly thereafter are rare and should raise the possibility of pyridoxine dependency or intoxication with local anesthetics. Some of the causes of neonatal seizures are listed below.

Etiology
A. Intracranial Disease:
1. Intraventricular, subarachnoid, or cerebral hemorrhage.
2. Hypoxia.
3. Cerebral edema (secondary to injury, hypoxia, or infection).
4. Kernicterus.
5. Cerebral venous thrombosis.
6. Arteriovenous fistula.
7. Infection (meningitis, encephalitis, abscess).
8. Brain malformation or masses.
9. Arterial emboli as complication of catheterization.

B. Generalized Disease:
1. Infection (sepsis with toxicity).
2. Metabolic—
   (1) Hypoglycemia.
   (2) Hypocalcemia.
   (3) Hypernatremia.
   (4) Maple syrup urine disease (convulsions rare before 2 weeks).
   (5) Pyridoxine dependency.
3. Toxic—
   (1) Maternal narcotic addiction.
   (2) Mepivacaine (Carbocaine) toxicity secondary to its use in paracervical anesthesia.

Treatment
Phenobarbital is an excellent anticonvulsant in the newborn, giving a good anticonvulsive effect at doses that do not cause respiratory depression. Give the first dose intramuscularly or intravenously to control convulsions. The dose is 8–10 mg/kg/day in 4 doses. Diazepam (Valium) may occasionally be required for control of status seizures but does not serve as a continuing anticonvulsant; the dose is 0.15–0.3 mg/kg, repeated if necessary in 10–20 minutes.

Holden KR, Freeman JM: Neonatal seizures and their treatment. Clin Perinatol 2:3, 1975.
Volpe J: Neonatal seizures. N Engl J Med 289:413, 1973.

6. KERNICTERUS
(Bilirubin Encephalopathy)

Kernicterus refers to the clinical syndrome and pathologic changes in the CNS secondary to deposition of unconjugated bilirubin in certain nuclei of the brain. As a rule, the risk of kernicterus becomes significant at serum bilirubin levels above 17–23 mg/100 ml. However, certain factors predispose to the development of kernicterus at lower serum levels. These factors mainly result in decreased albumin binding capacity for bilirubin (acidosis, low albumin levels, sulfonamide administration, elevated free fatty acid, etc).

The infant with kernicterus has severe hyperbilirubinemia, usually secondary to erythroblastosis but in some cases associated with jaundice due to other causes. There is a fairly sudden onset of lethargy and poor feedings; a weak or incomplete Moro reflex; a weak, high-pitched cry; and opisthotonos. In premature infants, slowed respiratory rate and apneic periods may be prominent findings. Apnea, respiratory arrest, and convulsions constitute the terminal episode. Fortunately, kernicterus has become extremely rare as technics for monitoring newborn infants have improved. Kernicterus can be prevented by close monitoring of unconjugated bilirubin concentrations and the initiation of appropriate treatment in jaundiced infants.

Towbin A: Cerebral hypoxic damage in the fetus and newborn: Basic patterns and their clinical significance. Arch Neurol 20:35, 1969.

● ● ●

General References

Andrews BF (editor): Symposium: The small-for-dates infant. Pediatr Clin North Am 17:1, 1970.

Assali NS (editor): *Pathophysiology of Gestation.* 3 vols. Academic Press, 1972.

Avery GB (editor): *Neonatology: Pathophysiology and Management of the Newborn.* Lippincott, 1975.

Cockburn F, Drillien CM (editors): *Neonatal Medicine.* Blackwell, 1974.

Korones SB: *High-Risk Newborn Infants: The Basis for Intensive Nursing Care.* Mosby, 1972.

Mustard WT & others (editors): *Pediatric Surgery,* 2nd ed. Year Book, 1969.

Schaffer AT, Avery ME: *Diseases of the Newborn,* 4th ed. Saunders, 1977.

Standards and Recommendations for Hospital Care of Newborn Infants, 5th ed. American Academy of Pediatrics, 1971.

Stave U: *Physiology of the Perinatal Period.* 2 vols. Appleton-Century-Crofts, 1970.

4...
Normal Childhood Nutrition & Its Disorders

H. Peter Chase, MD, & Donough O'Brien, MD, FRCP

In the early years of their emerging differentiation from the internists, children's physicians laid great stress on dietary manipulation as a means of treating disease and promoting optimal health and development. Advances in the understanding of fluid and electrolyte problems, the control of infectious disease, and formula reliability have tended to distract the interest of physicians from nutrition and its problems. Once again, however, the realization that undernutrition is the most important child health problem the world over; that it is far more prevalent in North America than was formerly thought to be the case; and that nutrition problems complicate many of the more serious children's diseases has done much to restore the science of infant and child nutrition to its proper place in the training and daily practice of pediatricians.

GENERAL NUTRITIONAL REQUIREMENTS & COMPOSITION OF FOODS

Requirements for various nutrients change during childhood depending on the growth rates of different tissues; they also vary considerably with sex, stage of maturation, physical activity, and body build. The nutritional needs during any growth period will depend on the nutritional status of the child at that time and on whether or not a given nutrient can be stored by the body. The recommended daily allowances (Table 4–1) may be used as guides for estimating the requirements at any age; however, differences in needs should be recognized for each child. The child's general health and conformity to established growth percentiles are the best indices of his nutritional status. A normal term infant, for example, will double his birth weight by 5 months and triple it by 12 months irrespective of birth weight percentile.

CALORIES

Total caloric requirements for children rise with age in a curve that roughly parallels the height and weight curves. Following the neonatal weight gain, caloric needs per unit of body weight begin to decline during early childhood. This pattern is similar to the decline in growth rate observed between 18 and 36 months of age. Appetite is a reliable index of caloric needs of most healthy children. During the neonatal period, growth is rapid, appetite tends to be good, and caloric intake rises smoothly. Toward the end of the first year, appetite declines with the decrease in growth rate and with increases in physical mobility, interests, and independence. The recommended caloric intakes for males and females at different ages are given in Table 4–1, but they can be approximated by adding 120 kcal/year of age to a base of 1000 kcal.

Caloric excess can be as undesirable as caloric deficiency. Important factors in considering the quantity of food an infant will voluntarily consume are the bulk of the food and the energy needs of the child. Intake also depends to some extent on the caloric concentration of the feeding. Human milk and most commercial formulas average 20 kcal/oz, but higher caloric densities of 24 or 27 kcal/oz are available for the low-birth-weight infant.

CARBOHYDRATES

The normal diet consists of approximately 46% calories as carbohydrate, 40% calories as fat, and 14% calories as protein. Carbohydrate intake may be as high as 90% of calories in the diets of people in the lower socioeconomic groups where its consumption is associated with a higher incidence of obesity. Humans have no set requirement for carbohydrate and it is not considered "essential," ie, survival is not dependent on its consumption. Carbohydrate provides about 4 kcal/gm consumed. Starch and sucrose are the major carbohydrates ingested from plant foods. The former is a polysaccharide which must be hydrolyzed to glucose prior to absorption. The greater part of ingested starch is converted to maltose by salivary amylase working in the mouth and stomach and by pancreatic amylase, which has similar activity in the intestine. The disaccharides then enter the intestinal mucosa where final hydrolysis and absorption or metabolism of the monosaccharides occurs.

Table 4–1. Recommended daily dietary allowances of the Food and Nutrition Board, National Academy of Sciences–National Research Council.[1] (Revised 1974.) *Designed for the maintenance of good nutrition of practically all healthy people in the USA.*

	Age (Years)	Energy (kcal)[2]	Protein (gm)	Fat-Soluble Vitamins				Water-Soluble Vitamins									Minerals							
				A Activity (RE)[3]	A (IU)	D Activity (IU)	E Activity[5] (IU)	C (mg)	Folacin[6] (µg)	Niacin[7] (mg)	Riboflavin (mg)	Thiamine (mg)	B6 (mg)	B12 (µg)	Biotin (mg)	Pantothenic Acid (mg)	Ca (mg)	P (mg)	I (µg)	Fe (mg)	Mg (mg)	Zn (mg)	Cu (mg)	Mn (mg)
Infants	0–0.5	kg × 117	kg × 2.2	420[4]	1400	400	4	35	50	5	0.4	0.3	0.3	0.3	0.5	3	360	240	35	10	60	3	0.6	2
	0.5–1	kg × 108	kg × 2	400	2000	400	5	35	50	8	0.6	0.5	0.4	0.3	0.5	3	540	400	45	15	70	5	0.6	2
Children	1–3	1300	23	400	2000	400	7	40	100	9	0.8	0.7	0.6	1	1.5	5	800	800	60	15	150	10	1	2.5
	4–6	1800	30	500	2500	400	9	40	200	12	1.1	0.9	0.9	1.5	3	10	800	800	80	10	200	10	1.5	3
	7–10	2400	36	700	3300	400	10	40	300	16	1.2	1.2	1.2	2	3	10	800	800	110	10	250	10	1.5	3
Males	11–14	2800	44	1000	5000	400	12	45	400	18	1.5	1.4	1.6	3	3	10	1200	1200	130	18	350	15	2	4
	15–18	3000	54	1000	5000	400	15	45	400	20	1.8	1.5	2	3	3	10	1200	1200	150	18	400	15	2	4
	19–22	3000	54	1000	5000	400	15	45	400	20	1.8	1.5	2	3	3	10	800	800	140	10	350	15	2	4
	23–50	2700	56	1000	5000		15	45	400	18	1.6	1.4	2	3	3	10	800	800	130	10	350	15	2	4
	51+	2400	56	1000	5000		15	45	400	16	1.5	1.2	2	3	3	10	800	800	110	10	350	15	2	4
Females	11–14	2400	44	800	4000	400	12	45	400	16	1.3	1.2	1.6	3	3	10	1200	1200	115	18	300	15	2	4
	15–18	2100	48	800	4000	400	12	45	400	14	1.4	1.1	2	3	3	10	1200	1200	115	18	300	15	2	4
	19–22	2100	46	800	4000	400	12	45	400	14	1.4	1.1	2	3	3	10	800	800	100	18	300	15	2	4
	23–50	2000	46	800	4000		12	45	400	13	1.2	1	2	3	3	10	800	800	100	18	300	15	2	4
	51+	1800	46	800	4000		12	45	400	12	1.1	1	2	3	3	10	800	800	80	10	300	15	2	4
Pregnant		+300	+30	1000	5000	400	15	60	800	+2	+0.3	+0.3	2.5	4	3	10	1200	1200	125	18+[8]	450	20	2	4
Lactating		+500	+20	1200	6000	400	15	80	600	+4	+0.5	+0.3	2.5	4	3	10	1200	1200	150	18	450	25	2	4

[1] The allowances are intended to provide for individual variations among most normal persons as they live in the United States under usual environmental stresses. Diets should be based on a variety of common foods in order to provide other nutrients for which human requirements have been less well defined.

[2] Kilojoules (kJ) = 4.2 × kcal.

[3] Retinol equivalents.

[4] Assumed to be all as retinol in milk during the first 6 months of life. All subsequent intakes are assumed to be one-half as retinol and one-half as β-carotene when calculated from international units. As retinol equivalents, three-fourths are as retinol and one-fourth as β-carotene.

[5] Total vitamin E activity, estimated to be 80% as α-tocopherol and 20% other tocopherols.

[6] The folacin allowances refer to dietary sources as determined by *Lactobacillus casei* assay. Pure forms of folacin may be effective in doses less than one-fourth of the recommended dietary allowance.

[7] Although allowances are expressed as niacin, it is recognized that on the average 1 mg of niacin is derived from each 60 mg of dietary tryptophan.

[8] This increased requirement cannot be met by ordinary diets; therefore, the use of supplemental iron is recommended.

The major disaccharides ingested are lactose (glucose + galactose), sucrose (glucose + fructose), and maltose (glucose + glucose). Milk contains primarily lactose, and intestinal lactase activity is indeed highest in young infants. Lactase activity falls after infancy to lower levels than sucrase or maltase activity and is most easily compromised following diarrhea, malnutrition, or other gastrointestinal insults. Restriction of lactose-containing formulas in diarrhea is thus physiologically wise. Black children and American Indian children normally have a lessening of lactase activity before adolescence and are thereafter unable to tolerate large quantities of milk products. Premature infants may also have a reduced ability to hydrolyze lactose.

Table 4—3. Limiting amino acids in major foods.

Food Protein	Limiting Amino Acid	Biologic Assessment (NPU*)
Egg	. . .	100
Whole milk	. . .	75
Wheat	Lysine	52
Rice	Lysine	67
Corn (maize)	Lysine and tryptophan	56
Beans (including soy)	Sulfur amino acids (methionine and cystine)	47
Sorghum	Lysine	56

*NPU = Net protein utilization.

PROTEIN

In contrast to carbohydrate, protein is essential for growth and life. There are 8 "essential" amino acids for man: leucine, isoleucine, valine, lysine, methionine, phenylalanine, tryptophan, and threonine. Histidine and perhaps taurine are also essential in infants. If one essential amino acid is missing, body protein catabolism will temporarily supply the missing amino acid for necessary protein formation and serum levels will rise coincidentally. Within 1—2 weeks, however, weight loss and protein malnutrition will follow. Protein malnutrition may also occur with seemingly adequate protein intake if caloric intake is low. The body's need for calories and energy takes precedence over protein needs, and the protein will be used for energy requirements. Protein provides about 4 kcal/gm consumed.

Requirements of the essential amino acids are shown in Table 4—2. It should be noted that lysine needs are relatively high and that it is this amino acid whose content is critically low in cereal protein. Egg white is considered to have the best balance of essential amino acids, and meat, milk, and fish follow with about 20% less effectiveness. Human requirements for protein are highest in infancy (Table 4—1) and de-

crease gradually thereafter. Increased protein needs exist during pregnancy and lactation and in periods of rapid growth and tissue repair. The recent Ten-State Nutrition Survey showed 13% of pregnant women to have low serum protein levels. Amino acid deficiencies of major food sources are shown in Table 4—3. A major currently developing area of food technology involves supplementation of these vegetable proteins with other proteins such as fish meal to provide complete proteins.

Proteins are hydrolyzed as a result of pepsin activity in the stomach, pancreatic trypsin digestion in the intestine, and peptidase digestion by the pancreatic and intestinal peptidases. The resultant amino acids may be further catabolized in the intestine or may be absorbed into the portal blood system. It is thought by some that the passage of large proteins through the intestinal mucosa results in allergies to those proteins. Protein malabsorption and leakage may occur in diseases such as intestinal lymphangiectasia.

Graham GG & others: Dietary protein quality in infants and children. Am J Clin Nutr 25:875, 1972.

FATS

It has been debated whether fats are essential to the human, but it is now believed that linoleic acid must be provided in the diet of small infants to ensure adequate growth and prevent a desquamating dermatitis. Fats provide about 9 kcal/gm of food consumed and represent both the most compact and most important energy stores because they are not solubilized in water. The type of fat and protein consumed in the USA has received much criticism in recent years. Even lean meat has approximately 40% fat between the muscle fibers, and animal protein carries primarily saturated fats. In the USA, 80% of protein consumed is animal protein, whereas preindustrialized societies usually obtain 80% of their protein from vegetable sources. Vegetable fats—except coconut oil—are pri-

Table 4—2. The essential amino acid requirements of infants and adults (mg/kg/day). (See also Table 35—12.)

	Infants	Adult men
Histidine	34	. . .
Isoleucine	110	10.4
Leucine	150	9.9
Lysine	135	8.8
Methionine (in presence of cystine)	45	3.9
Phenylalanine (in presence of tyrosine)	90	4.3
Threonine	87	6.5
Tryptophan	20	2.9
Valine	105	8.8

marily polyunsaturated. Increased consumption of polyunsaturated fats—in combination with reducing cholesterol intake—has been shown to reduce blood cholesterol levels, which may diminish the chances of coronary heart disease.

Triglycerides are emulsified by bile salts in the presence of mono- and diglycerides. Forty percent are then completely hydrolyzed by pancreatic and intestinal lipase; 40% are hydrolyzed to mono- and diglycerides; and 20% are unhydrolyzed. Long chain fatty acids ($> C_{16}$) are absorbed in the free state or as monoglycerides into the mucosal cell, where they are resynthesized into triglyceride before passing into the lymph. Medium chain ($C_{10}-C_{16}$) and short chain ($< C_{10}$) fatty acids may be absorbed into mucosal cells in any form as mono-, di-, or triglycerides or in the free state. Resynthesized in the mucosal cell into triglyceride, they pass into the portal blood. Short chain fatty acids also enter the portal blood and are attached to albumin.

Medium chain triglyceride (MCT) preparations have an obvious role in patients who for a variety of reasons cannot absorb long chain triglycerides.

Special restriction of dietary lipid in infancy is not indicated except in the obese.

VITAMINS

Vitamins are organic compounds which the body cannot make in adequate quantity for optimal health and which must be provided from external sources. The vitamins are divided into the fat-soluble vitamins—A, D, E, and K—and the water-soluble vitamins—vitamin C and the B complex. The fat-soluble vitamins are stored in the liver, and excess quantities can lead to toxicity. The water-soluble vitamins are not stored in the body in large amounts, and excess quantities—such as with vitamin C "megadosage" in cold prevention—just result in excessive excretion. Sources and recommended dietary allowances of the various vitamins are outlined in Tables 4–4 and 4–1, respectively.

Table 4–4 indicates which common foods are highest in selected nutrients and also provides a reference for quick calculation of the major nutrients of a day's diet. When these nutrients are adequate in the diet, other nutrients such as thiamine, riboflavin, and niacin are also present in adequate amounts.

Fomon SJ: *Infant nutrition,* 2nd ed. Saunders, 1974.
Williams SR: *Nutrition and Diet Therapy,* 2nd ed. Mosby, 1973.

INFANT FEEDING
Lula O. Lubchenco, MD

BREAST FEEDING

Advantages & Disadvantages of Breast Feeding

A. Advantages: Breast feeding has been encouraged mainly for its psychologic advantages, economy, and asepsis. For normal infants, the composition of human milk appears ideal and has the following advantages over cow's milk or formula: (1) The anti-infectious qualities of IgA and lysozyme in colostrum and of lactoferrin and transferrin in milk. This may also afford protection against necrotizing enterocolitis. (2) A lower osmotic load, especially in regard to sodium, potassium, and phosphorus. (3) A more efficient nutritional balance between iron, vitamin E, and unsaturated fatty acids. (4) A lower protein content with a higher whey:casein ratio. The importance of the higher taurine content is not yet accepted. (5) A possible long-term advantage in cardiovascular disease because the higher cholesterol content (compared to formula) may induce the production of enzymes required for cholesterol catabolism. (6) A higher vitamin C content. Nursing is of benefit to the mother in the postpartum period because it is associated with vigorous contraction of the uterine musculature and speeds the return of that organ to normal size and position.

B. Disadvantages and Contraindications: The only absolute contraindication to breast feeding is active tuberculosis in the mother. Breast feeding is not advisable if the mother has strong negative feelings about it.

There are temporary problems associated with nursing a weak, ill, or premature infant or one with cleft palate or lip. The mother may need to pump the milk from her breasts until the infant is able to nurse. Nursing mothers may experience discomfort from engorgement of the breasts and sore or cracked nipples in the first few days after delivery. There is an increased frequency of breast abscess in nursing mothers. It is not advisable to discontinue nursing if a breast abscess develops.

Management of Breast Feeding

When a mother wishes to nurse her infant, success or failure is related to the amount of factual information given to her and the emotional support of physicians, nurses, and family.

It is important for her to know that very few women are unable to nurse their babies. She should know that breast milk may look "weak or dilute," but if the infant is not satisfied the problem is one of supply and not quality. It is essential that she understand that milk production can be increased by frequent nursing and that the supply of milk lags behind the infant's demand for approximately 24 hours. She should know that if she substitutes supplementary feedings for nursing—especially in the first weeks after

Table 4—4. Vitamin, protein, and mineral content of foodstuffs.

VITAMIN A

10,000 IU vitamin A in:
  1 oz liver
  ½ cup dark greens
  ½ cup carrots, cooked

3000 IU vitamin A in:
  ½ cup broccoli
  ½ cup cantaloupe
  ½ cup sweet potatoes (1 medium)

1000 IU vitamin A in:
  1 medium tomato
  ½ cup canned tomato
  1 medium apricot
  ½ cup peaches (1 medium)
  ½ cup pumpkin
  ½ cup yellow squash
  ½ cup leaf lettuce

500 IU vitamin A in:
  1 large dark green lettuce leaf
  ½ cup head lettuce
  ½ cup light green vegetable (string beans, peas, lima beans)
  8 oz milk
  1 egg
  1 tbsp butter or margarine
  2 tbsp cream
  1½ oz cheddar cheese

IRON

3 mg iron in:
  3 tbsp cooked enriched or quick-cooking Cream of Wheat
  ½ cup cooked dried beans
  ½ cup dark greens
  1 oz liver
  1 tbsp dry baby cereal

1 mg iron in:
  1 oz meat, fish, fowl
  1 egg
  ½ cup cooked cereal
  1 tbsp molasses
  2 dried prunes
  1 cup broccoli
  9 brussels sprouts

0.5 mg iron in:
  2 dried apricot halves
  1 slice whole grain or enriched bread
  1 medium potato
  1 tbsp dried raisins
  1 serving other fruit or vegetable

CALCIUM

0.3 gm calcium in:
  8 oz milk
  4 oz evaporated milk
  1½ oz American cheese (1¾ inch cube)
  1 cup dark greens (except spinach, chard, beet greens*)
  1½ cup ice cream
0.3 gm calcium in remainder of diet

ASCORBIC ACID

50 mg vitamin C in:
  1 medium orange
  ½ cup orange juice
  ½ cup grapefruit or juice
  ½ cup any other citrus
  1 cup raw cabbage
  1 large raw tomato
  1 cup lightly cooked cabbage, cauliflower, broccoli, spinach, or other greens
  1 cup cantaloupe (½ melon)
  10 large raw strawberries
  1/3 medium raw pepper

20 mg vitamin C in:
  1 medium potato, baked, boiled, fried from raw
  ½ cup canned tomato or juice
  1 small sweet potato, baked

10 mg vitamin C in:
  1 cup other raw fruit or vegetable

5 mg vitamin C in:
  ½ cup other cooked fruit or vegetable
  2 tbsp ketchup
  20 pieces potato chips (1½ oz)

PROTEIN

7 gm protein in:
  1 egg
  1 oz meat, fish, or fowl
  1 oz cheese (1½ inch cube American, 2 tbsp cottage cheese)
  8 oz milk
  ½ cup cooked dried beans
  2 tbsp peanut butter

3 gm protein in:
  ½ cup cooked cereal
  1 cup dry cereal (1 large shredded wheat biscuit)
  2/3 cup ice cream
  ½ cup milk pudding
  1 slice bacon

2 gm protein in:
  1 slice bread
  1 serving cake, pie, or cookies
  4 soda crackers
  ½ cup gelatin dessert
  1 medium potato

1 gm protein in:
  1 serving fruit or vegetable

FOLIC ACID

0.4 mg in:
  1 cup soy flour
  4 oz beef liver

0.1 mg in:
  3½ oz asparagus

0.05 mg in:
  1 cup wheat flour
  1 cup beans (navy, lima, kidney)
  3½ oz broccoli
  3½ oz brussels sprouts
  3½ oz greens (spinach, beet, turnip)

*Calcium not well utilized in these because of oxalic acid.

birth—the supply of milk will decrease. Many working mothers find it possible to nurse their infants once milk production is well established.

Technic of Nursing

A. Breast Preparation Before Delivery: It is thought by some that nipple soreness can be minimized by preparation of the breasts prior to delivery. The method recommended is as follows: Cup one breast from below with the palm of the hand and, with a soft washcloth, rub the nipple 4 or 5 times. Then gently pull the nipple several times. This can be done once or twice daily.

B. Preparation for Nursing: A daily bath is all that is necessary for cleanliness of the breasts. When nursing, the mother should assume a comfortable position either lying down or sitting in a rocking or upright chair.

C. Nursing the Infant: The baby should be fed when he shows signs of hunger and should be offered both breasts at each feeding for maximum milk production. The infant usually nurses for about 10 minutes on the first side, completely emptying this breast, and then finishes the feeding on the opposite breast.

The rooting reflex is stimulated by touching the baby's cheek with the nipple (not pushing the mouth toward the breast). It is important to help the infant grasp the whole areola and to have the nipple well back in the baby's mouth.

The breast may need to be held away from the infant's nostrils once he begins sucking.

After a minute or two of nursing, the letdown reflex occurs and the baby may have difficulty swallowing the rapidly flowing milk. The letdown affects both breasts simultaneously.

When the infant has finished nursing, he usually releases the nipple. If not, suction should be broken by gently opening the baby's mouth before removing the breast. Burping the infant following feeding is usually done, but breast-fed infants do not swallow as much air as bottle-fed infants.

Colostrum

Colostrum is a yellow, alkaline breast secretion which may be present in the last few months of pregnancy and for the first 2—4 days after delivery. It has a higher specific gravity (1.040—1.060), a higher protein, vitamin A, and mineral content, and a lower carbohydrate and fat content than breast milk.

Transmission of Drugs & Toxins in Breast Milk

A. Drugs Secreted in Small Amounts: Alcohol, nicotine, caffeine, opiates, meperidine (pethidine), quinine, hyoscine, atropine, sulfonamides, penicillin, and laxatives (other than cascara) may be taken in moderation by the nursing mother. Small but not harmful amounts may be transmitted to breast milk. If the mother takes increased amounts of vitamin C, it will be transmitted to her milk. Traces of pesticides have been found in human milk but are not yet known to be harmful to the infant.

B. Drugs Secreted in Large Amounts: Barbiturates, salicylates, iodides, thiouracil derivatives, bromides, ergot, and cascara are transmitted in significant quantities. If the mother's intake is excessive, toxicity may be produced in the child.

C. Drugs That Interfere With Milk Production: Hormones used in birth control pills interfere with optimum milk production and occasionally cause breast engorgement in the infant. Nursing itself inhibits ovulation, but if pregnancy must be avoided other forms of contraception are recommended.

Weaning

The time at which the infant is ready for weaning varies from 6 months to 18 months or longer. The mother should be helped to recognize the signs of readiness for weaning and instructed to decrease the number of feedings as indicated. Most infants will take a cup at this time.

INFANT FORMULAS

A variety of satisfactory prepared formulas, modified from cow's milk, are available commercially (Table 4—5). Formulas may also be prepared from evaporated milk by the addition of water and carbohydrate. A mixture of 13 oz evaporated milk, 19 oz water, and 1½ oz carbohydrate (Karo Syrup) is satisfactory for most infants until they are ready to take whole milk.

Protein

Human milk consists of approximately 1.2% protein, whereas cow's milk contains 3.5% protein. Most commercial formulas are 1.5—1.7% protein. The quantity of protein a small premature infant should receive is still a matter of debate, although recent studies indicate that weight gains are probably similar in infants receiving 2.25—5 gm/kg/day. It has been suggested that growth in length and body maturation may be enhanced by a higher protein intake, whereas edema and low serum protein levels are more common with lower serum protein intake. In the future, the increasing cost of milk protein will probably lead to the introduction of milk substitute formulas based on soy and other vegetable proteins. These will have to contain a minimum of 1.8 gm/100 kcal of a protein nutritionally equivalent to casein.

Fats

Both human milk and cow's milk contain approximately 3.5% fat, and fats account for about 50% of the calories in either human or cow's milk. Thus, fat malabsorption should be considered in infants who fail to thrive. Human milk has more fat (10%) as the essential fatty acid linoleic acid than does cow's milk (2%). Human milk has a higher percentage of polyunsaturated fatty acids (41%) than cow's milk (23%). For-

Table 4–5. Normal and special infant formulas.*

	Manufacturer	CHO Source	Fat Source	Indications for Use	Comments (Nutritional Adequacy)
Milk and milk-based formulas					
Cow's milk Evaporated milk	Several brands	Lactose, sucrose	Butterfat	Feeding of full-term and premature infants with no special nutritional requirements.	Supplemented with iron and vitamins C and D if not fortified.
Commercial infant formulas					
SMA	Wyeth	Lactose	Oleo, coconut; safflower, and soy	Feeding of full-term and premature infants with no special nutritional requirements.	Supplemented with iron, 12 mg/liter.
Enfamil Ready to use Concentrated liquid Powder	Mead Johnson	Lactose	Coconut, soy	Feeding of full-term and premature infants with no special nutrition requirements.	Available fortified with 12 mg iron/liter.
Similac Ready to feed Concentrated liquid Powder	Ross	Lactose	Coconut, corn, soy	Feeding of full-term and premature infants with no special nutritional requirements.	Available fortified with 12 mg iron/liter.
Products for milk protein-sensitive infants ("milk allergy")					
Neo-Mull-Soy liquid	Syntex	Sucrose	Soy		Soy protein isolate.
Prosobee	Mead Johnson	Corn sugar,† sucrose	Soy		Soy protein isolate. Zero band antigen.
Isomil	Ross	Corn sugar,† sucrose, corn starch	Corn, coconut, soy		Soy protein isolate.
Meat base	Gerber	Modified tapioca starch	Sesame		
Elemental diets for tube feeding and products for oral supplements					
Vivonex	Eaton	Glucose, glucose oligosaccharides	Safflower oil	Used as a general dietary supplement or as a sole nutritional source in malabsorption.	Pure amino acid base. Also high in nitrogen.
Flexical	Mead Johnson	Sucrose, dextrin	20% medium chain triglycerides, 80% soy	Fat malabsorption.	
Ensure	Ross	Sucrose, corn syrup solids	Corn oil	Lactose intolerance.	Soy protein plus calcium and sodium caseinate.
Hycal	Beecham	Glucose			A flavored product for calorie supplementation only.
Polycose	Ross	Glucose polymers			A powdered or liquid calorie supplement.
Low-sodium formulas					
Lonalac powder	Mead Johnson	Lactose	Coconut	Management of children with congestive cardiac failure.	For long-term management, additional sodium must be given. Supplement with vitamins C and D and iron. Na = 1 mEq/liter.
Partially demineralized whey formulas					
Similac PM 60/40 Powder	Ross	Lactose	Coconut, corn	Use where a low-salt diet is indicated.	Relatively low solute load. Na = 7 mEq/liter.

*Committee on Nutrition, American Academy of Pediatrics: Commentary on breast feeding and infant formulas including proposed standards for formulas. Pediatrics 57:278, 1976. Committee on Nutrition, American Academy of Pediatrics: Nutritional needs of low birth weight infants. Pediatrics 60:519, 1977.

†Composed of glucose, maltose, and dextrins.

Table 4—5 (cont'd). Normal and special infant formulas.*

	Manufacturer	CHO Source	Fat Source	Indications for Use	Comments (Nutritional Adequacy)
Products for infants with malabsorption syndromes					
Vivonex	Eaton	Glucose, glucose oligosaccharides	Safflower oil	Elemental diet in chronic secretory diarrheas.	Pure amino acid base.
Portagen	Mead Johnson	Sucrose, maltodextrins	Medium chain triglycerides (coconut source) and corn oil.	Management of chyluria, intestinal lymphangiectasia, various forms of steatorrhea, biliary atresia.	Fat in medium chain triglycerides and corn oil.
Alacta (Available internationally but not in USA)	Mead Johnson	Lactose	Butterfat	Infants with poor fat tolerance or poor fat absorption.	Supplement with vitamins A, D, and C and iron. To increase calories, supplement with carbohydrates. Renal solute load is high if powder only is used to increase calories to 67 kcal/100 ml.
Nutramigen	Mead Johnson	Sucrose, tapioca	Corn	Feeding of infants and children intolerant to food proteins. Use in galactosemic patients.	Enzymatic hydrolysate of casein.
Pregestimil	Mead Johnson	Glucose, tapioca	Medium chain triglycerides (coconut and corn source)	Malabsorption syndromes, especially after diarrhea and in malnutrition.	Contains added iron and vitamins. Protein is enzymatically hydrolyzed milk protein.
Cho-Free	Syntex	None	Soybean oil	Infants intolerant to carbohydrate.	Carbohydrate-free soy oil and protein. Add carbohydrates to increase calories.
For infants with phenylketonuria					
Lofenalac	Mead Johnson	Corn sugar,† sucrose	Corn	Infants and children with phenylketonuria.	
Albumaid XP 3229	Milner Mead Johnson	Corn sugar,† sucrose, modified tapioca starch	Corn	Older children with phenylketonuria.	Very low phenylalanine content permits increased supplementation with normal foods.

†Composed of glucose, maltose, and dextrins.

Table 4—6. Composition and schedule of milk feedings for infants up to 1 year of age.*

Age (months)	0	1	2	3	4	5	6	7	8	9	10	11	12
Calories (kcal) per day†	130–100/kg (60–45/lb)						110–100/kg (50–45/lb)				100–90/kg (45–40/lb)		
Fluid per day (ml)	130–200/kg (2–3 oz/lb)				130–165/kg (2–2½ oz/lb)					130/kg (2 oz/lb)			
Number of feedings per day ‡	6 or 7		4 or 5				3 or 4				3		
Ounces per feeding	2½–4	3½–5	4–6	5–7	6–8	7–9							
Milk													
Evaporated	65 ml/kg (1 oz/lb) up to a total of 13 oz (1 can) daily												
Whole	130 ml/kg (2 oz/lb) up to a total of 28–32 oz daily												
Sugar per day	1–1½ oz					§	None						

*Modified and reproduced, with permission, from Silver HK, Kempe CH, Bruyn H: *Handbook of Pediatrics,* 12th ed. Lange, 1977.
†The larger amount should be used for the younger infant.
‡Will vary somewhat with individual babies.
§Decrease sugar by ½ oz every 2 weeks.

Table 4—7. Composition of milk and milk formulas.*

Percentage of Calories From	Human Milk	Cow's Milk	Diluted Cow's Milk + 10% CHO	Evap Milk 13 oz Water 19 oz CHO 1½ oz
Protein	8%	20%	10%	15%
Fat	50%	50%	25%	39%
CHO	42%	30%	65%	46%

*From: Nutritional needs for low birth weight infants. AAP. Nutrition Committee Memorandum.

mulas based on vegetable oils are also high in unsaturates.

There is no indication for routinely using low-fat milks at this time, and their use should be restricted to problems of obesity and known type II hypercholesterolemia. Premature infants have physiologic fat malabsorption, the cause of which is unknown. An initial study has suggested that medium chain triglycerides may be more effectively absorbed, but further research in this area is needed.

Carbohydrates

Table 4—7 shows that a higher percentage of calories are derived from carbohydrate when breast milk is consumed compared to cow's milk. Human milk contains about 7% carbohydrate compared to 4.5% for cow's milk. Lactose (galactose-glucose) is the major sugar in both. Small prematures may not have fully developed intestinal lactase activity and may develop osmotic diarrhea with a secondary low stool pH, dehydration, and acidosis. A mild form of incomplete lactose malabsorption can apparently also exist in prematures without these symptoms. Full-term infants have full intestinal activities of lactase, sucrase, and maltase. It is not yet known if small premature infants might gain weight better with carbohydrates other than lactose, although this would seem possible.

Ash

The ash content of milk refers to the minerals and includes primarily sodium, potassium, chlorine, calcium, and phosphate (Table 4—8). The ash content of cow's milk is approximately 3 times that of human milk. The high phosphate content of cow's milk is thought to be a cause of neonatal hypocalcemia. The osmolality of breast milk is about 116 mOsm/liter and that of cow's milk 307 mOsm/liter.

Table 4—8. Electrolyte content of infant foods (mEq/liter).

Food	Na$^+$	K$^+$	Ca^{++}	PO$_4^{\equiv}$	Cl$^-$
Human milk	7	14	17	9	12
Cow's milk	25	36	61	53	34
A typical commercial modified formula	17	23	42	37	19

Supplements

Nearly all milk products are fortified with vitamins A and D; therefore, only vitamin C is deficient and should be provided as a supplement (50 mg/day). The American Academy of Pediatrics has also recommended the general adoption of iron-fortified formulas. Underweight or overweight infants generally have the same food requirements as do infants of the same age with a normal weight. Undiluted whole milk or formulas providing equal parts of evaporated milk and water should not be used for infants under 1 month of age since these do not provide enough free water in the event of high environmental or body temperature. When given later, provide supplemental water.

Preparation of the Formula

Many companies which supply baby foods prepare instruction booklets for the mother which give the steps in preparation of the formula. The exact ingredients should be determined by the physician. The emphasis presently is on demand feeding, but the physician should make certain that the formulas are diluted correctly and that caloric needs are being met. An infant generally does not need more than 1 quart of whole milk or 1 large can of evaporated milk per day. One pint of whole milk per day is adequate for the older child who is eating a reasonable diet.

Sterilization of bottles and formulas is not usually necessary. In most city homes, the opened can is stored in the refrigerator and each bottle is diluted as required, using warm tap water. Bottles and nipples are washed in soap and water, rinsed, and dried. Where the water supply may not be clean, boiled water should be used. In situations where cleanliness is more difficult to maintain, powdered milks should be used and dissolved in boiled water.

Feeding the Baby

The bottle should be held, not propped, for 2 reasons: (1) There is a higher incidence of acute and recurrent otitis media in infants who suck bottles in the horizontal position. The short, wide eustachian tube of infants is at such an angle that mucus from rhinitis or nose allergy fills or obstructs the ducts to the middle ear very readily. Also, the eustachian tube orifice is opened during swallowing. (2) The emotional and physical satisfactions gained from being held are well known.

The nipple holes should be wide enough so that a drop of milk forms on the end of the nipple and drops off with little shaking of the cool bottle when turned upside down.

More water may be added to the formula if the infant consistently finishes each bottle, but be certain caloric intake is adequate.

The infant need not take all of every bottle.

The baby should be burped during and at the end of feeding.

Special Dietary Products

In recent years a variety of dietary products have

become available that have special therapeutic roles. These may be divided broadly into 3 categories:

A. Complete Formulas (Elemental Diets): These low-residue liquid products are complete foods which need no supplementation. They are variable mixtures of simple hexoses, hydrolysates or amino acid mixes, and oils with or without medium chain triglycerides. They are low in residue and require a minimum of pancreatic enzymes for absorption and are thus suitable for treating malnutrition, inflammatory bowel disease, and short bowel syndromes. The high osmolality may be a disadvantage.

B. Special Dietary Products to Be Used Only Under Medical Supervision: The dietary management of inborn errors of metabolism is dependent on a variety of products in which one or more components, usually an amino acid, is restricted or deleted. In that they are deficient in one or more essential nutrients and may well need further supplementation—eg, with minerals and vitamins—they must be prescribed only under the strictest nutritional supervision and with appropriate laboratory monitoring.

C. Modular Diets: The provision of individual components of complete nutrition is increasingly possible. Examples include medium chain triglyceride preparations such as Portagen for use in steatorrheas, amino acid mixtures such as Amin-Aid, a nitrogen supplement, for children on chronic dialysis with growth problems, and Polycose, a glucose polymer used for increasing calorie intake. Used under proper supervision, these items are useful in nutrition therapy, although their use in children is often restricted by their unattractive organoleptic properties.

Committee on Nutrition, American Academy of Pediatrics: Commentary on breast-feeding and infant formulas, including proposed standards for formulas. Pediatrics 57:278, 1976.

Committee on Nutrition, American Academy of Pediatrics: Nutritional needs of low-birth-weight infants. Pediatrics 60:519, 1977.

Committee on Nutrition, American Academy of Pediatrics: Special diets for infants with inborn errors of metabolism. Pediatrics 57:783, 1976.

Sherman JO, Hamly CA, Khachadurian AK: Use of an oral elemental diet in infants with severe intractable diarrhea. J Pediatr 86:518, 1974.

ASSESSMENT OF NUTRITIONAL STATUS

Conformity to established height and weight percentiles and a simple history of an adequate and well balanced intake are usually sufficient to determine that the child's nutritional status is normal. A clinical diagnosis of specific or generalized malnutrition should be supported by the dietary history and, when possible, by laboratory examinations. Normal and deficient biochemical levels are given in Table 4–9. Laboratory appraisals are of significant value in the detection of specific nutritional defects. In children whose nutritional needs are distorted by inborn errors, by illness, or by deprivation, appraisal by a nutritionist or dietitian may be needed.

Dietary information may be collected by using a food record, 24-hour recall, or dietary history.

Food Record

The 4- to 7-day food record is a helpful aid for teaching adequate nutrition, and conscientious mothers are good reporters. However, if the mother has many responsibilities, valid information is hard to obtain from a food record. In addition, the mother may be ashamed of or may feel threatened by revealing the child's normal eating habits and may "exaggerate" the record or temporarily offer more or better foods if the facts are being recorded. In older children and adolescents who tend to be overweight, recording is a useful exercise which may discourage overeating.

24-Hour Recall

The 24-hour recall is a verbal report of all foods eaten by the patient during the preceding 24 hours. The amounts of foods consumed on a typical day must be reported, including a detailed description (how cooked, what added, etc) and the times of the day. A typical day should be described. This information is then used as representative of normal intake during a given period.

Dietary History

The dietary history includes the questions "how often" and "how much" about all foods, including beverages, snacks, etc. The following questions are typically asked in taking a preliminary history. The answers may suggest the need for more detailed and complete data which can easily be acquired by a dietitian or nutritionist.

A. Formulas: What formula is the child now taking? Frequency of feeding? Amount per feeding? How is the formula mixed and put in the bottle?

B. Table Foods: What is the meal pattern? (Times and kinds of foods eaten throughout the day.) Are there particular likes and dislikes? Does he feed himself or show interest in the food? At what ages did he start cereal? fruit? vegetables? meat? Has the introduction of solid food been a problem?

OTHER FACTORS AFFECTING DIETARY INTAKE

A child's nutritional status or dietary intake cannot be examined or altered without looking at his family. The kind of food served in a family is affected

Table 4—9. Laboratory data in the interpretation of nutritional status in infants and young children.*

Hematologic Data

Hemoglobin, hematocrit	A concentration of hemoglobin of < 10 gm/100 ml in the ages 1—3 and < 11 gm/100 ml in ages 3—6 is presumptive evidence of iron deficiency anemia. Hematocrit at all ages should be > 33% in children living at or near sea level.
Serum transferrin saturation	< 7% indicates iron deficiency alone. < 16% indicates iron deficiency in the presence of additional evidence such as anemia and microcytosis.
MCHC	Should exceed 30% at all ages.
MCV	< 70 fl at age 0.5—2 years, < 73 fl at age 2—4 years, or < 75 at age 4—8 years indicates iron deficiency.
Serum ferritin	< 10 ng/ml indicates iron deficiency.
FEP (free erythrocyte protoporphyrin)	> 3 µg/gm hemoglobin indicates iron deficiency.

Biochemical Data

Estimation	Deficient or Low	Minimum Normal†	Estimation	Deficient or Low	Minimum Normal†
Serum alkaline phosphatase in IU/liter as an index of vitamin D deficiency	> 150	60—150	Urinary riboflavin, µg/gm creatinine		
Serum folacin, ng/ml	< 3.0	6.0	1—3 years	< 150	500
Serum protein, gm/100 ml			4—6 years	< 100	300
0—12 months	< 3.0	5.0	7—9 years	< 85	270
1—5 years	< 5.5	5.5	10—15 years	< 70	200
6—17 years	< 6.0	6.0	Urinary iodine, µg/gm creatinine	< 50	70
Serum albumin, gm/100 ml					
0—5 years	< 3.0	3.0	Blood urea nitrogen, mg/100 ml	< 9	10
6—17 years	< 3.5	3.5	Serum amylase, Close-Street units	< 6	6
Serum vitamin C, mg/100 ml					
0—12 months	< 0.15	0.3	Serum zinc		77 µg/100 ml by atomic absorption
1 year	< 0.15	0.2			
Plasma carotene, µg/100 ml					
0—5 months	< 10	10	Serum vitamin B₁₂		300 pg/ml
6—11 months	< 30	30	Serum vitamin E		0.5 mg/100 ml
1—17 years	< 40	40	Linoleic acid	< 5 ml/100 ml. Presence of 20:3ω9 on chromatogram. > 0.1 total fatty acids.	10 ml/100 ml
Plasma vitamin A, µg/100 ml					
0—5 months	< 10	20			
6 months—17 years	< 20	30			
Urinary thiamine, µg/gm creatinine					
1—3 years	< 125	176	Arachidonic acid	< 5 mg/100 ml	10 mg/100 ml
4—15 years	< 125	121			

*Zerfas AJ, Neumann CG: Office assessment of nutritional status. Pediatr Clin North Am 24:253, 1977.
†See also Chapter 38.

by cultural influences, food economics, and food preferences. From the first day of human life, ingestion of food is culturally structured. Foods eaten by individuals are seldom chosen for their nutritional value. Diet modifications must occur within the cultural framework of the family, and one must consider the psychologic need the particular food may be satisfying. Available money and the amount budgeted for food influence the purchasing power of a family. The food allotment is frequently sacrificed when a financial crisis occurs. Fluctuations in price and demands for increased quantities are more acutely felt in poorer families. Food assistance programs are available from the United States Department of Agriculture to families with limited incomes. Finally, a child's choice of foods is determined by his family experience, but new food habits may be acquired through association with peers and various educational programs.

COMMON PROBLEMS IN NUTRITION

Infancy

Power struggles are frequently set up around eating because it is one of the few areas in which a child can attempt control of parents. The 2 major reasons for such problems are lack of consistency and lack of patience on the part of the parents.

Likes and dislikes of tastes as well as food consistency are already present in the 1-year-old. Thus, although encouragement should be given to try new foods, they should not be forced on a child. As a child gets old enough to reason, games can be made of trying new foods, such as having 3 steps with a new food: "touch your tongue," "nibble a bit," and "eat it all."

Not infrequently, parents will expect a young child to reason like an adult, and this leads to problems. Quite often, if a child will try a new food, even though he thinks he won't like it, he may discover he does. Even so, the least success will be obtained with the domineering approach—"You must eat all of this." Fortunately, most children have a few favorite vegetables, fruits, and meats, and these can be offered until new tastes develop. If a mother is concerned that her child is not eating enough vegetables, fruits, etc, the physician can suggest polyvitamins as a temporary measure and encourage the mother to continue to patiently offer new foods but not to worry in the meantime.

Although it is important for the parent not to be overpowering, it is also important to be consistent. If a rule is made that dessert or snacks are not allowed unless a child tries the carrots or other food, it should be adhered to. If the child learns that he can get more food later whether or not he eats his dinner, he is on his way to winning his battle.

Children who lead active lives fortunately have feelings of hunger just as adults do. Thus, if nutritious foods are available, the child will choose some of these to eat. Parents have a major responsibility of having nutritious foods available and keeping "empty calorie" foods such as candy, soft drinks, and pastries at a minimum. If snacks are to be allowed, they should be foods with some nutritional value and not just calories. Fruits or vegetables can make good snack foods. A plate of fresh carrot sticks, cantaloupe on toothpicks, or sliced apples offered to a group of children will often encourage a child to try the new food even though he thought he didn't like it.

In Adolescence

Adolescent nutritional problems have received increased attention in recent years. Perhaps the greatest cause of nutritional deficiencies in adolescents is their fast-moving and demanding society. A teenager with a recent history of a 20 lb weight loss gave a history of rising at 6:15 a.m. to get to school by 7 a.m. His parents did not get up until after he had left for school, and he usually ate little or no breakfast. He finished school at 2 p.m. and stopped at home to grab a snack (both parents worked, and this stop was inconsistent and unsupervised) before going to work from 3 to 8 p.m. After work, he usually went to join friends. He was not eating one balanced meal in the day, and rapidly began to regain weight after changing his life schedule and eating patterns. It is presently estimated that over half of American teenagers eat little or no breakfast and have a generally inadequate diet. Studies have shown that children concentrate and learn better in school if they have had an adequate breakfast.

School breakfast and lunch programs are now providing an increasingly important portion of children's nutritional needs. This is particularly true among lower socioeconomic populations.

The national nutrition survey recently found that the sex and age group with the highest incidence of low hemoglobins and hematocrits was—suprisingly—adolescent boys. The reasons for this are uncertain but probably include inadequate nutrition as well as increased demands resulting from the large increase in muscle mass during adolescence.

Obesity is an important type of adolescent malnutrition. The major cause is excessive caloric intake for the daily work load, although hypoinsulinism or other metabolic problems accentuate the obesity or play an etiologic role in some cases. Fat cells are increasing in number throughout childhood, and it has been suggested that childhood obesity is associated with an increased number of adipocytes which remain into adulthood. This type of obesity is in contrast to adult onset obesity, which is associated with an increase in size of fat cells.

Adolescent overeating is frequently found in association with parental overeating, and nutritional and psychologic rehabilitation should involve the entire family. Complete starvation may result in acute weight loss, but this is usually regained later. The most hopeful approach involves group therapy combined with diet and exercise programs. Groups have the ability to make individuals aware of reality, improve self-esteem, and to raise the motivational level, all of which are important in treating obesity.

A problem of increasing frequency is inadequate nutrition during teenage pregnancies. Inadequate maternal weight gain is now recognized to be an important factor associated with the birth of small for gestational age infants and an increased neonatal mortality rate. The greatest hazard is with maternal weight gain under 10 lb; the recommended weight increase is now 20–30 lb. Prenatal vitamins, iron, and a well-balanced diet, with an adequate protein content, should be encouraged for a pregnant or lactating teenager.

Hirsh J, Knittle JL: Cellularity of obese and non-obese human adipose tissue. Fed Proc 29:1516, 1970.

Fad Dieting for Quick Weight Loss

Starvation studies show that weight lost is water and muscle, with little fat. Adherence to most fad diets for the length of time necessary for appreciable loss is impossible. Give valid nutrition information and explain that weight gain was slow and that weight loss may be slow. There is no magic method.

Diets for Athletes

The most effective diet for vigorous physical activity is a conventional balance of fat, protein, and carbohydrate with breakfast providing one-fourth to one-third of the day's needs. Coaches have stressed high-protein diets in the past, but research indicates that protein is not the fuel for working muscles. During mild exercise, fat is the prime fuel. As physical activity increases, carbohydrate becomes more important. Under extreme muscular effort, all muscle energy comes from carbohydrate.

Maximum dietary preparation several days prior to an athletic event is a normal balance of protein and fat with a high-carbohydrate intake. The high-carbohydrate intake improves the capacity for prolonged exercise when given in addition to the balanced diet. Food eaten immediately prior to the event must be readily digested. Fat takes longer to digest and should be kept to a minimum. Liquid meals of approximately 1000 calories providing 75% carbohydrate and 25% protein are preferable because they are more readily digested and will not induce vomiting, as a heavy protein and fat meal could.

Water should not be restricted during exercise, and players should be allowed to drink glucose in water or 0.2% sodium chloride solution throughout a game. Maintaining water balance is important for the athlete. One of the principal manifestations of dehydration is fatigue. This is true in cold weather as well as hot weather. The use of special commercial drinks for athletes has its basis in this fact.

Smith NJ: *Food for Sport.* Bull Publishing Co., 1976.

Vegetarian Diets

Many peoples of the world subsist on a diet considered by the more affluent to be a vegetarian diet. However, young people may try various types of vegetarian diets by choice. These diets may be categorized as *pure vegetarian* or *vegan diets,* which are not supplemented with any animal foods, dairy products, or eggs; *lactovegetarian diets,* which are supplemented with milk and cheese; or *lacto-ovo-vegetarian diets,* which are supplemented with milk, cheese, and eggs. The latter 2 diets can be quite adequate. The former, lacking complete proteins, may eventually prevent adequate nutrition, as may any extremely narrow choice of foods.

Young health food "addicts" are usually interested in nutrition but need enough basic knowledge to plan diets with their health foods and maintain a balance. Health food stores, though expensive, are a source of various vitamins and foods which are acceptable to these young people. They must be warned, however, that the fat-soluble vitamins can be taken in toxic amounts since they are stored in the body. Table 4–1 can be used as a guideline for dosage limitations of these nutrients.

So-called health foods are often stocked in chain groceries at cheaper prices than at the health food store. Since most food faddists cannot be persuaded to change their diet completely, it is well to know that most vegetarians who take a variety of fruits, vegetables, unrefined cereals, legumes, seeds, nuts, and dairy products have adequate intakes. It is the narrow diet which is restricted to a few foods and is high in carbohydrates that tends to be inadequate.

Committee on Nutrition, American Academy of Pediatrics: Nutritional aspects of vegetarianism, health foods, and fad diets. Pediatrics 59:460, 1977.

Megavitamin Therapy

The use of NAD, riboflavin, ascorbic acid, pyridoxine, calcium pantothenate, vitamin B_{12}, folic acid, and trace minerals in doses considerably in excess of the RDA has been advocated for childhood autism and learning disabilities.

While there are a number of rare dependency syndromes for which large doses of specific vitamins are indicated (eg, vitamin D in certain types of rickets; vitamin B_6 in some cases of homocystinuria), megavitamin therapy for learning disabilities is not justified on the basis of existing documented clinical results.

Committee on Nutrition, American Academy of Pediatrics: Megavitamin therapy for childhood psychoses and learning disabilities. Pediatrics 58:922, 1976.

Diseases & Nutrition

Most cases of severe malnutrition in the USA are secondary to the onset of other chronic diseases. Such diseases commonly include congenital bowel malformations or obstructions in infancy, malabsorption diseases such as cystic fibrosis, congenital heart disease, liver disease, ileitis or colitis, and many others. Intravenous hyperalimentation is being used with increased frequency in the treatment of neonatal bowel abnormalities and is discussed in Chapter 35. Elemental diets (Pregestimil, Vivonex), usually consisting basically of mixtures of amino acids, glucose, and medium chain triglycerides for optimal absorption and utilization, can be helpful nutritional supplements for many patients. Nutritionists working in hospitals should advise on nutrition in patients with chronic diseases.

DISORDERS OF NUTRITION

DISEASES OF GENERALIZED UNDERNUTRITION

Undernutrition has long been recognized as the single most important problem in child health the world over. It was considered to be rare in the USA, although recent investigations have shown that this is regrettably far from true. Occult undernutrition is not uncommon among the poor and usually takes the form of iron deficiency anemia. Vitamin A deficiency may be seen in special groups such as children of migrant farm workers; and vitamin C deficiency is common in children of American Indians. Severe malnutrition usually is a complex result of want and ignorance, with some element of the battered child syndrome. There is increasing evidence that intrauterine malnutrition in the last trimester or nutritional deprivation in the first year of life results in irrevocable impairment of normal intellectual development. The morbidity for infections and diarrheal diseases as well as overall mortality is increased in undernourished children.

Chase HP: The effects of intrauterine and postnatal undernutrition on brain development. Ann NY Acad Sci 205:231, 1973.

National Nutrition Survey: *Nutrition and Human Needs.* Part 3. US Government Printing Office, Washington, DC, 1969.

Sandstead HH & others: Nutritional deficiencies in disadvantaged preschool children. Am J Dis Child 121:455, 1971.

INFANTILE CALORIC UNDERNUTRITION
(Marasmus)

Marasmus is a syndrome of generalized undernutrition in infancy secondary to inadequate caloric intake. The term should be applied to children weighing less than 60% of the expected mean weight for age (Table 2–4) who have no edema. The causes are many and include underfeeding of breast milk, which in turn may be due to severe undernutrition in the mother or to various social, emotional, or economic causes. Improper preparation of formulas in areas where prolonged breast feeding is not practiced is also an important cause. Again, the basic operative factors may be ignorance or poverty. Other precipitating causes are prematurity with difficulty in feeding, infections, obstructive diseases of the oropharynx and upper gastrointestinal tract, disease of the mouth, malabsorption syndromes, inborn errors of metabolism, any serious organic disease, and maternal anxiety and insecurity. In the USA over half of the children hospitalized for "failure to thrive" in infancy are the victims of inadequate feeding.

Clinical Findings

A. Symptoms and Signs: The clinical picture depends to some extent on the causes as well as the severity and duration of undernutrition. Loss of subcutaneous fat (which can be quantitated with calipers) is striking and may be confused with dehydration, particularly if diarrhea complicates the history. Muscle wasting, particularly over the buttocks and in the extremities, is usually quite evident. The infant loses interest and acquires a pinched appearance, with sunken eyes. The abdomen may be somewhat distended, usually because of an enlarged liver which contains increased fat stores. Characteristically, there is no detectable edema, hair changes, or dermatosis.

B. Laboratory Findings: The diagnosis is a clinical one, and a 10- to 15-day in-hospital trial of adequate nutrition may be imperative in a young infant. The total serum protein and albumin should be checked as these may be low, even though the child is not edematous. The serum BUN level ($<$ 9 mg/100 ml) and amylase activity ($<$ 5 units/100 ml) are often low and will rise with rehabilitation. The hemoglobin ($<$ 10 gm/100 ml) may be low as a result of associated poor iron intake. It is important to follow the stool pH since disaccharidase deficiency is present in over half of cases and will lead to further problems. (Table 4–9.)

Treatment

Treatment consists of providing for adequate nutrition and treating the primary cause if there is one. Initial therapy should be aimed at intravenous restoration of adequate blood volume if the child is dehydrated. The milk formula should be diluted to give a lower osmotic load and should be lactose-free, since many of these children develop diarrhea when given a large lactose load. Disaccharide intolerance may last for several months after rehabilitation, although it usually disappears in the first month. Vitamins should be given during recovery because of the body's increased needs during rapid growth. It is frequently necessary to gradually increase the caloric intake to 150–200 calories/kg/24 hours before weight gain finally starts. If possible, the child should not be exposed to other children with infections during early rehabilitation because of the increased morbidity and mortality that results. Family counseling and close follow-up are very important.

Prognosis

Severely affected infants have a poor prognosis and frequently acquire secondary infections and adapt slowly to nutritional therapy. The ultimate height, weight, and head circumference are related to the timing, severity, and duration of the malnutrition. Low head circumference relates to poor brain growth and is important in estimating adult intellectual capacity.

Chase HP, Martin HP: Undernutrition and child development. N Engl J Med 292:933, 1970.

Rutishauser IHE, McCance RA: Caloric requirements for growth after severe undernutrition. Arch Dis Child 43:252, 1968.

Scrimshaw NS: Synergism of malnutrition and infection. JAMA 212:1685, 1970.

PROTEIN MALNUTRITION
(Kwashiorkor)

Kwashiorkor is a multiple deficiency disease due mainly to inadequate protein intake in the presence of an adequate or even high carbohydrate intake. The diagnosis specifically denotes children who are 60–80% of the expected mean weight for age and who also have edema. The frequent occurrence of caloric undernutrition with protein deficiency has resulted in the term "marasmic kwashiorkor," which applies to children who are less than the 60% of the expected mean weight for age and who have edema. As with infantile malnutrition, there may be a variety of underlying causes other than simple nonavailability of adequate protein. Moreover, in the early years of life, a balanced but calorie-deficient diet is less of a threat to life than an unbalanced but calorically sufficient diet.

A great variety of metabolic aberrations occur in kwashiorkor. There is fatty infiltration of the liver; glucose is not readily mobilizable by epinephrine; and hypoglycemia is common. The ratio of essential to nonessential amino acids in the plasma is decreased, and generalized aminoaciduria is frequently present. It has been shown that total body water is not increased but that there is a definite shift of intracellular water toward the extracellular space. Muscle biopsies consistently demonstrate increased Na^+ and decreased K^+ and Mg^{++} content. A malabsorption pattern is often seen, with morphologic small bowel changes and disaccharidase deficiency.

Kwashiorkor usually occurs in children 1−5 years of age. This coincides with weaning from breast milk, which provides sufficient proteins and calories. It can occur in the USA as a result of poverty or neglect as well as protein restriction imposed as part of the treatment for food allergies, but almost all cases occur in the underdeveloped tropical world where the staples are incomplete protein foods (rice, maize, cassaba, etc).

Clinical Findings

The principal manifestations of kwashiorkor are growth failure; edema, which is usually peripheral but which may involve the rest of the body; wasted muscles and persistence of subcutaneous fat; lethargy, lack of interest in the environment, and poor appetite; and sparse, silky hair, unusually light in color. Other common symptoms and signs include anemia, loose, foamy stools, hepatomegaly, and skin manifestations. The dermatologic expression of the disease includes dark-colored patches on a background of relatively normal skin and striae over areas of stretched skin. The patches are most often seen on the backs of the thighs, on the buttocks, and in moist skin areas, leaving areas of depigmentation when they peel off. Small skin ulcers are often present, especially over pressure points.

Prevention & Treatment

Kwashiorkor can be prevented by making sure that adequate proteins like whole dried fish meal, protein concentrates from soy, cottonseed, and peanut flours, lysine-fortified flour, and dried milk are available to deprived populations. Population control and improved agriculture are even more important.

Therapy consists initially of treating severe electrolyte imbalance and anemia. Blood and plasma in small amounts so as not to precipitate congestive heart failure are often beneficial. Antibiotics should be used as indicated for infections. Hypoglycemia may be severe and, when it occurs in association with hypothermia and coma, is a poor prognostic sign. The cause of the encephalopathy that occasionally is seen is not known, but it is apparently more frequent with too rapid rehabilitation.

Liquids are usually necessary for initial oral feedings, and, because of the multiple intestinal and pancreatic enzyme deficiencies, should consist of as simple a formula as possible. A lactose-free formula should always be used, and, when available, hydrolyzed proteins are probably better than whole protein. A protein of high biologic value (with high content of all essential amino acids) such as casein is essential. The protein should be reintroduced gradually, or the patient's condition may actually worsen. Formulas containing medium chain triglycerides (MCT) may reduce the steatorrhea, as lipases are not necessary for MCT absorption. Vitamin supplementation is also important.

Prognosis

The overall mortality in good hospitals is between 15 and 30%, and is even higher in severe cases. Hypothermia and encephalopathy are signs of a poor outcome. Congestive heart failure due to cardiac myopathy and rapid shifts of water and electrolytes during initial therapy may be fatal. Hypoglycemia is also considered by some to be a frequent cause of death.

The eventual height, weight, and intellectual attainment depend, as with marasmus, on the timing, severity, and duration of undernutrition. The brain is not apparently as severely affected by undernutrition after the first year of life as during the first year, when it is growing very rapidly.

Balmer S, Howells G, Wharton B: The acute encephalopathy of kwashiorkor. Dev Med Child Neurol 10:766, 1968.

Brinkman GG & others: Body weight composition in kwashiorkor. Pediatrics 36:94, 1965.

Gomez F & others: Malnutrition in infancy and childhood, with special reference to kwashiorkor. Adv Pediatr 7:131, 1955.

Kumar V & others: Alterations in blood biochemical tests in progressive protein malnutrition. Pediatrics 49:736, 1972.

Wharton B: Hypoglycemia in children with kwashiorkor. Lancet 1:171, 1970.

FAILURE TO THRIVE

The term "failure to thrive" is commonly applied to infants who, for a variety of reasons, show a striking lag in somatic growth. By far the most common cause is nutritional deprivation, and a meticulous nutritional history will elicit this. Nutritional problems in turn may reflect ignorance, poverty, or emotional conflicts over the child.

Organic causes for failure to thrive must also be considered. The list given in Table 24−1 for short stature can be used as a diagnostic guide.

VITAMIN DEFICIENCIES, DEPENDENCIES, & INTOXICATIONS

Vitamins are necessary organic substances which cannot be made in sufficient quantities by the body.

Vitamins A, D, E, and K make up the fat-soluble vitamins, and, with vitamin C, are the most frequent causes of vitamin deficiency in the USA. The fat-soluble vitamins are stored in the body tissues, in contrast to the water-soluble vitamins which are minimally stored and which are readily excreted in the urine. Toxicity from fat-soluble vitamins is more common than with water-soluble vitamins, and food supplementation has in consequence been more restricted. Deficiency states for fat-soluble vitamins are thus also more common. In addition, in any medical condition associated with fat malabsorption (undernutrition, celiac disease, sprue, cystic fibrosis), the fat-soluble vitamins are poorly absorbed.

1. FAT-SOLUBLE VITAMINS

VITAMIN A

Vitamin A is a fat-soluble alcohol derived in the animal body from certain of the carotenoid plant pigments, of which β-carotene is the most important. β-Carotene has a unique and specialized role in the photochemical basis of vision. The photosensitive pigment rhodopsin is formed from vitamin A and a protein called opsin. The general effect of vitamin A on cellular function is to reduce the stability of lysosomes; it has some influence also on sulfur metabolism by activating sulfate in mucopolysaccharide formation, and on steroid hormone production. It is considered important in the maintenance of epithelial membranes in the body.

Vitamin A is present in food primarily as the palmitate ester and is hydrolyzed to its free alcohol, retinol, in the intestine. Within intestinal cells, retinol is reesterified, primarily to palmitate, incorporated into the chylomicrons of the mucosa, and absorbed into the lymphatic system.

1. VITAMIN A DEFICIENCY

Clinical Findings

A. Symptoms and Signs: Night blindness and loss of visual acuity in poor light are early eye symptoms, followed by squamous metaplasia that produces dryness of the conjunctivas, xerophthalmia, and, very often, typical small gray-white patches called Bitot spots on the bulbar conjunctivas. As metaplasia progresses, the cornea becomes cloudy and soft (keratomalacia) and, eventually, secondarily infected and ulcerated, at which point corneal damage and loss of vision are irreversible except for the possibility of

corneal transplant. Hypertrophy or atrophy of tongue papillae occurs early in vitamin A deficiency. Follicular hyperkeratosis on the buttocks and extensor surfaces of the extremities is common, as are skin and upper respiratory tract infections also.

Vitamin A deficiency (serum level < 20 μg/100 ml) has been shown to be present in 2% of preschool children in the USA. In high-risk populations such as Mexican-Americans, one-third of preschool children have been shown to have levels under 20 μg/100 ml and over half have levels under 30 μg/100 ml. Vitamin A deficiency is common in children with kwashiorkor. Vitamin A levels are lower in sera of children born of mothers who have not received prenatal vitamin supplementation.

B. Laboratory Findings: The normal plasma vitamin A level in childhood has been suggested to be > 20 μg/100 ml or more prior to age 6 months and > 30 μg/100 ml or more thereafter. The mean value in preschool children in the USA has been determined to be 33 ± 7.6 μg/100 ml.

Serum carotene determination is a helpful test in cases of nutritional vitamin A deficiency or fat malabsorption. The normal levels are approximately 70 μg/100 ml at birth, rising to approximately 340 μg/100 ml at age 1. The levels fall to about 150 μg/100 ml at age 3½; thereafter, they are between 100 and 150 μg/100 ml. Since β-carotene is carried attached to β-lipoproteins, conditions in which β-lipoproteins are elevated, such as hypothyroidism, will be associated with high circulating levels of β-carotene.

Prevention & Treatment

The minimum requirement of vitamin A varies with age but is in the range of 2500 IU (750 μg)/day in the child under age 4 years and 5000 IU/day from age 4 on. Vitamin A has approximately equal concentrations in breast and cow's milk (53 and 34 μg/100 ml, respectively). Supplementation is of particular importance in premature infants with small intakes and poor hepatic stores. Table 4–10 lists the vitamin A content of some common foods. The recommended daily dose of vitamin A in cases of vitamin A deficiency is 25,000 IU for 1–2 weeks in conjunction with a high-protein diet. Prophylactic doses are then continued. It is usually necessary to replenish liver stores of vitamin A before the serum levels increase, which may take several weeks. It is also possible to treat deficiency with single massive doses. In cases of malabsorption, a water-miscible vitamin A preparation is given in twice

Table 4–10. Vitamin A content of some common foods.

Liver (2 oz fried)	37,000 IU
Carrots (1 large or 2 small)	11,000 IU
Sweet potato (1 small)	8,100 IU
Spinach (½ cup cooked)	7,300 IU
Cantaloupe (½ cup)	4,100 IU
Milk (1 cup, whole fresh)	340 IU

the recommended amount (5000–10,000 IU) as a minimum requirement.

Prognosis

When xerophthalmia is part of a malabsorption syndrome and treatment is early, effective, and sustained, the progress is good. If vitamin A deficiency is associated with general malnutrition, scarring and secondary infection of the cornea have occurred and subsequent blindness is common.

Chase HP: Nutritional status of preschool Mexican-American migrant farm children. Am J Dis Child 122:316, 1971.

McLaren DS & others: Xerophthalmia in Jordan. Am J Clin Nutr 17:117, 1965.

Olson JA: Metabolism and function of vitamin A. Fed Proc 28:1670, 1969.

Sandstead HH & others: Nutritional deficiencies in disadvantaged preschool children. Am J Dis Child 121:455, 1971.

Strikantia SG, Reddy V: Effect of a single massive dose of vitamin A on serum and liver levels of the vitamin. Am J Clin Nutr 23:114, 1970.

2. VITAMIN A TOXICITY

The requirement of a doctor's prescription in order to obtain high-potency vitamin A preparations in recent years has diminished but not abolished the incidence of toxicity. Patients may show peeling of the skin, particularly over the fingers and hands. Long bone pain is marked over the distal extremities, and the child may refuse to walk. Loss of appetite, hypertrophy and hyperemia of gums, skin pigmentation, and alopecia are also found. Signs and symptoms of pseudotumor cerebri occur and can last for several months after vitamin A is discontinued. Radiologically, there is evidence of subperiosteal new bone formation.

The only treatment is discontinuation of excessive doses of vitamin A. Clinical improvement begins within a few days, but a return of the bones to normal may not occur for several months.

Committees on Drugs and on Nutrition, American Academy of Pediatrics: The use and abuse of vitamin A. Pediatrics 48:655, 1971.

Lascari AD, Bell WE: Pseudotumor cerebri due to hypervitaminosis A: Toxic consequences of self medication for acne in an adolescent girl. Clin Pediatr 9:627, 1970.

VITAMIN D

Vitamin D is absorbed by the intestine in solution in triglyceride particles. It is then carried on an a_2 globulin to the liver, where it is converted to the more active forms 25-hydroxycholecalciferol (25-HCC) and 25-hydroxyergocalciferol. These forms are essential to

Table 4–11. A classification of rickets.

Essential calcium deficiency
Responsive to normal doses of vitamin D_3 or 25-HCC
Dietary vitamin D or calcium deficiency
Responsive to high doses of vitamin D_3, 25-HCC, or $1a$-HCC
Fat malabsorption syndrome
Chronic renal disease
Vitamin D dependency
Magnesium-dependent rickets
Essential phosphorus deficiency
The renal tubular dystrophies
X-linked dominant vitamin D resistance
Phosphate depletion from overuse of aluminum hydroxide gels
Essential matrix abnormalities
Metaphyseal dysostosis
Hypophosphatasia and pseudohypophosphatasia

normal bone physiology and to the maintenance of adequate concentrations of calcium and phosphorus within the extracellular fluid. They also appear to enhance the enzymatic processes necessary for the calcification of the bone matrix. In the presence of parathormone, vitamin D promotes the reabsorption of phosphate by kidney tubules and may increase the tubular reabsorption of amino acids. Sunlight promotes the endogenous synthesis of vitamin D.

The kidney is now known to form 1:25 dihydroxy HCC, a derivative of 25-HCC which is specifically active in promoting the synthesis of the calcium transport protein in the intestinal villus.

Rickets is a disorder of the deposition of hydroxyapatite in bone matrix and in preosseous cartilage at the zone of provisional calcification. By definition, it is conditional on active growth. Although first recognized in relation to vitamin D deficiency, rickets can also result from disorders of phosphate transport and of the bone matrix itself. The classification shown in Table 4–11 is appropriate in the light of present knowledge. Premature infants fed commercial formulas containing 400 IU vitamin D per liter may require additional vitamin D to prevent rickets.

De Luca M: Role of kidney tissue in metabolism of vitamin D. N Engl J Med 284:554, 1971.

Stamp TCB: Intestinal absorption of 25-hydroxycholecalciferol. Lancet 2:121, 1974.

Stamp TCB: Vitamin D metabolism: Recent advances. Arch Dis Child 48:2, 1973.

1. RICKETS DUE TO VITAMIN D DEFICIENCY AND VITAMIN D RESISTANCE

Essentials of Diagnosis

- History of insufficient dietary intake of vitamin D or of malabsorption.
- Listlessness, hypotonicity, and retarded motor development.

- Bony deformities clinically and on x-ray.
- Normal serum calcium, low serum phosphorus, elevated serum alkaline phosphatase.

General Considerations

Vitamin D deficiency rickets continues to be a significant problem in those parts of North America where there is little direct sunlight and where the milk supply is not fortified with vitamin D. Minor degrees of clinical rickets are common in underprivileged groups such as migrant farm workers, especially those with darkly pigmented skins, in bedridden children in institutions, and in areas where cow's milk is unfortified. Calcium deficiency rickets may be seen in families on vegan diets. Nowadays, however, the X-linked dominant form of vitamin D resistant rickets is the commonest type seen clinically.

Clinical Findings

A. Symptoms and Signs: Leg bowing in toddlers; beading of the ribs; widening of the wrists, knees, and ankles; frontal bossing, craniotabes, the development of Harrison's sulcus in the chest wall, and, very rarely, pathologic fractures. There also may be lethargy, hypotonicity, muscle pain, hyperextensibility of joints, and motor retardation followed, as the severity increases, by convulsions and tetany. A history of poor vitamin D intake or of exclusion from sunlight is usual.

B. Laboratory Findings: These include variable hypocalcemia and hypophosphatemia. Alkaline phosphatase levels are usually elevated except in generally malnourished children. Generalized aminoaciduria and some impairment of tubular hydrion excretion may also be present, as may minimal glycosuria.

C. X-Ray Findings: Cupping, fraying, and flaring are seen at the ends of the bones. Bony trabeculae lose their sharp definition, which accounts for the general decrease in skeletal radiodensity.

Differential Diagnosis

It should be possible on the basis of the history to differentiate rickets due to dietary deficiency of calcium or vitamin D or due to steatorrhea or chronic renal disease from that due to X-linked dominant phosphaturia. Other forms of phosphaturia (see p 519) must of course be excluded, and the most common of these is cystinosis. A routine look for aminoaciduria and for cystine crystals in the lens or the bone marrow is wise. A serum magnesium level will exclude magnesium-dependent rickets. In hypophosphatasia and pseudohypophosphatasia, the bone changes are similar to those observed in rickets, serum calcium levels may be elevated, there is vitamin D resistance and phosphoethanolaminuria, and serum alkaline phosphatase levels are low or normal. In hereditary metaphyseal dysostosis, the bone changes are also similar, but there are no biochemical changes, no response to vitamin D even in large doses, and the children are essentially healthy, albeit stocky and bowlegged. This last condition is also sometimes associated with neutropenia, hair hypoplasia, and pancreatic insufficiency.

Prevention

The addition of vitamin D to fluid milk, evaporated milk, and to special milk products and substitutes has helped eradicate vitamin D deficiency rickets in the USA.

Treatment

Vitamin D deficiency rickets is cured by vitamin D, 5000 IU orally every day for 4–5 weeks. Evidence of cure is rapid. Radiologic and biochemical signs of improvement appear after the first week of therapy.

The disturbance of calcium absorption in malabsorption syndromes is secondary to enteric losses of vitamin D with stool fat. For this reason, doubling the recommended prophylactic dose of vitamin D is usually sufficient; however, in certain cases of hepatobiliary disease, a true resistance to vitamin D has been described. Renal rickets is always complicated by hyperparathyroidism but may respond to 1α-hydroxycholecalciferol. Vitamin D resistance must be treated with phosphate solutions and is relatively unresponsive to vitamin D_3, 25-hydroxycholecalciferol, and 1,25-dihydroxycholecalciferol.

Castile RG & others: Vitamin D deficiency rickets. Am J Dis Child 129:964, 1975.

Chalmers TM & others: 1-alpha-hydroxycholecalciferol as a substitute for the kidney hormone 1,25-dihydroxycholecalciferol in chronic renal failure. Lancet 2:696, 1973.

Daeschner CW & others: Metaphyseal dysostosis. J Pediatr 57:844, 1960.

Fraser D: Hypophosphatasia. Am J Med 22:730, 1957.

Glorieux FH & others: Use of phosphate and vitamin D to prevent dwarfism and rickets in X-linked hypophosphatemia. N Engl J Med 287:481, 1972.

Goel KM & others: Florid and subclinical rickets among immigrant children in Glasgow. Lancet 1:1141, 1976.

Reddy V, Sivakumar B: Magnesium-dependent vitamin-D-resistant rickets. Lancet 1:963, 1974.

Scriver CR, Cameron D: Pseudohypophosphatasia. N Engl J Med 281:604, 1969.

2. VITAMIN D DEPENDENCY

Vitamin D dependency rickets has recently been differentiated as a form of vitamin D resistant disease which is probably due to a disorder in the formation or activity of the intestinally active polar dihydroxy form of 25-$(OH)D_3$, 1,25-$(OH)_2 D_3$. The clinical features appear in the first year of life and mimic closely those of vitamin D deficient rickets. In this condition, other siblings may be affected and there is usually a history of normal vitamin D ingestion. There is a prompt response with administration of about 40,000 IU of vitamin D per day, but none to normal daily requirements. The presence of hyperaminoacidemia and renal tubular acidosis distinguishes the condition from X-linked hypophosphatemic vitamin D resistant rickets. Differentiation from the complex Fanconi syndrome may be difficult. However, this form of tubular disease is always secondary to some other condition (eg, cystinosis) and also requires phosphate supplementation as well as vitamin D for treatment.

Fraser D & others: Pathogenesis of hereditary vitamin-D-dependent rickets. N Engl J Med 289:817, 1973.
Scriver CR: Vitamin D dependency. Pediatrics 46:361, 1970.

3. VITAMIN D INTOXICATION

Two forms of vitamin D intoxication are recognized. In the first, relatively small daily ingestion of vitamin D, ie, 5000 IU/day or less from oversupplemented foods, appears to have led to idiopathic hypercalcemia (see p 688) in sensitized children. The outbreaks occurred primarily in Britain, and the condition is now very uncommon in infancy.

In persons not resistant to vitamin D, ingestion of doses of the order of 1000–3000 IU/kg/day may lead to hypercalcemia together with nausea, anorexia, constipation, polyuria, and transient nitrogen retention. Later, nephrocalcinosis and irreversible renal failure can occur.

Treatment consists of immediate discontinuance of vitamin D.

Committee on Nutrition, American Academy of Pediatrics: The prophylactic requirement and toxicity of vitamin D. Pediatrics 31:512, 1963.
Seelig MS: Vitamin D and cardiovascular, renal, and brain damage in infancy and childhood. Ann NY Acad Sci 147:537, 1969.

VITAMIN E DEFICIENCY

Vitamin E is believed to be important in stabilizing biologic membranes. Deficiency in laboratory animals results in decreased reproductive ability, muscular dystrophy, and anemia. Vitamin E is widely distributed in foods eaten by man, particularly vegetable fats, plant seeds, nuts, egg yolk, and leafy vegetables.

Lack of vitamin E through absolute dietary deficiency or secondary to steatorrhea has been shown to result in hemolytic anemia in premature infants. Although reduced virility has not been described in humans, focal necrosis of striated muscle occurs in deficient individuals.

Premature infants fed on formulas with a vegetable oil fat source that is high in linoleic acid require 0.7 IU of vitamin E/100 kcal or 1 IU/gm of linoleic acid. This is particularly important with iron-fortified preparations if hemolytic anemia is to be avoided.

Symposium: Hematologic aspects of vitamin E. Am J Clin Nutr 21:1, 1968.

Symposium: Tocopherol. (2 parts.) Lipids 6:238, 281, 1971.
Underwood BA & others: Correlations between plasma and liver concentrations of vitamins A and E in children with cystic fibrosis. Bull NY Acad Med 47:34, 1971.

VITAMIN K

Vitamin K affects the rate of hepatic synthesis of prothrombin (factor II) and of factors VII, IX, and X. A large number of dietary components have biologic vitamin K activity, including green vegetables, soybeans, and fish. Intestinal bacteria also produce considerable quantities of vitamin K for absorption.

1. VITAMIN K DEFICIENCY

Vitamin K deficiency is most frequently found in newborn infants, particularly when breast-fed, since human milk contains only one-fourth (15 μg/liter) the vitamin K found in cow's milk. The incidence of severe bleeding in newborn infants given vitamin K is 0.3%, compared to 2–5% for infants not given vitamin K.

Diarrhea, oral antibiotics, fat malabsorption, some special formulas, and—since bile salts are important in vitamin K absorption—obstructive jaundice may lead to vitamin K deficiency. Bacterial colonization of the infant's intestine is frequently inadequate at age 24 hours, when maternal prothrombin disappears from the newborn infant's blood.

Newborn infants are usually given 1 mg of water-soluble vitamin K (eg, AquaMephyton) IM, which prevents the postnatal fall in factors II, VII, IX, and X and lessens the incidence of neonatal hemorrhage.

Committee on Nutrition, American Academy of Pediatrics: Vitamin K supplementation. Pediatrics 48:483, 1971.

2. VITAMIN K TOXICITY

Excessive administration of vitamin K, or administration of the fat-soluble forms, can result in hemolytic anemia. This may accentuate hyperbilirubinemia in the newborn infant.

2. WATER-SOLUBLE VITAMINS

Deficiencies of water-soluble vitamins are much less frequent in the USA because of the frequent fortification, particularly with B vitamins, of many foods. Most bread and wheat products are now routinely fortified with B vitamins.

There is less danger of toxicity from water-soluble vitamins because excesses can be excreted in the urine. However, deficiency states can also develop more quickly than with the fat-soluble vitamins because of the limited stores. Deficiencies of folate and vitamin B_{12} are discussed in Chapter 14.

THIAMINE DEFICIENCY

Thiamine (vitamin B_1) is an essential cofactor in the oxidative decarboxylation of pyruvic acid to acetyl-coenzyme A and of other a-keto acids. With magnesium, it activates transketolase in the regeneration of fructose-6-phosphate from ribulose-5-phosphate in the hexose monophosphate shunt. The vitamin is water-soluble and easily destroyed by heat; nevertheless, overt deficiency states are exceedingly rare in North America. Where deficiency does occur, the impact is predominantly on the heart and peripheral nerves. The myocardium shows fatty degeneration, and there is edema of the heart and interstitial tissues. Myelin and axonal degeneration is found in the peripheral nerves. Low red cell transketolase in 20% of underprivileged children in the USA offers some evidence of subclinical involvement in this group.

Clinical Findings

A. Symptoms and Signs: Symptoms are most likely to appear in early infancy, especially if the mother is providing thiamine-deficient breast milk. The infant becomes restless, has attacks of crying as though from abdominal pain, and may vomit breast milk. The vomiting may increase and be accompanied by abdominal distention, flatulence, constipation, and insomnia.

In the acute cardiac forms, there is tachycardia, gallop rhythm, dyspnea, cyanosis, cardiomegaly, hepatomegaly, and pulmonary edema. The condition is rapidly fatal unless treated. In endemic deficiency areas, cardiac failure of unknown cause should always be treated with thiamine. Less dramatic (but equally serious) is the meningitic form that starts with a bulging fontanel, head retraction, and dilated pupils and may go on to convulsions and coma.

In older infants a chronic form is common in which the symptoms are anorexia, weight loss, weakness, diarrhea, constipation, and edema. Peripheral palsies, which may include vocal cord paralysis, may be seen, and the stretch reflexes are usually absent. Ataxia is a common finding.

B. Laboratory Findings: A blood thiamine level under 4 μg/100 ml (normal: 10 ± 5 μg) is suggestive of thiamine deficiency, but perhaps the most helpful test is to show a level of thiamine in the milk of <7 μg/100 ml. Normal pasteurized cow's milk contains about 40 μg/100 ml.

Differential Diagnosis

The initial symptoms must be differentiated from pyloric stenosis and other high obstructions. The cardiac forms may be confused with fibroelastosis, congenital heart disease, Pompe's disease, and severe pneumonitis. A sterile CSF culture excludes pyogenic meningitis. Chronic thiamine deficiency must be distinguished from lead poisoning.

Prevention & Treatment

The disease can be prevented by a normal diet containing at least 0.4 mg of thiamine daily. In acute deficiency states, 25 mg of thiamine should be given IV, followed by 20 mg IM twice daily for 3 days and 10 mg orally daily for 6 weeks.

Prognosis

Complete recovery is expected provided an adequate thiamine intake can be assured.

Field CE: Infantile beriberi. Chap 8, pp 194–199, in: *Diseases of Children in the Subtropics and Tropics.* Trowell HC, Jelliffe DB (editors). Arnold, 1958.

Sadstead HH & others: Nutritional deficiencies in disadvantaged preschool children. Am J Dis Child 121:455, 1971.

THIAMINE DEPENDENCY SYNDROMES

Anomalies of the branched chain keto acid decarboxylase system (see p 960) are known to present as a number of traits. One of these is thiamine-dependent and responds to 10 mg/day of the hydrochloride.

Thiamine dependency has also been reported in a syndrome with optic atrophy and intermittent ataxia, lactic acidosis, and hyperalaninemia due to pyruvate decarboxylase deficiency.

Lonsdale D & others: Ataxia, hyperpyruvic acidemia, hyperalaninemia, hyperalaninuria. Pediatrics 43:1025, 1969.

Scriver CR: Vitamin-responsive inborn errors of metabolism. Metabolism 22:1319, 1973.

RIBOFLAVIN DEFICIENCY

Riboflavin (vitamin B_2) is a constituent of a number of flavoprotein enzymes involved in intermediary metabolism. As riboflavin phosphate, it is incorporated into Warburg yellow enzyme, cytochrome c reductase, and D-amino acid dehydrogenase. As the flavin adenine nucleotide it is the prosthetic group in glycine oxidase, xanthine oxidase, and diaphorase. Riboflavin is water-soluble and is a constituent of both animal and vegetable protein foods (eggs, meat, fish, beans, etc); therefore, riboflavin deficiency often accompanies protein malnutrition.

Breast milk and cow's milk provide adequate amounts of riboflavin, so that the disorder appears only in children on restricted protein intakes or in those with protein malabsorption. The characteristic triad of signs is sore red lips, seborrheic skin lesions with fissuring of the nasolabial folds and extending from the angle of the mouth, and a purplish-red smooth tongue with enlarged papillae. Corneal injection may also occur at the limbus, with eye pain, tearing, photophobia, and ultimately interstitial keratitis. Excretion of less than 125 μg of riboflavin per gram of creatinine in a random urine sample is suggestive of riboflavin deficiency.

The deficiency state can be prevented by a diet containing 0.6 mg riboflavin/1000 kcal. Treatment consists of giving riboflavin, 2 mg IM daily for 2 days, followed by 10 mg IM daily for 3 weeks. Thereafter, a diet containing adequate amounts of riboflavin must be maintained.

NICOTINIC ACID DEFICIENCY
(Pellagra)

Nicotinic acid (niacin) may be ingested from natural food sources or derived endogenously as one of the end products of the kynurenine pathway of tryptophan breakdown. The molecule is a component of nicotinamide adenine dinucleotide (NAD) and nicotinamide adenine dinucleotide phosphate (NADP), which act as hydrogen and electron transfer agents by reversible oxidation and reduction. Nicotinic acid is plentiful in most protein foods and in grains. The only critical diet is one in which there is a substantial content of highly milled maize, which also has a relatively low tryptophan content.

Pellagra tends to be associated with a state of chronic, difficult to define ill health. The most typical lesions are found on the exposed parts of the skin and are aggravated by sunlight and sometimes confused with sunburn. The lesions start as an erythema which then becomes darkly pigmented and progresses to a rough, sharply demarcated, fissured, scaly dermatosis with little tendency to desquamate. The mouth and tongue become red and painful and there is widespread gastrointestinal inflammation with dysphagia, nausea, vomiting, and attacks of diarrhea. Apathy is seen in childhood, but not the more severe psychoses that occur in adult pellagra.

The skin lesions may be confused with those of kwashiorkor. In kwashiorkor, however, the lesions tend not to be on the exposed extremities but around pressure sites in the groin and trunk. The diarrhea must be differentiated from that due to parasitic diseases (including amebiasis) and other infections.

Prevention & Treatment

The condition may be prevented by ensuring a nicotinamide intake of 6–10 mg/day orally, depending on age. Treatment consists of giving 10–25 mg of nicotinamide 3 times daily for 2 weeks, followed by a continuing adequate diet containing sufficient B complex vitamins.

PYRIDOXINE DEFICIENCY

Pyridoxine (vitamin B_6) deficiency was first produced artificially in 2 retarded infants. One developed a marked hypochromic anemia and the other, more characteristically, severe convulsions. Both infants responded promptly to intravenous pyridoxine and were ultimately stabilized on 150 μg/day orally. Shortly afterward, a group of infants given a proprietary liquid milk formula were observed to become hyperirritable between 6 weeks and 4 months of age. Generalized seizures followed which were treated successfully with oral pyridoxine or with a formula containing normal amounts of pyridoxine. A similar history was given by a mother whose breast milk was shown to contain unusually low amounts of pyridoxine. These infants all had normal interictal EEGs, showed no familial incidence of convulsions, and developed unexceptionally on a proper diet. Xanthurenic aciduria was apparent on tryptophan loading; the correction of this abnormality was notable in that greater amounts of pyridoxine were required for its correction than for control of the convulsions. Although pyridoxal phosphate is a coenzyme in a wide range of reactions, the key pyridoxal-dependent reaction in causing convulsions is thought to be that of the formation of gamma-aminobutyric acid from glutamic acid by glutamic acid decarboxylase.

For practical purposes, pyridoxine deficiency occurs only in infancy. It should be considered when convulsions or anemia is otherwise unexplained.

Complete recovery may be expected after the administration of 5 mg of pyridoxine IM followed by 0.5 mg daily by mouth for 2 weeks together with a normal dietary intake.

Coursin DB: Vitamin B_6 metabolism in infants and children. Vitam Horm 22:756, 1964.

THE PYRIDOXINE (VITAMIN B_6)
DEPENDENCY SYNDROMES

There are a number of rare inborn errors of metabolism in which the clinical picture or the abnormal biochemistry is ameliorated by large doses of pyridoxine, as the cofactor for the abnormal enzyme.

Some cases of infantile seizures respond promptly to 2–10 mg of pyridoxine orally, as do some cases of myoclonic epilepsy, although in the latter, treatment may need to be sustained with doses up to 100 mg/day orally.

Pyridoxine may also restore normal biochemical patterns in cases of homocystinuria, cystathioninuria, and kynureninase deficiency.

VITAMIN C DEFICIENCY

Essentials of Diagnosis

- Dietary history of an infant 6–12 months of age fed cow's milk and no citrus fruits or green vegetables.
- Fretfulness, anorexia, weight loss, and tenderness of the lower extremities. Legs held in the "frogleg" position.
- Hemorrhages in the gums, skin, or mucous membranes.

General Considerations

Scurvy is rare today even though a 10-state survey showed that 31% of children received less than 15 mg of vitamin C a day and 6% of infants had serum levels less than 0.3 mg/100 ml.

Structurally, ascorbic acid resembles monosaccharide sugars. Most animal species can synthesize ascorbic acid and thus have no dietary requirement for this vitamin. However, humans, other primates, and guinea pigs cannot metabolize glucose to ascorbic acid because of the absence of the enzyme L-gulonolactone oxidase.

Ascorbic acid has many metabolic roles. Because of its reversible oxidation-reduction capacity, it is active in microsomal electron transport. It is important in preventing depolymerization of collagen and in maintaining the integrity of ground substance. Ascorbic acid presumably has an effect on hematopoiesis since anemia usually accompanies scurvy.

By protecting the enzyme parahydroxyphenylpyruvic acid oxidase from inhibition by its substrate, tyrosine, vitamin C plays an essential role in the metabolism of tyrosine in the newborn period.

Large doses of vitamin C have achieved some notoriety in the prophylaxis and amelioration of the common cold. A recent double-blind study showed some evidence of benefit in a group of school-age girls.

Clinical Findings

Populations where breast feeding is in disfavor and where most newborns are fed cow's milk have a higher incidence of symptomatic scurvy. A history of a poor intake of fruits and vegetables is also suggestive. The time required for the development of scurvy after a grossly deficient diet is instituted is about 4–7 months. Certain groups such as the Navajo Indians are especially susceptible.

A. Symptoms and Signs: Nonspecific symptoms appear before any physical changes are evident. Irritability, weakness, anorexia, weight loss, and tenderness of the extremities, particularly of the legs, are common. In more advanced stages of the disease, the affected infant lies quietly in the frogleg position and may exhibit pseudoparalysis because the slightest motion causes severe pain. Small or large hemorrhages may occur anywhere in the body but are most frequent under the periosteum of the long bones, particularly the lower end of the femur and the proximal end of the tibia; this may not be detectable on x-ray until healing has begun with superficial calcification. Gastrointestinal, genitourinary, and meningeal bleeding have been reported occasionally in advanced stages. Hemorrhaging under the mucous membranes of the gums is common if teeth have erupted or are about to erupt. Conjunctival and tongue hemorrhagic lesions are also common. Costochondral beading, which differs from the rachitic rosary by its sharpness ("bayonet" deformity), often occurs.

B. Laboratory Findings: A fasting serum ascorbic acid level of < 0.1 mg/100 ml suggests scurvy. Levels in the 0.1–0.19 mg/100 ml range are considered "low." Samples must be assayed within 48 hours of collection. A more satisfactory procedure is to perform a tolerance test by giving ascorbic acid, 20 mg/kg IV as a 4% solution in normal saline. A 4-hour urine sample containing > 1.5 mg/100 ml rules out scurvy.

C. X-Ray Findings: The earliest x-ray changes appear at the sites of most active growth, eg, the knees, and are characterized by thickening and irregularity at the epiphyseal lines with a subepiphyseal zone of rarefaction. There is thinning of bone cortices and atrophy of the trabecular structure, causing increased transparency ("ground glass" appearance). Shadows of the subperiosteal hemorrhages give the affected long bones a club shape; they become more clearly outlined after several days of treatment, when bone formation is initiated in the periphery.

Differential Diagnosis

If there are no gum hemorrhages, the signs may resemble those of acute pyogenic arthritis. However, the radiologic evidence is distinctive.

Prevention & Treatment

Breast-fed infants ingest 20–50 mg/day (4.3 mg/100 ml) of ascorbic acid unless the mother's diet is very inadequate. Cow's milk contains lesser amounts of vitamin C. Attempts at adding vitamin C to proprietary formulas have succeeded despite the fact that vitamin C is extremely susceptible to oxidation and heat.

The therapeutic dose of ascorbic acid is 100 mg 3 times a day for infants and children. Infants should receive—in formula, citrus fruit juice, or green vegetables—35 mg of ascorbic acid daily.

Prognosis

Dramatic clinical improvement occurs within 24 hours after therapy with vitamin C is started. X-ray signs show some degree of amelioration within 10 days of the onset of therapy.

Miller JZ & others: Therapeutic effect of vitamin C. JAMA 237:248, 1977.

3. TRACE ELEMENTS

An increasing number of elements are known to be of nutritional importance to man and animals in trace quantities. In addition to iron and iodine, these include copper, zinc, chromium, manganese, cobalt, selenium, molybdenum, nickel, vanadium, tin, and silicon. The extent to which man may be at risk from nutritional deficiencies of these elements is not known, but it is apparent that specific trace deficiencies are of clinical importance in a variety of circumstances.

Copper Deficiency

Copper deficiency may occur in the following circumstances: (1) In premature infants, especially those fed on low-copper milk preparations, (2) In association with more generalized malnutrition states. (3) Secondary to intestinal malabsorption states or prolonged diarrhea. Milk is a poor source of dietary copper, and infants rehabilitated on a milk-based formula are at particular risk from copper deficiency. (4) In patients maintained on prolonged total parenteral alimentation without copper supplementation.

Osteoporosis is an early finding. Later skeletal changes include enlargement of the costochondral cartilages, cupping and flaring of long bone metaphyses, and spontaneous fractures of the ribs. The radiologic findings, which are attributable in part to a lack of copper amine oxidases and of ascorbic acid oxidase, may suggest a diagnosis of battering. Neutropenia and hypochromic anemia are other early manifestations. The anemia results in part from a lack of copper-containing ferroxidases, including ceruloplasmin, which are involved in the release of iron from body stores. The anemia is unresponsive to oral iron and in later stages to parenteral iron. Other clinical features that may be associated with copper deficiency include decreased pigmentation of skin and hair, dilated superficial veins, seborrheic dermatitis, anorexia, failure to thrive, diarrhea, hypotonia, and apneic episodes. Very severe CNS disease is present in Menkes' steely (kinky) hair syndrome, in which a profound copper deficiency state results from a specific X-linked inherited defect in the intestinal absorption of this element.

The diagnosis of nutritional copper deficiency is based on a combination of clinical findings (especially osteoporosis, neutropenia, and anemia), suggestive circumstances (eg, prematurity), and the presence of a low serum copper or ceruloplasmin level that is not attributable to other factors, (eg, hypoproteinemia). Copper deficiency can be treated with a 1% solution of copper sulfate (2 mg of the salt or 400 μg of elemental copper per day for infants). Preventive measures include copper supplementation of parenteral alimentation solutions to provide 30 μg of copper per kg body weight per day.

Ashkenazi A, & others: The syndrome of neonatal copper deficiency. Pediatrics 52:525, 1973.

Cordano A, Graham GC: Copper deficiency complicating severe chronic intestinal malabsorption. Pediatrics 38:596, 1966.
Danks DM & others: Menkes' kinky hair disease: Further definition of the defect in copper transport. Science 179:1140, 1973.
Danks DM & others: Menkes' kinky hair syndrome. Lancet 1:1000, 1972.
Graham GG, Cordano A: Copper deficiency and depletion in the malnourished infant. Johns Hopkins Med J 124:139, 1969.
Karpel JT, Peden VH: Copper deficiency in long-term parenteral nutrition. J Pediatr 80:32, 1972.

Zinc Deficiency

Zinc is an essential component of many metalloenzymes, including alkaline phosphatase and carbonic anhydrase. It is necessary for normal nucleic acid metabolism and protein synthesis. Human zinc deficiency was recognized first in Egypt and Iran, where it contributes to the dwarfism and delayed sexual maturation of "adolescent nutritional dwarfism." The large quantity of phytate in the diet of Iranian villagers impairs zinc absorption. Zinc deficiency may complicate intestinal malabsorption syndromes, and severe deficiency has been reported in a case of regional enteritis. Zinc depletion can also result from excessive loss of this element from chronic blood loss, excessive sweating, or hyperzincuria. The latter may occur in any catabolic state or when there is an increase in amino acid-liganded zinc in the serum, as in acute viral hepatitis. Other circumstances in which zinc deficiency has been identified include prolonged parenteral alimentation, sickle cell disease, and protein-calorie malnutrition.

Suboptimal zinc nutrition appears to be common in infants and young children in the USA, especially in those in poor families subsisting on inadequate diets. Clinical manifestations of zinc deficiency include failure to thrive in infancy, failure to achieve maximum growth potential, delayed sexual maturation, anorexia, impaired taste perception, pica, and impaired wound healing.

Support for a diagnosis of zinc deficiency is provided by a plasma zinc level of less than 70 μg/100 ml or a hair zinc level less than 70 μg/gm dry weight (there is some variation in normal levels at different laboratories). Hypozincemia without zinc depletion occurs in association with various infections and with raised estrogen levels. There is a very high incidence of low plasma and hair zinc levels during infancy in the USA. It is not known to what extent these low levels may or may not be accepted as normal in this age group.

Zinc deficiency can be treated with zinc sulfate, 5 mg (approximately 1 mg of elemental zinc) per kg body weight per day. Patients maintained on total parenteral alimentation for more than a few days should receive 30 μg of elemental zinc per kg per day added to their intravenous solutions.

Acrodermatitis enteropathica has been identified as an inborn error of zinc metabolism. The cardinal features of this autosomal, recessively inherited disease are skin lesions (commencing at the extremities and around the body orifices), diarrhea, and alopecia with onset in infancy shortly after weaning. These and other features of this disease, eg, failure to thrive, are attributable to the profound zinc deficiency that appears to result from an inherited defect in zinc absorption. Plasma zinc levels in the untreated disease state approximate 30 µg/100 ml or less. Rapid and sustained clinical improvement can be achieved with 50—100 mg of zinc sulfate orally twice daily.

Halsted JA & others: Zinc deficiency in man. Am J Med 53:277, 1972.

Hambidge KM & others: Low levels of zinc in hair, anorexia, poor growth, and hypogeusia in children. Pediatr Res 6:868, 1972.

Neldner KN, Hambidge KM: Zinc therapy of acrodermatitis enteropathica. N Engl J Med 292:879, 1975.

Sandstead HH: Zinc nutrition in the United States. Am J Clin Nutr 26:1251, 1973.

Chromium Deficiency

Trivalent chromium acts as a cofactor for insulin at the insulin-responsive cell membrane and is necessary for normal glucose tolerance. Chromium is one of the newly recognized essential trace elements, and present knowledge is limited with respect to human nutrition; however, suboptimal chromium nutrition may be common in the USA. In Turkey, Jordan, and Nigeria, chromium deficiency has been demonstrated in malnourished infants, in whom it is responsible, at least in part, for the impairment of glucose tolerance. Chromium deficiency has also been reported to be growth-limiting during the early recovery stage from protein-calorie malnutrition in Turkish infants. The deficiency can be corrected by a single dose of 180 µg of trivalent chromium administered as chromic chloride.

Gurson CT, Saner G: Effects of chromium on glucose utilization in marasmic protein-calorie malnutrition. Am J Clin Nutr 24:1313, 1971.

Gurson CT, Saner G: Effects of chromium supplementation on growth in marasmic protein-calorie malnutrition. Am J Clin Nutr 36:988, 1973.

Hambidge KM: Chromium nutrition in man. Am J Clin Nutr 27:505, 1974.

Hopkins L, Masas A: Improvement of CHO metabolism of malnourished infants by administration of chromium. Fed Proc 25:303, 1966.

Mertz W: Chromium occurrence and function in biological systems. Physiol Rev 49:163, 1969.

Cadmium Intoxication

Bone pain, osteomalacia, aminoaciduria, and glycosuria with multiple fractures have been reported as possible sequelae of cadmium intoxication.

Cadmium pollution and itai-itai disease. Lancet 1:382, 1971.

*   *   *

Hambidge KM: The clinical significance of trace element deficiencies in man. Proc Nutr Soc 33:249, 1974.

Underwood EJ: *Trace Elements in Human and Animal Nutrition.* Academic Press, 1971.

4. ESSENTIAL FATTY ACID (EFA) DEFICIENCY

Deficiency of linoleic acid has come to be increasingly recognized in recent years, particularly with the increased survival of infants after major bowel surgery. Linoleic acid is referred to either as an 18:2ω6 fatty acid, meaning that it has 18 carbons and 2 double bonds with the first at the 6 position from the methyl (omega) end, or as an 18:2Δ9,16 fatty acid, meaning that the 2 double bonds are in the 9 and 16 positions from the carboxyl (delta) end. Linoleic acid cannot be synthesized in the body and is thus an "essential" nutrient. Linolenic acid (18:3ω3) is required by some mammals but not, so far as is known, by humans.

Studies by Hansen and co-workers clearly demonstrated the need of human infants for linoleic acid. Infants were fed milks containing 0.04 to 7.3% linoleic acid, and all infants who received the lower quantity developed dry, scaly skin. Of 16 hospitalized infants, 4 of 5 with pneumonia, 3 of 4 with skin infections, and 6 of 7 with diarrhea were on fatty acid deficient diets. Premature infants are most severely affected because of their rapid growth and low fat stores. Growth failure is a common feature of EFA deficiency, and thrombocytopenia and poor wound healing have been described. Older children with cystic fibrosis or other fat malabsorption problems may also be EFA deficient.

Metabolism

Linoleic acid (18:2) is metabolized primarily first by desaturation and then by elongation to arachidonic acid (20:4). Prostaglandins are produced from arachidonic acid, and their importance is just now beginning to be appreciated in medicine.

Laboratory Diagnosis

The laboratory diagnosis of linoleic acid deficiency should be made by gas chromatography of plasma and red blood cell fatty acids. The latter represent membrane lipid and are more likely to be altered in chronic deficiency conditions such as cystic fibrosis. Normal values ± 2 SD are given below but should be determined for individual laboratories.

| | Percentage of Total Fatty Acids (± 2 SD) | |
	Linoleic Acid	Arachidonic Acid
Plasma	29.3 ± 10	9.4 ± 6
Red cells	14.1 ± 8	19.4 ± 7

Levels of 16:0 (palmitic), 18:0 (stearic), and 18:1 (oleic) acids are usually elevated with EFA deficiency.

In addition, a peak for a $20:3\omega9$ (5,8,11-eicosatrienoic) fatty acid may be detected which is considered diagnostic of linoleic acid deficiency. Prior to the availability of gas chromatography, EFA was often estimated using a triene/tetraene ratio, which is the ratio of the quantity of fatty acids with 3 double bonds to the quantity of fatty acids with 4 double bonds (primarily arachidonic acid). This ratio increases to a level above 0.6 with EFA deficiency as 20:3 compounds increase and arachidonic acid (made from linoleic acid) decreases.

Treatment

Three percent of calories should be provided as linoleic acid. Human milk has 5% of calories as linoleic acid, but cow's milk has only 1% and young infants may be borderline deficient if receiving only cow's milk. The deficiency is usually not great enough to impair growth or cause skin lesions. Safflower oil has 77% of fatty acids as linoleic acid, with corn oil at 57% and soy and cottonseed oils at 53%. Topical application of vegetable oils to the skin has been tried in some infants who could not ingest adequate quantities orally, but this is not always successful. When Intralipid is used to treat or prevent EFA deficiency, it should be remembered that it is usually used as a 10% solution and that 50% of the lipids are linoleic acid. Thus, 100 ml of a 10% solution would have 5 gm of linoleic acid, or 45 kcal, which would be 3% of the calories for a child receiving 1500 kcal/day. It should also be remembered that vitamin E requirements are increased when more polyunsaturates are given, especially in iron fortified formulas.

Elliott RB: A therapeutic trial of fatty acid supplementation in cystic fibrosis. Pediatrics 57:474, 1976.

Friedman Z & others: Rapid onset of essential fatty acid deficiency in the newborn. Pediatrics 58:640, 1976.

Hansen AE & others: Role of linoleic acid in infant nutrition: Clinical and chemical study of 428 infants fed on milk mixtures varying in kind and amount of fat. Pediatrics 31:171, 1963.

Holman RT: Essential fatty acid deficiency in humans. Page 127 in: *Dietary Lipids and Postnatal Development.* Raven, 1973.

• • •

General References

Committee on Nutrition, American Academy of Pediatrics: *A Handbook of Clinical Nutrition,* 1978.

Fomon SJ: *Infant Nutrition,* 2nd ed. Saunders, 1974.

Goodhart RS, Shils ME: *Modern Nutrition in Health and Disease.* 5th ed. Lea & Fibiger, 1973.

McLaren DS, Burman D: *Textbook of Pediatric Nutrition.* Churchill-Livingston, 1976.

Neuman CG, Jelliffee DB (editors): Symposium on nutrition in pediatrics. Pediatr Clin North Am 24:1, 1977. (Entire issue.)

Olsen RE: *Protein-Calorie Malnutrition.* Academic Press, 1975.

O'Neal RM, Johnson DC, Schaeffer AE: Guidelines for classification and interpretation of group blood and urine data collected as part of the National Nutrition Survey. Pediatr Res 4:103, 1970.

Owen GM & others: A study of nutritional status of pre-school children in the United States 1968–1970. Pediatrics 53 (Suppl):597, 1974.

Ten-State Nutrition Survey. Publication No. (HSM) 72–8134, Department of Health, Education, and Welfare. 1972.

Walt BK, Memle AL: *Composition of Foods–Raw, Processed, Prepared.* USDA Handbook No. 8, 1963.

Winick M: *Malnutrition and Brain Development.* Oxford Univ Press, 1976.

5...
Immunization

Vincent A. Fulginiti, MD

All pediatric immunizations are planned to prevent specific infectious diseases or their toxic manifestations. Thus, to achieve maximum effectiveness, the vaccines must be administered to the appropriate populations at the appropriate times in life when the individual is immunologically capable and has not yet been exposed to the natural disease. "Routines" of immunization are designed to simplify ordinary practice and to permit reasonable immunization scheduling. However, exceptions to the routine are dictated by peculiar local epidemiologic circumstances (eg, epidemics or absence of a disease in the community) and by individual differences in immunologic response or susceptibility to the adverse effects of specific products. Each immunization should be viewed as a balance between the risk of that disease in the individual and population and the potential adverse effects of the immunizing procedure. This chapter will attempt to present the "routine" as well as the tempering influences for each product and schedule.

Administration of vaccines and other biologic agents is not without intrinsic risk. For all products utilized there are expected side-effects and occasional adverse reactions. Each physician may be considered responsible for informing his patients (parents) of the risk of a given biologic as well as its benefits. The patient (parent) should also be informed about the risk of *no* immunization, ie, the risks of the natural disease. Although consent is implied in usual practice, some sentiment is developing for a requirement that written permission be obtained before any vaccine is administered. In some states such written "consent" is required for some immunizations. The Center for Disease Control (CDC) is developing standard information sheets for parental or patient use before written consent is obtained by the physician. Such forms were used in the national swine influenza vaccine campaign in 1975–1976. To the author's knowledge, there is no single authoritative method for documenting so-called "informed consent" in these circumstances. The prudent physician should discuss each vaccine with his patients, answer questions, and obtain some record of permission granted by the patient or parent for administration of the vaccine. It is anticipated that specific routine procedures may be adopted locally or nationally in the future.

Sources of Information

Recommendations for immunization change as experience accumulates and new products and new indications become available. Several sources of such information are available to the practitioner:

A. The American Academy of Pediatrics' *Red Book.* A useful, comprehensive guide to immunization practices. Distributed free to all Fellows of the Academy and available to others at the nominal cost of $6.00 from the Academy, PO Box 1034, Evanston, Illinois 60204. The *Red Book* is supplemented by special information published as needed in the *Academy Newsletter.*

B. *Control of Communicable Diseases in Man,* 12th ed. Benenson AS (editor). American Public Health Assoc., Washington DC, 1975. Similar to the "Red Book," this publication provides somewhat more detailed clinical and microbiologic information.

C. *Morbidity and Mortality Reports.* A weekly publication of the Center for Disease Control, Atlanta, Georgia, of the US Department of Health, Education, and Welfare—useful reports of the major notifiable diseases supplemented periodically with specific immunization recommendations of the Surgeon General and USPHS.

D. Local public health agencies—either through periodic publications or by special bulletins—make available immunization information, particularly of a local nature. Specific inquiry about requirements for foreign travel, special immunizations, etc can be handled at these agencies.

E. *Immunization Information for Foreign Travel,* a useful booklet formerly published by the Department of Health, Education, and Welfare (Publication No. 384), is no longer available from the Superintendent of Documents but may be consulted at the medical library.

STERILITY & SAFETY OF INJECTABLE VACCINE ADMINISTRATION

Avoidance of Bacterial Infection & Hepatitis

Most of the "sterile" or aseptic precautions are

recommended in order to prevent the introduction of unwanted infectious agents. Simple cleanliness and the use of sterilized equipment would suffice to prevent most bacterial infections. However, the more stringent precautions are designed to prevent hardier bacteria and the hepatitis agent from gaining access to the vaccinee.

The following steps are recommended:

A. Single-Unit Dosage: Where possible, single-unit disposable equipment should be used for immunizations. Plastic syringes or single-dose vaccine units are most desirable.

B. Sterilization of Equipment: If glass syringes are used, adequate sterilization procedures must be employed between individual patient usage. The following procedures are recommended by the American Academy of Pediatrics: (1) Autoclaving at a temperature of 121° C for a period of 15 minutes at 15 lb pressure. (2) Dry heat for 2 hours at 170° C or boiling for 30 minutes are also acceptable, but one must be certain that the time and temperature requirements are met.

C. Disinfection: For most procedures, it is sufficient to cleanse the intended injection site and the surface of the immunization container with a solution of 70% alcohol. Some prefer 2% tincture of iodine followed by 70% alcohol. Iodine burns have occurred when the tincture is not removed or is allowed to pool in contact with the skin. Our current feeling is that no skin preparation or, at most, gentle washing with soap and water is preferable preceding smallpox immunization.

Routes & Methods of Immunization

All adjuvant or "depot" antigens which contain alum, aluminum hydroxide or phosphate, mineral oil, etc should be administered *intramuscularly only*. Subcutaneous injection results in considerable irritation and pain and may lead to the so-called sterile abscess.

Intramuscular injections should be given into the anterolateral thigh (vastus lateralis muscle) or into the deltoid or triceps muscle mass (older children and adults). This is to avoid sciatic nerve damage, which may follow intragluteal injections.

One should always aspirate prior to injection to avoid intravascular administration.

Aqueous vaccines can be given either intramuscularly or subcutaneously—or, on occasion, intracutaneously.

Live vaccines should be given on occasions separated by at least 1 month unless an emergency situation dictates otherwise. This will minimize potential interference and additive effects such as fever, malaise, etc and will clarify the etiology of reactions should they occur. An exception to this practice is the use of *proved* live virus vaccine combinations. These preparations have been shown to be effective and safe, with no additive clinical effects.

The "jet gun" or compressed air injection of vaccines is useful for mass immunization. The advantages are ease of administration, rapidity of multiple injections, and greater acceptance. The units are expensive, and single dose administration units are not yet practical. This method may find greater favor with the development of improved, inexpensive equipment.

Host Factors in Safety of Immunizations

Only healthy children should be immunized. Febrile illnesses, incubation of a childhood exanthem, and any active infection are contraindications to immunization. The child who has a "cold" each time he presents for his routine immunizations poses a problem in completion of his primary series. Two alternatives exist to achieve adequate protection: (1) Have the child return between regularly scheduled visits when he is well. (2) Administer the vaccine. This requires judgment, as the child may have a minimal upper respiratory illness and will tolerate the procedure quite well.

Chronic illnesses in themselves are not necessarily contraindications; indeed, they may make immunizations more desirable or even mandatory. Caution must be exercised if CNS damage exists.

Chronic open skin diseases such as eczema must be regarded as absolute contraindications to smallpox immunization or contact with a newly vaccinated individual. Acute dermatitis or injury resulting in weeping surfaces again contraindicates vaccination or contact. If vaccination of a sibling or other contact is desirable, the affected child must be completely removed from the environment until the crust has separated and the vaccinee is free of virus.

Immunologic deficiency states are an absolute contraindication to live virus immunization. Whether congenital or acquired, these deficiency diseases expose the host to the danger of dissemination of the vaccine virus. Malignancies of the lymphatic system are frequently overlooked as predisposing the host to such complications. More and more children are being treated with corticosteroids and immunosuppressive agents. These drugs may induce a state of lowered immunologic reactivity, and live virus immunization at such times may result in generalized and frequently fatal infections.

Allergy to a component of the vaccine preparation is infrequent but often can be anticipated. Antibiotic allergies should be elicited by questioning and the antibiotic composition of various viral vaccines known. Many vaccines are prepared in eggs or in fowl tissues, and patients who are sensitive should not receive such preparations. A rough guide which is frequently advised is that if a child can eat a whole egg without adverse effects he can receive egg or fowl tissue prepared vaccines. Infrequently, patients are sensitive to the preservative included in the vaccine, eg, mercury.

THE IMMUNIZING ANTIGENS

Increasing numbers of vaccines, antisera, and gamma globulin preparations are becoming available. They differ significantly in their composition, form, stability, route of administration, and timing. It is essential that the practitioner carefully assess each preparation before he administers it to any patient. The brochure provided with the preparation is almost invariably complete in its description of the product and its proper use.

"Typical" Composition

The typical vaccine does not exist, but the following categories of components are found. The list is presented to point out the complexities of some vaccines and the difficulty in attributing an unusual reaction to a specific component. Immunization involves administering a complex product to a complex individual, and the result of this administration is complex.

A. **The Principal Antigen:** May be whole bacteria, bacterial products (toxins, hemolysins, etc), whole viruses, or substructures of viruses.

B. **Host-Derived Antigens:** Protein or other constituents of host tissue which are carried along with or intimately associated with the virus particles.

C. **Altered Antigens:** Distorted proteins and other substances may become incorporated into vaccines as a result of the complex changes associated with the effects of virus infection on the cells in which it is grown.

D. **Preservatives and Stabilizers:** A variety of chemical compounds are employed to prevent bacterial growth or to maintain the desired antigen in a stable form. Mercury compounds and glycine are typical examples.

E. **Antibiotics:** Trace amounts may be found in viral vaccines which must be prepared in antibiotic-containing media. Various antibiotics are employed, and the "same" vaccine prepared by different manufacturers may vary in the specific antibiotics used.

F. **Menstruum:** All vaccines are solutions or suspensions. The fluid phase may consist simply of saline solution or may be as complex as the tissue culture media employed in viral growth.

G. **Unwanted or Unknown Constituents:** Despite elaborate precautions in preparing vaccines, viruses or other antigens may be included which are not wanted or not even detectable.

H. **Adjuvants:** A variety of substances may be used to enhance the antigenic effect of the principal antigen. Such materials as alum, aluminum phosphate, and aluminum hydroxide are currently in use, and others (mineral oil, peanut oil, etc) may be employed in the future. These materials retain the antigen at the depot site and release it slowly, thus enhancing the response by prolonging contact.

Properties of Antigens

Antigens vary in their ability to produce the desired immunologic response; some do so weakly, and some strongly. For a given antigen, the response may be variable, with some individuals responding poorly and a few not at all. One should be aware of this phenomenon in assessing the clinical effects of a preparation. Some children who receive optimal immunizations will simply not respond and may contract the disease if exposed naturally. This should not condemn the particular antigen for all children, as it may protect the vast majority of recipients.

Adjuvant Vaccines

In general, depot type vaccines are preferred since they provide more prolonged immunity and greater antigenic stimulation and reduce the systemic effects observed with fluid antigens, which are rapidly absorbed. For example, DTP (diphtheria and tetanus toxoid and pertussis organisms) provides prolonged antitoxic immunity against diphtheria and tetanus. In addition, it enhances the antibody response to pertussis, particularly in early infancy. Fluid or aqueous preparations may achieve earlier immunity and are less likely to produce local reactions at the site of injection.

Gamma Globulin Preparations

A variety of gamma globulins are available for clinical use. Whatever the label, they are all essentially the same. They consist of roughly a 16% solution of a limited spectrum of serum proteins in the gamma range of electrophoretic mobility. They differ in their antibody content to a significant degree. Thus, tetanus immune globulin is a preparation obtained by pooling and concentrating donor plasma from individuals recently stimulated with tetanus toxoid, thus assuring a higher level of antitoxin than is found in other gamma globulins obtained from donors irrespective of their tetanus immunization status. This is true for all of the specifically labeled gamma globulins—they contain a standard level of the specific antibody desired, whereas randomly prepared lots do not.

Gamma globulins are intended only for intramuscular injection and should not be given intravenously since intravenous administration results in predictable anaphylactoid reactions. (An intravenous gamma globulin is now in preparation but as of this writing has not been marketed.)

The dosage of gamma globulin is not uniform but varies for each specific preparation and for the specific clinical circumstances of its use. One must learn these variables in order to use the antibody contained in the preparations effectively.

Intradermal testing with gamma globulin is unnecessary and may be misleading. The intradermal inoculation of gamma globulin may result in a wheal and flare reaction which does not indicate sensitivity to intramuscular administration. Thus, this method is not advised.

Whenever gamma globulin is administered simultaneously with an active immunizing antigen, one must be concerned about decreasing the effect of the antigen. This is due to the combination of the specific antibody in the gamma globulin with the antigen that occurs in the host after injection. It may be wise in some situations to administer additional doses of the antigen subsequently to ensure adequate stimulation. These special circumstances are pointed out in the specific immunization sections that follow.

Horse Serum Sensitivity

A major limiting factor in the use of antibody in the form of horse serum is the existence or development of horse serum sensitivity. This possibility must be considered each time the use of horse serum is contemplated. Appropriate medications to treat anaphylactic shock should be instantly available. The possibility of serum sickness developing later should be borne in mind.

To test for preexistent horse serum sensitivity, the following steps should be taken:

A. Allergic History: Elicit a careful history of prior administration of horse serum products and of any allergic reactions. Allergy in general is an indication for caution in administering horse serum.

B. Sensitivity Tests: Skin or conjunctival tests should be performed, bearing in mind that severe reactions may occur from the testing procedure itself and that the physician must be prepared to intercede.

1. Skin test—Give intradermally 0.1 ml of a 1:100 saline dilution of the serum to be used. In allergic indi-

viduals, reduce the dose to 0.05 ml of a 1:1000 dilution. The appearance of a wheal in 10—30 minutes indicates hypersensitivity.

2. Conjunctival test—One drop of a 1:10 dilution in saline is placed in the lower conjunctival sac and 1 drop of saline solution in the other eye as a control. A positive reaction consists of conjunctivitis and tearing in 10—30 minutes.

C. Desensitization: Table 5—1 outlines the subsequent procedure to be followed.

SPECIFIC IMMUNIZATIONS

DIPHTHERIA

Immunity against diphtheria is related to the levels of circulating antitoxin. Immunization may not prevent the carrier state. Occasionally, even well immunized individuals develop the disease, although morbidity is less and mortality rates are lower in such cases than in the nonimmunized. Protection is in excess of 85%. The major significant reservoirs of diphtheria in the USA today are the unimmunized, particularly older individuals whose immunity has waned and underprivileged children who have received no immunizations.

Vaccines Available

A. Combined Diphtheria-Tetanus-Pertussis (DTP): See below.

B. Diphtheria Toxoid: Recommended only when there is a specific contraindication to the combined preparations. It is usually given in 3 doses of 0.5 ml IM 4—6 weeks apart. A recall dose should be given 1 year later.

C. Diphtheria-Tetanus (DT) (Pediatric): This preparation contains full amounts of both diphtheria and tetanus toxoids and is indicated in those individuals who cannot be given pertussis vaccine. It is usually given in 3 doses of 0.5 ml IM 4—6 weeks apart with a booster 1—2 months later. Do not administer to adults because severe reactions may occur.

D. Diphtheria-Tetanus (Td) (Adult): This preparation contains one-twentieth the amount of diphtheria toxoid contained in DTP or in pediatric DT. It is designed for use after the age of pertussis immunization. This amount of diphtheria toxoid elicits a booster response but results in far fewer local reactions.

E. Diphtheria Toxoid (Fluid): An infrequently used preparation which does not contain alum.

F. Diphtheria Toxin for Schick Test: Intradermal inoculation of 0.1 ml will result in 10 mm or more of erythema and induration approximately 4 days after injection. Pseudoreactions reach their peak earlier and fade by the third or fourth day. If a reaction occurs, it

Table 5—1. Desensitization procedure in horse serum sensitivity.

History	Sensitivity Test	Procedure
−	−	IM dose can be given. For IV use, give 0.5 ml serum in 10 ml fluid first; if there is no reaction in 30 minutes, give the remainder of the dose as a 1:20 dilution.
+ or −	− +	If serum use is imperative, give 1 ml of 1:10 dilution subcut; if there is no reaction, proceed with 1 ml undiluted and if still no reaction proceed as above.
+	+	Serum should only be used if there is no alternative and it may be lifesaving. Begin with 0.05 ml of a 1:20 dilution subcut and increase every 15 minutes as follows if there is no reaction: 0.1 ml of 1:10, 0.3 ml of 1:10, 0.1 ml undiluted, 0.2 ml undiluted, 0.5 ml undiluted, and then the remainder of the dose. If an untoward reaction occurs at any stage, reduce the dose by half.

means that the individual has too little antibody to neutralize the toxin and is susceptible.

Schick test material may be difficult or impossible to obtain. If protection is questionable in a given individual, it is best to administer the vaccine.

Immunization Schedules

Diphtheria immunization should be initiated in early infancy. Three doses of toxoid, alone or in combination with tetanus and pertussis vaccines, are administered at 2, 4, and 6 months. A booster dose is required at 1½ years, at 4 years, at 14–16 years, and every 10 years thereafter (see Table 5–2). If it is desired to avoid pertussis immunization, then 3 doses of pediatric DT should be administered to children younger than 6 years. Older individuals should receive 2 doses of adult Td 8 weeks apart. In all cases, a booster dose should be administered 1 year later and at 10-year intervals.

Precautions

Diphtheria toxoid is associated with few side-effects in the pediatric age range. As it is a depot type vaccine, it should never be given by a route other than intramuscularly. In older children and adolescents, a reduced dose of diphtheria toxoid will ensure a low reaction rate and still provide effective immunization.

Antibody Preparations

A. **Diphtheria Antitoxin, Equine:** This material is prepared by hyperimmunization of horses and is available in vials containing 1000, 10,000, 20,000, and 40,000 units.

B. **Antitoxin Schedule:** Diphtheria antitoxin should be given as early as possible (half intramuscularly and half intravenously) in the following clinical situations: tonsillar, 20 thousand units IM; anterior nares, 10–20 thousand units; larynx, 20–40 thousand units; nasopharynx, 40–75 thousand units (dilute 1:20 in saline and administer slowly).

If the diagnosis has been delayed beyond 72 hours from the onset of symptoms and in very severe cases of diphtheria—especially those associated with considerable brawny edema of the neck—larger doses (80–120 thousand units) should be employed.

The unimmunized individual exposed to diphtheria who cannot be followed adequately should receive 10,000 units prophylactically.

Always test for horse serum sensitivity. Administer all antitoxin intravenously if symptoms are severe and the disease is life-threatening. The actual dose of antitoxin is less critical than early administration. If the patient has been ill more than 48 hours, increase the dose. *Note:* Never substitute antibiotic therapy for antitoxin therapy.

Table 5–2. Recommended schedules of active immunization.

Normal infants and children		Those not immunized in infancy	
2 months	DTP[1] and TOPV[2]	**Less than 6 years of age (cont'd)**	
4 months	DTP and TOPV	14–16 years of age	Td
6 months	DTP and TOPV*	Every 10 years therafter	Td
15 months	Measles, mumps, rubella[3]	**6 years of age and older but less than 18 years**	
~ 18 months	DTP and TOPV	Initial	Td and TOPV
4–6 years (school entry)	DTP and TOPV	1 month later	Measles, mumps, rubella
14–16 years	Td	2 months later	Td and TOPV
Every 10 years thereafter	Td	6–12 months later	Td and TOPV
Those not immunized in infancy		14–16 years of age	Td
Less than 6 years of age		Every 10 years thereafter	Td
Initial	DTP and TOPV	**Older than 18 years**	
1 month later	Measles, mumps, rubella	Substitute IPV[4] for TOPV and give boosters as directed	
2 months later	DTP and TOPV	by manufacturer.	
4 months later	DTP		
6–12 months later (or preschool)	DTP and TOPV		

*TOPV optional. Should be administered in areas anticipating importation of poliovirus, eg, southwest border states.

[1]**DTP:** Diphtheria and tetanus toxoid—alum precipitated or aluminum hydroxide adsorbed combined with suspension of pertussis bacilli or extracted pertussis bacillary antigens—to be administered IM.

[2]**TOPV:** Live polioviruses types I, II, and III in liquid form for oral administration. TOPV is preferred vaccine (American Academy of Pediatrics, Committee on Infectious Diseases of USPHA, Special Institute of Medicine Poliovirus Immunization Review Panel).

[3]**Measles, mumps, rubella:** All are live vaccines prepared in tissue culture and administered subcutaneously. Live measles vaccine may be administered alone if preferred, or in commercially available combinations (see text). If these vaccines are given separately, a 1-month interval between them should be observed. The only live measles vaccine available is further attenuated, which should *not* be given with gamma globulin. Whenever possible, tuberculin testing should be performed prior to measles virus vaccine administration (see text).

[4]**IPV:** Inactivated polioviruses types I, II, and III. Some experts feel it should be offered as a choice to all individuals. Most experts agree it is the preferred vaccine for the immunodeficient or immunosuppressed patient and as primary immunization for adults.

PERTUSSIS

Potent pertussis vaccines confer immunity upon infants given the full schedule. Attack rates can be reduced from 90% to less than 15%. One major problem is the need for early protection in infants since little or no maternal immunity is transferred. Although schedules in which immunization is started at 6—8 weeks of life result in a lower level of antibody than those beginning after 6 months of age, it is vital to begin immunization early, accepting a somewhat lesser immunologic effect for the earlier protection afforded. Furthermore, booster doses eliminate the difference between the early-immunized and the later-immunized.

England has experienced a continuing controversy concerning pertussis vaccine in the last decade. Analysis of the English experience is of interest since the principles can influence practice elsewhere in the world.

Pertussis in England was rampant prior to the introduction of vaccine in 1958. The incidence was reduced 50% by 1961, and the vaccine is believed to be responsible. Pertussis has continued to decrease in incidence since that time. There have been outbreaks, however, and many experts feel these episodes were related to fluctuating potency of the vaccines in use *plus* uneven application of vaccine.

Since 1968, the vaccines in use have been potent and the strains included have been appropriate to the types producing disease. An Expert Committee has concluded in 1977 that the vaccines in use are effective in protecting against pertussis.

Critics of pertussis vaccine in Britain have cited the toxicity of vaccine as unacceptable. The Expert Committee has concluded that the risk of serious sequelae is slight. Reported sequelae are frequent, but 2 factors suggest that these reactions are probably not related to pertussis vaccine: (1) the reactions are those that occur in the age group receiving pertussis vaccine among those who are uninoculated; and (2) the serious reactions cannot be attributed to pertussis vaccine directly since they are syndromes resulting from many other causes. In addition, pertussis itself has serious sequelae and a significant morbidity rate. Fully 10% of infants with pertussis are hospitalized in England, and the fatality rate remains unchanged in infants despite advances in medical care.

The comprehensive review conducted by the Joint Committee on Vaccination and Immunization of the Central Health Services Council and the Scottish Health Service Planning Council led to the conclusion that pertussis vaccine should be continued in routine infant immunization programs.

Outbreaks of pertussis in the USA are now being observed in preteen and teen-age children who received full infant immunization but were not boosted beyond the preschool years. We ordinarily refrain from pertussis immunization in older children because the reaction rate is high. Pertussis immunization must therefore be determined by the epidemiologic circumstances. In communities with high attack rates, one might wish to begin immunization in the newborn period and carry booster programs through the 12th year of age, recognizing that booster doses will be necessary in order to achieve a high level of immunity beyond the first few months of life. Untoward reactions in older children include severe fever, convulsions, and, rarely, encephalopathy. In communities where pertussis occurs rarely or never, ordinary scheduling suffices for adequate immunity. It would be unwise to abandon pertussis immunization completely since the child may move from an area of low incidence to one where the incidence is higher.

The best available data tend to indicate that pertussis immune globulin is unimportant in clinical practice. There is sound immunologic reason to doubt the efficacy of pertussis immune globulin. Injected IgG antibody should not be expected to prevent or treat an infection of the respiratory mucosa. From available data, it appears that the administration of erythromycin may afford the best prophylaxis in exposed susceptibles and is useful in bacteriologic cure in early pertussis. In well-established disease, reduction in the number of bacteria does not appear to influence the course of the disease.

Vaccines Available

A. Plain Pertussis Vaccine (Without Alum): Useful in epidemics for rapid protection. Administer 3 IM doses of 0.5 ml (4 NIH units) each at monthly intervals.

B. Adjuvant Pertussis Vaccine (With Alum, Aluminum Phosphate, or Aluminum Hydroxide): Give 3 IM doses of 0.5 ml (4 NIH units) each at monthly intervals for primary immunization. Within 8—12 months following primary immunization, whether plain or adjuvant pertussis vaccine, a booster dose of adjuvant vaccine should be used.

C. Diphtheria-Tetanus-Pertussis (DTP): See p 119.

Immunization Schedules

Pertussis immunization is usually started at 6—8 weeks of age with combined diphtheria-tetanus vaccine. Three doses at bimonthly intervals complete primary immunization. Booster doses should be administered 8—12 months after completion of the primary series. Ordinarily, pertussis immunization is maintained by boosters at approximately 18 months and 4 years of life (prior to starting school).

In areas of high endemicity, one may wish to start immunization with 0.5 ml of adjuvant pertussis vaccine on the second day of life in a healthy infant, with monthly doses at 1 and 2 months. An initial booster dose at 8—9 months of age and the regular boosters at 18 months and 4 years would complete the series. Additional boosters at 8 and 12 years could also be given. If this method is chosen, DTP could be given instead of adjuvant pertussis vaccine. If it is not, then DT (pediatric) should be administered in doses of 0.5 ml at monthly intervals for 3 doses early in infancy.

Precautions

Since pertussis vaccine is usually a depot antigen, it should only be given intramuscularly. Local and systemic reactions (tenderness, induration, and fever) are common, and many physicians prescribe aspirin routinely for 2–12 hours following immunization. Severe reactions are less common, and those involving the CNS least common. The occurrence of a severe febrile reaction or any CNS symptoms following pertussis immunization is an absolute contraindication to further doses. Pertussis vaccine should be administered to infants with CNS disease only after their first birthday—and then cautiously, in fractional doses.

Antibody Preparations

Pertussis immune globulin is available commercially. Almost all experts agree that it is of unproved value and do not recommend its use, either prophylactically or therapeutically. Some clinicians still resort to its use in young infants because of the high morbidity rate of the disease, with occasional deaths.

Although data are lacking, some experts suggest the administration of erythromycin (40 mg/kg/day) to exposed infants. There is evidence that erythromycin can eradicate the organism in established disease without necessarily influencing the course of illness.

TETANUS

Tetanus vaccine is one of the best immunizing agents available, conferring almost 100% protection in a fully immunized individual. A prolonged period of adequate immunity follows primary immunization, and booster doses are required only 10 years apart. Military personnel who received primary immunization in the 1940s maintained adequate serum antitoxin levels or were easily "boosted" by a single dose as long as 20 years later.

Vaccines Available

A. Plain Tetanus Toxoid (Fluid): This preparation is rapidly absorbed, resulting in more rapid immunization, but it is rarely needed.

B. Tetanus Toxoid, Aluminum Phosphate Adsorbed: The usual "booster" toxoid. Administer 0.5 ml IM as a booster; 3 doses spaced at monthly intervals provide primary immunization.

C. Tetanus-Diphtheria Toxoid (Pediatric and Adult): See Diphtheria, above.

D. Diphtheria-Tetanus-Pertussis (DTP): See next section.

Immunization Schedules

Three doses of 0.5 ml of an adjuvant tetanus toxoid suffice for primary immunization. Booster doses should be given 1 year later and every 10 years thereafter.

Management of injuries requires (1) early treatment, (2) adequate surgical care of the wound, (3) antibiotic therapy, if indicated, and (4) tetanus immunoprophylaxis. With minor injuries, prophylaxis is not necessary, although this may be an opportunity to start tetanus immunization in an unimmunized individual. In the case of injuries involving heavy contamination or extensive tissue destruction or delay in treatment, it is desirable to employ both tetanus immune globulin and recall tetanus vaccine in the previously immunized. With lesser injuries, tetanus immune globulin should not be given, but a booster (0.5 ml) dose of toxoid should be administered if a booster dose has not been given in the past 5 years. In the unimmunized, both tetanus immune globulin and tetanus toxoid should be given. It is imperative that full immunization subsequently be completed in the unimmunized.

Precautions

Tetanus toxoid is one of the safest immunizing antigens in the pediatric age range. Reactions are very infrequent and usually mild when they do occur, consisting only of local erythema and tenderness. More severe local reactions, sometimes accompanied by fever, are encountered in older individuals with repetitive doses of toxoid. Reduction in dosage reduces the risk of such reactions.

Antibody Preparations

A. Tetanus Immune Globulin, Human (Hyper-Tet): This is the preparation of choice. It has virtually no side-effects and is not immunologically removed from the circulation, ensuring prolonged antitoxin levels. It is supplied in 250 unit vials. The prophylactic dose is 250–500 units administered IM. The therapeutic dose is uncertain, but 3000–6000 units is the recommended initial dose. It is thought that this dose is sufficient, but in severe cases one may repeat it if the clinical response is unsatisfactory.

B. Tetanus Antitoxin, Equine: This preparation should not be used today because of the dangers of horse serum sensitization. (Whenever possible, human tetanus immune globulin should be used.)

The equine preparation is supplied in 1500, 3000, 20,000, and 40,000 unit vials. For prophylaxis against tetanus, give 5–10 thousand units. For therapy of tetanus, give 50–100 thousand units—preferably half intravenously and half intramuscularly (given simultaneously)—after testing for horse serum sensitivity.

C. Tetanus Antitoxin, Bovine: This preparation was formerly used for individuals sensitive to horse serum. It is available only from Merck Sharp & Dohme by special contact. It has largely been superseded by human tetanus immune globulin.

COMBINED DIPHTHERIA-TETANUS-PERTUSSIS (DTP) IMMUNIZATION

The most common and most practical method for immunizing infants and young children is the combination of diphtheria and tetanus toxoids with pertussis vaccine (DTP). The combination has the advantages of triple immunization simultaneously and in one injection plus the enhancement of pertussis vaccine potency by the adjuvant effect of the toxoids. It has the disadvantage of confusing the etiology of reactions since all 3 antigens are given at once.

Vaccines Available

A. Diphtheria and Tetanus Toxoids and Whole Pertussis Vaccine: This is a combination of the bacterial-suspension of pertussis plus the 2 toxoids. It is usually distributed in multiple dose vials. The individual dose is 0.5 ml IM.

B. Diphtheria and Tetanus Toxoids and Extracted Pertussis Antigen: Contains the 2 toxoids (as above) with a cell-free extract of pertussis organisms. The claim has been made that it causes fewer local and systemic reactions. However, the results of one study show that the reduced reaction rate is attributable solely to a lower incidence of local reactions and that the incidence of systemic reactions is not affected.

Immunization Schedules

Three 0.5 ml doses of vaccine are administered IM at bimonthly intervals, usually beginning at 2 months of age. A booster dose should be given at 18 months and again at 4–5 years. Thereafter, the pertussis component is eliminated and DT or Td preparations are utilized. (Exceptions are noted under Pertussis, above.)

Precautions

As for the individual components.

POLIOMYELITIS

Poliovaccines afford a high degree of protection to individuals adequately immunized against all 3 types. Both inactivated (killed, Salk) and attenuated (oral, live, Sabin) vaccines produce satisfactory immunity.

The advantages of inactivated vaccine (IPV) are that it cannot cause polio from the vaccine, the assurance that the vaccinee receives the vaccine, and simplicity of storage. The disadvantages include reduction in antibody titer and, presumably, immunity with the passage of time; the ability of wild poliovirus to grow in the intestinal tract of the vaccinee; and the need for repeated intramuscular injections.

The advantages of attenuated vaccine (OPV) include ease of administration (oral); prolonged immunity; intestinal immunity, which prevents wild poliovirus multiplication in the intestinal tract; a lesser risk of sensitization to vaccine constituents other than poliovirus; and its ability to limit epidemics by mass application. Its disadvantages include uncertainty of adequate immunization if the vaccinee vomits or if it is given early in life; the potential instability of types

3 and 1, which appear to have reverted to neurovirulence and have produced clinical polio in a few recipients or contacts of recipients; and the need for storage and maintenance at freezing temperatures.

In the past 3 years, considerable controversy has developed between those advocating IPV and those who support OPV. This controversy has erupted into the legislative and public domains, with the result that an Expert Committee of the Institute of Medicine was established to reconsider poliovaccine policy. The report issued in 1977 contains the following recommendations and findings:

(1) Continued use of OPV as the principal vaccine.

(2) IPV should be provided for persons with heightened susceptibility to infection (immunodeficient children and their siblings, immunosuppressed persons, adults undergoing initial vaccination, adults traveling to areas of high incidence of disease).

(3) OPV is acceptable for adults who have previously been immunized or if circumstances do not permit adequate intervals for IPV administration.

(4) IPV should be provided to any individuals who elect to receive it after being informed of the risks of OPV and the recommendation that it be administered. Such persons should be prepared to make a commitment to the full schedule of IPV immunization.

(5) One dose of OPV is recommended for all entrants into the seventh grade or equivalent. (Of course, a full series of trivalent OPV should be given to those who are unimmunized.)

(6) Any other immunization options were considered imprudent until at least 90% of persons are adequately immunized. Federal support was urged to accomplish this high rate of vaccine acceptance and use.

(7) These recommendations should be reviewed in 5 years, or sooner if a 90% immunization rate is achieved.

(8) Current consent forms should be modified to reflect the above recommendations. Specifically mentioned were (a) more information on IPV and (b) a statement about a person's right to request IPV.

Within the pediatric age range, it would appear that attenuated vaccine in its trivalent form represents the safest, simplest, and most effective immunizing material. Until the issues are completely resolved, primary and so-called "booster" doses of poliovaccine should be the trivalent attenuated type.

In epidemics, monotypic vaccine corresponding to the epidemic type should be administered in a mass, short-term campaign. This method will result in limiting the epidemic but should be followed with efforts to provide protection against the nonepidemic types.

Early problems with inactivated vaccine manufacture which permitted live polio or simian viruses to remain in supposedly inactivated lots are no longer existent. Inactivated vaccines are now free of any demonstrable viral agent prior to release.

Vaccines Available

A. Inactivated Poliovaccine: This is a formalde-hyde inactivated virus containing all 3 types (1, 2, and 3). The viruses are grown on monkey kidney tissue culture containing minute amounts of penicillin. Neomycin is added during manufacture to ensure sterility. The vaccine does not contain alum or any other adjuvant. The vaccine is supplied in 9 ml vials. The usual dose is 1 ml IM.

At this time (late 1977), IPV is not readily available. One Canadian firm manufactures IPV and has an outlet in the USA, but supplies have been limited to date.

B. Monovalent Attenuated Poliovirus Vaccine: This vaccine is supplied as the live attenuated virus, which is grown on monkey kidney tissue culture. The vaccines are monospecific, ie, they will confer protection only against the type administered. They must be stored at less than $0°$ C for maximum stability. If stored at ordinary refrigerator temperatures ($0-4°$ C), the vaccine must be used within 30 days; once the vial is opened, the period of use is reduced to 7 days. In order to ensure stability, the freezer compartment of most office refrigerators will suffice provided ice can be maintained continuously as a solid. The dose is 200–500 thousand $TCID_{50}$. (Consult manufacturer's brochure for exact dosage.)

C. Trivalent Attenuated Poliovirus Vaccine: This preparation is similar to the monovalent preparation except that it contains all 3 types of poliovirus in a single dose. Each dose contains more types 1 and 3 polioviruses than type 2 in order to prevent inhibition of the others by type 2. Storage and dosage considerations are similar to those outlined above for the monovalent vaccine. A new preparation of trivalent poliovirus vaccine grown in human fetal tissue (WI–38) was licensed in 1972 and is equivalent in characteristics to the monkey kidney tissue-grown preparation.

Immunization Schedules

Scheduling of polio immunization has undergone many revisions and a number of alternatives are available to the practitioner. A final and definitive schedule awaits long-term safety and immunity data. For the present, the following regimens are listed in the order of preference:

A. Trivalent Attenuated Vaccine Alone:

1. Infants—Three oral doses of trivalent vaccine are administered concurrently with DTP immunization at 2, 4, and 6 months of age. This regimen is followed by single doses of trivalent attenuated vaccine at 18 months and 4–6 years of age (just before entry into school).

2. Older children—Two oral doses of trivalent attenuated vaccine are administered 6–8 weeks apart. This regimen can be utilized in the unimmunized, in those whose previous immunization is uncertain, in those who have received monovalent attenuated vaccines, or in those previously immunized with inactivated vaccine. An additional dose of trivalent vaccine

should be given at entry into school or nursery school if this is 12 months or more following the initial series.

B. Monovalent Attenuated Vaccine:

1. Infants—Oral type 1 vaccine should be given first, followed in 6–8 weeks by type 3 and, in an additional 6–8 weeks, by type 2. This sequence is required to ensure that type 2 does not inhibit immunization· with types 1 and 3.* Subsequent doses are given as trivalent vaccine at ages 18 months and 4–5 years.

2. Older children—The schedule is the same as for infants. Trivalent "booster" doses are given at suggested ages only if feasible; if the child is older, give one trivalent dose 12 months after the primary series.

C. Inactivated Vaccine:

1. Infants—Give three 1 ml doses IM at monthly intervals. The vaccine can be given in combination with DTP if mixed immediately prior to injection. Alternatively, give at a different site as a separate injection. Booster doses are given 12 months later and at approximately 2-year intervals for as long as protection is considered necessary. Some prefer to give trivalent attenuated vaccine after infancy. Conversion to live vaccine by 3 doses, 2 months apart, is advised except in cases with immunologic deficiencies.

2. Older children, adolescents, and adults—If inactivated vaccine is the desired method of immunization, follow the recommendations in ¶ 1, but do not administer attenuated vaccine to individuals over age 18 as initial immunization. (See Institute of Medicine's recommendation on page 120.) Immunity may be maintained by 1 ml inactivated vaccine every 2 years, although exact schedules for booster doses are uncertain.

Precautions

Inactivated poliovaccine causes essentially no side-effects. It is an aqueous product and does not contain alum.

OPV (attenuated vaccine) is associated with a remote risk of paralytic disease. In normal infants the risk approximates one per 9 million doses. In siblings and other contacts of an immunized individual, the risk is somewhat higher, probably one per 6 million doses. The risk to immunodeficient individuals is much higher, but a precise figure cannot be established since the base denominator is not known.

Persons over 18 years of age should not receive the attenuated vaccine as an initial immunization. Known immunodeficient children or persons who are immunosuppressed should not receive OPV.

Antibody Preparations

Although much human gamma globulin is labeled polioimmune globulin, its use in the prevention of this disease is antiquated. Such labeling simply implies standardization of the preparation for its polio anti-

---

*This is in accord with American Academy of Pediatrics recommendations. The USPHS Advisory Committee on Immunization Practices recommends the sequence 2-1-3.

body content. It is true that polio can be prevented by the prophylactic use of gamma globulin, but there are no indications for its use for this purpose in modern medical practice.

MEASLES

Attenuated measles vaccine affords 95–100% protection against natural disease. Immunity appears to be long-lived—probably lifetime—but the exact duration will only be determined by continued observation.

Recent experience indicates that a sizable reservoir of susceptible persons exists despite the widespread use of measles vaccines in the last 14 years. Subpopulations in this reservoir include the following:

(1) Unimmunized persons at all ages—probably as high as 30–35%. Despite distribution of 88.5 million doses of vaccine since 1963, only 68.6% of children under 13 years of age had received vaccine by 1975.

(2) Individuals who received vaccine which was rendered inert by incorrect storage, handling, or administration. The size of this group is unknown.

(3) Individuals who received active live vaccine but failed to be immunized. There are several subgroups in this category:

(a) 3–5% who fail to be immunized—so-called "primary vaccine failures." This appears unavoidable with current vaccines, which are successful in 95–97% of the persons who receive it. There is no way of identifying such individuals.

(b) Infants immunized prior to 13 months of age, especially if gamma globulin was also administered. Failure of immunization in this group is probably the result of sustained maternal immunity. Estimates of the failure rate by age are as follows: 9 months of age, 35%; 12 months, 15–22%. There is controversy concerning the number of immunization failures at 12 months.

(c) Individuals given live vaccine after having received killed or inactivated vaccine. In many of these persons, the live vaccine was rendered inert in vivo by antibody developed after inoculation of killed virus.

(4) Recipients of inactivated vaccine, alone or in combination with live vaccine (so-called KKK or KL or KKL recipients). These children not only were unimmunized on a permanent basis but retain an unusual susceptibility to wild measles virus which causes severe disease on exposure ("atypical measles").

These observations have led to revision of live measles vaccine recommendations in 1977 by the American Academy of Pediatrics Committee on Infectious Diseases (Red Book Committee) and the Advisory Committee on Immunization Practices of the Public Health Services. These new recommendations will be detailed later.

Each of the attenuated vaccines is associated with a predictable febrile response and, in some instances, a morbilliform rash. The incidence of fever and rash is reduced by concomitant administration of measles immune globulin or by the use of further attenuated measles vaccine instead of the Edmonston attenuated strain (see below).

Inactivated measles vaccines are associated with relatively short-term immunity and a sufficient incidence of serious immunologic effects to warrant discontinuation of their use since 1965. Inactivated vaccines have demonstrated an altered reactivity to live measles virus, resulting in unusual local reactions to subsequent live virus administration and in a "new" disease—atypical measles—upon exposure to the wild virus, even 14 years after receipt of killed vaccine.

Vaccines Available

A. Attenuated Measles Virus Vaccine, Edmonston Strain (Enders Vaccine): The Edmonston virus, originally isolated in human cells, had been adapted to chick embryo tissue culture, in which the vaccine is prepared. This type of vaccine is no longer available.

B. Further Attenuated Measles Virus Vaccine (Schwarz or Moraten Strains): This product was prepared from Edmonston strain virus and passaged many additional times in chick embryo tissue culture. The result is further attenuation, with a lessened capacity for febrile and exanthematous reactions but apparent preservation of immunologic potency. The advantage of this vaccine is that it does not require simultaneous administration of measles immune globulin. The Moraten strain is the only currently available live virus vaccine.

C. Inactivated Measles Virus Vaccine: Two preparations were marketed for use; they are no longer available. One was prepared in monkey kidney tissue culture and the other in chick embryo tissue culture. The American Academy of Pediatrics has officially advised that their use be discontinued. For children already immunized, it is suggested that a subsequent dose of attenuated vaccine be used (see Immunization Schedules, below).

D. Combined Vaccines: Measles (rubeola) vaccine has been combined with rubella (German measles) virus alone, and also with both rubella and mumps viruses.

Immunization Schedules

Attenuated measles vaccine should be administered at 15 months of age. If vaccine is given earlier, a significant number of individuals fail to be immunized presumably as a result of sustained maternal immunity (see above).

In an epidemic situation, it is prudent to immunize infants 6–15 months of age, realizing that some will not be immunized. Such individuals must receive a second dose of vaccine after they attain a calendar age of 15 months. Second doses of live measles vaccine have not been associated with untoward effects, although experience is limited.

Children who have received live virus vaccine at 12 months of age pose a dilemma for the clinician.

Such children number in the millions, and it is deemed imprudent to reimmunize all of them because of the limited experience with 2 doses of live virus vaccine. However, in an epidemic situation, it is probably wise to reimmunize those who are at risk of exposure. It is hoped that this dilemma will be resolved by an intense immunization campaign which should reduce the incidence of minor epidemics of measles.

Considerable confusion occurs as a result of varying recommendations by national advisory groups, local health departments, legislative statutes, and individual expert opinion. The major problems with the new recommendation of 15 months for initiating live measles virus vaccine are listed below with suggested courses of action:

(1) Should individuals immunized in the past at less than 15 months but on or after 12 months of age be reimmunized? As stated above, *routine* reimmunization of all such individuals is not recommended for the following reasons:

(a) Millions of children are involved, and over 85% of them are already immune. To reach the approximately 15% who are not immune would require administration of a second dose of live vaccine to the 85% or more who are. Although second doses of live virus vaccine are thought to be safe, the data are insufficient to be certain.

(b) One modification of this negative recommendation is to reimmunize those at high risk of exposure to natural disease. Thus, if in a given year and a given community measles is epidemic, it may be prudent to administer live vaccine to individuals who received their primary immunization at 12 months of age.

(c) Another reason for not routinely immunizing such individuals is the controversy about the accuracy of the data implying failure of immunity in 15–22% of children immunized at 12 months of age. Some studies do not show this effect, and some experts dispute the new recommendation.

(2) Should individuals immunized prior to a specified year, usually 1965 or 1968, receive a second dose of live virus vaccine? This recommendation is being made by some health departments on the following bases: (a) Children immunized prior to these dates most likely received their primary immunization either at or before 12 months of age; or (b) gamma globulin was apt to have been administered with the live vaccine.

The routine use of a given year as the cutoff point for recommending reimmunization is not felt to be sound. Rather, the specific history (or records) of each child should be examined and a decision made based on the reasoning detailed above.

Gamma globulin administration is cited as a reason for reimmunization as a result of confused interpretation of the data. The following facts are known: (a) If gamma globulin was given with Edmonston virus (the original measles strain, not currently in use) at an appropriate dose and at a separate site, using a separate syringe, the child will be protected. This observation is supported by the long-term studies of Krugman and

coworkers in New York. (b) If gamma globulin was given in too large a dose, or mixed with live virus vaccine, or injected at the same site, it is possible that the vaccine was rendered ineffective. (c) If gamma globulin was given in the usual dose for the Edmonston strain but in conjunction with one of the further attenuated strains (Schwarz or Moraten), it is possible that the vaccine virus was inhibited. (d) If gamma globulin was given with live virus vaccine *prior to* 12 months of age, immunization may not have occurred.

Again, it is wise to review the specific record of each recipient in order to make a sound decision regarding the necessity for a second dose of live virus vaccine.

(3) Should rubella and mumps live virus vaccines also be given at 15 months of age? Although there is evidence that live mumps and rubella vaccines are fully effective when given at 12 months of age, for practical purposes it is recommended that they be given together with measles vaccine at 15 months of age. The advent of the combined vaccine MMR (Merck) has made this practical suggestion easily implementable. One can give a single product at 15 months of age and accomplish protection against all 3 viruses in 95% or more of recipients.

(4) What should be done with children whose history is unknown or confused? The prudent course to follow in instances where exact information concerning the timing and nature of the vaccines given is not available is to administer the appropriate vaccines as if no immunization had been given. The single precaution is in the instance of possible prior receipt of killed (inactivated) measles vaccine. In this circumstance, a local or systemic reaction may result (see below).

For individuals older than 15 months of age, a single dose of attenuated vaccine is sufficient. If the child has had natural measles but this is not certainly known, attenuated vaccine administration causes no untoward effects. Susceptible adolescents and adults have been immunized with no greater clinical symptoms than those seen in infants and children.

Further attenuated vaccine administration results in fever (5–15%) and rash (5%). No concomitant measles immune globulin need be given.

A special use of attenuated measles vaccine is in the just-exposed child. If attenuated vaccine is administered just prior to or on the day of exposure to natural disease in a susceptible child, the disease may be prevented by successful immunization. This is because the incubation period of the vaccine is approximately 7 days, in contrast to a 10-day period for the natural disease. However, if exposure has occurred one or more days previously, it is best to administer a preventive dose of measles immune globulin and to administer live virus vaccine 6–8 weeks later.

Inactivated measles virus vaccine is no longer available. A state of altered immunologic reactivity to live virus, attenuated or wild, appears to be induced in some vaccinees. This will result in induration, erythema, and tenderness at the site of subsequent attenuated virus vaccine in 6—50% of previous recipients of inactivated vaccine. Additionally, upon exposure to natural disease months or years after receiving inactivated vaccine, some children develop an atypical measles characterized by pneumonia with or without pleural effusion, a petechial rash, edema, and temperatures of 39.5—40.5° C (103—104.9° F). Because of the risk of atypical measles, children who have been immunized with inactivated vaccine should be given attenuated vaccine. Although this may result in a local reaction in some cases, the risk is acceptable in the face of potentially serious atypical measles.

Combinations of inactivated and attenuated vaccines are not recommended. All recipients of such combinations in the past should be regarded as inactivated vaccine recipients, and a second dose of attenuated vaccine should be administered as above.

One investigation of a large scale measles outbreak in a major city revealed a few instances of modified or atypical measles occurring in children who had previously been immunized with live virus vaccine. Although this finding has led to questions about the permanence and quality of immunity following live measles virus vaccine, the incidence of such reactions is very low and no firm recommendations can be derived at this time. Only continued observation of vaccinees and the passage of time will provide the definitive information needed to merit reappraisal of current policy. For the present, practice should be guided by the overwhelming accumulation of data that suggest that long-term, solid immunity follows the administration of live virus vaccine.

Acute encephalitis has occurred after live measles virus vaccine but with much lower frequency than following natural disease. The rate of all neurologic disorders occurring within 30 days of live measles virus vaccine is 0.99 cases per million doses. This compares with one case of encephalitis per 1000 cases of natural measles, or a 1000-fold reduction.

Subacute sclerosing panencephalitis (SSPE) has also been observed following live measles virus vaccine. It occurs about 20 times less frequently after vaccination than after the natural disease.

Precautions

Inactivated measles vaccine is not recommended. Its side-effects have been commented upon above.

Because attenuated measles vaccine has been associated with febrile convulsions, a history of febrile convulsions is a contraindication to its use. The vaccine has rarely been associated with CNS complications. As with any live vaccine, its administration to pregnant females and to infants and children with acquired or congenital immunologic deficiencies is contraindicated.

Vaccines prepared in chick embryo tissue should not be administered to children who cannot eat a whole egg without developing allergic symptoms.

Some children with proved egg allergy have been given chick embryo-grown measles vaccine under controlled circumstances without untoward effect. However, the number is small, and the recommendation is to *not* immunize such children except in very unusual circumstances.

Antibody Preparations

Measles immune globulin is human gamma globulin in which the measles antibody content is standardized at 4000 measles neutralizing units/ml. The dose for use in attenuated measles virus immunization is 0.01 ml/lb (0.025 ml/kg). In the prophylaxis of measles following natural exposure of a nonimmune individual, the dose is 0.1 ml/lb (0.25 ml/kg). This is the so-called preventive dose. Prevention of measles depends upon administration of an adequate dose early in the incubation period, usually within 6 days of exposure. The author believes the concept of modifying measles by administration of a smaller dose (0.02 ml/lb [0.05 ml/kg]) of gamma globulin following exposure is unwise. In the unimmunized susceptible, it is best to attempt protection with gamma globulin upon exposure and to administer attenuated vaccine 8—12 weeks later.

Grand MG & others: Clinical reactions following rubella vaccination. JAMA 220:1569, 1972.
Horstman DM: Rubella: The challenge of its control. J Infect Dis 123:640, 1971.

SMALLPOX*

Smallpox immunization confers virtually 100% protection within 6—12 months following successful immunization and gradually diminishing protection against disease thereafter. At 20 years after immunization, protection is virtually nil. However, once one is successfully immunized, protection against death, if the disease is contracted, is of a very high order. Repeat successful vaccinations at 1—4 year intervals aid in the maintenance of a high level of immunity.

A recent decision of the WHO Expert Committee on Smallpox makes the definition of successful takes easier. Reactions following primary immunization are considered *major* if there is evidence of a take 7 days later—a vesicular lesion at 7—10 days in a primary take, or a vesicle, pustule, or definite induration and congestion surrounding an ulcer or scab following revaccination. All other reactions are *equivocal* and an indication for revaccination. Almost everyone can be vaccinated; the few people in whom successful takes repeatedly fail into 2 categories: (1) those who are vaccinated by improper technic or with impotent vaccine, and (2) true nonreactors (rare). The former can be successfully vaccinated by an experienced person. The latter probably have had an active-passive immunization earlier and are truly resistant to reimmunization, although very rare instances defy explanation.

*Despite worldwide reduction in incidence of smallpox, which has confined it to a small area in Africa, this section is retained because the vaccine is still used occasionally.

Smallpox is endemic only in Ethiopia and Somalia; all the rest of the world is now smallpox free. Most of the Western world has eliminated the requirement for compulsory infant immunization and for a valid vaccination certificate for entry if travel has been limited to nonendemic regions. Smallpox vaccination is still indicated for all individuals resident in or traveling to or from endemic areas.

Vaccines Available

A. Calf Lymph Smallpox Vaccine: This preparation is derived from the dermal pulp of vaccinia virus-infected calves. The vaccine contains 100 million pock-forming units of vaccinia virus supplied either as a glycerinated aqueous preparation or freeze-dried (lyophilized). The dose is not a measured one but consists of enough virus to produce a localized skin infection when the skin underlying a drop of vaccine is scratched or multiply punctured.

B. "Avianized" Smallpox Vaccine: This product is derived from an egg-adapted vaccinia virus strain. It is as potent in titer as the calf lymph vaccine but produces milder vaccination reactions. Its use is as described under calf lymph vaccine.

Immunization Schedules

Smallpox vaccination as a routine compulsory immunization is no longer recommended. The World Health Organization, the USPHS Advisory Committee of Immunization Practices, and the Red Book Committee on the American Academy of Pediatrics are unanimous in this recommendation.

Precautions

See Vaccinia in Chapter 25.

Antibody Preparations

Vaccinia immune globulin (VIG) is human gamma globulin collected from young military recruits following vaccination. Its titer is variable but usually approximates 620 neutralizing antibody units—in comparison with a titer of 64 or less in randomly collected gamma globulin. It is used in complications of vaccination, and the dosage is variable (0.3—0.6 ml or more per kg body weight IM). (See Chapter 25.)

RUBELLA

Rubella is a benign disease of childhood. The major reason for immunization is to prevent rubella infection of pregnant females and subsequent fetal infection. In 1964, more than 20,000 infants died or were permanently handicapped as a result of intrauterine rubella infection.

Immunization is recommended by the various immunization advisory committees for all prepubertal children in the USA. In England and elsewhere, immunization is only recommended among women of childbearing age.

The efficacy of rubella immunization is conjectural at present. More than 96% of recipients develop demonstrable serum antibody, and short-term exposure trials have demonstrated protection against disease. However, reinfection with mild rubella virus occurs in individuals previously immunized, and it is not known whether a previously immunized pregnant female who is reinfected will transmit the virus to her fetus. Most virologists do not believe intrauterine infection will occur in the fetuses of previously immunized pregnant women because viremia has not been demonstrated.

Rubella virus is recoverable from the throat in more than 75% of recipients of vaccine. The virus is present in low titers, and except in a few instances transmission to a susceptible contact has not been observed. It thus appears unlikely that a susceptible pregnant woman will contract rubella from an immunized child, although the potential exists.

Arthritis and arthralgia have been observed in recipients of rubella virus vaccine. In children, the frequency is low. In adolescents and adults, over 10—30% of recipients have had this manifestation of immunization, parelleling the incidence in natural disease.

Peripheral neuritis, resulting in prolonged and painful neuromuscular syndromes, has been observed rarely in children who have received rubella vaccine. Two forms are thus far recognized: one affecting the upper extremities with severe, recurrent pain; and another affecting the lower extremities, resulting in a peculiar crouching posture. The exact significance and extent of these syndromes is not defined at present.

Vaccines Available

Several different preparations are now commercially available. The reader is advised to consult the manufacturers' brochures concerning specific instructions for administration.

Two recently licensed products with which experience is limited incorporate rubella virus with measles in one preparation and with measles and mumps in the other. There is no loss of antigenicity in these combinations, and they appear to be safe.

Immunization Schedules

Current policy is to administer rubella vaccine routinely in infancy and to attempt immunization of all susceptibles prior to pubescence. In addition, some experts advise identification of rubella susceptibility in postpubescent girls by antibody testing and subsequent live virus administration. If this approach is to be used, the following should be observed:

(1) Inform patient (and parent, where applicable) of risks of vaccine, including the occurrence of arthralgia and arthritis and the potential risk of fetal infection if pregnancy is current or occurs within 2 months.

(2) Obtain a negative pregnancy test.

(3) Advise a medically sound program of contraception for at least 2 months following vaccine administration.

Although rubella vaccine can be administered at

12 months of age, since the recommendation to change measles vaccine to 15 months has been made and since rubella vaccine is most practically (and frequently) given in combination with measles (MMR), it is most practical to administer it at 15 months of age.

Precautions

The usual precautions concerning live virus vaccines apply to rubella virus vaccine also. (See Measles, above.)

Rubella virus immunization may result in arthritic symptoms or in peripheral neuritis syndromes. These conditions postdate immunization by as much as 70 days, and the association may not be apparent unless sought.

There is a potential risk of decidual or fetal infection if a woman is pregnant at the time of receipt of rubella virus vaccine or becomes pregnant shortly thereafter (see Immunization Schedules, above).

Antibody Preparations

No specific rubella gamma globulin preparation exists. Standard pooled adult gamma globulin has been used in exposed pregnant females in an effort to prevent transplacental virus transmission. Results to date have been unsatisfactory with doses of 20–40 ml IM.

Center for Disease Control: Rubella virus vaccine: Recommendation of the Public Health Service Advisory Committee on Immunization Practices. Ann Intern Med 75:757, 1971.

MUMPS

Mumps is generally a benign disease which in most children either is asymptomatic or causes only mild to moderate symptoms. Infection may be accompanied by aseptic meningitis, pancreatitis, or orchitis or oophoritis. The gonadal complications are the major reasons for protecting adolescents and adults against mumps. An attenuated vaccine has recently become available which induces antibody in 98% of susceptible vaccinees, and early studies indicate almost complete protection for 1 year and possibly for 2 years. Further data on the duration of immunity will become available with continuing observation of vaccinees.

Inactivated vaccine confers only partial and short-lived immunity; it is not a very good immunizing agent.

Vaccines Available

A. Attenuated Mumps Vaccine, Jeryl-Lynn Strain: This vaccine is a chick embryo adapted mumps virus to which neomycin has been added. It is supplied as a freeze-dried (lyophilized) powder to be reconstituted according to the manufacturer's directions. Its stability is such that reconstituted vaccine must be used within 8 hours, preferably immediately. Storage of the dry powder is at ordinary refrigerator temperatures. The vaccine is light-sensitive and should be protected from sunlight. The dosage is 0.5 ml IM.

B. Combined Vaccine: Mumps vaccine has been combined with measles and rubella virus vaccines. In the combined vaccine, it appears to be antigenic and safe.

Immunization Schedules

Routine mumps vaccination in childhood is now recommended by the Committee on Infectious Diseases of the American Academy of Pediatrics. Mumps immunization has a lower priority than any of the others discussed above, but it is especially recommended that the following groups who have not had mumps should receive the vaccine: children approaching puberty; adolescents and adults, particularly males; institutionalized children; and children in large groups where epidemic mumps may disrupt normal routines. Routine use in children should be limited to those over age 1 and only after DTP and poliomyelitis immunizations are complete.

The introduction of combined measles-mumps-rubella vaccines has led to the practical abandonment of individual vaccine indications. For those physicians who choose not to use the triple vaccine routinely at 15 months of age, the separate products can be administered according to the specific recommendations listed for each component.

The susceptible exposed adolescent or adult poses a difficult problem. It has been estimated that oophoritis occurs in 5% of females with mumps and unilateral orchitis in 20–30% of males. Although sterility is an extremely uncommon result, the gonadal infection is an uncomfortable and incapacitating one. Current methods of prophylaxis are not reliable. Inactivated vaccine is of dubious value, and mumps immune globulin (see below) is said to reduce orchitis by 75% (although adequate studies are lacking). The best course appears to be to administer attenuated mumps vaccine prior to exposure. It has no value at or following exposure because antibody development requires 28 days.

Precautions

As with other live vaccines, mumps vaccine should not be given to pregnant females, to children with congenital or acquired immunologic deficiencies, or to egg-sensitive individuals (see Measles, above). No untoward reactions have been observed in a small number of adults given the vaccine.

Antibody Preparations

Mumps immune globulin is human gamma globulin obtained from hyperimmunized donors. The mumps antibody content is 20 times that of human mumps immune serum.

Mumps immune globulin is available. The author does not recommend its use since its efficacy has not been proved.

SPECIFIC IMMUNIZATIONS
FOR SPECIAL CIRCUMSTANCES

RABIES

In the USA, about 50,000 persons receive rabies immunization each year. The vast majority of these immunizations are unnecessary, but the disease is so feared and the circumstances surrounding many animal bites so uncertain that administration of the vaccine seems the safer course to follow. However, there is a predictable morbidity with rabies immunization, and if unnecessary immunizations are given too frequently the risk of complications of the vaccine or antiserum will outweigh the potential benefits. The physician must know the epidemiology of rabies in his area. A bite from a pet beagle is not equivalent to a similar bite from a stray street dog. In the first situation rabies is exceedingly unlikely, and in the second it is a distinct possibility. The often quoted WHO recommendations will not be repeated here since they are not applicable to most of the world and certainly not to most of the USA. The physician is referred to his state health department and to the USPHS for local information about rabies epidemiology in his area of practice.

Vaccines Available

A. Inactivated Rabies Vaccine, Animal Nervous Tissue Origin (Semple Vaccine): This is a sterile suspension of rabies virus in rabbit brain and spinal cord. The vaccine is prepared from animals 6 days after inoculation with fixed virus. The virus is then inactivated by phenol (Semple method) and supplied in individual dose ampules.

B. Inactivated Rabies Vaccine, Duck Embryo Tissue Origin: This consists of propiolactone inactivated virus to which various stabilizing agents are added plus thimerosal as a preservative. Antibody develops within 10–15 days after initiation of daily immunization. The vaccine is distributed as single dose vials with diluent in a package containing 14 doses. Follow the manufacturer's recommendations for storage, reconstitution, and dosage.

Vaccine Schedules

A. Preexposure Immunization: This is recommended for persons at high risk of exposure—veterinarians, laboratory technicians working with diagnostic specimens or rabies virus, deliverymen and others who are frequently bitten by dogs, spelunkers (cave explorers) exposed to bats in caves, etc. Two effective schedules are employed: (1) three injections of 1 ml subcut at weekly intervals, followed by 1 ml subcut in 5–6 months; (2) two injections of 1 ml subcut 1 month apart and then 1 ml subcut 7 months later. Booster doses of 1 ml are suggested every 1–2 years. Antibody titers must be determined, because immunization is not 100% effective.

B. Postexposure Immunization: Because the incubation period of rabies is often prolonged, postexposure immunization is feasible. The exact regimen used is empiric and largely based upon Pasteur's original schedule coupled with antibody stimulation data. The usual regimen is to give 14–21 subcutaneous injections of 1 ml each. Injections are usually given over the abdomen, each one in a different site. Severe bites or bites about the head and neck are indications for prolonging the daily injections to 21 days. In individuals who have been bitten by wild animals, it may be desirable to give twice daily doses of vaccine for 7 days and daily doses for 7 more days in an attempt to stimulate early antibody production. If the animal is healthy after 5 days, the injections should be discontinued. All other patients are treated for at least 14 days. If severe systemic reactions or neuroparalytic complications occur, the injections must be discontinued.

The most difficult decision is whom to immunize. The WHO guidelines are not universally applicable, and more harm than good may follow indiscriminate rabies immunization in an area where there is no risk of rabies. The practitioner must be guided by the rabies epidemiologic data in his area. Nevertheless, some general guidelines can be suggested.

1. Wild animal bites, particularly by skunks and bats, are absolute indications for rabies prophylaxis.

Frequently, therapy is delayed in the case of wild animal bites pending confirmation of rabies in the captured or killed animal. The author believes this is an unwise practice. Therapy should be started as soon after the bite as possible. One can always discontinue therapy if the animal is proved to be free of rabies, but lost time cannot be regained if the animal is rabid.

2. Pets seldom become infected unless exposed to a rabid animal. Pets with current rabies immunization are obviously not a risk.

3. Provoked bites in toddlers are seldom an indication for immunization, particularly if the animal is a pet.

4. Stray animals pose a special problem since they frequently cannot be found. The physician must depend upon current epidemiologic information and balance the risks of immunizing against the possibility of rabies.

5. Rodents are seldom infected with rabies.

6. If in doubt and the animal is impounded, begin immunization and discontinue the series after 5 days if the animal remains healthy. The complications of immunization are uncommon before the fifth day, and a rabid animal will not appear healthy 5 days after biting someone. If the animal sickens or dies, it is essential that adequate virologic examination be carried out by the local public health authorities.

Surgical Management & Antiserum

Adequate prophylaxis against rabies must include (1) extensive surgical (possibly chemical) debridement of the bites as quickly as possible after the episode (excisional surgery is best) and (2) concomitant use of human rabies immune globulin (see below). This recent improvement in rabies prophylaxis is most welcome. The use of potent human globulin avoids the risks of horse serum administration. Part of the dose can be administered at the wound site by infiltration at the edges of the bite and the remainder given intramuscularly. Although supplies of human rabies immune globulin appear sufficient for the anticipated need, on occasion it may be unavailable or a long delay may be encountered. In these instances, one should use the horse serum product, since the longer the interval between the rabid bite and administration of antibody, the less the protective effect. Whenever possible, human globulin should be used.

For maximal benefit, the immune globulin should be administered as soon as possible after the bite—ie, within 24 hours if possible and certainly within 72 hours. When passive antibody is used, additional doses of rabies vaccine (preferably avian type) should be given 10 and 20 days after the primary series.

Precautions

Approximately 1:6000 rabies immunizations with animal brain tissue result in neurologic sequelae. These consist of 3 clinical types: encephalitic, myelitic, and neuritic. The encephalitis has its onset suddenly 6—54 days following the first dose of vaccine. Chills, fever, headache, vomiting, and changes in mental state are observed. The myelitic and neuritic complications are paralytic, usually consisting of flaccid paralysis of the lower extremities. Its onset is more gradual. The neurologic sequelae are usually not fatal, although as many as 35% result in permanent residual deficits.

Duck embryo vaccine has been associated with 4 cases of neurologic sequelae in 90,000 14-day courses—a very low reaction rate. Much more common is the occurrence of tenderness, erythema, and induration at the site of inoculation. These local reactions tend to occur after the fifth day and may be associated with a flare-up at previous injection sites. Lymph node enlargement and tenderness can also be observed. Rarely, anaphylactic shock has occurred. Great caution should be exercised in persons with known egg allergy.

Antibody Preparations

Rabies immune globulin (human) is prepared from the plasma of human volunteers who have been actively immunized. It is identical to all human gamma globulin preparations. This is the preferred preparation for use in rabies prophylaxis. With adequate supplies, it should completely replace the horse serum preparations. It is available as Hyperab (Cutter) and is dispensed in 2 and 10 ml vials containing 150 IU/ml. The dosage is 20 IU/kg, administered as soon after the bite as possible. Up to half of the total dose can be infiltrated into the edges of the wound and the remainder given IM.

Rabies antiserum is horse serum containing 1000 units/ml of rabies neutralizing antibody. All of the precautions in administration of horse serum should be observed.

INFLUENZA VACCINE

Although some doubt the efficacy of influenza vaccines, most experts agree that protection in excess of 65—75% can be expected with their use. Non-epidemic influenza is a relatively unimportant cause of serious childhood respiratory infections. Epidemic or pandemic influenza may result in significant morbidity in very young infants and in individuals with chronic cardiac, pulmonary, metabolic, renal, or neurologic disease. Furthermore, institutionalized children may constitute a unique epidemiologic setting, facilitating rapid spread. These groups should be immunized regularly, but especially in epidemic years. Pandemic spread may require more broad-scale immunization of healthy infants and children, particularly when a new antigenic strain appears.

As a result of experience in 1976—1977 with swine influenza immunization, much was learned of the safety and efficacy of influenza vaccines in children. Whole virus vaccine appears to be too toxic for use in children. However, preparations of inactivated vaccine which have been chemically treated to "split" the virus into its highly antigenic surface antigens are apparently both safe and effective.

Vaccines Available

Influenza vaccine is chemically inactivated virus. There are 2 principal forms. The first consists of the entire virus (whole virus vaccine) and will not be further discussed as it is not recommended for children.

Further treatment of whole virus vaccine produces a highly concentrated surface antigen product—the so-called "split virus vaccine." This preparation currently contains antigens of the prevalent "A" strain of influenza—A/Victoria vaccine—and the expected "B" strains—B/Hong Kong.

The vaccine is an aqueous suspension and is administered intramuscularly.

Immunization Schedules

Routine immunization is not currently recommended. Only children at increased risk of influenza infection should receive the vaccine; these include children with chronic cardiovascular and respiratory diseases, malignant neoplasms, immunodeficiency syndrome, and immunosuppression. Other groups that may be eligible are those with chronic disabling neuralgia or metabolic and renal diseases.

Precise dosage information is given in Table 5—3.

Booster doses should be given yearly or at least within 3 years of primary immunization.

Side-Effects

Three types of side-effects and adverse reactions have been observed. They are more frequent with whole virus vaccine and neglible following split virus vaccine. Children with no prior influenza virus experience are more vulnerable to the toxic effects of influenza virus preparations.

Table 5–3. Influenza vaccine dosage by age, type of vaccine, and potency for 1977–1978.*

Age	Type of Vaccine	Dose	Potency†	Number of Doses Required
6 months–3 years	Split virus	0.15 ml	120	2
3 years–5 years	Split virus	0.25 ml	200	2
6 years–17 years	Split virus	0.5 ml	400	1

*All vaccines contain A/Victoria/75 and B/Hong Kong/72.
†Chick Cell Agglutinating (CCA) units.

(1) Toxic effects, presumably due to the viruses' innate toxicity, consist of fever, malaise, myalgia, etc, beginning 6–12 hours after immunization and lasting 1–2 days.

(2) Presumed allergic responses occurring within a short time after receiving the vaccine and consisting of immediate hypersensitivity or type I reactions—wheal and flare, urticarial lesions, and anaphylaxis. These are very rare and may be related to egg sensitivity, although no such relationship has been proved.

(3) Neurologic reaction—much more common in adults. Guillain-Barré syndrome has been observed infrequently after influenza immunization, occurring at a rate of ~10/million persons vaccinated. It also occurs in nonimmunized individuals. Permanent paralysis and even death have occurred.

Precautions

A history of severe reaction to influenza vaccine should preclude its readministration.

Egg-sensitive individuals should not receive the vaccine, as the virus is grown in hens' eggs.

Influenza vaccine is not absolutely contraindicated in pregnancy but should be avoided just like any procedure that is not essential.

PNEUMOCOCCAL VACCINE

Pneumococcal disease still accounts for many cases of otitis media, lower respiratory tract infection, and meningitis in infants and children. Although penicillin has resulted in marked reduction in morbidity and mortality rates from these diseases, some individuals are at very high risk. The immunodeficient child, the child with sicklemia, and the functionally and organically asplenic child all represent high-risk groups for abrupt, life-threatening pneumococcal disease. The disease encountered in these children is often fulminant and thus difficult to treat early and effectively. In addition, some pneumococci have been demonstrated to be resistant to penicillin and other commonly used antibiotics. These facts argue for the use of an effective vaccine, at least in selected groups of children.

In late 1977, a vaccine containing the purified capsular polysaccharide of 14 of the most common strains of pneumococci causing disease in humans was approved for use by the FDA.

Vaccine Available

Pneumovax (Merck) is a mixture of capsular polysaccharides of 14 types of pneumococci, including those that account for almost 83% of 3500 bacteremic infections in humans. The vaccine contains 50 µg of each component antigen. *Since this is a new product, the physician is advised to consult the product brochure for specific dosage and route of administration.* In experimental trials children were given 0.5 ml subcutaneously.

Immunization Schedule

At this point, pneumococcal vaccine cannot be recommended for routine use. The available data for the 14-type product are very limited in children. More information has been accumulated using an 8-type product in children.

The vaccine appears to be of low reactogenicity, although data in children are limited.

A single dose appears to be all that is required at present; the need for booster doses, if any, has not been established.

Currently, only children over 2 years of age with high risk of death following pneumococcal infections are candidates for vaccination. Amman and coworkers suggest that patients with functional and anatomic asplenia as well as those with sicklemia can receive this vaccine safely and respond with demonstrable antibody titers. The immunized children with sicklemia, in addition, had significantly fewer serious bacteremic pneumococcal infections than unimmunized age-matched children with sicklemia (8 infections with 2 deaths compared to no infections).

At present, the vaccine can only be recommended for children with sicklemia and functional or anatomic asplenia. More data are needed before recommendations can be made for other children.

Precautions

Adverse effects have been observed only rarely in the few children studied and reported thus far. Local pain and low-grade fever have been noted.

TUBERCULOSIS

BCG (bacille Calmette-Guérin) vaccine is an attenuated tuberculosis vaccine which is indicated for children in geographic areas or in social circumstances where the risk of infection is high. A positive tuberculin test indicates BCG will be ineffective and potentially dangerous. The vaccine should not be given to any child with acquired or congenital immunologic deficiency.

Immunization is accomplished by intracutaneous, superficial injection over the deltoid or triceps muscle. The dosage is 0.05 ml (newborns) or 0.1 ml (for all other children).

CHOLERA

For infants and children traveling to or resident in cholera endemic areas, 3 intramuscular or subcutaneous injections at weekly (or longer) intervals are advised. The dosage is as shown below. Booster doses appropriate to age must be given as often as every 6 months to maintain immunity.

	6 Months– 4 Years	5–9 Years	10 Years– Adult
First dose	0.1 ml	0.3 ml	0.5 ml
Second dose	0.3 ml	0.5 ml	1.0 ml
Third dose	0.1 ml	0.3 ml	0.5 ml

PLAGUE

Plague immunization is recommended for children residing in or traveling to endemic areas (particularly the Far East). Primary immunization is as follows:

	Age (in Years)			
	Less Than 1	1–4	5–10	Over 10
Day 0	0.1 ml	0.2 ml	0.3 ml	0.5 ml
Day 30	0.1 ml	0.2 ml	0.3 ml	0.5 ml
4–12 weeks later	0.04 ml	0.08 ml	0.12 ml	0.2 ml

YELLOW FEVER

Yellow fever vaccine is obtainable only from certain public health facilities. A single injection of 0.5 ml of a 1:10 dilution is given, with a similar booster dose every 6 years. For travel to certain areas, this immunization is mandatory. Consult authorities.

EPIDEMIC TYPHUS

Vaccination against epidemic typhus is recommended for persons traveling to endemic areas even though it is not required. The vaccine is given subcutaneously. The dosage is as follows:

	6 Months– 4 Years	5–9 Years	10 Years– Adult
First dose	0.2 ml	0.5 ml	1 ml
Second dose	0.2 ml	0.5 ml	1 ml
Third dose	0.2 ml	0.5 ml	1 ml

For children under 10 years of age the vaccine is given every 1–3 weeks; for those over age 10, the first 2 doses are separated by 1–3 weeks and the third is given 1 year later. Annual boosters are recommended.

IMMUNOPROPHYLAXIS & THERAPY

IMMUNE SERUM GLOBULIN (HUMAN) (ISG)

All human immune globulins currently available are similar in physical and chemical properties. All are prepared from pooled donor plasma (usually 1000 or more individual donors), are Cohn-fractionated, concentrated to a 16.5% solution, and have preservatives added. The generic term for such preparations is immune serum globulin (ISG). ISG contains principally IgG with only trace amounts of IgA, IgM, and other serum proteins. The IgG tends to aggregate on storage–a biologically significant phenomenon. Aggregated IgG behaves as antigen-antibody complexes and has produced anaphylaxis on entry into the bloodstream. For this reason, ISG must be administered intramuscularly and great care must be exercised to avoid injection directly into a vessel.

ISG can be very irritating because of its concentration. Doses larger than 5 ml must be split and injected deeply intramuscularly into separate large muscle masses.

The antibody content of a specific ISG depends upon the pool from which it is derived. Ordinary ISG contains those antibodies generally present in adults in large quantities–measles, hepatitis, pneumococcal, etc. ISG which has been prepared from selected donor pools is termed special immune globulin (SIG) and is labeled with the name of the disease which is to be prevented or treated, eg, tetanus immune globulin, rabies immune globulin. SIG has carefully calibrated amounts of antibody directed against a specific infectious agent. The use of the various specific SIG preparations is discussed elsewhere in this chapter.

Adverse effects of ISG or SIG are few. Pain on injection is usual, particularly with large doses. Rarely, so-called sterile abscesses may develop. Administration of ISG intravenously can result in anaphylactic shock due to aggregated IgG; rarely, anaphylaxis follows intramuscular administration of large doses if absorption is rapid. Individuals who receive ISG may develop antibodies against some components. For example, individuals lacking serum IgA (one in 800 of the general population; a higher rate in some disease states) will develop anti-IgA antibody directed against the trace amounts of IgA present in ISG. Subsequently, upon exposure to passive IgA such as occurs with blood transfusion, pyogenic reactions may occur. In similar fashion, antibody may develop against IgG in pooled ISG which is genetically different from the recipient's IgG. Subsequent administration of "foreign" IgG may result in reactions.

A potential adverse effect of ISG administration is anticipated but has not yet been demonstrated. Women who receive ISG may develop antibody directed against those types of immunoglobulin which are genetically different from their own. If, during a subsequent pregnancy, a woman who has received ISG has a fetus who possesses one of these different immunoglobulin types, it is conceivable that her preexistent antibody will suppress fetal immunoglobulin synthesis. Hypoimmunoglobulinemia may result in the fetus and be manifest after birth. This situation is analogous to Rh incompatibility. Thus far, this potential phenomenon has not been recognized, but it remains a threat which should moderate the indiscriminate use of ISG.

There are only 3 unequivocal indications for ISG administration: (1) as replacement therapy in IgG-deficient states, (2) in the prevention of measles, and (3) in the prevention of infectious hepatitis. All other uses are either unproved or unwarranted.

Replacement Therapy in IgG-Deficient States

Passive antibody can protect individuals incapable of IgG synthesis. Most conditions warranting such therapy are genetic immunodeficiencies; a few acquired states are associated with deficient IgG (see Chapter 15). The usual dose for initiating adequate IgG levels is 1.4 ml (220–240 mg)/kg body weight as a single dose. Subsequent doses are for maintenance; 0.6–0.7 ml/kg body weight every 3–4 weeks is usually sufficient. All of these doses are empiric, and some variation may be expected. The best guideline for adequacy of therapy is the absence of serious bacterial infections (eg, bacteremia, meningitis) in the individual patient. Serum immunoglobulin levels are unreliable in predicting the adequacy of ISG therapy. Infections of the mucosal surfaces may not diminish with ISG administration since the individuals being treated usually have secretory IgA deficiencies which are not repaired by ISG administration.

Administration of ISG will not benefit patients with neutrophil dysfunction, lymphocyte-mediated immune deficiency, complement deficiency, or any other non-IgG deficient condition.

Measles Prevention

See discussion on p 122.

Prevention of Infectious Hepatitis

Specific hepatitis immune globulin is still in the developmental stage, and the clinician must rely upon ISG to protect exposed susceptibles. Prophylaxis against infectious hepatitis (type A hepatitis) should be offered family contacts and individuals experiencing heavy or continuous exposure.

A. Family Contact Exposure: This is defined as any relationship in which individuals share living, eating, and toilet facilities. This includes many babysitters or other caretakers, lodgers, and members of some sports teams as well as blood relatives living together. This category usually does not include schoolmates, members of social groups, or casual contacts. The dose is 0.02–0.04 ml/kg body weight in a single dose. The expected duration of protection is 5 weeks.

B. Intense or Continued Exposure: This is defined as the kind of exposure experienced by persons who provide custodial care with maximal fecal exposure (eg, attendants in institutions for the mentally retarded or psychiatrically ill patients), health workers with repeated exposure to clinical cases, or travelers to endemic areas with primitive hygienic facilities.

The dose is 0.06 ml/kg body weight. With continued exposure, the same dose is repeated in 5–6 months. Continuous exposure for this length of time is probably associated with infection during the passive protection period, and further doses of ISG are unnecessary.

To date, ISG has proved unreliable in the prevention of serum hepatitis (type B HB_S Ag-positive hepatitis). ISG prepared since 1972 appears to have higher effective antibody levels against serum hepatitis. This may be related to selection of donors only from antigen-negative donors. Experts now suggest that post-1972 ISG can protect against minimal exposure such as pricking one's finger with a needle known to be contaminated with antigen-positive blood. The suggested dose is 5 ml.

Unproved, Unwarranted Use of ISG; the Abuse of Gamma Globulin

ISG should not be given when it is not indicated because it is painful and costly and in limited supply. The most common abuse is the administration of ISG to children with frequent upper respiratory coryzal symptoms, most frequently due to allergic disease. Without demonstrable IgG or antibody deficiency, there is no indication for the use of ISG in this common situation.

ISG has no place in the treatment of asthma, allergic rhinitis, and other allergic diseases, recurrent herpes simplex (hominis) infections, recurrent group A hemolytic streptococcal infections, most established bacterial infections, in children who fail to thrive, or as a last resort in incurable diseases.

There are some uses for ISG which are controversial or equivocal. Examples are patients with severe burns, susceptible varicella contacts, and pregnant women exposed to rubella. There are a few reports suggesting that ISG administration might be beneficial in the prevention of pseudomonas infection in severely burned young patients. Most available information does not support the use of ISG in burned patients.

Certain susceptible varicella contacts (newborn or young infants, patients with lymphatic malignancies) are given ISG in large doses to prevent chickenpox. ISG in large doses can modify varicella but does *not* prevent the disease. It is better to administer zoster immune globulin (ZIG) for this purpose (see p 728). Pregnant women who are susceptible to rubella and exposed in the first trimester pose a frustrating problem. If therapeutic abortion is not contemplated, there is no way to make certain that the fetus will be protected. Large doses (20–40 ml) of ISG have been administered, but there is no evidence that this protects the fetus and some data suggest that it does not.

•   •   •

General References

Arbeter AM & others: Measles immunity: Reimmunization of children who previously received live measles vaccine and gamma globulin. J Pediatr 81:737, 1972.

Barkin SZ, Barkin RM: Measles-mumps-rubella vaccine: Advance in immunization. Rocky Mt Med J 72:247, 1975.

Berg JM: Neurologic complications of pertussis immunization. Br Med J 2:24, 1958.

Bloom JL & others: Evaluation of a trivalent measles, mumps, rubella vaccine in children. J Pediatr 87:85, 1975.

Brickman HF, Beaudry PH, Marks MI: The timing of tuberculin tests in relation to immunization with live viral vaccines. Pediatrics 55:392, 1975.

Committee on Infectious Diseases: *Report,* 18th ed. American Academy of Pediatrics, 1978.

Deforest A & others: The effect of breast-feeding on the antibody response of infants to trivalent oral poliovirus vaccine. J Pediatr 83:93, 1973.

Eickoff TC: Immunization against influenza: Rationale and recommendations. J Infect Dis 123:446, 1971.

Fleet WF & others: Fetal consequences of maternal rubella immunization. JAMA 227:621, 1974.

Goldstein JA & others: Smallpox vaccination reactions, prophylaxis, and therapy of complications. Pediatrics 55:342, 1975.

John TJ: The effect of breast feeding on the antibody response of infants to trivalent oral poliovirus vaccine. (Correspondence.) J Pediatr 84:307, 1974.

Krugman RD & others: Improper handling of live virus vaccines in clinical practice. J Pediatr 85:512, 1974.

Krugman S: Present status of measles and rubella immunization in the United States: A medical progress report. J Pediatr 78:1, 1971.

Krugman S: Rubella immunization: A five-year progress report. N Engl J Med 290:1375, 1974.

Landrigan PJ, Witte JJ: Neurologic disorders following live measles-virus vaccination. JAMA 223:1459, 1973.

Mellman WJ & others: Depression of the tuberculin reaction by attenuated measles virus vaccine. J Lab Clin Med 61:3, 1963.

Rasmussen CM & others: Inadequate poliovirus immunity levels in immunized Illinois children. Am J Dis Child 126:465, 1973.

Rousseau WE & others: Persistence of poliovirus neutralizing antibodies eight years after immunization with live, attenuated-virus vaccine. N Engl J Med 289:1357, 1973.

Sanders DY, Cramblett HG: Antibody titers to polioviruses in patients ten years after immunization with Sabin vaccine. J Pediatr 84:406, 1974.

Weibel RE & others: Measurement of immunity following live mumps (5 years), measles (3 years), and rubella (2½ years) virus vaccines. Pediatrics 49:334, 1972.

Weibel RE & others: Persistence of immunity following monovalent and combined live measles, mumps and rubella virus vaccines. Pediatrics 57:467, 1973.

White WG & others: Duration of immunity after active immunization against tetanus. Lancet 2:95, 1969.

6 . . .
Ambulatory Pediatrics

Barton D. Schmitt, MD

This chapter offers guidelines for the conduct of 4 specific types of pediatric visit: (1) health maintenance care, (2) acute illness care, (3) chronic disease follow-up, and (4) consultation. Each type of visit requires a specific service that is different in many ways from the others. If the pediatrician and the staff can mentally classify the patients in this way and vary their approach accordingly, the delivery of pediatric care will become more logical and consistent.

This organization of ambulatory care has 3 general advantages: (1) The quality of care improves since the patient benefits from the comprehensiveness of care that only a systematic approach can ensure. (2) The practice of pediatrics becomes more enjoyable because the establishment of clear office guidelines and policies prevents many frustrations and much duplication of effort for the physician. (3) The cost of medical care is reduced by increasing the efficiency of health care delivery.

HEALTH MAINTENANCE VISITS*

OBJECTIVES

Health maintenance or health supervision visits are the key to preventive pediatrics. These visits involve 3 people: the physician, the parent, and the child. The child should assume a more active role in his own health care with each passing year. The visit has multiple purposes: responding to the parent's or child's current concerns, presenting age-appropriate anticipatory guidance, assessing growth and development, performing a physical examination, obtaining laboratory screening tests, and administering immunizations. A natural outcome of these visits is a deepening of family-physician rapport.

*In cooperation with Dr. Burris R. Duncan.

Samples of forms, flow sheets, etc discussed in this chapter may be found on pp 156–173. No permission is required to reproduce them.—*The Editors.*

PARENTAL CONCERNS

The first part of each well child visit should be directed toward dealing with the current concerns of the parent, usually the mother. Most expectant mothers have many questions which should be discussed with their pediatrician several weeks prior to delivery. The most frequent concerns include the arguments for and against breast feeding, preparation of the breasts if breast feeding is to be used, hospital policies about when the mother can hold her baby and begin his care, separation problems with the other children during the mother's confinement, and ways of decreasing sibling jealousy. It has been traditional for the first newborn office visit to take place at 6 weeks, probably because 6 weeks is the traditional time for the mother's first postdelivery obstetric visit. However, most mothers—particularly primiparas—have many questions and concerns well before this traditional interval after birth. A 2-week postpartal office visit is much more logical.

The early weeks and months are characterized by rapid change. The infant doubles his birth weight in the first 5 months and triples it within the first year. His length increases 50% in the first year, but it takes 4½ more years for it to increase another 50%. His head circumference increases 40% in 1 year, whereas in the next 17 years head circumference increases only another 16%. The newborn changes from a totally dependent, passive individual who sleeps 18–20 hours a day into a curious, mobile, independent, negative 2-year-old. This constant confrontation with change often causes anxiety, concern, and frustration in the parents. During the health maintenance visit the physician must encourage the parent to vent those feelings and he must be prepared to deal with them. Questions range from, "How frequently should I hold him?" to "Is it all right to spank children?" to "How old should he be before I should let him cross the street alone?" Many of the questions have no clear-cut answers. Many cannot be answered, but all should be discussed.

Alpert JJ & others: Delivery of health care for children: Report on an experiment. Pediatrics 57:917, 1976.

Heavenrich RM: Child health supervision—is it worth it? Pediatrics 54:52, 272, 1973.

Hoekelman RA: What constitutes adequate well-baby care? Pediatrics 55:313, 1975.

Korsch BM: How comprehensive are well child visits? Am J Dis Child 122:483, 1971.

Liptak GS, Hulka BS, Cassel JC: Effectiveness of physician-mother interactions during infancy. Pediatrics 60:186, 1977.

ANTICIPATORY GUIDANCE

Anticipatory guidance usually includes nutritional counseling, accident prevention, behavioral counseling, suggestions for developmental stimulation, sex education, dental recommendations, medical education, etc. A list of suggested topics to be discussed at particular ages is found on the Health Maintenance Encounter forms on pp 156 through 161. The significance of a dash or colon on these encounter forms is that a comment is required following that item. All anticipatory guidance advice is followed by the optimal age for discussion in parentheses. A check mark in the box that follows each of these advice items indicates that this counseling was done. These topics can be covered in a variety of ways. Some physicians prefer to discuss all the items with the parents personally; others prefer to delegate the discussion of these issues to an assistant, who might be either a nurse or a nonprofessional assistant; and still others use printed materials which can be supplemented by personal comments as the need arises.

American Academy of Pediatrics: *Standards of Child Health Care,* 2nd ed. Council of Pediatric Practice, 1972.

Browden J: Needs and techniques for counselling parents of young children. Clin Pediatr 9:599, 1970.

Illingworth RS: The prevention of accidents. Clin Pediatr 6:286, 1967.

Patterson GR, Gullion ME: *Living With Children.* Research Press, 1968.

EXAMINATION OF THE
PEDIATRIC PATIENT

The content of the physical examination of the well child depends upon the age of the child and the purpose for which the examination is done. The examination done in the delivery room or the first newborn office visit is far different from the preschool physical, and each is quite different from the examination required for participation in high school athletics.

1. EXAMINATIONS DURING INFANCY

Growth

A. Weight: An infant should gain 15–30 gm/day during the first 4 or 5 months of life. The newborn will regain his birth weight by age 10 days; at 2 weeks, he should weigh at least 60–120 gm more than his birth weight; and at 2 months he should weigh approximately 1500 gm (3.3 lb) more than he weighed at birth. This evaluation provides information about nutritional status, feeding and elimination, and the mother-child relationship.

B. Head Circumference: The head circumference at birth is frequently not accurate as a result of molding, scalp edema, or cephalhematoma, and is more accurate at the time of discharge. By 2 weeks of age, an exact measurement can be obtained as a reference point for further measurements of head circumference. By 2 months, the head circumference is in its steepest growth curve and should have increased about 4 cm.

C. Length: The newborn's length increases about 16% in the first 2 months of life from a mean of 50 cm to a mean of 58 cm.

Vision

Most newborns have the visual capacity to fix on a moving object as early as the first few minutes of life. Infants who do not follow a face at the first well child visit should be suspected of having a visual problem.

Hearing

A procedure for detection of congenital deafness is discussed in Chapter 11. Every physician who is responsible for the care of infants should develop similar screening programs in the hospital nursery and also check the infant's hearing at the 2 month visit by the use of squeak toys and bells which have as close to pure tone sounds as possible. The newborn may only respond by a flicker of his eyelids or by an abrupt arrest of movement. By 6 months of age, the infant should lateralize or turn toward the sound; by 12 months, the infant localizes sound which is lateral to and above or below the level of the ears.

Congenital Anomalies

Close attention to relatively minor malformations detectable by surface examination will alert the physician to the possibility of major internal malformations. In one important study (see Marden reference, below), 14% of newborns examined were found to have a single minor anomaly but no appreciable increase in the frequency of associated major abnormalities over the general newborn population; 0.8% of babies had 2 minor external defects which carried a 15% frequency of major internal abnormalities; and 0.5% with 3 or more minor anomalies had a 90% incidence of major defects. The minor abnormalities described in this study usually go undetected unless specifically looked for. Examples include lateral displacement of the inner epicanthic folds, downslanting or upslanting palpebral fissures, preauricular cutaneous tags or pits, incomplete helix development, absence of the lobulus of the pinna, low-set ears, simian crease, bridged palmar creases, short and broad nails, hypoplasia of the nails, clinodactyly of the fifth finger, deep dimples at bony promontories (elbows, sacrum), low posterior hairline, body hirsutism, multiple hair whorls, pectus excavatum, and short sternum. Attention should also be given at the 2-week visit to checking for several silent malformations, such as urine stream for lower urinary tract obstruction, stool pattern for Hirschsprung's disease, Ortolani's maneuver for congenital hip dislocation, femoral pulses for coarctation of the aorta, and inspection of the genitalia for cryptorchidism and imperforate hymen.

The Mother-Child Relationship

A very important question to ask of each new mother is, "Do you enjoy your baby?" The response is sometimes not congruent with what is observed as she handles her child. Many mothers will frankly admit they do not enjoy caring for the child but then feel guilty about that attitude. They need a listener and someone who can help them find ways to derive pleasure from their offspring. This must be done as early as possible; if it is not, the mother-child relationship may become more disturbed and the child will make life miserable for everyone around him or even be injured.

Early discussions should include what the parents expect from their child, whether the expectations are realistic, and how the parents resolve the difficulty when the child fails to meet those expectations.

Some mothers are highly maternal and others treat their newborns in a detached way. Observing an occipital bald spot and poor skin care tends to confirm an early suspicion of some disturbance in the mother-child relationship.

Anderson FP: Evaluation of the routine physical examination of infants in the first year of life. Pediatrics 45:950, 1970.

Bergstrom LB & others: A high risk registry to find congenital deafness. Otolaryngol Clin North Am 4:369, 1971.

Haggerty RJ & others: Symposium: Does comprehensive care make a difference? Am J Dis Child 122:467, 1971.

Marden PM, Smith DW, McDonald MJ: Congenital anomalies in the newborn infant, including minor variations. J Pediatr 64:357, 1964.

2. EXAMINATION BEFORE ENTERING SCHOOL

The preschool examination of the 4- or 5-year-old child should be designed to answer the basic question, "Is the child ready for school?" Listening to the child's chest at this examination is probably of far less importance than determining if he has any speech impediments, if his vision and hearing are normal, if his developmental age is commensurate with his chronologic age, if his attention span is adequate for learning, and

if his parents have adequately prepared him for the separation implied by entering school. This is not to say that these variables are not investigated prior to age 5; however, it is at the preschool examination that they are of greatest significance. See p 159 for a school readiness screening questionnaire.

Vision

Five to 10% of preschool children have some kind of visual impairment. The illiterate E chart, Snellen chart, or Allen cards can be used for checking visual acuity, and each eye should be tested separately. The 5-year-old child should have a visual acuity of 20/30 or better in both eyes, and there should be no more than a 2-line difference between the 2 eyes. Amblyopia ex anopsia affects 2–5% of children and must be detected early before permanent loss of vision occurs. Amblyopia is frequently secondary to strabismus, which can be detected by noting the position where light is reflected off both corneas or by using the more refined cover test (see Chapter 9).

Hearing

Hearing deficits occur in approximately 1% of young school children, and in 10% of those children the loss is profound and bilateral. Most children with hearing loss have recurrent purulent otitis media or serous otitis media. Even children with a single episode of otitis media may have some degree of hearing impairment for 3–6 months after the acute episode. Although the losses are generally not too severe, if they occur at an inopportune time they may be sufficient to prevent an early school-age child from learning phonics; hence, the effect of the loss may be carried on and magnified throughout much of the school years. If such losses are detected before entry into school, some of the learning problems and some of the behavior and discipline problems which occur secondary to poor attention might be averted. Detection of such problems is as much a part of preventive pediatrics as is the immunization routine. Audiologic screening tests can be performed by nonprofessional technicians and should be a part of the preschool examination.

Speech

The child entering school should be able to speak distinctly and clearly without difficulty. He should be able to answer questions and, after a period of getting acquainted, carry on a conversation with the physician about recent events or tell a story about something he has experienced. Poor speech may impair the child's general performance in school. An easily administered articulation test has been developed which can be used as a screening test to identify children who should be referred to a speech pathologist for definitive evaluation (see Drumwright reference, below).

Emotional Development & Behavior

The assessment of emotional development and behavior is an important part of the preschool examination. In one study, 42 physicians were observed conducting 673 well child clinic visits. On the average, they said fewer than 2 sentences per visit to the mother which were relevant to child behavior. Yet, when given the opportunity to respond to a questionnaire about behavior, 85% of mothers of preschool children (ages 1½–6 years) indicated one or more such concerns (mean of 3.5 concerns per child). A simple self-administered questionnaire (see Willoughby & Haggerty reference, below) is an effective and efficient device which not only indicates to the parent that the physician is interested in discussing behavioral problems and the emotional growth of the child but also helps the physician to concentrate on the areas of guidance which are most relevant to the mother's concerns. The 6 health maintenance encounter forms (pp 156–161) stress anticipatory guidance and counseling for behavioral aspects of pediatrics.

A number of easily administered developmental tests are available. The Denver Developmental Screening Test (see Chapter 2) is extremely helpful in the younger age groups. For a school entrance examination, the Peabody Picture Vocabulary Test and the Goodenough Draw-A-Man Test can be useful; both are easily administered in the physician's office by a nurse or a trained allied health worker. They should not be thought of as more than screening tests, but they can be used to identify children with developmental lags who may have difficulty in the early months of school as well as those who may need to be referred for psychologic evaluation.

Physical, emotional, and developmental maturation proceeds at different rates for different children. Some children are ready for school long before their fifth birthday; others are not nearly ready at that age. Some parents tend to push their children into experiences that are beyond their capacities at a given age. Children should begin their school experiences with successes; the child who starts with failure is often criticized and becomes discouraged and less interested in school, so that a pattern of failure may develop. The child may continue to lag behind and miss the early fundamentals of learning which are the basis for further education. Many children develop behavioral disorders and truancy simply because they cannot read and so are unable to understand what is going on in the classroom. Part of the physician's role is to help parents recognize physical, emotional, and developmental lags early so that corrective measures can be taken to prepare the child for school. If, despite these efforts, the child is not ready for school, the physician must advise the parents appropriately.

3. EXAMINATION OF THE TEENAGER*

The well child visit for the teenager who wants to participate in athletics or attend summer camp should

*See also Chapter 7, Adolescence.

be designed to elicit data about special concerns. Most such visits emphasize the physical status and immunologic status of the patient. The physician may perform mass examinations which merely fulfill a legal requirement that all participants should have "a physical." Physicians who examine professional athletes are interested in the player's strength, endurance, sensory perception, and judgment under game-simulated conditions, and the examination should assess those aspects. Unfortunately, however, the examination of the high school athlete is usually done with the student relaxed after sitting in the physician's office or standing in line at the school gymnasium and is apt to consist of nothing more than a "routine physical examination." The Cooper reference cited below describes an exercise test that can be used to measure a student's general physical fitness. The student is instructed to bring his gym shoes to the examination. He is given a stopwatch and told to run and walk as fast as he can for 12 minutes on the nearest track and report back to the physician the distance he has covered. His performance can be compared to standards listed in the reference. If this procedure is made a part of the routine yearly checkup, it can serve as a means of stimulating a teenager to increase his physical activity level.

Ideally, the adolescent should be given the opportunity to discuss problems which are of concern to him as an adolescent—rapid changes in sexual development, sexual drive, birth control, drugs, ambivalent feelings, and identity problems. He needs an understanding listener as much as he needs a physical examiner.

Allen CM, Shinefield HR: Automated multiphasic screening. Pediatrics 54:621, 1974.

American Academy of Pediatrics Committee on Children With Handicaps: Vision screening of preschool children. Pediatrics 50:966, 1972.

Cooper KH: *The New Aerobics.* Bantam Books, 1970.

Drumwright A & others: The Denver Articulation Screening Examination. J Speech Hear Disord 38:3, 1973.

Frankenburg WK & others: Training the indigenous nonprofessional. J Pediatr 77:564, 1970.

Grant WW: Health screening in school-age children. Am J Dis Child 125:520, 1973.

Willoughby JA, Haggerty RJ: A simple behavior questionnaire for preschool children. Pediatrics 34:798, 1964.

LABORATORY SCREENING TESTS

A health maintenance flow sheet (see p 162) is a helpful reminder to the nurse and physician that certain procedures, laboratory tests, developmental evaluations, and immunizations need to be done. All of these items can be initiated by the nurse or aide if the physician establishes the routine to be followed.

Blood

Iron deficiency anemia is found more often in lower socioeconomic populations and has its highest incidence in infants between 9 and 24 months of age. A routine hemoglobin or hematocrit is recommended in this age group and is particularly important in the child whose diet is low in iron-containing foods.

Some clinics advocate routine screening of all black children for sickle cell trait or disease. Sickle cell disease can be suspected on the basis of a routine hemoglobin determination. Sickle cell trait detection has led to misunderstanding in many parents and over-restriction of many children and might best be left until the late teenage years.

Screening for phenylketonuria should be done by blood test in the hospital nursery prior to the infant's discharge, and in many states such a test is required by law. A baby with this disorder who failed to ingest sufficient milk protein may have a negative test in the first few days of life. Therefore, most centers recommend a repeat PKU test at 10–14 days of age. Screening newborns for another treatable cause of mental retardation, congenital hypothyroidism, is also now recommended. A T_4 assay can be processed on cord blood.

Screening for lead poisoning is extremely important in areas where the child has access to lead-based paint or soil contaminated by lead. Children living in such cities should have a routine blood lead level performed at 18–24 months of age. This test should be repeated in children with pica.

Urine

Routine urinalysis has a low yield in the asymptomatic patient. In contrast to the adult population, it is unusual for a child to have asymptomatic diabetes, and proteinuria is a very infrequent presentation for a renal abnormality in an asymptomatic child. Transient orthostatic proteinuria is frequently found, but its significance has not been determined.

Urine cultures probably have a greater yield than microscopic examination of urinary sediment. Over half of children with significant bacteriuria have no pyuria. Significant bacteriuria has been found in 1% of infants 1–4 days of age; in 2% of infants between 4–12 months; and in 1–1.5% of school-age girls. If every girl had numerous urine cultures over a period of several years, up to 5% would be found to have a urinary tract infection. Several inexpensive methods are available to screen for bacteriuria (eg, Testuria).

The sexually active teenage female is becoming a commonplace pediatric problem. Such girls can benefit from yearly gonococcal cultures and Papanicolaou smears. Birth control counseling can also be offered at this time.

Bailey EN & others: Screening in pediatric practice. Pediatr Clin North Am 21:123, 1974.

Buist NR, Jhaveri BM: A guide to screening newborn infants for inborn errors of metabolism. J Pediatr 82:511, 1973.

Chisholm JJ: Screening for lead poisoning in children. Pediatrics 51:280, 1973.

Fost N, Kaback MM: Why do sickle screening in children? Pediatrics 51:742, 1973.

Galli ML: Recommendations for screening programs for congenital hypothyroidism. J Pediatr 89:692, 1976.

Hein K & others: The need for routine screening in the sexually active adolescent. J Pediatr 91:123, 1977.

Kunin CM: Emergence of bacteriuria, proteinuria, and symptomatic urinary tract infection among a population of school girls followed for 7 years. Pediatrics 41:968, 1968.

North AF: Screening in child health care: Where are we now and where are we going? Pediatrics 54:631, 1974.

IMMUNIZATIONS

A child's immunization status can be easily monitored on the health maintenance flow sheet (see p 162). It should be noted that the 15 month visit is for shots only in our clinic. A record of the child's immunizations should also be given to the parents and updated by the nurse as additional immunizations are given.

The details of routine immunization of children are presented in Chapter 5.

PARTICIPATION OF PARAMEDICAL PERSONNEL

A number of paramedical personnel (social workers, visiting nurses, nutritionists) as well as volunteer or semiprofessional women have been helping physicians take care of patients for many years. Only large clinics or group practices are able to employ and fully utilize such a variety of health workers. Some smaller pediatric offices have found it helpful to employ a social worker one-half day a week to help patients with serious emotional and social problems, since such patients would otherwise take up an inordinate amount of the physician's time.

In the past few years, many programs have been initiated to train new types of allied health workers and to make the actual work a person does more nearly commensurate with his training. Examples include pediatric nurse practitioners, chronic disease nurses, and community health workers. The Pediatric Nurse Practitioner (PNP) is a graduate nurse who has been given additional training which improves her skills as a nurse and equips her to take a complete history, to perform a physical examination which includes use of an otoscope and stethoscope, and to give well child guidance and counseling. Her role is to help the physician deliver health maintenance care and to distinguish the sick child from the well child and the abnormal finding from the normal one. The PNP is well accepted by parents, is able to answer parents' concerns about normal growth and development, and is accurate in her physical assessments. The time thus saved has allowed the pediatrician to spend more time with sick patients and to increase the total number of patients cared for.

In addition to these programs, Silver and others have trained an entirely new type of health worker, the Child Health Associate. This allied health worker, who has completed a minimum of 2 years of college and 3 years of pediatric training, is licensed to deliver all well child care and to diagnose and treat (under a physician's supervision) most acute ambulatory illnesses. His only responsibility for hospitalized patients involves healthy newborns. Help is thus available to the physician in caring for the expanding pediatric population. However, it is up to the doctor to utilize these deliverers of health care in an effective way, for he remains the one who is ultimately responsible for patient care.

Duncan B, Smith AN, Silver HK: Comparison of the physical assessment of children by pediatric nurse practitioners and pediatricians. Am J Public Health 61:1170, 1971.

Foye H, Chamberlin R, Charney E: Content and emphasis of well-child visits. Am J Dis Child 131:794, 1977.

Silver HK: A new primary-care medical practitioner. Am J Dis Child 126:324, 1973.

Silver HK, Igoe JB, McAtee PR: The school nurse practitioner: Providing improved health care to children. Pediatrics 58:580, 1976.

Silver HK, Ott JE: The child health associate: A new health professional to provide comprehensive health care to children. Pediatrics 51:1, 1973.

Townsend EH: The social worker in pediatric practice. Am J Dis Child 107:77, 1964.

Yankauer A & others: Pediatric practice in the United States: With special attention to utilization of allied health worker services. Pediatrics 45 (Suppl 3):521, 1970.

ACUTE ILLNESS VISITS

The episodic office visit for the child with an acute illness places special demands on the physician.

OBJECTIVES

Diagnosis and treatment of the chief complaint is the first priority for the parents, patient, and physician. Extenuating circumstances (eg, a crowded waiting room) rarely justify an incomplete work-up of an acute chief complaint.

Detection of problem patients who have a chronic disease or an undiagnosed chronic complaint is of nearly equal importance to the physician.

ASSESSING ACUTE ILLNESS

Optimal management of an acute illness mainly includes telephone triaging, office triaging, diagnosis, assessment of the need for hospitalization, home therapy, and a follow-up plan.

The detection of multiple problem patients is best accomplished by using a brief screening questionnaire, which should be completed on any new patient who makes his initial contact for sick care. Some parents have only crisis care available to their families (eg, in rural areas). Other parents have access to comprehensive health care but use only crisis care because their daily lives are beset with too many other problems (eg, urban slums). This situation is usually a byproduct of a disorganized poverty environment rather than a reflection of disinterest in preventive medicine. The screening questionnaire is unnecessary for patients already being followed for health maintenance care. It can be deferred if the patient has a true emergency problem. An example of a useful questionnaire is given on p 163.

The parent can complete this questionnaire while waiting to see the physician. Since it identifies only major problems, an affirmative answer to any of the first 4 questions should cause the physician considerable concern. In these cases, he should strongly recommend a follow-up appointment even if the parent has not requested ongoing health maintenance care.

Katcher AL: Efficient office practice. Pediatrics 59:533, 1977.

1. TELEPHONE TRIAGING & ADVICE

Does the Patient Need to Be Seen?

The physician himself is the person best qualified to give medical advice, both in the office and over the phone. However, talking with parents on the phone may take too much of a physician's time, so that delegation of this function to another member of the office team is desirable. Most of the questions are routine ones that require only routine answers. An office nurse is probably the best person to manage such routine medical calls. If the physician delegates this responsibility to her, he must first specifically train her for this role. For a nurse to be successful in giving medical advice, office policies should be standardized. Routine instructions for handling minor infections, minor injuries, reactions to immunizations, infant feeding problems, newborn care, and prescription refills are easy to communicate to parents if they are written down in an office protocol book. The protocol book should also clarify at what point each problem requires an office visit. This decision depends on (1) the type of symptom, (2) the duration of the symptom, (3) the age of the patient, (4) whether or not the patient acts "sick," (5) an assessment of the parents' anxiety, and (6) the presence of any underlying chronic disease. (For example, most patients under 1 year of age with diarrhea need to be examined in person.) After telephone baseline data are gathered, the nurse must be able to decide whether the child needs to be seen or not. She should err on the side of giving an appointment. For patients not seen, any pertinent telephone data should be entered on a temporary card file. If an office visit later becomes necessary, this data should be transferred to the patient's chart.

It is helpful if parents understand 2 general telephone rules: (1) the nurse will screen all calls from parents except emergency ones, and (2) calls regarding routine questions will only be accepted during office hours. Night calls should be restricted to urgent ones. Most routine calls come from overanxious, insecure mothers who need reassurance and acceptance, not criticism and abruptness. The conversation with the nurse should build the mother's confidence and independence. The mother can be asked what she had considered doing and have her approach strongly endorsed if it is at all reasonable. If parents are educated to be more medically independent, unnecessary visits will diminish, as will medical costs for society in general. However, the conversation should close with the feeling that telephone calls are considered an important aid in medical care and that the parent is free to call again.

The physician directly accepts some calls: (1) emergency calls from parents, (2) calls from other physicians, (3) calls regarding hospitalized patients, (4) long distance calls, (5) calls from a parent who "demands" to talk to the physician, and (6) calls where the nurse is unclear about what should be done. These exceptions to the rule are obvious. Parents reasonably expect their personal physician or his designated substitute to be readily available for emergencies, even if the "emergency" exists only from their viewpoint. The physician must be especially circumspect about calls after midnight, for they usually relate to psychosocial crises or urgent medical problems.

There are 4 other possible methods of dealing with telephone calls, any of which may serve as an alternative to having an office nurse give telephone advice: (1) The physician can accept calls continuously throughout the day. These interruptions are unacceptable to most physicians and parents. (2) The physician can have a telephone hour at the beginning and end of the day and accept only emergency calls at other times. The disadvantages of this approach are that some parents must then wait for answers to urgent questions and the physician wastes his time with many routine calls. (3) The physician may charge for telephone advice. This charge decreases the number of calls, but in the process it discourages important calls and thereby interferes with preventive pediatrics. (4) The physician can allow various nonmedical office personnel to protect him from telephone calls by accepting calls randomly themselves. This approach would result in inconsistent medical advice and could be dangerous. The physician is liable for phone advice.

Brown SB, Eberle BJ: Use of the telephone by pediatric house staff: A technique for pediatric care not taught. J Pediatr 84:117, 1974.

Greitzer L & others: Telephone assessment of illness by practicing pediatricians. J Pediatr 88:880, 1976.

Strain JE, Miller JD: The preparation, utilization, and evaluation of a registered nurse trained to give telephone advice in a private pediatric office. Pediatrics 47:1051, 1971.

Sturtz GS, Brown RB: Concerning A.G. Bell's invention. Clin Pediatr 8:378, 1969.

When Does the Patient Need to Be Seen?

Some patients must be seen immediately (eg, a foreign body in the eye). Others can be seen later the same day (eg, a cough that kept the patient awake much of the preceding night). Other patients can be scheduled 1–2 days later (eg, recurrent epistaxis). The nurse can make these decisions.

Where Should the Patient Be Seen?

Most sick patients can be seen in the physician's office by appointment. The physician can keep the first and last hour of each day plus at least 15 minutes out of each hour reserved for acute problems. Most of the first-hour appointments will be given to parents who call the physician during the preceding evening.

Another facility where patients can be seen for medical care is the hospital emergency room. This routing applies to patients who are highly likely to be admitted (eg, croup). Some physicians also send patients with poisonings, lacerations, or possible fractures to the nearest emergency room.

A third possibility is a house call. Most physicians consider this disadvantageous to themselves financially and to the patient medically since laboratory services are not available. A rare indication for a house call might be a particularly contagious disease that needs confirmation (eg, varicella). The physician could occasionally see such a patient in his office parking lot.

2. OFFICE TRIAGING & PROCEDURES

How Sick Is the Patient?

The nurse should screen every sick patient as soon as possible after he arrives at the office. She can think in terms of 3 general groups: emergency, contagious, and minor illness. Most patients have a minor illness (eg, cold, accident, earache) and can be seen at their appointed time. Some patients are contagious until proved otherwise and should quickly be moved from the waiting room to an isolated examining room (eg, febrile illnesses with rashes, lice, jaundice, possible pertussis). An attempt should be made to keep children with bronchiolitis or croup away from infants. When an office emergency (eg, febrile seizures or respiratory distress) is recognized by the nurse, she should notify the physician immediately. He can take appropriate emergency action, stabilize the patient, and arrange for transfer to the hospital if necessary (eg, an acidotic, dehydrated infant). (See Chapter 29.)

Russo RM & others: Triage abilities of nurse practitioner vs pediatrician. Am J Dis Child 129:673, 1975.

Preparation of the Patient for the Physician

The office aide can record the sick patient's temperature, height, and weight. The office nurse can record the chief complaint. Depending upon the symptom, the nurse can initiate the office's standing orders on laboratory procedures and symptomatic treatment listed below.

Initial Treatment & Laboratory Work-Up

A. Abdominal Pain: Take samples for urinalysis and urine culture; save stool specimen for occult blood testing.

B. Animal Bite: Wash out immediately with benzalkonium chloride for 10 minutes. Initiate the official reporting form, and call the county health department.

C. Cough: If present over 1 month, apply a tuberculin skin test.

D. Diarrhea: Take sample for stool culture if the stool contains blood or mucus or if diarrhea has persisted for more than 1 week at any age. For children under age 2, give 6 oz of 5% dextrose in water and record the naked weight on each visit. If child appears dehydrated, collect urine for specific gravity.

E. Earache: Give acetaminophen if in obvious pain. Obtain audiometrics if cooperative. If there is a possibility of mumps, isolate the patient.

F. Eye Injury: Obtain visual acuity test if child is over age 3. Place eye tray in the examining room.

G. Fever Over 39° C (102.2° F): Give acetaminophen in age-appropriate dose. Put the child in an examining room and assist the parent in undressing him. Initiate a sponge bath if temperature is > 40° C (104° F) despite drugs and the child is uncomfortable. Provide a bag for urine if not toilet-trained and save urine in refrigerator for analysis and culture. If unexplained fever has been present over 24 hours, do a white count and differential. If the baby is under 3 months old, notify the physician immediately.

H. Fractures: Notify the doctor immediately, obtain equipment to immobilize the site, and fill out the x-ray request.

I. Head Injury: Record vital signs and check the pupils for equal size and reaction to light.

J. Infectious Hepatitis Exposure: Record weights on persons who have had intimate contact with the patient in anticipation of giving gamma globulin, 0.03 ml/kg IM.

K. Lacerations: Wash thoroughly with hexachlorophene soap and water (at least 10 minutes). Check date of last tetanus shot and record. (The physician must decide if tetanus booster or antitoxin is needed.) Shave around the wound edges if necessary (but never shave eyebrows). Have parents sign consent for suturing.

L. Nasal Discharge (Purulent): Take material for culture.

M. Nosebleed: Instruct the parent or child on how to compress the bleeding site for 10 minutes. Check blood pressure and perform fingerstick for hematocrit.

N. Painful Urination (Burning or Frequency): Take sample for urinalysis, urine culture, and a gram-stained smear of unspun drop.

O. Pinworms: Record the approximate weights of all family members if the infection is a recurrent one (for calculation of dosage of medication).

P. Sore Throat: Take material for throat culture (contraindicated if the patient has croup).

Q. Streptococcal Sore Throat (Culture Positive): Inquire about penicillin allergy and record. Arrange for symptomatic family contacts to have throat cultures taken.

R. Vomiting: Record an accurate weight. Give patient emesis basin and sips of iced cola drink while waiting. If patient appears dehydrated, collect urine for specific gravity.

3. THE WORKING DIAGNOSIS

The physician makes the final decision about the patient's diagnosis and the severity of the disease. He may detect emergency conditions that were not obvious to his nurse (eg, shock or meningitis). His history-taking can be modified according to the chief complaint. A history of recent exposure to disease is often important. Severity can be partially assessed by inquiries about playfulness, energy, ability to sleep, and the mother's feelings about how sick her child is this time compared to other times. If a family of sick children is brought in, the physician should ask the mother which children she considers the sickest. The physical examination should also be mainly directed toward the chief complaint. A patient with a dog bite does not require a complete examination, but a patient with an earache must be checked for mastoid swelling and meningeal signs in addition to otoscopic examination.

Utilizing the conventional technics of history, physical examination, and laboratory tests, the physician will correctly diagnose the majority of acute chief complaints. However, unless he maintains a high index of suspicion and applies his keenest clinical judgment, he will occasionally miss a child with septicemia. Septic children usually present as unexplained fevers, but (unlike children with acute viral fevers) they often won't play or smile even with their parents. They frequently are physically exhausted and too weak to resist the physical examination, constantly irritable and unable to sleep, and respond paradoxically to cuddling by the mother. Irritability usually stems from pain or hypoxia. A less common finding in the toxic child is constant lethargy or sleepiness. This is difficult to assess because most sick children sleep more than normally. A child with suspected septicemia requires an intensive work-up and therapy in a hospital setting. Making this diagnosis requires the greatest vigilance by the pediatrician.

Russo RM & others: Outpatient management of the severely ill child. Am J Dis Child 124:235, 1972.

4. INDICATIONS FOR HOSPITALIZATION

For every acute problem, the physician must decide whether to treat the child at home or in the hospital. Overhospitalization is currently a greater problem in the USA than underhospitalization. In recent studies, at least 20% of hospitalizations were judged to be unnecessary. Overhospitalization takes 3 general forms: (1) Hospitalization for an acute illness sometimes occurs because the primary physician is uncertain of the diagnosis and prognosis. Reassurance in the face of such insecurity can often be gained by immediate consultation with a colleague. (2) Hospitalization is sometimes arranged for a diagnostic evaluation and tests because the patient has no outpatient insurance. Unless the parents are having serious financial difficulty, this custom is unethical. It is to be hoped that more realistic insurance coverage will make ambulatory studies equally reimbursable. (3) Periodic hospitalizations sometimes are ordered for routine reevaluations of a chronic disease. Even if the patient travels a great distance, this reevaluation can be done on an ambulatory basis if it is carefully planned in advance. The combined costs of the special studies plus hotel accommodations will be far less than hospitalization charges.

Unnecessary hospitalization carries 5 main problems or risks, the last one probably being the most serious: (1) Children under 3 years of age can experience separation problems. (2) The parents' confidence in caring for a sick child themselves is undermined. (3) There is a danger of cross-infection to the patient and others. (4) There is a risk of medical error, such as the wrong medication or wrong dosage. (5) Society sustains an endlessly rising cost for medical care.

If it is not clear whether or not an acutely ill child should be hospitalized, he should be observed in the office for several hours. This will allow time for any reassurance given to the mother to take effect and permits the physician to compare the patient at 2 points in time and determine whether he is improving or getting worse. This interval also helps one decide what to do when the mother's history and the physical examination are conflicting (eg, "recurrent vomiting" without dehydration, "no urination" without bladder distention). If necessary, another physician can be called in for consultation during this period.

A patient should be hospitalized if his problems fit into one of the following 3 groups of indications:

Major Emergencies

Some examples of obvious life-threatening conditions are shock, severe dehydration, coma, meningitis (bacterial or of unknown cause), respiratory distress, congestive heart failure, severe hypertension, acute renal failure, status epilepticus, and surgical emergencies.

Potentially Life-Threatening or Crippling Illnesses

Some patients are not in critical condition when first seen but require hospitalization because their problem may be rapidly progressive during treatment. If deterioration occurs in the hospital, emergency therapy can be rapidly instituted. Most of the entities in this group are caused by infection or trauma. Endogenous diseases rarely change this rapidly. Although absolute rules cannot be formulated for every situation, the following guidelines can be applied to most cases of acute illness. Obviously, these rules will have some exceptions. Also, the list is not complete (eg, chronic diseases are not listed).

These problems are listed according to body systems:

A. **Skin:**
   1. Cellulitis if less than 2 months old, omphalitis if less than 2 months old, erysipelas, toxic epidermal necrolysis, acute necrotizing fasciitis, in cavernous sinus drainage area, if underlying osteomyelitis is suspected, or if there is no response after 2 days of therapy.
   2. Suspected thrombophlebitis.
   3. Burns (second or third degree) involving more than 10% of surface area (> 15% if more than 1 year old), burns of perineal area, hand burns if they might need grafting, facial burns if they might need grafting, all inhalation burns, most electrical burns.
   4. Purpura with fever, without fever but unexplained, or without fever but progressive.

B. **Eyes:**
   1. Gonococcal conjunctivitis, bacterial keratitis.
   2. Eye injury if visual acuity is decreased.
   3. Papilledema.

C. **Ears, Nose, and Throat:**
   1. Acute otitis media if less than 1 month old.
   2. Mastoiditis.
   3. Sinusitis if overlying redness or edema is present.
   4. Nasal obstruction if less than 6 months old and an apneic episode has occurred.
   5. Epistaxis if uncontrolled, if hypertension is present, if there is bleeding elsewhere, or if anemia is present.
   6. Fluctuant tonsillar abscess.
   7. Retropharyngeal abscess.
   8. Diphtheria (any symptoms at any age).

D. **Respiratory System:**
   1. Epiglottitis (all cases).
   2. Viral laryngitis if there is stridor at rest, dyspnea, or drooling; if it is currently progressive; if there is a history of a previous bout with rapid progression; or if the patient is less than 1 year old (even if stridor occurs only with crying).
   3. Pertussis if symptomatic and the patient is less than 1 year old; or at any age with apnea, respiratory distress, a whoop, or weight loss.

4. Bronchiolitis if dyspneic, if it is progressive, or if fluid intake is poor.
5. Pneumonia if the patient is less than 1 month old; if bacterial pneumonia is suspected and the patient is less than 6 months old; if there is a history of apnea, cyanosis, or choking spells; with dyspnea (any age); with pleural effusion; if staphylococcal pneumonia is suspected (any age); if aspiration pneumonia is present; if fluid intake is poor; if there is underlying cystic fibrosis or congenital heart disease; or if there is no response after 2 days of therapy.
6. Suspected foreign body of the airway.
7. Hemoptysis if unexplained, if there is bleeding elsewhere, or if anemia is present.

E. **Cardiovascular System:**
1. Suspected subacute infective endocarditis.
2. Any myocarditis or pericarditis.
3. Acute hypertension.
4. Unexplained arrhythmias.

F. **Gastrointestinal System:**
1. Vomiting persisting over 24 hours or with dehydration.
2. Hematemesis if documented and not caused by swallowed blood.
3. Diarrhea if explosive in character, if there is abdominal distention, associated with Kussmaul respirations, suspected typhoid fever at any age, suspected acute shigella enteritis if less than 1 year old, suspected staphylococcal enterocolitis, moderate dehydration, or mild dehydration but with vomiting or if patient is less than 1 year old.
4. Melena or unexplained bright-red blood mixed in the stools.
5. Suspected appendicitis, peritonitis, or intussusception.
6. Abdominal trauma if penetrating injury has occurred or if damage to the spleen, liver, kidneys, pancreas, or intestines is suspected.
7. Toxic ileus.

G. **Urinary System:**
1. Pyelonephritis if patient is less than 1 year old, toxic, unimproved after 2 days of therapy, if underlying renal disease is present, or if recurrences have been frequent.
2. Acute edema, oliguria, or azotemia.
3. Hematuria with symptoms listed in (2), renal colic, and unexplained or posttraumatic gross hematuria.
4. Acute urinary retention.

H. **Genitalia:**
1. Vaginitis if associated with salpingitis.
2. Vaginal injury with sharp object.
3. Suspected testicular torsion.
4. Priapism.

I. **Skeletal System:**
1. Suspected osteomyelitis.
2. Arthritis if possibly septic or acute rheumatic fever.

3. Wringer injury if above the elbow, if a hematoma or avulsed skin is present, if a fracture or nerve injury is present, or if the peripheral pulse is diminished.

J. **Nervous System:**
1. Aseptic meningitis if the level of consciousness is depressed or there is a motor deficit.
2. Suspected tetanus.
3. Suspected epidural spinal abscess or brain abscess.
4. Febrile seizures if they continue more than 30 minutes, if there are persistent neurologic signs, or if the level of consciousness is decreased.
5. Head injury if the patient has been unconscious longer than 1 minute, if there are persistent neurologic signs, if the level of consciousness is decreased, if a seizure has occurred, if CSF rhinorrhea or otorrhea is present, if there is significant swelling over the middle meningeal artery, retinal hemorrhages, progressive headaches, or if abnormal or irregular vital signs are present.
6. Skull fractures—depressed, compound (ie, into air sinuses or overlying scalp laceration), across the middle meningeal artery or venous sinus, occipital fracture into the rim of the foramen magnum, or any fracture with an underlying bleeding disorder.
7. Suspected spinal cord trauma.
8. Acute muscle weakness.
9. Acute cognitive deterioration.
10. Suspected increased intracranial pressure.

K. **General:**
1. Suspected septicemia.
2. Poisoning if the patient is symptomatic (eg, respirations slow or irregular, drowsiness, etc), the agent or dosage is unknown, or the dosage is a potentially fatal one.
3. Suspected lead poisoning.
4. Unexplained mass.
5. Unexplained failure to thrive if the patient is less than 6 months old; failure to thrive at any age if neglect is suspected.
6. Unexplained hypoglycemia.

Duff RS & others: Use of utilization review to assess the quality of pediatric inpatient care. Pediatrics 49:169, 1972.
Gururaj VJ: Short stay in an outpatient department. Am J Dis Child 123:128, 1972.
Lovejoy FH & others: Unnecessary and preventable hospitalizations: Report on an internal audit. J Pediatr 79:868, 1971.

Psychosocial Indications for Hospitalization

Patients with acute psychosocial problems now comprise a larger proportion of hospitalized children than was formerly the case. Until society can provide alternative facilities for these crises, hospitalization will continue to fulfill this need. These indications fall into 3 general groups: parent, child, and disease problems.

A. Parent Problems:

1. Child abuse (eg, battering, failure to thrive secondary to neglect, or incest).
2. Incipient battering (eg, the parent has made a homicidal threat against his child).
3. Absent parents (eg, abandonment, emancipated minors without caretakers, or the parents themselves are hospitalized).
4. Physically exhausted parents (eg, no sleep for 2 nights).
5. Severely overanxious parents (eg, if the parents remain immobilized and extremely anxious after a careful explanation of their child's illness).
6. Neglectful parents who seem uninterested in their child's illness or therapy (eg, neglected eczema). This is a rare situation compared to overly anxious parents.
7. Intellectually incompetent parents (eg, a mentally retarded mother who can't reliably follow verbal or written instructions).
8. Emotionally disturbed parents who need psychiatric hospitalization treatment for their own problems (eg, a floridly psychotic mother).
9. Parent who is alcoholic or drug abuser.

B. Child Problems:

1. Suicide attempt—A short hospital admission allows time for the mental health worker to do his evaluation and the family to look seriously at their problems.
2. A destructive, dangerous child can be held on a pediatric ward pending placement. A dangerous adolescent will require a psychiatric setting.
3. Severe delirium (eg, if the parents cannot control it).
4. An incapacitating emotional symptom (eg, a severe conversion reaction such as paraplegia or blindness).

C. Disease Problems:

1. An incapacitating (but not life-threatening) physical disease (eg, severe Sydenham's chorea).
2. Initial diagnosis of a disease with a complex treatment regimen. The parents and patient deserve a careful, unhurried, and organized introduction to the complex home management of some chronic diseases (eg, diabetes mellitus).
3. Initial diagnosis of a fatal disease—This gives the family time to work through the impact phase (eg, leukemia).
4. Terminal care if the family does not want the child to die at home.
5. Chronic diseases that are exacerbated by family conflicts (eg, ulcerative colitis).
6. Hazardous home (eg, carbon monoxide or lead poisoning).

5. TREATMENT OF THE NONHOSPITALIZED PATIENT

Words are as necessary as drugs in the treatment of a sick child. The parents expect to be told their child's diagnosis and its causes, prognosis, and treatment. They also need to have their special concerns acknowledged and clarified. If this communication does not take place, the parents will often be dissatisfied with the quality of care being given, and their compliance with regard to medications, advice, and follow-up will probably be less than optimal.

If the child has a mild acute illness (eg, viral nasopharyngitis), the parent would be reassured by the following general types of comment:

Diagnosis

"David has a cold." The diagnosis should be conveyed in plain English, not in medical jargon. If the physician does not precisely mention his diagnosis to the parents, they may assume he was unable to arrive at one. (See also Ambiguous Diagnosis, below.)

Etiology

"It's due to a virus." This means to most parents that the infection is not serious. Some parents need an added statement that there was nothing they could have done to prevent it—eg, "Everyone is coming down with this."

Parents' Concerns

Mothers often do not listen to their physician's instructions until their own main concerns have been commented upon. These concerns are easily elicited by 3 questions: (1) "Why did you bring David to the clinic today?" (2) "What worried you most about him?" (3) "Why did that worry you?" After these concerns are out in the open, the physician is in an excellent position to clarify misconceptions. His reassurance can be specific—eg, "He doesn't have meningitis," or, "It won't turn into leukemia."

Treatment

In self-limited disease, the goal of medication is to keep the patient comfortable. The opportunities to use symptomatic medications far exceed those where specific medications are available. A useful list of common sense approaches to management (sometimes overlooked) is as follows: (1) An antipyretic is useful if the patient's fever causes discomfort. (2) Sedatives (eg, chloral hydrate) should be prescribed more often for the acutely restless child since his mother cannot easily function as a nurse without some sleep. (3) Codeine can be freely used for acute cough that interferes with sleep. (4) Advice about diet, bed rest, isolation, and mood are also appreciated by the parent. The patient can usually be allowed to select his own diet while he is sick. (5) Home bed rest is something each child may decide for himself in most cases. (6) Isolation within the family structure is rarely indicated since exposure has usually preceded the diagnosis. (7) Parents can be reassured about temporary emotional regression during an acute illness. A return to the previous level of maturity need not be encouraged until good health returns.

Prognosis

"David will probably feel better in 2 or 3 days. This is not a serious infection. If something new develops or his fever lasts over 3 days, give me a call." Nothing is gained by mentioning all the possible complications. Without promoting anxiety, the door to additional medical evaluation is quietly left open for any new problems that might arise.

Closing

"You're doing a fine job with David. Just hold the fort and he will be his old self in a few days." The visit should close on a positive note, even a compliment if possible. If the patient is older, an attempt can be made to boost his morale as well—eg, "This won't keep *you* out of action for long."

The Ambiguous Diagnosis

An unclear diagnosis presents special problems in communication with the parents. The physician must be honest about the inconclusive diagnosis and yet not unduly alarm the parents. "David's illness is not far enough along to be diagnosed exactly. Another day or so will be needed to pinpoint the problem. I can tell you a few things for certain. He is not in any serious trouble. He doesn't have meningitis. I definitely want to see him tomorrow. Call me sooner if there are any new developments."

Symptomatic therapy should also be prescribed.

Carey WB, Sibinga MS: Avoiding pediatric pathogenesis in the management of acute minor illness. Pediatrics 49:553, 1972.

Korsch B & others: Practical implications of doctor-patient interaction analysis for pediatric practice. Am J Dis Child 121:110, 1971.

Waller DA, Levitt EE: Concerns of mothers in a pediatric clinic. Pediatrics 50:931, 1972.

6. FOLLOW-UP OF THE NONHOSPITALIZED PATIENT

Most children with an acute illness do not require follow-up unless their clinical course worsens or is prolonged. However, if the child has an ambiguous diagnosis (eg, high fever of unknown origin) or an unpredictable course (eg, vomiting), daily follow-up is necessary. This protects both the patient and the physician. This follow-up can be accomplished by revisits, telephone calls, or a visiting nurse.

Revisits

Daily office visits are the best approach to the more serious problem. The weight of the infant with diarrhea and the degree of respiratory distress in a child with croup cannot be estimated over the phone. If a scheduled revisit appointment is not kept, the office clerk should immediately notify the physician. A phone call or home visit should be made on that same day. If transportation is a problem for the parent, a community service agency can usually arrange this. If the late results of laboratory tests indicate that an illness is quite serious and other attempts at contact fail, the police can be requested to locate the patient and bring him in (eg, a stool culture that grows salmonella in a 4-month-old infant).

Telephone Calls

A daily telephone call will suffice for milder problems when only historical follow-up data are needed (eg, vomiting or lethargy). Since these calls are essential to proper management, the physician or his nurse should make them. A daily telephone list can be kept and the charts pulled prior to calling. If the follow-up is felt to be important, parents should not be depended upon to initiate these calls since some may not be made. Telephone calls become the realistic choice of follow-up when long distances are a factor.

Visiting Nurse

Home management of wounds and burns is an appropriate role for a visiting nurse. Mothers of large families who have both a babysitter problem and a transportation problem appreciate this type of follow-up. Mothers with several sick children or who are themselves in poor health also benefit from home visits.

MEDICOLEGAL PROBLEMS

The management of acute illness offers the greatest potential for malpractice litigation in pediatrics. The physician is responsible not only for his own errors but for those of his nurse as well. Errors can be made in any of the areas previously discussed. An error in telephone triaging can result in a delay in diagnosis (eg, calling meningococcemia a viral exanthem, or arranging an appointment for the next day for scrotal pain that turns out to be testicular torsion). An error in underhospitalization can lead to death (eg, epiglottitis being treated on an outpatient basis). Errors in therapy may result in sciatic nerve palsy if an injection is given into an inappropriate quadrant of the buttocks, or acute rheumatic fever if penicillin is not given for a streptococcal sore throat because it was not cultured. Errors in follow-up can result in undiagnosed abdominal pain silently progressing to a ruptured appendix.

The physician should obtain parental consent forms for all medical procedures (eg, lumbar puncture, suturing) unless an emergency exists. Consultation should be sought whenever a physician is uncertain about what is happening with an acutely and possibly seriously ill patient.

The errors listed above are not difficult to prevent if the physician bases all of his medical decisions on what is best for the patient.

Brown RH: Consent. Pediatrics 57:414, 1976.

Conkling WS (Chairman): *An Introduction to Medical Liability for Pediatricians.* Task Force on Medical Liability of the Council on Pediatric Practice, 1975.

CHRONIC DISEASE FOLLOW-UP VISITS

Office visits for a child with known or potential chronic disease present special problems. There are 5 broad types of chronic disease, each being progressively more difficult to manage: (1) Potential chronic disease (eg, the small premature, the newborn who has recovered from hypoglycemia, or the older child who has recovered from meningitis). (2) Reversible chronic disease (eg, tuberculosis, eczema, or idiopathic thrombocytopenic purpura). (3) Static chronic disease (eg, cerebral palsy, deafness, or dwarfism). (4) Progressive chronic disease (eg, diabetes mellitus or sickle cell anemia). (5) Fatal disease (eg, leukemia or muscular dystrophy). These children usually receive excellent care when they are hospitalized. They should also receive the same kind of thoughtful care when they do not occupy a hospital bed or have an interesting complication.

OBJECTIVES

There are 2 primary objectives in the management of a chronic disease. The first is to counteract the effects of the disease to the extent possible. This requires the aggressive use of every available therapeutic modality that could be useful for the individual patient's problems. The second objective is to help the patient and his parents make a healthy emotional adjustment to the treatment regimen and to the effects of the disease that cannot be controlled. Except for matters relating to his disease, the child should be reared no differently than his healthy siblings. He should live as nearly normal a life as possible.

Chronic disease management is optimal when the following general aspects receive ongoing attention: continuity of care, frequent visits, problem-oriented records, chronic disease flow sheets, personal medical identification documents, a chronic disease patient registry kept in the office, and medical passport.

1. CONTINUITY OF CARE

The patient with a chronic disease may have multiple problems that are difficult to manage. If anyone deserves continuous medical care from one physician, this person does. Discontinuous care by several physicians often results in a confused and maladjusted patient. When the patient has a progressive or fatal disease, depression can occur. In such a situation, patients depend upon a single sustaining physician to help them maintain their tenuous hope for survival. Fragmented medical care usually accentuates a poor psychologic adjustment. When a physician agrees to care for a patient with a chronic disease, he should give his home phone number and encourage its use. If the physician is unable to see the patient personally, he can coordinate arrangements by telephone for the patient to be seen by another physician who has been fully briefed. If the patient is unable to contact his personal physician, he should be able to turn to a substitute physician who has been designated well in advance.

Becker MH & others: Continuity of pediatrician: New support for an old shibboleth. J Pediatr 84:599, 1974.

2. FREQUENT VISITS

The patient with a chronic disease should be contacted frequently. Monitoring the patient's disease and response to therapy is impossible without periodic visits or telephone communications. If his problem is stabilized, he should be seen personally at least every 6 months; 3-month intervals are better for progressive diseases. If the disease is in relapse, the patient may need to be seen daily.

3. PROBLEM-ORIENTED RECORDS

In addition to a personal physician, comprehensive care of the chronically ill patient depends upon good record-keeping. No physician's memory is absolutely reliable, and in any case the patient must have accurate office records when the physician is away from the city or after he dies. An excellent system of record-keeping has been developed and refined in a practice setting (see references, below). It has 4 components: the initial data base, the active problem sheet, the plan for each problem, and the progress notes which contribute to the continually expanding data base and problem list.

Initial Data Base

The conventional present illness, review of systems, past medical history, family history, psychosocial history, physical examination, and laboratory screening tests comprise the data base. Information from all accessible sources is used. (See Chapter 1.)

Active Problem Sheet

The active problem list is the keystone of this system. It lists all the patient's significant problems, including psychosocial ones. These problems are defined from the data base currently at hand. They can be expressed as an etiologic diagnosis (eg, rheumatic heart disease), a pathophysiologic state (eg, congestive heart failure), or a sign or symptom (eg, edema). When the therapy carries considerable risk, it should be defined as a problem (eg, corticosteroids or tracheostomy). An attempt is made to list the problems in order of priority. Each problem is then assigned a permanent number (see p 168). Thereafter, this number should precede any entry in the chart that concerns this problem. The active problem sheet should be kept in the front of the patient's chart where it serves as a table of contents. The dates should be date of onset or date of resolution. New problems are added as identified, and old problems are transferred to the "resolved or inactive" column when appropriate. Symptom problems should be reidentified as diagnosed problems when the data accumulated justify doing so. When a patient with multiple diseases is cared for by several physicians, the last column on the active problem list can be used to list the responsible physician for each problem. This technic is especially helpful for improving continuity of care in a large medical center.

The active problem list can become somewhat standardized if "#1" is always used for "health maintenance care" (or well child care) and "#2" is always used for "minor acute illnesses" (or temporary problems). (See p 168.) The latter category is a convenient place to bury self-limited minor illnesses that do not warrant being given individual permanent numbers. Examples are colds, coughs, gastroenteritis, conjunctivitis, mumps, viral exanthems, impetigo, diaper rash, insect bites, minor trauma, etc. Acute illnesses that can be serious (eg, pneumonia) or recurrent (eg, otitis media) obviously should receive separate numbers.

Plan for Each Problem

Each problem as listed in the active problem sheet needs an individual diagnostic, therapeutic, and educational plan. If the plans for all the problems are combined, omissions are likely to occur.

Progress Notes

Progress notes contain newly collected data, an analysis of the data, and a reassessment of the plan. These notes should always pertain to one of the problems on the active problem sheet and be so labeled both by number and by title, eg, as follows:

#4—Seizures

Subjective—Two seizures last week, lasting 1 minute and 5 minutes. Occurred at 7:00 a.m. and 10:00 a.m. No precipitating events apparent. Last seizure 3 months ago. No headaches or vomiting. Not drowsy from medication.

Objective—Neurologic examination and fundi normal. No nystagmus. Gingival hyperplasia —mild.

Assessment—Seizures still in poor control.

Plan—Continue phenobarbital, 30 mg tid; increase Dilantin to 50 mg tid. Reviewed reasons for strict compliance.

Bjorn JC, Cross HD: *Problem-Oriented Practice*. Modern Hospital Press, 1970.

Hurst JW, Walker HIC: *The Problem-Oriented System*. Medicom, 1972.

Weed LL: Medical records that guide and teach. (2 parts.) N Engl J Med 278:593, 652, 1968.

Weed LL: *Medical Records, Medical Education and Patient Care*. Case Univ Press, 1969.

4. THE CHRONIC DISEASE FLOW SHEET

There are many variables in the management of a chronic disease. The variables can become lost in the substance of the chart and relatively unavailable for comparison and interpretation. For a patient with a chronic disease or multiple problems, critical data from the progress note should be recorded on a chronic disease flow sheet which tabulates variables so that trends and correlations can be accurately determined. The long axis of the flow sheet has time intervals. Inpatient flow sheets maintained on a critically ill child usually monitor vital signs, intake and output, blood gases, and numerous chemical determinations. Outpatient flow sheets often contain none of the above. Although a specific flow sheet is designed for each chronic disease, the following variables are commonly present in the ambulatory management of most chronic diseases. An example of how to use a flow sheet for a patient with diabetes mellitus is shown on p 164. Recommended variables for constructing flowsheets for other common chronic disorders are listed on pp 165—167.

Disease Status

One must monitor the activity level of the disease to know whether therapy is being effective or not. Such activity can be evaluated through the history, physical findings, laboratory data, consultations, and hospitalizations. Variables so determined can be tabulated on the flow sheet.

A. Symptom Data: The frequency and duration of asthma attacks are the main determinants of the success of asthma therapy. Migraine headaches, seizure episodes, and psychogenic recurrent abdominal pain must also be monitored largely by attack rates.

B. Physical Findings: Childhood nephrosis must be followed by weighing the patient and observing the presence or absence of edema. Splenomegaly is an important variable in leukemia. Motor milestones are important in cerebral palsy.

C. Laboratory Data: Chest films are important for following tuberculosis, EEGs for seizures, liver enzymes for chronic active hepatitis, urine cultures for recurrent urinary tract infection, etc.

D. Data for Early Detection of Complications: Some chronic diseases have complications that are not preventable but respond much better to therapy if they are detected early. Warning signs of these complications should be listed on the flow sheet. Examples are head circumference measurements to detect early subdural effusions or hydrocephalus after meningitis, and blood pressure measurements to detect early hypertension in chronic renal disease. Once hypertension is discovered, it is no longer an anticipated complication but an indicator of disease activity.

E. Consultations: One of the patient's problems may be followed by another specialist. The primary physician should record under the dates of these visits the consultant's name and abbreviated conclusions on the flow sheet. The date will permit easy location of the consultation report in the chart when it is needed.

F. Hospitalizations: All hospitalizations should be recorded under the problem that they were required for. They usually represent a marker of increased activity of the disease.

G. Emotional Status: Emotional maladjustments are a frequent and often unnecessary side-effect of chronic diseases. The physician can prevent them in many instances by reviewing an emotional problem checklist on *every* visit. Some of the more common but unvoiced maladjustments are unnecessary restrictions, overprotectiveness, favoritism, school phobia, underdiscipline, and teasing by peers. This subject is more fully discussed in Chapter 23.

Treatment Regimen

Therapy may or may not be responsible for improvement in the patient's disease status. Examining the temporal relationship of one to the other allows a physician to decide if the treatment has been effective. A chronic disease flow sheet should supply this information.

A. Medications: All medications and dosages should be listed with the dates when started, when discontinued, and when the dosage is changed. The dosage may be increased because the patient has outgrown it or because his problem is not under optimal control (eg, increasing the dosage of digoxin in persistent congestive heart failure). New drugs should be added when previous drugs have been pushed to tolerance without adequate control (eg, adding alternate-day prednisone to daily aminophylline/ephedrine therapy in asthma). Any drug the patient is receiving should have at least one related variable listed under disease status that permits rapid assessment of the efficacy of the drug (eg, bowel movements per day recorded for the patient with ulcerative colitis on Lomotil).

B. Toxicity: If drugs with side-effects are being used, these problems should be anticipated. The bone marrow, kidney, or liver function tests that need monitoring should be recorded on the flow sheet, as well as the required frequency of testing. If the potential toxicity is high, the drug should also be recorded on the problem list. If sudden discontinuance of the drug could lead to a severe adverse reaction, this risk should be frequently discussed with the patient (eg, anticonvulsants).

C. Nondrug Therapy: Other methods of treatment besides drugs should be recorded on the flow sheet so that their effect on the course of the disease can also be estimated. Examples are specific food avoidance in recurrent urticaria or bubble bath avoidance in recurrent urinary tract infection. In static diseases, compensatory devices (eg, braces in cerebral palsy or hearing aids in deafness) should be listed as well as the recommended interval for routine checks of these devices. Reassurance and other forms of supportive psychotherapy will generally be given on every visit and need not be listed here.

D. Therapy for Prevention of Complications: Many chronic diseases have predictable and preventable complications if therapy is instituted in advance. If these are listed in the flow sheet, the physician will be certain to remind the parent of them on each visit. Examples are performing daily range of motion exercises to prevent contractures in rheumatoid arthritis, requesting penicillin prophylaxis before dental procedures to prevent subacute bacterial endocarditis in congenital heart disease, avoidance of altitudes over 10,000 feet to prevent a crisis in sickle cell disease, and carrying an antihypoglycemic food in the pocket at all times in diabetes mellitus.

E. Compliance With Therapy: The best treatment regimen is useless unless the patient complies with it. A check on the patient's compliance can be performed by inquiring about his degree of satisfaction or dissatisfaction with the medical care he has been receiving; asking if the medications have been difficult to take; or in some cases measuring blood or urine levels of the drugs (eg, aspirin or penicillin).

F. Disease Education Reviews: Patients may not cooperate with a therapeutic plan until they are intellectually and emotionally committed to it. Unless the family fully understands what they are expected to do, they cannot do it. Unless they understand priorities, they may unknowingly discontinue some critical element in the treatment program when the treatment program as a whole becomes frustrating. Optimal patient education is reached when the patient and his family know as much about the home treatment of the disease as the physician does and when they can make decisions about minor adjustments of treatment independently.

When facts regarding the disease and treatment are reviewed, one should begin with basic information even though it has been covered many times before. After the first session, the subject is reviewed by asking the patient questions. In the early years, the facts are covered with the patient and both parents present. If the father excludes himself from the medical care of his child, serious marital problems will usually develop. In the adolescent years, the review sessions should be done privately with the teenager. The patient's knowledge of his problems should be explored approximately every 6 months. In the period immediately following diagnosis, it should be covered on every visit for a few months.

G. School Notification: Each fall the physician should notify the school nurse about any patient that may have manifestations of his disease at school. This notification will prevent any emotional problems secondary to mishandling of the physical problem by the school. The patient with chronic heart or lung disease may need a gym excuse. He may need modified gym (eg, no gym on days of wheezing, or no rope-climbing in a seizure patient). Both the nurse and the teacher need to know how to respond to a seizure or insulin reaction in the classroom. The physician should have this listed on his flow sheet so that it is never overlooked. The parents of the patient's closest friends should also have this information, as should the baby-sitters.

Schmitt BD: The chronic disease flowsheet in ambulatory pediatrics. Pediatrics 51:722, 1973.

5. THE MEDICAL IDENTIFICATION CARD

The patient with a chronic disease should carry an identification card with his active problem list, his physician's telephone number, and his parents' telephone number recorded on it. If he has a disease that can result in sudden changes in consciousness (eg, insulin reaction in diabetes mellitus) or an allergy that could be fatal if it were violated (eg, penicillin allergy), he should obtain a medical identification bracelet or necklace. These can be ordered from Medic Alert Foundation, Turlock, California 95380.

6. CHRONIC DISEASE PATIENT REGISTRY

Every effort should be made to keep certain patients from becoming "lost to follow-up." People with chronic diseases (eg, those with rheumatic heart disease receiving prophylactic penicillin) fall into this group. To prevent the disappearance of any of these patients, the physician should keep them listed in a chronic disease patient registry. Their charts should have a special mark placed on the corner of the cover to show that they are special high-risk patients. These patients should be sent a reminder card 1 week prior to appointments. If the parent cancels an appointment and promises to call back and make another one, the patient's name should be placed on a critical phone call list which automatically goes into effect if the appointment is not remade within 2 weeks. If the patient misses an appointment, the physician should be notified that same day and he should call the patient. If the parent has no phone, a letter should be sent. If there is no response to the letter, a visiting nurse referral should be sent. This usually returns the patient to his physician or shows that the family has changed physicians. If the family does not wish further medical care from anyone and the patient's disease is life-threatening but treatable (eg, tuberculosis or chronic pyelonephritis), the physician should report the case to the child protective services in his community. Since this is an example of medical care neglect, a court order will be issued for treatment of the child. The physician should assume the personal responsibility to follow indefinitely and tenaciously any high-risk patient until transfer of care occurs.

7. THE MEDICAL PASSPORT

Every year, 20% of American families move. Some of them have children with chronic diseases. Nothing is more frustrating for a physician than to receive a complicated new patient with no past records. Legally, the records belong to the physician; but morally, the records belong to the patient. When he moves, he should carry with him a copy of his active problem list, chronic disease flow sheet, health maintenance flow sheet, consultation reports, hospital discharge summaries, pertinent x-ray reports, and a covering letter. The original copies should never be sent because they may be lost. The physician should also give the family the names of 2 or 3 pediatricians they might use in the city they are moving to. These may be personal acquaintances or selections he has made from the *Directory of Medical Specialists.*

CONSULTATIVE VISITS

The physician must know how to act as a consultant when he is qualified and how to seek consultation when he needs it. The practicing pediatrician is still the best consultant for most pediatric problems.

OBJECTIVES

The usual purpose of a consultation is the evaluation of an undiagnosed problem followed by therapeutic recommendations. Some referrals are for treatment advice only. A secondary goal of consultation is to provide the referring physician with a continuing medical educational experience.

THE PEDIATRICIAN IN THE ROLE OF CONSULTANT

Referring Source

A. Self-Referral: Although not technically a consultation, some problems require the same kind of intensive approach that is needed when consulting with a colleague. A problem requiring a careful diagnostic evaluation may be detected during a well child visit or a sick child visit. These "big" problems are often not mentioned by the parent until the end of the visit or may be detected by a screening questionnaire. The physician should reschedule such a patient to himself. These diagnostic evaluations can keep practice stimulating. If the physician is "rusty" about the work-up of a particular problem, he will have time to review the literature prior to the appointment.

B. Physician Referral: Family practitioners or other specialists occasionally refer patients to a pediatrician for consultation. Within the pediatric community, some pediatricians refer patients to other physicians who have a subspecialty "interest" or expertise with a specific disease. This is more common within a group practice.

C. Nonphysician Referral: A physician who is well thought of receives referrals from dentists, school officials, psychologists, social workers, nurses, and previous patients. Some of these referred patients will require a consultation type visit.

Appointments

Consultations usually require 1-hour appointments. Some require 2 such visits to complete the evaluation. The average pediatrician will need to have 2–5 of these 1-hour appointments blocked out on his schedule each week. The visit will be considerably more productive if a screening questionnaire is completed in advance (see pp 168–171). This questionnaire delineates the patient's physical, intellectual, and emotional problems and serves as his initial data base. The psychosocial portion is different for each of 3 age groups. The physician will then have a tentative problem list at hand before he sees the patient.

These long appointments are easily arranged when the patient is referred by another professional because a telephone call or letter usually precedes the patient. However, a patient with almost any problem requiring a careful evaluation can walk into a physician's office at any time and the physician must have a logical response to such situations. When the mother of a 10-year-old patient who is being seen for acute otitis media mentions that her child has experienced 4 years of encopresis or 6 months of "staring spells" at school, the busy physician may feel under some pressure to make a quick recommendation. He may be tempted to do a 5-minute work-up, order some laboratory tests, do a piecemeal work-up over several short visits, or hospitalize the patient for a work-up. He may decide to disregard the complaint or minimize its importance. None of these approaches are in the patient's best interests. Long-standing diagnostic dilemmas require a comprehensive assessment which takes at least an hour. Most such evaluations can be done on an ambulatory basis. Shortcuts can lead to tentative conclusions, unconvinced parents, postponement of the indicated work-up, "doctor shopping," secondary gain for the patient, and an unresolved problem.

The first visit can serve a useful purpose. One can tell the parents that their child's problem is complicated and deserves a complete evaluation. A few screening laboratory tests such as a blood count and erythrocyte sedimentation rate may be ordered. The parent can fill out the screening data questionnaire. A release can be signed for hospital discharge summaries, prior consultation reports, laboratory test results (especially any tests that were dangerous, painful, or expensive), school reports, and growth information. These data will make the consultation visit more meaningful and avoid duplication of effort. Unlike hospitalized consultations, an immediate appointment is rarely needed and the patient can be rescheduled for the following week or later if more time is needed to accumulate data.

Extent of Services

When the patient is referred by the parents or a nonphysician, the request is usually for total care. When the patient is referred by a physician, there are 5 possible degrees of service the consulting physician can offer. If the referring physician does not specify precisely what is needed, the consulting physician may either ask him or assume that this cannot be predicted in advance and must await the results of the evaluation.

A. Evaluation Only: The consultant can do a diagnostic evaluation on a patient and tell the parents nothing except that he will discuss his findings with their primary physician. Parents generally dislike this. They have paid for the consultation, and they want to hear something from the expert personally. Common courtesy would suggest they are correct.

B. Evaluation and Interpretation: After the evaluation is completed, the consultant usually explains his findings regarding diagnosis and etiology to the family. If he mentions recommendations for therapy, it should only be in very general terms and with the clear understanding that the referring physician will be coordinating the therapy. The patient should then be returned to the referring physician, who will make specific therapeutic recommendations to the family. A specific return appointment date with the referring physician should be given. This is the usual type of referral process for a patient with a chronic disease. The consultant may be called upon periodically to reassess the response to therapy and to offer revised recommendations.

C. Evaluation and Treatment of an Isolated Problem: Sometimes the referring physician desires the consultant to completely manage the referred problem. This usually happens with treatable problems that will only require 3–6 visits (eg, recurrent headaches, breathholding spells, ringworm, Sydenham's chorea). The consultant should clearly define and support the referring physician's role as the continual provider of health supervision and acute illness care during this period of time. When the referred problem is resolved, the patient should be returned to the referring physician for complete care. A single follow-up visit to the consultant in approximately 1 year is usually acceptable. Sometimes a letter from the parent will suffice to supply the consultant with the progress report he desires.

D. Total Health Care: Occasionally a physician refers a patient to a consultant for a diagnostic problem plus all future medical care. This usually occurs when a family is having financial problems or has recently moved. The former patient is best referred to a community hospital-based consultant rather than a private one. When the diagnostic problem is minimal and the psychosocial problems maximal, this is commonly known as a "dump" and does not constitute a true consultation.

E. Evaluation and Referral for Additional Consultation: The patient's problem may require the expertise of a pediatric subspecialist (eg, pediatric hematologist). Before the step is taken, the original physician must be recontacted to obtain his permission for further consultation. Sometimes he will prefer to choose his own subspecialist, but usually he will appreciate the pediatrician's advice about the best expert on the patient's disorder.

Barness LA & others: Computer-assisted diagnosis in pediatrics. Am J Dis Child 127:852, 1974.
Swender PT & others: Computer-assisted diagnosis. Am J Dis Child 127:859, 1974.

Correspondence With the Referring Source

Communication is the key to a satisfactory referral process. The consulting physician is mainly responsible for this aspect of consultation. The referring physician should not have to contact the consultant to obtain his results. The following suggestions might be considered guidelines to the appropriate format for completing the process diplomatically.

A. Acknowledgement of the Referral: As soon as a referral letter is received, the consulting physician should send the referral source a brief note acknowledging the referral. Additional information can also be requested at this time: "Thank you for your recent referral letter on David Jones. I have sent the parents a screening data questionnaire. As soon as it is returned, he will be scheduled for a full evaluation. I will be in contact with you regarding the results. Best regards."

B. The Consultation Report: This report should be sent promptly. The content of the final report depends on the referring source. School officials do not want to know medical details; they usually just want to know if the patient is physically healthy or, if not, what their responsibility is. A referring physician expects a full report that will help him treat the patient. Recommendations should therefore be specific

(drugs, dosages, other forms of therapy, duration of therapy, specific laboratory tests, the recommended frequency of these tests, etc). A copy of or reference to a recent review article on the subject will also be appreciated.

This evaluation should be typed as a formal consultation report. It should not contain personal comments or resemble a letter. When written in this style, it can serve as an official evaluation report for anyone who might request a copy of it in future years. To make this communication to the referring physician more personal, it should be accompanied by a covering letter: "It was a pleasure to see David Jones today. A complete summary of his evaluation is included. The recommendations may need to be modified in the light of your previous experience with this family. As you well know, the marital situation is very stormy. It would be a privilege to see David again if you feel the need arises."

C. Phone Call to the Referring Physician: Most referring physicians prefer a consultation report to a phone call because the former can become a permanent part of the patient's record. Selected cases require a brief telephone report in addition to the written consultation report. These cases include situations where the patient needs to return to the referring physician before a consultation report can be sent, where the patient needs to be referred to an additional specialist, or where a question exists about proper disposition.

D. Return Appointment With the Referring Physician: At the end of the consultation, the consultant should tell the parents when he next wants them to see their primary physician regarding the referred problem. This interval is usually 1–2 weeks. Also, positive comments about the referring physician's competence and judgment should be made so that his reputation is enhanced by the referral process. The parents must feel confident that their primary physician can provide the necessary follow-up care. If the referring physician had tentatively made the correct diagnosis prior to referral, the consultant's corroboration should be made clear to the parents and also recorded in the consultation report.

Fees for Services Rendered

Many pediatricians are reluctant to charge adequately for their time. This seems illogical since an ambulatory consultation can prevent the high cost of an unnecessary hospital work-up. Even if ambulatory insurance does not cover the full cost of such an evaluation, the pediatrician should bill for these evaluations as "office consultations" and charge for the time allotted. His hour is worth the same whether it is spent with one consultation or several well or sick children.

THE PEDIATRICIAN IN THE ROLE OF REFERRING PHYSICIAN

Indications for Referral

There are generally 8 indications for seeking consultation. The last 2 are primarily to help the parents deal with realities.

A. The Pediatrician Is Uncertain of the Diagnosis: Referral for a diagnostic evaluation is a time-honored indication. A diagnostic dilemma should not be allowed to continue unresolved, especially if some of the possible causes are life-threatening. The ambulatory consultation is preferable to hospitalization.

B. The Treatment Requires Special Technical Expertise: When the physician knows the diagnosis but treatment is outside of his specialty, he should refer (eg, surgery).

C. The Treatment Is Nonmedical: The physician with a holistic approach to his patient's health will not infrequently need the services of psychiatrists, psychologists, social workers, educators, speech therapists, and other professionals to treat the problems he detects within their special fields.

D. The Treatment Is Complex: A physician no longer needs to say he doesn't know how to treat a certain disease because he can look up the currently recommended therapy in several textbooks. However, every pediatrician must know his limitations. The treatment of some diseases is so complex that the physician unfamiliar with it should refer (eg, cystic fibrosis, muscular dystrophy, leukemia).

E. Conventional Treatment Is Not Effective: When the patient is not doing as well as expected, 2 heads are better than one. Even with diseases that the physician has successfully treated many times, an atypical problem may arise that requires a fresh opinion (eg, recalcitrant seizures). A phone consultation with the appropriate subspecialist will sometimes solve the problem.

F. The Problem Is a Medicolegal One: Parents bring in children with injuries for which they are suing a physician or other person. The pediatrician's main task is to decide if the alleged disability or defect is real. If the injury proves to be significant, the physician can help the family find an expert consultant whose testimony will stand up in court (eg, an orthopedist for a hand injury). If the physician feels that the parents are exaggerating the child's disability for financial gain, he should declare the child healthy and suggest that he return to full activity without confronting the family about his suspicions.

G. The Parents Insist on Overtreatment: The pediatrician can help the family accept his recommendations for avoiding aggressive intervention by suggesting consultation. There are honest differences of opinion about the indications for tonsillectomy, "corrective" shoes, hyposensitization, etc. If the pediatrician is certain that the patient's interests will be best served by a supporting opinion from another doctor, he should choose consultants who share his philosophy and communicate in advance that he wishes the consultant to discourage an escalation of therapy. Consultants sometimes assume that the intention of the referring physician is to have them provide special equipment rather than special advice, and they are reluctant not to comply.

H. The Parents Are Thinking About a Consultation: When the parents have to ask for a consultation or obtain one without telling their physician, the pediatrician has waited too long. He should recognize that such an attitude is developing when parents criticize him, question his judgment, or seem angry. The parents' tendency to deny the prognosis can be anticipated with certain diseases (eg, fatal diseases and mental retardation). This denial should be respected if it does not interfere with therapy.

A rare or fatal disease is not intrinsically an indication for referral. Some physicians automatically seek "confirmation" of a diagnosis they already know or "approval" of a treatment regimen they are already familiar with. The physician who is confident of his knowledge about a particular disease does not reassure the family by hiding his competence.

Method of Referral

A. Obtain Permission From the Family: The family will usually agree to a referral if the reason for it is made clear. Patients sometimes feel that a referral means they are being abandoned by their physician. The referring physician must make it clear that he will remain available for primary medical care. The family should also be told in advance that the consultation will cost more than a regular visit but that it will be worth more.

B. Help the Family Choose a Consultant: The physician should maintain a file listing the best consultants in his community and at the nearest medical center. The parents can be given the names of 2 or 3 competent physicians. If one is outstanding, the pediatrician should not be reluctant to state his preference. If the parents suggest someone they have heard of but whom the physician feels is unqualified, the pediatrician should tell them he does not consider the person they mention an expert on their particular problem. It often happens that only one subspecialist is available in a given community (eg, oncologist) and no choice exists.

C. Make an Appointment for the Family: After the family has agreed to the referral, the physician can ask his secretary to arrange an appointment for them. This increases compliance. If the case is particularly complicated, a long consultation visit should be requested.

D. Send a Referral Letter: A referral letter should be sent immediately so that it will arrive well in advance of the appointment with the consultant. All pertinent information, such as copies of previous evaluations, hospital discharge summaries, and laboratory results, should be included. If time is short, the consultant can be prepared for the visit by phone and pertinent data can be sent along with the patient.

E. Specify the Service Requested: The specific questions to be answered and the future role of the referring physician should be clarified if possible in the referral letter.

Williams TF, MacKinney LG: Consultation-referral process. In: *Ambulatory Pediatrics.* Green M, Haggerty RJ (editors). Saunders, 1968.

QUALITY CONTROL OF AMBULATORY PEDIATRIC CARE

At a time when the consumer, third-party payers, and physicians themselves are alarmed at rising health care costs, all concerned should attempt to develop some kind of reliable quality control. In general, "organized medicine" has in the past been incapable of effectively penalizing any but the most flagrant examples of medical incompetence. The medical societies and academies are now attempting to develop a system of "peer review" which will at least ensure the consumer that the services billed for are appropriate and properly priced. This concept of peer review or medical audit can be implemented by a group of physicians for the purposes of self-education as well as the continual improvement of quality.

In any good hospital with an interested staff—especially where house staff are present—quality control is almost a built-in feature. Frequent reassessment of the inpatient's status by the physician, plus constant review by other medical and paramedical personnel, make "peer review" an ongoing process.

Care of ambulatory patients, on the other hand, usually is not reviewed systematically. The following is a suggestion for developing a program that will both improve the quality of ambulatory practice and make it more challenging and satisfying.

Physicians can attempt to schedule 1 hour a week for chart review. Several pediatricians should be present to make this a maximal learning experience. In group practice, the participants are already available. The pediatrician in solo practice can meet with the one or 2 pediatricians with whom he shares night calls. The group can focus on random charts or on selected charts that cover a specific problem. The latter method requires an office data retrieval system.

CHART REVIEWS

Health Maintenance Chart Review

The delivery of comprehensive health maintenance care can be easily audited by reviewing the health maintenance flow sheet (see p 162). Since the

nursing staff is primarily responsible for filling out these flow sheets, this type of review is largely a check on their ability to comply with office protocol and need not be done very often. The office protocols themselves require periodic review and revision.

Acute Illness Chart Review

Acute illness charts can be audited for completeness in diagnosis and therapy of the chief complaint. The following questions can be asked: (1) Was the diagnosis valid? Validity is substantiated if the chart contains adequate historical, physical, or laboratory data to document the diagnosis. (2) Was the therapy optimal? (3) Was the follow-up plan optimal? Charts of patients with a specific acute illness (eg, acute lymphadenitis, streptococcal pharyngitis, or infectious hepatitis) can be pulled and audited to test the group consensus about therapy and follow-up.

Chronic Disease Chart Review

Examination of the chronic disease flow sheet (see p 164) is an easy way to audit chronic disease management. If no such flow sheet exists, the variables recommended above for monitoring chronic disease can be assessed as one reviews the entire chart. This process could then result in the formation of a chronic disease flow sheet for that patient. Chart review sessions can be more educational if only one chronic disease is considered each time and if an "expert" on that disease is present. The expert can be an actual subspecialist or a member of the group who has reviewed the literature or attended a workshop on this disease.

Diagnostic Problem Chart Review

An easy way to review consultations is to criticize the consultation report. The following questions can be asked: (1) Was the data base adequate? (2) Were all the active problems identified? (3) Was the diagnostic plan for each problem optimal? (4) Were the final diagnoses valid? (5) Was the recommended therapy for each diagnosis optimal? (6) Was the role of the referring physician clarified and honored? If these consultations are concerned with general pediatric problems, an outside consultant will usually not be required.

Brook RH, Appel FA: Quality-of-care assessment: Choosing a method for peer review. N Engl J Med 288:1323, 1973.
Coulter LW: Peer review: Tutor or judge? JAMA 230:1161, 1974.
Haggerty RJ: Quality assurance: The road to PSRO and beyond. Pediatrics 54:90, 1974.
Meyers A: Audit of medical records from pediatric specialty clinics. Pediatrics 51:22, 1973.
Osborne CE, Thompson HC: Criteria for evaluation of ambulatory child health care by chart audit: Development and testing of a methodology. Pediatrics 56 (Suppl):625, 1975.
Peterson P: Teaching peer review. JAMA 224:884, 1973.
Starfield B & others: Private pediatric practice: Performance and problems. Pediatrics 52:344, 1973.

MEDICAL CARE COMPLIANCE

Correct diagnoses and optimal therapeutic recommendations can be ensured by the voluntary type of peer review discussed above. An aspect of the quality of care which is not easy to assess by chart review but which needs to be borne in mind is patient compliance. Superb recommendations do not guarantee anything. Medical care does not become effective until the parent accepts the diagnosis and carries out the therapeutic recommendations. These matters could be considered beyond the physician's control, but he has some influence over them. A parent's compliance often reflects her satisfaction with the medical care being given. Until there is a better understanding of missed follow-up appointments, missed referrals, missed laboratory tests, ungiven medications, unfollowed advice, and unkept home records, even the best conceived therapeutic goals will often not be achieved.

Charney E: Patient-doctor communication: Implications for clinicians. Pediatr Clin North Am 19:263, 1972.
Fink D & others: Effective patient care in the pediatric ambulatory setting: A study of the acute care clinic. Pediatrics 43:927, 1969.
Rogers KD: Effectiveness of aggressive follow-up on Navajo infant health and medical care use. Pediatrics 53:721, 1974.
Stanfield B, Scheff D: Effectiveness of pediatric care: The relationship between processes and outcome. Pediatrics 49:547, 1972.

PRACTICAL TIPS FOR AMBULATORY CARE

A number of problems arise which may be perplexing both to the patient and to the physician in the daily care of ambulatory patients. Some of these apparently complex problems have rather simple solutions.

FOREIGN BODIES

Metallic Foreign Body in the Soft Tissues

Tape a straight pin with the point over the site where the metallic object entered the skin. Then obtain an x-ray of the area. An exact measurement can then be obtained to locate the foreign body in relation to the straight pin. Located in this manner, the foreign body can be removed with minimal exploration.

Inlow PM: "Tip of the Month." Consultant 7(6):27, 1967.

Splinters Under the Nails

Using a single-edged razor blade or a sharp thin scalpel, the nail can be gently shaved over the distal end of the splinter until the splinter is exposed. The sliver can then be easily pulled out with a pair of fine-pointed tweezers.

Mikelionis J: "Tip of the Month." Consultant 5(2):28, 1965.

Imbedded Fishhook

Fishhooks can be removed (eg, from a finger) without local anesthesia or wirecutters by bringing them back through their point of entry. A piece of fishline is looped around the curve of the fishhook. The 2 strands of the fishline are wrapped tightly about the physician's forefinger about 1 foot from where it is looped around the hook. The patient's finger is held against a firm surface to stabilize it. The free shank of the fishhook is pressed against the patient's finger with the physician's free hand until the barb is disengaged and the barb's long axis is parallel to the line of intended expulsion. With the string in this same axis, a quick yank expels the hook immediately.

Another technic described in the second reference can be performed without yanking. An 18-gauge needle is inserted into the wound through the point of entry. After the needle bevel is locked firmly over the barb, the fishhook and needle can be slowly withdrawn through the original wound as a unit.

Friedenberg S: Removing an imbedded fishhook. Hosp Physician 7(8):48, August 1971.
Longmire WT: Another twist on a fishhook. Emergency Med 3(7):98, July 1971.

Feasting Ticks

Most imbedded ticks will withdraw when covered with alcohol, nail polish, mineral oil, or an ointment. Occasionally, a needle can be inserted between the tick's jaws and used to pry loose his grip. If the above methods fail, the following definitive method can be employed. Pick up the body of the tick with a pair of forceps. Apply gentle traction so that the skin is tented up at the site where the tick is imbedded. Then take a number 11 scalpel blade (or a razor blade) and quickly cut away the superficial layer of dermis in which the tick has buried its jaws. Brief pressure will stop the bleeding. This method of extracting the tick is relatively painless and ensures removal of the head.

The Zipper-Entrapped Penis

A young child in a hurry to urinate can inadvertently catch his penis in his zipper. A zipper is composed of 2 rows of zipper teeth plus a zipper fastener in the middle. The zipper fastener is composed of an upper and a lower plate. The plates are joined by a U-shaped median bar. This U-shaped bar should be cut with side-cutters or wire-cutters. After this is done, the zipper fastener will come apart, and this will usually free the skin. If the skin remains attached to the zipper teeth, these can be separated by grasping them on both sides and using a circular motion, rotating the 2 sides away from each other.

Thomson GH: Removing zippers from chins and penises. Hosp Physician 9(6):58, 1973.

Ring on a Swollen Finger

Pass a piece of string under the ring and then wind the distal end of the string in close loops tightly from the distal edge of the ring past the knuckle. Exert a slow, firm pull on the proximal end of the string. The edema passes underneath the ring and the ring is slowly pulled distally as the cord unwinds.

Another method of removing a ring without cutting it is to place 2 or 3 hairpins between the finger and the ring. The hairpins then serve as a track over which the ring quite easily slides off.

If there is a dentist's office nearby, another way the ring might be removed is to have the dentist cut it off with a carborundum disk attached to his drill. The flesh of the finger must be protected by an inserted strip (eg, a tongue blade segment).

Burgoon EB: "Tip of the Month." Consultant 4(4):8, 1964.
Steier M: Resident and Staff Physician. 20(8):27, 1974.

Hair Wrapped Around a Digit

A piece of fine hair wrapped about an infant's digit and left unnoticed can cause severe edema or even amputation. Removal of the hair is usually difficult because it cannot be readily grasped. Application of a liquid hair remover (eg, Nair) will usually dissolve the hair within 15 minutes.

Douglas ED: (Correspondence.) J Pediatr 91:162, 1977.

Gum in the Hair

An easy and nontraumatic way to remove gum from children's hair is by rubbing the gum with peanut butter until the hairs are freed from the gum. This technic is far superior to pulling or cutting the gum out of the hair.

Tar on the Skin

Tar can be removed by applying ice to it for 1 or 2 minutes. The ice causes the tar to become quite hard and nonsticky, so that it can be easily peeled from the skin. Hydrocarbon solvents merely soften the tar and smear it around, and they are painful if a wound is present.

Bostrom PD: "Tip of the Month." Consultant 8(1):12, 1968.

Fiberglass Itch

The small glass spicules from fiberglass can be removed by applying hypoallergenic tape to the affected areas and leaving it on for 15–20 minutes. This allows the spicules to become firmly attached to the tape and removed as the tape is peeled away. A corticosteroid cream applied twice daily for 1–2 days may be helpful after the treatment. This treatment is also helpful for some plant stickers (eg, cactus, stinging nettle).

Tompkins RR: "Tip of the Month." Consultant 12(2):88, 1972.

LACERATIONS

Wound Cleaning in a Resistant Child

The wound can be covered with gauze saturated with 1% lidocaine for 15 minutes, which will cause momentary discomfort. The area will then be relatively anesthetized, and vigorous wound cleaning will be tolerated. The subcutaneous injection of additional lidocaine after the wound is cleaned will also be better tolerated.

Avoiding Unwanted Tattoos

Dirty abrasions of the knee, face, and elbow can result in permanent tattooing if all foreign particulate matter, especially carbon particles, is not meticulously removed. The area should be anesthetized as described above and then scrubbed gently with an antibacterial cleanser using a soft surgical nail brush. Some contaminated pieces of skin may need debridement.

Diefenbach WC: "Tip of the Month." Consultant 17(5):34, 1977.

Laceration Closure in a Frightened Child

Wounds can often be closed without local anesthesia or sutures by using microporous adhesive tape (Steri-Strip). The skin adjacent to the laceration is made tacky with tincture of benzoin. The 1/8-inch strips of tape are applied in either a parallel or crisscross pattern. This microporous tape is a decided improvement over "butterfly" tape.

Abramo A: Recent results with sutureless wound closure in children. Am J Dis Child 110:42, 1965.

Suture Removal

There is a way to avoid having to dig imbedded sutures out of the skin of a struggling child. At the time the laceration is closed, a straight needle threaded with silk can be passed under each suture used for skin closure. The ends of this silk suture can be tied together, leaving a loose loop. At the time of removal, picking up this loose loop will lift up the sutures which have been used to close the wound. The scissors can then be easily slid underneath the sutures for snipping.

Floyd BG, McKnight CA: "Tip of the Month." Consultant 10(4):35, 1970.

Traumatic Amputations

When a patient loses a significant piece of his skin (eg, a fingertip) in an accident, the skin should be placed in cold normal saline solution and sent with the patient to a plastic surgeon.

BLUNT TRAUMA

Subungual Hematomas

The painful pressure secondary to a subungual hematoma can easily be relieved by applying a red-hot paper clip or other thick wire to the nail surface. The paper clip is held by a clamp. A hole is quickly burrowed through the nail and the blood is allowed to escape. This "hot iron" approach can be very frightening for a child. If there is a dentist's office nearby, it is preferable to have the dentist bore a hole quickly through the nail with a high-speed drill.

Traumatic Tooth Avulsion

Reimplantation of a tooth is possible only with the permanent teeth. The physician or parent should attempt to replace the avulsed tooth in its socket prior to going to the dentist. If this proves impossible, the tooth should be placed in cold normal saline solution and sent with the patient to his dentist.

Bernick SM: What the pediatrician should know about children's teeth: Dental emergencies. Clin Pediatr 9:487, 1970.

INJECTIONS

Painful Rabies Vaccine Injections

The local pain that occurs with daily rabies vaccine injections can be relieved by adding 1 ml of 2% lidocaine (Xylocaine) to the syringe.

Baehren PF: Pain and rabies vaccine. Clin Pediat 10:298, 1971.

Inadvertent Subcutaneous Injections

When intramuscular agents are given subcutaneously by mistake, complications can result. The location of the needle point can be rapidly assessed by trying to wiggle it prior to injection. If it is in a muscle mass, the needle point will be relatively fixed. If it is in the subcutaneous fatty tissues, it can be felt to move freely.

Schmitt BD: "Tip of the Month." Consultant 12(6):113, 1972.

MISCELLANEOUS PROCEDURES

Genital Labial Adhesions

Labial adhesions can usually be separated by introducing a probe into any opening remaining in the introitus and then tearing the adhesions. This method is only acceptable for thin adhesions. An ointment should be applied to the newly separated surfaces for several days to prevent them from resealing. A nontraumatic method for separating thicker labial adhesions is application of estrogen cream to the medial line for 3 or 4 days.

Hiccup

One teaspoonful of ordinary white granulated sugar swallowed "dry" will result in immediate cessation of hiccup in almost all patients. If the hiccups recur, this method will again be effective.

Engleman EG & others: Letters to the editor. N Engl J Med 285:1489, 1971.

Painful Bee Stings or Other Insect Bites

A dash of meat tenderizer (papain powder) and a drop of water massaged into the sting site for 5 minutes quickly relieves the pain. If these ingredients are not available, an ice cube often helps.

Forrer GR: "Tip of the Month." Consultant 12(9):121, 1972.

Paraphimosis

In this condition, the foreskin has become retracted and trapped behind the corona. Manual reduction can usually be achieved by placing the tips of the index and middle fingers of one hand behind the swollen foreskin, the thumb of the other hand over the urethral meatus, and applying gradual pressure. The foreskin will usually return to its normal position after this technic has been applied continuously for 4–5 minutes. If this approach fails, a urologist should be consulted for an emergency dorsal slit.

Postcircumcision Skin Tags

Parents occasionally bring their baby in during the first month of life because the foreskin has an irregular skin tag. A clamp can be applied along the desired line of cleavage for 1 minute. After the clamp is removed, an iris scissors can be used to cut along the crushed skin line without causing any significant bleeding.

Schmitt BD: "Tip of the Month." Consultant 12(5):91, 1972.

Umbilical Granulomas

Umbilical granulomas usually respond to alcohol cleansing. If a pinch of table salt is placed in the umbilical area after alcohol cleansing once a day for 3 days, the desiccant effect of the salt will rapidly shrink the granuloma.

Schmitt BD: "Tip of the Month." Consultant 12(8):91, 1972.

University of Colorado Medical Center   Name _____

PEDIATRIC HEALTH MAINTENANCE   Date of Birth _____

Birth through 3 months   Hosp. No. _____

Health Maintenance Visit   Date _____

Parent's concerns

Newborn data base
   Birth weight _____   Gestational age _____
   Pregnancy or delivery problems   Neonatal problems

Growth (comment on growth curve)

Feeding advice
   Formula _____   oz/24 hours _____
   Breast feeding: Frequency _____   min/feeding _____
   Vitamins _____   Iron _____
   Solids _____
   Feeding problems _____
   Advice: Introduce bottle in breast fed (2w) ☐   Introduce fluids other than milk (2m) ☐

Developmental status
   Stimulation advice: Hold baby (2w) ☐   Talk to baby (2m) ☐

Child rearing advice
   Sleep pattern _____
   Crying or colic _____
   Mother-child interaction _____
   Sibling rivalry (2w) _____

Family status
   Advice: Paternal involvement, family planning (2w) ☐   Utilize sitter (2m) ☐

Accident prevention advice
   Car seats, crib safety (2w) ☐   Rolling over (2m) ☐

Medical advice
   Discuss symptoms of major illness ☐   Demonstrate use of bulb syringe for nose (2w) ☐
   Temperature taking, Tylenol and fever handout (2m) ☐

Intercurrent illness

University of Colardo Medical Center

PEDIATRIC HEALTH MAINTENANCE

4 months through 14 months

Health Maintenance Visit

Name _____

Date of Birth _____

Hosp. No. _____

Date _____

Parent's concerns

Growth (comment on growth curve)

Feeding advice
Formula _____ oz/24 hours _____
Breast feeding: Frequency _____ min/feeding _____
Vitamins _____ Iron _____
Solids _____
Feeding problems _____
Advice: No bottles in bed; introduce solids, spoon, cup (4m) ☐
    Confirm intake of iron-rich solids (6m) ☐ Introduce finger foods, confirm on 3 meals/day (9m) ☐
    Entirely on table foods. Phase out bottle by 18m (12m) ☐

Developmental status
Stimulation advice: Toys for reaching (4m) ☐ Avoid confining baby equipment (6m) ☐
Repeat baby's sounds (9m) ☐ Name objects and pictures for baby (12m) ☐

Child rearing advice
Sleep pattern _____
Behavior problems _____
Advice: Sleeps through the night (4m) ☐ Normal separation anxiety (6m) ☐
    Discipline: Use negative voice and eye contact rather than physical punishment (9m) ☐
    Don't punish for normal exploratory behavior, discuss positive strokes for good behavior (12m) ☐

Family status

Accident prevention advice
Safe toys (4m) ☐ Stairs and gates, drowning in bathtub (9m) ☐
Electrical cords (6m) ☐ Ipecac and poison talk (12m) ☐

Medical advice
Teething myths (6m) ☐ Shoes (9m) ☐ Use of 911 (12m) ☐

Intercurrent illness

University of Colorado Medical Center   Name _____

PEDIATRIC HEALTH MAINTENANCE   Date of Birth _____

15 months through 3 years   Hosp. No. _____

Health Maintenance Visit   Date _____

Parent's concerns

Growth (comment on growth curve)

Diet
    Milk _____ oz/24 hours
    Eating problems _____
    Advice: Entirely on table foods, off all bottles (18m) ☐
    Physiologic anorexia, protein intake (2y) ☐

Developmental status
    Advice: Read to child (1½, 2) ☐   Listen to child (2) ☐   TV rules (3) ☐

Child rearing advice
    Sleep problems _____
    Behavior problems _____
    Frequency of spanking _____
    Advice: Don't punish for normal negativism (1½) ☐   Discuss toilet training (1½) ☐
       Discuss positive "strokes" for good behavior (2) ☐   Review progress of toilet training (2, 3) ☐
       Emphasize consistency in discipline and use of time-out room (2, 3) ☐

Family status

Accident prevention advice
    Scalds, aspiration foods (1½) ☐   Street/garage safety (2) ☐
    Drowning in ditch and pools (3) ☐

Dental advice
    Brushing frequency _____
    Advice: Avoid snacks that cause cavities (1½) ☐   Use fluoride toothpaste (2) ☐
    Brushing technics (3) ☐

Intercurrent illness

University of Colorado Medical Center

PEDIATRIC HEALTH MAINTENANCE

4 years through 5 years

Health Maintenance Visit

Name _____

Date of Birth _____

Hosp. No. _____

Date _____

To be completed by parent   Check correct answer

School readiness:

1. Does your child pay good attention when you read him a story?	Yes	No
2. Can your child play quietly by himself for over ½ hour?	Yes	No
3. Does your child mind adults and follow instructions?	Yes	No
4. Does your child speak clearly enough for others to understand?	Yes	No
5. Does your child object to being left with a sitter?	No	Yes
6. Can your child dress himself?	Yes	No
7. Does your child ever wet or soil himself during the day?	No	Yes

To be completed by physician or nurse

Parent's concerns

Growth (comment on growth curve)

Diet

School readiness
Problems detected by above questions _____
Development: PDQ (4, 5) Score _____   Weak category _____
  DDST (if fails PDQ) Result _____
  Articulation: DASE (4) Score _____   Percentile _____
Advice: Preschool if any problems (4) ▢

Accident prevention advice
Adult seat belts, petting dogs (4) ▢   Crossing street, trampoline (5) ▢

Dental advice
No daytime thumbsucking (4) ▢   No nighttime thumbsucking (5) ▢
Frequency of brushing _____ Type of toothpaste _____

Intercurrent illness

University of Colorado Medical Center   Name _____

PEDIATRIC HEALTH MAINTENANCE   Date of Birth _____

6 years through 11 years   Hosp. No. _____

Health Maintenance Visit   Date _____

Parent's concerns

Diet

School
   Name of school _____   Grade _____
   Academic performance _____
   Attendance _____
   Behavior _____
   Advice: Child's responsibility for schoolwork (6) ☐   Adult at home before and after school (6, 10) ☐

Behavior
   Behavior problems _____
   Chores _____
   Friends _____
   Advice: TV less than 2 hrs/day (6) ☐   One sport or club (8, 10) ☐

Family status

Sex education
   Discuss puberty and menarche before Jr. High School (10) ☐
   Menstrual status (10 ♀) _____

Accident prevention advice
   Bicycle safety (6) ☐   Swimming lessons (8) ☐
   Fires, matches (10)

Dental advice
   Frequency of brushing _____ Type of toothpaste _____
   Dental referral (6) ☐

Intercurrent illness

University of Colorado Medical Center   Name _____

PEDIATRIC HEALTH MAINTENANCE   Date of Birth _____

12 years through 17 years   Hosp. No. _____

Health Maintenance Visit   Date _____

Parent's concerns

Adolescent's concerns

Growth (comment on growth curve)

Diet

School
   Name of school _____   Grade _____
   Academic performance _____
   Attendance _____
   Behavior _____
   Career plans _____

Behavior
   Free time/friends _____
   Chores/job _____
   Person to confide in _____
   Predominant mood _____
   Advice: Discuss values of babysitting (12) ☐   Discuss drugs and alcohol (12, 16) ☐
       Discuss smoking (14) ☐

Family status
   Advice: Discuss independence and parent's trust (16) ☐

Sex education
   Dating, contraception, venereal disease, masturbation (14) ☐   Marriage (18) ☐
   Sexual activity (14, 16, 18) _____

Accident prevention advice
   Firearms (12) ☐   Cycling safety (14) ☐   Driving safety, water safety (16) ☐
   Motorcycles, seat belts (18) ☐

Dental advice
   Frequency of brushing _____ Type of toothpaste _____

Medical advice
   Acne ☐   Personal hygiene (14) ☐   Teach self examination of breasts (16?) ☐

Intercurrent illness

University of Colorado Medical Center   Name _____

PEDIATRIC OPD   Hosp. No. _____

Health Maintenance Flowsheet   Date of Birth _____

Directions: Record date only for all immunizations.
Record value for head circumference, height, weight, BP, PKU, and Hct.
Record N (normal) or ABN (abnormal) for all other items.

	2 wk	2 mo	4 mo	6 mo	9 mo	12 mo	15 mo	18 mo	2 yr	3 yr	4 yr	5 yr	6 yr	8 yr	10 yr	12 yr	14 yr	16 yr	18 yr
Today's date																			
Head circ.																			
Height (cm)																			
Weight (kg)																			
BP																			
Dental caries screen																			
DPT (dT after 6 years)																			
OPV																			
Measles-rubella																			
Mumps																			
TB																			
PDQ (DDST if fail PDQ)																			
Speech (DASE)																			
Hearing[1]																			
Vision[2]																			
Color vision																			
PKU retest																			
Hct																			
Urine dip-stick																			
Urine culture ♀																			
VDRL/GC[3]																			
Pap smear[4]																			

[1] Listen to soft sounds (2m)
   Turns to sound (6m)
   Audiometrics (4y)

[2] Red reflex (2w)
   Regards smiling face (2m)
   Follows past midline (4m)
   Corneal light reflection test (6m)
   Visual acuity (3y)

[3] Sexually active patients
[4] If pelvic exam is done for other reason

University of Colorado Medical Center

ACUTE ILLNESS CLINIC

Name_____

Hosp. No._____

Date_____

Brief Screening Questionnaire for Major Problems in New Patients

We realize you are here because your child is sick. We will concentrate on that problem today. Please answer the following questions to help us decide what **other** medical care your child may need.

Circle One

1. Does your child have any important physical problems? . . . . No   Yes
2. Does your child have any important emotional problems? . . . . No   Yes
3. Does your child have any important school problems? . . . . No   Yes
4. Does your child have any other medical problem you would like evaluated? . . . . No   Yes
If the answer to 1, 2, 3, or 4 is Yes, list the problems below.

5. Has your child ever been hospitalized? . . . . No   Yes
If Yes, list date, hospital, and diagnosis below.

6. Is your child allergic to any medicines? . . . . No   Yes
If Yes, which ones?

7. Would you like future well child care at our office? . . . . No   Yes
8. Does your child receive his well child care elsewhere? . . . . No   Yes
If Yes, where?

University of Colorado Medical Center

DIABETES MELLITUS FLOW SHEET

Name _____
Hosp. No. _____
Date _____

Dates:	Baseline Data	22 Apr 71	6 May 71	10 June 71	5 Aug 71	7 Oct 71	13 Oct 71	4 Nov 71	
DISEASE STATUS									
Hypoglycemia —frequency	3-4x/m.	"	2	0	3	1	1	1	
—time of day	Usually 11 AM	"	11 AM 4 PM	—	Various	10 AM	11 AM	4 PM	
—severity	Rarely a seizure	"	Mild	—	Mild	Mild	Seizure	Mild	
—pptg. event	?	"	Mother forbade snack	—	Exercise at camp	Gym	Took 10u. extra insulin	Sports	
Ketosis —frequency	0-1x/m.	"	0	0	0	1	0	0	
—duration		"	—	—	—	8 hrs	—	—	
—pptg. event		"	—	—	—	URI	—	—	
Weight/BP	—	85 88/62	85 —	86	88 96/70	87	88	88	
Fundi/liver	—	OK 0	—	—	OK 0	—	—	—	
Urine gluc./acet.	—	0 / 0	1+ / 0	3+ / 0	1+ / 0	4+ / large	1+ / 0	2+ / 0	
Blood gluc./acet.	highly variable	—	—	—	—	410 / small	—	—	
Hospitalizations	5x in last 4 yrs.	—	—	—	—	No	—	—	
Emotional status	Depressed	"	"	Improved	Happy	OK	OK	OK	
TREATMENT REGIMEN									
Insulin —type	Reg/NPH	"	"	"	"	"	"	"	
—dosage	14/20	10/20	"	"	"	"	"	"	
—SC dystrophy	buttocks hypertrophy	"	"	"	"	"	"	"	
Rotates sites	all into buttocks	discontinue buttocks	Done	75% into @ thigh	OK	"	"	"	
Diet type	ADA exchange	Unmeasured Diet	Mother resistant	OK	"	"	"	"	
Snacks	Variable	3 snacks	Mother resistant	OK	"	Raisins before gym	OK	"	
Carrying food/ Glucagon at home	No /Yes	Advice given / "	No / "	Yes / "	No / "	Yes / "	" / "	" / "	
Rx compliance —gives shot	Mother gives 100%	Pt. to give shots	90% by pt.	10% by pt.	100% by pt. Camp helped	"	"	"	
—checks urine	Yes	Same	"	"	"Forgot" records	Same	No	Only when symptomatic	
Camp/ID card	No/No	Rec./given	— /yes	Camp form / "	— / "	— / "	— / "	— / "	
Education (time spent)	—	1 hour	1 hour	30 mins	15 mins	15 mins	20 mins	10 mins	

EXAMPLES OF VARIABLES FOR CHRONIC DISEASE FLOW SHEETS*

Acute Glomerulonephritis

A. Disease Status: Gross hematuria, headaches, weight/BP, signs of CHF edema (sites, duration), impetigo, microscopic hematuria, casts, proteinuria, 24-hour urine protein, creatinine clearance, BUN/creatinine, Hct/ESR, throat culture, complement fixation, hospitalization, consultations.

B. Treatment Regimen: Penicillin, activity restriction.

Allergic Rhinitis

A. Disease Status: Exacerbations (dates, nose symptoms, eye symptoms, place of onset, response to drug), nasal turbinates, nasal polyps, mouth breather, conjunctiva, allergic shiners, nasal smear for eosinophils, allergens (by history, by skin test), sinus films, consultations.

B. Treatment Regimen: Decongestants, vasoconstrictor nosedrops, vasoconstrictor eyedrops, avoidance of allergens, avoidance of triggers, environmental control checks, hyposensitization, treatment compliance, education (time spent).

Asthma

A. Disease Status: Attacks (frequency, duration, response to drug, pptg. event), exercise tolerance, height/weight, lung auscultation, chest x-ray, consultations, hospitalization (duration, resp. failure), emotional status.

B. Treatment Regimen: Theophylline orally (amount, mg/kg/dose), theophylline rectally, nebulizer (type and dosage), adrenaline/Sus-Phrine, antibiotics, hydration, hyposensitization, gym restrictions, environmental control checks,[1] treatment compliance, education (time spent).

[1] Allergens identified by history; allergens identified by skin test; nonallergenic triggers.

Atopic Dermatitis

A. Disease Status: Exacerbations (dates, site, severity, pptg. event, response to drug), skin findings, excoriations, infected clinically, cultures, consultations, emotional status.

B. Treatment Regimen: Steroid cream, occlusive dressings, skin hydration, lubricating creams, nonallergenic soap, antihistamines h.s., antibiotics, protec. cloths/cut fingernails, avoidance,[1] treatment compliance, education (time spent).

[1] Avoid allergens, nonspecific irritants, vaccinia, herpes simplex.

Chronic Serous Otitis Media

A. Disease Status: Bout of AOM (right, left), TM appearance (right, left), TM mobility (right, left), Weber test, audiometrics (right, left), mastoid films (right, left), consultations.

B. Treatment Regimen: Decongestants, antibiotics, chewing exercises, myringotomy, polyethylene tubes, adenoidectomy, evidence for allergy, feeding position (infant), treatment compliance, education (time spent).

Constipation

A. Disease Status: Usual BMs (frequency, consistency, size, pain, blood), soiling (amount/day, place of occurrence), days without soiling/week, abdominal exam, rectal exam, fissure, barium enema, consultations.

B. Treatment Regimen: Mineral oil, cathartic, enemas, suppositories, vitamins, diet, praise, rewards, treatment compliance (takes meds, sits on toilet, releases BMs).

Diabetes Mellitus

A. Disease Status: Hypoglycemia (frequency, time of day, severity, pptg. event), ketosis (frequency, duration, pptg. event), weight/BP, fundi/liver, urine gluc./acet., blood gluc./acet., hospitalizations, emotional status.

B. Treatment Regimen: Insulin (type, dosage, SC dystrophy), rotates sites, diet type, snacks, carrying food/glucagon at home, treatment compliance (gives shot, checks urine), camp/ID card, education (time spent).

Enuresis

A. Disease Status: Nights (total dry, dry without awakening, dry in a row, nocturia, depth of sleep), days (frequency—hrs., urgency, wetting, ability to wait), polydipsia, consultations.

B. Treatment Regimen: Voids at bedtime, minimal fluids after 6:00 p.m., awakened by parents, bladder stretching (maximum ounces, average ounces), stream interruption, praise, rewards, overnights, drugs (type, dosage, toxicity), treatment compliance.

Failure to Thrive

A. Disease Status: Milk/day (oz), solids/day, calo-

* Some of the abbreviations in the text that follows may be unfamiliar to the reader: acet. = acetone; AOM = acute otitis media; ASO = antistreptolysin O; BE = barium enema; BM = bowel movement; BP = blood pressure; BUN = blood urea nitrogen; cath. = catheter; CCMS = clean catch midstream; CHF = congestive heart failure; Cr = creatinine, DDST = Denver Developmental Screening Test; ESR = erythrocyte sedimentation rate; gluc. = glucose; Hct = hematocrit; hpf = high-power field; h.s. = at bedtime; ID = identification; med = medication; MHC = mental health clinic; PHN = public health nurse; pptg. = precipitating; protec. = protective; resp. = respiratory; retics. = reticulocytes; RF = rheumatoid factor; ROM = range of motion; SC = subcutaneous; TM = tympanic membrane; UGI = upper gastrointestinal; UTI = urinary tract infection.

ries/kg/day, vomiting/diarrhea, weight gain (oz/week), height/head circumference, ability to suck, signs of trauma, hygiene neglect, mother-child interaction, DDST, broken appts., consultations, hospitalizations (dates/wt gain, parental visits).

B. Treatment Regimen: Diet (type, calories/kg/day), nutritionist, crisis phone number, PHN status, child welfare status, court (dates, decisions).

Hyperactive Child

A. Disease Status: Parent report (hyperactivity,[1] attention span,[2] aggression), school report (hyperactivity, attention span, aggression), academic performance, office activity level, office attention span, consultation.

B. Treatment Regimen: Stimulants (size, dosage, weight, side-effects), dangerous drug check, trial without medication, home behavior modification program, special classroom, treatment compliance, school note, counseling (time spent).

[1] At different places—home, neighbor's house, stores, church, car, etc.
[2] With different activities—TV, toys, games, books, etc.

Inflammatory Bowel Disease

A. Disease Status: Flare-ups (dates, BMs/day, amount of blood, cramps, pptg. event, response to drug), weight/height, abdominal tenderness, rectal exam, extraintestinal signs, Hct/ESR/stool Hematest, sigmoidoscopy/biopsy, x-rays (BE/UGI), hospitalizations, consultations, emotional status.

B. Treatment Regimen: Azulfidine, steroids (oral), steroids (enema), iron, antidiarrhea agent, sedatives, treatment compliance.

Migraine Headache

A. Disease Status: Attacks (frequency, aura, duration, interference with activity, vomiting, place of onset, pptg. event, response to drug), neurologic exam, fundi/cranial bruit, consultations, emotional status.

B. Treatment Regimen: Analgesic (type, dosage, toxicity), ergotamine (type, dosage, vomiting), carrying drug on person, dangerous drug control, rest and dark room, treatment compliance, school note, education (time spent).

Nonaccidental Trauma

A. Disease Status: Signs of trauma, alleged cause, weight/head circumference, fundi, photographs, trauma x-rays, hygiene neglect, mother-child interaction, DDST, broken appts., crises and outcome, consultations, hospitalizations (dates, parental visits).

B. Treatment Regimen: Crisis phone number, PHN status, child welfare status, therapist (MHC, lay, group, etc), court (dates, decisions), day care/foster home.

Peptic Ulcer

A. Disease Status: Flare-up of ulcer (dates, frequency of pain, severity, vomiting, hematemesis/me-lena, pptg. event, response to food, response to antacid), weight/height, epigastric tenderness, Hct/stool Hematest, upper GI x-ray, hospitalizations, consultations, emotional status.

B. Treatment Regimen: Antacids, diet, snacks, anticholinergics, avoidance of aspirin, extra rest, sedatives, treatment compliance, education (time spent).

Rheumatic Heart Disease

A. Disease Status: Disability level, height/weight, resting pulse, cardiac exam, signs of CHF, chest film, ECG, ESR/ASO, throat culture, strep in family, consultations, hospitalizations (dates, type of flare-up, cause), emotional status.

B. Treatment Regimen: Aspirin (size, amount, mg/kg/day, serum level, toxicity), prophylactic penicillin, activity restrictions, treatment compliance.

Rheumatoid Arthritis

A. Disease Status: Flare-ups (dates, fever, response to drug), remission (pain, disability level), weight, height, active arthritis (site, size, ROM, swelling, heat, etc), slit lamp, Hct/ESR/RF, x-rays, consultations, hospitalizations, emotional status.

B. Treatment Regimen: Aspirin (amount, mg/kg/day, serum level, toxicity), ROM exercises twice a day, gym restrictions, treatment compliance.

Seizures

A. Disease Status: Attacks (frequency, dates and times, aura, type and duration, postictal condition, pptg. event), weight/fundi, neurologic exam, EEG, consultations, hospitalizations, emotional status.

B. Treatment Regimen: Drug #1 (type, dosage, mg/kg/day, toxicity), drug #2 (type, dosage, mg/kg/day, toxicity), medical restrictions,[1] treatment compliance, ID card, education (time spent).

[1] Modified gym, swimming with supervision, avoiding heights and cycling on major roads.

Sickle Cell Disease

A. Disease Status: Pain crisis (frequency, duration, site, pptg. event, response to drug), infection, disability level, height/weight, jaundice/spleen, Hct/WBC, retics. (%)/sickled (%), bilirubin (indirect), Howell-Jolly bodies, hospitalizations, emotional status.

B. Treatment Regimen: Alkali, hydration, antibiotics, transfusions, analgesic, gym restrictions, preventive measures,[1] treatment compliance, education (time spent).

[1] Avoid cold water, dehydration, physical exhaustion, altitudes over 10,000 ft.

Sydenham's Chorea

A. Disease Status: Disability (eating, dressing, toileting, sleeping), speech, handwriting, facial grimaces, gait, sustained postures, heart exam, ESR/ASO, throat culture, hospitalizations, consultations, emotional status.

B. Treatment Regimen: Thorazine (size, dosage, toxicity), prophylactic penicillin, occupational therapy, treatment compliance, education (time spent).

Urinary Tract Infection

A. Disease Status: Early UTI symptoms, weight/ BP, UTI signs, urine stream, urinalysis (WBC/hpf,[1] bacteria/hpf,[2] casts/hpf, sp. gr./pH), urine culture (collec. meth.,[3] colony count, organism, antibiotic sensitivities), verification of UTI,[4] Cr/BUN, x-rays, consultations, hospitalizations.

B. Treatment Regimen: Antibiotics (type, mg/kg/ day, toxicity), acidifying agent, preventive measures,[5] treatment compliance, education (time spent).

[1] 5 ml spun 3 min × 3000 rpm
[2] 1+ = 1–10 bacteria/hpf
   2+ = 10–100 bacteria/hpf
   3+ = innumerable, loosely packed/hpf
   4+ = innumerable, closely packed/hpf
[3] CCMS, cath, suprapubic
[4] CCMS: > 10⁵ of single organism on 2 specimens
   Cath (exclude 1st 5 ml): > 10³
   Suprapubic: any growth
[5] Hydration
   Frequent voiding
   Perineal hygiene
   Avoidance of bubble bath

University of Colorado Medical Center

PROBLEM LIST

Name _____

Hosp. No. _____

Date of Birth _____

Problem Number	Date of Onset	Problem (Active)	Date of Resolution	Responsible Physician
1	1958	Health maintenance		Dr. R. Jones
2	1958	Minor acute illness		Dr. R. Jones
3	1964	Diabetes mellitus		Dr. R. Jones
4	1966	Grand mal seizures		Dr. R. Jones
5	Sept 1969	School phobia		Dr. R. Jones
6	Feb 1970	Recurrent epistaxis	May 1970	Dr. R. Jones
7	Aug 1970	Scoliosis		Dr. B. Craig (Orthopedics)

University of Colorado Medical Center

PEDIATRIC REFERRAL CLINIC

Name _____

Hosp. No. _____

Date of Birth _____

–1–

Date _____

Reason for Referral (to be completed by a parent)

Describe your child's current problem (or problems).
Be as brief as possible.
Include approximate dates whenever possible.

–2–

PHYSICAL SCREENING DATA

A. Review of Systems

Circle any of the following symptoms that apply to your child.

1. **General:** poor appetite excessive appetite excessive thirst
overweight underweight weight loss too tall too short
difficulty in sleeping excessive sleeping confusion loss of memory
no energy excessive energy fevers

2. **Skin:** rash acne unexplained lump easy bruising
dandruff itching

3. **Eyes:** eye pain blurred vision crossed eyes wears glasses

4. **Ear-Nose-Throat:** earaches decreased hearing sneezing attacks
frequent nosebleeds bad teeth mouth breathing
difficulty in swallowing

5. **Respiratory:** hoarseness cough wheezing difficulty in breathing
"shortness of breath" attacks

6. **Cardiovascular:** chest pain heart murmur high blood pressure

7. **Gastrointestinal:** abdominal pains nausea vomiting
frequent indigestion diarrhea constipation blood in stools
stools in underwear (soiling)

8. **Urinary:** painful urination frequent urination weak urine stream
daytime wetting bedwetting

9. **Skeletal:** bone pain back pain limp swollen joints
frequent accidents

10. **Neuromuscular:** headache migraine weakness paralysis
numbness clumsiness loss of balance dizziness
unexplained movements or jerks convulsions staring spells
fainting breathholding spells unexplained "attacks"

11. If your daughter has started her menstrual periods, complete the following:
When did they begin? Month _____ Year _____
Circle if any of the following apply:
painful periods excessive bleeding other menstrual problems

12. Do you feel that any of your child's symptoms are caused by stress or worry? No ____ Yes ____

13. Do you feel that your child is physically delicate? No ____ Yes ____

(This medical information is confidential.)

University of Colorado Medical Center

PEDIATRIC REFERRAL CLINIC

Name _____

Hosp. No. _____

Date of Birth _____

—3—

B. Past Medical History

    1. Newborn: How much did your baby weigh at birth?   _____ lb, _____ oz

        How long did your pregnancy last?   _____ (weeks or months)

        Did your baby have any complications at birth or in the first days of life?   No _____   Yes _____

    2. Hospitalizations: Has your child ever been hospitalized?   No _____   Yes _____

                If Yes, list the approximate dates, hospital, and reason for admission.

    3. Other illness: Has your child had any important illnesses for which he/she was **not** hospitalized?

                                                            No _____   Yes _____

                If Yes, list the approximate dates and the type of illness.

    4. Allergies: *Circle* any of the following allergies your child has:

            asthma   nose allergy   eye allergy   eczema   hives

            drug allergy   food allergy

    5. Medications: Is your child on any daily medication?   No _____   Yes _____

                If Yes, list the drug and the amount per day.

University of Colorado Medical Center

PEDIATRIC REFERRAL CLINIC

Name _____

Hosp. No. _____

Date of Birth _____

–4–

C. Family History

1. Are there any inherited diseases that run in your family?   No _____ Yes _____

2. Are there any family problems that might be related to your child's symptoms?   No _____ Yes _____

3. List below the name and age of each person who lives in your house. (If any of the people have a medical problem, mention it.)

_____

_____

_____

_____

_____

_____

_____

_____

_____

_____

_____

_____

D. Past Medical Work-Up

1. *Circle* any of the following people that your child has already seen for his or her problem. Ask that person to send us a copy of the results.

family physician	pediatrician	osteopath
neurologist	psychologist	psychiatrist
chiropractor	any other specialist	

2. Has your child already undergone any expensive tests for his or her problem?   No _____ Yes _____

   If Yes, please request that copies be sent to us.

University of Colorado Medical Center   Name _____

PEDIATRIC HEALTH MAINTENANCE   Birthdate _____

6—12 Years Old   Today's date _____

COMPREHENSIVE QUESTIONNAIRE ON BEHAVIOR AND DEVELOPMENT

To be completed by a parent.
This medical information is confidential.

A. Speech and Self-Care (Circle yes or no)

Yes	No	1. Did your child walk alone across the room by 18 months?
Yes	No	2. Speak in sentences by age 3?
Yes	No	3. Tie shoestrings alone by age 6?
Yes	No	4. Develop as quickly as brothers and sisters?
No	Yes	5. Have a problem with pronouncing words?
No	Yes	6. Stutter?
Yes	No	7. Bathe without assistance?
Yes	No	8. Go to other children's homes alone?
No	Yes	9. Have difficulty separating from parents when starting school?
Yes	No	10. Have some chores?

B. Mood (Circle yes or no)

No	Yes	1. Is your child often tense?
No	Yes	2. Does your child worry a lot?
Yes	No	3. Is your child able to talk about what's bothering him or her?
No	Yes	4. Often unhappy?
No	Yes	5. Often angry?

C. School

1. Name of school _____

   Address _____   Telephone number _____

   Name of teacher _____   Grade _____

2. How many days has your child missed so far this year?

   How many total days did your child miss last year?

3. Circle any of the following that you have been told apply to your child:

mentally retarded	slow learner	low normal intelligence
brain damaged	cerebral palsy	perceptual-motor problems
reading problems		other learning problems

Yes	No	4. Does your child get along well in school?
No	Yes	5. Have difficulties with schoolwork?
No	Yes	6. Has your child ever repeated a grade? If yes, which one?
No	Yes	7. Ever been in special classes?
No	Yes	8. Is something upsetting the child and interfering with schoolwork?
No	Yes	9. Does your child need pressure to do homework?
No	Yes	10. Seem to have "given up" in school?
Yes	No	11. Is your child doing as well in school as brothers and sisters?
No	Yes	12. Does your child get into any trouble with classroom misbehavior?
No	Yes	13. Has your child ever been suspended for a while from school?

D. Friends (Circle yes or no)

Yes	No	1. Does your child get along well with children of about the same age?
No	Yes	2. Have trouble keeping friends?
No	Yes	3. Fight a lot with other children?
No	Yes	4. Has your child ever hurt anyone while fighting?
No	Yes	5. Prefer to play alone?
Yes	No	6. Have a real close friend?
No	Yes	7. Is there any aspect of sex education or behavior you would like to discuss?

E. Discipline (Circle yes or no)

No	Yes	1. Is your child a difficult one? Does he or she often break the rules?
No	Yes	2. Is your child impossible to deal with?
Yes	No	3. Does your child have many good points?
No	Yes	4. Need to be spanked frequently?
Yes	No	5. Care whether spanked or not?
No	Yes	6. Do you ever use a paddle or belt in spanking?
		7. How many times a day does your child need to be corrected?
		8. What type of discipline works best?

F. Behavior: Circle any of the following behaviors that are present in your child:

Hyperactive	Very shy	Runs away	Gets teased
Has tics	Homesick	Sexual problems	Destructive, damages property
Sets fires	Sleep problem	Eating problem	Highly conscientious
Tried drugs	Skips school	Masturbates	Juvenile delinquency
Suicide attempt	Cries excessively	Very stubborn	Repeated accidents
Defiant	Temper tantrums	Sucks thumb	Swears
Bites nails	Has fears	Bites	Has nightmares
Hurts animals	Lies	Steals	BMs in underwear
Daytime wetting	Bedwetting	Frequent pains	

G. Family Difficulties: The following questions are about the parents rather than the child. You do not have to answer them if you do not wish to. However, difficulties in any of these areas probably have an effect on your child. (Circle yes or no)

No	Yes	1. Are there lots of stresses on your family?
No	Yes	2. Any serious disagreements in the marriage?
No	Yes	3. Any recent separations between the parents?
No	Yes	4. Does either parent have a violent temper?
No	Yes	5. Was either parent ever hospitalized for psychiatric difficulties?
No	Yes	6. Is either parent currently receiving counseling?
No	Yes	7. Is either parent currently having difficulty with drugs or alcohol?
No	Yes	8. Any recent deaths or serious illness in the family?

Developed by Barton Schmitt, MD, Department of Pediatrics, University of Colorado Medical Center, 1970 (revised November, 1975).

● ● ●

General References

American Academy of Pediatrics: *Standards of Child Health Care,* 2nd ed. Council of Pediatric Practice, 1972.

Charney E: Primary care pediatrics. Pediatr Clin North Am 21:3, 1974. [Entire issue.]

Crook WG: Changing patterns in child health care. Pediatr Clin North Am 16:771, 1969.

Green M, Haggerty RJ (editors): *Ambulatory Pediatrics.* Saunders, 1968.

Helfer RE (editor): *Advances in Ambulatory Pediatrics.* Year Book, 1973.

Illingworth RS: *The Treatment of the Child at Home.* Blackwell, 1971.

Medovy H: School health problems. Pediatr Clin North Am 12:851, 1965.

Steigman AJ, Hammond K: Office practice and procedures. Pediatr Clin North Am 8:1, 1961.

7...
Adolescence

Henry E. Cooper, Jr., MD, & Ida Nakashima, MD

Adolescence is the period of growth and development during which the child grows to adulthood. The upper developmental limit of adolescence is unclear since there are no objective physiologic events that can be used to define its termination. Physiologic and psychologic changes during this period prepare the individual for mature adult biologic and emotional functioning.

Chronologically, adolescence extends from about 12–13 years of age to the early 20s, with wide individual and cultural variations. Adolescence tends to begin earlier in girls than in boys and to end earlier in both in some cultures.

Puberty is a more restricted term for the biologic and physiologic changes associated with physical and sexual maturation. Although the gross observable changes of puberty may not manifest themselves clinically until the second decade, subtle physiologic changes may occur as early as 8 years of age. Pubescence is the time during which the reproductive functions mature; it also includes the appearance of secondary sex characteristics as well as the physiologic maturation of the primary sex organs. In general, puberty is reached when full reproductive maturity has been achieved.

PHYSICAL CHANGES DURING ADOLESCENCE

Because the age at onset of the physical and emotional changes characteristic of adolescence is variable, it is convenient to assess the stage of development of adolescent children in terms of degree of maturation and physiologic changes. A prominent feature of adolescence is accelerated growth rate. The adolescent growth spurt occurs in all developing children but is quite variable in time of onset, duration, and extent. The adolescent spurt begins earlier in girls than in boys, usually between 11 and 14 years; in boys, the growth spurt begins, on the average, between the ages of 12 and 16 years. In boys this growth spurt accounts for a gain in height of 10–30 cm (4–12 inches) and a gain in weight of 7–30 kg (15–65 lb). The age of maximum velocity of growth may be anywhere between the ages of 12 and 17. In girls the growth spurt is usually slower and less extensive and accounts for a gain of 5–20 cm (2–10 inches) in height and 7–25 kg (15–55 lb) in weight. Every organ system seems to be involved, but all organs do not grow at the same rate. One exception is the brain, which does not seem to change appreciably in size after age 10 although an increase in head diameter does occur. Lymphatic tissue increases in size from birth and begins to decrease during adolescence, usually at about the time of the growth spurt.

The adolescent growth spurt usually proceeds in a fairly orderly sequence. Leg length usually begins to increase first, and the legs are the first to reach adult length. After a few months, there is an increase in hip width and chest breadth. Shoulder width increases a few months later, and this is followed by an increase in the length of the trunk and the depth of the chest. A great part of the change in weight and muscle mass tends to occur after the bone growth spurt. During the early adolescent period—especially in boys—there may be an increase in subcutaneous fat before the height spurt occurs. This fat is usually lost 1–2 years later and returns with the onset of the skeletal growth spurt.

The rate and onset of the adolescent growth spurt may be influenced by many factors, including sex, racial origin, nutrition, and illness. In children who mature early, this spurt may proceed faster than in those who mature late. The most important determinant of the time of onset and rate of growth seems to be the genetic heritage. Over the past 100 years, there has been a spectacular acceleration of statural size and biologic maturation. In both the USA and Western Europe, there has been an increase in the height of adolescents of the same age during the 20th century. Acceleration of biologic maturity is manifested by the decreasing average age at menarche in girls that has been observed in many areas of the world.

Along with changes in body size, the adolescent assumes the adult physique of his or her sex. The outstanding features are changes in subcutaneous fat distribution, differences in relative bulk growth of the arms, shoulders, and pelvis, and the appearance of secondary sex characteristics. The hormonal changes that occur in the adolescent bring about an increase, in men, in shoulder breadth, leg length, and arm length, particularly the forearm. In girls there is an increase in the width of the hips and a change in the size of the bony pelvis. Girls have a greater amount of subcutaneous fat before adolescence and during the growth spurt, associated with little spurt in bone diameter. In contrast, males have an increase in muscle mass and bone diameter and a smaller increase in subcutaneous fat. (The approximate pattern of appearance of sex characteristics is shown in Tables 2–9 and 2–10.)

PHYSIOLOGIC CHANGES DURING ADOLESCENCE

Hormonal Changes

Hormones are known to have an important influence on the adolescent growth spurt and the physiologic changes during adolescence. Although the origin of the triggering mechanism of adolescence and puberty is not definitely known, it appears to be a response of the anterior pituitary to a stimulus from the hypothalamus. Evidence presently indicates that with maturation there is a decreasing sensitivity to the inhibition by gonadal sex hormones of the hypothalamus and other CNS centers. This causes an increase in hypothalamic releasing factors, a subsequent increase in pituitary tropic hormones, and a resultant increase in gonadal and sex hormones. During midpuberty there is also a stimulating effect of requisite amounts of estrogens on the hypothalamus, causing an increase in luteinizing hormone.

The gonadotropic hormones—follicle-stimulating hormone (FSH) and luteinizing hormone (LH), including luteotropic hormone (LTH)—are the major hormones elaborated.

Urinary gonadotropin levels in early childhood are less than 6 mouse units/day; they rise during adolescence to reach adult levels of 6–52 units/day. Illness, nutritional disturbances, or emotional disorders may cause a decline in the amount of gonadotropin produced.

A. Female Hormones: Estrogens and progesterone are produced by the ovaries, the testes, and the adrenals. In the female, the estrogen originates in the graafian follicles; in the male, in the testes and adrenals. Estrogen produced before pubescence is probably of adrenal origin. In girls, the amount of estrogen produced increases after approximately age 11, but in boys there is no increase during puberty. The secretion of estrogens assumes a cyclic pattern starting approximately 2 years before menarche. The female secondary sex characteristics, stimulated by estrogen production, are enlargement of the uterus and ovaries, development of the breasts, labia minora, and fallopian tubes, increase in vaginal acidity, and cornification of the vaginal epithelial cells. Progesterone is produced in the corpus luteum, adrenal cortex, and testes. It is excreted principally as pregnanediol, seems to act primarily on the female genital tissues, and participates in the development and function of the breasts. There appears to be no change in excretion of pregnanediol with age, nor is there any sex difference save for a premenstrual increase in pregnanediol excretion which is thought to be evidence of ovulation.

B. Male Hormones: In males, androgenic hormones are produced by the adrenal cortex (two-thirds) and testes (one-third); in females, androgens are produced only by the adrenal glands. Some of the earliest changes of adolescence are a by-product of androgen stimulation. A sharp increase in urinary 17-ketosteroids is noted at around 7–9 years of age, the increase being maintained until puberty. The prepubertal rise is noted in both boys and girls, but is greater in boys at about 10–12 years of age. The androgens are believed to be responsible for the growth spurt during adolescence and for the increase in muscular development. In girls, androgens are believed to be responsible for the growth of the labia majora and clitoris, the appearance of axillary and pubic hair, and the stimulation of the sebaceous glands, with resultant seborrhea and acne. In boys, androgens stimulate the growth of the penis, scrotum, testes, prostate, and seminal vesicles and are responsible for the increase in sebaceous secretion, the appearance of pubic, axillary, and facial hair, and the enlargement of the larynx with deepening of the voice. Measuring the urinary 17-ketosteroids is a widely used method of determining androgen production.

C. Other Hormones: Adrenal corticosteroids are excreted in gradually increasing amounts from birth to maturity, and in adults the amount is dependent upon body size and appears to have no relation to age and sex. The 17-hydroxycorticosteroids may show a rise starting at about 15 years of age in both males and females, and this rise may also be accounted for by increase in size.

Thyroid hormone may decline slightly after puberty, reaching its lowest point in the greatest period of sexual maturation. The degradation rate of thyroxine during adolescence does not seem to differ significantly from that of the younger child or adult. Parathyroid hormone may increase slightly during adolescence.

Other Physiologic Changes

(1) By about age 16, adult levels of extracellular water are achieved (25% of total body weight) in both sexes.

(2) Hemoglobin rises slightly in both sexes, but the rise is greater in boys.

(3) Blood pressure rises and heart size increases.

(4) Pulse rate decreases.

(5) Strength, speed, and stamina increase in both sexes.

(6) Blood alkaline phosphatase levels fall rapidly at the end of the height spurt, attaining adult levels after bone growth ceases.

Berenberg SR (editor): *Puberty.* H E Stenfert-Kroese BV, 1975.

Donovan BT, Van Der Werff Ten Bosch JJ: *Physiology of Puberty.* Arnold, 1965.

Grumbach M, Grane G, Mayer F: *Control of the Onset of Puberty.* Wiley, 1974.

Heald FP, Dangela M, Brunschuyler P: Physiology of adolescence. (4 parts.) N Engl J Med 268:192, 243, 299, 361, 1963.

Root AW: Endocrinology of puberty. 1. Normal sexual maturation. J Pediatr 83:1, 1973.

Tanner JM: *Growth at Adolescence,* 2nd ed. Blackwell, 1962.

Villee DB: *Human Endocrinology.* Saunders, 1975.

Visser HKA: Some physiological and clinical aspects of puberty. Arch Dis Child 48:169, 1973.

Wilkins L: *The Diagnosis and Treatment of Endocrine Disorders in Childhood and Adolescence,* 3rd ed. Thomas, 1965.

PSYCHOLOGIC CHANGES DURING ADOLESCENCE

Cognitive Development

Until age 11–12, the child uses concrete operations in problem solving. At adolescence the ability to think scientifically blossoms. The adolescent begins to form hypotheses and to test them in reality or in thought in solving a problem. By the time he is 15, he is able to use logical operations and formal logic in solving problems just as an adult is able to do. The development of formal thought operations allows the adolescent to conceptualize the thoughts of others, and this appears to be the basis of egocentrism during adolescence. Because he is unable to differentiate his thought foci from others and because of his self interest brought on by pubertal changes, the adolescent develops an egocentrism that is characterized by his belief that he is being observed by all others. Indeed, he frequently feels "on stage," and this accounts for the frequently observed self-consciousness of many teenagers. This egocentrism subsides as the feelings that led to it are resolved. The resolution comes as the adolescent determines that his own thoughts are distinct and different from the thoughts of others and he sees himself realistically and not as the center of attention of others. With this realization he also begins to recognize the feelings of others and integrate them with his own.

Ego Development

The combination of accelerated growth, physiologic changes, cultural expectations, and the boy's or girl's own inner drives brings about certain characteristics commonly associated with adolescence. In addition to developing the capacity for scientific and abstract thought, the adolescent faces the task of acquiring appropriate feelings and attitudes toward sex and developing an identity of his own.

The awakening of sexual interest and the increase in body awareness and sexual drive may cause the adolescent and his parents to become confused and anxious. The growing individual may find the prospect of adult responsibility difficult, and there may be marked vacillations between childish and adult behavior. These behavior swings may further puzzle the adolescent and his parents and may lead to physical and behavioral symptoms. The rapidly shifting interests assumed by adolescents are to be regarded as experimental attempts to understand life. There may be great concern about the physical adequacy of the developing body, and anxiety caused by fears of physical imperfection may be too overwhelming to be verbalized. This denial can usually be overcome by an understanding adult, particularly a physician.

Concern about body changes may cause a feeling of strangeness in a child who formerly felt comfortable about his physical self. It may produce many fantasies about both the external and internal functions of the body. This concern may cause the child to complain of symptoms, and he may become a "hypochondriac." However, the physician must beware of assuming that all complaints are of emotional origin; a careful examination is always required to rule out disease.

With maturation and the attempt to establish a personal identity, the adolescent strives for independence. Early adolescence is the time for testing parental controls and discipline and renouncing parental standards in preparation for breaking close ties with the parents. The adolescent is vociferous in his attempts to act without the direction of adults, particularly his parents. However, the psychologic changes that are taking place may make independent action even more difficult than in past stages of development, and the boy or girl may appear to be compulsive in his behavior and confused about his goals. During this period he is driven to experiment with new ideas and experiences free of adult supervision. When he meets challenges or obstacles he finds difficult to cope with, he turns to adults for guidance and support. This return to a state of dependency is usually appropriate to the reality situation. If the parents fail to provide adequate reassurance and comfort during these intervals of necessary dependency, the adolescent may seek relief in earlier patterns of childlike behavior and methods of handling anxiety. With appropriate parental support, he will be able to give up his immature behavior. However, he may regard the regressive episode as a defeat in his attempts to achieve adulthood. He protests the regression but wishes to avoid self-blame and to deny his own weakness. Consequently, he blames his parents or other adults who are aware of his period of regression. This "scapegoat" role is important for the adolescent as he strives for independence.

As the adolescent begins to break away from parental influence, the peer group attains increasing importance and may even dominate the adolescent's thinking and behavior. In the group the adolescent finds a sense of security that is a source of comfort in dealing with conflicts. He achieves status and a sense of productivity or achievement simply by belonging to the group. In return, he must accept group standards of dress and behavior and the group's attitude toward authority, education, etc. Although membership in a particular group is determined partly by age and intellectual ability, emotional empathy is just as important. The group is usually composed of individuals at the same stage of emotional development. As an individual matures emotionally, he may give up one group to join another more in harmony with his changing interests and goals. The peer group may be unacceptable to the parents for political or social reasons, but association with such a group is probably a necessary part of the adolescent's experimentation with alternative styles of life.

Emerging Sexual Identity

The process of developing a sexual identity during adolescence is related to the development of the primary sex organs and secondary sexual characteristics. At this time, sexual feelings, drives, and fantasies are increased. Dealing with these feelings may bring the adolescent into direct conflict with previously learned attitudes toward sex. Interest in sexual matters may be reflected in curiosity about sex, much seeking of sex information, sexual overtones in conversation, sexual daydreaming, fantasies about heterosexual relationships, and masturbation. During the early phase of heterosexual concerns, there may be an initial retreat into the safety of associations with the same sex. This "homosexual" activity may occur between individuals and in groups. Boys may practice mutual and group masturbation. Similar behavior in girls may include hand-holding, kissing, breast fondling, and mutual masturbation. Such behavior in adolescents does not necessarily lead to sexual deviation or homosexuality in adulthood and should not be stigmatized as abnormal. Homosexual behavior at this age is a way of coping with the anxieties of emerging sexual feelings. Adolescents may express physical sexual urges through body contact, kissing games, and playful roughhousing behavior.

Adolescents express their sexual drive in a variety of patterns of behavior. Some may be so threatened by their emerging sexual drives that they may suppress all expression of sexuality and persist in early childhood behavior. Others may avoid contact with others of both sexes in order to control their own sexual feelings. Still others seem to have little trouble with sexuality and welcome the opportunity for dating and heterosexual social activities. The "boy crazy" girl or "girl crazy" boy may be involved in such activities in order to overcome fears of homosexuality, or he or she may really be ready for and able to accept a heterosexual relationship.

The Implications of Adolescence for Medical Practice

The physician can play an important role in encouraging and facilitating adolescent development. He can serve as a source of understanding and interest, and provides the opportunity to express feelings and attitudes and to ask questions without criticism or embarrassment. Ample time should be scheduled so that the adolescent and his parents can express their concerns and ask about anything that is puzzling to them. Visits should also be managed so that the physician can focus separately upon problems presented by the parents and by the child. Parents should be informed of the normal physical and emotional changes that occur during adolescence.

The physical examination should be performed with consideration for the shyness and the need for privacy that is characteristic of this age group. Drapes should be used during the examination, and chaperoning is essential during the examination of girls. Vaginal examination during adolescence should be avoided except upon definite medical indication. A useful technic is to conduct a review of systems during the examination. It is important that the physician carefully discuss with the patient any diagnostic procedures used and that the physical findings be interpreted to the patient.

Overidentification with the adolescent or the parents should be avoided. A sure understanding of the social and cultural influences acting on the parents and on the adolescent is necessary so that the parents can confidently set limits and maintain discipline in the home and the community.

Elkind D: Egocentrism in adolescence. In: *Contemporary Issues in Adolescent Development.* Conger JJ (editor). Harper & Row, 1975.

Fine LL: What's a normal adolescent? Clin Pediatr (Phila) 12:1, 1973.

Gallagher JR: *Medical Care of the Adolescent,* 2nd ed. Appleton-Century-Crofts, 1966.

Josselyn IM: *The Adolescent and His World.* New York Family Service Association of America, 1957.

Normal Adolescence. Group for the Advancement of Psychiatry. Vol VI, Report No. 68, Feb 1968.

Solnit AJ, Prevence SA (editors): *Modern Perspectives in Child Development.* Internat Univ Press, 1963.

GROWTH PROBLEMS DURING ADOLESCENCE

DELAYED ADOLESCENCE

Essentials of Diagnosis

- Delay in growth spurt and appearance of secondary sex characteristics.
- Absence of endocrinopathies.

General Considerations

Delayed adolescence is more common in boys than in girls.

The timing, extent, and pattern of pubertal changes vary widely with different individuals. In the evaluation of delayed puberty, developmental age is more reliable than chronologic age. Developmental age may be based on x-ray determination of skeletal age and on standards of development of secondary sex characteristics. Determination of sexual maturity may be based on the following.

A. Genital Development in Males:

Stage 1: Preadolescent.

Stage 2: Beginning enlargement of the scrotum and testes; reddening of the scrotum, and changes in its texture.

Stage 3: Penile enlargement with increase in length and further growth of the scrotum and testes.

Stage 4: Further increase in penile size; growth in breadth and development of the glans. Further enlargement of the testes and scrotum and continued darkening of the scrotal skin.

Stage 5: Adult genitalia in size and shape.

B. Pubic Hair Development in Males and Females:

Stage 1: Preadolescence, with the vellus over the pubic area no more profuse than that on the abdomen.

Stage 2: Sparse growth of long, slightly pigmented, downy hair which is straight or only slightly curled, and appearing usually at the base of the penis or along the labia.

Stage 3: Pubic hair is darker, coarser, and more curly, and the hair is spreading sparsely over the pubic area.

Stage 4: Further spread of the pubic hair, still considerably less than in the adult, and no extension of hair bilaterally up to the middle of the thighs.

Stage 5: Adult in amount and type of hair.

C. Breast Development in Females:

Stage 1: Preadolescent, with coloration of the papillae only.

Stage 2: Breast bud stage; breasts and papillae are elevated above the chest in a small mound, with enlargement of the areolar diameter.

Stage 3: Further elevation and enlargement of the breasts and areolas but no separation of the contours.

Stage 4: The areolas and papillae project from the breast to form a secondary mound.

Stage 5: Adult stage; projection of the papillae only, with recession of the areolas into the general breast contour.

Variations in the pubertal changes occur both within and between the groups, boys and girls. Boys may take 1.8–4.7 years to proceed from stage 2 to stage 5 in genital or pubic hair development. Some boys may move from stage 2 to stage 5 in less time than others go from one stage to the next. The peak height velocity in boys usually occurs 2 years later than in girls and generally occurs in stage 4 genital or pubic hair development. Many girls may have their peak height velocity in stage 2 of breast development. Thus, the short boy within the early stages of development may still have considerable growth to come. This is not true for girls.

Girls may take 1.5–8 years in passing from stage 2 to stage 5 breast development and 1.5–3 years from stage 2 to stage 5 pubic hair development. Some girls may progress to stage 3 or 4 breast development before pubic hair stage 2 is reached. Alternatively, pubic hair may progress to stage 3 or 4 before breast development starts. Most girls have their menarche at stage 3 or 4 breast and pubic hair development. The peak height velocity usually occurs just before the menarche.

Marshall WA, Tanner JM: Variations in the pattern of pubertal changes in boys. Arch Dis Childhood 45:13, 1970.

Marshall WA, Tanner JM: Variations in the pattern of pubertal changes in girls. Arch Dis Childhood 44:291, 1969.

Clinical Findings

A. Symptoms and Signs: Puberty may be delayed until as late as 18–19 years, but most children reach puberty by 15 or 16 years of age. There may be no symptoms except for psychologic problems caused by teasing, exclusion from athletic and social activities, or just a feeling of difference from others. The psychologic import of delayed adolescence may be manifested as poor school work, delinquent behavior, withdrawal, or paranoid tendencies.

The physical examination shows that there is a lag behind children of the same age in body weight, muscular development, stage of sexual maturity, and psychosocial development. The history may show that growth retardation has been evident throughout childhood or that another family member has exhibited the same pattern of development.

B. Laboratory Findings: Endocrinologic studies are unrevealing. Skeletal age may show a delay of 2–4 years which has existed throughout preadolescence. Urinary 17-ketosteroids or FSH and serum LH are usually at adolescent levels.

Treatment

Observation at intervals will reveal that somatic growth and sexual maturation do occur, but late. A series of visits should be scheduled so that the physician can give continued interest and reassurance. Signs of poor psychologic adjustment should be observed for and handled appropriately when they occur.

A. Males: In boys 17 years old or more, if pubertal development is considerably retarded, if no progress toward maturity is evident, and if the physician's efforts to give reassurance and support are to no avail, it is probably wise to start hormone therapy to stimulate growth. Chorionic gonadotropin, 2000–4000 units IM twice a week for 3–6 months, usually produces rapid somatic growth and initiates the development of secondary sex characteristics. After one course of therapy, maturation will often continue to progress. If this does not occur after 3–6 months, a second course of treatment may be given.

B. Females: There is no completely reliable means of initiating puberty in girls with delayed adolescence. In some cases, pubertal changes will begin after a course of continuous estrogen therapy for 2–3 months followed by cyclic estrogen-progesterone treatment for a few more months. Diethylstilbestrol, 1–2 mg daily orally, is given for 2–3 months, during which time feminization will occur. This is followed by diethylstilbestrol, 1–2 mg orally daily for 21 days, adding medroxyprogesterone, 10 mg orally daily on the 15th through the 21st day, and then withdrawing both. In 3–5 days, vaginal bleeding will occur. The treatment is then resumed starting on the third day of bleeding. This is usually carried out for about 6 months. Chorionic gonadotropin is contraindicated because of the cystic ovarian changes it produces.

Prognosis

In all cases of delayed adolescence due to a slow growth pattern, the patient will eventually undergo pubertal changes. Once started, maturation occurs in a rapid spurt or as a gradual development, and average adult height is eventually attained.

Bayley LM, Bayley N: *Growth Diagnosis: Selected Methods for Interpreting and Predicting Physical Development from One Year to Maturity.* Univ of Chicago Press, 1965.

Gallagher JR, Heald FP, Garell DC: *Medical Care of the Adolescent,* 3rd ed. Appleton-Century-Crofts, 1976.

Hubble D: *Pediatric Endocrinology.* Davis, 1969.

Kulin HE, Reiter EO: Delayed sexual maturation, with special emphasis on the occurrence of the syndrome in the male. In: *Control of the Onset of Puberty.* Grumbach MM, Grave GD, Mayer FE (editors). Wiley, 1974.

Wilkins L: *The Diagnosis and Treatment of Endocrine Disorders in Childhood and Adolescence,* 3rd ed. Thomas, 1965.

OVERGROWTH & INCREASED HEIGHT

In some adolescents, the rate of change in height prior to puberty suggests that they may have excessive height as adults. In girls, this may be a cause of great anxiety and may be a severe social handicap. When the question arises, height prediction tables should be used to estimate the probable adult height. In general, patients with advanced bone development have less growing time and may stop growing before they become too tall. If the probability of excessive adult height is great and hormonal intervention is being considered, thorough interviews are necessary before treatment is started in an attempt to encourage the patient to accept her body. The indications for hormone therapy are a family history of excessive tallness, a skeletal age that by age 10 is less than normal or normal, and a probable adult height of over 6 feet as estimated by reference to prediction tables.

Treatment is instituted about 1 year before the predicted time of menarche and after secondary sex characteristics have become manifest. The more advanced the bone age at the time therapy is started, the less effective the treatment in reducing height gain. When the bone age has reached 15 years, the effectiveness of treatment is nil. Reported reductions from predicted heights started before growth is completed range from 1–4 inches. Conjugated estrogenic substances (Premarin), 12.5 mg orally, or diethylstilbestrol, 2 mg orally, is given for 21 days, with medroxyprogesterone, 10 mg orally, added on days 15 through 21, and both drugs are then withdrawn. The cycle is then repeated on the third day of vaginal bleeding which occurs following withdrawal. Treatment is continued for approximately 1 year, at which time there is usually evidence of considerable advance of bone age

or evidence of epiphyseal closure. Menorrhagia occasionally occurs during treatment but may be controlled by increasing the dose of diethylstilbestrol to 3 mg/day during the first 5 days of treatment. Pigmentation may occur, particularly over the breasts, nipples, and labia.

The effectiveness of and need for estrogen therapy in preventing excessive height is not universally agreed upon. Some data suggest that estrogens slow growth but may not significantly influence adult height.

Fraser SD, Smith FG Jr: Effect of estrogens on mature height in tall girls: A controlled study. J Clin Endocrinol 28:416, 1968.

Kuhn N & others: Estrogen treatment in tall girls. Acta Paediatr Scand 66:161, 1977.

Wettenhall HN, Cahill C, Roche AF: Tall girls: A survey of management and treatment. Pediatrics 86:602, 1975.

Zachman M & others: Estrogen treatment of excessively tall stature in girls. Helv Pediatr Acta 30:11, 1975.

GYNECOMASTIA

Enlargement of one or both breasts in boys occurs frequently during puberty and occasionally in the preadolescent years and may cause great anxiety. It may be differentiated from gynecomastia due to Klinefelter's syndrome, liver disease, severe malnutrition, obesity, and feminizing endocrinopathies, particularly carcinoma of the testis.

The cause of physiologic gynecomastia during adolescence is not known, but it is postulated that testicular or adrenal androgens may be converted to estrogens which stimulate enlargement.

Benign adolescent breast hypertrophy presents as mild to moderate enlargement of one or (usually) both breasts. It is palpable as a firm, sometimes slightly tender mass 1–2 cm in diameter just beneath the areola, and may be associated with hyperesthesia of the nipple. It occurs frequently in boys who have well developed testes and are virilizing rapidly.

Gynecomastia is usually transitory and subsides spontaneously after about 6 months. When enlargement is considerable, it may persist for years.

In a few cases, gynecomastia which is not associated with endocrine disfunction may present as unilateral or bilateral breast enlargement typical of the developing female pattern. The breasts may be diffusely enlarged, but much more so in the subareolar area, with no tenderness, and may become pendulous, with enlargement and hyperpigmentation of the areolas. These boys may have normal male secondary sex characteristics in all other respects. This type of gynecomastia causes great embarrassment and anxiety and may seriously impair psychologic development.

Treatment of both types usually consists of assurance that the "growth" is benign and transitory.

In extensive and pendulous enlargement, plastic

surgery is indicated for psychologic and cosmetic reasons. The patient must be reassured about physical integrity and normal masculinity.

In patients who have residual gynecomastia following correction of endocrine disorders, plastic surgery may be indicated for cosmetic reasons.

Ginsburg J: Gynaecomastia. Practitioner 203:166, 1969.

LaFranchi SH & others: Pubertal gynecomastia and transient elevation of serum estradiol levels. Am J Dis Child 129:927, 1975.

Latorre H, Kenny F: Idiopathic gynecomastia in seven preadolescent boys. Am J Dis Child 126:771, 1973.

Nydick M & others: Gynecomastia in adolescent boys. JAMA 178:449, 1961.

OBESITY

Obesity, beyond the temporary prepubertal accumulation of subcutaneous fat in most girls and some boys, is becoming more common in the USA and Western Europe, possibly related to the dynamics of affluence and patterns of overeating. Although endocrine factors were formerly felt to be prominently involved in many cases of obesity, they appear now to be only rarely influential. Most cases result basically from an excess of intake over output of calories as a result of hyperphagia, usually in families with tendencies toward overeating. Psychosocial, genetic, environmental, and metabolic factors, especially hyperinsulinism, are well documented contributing causes. A small number of cases are associated with a variety of organic diseases (Table 7–1).

From the psychosocial point of view, seriously obese children and adolescents fall into 2 major groups: reactive and developmental. The reactive type is characterized by obesity, overeating, and underactivity in response to an emotionally traumatic experience such as the death of a parent or sibling, the break-up of a family through divorce, or school failure. Such children tend to use food for emotional purposes as a substitute for more basic emotional gratifications. Supportive psychotherapeutic or environmental measures, often with the aid of psychiatric consultation, may be fairly helpful in this group, although some children from more disturbed families require intensive psychotherapy to relieve persistent depression or other manifestations.

The developmental type of obesity usually has its origins in strong family tendencies toward obesity and overeating, representing a disturbed way of life (family frame) involving the whole family. The mother usually dominates and overprotects the child, and the father plays a relatively passive role; both parents, however, may unconsciously use one particular child to satisfy their own emotional needs or compensatory tendencies. Often the child is overvalued by the parents, sometimes because of the death of a previous child,

Table 7–1. Etiologic classification of obesities.

Genetic Origin
  Laurence-Moon-Biedl syndrome
  Prader-Willi syndrome
  Glycogen storage disease
  Familial hypoglycemosis
Hypothalamic Origin
  Diencephalic
  Panhypopituitarism and narcolepsy
CNS Origin
  Postfrontal lobotomy
  Cortical lesions (frontal lesions in particular)
Endocrine Origin
  Insulin-producing adenoma of islets of Langerhans
  Diabetes
  Chromophobe adenoma of pituitary gland
  Hyperadrenocorticism (Cushing's syndrome; iatrogenic due to corticosteroid administration)
  Klinefelter's syndrome
  Turner's syndrome
  Male hypogonadism
  Castration
Miscellaneous Causes
  Immobilization
  Psychic disturbances
  Social and cultural pressure

and overfeeding may represent an attempt to deal with guilt. The child is often large at birth, soon becomes obese with overfeeding, and continues to be obese from early infancy on. After early demanding behavior, the child usually becomes passive, oversubmissive, overdependent, and immature.

In such children, feelings of helplessness, despair, and a tendency to withdraw from social interaction often become associated with a tendency to overeat and patterns of inactivity. Food may be used to ward off depression or feelings of hostility; eating or chewing may acquire unconscious symbolic significance as a conversion symptom, or patterns of "addiction" to food may result. Although obesity is a social handicap, some children or adolescents may hide behind the "wall of weight" and ward off sexual conflicts with the feeling that they are ugly or unattractive. Too rapid reduction in weight may produce a "dieting depression" or even a psychotic picture in some markedly obese and seriously disturbed person.

Clinical Findings

Evaluation of the obese patient must include height and weight histories of parents and siblings, eating habits, quality and timing of appetite and hunger patterns, the duration of the obesity, and, when possible, height and weight plotted longitudinally. In experienced hands, the use of skinfold calipers can give an objective measurement of obesity (Pediatrics 42:538, 1968). The history should also include information about family attitudes, the patient's feelings about himself, previous weight reduction attempts, physical activities engaged in, and the general adjustment pattern of the patient. A careful history and physical examination will help to distinguish between exogenous obesity and other, organic causes of increased subcutaneous tissue such as Cushing's syndrome or hypothyroidism. A common error is failure to realize that children with hypothyroidism may be thin rather than fat, and that the excess weight gain with hypothyroidism is myxedema rather than fat. Many patients with exogenous obesity are inappropriately treated with thyroid medication for this reason.

Treatment

The treatment of obesity must be individualized. Only in very rare cases do psychologic factors preclude attempts at weight reduction. The patient-doctor relationship is of paramount importance because treatment must continue over a long time with repeated interviews. The physician must be able to give the patient a feeling of personal worth and an optimistic outlook for the future.

A. Diet: Dietary control should be attempted. As a rule, it should be introduced and discussed after several visits. The physician's attitude should be one of sympathy rather than criticism of failure to adhere to the diet, and the relationship with the patient must not be jeopardized by insisting that the patient lose weight "for the doctor." In early adolescence, during the growth spurt, good nutrition must be maintained; the diet should include adequate proteins and calcium and fewer concentrated sweets and fats. Since a marked reduction in food intake may affect linear growth, the recommended minimum daily caloric intake during early adolescence should be 1200 kcal for girls and 1400 kcal for boys. Older adolescents may be given diets containing as little as 1000 kcal/day as long as 20% of it is protein and vitamin and mineral requirements are met.

The caloric intake should be spread over 3 meals a day. Raw carrots, celery, and raw vegetables may have the effect of slowing the course of meals and allowing satiety to occur. Artificial sweeteners may be substituted for sugar in beverages.

B. Anorexigenic Drugs: The anorexigenic drugs (amphetamines and related compounds) are of limited value in the treatment of obesity. There is no indication for their use in the patient who eats too much even when not hungry. They may be helpful for the patient who is too hungry on a low-calorie diet. If there is excessive hunger, small doses of dextroamphetamine (5–10 mg) may be given 30 minutes prior to the estimated peak of hunger. In general, the effective duration of amphetamine treatment is usually 6–8 weeks. The patient must be aware that this is an adjunct to therapy and that the responsibility for correction of obesity cannot be delegated to the drug. Other drugs used as anorectics include clortermine, fenfluramine, and mazindol. These compounds appear to be comparable to amphetamines in producing a de-

crease in appetite, but they also tend to lose their effectiveness after several weeks of use and are useful only as short term adjuncts to a diet-based treatment program.

C. Exercise: The obese adolescent must be encouraged to exercise at least 1 hour a day during the week and 2–4 hours a day during weekends and when school is not in session. The type of exercise makes no difference as long as it is done consistently and intensely. The physician may suggest new activities and interests which might not only create an interest in exercise but also gain for the patient recognition, friends, and the satisfaction of accomplishment.

D. Surgery: Operations being attempted for the control of obesity include (1) ileal-jejunal bypass and (2) gastric pouch construction. Both of these procedures have been recommended only for morbidly obese patients in whom all other medical approaches have failed and in whom the risk of or the complications of the obese state are severe. Following surgery, weight losses of 75–100 pounds are reported; however, the weight loss usually stabilizes after 18 months, and many of the very obese patients remain smaller but still obese. The complications of surgery may be severe and include enteritis, kidney stones, gallstones, and liver dysfunction. Surgery for obesity during adolescence should be regarded as an extreme remedy to be recommended only rarely. Further investigation is needed.

E. Other Measures: A useful adjunct in the management of obese girls is grooming tips and "figure" control advice to promote self-esteem. Obesity clubs and summer camps may be of some help.

Complications

Most of the complications of obesity during adolescence are psychosocial ones. Respiratory difficulties (Pickwickian syndrome), hypertension, and cardiovascular complications may occur, and menstrual disorders in young girls. Many of these difficulties can be relieved by weight reduction. The psychologic concomitants of obesity may represent disturbances in emotional development during early life, a manifestation of the adjustment reaction to obesity, or an interplay of both. Transient or prolonged psychic stress may lead to increased food intake and an increase in subcutaneous fat. Patients with long-standing obesity frequently show extreme passivity, poor self-esteem, fear of social gatherings, and passive-aggressive personality traits. Because of their inability, real or imagined, to compete with peers in physical and social activities, they may withdraw. This makes them more unacceptable to their peers, and the sedentary activities in which they engage may contribute to their obesity.

Prognosis

The prognosis in long-standing severe obesity is poor for weight reduction, but these patients can be helped to lead a more normal life by accepting their obesity. Patients whose subcutaneous fat tissue increases to excessive amounts after 9 years of age are usually less obese; with careful management, about half of these can achieve average weight as adults.

Bray GA: *The Obese Patient*. In: *Major Problems in Internal Medicine*. Vol 9. Saunders, 1976.

Bruch H: The treatment of eating disorders. Mayo Clin Proc 51:266, 1976.

Faloon WW: Ileal bypass for obesity: Postoperative perspective. Hosp Pract 12:73, Jan 1977.

Garn SM, Clark DC: Trends in fatness and the origins of obesity. Pediatrics 57:443, 1976.

Mayer J: Some aspects of the problem of regulation of food intake and obesity. (3 parts.) N Engl J Med 244:610, 722, 731, 1966.

Nutrition Committee of the American Academy of Pediatrics: Obesity in childhood. Pediatrics 40:455, 1967.

Soper RT & others: Gastric bypass for morbid obesity in children and adolescents. J Pediatr Surg 10:51, 1975.

GYNECOLOGIC PROBLEMS IN ADOLESCENCE

MENSTRUAL DISORDERS DURING ADOLESCENCE

1. DYSMENORRHEA

General Considerations

Dysmenorrhea, or painful menstrual periods, is one of the most common menstrual complaints among adolescent girls. It is divided into 2 types: primary dysmenorrhea, for which no pelvic disease can be demonstrated; and secondary dysmenorrhea, which is associated with organic pelvic disorders such as endometriosis, adenomyosis, uterine myomas, polyps of the cervix or uterus, chronic pelvic infections, or an intrauterine device.

The reported incidence of dysmenorrhea varies from 3% to as high as 80% depending on the population studied and the criteria used. A study of 1606 high school girls showed that 10% of them had pain severe enough to keep them home from school.

Primary dysmenorrhea accounts for the vast majority of cases of pelvic pain in this young age group at a time when anovulatory menses, usually painless, are common. The pain is thought to be related to the secretion of progesterone following ovulation and begins on the first day, lasting a few hours to days. It is sharp and colicky, centered in the lower abdomen, and can radiate to the back and lower thighs. Nausea, vomiting, and syncope may accompany severe pain.

Etiology

The cause of primary dysmenorrhea is still unclear, although recent evidence strongly suggests that prostaglandin F_{2a}, primarily produced in the endometrium, particularly in the secretory phase of the menstrual cycle, causes menstrual cramps and uterine contraction. Both indomethacin and aspirin inhibit prostaglandin synthesis. For this reason, indomethacin, 25 mg 3 times a day, has been administered to patients at the onset of menses and continued for 2–3 days with mixed results, some women experiencing relief and others noting no change. Further clinical study and trial seem indicated for this mode of therapy.

Diagnosis

A careful history and physical examination, including a pelvic examination to rule out organic causes of pelvic pain, are essential before a diagnosis of primary dysmenorrhea can be justified. It is helpful to assess the girl's degree of understanding of the physiology of the menstrual cycle and related body functions. Secondary gains from being unwell include special care and concern from the mother or a legitimate excuse for staying home from school. It should be determined whether the girl has been brought up to expect menses to be a miserable experience.

Treatment

Reassurance and education can do much to allay anxiety arising from a distorted misunderstanding of menstruation. Mild dysmenorrhea usually responds to simple aspirin analgesics, propoxyphene (Darvon), or phenobarbital and belladonna compounds every 6 hours. If cramps are severe, aspirin with codeine, 30 mg every 6 hours, is helpful if started before the cramps become really painful. Vomiting may be controlled with prochlorperazine (Compazine), 5–10 mg orally every 4 hours, starting at the beginning of the menstrual period. If the patient vomits the pills, chlorpromazine (Thorazine), 25 mg rectally every 6 hours, may be used.

If severe, incapacitating dysmenorrhea does not respond to these measures, a trial of oral contraceptives may be instituted for a period of 3–6 months. Menses are often less painful after oral contraceptives are discontinued, and analgesics may then be adequate to control discomfort. Although a patient's symptoms may seem to be secondary to a relative or functional cervical stenosis, cervical dilatation affords only temporary relief from dysmenorrhea and should not be done routinely.

2. PREMENSTRUAL TENSION

Premenstrual tension syndrome usually occurs in older teenagers. It is characterized by irritability, depression, headache, abdominal bloating, and enlarged, tender breasts, often with a weight gain of 3–5 lb beginning 4–7 days before onset of menses. It is thought to be causally related to edema resulting from sodium retention perhaps associated with elevated estrogen and progesterone levels.

Again, reassurance and education about the menstrual cycle are helpful. Small doses of hydrochlorothiazide (Hydro-Diuril), eg, 25 mg daily for 3 days before and 2 days during menses, may provide substantial relief of headache and irritability.

Emans SJH, Goldstein DP: *Pediatric and Adolescent Gynecology.* Little, Brown, 1977.

Halbert DR & others: Dysmenorrhea and prostaglandins. Obstet Gynecol Surv 31:77, 1976.

Oriatti MD: Dysmenorrhea. Pediatr Ann 4:60, 1975.

Willson JR, Beecham CT, Carrington ER: *Obstetrics and Gynecology,* 5th ed. Mosby, 1975.

3. DYSFUNCTIONAL UTERINE BLEEDING
(Metropathia Hemorrhagica)

Essentials of Diagnosis

- Irregular, noncyclic bleeding.
- Absence of systemic and pelvic disorders.
- Occurs after menarche and before regular ovulation is established.

General Considerations

Most abnormal bleeding problems in this age group fall into the category of dysfunctional uterine bleeding. This disorder is thought to be caused by the abnormal persistence of unruptured follicles, with consequent absence of functioning corpora lutea and with hyperplasia of the endometrium resulting from continuous and excessive estrogenic stimulation. Irregularity in timing and amount of flow may continue for 1–4 years following menarche. Basically, dysfunctional bleeding refers to abnormal uterine bleeding not due to pregnancy, neoplasm, trauma, infections, or blood dyscrasias; it is therefore a diagnosis of exclusion. Appropriate history, physical examination—including pelvic examination—and indicated laboratory studies must be completed before arriving at this diagnosis.

Differential Diagnosis

Dysfunctional uterine bleeding must be differentiated from complications of pregnancy (ectopic pregnancy, abortion, and hydatidiform mole); malignancies of the pelvic organs; benign lesions of the pelvic organs (cervicitis, cervical and endometrial polyps, chronic endometritis, vaginal adenosis, and salpingitis); systemic disorders (blood dyscrasias, anticoagulant therapy, chronic anemias); irregular bleeding caused by sporadic and spotty ingestion of birth control pills and occasionally by use of intrauterine devices; and functional factors (polycystic ovarian syndrome, thyroid disorders, psychotropic drugs, obesity, and emotional stress).

Laboratory Data

A pregnancy test on urine, complete blood count, platelet count, and Papanicolaou smear with maturation index should be obtained.

Treatment

Simple reassurance after a thorough evaluation may relieve a great deal of anxiety; a policy of watchful waiting should be maintained. If the blood count indicates anemia, oral iron therapy may be started. If bleeding has persisted more than 7 days, progesterone in oil, 100 mg IM, or medroxyprogesterone (Provera), 10 mg/day orally for 5 days, may be given. This produces secretory endometrium with increased bleeding within 3–5 days, followed by cessation of bleeding. Frequently, the girl's next menses will be normal with no further irregularities. If the problem persists, medroxyprogesterone (Provera), 50 mg orally, may be given at the end of 28 days for 3 menstrual cycles.

In persistent cases, cyclic hormones may be used, particularly those with progestational activity. These adolescent patients may also be relatively hypoestrogenic in the sense that heavy bleeding and incomplete sloughing have left the endometrium irregular and denuded.

Sequential preparations were removed from the market in the USA in June 1976 because it was determined that their prolonged use was associated with an increased risk of thromboembolism and endometrial cancer. Therefore, combination products such as Ortho-Novum 2 mg (norethindrone 2 mg with mestranol 0.1 mg) or Enovid-E (norethynodrel 2.5 mg with mestranol 0.1 mg), which have relatively high estrogen (mestranol) content, can be used for 2–3 months before a 6-month course of medroxyprogesterone acetate (Provera) is started.

Dilatation and curettage may be required if excessive bleeding persists, but this is a rare occurrence.

Prognosis

Patients should be followed carefully, as Southam & Richert have indicated that many of them continue to have recurrent problems, particularly if menstrual irregularity persists beyond 10 years.

Emans SJH, Goldstein DP: *Pediatric and Adolescent Gynecology.* Little, Brown, 1977.

FDA Drug Bulletin. Page 26, June-July 1976.

Gailey TA, McDonough PG: Atypical uterine bleeding. Pediatr Ann 4:66, 1975.

Novak ER, Jones GS, Jones HW: Page 323 in: *Gynecology.* Williams & Wilkins, 1971.

Southam AL, Richert RM: The prognosis for adolescents with menstrual abnormalities. Am J Obstet Gynecol 94:637, 1966.

4. PRIMARY AMENORRHEA

Primary amenorrhea is defined as failure of menarche to occur; it may be difficult to differentiate from delayed menarche.

Etiology

A. Physiologic Causes: Amenorrhea may have a

physiologic cause, eg, delayed menarche or, rarely, pregnancy.

B. CNS or Hypothalamic-Pituitary Causes: Causes in this category include congenital disorders such as panhypopituitarism and Laurence-Moon-Biedl syndrome (which would, however, have been noted long before puberty). Another possibility is hypogonadotropic hypogonadism, also rare, in which there are decreased levels of LH and FSH and in which the primary defect is not in the gonads. Prepubertal polycystic ovaries are also a possibility. Neoplastic causes include suprasellar and intrasellar tumors, such as craniopharyngioma and gliomas.

C. Psychogenic Causes: Anorexia nervosa is the only psychogenic cause of primary amenorrhea in adolescent girls.

D. Genetic Causes: Genetic causes to be considered are Turner's syndrome and variants (about 30% of all girls with primary amenorrhea have this condition), adrenogenital syndrome, testicular feminization syndrome, and true hermaphroditism.

E. Endocrine Abnormalities: Endocrine abnormalities causing primary amenorrhea include hypothyroidism, diabetes mellitus, Cushing's syndrome, and functioning ovarian tumors.

F. Anatomic Causes: Anatomic causes include imperforate hymen, vaginal agenesis, congenital absence of the uterus and vagina, and atresia of the uterine cervix.

G. Miscellaneous Causes: These include chronic debilitating conditions and autoimmune disorders.

Diagnostic Evaluation

It is necessary to obtain a careful history and physical examination, including a pelvic examination. The physician must look for absent, poor, or well-developed secondary sexual characteristics and for ambiguous or abnormal genitalia. Other recommended procedures are buccal smear for chromatin-positive Barr bodies, vaginal smear for estrogen effect, bone age films, thyroid function tests, and measurement of urinary 17-ketosteroid and FSH levels.

Skull x-rays, visual field tests, and an EEG are indicated if a suprasellar or intrasellar tumor is suspected. If warranted, perform a pneumoencephalogram and arteriograms. Laparoscopy and gonadal biopsy are done if test results justify such procedures.

The management of primary amenorrhea depends on the cause.

De Koos EB: Primary amenorrhea. Pediatr Ann 4:22, 1975.
Dewhurst CS: Amenorrhea and the pediatrician. Pediatr Clin North Am 19:605, 1972.

5. SECONDARY AMENORRHEA

Secondary amenorrhea is cessation of menses following onset of menarche. It is the absence of spontaneous bleeding for an interval of at least 120 days.

Etiology

The most common cause of secondary amenorrhea in adolescence is pregnancy. Temporary cessation of menses also frequently occurs when birth control pills are stopped. Amenorrhea in such cases may last 2–3 months.

A. Ovarian Causes: These include ovarian neoplasms such as granulosa cell tumors, which secrete estrogen and produce a prolonged proliferative phase of the endometrium. Androgen-producing tumors may result in virilization. Another possibility is polycystic ovarian disease—exemplified by Stein-Leventhal syndrome—with anovulatory cycles, unopposed estrogen production, and mild masculinization, often in an obese, hairy girl. Premature ovarian failure with signs of estrogen deficiency including hot flashes, breast atrophy, and vaginal irritation should also be considered. A rare cause is autoimmune disease in association with hypoadrenocorticalism and hypoparathyroidism.

B. Nonovarian Causes:

1. Psychogenic causes—Amenorrhea may be triggered by environmental or emotional trauma.

2. Nutritional deficiencies—Amenorrhea may be produced by "crash diets" and may occur with anorexia nervosa, sometimes months before significant weight loss occurs.

3. Organic brain disease—Causes of amenorrhea include suprasellar and intrasellar tumors.

4. End organ disease—Amenorrhea may be a by-product of end organ disease following overvigorous curettage or severe uterine infection postoperatively. Cervical stenosis or the development of synechias may also result from uterine surgery.

5. Systemic illness—Causes in this category include thyroid disorders or adrenal disease. The increased cortisol secretion in Cushing's syndrome may produce secondary amenorrhea before the onset of classical symptoms. Addison's disease is a rare cause of secondary amenorrhea.

Diagnostic Evaluation

Diagnostic procedures include a careful history and physical examination (including pelvic examination), a fern test on cervical mucus, and an examination of vaginal cells for maturation index.

A progesterone withdrawal test may also be administered in which the patient receives progesterone in oil, 100 mg IM, or takes medroxyprogesterone acetate (Provera), 10 mg/day orally for 5 days. Withdrawal bleeding should occur in 5–7 days. Bleeding shows that a source of estrogen exists and that the uterine cavity, cervix, and vagina are patent and functional. If bleeding does not occur following this therapeutic test, total urinary gonadotropins and plasma FSH and LH should be measured. If gonadotropins are low, pituitary tumor should be considered as a cause, and visual field tests, thyroid function tests, and skull films of the sella should be ordered.

Urinary 17-ketosteroids and 17-hydroxycorticosteroids are not very helpful in the absence of clinical evidence of adrenocortical malfunction.

Laparoscopy and gonadal biopsy usually serve to confirm the diagnosis after a patient has undergone other diagnostic procedures.

Treatment

Normal cyclic menses are spontaneously resumed in only 50% of adolescents with secondary amenorrhea, and a large proportion will be relatively infertile as adults.

Depending on the cause, surgical removal of ovarian tumors or wedge resection of the ovary (in polycystic ovarian disease) may be required. Documented evidence of thyroid or adrenal disease calls for appropriate treatment as does any chronic systemic illness.

Use of oral contraceptives to regulate menses is discouraged, as the incidence of "post-pill" amenorrhea is probably highest in those patients who have had some type of menstrual irregularity prior to starting the pill.

For the adolescent with persistent amenorrhea but with adequate estrogen stimulation, the administration of progestins is recommended in the form of oral medroxyprogesterone acetate (Provera), 10 mg daily for 5 days every 6 weeks for 3 cycles, then stopped for 3 months to allow the patient to resume spontaneous function.

Grodin JM: Secondary amenorrhea in adolescents. Pediatr Clin North Am 19:621, 1972.

VULVOVAGINITIS

1. GONORRRHEA

Over 800,000 cases of gonorrhea were reported in 1973, the highest number ever reported since the US Public Health Service began keeping records. Since many cases of this disease are not detected and many of those treated are not reported, the Public Health Service estimates that the actual number of cases in 1973 totaled at least 2.5 million. The reported incidence of all cases of gonorrhea was highest among women in the age group from 20–24 years. Women 15–19 years of age had the second highest incidence, and the incidence of disseminated infection (salpingitis, arthritis) was greatest among the latter group.

Clinical Findings

An acute purulent endocervical discharge is readily visible with the vaginal speculum. The gonococcus tends to ascend through the endometrial cavity just after the menstrual flow to reach the oviducts. The patient may have chills and fever to 39.5° C (103.1° F) and may complain of severe bilateral lower abdominal pain with rebound tenderness. The white blood cell count is elevated, and the sedimentation rate may rise to 60–110 mm/hour.

Up to 85% of infections in females and 10–40% in males may be asymptomatic. Screening cervical cultures show that the rate of asymptomatic gonorrhea varies from 0.2–13% in adult women, depending on the setting. However, a study of girls in homes for delinquent teenagers revealed an asymptomatic rate of 10–12%. Routine cervical cultures will identify approximately 70–85% of cases of gonorrhea. A sterile swab is inserted into the cervical os, allowed to rest there for a few seconds, and then plated directly on Thayer-Martin medium.

Pelvic examination may reveal marked tenderness on bimanual examination, particularly with manipulation of the cervix.

Differential Diagnosis

For the patient with vaginal discharge, a wet preparation may show yeast or trichomonads, but these may be present in addition to the gonococcus. For a patient with fever and abdominal pain, appendicitis and acute pyelitis must be considered. Ectopic pregnancy, endometriosis, and ruptured ovarian cyst must also be considered as possible causes of the symptoms.

Treatment

Any of the following regimens is effective:

1. Aqueous procaine penicillin G, 4.8 million units IM simultaneously with 1 gm probenecid orally.

2. Ampicillin, 3.5 gm orally simultaneously with 1 gm probenecid.

3. Spectinomycin (Trobicin), 2 gm IM for both females and males.

4. Tetracycline, 1.5 gm orally immediately, followed by 500 mg 4 times daily for 4 days for a total of 9.5 gm.

A serologic test for syphilis should be obtained when gonorrhea tests are done, and a second culture should be taken 7–10 days following treatment. All sexual partners should be treated as well.

Altchek A: Adolescent vulvovaginitis. Pediatr Clin North Am 19:735, 1972.
American Social Health Association: Page 12 in: *Today's V.D. Control Problem*. 1974.
Colorado Communicable Disease Bulletin. Vol 2, No. 38, Sept 21, 1974.
Dans P: Gonococcal anogenital infection. Clin Obstet Gynecol 18:103, 1975.
Emans SJH, Goldstein DP: Page 113 in: *Pediatric and Adolescent Gynecology*. Little, Brown, 1977.

2. PEDICULOSIS PUBIS
(Crab Lice)

Pediculosis pubis is spread by close contact, by exchanging blankets and clothing, and even occasionally by toilet seats. It is suspected when the patient complains of pubic and vulvar itching or when pruritic dermatoses are present.

The adult louse (about 1–2 mm in length) is attached to pubic hairs close to the skin and looks much like a brown dandruff flake. It may be carefully detached with a pair of fine forceps, placed on a glass slide with a drop of water under a coverslip, and examined at low power. The pubic louse is a 6-legged hairy insect filled with red blood corpuscles. Oval white nits about 0.5 cm in size are attached to the hair shaft and resemble grains of rice.

Treatment

The treatment of choice is 1% gamma benzene hexachloride (Gamene, Kwell). The patient should use it as a 4-minute shampoo and should follow it with the use of a fine-tooth comb to remove remaining nits. The shampoo may be repeated in 24 hours but should not be used more than twice a week.

This preparation may also be used as a lotion in the pubic area. After thorough cleansing, it is applied, left on overnight, and then washed off. The treatment may be repeated in 4 days.

Older successful remedies included 25% benzyl benzoate lotion and DDT powder.

All bedding, towels, and clothes should be washed in very hot water or dry cleaned.

The adult louse dies in 24 hours if separated from the human host, and nits hatch in 7–9 days.

3. CANDIDAL VULVOVAGINITIS

Candida albicans is one of the most frequent causes of vulvovaginitis and sometimes one of the most difficult to treat. Usually the patient complains of intense itching and a feeling of being "scalded" when urine touches the vulva. Vaginal discharge, when present, is thick and curdy. The labia are beefy red, swollen, dry, and painful on examination. There may be redness and excoriation of the inner thighs and perianal area.

A wet preparation using a cotton-tipped swab to collect discharge, with 0.5 ml normal saline and 1 drop of green food coloring for better visibility on a glass slide with a coverslip, will show yeastlike budding cells and hyphae. An alternative procedure is to use 1 drop of KOH with 1 drop of the discharge to dissolve pus cells, but these are usually not numerous.

Treatment

Sitz baths may be used if symptoms are severe. Medication consists of Mycolog Cream (neomycin sulfate, gramicidin, and triamcinolone acetonide), applied locally to relieve swelling and inflammation, and nystatin vaginal suppositories, one inserted in the morning and one at bedtime, for 14 days.

Alternative methods of treatment are Sporostacin Vaginal Cream (chlordantoin, 1%, and benzalkonium chloride, 0.05%), 1 applicatorful intravaginally daily for 14 days; candicidin (Candeptin) vaginal ointment, tablets, or capsules, one applicatorful, tablet, or capsule inserted intravaginally twice a day for 14 days; or miconazole nitrate (Monistat), 2% vaginal cream, 1 applicatorful at bedtime for 14 days. Since a small amount is absorbed from the vagina, miconazole nitrate should not be used in pregnant women.

For resistant or recurrent cases, further laboratory tests may be required. Fasting blood sugar or 2-hour postprandial blood sugar tests may be done. If results are abnormal, a glucose tolerance test should be obtained. A complete blood count to rule out leukemia should be performed. The patient should discontinue birth control pills and should take oral nonabsorbable nystatin, 1 tablet daily for 10 days, to decrease yeast cell organisms in the colon and to eradicate an anal source of reinfection. The patient should cleanse the vaginal area, should wear cotton panties, and should avoid tight panty hose or pants. The male carrier should be treated with nystatin cream. The course of treatment should be repeated. Nystatin should be inserted intravaginally daily or every other day for 2–3 months.

4. *TRICHOMONAS VAGINALIS* VULVOVAGINITIS

The life cycle of *Trichomonas vaginalis* is unknown. Vulvovaginal infection with this organism is uncommon before menarche but has been reported in children. It appears to be spread by coitus and is found in nature only in the human female vagina. The infection produces a profuse, thin, yellow-green frothy discharge (often with a peculiar "mousy" odor) that may appear several days following intercourse with a particular male partner. There may be associated itching, pain, and burning of the vulvar area. On speculum examination, typical "strawberry spots"—red punctate mucosal hemorrhages in the cervix—are seen, with a bubbly discharge in the posterior fornix.

Examination of the discharge under high power using the wet preparation technic will reveal pear-shaped motile organisms with whipping flagella, larger than the numerous pus cells. Mixed infections of *Candida albicans,* trichomonas, and gonorrhea are common.

Treatment

Treatment consists of metronidazole (Flagyl) given orally in a single dose of 2 gm (8 tablets). This dosage has been shown to be 85–90% effective in eradicating trichomonas. The traditional regimen, ie, 250 mg 3 times daily for 10 days, may be used for cases unresponsive to the single dose. The patient should be warned that a large intake of alcohol while on this medication may produce severe abdominal cramping, vomiting, and flushing (disulfiram-like effect). Metronidazole is contraindicated in patients with blood dyscrasias and in pregnancy.

Controversy has arisen over the use of oral metronidazole because of its reported carcinogenic effects in rodents and its mutagenic effects in bacteria in high doses. The single-dose treatment should decrease such risks.

Metronidazole vaginal suppositories, one inserted daily for 10 days, can be used instead of the oral preparation during pregnancy. However, when these are not available, Tricofuron Vaginal Suppositories (furazolidone-nifuroxime) may be used, one in the morning and one at bedtime for the first week and then one at bedtime for another week.

The male partner, who harbors the parasite in the prostate and urethra, should also be treated with metronidazole as above.

Cowdrey SC: Hazards of metronidazole. (Correspondence.) N Engl J Med 293:454, 1975. [And reply by Dykers JR.]

Dykers JR: Single-dose metronidazole for trichomonal vaginitis. N Engl J Med 293:23, 1975.

Hayward MJ, Roy RB: Two-day treatment of trichomoniasis in females: Comparison of metronidazole and nimorazole. Br J Vener Dis 52:63, 1976.

Metronidazole (Flagyl). Med Lett Drugs Ther 17:53, 1975.

Morton RS: Metronidazole in single-dose treatment of trichomoniasis in males and females. Br J Vener Dis 48:525, 1972.

5. *CORYNEBACTERIUM VAGINALE* VULVOVAGINITIS

Corynebacterium vaginale (formerly *Haemophilus vaginalis*), a short rod-shaped bacillus, thrives in an estrogenic vagina. It is one of the few bacilli which causes vaginitis and is spread chiefly by coitus. It produces a gray, homogeneous, malodorous discharge and mild pruritus. Microscopic examination of the wet preparation shows "clue cells," superficial vaginal cells with a stippled or granulated look due to *C vaginale*. There are few pus cells. Gram's stain reveals masses of small gram-negative *C vaginale*.

Treatment

Sulfonamide preparations such as Sultrin (triple sulfa) vaginal cream or tablets, or AVC (sulfanilamide) or Furacin (nitrofurazone), both available as both vaginal cream and suppositories, used nightly for 10 days, are effective against this infection. Tetracycline vaginal suppositories may be inserted at bedtime for 10 days. Since this may encourage candidal growth, nystatin suppositories may be used concomitantly.

Since the infection can be transmitted by sexual intercourse, the male partner should be treated with ampicillin, 500 mg 4 times daily for 5 days, or with tetracycline, 250 mg 4 times daily for 5 days.

6. VULVOVAGINITIS DUE TO HERPES SIMPLEX TYPE 2

Herpes simplex infection is characterized by sudden onset of localized pain, burning, and itching in the perineal area, and dysuria. There may be unilateral or bilateral tender inguinal nodes. This condition begins as a localized vulvar cluster of skin vesicles on an erythematous base which ruptures in 1–3 days, resulting in painful ulcerations. The ulcers persist from 3 days to 2 weeks—occasionally longer—and then clear spontaneously without a trace.

Herpes simplex infection may occasionally cause cystitis with dysuria and urinary retention. If urinary symptoms are pronounced and bacterial cultures are negative, viral cystitis should be considered.

Previous infection with herpesvirus hominis type 1 may give some immunity.

Direct smears may be made of the lesion by scraping the ulcer base with a scalpel and smearing the material on a glass slide. After staining with Wright's or Giemsa's stain, the smear may show giant multinucleated cells and inclusion bodies. Such giant cells may also be seen on Papanicolaou smears, and about two-thirds of cases may be diagnosed by these smears.

The virus can be transmitted by sexual intercourse and is now the second most common venereal disease. Exacerbations may recur as frequently as every 3 months, although the cause is unknown. However, some exacerbations occur just before menses, with emotional stress, with fever, and with upper respiratory infections.

Both epidemiologic and investigative studies strongly implicate herpesvirus type 2 in the etiology of squamous cell cancer of the cervix. A higher incidence of cervical cancer appears in women who begin sexual intercourse at an early age, whose first marriage and first pregnancy occur in early youth, and who have large numbers of sexual partners, many marriages, and multiple "live births."

Follow-up studies of patients with confirmed herpes infection indicate that they develop serious anaplastic changes at a higher rate than the general population. A virus-specific protein antigen has been isolated experimentally and shown to react with antisera from cancer patients.

Because of the risk of disseminated herpes in the newborn, pregnant patients at term with active herpes infections should be delivered by cesarean section.

Treatment

Symptomatic relief is the primary aim of treatment, as there is no cure. Patients with genital herpes are miserable, with pain, dysuria, and local swelling.

Sitz baths twice daily can afford immediate relief. Burow's soaks may be used locally. Fresh tea bags applied to the genital area can help reduce pain and swelling. Local anesthetic ointment such as lidocaine, 2.5%, may help decrease discomfort, particularly with voiding.

Photodynamic inactivation of herpesvirus by the topical application of supravital dyes such as neutral red or proflavine was initially reported to produce symptomatic improvement and a reduced recurrence of herpetic lesions. These earlier observations have not been confirmed in placebo-controlled studies, and this therapy is no longer used.

Alford CA, Whitley RJ: Treatment of infections due to herpes virus in humans: A critical review of the state of the art. J Infect Dis 133 (Suppl):A101, 1976.

Amstey MS: Genital herpesvirus infection. Clin Obstet Gynecol 18:89, 1975.

Jawetz E, Melnick JL, Adelberg EA: Herpesvirus family. Chap 38 in: *Review of Medical Microbiology,* 12th ed. Lange, 1976.

Myers MG & others: Failure of neutral-red photodynamic inactivation in recurrent herpes simplex infections. N Engl J Med 293:945, 1975.

7. CONDYLOMATA ACUMINATA

Condylomata acuminata or genital warts used to be a rare condition in adolescents but is now being seen with increasing frequency. These warts are thought to be caused by a virus similar to that causing warts on the hand. The genital warts are believed to be spread by sexual intercourse or other forms of close physical contact.

The warts are dry, single or (frequently) multiple, and may appear in linear streaks bilaterally in the groove between labia minora and majora. These growths may cover the vulva, the distal vagina, the perianal area, and the anorectal mucosa. They may bleed from abrasion or tearing and are worse with pregnancy.

Treatment

The first objective of treatment is to clear up any vaginal discharge regardless of the cause, since the presence of moisture and irritation seems to encourage the growth of warts.

The lesions should be daubed with podophyllum resin, 25% in tincture of benzoin. Care should be taken to avoid uninvolved skin, as podophyllum resin is extremely caustic. Unaffected areas may first be covered with a protective layer of petrolatum. Only a few lesions are treated at a time if they are numerous.

The patient should wait for at least 2 hours following treatment and then take a sitz bath. The lesions slough off in 2–4 days. If too much podophyllum resin is applied, the patient will have severe constant pain for up to 2 days. The patient should return in 1–2 weeks for repeat treatment if necessary.

If the warts keep recurring, and especially if their gross appearance changes, a biopsy should be done, as the warts have a tendency toward malignant change.

Large lesions over 1 cm in size should be removed by excision or electrofulguration.

8. VAGINAL FOREIGN BODY

Inserted either purposely or accidentally, a foreign body in the vagina may produce a foul, purulent discharge within a few days. The most common foreign body in this age group is a menstrual tampon. Vaginal wall irritation and discharge will clear spontaneously within a day or two. Less frequently, articles used for masturbation, such as a candle, a lipstick case, or a root vegetable, may be found.

Deodorant vaginal spray may occasionally cause pain and edema.

CONTRACEPTION

Not only venereal disease and vaginitis but also unplanned and unwanted pregnancies are among the consequences of sexual activity. Because such accidental pregnancies can be so disruptive and destructive for the unwed teenage girl, contraception should be strongly advised as a preventive measure for the girl who is sexually active.

Considerable evidence suggests that teenage girls begin sex life first and seek contraception later, often after having missed a menstrual period. A recent study in Los Angeles of 502 unwed nonpregnant girls under age 18 showed that only 4% had never had sex, and 63% had never used any form of contraception.

Teenage girls tend to be quite confused about reproduction. For example, one-third believed that a girl was most likely to become pregnant before, during, or immediately after her menses (ie, the "safest time" would then be in midcycle).

Counseling relating to sexual activity is an essential part of contraceptive advice. It is important to explore the relationship the girl has with her sexual partner. Is the desire to have sex a natural outgrowth of a stable and loving relationship? Or is the girl using sex to hold the boy's interest and affection? Many emotionally deprived girls engage in sex because it provides them with a feeling of warmth and closeness to someone. Their sexual activity derives from pregenital needs for being held and fondled. Sexual intercourse may also be a result of peer pressure and a means of gaining acceptance by a particular group. The love of risk-taking and desire for experimentation, so characteristic of adolescence, may push teenagers into trying sexual intercourse. Adolescents also tend to feel immune to risk, feeling that "someone else may get pregnant but I won't," which may lead to an unwanted pregnancy.

The risks of pregnancy and venereal disease, as well as of other less serious sexually transmitted conditions (eg, vulvovaginitis), should be discussed in a straightforward and nonjudgmental manner. Is she ready for the hazards, the stresses, and the strains that having sex can place on a young girl? Or would she rather avoid these pressures, at least for the present?

The girl should be helped to build up her self-esteem and self-respect so that she can feel she does not have to succumb to individual or group pressure regarding sexual activity. She should feel that having sex is her own decision and that she is ready to accept responsibility for it. The physician should remember that this is an age of rebellion and testing-out behavior, and the final decision to use contraception, after a full discussion of pros and cons, should be left to the girl.

If the girl expresses a desire for contraception, the physician then discusses all the methods used, including rhythm, withdrawal, condom, vaginal foam, diaphragm, birth control pills, and intrauterine devices; the physician also tries to perceive any fears, anxieties, or misconceptions she may have about any of the birth control methods.

Use of Birth Control Pills

Before prescribing birth control pills, the physician should obtain a medical history in order to rule out recent hepatitis, thrombophlebitis, migraine headaches, undiagnosed genital bleeding, and any history of breast or genital neoplasms. If any of these exist, oral contraceptives are contraindicated and alternative methods of birth control should be suggested. The physician should also perform a physical examination that includes blood pressure, examination of the breasts, pelvic examination, Papanicolaou smears, culture for gonococci, and wet smear for trichomonas and yeast. The girl is asked to return in 6 weeks following her first menstrual period after starting birth control pills; at 6 months; and again at 1 year, when the initial examination is repeated, in addition to the Papanicolaou smears, gonococcal culture, and wet smear.

The girl should start on estrogen-progestogen compounds with relatively little estrogen effect, such as Norinyl 1/50, Norlestrin 1 mg with iron, or Ovral, all of which contain 0.05 mg of estrogen and 1 mg of progestogen per tablet. The pills should be prescribed in 28-day packs; they are begun on day 5 of the menstrual cycle, with the girl taking one tablet a day. The girl should have a menstrual period between days 21—28. These tablets contain no gonadal steroids. When the girl finishes the 28th tablet, she opens the next 28-day pack. Since teenagers are notorious for taking medicines in an irregular and erratic manner, the 28-day pack is more likely to ensure daily usage (and consequently protection) than the 21-day pack, which requires a wait of 7 days before beginning the next packet.

Compounds containing less than 0.05 mg of estrogen are not prescribed because they tend to cause more breakthrough bleeding and have a higher failure rate.

Diabetes and epilepsy are usually not contraindications to the use of birth control pills. It is felt that the hazards of pregnancy far outweigh the risks of taking contraceptive pills.

Fluid retention can be treated with hydrochlorothiazide, 25 mg/day orally for the first 2—3 days of the menstrual period.

Complications

Breakthrough bleeding, ie, bleeding which occurs at any time in the cycle except days 21—28, is probably the most common complication. If the bleeding occurs in the early part of the cycle, estrogenic stimulation is probably inadequate and the girl can be changed to a compound containing an increased amount of estrogen; such as Norinyl 1/80 or Ortho-Novum 1/80. If breakthrough bleeding occurs late in the cycle, progestogen effect may be lacking, and a compound containing more of this steroid may be prescribed, such as Norlestrin 2.5/50. However, menometrorrhagia may occur only in the first one or 2 cycles on contraceptive pills, and the girl should be urged to take them through the first 2 cycles before initiating a change.

Birth control pills are often taken sporadically by girls who "forget" to take them, which can result in erratic, irregular spotting and bleeding. The actual days when pills were taken should be determined as closely as possible. If this is impossible, it is better to have the girl discontinue her pills for the rest of the month and wait until she has a normal menstrual period. She should be advised to use alternative methods of protection such as vaginal foam and a condom until her period does occur.

Since accidental pregnancies can occur after such sporadic intake of birth control pills, a girl with such a history and irregular bleeding should always have a pelvic examination and a pregnancy test. With the emergence of VACTERL anomalies (*v*ertebral, *a*nal, *c*ardiac, *t*racheal, *e*sophageal, *r*enal, and *l*imb defects) in infants born to mothers who ingested progestogen-estrogen compounds early in the course of pregnancy, there is much concern about the possible teratogenic role of these compounds. Available data suggest that these anomalies occur at a low frequency rate and that the compounds probably act on predisposed persons.

Sore breasts and nausea often occur with the first cycle and usually diminish with subsequent cycles. If nausea is a problem, the girl can be advised to take her pills at bedtime.

If rising blood pressure is noted when the girl returns at her regular 6 weeks revisit, other causes of hypertension should be considered and ruled out with appropriate laboratory tests. Contraceptive steroids should be discontinued and other methods of birth control used.

Severe headaches in themselves are a contraindication to the use of birth control pills. However, painful and disabling headaches can occur after a girl starts on contraceptive steroids even in the absence of a previous history of headaches. A careful history and neurologic examination must be done to rule out migraine headaches. If the headaches are of the migrainous variety, the steroids should be discontinued immediately.

Use of Intrauterine Devices

Among intrauterine devices, the copper 7 is particularly acceptable among nulliparous females because of easy insertion, fewer complications, and excellent contraceptive protection, comparable to the protection afforded by oral contraceptive steroids. However, it must be replaced every 2 years. Where feasible, the plastic loop and coil may be used.

Use of Vaginal Foam

Vaginal foam and the condom used together provide very effective contraception. The condom has the added advantage of protecting against venereal disease. However, the tandem use of foam and condom does require some forethought and preparation and, for this reason, is not popular among the teenage group. The condom alone, however, is one of the most widely used devices.

Forschner DS, Baroff S, Cooper D: Sexual experience of younger teenage girls seeking contraceptive assistance for the first time. Fam Plann Perspect 5:223, 1973.

Lane ME: Contraception for adolescents. Fam Plann Perspect 5:19, 1973.

Nelson JH: Clinical evaluation of side effects of current oral contraceptives. J Reprod Med 6:43, 1971.

Oster G, Salgo MP: The copper intrauterine device and its mode of action. N Engl J Med 293:432, 1975.

·   ·   ·

RESPONSE TO ILLNESS DURING ADOLESCENCE

Any severe illness during adolescence involves the risk of impaired development or emotional disorganization that may interfere with effective functioning in later life. Factors that seem to determine the ability of a boy or girl to cope with his state of illness are as follows: (1) Severity and duration of the illness. (2) Psychosexual, social, and physiologic development of the individual. (3) Adaptive capacity of the individual and his family. (4) Past and present nature of the parent-child relationship. (5) Nature of the illness and the meaning it has for the patient and his family.

Types of reaction to illness during adolescence may range from acceptance of the illness (with a realistic view of symptoms and treatment) to regressive behavior and denial of the existence of illness. The intensity of the reaction may be tempered or increased by the patient's prior experience with a similar illness in his own life or in the lives of meaningful persons within his environment, and by the attitudes of others toward the illness. The ability to adapt to the illness will depend upon biologic factors, intellectual endowment, the abilities of tissues and organs to respond normally, and the psychosocial status of the patient and his family.

The nature of the illness may determine the extent of the reaction. Important in this regard are the following: (1) The organ system involved. Most anxiety is attached to illnesses which involve the organs of the vital functions and the genitalia. (2) Symptomatology. Pain and loss of control of body function may be highly stressful and make adaptation difficult. (3) Type of care involved. The adolescent frequently finds it difficult to submit to the types of body manipulations that are sometimes necessary in treatment. (4) Duration of the illness and the prognosis for life or residual handicap.

The initial impact at onset of illness may elicit an aggressive response with various symptomatic manifestations, unrealistic fear, or denial. There may then be a period of depression, eating disturbances, hostility toward the physician or health care agency, and, later, a period of self-pity related to the handicapping nature of the illness. Adaptation involves acceptance of the situation and the evolution of constructive attitudes which permit planning in mastering stress and overcoming difficulties.

In illnesses which require prolonged care or which threaten temporary or permanent handicaps, a more intense reaction occurs. Diabetes, epilepsy, asthma, or hemophilia may significantly influence personality development, and this may itself interfere with medical care and attempts to plan for vocational, educational, and social adjustment. Chronic illness may elicit a variety of reactions, ranging from overdependence and passivity and an attempt to derive secondary gain to overindependence and aggressive behavior and strong denial of the illness. Some patients have a realistic attitude; others have a great need to deny the complications of their disease and may resist the physician's attempts at treatment.

Paralleling the patient's reactions are those of the parents. Parents may blame the physician for the child's illness and may unconsciously push the child physically and emotionally beyond his capacities for adjustment; or they may reject the patient because of the discrepancy between what he is and what they hoped he would be. The physician should help the parents to adapt and realistically help the child by permitting both an appropriate dependency and continued development within the limits of the illness.

The management of the ill adolescent demands the physician's interest and understanding and the establishment of a therapeutic doctor-patient relationship. By providing a setting where the patient can be heard and accepted and where his concerns about illness can be aired and interpreted, the physician can establish this relationship. In prolonged and handicapping illnesses the physician may need to call upon all possible resources—including educational, social, paramedical, and community agencies—to help the patient and the family adapt.

When hospitalization is required, the reaction to the hospital as well as the illness must be dealt with. The hospital setting must be one in which development can continue to the greatest possible extent, and the patient should be returned to home and school at the earliest possible time.

In his therapeutic relationship with the patient, the physician attempts to provide information and understanding to correct misconceptions and to interpret the handicap and illness. The physician should impart an attitude of optimism for future success and should not hesitate to discuss career goals and vocational possibilities in realistic terms. Since many patients frequently test the doctor-patient relationship by being angry at the physician, not cooperating in treatment programs, and in other ways, the physician should be prepared to respond with understanding and without anger or hostility.

Psychologic and psychiatric examinations may be necessary before medical care can be effectively administered, and collaborative care with a psychiatrist or psychologist may be indicated.

EMOTIONAL PROBLEMS DURING ADOLESCENCE

Adolescents may be brought to or may come to the physician with complaints of emotional or behavioral disorders. The initial complaints may be manifestations of emotional stress. An effort must be made to evaluate the extent of the problem and the type and amount of treatment necessary. Many common emotional problems of adolescence can be handled by the pediatrician who has an appropriate orientation to development during adolescence. In many instances the pediatrician will have the advantage of having known the child and the family for many years.

The evaluation and management of emotional problems during adolescence requires the establishment of a good patient-doctor relationship. The physician should schedule adequate time for visits so that he can show his serious interest in and respect for the adolescent as a developing person. This will permit the adolescent to verbalize his own feelings and attitudes and help him to accept counseling. Initial interviews should be carried out unhurriedly, and the physician must resist the impulse to get to the heart of the problem quickly. The medical history should be designed to gather information (in an unobtrusive manner) about the patient's social and interpersonal interrelationships. The history may also reveal personal habits and dream material that will be valuable in understanding the problem. Some adolescents find it difficult to verbalize their concerns and feelings and have to be drawn out with questions. Frequent reassurance is often needed to solidify the patient-doctor relationship.

If a disorder seems to be predominantly emotional, it is often helpful to point this out and to assure the patient of the physician's willingness to help solve the problem. Excessive prying is to be avoided, but the patient should be permitted to talk while the physician asks appropriate questions and makes comments as the occasion arises. The physician does not need to adhere to the classical 1-hour visit each week; shorter visits at intervals of up to 3 weeks are often sufficient. Psychologic or psychiatric consultation may be necessary for evaluating the problem and determining what treatment is required. It is also helpful if the physician has a psychologic or psychiatric colleague with whom special problems can be discussed. Discussions with school authorities or other community agencies with whom the patient has been related will be valuable in the diagnosis and treatment, but the patient's permission must be obtained before anyone outside the family is approached.

Parents should be seen in separate interviews so that their evaluation of the problem, attitudes, and questions may be heard. Conflicts between the adolescent and his parents can sometimes be resolved in this way.

If the physician feels that psychiatric care is required, appropriate referral is indicated. In doubtful cases, psychiatric evaluation can serve as a basis for continued management by the pediatrician. The decision on whether to refer or not often depends upon such factors as the number of emotional problems carried in the practice, availability of time, and the physician's ability to manipulate forces in the environment when these are playing a prominent role in the patient's problem.

Hollender MH (editor): *The Psychology of Medical Practice.* Saunders, 1958.

Korsch BM: *Psychologic Principles in Pediatric Practice: The Pediatrician and the Sick Child.* Year Book, 1958.

● ● ●

General References

Adolescent Newsletter. Society for Adolescent Medicine. [Semi-annual. Current publications in adolescent medicine.]

Barnes HV (editor): Adolescent medicine. Med Clin North Am 59:1279, 1975. [Entire issue.]

Chapman AH: *Management of Emotional Problems of Children and Adolescents.* Lippincott, 1965.

Cohen MI & others: Perspectives on adolescent medicine: Concepts and program design. Acta Paediatr Scand (Suppl) 256:8, 1975.

Conger JJ: *Adolescence and Youth: Psychological Development in a Changing World.* Harper & Row, 1973.

Daniel WA Jr: *The Adolescent Patient.* Mosby, 1970.

Gallagher JR, Heald FP, Garell DC: *Medical Care of the Adolescent,* 3rd ed. Appleton-Century-Crofts, 1976.

Garell DC (editor): *Symposium on Adolescent Medicine.* Pediatr Clin North Am 20:4, 1973.

Hofmann AP: *The Hospitalized Adolescent: A Guide to Managing the Ill and Injured Youth.* NY Free Press, 1976.

Lopez RI: *Adolescent Medicine.* Vol 1. Spectrum Publications, 1976.

Masterson JF Jr: *The Psychiatric Dilemma of Adolescence.* Little, Brown, 1967.

Millar HEC: *Approaches to Adolescent Health Care in the 1970's.* Department of Health, Education, & Welfare Publication No. (HSA) 75-5014, 1975.

Muus RE: *Theories of Adolescence,* 3rd ed. Random House, 1975.

8 . . .
Skin

William L. Weston, MD

GENERAL PRINCIPLES OF DIAGNOSIS

Examination of the skin requires that the entire surface of the body be inspected and palpated. The skin offers many clues to internal disorders and must be scrutinized with the same care required for auscultation of diastolic murmurs. "The skin does not lie" and may provide answers to puzzling problems of diagnosis.

Terminology of Skin Lesions

The sometimes difficult language of dermatology prevents many students of medicine from accurately describing cutaneous eruptions. The word "rash" is too vague to be useful and should be qualified appropriately. The following terminology should be mastered by all physicians.

A. Primary Lesions (the First to Appear):

1. Macule—Any circumscribed color change in the skin that is flat. *Examples:* White (vitiligo), brown (café-au-lait spot), purple (petechia).

2. Papule—A solid elevated area < 1 cm in diameter whose top may be pointed, rounded, or flat. *Examples:* Acne, warts, small lesions of psoriasis.

3. Plaque—A solid, circumscribed area > 1 cm in diameter, usually flat-topped. *Example:* Psoriasis.

4. Vesicle—A circumscribed, elevated lesion < 1 cm in diameter and containing clear serous fluid. *Example:* Blisters of herpes simplex.

5. Bulla—A circumscribed, elevated lesion > 1 cm in diameter and containing clear serous fluid. *Example:* Bullous erythema multiforme.

6. Pustule—A vesicle containing a purulent exudate. *Examples:* Acne, folliculitis.

7. Nodule—A deep-seated mass with indistinct borders that elevates the overlying epidermis. *Examples:* Tumors, granuloma annulare. If it moves with the skin on palpation, it is intradermal; if the skin moves over the nodule, it is subcutaneous.

8. Wheal—A circumscribed, flat-topped, firm elevation of skin resulting from tense edema of the papillary dermis. *Example:* Urticaria.

B. Secondary Changes:

1. Scales—Dry, thin plates of keratinized epidermal cells (stratum corneum). *Examples:* Psoriasis, ichthyosis.

2. Lichenification—Dry, leathery thickening of skin with deep and exaggerated skin lines and a shiny surface resulting from chronic rubbing of the skin. *Example:* Atopic dermatitis.

3. Erosion—A moist, circumscribed, slightly depressed area representing a blister base with the roof of the blister removed. *Examples:* Burns, bullous erythema multiforme. Most oral blisters present as erosions.

4. Crust—Dried exudate of plasma on the surface of the skin following acute dermatitis. *Examples:* Impetigo, contact dermatitis.

5. Fissure—A linear split in the skin extending through the epidermis into the dermis. *Example:* Angular cheilitis.

6. Scar—A flat, raised, or depressed area of fibrotic replacement of dermis or subcutaneous tissue. *Examples:* Acne scar, burn scar.

C. Configuration of Lesions: Clues to diagnosis may be obtained from the characteristic morphologic arrangement of primary or secondary lesions.

1. Annular (circular)—Annular nodules represent granuloma annulare; annular papules are more apt to be due to dermatophyte infections.

2. Linear (straight line)—Linear papules represent lichen striatus; linear vesicles, incontinentia pigmenti; linear papules with burrows, scabies.

3. Grouped—Grouped vesicles occur in herpes simplex or zoster.

D. Special Types of Lesions:

1. Iris—Annular lesion with 3 circles of different color change—an outer circle of red, then white, and an inner blue circle. *Example:* Erythema multiforme.

2. Comedo—An open comedo (blackhead) is a 1–2 mm papule with a black crater in the center representing oxidized melanin within keratinous plugging of the pilosebaceous orifice. A closed comedo (whitehead) is a 1–2 mm papule with white contents representing a superficial cyst in a pilosebaceous follicle.

3. Burrow—A linear papule diagnostic of scabies.

4. Telangiectasia—A persistent dilatation of individual skin venules. *Example:* Spider angioma.

GENERAL PRINCIPLES OF TREATMENT OF SKIN DISORDERS

PERCUTANEOUS ABSORPTION & THE ROLE OF WATER

Some skin disorders can be treated in different ways by different practitioners and with varying degrees of success. In this section we will deliberately exclude many therapies, including a few time-honored ones, in order to present a rational approach to the treatment of skin disease.

Treatment should be simple and aimed at preserving or restoring the physiologic state of the skin. It is essential to keep in mind that one is treating the child and not the anxious parent or grandparent. Topical therapy is often preferred because medication can be delivered in optimal concentrations at the exact site where it is needed.

Water is an important therapeutic agent that is often forgotten (it is the active ingredient in Burow's solution, calamine lotion, potassium permanganate, and tannic acid soaks). When skin is optimally hydrated, it is soft and smooth (Table 8–1). This occurs at approximately 60% environmental humidity. Since water evaporates readily from the cutaneous surface, the skin (stratum corneum of the epidermis) is dependent on the water concentration in the air, and sweating contributes little. However, if we prevent sweat from evaporating (eg, axilla, groin), the environmental humidity is increased and so is the hydration of the skin. As environmental humidity falls below 15–20%, the stratum corneum shrinks and cracks; the epidermal barrier is lost and allows irritants to enter the skin and induce an inflammatory response. Replacement of water will correct this if the water is not allowed to evaporate. Therefore, in treating dry and scaly skin, one would soak the skin in water for 5 minutes and then add a barrier to prevent evaporation. Oils and ointments prevent evaporation for 8–12 hours. Thus, oils and ointments must be applied once or twice a day. In areas already occluded (axilla, diaper area), ointments or oils will merely increase retention of water and should not be used.

Overhydration (maceration) can also occur. As environmental humidity increases to 90–100%, the number of water molecules absorbed by the stratum corneum increases and the tight lipid junctions between the cells of the stratum corneum are gradually replaced by weak hydrogen bonds (water); the cells eventually become widely separated, and the epidermal barrier falls apart. This occurs in immersion foot, diaper areas, axillas, etc. It is desirable to enhance evaporation of water in these areas. Exposure to less humidity and the use of powders (talcum) that take up extra water are indicated in maceration.

Evaporation of water is also cooling, vasocon-

Table 8–1. Bases used for topical preparations.

Base	Combined With	Uses
Liquids		Wet dressings; relieve pruritus, vasoconstrict.
	Powder	Shake lotions, drying pastes; relieve pruritus, vasoconstrict.
	Grease and emulsifier; oil in water	Vanishing cream: penetrates quickly (10–15 minutes) and thus allows evaporation.
	Excess grease and emulsifier; water in oil	Emollient cream: penetrates more slowly and thus retains moisture on skin.
Grease		Ointments: occlusive (hold material on skin for prolonged time) and prevent evaporation of water.
Powder		Enhances evaporation.

(1) Most greases are triglycerides such as Aquaphor, petrolatum, Eucerin (equal parts of Aquaphor and water), Hydrosorb, Plastibase, Polysorb.

(2) Oils are fluid fats (Alpha-Keri, Lubath, olive oil, mineral oil).

(3) True fats, such as lard or animal fats, contain free fatty acids that increase in amount upon standing and cause irritation.

(4) Ointments (Aquaphor, petrolatum, Crisco, Fluffo) should not be used in intertriginous areas such as the axillas, between the toes, and in the perineum because they increase maceration. Lotions or creams are preferred in these areas.

(5) Oils and ointments hold medication on the skin for long periods of time and are therefore ideal for barriers or prophylaxis and for dried areas of skin. Medication gets into the skin more slowly from ointments.

(6) Creams carry medication into skin and are preferable for intertriginous dermatitis. Over thickened lesions, preventing rapid evaporation of water by covering with Saran Wrap for 8–12 hours at a time will further enhance penetration of the medication.

(7) In the scalp, solutions or lotions should be used.

strictive ("gets the red out"), and antipruritic—all desirable objectives in the management of itchy, red skin.

WET DRESSINGS

By placing the skin in an environment where the humidity is 100% and allowing the moisture to evaporate to 60%, pruritus is relieved. Evaporation of water stimulates cold-dependent nerve fibers in the skin—thereby, theoretically, tying up the circuits so that the itching sensation coming through the pain fibers will not reach the CNS. It also is vasoconstrictive, which helps reduce the erythema and also decreases the inflammatory cellular response.

Wet dressings are applied as follows: For use on the extremities one can use a 4-inch roll of 20/12 mesh gauze. (Five yards is usually sufficient.) Parke-Davis gauze comes in 100-yard rolls. For the trunk, 18-inch gauze, 20/12 mesh, made by Curity, may be used. An alternative is the "2 long john" technic, using a pair of wet cotton long-sleeved and long-legged underwear covered by a dry pair.

Warm but not hot water is used, and the gauze or long johns are soaked in the water and then wrung out until no more drops come out. The dressings are then wrapped around the extremities and fastened with a safety pin. The wet dressings are then covered with dry flannel or dry long johns, which will slow down the evaporation process but not completely retard it, so that the wet dressings need only be changed every 3 or 4 hours.

TOPICAL CORTICOSTEROIDS

Topical corticosteroids (Table 8–2) can also be used under wet dressings. Fluocinolone acetonide cream (Fluonid, Synalar 0.01%) is made specifically for this purpose. If steroids are to be used, the wet dressings are removed completely and the steroids are replaced every 4–6 hours. Treatment for 24, 48, or 72 hours is

Table 8–2. Topical corticosteroids.

It is better to select one preparation from each of the less potent categories (1–3) and get to know them well.

Topical Corticosteroids	Concentration
Group 1: Relative potency = 1	
Hydrocortisone	1.0%
(1) Compounded	
(2) Ready-made	
Group 2: Relative potency = 1–5	
Triamcinolone acetonide (Kenalog quarter strength)*	0.025%
Flurandrenolone (Cordran half strength)*	0.025%
Fluocinolone (Synalar half strength)*	0.01%
Group 3: Relative potency = 5–10	
Methylprednisolone acetate (Medrol)	0.25%
Betamethasone acetate (Celestone)	0.2%
Triamcinolone acetonide (Kenalog, Aristocort)	0.1%
Betamethasone valerate (Valisone)	0.1%
Dexamethasone (Decadron)	0.1%
Flurandrenolone (Cordran)	0.05%
Flumethasone pivalate (Locorten)	0.03%
Fluocinolone acetonide (Synalar, Fluonid)	0.025%
Group 4: Relative potency = 10–100+	
Fluocinonide (Lidex)	0.05%
Fluocinolone (Synalar HP)	0.2%
Triamcinolone acetonide (Aristocort)	0.5%

*To be used with wet dressings.

Note: The only common skin disease in children for which high-potency steroids are indicated is psoriasis. Dermatitis does not require such potent medication. Use of these medications on the face will lead to a severe acne-like eruption with telangiectasia called perioral dermatitis; in the axillas and groin, striae may result, and in other areas atrophy and telangiectasia. Always select the least potent steroid that is effective (groups 1 to 3).

usually sufficient to completely clear a severe generalized dermatitis. Prolonged use of this treatment will result in a significant systemic absorption of steroids. Establishing a higher concentration of corticosteroid drug in the skin by topical rather than systemic therapy will result in marked clearing. Because of the high concentration of steroids remaining in the skin, the mainstay of treatment of chronic forms of atopic dermatitis is application of topical corticosteroid preparations (Table 8–2).

DISORDERS OF THE SKIN IN NEWBORNS

TRANSIENT DISEASES IN THE NEWBORN

No treatment is required for any of the following disorders, though treatment may be given as noted below.

Milia

Multiple white papules 1 mm in diameter scattered over the forehead, nose, and cheeks are present in up to 40% of newborn infants. Histologically, they represent superficial epidermal cysts filled with keratinous material associated with the developing pilosebaceous follicle. Their intraoral counterparts are called Epstein's pearls and are even more common than facial milia. All of these cystic structures spontaneously rupture and exfoliate their contents.

Bhaskar SN: Oral lesions in infants and newborns. Dent Clin North Am 35:421, 1966.
Gordon J: Miliary sebaceous cysts and blisters in the healthy newborn. Arch Dis Child 24:286, 1949.

Sebaceous Gland Hyperplasia

Prominent yellow macules at the opening of each pilosebaceous follicle, predominantly over the nose, represent overgrowth of sebaceous glands in response to the same androgenic stimulation that occurs in adolescence.

Acne Neonatorum

Open and closed comedones, erythematous papules, and pustules identical in appearance to adolescent acne may occur in infants. These are found over the forehead, cheeks, and chin. The lesions may be present at birth but usually do not appear until 3–4 weeks of age. Spontaneous resolution occurs over a period of 6 months to a year or sometimes less. Rarely, neonatal acne may be a manifestation of a virilizing syndrome.

Tromovitch TA, Abrams AA, Jacobs PH: Acne in infancy. Am J Dis Child 106:230, 1963.

Harlequin Color Change

A cutaneous vascular phenomenon unique to neonates occurs when the infant (particularly one of low birth weight) is placed on one side. The dependent half develops an erythematous flush with a sharp demarcation at the midline, and the upper half of the body becomes pale. The color changes usually subside within a few seconds after the infant is placed supine but may persist for as long as 20 minutes.

Mortenson O, Stougard-Andresen P: Harlequin color change in the newborn. Acta Obstet Gynecol Scand 38:352, 1959.

Mottling

A lace-like pattern of dilated cutaneous vessels appears over the extremities and often the trunk of neonates exposed to lowered room temperature. This feature is transient and usually disappears completely upon rewarming.

Erythema Toxicum

Up to 50% of term infants develop erythema toxicum. Usually at 24—48 hours of age, blotchy erythematous macules 2—3 cm in diameter appear, most prominently on the chest but also on the back, face, and extremities. These are occasionally present at birth but rarely have their onset after 4—5 days of life. The lesions vary in number from 2—3 up to as many as 100. Incidence is much higher in term infants than in premature ones. The macular erythema may fade within 24—48 hours or may progress to develop urticarial wheals in the center of the macules or, in 10% of cases, pustules. Examination of a Wright-stained smear of the lesion will reveal numerous eosinophils. This may be accompanied by peripheral blood eosinophilia of up to 20%. All of the lesions fade and disappear by 5—7 days.

Finlay HVL, Bound JP: Urticaria neonatorum (erythema toxicum neonatorum). Arch Dis Child 28:404, 1952.
Levy HL, Cothram F: Erythema toxicum neonatorum present at birth. Am J Dis Child 103:617, 1962.

Sucking Blisters

Bullae, either intact or in the form of an erosion representing a blister base without inflammatory borders, may occur over the forearms, wrists, thumbs, or upper lip. These presumably result from vigorous sucking in utero. They resolve without complications.

Murphy WF, Langley AL: Common bullous lesions presumably self-inflicted—occurring in utero in the newborn infant. Pediatrics 32:1099, 1963.

Miliaria

Obstruction of the eccrine sweat ducts occurs often in neonates and produces one of 2 clinical pictures depending upon the level of obstruction. *Miliaria crystallina* is characterized by tiny (1—2 mm) superficial grouped vesicles without erythema over intertriginous areas and adjacent skin (eg, neck and upper chest). Obstruction occurs in the stratum corneum portion of the eccrine duct. More commonly, obstruction of the eccrine duct deeper in the epidermis results in erythematous grouped papules in the same areas and is called *miliaria rubra*. Rarely, these may progress to pustules. Heat and high humidity predispose to eccrine duct pore closure. Removal to a cooler environment is the treatment of choice.

Perlstein MA: Evaluation of certain preparations for care of the skin of newborn infants. Am J Dis Child 75:385, 1948.

Subcutaneous Fat Necrosis

Reddish or purple, sharply circumscribed, firm nodules occurring over the cheeks, buttocks, arms, and thighs and occurring between day 1 and day 7 in infants represent subcutaneous fat necrosis. Cold injury is felt to play an important role. These lesions resolve spontaneously over a period of weeks, although, like all instances of fat necrosis, they may calcify.

Marks MB: Subcutaneous adipose derangements of the newborn. Am J Dis Child 104:122, 1962.

Sclerema

Premature newborns, especially those who suffer metabolic alterations (eg, metabolic acidosis, hypoglycemia, hypothermia), are susceptible to a diffuse hardening of the skin so that it becomes shiny and feels tight. Severe cold injury in undernourished infants is assumed to be the cause, and these infants do poorly.

Treatment consists of protecting the infant from undue exposure to cold and repairing metabolic and nutritional deficiencies.

Anagnostakis A & others: Sclerema neonatorum. Pediatrics 53:24, 1974.
Kellum RE, Ray TL, Brown GR: Neonatal cold injury: Evidence of defective thermogenesis due to impaired norepinephrine release. Arch Dermatol 97:372, 1965.

BIRTHMARKS

Birthmarks may involve an overgrowth of one or more of any of the normal components of skin: pigment cells, blood vessels, lymph vessels, etc. A nevus is a hamartoma of highly differentiated cells that retain their normal function (see Table 8—3).

Note: All tissue excised should be submitted for pathologic examination.

1. PIGMENT CELL BIRTHMARKS

Mongolian Spot

A blue-black macule found over the lumbosacral

Table 8—3. Classification of nevi in neonates and infants.

Dermal nevi
  Pigment cell (melanocytic)
    Mongolian spot
    Café-au-lait spot
    Junctional nevus
    Compound nevus
    Intradermal nevus
    Giant hairy nevus
    Blue nevus
    Spindle and epithelioid cell nevus (juvenile melanoma)
  Vascular
    Capillary
      Flat hemangiomas
        Salmon patch
        Port wine stain
    Capillary and venous raised hemangiomas
      Strawberry hemangiomas
      Cavernous hemangiomas
    Lymphangiomas
      Lymphangioma circumscriptum
      Cystic hygroma
  Connective tissue nevi
    Collagenoma
    Juvenile elastoma
  Fat tissue
    Lipoma
    Nevus lipomatosis superficialis
Epidermal nevi
  Epidermal nevus (nevus unius lateris, ichthyosis hystrix)
  Pilosebaceous
    Nevus sebaceous
    Nevus comedonicus
  Apocrine
    Nevus syringocystadenoma papilliferum

---

area in 90% of American Indian, black, and Oriental babies is called a mongolian spot. These are occasionally noted over the shoulders and back and may extend over the buttocks. Histologically, they consist of spindle-shaped pigment cells located deep in the dermis. These lesions fade somewhat with time, but some traces may persist into adult life.

Jacobs A, Walton R: The incidence of birthmarks in the neonate. Pediatrics 58:218, 1976.

Café-au-Lait Spot

A café-au-lait spot is a light brown, oval macule (dark brown on black skin) that may be found anywhere on the body. Ten percent of white and 22% of black children have café-au-lait spots greater than 1.5 cm in their longest diameter. These lesions persist throughout life and may increase in number with age. The presence of 6 or more café-au-lait macules greater than 1.5 cm in their longest diameter may represent a clue to neurofibromatosis. Patients with Albright's syndrome also have increased numbers of café-au-lait macules. Although it has recently been suggested that the melanocytes of café-au-lait macules in neurofibro-

matosis contain giant pigment granules, this is not often the case in children, and their absence does not rule out neurofibromatosis.

Junctional & Compound Nevi

Dark brown or black macules, usually few in number at birth but becoming more numerous with age, represent junctional nevi. Histologically, these lesions are large clones of melanocytes at the junction of the epidermis and dermis. With aging, they may become raised (papules) and contain intradermal melanocytes, creating a compound nevus. Often the surface becomes irregular and roughened.

There is controversy about whether junctional and compound nevi are precancerous. Seventy to 80% of melanomas arise on skin that previously contained no pigmented lesion, so the question is not whether junctional nevi are more likely to produce melanoma than normal skin but whether the pigmented lesion really is a junctional nevus or has been a melanoma all along.

Lesions with variegated colors (red, white, blue), notched borders, and nonuniform, irregular surfaces should arouse a suspicion of melanoma. Ulceration and bleeding are advanced signs of melanoma.

If melanoma is a possibility, excisional biopsy for pathologic examination is the treatment of choice.

Kopf AW, Bart RS, Rodriguez-Sains RS: Malignant melanoma: A review. J Dermatol Surg Oncol 3:43, 1977.
Trozak DJ, Rowland WD, Hu F: Metastatic malignant melanoma in prepubertal children. Pediatrics 55:191, 1975.

Intradermal Nevi & Blue Nevi

Brown to blue solitary papules with smooth surfaces represent intradermal nevi. When pigmentation is present deeper in the dermis, the lesions appear blue or blue-black and are called blue nevi.

Spindle & Epithelioid Cell Nevi (Juvenile Melanoma)

A reddish-brown solitary nodule appearing on the face or upper arm of a child represents a spindle and epithelioid cell nevus. The name melanoma is misleading because this tumor is biologically benign. Histologically, it consists of pigment-producing cells of bizarre shape with numerous mitoses.

Treatment consists of excision.

Coskey RJ, Mehregan A: Spindle cell nevi in adults and children. Arch Dermatol 108:535, 1973.

Giant Pigmented Nevi (Bathing Trunk Nevus)

An irregular dark brown to black plaque found over a large percentage of the body surface represents a giant pigmented nevus. Exactly how large is "giant" is unclear from the literature. Often they are of such size as to cover the entire trunk (bathing trunk nevi). Histologically, they are compound nevi. Transformation to malignant melanoma has been reported in as many as 10% of cases in some series, although the true incidence is probably somewhat less. Malignant change may occur at birth or at any time thereafter.

Because of the possibility of melanoma, it is currently recommended that the entire lesion be excised if feasible. If not, small excisional biopsies of raised areas should be performed.

Mark GJ & others: Congenital melanocytic nevi of the small and garment type. Hum Pathol 4:395, 1973.

2. VASCULAR BIRTHMARKS

Flat Hemangiomas

Flat birthmarks can be divided into 2 types: those that are orange or light red (salmon patch) and those that are dark red or bluish red (port wine stain).

A. Salmon Patch: The salmon patch (nevus flammeus) is a light red macule found over the nape of the neck, upper eyelids, and glabella. Fifty percent of infants have such lesions over their necks. Eyelid lesions fade completely within 3–6 months and glabellar lesions by age 5 or 6; those on the nape of the neck fade somewhat but may persist into adult life.

B. Port Wine Stain: Port wine stains are dark red or purple macules appearing unilaterally on the side of the face or an extremity. A port wine stain over the face may be a clue to *Sturge-Weber syndrome*, which is characterized by seizures, mental retardation, glaucoma, and hemiplegia. Most babies with unilateral port wine stains do not have Sturge-Weber syndrome. If the angioma is in the distribution of the ophthalmic branch of the trigeminal nerve or hemihypertrophy of that side of the face exists, Sturge-Weber syndrome is more likely.

Similarly, a port wine hemangioma over an extremity may be associated with hypertrophy of the soft tissue and bone of that extremity called the *Klippel-Trenaunay syndrome.*

The only treatment for port wine stain is the use of cosmetic coverings such as Covermark.

Alexander GL, Norman RM: *The Sturge-Weber Syndrome.* J. Wright & Sons (Bristol), 1960.
Brooksaler F: The angioosteohypertrophy syndrome. Am J Dis Child 112:161, 1966.
Jacobs AH, Walton RG: The incidence of birthmarks in the neonate. Pediatrics 58:218, 1976.

Strawberry Hemangioma

A red, rubbery nodule with a roughened surface is a strawberry nevus. The lesion is often not present at birth but is represented by a permanent blanched area on the skin that is supplanted at 2–4 weeks of age by red nodules. Histologically, these are often mixtures of capillary and venous elements, and, although a deep nodule (cavernous hemangioma) may be part of the strawberry lesion, the biologic behavior is the same. Fifty percent resolve spontaneously by age 5; 70% by age 7; 90% by age 9; and the rest by adolescence.

Strawberry hemangiomas resolve, leaving only redundant skin, and uncomplicated ones are best treated by watchful waiting. Complications include superficial ulceration and secondary pyoderma, which are treated by topical antiseptics and observation.

Complications that require treatment are (1) thrombocytopenia (platelet trapping with the lesion—*Kasabach-Merritt syndrome*); (2) airway obstruction (hemangiomas of the head and neck are often associated with subglottic hemangiomas); (3) visual obstruction (with resulting amblyopia); and (4) cardiac decompensation (high-output failure). In these instances, the treatment of choice is prednisone, 1–2 mg/kg/day orally every other day for 4–6 weeks.

Hidano A, Nakajima S: Earliest features of the strawberry mark in the newborn. Br J Dermatol 87:158, 1972.
Lasser AE, Stein AF: Steroid treatment of hemangiomas in children. Arch Dermatol 108:565, 1973.
Shim WKT: Hemangiomas of infancy complicated by thrombocytopenia. Am J Surg 116:896, 1968.
Simpson JR, Lond MB: Natural history of cavernous hemangiomata. Lancet 2:1057, 1959.

Lymphangiomas

Lymphangiomas are rubbery, skin-colored nodules occurring in the parotid area (cystic hygromas) or on the tongue. They often result in grotesque enlargement of soft tissues.

Surgical excision is the only treatment available, although the results are not satisfactory.

Flanagan BP, Helwig EB: Cutaneous lymphangioma. Arch Dermatol 113:24, 1977.
Peachey RDG, Lim CC, Whimster IW: Lymphangioma of skin: A review of 65 cases. Br J Dermatol 83:519, 1970.

3. EPIDERMAL BIRTHMARKS

Nevus Unius Lateris, Ichthyosis Hystrix

Linear or groups of linear, warty, papular, unilateral lesions represent overgrowth of epidermis since birth. These areas may range from dirty yellow to brown or may be darkly pigmented. The histologic features of the lesions include thickening of the epidermis and elongation of the rete ridges and hyperkeratosis. Clinically, the lesions may be associated with focal motor seizures, mental subnormality, and skeletal anomalies.

Treatment with topical tretinoin (retinoic acid [Aberel, Retin-A]) 0.05%, once or twice daily will keep the lesions flat.

Dupte A, Christol G: Inflammatory linear verrucose epidermal nevus. Arch Dermatol 113:767, 1977.
Solomon LM, Fretzin DF, Dewald RL: The epidermal nevus syndrome. Arch Dermatol 97:273, 1968.

Nevus Comedonicus

The lesion known as nevus comedonicus consists of linear groups of widely dilated follicular openings plugged with keratin, giving the appearance of localized noninflammatory acne. The treatment of choice is surgical removal. If this is not feasible, topical retinoic acid is helpful.

Leppard J, Marks R: Nevus comedonicus. Trans St Johns Hosp Dermatol Soc 59:45, 1973.

Nevus Sebaceus

The nevus sebaceus of Jadassohn is a hamartoma of sebaceous glands and underlying apocrine glands that is diagnosed by the appearance at birth of a yellowish, hairless, smooth plaque in the scalp or on the face. These may be contiguous with an epidermal nevus on the face and constitute part of the linear epidermal nevus syndrome.

Histologically, nevus sebaceus represents an overabundance of sebaceous glands without hair follicles. At puberty, with androgenic stimulation, the sebaceous cells in the nevus divide, expand their cellular volume, and synthesize sebum, resulting in a warty mass.

Because 15% of these lesions become basal cell carcinomas after puberty, excision is recommended before puberty.

Lovejoy FH Jr, Boyle WE Jr: Linear nevus sebaceous syndrome: Report of 2 cases and a review of the literature. Pediatrics 52:382, 1973.
Wilson-Jones E, Heyl T: Naevus sebaceus. Br J Dermatol 82:99, 1970.

4. CONNECTIVE TISSUE BIRTHMARKS
(Juvenile Elastoma, Collagenoma)

Connective tissue nevi are smooth, skin-colored papules 1—10 mm in diameter that are grouped on the trunk. A solitary, larger (5—10 cm) nodule is called a *shagreen patch* and is histologically indistinguishable from other connective tissue nevi which show thickened, abundant collagen bundles with or without associated increases of elastic tissue. Although the shagreen patch is a cutaneous clue to tuberous sclerosis, the other connective tissue nevi occur as isolated events.

These nevi remain throughout life, and no treatment is necessary.

Staricco RG, Mehregan AJ: Nevus elasticus and nevus elasticus vascularis. Arch Dermatol 84:943, 1961.

HEREDITARY SKIN DISORDERS

The Ichthyoses

Ichthyosis is a term applied to several heritable diseases characterized by the presence of excessive scales on the skin. The nomenclature of this group of diseases is confusing. Table 8—4 divides ichthyoses into 2 major types—those with increased retention of scales and those with excessive production of scales—with 2 subtypes in each category.

Treatment consists of control of scaling through the use of a-hydroxy acids—5% pyruvic, citric, lactic, or salicylic acid in petrolatum applied once or twice daily. Restoring water to the skin is also very helpful.

Van Scott ET, Yu RJ: Control of keratinization with a-hydroxy acid and related compounds. Arch Dermatol 110:586, 1974.

Epidermolysis Bullosa

The diagnostic feature of this group of diseases is the formation of hemorrhagic blisters in response to slight trauma. They can be divided into scarring and nonscarring types (Table 8—5).

Treatment usually consists of (1) systemic antibiotics for infection; (2) protective dressings of petrolatum or zinc oxide; and (3) cooling the skin. In disease involving the hands and feet, reducing skin friction with 5% glutaraldehyde every 3 days is helpful.

Table 8—4. Four major types of ichthyosis.*

Name	Age at Onset	Clinical Features	Histology	Inheritance
Ichthyosis with normal epidermal turnover				
Ichthyosis vulgaris	Childhood	Fine scales, deep palmar and plantar markings	Decreased to absent granular layer, hyperkeratosis	Autosomal dominant
X-linked ichthyosis	Birth	Palms and soles spared; thick scales that darken with age; corneal opacities in patients and carrier mothers	Hyperkeratosis	X-linked
Ichthyosis with increased epidermal turnover				
Epidermolytic hyperkeratosis	Birth	Verrucous, yellow scales in flexural areas and palms and soles	Hyperkeratosis, vacuolated reticular spaces in epidermis	Autosomal dominant
Lamellar ichthyosis	Birth; collodion baby	Erythroderma, ectropion, large coarse scales; thickened palms and soles	Hyperkeratosis, many mitotic figures	Autosomal recessive

*Reproduced, with permission, from Frost P, Weinstein GD: Ichthyosiform dermatoses. In: *Dermatology in General Medicine.* Fitzpatrick TB (editor). McGraw-Hill, 1971.

Table 8–5. Types of epidermolysis bullosa.

Name	Age at Onset	Clinical Features	Histology	Inheritance
Nonscarring types				
Epidermolysis bullosa simplex	Birth	Hemorrhagic blisters over the lower legs; cooling prevents blisters	Disintegration of basal cells	Autosomal dominant
Recurrent bullous eruption of the hands and feet (Weber-Cockayne syndrome)	First few years of life	Blisters brought out by walking	Cytolysis of suprabasal cells; dyskeratotic cells	Autosomal dominant
Junctional bullous epidermatosis (Herlitz disease)	Birth	Erosions on legs, oral mucosa; severe perioral involvement	Separation between plasma membrane of basal cells and PAS-positive basal lamina	Autosomal recessive
Scarring types				
Epidermolysis bullosa dystrophica, dominant	Infancy	Numerous blisters on hands and feet; milia formation	Separation of PAS-positive basal lamina; anchoring fibrils lost	Autosomal dominant
Epidermolysis bullosa dystrophica, recessive	Birth	Repeated episodes of blistering, secondary infection and scarring—"mitten hands and feet"	Separation below PAS-positive basal lamina; anchoring fibrils lost	Autosomal recessive

Jarrett M: Diagnosis and treatment of epidermolysis bullosa. South Med J 69:113, 1976.

Incontinentia Pigmenti

Linear blisters in the newborn represent incontinentia pigmenti. These are replaced by hypertrophic, linear, warty bands within several months, followed by swirling brown hyperpigmentation. Most cases are felt to be X-linked dominant, lethal to the male. Mental retardation and seizures were reported in as many as 30% of cases in one series, but the true incidence is probably much less.

Carney RG Jr: Incontinentia pigmenti. Arch Dermatol 112:535, 1976.

COMMON SKIN DISEASES OF INFANTS, CHILDREN, & ADOLESCENTS

ACNE

Obstruction of the sebaceous follicle is a mechanism common to all forms of acne. The sebaceous follicles are those that have abundant sebaceous glands and no hair. The obstruction (plugging) is due to excessive scale production by the follicular wall. Obstruction at the follicular orifice results in a wide patulous opening (open comedo, blackhead). Obstruction at the neck of the sebaceous follicle just below the epidermis results in a subepidermal papule (closed comedo, whitehead). Closed comedones are the lesions that become inflamed, resulting in inflammatory papules, pustules, or cysts. Rupture of the wall of the obstructed follicle due to bacterial enzymes or mechanical trauma will result in an inflammatory lesion.

Typical adolescent acne has its onset between the ages of 8 and 10. It is characterized by many different types of lesions present at one time (open and closed comedones, inflammatory papules, and pustules). In drug-induced acne secondary to ingestion or other exposure to antigens, corticosteroids, or hydantoins, all lesions are usually in the same state at the same time and there is extensive involvement of the abdomen, lower back, arms, and legs.

Treatment

A. Topical Keratolytic Agents: The mainstay of acne therapy is the use of potent topical keratolytic agents applied to the skin to relieve follicular obstruction. Two classes of agents have been found to be most effective for this purpose: (1) Tretinoin (retinoic acid) cream, 0.05%, a potent keratolytic agent, is applied to acne-bearing areas of skin once daily. (2) The benzoyl peroxide gels in 5% concentration also are potent keratolytic agents. The combination of tretinoin cream in the morning and benzoyl peroxide gel in the evening will control 85% of cases of adolescent acne.

B. Systemic Antibiotics: Antibiotics that are concentrated in sebum (tetracycline, erythromycin) are effective in inflammatory acne. The usual starting dose is tetracycline, 500 mg once daily, taken on an empty stomach (nothing to eat for 1 hour before or after). The drug should be continued for 2–3 months until the acne lesions are suppressed.

C. Suggested Treatment Program:

1. Comedones only—Use either tretinoin 0.05% cream or benzoyl peroxide gel 5% once a day.

2. Comedones plus inflammatory papules and a few pustules—Tretinoin 0.05% cream in the morning and benzoyl peroxide gel 5% at bedtime.

3. Comedones plus pustules plus cysts—Both keratolytics plus tetracycline, 0.5—1 gm/day.

Cunliffe W, Cotterill J: *The Acnes.* Saunders, 1976.

Knutson DD: Ultrastructural observations in acne vulgaris: The normal sebaceous follicle and acne lesions. J Invest Dermatol 62:288, 1974.

Price VH: Testosterone metabolism in the skin. Arch Dermatol 111:1496, 1975.

BACTERIAL INFECTIONS OF THE SKIN
(Pyoderma)

Impetigo

Erosions covered by honey-colored crusts are diagnostic of impetigo. Group A streptococci are the important pathogens in this disease, which histologically consists of superficial invasion of bacteria into the upper epidermis, forming a subcorneal pustule.

Although topical antibiotics may effect a clinical cure, parenteral penicillin or oral penicillin for 10 days is necessary to eradicate the streptococci. The risk of nephritogenic strains varies considerably from area to area, but an active program of treatment of patients and contacts with systemic penicillin will significantly reduce the incidence of acute glomerulonephritis in endemic areas.

Ferrieri P, Dajani AS, Wannamaker LW: Benzathine penicillin in the prophylaxis of streptococcal skin infection. J Pediatr 83:572, 1973.

Ferrieri P & others: The natural history of impetigo. J Clin Invest 51:2851, 1972.

Wannamaker LW: Impetigo contagiosa. Prog Dermatol 7:11, 1974.

Ecthyma

Ecthyma is a firm, dry crust, surrounded by erythema, that exudes purulent material. It represents deep invasion by the streptococcus through the epidermis to the superficial dermis.

Treatment is with systemic penicillin.

Cellulitis

Cellulitis is characterized by erythematous, hot, tender, ill-defined plaques accompanied by regional lymphadenopathy. Histologically, this disorder represents invasion of microorganisms into the lower dermis and sometimes beyond, with obstruction of local lymphatics. Streptococci and staphylococci are common offending organisms, although a bluish cellulitis is diagnostic of *Haemophilus influenzae.*

Septicemia is common, and treatment with the appropriate systemic antibiotic is indicated.

Rasmussen JE: *Haemophilus influenzae* cellulitis. Br J Dermatol 88:547, 1973.

Folliculitis

A pustule at a follicular opening represents folliculitis. If the pustule occurs at eccrine sweat orifices, it is correctly called *poritis.* Staphylococci and streptococci are the most frequent pathogens.

Treatment consists of measures to remove follicular obstruction—either cool wet compresses for 24 hours or keratolytics such as are used for acne.

Abscess

An abscess occurs deep in the skin, at the bottom of a follicle or an apocrine gland, and is diagnosed as an erythematous, firm, acutely tender nodule with ill-defined borders. Staphylococci are the most common organisms.

Treatment consists of incision and drainage and systemic antibiotics.

Fritsch WC: Therapy of impetigo and furunculosis. JAMA 214:1862, 1971.

Scalded Skin Syndrome

This entity consists of the sudden onset of bright red, acutely painful skin, most obvious periorally, periorbitally, in the flexural areas of the neck, the axillas, the popliteal and antecubital areas, and the groin. The slightest pressure on the skin results in severe pain and separation of the epidermis, leaving a glistening layer (the stratum granulosum of the epidermis) beneath. The disease is due to a circulating toxin (exfoliatin) elaborated by group II staphylococci (types 71, 55, 3A, 3B, and 3C). The site of action of exfoliatin is the intercellular area of the granular layer, resulting in a separation of cells.

Scalded skin syndrome includes *Ritter's disease* of the newborn, toxic epidermal necrolysis, and the mildest form, staphylococcal scarlet fever. (See also next section.) In all of the forms of this entity, the causative staphylococci may not be isolated from the skin but rather from the nasopharynx, an abscess, blood culture, etc.

Treatment consists of systemic administration of antistaphylococcal drugs, eg, dicloxacillin, 25—50 mg/kg/day orally, or methicillin, 200—300 mg/kg/day IV. No topical therapy is necessary or warranted.

See references below.

Bullous Impetigo

Still a fourth form of scalded skin syndrome is bullous impetigo. All impetigo is bullous, with the blister forming just beneath the stratum corneum, but in "bullous impetigo" there is, in addition to the usual erosion covered by a honey-colored crust, a border filled with clear fluid. Staphylococci may be isolated from these lesions, and systemic signs of circulating exfoliatin are absent. "Bullous varicella" is a disorder that represents bullous impetigo in varicella lesions.

Treatment with dicloxacillin, 25—50 mg/kg/day orally for 5—6 days, is effective. Application of cool compresses to debride crusts is a helpful symptomatic measure.

Elias PM, Fritsch P, Epstein EH Jr: Staphylococcal scalded skin
  syndrome. Arch Dermatol 113:207, 1977.

FUNGAL INFECTIONS OF THE SKIN

1. DERMATOPHYTES

Dermatophytes become attached to the superficial layer of the epidermis, nails, and hair, where they proliferate. They grow mainly within the stratum corneum and do not invade the lower epidermis or dermis. Release of toxins from dermatophytes, especially those whose natural host is animals or soil, eg, *Microsporum canis* and *Trichophyton verrucosum*, results in dermatitis.

Classification & Diagnosis

A. Tinea Capitis: Thickened, broken-off hairs with erythema and scaling of underlying scalp are the distinguishing features of tinea capitis. Pustule formation and a boggy fluctuant mass on the scalp occur in *M canis* and *Trichophyton tonsurans* infections. This mass, called a *kerion,* represents an exaggerated host response to the organism.

B. Tinea Corporis: Tinea corporis presents either as annular marginated papules with a thin scale and clear center or as an annular confluent dermatitis. The most common organisms are *Trichophyton mentagrophytes* and *M canis.* The diagnosis is made by scraping thin scales from the border of the lesion, dissolving them in 20% KOH, and examining for hyphae.

C. Tinea Cruris: Symmetric, sharply marginated lesions in inguinal areas are seen with tinea cruris. The most common organisms are *Trichophyton rubrum, T mentagrophytes,* and *Epidermophyton floccosum.* Scrapings taken from the border should be examined under the microscope with 20% KOH for dermatophytes.

D. Tinea Pedis: The diagnosis of tinea pedis in a prepubertal child must always be regarded with skepticism; atopic feet or contact dermatitis is a more likely diagnosis in this age group. Tinea pedis is seen most commonly in postpubertal males with blisters on the instep of the foot. Fissuring between the toes is occasionally seen. Microscopic examination of thin scales or the undersurface of the blister roof confirms the diagnosis.

E. Tinea Unguium (Onychomycosis): Loosening of the nail plate from the nail bed (onycholysis), giving a yellow discoloration, is the first sign of fungal invasion of the nails. Thickening of the distal nail plate then occurs, followed by scaling and a crumbly appearance of the entire nail plate surface. *Trichophyton rubrum* and *T mentagrophytes* are the most common causes. The diagnosis is confirmed by KOH examination. Usually one or 2 nails are involved. If every nail is involved, psoriasis or lichen planus is a more likely diagnosis than fungal infection.

Treatment

The treatment of dermatophytosis is quite simple: *If hair or nails are involved, griseofulvin is the treatment of choice.* Topical antifungal agents do not enter hair or nails in sufficient concentration to clear the infection. The absorption of griseofulvin from the gastrointestinal tract is enhanced by a fatty meal, so that whole milk or ice cream taken with the medication increases absorption. The dosage of griseofulvin is 10—20 mg/kg/day. With hair infections, it should be continued for a minimum of 6 weeks; in nail infections, for a minimum of 3 months. It is supplied in capsules containing 250 mg or as a suspension containing 125 mg/5 ml. The side-effects are few, and the drug has even been used successfully in the newborn period.

The treatment of kerion includes suppression of the exaggerated inflammatory response with steroids. Either repository steroids injected into the lesion or prednisone, 1.5 mg/kg orally every other morning for 1 month, will prevent scarring and alopecia.

Tinea corporis, tinea pedis, and tinea cruris can be treated effectively with topical medication after careful inspection to make certain that the hair and nails are not involved. The most consistently effective topical agent is tolnaftate (Tinactin) cream or 1% powder, applied 2—3 times a day until the eruption has cleared. Treatment should be continued for 1 week after the eruption has disappeared. Haloprogin (Halotex), miconazole (Micatin), and clotrimazole (Lotrimin) are useful alternatives.

Animal ringworm. (Leading article.) Br Med J 1:405, 1977.
Blank H: Antifungal and other effects of griseofulvin. Am J
  Med 39:831, 1965.

Table 8—6. Clinical features of tinea capitis.

Most Common Organisms	Clinical Appearance	Microscopic Appearance in KOH
Trichophyton tonsurans (60%)	Hairs broken off 2—3 mm from follicle; "black dot"; no fluorescence	Hyphae and spores within hair
Microsporum canis (35%)	Thickened broken-off hairs that fluoresce yellow-green with Wood's lamp*	Small spores outside of hair; hyphae within hair
Microsporum audouini (5%)	Thickened broken-off hairs that fluoresce yellow-green with Wood's lamp*	Small spores outside of hair; hyphae within hair

*Select fluorescent hairs for examination in KOH and culture.

2. TINEA VERSICOLOR

Tinea versicolor is a superficial infection caused by *Malassezia furfur,* a yeast-like fungus. It characteristically causes polycyclic connected hypopigmented macules and very fine scales in areas of sun-induced pigmentation. In winter, the polycyclic macules appear reddish-brown.

Treatment consists of application of selenium sulfide (Selsun), full-strength suspension, or 25% sodium thiosulfate (Tinver). Selenium sulfide should be applied to the whole body and left on overnight. Treatment can be repeated again in a week and then monthly thereafter. It tends to be somewhat irritating, and the patient should be warned about this difficulty.

Albright SD, Hitch JM: Rapid treatment of tinea versicolor with selenium sulfide. Arch Dermatol 92:460, 1966.

McGinley KJ, Lantis LR, Marples RR: Microbiology of tinea versicolor. Arch Dermatol 102:168, 1970.

3. *CANDIDA ALBICANS*

In addition to being a frequent invader in diaper dermatitis, *C albicans* also infects the oral mucosa, where it appears as thick white patches with an erythematous base *(thrush);* the angles of the mouth, where it causes fissures and white exudate *(perlèche);* and the cuticular region of the fingers, where thickening of the cuticle, dull red erythema, and distortion of growth of the nail plate suggest the diagnosis of candidal paronychia. *C albicans* is able to penetrate the stratum corneum layer and locally activate the complement system.

Nystatin (Mycostatin) is the drug of first choice for *C albicans* infections. It is supplied as an ointment or a cream, as an oral suspension, and as vaginal tablets. In diaper dermatitis, the cream form can be applied every 3–4 hours. In oral thrush, the suspension should be applied directly to the mucosa with the mother's finger or a cotton-tipped applicator, since it is not absorbed and acts topically. In candidal paronychia, nystatin is applied over the area, covered with Saran Wrap, and left on overnight after the application is made airtight.

Haloprogin (Halotex) is an effective alternative.

Carter VH, Olansky S: Haloprogin and nystatin therapy for cutaneous candidiasis. Arch Dermatol 110:81, 1974.

Ray TL, Wuepper KD: Experimental cutaneous *Candida albicans* infections in rodents: Role of complement. Clin Res 23:228A, 1975.

VIRAL INFECTIONS OF THE SKIN

Herpes Simplex

Grouped vesicles or grouped erosions suggest herpes simplex. The microscopic finding of epidermal giant cells after scraping the vesicle base with a No. 15 blade, smearing on a slide, and staining with Wright's stain (Tzank smear) suggests herpes simplex or varicella-zoster. In infants, lesions due to herpes simplex type 1 are seen on the gingiva and lips, periorbitally, or on the thumb in thumb suckers. Recurrent erosions in the mouth are usually aphthous stomatitis in children rather than recurrent herpes simplex. Herpes simplex type 2 is seen on the genitalia and in the mouth in adolescents. Herpes simplex infection of the genitalia is now the second most common venereal disease. Cutaneous dissemination of herpes simplex occurs in patients with atopic dermatitis *(eczema herpeticum, Kaposi's varicelliform eruption).*

Since the herpes simplex virus has already proliferated and destroyed cells even in the papular (prevesicular) stage, it is not surprising that all attempts at treatment have had disappointing results. Sterilely rupturing the vesicles and drying the lesions out with frequent (every hour while awake) applications of 70% alcohol will shorten the course of the disease and relieve pain. Other drying agents such as flexible collodion (containing ether) may also provide symptomatic relief. In theory, it may also prevent exogenous reinfection.

Spruance SL & others: The natural history of recurrent herpes labialis. N Engl J Med 297:69, 1977.

Varicella-Zoster

Grouped vesicles in a dermatome on the trunk or face suggest herpes zoster. Zoster in children is not painful and usually has a mild course. In patients with compromised host resistance, the appearance of an erythematous border around the vesicles is a good prognostic sign. Conversely, large bullae without a tendency to crusting imply a poor host response to the virus. Varicella-zoster and herpes simplex lesions undergo the same series of changes: papule, vesicle, pustule, crust, slightly depressed scar. Varicella therefore appears in crops, and many different stages of lesions are present at the same time.

Itching is usually the only symptom, and cool baths as frequently as necessary or drying lotions such as calamine lotion are sufficient to relieve symptoms.

Luby JP: Varicella-zoster virus. J Invest Dermatol 61:212, 1973.

Rogers RS, Tindall JP: Herpes zoster in children. Arch Dermatol 106:204, 1972.

Virus-Induced Tumors

A. Molluscum Contagiosum: Molluscum contagiosum consists of umbilicated, white or whitish-yellow papules in groups on the genitalia or trunk. They are common in sexually active adolescents as well as in infants and preschool children. Crushing a lesion between glass slides followed by microscopic examination after staining with Wright's stain will demonstrate epidermal cells with inclusions. Molluscum contagiosum is a poxvirus that induces the epidermis to proliferate, forming a pale papule.

Removal of the lesion with a sharp curet or knife is curative. This therapy may leave a small scar, and one must weigh the advantage of removal of lesions that will disappear in 2 or 3 years.

B. Warts: Warts are skin-colored papules with irregular (verrucous) surfaces. They are intraepidermal tumors caused by infection with human papilloma virus. This DNA virus induces the epidermal cells to proliferate, thus resulting in the warty growth. If the wart virus stimulus is small, the result is a flat wart. If the stimulation is great, the cells proliferate and thicken, causing the skin to fold upon itself and giving rise to an irregular (verrucous) surface. This verrucous surface is seen on isolated warts on the body called verruca vulgaris, in plantar warts (verruca plantaris), and often in venereal warts (condyloma acuminatum). It is thought that the same wart virus is responsible for all of these varied lesions.

No therapy for warts is ideal, and some types of therapy should be avoided because the recurrence rate of warts is high. Flat warts generally require no treatment. They may be considered a mild wart virus infection, and since they usually disappear within 6–9 months they are best left alone. This holds true especially for all flat warts on the face. A good response has been reported to 0.05% tretinoin (Retin-A) cream applied once daily for 3–4 weeks.

The best treatment for the solitary *common ("vulgaris") wart* is to freeze it with liquid nitrogen. The liquid nitrogen should be allowed to drip from the cotton-tipped applicator onto the wart without pressure. Pressure exaggerates cold injury by causing vasoconstriction and may produce an undesirable deep ulcer and scar. Liquid nitrogen is applied by drip until the wart turns completely white and stays white for 20–25 seconds. Small plantar warts usually need not be treated. Large and painful ones are treated most effectively by applying 40% salicylic acid plaster cut with a scissors to fit the lesion. The sticky brown side is placed against the lesion, taped on securely with adhesive tape, and left on for 5 days. After 5 days, the bandage is removed and the white necrotic warty tissue can be gently rubbed off with the finger and a new salicylic acid plaster applied. This procedure is repeated every 5 days and the patient is seen every 2 weeks, and most plantar warts resolve in 2–4 weeks when treated in this way.

Sharp scalpel excision, electrosurgery, and radiotherapy should be avoided, since the resulting scar often becomes a more difficult problem than the wart itself and may result in recurrence of the wart in the area of the scar.

Condyloma acuminatum is best treated with 25% podophyllum resin (podophyllin) in alcohol. This should be painted on the lesions with a warning that it be washed off after 4 hours. Re-treatment in 7–10 days may be necessary. A condyloma not on the vulvar mucous membrane but on the adjacent skin should be treated as a common wart and frozen.

For isolated warts and periungual warts, cantharidin (Cantharone) is effective and painless in children. It causes a blister and sometimes is difficult to control. An undesirable complication is the appearance of warts along the margins of the cantharidin blister. Cantharidin is applied to the skin, allowed to dry, and covered with occlusive tape such as Blenderm for 24 hours.

No wart therapy is immediate and definitive, and recurrences are reported in 20–30% of cases even with the best care.

Binney ML & others: Warts. Br J Dermatol 94:667, 1976.

Noyes WF: Verrucae: Virus structure, localization of antigens and comparison with the Shope papilloma. Cancer Res 28:1321, 1968.

Oriel JD, Almeida JD: Demonstration of virus particles in human genital warts. Br J Vener Dis 46:37, 1970.

Postlewaite R: Molluscum contagiosum: A review. Arch Environ Health 21:432, 1970.

Pyrhonen S, Johansson E: Regression of warts. Lancet 1:92, 1975.

INSECT INFESTATIONS
(Zoonoses)

Scabies

Scabies is suggested by the appearance of linear burrows about the wrists, ankles, finger webs, areolas, anterior axillary folds, genitalia, or face (in infants). Often one sees excoriations, honey-colored crusts, and pustules from secondary infection. Identification of the female mite or her eggs and feces is necessary to confirm the diagnosis. Slice off an unscratched papule or burrow with a No. 15 blade and examine microscopically in either immersion oil or 10% KOH to confirm the diagnosis. In a child who is scratching a lot, scrape under the fingernails. Examine the parents for unscratched burrows.

We are currently undergoing a pandemic of scabies. Gamma benzene hexachloride (Gamene, Kwell) is an excellent scabicide. However, since gamma benzene hexachloride is concentrated in the CNS and CNS toxicity from systemic absorption in infants has been reported, the following restricted use of this agent is recommended: (1) For adults and older children, one treatment of gamma benzene hexachloride lotion or cream applied to the entire body and left on for 4 hours, followed by shower, is sufficient. (2) Infants tend to have more organisms and many more lesions, and therapy should be repeated every 5–7 days for 4 or 5 treatments. All family members should be treated simultaneously.

Fernandez N, Torres A, Ackerman AB: Pathologic findings in human scabies. Arch Dermatol 113:320, 1977.

Hurwitz S: Scabies in babies. Am J Dis Child 126:226, 1973.
Solomon LM & others: Gamma benzene hexachloride toxicity. Arch Dermatol 113:353, 1977.

Pediculoses (Louse Infestations)

Excoriated papules and pustules with a history of severe itching at night suggest infestation with the human body louse. This louse may be discovered in the seams of underwear but not on the body. In the scalp hair, the gelatinous nits of the body louse adhere tightly to the hair shaft. The pubic louse may be found crawling among pubic hairs, or blue-black macules may be found dispersed through the pubic region (maculae ceruleae). The pubic louse is often seen in the eyelashes of newborns.

Gamma benzene hexachloride (Gamene, Kwell) is the treatment of choice. Since gamma benzene hexachloride is concentrated in the central nervous system and CNS toxicity from systemic absorption in infants has been reported, the following modification in the use of gamma benzene hexachloride is recommended: For head lice, a shampoo preparation is left on the scalp for 5 minutes and rinsed out thoroughly. The hair is then combed with a fine-tooth comb to remove nits. This may be repeated in 24 hours. Gamma benzene hexachloride cream or lotion applied to the body for 4 hours may be necessary for body lice, but washing the clothing in boiling water followed by ironing the seams with a hot iron usually eliminates the organisms.

Gamma benzene hexachloride cream or lotion applied to the pubic area for 24 hours is sufficient to treat pediculosis pubis. It may be repeated in 4–5 days.

Ackerman AB: Crabs: The resurgence of *Phthirus pubis*. N Engl J Med 228:950, 1968.

Papular Urticaria

Papular urticaria is characterized by grouped erythematous papules surrounded by an urticarial flare and distributed over the shoulders, upper arms, and buttocks in infants. These lesions represent delayed hypersensitivity reactions to stinging or biting insects and can be reproduced by patch testing with the offending insect. Dog and cat fleas are the usual offenders. Less commonly, mosquitoes, lice, scabies, and bird and grass mites are involved. The sensitivity is transient, lasting 4–6 months.

The logical therapy is to remove the offending insect. Spraying or dusting the dog or cat with Raid, Off, or similar insecticide products may be necessary. Topical corticosteroids and oral antihistamines will control symptoms.

Gouck HK: Papular urticaria. Arch Dermatol 93:112, 1966.
Massie FS: Papular urticaria: Etiology, diagnosis and management. Cutis 13:980, 1974.

DERMATITIS
(Eczema)

The terms dermatitis and eczema are currently used interchangeably in dermatology, although the etymologic implication of eczema is "a boiling over" and the term originally denoted an acute weeping dermatosis. All forms of dermatitis, regardless of cause, may present with acute edema, erythema, and oozing with crusting, mild erythema alone, or lichenification. Lichenification is diagnosed by thickening of the skin with a shiny surface and exaggerated, deepened skin markings. It is the response of the skin to chronic rubbing or scratching.

Although the lesions of the various dermatoses are histologically indistinguishable, clinicians have nonetheless divided the disease group called dermatitis into several categories based on known causes in some cases and differing natural histories in others.

Atopic Dermatitis

Atopic dermatitis is not a clearly defined clinical entity but a general term for chronic superficial inflammation of the skin that can be applied to a heterogeneous group of patients. Many (not all) patients go through 3 clinical phases. In the first, infantile eczema, the dermatitis begins on the cheeks and scalp and frequently expresses itself as oval patches on the trunk, later involving the extensor surfaces of the extremities. The usual age at onset is 2–3 months, and this phase ends at age 18 months to 2 years. Only one-third of all infants with atopic eczema progress to phase 2—childhood or flexural eczema—in which the predominant involvement is in the antecubital and popliteal fossas, the neck, the wrists, and sometimes the hands or feet. This phase lasts from age 2 years to adolescence. Some children will have involvement of the soles of their feet *only*, with cracking, redness, and pain—the so-called *atopic feet*. Only a third of children with typical flexural eczema will progress to adolescent eczema, which is usually manifested by hand dermatitis only. Atopic dermatitis is quite unusual after age 30.

Atopic dermatitis has no known cause, and, despite the high incidence of asthma and hay fever in these patients (30%) and their families (70%), evidence for allergy beyond this hereditary association is limited to testimonials. The case for food and inhalant allergens as causes of atopic dermatitis is not strong enough to warrant further discussion in this text.

A few patients with atopic dermatitis have immunodeficiency with recurrent pyodermas, unusual susceptibility to herpes simplex and vaccinia virus, hyperimmunoglobulinemia E, defective neutrophil and monocyte chemotaxis, and impaired T lymphocyte function.

A faulty epidermal barrier may predispose the patient with atopic dermatitis to itchy skin. Inability to hold water within the stratum corneum results in rapid evaporation of water, shrinking of the stratum corneum, and "cracks" in the epidermal barrier. Such skin forms an ineffective barrier to the entry of various irritants—and, indeed, it may be clinically useful to regard atopic dermatitis as a primary irritant contact dermatitis and simply tell the patient that he has "sensitive skin." Chronic atopic dermatitis is frequently secondarily infected with *Staphylococcus aureus* or *Streptococcus pyogenes.*

A. Treatment of Acute Stages: Application of wet dressings and topical corticosteroids is the treatment of choice for acute, weeping atopic eczema. Fluocinolone (Synalar), 0.01% cream, designed for use under wet dressings, is applied 4 times daily and covered with wet dressings as outlined on p 194. Systemic antibiotics chosen on the basis of appropriate skin cultures may be necessary since, in the acute phases, atopic dermatitis is often secondarily infected with *S aureus* or streptococci.

B. Treatment of Chronic Stages: Treatment is aimed at avoiding irritants and restoring water to the skin. No soaps or harsh shampoos should be used, and the patient should avoid woolen clothing or any rough clothing. Restoring water to the skin is important in atopic dermatitis. This can be accomplished by 2 "drip-dry" baths daily, less than 5 minutes each, after which lubricating oils or ointments are applied. Alpha-Keri bath oil or Keri lotion (both lanolin base preparations) will suffice, as will Nutraderm or Lubriderm lotion (oil in water emulsion bases). Plain petrolatum and lards are often too greasy and may cause considerable sweat retention. Liberal use of Cetaphil lotion as a lubricant 4 or 5 times a day according to the modified Scholtz regimen is also satisfactory as a means of lubrication. A bedroom humidifier is often helpful. Topical corticosteroids should be limited to the less potent ones. Hydrocortisone ointment, 1% twice daily, is often sufficient. There is *never* any reason to use high-potency corticosteroids in atopic dermatitis. In super-infected atopic dermatitis, systemic antibiotics for 10–14 days (erythromycin, 40 mg/kg/day; dicloxacillin, 50 mg/kg/day) are necessary.

Treatment failures in chronic atopic dermatitis are most often due to patient noncompliance. This is a frustrating disease for parent and child.

Hill HR, Quie PG: Raised serum IgE and depressed neutrophil chemotaxis in 3 children with eczema and recurrent bacterial infections. Lancet 1:183, 1974.
Leyden JL: *Staphylococcus aureus* in the lesions of atopic dermatitis. Br J Dermatol 90:525, 1974.
Möller H: Atopic winter feet in children. Acta Derm Venereol (Stockh) 52:401, 1972.
Norins AL: Atopic dermatitis. Pediatr Clin North Am 18:801, 1971.
Rajka G: *Atopic Dermatitis.* Saunders, 1975.

Nummular Eczema

Nummular eczema is diagnosed by numerous symmetrically distributed coin-shaped ("nummular") patches of dermatitis, principally on the extremities. These may be acute, oozing, and crusted or dry and scaling. The disease lasts 9 months to 1 year. The dif-ferential diagnosis should include tinea corporis and atopic dermatitis.

The same topical measures should be used as for atopic dermatitis, though treatment is often more difficult.

Hellgren L, Mobacken H: Nummular eczema: Clinical and statistical data. Acta Derm Venereol (Stockh) 49:189, 1969.
Krueger GG & others: IgE levels in nummular eczema and ichthyosis. Arch Dermatol 107:56, 1973.

Primary Irritant Contact Dermatitis (Diaper Dermatitis)

Contact dermatitis is of 2 types: primary irritant and allergic eczematous. Primary irritant dermatitis develops within a few hours, reaches peak severity at 24 hours, and then disappears. Allergic eczematous contact dermatitis (see below) has a delayed onset of 18 hours, peaks at 48–72 hours, and often lasts as long as 2 or 3 weeks, even if exposure to the offending antigen is discontinued.

The most common form of primary irritant contact dermatitis seen in pediatric practice is *diaper dermatitis,* which is due to prolonged contact of the skin with a combination of urine and feces with their irritating chemicals such as urea and intestinal enzymes. The diagnosis of diaper dermatitis is based on the picture of erythema and thickening of the skin in the perineal area and the history of skin contact with urine or feces.

Treatment consists of changing diapers frequently to prevent prolonged contact with urine and feces. Rubber or plastic pants serve as occlusive dressings and prevent the evaporation of the contactant and enhance its penetration into the skin; they should be avoided as much as possible. Talcum powder as a hygroscopic agent is useful in taking up irritant from the skin. Cornstarch should not be used since it is a medium in which *Candida albicans* flourishes. In 80% of cases of diaper dermatitis lasting more than 4 days, the affected area is colonized with *C albicans* even before the classical signs of a beefy red, sharply marginated dermatitis with satellite lesions appear.

Treatment of long-standing diaper dermatitis should include application of nystatin (Mycostatin) cream with each diaper change. In extremely inflammatory diaper dermatitis, 1% hydrocortisone cream should be alternated with nystatin cream at every other diaper change.

Dixon PN, Warin RP, English MP: Alimentary *Candida albicans* and napkin rashes. Br J Dermatol 86:458, 1972.
Montes LF & others: Microbial flora of infants' skin. Arch Dermatol 103:640, 1971.

Dyshidrotic Eczema; Hand Eczema

Dyshidrotic eczema consists of vesicles along the lateral margins of the fingers and on palmar surfaces that break down and become erythematous and scaly. Adolescents are most commonly affected. Primary irritants, such as soap, are an important cause.

Treatment involves frequent lubrication (4–5 times a day) of the hands with Nutraderm or Lubriderm lotion (oil in water emulsion bases) and avoidance of irritating agents. Topical corticosteroids at night under white dermal cotton gloves are a useful symptomatic measure. White dermal cotton gloves are soft, come 12 to a box for approximately 50 cents, and can be moistened at night to serve as cool compresses.

Bettley FR: Hand eczema. Br Med J 2:151, 1964.

Garcia-Perez A, Martin-Pascual A, Sanchez-Misiega A: Chrome content in bleaches and detergents. Acta Derm Venereol (Stockh) 53:353, 1973.

Lichen Simplex Chronicus (Localized Neurodermatitis)

Lichen simplex chronicus is a sharply circumscribed single patch of lichenification usually found on the back of the neck in adolescent girls. The patients produce the morphologic skin changes by chronic rubbing and scratching.

Treatment of the thickened lesions is with topical corticosteroids. Because the epidermal barrier has thickened, penetration of topical corticosteroids is poor. Penetration can be enhanced in several ways. Airtight occlusion with plastic dressings (eg, Saran Wrap) overnight over topical corticosteroids is useful, or flurandrenolide (Cordran) tape impregnated with corticosteroids will penetrate the lesion. Covering the lesion will also prevent scratching of the area.

Allergic Eczematous Contact Dermatitis (Poison Ivy Dermatitis)

Children often present with acute dermatitis with blister formation, oozing, and crusting. Blisters are often linear and of acute onset. Plants such as poison ivy, poison sumac, and poison oak cause most cases of allergic contact dermatitis in children.

Allergic contact dermatitis has all the features of delayed type (T lymphocyte – mediated) hypersensitivity. Although many substances may cause such a reaction, nickel sulfate (metals), potassium dichromate, thimerosal (Merthiolate) (preservative in cosmetics and cream), neomycin, and formaldehyde (in clothing) are the most common causes. The true incidence of allergic contact dermatitis in children is not known.

Treatment of contact dermatitis is with topical corticosteroids in localized areas or, in severe generalized involvement, with prednisone, 1–2 mg/kg/day orally for 14–21 days.

Levis WR, Whalen JJ, Miller AE: Studies on the contact sensitization of man with simple chemicals. J Invest Dermatol 62:2, 1974.

Malten KE: Cosmetics, the consumer, the factory worker and the occupational physician. Contact Dermatol 1:16, 1975.

Rudner EJ & others: The frequency of contact dermatitis in North America. Contact Dermatol 1:277, 1975.

Seborrheic Dermatitis

Seborrheic dermatitis consists of an erythema-tous scaly dermatitis accompanied by overproduction of sebum occurring in areas rich in sebaceous glands, ie, the face, scalp, and perineum. This common condition occurs predominantly in the newborn and at puberty, the ages at which hormonal stimulation of sebum production is maximal. Although it is tempting to speculate that the overproduction of sebum causes the dermatitis, the exact relationship is unclear.

Seborrheic dermatitis on the scalp in infancy is often confused with atopic dermatitis, and only after other areas are involved or flexural involvement occurs is it clear that the diagnosis is atopic dermatitis. Psoriasis also occurs in seborrheic areas in older children and should always be considered in the differential diagnosis.

Seborrheic dermatitis responds well to topical corticosteroids; 1% hydrocortisone cream 3 times daily is often sufficient to control this disorder.

Dandruff

Physiologic scaling or mild seborrhea, in the form of greasy scalp scales, can easily be treated by daily or alternate-day shampoos with cream rinse shampoos or selenium sulfide.

Leyden JJ & others: Role of microorganisms in dandruff. Arch Dermatol 112:333, 1976.

Dry Skin (Asteatotic Eczema, Xerosis)

Newborns and older children who live in arid climates are susceptible to dry skin, characterized by large cracked scales with erythematous borders. The stratum corneum is dependent upon environmental humidity for its water, and below 30% environmental humidity the stratum corneum loses water, shrinks, and cracks. These cracks in the epidermal barrier allow irritating substances to enter the skin, predisposing to dermatitis.

Treatment consists of increasing the water content of the skin's immediate external environment. House humidifiers are very useful. Two 5-minute baths a day with immediate application of oils (Alpha-Keri, Domol) or ointments (petrolatum, Aquaphor) will allow the skin to retain water. Frequent soaping of the skin impairs its water-holding capacity and serves as an irritating alkali, and all soaps should therefore be avoided. Frequent use of emollients on the skin should be a major part of therapy. Eucerin (hydrophilic petrolatum in water), Lubriderm or Nutraderm (oil in water emulsion bases), and Cetaphil lotion are all helpful in this regard.

Warin AP: Eczema craquelé as the presenting feature of myxoedema. Br J Dermatol 89:189, 1973.

Polymorphous Light Eruption

The appearance of vesicular, eczematous, or urticarial lesions in sun-exposed areas (cheeks, nose, chin, dorsum of the hands and arms) in the springtime should suggest a diagnosis of polymorphous light eruption. Confirmation can be made by skin biopsy demonstrating dense lymphocytic infiltrates in the dermis or by reproducing the lesion by daily exposure to artificial ultraviolet light. In American Indians it is inherited as an autosomal dominant. Onset is usually at age 5 or 6, and spontaneous improvement occurs at puberty. The first rays of sunlight of sufficient energy reaching the earth's surface in early spring induce the disease. As summer progresses, the skin thickens in response to sunlight, less ultraviolet energy enters the skin, and the disease subsides. The differential diagnosis includes erythropoietic protoporphyria, in which patients experience severe pain and itching after 5 or 10 minutes of exposure to the sun but do not develop significant skin lesions except for small papules over the dorsum of the hand; and photodermatitis from plants (psoralens) or drugs, eg, thiazide diuretics, antihistamines, phenothiazine tranquilizers, tetracyclines, and sulfonamides.

Treatment of the dermatitis with topical corticosteroids, eg, 1% hydrocortisone cream to the face 3 times daily, and daily use of sunshield (5% PABA; Presun) applied at bedtime and each morning are sufficient.

Birt AR, Davis AR: Hereditary polymorphic light eruption. Int J Dermatol 14:105, 1975.
Frain-Bell W: The photosensitive child. Trans St Johns Hosp Dermatol Soc 59:159, 1973.

COMMON SKIN TUMORS

If the skin moves with the nodule on lateral palpation, the tumor is located within the dermis; if the skin moves over the nodule, it is subcutaneous. Table 8–7 lists the tumors according to these categories.

Granuloma Annulare

Circles or semicircles of nontender intradermal nodules found over the lower legs and ankles, the dorsum of the hands and wrists, and the trunk, in that order, suggest granuloma annulare. Histologically, the disease appears as a central area of tissue death (necrobiosis) surrounded by macrophages and lymphocytes.

No treatment is necessary. Lesions resolve spontaneously within 1 or 2 years.

Table 8–7. Common skin tumors.

Intradermal	Intradermal (cont'd)
Granuloma annulare	Lymphangioma
Dermatofibroma	Hemangioma
Epidermal inclusion cyst	Hair and sweat gland hamartomas
Neurofibroma	
Neuroma	**Subcutaneous**
Leiomyoma	Lipoma
Calcifying epithelioma	Rheumatoid nodule
Melanocytic nevus	Osteoma
Pyogenic granuloma	

Wells RS, Smith MA: The natural history of granuloma annulare. Br J Dermatol 75:199, 1963.

Pyogenic Granuloma

Rapid growth of a dark red papule with an ulcerated and crusted surface over 1–2 weeks following skin trauma suggests pyogenic granuloma. Histologically, this represents excessive new vessel formation with or without inflammation (granulation tissue). It is neither pyogenic nor granulomatous but should be regarded as an angioma.

Excision is the treatment of choice.

Leyden JJ, Master GH: Oral cavity pyogenic granuloma. Arch Dermatol 108:226, 1973.
Ronchese F: Granuloma pyogenicum. Am J Surg 109:430, 1965.

PAPULOSQUAMOUS ERUPTIONS

Pityriasis Rosea

Erythematous papules that coalesce to form oval plaques preceded by a large oval plaque with central clearing and a scaly border (the herald patch) establish the diagnosis of pityriasis rosea. The herald patch has the appearance of ringworm and is often treated as such. It appears 1–30 days before the onset of the generalized papular eruption. The oval plaques are parallel in their long axis and follow Langer's lines of skin cleavage. In whites, the lesions are primarily on the trunk, accentuated in the axillary and inguinal areas. In blacks, lesions are primarily on the extremities. This disease is common in school-age children and adolescents and is presumed to be viral in origin. It lasts 6 weeks and may be pruritic the first 7–10 days. The major differential diagnosis is secondary syphilis, and a VDRL test should be done on such patients (see Table 8–8). A chronic variant of this disease may last 2 or 3 years and is called *chronic parapsoriasis* or *pityriasis lichenoides chronicus*.

Exposing the skin to sunlight until a mild sunburn occurs (slight redness) will hasten the disappearance of lesions. Ordinarily, no treatment is necessary.

Plemmons JA: Pityriasis rosea: An old therapy revisited. Cutis 16:120, 1975.
Vollum DI: Pityriasis rosea in the African. Trans St Johns Hosp Dermatol Soc 59:269, 1973.

Psoriasis

Psoriasis is characterized by erythematous papules covered by thick white scales. Guttate (drop-like) psoriasis is a common form in children that often follows an episode of streptococcal pharyngitis by 2–3 weeks. The sudden onset of small (3–8 mm) papules, predominantly over the trunk, that quickly become covered with thick white scales, is characteristic of guttate psoriasis. Chronic psoriasis is marked by thick, large

Table 8–8. Papulosquamous eruptions in children.

Psoriasis
Pityriasis rosea
Secondary syphilis
Lichen planus
Chronic parapsoriasis
Pityriasis rubra pilaris
Tinea corporis
Dermatomyositis
Lupus erythematosus

Nyfors A, Lemholt K: Psoriasis in children. Br J Dermatol 92:437, 1975.
Parrish JA & others: Photochemotherapy of psoriasis with oral methoxsalen and longwave ultraviolet light. N Engl J Med 291:1207, 1974.
Perry HO, Soderstrom CW, Schulze RW: The Goeckerman treatment of psoriasis. Arch Dermatol 98:178, 1968.

(5–10 cm) scaly plaques over the elbows, knees, scalp, and other sites of trauma. Pinpoint pits in the nail plate are seen as well as yellow discoloration of the nail plate resulting from onycholysis. Thickening of all 20 fingernails and toenails is an uncommon feature. The sacral and seborrheic areas are commonly involved. Psoriasis has no known cause and demonstrates active proliferation of epidermal cells with a turnover time of 3–4 days versus 28 days for normal skin. These rapidly proliferating epidermal cells are producing excessive stratum corneum, giving rise to thick opaque scales. Papulosquamous eruptions that present problems of differential diagnosis are listed in Table 8–8.

Treatment

All therapy is aimed at diminishing epidermal turnover time. Sunlight or artificial ultraviolet light (UVL) alone will produce some improvement. Coal tar enhances the effect of UVL and hastens the disappearance of psoriatic lesions. Bathing with a bath product containing tar (eg, Balnetar) at night, followed by UVL the next day, may be sufficient in mild cases. In more severe psoriasis, 2% crude coal tar in petrolatum should be applied after the bath. The new tar gels (Estar gel, Psorigel) avoid staining properties and are most efficacious. They are applied twice daily for 6–8 weeks.

Crude coal tar therapy is messy and stains bedclothes, and patients may prefer to use topical corticosteroids. Penetration of topical corticosteroids through the enlarged epidermal barrier in psoriasis requires that more potent preparations be used, eg, fluocinonide (Lidex, Topsyn), 0.05%, or triamcinolone (Aristocort, Kenacort), 0.5%, 4 times daily. A successful alternative is to add a keratolytic agent to the topical corticosteroid to help remove scales and enhance penetration of the steroid. A cream consisting of salicylic acid, 2%, in fluocinonide, 0.05%, 4 times daily, is effective.

Scalp care using a tar shampoo (Polytar, Sebutone, Zetar, many others) requires leaving the shampoo on for 5 minutes, washing it off, and then shampooing with commercial shampoo to remove scales. It may be necessary to shampoo daily until scaling is reduced.

More severe cases of psoriasis are best treated by a dermatologist using the Goeckerman regimen.

Jacobs AH, Farber EM: Infantile psoriasis. In: *Psoriasis: Proceedings of the Second International Symposium*, Yorke, New York, 1977.

Lichen Planus

Lichen planus consists of pruritic, light purple, flat-topped, many-sided papules, predominantly on the lower legs, penis, wrists, and arms. A white lacy pattern in the buccal mucosa is often seen. Pruritus may be severe.

If pruritus is mild, no treatment is necessary, and the disease will disappear in 6–12 months. With severe pruritus, a trial of antihistamines, eg, diphenhydramine, 5 mg/kg/day, or hydroxyzine, 2 mg/kg/day orally, is warranted. Rapid relief of pruritus and disappearance of the lesions can be achieved by administering prednisone, 1 mg/kg/day orally for 3–4 weeks.

Altman J, Perry HO: The variation and course of lichen planus. Arch Dermatol 84:179, 1961.
Black MM, Wilson-Jones E: The role of the epidermis in the histopathogenesis of lichen planus. Arch Dermatol 105:81, 1972.

HAIR LOSS
(Alopecia)
(See Table 8–9.)

Hair loss in children imposes great emotional stress on the parent and doctor—often more so than on

Table 8–9. Other causes of hair loss in children.*

Hair loss with scalp changes
  Nodules and tumors:
    Nevus sebaceus
    Epidermal nevus
  Thickening:
    Linear scleroderma
      (morphea) (en coup de sabre)
    Burn
  Atrophy:
    Lupus erythematosus
    Lichen planus
Hair loss with hair shaft defects (Hair fails to grow out enough to require hair cuts):
  Monilethrix—alternating bands of thin and thick areas
  Trichorrhexis nodosa—nodules with fragmented hair
  Trichorrhexis invaginata (bamboo hair)—intussusception of one hair into another
  Pili torti—hair twisted 180 degrees, brittle
  Pili annulati—alternating bands of light and dark pigmentation

*Price VH: Office diagnosis of hair shaft defects. Cutis 15:231, 1975.

the child. A 60% hair loss in a single area is necessary before hair loss can be detected clinically. Examination should begin with the scalp to determine if there are color changes or infiltrative changes. Hairs should be examined microscopically for breaking, structural defects, and, finally, to see if growing or resting hairs are being shed. Placing removed hairs in mounting fluid (Permount) makes them easy to examine.

Alopecia Areata

Loss of every hair in a localized area is called alopecia areata. This is the most common cause of hair loss in children. An immunologic pathogenetic mechanism is suspected because dense infiltration of lymphocytes precedes hair loss. Ninety-five percent of children with alopecia areata completely regrow their hair within 12 months, though as many as 40% may have a relapse in 5 or 6 years. A rare and unusual form of alopecia areata begins at the occiput and proceeds along the hair margins to the frontal scalp. This variety, called *ophiasis,* often results in total scalp hair loss or *alopecia totalis.* The prognosis for regrowth in ophiasis is poor.

No treatment is indicated for alopecia areata. Systemic corticosteroids given to suppress the inflammatory response will result in hair regrowth, but the hair will fall out again when the drug is discontinued. In children with alopecia totalis, a wig is most helpful.

Gip L, Lodin A, Molin L: Alopecia areata: A follow-up investigation of outpatient material. Acta Derm Venereol (Stockh) 49:180, 1969.
Winter AJ, Kern F, Blizzard RM: Prednisone therapy for alopecia areata. Arch Dermatol 112:1549, 1976.

Trichotillomania

Traumatic hair-pulling causes the hair shafts to be broken off at different lengths, an ill-defined area of hair loss, petechiae around follicular openings, and a wrinkled hair shaft on microscopic examination. This may be merely habit or the result of severe anxiety in the child. Eyelashes and eyebrows rather than scalp hair may be pulled out.

Treatment aimed at reducing anxiety is sometimes helpful, and this symptom should suggest the need for investigating the family for severe psychopathologic disturbance.

Muller S, Winkelmann RK: Trichotillomania. Arch Dermatol 105:535, 1972.
Stephenson PS: Eyelash pulling: A rare symptom of anxiety. Clin Pediatr (Phila) 13:147, 1974.

REACTIVE ERYTHEMAS

Erythema Multiforme

The iris lesion, usually found on the hands and feet, is diagnostic of erythema multiforme. It consists of a series of concentric circles—red, white, and blue from outside to inside—corresponding to vasodilatation, edema, and leakage of red cells. As the name multiforme implies, other types of lesions also appear, from pruritic erythematous half-circles and polycyclic erythema to urticaria to severe bullae and erosions. It is convenient to think of erythema multiforme in terms of varying stages of cutaneous blood vessel injury; vasodilatation, edema, leakage of red blood cells, and thrombosis with overlying subepidermal bulla formation. The severe bullous type may be limited to mucous membranes only with large erosions. Many agents have been thought to be responsible for this reaction pattern in the skin—but sulfonamide drug reactions and herpes simplex and mycoplasma infections are most commonly involved (Table 8–10).

Table 8–10. Common skin reactions associated with frequently used drugs.

Drug	Common Reactions
Aspirin	Urticaria rarely; purpuric eruptions.
Anti-infective agents	
Erythromycin	Urticaria.
Griseofulvin	Exanthematous eruptions; rarely, cold urticaria or photodermatitis.
Lincomycin (Lincocin)	Urticaria or exanthematous eruptions.
Penicillin and synthetic penicillins	Serum sickness, urticaria, exanthematous eruptions, anaphylactic shock. Ampicillin causes a high incidence of exanthematous eruption in patients with infectious mononucleosis.
Streptomycin	Exanthematous eruptions, urticaria, stomatitis.
Sulfonamides	Urticaria, erythema multiforme, exanthematous eruptions, Stevens-Johnson syndrome, photodermatitis.
Tetracycline	Exanthematous eruptions, urticaria; rarely, bullous eruptions. Demeclocycline (Declomycin) can cause phototoxic reactions.
Antihistamines	Exanthematous eruptions, urticaria, photodermatitis.
Barbiturates	Maculopapular eruptions, urticaria, erythema multiforme, Stevens-Johnson syndrome, bullous eruptions.
Chlorothiazides	Exanthematous eruptions, urticaria, photodermatitis, hemosiderosis of the lower extremities, leading to development of petechiae with resultant pigmentation (Schamberg's phenomenon).
Cortisone and derivatives	Acneiform drug reactions on trunk—pustular, purpuric eruptions.
Insulin	Urticaria, erythema at injection site.
Iodides (cough syrups, antiasthma preparations)	Acneiform pustules over trunk, granulomatous reaction.
Phenytoin	Exanthematous eruptions usually in first 3 weeks of treatment; gingival hyperplasia, hypertrichosis.
Prochlorperazine	Urticaria, pruritus, photosensitive dermatitis.

There are obviously many agents that have not yet been identified. The natural history in the mild form is spontaneous healing in 10—14 days, but the severe bullous, mucous membrane form *(Stevens-Johnson syndrome)* may last 6—8 weeks if untreated.

Treatment is symptomatic in uncomplicated erythema multiforme. Removal of offending drugs is an obvious necessary measure. Oral antihistamines such as hydroxyzine, 2 mg/kg/day orally, are useful. Cool compresses and wet dressings relieve pruritus.

Kauppinen K: Cutaneous reactions to drugs. Acta Derm Venereol (Stockh) 52 (Suppl):68, 1972.
Rasmussen JE: Erythema multiforme in children. Br J Dermatol 95:181, 1976.

Erythema Nodosum

Erythema nodosum consists of painful, erythematous nodules on the anterior lower legs. In streptococcal infections, coccidioidomycosis, histoplasmosis, and tuberculosis, the onset of erythema nodosum parallels the appearance of cell-mediated immunity. Streptococcal infections and birth control pills are the most common causes of this panniculitis in the USA.

Treatment consists of removal of the offending drug or eradication of infection. Topical corticosteroids afford some relief, but prednisone, 1—2 mg/kg/day orally, may be necessary for 2—3 weeks.

Blomgren SE: Conditions associated with erythema nodosum. NY State J Med 72:2302, 1972.
Fine RM, Meltzer HD: Chronic erythema nodosum. Arch Dermatol 100:33, 1969.

MISCELLANEOUS SKIN DISORDERS ENCOUNTERED IN PEDIATRIC PRACTICE

Aphthous Stomatitis

Recurrent erosions on the gums, lips, tongue, palate, and buccal mucosa are often confused with herpes simplex. A smear of the base of such a lesion stained with Wright's stain will aid in ruling out herpes simplex by the absence of epithelial giant cells. A culture for herpes simplex is also useful in this difficult differential diagnostic problem. It has been shown that recurrence of aphthous stomatitis correlates positively with lymphocyte-mediated cytotoxicity.

There is no specific therapy for this condition. Topical steroids in a base that adheres to mucous membrane (Kenalog in Orabase) may provide some relief. In severe cases that interfere with eating, prednisone, 1 mg/kg/24 hours orally for 3—5 days, will suffice to abort an episode.

Cooke BE: Recurrent oral ulceration. Br J Dermatol 81:159, 1969.
Rogers RS, Sams WM Jr, Shorter RG: Lymphocytotoxicity in recurrent aphthous stomatitis. Arch Dermatol 109:361, 1974.

Corns & Calluses

Thickened areas of epidermis in response to repeated or prolonged friction or pressure are called either corns or calluses. Corns are clearly demarcated and painful, whereas calluses have ill-defined margins and are not tender. A painful corn may overlie an exostosis, and one should get an x-ray of that digit.

Treatment begins with removing the cause of friction or pressure, if possible, such as ill-fitting shoes. Local therapy consists of paring down the lesion with a razor blade or No. 15 knife blade and covering it with a cut-to-size piece of 40% salicylic acid plaster. Cover firmly with adhesive tape to prevent loosening due to sweating. The plaster should not be allowed to get wet. It can be removed every 5 days and the dead skin gently removed. The plaster may then be put in place.

Bennett RG, Gammer S: Painful callus of the thumb due to phalangeal exostosis. Arch Dermatol 108:826, 1973.
Montgomery RM: Corns, calluses and warts: Differential diagnosis. NY State J Med 63:1531, 1963.

Morphea (Linear Scleroderma)

Morphea is characterized by the appearance, anywhere on the body, of well circumscribed, shiny, white, firmly bound-down skin. It is particularly cosmetically deforming on the face. A light purple border is indicative of an early lesion or continuing activity. Skin biopsy reveals replacement of subcutaneous fat with thickened collagen fibers. The lesions tend to burn themselves out in 3—5 years. It may be difficult to differentiate morphea from lichen sclerosis et atrophicus, which has similar white patches that occur primarily on the upper back and genitalia. Histopathologic differentiation is often necessary and may be difficult.

Lesions that are not cosmetically disturbing should not be treated. Lesions on the face may be cleared by injections of repository steroids, eg, triamcinolone acetonide diluted 1:4 with saline to make 2.5 mg/ml and injected through a 30-gauge needle. Less than 1 ml should be injected. Complications of local corticosteroid injection include atrophy, depigmentation, ulceration, and infection; therefore, this therapy should be reserved for unusual circumstances.

Curtis AC, Jansen TG: The prognosis of localized scleroderma. Arch Dermatol 78:749, 1958.

Necrobiosis Lipoidica Diabeticorum

A depressed yellow area with telangiectasia surrounded by an erythematous nodular border found on the anterior lower leg is diagnostic of necrobiosis lipoidica diabeticorum. Histopathologically, one sees atrophy of the epidermis and a palisading granuloma of lymphocytes and macrophages surrounding an area of homogenized devitalized dermis. These are most often found in diabetics but can be seen in nondiabetic children.

No treatment is known.

Muller SA, Winkelmann RK: Necrobiosis lipoidica diabeti-
    corum: A clinical and pathological investigation of 171
    cases. Arch Dermatol 93:272, 1966.

CUTANEOUS SIGNS OF SYSTEMIC DISEASES

·   ·   ·

Table 8–11 describes cutaneous signs of various systemic diseases in infants and children.

Table 8–11. Cutaneous signs of systemic disease in infants and children.

Sign	Disease
Acne-like erythematous papules in mid face and white ash-leaf macules on trunk, shiny thickened patch on back, subungual fibromas	Tuberous sclerosis
Pruritic blisters on buttocks, elbows, knees, and scapula	Dermatitis herpetiformis (celiac disease)
Café-au-lait macules	Neurofibromatosis, Albright's disease
"Chicken skin"—yellow rows of soft papules with wrinkled valleys in between in neck, axilla, groin	Pseudoxanthoma elasticum
"Dirty" neck and axillas (hyperpigmented, velvety flexural papules)	Acanthosis nigricans and obesity (endocrinopathies)
Eczematous erosions around the mouth, eyes, perineum, fingers, and toes; alopecia and diarrhea	Acrodermatitis enteropathica (zinc deficiency)
Erythematous, isolated papules on elbows, knees, buttocks, face	Papular acrodermatitis (antigen-positive hepatitis)
Erythematous, truncal macules with central pallor	Juvenile rheumatoid arthritis
Erythematous, flat-topped papules over knuckles	Dermatomyositis
Hemorrhagic (1–2 mm) macules on lips, tongue, palms (epistaxis, gastrointestinal bleeding)	Hereditary hemorrhagic telangiectasia (Osler-Weber-Rendu syndrome)
Hyperpigmentation in palmar creases, knuckles, scars, buccal mucosa, linea alba, scrotum	Addison's disease
Linear or oval vesicles on hands or feet, erosions on soft palate, tonsillar pillars	Hand, foot, and mouth syndrome (Coxsackie A16 and others)
Palpable purpura	Vasculitis
Pigmented macules on oral mucosa	Peutz-Jeghers disease (benign small intestinal polyps)
Purpuric lakes	Purpura fulminans—disseminated intravascular coagulation
Purpuric pustules on hands and feet	Gonococcemia
Purpuric (petechiae) seborrheic dermatitis	Histiocytosis X
Sebaceous (multiple) cysts on face and trunk	Gardner's syndrome (premalignant polyps of colon and rectum)
Stretchy skin; healing with large purple scars	Ehlers-Danlos syndrome
Tight, hard skin, telangiectases, hypo- and hyperpigmentation	Scleroderma
Ulcers with undermined, liquifying borders	Pyoderma gangrenosum (ulcerative colitis, regional enteritis, rheumatoid arthritis)
Vitiligo (completely depigmented macules with hyperpigmented borders)	Pernicious anemia, Hashimoto's thyroiditis, Addison's disease, diabetes mellitus
Yellow papules (lower eyelids, joints, palms)	Xanthomas, hyperlipidemias

●   ●   ●

General References

Braverman IM: *Skin Signs of Systemic Disease*. Saunders, 1970.
Odland GF: *The Skin*. Univ of Washington Press, 1971.
Solomon LS, Esterly NB: *Neonatal Dermatology*. Saunders, 1973.

Weinberg S, Leider M, Shapiro L: *Color Atlas of Pediatric Dermatology*. McGraw-Hill, 1975.

9 . . .
Eye

Philip P. Ellis, MD

GROWTH & DEVELOPMENT OF THE EYE

Although the eye is not completely developed at birth, it is a relatively large functioning sensory organ in the newborn. The postnatal growth of the eye and the brain are comparable. By the end of the fourth year, the eye has attained about 70% of its adult volume. Subsequent growth is much slower, until about age 10–12 years, when adult proportions are reached.

The average anteroposterior diameter of the newborn infant's eye is approximately 16.5 mm (the average adult diameter of the eye is slightly over 24 mm). The cornea is comparatively large, with an average transverse diameter of 10 mm; by the second year of life, the average adult corneal diameter of 12 mm is reached. The cornea in the newborn is relatively flat, and the iris contains little pigment and appears to have a bluish color. As pigment forms, the color of the iris becomes more distinct. By the age of 6 months, it is usually possible to determine whether the irides will become brown or remain blue.

The lens in the newborn infant's eye is quite spherical compared to that in the adult eye. This helps to overcome some of the hyperopia (farsightedness) resulting from the comparative shortness of the eyeball and the relative flatness of the cornea. At birth, approximately 75–80% of children are hyperopic. Hyperopia may increase for the first 7 or 8 years of life and then frequently diminishes. This contrasts to myopia (nearsightedness), which does not usually develop until age 8–10 years and then increases until 20–30 years of age.

The macula in the retina is poorly developed at birth, and this is a major factor in the poor vision of newborns. Full development of the macula does not occur until about 6 months of age. The periphery of the retina is not as well developed as the remainder. Peripheral vascularization is not complete until about the time of term delivery.

Myelination of the optic nerve is incomplete at birth; further myelinization continues until about the fourth month of life. The sclera is relatively thin, and the underlying uvea is what causes the blue color of the newborn sclera. Scleral fibers soon thicken to give a whiter appearance to the eye.

The orbit is almost round at birth. By the first year of life, orbital volume is doubled, and by the sixth year it is redoubled. The lacrimal gland is poorly developed at birth, which accounts for the paucity of tears when the newborn cries. The nasolacrimal duct is usually patent at birth, but in many infants the distal end remains plugged for several months (see discussion under lacrimal apparatus).

Movement of the eyes is not well developed for the first few months of life; the ability to follow an object is usually well established by age 3–4 months. Binocular visual responses begin to develop between the ages of 4–6 months and become firmly established during the second 6 months of life. Persistent deviation of an eye after age 3–4 months should always be investigated by an ophthalmologist.

Harley RD (editor): *Pediatric Ophthalmology.* Saunders, 1975.

GENERAL PRINCIPLES OF DIAGNOSIS

A careful history is essential in establishing an accurate diagnosis of an ocular disorder. The history should include time and rate of onset of the presenting symptoms, associated symptoms, past history of eye disorders and treatment, and pertinent family and social history. However, many eye problems, such as poor vision in one eye, are asymptomatic and are discovered only on testing of visual acuity or other objective diagnostic methods.

COMMON NONSPECIFIC SYMPTOMS & SIGNS

Tearing

In infants, tearing is usually due to nasolacrimal duct obstruction. Tearing may also be associated with local inflammatory and allergic and viral diseases, and with glaucoma.

Discharge

Purulent discharge is usually associated with bacterial infections. Mucoid discharge is usually associated with chemical irritations, some viral infections, or allergic conditions; it may be secondary to obstructions of the nasolacrimal duct.

Pain

Pain in or about the eye may be due to foreign bodies in the cornea or conjunctiva, corneal abrasions, acute infections of the lid, orbital cellulitis, acute dacryocystitis, acute iritis, or glaucoma. Refractive errors seldom produce headaches in young children. Large refractive errors or poor convergence may produce headaches in older children, particularly those who read a good deal.

Poor Vision

In infants, poor vision is usually due to a serious ophthalmologic or neurologic disorder such as congenital nystagmus, corneal or lenticular opacities, disorders of the retina, optic nerve and CNS abnormalities, or very high myopia. In older children, the development of poor vision is often associated with refractive errors. Unilateral poor vision is usually associated with strabismus or large unequal refractive errors between the 2 eyes (anisometropia).

The approximate visual acuity of a 1-year-old child is 20/100; a 2-year-old has approximately 20/60 vision. By age 4–5 years, a visual acuity of about 20/20 has developed.

Leukocoria

A white spot in the pupil is a serious finding which may be due to congenital cataract, retrolental fibroplasia, retinal dysplasia, intraocular infection, retinoblastoma, or persistence and hyperplasia of primary vitreous.

EXAMINATION

Visual Acuity

Routine testing of visual acuity should be a part of every general physical examination. It is the single most important test of visual function. In children 4 years old or older, satisfactory visual acuity tests can usually be obtained with the use of Snellen test cards or illiterate E charts. In using the latter, the child is asked to point in the direction of the "feet" of the figure E. Because of distractions in the office, children are sometimes unable to perform this test adequately; special illiterate E cards may be sent home só that the parents can test the vision at home under better circumstances. The mother, with her interest, can repeat the test at her leisure, and the final result is usually more accurate than testing done in the office by the pediatrician or the nurse.

Visual acuity is difficult to evaluate in infants. One can observe whether an infant will follow a light or a bright attractive object in different directions of gaze. Each eye is tested separately. If the infant fails to respond to such testing, one can observe the pupillary responses for reaction to direct light stimulus, which depend upon a functioning retina and optic nerve. However, cortical blindness can exist with preservation of pupillary light reflexes. Optokinetic nystagmus (slow pursuit movements in the direction of a moving stimulus and quick saccadic movements in the reverse direction; "railway nystagmus") indicates that there are functioning neural receptors in the retina and intact neural pathways. Threat reflexes, such as swiftly bringing an object in the direction of the patient's eyes and observing whether he blinks, are sometimes used to determine if there is a gross deficiency in visual acuity. The difficulty with this test is eliminating the rush of air that can produce corneal sensation and a reflex blink.

Poor visual acuity due to refractive errors in older children can be differentiated from poor vision due to other diseases by a pinhole test. If the reduced visual acuity is due to a refractive error, placement of a pinhole before this eye in line with the pupil will result in improved vision.

External Examination

External examination should include general inspection of the lids and eyeballs, noting their prominence, size, and position as well as any growths, inflammations, discharge, or vascular injection. Forward protrusion (exophthalmos) or retraction (enophthalmos) of the globe should be noted. Unusual size of the globes as indicated by megalocornea or microphthalmos should be noted. The positions of the lids in relation to the globe and the coverage of the lids over the closed eyes should be observed. Normally, with the eyes open, the lower lid margin is at the lower border of the cornea in the forward position of gaze, and the upper lid should cover approximately 2 mm of the cornea. Any drooping of the upper lid (ptosis) or retraction of the eyelids should be noted. The lid margins should be inspected to see if they are against the globes in proper alignment, or whether there is ectropion (turning outward of the lid margins) or entropion (turning inward). The distribution of the lashes and their position should be studied. The lid margins should be inspected for inflammation, crusting, and patency of the lacrimal puncta. If a conjunctival foreign body is suspected, the lids should be everted and the palpebral as well as the bulbar conjunctivas inspected. The upper lid may be everted by pulling the lid forward (grasping the lashes), placing a small applicator behind the tarsal area, and gently pressing down on the lid (Fig 9–1). The maneuver is facilitated if the patient looks downward. If a corneal abrasion or foreign body is suspected or if there is sudden unexplained pain in the eye, sterile fluorescein solution should be instilled into the conjunctival cul-de-sac and the cornea observed to see if there is any staining. Pupillary light reflexes should be tested for each eye, and both direct and consensual reflexes noted.

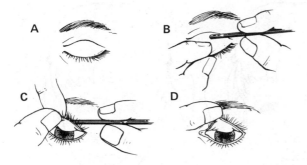

Figure 9–1. Eversion of the upper lid. *A:* The patient looks downward. *B:* The fingers pull the lid down and a rod is placed on the upper tarsal border. *C:* The lid is pulled up over the rod. *D:* The lid is everted. (Redrawn and reproduced, with permission, from Liebman SD, Gellis SS [editors]: *The Pediatrician's Ophthalmology.* Mosby, 1966.)

Corneal sensitivity may be tested by touching the cornea gently with a fine wisp of cotton. If corneal sensation is intact, a brisk blink reflex will result.

Extraocular Muscles

The position of the eyes should be observed by inspection. As a rule there is little difficulty in telling whether gross strabismus is present. A quick estimation of the alignment of the eyes can be made by the corneal light reflection technic (Hirschberg test). The light reflection should come from corresponding parts of each cornea when a light is shone into the eyes. If there is lateral displacement of the light reflection, esotropia (internal deviation) of the eye is present (Fig 9–2). If the light reflection is displaced nasally, exotropia (outward deviation) is present. A more refined method of judging alignment of the eyes is by means of the cover test. In this test the patient is instructed to look at an object and one eye is then covered. If the uncovered eye has been looking straight forward at the object, there will be no shift in movement of this eye. If, however, the eye has been turned either inward or outward, then a corresponding corrective movement will be made with this eye to align the object in the visual gaze (Fig 9–3). The other eye is then similarly tested. The eye under cover should also be observed to see whether there is inward or outward movement,

indicating the presence of a phoria, or a tendency for ocular deviation. If the eye remains in the deviated position after removing the occluder, a tropia (deviation of the eyes not corrected by the fusion mechanism) rather than a phoria (deviation that is corrected by the fusion mechanism) is present.

The cardinal positions of gaze should be checked. An object or light is shown to the infant, and his ability to follow the movement of the object in different directions is tested. If marked strabismus or muscle paralysis is present, there may be limitation of movement in one direction of gaze. To determine whether true paresis of an extraocular muscle is present, the nondeviating eye should be covered and the ocular movement of the uncovered eye tested in all directions of gaze.

Nystagmus

If nystagmus is present, its characteristics should be observed and the movements classified, first by rate or variation in rate of movement and then by direction. *Pendular (undulatory) nystagmus* consists of excursions that are equal in each direction of gaze; this type of nystagmus is usually observed in children with poor vision and is usually ocular in origin. *Jerking (rhythmic) nystagmus* is characterized by a slow component followed by a quick corrective component; it may be congenital, physiologic (at the extreme positions of gaze), due to inner ear disease, or secondary to CNS disease. *Congenital nystagmus* is a type of jerking nystagmus that is usually not associated with other neurologic disorders. The nystagmus is present in all directions of gaze, but it is usually minimized when the patient turns his eyes lightly to one side or the other.

Nystagmus is further classified according to the direction of movement (horizontal, rotatory, vertical, or mixed). Rotatory and vertical nystagmus result from brain stem disorder. Spasmus nutans is a disorder in which vertical head-nodding is associated with nystagmus; the nystagmus is usually horizontal but may be vertical. The condition occurs in small infants and usually disappears within the first 2 years of life.

Measurement of Intraocular Tension

The only satisfactory method of measuring ocular tension is with a tonometer. Tactile tension, particularly in infants, is totally unreliable.

If glaucoma is suspected, the intraocular tension should be measured with a tonometer. In infants, general anesthesia is usually required, although in selected cases chloral hydrate sedation and topical corneal anesthesia may be used. In children 6–7 years of age, intraocular tensions can usually be measured with a tonometer after topical anesthesia. Intraocular tensions should be measured in any child with enlarged or hazy corneas or traumatic hyphema (blood in the anterior chamber).

Ophthalmoscopic Examination

Satisfactory ophthalmoscopic examination of the infant eye can be accomplished only after pupillary dilatation. The combined use of 5% homatropine and

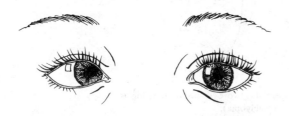

Figure 9–2. Lateral displacement of light reflection showing esotropia (internal deviation) of the right eye. Nasal displacement of the reflection would show exotropia (outward deviation).

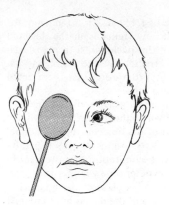

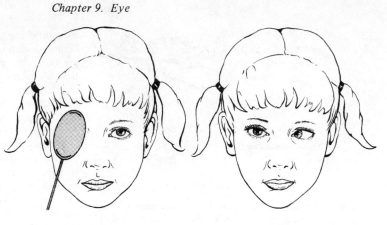

The eyes of a child with severe amblyopia may not be able to fixate an object even when the good eye is covered. Vision of such an eye is 20/200 or less.

If the child with an amblyopic eye will fix only when the good eye is covered but does not hold fixation when the cover is removed, vision of the poor eye is usually from 20/100 to 20/50.

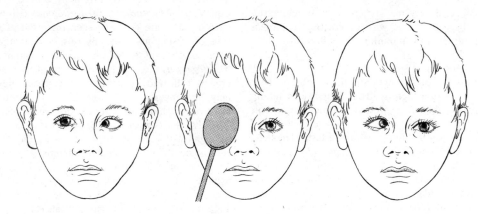

If covering the fixing eye causes fixation with the other eye, and if this second eye maintains fixation for some time even when the cover is removed, the second eye will usually have vision between 20/50 and 20/30.

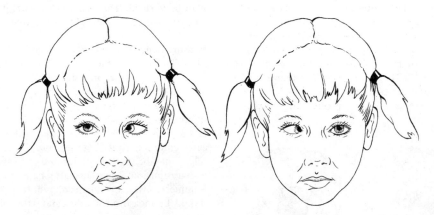

Spontaneous alternation of fixation between the two eyes occurs if vision is equal (no suppression amblyopia).

Figure 9–3. Estimation of visual acuity in amblyopia. (Modified slightly. Redrawn and reproduced, with permission, from Havener WH: *Synopsis of Ophthalmology,* 4th ed. Mosby, 1975.)

2.5% phenylephrine or 0.2% cyclopentolate with 1% phenylephrine (Cyclomydril) instilled 2–3 times at intervals of 10–15 minutes usually gives satisfactory pupillary dilatation. In children 2 years of age and older, 1% cyclopentolate (Cyclogyl) instilled twice at 5–10 minute intervals gives good pupillary dilatation.

It is important to study all of the structures in the eye with the ophthalmoscope, including the cornea, lens, and vitreous as well as the optic disk and retina. In the infant eye the optic disk appears paler than in the adult eye. The foveal light reflection is absent. The periphery of the fundus is gray. The peripheral retinal vessels are not well developed.

Refraction

Cycloplegia is necessary to perform satisfactory refractions in infants and small children. The topical instillation of 1% cyclopentolate (Cyclogyl) or 5% homatropine is usually adequate. More complete cycloplegia can be obtained with 0.5–1% atropine instilled 2–3 times a day for 3 days, but this is seldom necessary. Retinoscopy is performed with trial lenses. After the child is 7 or 8 years of age, subjective methods of refraction can be used in addition to retinoscopy.

Visual Fields

It is virtually impossible to judge visual fields in infants. One can sometimes estimate gross restriction of peripheral visual fields by covering one eye and directing the infant's gaze to an object. A second object is brought in from the side, and the infant is observed to see when he will first shift his direction of gaze to the new object. Different types of toys and colored lights can be used for the visual test objects.

Perimetry examination of visual fields in children is easier to perform than tangent screen examination. When a child is 6 or 7 years of age, satisfactory perimetric examinations can usually be performed. In this test, attractive toys and large test objects are brought in along the perimetry arm.

Gay AJ & others: *Eye Movement Disorders.* Mosby, 1974.

Harley RD (editor): *Pediatric Ophthalmology.* Saunders, 1975.

Harrington DO: *The Visual Fields: A Textbook and Atlas of Clinical Perimetry,* 4th ed. Mosby, 1976.

Hospital For Sick Children, Toronto: *The Eye in Childhood.* Year Book, 1967.

Liebman SD, Gellis SS (editors): *The Pediatrician's Ophthalmology.* Mosby, 1966.

Parks MM: *Ocular Motility and Strabismus.* Harper & Row, 1975.

GENERAL PRINCIPLES OF TREATMENT OF OCULAR DISORDERS

For diseases of the anterior segment of the eye, topical medication is effective. For diseases of the posterior segment of the eye and for diseases of the orbit, systemic medication is necessary. In many instances (eg, severe intraocular infections or uveitis), the combined use of topical and systemic medication is required.

The intraocular penetration of topically applied drugs depends upon their solubility in fat and water. The epithelium of the cornea presents a barrier to medications that are not fat-soluble. The alkaloids, the corticosteroids, and some of the anesthetics penetrate the eye quite easily after topical application to the cornea. Most antibiotics do not penetrate the eye when topically applied.

The degree of intraocular penetration of systemically administered drugs depends upon their ability to pass the blood-aqueous and blood-vitreous barriers. In the normal eye most systemically administered antibiotics do not penetrate the barriers. In the inflamed eye the barriers are broken down, and drugs penetrate in much better concentrations. Systemically administered corticosteroids penetrate the eye quite easily. Certain drugs such as mannitol and glycerol do not cross the blood-aqueous barrier and therefore are valuable in the temporary treatment of acute glaucoma because an osmotic gradient is produced in which the blood is hypertonic to the aqueous and vitreous.

Solutions Versus Ointments

Topical ophthalmic preparations may be administered either as solutions or as ointments. In children, ointments have several advantages over solutions: They are not washed away with the tears; they are quite comfortable upon initial instillation; there is less absorption into the lacrimal passage; and, since the contact time in the eye is much longer, they can be used less frequently. The chief disadvantage of ointments is that they produce a film over the eye and thus interfere with vision. The advantages of solutions are that they do not interfere with vision and cause fewer contact dermatitis reactions than ointments. The chief disadvantage of solutions is that they must be instilled at frequent intervals.

Topical Corticosteroids

The corticosteroids are effective in many eye diseases, including allergic blepharitis and conjunctivitis, vernal conjunctivitis, phlyctenular keratoconjunctivitis, mucocutaneous conjunctival lesions, contact dermatitis of the eyelids and conjunctivas, interstitial keratitis, and many forms of iritis and iridocyclitis. Weaker steroid preparations such as 1% medrysone, 0.5–1.5% hydrocortisone, and 0.125% prednisolone are usually adequate for the management of allergic reactions of the conjunctiva and eyelids.

Many complications follow long- and short-term administration of topical corticosteroids. Among these are increased incidence or aggravation of herpes simplex keratitis and fungal ulcers of the cornea, decreased healing of corneal abrasions and wounds, glaucoma, and cataract formation. The incidence of complications increases with the use of the more potent

Table 9—1. Topical chemotherapeutic and antibiotic agents.

Drug	Trade Name	Solution	Ointment
Amphotericin B	Fungizone	1.5—5 mg/ml*	
Bacitracin	Baciguent	250—1000 units/ml†	500 units/gm
Chloramphenicol	AntiBiOpto Chloromycetin Chloroptic Econochlor Optochlor	2.5—5 mg/ml	10 mg/gm
Colistin	Coly-Mycin	1.2 mg/ml*	1—2 mg/gm
Erythromycin	Ilotycin	5 mg/ml*	5 mg/gm
Gentamicin	Garamycin	3 mg/ml	3 mg/gm
Neomycin	Myciguent	2.5—5 mg/ml†	5 mg/gm
Nystatin	Mycostatin	100,000 units/ml†	100,000 units/gm
Polymyxin B	Aerosporin	1 mg/ml†	2 mg/gm
Streptomycin		50 mg/ml*	
Sulfacetamide sodium	Many	100—300 mg/ml	100 mg/gm
Sulfisoxazole	Gantrisin	40 mg/ml	40 mg/gm
Tetracycline group	Many	5—10 mg/ml	5—10 mg/gm

*Not commercially available.

†Available commercially only in combined drug preparations.

corticosteroid preparations such as 0.1% dexamethasone, 1% prednisolone, 0.1% triamcinolone, and 0.1% betamethasone. The use of these agents generally should be reserved for the treatment of severe intraocular inflammation. Any eye disorder severe enough to require prolonged topical corticosteroid therapy should be treated by an ophthalmologist.

Topical Antibiotics & Chemotherapeutic Agents

Ideally, the infecting organism should be identified and its antibiotic sensitivity established before specific antibiotic therapy is started. This is often impractical, however, and topical antibiotics are in most cases instituted empirically. If possible, those antibiotics should be used that are seldom employed systemically in order to decrease the risk of hypersensitivity reactions. For this reason, neomycin, bacitracin, and polymyxin (or mixtures) are frequently used in the treatment of conjunctivitis. Broad spectrum antibiotics and sulfacetamide or sulfisoxazole seldom produce sensitivity. Topical penicillin therapy should be avoided if possible.

In Tables 9—1 and 9—2 are listed the commonly used topical chemotherapeutic and antibiotic ophthalmic agents.

Mydriatics & Cycloplegics

Mydriatics are agents that dilate the pupil without paralyzing the ciliary muscle of accommodation. They are useful for ophthalmoscopic examination and in preventing and breaking posterior synechias (adhesions of the iris to the lens). The commonly used mydriatics are phenylephrine, 2.5—10%; hydroxyamphetamine, 1%; and eucatropine, 5%. The duration of effect of the mydriatics is only a few hours.

Cycloplegic drugs are agents that produce paralysis of accommodation as well as pupillary dilatation. They are used in refraction and in the treatment of

acute inflammatory conditions of the iris and ciliary body. The more commonly used cycloplegics are atropine, 0.25—2%; homatropine, 2—5%; scopolamine, 0.2%; cyclopentolate, 1—2%; and tropicamide, 1%.

Atropine is the most powerful cycloplegic; its effect may last for as long as 14 days. Scopolamine has an effect which lasts 2—5 days, whereas the effects of homatropine are usually gone within 48 hours. Cyclopentolate and tropicamide produce more rapid cycloplegia than the other agents, but their effect is usually gone within 24 hours. Each drop of 1% atropine contains approximately 0.5 mg of atropine. If 1% atropine drops were instilled into each eye and total absorption occurred, a toxic reaction would result. When instilling atropine into the eyes of infants, exert pressure over the lacrimal sac to prevent the drop from reaching the nasal mucosa, where it could be absorbed; alternatively, the head may be tipped so that the excess of medication will run out of the side of the eye.

Table 9—2. Combinations of anti-infective drugs.

Drugs	Trade Name
Bacitracin and neomycin	Bacimycin
Bacitracin and polymyxin B	Polysporin
Bacitracin (gramicidin), neomycin, and polymyxin B*	Mycitracin, Neosporin, Neo-Polycin, Polyspectrin SOP, Pyocidin
Chloramphenicol and polymyxin B	Chloromycetin-Polymyxin B
Oxytetracycline and polymyxin B	Terramycin-Polymyxin B
Neomycin and polymyxin B	Polyspectrin, Statrol

*Some commercial preparations utilize gramicidin in place of bacitracin.

Topical Anesthetics

The most commonly used local anesthetics are proparacaine, 0.5%; benoxinate, 0.4%; and tetracaine, 0.5%. Topical anesthetics may be used before the removal of a conjunctival or corneal foreign body. They may be necessary to relieve the blepharospasm induced by a chemical injury before satisfactory irrigation and examination of the eye can be accomplished. They should never be prescribed for home use, since they might mask a serious ocular disorder or result in corneal ulceration.

Sterility of Topical Medication

Any ophthalmic medication may become contaminated. This is particularly true of solutions of fluorescein, which frequently become infected with *Pseudomonas aeruginosa.* It is well to discard all old ophthalmic solutions and any container whose tip has been touched by the examiner's hand or by the patient's eyelids. In the case of fluorescein, single use disposable solution or impregnated filter paper strips should be employed.

Baum JL: The eye. In: *Current Pediatric Therapy,* 7th ed. Gellis S, Kagan B (editors). Saunders, 1975.
Ellis PP: *Ocular Therapeutics and Pharmacology,* 5th ed. Mosby, 1977.

OCULAR INJURIES

FOREIGN BODIES

Conjunctival Foreign Body

A conjunctival foreign body can usually be removed with a moist cotton applicator. A common site for foreign bodies is the furrow immediately behind the margin of the upper lid. Eversion of the upper lid, as described above, is necessary to visualize these foreign bodies.

Corneal Foreign Body

Superficial corneal foreign bodies usually can be removed without difficulty. A sterile topical anesthetic should be instilled into the eye and an attempt made to wipe away the foreign body with a moistened cotton applicator. If this is not successful, a blunt spud or small sterile dull hypodermic needle (No. 20) can be used. Care must be taken not to injure the deeper layers of the cornea; if the foreign body is deeply embedded in the stroma, the patient should be referred to an ophthalmologist. All rust rings of foreign bodies should be removed primarily. An antibiotic ointment should be instilled, and the eye should be patched until epithelialization of the cornea has occurred. The patient should be reexamined within 24 hours to make certain that infection has not occurred.

Intraocular Foreign Body

Intraocular foreign bodies are serious injuries which may not be suspected on initial examination. The usual history is that the patient was pounding on a metallic object with a hammer when something flew up into his eye. Examination may show a perforating wound of the cornea, a hole in the iris, and an opaque lens. However, the foreign body may be so small that little evidence of penetration is seen. An x-ray of the eye may be necessary to rule out the possibility of foreign body. If there is any question of a foreign body, the patient should be referred to an ophthalmologist, since removal of these foreign bodies is extremely difficult. The visual prognosis is poor.

Haik GM, Coles WH, McFetridge EM: *Intraocular Injuries.* Lea & Febiger, 1972.
Paton D, Goldberg MF: *Management of Ocular Injuries.* Saunders, 1976.
Runyan TE: *Concussive and Penetrating Injuries of Globe and Optic Nerve.* Mosby, 1975.
Zagora E: *Eye Injuries.* Thomas, 1970.

INJURIES OF THE EYELIDS

Ecchymosis

Severe ecchymosis of the eyelids should be treated first with cold compresses to reduce hemorrhage and swelling. After 24–48 hours, hot packs will speed absorption of extravasated blood.

Lacerations

Lacerations of the eyelids should be sutured primarily. When the laceration involves the lid margin, particularly the lower lid, it is imperative that the margins be sutured as evenly as possible to prevent development of a notch. Such patients should be referred to an ophthalmologist. Lacerations involving the medial portion of the eyelids should be examined to rule out injury to the lacrimal canaliculi. If the canaliculi are cut, they should be repaired at the time of primary closure of the lid laceration, since delayed attempts to repair cut canaliculi are rarely successful.

Tenzel RR: Trauma and burns. Int Ophthalmol Clin 10:55, 1970.
See Paton & Goldberg and Zagora references, above.

CORNEAL INJURIES

Corneal Abrasions

Corneal abrasions usually produce severe discomfort. The diagnosis is made by instilling fluorescein into the eye and observing the cornea for staining.

Treatment consists of the instillation of a mild cycloplegic such as 5% homatropine or 1% cyclopentolate (Cyclogyl), the application of antibiotic ointments, and firm patching of the eye for 24—48 hours until the epithelium has healed.

Corneal Lacerations

Corneal lacerations should be referred to an ophthalmologist for primary suturing. The patient should be observed for the development of intraocular infection. Systemic antibiotics and tetanus toxoid are indicated if the perforation occurred with a contaminated object.

See Paton & Goldberg and Zagora reference, p 219.

HYPHEMA

Hyphema (blood in the anterior chamber) is a common contusion injury in children. It is a serious injury requiring hospitalization. Secondary bleeding is frequent and occurs usually within 6 days after the primary bleeding. Patients with hyphema should be examined for the development of glaucoma. Ophthalmoscopy should also be attempted to ascertain whether there has been more extensive injury to the posterior part of the eye.

Treatment consists of bed rest, eye bandages, and sedatives. Binocular bandages are advisable, but if they produce excitement they may be omitted. Recent studies have suggested that bed rest and monocular patches are as effective as binocular patches in mild or moderate hyphemas. However, in severe hyphemas, binocular patches are preferred. No pupillary dilating (mydriatic) or pupillary constricting (miotic) drops should be used. If glaucoma develops, the use of carbonic anhydrase inhibitors, intravenous urea or mannitol, or oral glycerol is indicated initially. If this does not control the glaucoma, surgical removal of the blood clot by irrigation with saline or fibrinolysin is indicated.

Another complication of hyphema is blood staining of the cornea. This occurs only if the hemorrhage remains for a long period; it may occur whether or not glaucoma develops.

Edwards WC, Layden WE: Monocular versus binocular patching in traumatic hyphema. Am J Ophthalmol 76:359, 1973.
Fritch CD: Traumatic hyphema. Ann Ophthalmol 8:1223, 1976.
Pilger IS: Medical treatment of traumatic hyphema. Surv Ophthalmol 20:28, 1975.
Read J, Goldberg MF: Comparison of medical treatment for traumatic hyphema. Trans Am Acad Ophthalmol Otolaryngol 78:799, 1974.

BURNS

Burns of the eyelids should be treated in essentially the same way as burns of the skin elsewhere. It is important to protect the eyeballs from infection and exposure. Since burns frequently become contaminated with pseudomonas organisms which can produce severe corneal ulceration, an antibiotic preparation containing either colistin, gentamicin, or polymyxin B should be instilled into the eyes 3—4 times a day. As the burns begin to heal, cicatricial ectropion with corneal exposure may develop. To prevent corneal exposure, ointments should be applied inside the eyelids. Plastic surgery usually is necessary to correct cicatricial ectropion.

Chemical burns of the cornea and conjunctiva should be treated initially with thorough irrigation with any clean nonirritating fluid. This may be tap water, saline or boric acid solution, or whatever is available. It may be necessary to instill topical anesthetics into the eye to relieve blepharospasm before irrigation can be accomplished. After irrigation the eye should be inspected for retained chemical particles, which can be removed with a moistened cotton applicator. The extent of the damage is then determined. A weak acid solution such as 0.5% acetic acid may be used to irrigate the eye burned with alkali. In the case of acid burns, 3% sodium bicarbonate may be used for irrigation. In no case should a delay occur while waiting for a certain irrigating solution. If the burn involves the cornea, the eye should be dilated with 1% atropine or 5% homatropine after irrigation. An antibiotic ointment should be instilled and the eye patched. Any patient who has suffered a severe chemical burn of the eye should be hospitalized and should be seen by an ophthalmologist.

Ultraviolet burns of the cornea usually cause severe pain and tearing. There is a history of exposure to ultraviolet light (eg, a welder's arc, snow on the ski slopes, sunlamp or treatment lamp). Symptoms develop 10—12 hours after exposure. Examination shows superficial corneal edema and pinpoint areas that stain with fluorescein. Treatment consists of the application of a topical anesthetic every 5—10 minutes until the pain is relieved. After pain has subsided, an antibiotic or an antibiotic-corticosteroid ointment is instilled into the eye and the eye is patched. Systemic analgesics and sedatives are then prescribed. Recovery is usually prompt and complete within 48 hours. (*Note:* Topical anesthetics should never be sent home with the patient.)

Retinal burns with permanent loss of vision may occur as a result of exposure to strong infrared light such as from observing an eclipse. If this is suspected, the patient should be referred to an ophthalmologist.

Brown SI, Tragakis MP, Pearce DB: Treatment of the alkali-burned cornea. Am J Ophthalmol 74:316, 1972.
Lemp MA: Cornea and sclera: Annual review. Arch Ophthalmol 94:473, 1976.
See Paton & Goldberg reference, p 219.

FRACTURES OF THE ORBIT

Fractures of the orbit with any degree of displacement of the bones should be surgically reduced. The technics of surgery depend upon the location and extent of the fracture. If the fractures are not satisfactorily reduced, complications occur which include displacement of the globe, enophthalmos, and diplopia. Any injury that is severe enough to cause an orbital fracture may cause further skull fractures and intracranial and intraocular damage. The patient should be studied for these possibilities.

Blowout fractures generally result from blunt injury such as a blow from a ball or fist. The bones of the orbital rim usually remain intact, but there is a blowout of the floor of the orbit (rarely, the medial wall of the orbit) with herniation of the orbital contents into the blowout site. Blowout fractures should be suspected if there is evidence of diplopia in any direction of gaze or if there is limitation of ocular movement, particularly upward. Hypesthesia of the skin in the distribution of the infraorbital nerve is present in about 30% of patients. Blowout fractures are not always seen on routine x-rays of the orbit. Tomograms and other special diagnostic radiologic technics are sometimes necessary to demonstrate this fracture. Surgical treatment is usually required.

Bleeker GM, Lyle TK (editors): *Fractures of the Orbit.* Williams & Wilkins, 1970.
Emery JM & others: Management of orbital floor fractures. Am J Ophthalmol 74:299, 1972.
Greenwald HS & others: A review of 128 patients with orbital fractures. Am J Opthalmol 78:655, 1974.

CONTUSION OF THE GLOBE

In addition to the hyphema mentioned above, contusions of the globe may result in dislocation of the lens, hemorrhage into the vitreous, retinal edema and hemorrhage, retinal detachment, choroidal hemorrhage, choroidal rupture, and rupture of the eyeball. The diagnosis of these conditions is based upon (1) changes in visual acuity and (2) direct observation with the ophthalmoscope and slit lamp. If the fundus can be visualized well and if visual acuity is good, there is little likelihood that any significant damage to the posterior part of the eye has occurred. However, complications such as retinal detachment or dislocation of the lens may not appear until weeks after the initial injury.

Cherry PMH: Rupture of the globe. Arch Ophthalmol 88:498, 1972.
Eagling EM: Ocular damage after blunt trauma to the eye. Br J Ophthalmol 58:126, 1974.
See also Zagora reference, p 219.

REFRACTIVE ERRORS

Myopia (nearsightedness) is easily diagnosed; distant objects are blurred. Near vision is not usually impaired except in very high myopia. Frequently the patient squints his eyes in order to form a physiologic pinhole to improve visual acuity.

The diagnosis of *hyperopia* or *farsightedness* in children is more difficult. Children are able to accommodate much more effectively than adults and thus overcome their hyperopia. Sometimes there are associated symptoms of eyestrain or headaches after prolonged periods of close work. Children with severe farsightedness may have internal deviations of the eyes (esotropia).

Astigmatism produces distorted vision. Children will attempt to overcome the blurry vision by squinting their eyes and forming a pinhole. Children with severe astigmatism may complain of eyestrain and headaches.

Treatment of significant refractive errors consists of the proper fitting of lenses. Small degrees of hyperopia need not be corrected in children. Full correction of myopia is indicated. The use of bifocals in myopic children does not appear to prevent the progressive type of myopia. Other forms of treatment such as the use of cycloplegics, "eye exercises," or certain diets do not appear to influence the progression of myopia.

Contact lenses are seldom indicated in children. They have been purported to reduce the progression of myopia, but there is little evidence for this view. The exception is the child with unilateral aphakia (absence of the lens), severe anisometropia (difference of refractive errors in the 2 eyes), corneal scarring producing an irregular astigmatism, or keratoconus.

Duke-Elder S, Abrams D: *Ophthalmic Optics and Refraction.* Mosby, 1970.
Michaels DD: *Visual Optics and Refraction: A Clinical Approach.* Mosby, 1975.
Prakash P, Agarwal LP, Gupta SB: Refractive error in children. J Pediatr Ophthalmol 8:42, 1971.
Sloan AE: *Manual of Refraction,* 2nd ed. Little, Brown, 1970.

STRABISMUS
(Squint)

Approximately 5% of children have strabismus. The eyes may deviate inward (esotropia), outward (exotropia), upward (hypertropia), or downward (hypotropia). Strabismus is comitant if the same degree of deviation exists in all fields of gaze and noncomitant if the angle of deviation changes in the various directions of gaze. The terms tropia and phoria are both used to describe abnormal positions of the eye; tropias are manifest deviations, whereas phorias are latent deviations which become manifest only if fusion or binocular vision is broken up.

Strabismus is usually first observed either shortly after birth or at the age of 2—3 years; rarely, the onset is at a later age. Infants do not develop coordinated eye muscle movements until about 4—5 months of age.. An occasional infant is observed to have temporary deviation of the eyes, and realignment subsequently occurs. Any child who has a deviation that persists for several months or who develops a deviation after the age of 6 months should be investigated for the cause of the strabismus.

The diagnosis of strabismus is frequently made by simple inspection. If the eyes are deviated considerably, the diagnosis is evident. If there is only a slight deviation or if there is a questionable deviation because of wide epicanthal folds (pseudostrabismus) with more of the white of the eye being exposed temporally than nasally, the diagnosis is established by the corneal light reflection technic (Fig 9—2) or the cover test (Fig 9—3), as described above. Strabismus may also be suspected on the basis of marked reduced visual acuity in one eye. Children with head tilt may have strabismus with very little apparent displacement of the eyes.

During visual development diplopia occurs if alignment of the eyes is such that the object viewed does not fall on corresponding parts of the retina. To avoid diplopia, the child learns to suppress the vision in the deviating eye. If one eye continually deviates, then suppression is always in this eye, with the result that macular vision never develops. The term *amblyopia ex anopsia* or *suppression amblyopia* is applied to this condition. Visual screening examination of preschool children is important in diagnosing early suppression amblyopia.

Paralytic or noncomitant strabismus may result from CNS diseases or anatomic maldevelopments of the ocular muscles. The sudden onset of paralytic strabismus in any child should prompt examination for CNS disease.

Treatment

Children do not outgrow strabismus. Early treatment is important and should be given by an ophthalmologist. Treatment is directed toward the development of good visual acuity in each eye, realignment of the eyes in good cosmetic position, and functional cures with the establishment of binocular vision. The following steps are considered in the treatment of strabismus: (1) Careful ophthalmoscopic examination to rule out an organic intraocular cause for the deviation, eg, congenital cataracts, tumors, optic nerve atrophy. (2) Cycloplegic refraction and prescription of lenses. (3) Occlusion of the good eye to develop macular vision in the bad eye. (4) Surgery to align the eyes if glasses are unsuccessful in correcting the deviation.

Early surgery (ages 9—24 months) with alignment of the eyes is more likely to result in a functional cure than surgery performed at age 4—5 years or later.

Orthoptic exercises are of value in establishing binocular vision if the visual axes are nearly aligned. They are also of value in certain forms of intermittent strabismus. *Pleoptics* is a new orthoptic technic of stimulating macular vision in children with suppression amblyopia. These technics are of greatest value for children who do not respond to occlusive therapy. The value of pleoptics is not yet fully established; it appears that some children are able to develop useful macular vision with this form of therapy.

Burian HM, Von Noorden GK: *Binocular Vision and Ocular Motility: Theory and Management of Strabismus.* Mosby, 1974.

Helveston EM: Strabismus: Annual review. Arch Ophthalmol 93:1205, 1975.

Parks MM: *Ocular Motility and Strabismus.* Harper & Row, 1975.

Von Noorden GK, Maumenee AE: *Atlas of Strabismus,* 2nd ed. Mosby, 1973.

PTOSIS

Ptosis is a drooping of the upper eyelid. It may be congenital or acquired and unilateral or bilateral.

Congenital ptosis usually results from incomplete development of the levator muscle. Occasionally it is associated with third cranial nerve trauma at the time of birth, in which case other abnormalities of ocular movement are often present.

Acquired ptosis may be traumatic in origin, may follow inflammation or scarring of the eyelids, or may present as a sign of some neurologic disorder. When ptosis is a sign of myasthenia gravis, an injection of edrophonium chloride (Tensilon) will produce prompt improvement. (See Chapter 21.)

The treatment of congenital ptosis is surgical. The operation is usually performed at the age of 3—4 years. Rarely, the surgery should be done earlier if the eyelid covers the pupil completely and prevents development of normal vision. The treatment of acquired ptosis depends upon the origin, but primary consideration should be directed toward treating any basic underlying disease.

Beard C: *Ptosis,* 2nd ed. Mosby, 1976.

GLAUCOMA

Primary Glaucoma

Primary congenital glaucoma (hydrophthalmos) is due to an abnormal development of the aqueous drainage structures; it may be present at birth or may develop within the first 2 years of life. Diagnosis is based upon (1) enlarged corneas that are frequently edematous and show linear white opacities (breaks in Descemet's membrane), (2) symptoms of photophobia and tearing, and (3) increased intraocular pressure. Since the coats of the eye of an infant are not so rigid as those of an adult, increased intraocular pressure results in stretching of the corneal and scleral tissues.

Early surgery is essential. Medical therapy is of little value. Surgery is successful in controlling intraocular pressure in about 75% of cases. Without treatment, permanent blindness occurs at an early age.

Glaucoma may be associated with other developmental anomalies. These include aniridia, posterior embryotoxon (failure of reabsorption of the mesodermal tissue in the periphery of the iris and drainage angle), Sturge-Weber disease, Lowe's syndrome, Marfan's syndrome, Hurler's syndrome, neurofibromatosis, homocystinuria, and congenital rubella syndrome.

Secondary Glaucoma

Secondary glaucoma may be due to many causes. The mechanism of this type of glaucoma is usually an obstruction of the aqueous outflow channels. The various causes include lens dislocation, hemorrhage into the eye, iritis, tumors (including retinoblastoma), retrolental fibroplasia, and xanthogranulomas in the iris. Treatment of these conditions is complicated, and the patient should be referred to an ophthalmologist.

Kolker AE, Hetherington J Jr: *Becker-Shaffer's Diagnosis and Therapy of the Glaucomas,* 4th ed. Mosby, 1976.
Kwitko ML: *Glaucoma in Infants and Children.* Appleton-Century-Crofts, 1973.
New Orleans Academy of Ophthalmology: *Symposium on Glaucoma.* Mosby, 1975.
Shaffer RN, Weiss DI: *Congenital and Pediatric Glaucomas.* Mosby, 1970.

CATARACTS

A cataract is an opacity of the lens; it consists of precipitated lens protein. Cataracts may be unilateral or bilateral and partial or complete; considerable variation exists in the extent, position, shape, and density of cataract formation. They may be congenital and associated with other congenital anomalies. They can occur as a result of maternal rubella during the first trimester of pregnancy. Cataracts may be secondary to ocular trauma, or associated with systemic diseases such as diabetes mellitus, galactosemia, atopic dermatitis, Marfan's syndrome, or Down's syndrome. They may also be due to long-term systemic corticosteroid therapy.

The symptoms vary considerably according to location and extent. Vision may be affected very slightly, or considerable reduction in vision can occur. White spots may be observed in the pupil. In a few cases, strabismus or pendular nystagmus is present.

The diagnosis is made by inspection with a flashlight or by examination with an ophthalmoscope or slit lamp. In some cases cataracts can be observed only when the pupils are dilated.

Surgical lens extraction (before age 6 months) is indicated if the cataracts are bilateral and sufficiently dense that vision cannot develop. If cataracts are not dense enough to interfere with visual development, surgery should be deferred since some congenital cataracts do not progress. Surgery is indicated when visual loss is a serious handicap to the child.

Jaffe NS: *Cataract Surgery and Its Complications,* 2nd ed. Mosby, 1976.
Kirsch RE: The lens: Annual review. Arch Ophthalmol 93:284, 1975.
Scheie HG, Rubinstein RA, Kent RB: Aspiration of congenital or soft cataracts: Further experience. Am J Ophthalmol 63:3, 1967.
Sheppard RW, Crawford JS: The treatment of congenital cataracts. Surv Ophthalmol 17:340, 1973.
Weiss DI, Ziring PR, Cooper LZ: Surgery of the rubella cataract. Am J Ophthalmol 73:326, 1972.

DISEASES OF THE EYELIDS

HORDEOLUM

External hordeolum (sty) is a staphylococcal abscess of the sebaceous glands of the lid margin. Symptoms consist of localized tenderness, redness, and swelling. Internal hordeolum is an acute infection of the meibomian glands that usually points conjunctivally.

Treatment of both types consists of warm moist compresses 3–4 times a day. Instillation of an antibiotic or sulfonamide ophthalmic ointment 4–5 times a day is useful during the acute stage. Treatment should be continued for several days after the lesion has subsided in order to reduce the likelihood of a recurrence.

Spontaneous rupture frequently occurs, but if it does not the lesion should be incised when it becomes large and pointed. The removal of an eyelash will promote drainage of an external hordeolum.

Locatcher-Khorazo D, Seegal BC: *Microbiology of the Eye.* Mosby, 1972.
Vaughan D, Asbury T: *General Ophthalmology,* 8th ed. Lange, 1977.

CHALAZION

Chalazion is a granulomatous inflammation of the meibomian glands. The cause is not known. Symptoms consist of slight discomfort in the eyelid and a slight redness and a lump on the conjunctival surface of the lid overlying the involved meibomian gland. Local excision is usually necessary, but chalazions do occasionally disappear after treatment with warm moist compresses.

See Vaughan & Asbury reference, p 223.

BLEPHARITIS
(Granulated Eyelids)

Chronic inflammation of the lid margins may be seborrheic (nonulcerative), staphylococcal (ulcerative), or a combination of the 2 types. Symptoms are redness, burning, itching, and crusting of the lid margins. In the staphylococcal type the scales are dry; small ulcerative lesions of the skin are observed; and the eyelashes may fall out. In the seborrheic type the scales are oily; seborrhea of the scalp is usually present as well.

Treatment of staphylococcal blepharitis consists of the instillation of antibiotic or sulfonamide ophthalmic ointment into the eye twice a day. Treatment should be continued for a week or so after all symptoms have disappeared. The crusts on the lids should be gently removed with a moist cotton applicator before the ointment is instilled. The treatment of seborrheic blepharitis consists of controlling scalp seborrhea if it exists, removing the scales along the lid margins with a moist cotton applicator, and instilling sulfacetamide or an antistaphylococcal antibiotic ophthalmic ointment.

Other useful treatments are the careful application of 2.5% ammoniated mercury ointment, 1% silver nitrate solution, or 0.5% selenium sulfide (Selsun) ointment to the lid margins.

Scheie HG, Albert DM: *Textbook of Ophthalmology,* 9th ed. Saunders, 1977.
Thygeson P: Complications of staphylococcic blepharitis. Am J Ophthalmol 68:446, 1969.
See also Locatcher-Khorazo & Seegal reference, p 223.

DISEASES OF THE CONJUNCTIVA

CONJUNCTIVITIS

Conjunctivitis is the most common of all pediatric ocular disorders. It is usually due to bacterial, viral, or fungal infections. Less commonly it may result from an allergic reaction or physical or chemical irritation. Symptoms consist of redness of the conjunctiva, foreign body sensation, a mucoid or purulent discharge, and sticking together of the eyelids in the morning. Vision is not affected. The cornea, anterior chamber, and intraocular pressure are normal.

Bacterial Conjunctivitis

The most common causes of bacterial conjunctivitis are the pneumococcus, *Staphylococcus aureus,* Koch-Weeks bacillus, and hemolytic streptococci. There may be associated bacterial infections elsewhere in the body. Conjunctival membranes (diphtheritic conjunctivitis) or pseudomembranes (streptococcal conjunctivitis) may be present. Discharge, usually a prominent feature of bacterial conjunctivitis, is purulent or mucopurulent in character.

The causative organism should be identified, if possible, by obtaining smears and cultures. Empirical treatment with broad spectrum antibiotics or sulfonamide ophthalmic ointments instilled into the eye 4–5 times a day usually results in improvement within 48–72 hours. If improvement does not occur, it is important to make an etiologic diagnosis if this has not been done earlier. Bacterial conjunctivitis is usually a self-limited disease, but secondary corneal infection and ulceration occur rarely.

Inclusion Conjunctivitis (Swimming Pool Conjunctivitis)

This disease is due to the same organism that produces inclusion conjunctivitis in the newborn. It is characterized by conjunctival redness, clear or mucoid discharge, and follicles in the lower palpebral conjunctiva. Treatment consists of the local application of sulfonamide or tetracycline 4–5 times a day.

Trachoma

Trachoma is infection of the conjunctiva with a bacterium formerly thought to be a large atypical virus but now reclassified as a bacterium of the genus Chlamydia. The disease is usually associated with poor hygiene and poor economic conditions. It is a major cause of blindness in the world but is rare in the USA except among American Indians.

In the early stages, trachoma is characterized by a catarrhal type of reaction with diffuse redness, mild irritation, and a thin watery discharge. Subsequently the conjunctiva becomes thickened, with papillary hypertrophy and formation of follicles, particularly in the tarsal region of the upper lids. Scarring of the conjunctiva develops later, and there is corneal vascularization and opacification.

Local therapy can probably control trachoma adequately, but systemic therapy is usually recommended also. Systemic sulfonamides and tetracyclines are the agents most commonly used. For children over 9 years of age in whom dentition is complete, a 21-day course of oral tetracycline is given. Doxycycline is preferred since administration is required only once a day. The drug of choice is sulfisoxazole (Gantrisin), administered by mouth in a dose of 100 mg/kg body weight daily in 4 divided doses for 1 week, followed by 60 mg/kg body weight for an additional 2 weeks. It is sometimes necessary to repeat this treatment after 1 week without medication. The local treatment of choice is 1% tetracycline ointment applied twice a day, 6 days a week for 10 weeks. Since recurrences are common, follow-up evaluation is important.

Viral Conjunctivitis

Viral conjunctivitis is frequently due to infection with one of the adenoviruses and may be associated with pharyngitis and preauricular adenopathy. The conjunctiva is quite hyperemic and shows follicular reaction. There is a thin watery discharge. The condition usually lasts 12–14 days. No treatment is of value. Sulfonamide preparations or broad spectrum antibiotics are instilled locally to prevent secondary infection.

Vaccinial Conjunctivitis

This form of conjunctivitis usually results from auto-inoculation from a recent smallpox vaccination site. Treatment consists of the use of 0.5% idoxuridine (IDU) ophthalmic ointment (Stoxil) instilled into the eye 4 times a day. Vaccinia immune globulin (VIG), 0.3 ml/lb body weight, IM, may be given to ameliorate a severe reaction. No more than 5 ml of this serum should be given in one site. If no response occurs within 48 hours, VIG treatment should be repeated.

Leptothrix Conjunctivitis

Leptothrix conjunctivitis is characterized by small gray necrotic lesions on the palpebral conjunctiva. There is usually a history of contact with a cat. The course is protracted. Improvement may follow local excision of the necrotic areas.

Actinomyces Infections

Actinomyces species may produce conjunctivitis. The conjunctivitis is usually on the nasal side of the conjunctiva, and is frequently associated with inflammation of the lacrimal canaliculi. The organisms are susceptible to penicillin and broad spectrum antibiotics. If an infection exists in the canaliculi, this must be cleared before cure can result.

Allergic Conjunctivitis

Allergic conjunctivitis produces symptoms of itching, lacrimation, mild redness, and a stringy mucoid discharge. Eosinophils may be seen on scrapings from the conjunctiva. For acute cases of conjunctivitis, local 1.5% hydrocortisone ophthalmic ointment or its equivalent instilled into the eye 3–4 times a day is quite effective. For chronic forms of allergic conjunctivitis, an attempt should be made to isolate the offending allergen and to eliminate contact with it. Desensitization to the allergen can be carried out if elimination of contact is not possible. Temporary symptomatic relief may be obtained with the use of topical ophthalmic solutions containing vasoconstricting agents and antihistamines.

Phlyctenular Keratoconjunctivitis

Phlyctenular keratoconjunctivitis appears as elevated clear nodules, situated near the limbus, with surrounding hyperemia. The disease has been associated with a hypersensitivity reaction to tuberculin; phlyctenules may also develop as a hypersensitivity reaction to other bacterial products or other antigens.

Treatment consists of the local application of corticosteroids. Systemic tuberculosis should be ruled out.

Vernal Conjunctivitis

This form of conjunctivitis is seen in patients ages 5–20. It tends to be seasonal and becomes less severe with age. Symptoms consist of lacrimation, itching, stringy discharge, and giant "cobblestone" papillary hypertrophy in the tarsal conjunctiva or grayish elevated areas at the limbus. Many eosinophils are seen in the scraping of the lesions.

Treatment consists of the local application of corticosteroid ointment several times a day. Severe cases may require more extensive therapy, but this should be conducted by an ophthalmologist.

Ophthalmia Neonatorum

Ophthalmia neonatorum is inflammation of the conjunctiva of the newborn. It may be due to bacterial infection (gonococcal, staphylococcal, pneumococcal, or chlamydial [inclusion blennorrhea]) or to chemical irritation (silver nitrate). Bacterial conjunctivitis appears 2–5 days after birth; inclusion conjunctivitis appears 5–10 days after birth. Conjunctivitis associated with silver nitrate usually is evident within the first 24–48 hours after birth. A definite diagnosis is established by smears and cultures of the material taken from the conjunctiva. Conjunctivitis due to silver nitrate is sterile, although secondary bacterial infections may occur.

In most states in the USA, chemical (1% silver nitrate) or antibiotic prophylaxis of the newborn eye is required. These laws are highly variable in the different states. Various antibiotics such as penicillin, tetracyclines, or bacitracin are currently used for prophylaxis of gonococcal ophthalmia.

It is most important to treat gonococcal conjunctivitis vigorously, since in untreated or inadequately treated cases corneal ulceration and perforation can occur. The treatment of gonococcal conjunctivitis consists of topical application of either penicillin, erythromycin, or tetracycline drops into the eye every 2 hours and penicillin G, 30,000 units/kg of body weight daily IM, or systemic tetracycline therapy. If one eye is uninvolved, it should be covered with a shield to prevent contamination from the involved eye. The purulent discharge should be irrigated from the conjunctiva with normal saline and allowed to drain toward the outer edge of the eyelids away from the other eye. Cold compresses may be of value in relieving the marked swelling of the eyelids.

Other types of bacterial conjunctivitis of the newborn should be treated by the instillation of appropriate antibiotic ointments 4 times a day. Inclusion blen-

norrhea is treated by the local instillation of sulfacetamide or tetracycline ointment 4 times a day.

In all cases of conjunctivitis, treatment should be
continued for a few days after the symptoms have subsided to prevent early recurrences.

Dawson CR: Lids, conjunctiva and lacrimal apparatus: Eye in-
    fections with Chlamydia. Annual review. Arch Ophthal-
    mol 93:854, 1975.
Golden B (editor): *Ocular Inflammatory Disease.* Thomas,
    1974.
Mordhorst CH, Dawson C: Sequelae of neonatal inclusion con-
    junctivitis and associated disease in parents. Am J Oph-
    thalmol 71:861, 1971.
Thompson TR, Swanson RE, Wiesner PJ: Gonococcal ophthal-
    mia neonatorum. JAMA 228:186, 1974.
Thygeson P, Dawson CR: Trachoma and follicular conjunctivitis
    in children. Arch Ophthalmol 75:3, 1966.
See also Locatcher-Khorazo & Seegal and Scheie & Albert refer-
    ences, p 223 and 224.

MUCOCUTANEOUS DISEASES

Conjunctival lesions may be associated with
mucocutaneous diseases, including erythema multiforme, Stevens-Johnson syndrome, Reiter's syndrome,
and Behçet's syndrome. The conjunctival involvement
consists of erythema, vesicular lesions which frequently rupture, membrane formation, and the development
of symblepharon (adhesions) between the raw edges of
the bulbar and palpebral conjunctiva. Goblet cells in
the conjunctiva are destroyed in the cicatricial process.
This decreases the mucus secretion which is essential
for the spread of tears over the cornea. Keratitis sicca
(corneal drying) may result.

Treatment of the conjunctival lesions associated
with these conditions is symptomatic, ie, soothing eye
drops and compresses. Topical steroids are helpful in
the acute stages in diminishing the intensity and complications of the acute inflammatory phase. Antibiotics
are of no benefit except for prevention of secondary
infection. Erythema multiforme and Stevens-Johnson
disease may be precipitated by sulfonamide and antibiotic therapy. Topical antibiotic therapy may be used
when secondary bacterial infection occurs; care must
be taken to choose an antibiotic to which the patient is
not sensitive. The use of topical lubricants and the
application of soft contact lenses may prevent corneal
drying and ulceration.

Arstikaitis MJ: Ocular aftermath of Stevens-Johnson syndrome.
    Arch Ophthalmol 90:376, 1973.
Grayson M, Keates RH: *Manual of Diseases of the Cornea.*
    Little, Brown, 1969.
Sampson WG & others: Symposium on soft contact lenses.
    Trans Am Acad Ophthalmol Otolaryngol 78:383, 1974.
See also Golden and Scheie & Albert references, above.

DISEASES OF THE CORNEA

CORNEAL ULCERS

Corneal ulcers are serious ocular disorders. They
may follow corneal injury or conjunctivitis or may be
associated with systemic infections. Corneal ulcers are
usually diagnosed by simple inspection. There is loss of
anterior substance of the cornea with surrounding
opaque gray or white necrosis. Corneal ulcers may be
peripheral or central. Several ulcers may be present in
the same eye. The area of ulceration stains with fluorescein. A serious effort should be made to determine
the etiology of any corneal ulcer. Cultures and scrapings should be taken, and if bacterial organisms are
found sensitivity tests should be performed.

Bacterial Corneal Ulcers

Central bacterial corneal ulcers are due to infections with pneumococci, hemolytic streptococci, *Pseudomonas aeruginosa,* and, less commonly, gram-
positive and gram-negative rods. Marginal corneal
ulcers may develop as a result of bacterial sensitivity,
most commonly to staphylococcal infections.

Treatment should be started immediately, before
sensitivity tests are completed. Subsequently, the antibiotic can be changed if necessary. For mild superficial
bacterial ulcers, the topical use of antibiotic drops or
ointment at frequent intervals is usually satisfactory.
Until the susceptibility of the organism is known, it is
well to start the patient on an ophthalmic antibiotic
preparation which includes neomycin, bacitracin, and
polymyxin B, or else a broad spectrum antibiotic.
Cycloplegic drops should be used to relieve the iridocyclitis that accompanies bacterial ulcers. In more
severe corneal ulcers which involve the deeper portions
of the stroma, more intensive antibiotic therapy should
be given. Antibiotics should also be given subconjunc-
tivally and systemically. Corticosteroids should not be
given topically, since they interfere with the healing
process and might exaggerate an infection that was not
susceptible to the treatment being used.

Marginal corneal ulcers respond to topical steroids. If a staphylococcal infection of the conjunctiva
or eyelids is present, it should be treated with appropriate antibiotics.

Viral Corneal Ulcers

A. Herpes Simplex Ulcer (Dendritic): Herpes
simplex keratitis is becoming a more common corneal
disease in children. Lesions in the cornea may or may
not be associated with herpes labialis. Corneal involvement is frequently precipitated by the topical application of corticosteroids and less commonly with the
systemic use of corticosteroids. In the initial infection
the lesion has the appearance of a dendrite (Fig 9–4).
There are one or more branching vesicular lesions
involving the anterior part of the cornea. These vesicles

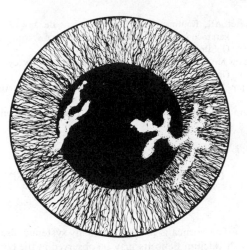

Figure 9–4. Dendritic type of lesion seen in herpes simplex keratitis. (Reproduced, with permission, from Vaughan D, Asbury T: *General Ophthalmology*, 8th ed. Lange, 1977.)

rupture. Subsequently, deeper involvement of the cornea may occur. Iritis may also develop as a complication.

Treatment of acute herpes infections of the cornea consists of the topical application of idoxuridine (IDU) applied as an 0.5% ointment (Stoxil) 4 times a day, or as an 0.1% solution (Herplex, Stoxil) hourly during the day and every 2 hours at night. The eye is usually more comfortable if the pupil is kept dilated with 1% atropine or 5% homatropine. Mechanical denuding of the corneal epithelium is also an effective method of treating fresh cases of superficial herpes simplex keratitis. This should be performed by an ophthalmologist. Deeper involvement of the cornea may represent a hypersensitivity reaction, and the use of topical corticosteroids in conjunction with IDU sometimes improves the condition. However, this type of therapy should be undertaken only by an ophthalmologist, since the use of corticosteroids in an active herpes infection can lead to rapid deterioration of the cornea. The topical application of vidarabine (Vira-A) in 3% ointment several times a day is frequently effective in controlling herpes simplex keratitis in patients in whom topical idoxuridine is unsuccessful.

B. Vaccinial Infection: Vaccinial keratitis is usually secondary to auto-inoculation from the site of a recent vaccination. It may also occur as a result of vaccine being splashed into the eye. The treatment of choice is the application of idoxuridine drops or ointments. Drops are employed in 0.1% concentration (Herplex, Stoxil) every hour during the day and every 2 hours at night. Ointment is applied in 0.5% concentration (Stoxil) 4 times a day. Vidarabine, applied as 3% ointment (Vira-A) 4 times a day, is also effective.

C. Herpes Zoster Infection: Herpes zoster keratitis is associated with zoster infection of the first branch of the trigeminal nerve. The involvement of the cornea is usually deep. Relief is obtained with the use of topical corticosteroids. Cycloplegic drops should be used for relieving the iridocyclitis which accompanies herpes zoster infection. The physician must be certain of the diagnosis of herpes zoster before employing topical corticosteroids, since other viral diseases of the cornea are aggravated by these agents.

Fungal Corneal Ulcers

Mycotic corneal infections are difficult to diagnose. Usually there is a history of recent trauma or foreign body. Frequently the ulcerated cornea shows surrounding satellite lesions; hypopyon (pus in the anterior chamber) may be present. Fungal corneal ulcers are rare, but their incidence seems to be increasing, possibly from the widespread use of topical corticosteroid and broad spectrum antibiotic medications. Whenever a diagnosis of mycotic corneal ulceration is suspected, cultures and sensitivity tests should be obtained.

Until recently, the only effective topical agents for the treatment of fungal keratitis were nystatin (Mycostatin) and amphotericin B (Fungizone). The nystatin drops are effective against most strains of candida and are employed in a concentration of 100,000 units/ml. Amphotericin B ophthalmic drops are effective against candida and several other fungi; they have been used in concentrations varying from 1.5–5 mg/ml. A more promising drug for topical use is pimaricin, which will soon be commercially available; it is effective as a 5% suspension or 1% ointment against a wide range of fungi. All of the drugs mentioned above should be instilled into the eye at frequent intervals. All of these drugs fail to penetrate the deeper structures of the cornea and anterior chamber and are mainly effective against superficial fungal corneal ulcers. For deep fungal infections of the cornea, it may be necessary to employ subconjunctival or systemic amphotericin B or systemic flucytosine.

DeVoe A: Corneal disorders in children. In: *Symposium on the Cornea*. New Orleans Academy of Ophthalmology. Mosby, 1972.

Hyndiuk R & others: Adenosine arabinoside in idoxuridine unresponsive and intolerant herpetic keratitis. Am J Ophthalmol 79:655, 1975.

Jones BR: Principles in the management of oculomycosis. Am J Ophthalmol 79:719, 1975.

O'Day DM & others: Vidarabine therapy of complicated herpes simplex keratitis. Am J Ophthalmol 81:642, 1976.

Pavan-Langston D, Buchanan RA, Alford CA Jr (editors): *Adenine Arabinoside: An Antiviral Agent.* Raven, 1975.

Wellings PC & others: Clinical evaluation of trifluorothymidine in the treatment of herpes simplex corneal ulcers. Am J Ophthalmol 73:932, 1972.

Wood TO, Williford W: Treatment of keratomycosis with amphotericin B 0.15%. Am J Ophthalmol 81:847, 1976.

ALLERGIC REACTIONS

Allergic reactions in the cornea may involve either the superficial epithelial or deeper stromal layers. Most forms of deep keratitis probably represent hypersensitivity reactions. The allergen may be airborne, or it may enter the cornea by way of the circulation in the limbus. Treatment consists of determining the offending agent, if possible, and then eliminating its contact with the patient. Topical corticosteroids usually give considerable relief.

Interstitial Keratitis

Interstitial keratitis is an acute immune reaction in the cornea usually associated with congenital syphilis. Symptoms consist of intense photophobia, tearing, pain, and decreased vision. On examination the cornea has a diffuse opaque appearance. Fine vessels may be noted in the stroma. There may be aggregates of these vessels which appear as orange-red areas (salmon patches). Other evidence of congenital syphilis may also be present. Serologic tests are often negative.

Interstitial keratitis may be associated with other diseases such as tuberculosis and the autoimmune disorders, and any such contributing condition should be ruled out.

Treatment consists of the use of topical steroids and cycloplegics for relief of symptoms. If active syphilis is present, it should be appropriately treated.

Aronson SB, Elliott JH: *Ocular Inflammation.* Mosby, 1972.
Schwartz B (editor): *Syphilis and the Eye.* Williams & Wilkins, 1970.
Thygeson P: The immunology and immunopathology of corneal infection. Trans Pac Coast Otoophthalmol Soc 57:357, 1976.
Waring GO & others: Alterations in Descemet's membrane in interstitial keratitis. Am J Ophthalmol 81:773, 1976.
See also Grayson & Keates reference, p 226.

CORNEAL DRYING & EXPOSURE

Keratoconjunctivitis Sicca

This rare condition results from a lacrimal gland insufficiency. The treatment of choice is tear replacement with artificial tears (eg, methylcellulose), 0.5–1% solution as necessary to keep the cornea moist.

Exposure Keratitis

Exposure keratitis may develop after facial nerve palsies or after a period of unconsciousness during which the eyes are exposed. Treatment is similar to that described above.

Neuroparalytic Keratitis

Neuroparalytic keratitis is seen after damage to the ophthalmic division of the trigeminal nerve. It is treated by tear replacement (see Keratoconjunctivitis Sicca, above).

Familial Dysautonomia (Riley-Day Syndrome)

In this condition there is a deficiency of tears, and corneal drying can occur. Tear replacement (see Keratoconjunctivitis Sicca, above) is indicated.

Gasset AR, Kaufman HE: Hydrophilic lens therapy of severe keratoconjunctivitis sicca and conjunctival scarring. Am J Ophthalmol 71:1185, 1971.
Lemp MA: Tear substitutes in the treatment of dry eyes. Int Ophthalmol Clin 13:145, 1973.
Lemp MA, Holly FJ: Ophthalmic polymers as ocular wetting agents. Ann Ophthalmol 4:15, 1972.
Norn MS: *External Eye: Methods of Examination.* Scriptor, 1974.

CORNEAL INVOLVEMENT IN OTHER SYSTEMIC DISEASES

The cornea is involved in many systemic diseases. Small calcium deposits may be observed in the corneas of patients with hyperparathyroidism. Cystine crystals are observed in patients with renal rickets (cystinosis). Excessive intake of vitamin D may lead to calcification of the anterior part of the cornea in a band opacity of the exposed portion of the cornea. Deficiency of vitamin A may lead to drying (xerosis) and softening (keratomalacia) of the cornea. Corneal ulceration may occur in patients with severe debilitating diseases such as dysentery. Corneal opacities may occur in children with Hurler's disease (gargoylism).

In all of these conditions it is important to recognize the underlying disease and treat appropriately.

Poirier RH, Hyndiuk RA: Diagnosis and therapy of corneal disease. In: *Gordon's Management of Ocular Disease,* 2nd ed. Dunlap EA (editor). Harper & Row, 1976.
Zimmerman TJ, Hood I, Gasset AR: Adolescent cystinosis. Arch Ophthalmol 92:265, 1974.
See also Grayson & Keates reference, p 226.

UVEITIS

Inflammation of the uveal tract may present anteriorly as iritis or cyclitis (inflammation of the ciliary body), or as posterior inflammations (choroiditis). Uveitis may be associated with other ocular diseases, such as corneal ulceration, keratitis, hypermature cataracts, necrotic intraocular tumors, or optic neuritis.

Uveitis may be classified as exogenous or endogenous. Exogenous uveitis follows the accidental introduction of pathogenic organisms or a foreign substance into the eye. Endogenous uveitis is a result of various systemic processes.

Uveitis may also be classified as suppurative or nonsuppurative according to the type of tissue reaction. Nonsuppurative uveitis, which is the more common form, may further be divided into granulomatous and nongranulomatous types. Nongranulomatous uveitis usually involves the iris and ciliary body and produces symptoms of photophobia, pain, redness, and blurred vision. The pupil is small and often irregular. There is circumcorneal injection. On examination with a slit lamp, cells in the anterior chamber and fine precipitates on the posterior surface of the cornea may be observed. Granulomatous uveitis may involve the iris, ciliary body, or choroid. Pain, redness, and photophobia are not ₅o prominent as in the nongranulomatous form. Vision may be markedly disturbed, particularly if the involvement is in the macular area. On ophthalmoscopy the vitreous may be quite hazy. Active lesions of choroiditis may be seen as swollen, white, indistinct irregular patches. As the choroiditis subsides, pigmentary changes may take place.

Uveitis presents a complex problem. The endogenous nonsuppurative form may be associated with systemic disease. Among the more common associated diseases are toxoplasmosis, histoplasmosis, tuberculosis; sarcoidosis, polyarteritis, rheumatoid arthritis, and other collagen diseases; bacterial infections of the sinuses or teeth; food and pollen allergies; and viral diseases such as mumps, measles, chickenpox, influenza, herpes simplex, and herpes zoster. The relationship between systemic disease and uveitis may be incidental. There is pathologic evidence that the choroid and retina may be invaded with toxoplasma and *Mycobacterium tuberculosis.* However, aside from these specific instances, causative organisms have not been found to enter the uveal tissue. There is accumulating evidence that most cases of uveitis are due to an immune reaction.

Treatment

If systemic disease is present, it should be appropriately treated. However, successful treatment of systemic disease does not always result in a cure of the uveitis. Nonspecific treatment of uveitis consists of the use of cycloplegics to dilate the pupil and to relieve the ciliary and iris spasm. Atropine, 1–2% solution, or scopolamine, 0.25% solution, should be used 2–3 times daily. In addition, the topical use of 10% phenylephrine hydrochloride is indicated to widely dilate the pupil. Corticosteroids should be used unless they are contraindicated by the presence of a specific bacterial or viral infection. For inflammations of the anterior uveal tract, topical and subconjunctival corticosteroids are useful in reducing the inflammation. For posterior uveitis, systemic corticosteroids should be used.

The management of uveitis is difficult. Many complications can occur, including glaucoma, cataract, and retinal detachment. Therefore, these cases should be managed by an ophthalmologist.

Mazow ML: Diagnosis and management of uveitis and complications in children. J Pediatr Ophthalmol 10:167, 1973.
O'Connor GR: The uvea: Annual review. Arch Ophthalmol 93:675, 1975.
Schlaegel TF: *Essentials of Uveitis.* Little, Brown, 1969.
Smith RE, Godfrey WA, Kimura SJ: Complications of chronic cyclitis. Am J Ophthalmol 82:277, 1976.

SYMPATHETIC OPHTHALMIA

Sympathetic ophthalmia is a special form of bilateral granulomatous uveitis. It follows a penetrating ocular injury of the uveal tract. It may occur at any time from 10 days after injury to many years later, but it usually presents within the first 2–4 months after initial injury. The etiology of sympathetic ophthalmia is not understood, but it probably represents a hypersensitivity response to uveal pigment. The diagnosis is based on a history of an injury to one (exciting) eye with the subsequent development of uveitis in the other (sympathizing) eye.

Treatment consists of the use of systemic and topical corticosteroids and topical cycloplegics. Long-term therapy is usually necessary, and maintenance doses of steroids are usually indicated to prevent a flare-up of this condition. The disease can be averted by early enucleation of the exciting eye, which has received a severe injury to the ciliary body and which has become visually useless.

See Schlaegel reference, above.

DISEASES OF THE RETINA

RETROLENTAL FIBROPLASIA (RLF)
(Retinopathy of Prematurity)

Retrolental fibroplasia is a primary bilateral retinal vascular disorder of premature infants. The disease occurs almost exclusively in prematures with a birth weight under 1500 gm who have received excessive amounts of oxygen therapy during the first 10–14 days of life. For several years, after the role of oxygen in the development of retrolental fibroplasia was established, the disease became almost extinct. Recently, therapy employing high concentrations of oxygen to treat respiratory distress syndrome in prematures has again been used and, possibly as a result, retrolental fibroplasia is being seen with increasing frequency.

In general, peripheral vascularization of the retina is not complete until about 2 weeks after full-term birth. However, this is variable; some eyes have complete vascularization at 8 months' gestational age. Until retinal vascularization is complete, the peripheral immature vessels, which are immediately posterior to the demarcation site of vascular to avascular retina, are extremely sensitive to hyperoxia and respond by vasoconstriction and obliteration. When oxygen concentrations are subsequently reduced, the retinal vessels in the posterior pole often dilate as a result of peripheral vascular shunts formed near the site of vaso-obliteration. These shunts may take the form of neofibrovascular membranes on the surface of the retina or may extend into the vitreous cavity. Tractional retinal detachments may occur. In advanced stages, the retrolental space is filled with fibrovascular and retinal tissues, the anterior chambers are shallow, and the eyes are small and blind. In incomplete forms, myopia and strabismus are often observed; retinal detachment may occur as a late complication in the teenage years. Up to 85% of acute cases of retrolental fibroplasia regress as vascularization to the peripheral aspect of the retina is completed in a near normal manner.

It is essential that pediatricians be aware of the relationship of oxygen therapy to the development of retrolental fibroplasia—not only the concentration of oxygen but also the duration of oxygen treatment and the degree of prematurity. The generally accepted safe concentration of oxygen is less than 40%, but this is subject to the other variables noted above. Many experts believe an arterial blood oxygen level over 70 mm Hg is inadvisable.

All premature infants receiving high concentrations of oxygen therapy should be followed as closely as possible to make certain that arterial blood oxygen levels do not remain excessively high for any period of time. Changes in the immature retinal vessels appear to be related not only to high arterial blood oxygen levels but also to the duration of exposure of hyperoxia. All prematures should have a careful ophthalmoscopic examination prior to discharge. If signs of retrolental fibroplasia are found, a follow-up ophthalmoscopic examination is needed after discharge and the parents should be counseled.

Flynn JT & others: Retrolental fibroplasia: Clinical observations. Arch Ophthalmol 95:217, 1977.

Kingham JD: Acute retrolental fibroplasia. Arch Ophthalmol 95:39, 1977.

Kushner BJ & others: Retrolental fibroplasia: Pathologic correlation. Arch Ophthalmol 95:29, 1977.

Patz A: Oxygen administration in the premature infant: A two-edged sword. Am J Ophthalmol 63:351, 1967.

Patz A: Retrolental fibroplasia. Surv Ophthalmol 14:1, 1969.

Ryan SJ Jr, Smith RE (editors): Selected Topics on the Eye in Systemic Disease. Grune & Stratton, 1974.

RETINAL DETACHMENT

Detachment of the retina in children is usually associated with severe ocular trauma or with high myopia. In the latter condition there are degenerative changes in the periphery of the retina which lead to subsequent separation of the retina. The diagnosis is established by a history of progressively more severe blurred vision. The visual disturbance may start with the sensation of flashing lights, or the patient may observe a dark cloud coming in from one section of the visual field. On ophthalmoscopy the area of detachment appears elevated and gray. The retinal vessels appear darker, and the retina is seen with increased convex dioptric power in the ophthalmoscope.

The only treatment is surgical repair.

Arentsen JJ, Welch RB: Retinal detachment in the young individual: A survey of 100 cases seen at the Wilmer Institute. J Pediatr Ophthalmol 11:198, 1974.

Tasman W (editor): Retinal Diseases in Children. Harper, 1971.

Tasman W: The retina and optic nerve: Annual review. Arch Ophthalmol 94:1201, 1976.

RETINOBLASTOMA

Retinoblastoma is a comparatively rare malignant tumor of children. It usually appears before the third year of life, although rare cases have been reported with onset in adolescence. Retinoblastoma is a hereditary disease due to mutation of an autosomal dominant gene. Patients who have survived retinoblastoma have about a 50% chance of transmitting retinoblastoma to their offspring. Approximately 25% of cases are bilateral.

The presenting symptom is usually a white spot in the pupil. Strabismus may be present. If the tumor becomes very large, glaucoma may occur, with a steamy cornea and red eye. Occasionally retinoblastoma ruptures through the globe and results in a painful red eye. The diagnosis is usually made by ophthalmoscopic examination. To accomplish ophthalmoscopy, wide pupillary dilatation is essential; general anesthesia is often necessary. The tumor appears as a solid yellow or white elevated mass. A small section of the eye may be involved, or the entire eye may be filled with tumor.

Treatment consists of enucleation of the involved eye in unilateral cases, although in selected cases small tumors are sometimes treated with x-ray or cryotherapy. If there is involvement of both eyes, the more severely involved eye should be enucleated and the other eye treated with x-ray therapy together with chemotherapy. Cryotherapy is sometimes employed for treatment of small peripheral lesions.

Since cases of retinoblastoma follow a strong hereditary pattern, parents of an affected child should be advised that other children might also suffer from this disease.

Bedford MA, Bedotto C, MacFaul PA: Retinoblastoma: A study of 139 cases. Br J Ophthalmol 55:19, 1971.

Henderson JW: Orbital Tumors. Saunders, 1973.

Hyman GA & others: Combination therapy in retinoblastoma. Arch Ophthalmol 80:744, 1968.

Nussbaum R, Puck J: Recurrence risks for retinoblastoma: A model for autosomal dominant disorders with complex inheritance. J Pediatr Ophthalmol 13:89, 1976.

Ramirez LD, de Buen S: Clinical and pathologic findings in 100 retinoblastoma patients. J Pediatr Ophthalmol 10:12, 1973.

Reese AB: Tumors of the Eye, 3rd ed. Harper & Row, 1976.

OPTIC NEURITIS

Optic neuritis may involve only the head of the nerve (papillitis) or the orbital portion of the nerve (retrobulbar neuritis). Optic neuritis may occur in association with generalized infectious diseases, demyelinating diseases, blood dyscrasias, or metabolic diseases, or may be due to exposure to toxins or drugs or extension of inflammatory disease such as sinusitis or meningitis. Clinically, there is an acute loss of vision. Involvement may be of one or both eyes; in children the disease is frequently bilateral. Central visual defects are present. There may be some discomfort in the eyes on movement of the globes. On ophthalmoscopic examination, papilledema may be present or the disks may appear normal.

Optic neuritis in children is usually a self-limited disease, and the visual prognosis is generally favorable. If the cause can be determined, it should be treated. Systemic corticosteroid therapy has been advocated, but its effectiveness has not been established.

The presence of papilledema may be a sign of increased intracranial pressure. The differentiation between optic neuritis and papilledema secondary to increased intracranial pressure is not always easy. In general, papilledema due to increased intracranial pressure does not produce a severe loss of vision, and there often are associated neurologic signs.

Kennedy C, Carrol FD: Optic neuritis in children. Trans Am Acad Ophthalmol Otolaryngol 64:700, 1960.

Lessell S: Neuro-ophthalmology: Annual review. Arch Ophthalmol 93:434, 1975.

See also Walsh & Hoyt reference, p 232.

DISEASES OF THE ORBIT

ORBITAL CELLULITIS

Orbital cellulitis is characterized by proptosis; swelling, redness, and congestion of the eyelids, orbital tissues, and bulbar conjunctiva; discomfort; and frequently fever. A distinct magenta discoloration of the skin of the eyelids is present in cases of *H influenzae* infection. In children, orbital cellulitis is usually due to bacterial infection. There may be associated infections elsewhere in the body, particularly in the sinuses. Treatment consists of hot packs and the vigorous use of systemic antibiotics; a favorable response is usually obtained within 48–72 hours.

Trokel SL: The orbit: Annual review. Arch Ophthalmol 91:228, 1974.

Watters EC & others: Acute orbital cellulitis. Arch Ophthalmol 94:785, 1976.

ENDOCRINE EXOPHTHALMOS

This condition is relatively uncommon in children. It may be unilateral or bilateral. Exophthalmos is the principal presenting sign. There may be retraction of the upper lids or swelling of the lids. Injection and swelling of the conjunctiva may be present, and there may also be some extraocular muscle weakness.

Treatment consists of management of the underlying thyroid disturbance. Severe ocular involvement in the form of exposure keratitis, glaucoma, or decreased visual acuity should be treated by an ophthalmologist.

Kramar P: Management of eye changes of Graves' disease. Surv Ophthalmol 18:369, 1974.

Mausolf FA (editor): *The Eye and Systemic Disease*. Mosby, 1975.

See also Trokel reference, above.

ORBITAL TUMORS

Orbital tumors are rare in children. The most common primary tumors are hemangiomas, neurofibromas, gliomas of the optic nerve, dermoids, rhabdomyosarcomas, and tumors of the lacrimal gland. Neuroblastoma and lymphoma may spread into the orbit. The presenting symptoms are exophthalmos, congestion of the globe and lids, extraocular muscle weakness, and displacement of the globe. Optic nerve gliomas may show enlargement of the optic foramen on x-ray examination.

Each case should be carefully evaluated. Treatment includes surgical removal, x-ray therapy, or the use of alkylating agents in certain cases. For certain benign tumors, it is often better not to attempt total removal of the lesion.

Sagerman RH, Tretter P, Ellsworth RM: Orbital rhabdomyosarcoma in children. Trans Am Acad Ophthalmol Otolaryngol 78:602, 1974.

Youssefi B: Orbital tumors in children. J Pediatr Ophthalmol 6:177, 1969.

See also Henderson and Reese references, above.

ORBITAL PSEUDOTUMOR

Pseudotumor of the orbit is uncommon in children. It is an inflammation of the orbital tissues, sometimes granulomatous in character but usually unrelated to any specific granulomatous disease. The histopathologic picture is highly variable but often shows lymphocytic aggregates, perivascular inflammation, and plasma cells. As a rule only one orbit is affected, but in about 25% of cases the other orbit is involved also. The symptoms may develop suddenly, or slowly over a period of months. Swelling of the eyelids and conjunctiva often precedes the development of proptosis and diplopia. The diagnosis is usually made by exclusion of other causes of swelling and proptosis: neoplasms, endocrine exophthalmos, orbital cellulitis, etc. Spontaneous remission often occurs. However, dramatic improvement usually follows systemic corticosteroid therapy.

Heersink B, Rodrigues MR, Flanagan JC: Inflammatory pseudotumor of orbit. Ann Ophthalmol 9:17, 1977.

DISEASES OF THE LACRIMAL APPARATUS

DACRYOSTENOSIS

In a significant number of babies the nasolacrimal duct fails to completely canalize at the time of birth; the obstruction is usually at the nasal end of the nasolacrimal duct. Symptoms consist of persistent tearing and often mucoid discharge in the inner corner of the eye.

Most cases subside without treatment. The obstruction usually opens spontaneously, and relief of symptoms occurs. Massage over the lacrimal sac with expression toward the nose may be helpful in establishing the patency. If a cure does not result within the first few months of life, probing of the nasolacrimal duct should be performed by an ophthalmologist.

Kohler U, Muller W: The treatment of stenoses of the lacrimal passages in infants and children. Ophthalmologica 159: 136, 1969.
Mirecki R: Late results after intranasal dacryocystorhinostomy in infants. J Pediatr Ophthalmol 8:38, 1971.
Veirs ER: *Lacrimal Disorders: Diagnosis and Treatment.* Mosby, 1976.
Veirs ER (editor): *The Lacrimal System: The First International Symposium.* Mosby, 1971.

DACRYOCYSTITIS

Dacryocystitis is usually secondary to obstruction of the nasolacrimal duct. There is resultant stasis of the tears in the sac, with secondary bacterial infection. Symptoms consist of tearing and mucopurulent discharge. There may be acute inflammation in the region of the lacrimal sac. Occasionally the sac may rupture to the skin surface.

If possible, cultures should be obtained and the organism identified. For mild cases, expression of the contents of the lacrimal sac followed by instillation of topical antibiotics in the region of the lacrimal puncta may be effective. More severe cases should also be treated with systemic antibiotics. Irrigation of the canaliculi and lacrimal sac with antibiotic solution is a more successful method of delivering adequate concentrations of antibiotics to the area of infection. Once the infection has subsided, an attempt should be made to establish the passage of tears. The nasolacrimal duct should be probed under general anesthesia if the system does not permit passage of fluid irrigated through the canaliculi.

See Kohler and Veirs references, above.

DACRYOADENITIS

Inflammation of the lacrimal gland may be associated with systemic disorders such as mumps or sarcoidosis. More rarely, infections of the lacrimal gland may be secondary to tuberculosis and syphilis.

Treatment should be directed toward the specific disease, if present; otherwise, symptomatic treatment should be used. Local applications of heat or cold over the lacrimal gland may give relief. Bed rest and salicylate analgesics are also useful. Systemic corticosteroids may reduce inflammation, but the use of steroids in any viral infection is risky.

Boniuk M: Eyelids, lacrimal apparatus and conjunctiva: Annual review. Arch Ophthalmol 90:239, 1973.
See Veirs references, above.

●   ●   ●

General References

Burian HM, Von Noorden GK: *Binocular Vision and Ocular Motility: Theory and Management of Strabismus.* Mosby, 1974.

Dunlap EH (editor): *Gordon's Medical Management of Ocular Disease,* 2nd ed. Harper & Row, 1976.

Ellis PP: *Ocular Therapeutics and Pharmacology,* 5th ed. Mosby, 1977.

Goldberg MF (editor): *Genetic and Metabolic Eye Disease.* Little, Brown, 1974.

Harley RD (editor): *Pediatric Ophthalmology.* Saunders, 1975.

Havener WH: *Ocular Pharmacology,* 3rd ed. Mosby, 1974.

Havener WH: *Synopsis of Ophthalmology,* 4th ed. Mosby, 1975.

Hospital for Sick Children, Toronto: *The Eye in Childhood.* Year Book, 1967.

Hughes WF (editor): *Year Book of Ophthalmology.* Year Book, 1976.

Kaufman HE (editor): *Ocular Anti-inflammatory Therapy.* Thomas, 1970.

Keeney AH: *Ocular Examination: Basis and Technique,* 2nd ed. Mosby, 1976.

Liebman SD, Gellis SS (editors): *The Pediatrician's Ophthalmology.* Mosby, 1966.

Moses RA (editor): *Adler's Physiology of the Eye: Clinical Applications,* 6th ed. Mosby, 1975.

Newell FW, Ernest JT: *Ophthalmology: Principles and Concepts,* 3rd ed. Mosby, 1974.

Ryan SJ Jr, Smith RE (editors): *Selected Topics on the Eye in Systemic Disease.* Grune & Stratton, 1974.

Scheie HG, Albert DM: *Textbook of Ophthalmology,* 9th ed. Saunders, 1977.

Sloane AE: *Manual of Refraction,* 2nd ed. Little, Brown, 1970.

Vaughan D, Asbury T: *General Ophthalmology,* 8th ed. Lange, 1977.

Walsh FB, Hoyt WF: *Clinical Neuro-ophthalmology,* 3rd ed. 3 vols. Williams & Wilkins, 1969.

10 ...
Teeth

Olof H. Jacobson, DDS

The primary teeth begin to develop by the sixth week of embryonic life; the permanent teeth, by the fourth or fifth month in utero. (Table 2–12 summarizes the sequence of calcification, eruption, and shedding of the teeth.)

ERUPTION OF THE TEETH

Because eruption of teeth is an easily observable part of general growth and development, the progress of tooth eruption may serve as an indicator of the physical condition of a growing individual. Only those cases that are not within the range of normal variation or are clearly not due to a familial tendency should be considered abnormal. Retarded eruption is more frequent than accelerated eruption and may be due to local or systemic causes.

Normal Eruption

As the teeth penetrate the gums, the infant may become irritable and have increased salivation, but "teething" does not cause systemic disturbances. Bacterial invasion through a break in the tissue or under a gingival flap covering the teeth may cause inflammation. Gentle irrigation often helps to relieve inflammation around a gum flap. Gingival incision is rarely indicated. A blunt, firm object or cracked ice wrapped in soft cloth may hasten eruption and relieve pain as the child chews on it.

Abnormal Eruption

Local causes such as premature loss of primary teeth and loss of space by a shift of neighboring teeth may retard eruption or cause impaction of some permanent teeth. Construction of a space maintainer by a dentist is often indicated.

In about 4% of normal individuals, one or more permanent teeth may fail to develop. A family history of similar problems can often be elicited. The third molars are most frequently missing, followed by the upper lateral incisors and the lower second premolars. Congenital absence of teeth in the primary dentition is rare.

Supernumerary teeth appear occasionally, most often in the upper incisor area. Extraction is the treatment of choice, at the discretion of the dentist.

Natal teeth (teeth present at birth or erupting shortly thereafter) may be part of the primary dentition or may be supernumerary teeth. Ordinarily, they should be removed since they present difficulties with nursing and may irritate the infant's lips and tongue. Roentgenograms should be taken by the dentist to prevent the removal of primary teeth. Extraction should not be undertaken arbitrarily because of the risk of bleeding and because these teeth may not be supernumeraries, but consideration should always be given to the danger that these teeth could be aspirated or swallowed. The teeth are easily removed with forceps or by ligation. No extraction should be undertaken until after the tenth postnatal day to avoid excessive hemorrhage. Administration of vitamin K may be indicated.

If a delay in eruption of the entire primary or permanent dentition is observed, hereditary, systemic, and nutritional factors should be evaluated. Hypopituitarism, hypothyroidism, cleidocranial dysostosis, and rickets must be considered. Local causes such as malposition of teeth, supernumerary teeth, cysts, over-retained teeth, and ankylosis may be responsible for failure of eruption of single teeth or small groups of teeth.

Early loss of primary teeth is the most common cause of premature eruption of permanent teeth. If the entire dentition is advanced, an endocrine disorder such as hyperpituitarism must be considered.

Ectopic Eruption

If the jaw size is inadequate or if a permanent tooth is out of position, a tooth may attempt to erupt into the position of its neighbor. This is most common in the upper first permanent molar and occasionally in the lower first permanent molar and the upper permanent cuspid. The molars are tipped mesially, so that they engage the second primary molar. The result is that eruption ceases or pressure resorption causes partial or complete loss of the second primary molar roots. The latter results in premature loss of the primary tooth, which could lead to subsequent impaction of the succedaneous premolar when its time to erupt comes. The dentist can often correct the path of eruption of the permanent tooth and guide it into proper position. If the primary tooth is lost, a space maintainer or space regainer should be placed. Maxillary cuspids frequently tend to erupt in improper position, resulting in pressure resorption of the roots of adjacent teeth or malocclusion. Visits to the pedodontist (at intervals specified by him) and appropriately timed x-ray examination and orthodontic consultation can frequently prevent or minimize problems arising from ectopic eruption.

IMPACTIONS

Impactions are teeth which are so closely lodged in the alveolar bone that they are unable to erupt. Common usage has applied the term to any tooth which remains within its alveolus and does not erupt. Although there are hereditary patterns leading to impacted teeth, the causative factors of most concern are prolonged retention of primary teeth, localized pathologic lesions, and shortening of the length of the arch.

The teeth most commonly involved are the third molars and maxillary cuspids. Impacted third molars should be removed early, when surgery is less traumatic and healing is more rapid. Surgery and orthodontics are required for both aesthetic and functional reasons in the case of maxillary cuspids because of their anterior position in the mouth.

The possible formation of dentigerous cysts is the most serious consequence of failure to remove impacted teeth, although pain and malocclusion may also result.

NORMAL OCCLUSION

Normal (class I) occlusion is defined as the circumstance wherein the mesio-buccal cusp of the upper first permanent molar occludes in the buccal groove of the lower first permanent molar. The 3 broad classifications of occlusion are illustrated in Fig 10–1.

Class II occlusion presents a retrognathic posture, whereas class III occlusion causes prognathism. There are several subclassifications, but these are of most interest to the orthodontist. In addition, in normal occlusion, the lower teeth occlude lingually to the uppers.

MALOCCLUSION

Malocclusion may be the result of genetic factors causing abnormal dimensional discrepancies between the jaws and teeth; premature loss of primary or permanent teeth; harmful oral habits such as thumb or finger sucking or tongue thrusting; or "pillowing"

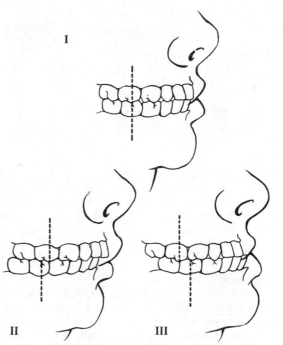

Figure 10–1. Types of occlusions.

(pressure induced by habitually sleeping on the stomach or supporting the head with the hand or fist). If bad habits can be controlled by age 4 or 5 years, physiologic growth may correct malocclusions due to this cause.

Prevention

Speech therapists can sometimes establish normal swallowing habits, eliminating tongue thrust. Thumb or finger sucking is often outgrown. It was once thought that the child was comforted by sucking and that it should be ignored since he might develop more pernicious habits or sustain psychologic trauma if made to stop. Dentists are now beginning to feel that these habits should be stopped early. Thumb or finger sucking starts with a psychologic need and then becomes a habit. The trauma to a 5- or 6-year-old child from being deprived of the comfort of sucking is considered to be less than the trauma to a teen-ager wearing orthodontic appliances as he undergoes the changes of puberty—not to mention the cost of orthodontic treatment. Sucking often occurs when the child is bored or tired or has nothing else to do with his hands, as when watching television. The dentist may construct a "crib" that is inserted in the mouth and breaks the suction seal or reminds the child that he is sucking. Mittens or bitter chemicals may be helpful, although eye contamination with chemicals may be dangerous or painful. Constant reminders by siblings or parents or appeals to the child's vanity are often successful.

Habits contributing to malocclusion must be eliminated before orthodontic therapy can be successful.

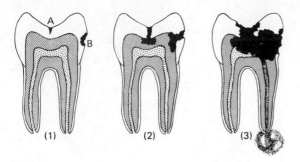

Figure 10—2. Stages of caries. (1) Initial decalcification and penetration of the enamel. (2) Invasion of the dentin (note rapid spread because dentin is relatively softer than enamel). (3) Pulpal involvement with periapical abscess. A, pit and fissure carries; B, smooth surface carries.

Treatment

Orthodontic treatment is usually most successful when started at about the time the last primary teeth are shed and before growth ceases, ie, in the early teens. In extreme cases, early consultation—when the permanent incisors and molars are starting to erupt—is advisable.

Increasing demand by society for comprehensive dental care is placing a tremendous burden on the orthodontist. As a result, many general dentists and pedodontists are providing interceptive care with extraction of appropriate primary teeth and the use of removable appliances to correct minor malocclusions.

DENTAL CARIES

Dental caries is one of the most common chronic diseases of man, occurring in over 50% of 3-year-olds and almost all adults. It has been defined as a disease of the calcified tissues of the teeth which is characterized by destruction beginning on the surface of the tooth in areas of predeliction and progressing inward toward the pulp. The destruction involves (1) decalcification of the inorganic portion and (2) disintegration of the organic substance of the tissue. The decalcification is caused by acids resulting from the action of acidogenic bacteria on refined carbohydrates, particularly sucrose. Three factors are necessary for the development of caries: a tooth, bacteria, and dental plaque. The incidence of caries in children at various ages is as follows: age 1 year, 5%; 2 years, 10%; 3 years, 40%; 4 years, 55%; and 5 years, 75%.

Three groups of bacteria play a role in producing dental decay: (1) Acidogenic and aciduric organisms, which produce the acids upon the tooth surface necessary to decalcify the hard tissues. *Lactobacillus acidophilus* and certain streptococci are encountered most frequently. (2) Proteolytic organisms which digest the organic matrix after decalcification. (3) Leptotrichia and leptothrix, which form plaques on the

smooth surface of the teeth, thus serving to harbor and protect the other organisms; these bacteria are thought to play no primary role in the production of decay.

Two processes are always operating on the enamel surfaces: acid production by bacteria and acid neutralization by the saliva. The rate of acid formation is of importance in caries susceptibility. In some individuals, acid is formed so rapidly that the buffering action of saliva cannot neutralize it. The effectiveness of the buffering action also varies in different individuals.

In certain systemic conditions—and possibly in some emotional states—the quality and quantity of saliva may be altered. This in turn may result in an increase in caries activity. Children and adults suffering from chronic debilitating diseases often show an increase in caries activity. The arrangement of teeth in the arch, their anatomy, and dietary factors may also contribute to the development of caries.

A genetic factor directly related to caries resistance has been established in laboratory animals. In humans, protection from caries seems to be a familial characteristic—as does increased susceptibility also.

Prevention

Dental caries can be controlled in most instances by the following measures:

(1) Frequent observation by a dentist, starting when all of the primary teeth have erupted or at least by age 3. The frequency should be determined by the dentist, depending on the individual child.

(2) Prompt removal of all active decay.

(3) Thorough brushing and rinsing after each meal and after snacks. If brushing is impossible, vigorous rinsing is advisable.

(4) Elimination of all concentrated sugars between meals and keeping the ingestion of sweets at mealtimes to a minimum. Carbohydrates, particularly in forms which cling (taffy, caramels) or have prolonged contact (hard candy, suckers, chewing gum) provide an ideal substrate for the production of tooth-destroying acids by bacteria. Excessive ingestion of sweetened soft drinks and juices can also be harmful. Sugars ingested at mealtimes are less harmful since the acid is buffered by other foods and saliva. The pediatrician should never give candy or gum to his patients as a reward. Inexpensive toys or rings provide a welcome and noncariogenic substitute.

(5) Provision of adequate roughage in the diet for its detergent effect. Such foods as apples, raw carrots, and celery tend to cleanse the surfaces of the teeth as they are masticated. Small children should not be allowed to fall asleep with a bottle of milk or to hold one in the mouth for prolonged periods during the day. A recognizable caries pattern of the primary dentition can often be related to this practice.

(6) Application of topical fluorides, except in areas where fluoride is already present in large amounts (over 3–4 ppm) in the community water supply. Fluoridation of the community water supply is the most effective preventive measure against dental caries, especially from birth to age 10–12. Children born and

raised in an area where the water contains 1–1.5 ppm fluoride have 60% less decay than children in areas where the fluoride content is low.

(7) The use of fluoridated toothpastes. The ADA Council on Dental Therapeutics has classified Crest toothpaste (stannous fluoride) and Colgate Dental Cream (monofluorophosphate) in group A, which consists of accepted products which will be listed in Accepted Dental Remedies. Certain other fluoridated toothpastes have been classified in group B, indicating that there is not sufficient evidence to justify present acceptance but that there is reasonable evidence of their usefulness and safety.

PREVENTIVE DENTISTRY

An exciting application of the foregoing is being incorporated into many dental practices today.

Under the supervision of the dentist, trained auxiliary personnel are instructing the patient and the parent in the proper methods of toothbrushing and flossing. Disclosing wafers and solutions containing erythrosine are used to reveal plaque deposits and debris that have been missed by ineffective or nonexistent brushing. An explanation of the role of plaque and bacteria in decay and periodontal disease and the importance of oral health to the overall health of the individual is also provided. Cultures of saliva reveal the presence of high bacterial counts which correlate with a high incidence of caries.

Many dentists are also providing nutritional counseling, evaluating the patient's diet and suggesting a more healthy, balanced diet which will improve general health. The use of visual aids and regular return visits are proving that dentistry now has the knowledge to provide a truly preventive service.

The pediatrician can contribute to his patient's oral and general health by (1) recommending early and regular visits to the dentist, (2) acquainting himself with normal and abnormal eruption, occlusion, and tooth form and number, and (3) learning the implications of various soft tissue lesions.

While fewer specific preventive measures are available to the dentist as compared to the physician, increased demand for oral health through education and prepaid dental plans can conceivably lead to a significant reduction in oral disease. Dental research is revealing methods which, with patient cooperation, can achieve this end.

ACCIDENTS TO THE TEETH

Trauma to the teeth may result in fractures of varying degrees of severity. Damaged teeth should be treated by the dentist as soon after the accident as possible to minimize the possibility of loss of tooth vitality and thus avoid the later need for pulpotomy (on primary teeth) or endodontic procedures (on permanent teeth). Loosened teeth will frequently stabilize and survive if they are repositioned and splinted for a time.

Evulsed teeth should be kept moist and handled very carefully until they can be replanted and stabilized. The patient or the parent should be encouraged to replant the tooth as soon as possible, since time is the most important factor in survival. The tooth should be rinsed gently before replantation so as not to remove remnants of the adhering periodontal membrane.

Endodontic therapy is always necessary in the case of an evulsed tooth, and tetanus immunization and antibiotic therapy (penicillin) are usually advisable, especially if the teeth have become contaminated while out of the mouth. The prognosis for replantation of evulsed permanent teeth depends on the time elapsed before replantation and the degree to which closure of the root apex has progressed. If these teeth are retained for 6–8 years (until the growth of the jaws is completed), more effective and aesthetic prosthetic devices can be employed. Loss of teeth in the young child adversely affects the development of proper occlusion.

If trauma causes intrusion of the teeth, primary treatment should be directed toward treatment of the soft tissues. Intruded teeth usually reerupt within a month. Most will be retained but will become nonvital, and some will be shed prematurely. Intrusion of primary teeth may cause moderate to severe damage to the developing permanent tooth.

STAINING OF THE TEETH

Hemolytic disease of the newborn may be followed by yellow-green to black staining of enamel and dentin and hypoplasia of the enamel of the primary teeth.

Tetracyclines administered to women in the third trimester of pregnancy, to nursing mothers, or to the infant or child during the period of tooth formation may cause yellow-gray, bright yellow, gray-brown, or dark brown discoloration of teeth forming at the time of exposure to the drug. Under ultraviolet light a yellow to yellow-brown fluorescence is noted, peaking at 340–370 nm.

Mottled enamel is found in persons whose tooth-formative years are spent in an area where the fluoride content of the drinking water is greater than 2 ppm. Mottling varies from small whitish spots to severe brownish discoloration and hypoplasia if the fluoride concentration is greater than 5 ppm.

There are many other varieties of staining, extrinsic and intrinsic, involving a great variety of agents and causes.

DISEASES & DISORDERS OF THE ORAL SOFT TISSUES

Periodontitis

Periodontitis is rare in children. It should alert the clinician to its systemic implications.

Hypophosphatasia, cyclic neutropenia, histiocytosis X, leukemia, scurvy, and vitamin D deficiency should be suspected when periodontal destruction occurs in children.

Children with Down's syndrome are extremely prone to develop periodontitis. Scrupulous home care (brushing) and, occasionally, ascorbic acid therapy (100–300 mg/day) seem to be useful. In spite of all measures, some of these children inevitably lose their teeth to periodontal disease.

Almost every adult suffers from periodontal disease to varying degrees. This destruction of the dental supporting structures is the leading cause of tooth loss in individuals over 35 years of age. The course of the disease is usually established during childhood, but the overt signs of periodontal disease do not usually appear until after puberty. Prior to puberty, the principal expression of an irritation in the dental supporting structures is gingival inflammation at the marginal areas. Except in conjunction with systemic diseases, this inflammation is usually due to local causes, especially poor oral hygiene.

Missing teeth, malocclusions, poor oral hygiene, and poor dietary habits all contribute to the production of periodontal disease, but the exact cause is not completely understood. Research with germ-free and gnotobiotic animals indicates that the bacterium *Odontomyces viscosus* colonizes at the gingival crevice and exudes a levan polymer to form a specific type of plaque material. With accumulations of this material, destruction of alveolar bone is observed. Traumatic occlusion, impaction of food, and other factors must also be considered.

Gingivitis

A distressingly high percentage of children exhibit the simple forms of gingivitis which involve the marginal gingivae and interdental papillae. Instruction in good oral hygiene and eating habits will usually eliminate the symptoms in young children and decrease the number of teeth lost to more severe forms of periodontal disease in later life.

Gingival Enlargement

Painless hyperplasia of the entire gingiva, sometimes so extensive that the teeth are entirely covered, may occur after prolonged administration of phenytoin. The degree of enlargement seems to be related directly to oral hygiene. Therapy should be directed toward improved home care. The tissue may be removed surgically but will almost always recur unless another drug is substituted or scrupulous care of the mouth is maintained.

Necrotizing Ulcerative Gingivitis

This disease goes by many names—NUG, trench mouth, Vincent's infection, fusospirochetal gingivitis, ulceromembranous gingivitis, etc. It is an acute gingival inflammation characterized by red, swollen gingivae, necrosis beginning in the interdental papilla and extending along the gingival margins, pain, hemorrhage, a necrotic odor, and, often, a pseudomembrane. The tongue may be coated, and salivary flow increases. The mucosa may become involved. It may occur as a response to many factors, including poor mouth hygiene, inadequate diet and sleep, and various other diseases such as mononucleosis, nonspecific viral infections, bacterial infections, oral thrush, blood dyscrasias, and diabetes mellitus. The presence of fusiform and spiral organisms is of no importance as they occur in about one-third of clinically normal mouths and are absent in some cases of necrotizing ulcerative gingivitis.

Management depends upon ruling out underlying systemic factors and treating the signs and symptoms as indicated with systemic antibiotics (penicillin), oxygenating mouth rinses, analgesics, rest, and appropriate dietary measures. The patient should be referred to a dentist for gentle, thorough cleansing of the teeth. It is extremely doubtful that the disease is communicable.

Herpetic Infection

Herpetic gingivitis results from infection of the gums with herpes simplex virus. Primary infection usually occurs in childhood. The disease is manifested by red, swollen, tender gingivae and oral mucosa without necrosis of the interdental papillae or gingival margins. The lips are usually swollen and dry. Localized herpetic lesions may be present. The disease is highly infectious and may be mistaken for necrotizing ulcerative gingivitis. The absence of a fetid odor, the lack of gingival necrosis, and the presence of a high temperature in the herpetic infection are the chief differential points. The disease runs its course in about 2 weeks.

Herpetic stomatitis is a vesicular disease of the mouth caused by herpes simplex virus. The term is also used for the secondarily infected ulcerations that follow the vesicles. The lesions have also been called aphthae, canker sores, and dyspeptic ulcers. Once a patient has had primary herpetic gingivostomatitis (see above), the virus remains in the cells, apparently without attacking the host. Whenever host resistance is lowered by trauma, infection, menstruation, allergy or sensitivity, psychic factors, or dietary deficiencies, the virus becomes active. The first lesion (the vesicle) soon ruptures inside the mouth and becomes secondarily infected. The typical lesion has a yellow, ulcerated center and a bright-red areola, is very painful, and heals in about 10–14 days. Several lesions may coalesce.

Classically, these lesions have been treated by caustics such as phenol, silver nitrate, chromic acid, and alum. These delay healing, although they do cauterize nerve endings and relieve pain. For solitary lesions, tetracycline pastes have proved effective in reducing secondary infection, relieving pain, and hastening healing.

PULPITIS

Pulpitis may be acute or chronic. It may be caused by infection or by physical, thermal, chemical, or electrical trauma. Pulpal invasion by mixed bacteria from the oral cavity is the most common cause. The invading bacteria are usually streptococci or staphylococci, although other forms of bacteria and fungi or viruses may be active causes. When the bacteria enter a tooth from the blood stream after they are attracted to a pulp injured by operative trauma, heat, or other noninfectious causes, the resulting pulpitis is termed anachoretic pulpitis.

Acute Pulpitis

The pulp shows dilatation of blood vessels and cellular infiltration. PMNs predominate and may be in abscess form or diffusely distributed. In its early phases, severe paroxysms of pain occur, often spontaneously and at night. Initially, cold will elicit pain; as the pulpitis passes its earliest phases, heat will cause pain. The tooth responds to the electric pulp tester at lower than average levels early in the disease and at higher levels in later phases. In these earlier phases, the patient can locate the offending tooth. As the pulpitis becomes more severe and extensive, the pain is agonizing, lancinating, and radiating. The application of heat causes excruciating pain which may be partially relieved by tepid or cool water. The pain may be referred to other regions of the face, and the patient cannot locate the tooth and may not even be able to localize the pain to one general region of the jaw. An incisional opening into the pulp may permit the escape of pus and bring immediate relief. Acute pulpitis may cause fever, headache, and malaise.

Acute pulpitis may be resolved if well localized and treated by removing its cause and applying obtundents (eg, eugenol) or in selected cases by pulpotomy and use of agents such as calcium hydroxide. It may become chronic, or the pulp may become necrotic. In most instances, removal of the pulp or of the tooth is the treatment of choice. Acute pulpitis may lead to periapical inflammation.

Chronic Pulpitis

In chronic pulpitis the pulp shows dilatation of vessels and infiltration by plasma cells and lymphocytes. There are often no symptoms, but at times there may be a dull throbbing pain when the subject lies down or takes hot foods. The tooth usually responds slowly to cold and to electric pulp tests. The application of heat may elicit pain. Pain may be referred. Occasionally, the patient may remember having an acute pain (at the time of acute pulpitis). Chronic pulpitis may progress and necrosis ensue without causing any symptoms. It may act as a source of bacteria or toxins which may spread to remote areas of the body. Any search for possible foci should include tests for chronic as well as for acute pulpitis.

Chronic pulpitis may become acute, or the pulp may become necrotic or calcify. Chronic pulpitis does not usually resolve without treatment, although it could conceivably repair itself with no symptoms ever giving a clue to its presence.

Treatment is by pulp extirpation, apicoectomy, or extraction, as determined by local, general, and socioeconomic factors.

PERIAPICAL PATHOSIS

The periapical tissue may become inflamed as a consequence of pulpitis, trauma (a blow, or occlusal or habitual trauma), or injury caused by drugs used in endodontic therapy. Following traumatic or chemical injury, bacteria may become localized from the blood stream by anachoresis. The periapical region may be resorbed or sclerosed with or without inflammation.

Acute Periapical Periodontitis

Also referred to as dento-alveolar abscess, this condition begins when infection from the pulp reaches the periodontal membrane or when the membrane is injured by other means. The severity of the injury (or virulence of the organisms) and the resistance of the tissue will determine whether the inflammation is acute or chronic. A chronic periapical inflammation may become acute, and vice versa. If the inflammation progresses, an abscess forms and the surrounding bone may begin to resorb. The inflammation spreads into the bone marrow. For these reasons, periapical periodontitis is a periostitis, an osteitis, and a focal osteomyelitis.

As a result of edema, the tooth is elevated in its socket. The tooth is sore to percussion, and the patient attempts to limit mastication on the side of the jaw involved. Pain on percussion is the most reliable sign. If the inflammation is due to trauma, relieving the traumatic cause may permit resolution of the inflammation. If infection is present, drainage is essential. Drainage may be accomplished by endodontic therapy, incision, or extraction. If infection is not treated, it may progress to form a distinct dentoperiosteal abscess. At this stage, there is pulsation and severe pain, which is increased on pressure. The patient attempts to keep the teeth out of occlusion. Opening of the pulp canal or extraction of the tooth permits the escape of yellow, creamy pus. The patient feels almost immediate relief, and the condition may resolve in a short time or become chronic.

Fistula

If no treatment is given for infected periapical periodontitis, the infection spreads. In about 3–5 days, the infection will point to as far as the cortical layer of bone, the bone is perforated, and a subperiosteal abscess forms. If the abscess is located subgingivally, it forms a parulis ("gum boil"). These subperiosteal abscesses give rise to a new series of painful symptoms until they rupture and evacuate. One sign of

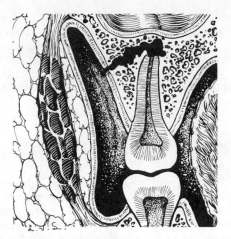

Figure 10—3. Fistula to buccal gingiva.

periapical periodontitis is redness, swelling, and tenderness over the root in the labial or buccal region.

When the periosteum and overlying skin or mucosa are penetrated, the abscess evacuates, the patient has relief, and acute symptoms subside. The fistula through which the abscess drained may form at various places opening onto the gingiva (Fig 10—3), the palate, or the skin. Drainage into the mouth is more common than through the skin. In the case of upper posterior teeth, the fistula may occasionally go into the maxillary sinus.

Acute dento-alveolar abscess is often accompanied by cellulitis of the face. If the cause is removed (infected tooth or pulp), the cellulitis usually subsides and the periapical lesion may heal by granulation. The use of local or systemic broad spectrum antibiotics may be necessary to promote healing. Without treatment, the infection may spread, resulting in osteitis or osteomyelitis, Ludwig's angina, cavernous sinus thrombosis, general toxicity, and possibly death. Infection may become chronic and remain as a potential source of future acute attacks and of toxins and bacteria.

Treatment is directed 'at removal of the cause, aiding the tissue in its inflammatory response, and minimizing chemical (drug) injury.

DENTISTRY FOR THE MENTALLY & PHYSICALLY HANDICAPPED

Increasing social awareness is dictating an increase in diagnostic and treatment services for mentally and physically handicapped children. Unfortunately, dental considerations are often given a low priority or overlooked altogether in the treatment of these individuals.

In the last decade, increasing emphasis has been placed on dental treatment for the handicapped. The mentally retarded, who often cannot communicate, exhibit improved behavior and achieve higher goals in habilitation programs when their mouths are kept free of pain and infection. Furthermore, their overall physical condition is often improved when a focus of infection is contained or eliminated.

To attempt orthodontic treatment or the construction of dentures for any but the mildly retarded is folly. Extensive bridgework on the anterior teeth of an uncontrolled epileptic is futile. Indeed, the hyperplastic tissue associated with the administration of phenytoin may protect the teeth in a manner similar to an athlete's mouthguard, contraindicating gingivectomy until seizures are controlled.

Prevention is of particular importance in the care of the mentally and physically handicapped. Devoting a few minutes a day to plaque removal to minimize dental caries and periodontal disease is far more practical than resorting to general anesthesia to restore a totally neglected mouth. Since many of these individuals lack the dexterity to care for their mouths or the ability to realize the importance of doing so, this duty may have to be performed by others such as a nurse, parent, or teacher. Proper dietary supervision with minimal ingestion of sweets also is of great importance. Early referral and regular visits to a dentist familiar with the problems of the handicapped and education in plaque control for those in charge of the care of the handicapped will alleviate many problems and help these patients to achieve their full potential in society.

●   ●   ●

General References

Baer PN, Benjamin SD: *Periodontal Disease in Children and Adolescents.* Lippincott, 1974.

Bernier JL, Muhler JC: *Improving Dental Practice Through Preventive Measures,* 3rd ed. Mosby, 1975.

Curzon MED: Dental implications of thumbsucking. Pediatrics 54:3, 1974.

Ellis RG, Davey KW: *The Classification and Treatment of Injuries to the Teeth of Children,* 5th ed. Year Book, 1970.

Finn SB: *Clinical Pedodontics,* 4th ed. Saunders, 1973.

McDonald RE: *Denistry for the Child and Adolescent,* 2nd ed. Mosby, 1974.

Moyer RE: *Handbook of Orthodontics,* 3rd ed. Year Book, 1973.

Nowack AJ: *Dentistry for the Handicapped Patient.* Mosby, 1976.

Pindborg JJ: *Atlas of Diseases of the Oral Mucosa.* Saunders, 1968.

Polson AM: Gingival and periodontal problems in children. Pediatrics 54:2, 1974.

White GE: *Dental Caries, A Multifactorial Disease.* Thomas, 1975.

11 . . .
Ear, Nose, & Throat

Barton D. Schmitt, MD

THE EAR

ACUTE SUPPURATIVE OTITIS MEDIA

Essentials of Diagnosis
- Earache.
- Fever.
- Red, bulging tympanic membrane.

General Considerations

Acute otitis media is an infection of the middle ear which is usually preceded by an upper respiratory infection. Young children are most commonly affected, possibly because they have an increased incidence of colds and shorter eustachian tubes.

Several tympanocentesis studies have been done on bulging eardrums in children. The organisms most frequently recovered are pneumococci (40%); *Haemophilus influenzae* (25%); and beta-hemolytic streptococci (5%). Sterile cultures, presumably viral, account for 30%. The incidence of *H influenzae* infection decreases to approximately 10% at age 5. *Staphylococcus epidermidis* has recently been demonstrated to be the cause of perhaps 5% of cases of acute suppurative otitis media. It is of interest that Halsted (see references) found all of his cultures from aspirates of flat, inflamed tympanic membranes to be sterile; where only the pars flaccida was bulging, he found a 20% incidence of bacterial infections; and where the entire eardrum was bulging, he recovered bacteria in 70%. In a study of predominantly hospitalized infants in the first 6 weeks of life, Bland found the major organisms in acute otitis media to be *Escherichia coli, Staphylococcus aureus,* and *Klebsiella pneumoniae.* Tetzlaff studied acute otitis media in predominantly outpatient babies in the first 6 weeks of life and found only 18% of the pathogens to be coliform organisms.

Clinical Findings

A. Symptoms and Signs: The major symptom of otitis media is earache. A young child may demonstrate his pain solely by increased irritability and difficulty in sleeping. Tugging at the ear is sometimes a useful sign, though it can be falsely positive. Rhinorrhea and fever are often present. *H influenzae* is more likely than other organisms to be associated with low-grade fever, minimal pain, and a mildly bulging eardrum.

The mainstay of diagnosis is the appearance of the tympanic membrane. It is usually flaming and diffusely red. In early cases, the bulging is limited to the pars flaccida. Later, the entire eardrum bulges outward, giving a doughnut-like appearance. On examination by pneumatic otoscopy, the bulging eardrum will be immobile. In about 20% of cases, the drum has spontaneously ruptured and there is a cloudy to purulent discharge in the ear canal, making examination of the eardrum difficult. Beta-hemolytic streptococcus is the most common cause of spontaneous perforation of the tympanic membrane. Cerumen that has melted with high fever or tears that have run into the ear canal can cause confusion with middle ear discharge.

B. Laboratory Findings: Nasopharyngeal and throat cultures correlate poorly with the organism found by tympanocentesis. Therefore, these cultures are not indicated. If perforation has occurred, it is useful to culture the discharge, using a nasopharyngeal culture swab. If the discharge has been present for over 8 hours, the likelihood of demonstrating the organism is small, since it frequently is overgrown with saprophytes. Lumbar puncture is indicated if the child has meningeal signs, a bulging fontanel, or is superirritable in addition to having an inflamed eardrum.

Differential Diagnosis

Not all earaches are caused by acute otitis media. Mumps, toothaches, otitis externa, a foreign body in the ear canal, hard cerumen, etc can all present with a chief complaint of earache. Injected vessels at the drum periphery and along the malleus are frequently over-diagnosed as "early otitis media." These can occur with fever or crying, both of which can cause a flushed tympanic membrane as well as a flushed face. Cleaning wax from the ear canal can cause reactive hyperemia of the same vessels. This degree of injection is also seen in the common cold. Such an eardrum may be red, but it will be mobile and not require treatment. Since acute otitis media is the most common complication of a cold, an infant with a cold and fever must never be sent home without examination of the eardrums. Cerumen removal will often be necessary (see p 247).

Complications

Without treatment, the tympanic membrane can proceed to pressure necrosis and spontaneous rupture, resulting in a sizeable perforation. More serious complications such as mastoiditis, meningitis, and cerebral thrombophlebitis can occur. These complications are not likely to occur if appropriate and prompt treatment is given.

Treatment

A. Specific Measures:

1. Systemic antibiotics—In older children (5 and over), the drug of choice for acute otitis media is penicillin, which can be given orally (50 mg/kg/day) or IM. In younger children (under age 5), in whom the incidence of *H influenzae* infection is high, the preferred drug is ampicillin, 75 mg/kg/day orally for 10 days. Ampicillin has the disadvantages of causing rashes and diarrhea and also being more expensive. Therefore, penicillin can be used in these younger children if combined with sulfisoxazole, 150 mg/kg/day orally for 10 days.

If the patient is allergic to penicillin, he can be treated adequately with erythromycin, 40 mg/kg/day orally for 10 days, plus sulfisoxazole as above. Hetacillin has no advantage over ampicillin, since it is converted to the latter in the blood stream and the frequency of rash and diarrhea is the same. Tetracyclines are contraindicated for ear infections because about 50% of pneumococci and streptococci are resistant to these drugs and because they cause staining of the tooth enamel.

Infants in the first 2 months of life with acute otitis media should receive myringotomy to identify the organism. If they are quite ill, they should be hospitalized and given ampicillin and kanamycin pending the results of cultures. If they look healthy, ampicillin will suffice, but they must be followed closely.

2. Antibiotic eardrops—If the eardrum has been perforated, there is usually a cloudy to watery material in the ear canal and antibiotic eardrops are not required. However, the child with considerable purulent drainage from the ear may profit from this adjunctive therapy. The purulent material should be removed by gentle suction, using a syringe and a short plastic tubing such as can be made by cutting a scalp vein needle set. Normal saline solution can be instilled without force and then removed. After this type of cleansing has eliminated the pus, antibiotic eardrops such as polymyxin B-bacitracin can be instilled 3 times a day. The child should be held with head sideways and stationary for a few minutes after drops are instilled.

B. General Measures:

1. Analgesics and antipyretics—An irritable child with an earache requires aspirin or even codeine to help him sleep through the first night while on treatment. Young children can be given codeine, 0.5 mg/kg/dose, up to 4 times a day. Codeine is available in several cough medicines in a concentration of 10 mg/tsp. Antipyretics for fever control may be required during the first 1 or 2 days.

2. Oral decongestants—Antihistamine-vasoconstrictor combinations are proved to be ineffective in the treatment of otitis media. They are probably indicated only if the patient has an associated history of allergic rhinitis.

3. Reassurance—Some parents are overly concerned about ear infections and their complications. Reassurance should be given as required. There is no danger of hearing loss as long as the prescribed medicines are taken as directed. The child can be allowed to go outside and need not cover his ears. Mountain travel is permitted. Swimming is permitted if perforation is not present.

4. Unwarranted measures—Vasoconstrictor nosedrops are of no value, since it is nearly impossible to deliver them to the entrance of the eustachian tube. Analgesic eardrops have never been proved to be effective for the relief of pain and have the disadvantage of obscuring the field of vision if the tympanic membrane needs to be reexamined.

C. Myringotomy:

The most common pitfall in therapy is not doing a myringotomy when it is indicated. In a child with an acutely bulging eardrum, myringotomy is indicated if the patient has severe pain (as evidenced by screaming) or if recurrent vomiting is associated with his ear infection. In these circumstances, myringotomy is more effective than analgesics or antiemetics. This procedure is described in detail on p 247.

D. Follow-Up Care:

Parents are routinely advised to return after 48 hours if there is any persistence of fever, pain, or purulent drainage at that time. If this does happen and the patient has received penicillin alone, the most likely problem is that the infecting organism is *H influenzae*. In this case, sulfisoxazole should be added to the treatment regimen. Another possibility is that a middle ear abscess is present which must be incised and drained via a myringotomy incision. Culture and sensitivity study of the middle ear pus will also identify rare cases of ampicillin-resistant strains of *H influenzae* or penicillin-resistant strains of *S epidermidis*. The third possibility is that the patient has a complication such as meningitis. A common cause of persistent pain alone is an abrasion of the ear canal from a speculum or an ear curet.

An appointment should be given routinely for the last day of treatment (10–14 days). The tympanic membrane is assessed at that time for normal appearance and mobility. Children over age 6 are also followed until the audiogram returns to the normal range. About 10% of patients still have signs of active infection on this visit, and antibiotics are continued for 1–2 weeks longer. If mobility or hearing is abnormal (another 10%), the patient must be followed for the development of chronic serous otitis media.

Prognosis

With treatment, suppurative complications such as mastoiditis are rare. Although temporary hearing loss is common, permanent deficits are probably unrelated to acute otitis media when appropriately treated.

Bass JW & others: Antimicrobials in the treatment of acute otitis media. Am J Dis Child 125:397, 1973.

Bland RD: Otitis media in the first six weeks of life: Diagnosis, bacteriology and management. Pediatrics 49:187, 1972.

Feigin RD & others: Assessment of the role of *Staphylococcus epidermidis* as a cause of otitis media. Pediatrics 52:659, 1973.

Halsted C & others: Otitis media. Am J Dis Child 115:542, 1968.

Howie VM & others: Otitis media: A clinical and bacteriological correlation. Pediatrics 45:29, 1970.

Rowe DS: Acute suppurative otitis media. Pediatrics 56:285, 1975.

Shurin PA & others: Otitis media caused by non-typable, ampicillin-resistant strains of *Haemophilus influenzae.* J Pediatr 88:646, 1976.

Tetzlaff TR & others: Otitis media in children less than 12 weeks of age. Pediatrics 59:827, 1977.

RECURRENT ACUTE SUPPURATIVE OTITIS MEDIA

Some patients develop suppurative acute otitis media with almost every cold. With appropriate antibiotic treatment, the tympanic membrane returns to a nearly normal appearance and mobility between bouts, but a recurrence follows quickly. These otitis-prone patients often have their first bout before 1 year of age. A practical working definition for this problem is a child who experiences 3 or more ear infections in a 6-month period.

Prophylactic antibiotics are a safe and usually effective solution to this problem. Benzathine penicillin G can be given IM in a 0.6 to 1.2 million unit dosage at monthly intervals. An alternative regimen is to give ampicillin orally as a single daily dose, or sulfisoxazole, 500 mg orally twice daily. This regimen is continued for 3 or 4 months, during which time the eustachian tube and middle ear usually undergo complete healing. If this method of treatment does not succeed, a more vigorous evaluation as described in the section on chronic serous otitis media can be initiated. Adenoidectomy has been advocated for this problem but is rarely helpful.

Maynard JE: Otitis media in Alaskan Eskimo children: Prospective evaluation of chemoprophylaxis. JAMA 219:597, 1972.

Perrin JM & others: Sulfisoxazole as chemoprophylaxis for recurrent otitis media. N Engl J Med 291:644, 1974.

ACUTE BULLOUS MYRINGITIS

In this condition, bullae form between the outer and middle layers of the tympanic membrane. In the past, this was considered to be always due to viral infections. More recent studies demonstrate that 50–75% of these patients have an underlying suppurative acute otitis media. The organisms are very similar to those found in isolated suppurative acute otitis media with the exception that *Mycoplasma pneumoniae* is occasionally involved in older children.

The patient usually complains of ear pain on the involved side. Examination of the ear reveals 1–3 bullae that may cover 20–90% of the drum surface. They are thin-walled and often sagging in appearance. They often contain a straw-colored fluid. There is minimal erythema.

Antibiotics are prescribed as for acute suppurative otitis media. Analgesics are sometimes indicated. The bullae do not have to be opened unless they are causing significant pain. They can be easily opened by nicking with a myringotomy knife or spinal needle.

Follow-up care is the same as that described for acute suppurative otitis media.

Coffey JD: Otitis media in the practice of pediatrics. Pediatrics 38:25, 1966.

Feingold M & others: Acute otitis media in children. Am J Dis Child 111:361, 1966.

Sobeslavsky O & others: The etiological role of *Mycoplasma pneumoniae* in otitis media in children. Pediatrics 35:652, 1965.

ACUTE BAROTITIS

Sudden changes in barometric pressure, as can occur with diving or flying, can lead to an acute serous effusion into the middle ear cavity. The history itself is diagnostic. The patient comes in complaining of severe pain and loss of hearing in the affected ear. Otoscopic examination usually reveals a hemorrhagic tympanic membrane.

The process is self-limited, lasting for 2–3 days. The principal therapeutic agent is an analgesic, usually codeine. Decongestants are also prescribed, but antibiotics are not necessary. The prognosis is excellent.

ACUTE TRAUMA TO THE MIDDLE EAR

Head injuries, a blow to the ear canal, blast injuries, or the insertion of pointed instruments into the ear canal can lead to perforation of the tympanic membrane or hematoma of the middle ear. Silverstein reported 50% of serious penetrating wounds of the tympanic membrane to be due to parental use of a cotton-tipped swab. Treatment of middle ear hematomas consists mainly of watchful waiting. Prophylactic antibiotics are not necessary unless signs of superimposed infection appear. The prognosis for unimpaired hearing depends upon whether or not the ossicles are dislocated or fractured in the process. The patient needs to be followed by audiometrics until his hearing has returned to normal.

Traumatic perforations of the tympanic membrane often do not heal spontaneously and should be referred immediately to an otolaryngologist. Early debridement and placement of a graft virtually assure closure.

Silverstein H & others: Penetration wounds of the tympanic membrane and ossicular chain. Trans Am Acad Ophthalmol Otolaryngol 77:125, 1973.

ACUTE SEROUS OTITIS MEDIA

Transient eustachian tube obstruction can occur in the absence of middle ear infection. This phenomenon usually occurs during colds or bouts of allergic rhinitis. It can also follow overly vigorous noseblowing. The patient complains of a stuffy ear or a crackling sensation in his ear. Otoscopic examination reveals serous fluid in the middle ear with an air-fluid level or, more commonly, just scattered air bubbles. The amount of air depends on the current patency of the eustachian tube.

Treatment consists of an oral antihistamine-decongestant and frequent use of chewing gum. Antibiotics are not necessary.

The process usually resolves in 4–7 days. The patient needs weekly follow-up until eardrum mobility has returned to normal. If suppurative otitis media develops—as evidenced by the sudden onset of fever or pain—he should be seen promptly.

CHRONIC SEROUS OTITIS MEDIA

Essentials of Diagnosis
- Painless hearing loss.
- Dull, immobile tympanic membrane.
- Fifteen to 30 dB hearing loss.

General Considerations
Chronic serous otitis media is present when the middle ear is persistently filled with sterile fluid. The main cause is a complete eustachian tube obstruction. The closure of the eustachian tube creates a vacuum in the middle ear after the air is reabsorbed, and secretions from goblet cells and transudate from the adjacent capillaries fill the space. Since superimposed infection can occur, there is some overlap between this problem and recurrent suppurative otitis media.

Clinical Findings
A. Symptoms and Signs: The patient usually complains of a hearing loss or at least a feeling of fullness in the ear. If he is older, he may state that it feels as if he were talking inside a barrel. In the preverbal child, this condition is usually not suspected unless it occurs bilaterally. Unlike acute suppurative otitis media, there is minimal pain.

Physical examination reveals a dull, opaque eardrum. The drum is usually quite pale, although in severe cases it may have a bluish tint. In long-standing cases, the tympanic membrane is retracted. When the eardrum becomes retracted, the position of the right malleus changes from 7 o'clock to 9 o'clock. Air bubbles are not present. Their occurrence indicates that the problem is not chronic and that the eustachian tube dysfunction is intermittent.

The essential finding in this disorder is lack of tympanic membrane mobility or, more commonly, a markedly diminished, sluggish movement on examination with the pneumatic otoscope. The physician must be able to operate this instrument in order to elicit this diagnostic sign. It has a closed head connected to a piece of tubing with a rubber suction bulb at the end. If the largest ear speculum that will fit the patient's ear canal is used, an airtight seal can be made. When the rubber ball is squeezed with the operator's hand, the normal tympanic membrane flaps briskly. In this disorder, it does not. It should be obvious that the perforated tympanic membrane also does not move.

B. Audiologic Examination: An audiogram is helpful for confirming this diagnosis. In the usual form, a 15—30 dB air conduction loss will be present in the involved ear, with normal bone conduction. In the severe form, the hearing loss may range from 30—50 dB. A tympanogram as recorded on an impedance bridge instrument will demonstrate decreased compliance. The place of the tympanometer in private practice is controversial. While pneumatic otoscopy gives similar results, the tympanometer is more accurate in uncooperative children and those with stenotic ear canals. However, the instrument is unreliable with children under age 7 months. Its value in audiology clinics and teaching settings is unquestioned. A Weber test with a tuning fork centered on the forehead will lateralize to the involved ear.

Contributing Factors
Most cases of chronic serous otitis media are due to primary congenital eustachian tube dysfunction. Treatment is difficult and is described below. On occasion, a contributing factor may be uncovered.

(1) Allergic rhinitis can precipitate this disorder. Allergic rhinitis is diagnosed by the presence of frequent episodes of clear nasal discharge, sneezing, nasal itching, and over 20% eosinophils on a stained smear of nasal discharge.

(2) Recurrent acute suppurative otitis media, if inadequately treated, may convert to chronic serous otitis media.

(3) A supine feeding position can occasionally lead to chronic serous otitis media in infants. Bottle-propping should be discontinued and the child fed in a more erect posture.

(4) Certain congenital malformations can lead to recurrent ear problems. Chronic serous otitis media is seen in 90% of children with cleft palate and 40% of children with submucous clefts. Cystic fibrosis and Turner's syndrome also predispose to recurrent ear problems.

(5) Adenoidal hyperplasia can occasionally block the exit of the eustachian tubes.

(6) Nasopharyngeal neoplasms can also produce eustachian tube obstruction.

(7) Hypothyroidism must also be considered.

When a chronic serous otitis media has been present for 1 month, the contributing factors mentioned above should be investigated. Essential laboratory work would include a nasal smear for eosinophils and a lateral film of the nasopharynx to rule out the presence of large adenoids or a tumor at this site.

Complications

Serious sequelae can occur in untreated chronic serous otitis media, but the number of children who progress to such complications is probably small. The longer the condition lasts, the more viscous the fluid in the middle ear becomes. The extreme form of this disorder is called adhesive otitis media ("glue ear"). This form gives retraction pockets and significant hearing losses. Rarely, a cholesteatoma can form despite the absence of a perforation.

Treatment

A. General Measures:

1. Oral decongestants—Recent studies have shown that oral decongestants are not effective at preventing or treating chronic serous otitis media. They should only be given a clinical trial in patients with underlying allergic rhinitis.

2. Autoinflation of the eustachian tube—If the child is cooperative, he can be taught to "pop" his ears several times a day. This requires a build-up of positive pressure in the nasopharynx to overcome the closed eustachian tube. In the child aged 3–6, this can sometimes be done by having him blow up a toy balloon while holding his nose firmly. The child over age 6 can often be taught to puff out his cheeks during a Valsalva maneuver while keeping his lips closed. The nostrils are also kept closed. The elevated pressure will sometimes include the nasopharynx. If not, this process can be enhanced by teaching the child to swallow while maintaining this pressure. Liberal use of chewing gum may be of some value in all ages.

3. Reassurance—The parents may be reassured that this is not a lifelong process and that the temporary manifestations can be helped in most cases. Some children with this problem have been punished because they have asked their parents to repeat statements or because they show speech regression. The parents must be reassured that there is no intentional element to these symptoms. The teacher should be informed that the child has some difficulty hearing and should be allowed to sit in the front row.

B. Follow-Up Care and Evaluation for Surgery: It is not clear how long the child should be followed to see if spontaneous resolution occurs before surgery is resorted to. The following indications for referring a patient are a composite of current practices in this country. The problem should be reviewed at least every month. If the condition is bilateral, affects hearing, and the child attends school, he should be referred for surgery if the findings persist for 1 month. If the condition is bilateral and affects hearing but the child does not attend school, he should be referred after 2 months. If the condition is unilateral, he can be referred for surgery after 4 months or perhaps only if the tympanic membrane becomes retracted.

C. Surgical Treatment: Myringotomy followed by insertion of polyethylene flanged ventilation tubes (tympanostomy tubes) has given excellent results in this disorder as long as the tubes are in place. The tubes permit pressure equalization and drying of the middle ear cavity without a functional eustachian tube. This procedure can be done in an outpatient setting by an otolaryngologist. Some suggest that tubes should not be placed until the results of myringotomy alone have been assessed. Possible side-effects of tympanostomy tubes are chronic perforations, cholesteatoma, secondary infection, mastoiditis, dislocation of the tube into the middle ear cavity, and the risks of anesthesia. Removal of the adenoids is rarely helpful.

Prognosis

Many children with chronic serous otitis media improve spontaneously. The condition is virtually unknown beyond age 12. Most of those who have a tympanostomy tube inserted also have a good outcome. The tube is extruded on the average of 6 months after insertion. The tympanic membrane nearly always heals over, and the eustachian tube often becomes functional. In occasional cases, the tubes need to be replaced. Kilby & others (see reference below) inserted tubes on only one side in children with bilateral serous otitis media. At 2-year follow-up, the recurrence of fluid and the persistence of hearing deficits was the same for both the treated and untreated ears.

Dees SC: Secretory otitis media in allergic children. Am J Dis Child 124:364, 1972.

Fraser JG: Secretory otitis media in children. Clin Pediatr (Phila) 10:261, 1971.

Kilby D, Richards SH, Hart G: Grommets and glue ears: Two-year results. J Laryngol Otol 86:881, 1972.

Mortimer EA Jr: Impedance audiometry: Is it a wise investment? Pediatrics 58:151, 1976.

Olson A & others: Prevention and therapy of serous otitis media by oral decongestant: A double blind study in pediatric practice. Ambulatory Pediatr Assoc Abstracts, p 24, 1976.

Paradise JL: On tympanostomy tubes: Rationale, results, reservations, and recommendations. Pediatrics 60:86, 1977.

Paradise JL, Bluestone CD: Early treatment of the universal otitis media of infants with cleft palate. Pediatrics 53:48, 1974.

Paradise JL & others: Tympanometric detection of middle ear effusion in infants and young children. Pediatrics 58:198, 1976.

CHRONIC PERFORATION OF THE TYMPANIC MEMBRANE

Essentials of Diagnosis

- Painless otorrhea, intermittent or persistent.
- Perforated tympanic membrane.
- Conductive hearing loss of 20—40 dB.

General Considerations

A perforation of the tympanic membrane can be considered chronic if it lasts for longer than 1 month. Most perforations seen with acute suppurative otitis media heal within 2 weeks. Chronic perforations usually can be prevented by aggressive early treatment of acute otitis media. Reinfections of the exposed middle ear cavity are the most common finding in this disorder.

Clinical Findings

A. Symptoms and Signs: A perforation is always present. If no infection is present, the middle ear cavity is seen to contain thickened, inflamed mucosa. If superimposed infection is present, serous or purulent drainage will be seen and the middle ear cavity may contain granulation tissue or even polyps. A conductive hearing loss will usually be present depending on the size of the perforation.

The site of perforation is important. Central perforations are usually relatively safe from cholesteatoma formation. Peripheral perforations, especially in the pars flaccida, impose a risk of development of cholesteatoma because the ear canal epithelium adjacent to the perforation may invade it. The condition is almost always painless.

B. Laboratory Findings: Any discharge that is present should be cultured before treatment is initiated. Sensitivity tests are often necessary because the most common organisms are pseudomonas, *Escherichia coli,* and staphylococci. A PPD test should be done to rule out tuberculosis.

C. X-Ray Findings: Mastoid films are helpful if a superimposed mastoiditis is suspected.

Complications

This disorder can have serious complications, but they are rare with proper therapy. They occur mainly in unattended cases of superinfected, chronically perforated eardrums. Cholesteatoma is the most common complication and can be suspected if the discharge is foul-smelling and if a white, oily mass is seen within the perforation. The associated perforation may be pinpoint in size. If the discharge does not respond to 2 weeks of aggressive therapy, granulations or mastoiditis are probably present. Serious CNS complications such as extradural abscess, subdural abscess, brain abscess, meningitis, labyrinthitis, or lateral sinus thrombophlebitis can occur with extension of this process. Therefore, patients with facial palsy, vertigo, or other CNS signs should be referred immediately. Otogenous tetanus is another possible sequela.

Treatment

A. Specific Measures: If a serous discharge is present, antibiotic eardrops such as polymyxin B-bacitracin (Polysporin) should be instilled 2—3 times daily. This should be continued for 1 week after the discharge has resolved. Since neomycin ear drops are ototoxic, they should be avoided because they may cross the round window and damage hearing. If the discharge is purulent or foul-smelling or if systemic signs are present, systemic antibiotics should also be prescribed. Penicillin can be given at the outset and another drug substituted depending on the culture results. This can be continued for 2 weeks. It is very important to instill antibiotic eardrops immediately if there is any recurrence of discharge.

B. Surgical Treatment: Repair of the defect in the tympanic membrane is rarely successful during the time period when children have frequent colds and recurrent eustachian tube dysfunction. Therefore, tympanoplasty is usually deferred until age 9—12. The patient should be referred for this procedure earlier if perforations are bilateral and neither has resolved spontaneously by 2 months. The associated hearing loss in bilateral cases may be an intolerable handicap, especially in a school-age child. If drainage persists despite treatment, the patient must be referred to an otologist to rule out cholesteatoma, mastoiditis, or other complication.

C. Follow-Up Care: The patient should be seen once a week until the discharge has cleared. Thereafter, he should be seen about once every 3 months until surgery has been done. This follow-up is imperative to prevent any serious complications.

D. Prevention of Recurrences:

1. Prophylactic eardrops—For the 1-month period following any flare-ups of otorrhea, eardrops consisting of 1:1000 thimerosal (Merthiolate) solution (not tincture) should be instilled in each ear once daily.

2. Bathing—Before bathing and hairwashing, cotton plugs should be put in the ear and the surface completely covered with petrolatum ointment.

3. Swimming—Swimming should be discouraged unless it is a matter of great importance to the patient, in which case it can be continued using custom-fitted ear molds plus a bathing cap for girls or a scuba cap for boys. Diving, jumping into the water, and underwater swimming must be absolutely forbidden.

4. Unwarranted measures—The constant use of a cotton plug in the ear canal increases the risk of superinfection. Exposure to air is helpful.

Prognosis

With treatment, 80—90% of perforations heal spontaneously by 1 year. The remainder require careful follow-up. With proper care, these patients will be in good condition for tympanoplasty at age 9—12.

Felder H: Chronic otitis media in children. Pediatr Ann 5:474, 1976.

Fischer GW & others: Otogenous tetanus: Sequelae of chronic ear infections. Am J Dis Child 131:445, 1977.

Frederickson J: Otitis media and its complications. Arch Oto-
laryngol 90:387, 1969.
MacAdam AM & others: Tuberculous otomastoiditis in children.
Am J Dis Child 131:152, 1977.

MASTOIDITIS

Infection of the mastoid antrum and air cells typically occurs 1 week following an episode of untreated
or improperly treated acute suppurative otitis media.
The organisms are usually similar to those that cause
acute otitis media. Mastoiditis is unusual before age 2,
when air cells begin to develop.

Clinical Findings

The principal complaints are usually postauricular
pain and fever. On examination, the mastoid area is
often indurated and reddened. In the late stage, it may
be fluctuant. The earliest finding is severe tenderness upon mastoid percussion. Acute otitis media is
almost always present. Late findings are a pinna that is
pushed forward by postauricular swelling and an ear
canal that is narrowed in the posterior superior wall
because of pressure from the mastoid abscess.

This condition cannot be diagnosed on the basis
of x-rays alone. In the acute phase, there is diffuse
inflammatory clouding of the mastoid cells as in every
case of acute suppurative otitis media. Only later is
there evidence of bony destruction and resorption of
the mastoid air cells.

Treatment & Prognosis

The patient must be hospitalized because this disorder represents osteomyelitis at this site. Initial treatment should include parenteral penicillin for 7–10
days. Myringotomy (see below) should be performed
before initiating therapy in order to obtain material for
culture and also to relieve the pressure in the middle
ear-mastoid space. If the patient's condition worsens
initially or is unresponsive after 7 days, consultation
should be obtained regarding the advisability of simple
mastoidectomy. Oral antibiotics should be continued
for 4–6 weeks after the patient is discharged.

The prognosis is good if treatment is started early
and continued until the process is inactive.

· · ·

MYRINGOTOMY & TYMPANOCENTESIS

Tympanocentesis (placement of a needle through
the tympanic membrane) is mainly a diagnostic procedure, since the hole closes over quickly and provides
little sustained drainage. Tympanocentesis is helpful in
(1) acute otitis media in a patient under 2 months,

because the pathogens may be gram-negative; (2) acute
otitis media in a patient with compromised host resistance, because the organism may be unusual; and (3)
painful bullae of the tympanic membrane.

Myringotomy involves incision of the drum with a
myringotomy knife, leaving a flap through which
drainage fluid may escape. This procedure is helpful
for both diagnostic and therapeutic purposes. Myringotomy is indicated (1) when a patient on an initial
visit with bulging acute suppurative otitis media has
severe pain or vomiting, since both symptoms are
relieved by myringotomy; (2) when pain and fever fail
to resolve after 48 hours of antibiotic treatment, since
a middle ear abscess or resistant organism probably
exists; and (3) for acute mastoiditis, because it is important to permit drainage as well as to identify the
particular organism.

Technic of Myringotomy.

A. Premedication: In the conditions mentioned,
the pain from a myringotomy is only slightly greater
than the pain that already exists from acute inflammation of the tympanic membrane. Therefore, no premedication is generally indicated. If the patient is extremely difficult to hold, he may be premedicated with
1 mg/kg meperidine IM. Some authors recommend premedication as for cardiac catheterization. Others recommend local anesthesia with lidocaine to the 4 quadrants of the ear canal.

B. Restraint: The patient must be completely
immobile while the incision is being made. A papoose
board or a sheet can be used to immobilize the body.
An extra attendant is required to hold the patient's
head steady.

C. Site: With an open-headed operating otoscope,
the operator carefully selects his target. This is generally in the posterior-inferior quadrant. This site prevents
disruption of the ossicles during the procedure.

D. Incision: The knife is lowered slowly until it
touches the surface of the tympanic membrane at the
chosen site. A quick 2- to 3-mm incision is then made,
leaving a curved flap in the area indicated.

E. Culture: The myringotomy knife tip should be
wiped on a cotton swab moistened with a few drops of
normal saline. The material is then placed on a sheep
blood agar plate, chocolate agar plate, and a slide for
Gram staining.

Technic of Tympanocentesis

Steps A, B, and C are as described above.

In this procedure, the operator needs 2 assistants,
one to hold the patient's head immobile and the other
to operate a syringe. The syringe is attached to a piece
of extension tubing which in turn is attached to a 3½
inch spinal needle (No. 18 or No. 20) with a short
bevel. The needle is bent at a right angle so that the
end of it is out of the operator's line of vision. The
operator moves the needle toward the posterior-inferior
quadrant and inserts it through the tympanic membrane. Then the assistant provides suction so that the
middle ear secretions can be withdrawn for culture.

Roddey OF: Myringotomy in acute otitis media: A controlled study. JAMA 197:127, 1966.

Stool SE: Myringotomy: An office procedure. Clin Pediatr (Phila) 7:470, 1968.

Kravitz H & others: The cotton-tipped swab: A major cause of ear injury and hearing loss. Clin Pediatr (Phila) 13:965, 1974.

. . .

CERUMEN REMOVAL

Cerumen removal is an essential skill for anyone who treats ear problems. Cerumen often prevents adequate visualization of the tympanic membrane. Impacted cerumen can also cause itching, pain, hearing loss, or otitis externa. If cerumen impinges on the eardrum, a chronic cough may be triggered and will persist until the cerumen is removed. The most common cause of impacted cerumen is the use of cotton-tipped swabs by parents in misguided attempts to clean the ear canal. Parents need specific advice that earwax will come out by itself, and they should never put anything into the ear canal to hurry the process.

The technic of removal depends on the consistency of the earwax. All the procedures described below require careful immobilization to prevent injury of the ear canal.

(1) Very soft cerumen: Semiliquid earwax can be removed with cotton twisted on toothpicks or paper clips. Several passages with clean cotton are usually necessary. Nasopharyngeal culture swabs are an expensive substitute.

(2) Average cerumen: Sticky cerumen will adhere to an ear curet. A piece of this consistency can sometimes be removed by embedding the ear curet in it. If this technic fails, irrigation as described below should be instituted.

(3) Hard cerumen: Very hard cerumen may adhere to the ear canal wall and cause considerable pain or bleeding if one attempts to remove it with a curet. This type of wax should be softened before irrigation with Cerumenex or a few drops of detergent. After 20 minutes, irrigation can be started with water warmed to 35−38° C (95−100.4° F) to prevent vertigo.

An easy-to-assemble ear syringe consists of a 12 ml plastic syringe plus a piece of small plastic tubing. The tubing can be made from any scalp vein needle set by cutting off the needle about 3 inches from the female connector. The front end of the tubing is placed in the canal, behind the cerumen if possible, and the water is ejected with maximal pressure on the syringe plunger. The advantage of this technic is that the very small tubing may be inserted into the ear canal itself and the water stream is thus directed in the proper direction without interfering with reflux.

A commercial Water Pik is also an excellent device for removing cerumen, but it is important to set it at a low power (2 or less) to prevent any damage to the intact tympanic membrane.

A perforated tympanic membrane is a contraindication to any form of irrigation.

EAR CANAL FOREIGN BODY

Numerous objects can be inserted into the ear canal by a child. An insect in the ear should be killed with alcohol solution (gin will do for telephone advice). The patient should be immobilized on a papoose board with his head firmly grasped by an assistant.

An attempt should be made first to remove a foreign body by straightening the ear canal by pulling on the pinna and gently shaking the child's head. If a smooth object such as a bead is present, a cotton-tipped applicator with collodion should be inserted and placed against the object for 1−2 minutes, after which time it can be removed. An object with an irregular surface can perhaps be removed with a bayonet forceps. A right-angled hook or ear curet can sometimes be inserted past the object and withdrawn, pushing the object ahead of it.

If these methods fail, irrigation can be attempted. The stream should be directed past the object so that as it rebounds against the tympanic membrane it flushes the object out. Another approach for smooth objects is to use a suction machine. The end of the rubber tubing forms a better seal with the foreign body if it is first coated with petrolatum.

Irrigation with water is contraindicated with vegetable materials because they swell on contact with water. They can be irrigated with a 70% alcohol solution. Tissue paper also becomes difficult to remove if wet.

If the object is large or wedged in place, the patient should be referred to an otolaryngologist early rather than risk damage to the eardrum or ossicles.

Cunningham DG, Zanga JR: Myiasis of the external auditory meatus. J Pediatr 84:857, 1974.

Merkel BM: Foreign bodies in the ear canal. J Iowa Med Soc 47:744, 1957.

Stool SE, McConnell CS: Foreign bodies in pediatric otolaryngology: Some diagnostic and therapeutic pointers. Clin Pediatr (Phila) 12:113, 1973.

OTITIS EXTERNA

Otitis externa is an inflammation of the skin lining the ear canals. The most common cause is accumulation of water in the ear, leading to maceration and desquamation of the lining and conversion of the pH from acid to alkaline (eg, from swimming or frequent showers). Other causes are trauma to the ear canal from using cotton-tipped applicators to clean it or poorly fitted ear plugs for swimming; contact dermatitis due to hair sprays, perfumes, or self-administered eardrops; and chronic drainage from a perforated tympanic membrane. The superimposed infections are often due to *Staphylococcus aureus* or *Pseudomonas aeruginosa*.

Clinical Findings

The patient usually complains of pain and itching in the ear, especially with chewing or pressure on the tragus. Movement of the pinna or tragus causes considerable pain. Drainage is minimal. The ear canal itself is grossly swollen, and the patient resists any attempt to insert an ear speculum. Debris is also noticeable in the ear canal. It is often impossible to visualize the tympanic membrane. The hearing is normal unless complete occlusion has occurred.

Treatment

Topical treatment usually suffices. The crucial initial step is removal of the desquamated epithelium and moist cerumen. This debris can be irrigated out using warm half-strength white vinegar or warm Burow's solution (1 packet of Domeboro Powder to 250 ml tap water). Once the ear canal is open, a combination of antibiotic-corticosteroid eardrops (eg, Cortisporin) is administered 3–4 times daily. The corticosteroid is needed to reduce the severe inflammatory response. The insertion of a wick is painful and usually unnecessary. A follow-up visit in 1 week to document an intact tympanic membrane is imperative.

Oral antibiotics are indicated if any signs of invasiveness are present such as fever, cellulitis of the auricles, or tender postauricular lymph nodes. Penicillin is an appropriate initial drug while awaiting the results of culture of the ear canal discharge. Analgesics—sometimes codeine—may be required temporarily. Children predisposed to this problem should instill 2–3 drops of 1:1 white vinegar/70% ethyl alcohol into their ears before and after swimming. During the acute phase, swimming should be avoided if possible. A cotton earplug is not helpful and may be harmful.

Hoadley AW & others: External otitis among swimmers and nonswimmers. Arch Environ Health 30:445, 1975.

McDonald TJ, Neel HB III: External otitis. Postgrad Med 57:95, May 1975.

EAR CANAL FURUNCLE

A furuncle in the outer cartilaginous portions of the ear canal is most often caused by *Staphylococcus aureus*. The patient usually complains of pain in the outer part of the ear opening and resists insertion of a speculum. A small red lump will be noticed by simply looking through the otoscope with a large speculum that is not inserted. Treatment consists of topical bacitracin ointment. When the furuncle has pointed, incision and drainage should be carried out, usually with a

needle. Spread of this infection is rare; if it occurs, dicloxacillin, 25 mg/kg/day orally, should be added to the regimen. Recurrences point to manipulation of the ear canal (eg, with dirty fingernails).

EAR CANAL TRAUMA

Children may insert sticks or other objects into the ear canal. This normally results in abrasion of the ear canal with more bleeding than might be suspected. Parents cause similar injuries by overzealous attempts to remove earwax. It is mandatory that the tympanic membrane be examined. If it is free of injury, no treatment is necessary since the abrasions heal readily.

HEMATOMA OF THE PINNA

Trauma to the earlobe can result in the formation of a hematoma between the perichondrium and cartilage. If this is unattended, it can cause pressure necrosis of the underlying cartilage and result in a boxer's "cauliflower ear." To prevent this cosmetic handicap, these patients should all be referred to a surgeon for aspiration and the application of a carefully molded pressure dressing.

PIERCED EAR PROBLEMS

The most common complication of ear-piercing is superimposed infection, usually with *Staphylococcus aureus*. A small abscess develops at the site, and purulent material drains from both sides of the perforation. The infection usually stems from the use of contaminated needles or posts (eg, keeping the channel open with a piece of straw). This localized infection can occasionally progress to life-threatening staphylococcal septicemia. Other potential complications are viral hepatitis, erysipelas, and keloid formation.

Treatment of a primary infection requires removal of the foreign body (the earring); dicloxacillin, 25 mg/kg/day orally for 5 days while awaiting results of the culture; and local bacitracin ointment. Infections acquired later can often be aborted with bacitracin ointment applied to the posts and reinserted 3 times a day.

Especially if they are made of nickel, earrings can occasionally cause dermatitis of the earlobe. If this is suspected, the earrings should be removed and replaced with 14 K gold or stainless steel earrings and topical corticosteroids applied to the posts several times a day.

A serious complication of pierced ears is to have the earring post grasped by a child in play and completely pulled through the earlobe, leaving a jagged laceration. The scar that develops can lead to deformity of the earlobe and may require plastic surgery. For this reason, the ears should not be pierced until the child is at least 8 years of age. Ideally, the child should give consent for this procedure and be a teenager before it is performed. The physician can train the office nurse to pierce ears under aseptic conditions with equipment purchased from a surgical supply house. This would prevent the majority of primary infections that occur.

Cortese TA, Dickey RA: Complications of ear piercing. Am Fam Physician 4:66, Aug 1971.
Johnson CJ & others: Earpiercing and hepatitis. JAMA 227:1165, 1974.
Lovejoy FH: Life-threatening staphylococcal disease following ear piercing. Pediatrics 46:301, 1970.

CONGENITAL EAR MALFORMATIONS

Agenesis of the external ear canal results in deafness that requires evaluation in the first month of life by hearing specialists and an otolaryngologist.

"Lop ears" (Dumbo ears) lead to much teasing and ridicule. To prevent the secondary emotional problems, these can be corrected at age 5 or 6 by plastic surgery. The ear is of approximately adult size by then, and there is little risk of affecting growth.

An ear is low-set if the upper pole is below eye level. This condition is often associated with renal malformations (eg, Potter's syndrome), and an intravenous urogram is helpful.

Preauricular tags, ectopic cartilages, fistulas, sinuses, or cysts require surgical correction, mainly for cosmetic reasons. Most preauricular pits are asymptomatic. If one should become infected, it should be treated with antibiotics and referred to an otolaryngologist for eventual resection. Children with any of the above findings should have their hearing tested.

Jaffe BF: Pinna anomalies associated with congenital conductive hearing loss. Pediatrics 57:332, 1976.
Klein DR: Prominent ears in children. GP 36:126, Aug 1967.

HEARING DEFICIT

At least 2% of school children have some degree of hearing loss. One in every 2000 children is deaf or severely hard of hearing. In the preschool and school years, more than 90% of hearing losses are due to middle ear problems. In most instances, these are improvable or even completely curable. The early detection and proper management of hearing loss is one of the most urgent duties of any physician who cares for small children.

The classification of hearing deficits according to severity is based on the average hearing in the speech range, 500–2000 hertz (Hz), in terms of decibel units. *Normal hearing* in children is defined as ability to hear in the 0–20 decibel (dB) range. *Mild hearing loss* is ability to hear only in the 20–40 dB range; these children require some special treatment, whether it be preferential seating, lip reading training, or hearing aids. *Moderate hearing loss* is ability to hear only in the 40–65 dB range; these children can hear normal conversation only if they are fitted with a hearing aid. *Severe hearing loss* is ability to hear only in the 65–85 dB range, and *profound hearing loss* is ability to hear only 85 dB and over; these children will be dependent on visual communication for their language learning.

There are 2 types of hearing loss: conductive and sensorineural. *Conductive hearing loss* involves only the middle ear structure (tympanic membrane, ossicles, and eustachian tube). *Sensorineural hearing loss* involves the organ of Corti or the eighth nerve system. Central hearing problems do not result in a loss of hearing acuity but in integration disorders at the midbrain or cortical level. Conductive problems cause at most a 65 dB loss and are more treatable.

Detection of Hearing Deficits

The main role of the pediatrician in hearing deficits is to detect the difficulty as early as possible. The most critical period for learning language is the first 2 years of life. If hearing problems are not detected until after this time, lost ground in language development is never fully regained. Screening tests that vary according to age should be part of routine office practice.

A. Newborn Screening: The newborn screening procedure that is recommended by the Joint Committee on Newborn Screening* is the 5-point High-Risk Register for Deafness. The 5 categories are as follows: (1) History of genetically determined childhood hearing impairment. (2) Rubella or other nonbacterial intrauterine fetal infection (eg, cytomegalovirus, herpes simplex). Deafness may be the only finding in congenital rubella. (3) Defects of ear, nose, or throat: malformed, low-set, or absent pinnas; cleft lip or palate (including submucous cleft); and any residual abnormality of the otorhinolaryngeal system. (4) Birthweight less than 1500 gm. (5) Any indirect bilirubin concentration that is potentially toxic (usually over 20 mg/100 ml in full-term infants). Arrangements for audiologic follow-up should be made for these infants before discharge from the newborn nursery.

Testing of all newborns with an acoustic stimulus (eg, the Warbler) for an arousal response rarely uncovers a baby with severe hearing loss that is not detected by the High-Risk Register for Deafness. Therefore, routine auditory screening of newborns is

---

*The Joint Committee is composed of representatives from the Academy of Pediatrics' Committee on Fetus and Newborn; from the Academy of Ophthalmology and Otolaryngology's Committee on Hearing and Equilibrium; and from the American Speech and Hearing Association.

probably uneconomical and unwarranted. Only babies on the High-Risk Register need screening for severe hearing loss in the newborn nursery.

B. Infant Screening: The pediatrician should have noisemakers in the office that allow him to screen his patients' hearing. High frequencies can be tested with a squeaky toy or small bell, and middle frequencies with a rattle or piece of tissue paper. While the baby is distracted with a visual stimulus such as a toy or brightly colored object, the noisemaker is sounded outside his field of vision. Normal responses are as follows: at 4 months, there is a widening of the eyes, a cessation of previous activity, and possibly a slight turning of the head in the direction of the sound; at 6 months, the head turns toward the sound; at 9 months or older, the child should usually be able to locate a sound originating below him as well as turn to the appropriate side; after 1 year, he should be able to locate sound whether it is below or above him.

Many hearing tests give *false normal results,* eg, banging pots together or "hearing" a low-flying airplane. Most children with significant hearing deficits have residual hearing and will respond to very loud noises. However, they are educationally and socially deaf if they cannot hear normal speech sounds.

C. Screening of Older Children: At age 3, a child can begin to be tested with a pure tone audiometer. As previously stated, the most important frequencies to test are 500 Hz, 1000 Hz, and 2000 Hz. For the younger preschool child, the testing must be made into a game. The child is told that the earphones are a telephone and that he will hear some telephone bells. Whenever he hears the bell, he is to place a block on a block tower, a peg in a pegboard, etc. The younger child can often cooperate in this type of screening. By age 4, the child can be taught to raise his hand whenever he hears the pure tone. An audiometer of this type should be present in every pediatrician's office, and one of the assistants should be taught to operate it in such a way as to achieve consistently accurate results. If a soundproof room is not available and ambient noise is present, the screening can be done at 1000, 2000, and 4000 Hz at a level of 25 dB. These frequencies will not be masked out by ambient noise the way 500 Hz is masked.

If an audiometer is unavailable for any reason, the whisper test can be substituted to assess hearing. The examiner can whisper commands into the child's ear (eg, "Point to the door") or whisper words that the child is requested to repeat. The obvious advantage of the whisper test is that it measures the response to the human voice.

Referral

When a physician suspects a chronic hearing deficit, referral to an audiologist who can do precise testing should be arranged. If the hearing deficit is confirmed, the patient should be referred to an otolaryngologist for examination in an attempt to determine the cause of the hearing loss. The following 5 categories of patients should be referred to an audiologist:

A. High-Risk Newborn Patients: Newborn infants who fall into a high-risk category for deafness should be referred to a suitable facility for audiologic testing and evaluation by 2 months after discharge from the newborn nursery (see Newborn Screening, above). Even if hearing is found to be normal, infants in categories (1) and (2) should receive additional hearing screening evaluations at the physician's office to guard against impairments of delayed onset.

B. High-Risk Older Patients: (1) Children with syndromes often or sometimes associated with deafness (eg, albinism, Waardenburg's syndrome, osteogenesis imperfecta, Hurler's syndrome, Alport's syndrome, Treacher-Collins syndrome, Klippel-Feil syndrome). (2) Any patient who has recently recovered from a major CNS insult (eg, meningitis, encephalitis).

C. Screening Test Failures: If the infant fails any of the office screening tests described above, he needs more sensitive tests to clarify his status.

D. Suggestive Symptoms in Infants:

1. Parents are concerned—Most mothers of deaf children have some suspicion of the problem by the time the child is 6 months old and sometimes earlier. When the parent suspects hearing impairment, a reliable hearing test must be given.

2. No awakening to sound—A normal sleeping infant sometimes awakens to noise in other parts of the house. If this has not happened, the mother should be asked to be alert for it and report upon it at the next well baby visit. If it does not occur, the child requires referral.

E. Speech Delays: Before any child is labeled as having mental retardation, autism, auditory agnosia, or developmental speech delay, he requires a valid hearing test. Verbal communication depends on hearing. If the patient is old enough to cooperate with pure tone audiometry and the results are normal, he does not need referral to an audiologist.

It is a common occurrence in pediatrics to see a patient who has been referred for failing a school audiometric test and to find a cerumen-encased foreign body impacted in the ear canal. Removal immediately restores full hearing. Referral to an audiologist should be preceded by otoscopic examination.

Prevention

There are several causes of hearing deficits and deafness that can be prevented by proper pediatric care. Erythroblastosis and hyperbilirubinemia should be prevented by RhoGam or controlled by exchange transfusions. Mumps immunization should prevent unilateral deafness due to this cause. Congenital rubella should be prevented to some extent by the use of rubella vaccine.

Ototoxic drugs should be used with reluctance. Systemic neomycin, vancomycin, and dihydrostreptomycin are rarely if ever indicated. Kanamycin is a useful drug, but the dosage should be carefully monitored, especially when the patient has renal insufficiency.

Meningitis must be diagnosed and treated aggressively. Chronic serous otitis media and chronic perforation of the tympanic membrane require vigorous treatment to prevent long-term damage to hearing. Firecrackers or other fireworks that can cause deafness should be forbidden. High-decibel rock concerts carry some risk for the musicians involved. They should wear ear protectors that lower noise levels to the 100 dB level.

Treatment

Treatment of hearing deficit is mainly a problem for the audiologist. Children can be fitted with hearing aids as early as 1 month of age. Special technics for stimulation, visual communication, speech therapy, and early enrollment in school require the coordination of professionals specially trained in this field.

Bergstrom L & others: A high risk registry to find congenital deafness. Otolaryngol Clin North Am 4:369, 1971.

Downs M: Audiological evaluation of the congenitally deaf infant. Otolaryngol Clin North Am 4:347, 1971.

Downs MP, Silver HK: The "A.B.C.D.'s" to "H.E.A.R." Early identification in nursery, office, and clinic of the infant who is deaf. Clin Pediatr (Phila) 11:563, 1972.

Holm VA, Thompson G: Selective hearing loss: Clues to early identification. Pediatrics 47:447, 1971.

McMahon J & others: The Committee on Children with Handicaps: The physician and the deaf child. Pediatrics 51: 1100, 1973.

Northern JL, Downs MP: *Child Audiology.* Williams & Wilkins, 1974.

Rupp RR, Koch LJ: Effects of too loud music on human ears. Clin Pediatr (Phila) 8:60, 1969.

Rupp RR, Wolski W: Hearing testing in young children. Clin Pediatr (Phila) 8:263, 1969.

THE NOSE & PARANASAL SINUSES

ACUTE VIRAL RHINITIS
(Common Cold)

The common cold is the most frequent infectious disease of man, and the incidence is higher in early childhood than in any other period of life. Closely similar upper respiratory infections may be caused by perhaps 100 different viruses such as adenoviruses, influenza virus, parainfluenza virus, respiratory syncytial virus, coxsackieviruses, etc. Minor epidemics occur during the winter months and spread rapidly among susceptible people. The peak month (September) coincides with the opening of schools.

Clinical Findings

The patient usually experiences a sudden onset of clear or mucoid rhinorrhea plus a fever. Mild sore throat and cough also frequently develop. Although the fever is usually low-grade in older children, in the first 5 or 6 years of life it can be as high as 40.6° C (105° F). The nose and throat are usually inflamed. Several members of a family are often sick simultaneously.

Complications

Acute suppurative otitis media is the most common complication and is often heralded by return of fever or crying. Other complications due to superinfection are purulent rhinitis, purulent conjunctivitis, pneumonia, and pyogenic adenitis. Common nonpyrogenic complications are sinusitis, bronchitis, croup, and bronchiolitis.

Treatment

Treatment is largely symptomatic. Aspirin or acetaminophen is helpful for fever, sore throat, or muscle aches. A stuffy, congested nose can be treated with normal saline nosedrops, 3 drops in each nostril, in the supine position with the neck hyperextended. After several minutes, a soft rubber bulb syringe can be used to remove the secretions of the infant who cannot blow his nose. If this fails and the stuffy nose still interferes with feeding or sleep, phenylephrine (Neo-Synephrine), 0.125%, or xylometazoline (Otrivin), 0.05%, 2 drops every 4 hours as necessary, can be used in children under 2 years of age. Children over 2 years of age can use 0.25% phenylephrine drops. Drops should be discontinued after 1 week to prevent a rebound vasomotor rhinitis. If there is significant rhinorrhea, an antihistamine decongestant such as triprolidine-pseudoephedrine (Actifed) can be used; but it is of unproved value.

Antibiotics do not prevent superinfection and should not be used. Vaporizers and humidifiers have no proved value and should not be routinely prescribed, especially if the parents cannot easily afford them.

The prognosis is excellent. In the usual cold, the fever lasts for less than 3 days and the other symptoms persist for less than 1 week.

Douglas R: Pathogenesis of rhinovirus common colds in human volunteers. Ann Otol Rhinol Laryngol 79:563, 1970.

Lampert RP & others: A critical look at oral decongestants. Pediatrics 55:550, 1977.

West S & others: A review of antihistamines and the common cold. Pediatrics 56:100, 1975.

ACUTE PURULENT RHINITIS

A purulent nasal discharge that persists for several days usually represents bacterial superinfection of a common cold. Any discharge that is profusely purulent for 1 day or intermittently purulent for over 4 days should be treated. The common cold may also be associated with some mucopurulent discharge, but usually intermittently and worse upon awakening in the morning. The most likely organisms are pneumococcus, *Haemophilus influenzae,* beta-hemolytic streptococci, and *Staphylococcus aureus.* Rare causes are meningitis and syphilis.

Parents usually complain that their child's cold has become worse. Besides the finding of a purulent discharge, there are often adherent yellow crusts in the nares. The underlying nasal mucosa, if it is visible, is inflamed. Beta-hemolytic streptococcus is the most likely organism if there is crusting around the nares that resembles impetigo, redness of the skin below the nares, or a blistering distal dactylitis. Purulent material should be taken for culture and Gram staining before therapy is started.

Without treatment, this process can progress to acute otitis media, purulent sinusitis, pneumonitis, or even septicemia.

Oral penicillin for 5 days will cure most of these patients. If streptococci are cultured, the penicillin should be continued for 10 days. Occasionally, dicloxacillin or ampicillin will be needed because of culture results.

The purulent material should be removed as completely as possible with cotton-tipped applicators and a washcloth and soap. Bacitracin ointment should be applied, especially if nasal impetigo exists.

If the problem recurs after adequate treatment, the patient should be referred to an otolaryngologist to rule out the possibility of a foreign body. If the discharge is foul-smelling, this becomes especially likely. The response to treatment is excellent in the majority of cases.

Hays GC, Mullard JE: Can nasal bacterial flora be predicted from clinical findings? Pediatrics 49:596, 1972.

PERSISTENT RHINITIS IN NEWBORNS

Rhinorrhea or nasal congestion in a young infant may be due to various causes.

About half of newborns are obligate nasal breathers, and if the nose becomes congested they have difficulty with air exchange and may become irritable and dyspneic. The problem is worse during feeding because the baby's oral airway is then completely useless. These babies gradually learn to become mouth breathers as well as nasal breathers by age 5 or 6 months.

Differential Diagnosis & Treatment

A. Transient Idiopathic Stuffy Nose of the Newborn: Many babies have unexplained, transient (about 3 weeks) stuffy noses with mucoid or clear discharge that bubbles during feeding. The cause is not known. The diagnosis is made by exclusion. Normal saline nosedrops can be instilled and, after several minutes, removed with cotton-tipped applicators or gentle suction on a rubber bulb syringe. If the problem interferes

with feeding, this can be preceded by 2 drops of 0.125% phenylephrine (Neo-Synephrine) for several days.

B. Reserpine Side-Effects: If the mother is taking reserpine and the drug is in her blood at an effective level during labor, the newborn may have a profoundly stuffy nose. Treatment is as above.

C. Chemical Rhinitis: This may be due to overtreatment of idiopathic stuffy nose with topical vasoconstrictors. The irritative nosedrops should be discontinued. The patient can be helped with oral decongestants for 2 days.

D. Pyogenic Rhinitis: Babies with pyogenic rhinitis can have a clear or mucoid discharge rather than the purulent discharge seen in older children. The diagnosis is based on cultures of nasal discharge. Treatment is as outlined above.

E. Congenital Syphilis: The onset is usually before 6 weeks of age. The diagnosis is established by checking the serology done on the mother during the prenatal period. If other signs besides the nasal discharge exist, such as an unresponsive skin rash or hepatosplenomegaly, additional serologic testing should be performed on the baby. Treatment is discussed in Chapter 26.

F. Hypothyroidism: See Chapter 24.

G. Choanal Atresia: This occurs bilaterally in 25% of affected children and unilaterally in 75%. Bilateral cases can cause severe respiratory distress—even apnea at birth if the child is an absolute nasal breather. Both types eventually present with a chronic nasal discharge because the normal sinus and nasal secretions can escape only anteriorly. A No. 8 soft rubber catheter should be passed through the nose and visualized in the oropharynx. If this cannot be accomplished, a diagnosis of choanal atresia should be confirmed by radiographic study.

An oral airway should be placed immediately if the infant has bilateral choanal atresia. A dentist can fashion a comfortable airway to tide the patient over until mouth breathing is established. Feeding by syringe or medicine dropper is preferred. An otolaryngologist should decide on the optimal timing for definitive surgery, but it is usually 1 year of age.

H. Nasal Fracture Secondary to Birth Trauma: Physical examination should reveal subluxation of the nasal septum occluding the nasal passages. The infant should be referred to an otolaryngologist for reduction.

Connelly JP: Choanal atresia. Part I. Medical aspects of this serious anomaly. Clin Pediatr (Phila) 4:65, 1965.

RECURRENT RHINITIS IN THE OLDER CHILD

This problem is all too frequent in the office practice of pediatrics. A child is brought in with the chief complaint that he has "one cold after another," "constant colds," or, "He is always sick." Such a patient may be in the office on almost a weekly basis. Although the problem is frustrating, the differential diagnosis is rather simple.* Approximately two-thirds of these children have recurrent colds, and another one-third have allergic rhinitis.

Differential Diagnosis & Treatment

A. Common Cold: The most common cause of recurrent runny nose is repeated viral upper respiratory infections. The onset is usually after 6 months of age. The bouts of rhinorrhea are usually accompanied by fever. Cultures are negative for bacteria. There is some evidence for contagion within the family or peer group in most of these cases. The nasal mucosa during attacks is often inflamed.

The most common reason for presentation is that the parents are overly concerned because they do not understand that the average child has approximately 8 colds a year in the preschool period. Or the patient may be overly exposed to viruses because he has a sibling at school who brings home many pathogens or because he is frequently left with large numbers of children at a day care center or with a baby-sitter.

Treatment consists of specific reassurance and concerned follow-up. The parents can be told their child's general health is good, as evidenced by his adequate weight gain and robust activity level; that the prognosis is good in that he will not have this number of colds for more than a few years; that the body's exposure and response to colds is building up his antibody supply; and that this problem is not their fault and that they are doing a good job as parents.

B. Allergic Rhinitis: The onset of "hay fever" is usually after 2 years of age—after the child has had adequate exposure to allergens. There is no fever or contagion among close contacts. The attacks include frequent sneezing, rubbing of the nose, and a profuse clear discharge. The nasal turbinates are swollen. The nasal smear demonstrates over 20% of the cells to be eosinophils. Nasal secretions should be collected only when the patient is symptomatic. Between attacks or after receiving antihistamines, the eosinophil smear may be falsely negative.

Oral decongestants and antihistamines should be tried until the right drug and dosage are found to give the optimal effect. Avoidance (especially of pets) and environmental controls should be initiated. If the symptoms persist, the patient should be referred to an allergist for evaluation and possibly hyposensitization.

A full discussion of allergic rhinitis is found in Chapter 32.

C. Chemical Rhinitis: Prolonged use of vasoconstrictor nosedrops beyond 7 days results in a rebound

reaction and secondary nasal congestion. The offending nosedrops should be discontinued.

D. Vasomotor Rhinitis: Some children react to sudden changes in environmental temperature with prolonged congestion and rhinorrhea. Air pollution may be a factor. Oral decongestants can be used periodically to give symptomatic relief.

Complications

Because this problem is such a nuisance, iatrogenic overtreatment is the most common complication.

Giving human gamma globulin injections is the most common error made in this disorder. The injections may be initiated without determining the serum IgG level or as a consequence of misinterpreting the results by comparing them with adult levels rather than with norms for age. Many studies show that human gamma globulin injections do not benefit patients with frequent upper respiratory infections. In addition to being painful and expensive, they may cause anaphylaxis or isoimmunization. Other worthless approaches to this problem include bacterial vaccines, prophylactic antibiotics, and tonsillectomy and adenoidectomy. The effectiveness of high doses of vitamin C in reducing the symptoms and duration of colds is promising but still controversial. Patients are not infrequently kept home from school, trips, athletic practices, parties, etc with little indication. As long as they do not have a fever or severe symptoms, they can attend these functions. They should be given suitable medications for symptomatic relief of mild symptoms so that they can participate normally in these important events of childhood. The risk to other children is almost irrelevant because these infections are contagious even during the incubation period and the best time to have them and develop immunity is during childhood.

Coulehan JL & others: Vitamin C prophylaxis in a boarding school. N Engl J Med 290:6, 1974.

McCammon RW: Natural history of respiratory tract infection patterns in basically healthy individuals. Am J Dis Child 122:232, 1971.

Miller DL & others: Allergic diseases of the nose and middle ear in children. Pediatr Ann 5:482, 1976.

MOUTH BREATHING SECONDARY TO NASAL OBSTRUCTION

A child is sometimes brought in with the complaint that, "He always breathes through his mouth," "He snores," etc. With the mouth covered, each nostril should be tested individually for patency. One or both nostrils may be so severely occluded that adequate air exchange cannot occur. Even when the nasal passages are not completely occluded, the patient may prefer to breathe through the mouth because it is more comfortable. With complete obstruction, a constant nasal discharge ensues because the normal sinus and nasal secretions can escape only anteriorly.

Note: An excessively ordered test is serum immunoelectrophoresis. Children with immune defects do not have an increased number of colds. Therefore, immunoglobulin tests are worthless unless the patient suffers from recurrent pneumonia, recurrent sinusitis, or recurrent adenitis.

Differential Diagnosis

A. Large Adenoids: Large adenoids can be suspected if the soft palate is depressed or has limited elevation, the patient has hypernasal speech, or possibly if the tonsils are huge. They can be diagnosed more precisely by digital palpation or by lateral soft tissue films of the nasopharynx.

B. Nasal Polyps: Polyps appear as glistening, gray to pink, jelly-like masses that are prominent just inside the anterior nares and occur singly or in clusters. They are most common in severe allergic rhinitis. They also occur in cystic fibrosis. One must be careful not to mistake the turbinates for polyps.

C. Other Causes: Persistent mouth breathing may be due to obstruction by nasopharyngeal tumor, meningocele or encephalocele herniated into the nasal cavity, or any of the disorders listed above under recurrent rhinitis which have become persistent.

Complications

Most children with prolonged mouth breathing eventually develop dental malocclusion and what has been termed an adenoidal facies. The face is pinched and narrow in appearance because normal maxillary bone development is not stimulated. If nasopharyngeal tumors, meningoceles, or encephaloceles are not diagnosed early, they can cause considerable destruction or may even become incurable.

Treatment

All patients with documented mouth breathing should be referred to an otolaryngologist for definitive evaluation and treatment. Polyps should never be removed until a meningocele has been ruled out.

Brown G: Nasal polyposis. Postgrad Med J 45:680, 1969.

ACUTE SINUSITIS

Essentials of Diagnosis

- Facial pain.
- Percussion tenderness over the sinuses.
- Postnasal drip.
- Nasal secretions induced by sniffing.

General Considerations

Sinusitis occurs when the sinus ostia are occluded and the sinus secretions accumulate. If the obstruction is intermittent, the sinus secretions drain periodically. The most common cause is the common cold, which results in edema and obstruction of the sinus ostia. In most cases, there is no superinfection of the sinus secretions because the posterior two-thirds of the nose are normally sterile. In cases in which superinfection occurs, the organisms are pneumococci, *Staphylococcus aureus, Haemophilus influenzae,* and beta-hemolytic streptococci.

The ethmoid sinus is the only one that is significantly developed at birth. The maxillary sinus is rudimentary at birth and visible on x-ray by 6 months. The frontal sinus is not visible until 3—9 years of age. Clinical ethmoiditis does not usually occur until 1 year of age. About half of cases occur between 1 and 5 years of age, during which time the most common sign is orbital cellulitis. Maxillary sinusitis is not usually seen clinically before 6 years of age. Frontal sinusitis is unusual before 10 years of age.

Clinical Findings

A. Symptoms and Signs: The most common finding is a sense of fullness or facial pain overlying the involved sinus. Ethmoiditis causes retro-orbital pain; maxillary sinusitis causes upper molar or zygomatic pain; and frontal sinusitis causes pain above the eyebrow. The patient usually also complains of an intermittent, profuse discharge persisting after resolution of the upper respiratory infections and may complain of a postnasal drip on swallowing.

Physical examination reveals percussion tenderness overlying the sinusitis. In ethmoiditis, the tenderness is elicited by pressing medially on the inner canthus of the eye. Tenderness of the eyeball may also be present. Maxillary sinusitis reveals percussion tenderness over the maxillary bone. Frontal sinusitis reveals tenderness when pressing upward on the floor of the supraorbital ridge. If the sinus is partially open, a convincing piece of evidence for the presence of retained sinus secretions is the reaccumulation of nasal secretions every time the patient sniffs or the drainage is aspirated. This finding can be accentuated by the introduction of a vasoconstrictor. The oropharynx reveals a purulent discharge after each swallow. Fever is occasionally present. Transillumination of the sinuses is difficult to perform and not very helpful. In those cases in which the sinuses are superinfected, fever and purulent rhinitis are usually present.

B. Laboratory Findings: A culture of fresh discharge is obtained by blowing the nose. If the patient is hospitalized because of complications, a blood culture should be obtained.

C. X-Ray Findings: In most cases, the clinical findings are so classic that x-rays are not needed. If the diagnosis is unclear, sinus films should be obtained. Positive films will show clouding of the involved sinuses or air-fluid levels if the obstruction is intermittent. It is notable that x-ray findings positive for sinusitis may be found in asymptomatic patients with colds or nasal allergies. Sinus x-rays are mainly indicated in children with facial swelling of unknown cause or with severe acute sinusitis, to document the degree of destructive bony changes—or in children with chronic or recurrent sinusitis.

Differential Diagnosis

In the infant, acute ethmoiditis may go undiagnosed for several days with a fever of unknown origin. Recognition occurs when overlying redness appears. In older children, the main diagnostic problem is confusion with headaches due to other causes. An uncommon cause of maxillary sinusitis is extension of a peri-apical abscess of an upper molar.

Complications

Untreated ethmoiditis not uncommonly presents as an abscess of the inner canthus or a periorbital abscess. Occasionally, this can progress to a retro-orbital abscess or even cavernous sinus thrombosis, which has a dire prognosis. The most common compli-cation of frontal sinusitis is osteomyelitis of the frontal bone. The most common maxillary complication is cel-lulitis of the cheek. Other possible complications are meningitis and frontal lobe abscess.

Treatment

A. Specific Measures:

1. Topical decongestants—The key to good thera-peutic results in most cases of sinusitis without super-infection is adequate drainage of the sinus.

The child can initially attempt to open the ostia by inhaling steam. This can be accomplished by breath-ing the vapors coming from a basin of very hot water while a towel is placed around the head like a tent.

The application of 0.25% phenylephrine (Neo-Synephrine) nosedrops every 4 hours can often induce adequate drainage. The nose should first be cleared by sniffing in the older child or by using a nasal aspirator for infants. The nosedrops must be delivered to the sinus ostia. The correct position for the child to be in when the nosedrops are placed is with the head low and turned slightly toward one side. A nasal spray does not provide adequate delivery of the medication. This medication cannot be used for more than 7 days because of the risk of rebound edema.

2. Oral decongestants—Systemic decongestants combined with antihistamines (eg, Actifed, Dimetapp) provide an added measure of relief for closed ostia. These are especially helpful for patients with under-lying allergies. They should be continued for 2 days after symptoms have subsided.

3. Oral antibiotics—In those occasional cases where superinfection is confirmed, ampicillin should be added to the treatment regimen in a dosage of 75 mg/kg/day orally for 1 week.

4. Treatment of complications—Patients with evi-dence of invasive infection or any of the complications listed above should be immediately hospitalized. Intra-venous ampicillin and methacillin should be initiated until culture results become available.

B. General Measures:
A patient will often need aspirin or even codeine temporarily to permit sleep until drainage of the obstructed sinus is achieved. The application of ice over the sinus may help to relieve pain.

Dryness of the mucous membranes—as occurs in many overheated homes in the winter if adequate humidification is not provided—can contribute to the obstruction. A humidifier in the patient's room and periodic warm showers may be of value. A child with sinusitis can be permitted to swim. Diving should be temporarily restricted unless noseplugs are used.

C. Surgical Treatment:

1. Lavage of the sinuses—If the patient has inca-pacitating initial pain or persistence of significant pain beyond several days, he should be referred to an otolaryngologist for lavage of the involved sinus.

2. External drainage—In complicated cases admit-ted to the hospital, ENT consultation should always be obtained. Although it is controversial, some feel that external drainage of the abscess is as important as anti-biotic therapy.

D. Follow-Up Care:
The patient should be seen at least once a week after treatment has been started. If the drainage has become purulent, a sample should be taken for culture and the patient started on antibiotics. If the sinusitis is unresponsive but considered sterile, the patient should be referred to an otolaryngologist for lavage and other measures.

Prognosis

Acute sinusitis is usually a mild, self-limited dis-ease which lasts for less than 1 week. Therapy as out-lined above usually provides partial to complete relief of symptoms during that week.

Evans FO Jr & others: Sinusitis of the maxillary antrum. N Engl J Med 293:735, 1975.

Haynes RE, Cramblett HG: Acute ethmoiditis: Its relationship to orbital cellulitis. Am J Dis Child 114:261, 1967.

Kogutt MS, Swischuk LE: Diagnosis of sinusitis in infants and children. Pediatrics 52:121, 1973.

McLean DC: Sinusitis in children. Clin Pediatr (Phila) 9:342, 1970.

Smith CH: Sinusitis in children: A simple diagnostic test. Clin Pediatr (Phila) 3:489, 1964.

RECURRENT SINUSITIS

Frequent episodes of sinusitis occur in a small group of patients. The most common cause is allergic rhinitis. The second most common cause—especially of frontal sinusitis—is diving or jumping into water feet first. The remaining cases are caused by pressure against the ostia by a septal deviation, nasal malforma-tion, a polyp, or a foreign body. In cases of recurrent pyogenic pansinusitis, poor host resistance (eg, an im-mune defect or cystic fibrosis) must be ruled out by immunoglobulins and a sweat chloride test. If allergies and diving do not offer a sufficient explanation of the problem, the patient should be referred to an otolaryn-gologist for complete evaluation.

Davison F: Chronic sinusitis and infectious asthma. Arch Otolaryngol 90:202, 1969.

Jaffe BF: Chronic sinusitis in children. Clin Pediatr (Phila) 13:944, 1974.

RECURRENT EPISTAXIS

Most children have a few isolated nosebleeds, but recurrent nosebleed usually warrants a visit to the pediatrician. The nose is a very vascular structure. In most cases, epistaxis is due to mild trauma to the anterior portion of the nasal septum (Kiesselbach's area), sometimes as a result of falls or fistfights but usually due to vigorous rubbing, noseblowing, or nosepicking.

Clinical Findings

A. Symptoms and Signs: The frequency of nosebleeds may be once a month to several times a day. If they are profuse, subsequent hematemesis or tarry stools may be reported. Examination of Kiesselbach's area reveals a red, raw surface with fresh clots or old crusts. There will often be blood under the fingernails.

B. Laboratory Findings: A baseline hematocrit is indicated in most patients. The true degree of anemia following a severe nosebleed may not be evident until 6–12 hours after bleeding has ceased.

Most patients do not need a bleeding work-up, but bleeding tests are indicated if any of the following are present: a family history of a bleeding disorder, a past medical history of easy bleeding, bleeding at other sites, bleeding that lasts for over 20 minutes or will not clot with the usual therapy, onset before age 2, or a drop in the hematocrit due to epistaxis.

Differential Diagnosis

Although most cases of epistaxis occur following trauma to the normal nose, several contributing factors must be ruled out. If they are present, specific treatment will be needed.

A. Allergic Rhinitis: Boggy, inflamed mucosa is predisposed to epistaxis. This diagnosis is confirmed by a nasal smear for eosinophils. In such a case, antihistamines may help to decrease the amount of nasal pruritus and subsequent rubbing.

B. Chronic Bleeding Disorder: Numerous bleeding disorders (eg, von Willebrand's disease, thrombocytopenia) may present as recurrent epistaxis. A history of easy bleeding with circumcision, tonsillectomy, lacerations, venipuncture, or tooth eruption points to this type of disorder. A family history of hemophilia or other bleeding tendencies is suggestive. A history of spontaneous bleeding at other sites—gastrointestinal tract, hemarthrosis, menorrhagia, petechiae with crying, etc—or current physical findings of bleeding at other sites is suggestive. The presence of hepatomegaly or splenomegaly is also suggestive. These patients require bleeding screens.

C. Aspirin: Recent studies reveal that ingestion of normal doses of aspirin can interfere with platelet aggregation or adhesiveness, so that prolonged bleeding can result. The abnormal bleeding time is confirmatory.

D. Vascular Malformation: Kiesselbach's area must be carefully examined for telangectasia, hemangiomas, or varicosities.

E. Hypertension: High blood pressure may predispose to prolonged nosebleeds.

F. Nasopharyngeal Angiofibroma: This tumor of adolescent males often presents with epistaxis. Bleeding confined to the back of the throat makes the elimination of this diagnosis mandatory. Lateral soft tissue films of the nasopharynx are diagnostic.

Complications

Unless an underlying bleeding disorder exists, the only complication of nosebleed is mild anemia. The latter is unusual and responds to iron therapy.

Treatment

A. Immediate Treatment: This approach can be carried out in the office or given as phone advice. The patient should sit up and lean forward so that he does not swallow the blood. The nose is pinched, with pressure over the bleeding site being maintained for 10 minutes by the clock. If bleeding continues, pressure is not being applied to the right spot, and it should be changed.

If this is not effective, clots should be removed by suction or blowing the nose. A pledget wet with 0.25% phenylephrine (Neo-Synephrine) nosedrops, 1% lidocaine (Xylocaine) with 1:1,000 epinephrine—or the most potent topical vasoconstrictor of all, 1% cocaine—is inserted into the nose. Pressure is again applied for 10 minutes. Rarely does this technic fail.

A different approach involves the insertion of a small piece of gelatin sponge (Gelfoam) or topical thrombin over the bleeding site. The insertion of a wedge of salt pork into the bleeding nostril is still another approach.

B. Preventive Treatment: The friability of the nasal vessels can be decreased with daily application of petrolatum by cotton-tipped applicator. Conjugated estrogen (Premarin) cream has also been advocated (by Chanin) for this purpose. The lubricants are applied daily until 5 days have passed without a nosebleed, then weekly for 1 month, and are resumed only if the nosebleeds recur. In a very dry environment, humidification of the patient's room may be helpful. Aspirin should be avoided.

C. Reassurance: Parents need reassurance regarding the amount of blood lost. It always looks like more than it actually is. A normal hematocrit is usually comforting to the parents. The child should not be blamed regarding this problem. The parents should be told that simply rubbing a dry nose can cause nosebleeds.

D. Unwarranted Treatment: Electrocautery is contraindicated because it is painful and frightening to the child. Both electrocautery and chemical cautery can cause destruction of the septal tissue, resulting in scarring and an increased tendency for later bleeding.

Prognosis

Once home treatment and prophylaxis are mastered, nosebleeds become an insignificant problem for most families. In unusual cases where posterior bleeding occurs, the child must be referred to an otolaryn-

gologist for a posterior pack, evaluation for nasopharyngeal lesions, and possibly a transfusion.

Chanin A: Prevention of recurrent nosebleeds in children. Clin
     Pediatr (Phila) 11:684, 1972.
Hathaway WE: Bleeding disorders due to platelet dysfunction.
     Am J Dis Child 121:127, 1971.
Simonton K: The emergency treatment of nosebleed. J Okla
     State Med Assoc 62:135, 1969.

NASAL FURUNCLE

A nasal furuncle is an infection of a hair follicle in
the anterior nares. Hair plucking or nosepicking can
provide a route of entry. The most common organism
is *Staphylococcus aureus.* The diagnosis is made by
finding an exquisitely tender, firm, red lump in the
anterior naris. Treatment includes dicloxacillin, 50
mg/kg/day orally for 5 days. The lesion should be
gently incised and drained as soon as it points, usually
with a needle. Topical bacitracin ointment may be of
additional value. Since this lesion is in the drainage
area of the cavernous sinus, the patient should be followed closely until healing is complete. Parents should
be advised never to pick or squeeze a furuncle in this
location, nor should the physician. Associated cellulitis
or spread requires hospitalization for intravenous antibiotics.

Some patients with recurrent skin abscesses as
well as nasal furuncles are nasal carriers of *S aureus.*
Resolution of the skin problem will often be unsuccessful until the nasal carrier state is eradicated by
systemic antibiotics, topical antibiotics, and recoloni-
zation of the nasal mucosa with a nonpathogenic
staphylococcus.

Fine RN & others: Bacterial interference in treatment of recur-
     rent staphylococcic infections in a family. J Pediatr
     70:548, 1967.

NASAL SEPTUM SUBLUXATION

About 5% of newborn infants have a subluxation
of the quadrangular cartilage of the septum. The tip of
the nose deviates to one side, and the inferior septal
border deviates to the other. There is also leaning of
the columella and instability of the nasal tip. In the
delivery room, reduction should be accomplished by
lifting up the inferior border of the septum and replacing it in the septal groove of the floor of the nose. If
any question regarding the procedure exists, an otolaryngologist should be consulted. This disorder must be
distinguished from the more common transient flattening of the nose caused by the birth process.

Jazbi B: Nasal septum deformity in the newborn. Clin Pediatr
     (Phila) 13:953, 1974.

Silverman SH & others: Dislocation of the triangular cartilage of
     the nasal septum. J Pediatr 87:456, 1975.

NASAL FRACTURE

Most blows to the nose result in swelling and
hematoma without a fracture. A persistent nosebleed
after trauma suggests nasal fracture. Crepitus or instability of the nasal bones is diagnostic of fracture, as is
marked deviation of the nose to one side. If the parents feel that the appearance of the nose has changed 3
days after injury when the edema has resolved, this
should be taken as strong evidence for fracture. X-rays
are not usually helpful since they are negative in half
of fractures.

Patients with suspected nasal fracture should be
referred to an otolaryngologist for definitive therapy.
In general, x-rays are warranted only in the patients
who have clinical suggestion of a fracture.

Goode RL, Spooner TR: Management of nasal fractures in
     children. Clin Pediatr (Phila) 11:526, 1972.
Hadley R: Nasal injuries in children. NY State J Med 69:281,
     1969.

NASAL SEPTUM HEMATOMA

After nasal trauma, it is essential to examine the
inside of the nose with a nasal speculum. Hematoma of
the nasal septum imposes a considerable risk of pressure necrosis and resorption of the cartilage, leading to
septal perforation or a saddle-back nose in adulthood.
This diagnosis is confirmed by the abrupt onset of
nasal obstruction following trauma and the presence of
a widened nasal septum.

Treatment consists of prompt referral to an otolaryngologist for evacuation of the hematoma and
packing of the nose.

NASAL SEPTUM ABSCESS

A nasal septal abscess usually follows nasal trauma or a nasal furuncle. The symptoms include fever,
nasal tenderness, and nasal occlusion. Physical findings
reveal a fluctuant gray septal swelling, usually bilateral.
The possible complications are the same as for nasal
septal hematoma plus septicemia, meningitis, or cavernous sinus thrombosis.

Treatment consists of immediate hospitalization,
incision and drainage by an otolaryngologist, and intravenous antibiotics.

Segal S & others: Bacterial meningitis secondary to abscess of
     the nasal septum. Pediatrics 60:102, 1977.

FOREIGN BODIES OF THE NOSE

Most objects inserted into the nose are detected by the parent soon after insertion, and the child is brought in acutely. Occasionally, a nasal foreign body is detected only after purulent rhinitis occurs. To prepare for removal, the nose should be suctioned and opened fully with a topical vasoconstrictor. The child's head should be held firmly to prevent movement and secondary injury during the removal. The position of the head should be forward to prevent aspiration of the foreign body into a bronchus. A nasal speculum is sometimes helpful.

There are many ways to remove nasal foreign bodies. The obvious first maneuver is to have the child blow his nose vigorously if he is old enough. If the object is round, such as a bead, collodion on a cotton-tipped applicator can be placed against it and left there for 1 or 2 minutes, after which it will usually be dry enough to remove the object. Irregular objects can sometimes be grasped with a bayonet forceps. If there is room to go past the object, a right-angled hook can be inserted and withdrawn, pushing the object ahead of it. If these technics are not successful and there is some space between the object and the side of the nose, a lubricated No. 8 Bardex Foley catheter can be inserted. When the balloon is past the object, it can be inflated and then used to extract the object.

With the head tilted over a large basin, the noninvolved nostril can be flushed rapidly with normal saline from a nasal bulb syringe. The fluid will wash around to the involved side and in most cases will force the object out. Closing the uninvolved nostril and placing one's mouth over the patient's mouth to administer a sudden blast of air will force the foreign body out if enough pressure is exerted. If the object seems inaccessible, is wedged in, or is quite large, the patient should be referred to an otolaryngologist without worsening its position through futile attempts.

Goff WE: "Tip of the Month." Consultant 13(1):144, 1973.
Rees AC: "Tip of the Month." Consultant 10(2):12, 1970.
Stool SE, McConnell CS: Foreign bodies in pediatric otolaryngology. Clin Pediatr (Phila) 12:113, 1973.

THE THROAT

ACUTE STOMATITIS

Recurrent Aphthous Stomatitis ("Canker Sore")

The main finding is multiple small, very painful ulcers on the inside of the lips and throughout the remainder of the mouth. There is usually no associated fever or cervical adenopathy. The ulcers last 1–2 weeks. They may recur numerous times throughout a patient's life span. The cause is not known, although an allergic or autoimmune basis is suspected. It is important to rule out any offending agents that could be avoided (chocolate, tomatoes, etc). These lesions are commonly misdiagnosed as herpes simplex.

Treatment consists of topical corticosteroids, either in a dental paste—eg, triamcinolone acetonide, 0.1% (Kenalog in Orabase)—or in a mouthwash administered 4 times a day. Pain can be symptomatically improved by a bland diet, avoiding salty or acid foods, switching from a bottle to a cup in infants, 2% viscous lidocaine (Xylocaine) prior to meals, and aspirin or even codeine at bedtime. Measures that are unwarranted and sometimes harmful are smallpox vaccine, systemic antibiotics, lactobacillus-containing agents, and astringents.

Herpes Simplex Gingivostomatitis

Approximately 1% of children who have their first encounter with the herpes simplex organism develop multiple small ulcers of the buccal mucosa, anterior pillars, inner lips, tongue, and especially the gingiva, with associated fever, tender cervical nodes, and generalized inflammation of the mouth. This disorder lasts 7–10 days. The symptoms interfere mainly with eating and drinking. The primary disorder does not recur; herpes simplex recurs only in the form of cold sores which are found mainly at the labial mucocutaneous juncture. A throat culture is recommended to rule out streptococcal infection and a white blood count to rule out agranulocytic mucosal lesions.

Treatment is symptomatic as described for Recurrent Aphthous Stomatitis (above), with the exception that corticosteroids are contraindicated because they may result in spread of the infection. The patient must be followed closely. Dehydration occasionally ensues despite liberal offerings of cold fluids, in which case the patient must be hospitalized so that intravenous fluids can be administered. Herpetic laryngotracheitis is a rare complication.

Stevens-Johnson Syndrome

The bullous form of erythema multiforme should be considered whenever there are vesicles and ulcers of the lips and oral mucosa with similar lesions on the conjunctiva and genitalia. In addition, most of these patients have a generalized erythema multiforme rash plus high fever and severe prostration. (For full discussion, see p 210.)

Thrush of Mouth

Oral candidiasis mainly affects babies who are being bottle-fed and occasionally older children who are in a debilitated state. *Candida albicans* is a saprophyte that normally is not invasive unless the mouth is abraded. The use of broad spectrum antibiotics may be a contributing factor. The symptoms include soreness of the mouth and refusal of feedings. Lesions consist of white curdlike plaques predominantly on the buccal mucosa. These plaques cannot be washed away after a water feeding.

Specific treatment consists of use of nystatin (Mycostatin) oral suspension, 1 ml 4 times a day for 1 week. This should be preceded by attempts to remove any large plaques with a moistened cotton-tipped applicator. The child should be fed temporarily with a spoon and cup to eliminate the pain, continued abrasion, and possible contamination from nipple feedings.

Oral Syphilis

The primary chancre can occur on the lips or in the oral cavity. Secondary syphilis can present as mucous patches on any part of the oral cavity. These have a gray, slimy, concentric appearance and can occur in various sizes. Both of these lesions can be diagnosed by darkfield examination. By the time mucous patches are present, the serologic test for syphilis will be positive. Syphilis is discussed more fully in Chapter 26.

Traumatic Oral Ulcers

Ulcers are a nonspecific response of the oral mucosa to trauma. Mechanical trauma most commonly occurs on the buccal mucosa secondary to accidentally biting it with the molars. Thermal trauma such as can occur from eating very hot foods can also cause ulcerative lesions. Chemical ulcers can be produced by mucosal contact with aspirin, caustics, etc. These lesions usually need no treatment. The pain subsides in 2 or 3 days.

Burket LW: Oral lesions: Local or systemic? Consultant 12 (8):45, 1972.

Cohen L: Chronic oral ulceration. J Oral Med 25:7, 1970.

Fermaglich DR, Fermaglich LF: Tracheostomy in primary herpetic gingivostomatitis. J Pediatr 82:884, 1973.

Samitz MH, Weinberg RA: Recurrent aphthous stomatitis. Postgrad Med 39:221, 1966.

ACUTE VIRAL PHARYNGITIS & TONSILLITIS

Over 90% of cases of sore throat and fever in children are due to viral infections. Most children develop associated rhinorrhea and mild cough and in fact are having a cold and nothing more. The findings seldom give any clue to the particular viral agent, but 6 types of viral pharyngitis are sufficiently different to permit the clinician to make an educated guess about the specific cause.

Clinical Findings

A. Infectious Mononucleosis: The findings are an exudative tonsillitis, generalized cervical adenitis, and fever, usually in a teenage patient. A palpable spleen or axillary adenopathy adds weight to the diagnosis. The presence of more than 20% atypical lymphocytes on a peripheral blood smear or a positive mononucleosis spot test confirms the diagnosis. This diagnosis is often not considered until a patient with a presumptive diagnosis of streptococcal pharyngitis has failed to respond to 48 hours of treatment with penicillin.

B. Herpangina: Herpangina ulcers are found on the anterior pillars and sometimes on the soft palate and uvula. There are no ulcers in the anterior mouth as seen in herpes simplex. Fever is present. The disease lasts up to a week. Herpangina is caused by several members' of the Coxsackie A group of viruses, and a patient can have up to 5 bouts of herpangina in his lifetime.

C. Lymphonodular Pharyngitis: (Coxsackie A10.) The classic finding is small, yellow-white nodules in the same distribution as the small ulcers in herpangina. In this condition, the nodules do not ulcerate.

D. Hand, Foot, and Mouth Disease: This entity is caused by Coxsackie A5, A10, and A16. Ulcers occur on the tongue and oral mucosa. Vesicles, which usually do not ulcerate, are found on the palms, soles, and interdigital areas.

E. Pharyngoconjunctival Fever: This disorder is caused by an adenovirus. Exudative tonsillitis, conjunctivitis, and fever are the main findings.

F. Rubeola: The prodrome of measles looks like any nonspecific viral respiratory infection until one closely examines the buccal mucosa and the inner aspects of the lower lip. Small white specks the size of salt granules on an erythematous base (Koplik's spots) found at these sites are pathognomonic of measles.

Treatment

The treatment of acute viral pharyngitis is strictly symptomatic. Older children can gargle with warm hypertonic salt solution. Younger children can suck on hard candy (especially butterscotch). Analgesics and antipyretics are sometimes helpful. Antibiotics are contraindicated.

Alpert JJ & others: Failure to isolate streptococci from children under age 3 with exudative tonsillitis. Pediatrics 38:633, 1966.

Moffet HL & others: Nonstreptococcal pharyngitis. J Pediatr 73:51, 1968.

ACUTE STREPTOCOCCAL PHARYNGITIS & TONSILLITIS

Approximately 10% of children with sore throat and fever have a streptococcal infection. Untreated streptococcal pharyngitis can result in acute rheumatic fever, glomerulonephritis, and suppurative complications (eg, cervical adenitis, peritonsillar abscess, otitis media, cellulitis, and septicemia). Whereas vesicles and ulcers are suggestive of viral infection, and petechiae and a tonsillar exudate are suggestive of streptococcal infection, the only way to make a definitive diagnosis is by obtaining a throat culture. A throat culture can be read 18 hours after being placed in an incubator. The bacteriology involved is simple, and an inexpensive office incubator is available. Office throat cultures are essential to the rational treatment of pharyngitis. A fuller discussion of the diagnosis and treatment of streptococcal infections is found in Chapter 26.

Battle CU, Glasgow LA: Reliability of bacteriologic identification of β-hemolytic streptococci in private offices. Am J Dis Child 122:134, 1971.

Breese BB: Culturing beta-hemolytic streptococci in pediatric practice. J Pediatr 75:164, 1969.

Hable KA & others: Bacterial and viral throat flora. Clin Pediatr (Phila) 10:199, 1971.

Sprunt K & others: Identification of *Streptococcus pyogenes* in a pediatric outpatient department. Pediatrics 54:718, 1974.

RECURRENT PHARYNGITIS

School-age children are occasionally brought to a physician with a complaint of recurrent or persistent sore throat. Fever and other systemic manifestations are usually absent. There are 3 common causes of this problem.

Mouth breathing leads to dryness and irritation of the throat, especially in areas of low humidity. Occasionally, a child will even complain upon awakening that his lips are stuck to his teeth. The causes of mouth breathing (see p 254) should be investigated. Symptomatic treatment consists of good hydration and environmental humidification.

Postnasal drip due to chronic sinusitis can lead to continuous irritation of the throat. Examination reveals mucopurulent secretions descending from the nasopharynx after the patient sniffs. The irritation is largely due to repeated clearing of the throat. Treatment is described on p 256.

School phobia. These children are brought in repeatedly for sore throats, but physical examination reveals a normal oropharynx and tonsillar area. The diagnosis is made by asking the parent if the problem has been interfering with the child's school attendance. The answer will be affirmative and completely out of keeping with the degree of symptoms. Management is described in Chapter 23.

PERITONSILLAR ABSCESS
(Quinsy)

Tonsillar infection occasionally penetrates the tonsillar capsule and spreads to the surrounding tissues. If untreated, necrosis occurs and a tonsillar abscess forms. This can occur at any age. The most common cause is the beta-hemolytic streptococcus.

The patient complains of a severe sore throat even before the physical findings become marked. A high fever is usually present. The process is almost always unilateral. The soft palate and uvula on the involved side are edematous and displaced forward toward the uninvolved side. In severe cases there is trismus, dysphagia, and finally drooling. The quality of the voice is severely impaired by the fixation of the soft palate. A serious complication of inadequately treated peritonsillar abscess is a lateral pharyngeal abscess. This leads to' fullness and tenderness of the lateral neck. Without intervention, the lateral pharyngeal abscess eventually threatens life by airway obstruction or carotid artery erosion.

Aggressive treatment in early cases of peritonsillar abscess will usually abort the process and prevent suppuration. The drug of choice is procaine penicillin by daily injection plus oral penicillin 4 times a day in high doses. Daily follow-up is critical to detect the case that has progressed to an abscess. If the initial swelling is marked, if fluctuation develops, or if symptoms fail to respond to 48 hours of antibiotics, the patient should be hospitalized. An otolaryngologist should be consulted to perform incision and drainage. A needle is introduced into the abscess to locate the space, and the incision is then made along the needle shaft. This procedure should be done with the patient's head in a lowered position to prevent aspiration of the purulent drainage. Material should be taken for culture. Recurrent peritonsillar abscesses are so uncommon that routine tonsillectomy for a single bout is not indicated.

Rubinstein E & others: Peritonsillar infection and bacteremia caused by *Fusobacterium gonidiaformans*. J Pediatr 85: 673, 1974.

RETROPHARYNGEAL ABSCESS

Retropharyngeal nodes drain the adenoids and nasopharynx and can become infected. The most common organism is the beta-hemolytic streptococcus. If this pyogenic adenitis goes untreated, a retropharyngeal abscess forms. The process occurs almost exclusively during the first 2 years of life. Beyond this age, retropharyngeal abscess usually results from superinfection of a penetrating injury of the posterior wall of the oropharynx.

The diagnosis should be strongly suspected in an infant with fever, respiratory symptoms, and neck hyperextension. Dysphagia, dyspnea, and gurgling respirations are also found and are due to the impingement by the abscess. Prominent swelling on one side of the posterior pharyngeal wall confirms the diagnosis. Swelling usually stops at the midline because a medial raphe divides the prevertebral space. Lateral neck soft tissue films provide additional confirmation if needed.

Retropharyngeal abscess is a surgical emergency. Immediate hospitalization is required. A surgeon should incise and drain the abscess to prevent its extension. The head should be kept down during incision to prevent aspiration of purulent material. Intravenous hydration and antibiotics should be instituted before surgery. Penicillin is the drug of choice pending the results of stained smear examination.

Janecka IP, Rankow RM: Fatal mediastinitis following retropharyngeal abscess. Arch Otolaryngol 93:630, 1971.

Wright NL: Cervical infections. Am J Surg 113:379, 1967.

LUDWIG'S ANGINA

Ludwig's angina is a rapidly progressive cellulitis of the submandibular space. The submandibular space extends from the mucous membrane of the tongue to the muscular and fascial attachments of the hyoid bone. The initiating factor in over half of cases is dental disease, including abscesses and extraction. Some patients have a history of lacerations and injuries to the floor of the mouth. The most common organism is the group A streptococcus, but other pathogens have been recovered.

The presenting symptoms are fever and a prominent swelling of the tongue. The tongue is not only enlarged but also commonly tender and erythematous. Upward displacement of the tongue may cause dysphagia and drooling. Laboratory evaluation includes blood cultures and hypopharyngeal aspiration to attempt to identify the specific pathogen.

Treatment consists of giving high dosages of intravenous ampicillin and methacillin until the results of cultures and sensitivity tests are available. Since the most common cause of death in Ludwig's angina is sudden airway obstruction, the patient must be followed closely in the intensive care unit and intubation provided for any progressive respiratory distress.

Barkin RM & others: Ludwig angina in children. J Pediatr 87:563, 1975.

Gross SJ & others: Ludwig angina in childhood. Am J Dis Child 131:291, 1977.

ACUTE CERVICAL ADENITIS

Essentials of Diagnosis

- Large, tender, unilateral cervical mass.
- Fever.
- Moderate to marked leukocytosis.

General Considerations

Local infections of the ear, nose, and throat can spread to the regional node and cause a secondary inflammation there. The most commonly involved node is the jugulodigastric node, which drains the tonsillar area. The problem is most prevalent among preschool children.

A classic case involves a large, unilateral, solitary, tender node. About 70% of these cases are due to beta-hemolytic streptococci, 20% are due to staphylococci, and the remainder may be due to viruses. Surgeons report a higher incidence of staphylococcal infection, but they see a greater proportion of atypical cases that have failed to respond to penicillin therapy or those that require incision and drainage.

The most common site of invasion is from pharyngitis or tonsillitis. Other entry sites for pyogenic adenitis are periapical dental abscess (usually producing a submandibular adenitis), impetigo of the face, infected acne, or otitis externa (usually producing a preauricular adenitis).

Clinical Findings

A. Symptoms and Signs: The patient is brought in with the chief complaint of a swollen neck or face. He usually has a sustained high fever, especially in staphylococcal infections. The mass is often the size of a walnut or even an egg. It is taut, firm, and exquisitely tender. If left untreated, it may develop an overlying erythema. The exact size of the node should be measured for future follow-up. Each tooth should be examined for a periapical abscess and percussed for tenderness. A protective torticollis is sometimes present.

B. Laboratory Findings: The white count is usually about 20,000/cu mm with a shift to the left. The combination of leukocytosis and a positive throat culture or an elevated ASO titer identifies the streptococcus in approximately two-thirds of cases where it is present. A tuberculin skin test should be started.

Differential Diagnosis

The causes of cervical adenopathy are numerous. Five general categories can be distinguished on the basis of the clinical findings.

A. Acute Unilateral Cervical Adenitis: See above.

B. Acute Bilateral Cervical Adenitis: Painful and tender nodes are present on both sides, and the patient usually has fever.

1. Infectious mononucleosis—This diagnosis can be aided by the finding of over 20% atypical cells on the white blood cell smear and a positive mononucleosis spot test. Toxoplasmosis and cytomegalovirus infections can imitate this disorder.

2. Tularemia—There will be a history of wild rabbit or deerfly exposure.

3. Diphtheria—Only occurs in nonimmunized children.

C. Subacute or Chronic Adenitis: In this condition, an isolated node usually exists, but it is smaller and less tender than the acute pyogenic adenitis described previously.

1. Nonspecific viral pharyngitis—This acounts for about 80% of cases in this category.

2. Beta-hemolytic streptococci—The streptococcus can occasionally cause a low-grade cervical adenitis; the staphylococcus never does.

3. Cat scratch fever—The diagnosis is aided by the finding of a primary papule in approximately 60% of cases. Cat scratches are present in over 90% of cases. The node is usually mildly tender.

4. Atypical mycobacteria—The node is generally nontender and submandibular. A history of drinking unpasteurized milk is helpful. A falsely positive PPD is diagnostic. A PPD-standard gives 5–10 mm of induration, whereas the PPD-Battey gives greater than 10 mm of induration. If skin tests for atypical mycobacteria are not available, the OT (old tuberculin) test can be substituted.

D. Cervical Node Cancers: These tumors usually are not suspected until the adenopathy persists despite treatment. Classically, the nodes are painless, nontender, and firm to hard in consistency. They may occur as a single node, unilateral multiple nodes in a chain, bilateral cervical nodes, or generalized adenopathy. Cancers which may present in the neck are Hodgkin's disease, lymphosarcoma, fibrosarcoma, thyroid malignancies, leukemia, and cancers which have an occult primary in the nasopharynx (eg, rhabdomyosarcoma).

E. Imitators of Adenitis: Several structures in the neck can become infected and resemble a node.

1. Mumps—The most common pitfall in diagnosis is mistaking mumps for adenitis. However, mumps crosses the angle of the jaw, is associated with preauricular percussion tenderness, is bilateral in 70% of cases, and there is frequently a history of exposure to mumps. Submandibular mumps can present a diagnostic dilemma.

2. Thyroglossal duct cyst—When superinfected, this congenital malformation can become acutely swollen. Helpful findings are the fact that it is in the midline, located between the hyoid bone and suprasternal notch, and moves upward when the patient sticks out his tongue or swallows.

3. Branchial cleft cyst—When superinfected, this can become a tender mass, 3–5 cm in diameter. Aids to diagnosis are the fact that the mass is located along the anterior border of the sternocleidomastoid muscle and is smooth and fluctuant as a cyst should be. Occasionally, it is attached to the overlying skin by a small dimple or a draining sinus tract.

4. Ranula—This sublingual retention cyst can be mistaken for a submental node (see p 267).

5. Sternocleidomastoid muscle hematoma—This cervical mass is noted at 2–4 weeks of age. On close examination it is found to be part of the muscle body and not movable. An associated torticollis is usually confirmatory.

Complications

The most common complication in the untreated case is suppuration of the node with eventual pointing and exterior drainage. In the preantibiotic era, extension sometimes occurred internally, resulting in jugular vein thrombosis, carotid artery rupture, septicemia, and compression of the esophagus or larynx. Poststreptococcal acute glomerulonephritis has also been reported.

Treatment

A. Specific Measures: Penicillin is the drug of choice unless *Staphylococcus aureus* is suspected. Oral penicillin can be given for 10 days. Daily procaine penicillin injections should also be given until improvement occurs. Dicloxacillin should be started initially if the patient is less than 6 months of age or the node is already fluctuant or erythematous. The patient should be referred to a dentist if a periapical abscess is suspected. These patients should also be covered with antibiotics for the associated facial cellulitis or submandibular adenitis.

B. General Measures: Analgesics (even codeine) are necessary during the first few days. Patients may receive significant relief from application of cold compresses or an ice cube to the inflamed node.

C. Surgical Treatment: Early treatment with antibiotics prevents most cases of pyogenic adenitis from progressing to suppuration. However, once fluctuation occurs, antibiotic therapy alone is not sufficient treatment. When fluctuation or pointing is present, the primary physician should incise and drain the abscess. This can easily be done as an outpatient procedure. Hospitalization is required only if the patient is toxic, dehydrated, dysphagic, or dyspneic.

D. Follow-Up Care: The patient must be seen daily. A good response includes resolution of the fever and improvement in the tenderness after 48 hours of treatment. Reduction in size of the nodes may take several more days. If there is no improvement in 48 hours and the PPD test is negative, it can be safely assumed that the infecting organism is penicillin-resistant *S aureus* and dicloxacillin, 50 mg/kg/day orally, should be added to the treatment regimen. Aspiration of the node with an 18-gauge needle and 0.5 ml of normal saline in the syringe to obtain material for Gram-stained smear, culture, and sensitivity tests is helpful at this stage. Aspirated material should be cultured aerobically and anaerobically.

E. Treatment of Nonpyogenic Adenitis:

1. Cat scratch fever and atypical mycobacteria—Treatment is described in Chapter 26.

2. Persistent unexplained node—As previously mentioned, cancer of the cervical node is usually asymptomatic. The patient with a cervical node that has been enlarging for more than 2 weeks despite treatment or is still large and unchanged in size for more than 2 months should be referred to a surgeon for biopsy.

3. Branchial cleft cyst and thyroglossal duct cyst—If superinfected, these lesions should be treated with penicillin for 10 days as described above. After the infection clears, the patient should be referred to a surgeon for definitive excision of the cyst.

Prognosis

With appropriate treatment, the prognosis is excellent. After the infection clears, the node may remain palpable for several months but will gradually decrease in size unless it is scarred. Recurrent pyogenic adenitis is rare. When it occurs, it is usually due to diseases such as chronic granulomatous disease of childhood or an immunologic disorder.

Barton LL, Feigin RD: Childhood cervical lymphadenitis: A reappraisal. J Pediatr 84:846, 1974.

Boyce JM & others: Nosocomial staphylococcal cervical lymphadenitis in infants: Report of an outbreak. Pediatrics 57:854, 1976.

Buckingham JM, Lynn HB: Bronchial cleft cysts and sinuses in children. Mayo Clin Proc 49:172, 1974.

Dajani AS & others: Etiology of cervical lymphadenitis in children. N Engl J·Med 268:1329, 1963.

Jaffe BF, Jaffe N: Head and neck tumors in children. Pediatrics 51:731, 1973.

May M: Neck masses in children: Diagnosis and treatment. Pediatr Ann 5:517, 1976.

Wright NL: Cervical infections. Am J Surg 113:379, 1967.

.　　.　　.

TONSILLECTOMY & ADENOIDECTOMY (T&A)

Removal of the tonsils and adenoids has been described as an American ritual. Although about 30% of American children have their tonsils and adenoids removed, only 1–2% of children have adequate medical indications for this procedure.

Besides being usually unnecessary, the procedure carries considerable risk. The mortality rate under good conditions is still one death per 15,000 operations. Postoperative bleeding occurs in approximately 5% of cases and requires transfusion or suturing of the tonsillar bed. Some children with previously normal speech develop hypernasal speech. The emotional hazards of hospitalization and surgery in a child under 5 years of age have been well documented. In terms of economics, the $200 million annually spent on this procedure could be better spent in other ways. Lastly, there are still questions regarding the role of tonsils in immunologic memory and disease prevention.

Invalid Reasons for T&A

The following conditions account for the removal of over 95% of tonsils and adenoids.

A. "Large Tonsils": Many parents feel that large tonsils mean bad tonsils. It is unfortunate that the peak incidence of infections correlates so well with tonsillar size. Normal lymphoid atrophy occurs spontaneously after age 8. The parent should be reassured that the patient's tonsils are within normal range. It is very important at well child check-ups not to call a child's tonsils "big" or "bad."

B. Recurrent Colds and Sore Throats: T&A does not decrease the incidence of viral respiratory infections. Parents must be reassured that these infections are a natural event at this age and that contacts eventually give the patient increased immunity.

C. Recurrent Streptococcal Pharyngitis: At one time, repeated episodes of "strep throat" were considered an indication for tonsillectomy. However, it has been shown in several studies that the incidence of streptococcal infections does not decrease after the tonsils have been removed. Moreover, the future diagnosis of streptococcal infections is made difficult by the lack of tonsillar exudates.

D. Parental Pressure: Some parents place great demands on their doctor for a T&A and must be skillfully reeducated.

E. School Absence: For the child who misses school for vague symptoms, removing the tonsils will not relieve the school phobia.

F. "Chronic Tonsillitis": Such a tonsil is allegedly so diseased that even antibiotics cannot eliminate the infections. It is unclear whether this condition even exists. If it does, it is certainly very rare.

G. Miscellaneous Conditions: Poor appetite, allergic rhinitis, asthma, unexplained fevers, and halitosis are not indications for tonsillectomy.

Indications for Adenoidectomy:

A. Persistent Nasal Obstruction: Mouth breathing can have many causes (see p 254). However, if this problem is due to large adenoids, they should be removed to prevent an adenoidal facies.

B. Recurrent Otitis Media: Most cases of recurrent suppurative otitis media can be treated with prophylactic antibiotics. Most cases of chronic serous otitis media are not due to large adenoids. Adenoidectomy may be indicated if tympanostomy tubes have failed and the patient has huge adenoids.

C. Snoring: If the patient experiences continual nighttime snoring and daytime snorting, he should have his adenoids removed if they appear to be the cause.

Indications for Tonsillectomy

A. Persistent Oral Obstruction: Intermittent oral obstruction and dysphagia can occur as a result of inflammation and swelling of the tonsils. If the problem is persistent and the tonsils are seen to almost touch in the midline, tonsillectomy should be performed. This is especially likely to happen in people who have small oral cavities to begin with.

B. Recurrent Peritonsillar Abscess: This problem implies that the tonsil is no longer inhibiting the spread of infection and needs to be removed.

C. Recurrent Pyogenic Cervical Adenitis: Again, the tonsil is no longer acting as an effective barrier to the spread of infection.

D. Suspected Tonsillar Tumor: The prominent unilateral tonsil, especially if it is enlarging, may be removed with the presumptive diagnosis of tonsillar neoplasm. This is a grave diagnosis to miss.

Indications for Combined T&A

A. Cor Pulmonale: A patient with adenoidal hypertrophy can develop chronic hypoxia which leads to pulmonary hypertension and finally to cor pulmonale and right-sided heart failure. This is a rare but serious complication that is definitely helped by T&A, sometimes on an emergency basis.

B. Sleep Apnea Syndrome: These children all have loud snoring interrupted by 30- to 60-second apneic episodes. Many are referred because of excessive daytime sleepiness and worsening school performance. Most of these children have obstructive apnea rather than central apnea. Their symptoms are reversed by T&A.

C. Recurrent Aspiration Pneumonia: The patient with huge tonsils, muffled speech, and gurgling respirations may occasionally present with repeated aspiration pneumonia.

Contraindications to T&A

A. Short Palate: A child with a cleft palate, submucous cleft palate, or bifid uvula should not have his adenoids removed because of the risk of aggravating the velopharyngeal incompetence and causing hypernasal speech.

B. Bleeding Disorder: If a chronic bleeding disorder is present, it must be diagnosed and compensated for before a T&A.

C. Acute Tonsillitis: T&A should be postponed until an acute tonsillitis is resolved. This guideline may prevent a superinfection of the wound.

D. Polio Season: T&A during polio season in a susceptible population leads to an increased risk of bulbar poliomyelitis. Wide-scale use of poliovaccine can eliminate this hazard.

Management of Parental Pressure

If parents are dissatisfied with the kind of treatment they are receiving, they can "doctor-shop" until they find someone who will remove their child's tonsils. This can be prevented by the following approach:

The parents' complaint must be taken seriously. All of the reasonable indications for T&A must be competently investigated. The ENT examination must be performed carefully, and the parents must be assured that there are some valid reasons to take out the tonsils but only when the benefit outweighs the risk, discomfort, inconvenience, and expense.

The parents can then be reassured that their child is basically healthy. The prognosis for spontaneous involution of the tonsils and adenoids and a lower incidence of respiratory infections in years to come can be offered. In addition, it can be mentioned that the risk of taking the tonsils out is considerably greater than the risk of leaving them in.

If the parents are still unconvinced, a consultation is in order. Since it is in the child's best interest, an otolaryngologist should be chosen who shares the pediatrician's viewpoint on this subject.

Caylor GG: Heart failure due to enlarged tonsils and adenoids. Am J Dis Child 118:708, 1969.

Chamovitz R & others: The effect of tonsillectomy on the incidence of streptococcal respiratory disease and its complications. Pediatrics 26:355, 1960.

Evans HE: Tonsillectomy and adenoidectomy: Review of published evidence for and against T&A. Clin Pediatr (Phila) 7:71, 1968.

Guilleminault C & others: Sleep apnea in eight children. Pediatrics 58:23, 1976.

Mawson S & others: A controlled study evaluation of adenotonsillectomy in children. (2 parts.) J Laryngol 81:777, 1967; 82:963, 1968.

Paradise JL: Why T&A remains moot. Pediatrics 49:648, 1972.

Shaikh W & others: A systematic review of the literature on evaluative studies of tonsillectomy and adenoidectomy. Pediatrics 57:401, 1976.

DISORDERS OF THE LIPS

Labial Sucking Tubercle

A small baby may present with a small callus in the middle of his upper lip. It usually is asymptomatic and disappears after cup feeding is initiated.

Cold Sores

A favorite site of recurrent herpes simplex infections is the mucocutaneous juncture of the lip. Lesions rapidly proceed from papular to vesicular to a crusted stage. They cause considerable pain and some burning. There is usually no fever. Recurrent bouts tend to involve the same site.

Treatment of these lesions is symptomatic. Superinfection is rare. One or 2 applications of rubbing alcohol to the vesicles after they have been opened with a sterile needle may dry them up and shorten the clinical course from 10 days to 3 days. Idoxuridine applied hourly to very early lesions may abort them, but this treatment is expensive and impractical. If the lesions are precipitated by sun exposure, they can often be prevented by the frequent use of sunscreen lotions. Injection of smallpox vaccine into the site of the lesion is not helpful and can cause scarring.

Cheilitis

Dry, cracked, scaling lips are usually due to sun or wind exposure. Licking the lips accentuates the process, and the patient should be warned of this. Liberal use of lip balms gives excellent results.

Perlèche

The angle of the mouth may become fissured and raw. This most commonly happens in children who drool or lick the sides of the mouth, establishing a macerated area. The most common pathogen is *Candida albicans.* Riboflavin deficiency is a rare cause. The lesions respond well to nystatin (Mycostatin) cream. Occasionally, a corticosteroid must be added.

DISORDERS OF THE TONGUE

Geographic Tongue (Benign Migratory Glossitis)

This condition of unknown cause is marked by circular or elliptical smooth areas on the tongue devoid of papillae and surrounded by a narrow ring of hyperkeratosis. The pattern can change from day to day.

The lesions are painless and may last months to years. This puzzling disorder is benign, uncommon after age 6, and requires no treatment.

Fissured Tongue (Scrotal Tongue)

This condition is marked by numerous irregular fissures on the dorsum of the tongue. It occurs in approximately 1% of people and is usually a dominant trait. It is also frequently seen in children with trisomy 21 and other retarded patients who have the habit of chewing on a protruded tongue.

Coated Tongue (Furry Tongue)

The tongue normally becomes coated if mastication is impaired and the patient is on a liquid or soft diet. Mouth breathing, fever, or dehydration can accentuate the process.

Macroglossia

Tongue hypertrophy and protrusion may be a clue to Beckwith's syndrome, glycogen storage disease, cretinism, Hurler's syndrome, lymphangioma, or hemangioma. In trisomy 21, the normal-sized tongue protrudes because the oral cavity is small.

ORAL TRAUMA

Puncture wounds of the floor of the mouth and soft palate are not uncommon in children. Most could be prevented if children were forbidden to play with sticks or pencils in their mouths. Treatment includes a tetanus booster if one has not been given in the previous 5 years. Prophylactic antibiotics are not helpful, but the patient should be seen after 48 hours to rule out the possibility of superinfection.

Lacerations of the lip require precise closure and alignment of the mucocutaneous juncture. Lacerations of the buccal mucosa usually heal without suturing. Most tongue lacerations heal without suturing; if they involve the edges of the tongue and are large enough to cause gaping of the wound, black silk sutures must be placed, sometimes under general anesthesia.

HALITOSIS

"Bad breath" is a puzzling and distressing complaint. In most cases it is due to acute stomatitis or pharyngitis. In children, there are 2 common causes of chronic halitosis: continual mouth breathing (see p 254) and thumb-sucking or blanket sucking. Unusual causes of foul breath are a nasal foreign body, esophageal diverticulum, gastric bezoar, bronchiectasis, or a lung abscess. In older children, the presence of orthodontic devices or dentures can cause halitosis if good dental hygiene is not maintained. Also, offensive skin odors (eg, dirty feet) of long duration can become absorbed and excreted through the lungs. Mouthwashes and chewable breath fresheners give limited improvement. The cause must be uncovered to help the patient with chronic halitosis.

SALIVARY GLAND DISORDERS*

Suppurative Parotitis

Pyogenic parotitis is an unusual clinical disorder found predominantly in newborns and debilitated older patients. The parotid gland is swollen, tender, and often reddened. The diagnosis is made by expression of purulent material from Stensen's duct. The material should be smeared and cultured. Fever and leukocytosis may be present.

Treatment includes hospitalization and intravenous methicillin, because the most common organism is *Staphylococcus aureus*. If fluctuation occurs and drainage through Stensen's duct is impaired, aspiration of the pus with an 18-gauge needle can avoid the necessity for incision and drainage. This may have to be repeated 3 or 4 times.

Recurrent Idiopathic Parotitis

Some children experience repeated episodes of parotid swelling that lasts 1−2 weeks and then resolves spontaneously. There is usually mild pain and often no fever. The process is most often unilateral, which weighs heavily against an autoimmune process as the underlying cause and points instead to some sort of obstructive process. Serum amylase is normal, which speaks against a diagnosis of viral parotitis as can occur with mumps, parainfluenza, and other viral infections. As many as 10 episodes may occur from age 2 on. The problem usually resolves spontaneously at puberty.

Treatment includes analgesics if pain is present. A 4-day course of corticosteroids can be recommended if it can be initiated early in an attack (see Gellis reference, below). A second attack of parotid swelling without fever should result in referral to an otolaryngologist for a sialogram to rule out calculus of Stensen's duct. The usual finding is sialectasis. The sialogram seems to improve as the recurrence rate diminishes.

Pneumoparotitis

Children with pneumoparotitis complain of a sudden onset of pain and swelling in the parotid area. A history of playing a musical wind instrument or blowing up balloons for a party confirms the diagnosis. The cause of this transient condition is inflation of the parotid gland secondary to sudden increased intraoral pressure.

Tumors of the Parotid

Mixed tumors and hemangiomas can present in

*Mumps is discussed in Chapter 25.

the parotid gland as a hard or persistent mass. Such a patient should be referred to a surgeon.

Ranula

A ranula is a retention cyst of a sublingual salivary gland. It is found on the floor of the mouth to one side of the lingual frenulum. Ranula has been described as resembling a frog's belly since it is thin-walled and contains a clear bluish fluid. Referral to an otolaryngologist for marsupialization is indicated.

David RB & others: Suppurative parotitis in children. Am J Dis Child 119:332, 1970.

Gellis SS: Editorial on recurrent parotitis. Page 169 in: *Yearbook of Pediatrics.* Year Book, 1970.

Habel DW: Recurrent swelling of the parotid gland. Postgrad Med 48:116, Aug 1970.

Leake D & others: Neonatal suppurative parotitis. Pediatrics 46:202, 1970.

Redpath T: Congenital ranula. Oral Surg 28:542, 1969.

Saunders HF: Wind parotitis. N Engl J Med 289:689, 1973.

ORAL CONGENITAL MALFORMATIONS

Tongue-Tie

The tightness of the lingual frenulum varies greatly among normal people. A short frenulum prevents both protrusion and elevation of the tongue. A puckering of the midline of the tongue occurs with tongue movement. The condition in no way interferes with the ability to nurse. It is unlikely that it interferes with the ability to speak, since even children with ankyloglossia have normal speech.

Treatment consists of reassurance. Although there is no evidence to support it, clipping of the frenulum is sometimes recommended if the tongue does not protrude beyond the teeth or gums. If this degree of tongue-tie is associated with impairment of rapid articulation, the patient should be referred to an otolaryngologist for correction. Casual frenulum clipping can result in significant bleeding from a cut lingual artery or injury to the orifices of Wharton's duct.

Catlin FI, DeHaan V: Tongue-tie. Arch Otolaryngol 94:548, 1971.

Horton CE & others: Tongue-tie. Cleft Palate J 6:8, 1969.

Cleft Lip & Cleft Palate

Cleft lip or palate (singly or together) is found in one in 800 live births. They are readily diagnosed in the newborn nursery. Treatment requires a multidisciplined team approach—plastic surgeons, otolaryngologists, audiologists, speech therapists, orthodontists, and prosthodontists. Cleft lip repair is usually withheld until the child weighs over 12 lb. Cleft palate repair is usually performed at 18 months of age; this is essential to permit normal speech development, which should begin at this time. Occasionally, the palate is short and results in nasal speech. A permanently constructed flap of tissue from the posterior pharyngeal wall may be of benefit.

Cleft palate causes eating problems and poor weight gain due to nasal regurgitation or lung aspiration of milk. Best results are obtained by feeding the baby with a cup or special compressible feeder (see Paradise reference, below). The sitting position is optimal for feeding. Cleft palate nipples are usually no more effective than standard nipples. Approximately 90% of children with cleft palate have chronic otitis media and must be carefully followed for this problem. Some otolaryngologists recommend prophylactic tympanostomy tubes.

Bergstrom L, Hemenway WG: Otologic problems in submucous cleft palate. South Med J 64:1172, 1971.

Paradise JL, McWilliams BJ: Simplified feeder for infants with cleft palate. Pediatrics 53:566, 1974.

Schilli W & others: A general description of 315 cleft lip and palate patients. Cleft Palate J 7:573, 1970.

Bifid Uvulas

A bifid uvula can be a normal finding. However, there is a close association between this and submucous cleft palate. A submucous cleft can be diagnosed by palpation of the hard palate. In this condition, the posterior bony portion of the hard palate is absent. These children have a 40% risk of developing chronic serous otitis media. They also are at risk of incomplete closure of the palate, resulting in nasal speech.

High-Arched Palate

A high-arched palate is usually a genetic trait of no consequence. It is also seen in children who are chronic mouth breathers. Some rare causes of high-arched palate are congenital disorders such as Marfan's syndrome, Treacher Collins syndrome, and Ehlers-Danlos syndrome.

Pierre Robin Syndrome

This congenital malformation is characterized by the triad of micrognathia, cleft palate, and glossoptosis. These children present as emergencies in the newborn period because of infringement on the airway by the tongue. The main objective of treatment is to prevent asphyxia until the mandible becomes large enough to accommodate the tongue. In some cases, this can be achieved by leaving the child in a prone position while unattended. In severe cases, a custom-fitted oropharyngeal airway or large suture through the base of the tongue that is anchored to the soft tissue in front of the mandible is required. The child requires close observation until he outgrows this problem.

Gunter G & others: Early management of the Pierre Robin syndrome. Cleft Palate J 7:495, 1970.

Hawkins DB, Simpson JV: Micrognathia and glossoptosis in the newborn. Clin Pediatr (Phila) 13:1066, 1974.

• • •

General References

Birrell JF: *The Ear, Nose and Throat Diseases of Children.* Davis, 1960.

Dale DMC: *Applied Audiology for Children,* 2nd ed. Thomas, 1967.

Proctor DF: *The Nose, Paranasal Sinuses and Ears in Childhood.* Thomas, 1963.

Stool SE, Belafsky ML: *Pediatric Otolaryngology: Current Problems in Pediatrics.* Yearbook, 1971.

Strome M: *Differential Diagnosis in Pediatric Otolaryngology.* Little, Brown, 1976.

Wilson JG: *Diseases of the Ear, Nose and Throat in Children,* 2nd ed. Grune & Stratton, 1962.

12...

Respiratory Tract & Mediastinum

John G. Brooks, MD, Ernest K. Cotton, MD, William H. Parry, MD

INTRODUCTION

The diagnosis and treatment of pulmonary diseases in children are enhanced by an understanding of the relevant pathophysiology. Basic normal and abnormal anatomic patterns and physiologic mechanisms are outlined in this chapter, and the diseases are classified according to the structures they involve.

ANATOMY & DEVELOPMENT

The air-containing component of the respiratory system includes the upper airway (above the glottis), larynx, trachea, bronchi, bronchioles (characterized by the absence of cartilage in the wall), terminal bronchioles (the smallest airways supplied primarily by the bronchial circulation), respiratory bronchioles (largest airways into which alveoli open directly, and the largest airways perfused primarily by the pulmonary circulation), alveolar ducts, and alveoli. The embryonic lung bud arises from the primitive endodermal tube in the fourth week of gestation and progresses by asynchronous dichotomous branching to form all conducting airways (terminal bronchioles and all larger airways) by the end of the fourth month of gestation. By about 28 weeks, after further airway growth and pulmonary capillary proliferation, gas exchange resulting from juxtaposition of terminal air spaces and pulmonary capillaries is normally sufficient to support life. Subsequently, terminal airway stability, which is dependent on the presence of surfactant, becomes the principal respiratory factor limiting viability. Although birth initiates major changes in respiratory function, its impact on lung morphology is minor. Between the end of the third trimester and 8–12 years of age, all alveoli are formed. Subsequently, there are further increases in alveolar complexity and size until about 18 years of age. During infancy and childhood, cartilaginous support of the larynx, trachea, and bronchi continues to develop along with airway smooth muscle and more pathways for collateral ventilation. During this period also, the upper airway becomes better stabilized (less vulnerable to spontaneous obstruction by the tongue and other pharyngeal tissues); the larynx becomes 1–2 cervical vertebrae lower, the respiratory muscles stronger, and the chest wall less compliant. Functional changes in the respiratory system include the end of obligate nasal breathing at about 2–4 months of age, change of the part of the airway with the smallest cross-sectional area from the level of the cricoid cartilage to the level of the vocal cords at about 5 years of age, and a significant decrease in the amount of total airway resistance that is due to the peripheral airways as compared to that due to the central airways at about 4–5 years of age. Some of these alterations, with the relatively small diameter of all airways in infants and young children, partially explain the tendency of these patients to develop significant respiratory distress with diseases such as croup and bronchiolitis, which would cause far fewer signs and symptoms in adults. Because of the sparseness of airway smooth muscle in normal young infants, bronchospasm is rare in the first 6 months of life, although it can occur.

Murray JF: *The Normal Lung: The Basis for Diagnosis and Treatment of Pulmonary Disease.* Saunders, 1976.

Pang LM, Mellins RB: Neonatal cardiorespiratory physiology. Anesthesiology 43:171, 1975.

Scarpelli EM: *Pulmonary Physiology of the Fetus, Newborn, and Child.* Lea & Febiger, 1975.

Smith CA, Nelson NM: *Physiology of the Newborn Infant.* Thomas, 1974.

Thurlbeck WM: Postnatal growth and development of the lung. Am Rev Respir Dis 111:803, 1975.

PHYSIOLOGY

The caliber of airways and pulmonary vessels is controlled by mechanical, humoral, and neural reflex mechanisms. Changes in caliber may or may not be uniform throughout the lung. When only some of the airways and blood vessels are involved, the distribution may be regional or anatomic (ie, affecting only certain sizes or types of airways or vessels). All intrapulmonary structures are connected by a connective tissue network which is important for transmitting mechanical forces throughout the lung (eg, negative pleural pressure opens alveoli and other airways during inspiration). This network (especially the elastic tissue) exerts radial traction on airway walls (and to a lesser extent the vessel walls), and this tethering action is important in maintaining normal lumen patency. The greatest alterations of airway caliber usually result from humoral or neural influences on airway smooth muscle. There is normally some resting tone of airway smooth muscle. Some endogenous bronchoconstrictors are acetylcholine, histamine, bradykinin, prostaglandin F_{2a}, serotonin, and significant hyper- or hypocapnia. Bronchodilatation is caused by β-adrenergic agonists and prostaglandins of the E series. Stimulation of pulmonary irritant receptors, which are located very superficially in the respiratory mucosa throughout most of the conducting airways, causes bronchoconstriction by a vagally mediated reflex. The irritant receptors may be stimulated by ether, cigarette smoke, sulfur dioxide, ammonia, dust particles, or mechanical deformation by a catheter, bronchoscope, or endotracheal tube, or by rapid inflations or deflations of the lung. Most changes in pulmonary vascular tone are humorally mediated. The wide variety of endogenous pulmonary vasoconstrictors again include histamine, angiotensin, fibrinopeptides, prostaglandin F_{2a}, and alveolar hypoxia. Pulmonary vasodilatation may likewise be caused by bradykinin, glucagon, E series prostaglandins, β-adrenergic agonists and acetylcholine.

Airway secretions are generally increased by irritant stimulation through a vagally mediated reflex or directly by parasympathomimetic agonists.

Gold WM: Neurohumoral interactions in airways. In: Symposium on cardiorespiratory function. Am Rev Respir Dis 115, No. 6 (Part II), p 127, 1977.

Nadel JA: Autonomic control of airway smooth muscle and airway secretions. In: Symposium on cardiorespiratory function. Am Rev Respir Dis 115, No. 6 (Part II), p 117, 1977.

Paintal AS: Thoracic receptors connected with sensation. Br Med Bull 33:169, 1977.

DIAGNOSTIC AIDS

1. PHYSICAL EXAMINATION OF THE RESPIRATORY SYSTEM

What constitutes an appropriate physical examination of the respiratory system of a child depends to some extent upon the age and cooperation of the patient. For example, chest percussion is of limited value in infants but is an important part of the chest examination in older children. In general, however, every examination should include inspection, percussion, and auscultation. One should inspect the nares for patency (passing a small soft catheter through the nares into the posterior pharynx rules out choanal

atresia), the posterior pharynx for obstructing lesions (eg, large or displaced tonsils), and the neck for masses and central position of the trachea. The chest should be observed for abnormal shape (eg, pectus excavatum or carinatum, scoliosis, or increased anterior-posterior diameter), asymmetry, and chest wall retractions. The nail beds, the lips, and the mucous membranes of the mouth should be inspected for pallor or cyanosis, and the digits should be examined for clubbing. The patient's height and weight should be carefully measured and plotted on a growth chart.

By means of auscultation, the examiner should assess the amount and symmetry of air entry and the character of breath sounds. An early sign of airway obstruction may be relative prolongation of expiratory sounds. Rhonchi (coarse, discontinuous, and lower-pitched) indicate large airway obstruction, usually by mucus. Rales (high-pitched, fine crackles) are usually inspiratory and indicate narrowing of small airways. Expiratory wheezes can be due to narrowing of large or small airways.

Cardiac auscultation should be performed to detect murmurs or increased intensity of the pulmonary valve closure sound (P_2), indicating pulmonary hypertension. Increased lung volume due to trapped gas often lowers the diaphragm and causes the edge of the liver to be palpable below the right costal margin.

Godfrey S & others: Clinical and physiological associations of some physical signs observed in patients with chronic airways obstruction. Thorax 25:285, 1970.

Waring WW: The history and physical examination. Chap 3 in: *Pulmonary Disorders.* Kendig EL (editor). Saunders, 1972.

2. PULMONARY FUNCTION TESTING

Pulmonary function testing can provide important diagnostic and prognostic information in the management of children with pulmonary disease. Such studies are helpful in differentiating obstructive from restrictive lung disease (Table 12–1). Obstructive lung disease is far more common than restrictive lung disease in children, and pulmonary function testing is useful in determining the site of obstruction as well as

Table 12–1. Pulmonary function tests in obstructive airway disease and restrictive lung disease. (N = normal.)

	Obstructive	Restrictive
Forced vital capacity (FVC)	↓	↓
Total lung capacity (TLC)	N or ↑	↓
Residual volume (RV)	↑	N or ↓
Timed vital capacity in 1 second as percent of FVC (FEV$_1$)	↓	N
Forced expiratory flow from 25–75% of FVC (FEF$_{25-75}$)	↓	N or ↓

its reversibility. The effects of a particular therapeutic regimen can be quantitatively evaluated with pulmonary function testing. Such tests are also helpful in objectively following the course and severity of many pulmonary diseases. Finally, preoperative pulmonary function evaluation of patients with lung disease can help evaluate the risk of anesthesia as well as assisting in the planning of postoperative respiratory care.

The most useful pulmonary function tests are arterial blood gas sampling, spirometry during quiet breathing, and measurement of maximal forced expirations. The first is appropriate in any age group; the latter two, like other more sophisticated pulmonary function tests, require a cooperative subject and therefore are appropriate only in children over 5–7 years of age.

Spirometry provides a measure of the vital capacity, ie, the maximum volume of air that can be taken into or forced out of the lungs; the forced expired volume exhaled in the first second of a maximum expiration (FEV_1), usually expressed as a percent of the total forced vital capacity (normal, $\geqslant 80\%$); and maximal flow rates at a variety of lung volumes. The maximum flow rate at high lung volumes (peak expiratory flow rate, PEFR) is an indication of respiratory muscle strength, degree of effort and cooperation, and large airway caliber. FEV_1 is primarily an index of larger airway caliber. Small airway function is reflected in the contour of the flow volume loop and the maximum flows at low lung volumes, eg, the average forced expiratory flow over the middle half of expiration (FEF_{25-75}). Absolute lung volumes (functional residual capacity, FRC; residual volume, RV), measured either by gas dilution technics or body plethysmography, are often elevated with small airway disease and are decreased in restrictive lung disease. The carbon monoxide diffusing capacity of the lung is a general reflection of pulmonary blood volume.

One approach to interpretation of pulmonary function tests is first to determine whether the vital capacity is normal or diminished. If diminished, is the abnormality due to a decrease in total lung capacity (TLC), as would be seen in restrictive disease, or to elevation of RV due to obstructive disease? A summary of pulmonary function tests in obstructive and restrictive lung disease is presented in Table 12–1. Having made the initial distinction between restrictive and obstructive disease, it is important to inspect the remainder of the pulmonary function results for internal consistency. If obstructive disease is suggested, there must be other evidence of small airway disease such as a decrease in the FEF_{25-75}. In contrast, in restrictive lung disease the maximum expiratory flow rates should be relatively normal. Inconsistency in the results of the different tests may indicate a poor or inconsistent effort on the part of the patient. Failure to expire to a true residual volume is one of the most common sources of error due to lack of cooperation among pediatric patients. If obstructive disease is identified, the patient should inhale a bronchodilator, and pulmonary function tests should be repeated after

about 20 minutes to look for evidence of reversibility of the airway obstruction. Probably the most reliable pulmonary function tests in young children are arterial blood gas measurements and FEV_1.

Arterial Blood Gases

Measurement of arterial oxygen tension (Pa_{O_2}), CO_2 tension (Pa_{CO_2}), and pH is an excellent means of assessing the gas exchange function of the lungs. Arterial sites for obtaining blood percutaneously, in decreasing order of desirability, are the radial, brachial, dorsalis pedis, posterior tibial, temporal, and femoral arteries. The femoral artery is least desirable because of the risk of serious complications. In order to minimize the deviation from steady state conditions caused by the arterial puncture, the site should be infiltrated with local anesthesia about 5–10 minutes before the arterial sample is drawn. When direct arterial sampling is not possible, "arterialized" capillary blood can be obtained. If the patient has adequate peripheral perfusion and if proper technic is used, the values are quite reliable for pH, P_{CO_2}, and base excess. The reliability of the oxygen measurement depends on the Pa_{O_2}. The proper technic for a capillary sample from the heel involves heating the extremity with warm towels for 10 minutes prior to the puncture and then making a sufficiently deep stab wound to ensure good blood flow. The free-flowing blood should be collected in a capillary tube as close as possible to the bleeding site without air bubbles collecting in the tube.

Normal blood gas values for sea level and for Denver, Colorado (altitude 5280 feet) are listed in Table 12–2. The amount of fixed shunting (including both intrapulmonary and intracardiac shunts) can be estimated by measuring Pa_{O_2} with the patient breathing 100% oxygen.

Transcutaneous measurement of Pa_{O_2} and Pa_{CO_2} will soon be clinically feasible and will allow for continuous monitoring of steady state blood gases.

Avery ME, Fletcher BD: Chap 6 in: *The Lung and Its Disorders in the Newborn Infant.* Saunders, 1974.

Bates DV, Macklin PT, Christie RV: *Respiratory Function and Disease.* Saunders, 1971.

Hjalmarson O: Mechanics of breathing in newborn infants with pulmonary disease. Acta Pediatr Scand Suppl 247, 1974.

Huch R & others: Transcutaneous P_{O_2} monitoring in routine management of infants and children with cardiorespiratory problems. Pediatrics 57:681, 1976.

Hunt CE: Capillary blood sampling in the infant: Usefulness and limitations of 2 methods of sampling compared with arterial blood. Pediatrics 51:501, 1973.

Table 12–2. Normal arterial blood values with $F_{IO_2} = 0.21$ (room air).

	Pa_{O_2} (mm Hg)	Pa_{CO_2} (mm Hg)	pH
Sea level	85–95	36–42	7.38–7.42
Denver	65–75	35–40	7.36–7.40

Jones RWA & others: Arterial oxygen tension and response to oxygen breathing in differential diagnosis of congenital heart disease in infancy. Arch Dis Child 51:667, 1976.

Polgar G: Pulmonary function testing for pediatric chest diseases. Pediatr Ann 6:526, 1977.

Polgar G, Promadhat V: *Pulmonary Function Testing in Children*. Saunders, 1971.

Williams HE, Phelan PD: Chap 17 in: *Respiratory Illness in Children*. Blackwell, 1975.

3. COLLECTION OF MATERIAL FOR CULTURE

Much pediatric pulmonary disease is of infectious etiology. A variety of technics are available for collection of material suitable for culture. There is a poor correlation between organisms grown from cultures of the nose or throat and those infecting the lower airway. Therefore, material from below the larynx should be obtained for culture to identify organisms in the lower airways. Expectorated sputum is the easiest material to obtain in cooperative patients, although it will be contaminated with upper airway organisms. A smear of sputum or other material collected should be prepared, appropriately stained, and examined with a microscope for the presence of organisms and inflammatory cells. Sputum expectoration may be encouraged or increased by chest percussion and postural drainage or by inhalation of ultrasonic mist for 10–15 minutes. In patients who are unable to expectorate sputum for collection, direct tracheal suction is useful—performed either blindly or under direct vision using a laryngoscope, Magill forceps, or a bronchoscope. This can be done through an endotracheal tube, which has the advantage of less contamination by mouth and pharyngeal flora but the disadvantage of further limiting the size of the suction catheter that can be used. A transtracheal route (percutaneous introduction of the catheter through the cricothyroid membrane) is usually not recommended in children, particularly in young children. Brush biopsy and transbronchial biopsy are additional methods by which to obtain material for culture from the lower airway, using a bronchoscope. These latter technics are most applicable in older children.

Direct needle aspiration of the lung is a useful procedure in children of all ages. This procedure should be performed with a No. 20- to 22-gauge needle attached to a glass syringe rinsed with normal saline to create an airtight seal, following local anesthesia of the appropriate area of the chest wall. Rapid introduction, over the top of the rib, into the lung parenchyma and aspiration during withdrawal of the needle will recover enough material for culture. The patient should refrain from breathing during the brief period while the needle is in the chest.

An area of relatively acute disease should be identified on the chest x-ray and an effort should be made to aspirate from that area if it is accessible and not adjacent to another major organ such as the heart or liver. Fluoroscopy is occasionally helpful in directing the needle.

The major complications of this procedure are hemoptysis and pneumothorax, but these are uncommon when the procedure is performed properly. Patients with pulmonary hypertension or obstructive airway disease with hyperaeration are at increased risk of morbidity.

Bartlett JG: Diagnostic accuracy of transtracheal aspiration bacteriologic studies. Am Rev Respir Dis 115:777, 1977.

Epstein RL: Constituents of sputum: A simple method. Ann Intern Med 77:259, 1972.

Garcia D & others: Lung puncture aspiration as a bacteriologic diagnostic procedure and acute pneumonias of infants and children. Clin Pediatr 6:346, 1971.

Klein JO: Diagnostic lung puncture in the pneumonias of infants and children. Pediatrics 44:486, 1969.

Mimica I & others: Lung puncture in the etiologic diagnosis of pneumonia: The study of 543 infants and children. Am J Dis Child 122:278, 1971.

Zavala DC: The diagnosis of pulmonary disease by non-thoracotomy techniques. Chest 64:100, 1973.

4. RADIOGRAPHIC PROCEDURES

The chest x-ray is important in diagnosis and management of pediatric lung disease, and newer high-speed exposure technics significantly reduce the radiation exposure from such films. Both frontal and lateral chest x-rays should be obtained in most cases for optimal interpretation and localization. Hyperaeration, for example, is best assessed on a lateral film by loss of diaphragmatic convexity. Lateral decubitus chest x-rays are useful in assessing the presence and extent of pleural air or fluid as well as the mobility of pleural fluid. Forced expiratory chest x-rays can demonstrate localized obstruction to expiration causing trapped air, as can be caused by an aspirated foreign body. Such trapped air may show no abnormality on inspiratory chest x-ray, whereas on a forced expiratory film there may be mediastinal shift toward the contralateral side and increased radiolucency over the affected area. The forced expiratory film can be obtained even in young uncooperative subjects if a technician wearing a lead glove presses on the immobilized child's epigastrium as the child exhales. The barium swallow is useful for evaluation of possible vascular rings, H type tracheoesophageal fistulas, chalasia, and pharyngeal incoordination. The larger airways and the upper airway can be effectively evaluated by higher penetration chest x-rays, ie, air contrast studies of the airway, often done in association with fluoroscopy. Evaluation of mediastinal masses and large airways may be enhanced by tomograms. Ventilation and perfusion scans using radioactive xenon- and technetium-labeled albumin, respectively, provide crude assessments of regional ventilation and perfusion. Regional differences in wash-in and washout rates of ventilation can be assessed in this manner. A much more precise evaluation of the pulmonary vascular bed is obtained with a pulmonary angiogram.

Bronchography is associated with a high morbidity rate in the pediatric age range and is rarely indicated.

Caffey J: *Pediatric X-ray Diagnosis,* 6th ed. Year Book, 1972.

Godfrey S & others: Unilateral lung disease detected by radioisotopic scanning in children thought to have asthma. Br J Dis Chest 71:7, 1977.

Lallemand D & others: Laryngo-tracheal lesions in infants and children: Detection and follow-up studies using direct radiographic magnification. Ann Radiol (Paris) 16:293, 1973.

Slovis TL: Noninvasive evaluation of the pediatric airway: A recent advance. Pediatrics 59:872, 1977.

Wesenberg RL: *The Newborn Chest.* Harper & Row, 1973.

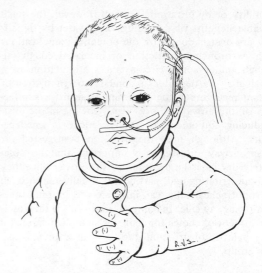

Figure 12—1. Nasal cannula for oxygen administration to infants.

GENERAL METHODS OF THERAPY FOR LUNG DISEASE

Effective treatment of lung disorders should be based on the physiologic alterations that occur during the disease process. Several general therapeutic and prophylactic modes of therapy, each directed toward a particular physiologic function or malfunction, are discussed below.

Mellins R: Respiratory care in infants and children: Report of Ad Hoc Committee American Thoracic Society. Am Rev Respir Dis 105:461, 1972.

Pierce AK, Saltzman HA: Conference on the scientific basis of respiratory therapy. Am Rev Respir Dis 110 (Suppl), 1974.

OXYGEN THERAPY

Oxygen therapy is defined as delivering an inspired oxygen concentration of greater than 21%. It is indicated when arterial blood gas determinations show that the arterial oxygen tension is low. The inspired gas, delivered by nasal cannula, mask, or hood, should be sufficiently enriched with oxygen to maintain an arterial oxygen tension of 65–85 mm Hg. Such inspired gas should always be humidified and should usually be warmed; supersaturation is usually not desirable. Oxygen tents are usually not able to deliver concentrations of oxygen greater than 25–30% unless the tent is tightly sealed, which interferes with nursing care. For these reasons, oxygen tents are rarely indicated.

Nasal prongs are useful for children. For infants, a nasal cannula can be constructed from a soft rubber or polyvinyl tubing which should be taped just inside the nares (Fig 12–1). With nasal prongs or a nasal catheter, an effective inspired oxygen concentration of up to 30–40% can usually be maintained. When nasal obstruction is present or a higher concentration of oxygen is required, a face mask or some other mode of delivery is necessary. The flow through a nasal catheter or prongs usually should not exceed 3 liter/minute in children and less in infants. The lowest effective amount of increased inspired oxygen should be delivered in order to minimize the risk of pulmonary oxygen toxicity.

Arterial blood gases must be measured in most patients receiving oxygen therapy. Some infants and children with chronic lung disease (eg, bronchopulmonary dysplasia or end-stage cystic fibrosis) can be treated at home with low-flow oxygen if the family can understand and accept certain responsibilities and possible complications.

Farney RJ & others: Oxygen therapy: Appropriate use of nebulizers. Am Rev Respir Dis 115:567, 1977.

Friedman SA & others: Oxygen therapy, evaluation of various air-entraining masks. JAMA 228:474, 1974.

Indyk L: P_{O_2} in the seventies. Pediatrics 55:153, 1975.

Pinny MA, Cotton EK: Home management of bronchopulmonary dysplasia. Pediatrics 58:856, 1976.

MIST THERAPY

The most effective and safe expectorant and mucolytic agent for airway secretions is water, given systemically. Small amounts of water may be deposited in the lower airway by inhalation of air of high humidity or by ultrasonic aerosol. However, the small possible benefits of delivering extra water by the airway are overshadowed by the potential complications such as bronchoconstriction or increased cough (although under some circumstances stimulation of a cough may be desirable) secondary to stimulation of irritant receptors in the upper and large airways, infection of the airway by organisms growing in the mist-producing equipment, or fluid overload in small patients. Although mist therapy is not suggested for lower airway disease, it is important that no completely dry gases be delivered to the airway since they also are irritating and, particularly if delivered through an endotracheal tube, can interfere with normal function of airway cilia. In contrast, mist aerosol therapy is a treatment of choice for acute inflammatory laryngeal or subglottic obstruction due to viral or postextubation croup.

Harris TM & others: An evaluation of bacterial contamination of ventilator humidifying systems. Chest 63:922, 1973.

Hayes SB, Robinson JS: An assessment of methods of humidification of inspired gas. Br J Anaesth 42:94, 1970.

Rosenblut M, Chernick V: Influence of mist tent therapy on sputum viscosity and water content in cystic fibrosis. Arch Dis Child 49:606, 1974.

Taussig LM: Mists and aerosols: New studies, new thoughts. J Pediatr 84:619, 1974.

Walker JEC, Well RE: Heat and water exchange in the respiratory tract. Am J Med 30:259, 1961.

BRONCHODILATOR INHALATION THERAPY

Bronchoconstriction and the resultant impaired respiratory function can result from a wide variety of intrinsic and extrinsic stimuli. Many bronchodilator agents are available, and those which are most used clinically can be divided into 4 classes: (1) beta-adrenergic agonists, (2) methylxanthines, (3) parasympatholytic agents, and (4) corticosteroids. These drugs are used most commonly in the treatment of asthma (see p 914), but some patients with other types of acute (eg, bronchiolitis) or chronic (eg, cystic fibrosis) lung disease may benefit from bronchodilator therapy.

The remainder of this discussion will deal only with inhaled adrenergic agonist drugs. Aerosolized adrenergic agonist agents may be delivered from a prepackaged pressurized canister (most include a fluorocarbon propellant, which may increase myocardial sensitivity to the potential arrhythmogenic complications of these agents). Such canisters have the disadvantage of being very easy for the patient to abuse by too frequent use, thus risking overdosage and death. A safe but less convenient means of delivery is by a reusable nebulizer (eg, DeVilbiss No. 40), where the drug solution is aerosolized by continuous gas flow from a tank of compressed gas or from a portable gas compressor. The nebulized drug should be inhaled slowly and deeply. In many patients the nebulizer should be driven by 40% or 100% oxygen to counteract the potential or real arterial hypoxemia caused by the pulmonary vasodilating effect of the adrenergic agonists and the resultant increase in venous admixture from increased perfusion of poorly ventilated areas of the lung. When possible, an improvement in pulmonary function after bronchodilator inhalation should be quantitatively documented before initiating a regular program of bronchodilator therapy. Such pulmonary function studies should include measurement of both maximal expiratory flow rates and absolute lung volumes, since improvement may be evident in only one of these categories. Bronchodilator inhalation is frequently used prior to chest percussion.

Infants or uncooperative children may be given the necessary few breaths of aerosol by placing a feeding nipple with the tip cut off over the end of a canister nebulizer, holding the nose, and administering the drug at the beginning of an inspiration. Continuous breathing of a 1:4 or 1:8 mixture of bronchodilator in distilled water is also effective. There is no evidence that better distribution of the aerosol can be obtained with delivery by intermittent positive pressure breathing (IPPB) than with active deep breathing. A patient who will not cooperate for active breathing is unlikely to cooperate for IPPB. Delivery of a drug by inhalation by any means has the disadvantages that most of the aerosol is deposited in the upper airway, and the aerosol that does reach the smaller airways is preferentially directed toward the well-ventilated areas and away from those that are poorly ventilated, ie, those in most need of bronchodilatation.

All currently available beta-adrenergic agonists have both $beta_1$ activity (eg, inotropic and chronotropic cardiac effects; decreased intestinal motility); and $beta_2$ activity (eg, relaxation of airway and arteriolar smooth muscle; skeletal muscle tremor), although some newer agents such as metaproterenol, terbutaline, and salbutamol have more $beta_2$ selectivity than isoproterenol and isoetharine. In addition, these newer agents have longer durations of action (3–5 hours). Further discussion of other bronchodilator agents is included in the section on asthma (see p 914).

Campbell AD, Soika LF: Selective beta-2 receptor agonists for the treatment of asthma: Therapeutic breakthrough or advertising ploy? J Pediatr 89:1020, 1976.

Chang N, Levison H: Effect of a nebulized bronchodilator administered with or without IPPB on ventilatory function in children with cystic fibrosis and asthma. Am Rev Respir Dis 106:867, 1972.

Dolovich MB & others: Pulmonary aerosol deposition and chronic bronchitis: Intermittent positive pressure breathing vs quiet breathing. Am Rev Respir Dis 115:397, 1977.

Moore RB, Cotton EK: The effect of intermittent positive pressure breathing on airway resistance in normal and asthmatic children. J Allergy Clin Immunol 49:137, 1972.

Murray FJ: Review of the state of the art in intermittent positive pressure breathing therapy. Am Rev Respir Dis 110:193, 1974.

Sackner MA: Bronchodilator agents. Clin Notes Respir Dis 15:3, Summer 1976.

PULMONARY PHYSIOTHERAPY

Postural drainage and chest percussion are used to aid in the removal of material such as mucus and aspirated matter from the lungs. They are accomplished by positioning a patient so that the involved segment is uppermost. The therapist then percusses over the involved area with a cupped hand and relaxed wrist and elbow. There is a slightly different optimal body position for drainage of each lung segment into a major airway. It is important that the therapist be aware of normal lung anatomy and position the patient accordingly. For generalized disease, percussion should be done with the patient in the different positions shown in Fig 12–2. While infants and small children can often be effectively positioned in the therapist's lap or across the therapist's legs, pillows or padded boards are most effective for positioning older children. Some material such as a shirt or towel over the skin being percussed will minimize chest wall tenderness. Care should be taken to avoid trauma to the liver, kidneys, or spleen. The time spent percussing each lung area depends on the extent of lung involvement and the cooperation and tolerance of the child. When there is general lung disease, 1 or 2 minutes should be spent in each position, not to exceed a total of about 15 minutes for the whole treatment. If only one lung area is involved, 2–3 minutes in that position is sufficient. The frequency of treatments may vary from every 2 hours to once or twice daily. If possible, treatments given only once daily should be given in the morning shortly after the patient awakens.

When the cough reflex is weak or absent, mechanical suction should be readily available in order to assist with removal of secretions from the upper or large airways. All patients should be encouraged to expectorate the sputum rather than swallowing it. In patients with significant lung disease, body positioning and chest percussion may cause significant decreases in arterial oxygenation, so that such patients should receive supplemental inspired oxygen during and for a short period after such treatments.

Regular exercise is encouraged in patients with chronic lung disease, as the associated deep breathing may precipitate cough and enhance removal of lung secretions. Mechanical chest percussors are available and are useful for older children and adults.

There are several ways to stimulate a child to cough and breathe deeply. The best way is simply for a parent or nurse to verbally encourage the child, and to assist the patient by frequent changes of position and by placing the child's hands on his chest so he can feel when his chest expands. This takes time, patience, and imagination. Devices that may be helpful in encouraging large inspirations to counteract atelectasis are blow bottles, balloons, and incentive spirometers. Large forced inspirations or forced expirations will often stimulate cough and thus enhance clearance of mucus.

Blow bottles consist of a closed system of 2 bottles connected by a tube that nearly reaches the bottom of each tube. Colored fluid in one bottle is transferred to the other bottle when the patient blows on a second tube emerging from the top of the bottle. The child must be encouraged to inhale and exhale as fully as possible, since nothing is gained by exhaling in short puffs. Some supervision and instruction are essential. Balloons are used in the same way as blow bottles.

In some patients who cough poorly, deep pharyngeal suctioning may stimulate cough and assist in removal of secretions from the large airways. This method, as well as direct tracheal suctioning, can cause laryngospasm and thus should be used only in intensive care units by experienced personnel.

Chopra SK & others: Effects of hydration and physical therapy on tracheal transport velocity. Am Rev Respir Dis 115:1009, 1977.

Holsclaw DS, Tecklin JS: A critical evaluation of bronchial hygiene in pediatric pulmonary disease. Pediatr Ann 6:550, 1977.

Mellins RB: Pulmonary physiotherapy in the pediatric age group. Am Rev Respir Dis 110:137, 1974.

Pinney M: Postural drainage for infants: A better approach. Nursing 2:45, 1972.

MECHANICAL VENTILATION

Mechanical ventilators can generally be classified as either volume-limited or pressure-limited. The volume-limited ventilator produces a preset volume, and that entire volume minus the compression volume (the volume lost as a result of gas compression in the ventilator tubing circuit) is transferred to the patient provided there are no leaks in the ventilator circuit. Examples are the Ohio 560, the Bennett MA 1 ventilator, the Bourns LS-104 infant volume ventilator, and the Emerson volume ventilator. When very high inspiratory pressures are required because of markedly decreased lung compliance or increased airway resistance, a volume-limited ventilator may be necessary for adequate ventilation of the patient. Volume-limited ventilators do not compensate for variable leaks in the circuit (eg, around the endotracheal tube) but do deliver a constant tidal volume in patients with changing lung mechanics.

The pressure-limited ventilator inflates the patient's lung to a certain preset pressure; once this pressure is reached, expiration may begin or the inspiratory pressure may be held constant, but there is no further lung inflation. This type of ventilator will compensate for changing leaks in the circuit but will not deliver a constant tidal volume with changing lung mechanics. Most patients can be adequately ventilated with either a pressure-limited or a volume-limited ventilator. The pressure-limited ventilators with a continuous flow through the circuit are generally less expensive and often more versatile, particularly with small patients.

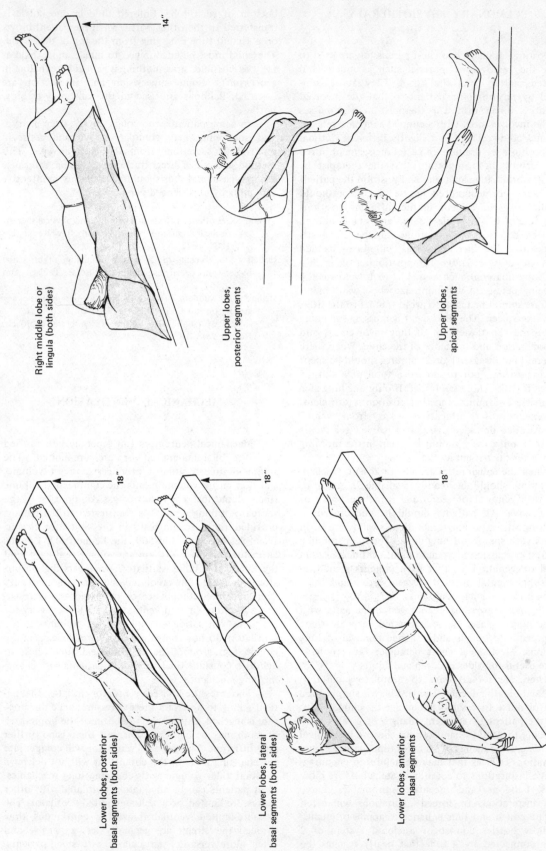

Figure 12–2. Body positions for pulmonary drainage.

All mechanical ventilation systems should have an apparatus for humidification and adjustments of oxygen concentration in the inspired gas as well as appropriate high- and low-pressure alarms for the patient circuit. It is essential that an accurate pressure gauge be properly functioning and easily visible to display a continuous recording of the patient circuit pressure. Finally, it is essential that safety pressure popoffs be available and properly set.

Technics of setting up the ventilator and attaching the patient:

(1) Set up the ventilator as described below, while assisting the patient's ventilation with a manual resuscitation device as necessary.

(2) Adjust the tidal volume or inspiratory and expiratory pressure limits to the estimated requirement. An average starting tidal volume is 10 ml/kg. For normal lungs, inspiratory and expiratory pressures of 16–18 cm water and 2 cm water, respectively, are appropriate starting pressures. These settings must be increased or decreased depending on the arterial blood gases.

(3) Adjust inspiratory time and expiratory time to produce the desired respiratory rate. An appropriate beginning respiratory rate would be 14–24 breaths/minute, depending on the patient's age. A normal inspiratory time is about 0.3–0.6 second, depending on the age of the patient. Prolonged inspiratory times are likely to improve arterial oxygenation but may interfere with pulmonary circulation and cardiac output. It is important that adequate time (at least 0.4–0.5 second) be available for expiration.

(4) Adjust inspired oxygen concentration.

(5) Fill and set humidifier.

(6) Adjust inspiratory flow rate. Slower rates should be used for smaller patients and for patients with significant obstructive airway disease.

(7) Make sure that all warning devices and safety popoffs are set and working.

(8) Attach patient to the ventilator.

(9) Observe movement of patient's chest and auscultate to check for good ventilation of both lungs.

(10) Measure arterial blood gases and pH at regular intervals.

Controlled Ventilation

The ventilator controls both the rate and depth of ventilation, and there is no way for the patient to take spontaneous breaths between the mandatory delivered breaths. For this reason, there may be incoordination of the patient's spontaneous breathing attempts and the ventilator-delivered breaths. This can only be remedied by decreasing the patient's respiratory drive or ability to breathe. The former is achieved by mildly hyperventilating the patient or by the administration of narcotics to depress the respiratory center. The latter method involves administration of muscular blocking agents (eg, gallamine). Paralysis of patients being mechanically ventilated should be performed only when very close observation of the patient is available, because of the risk of ventilator failure or the patient becoming disconnected from the respirator.

Assisted Controlled Ventilation

The small negative pressure generated by the beginning of a patient's respiratory effort triggers the delivery of a full preset tidal volume or inspiratory pressure to the patient. Thus, the patient controls the rate but not the depth of ventilation. Incoordination of ventilator effort and patient effort is less likely with this mode of ventilation, but hyperventilation is a relatively common problem.

Intermittent Mandatory Ventilation (IMV)

The ventilator is set to deliver a certain rate and depth of mandatory breaths. In addition, however, there is a mechanism to provide fresh gas in the patient circuit to allow the patient to take spontaneous breaths of any rate or depth in between the mandatory breaths. Some newer ventilators have synchronized IMV (SIMV), meaning that the mandatory breaths are delivered at the time of an inspiratory effort by the patient if such an effort is made within the appropriate time period for a mandatory breath. This mode of ventilation is helpful in gradually decreasing the rate of mandatory breaths as less mechanical ventilatory support is required and the patient is able to perform more effective spontaneous ventilation.

Positive End-Expiratory Pressure (PEEP)

A positive end-expiratory pressure can be maintained throughout the expiratory period when a patient is receiving mechanical ventilation by any of the 3 above modes. This method helps minimize alveolar volume loss during expiratory pauses and thus decreases the tendency toward atelectasis and the resultant venous admixture. PEEP is indicated in most conditions where mechanical ventilation is required for alveolar or small airway instability or collapse. It is not indicated for problems of large airway obstruction or when gas trapping is a major problem.

Continuous Positive Airway Pressure (CPAP)

The apparatus shown in Fig 12–3 is one means of delivering continuous positive pressure to the airway. CPAP refers to a relatively constant positive airway pressure in the absence of any mandatory, mechanically delivered tidal volumes. The indications are similar to those for PEEP. Nasal prongs, a nasopharyngeal tube, or a facemask can be used instead of an endotracheal tube for application of the positive airway pressure.

Negative Pressure Ventilation

Negative pressure modes of mechanical ventilation analogous to those positive pressure methods listed above can be used for respiratory support in infants and children. Negative pressure ventilation avoids the complications of endotracheal intubation but has the disadvantage of making nursing care and other access to the patient more difficult, and it is difficult to generate large transpulmonary pressures. Temperature control and actual trauma to the patient are problems in very small infants.

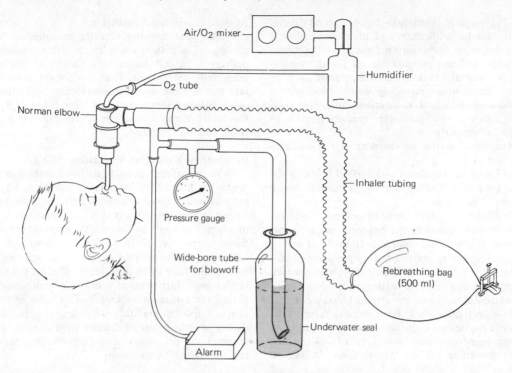

Figure 12—3. Equipment for continuous positive pressure breathing.

Buyukpamukcu N, Hicsonmez A: The effect of CPAP upon pulmonary reserve and cardiac output under increased abdominal pressure. J Pediatr Surg 12:49, 1977.

Gregory GA: Respiratory care of newborn infants. Pediatr Clin North Am 19:311, 1972.

Kirby RR & others: High level positive end expiratory pressure (PEEP) in acute respiratory insufficiency. Chest 67:2, 1975.

Muchin WW & others: *Automatic Ventilation of the Lungs.* Blackwell, 1969.

Sanyal SK & others: Continuous negative chestwall pressure as therapy for severe respiratory distress in an older child: Preliminary observations. J Pediatr 85:230, 1974.

Suter PM, Fairley HB, Isenberg MD: Optimum end-expiratory airway pressure in patients with acute pulmonary failure. N Engl J Med 292:6, 1975.

Wung JT & others: CDP: A major breakthrough! Pediatrics 58:783, 1976.

Zwillich CW & others: Complications of assisted ventilation. Am J Med 57:161, 1974.

ENDOTRACHEAL INTUBATION

Endotracheal tubes are available in a variety of shapes and sizes. The sizes refer to the internal diameter of the tube and range from about 2.5—9.5 mm. Only tubes made of inert polyvinyl chloride should be used. The correct tube size is that which comfortably passes through the vocal cords and the area of the cricoid cartilage. Generally, a tube which will pass through the external nares will also pass through the cords and subglottic area. For an approximate guide to the endotracheal tube sizes appropriate for infants and children, see Table 12—3.

There are 3 main types of endotracheal tube. The straight tube (Magill), which has the same diameter throughout its entire length, is best for most situations. This tube is available with a side and end hole at the distal end of the tube, but this variety should not be used as it may increase the risk of complete tube obstruction from a blood clot or mucous plug which originates in the sidehole. The Cole tube has a significantly narrower diameter at the distal end. It is classified by the diameter of the narrow part. This type of tube is generally available only in small sizes and is useful only for brief intubations in newborns or young infants to avoid passing the endotracheal tube too far into the airway. The shoulder (site of increase in diameter) of the tube will not pass through the vocal cords. This stabilizes the tube but may also injure the vocal cords. For this reason, it should be left in place for

Table 12—3. Recommended endotracheal tube sizes.

Age	Internal Diameter (mm)
Premature (< 1 kg)	2.5
Premature (1—2.5 kg)	3.0
Newborn (2.5—4.0)	3.5
1—12 months	4.0
1—3 years	4.5
3—10 years	5—5.5

only a short time and then changed to a straight (Magill) tube. The appropriate length of the tube should be estimated by holding the tube alongside the patient's airway; before the intubation, the tube should be shortened, leaving only a little extra length. Tubes of 5 mm internal diameter or larger are available with or without cuffs. A cuffed tube is indicated in a patient with excessive upper airway secretions or hemorrhage to prevent the spread of these materials into the lung or when very high pressures may be required for ventilation to minimize the air and pressure leak around the tube. The cuff does not prevent spread of infection to the lower airway. Only tubes with soft, low-pressure cuffs should be used. When cuff inflation is necessary, the smallest possible volume of air should be used. Cuff pressures can be monitored using a blood pressure manometer and should never exceed 30 cm water. All intubations should be performed by experienced personnel. The following equipment should be available for successful intubation:

(1) Suction machine producing an adequate negative pressure, equipped with a tonsil suction and a wide-bore suction catheter.

(2) Self-inflating bag capable of delivering 100% oxygen.

(3) Laryngoscope in good working order. Prior to intubation, the bulb and battery should be checked and the bulb tightened.

(4) Either a straight or curved laryngoscope blade may be used depending on the preference of the intubator. At least 2 sizes of blades should be available.

(5) McGill forceps if nasal intubation is to be performed.

(6) A cardiac monitor or stethoscope to monitor heart rate and rhythm during intubation.

(7) Endotracheal tube of the correct diameter and length (Table 12–3) and a tube smaller than the estimated size should also be available. If it is possible that the airway might be severely obstructed (as in croup), a very small tube should be available.

(8) Tracheostomy set.

Intubation Technic

When all equipment has been assembled and checked, the patient should be positioned so the intubator can be at the patient's head, with the patient's head and shoulders straightly aligned in the neutral position. The person performing the procedure should be seated or kneeling in a comfortable position so that his or her head is just above the head of the patient. The patient's head (not the shoulders) must be placed on a small pillow or roll in the "sniff position" (Fig 12–4). The position of the head on the pillow depends on the patient's age. In the adult, the head is rotated back; in the child, the head is in a more horizontal position; and in the infant, the glottis can often be observed better with the neck slightly flexed. Either the oral or the nasotracheal route may be used depending on the preference and skills of the intubator. Intubation should usually be performed with the

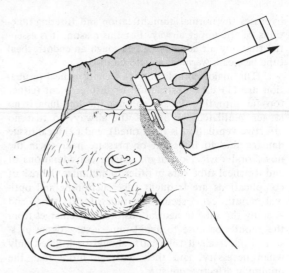

Figure 12—4. Position of head and neck for intubation.

patient awake and breathing spontaneously. The patient should breathe 100% oxygen for several minutes prior to the intubation attempt. The posterior pharynx should be maximally suctioned and the patient then reoxygenated. It is sometimes helpful to put some tape on the convex surface of the laryngoscope blade in order to minimize the chance of the tongue slipping across the blade. The laryngoscope blade is introduced on the right side of the patient's mouth and then brought into the mid position. Throughout the period of intubation, oxygen should be given to the patient by a catheter at the mouth, down the back of the laryngoscope, or down the endotracheal tube. It is very important to identify the anatomy of the larynx and observe the endotracheal tube pass through the vocal cords. If there is difficulty observing the larynx, gentle external pressure on the thyroid cartilage will often improve visualization. The tube should be passed through the larynx to a distance approximately midway between the vocal cords and the carina. After intubation, several breaths of positive pressure ventilation should be delivered while the chest is auscultated to ensure equal breath sounds in each hemithorax. It is best to listen in each axilla and then over the stomach to rule out accidental esophageal intubation. If breath sounds are decreased on the left side, the tube should be slowly withdrawn, with continuous auscultation until the breath sounds improve on the left, unless there is some intrinsic problem of the left lung which would cause decreased breath sounds. When it is properly positioned, the endotracheal tube should be securely fastened in place. A variety of methods are available for fastening either oral or nasotracheal tubes, perhaps the quickest being a piece of tape which totally encircles the head. If this method is used, it is useful to apply backing to part of the tape so that it does not stick to the hair. Finally, tube placement should be verified by chest x-ray.

It is important to note that an endotracheal tube

bypasses the normal humidification and filtering functions of the upper airway. For this reason, it is essential that any air administered through an endotracheal tube be clean, warmed, and humidified.

The major complications of endotracheal intubation are (1) tube obstruction or displacement (either too far into the airway, so that the left lung is no longer ventilated, or out of the airway, so that no effective ventilation is performed); and (2) local tissue damage due to infection or pressure necrosis in the nose, oral cavity, or larynx. Major considerations of endotracheal tube care in order to minimize the risk of complications are frequent tube suctioning and optimal mouth care, secure fixation of the tube, and keeping the tube in neutral position as it emerges from the mouth or nose to avoid unnecessary tissue pressure. Endotracheal tube cuffs should be inflated only when necessary, and then with no more than the minimum effective pressure.

Aberdeen E, Downes JJ: Artificial airways in children. Surg Clin North Am 54:1155, 1974.

Gregory GA: Respiratory care of newborn infants. Pediatr Clin North Am 19:311, 1972.

Jennings PB, Alden ER, Brenz RW: Teaching pediatric intubation. Pediatrics 52:284, 1974.

TRACHEOSTOMY

Tracheostomy should always be performed as an elective procedure, preferably in an operating room. Whenever possible, tracheostomies should be done over a previously placed endotracheal tube under controlled conditions. Occasionally, tracheostomy is required as an urgent lifesaving procedure.

Emergency Cricothyroidotomy

An incision is made between the cricoid and thyroid cartilages into the trachea in the subglottic area. A tracheostomy tube or other improvised airway is then introduced. Such a tube placed through the cricothyroid membrane is within a few millimeters of the true vocal cords. Therefore, it must be removed within 24 hours and replaced by a regular tracheostomy performed under optimal conditions. A well-designed instrument for cricothyroidotomy is the cricothyroidotomy scissors.

Elective Tracheostomy

This procedure requires that an airway first be established by endotracheal tube or bronchoscope. The procedure should be done in the operating room with adequate light, suction, instrumentation, and anesthesia. If an attempt is made to perform this procedure over an obstructed airway, pneumomediastinum and pneumothorax may result because of the marked negative intrathoracic pressure.

Local anesthesia is adequate since the agitated,

hypoxic child usually goes to sleep following placement of the endotracheal tube or bronchoscope. The diameter of a tracheostomy tube should be approximately two-thirds that of the trachea. Newer Teflon tubes are best for general use. The advantages of the Teflon tube over the older silver tube are its movable flange, which decreases the chance of accidental extubation; its softness, which decreases the risk of tissue erosion or necrosis; and its thin wall, which increases the internal diameter. The smaller sizes of Teflon tube have no inner cannula, but their inner surface has only a very slight tendency to accumulate secretions to the point of airway obstruction.

Tracheostomy Care

Constant vigilance by experienced nurses is necessary in the care of children with tracheostomies. Tracheostomy tubes may become displaced from the trachea into the soft tissues of the neck. This problem must be recognized immediately and the tube replaced, although effective ventilation through the upper airway by means of a bag and mask can be lifesaving when a tube is displaced before it is replaced. "Stay" sutures placed in the tracheal cartilage at the time of tracheostomy aid greatly in locating the stoma in cases of accidental decannulation of a fresh tracheostomy.

The necessary equipment (adequate suction, sterile suction catheter and glove, self-inflating resuscitation bag, appropriate size face mask, and extra, appropriate size tracheostomy tube) and personnel must be at hand if tracheostomy in small children is to successfully reduce the number of childhood deaths due to upper respiratory problems. Infants less than 1 year of age are at increased risk of tracheostomy tube obstruction and death. Regular tube suctioning is of key importance to minimize this risk.

Decannulation

In decannulation, the tube should be replaced with progressively smaller sizes and finally blocked for 24 hours before completely removing the tube. The external fistula closes within several days. Painstaking and persistent effort is necessary in decannulation of children under 1 year of age.

Aberdeen E, Downes J: Artificial airways in children. Surg Clin North Am 53:1155, 1973.

Bush GH: The management of the retained tracheostomy tube. Anaesth Intensive Care 4:113, 1976.

Hawkins D, Williams EH: Tracheostomy in infants and young children. Laryngoscopy 86:331, 1976.

Lynn H, VanHeerden JA: Tracheostomy in infants. Surg Clin North Am 53:945, 1973.

Wright L & others: Behavioral tactics for reinstating natural breathing in infants with tracheostomy. Pediatr Res 3:275, 1969.

DISORDERS OF THE CONDUCTING AIRWAYS

Abnormalities of the conducting airways (pharynx, larynx, trachea, bronchi, and bronchioles) produce signs and symptoms secondary to airway obstruction. The major signs of airway obstruction are stridor, rhonchi, wheezing, and prolongation of inspiratory or expiratory time. Obstruction of the extrathoracic airway results in greater obstruction to inspiration than to expiration, while obstructive lesions of the intrathoracic airway cause greater expiratory than inspiratory obstruction. The increase in obstruction is due to dynamic compression of the airways during that phase of respiration. Therefore, an assessment at the time of physical examination and history-taking of the relative severity of airway obstruction during inspiration as compared to expiration can be very helpful in localizing the primary obstructive disorder.

CONGENITAL ABNORMALITIES OF THE LARYNX

With the exception of atresia, laryngeal malformations are characterized by the development of a weak, sometimes hoarse cry and varying degrees of stridor. Congenital obstructive laryngeal lesions may cause symptoms of primarily inspiratory obstruction from the time of birth, or the infant may be relatively free of symptoms until the time of his first upper respiratory infection. The additional airway narrowing due to the infectious inflammation of the respiratory epithelium may precipitate significant respiratory difficulty. The clinical findings in patients with congenital laryngeal malformations are likely to include inspiratory stridor, intercostal and supraclavicular retractions which are worse with crying, and a hoarse cry. The diagnostic evaluation should include a careful history and physical examination, anterior-posterior and lateral x-rays of the chest, lateral soft tissue x-rays of the neck, and fluoroscopic examination of the upper airway and of the contrast-filled esophagus to rule out an anomalous vessel that might be compressing the upper trachea. Pulmonary function tests performed on patients with fixed upper airway narrowing who are old enough to cooperate (ie, over 6 years of age) demonstrate decreased peak flow rates (more marked on inspiration than on expiration). The definitive diagnosis is usually made by direct laryngoscopy. Treatment of congenital laryngeal malformations is usually directed at correction of the primary abnormality when possible and maintenance of an adequate airway at all times. Inspiratory obstruction due to a wide variety of causes is likely to be ameliorated by extension of the neck and by placing the infant in a prone position. Other congenital causes of inspiratory stridor which should be considered in the differential diagnosis include macroglossia, micrognathia, upper airway cysts, nasal obstruction, and congenital subglottic stenosis or subglottic hemangioma.

Alcala H, Dodson WE: Syringobulbia as a cause of laryngeal stridor in childhood. Neurology 25:875, 1975.

Ferguson CF: Congenital abnormalities of the infant larynx. Otolaryngol Clin North Am 3:185, 1970.

Holinger PH, Brown WT: Congenital webs, cysts, laryngoceles and other anomalies of the larynx. Ann Otol Rhinol Laryngol 76:744, 1967.

LeRoux BT & others: Thoracocervical cysts as a cause of stridor. Thorax 29:564, 1974.

1. CONGENITAL LARYNGEAL STRIDOR
(Laryngomalacia)

Congenital laryngeal stridor is a usually benign entity due to minor developmental variations of the larynx. There may be an unusually shaped ("omega-shaped" [Ω]) and long epiglottis which falls posteriorly during inspiration, causing partial obstruction, or particularly short aryepiglottic folds, or unusually large, mobile arytenoid cartilages which move forward during inspiration and cause obstruction. The diagnosis is made by exclusion and by direct laryngoscopy and accounts for more than 75% of all laryngeal problems of infants. The onset of the inspiratory stridor is usually within the first week of life, although it may be delayed for several months. The stridor has usually disappeared by 12–18 months, although occasionally it may persist for several years. Such infants are usually not hoarse and only very rarely become cyanotic. There may be feeding difficulties (vomiting after feeding) and an increased incidence of early speech problems.

Since this is usually a benign, self-limited disorder, specific treatment is rarely required. Some infants may require hospitalization at the time of an upper respiratory infection owing to increased severity of the respiratory obstruction. In the very unusual case, tracheostomy is required because of chronic upper airway obstruction, usually during the second year of life.

Cox MA & others: Reversible pulmonary hypertension in a child with respiratory obstruction and cor pulmonale. J Pediatr 87:190, 1975.

McSwiney PF, Cavanagh NPC, Languth P: Outcome in congenital stridor (laryngomalacia). Arch Dis Child 52:215, 1977.

2. LARYNGEAL WEB

A laryngeal web is a triangular membrane, often concave posteriorly, in the anterior portion of the larynx. The membrane is usually attached to the superior surface of the true vocal cords. In other instances, apparent fusion of the anterior part of the true or false cords produces a weblike structure.

The onset of inspiratory stridor, if the web is large enough, is usually at birth. Affected infants have weak, occasionally hoarse cries.

Conservative treatment is usually adequate. Repeated gentle dilatation with laryngeal dilators may be appropriate. One should always be prepared to perform a tracheostomy following each dilatation, since the procedure may precipitate increased laryngeal edema and further obstruction. Simple incision of the web may be followed by re-formation. In older children, a thin sheet of Teflon can be placed within the larynx and between the "leaves" of the divided web. This is attached to the thyroid cartilage and allowed to remain in place until complete epithelialization has taken place.

3. LARYNGOCELE

This congenital lesion is seldom clinically apparent at birth. A defect in the muscular wall of the larynx allows the inflation of an air-filled cyst. This cyst presents in the neck when the intralaryngeal pressure is elevated and may cause upper airway obstruction.

4. LARYNGEAL CYSTS

A true laryngeal cyst is differentiated from laryngocele because it secretes fluid. It is rare in infancy but may present as a localized swelling in the neck which increases with crying or may impinge on the airway from the laryngeal ventricle. The cyst is usually sessile, with a thin glistening wall. In addition to the signs and symptoms of inspiratory obstruction, there may be dysphagia. Laryngeal cysts must be differentiated from internal thyroglossal duct cysts at the base of the tongue. Occasionally, laryngeal cysts may be eliminated by repeated aspiration, but much more frequently surgical removal of the cyst wall, as completely as possible, is necessary to eliminate recurrence.

Shackelford GD, McAlister WH: Congenital laryngeal cyst. Am J Roentgenol Radium Ther Nucl Med 114:289, 1972.

5. LARYNGOTRACHEOESOPHAGEAL CLEFT

This unusual congenital anomaly results from failure of posterior cricoid fusion during embryologic formation of the tracheoesophageal septum, leaving the larynx and part of the trachea open posteriorly. Affected patients are likely to have inspiratory stridor owing to poor laryngeal support and frequent aspiration of secretions and food. The cry is often very weak; there may be frequent cyanotic episodes due to aspiration; and recurrent or persistent pneumonitis is common. Weight gain is poor as a result of severe feeding problems and chronic lung disease.

The diagnosis of this entity can be very difficult. The diagnostic workup should include a barium swallow with fluoroscopy, direct laryngoscopy, esophagoscopy, and bronchoscopy. These patients should be fed by gastric tube. Corrective surgery has been successful in a few patients. Before surgery is attempted, the patient's nutritional status should be carefully attended to and intensive pulmonary therapy instituted. Tracheostomy or gastrostomy may be helpful in rehabilitation.

Beazer R & others: Laryngotracheo-esophageal cleft. Arch Dis Child 48:912, 1973.

Blumber JB & others: Laryngotracheo-esophageal cleft: The embryologic implications. Review of the literature. Surgery 57:559, 1965.

6. VOCAL CORD PARALYSIS

Vocal cord paralysis may be unilateral or bilateral and congenital or acquired. Vocal cord paralysis at birth is usually a laryngeal manifestation of a significant anomaly of another organ system. Bilateral cord paralysis may rarely be an isolated finding in an otherwise normal infant but more frequently is associated with birth trauma, cerebral agenesis, severe retardation, or meningomyelocele. Unilateral cord paralysis, whether congenital or acquired, is more common on the left than on the right because of the longer course of the left recurrent laryngeal nerve in the thorax and its anatomic proximity to major thoracic structures. The clinical presentation is similar to that of other congenital obstructive lesions of the upper airway. The amount of obstruction depends primarily on the severity of the paresis or paralysis. An artificial airway is rarely required with unilateral paralysis but frequently is required with bilateral paralysis. The diagnosis is established by direct laryngoscopy. Care must be taken to avoid artifactual fixation of one vocal cord (particularly the right) by the laryngoscope blade during the examination. The prognosis depends primarily on the associated anomalies.

Hagan PJ: Vocal cord paralysis. Ann Otol Rhinol Laryngol 72:206, 1963.

CROUP SYNDROME

Croup syndrome consists of inspiratory stridor and cough, usually of relatively acute onset. There may be associated hoarseness. This syndrome may be caused by a variety of inflammatory conditions of the upper airway in the region of the larynx. There may be underlying noninflammatory abnormalities of the upper airway such as vocal cord paralysis or congenital laryngeal stridor. Occasionally the syndrome may be caused entirely by noninflammatory problems such as an aspirated foreign body which is lodged in the extrathoracic airway, most likely at the level of the larynx or the cricoid cartilage. Croup syndrome can be due to hypocalcemic laryngeal tetany, or it may be one manifestation of the more generalized allergic response, as in angioneurotic edema. There may be a truly allergic form of croup (spasmodic) in the absence of other atopic symptoms. The differential diagnosis should also include the functional obstruction referred to as Munchausen's stridor. However, infection is the cause of croup syndrome in most cases (see Table 12–4). Viral croup is most common and bacterial croup is most serious. Rubeola and diphtheria can cause significant croup, but this is rarely seen.

1. VIRAL CROUP
(Laryngotracheobronchitis)

Viral croup most commonly affects children between 3 months and 3 years of age, characteristically occurs during the late fall or early winter, and is usually caused by the parainfluenza virus. It can also be caused by respiratory syncytial virus, influenza virus, rubeola virus, or adenoviruses. Although there is likely to be inflammation of the respiratory mucosa of all the connecting airways, the major cause of symptoms is inflammation and edema in the subglottic area, particularly at the level of the cricoid cartilage, which can cause significant narrowing of the airway at that point.

Clinical Findings

A. Symptoms and Signs: The onset is usually gradual, with a history of several days of symptoms of upper respiratory tract infection prior to the onset of barking cough and then inspiratory stridor. There are generally only mild elevations of temperature and white blood count, and the child does not appear toxic. If the lower respiratory tract is significantly involved, wheezing may be present. As the laryngeal obstruction progresses, stridor becomes associated with suprasternal, subcostal, and intracostal retractions. Auscultation may reveal decreased breath sounds. The child may become anxious and restless as hypoxemia develops. Cyanosis is a late sign and may herald complete airway obstruction. A decrease in the intensity of the inspiratory stridor may indicate improvement or may indicate significant deterioration of the patient with decreased inspiratory effort and increased inspiratory obstruction.

B. Laboratory Findings: The white blood count seldom increases to greater than 15,000/cu mm, and there is usually no significant leftward shift. Virus isolation studies have epidemiologic but not diagnostic usefulness. Blood cultures are rarely positive.

C. X-Ray Findings: X-rays of the cervical trachea demonstrate fixed circumferential subglottic narrowing. Chest x-ray is usually normal.

Complications

The principal complication in patients with viral croup is asphyxia secondary to laryngeal obstruction. Other complications are related to misadventures in attempting to supply an airway in an emergency situation and complications associated with management of a tracheostomy or endotracheal tube after an airway has been provided. A particularly traumatic tracheal intubation may convert a reversible subglottic narrowing into a fixed, nonreversible subglottic stenosis.

Treatment

A. Outpatient Management: Most patients who have no inspiratory stridor at rest may be treated at home. The parents should be instructed about the signs and symptoms of increasing airway obstruction (eg, tachypnea, cyanosis, increased retractions, or increased anxiety). Cool mist is a useful home treatment for mild croup. A heavy mist generated by running the shower in the bathroom with the doors closed will often afford significant relief.

B. Hospital Management: Any patient with an acute onset of inspiratory stridor at rest should be

Table 12–4. Croup syndrome.

	Bacterial Croup (Epiglottitis)	Viral Croup (Laryngotracheobronchitis)
Common cause	*Haemophilus influenzae*	Parainfluenza virus; respiratory syncytial virus
Most common age range	3–7 years	Less than 3 years
Seasonal occurrence	None	Late fall, winter
Clinical onset	Rapidly, acutely ill	Preceded by rhinitis and cough for several days
Dysphagia	Marked; may be drooling	None
Fever	> 39.4° C (103°F)	Variable, usually < 39.4° C (103° F)
White blood count	High (> 18,000/cu mm)	Usually normal
Criteria for diagnosis	"Cherry-red" epiglottis on direct visualization	Clinical presentation and exclusion of other diagnoses
Treatment	Ampicillin intravenously, artificial airway	Cool mist; racemic epinephrine

admitted to the hospital for therapy and close observation. Cool mist therapy is the most generally accepted treatment for viral croup and can be administered in either a high humidity room or a clear plastic mist tent. Large particle mist is probably most effective. Some croup patients have such severe dyspnea that they do not take adequate fluids orally, and in such cases intravenous hydration is necessary. It is helpful to monitor the urine specific gravity to ensure adequate hydration. All patients should be closely observed for signs of increasing hypoxia and impending respiratory failure. It is important to minimize any unnecessary anxiety, since increased anxiety results in increased inspiratory effort, which in turn increases the airway obstruction (dynamic compression), and increased oxygen consumption, all of which may worsen the patient's condition. Significant persistent inspiratory stridor can often be transiently ameliorated or eliminated with racemic epinephrine delivered by intermittent positive pressure breathing. A mixture of 0.5 ml of racemic epinephrine in 3.5 ml of preservative-free sterile water is nebulized by an IPPB machine driven by 40% oxygen. Many young patients will resist the IPPB initially, but after 1 minute or so they will breathe in phase with the machine as they realize that the machine overcomes much of their inspiratory difficulty. Particularly during this initial period, it is important to adequately restrain the infant and prevent any leak of pressure around the face mask. Since significant inspiratory stridor may return 1–2 hours after racemic epinephrine treatment, such therapy is appropriate only for hospitalized patients.

All croup patients who have significant obstruction have some degree of hypoxemia. For this reason, 25–30% oxygen is often administered.

Pharmacologic sedation should not be given to patients with viral croup unless an artificial airway is in place. Having the mother or some other familiar person close to the young patient is often the most effective form of sedation.

The use of corticosteroids is controversial. However, a brief course—eg, 0.5 mg/kg/day of dexamethasone (Decadron) or comparable agent in 4 divided doses for 1–3 days—may be beneficial in cases of severe croup.

If the usual medical measures are unsuccessful in relieving respiratory distress and if the patient remains restless, agitated, and has progressively increasing cyanosis and decreasing air entry, an artificial airway must be provided. Some centers use arterial or capillary blood gas analysis as an indication of the need for an artificial airway. However, the authors have avoided blood gas measurements since the procedure increases the agitation of the patient.

Endotracheal intubation is the generally recommended means of establishing an artificial airway. Intubation should be performed under controlled and optimal circumstances. Once the decision to provide an artificial airway has been made, the child should be given high concentrations of oxygen while arrangements are being completed. A small endotracheal tube should be used to reduce trauma to the glottis and the subglottic area. Optimal endotracheal tube care is mandatory and consists of careful suctioning, postural drainage and chest percussion, and humidification of inspired air. The patient can usually be extubated in 3–5 days, when he is able to breathe easily around the endotracheal tube.

Prognosis

Most children do not progress beyond the stage of cough, stridor, and mild retractions, and the disease usually resolves completely in 3–7 days.

Hamilton AG & others: Laryngeal oedema due to hereditary angioedema. Anaesthesia 32:265, 1977.

Newth CJL & others: The respiratory states of children with croup. J Pediatr 81:1068, 1972.

Patterson R & others: Munchausen's stridor: Nonorganic laryngeal obstruction.Clin Allergy 4:309, 1974.

Taussig LM & others: Treatment of laryngotracheal bronchitis (croup). Am J Dis Child 129:790, 1974.

Travis KW & others: Pulmonary edema associated with croup and epiglottitis. Pediatrics 59:695, 1977.

2. EPIGLOTTITIS
(Bacterial Croup)

Epiglottitis is the most serious form of croup syndrome and generally affects children between the ages of 3–7 years, with no particular seasonal distribution. The course is rapidly progressive and fulminant. The most common pathogen is *Haemophilus influenzae* type B, although beta-hemolytic streptococci and pneumococci have been implicated in rare cases. See Table 12–4 for a comparison of the clinical presentation of epiglottitis with that of viral croup.

Clinical Findings

A. Symptoms and Signs: The onset is abrupt over a period of only a few hours. Young children often present with high fever and respiratory distress; older children may appear toxic and in addition complain of difficulty in swallowing and severe sore throat. Because of extreme dysphagia, pooling of secretions in the posterior pharynx and drooling are prominent signs. Since the marked inflammation involves primarily the epiglottis and arytenoid cartilages, the patient may have a muffled voice but may not be hoarse. There is usually a high fever (> 38.4° C [103° F]), and the patient appears toxic or even shocky. Within a few hours after the onset of symptoms, the child may be in marked respiratory distress with severe inspiratory stridor and retractions. The pharynx is likely to be inflamed, and there may be excessive pharyngeal secretions. The diagnosis is made by direct visualization of the markedly enlarged, friable, "cherry-red" epiglottis with a tongue blade or laryngoscope. Direct visualization must be undertaken with great caution because stimulation of the epiglottis has produced abrupt laryngospasm and death. The tongue blade is less invasive and can be used with the patient in the characteristic sitting position with the neck extended, which is the position of choice for these patients in order to maximize the patency of the upper airway. The disadvantage of the tongue blade method is that it is impossible to visualize the arytenoid cartilages, and occasionally the inflammation may be localized to this site. Direct visualization with a laryngoscope has the advantage that the anatomy can be much more clearly seen (especially the arytenoid cartilages), but this method may precipitate laryngospasm and is usually performed with the patient supine, which may cause the epiglottis to totally obstruct the airway. No throat culture should be obtained until epiglottitis has been ruled out or until an artificial airway is in place, since this maneuver may also precipitate laryngospasm. Any attempt to visualize the laryngeal area should be preceded by administration of 100% oxygen.

B. Laboratory Findings: Leukocytosis of more than 15,000 white blood cells/cu mm and a leftward shift of the differential count is usually present. Blood cultures are usually positive for *H influenzae* type B.

C. X-Ray Findings: Lateral x-rays of the soft tissues of the neck may be of value in confirming the enlargement of the epiglottis without resorting to direct visualization. This technic is particularly applicable when experts in intubation are not immediately available. The patient with suspected epiglottitis should always be accompanied to the x-ray department for such an examination in case total airway obstruction should develop.

Treatment

When the diagnosis of epiglottitis is suspected, one of the above methods of confirming the diagnosis should be employed. Once the diagnosis is established, steps should be taken to introduce an artificial airway. Preparations should be made for controlled intubation, preferably in an operating room, with a tracheostomy set available. Because of the marked swelling and friability of the tissue, intubating such a patient is extremely difficult. The person most skilled in performing intubation should perform this procedure. While preparation is being made for controlled intubation, an intravenous line should be established and antibiotic therapy started by that route. Ampicillin (300 mg/kg/day in 6 divided doses) is the treatment of choice. In penicillin-sensitive patients, chloramphenicol may be employed.

Racemic epinephrine should not be used to treat this condition. A smaller than usual endotracheal tube should be used for this difficult intubation.

Prognosis

The inflammation usually subsides rapidly after the initiation of antibiotic therapy. The patient should be extubated when he can breathe around the endotracheal tube and when direct visualization demonstrates marked decrease in the epiglottic swelling. This usually occurs after 48–72 hours of intubation. If an artificial airway is not provided promptly, the mortality rate may be as high as 50%.

Battaglia JD, Lockhart CH: Management of acute epiglottitis by nasotracheal intubation. Am J Dis Child 129:334, 1975.

Molteni RA: Epiglottitis: Incidence of extraepiglottic infection. Report of 72 cases and review of the literature. Pediatrics 58:526, 1976.

Oh TH, Motoyama EK: Comparison of naso-tracheal intubation and tracheostomy in management of acute epiglottitis. Anesthesiology 46:214, 1977.

Rapkin RH: Simplicity and reliability of radiograph of the neck in the differential diagnosis of the croup syndrome. J Pediatr 80:96, 1972.

OTHER ACQUIRED ABNORMALITIES OF THE EXTRATHORACIC AIRWAY

1. UPPER AIRWAY OBSTRUCTION DUE TO ENLARGED TONSILS & ADENOIDS

The syndrome of chronic hypoventilation, particularly during sleep, and cor pulmonale, sometimes associated with daytime somnolence in children, is most commonly caused by marked enlargement of tonsillar and adenoidal lymphoid tissue in the posterior pharynx. A similar clinical picture can rarely develop with other causes of chronic upper airway obstruction such as laryngomalacia or micrognathia. The marked upper airway obstruction results in a great increase in the work of breathing and the gradual development of hypoventilation with CO_2 retention and associated hypoxemia. The low oxygen saturation causes pulmonary vasoconstriction, increased right ventricular work, and eventually cor pulmonale. Most children with this problem are between the ages of 3 months and 9 years of age; there is predominance of males over females of 3:1, and patients often have a history of recurrent pulmonary infections, somnolence, snoring, and mouth breathing.

Clinical Findings

These patients will usually have a rattly, low-pitched inspiratory stridor which is worse when supine. Tonsillar and adenoidal tissues are enlarged. There is likely to be accentuation of the pulmonary valve component of the second heart sound, a cardiac gallop, and often a cardiac murmur (especially of tricuspid insufficiency). Ten percent of these patients will have digital clubbing.

Chest x-ray demonstrates an enlarged cardiac silhouette, and there is often pulmonary edema. Such patients are often misdiagnosed as having myocarditis. X-rays of the soft tissues of the neck demonstrate large tonsils in many cases which significantly narrow the airway.

ECG will demonstrate right axis deviation, right atrial hypertrophy, and right ventricular hypertrophy.

Arterial blood gases may demonstrate CO_2 retention and hypoxemia, and there may be an elevated serum bicarbonate concentration as compensation for the chronic respiratory acidosis.

When this diagnosis is suspected in outpatients, it is appropriate to examine a chest x-ray and ECG and determine the serum bicarbonate to look for any evidence of chronic hypoventilation.

Treatment

If the significance of the upper airway obstruction is in doubt, a nasopharyngeal airway can be placed, and this should afford significant relief. The definitive treatment is tonsillectomy and adenoidectomy. Oxygen therapy and sedation should be used very cautiously since there may be depressed ventilatory drive. Assisted ventilation may be necessary for several days after surgery because of excessive secretions, upper airway edema, and persistent congestive heart failure.

Prognosis

There is significant clinical improvement after tonsillectomy and adenoidectomy, and probably gradual increase in respiratory drive. The pulmonary hypertension is probably completely reversible in most cases.

Cogswell JJ, Easton DM: Cor pulmonale in the Pierre Robin syndrome. Arch Dis Child 49:905, 1974.

Cox MA & others: Reversible pulmonary hypertension in a child with respiratory obstruction and cor pulmonale. J Pediatr 67:192, 1965.

Ingram RH, Bishop JB: Ventilatory response to carbon dioxide after removal of chronic upper airway obstruction. Am Rev Respir Dis 102:645, 1970.

Kravath RE & others: Hypoventilation during sleep in children who have lymphoid airway obstruction treated by nasopharyngeal tube and T and A. Pediatrics 59:865, 1977.

Kryger M & others: Diagnosis of obstruction of the upper and central airways. Am J Med 61:85, 1976.

Levin DL & others: Cor pulmonale secondary to upper airway obstruction in nine patients. Chest 68:166, 1975.

2. SUBGLOTTIC STENOSIS

Narrowing of the subglottic airway (from the level of the cricoid cartilage up to just below the vocal cords) can be either congenital, due to an abnormality of development, or acquired. Infants with congenital subglottic stenosis usually have inspiratory stridor from the time of birth, although milder cases of congenital or acquired stenosis may only have recurrent attacks of "croup." In any case, the voice and cry are usually normal except for inspiratory stridor. Acquired stenosis is usually secondary to trauma associated with the insertion or presence of an endotracheal tube. There is an increased risk of developing subglottic stenosis when the traumatized subglottic area is or becomes infected. The risk is minimized by using a small

endotracheal tube, performing controlled gentle intubation, and using an endotracheal tube made of polyvinyl chloride.

The treatment of subglottic stenosis may involve tracheostomy, repeated dilatation or cauterization of the narrowed airway (or both), or, occasionally, surgical resection. The differential diagnosis, particularly when there is asymmetric or unilateral narrowing, should include subglottic tumors such as hemangioma.

Kim SH, Hendren WH: Endoscopic resection of obstructing airway lesions in children. J Pediatr Surg 11:431, 1976.

Rodgers BM & others: Endobronchial cryotherapy in the treatment of tracheal strictures. J Pediatr Surg 12:443, 1977.

3. LARYNGEAL FRACTURE

Laryngeal fractures and soft tissue injuries in children are commonly the result of the child's being hurled against the dashboard of a car as the result of sudden deceleration. If the larynx is crushed, the airway may be completely obstructed so that immediate tracheostomy is required to prevent death. If the child survives the immediate postinjury period, careful observation is necessary during the ensuing 48 hours since edema and expansion of hematomas may compromise the airway.

After attention has been paid to the airway, the important considerations in injuries of this type are debridement and closure of lacerations and treatment of any intracranial complications. The physician is commonly misled at this point by his inclination to be conservative. Expectant treatment is just as inappropriate for the fractured larynx as it is for fracture-dislocation of the tibia. If normal function is to be restored, reduction of laryngeal fractures is usually necessary.

4. GLOTTIC & SUBGLOTTIC TUMORS

Papilloma and subglottic hemangioma are the most common tumors of the laryngeal area in infants and young children. Both may be present at birth and may present with inspiratory stridor. Subglottic lymphangioma can also occur but is very rare.

Papilloma

The most common laryngeal tumor in pediatrics is papilloma. It most often presents between 2–4 years of age. It is histologically benign, consisting of proliferation of stratified squamous epithelium with a central core of connective tissue and very little vascular supply. There are usually multiple papillomas, and they typically disappear about the time of puberty. If they do persist into adulthood, spontaneous remission becomes less likely and the possibility of malignant degeneration exists. The papillomas most commonly involve the cords and the anterior commissure but may extend to other glottic and subglottic structures and occasionally farther down the airway.

A typical presentation is with croupy cough and persistent hoarseness. There is progressive evidence of upper airway obstruction and occasionally lower airway obstruction, when there is more extensive distribution of the papillomas.

Treatment consists of repeated superficial excision until the problem spontaneously subsides. These tissue growths do not metastasize but do tend to recur frequently even after repeated excision. It is of key importance to maintain an adequate airway at all times.

Fechner RE & others: Invasive laryngeal papillomatosis. Arch Otolaryngol 99:147, 1974.

Gorrell DS: Laryngeal papillomata in children. Can Med Assoc J 67:425, 1952.

Smith L, Gooding CA: Pulmonary involvement in laryngeal papillomatosis. Pediatr Radiol 2:161, 1974.

Subglottic Hemangioma

Hemangiomas of the larynx in the infant are usually subglottic and tend to present early in life with signs of airway obstruction, usually without hoarseness. The hemangioma is sessile, soft and compressible, and usually not notably blue or red. In half of patients with subglottic hemangioma there are associated skin hemangiomas. Over 90% of isolated subglottic hemangiomas present before 6 months of age.

Most subglottic hemangiomas tend to regress and totally disappear within the first several years of life. Tracheostomy may be required while waiting for the hemangioma to regress spontaneously.

Ferguson CF: Congenital abnormalities of the infant larynx. Otolaryngol Clin North Am 3:185, 1970.

INTRATHORACIC AIRWAY OBSTRUCTION*

1. FOREIGN BODY ASPIRATION

Essentials of Diagnosis
- Sudden onset of coughing and wheezing.
- Localized wheezing and decreased air entry.
- Localized air trapping on forced expiratory chest x-ray.

General Considerations

Children between 6 months and 4 years of age are at particularly high risk for aspiration of any small object to which they have access such as seeds, grasses,

*Status asthmaticus is discussed in Chapter 32.

nuts, pins, or pebbles. The key to making this diagnosis, once it is suspected, is to take a very careful history in order to document the episode of choking associated with the onset of wheezing and chronic cough. There is often a history of playing with or near (or eating) some small object.

Clinical Findings

Aspiration of the foreign body classically precipitates an acute episode of choking, gagging, coughing, and wheezing, which in some instances may be associated with severe respiratory distress depending on the location of the foreign body in the airway. If the foreign body is not coughed out or if treatment is not initiated at that time, a period of several days with diminished symptoms may occur followed by recurrence of wheezing and persistent cough. The foreign body initially functions as a ball valve obstruction, which may cause localized hyperinflation; later, however, the foreign body and the associated mucosal inflammation may completely obstruct the airway, causing distal atelectasis. Trapping of secretions behind the foreign body may occur at any time, and they may become infected. Recurrent or persistent pneumonia, always occurring in the same area of the lung, may be due to a retained foreign body. If the foreign body remains in the airway for a long period with persistent distal pneumonia, bronchiectasis or lung abscess may develop in the distal airways.

A. Symptoms and Signs: Physical examination of the chest will usually reveal asymmetric auscultatory findings, ie, decreased breath sounds over the affected lung, often associated with inspiratory rhonchi and expiratory wheezing, particularly in the first few hours after aspiration. There may be increased or decreased resonance to percussion over the affected area. Occasionally the foreign body may lodge in the extrathoracic (larynx or high trachea) airway and cause signs of severe respiratory distress. When the foreign body comes to rest in a lower airway, there may be tracheal shift and asymmetric chest movement and aeration.

B. X-Ray Findings: The foreign body itself is usually radiolucent and therefore not seen on chest x-ray. If, as in the early stages after aspiration, the foreign body is functioning primarily as a ball valve obstruction, there may be localized hyperinflation. In such cases, however, the chest x-ray is most likely to be normal if taken during full inspiration, but a film during forced expiration will show localized hyperinflation with mediastinal shift away from the affected side. A forced expiratory film can be obtained in a patient of any age by manual pressure on the abdomen during a spontaneous expiration. If the foreign body has completely obstructed an airway, there will be distal resorption of air with resultant atelectasis and volume loss seen on the chest x-ray. This is particularly likely if the foreign body has been in place for several weeks. In such cases there will be no localized hyperinflation on the forced expiratory chest x-ray. If the signs, symptoms, and history are strongly suggestive of an aspirated foreign body, this diagnosis should be persued by bronchoscopy even if repeated inspiratory and expiratory films are normal.

Prevention

Small objects such as beads, buttons, and certain foods (nuts, seeds, popcorn) must be kept out of the reach of small children. It is important to prevent children from running with food or other small objects in their mouths and to discourage siblings from force feeding infants in play.

Treatment

All patients with suspected acute foreign body aspiration should be admitted to the hospital. Recent improvements in bronchoscope optics have made bronchoscopy a much safer procedure and therefore the treatment of choice for most aspirated foreign bodies. Bronchoscopy for foreign body in children is, however, a difficult and potentially hazardous procedure and therefore must be performed by an experienced and skilled bronchoscopist. The urgency with which treatment must be initiated and the recommended treatment depends to some degree on the location of the foreign body in the airway and the degree of the patient's respiratory distress. A foreign body located at or above the carina requires immediate emergency bronchoscopy. When the foreign body is lodged in a main stem bronchus, bronchoscopy should be performed as soon as convenient and certainly within 12–24 hours. A foreign body in a more distal airway can be treated by bronchoscopy or by a 48-hour trial of vigorous pulmonary therapy, to be followed by bronchoscopy if this technic is unsuccessful. Vigorous pulmonary therapy consists of hourly chest percussion over the affected area of the lung while the patient is awake and several times during the night. The chest percussion is preceded by having the patient inhale a nebulized bronchodilator. The patient should breathe oxygen while chest percussion is being administered.

Once the foreign body has been removed by either method, pulmonary therapy must be continued every 4–6 hours for 1–2 weeks, or longer if necessary, until physical examination and chest x-ray show that a normal physiologic and anatomic status has been restored.

Prognosis

The chance of complete recovery is excellent if the patient survives the acute episode and if the foreign body is removed within a short period. Foreign bodies that remain in place for many weeks can cause distal bronchiectasis or lung abscess.

Abdulmajid OA & others: Aspirated foreign bodies in the tracheal bronchial tree: Report of 250 cases. Thorax 31:635, 1976.

Law D, Kosloske AM: Management of tracheal bronchial foreign bodies in children: A reevaluation of postural drainage and bronchoscopy. Pediatrics 58:326, 1976.

Williams HE, Phelan PD: The "missed" inhaled foreign body in children. Med J Aust 1:625, 1969.

2. ANATOMIC NARROWING OF THE INTRATHORACIC TRACHEA & BRONCHI

The airway can be narrowed by intrinsic tumors, acquired or congenital fixed stenosis, extrinsic compression by aberrant blood vessels, or dynamic compression from altered transmural pressure gradients across the airway wall due to primary obstruction of more peripheral airways. Extrinsic compression of the airway can also be caused by mediastinal masses (Table 12–5).

Clinical Findings

Patients with fixed narrowing of the larger intrathoracic airways may present with a croup-like cough and, generally, more expiratory than inspiratory difficulty. An expiratory wheeze is frequently heard. There is often a history of recurrent, possibly localized pneumonia and increased respiratory distress with apparently mild respiratory infections. Chest x-ray may show localized or diffuse parenchymal infiltrates and possibly a mediastinal mass. (Many mediastinal masses do not cause airway narrowing.) Tomograms of the airway and high kilovoltage x-rays which better delineate the tracheobronchial air column may demonstrate a localized airway narrowing. When the airway obstruction is due to functional dynamic compression and not to a fixed anatomic narrowing, the small lumen may be demonstrable only during a forced expiratory maneuver. Pulmonary function tests may demonstrate decreased maximal inspiratory and expiratory flow rates if the narrowing is fixed. When the intrathoracic narrowing is due to dynamic compression, the peak expiratory but not the peak inspiratory

Table 12–5. Differential diagnosis of mediastinal mass according to anatomic location.

Superior mediastinum	Anterior mediastinum
Cystic hygroma	Thymoma
Vascular tumors	Thymic hyperplasia
Neurogenic tumors	Thymic cyst
Thymic tumors	Teratoma
Teratoma	Vascular tumors
Hemangioma	Lymphoma
Mediastinal abscess	Intrathoracic thyroid
Aortic aneurysm	Pleuropericardial cyst
Intrathoracic thyroid	Lymphadenopathy
Esophageal lesions	
Middle mediastinum	**Posterior mediastinum**
Lymphoma	Neurogenic tumors
Granuloma	Gastrointestinal tract
Hypertrophic lymph nodes	duplications
Bronchogenic cyst	Thoracic meningocele
Gastrointestinal tract duplication	Aortic aneurysm
Metastases	
Pericardial cyst	
Aortic aneurysm	
Anomalies of great vessels	

flow will be decreased. If localized intrinsic narrowing is strongly suspected but cannot be proved, diagnostic bronchoscopy may be indicated. The presence of a bronchoscope in the airway may significantly alter intrapulmonary pressure gradients, so that a significant functional dynamic compression of the airway may not be evident. Bronchography is a dangerous procedure in young children and is only rarely necessary. An esophagogram or angiograms may be helpful in defining the cause of some types of large airway obstruction.

Treatment

The appropriate treatment depends on the specific type of airway obstruction. Some intrinsic obstructions to the larger intrathoracic airways, such as acquired tracheal or bronchial stenosis, can be successfully treated by endoscopic electrocoagulation or by total resection and end-to-end reanastomosis of the proximal and distal airway segments.

Agosti E & others: Generalized familial bronchomalacia. Acta Pediatr Scand 63:616, 1974.

Feist JH & others: Acquired tracheomalacia: Etiology and differential diagnosis. Chest 68:340, 1975.

Kim SH, Hendren WH: Endoscopic resection of obstructing airway lesions in children. J Pediatr Surg 11:431, 1976.

Landing BH, Wells TR: Tracheal bronchial anomalies in children. In: *Perspectives in Pediatric Pathology.* Vol 1. Rosenberg HS, Bolande RP (editors). Year Book, 1973.

Wolman JJ: Congenital stenosis of the trachea. Am J Dis Child 61:1263, 1941.

3. TRACHEOMALACIA

The trachea of the newborn and young infant is significantly more compliant and therefore more compressible than that of the adult because of incomplete development of airway cartilage and other supportive tissue. Nonetheless, pathologic "tracheomalacia" in the absence of other lung disease is probably very rare. Tracheal collapse may occur in any patient with obstruction in smaller airways which necessitates forced expiration to empty the lungs. The positive intrathoracic pressure thus developed causes "dynamic compression" of the larger intrathoracic airway. Other causes of tracheal compression (eg, vascular ring) must be ruled out. There are rare cases of acquired or congenital defects of one or more tracheal rings which can cause a true isolated "tracheomalacia."

Treatment in most cases of "tracheomalacia," ie, those secondary to other airway disease, should be directed toward correction of the small airway disease. An artificial airway is rarely required.

Wittenborg MH & others: Tracheal dynamics in infants with respiratory distress, stridor, and collapsing trachea. Radiology 88:653, 1967.

4. VASCULAR RING

Tracheobronchial compression by anomalous blood vessels will usually cause symptoms within the first year of life if at all. There may be associated congenital cardiac disease. The symptoms of the obstruction are most commonly a persistent expiratory wheeze and noisy breathing, often with recurrent pneumonias and persistent cough. Patients with vascular rings may assume an opisthotonos position to optimize the airway. Rarely, such compression of the airway may present with apneic episodes. There may be associated difficulty with swallowing. The chest x-ray is likely to show persistent or recurrent increased bronchovascular markings, and occasionally there may be evidence of airway indentation. An esophagogram is diagnostic in the great majority of cases of vascular ring. Occasionally, bronchoscopy with or without pulmonary or systemic angiography is indicated to confirm or clarify the diagnosis. The more common vascular anomalies which may compress the trachea are (1) right aortic arch with left ligamentum arteriosum or patent ductus arteriosus, (2) double aortic arch, (3) anomalous innominate or left carotid artery, and (4) aberrant right subclavian artery.

All patients in whom vascular ring causes significant symptoms should have surgical correction if possible. Many infants have prolonged persistence of symptoms of expiratory obstruction even after surgical correction, suggesting a permanent abnormality of airway development, possibly secondary to the initial presence of the vascular anomaly.

Fearon B, Shortreed R: Tracheal bronchial compression by congenital cardiovascular anomalies in children: Syndrome of apnea. Ann Otol Rhinol Laryngol 72:949, 1963.

Godtfredsen J & others: Natural history of vascular ring with clinical manifestations: A follow-up study of 11 unoperated cases. Scand J Thorac Cardiovas Surg 11:75, 1977.

Hallman GL, Cooley DA, Bloodwell RD: Congenital vascular ring. Surg Clin North Am 46:885, 1966.

Keith HH: Vascular rings and tracheobronchial compression in infants. Pediatr Ann 6:91, 1977.

Stanger P & others: Anatomic factors causing respiratory distress in acyanotic congenital heart disease. Pediatrics 43:760, 1969.

Zdesbska E & others: Early diagnosis and surgical treatment of children with congenital vascular ring and accompanying heart lesions. J Pediatr Surg 12:121, 1977.

5. BRONCHITIS

Bronchitis may be acute or chronic, infectious (viral, bacterial [including mycoplasmal], or fungal), or due to chemical or mechanical irritation of the bronchial epithelium. Bronchitis as an isolated clinical entity is uncommon in childhood.

Clinical Findings

A. Symptoms and Signs: There is generally a dry, hacking, nonproductive cough for the first 4–6 days, after which the cough is likely to become productive. Fever, if present, is usually low-grade. Chest pain aggravated by coughing may develop. There are likely to be diffuse rhonchi, particularly during expiration. After 7–10 days, mucus production usually decreases and the cough gradually disappears.

B. Laboratory Findings: The white blood count is apt to be normal or only slightly elevated. Pulmonary function tests reveal a variable amount of airway obstruction which is usually not reversible with bronchodilator inhalation.

C. X-Ray Findings: The chest x-ray shows increased bronchovascular markings in chronic bronchitis and in some cases of acute bronchitis, but it may be normal.

Treatment

The general treatment for all types of bronchitis includes postural drainage and chest percussion preceded by bronchodilator inhalation, avoiding inhalation of irritants such as cigarette smoke and significant environmental pollution. Expectorants have no proved benefit. Cough suppressants are contraindicated since coughing is necessary to clear secretions. Mist or high humidity offers symptomatic relief but does not shorten the course of the disease. Antibiotics should be used in bronchitis due to bacterial infection.

Colley JRT, Reed DD: Urban and social origins of childhood bronchitis in England and Wales. Br Med J 2:213, 1970.

Pearlman ME & others: Nitrogen dioxide and lower respiratory illnesses. Pediatrics 47:391, 1971.

6. BRONCHIECTASIS

Essentials of Diagnosis

- Chronic cough and sputum production (worse in morning).
- Persistent localized pulmonary abnormality.

General Considerations

Bronchiectasis is chronic dilatation and infection of one or more bronchi. It usually begins in early childhood and may be generalized or localized to one or 2 lobes. The incidence in the general population is less than 0.5%. The lower lobes are more commonly affected than the upper lobes. The disease may be classified as cylindric, varicose, or saccular depending on the nature and severity of the bronchiectatic changes on bronchography or histologic examination. The prognosis in terms of reversibility of the lesions relates to this classification. In cylindric bronchiectasis, the bronchi are dilated but retain regular, smooth outlines. In varicose bronchiectasis, there is both irregular dilatation and constriction of bronchi. In saccular bronchiectasis, which carries the worse prognosis, the bronchi are widely dilated with increasing diameter in more distal airways. The airways tend to end in large blind sacs.

Bronchiectasis may occur in association with a variety of primary abnormalities or may be secondary to different lung insults. Some episodes of acute pneumonia due to adenovirus types 7 or 21, rubeola, pertussis, and, less frequently, *Haemophilus influenzae* type B, pneumococci, or *Staphylococcus aureus* may be followed by chronic recurrent symptoms of bronchiectasis rather than resolution, which is the typical outcome. Tuberculous pneumonia may also cause bronchiectasis.

Bronchiectasis may develop secondary to chronic or recurrent lower respiratory tract infections in patients with cystic fibrosis, immunodeficiency syndromes, recurrent aspiration, bronchial stenosis, congenital deficiencies of the bronchial cartilage, pulmonary lobar sequestration, or bronchogenic cyst. Occasionally, localized bronchiectasis may develop in a chronically collapsed lobe due (for example) to an unrecognized aspirated foreign body, a mucous plug, or right middle lobe syndrome.

Some cases are probably congenital in origin and have been postulated to result from an arrest of bronchial development leading to the formation of cysts which become infected.

The association of bronchiectasis and sinusitis with dextrocardia is known as *Kartagener's syndrome.* The cause of the coexistent sinus and bronchial disease (with or without dextrocardia) is unknown, although a generalized mucosal defect has been postulated. The complete Kartagener's syndrome has a high familial incidence but appears in only one generation.

Clinical Findings

A. Symptoms and Signs: The severity of the clinical manifestations of bronchiectasis varies widely. Most children with this disease appear healthy. There is likely to be a chronic productive cough, worse in the morning, which is often triggered by vigorous exercise. The sputum varies from white to gray in color, and in older children it may be foul-smelling and purulent. There may be a history of recurrent lower respiratory tract infections and dyspnea on exertion. Some children develop hemoptysis and bronchospasm. Digital clubbing appears in 25–50% of patients and does not necessarily relate to severity. There may be associated sinusitis, producing copious nasal and postnasal drainage, and headache. There are likely to be recurrent or low-grade persistent fevers and moist rales over the involved area of lung. There may also be rhonchi, decreased air entry, and dullness to percussion over the bronchiectatic area.

B. Laboratory Findings: Sputum culture usually reveals a mixed flora of bacteria, with *H influenzae* being the most common. Pulmonary function testing reveals decreased maximal expiratory flow rates (particularly at lower lung volumes), elevated pulmonary resistance, reduced dynamic lung compliance, and increased lung volumes indicating gas trapping. These findings not only reflect the localized disease but also indicate that many patients have generalized small airway disease.

C. X-Ray Findings: The plain chest film is almost always abnormal in patients with bronchiectasis. Radiologic abnormalities may range from mildly increased bronchovascular markings to cystic changes or complete lobar collapse. Bronchograms may help determine whether disease is localized or diffuse; however, a normal bronchogram does not necessarily rule out bronchiectasis. Since bronchograms can be very dangerous in children, they should be performed with great care and only if surgery is seriously considered, ie, to support an impression of localized disease. They should not be performed until the patient has received maximal medical therapy for at least 3–6 months. A bronchogram will allow for classification of the bronchiectasis as cylindric, varicose, or saccular. In some cases, high penetration chest x-rays will allow for the diagnosis of bronchiectasis without a bronchogram.

Complications

Complications include brain or lung abscess, emphysema, bronchopleural fistula, hemoptysis, cor pulmonale, and amyloidosis.

Prevention

Pneumonia should be treated with appropriate antibiotics in adequate dosages and vigorous pulmonary physiotherapy. All children should receive adequate immunizations for pertussis and rubeola.

Treatment

A thorough search for underlying causes of bronchiectasis should include repeated sputum cultures, evaluation of the immune system, sweat test, Mantoux test, sinus x-rays, and in some cases forced expiratory chest films and bronchoscopy. Systemic antibiotics should be selected on the basis of bacterial culture results and administered for at least 2–4 weeks. Optimal pulmonary physiotherapy is essential and consists of bronchodilator inhalation followed by postural drainage and chest percussion to the affected lobe or lobes. This should be performed at least 2–4 times daily. Patients with evidence of acute reversibility of airway obstruction following bronchodilator inhalation may benefit by chronic aminophylline therapy. Sinusitis should be vigorously treated.

Surgical removal of one or 2 lobes which have severe saccular bronchiectasis may be indicated if optimal medical therapy for at least 9–12 months has been without benefit and if the rest of the lung appears to be entirely normal. Only a very few children with bronchiectasis are appropriate candidates for lobectomy.

Prognosis

The prognosis for patients with bronchiectasis depends on the cause, the severity, and the distribution of the bronchiectasis. Cylindric bronchiectasis is potentially reversible and is frequently present transiently after acute episodes of pneumonia, even in normal patients. The saccular type of bronchiectasis involves irreversible tissue destruction. Some patients will improve significantly after lobectomy or treatment of sinusitis, and most patients will show some improvement with optimal medical management. Most children with this disease are quite well controlled and lead relatively normal lives. Patients in whom the bronchiectasis is associated with immunologic deficiency or cystic fibrosis have the poorest prognosis. In some cases, the disease clears entirely by adolescence.

Holmes LB & others: A reappraisal of the Kartagener's syndrome. Am J Med Sci 255:13, 1968.

Kartagener M, Stucki T: Bronchiectasis with situs inversus. Arch Pediatr 79:193, 1962.

Landau LI & others: Ventilatory mechanics in patients with bronchiectasis starting in childhood. Thorax 29:304, 1974.

Sanderson JM & others: Bronchiectasis: Results of surgical and conservative management: A review of 393 cases. Thorax 29:407, 1974.

Williams HE & others: Generalized bronchiectasis due to extensive deficiency of bronchial cartilage. Arch Dis Child 47:423, 1972.

7. ACUTE BRONCHIOLITIS

Essentials of Diagnosis

- Rhinitis, cough, and expiratory wheeze.
- Tachypnea.
- Pulmonary hyperaeration on chest x-ray.

General Considerations

Acute bronchiolitis is a potentially serious disease that characteristically occurs during the winter months in children under 2 years of age. The widespread bronchiolar inflammatory exudate, mucosal edema, and resultant narrowing of the airway can be due to either infection or allergy or a combination of the two. An allergic component is particularly likely to be present in infants with recurrent acute bronchiolitis or a strong personal or family history of allergy. Respiratory syncytial virus (RSV) is by far the most frequent causative organism, but parainfluenza viruses, adenoviruses, and influenza viruses can cause the same clinical picture. All patients with bronchiolitis have some degree of hypoxemia, which may become severe. Occasionally there may be CO_2 retention. The hypoxemia may persist for 4–6 weeks after the child has begun to improve clinically.

Clinical Findings

A. Symptoms and Signs: After 1–2 days of mild rhinitis, the infant gradually develops increasing cough, expiratory wheeze, and respiratory distress. The respiratory rate becomes rapid, with shallow respiratory excursions. There may be intercostal, subcostal, and suprasternal retractions on inspiration, nasal flaring, and intermittent cyanosis. Chest auscultation reveals diffuse rales, expiratory wheezes, decreased breath sounds, and prolonged expiratory time. Pulmonary hyperinflation due to air trapping may produce an increase in chest diameter and depression of the diaphragm, resulting in displacement of the edge of the liver below the right costal margin. The easily palpable liver should not be confused with cardiac failure, which may or may not be present.

Some infants with respiratory syncytial virus infection may present with significant apneic episodes early in the course of the disease, requiring mechanical ventilation. Coexisting findings of bronchiolitis are usually present in these patients.

B. Laboratory Findings: The white blood count is usually normal—an important point in the differentiation of acute bronchiolitis from pneumonia and pertussis. In allergic infants, nasal and peripheral eosinophilia may be present. Immunofluorescent staining of nasal secretions is likely to be positive for respiratory syncytial virus.

C. X-Ray Findings: The chest x-ray reveals hyperinflation (loss of posterior diaphragmatic upward convexity on lateral x-ray and increased lucency of lung fields). There may be increased bronchovascular markings and very mild infiltrates.

Differential Diagnosis

In small infants it may be difficult or impossible to differentiate bronchiolitis from bronchopneumonia. Fever is high in bronchopneumonia, as is the neutrophil count. Pertussis may be clinically similar to bronchiolitis except that white counts over 15,000/cu mm and marked lymphocytosis are unusual in bronchiolitis but common with pertussis.

Asthma can occur in infants, and the differentiation from bronchiolitis may be difficult at the time of the first illness. A positive family history for allergy, repeated attacks, nasal or peripheral eosinophilia, and immediate response to a bronchodilator suggest that an allergy may be partly responsible for the wheezing.

In severe cases, an erroneous diagnosis of heart failure may be made. Growth retardation, enlarged heart (rare in bronchiolitis), and cardiac murmurs indicate heart disease.

Complications

The principal complication is secondary bacterial infection. Pneumothorax and mediastinal emphysema have been reported. Respiratory failure may occur.

Treatment

Hospitalization is recommended for infants with bronchiolitis who meet *any* of the following criteria: (1) less than 2 months of age, (2) a history or presence of cyanosis, (3) a history of a previous severe attack of wheezing, (4) a resting respiratory rate of $\geqslant$ 60/minute, (5) arterial P_{CO_2} > 45 mm Hg, or (6) arterial P_{O_2} < 60 mm Hg with the infant breathing room air. It is important that arterial blood gases be measured since a patient with bronchiolitis who meets any of the above

criteria will be hypoxemic. The inspired gas should be humidified and enriched with sufficient oxygen to maintain an adequate arterial P_{O_2}. Infants with bronchiolitis may be dehydrated owing to inadequate fluid intake. The treatment should be directed toward achieving and maintaining a state of normal hydration, carefully following fluid intake and urine output as well as urine specific gravity. It is important to avoid overhydration since this might contribute to pulmonary edema and thus further impair respiratory function. Chest percussion and postural drainage preceded by bronchodilator inhalation may be helpful in some patients with bronchiolitis.

Since allergic mechanisms may be responsible for part of the airway obstruction in some infants with acute bronchiolitis, a trial of epinephrine 1:1000 solution, 0.01 ml/kg subcut, with or without theophylline, 2–4 mg/kg orally every 6 hours, should be tried.

Antibiotic therapy is indicated in more severe cases of bronchiolitis and those where secondary bacterial infection is strongly suspected. High fever, significant infiltrates on chest x-ray, significant elevation of the white blood count with a leftward shift of the differential count, respiratory failure, or positive bacterial cultures are indications for parenteral antibiotics.

Endotracheal intubation and mechanical ventilation are required for occasional infants who develop respiratory failure. Apnea or respiratory acidosis with a pH of less than 7.25 or inability to maintain the arterial P_{O_2} above 60 mm Hg is a generally accepted indication for intubation and ventilation. The time course and progression of the disease may necessitate modification of these guidelines.

There is no evidence that exogenous corticosteroids influence the course of this disease. Pharmacologic sedation should not be used unless the patient is intubated and receiving assisted ventilation.

Prognosis

Acute symptoms of bronchiolitis usually last 2–7 days, with total resolution of the disease by 7–10 days. With prompt optimal therapy, the prognosis is usually excellent. Far less than 1% of infants with bronchiolitis will die of respiratory failure. About half of infants with bronchiolitis will have subsequent episodes of wheezing and are very likely atopic.

Downes GJ & others: Acute respiratory failure in infants with bronchiolitis. Anesthesiology 29:426, 1968.

Kettan M & others: Pulmonary function abnormalities in symptom-free children after bronchiolitis. Pediatrics 59:683, 1977.

Wohl MEB & others: Resistance of the total respiratory system in healthy infants and infants with bronchiolitis. Pediatrics 43:495, 1969.

Workshop on bronchiolitis. Pediatr Res 11:209, 1977.

8. BRONCHIOLITIS OBLITERANS
(Bronchiolitis Fibrosa Obliterans)

Bronchiolitis obliterans, quite rare in children, can be diagnosed with certainty only by microscopic examination of lung tissue. A major insult to the lower respiratory tract is the most common cause, and the chief pathologic features are extensive damage to the bronchiolar wall with obstruction of the lumen by organized exudate and polypoid masses of granulation tissue. Distal to the bronchiolar obstruction, there may be air trapping or marked accumulation of fat-filled phagocytes. Ultimately, the involved bronchioles may be replaced by fibrous scars. There may be an associated interstitial pneumonia.

Bronchiolitis obliterans may occur following inhalation of toxic gases, lower respiratory tract infections (influenza, rubeola, pertussis, and adenovirus type 21), or inhalation of foreign bodies. In some cases, the cause is not known.

The most common symptoms are cough, dyspnea, chest pain, malaise, sputum production, and sometimes hemoptysis. Rales are commonly heard on chest auscultation. Chest x-ray abnormalities are variable and may include nodular densities, alveolar opacities, or occasionally hyperinflation. Pulmonary function studies may demonstrate either restrictive or obstructive disease.

Some children with bronchiolitis obliterans may benefit by steroid therapy. In some cases, antibiotic therapy is indicated.

Becroft DMO: Bronchiolitis obliterans, bronchiectasis, and other sequelae of adenovirus type 21 infection in young children. J Clin Pathol 24:72, 1971.

Gosnick BB, Friedman PJ, Liebow AA: Bronchiolitis obliterans: Roentgenologic-pathologic correlation. Am J Roentgenol Radium Ther Nucl Med 117:816, 1973.

9. ATELECTASIS

Nonaeration of part of the lung is usually due either to complete obstruction of a conducting airway, with resorption of all distal air, or to instability and collapse of terminal air spaces, often associated with inadequate surfactant, as in hyaline membrane disease or "shock lung." The extent of nonaeration or lung collapse may vary from one entire lung or more to an involvement of only very distal air spaces in localized or diffuse distribution. With segmental or lobar atelectasis, the primary larger airway obstruction may be either intrinsic or extrinsic. Intraluminal obstruction of a major airway may be caused by a mucous plug, tumor, or aspirated food, foreign body, or vomitus. Airway obstruction due to extrinsic compression is usually due to an enlarged lymph node, usually associated with infection or cancer. Enlarged or aberrant major blood vessels occasionally cause marked extrinsic compression of an airway sufficient to result in distal atelectasis. In addition, atelectasis can occur as a result of direct local parenchymal compression (eg, secondary to lobar emphysema or pleural effusion), chronic shallow respiration (eg, secondary to diaphragmatic paralysis or muscular dystrophy), mucosal inflammation, or endobronchial tuberculosis. Atelectasis is a common finding in patients with cystic fibrosis and asthma. Allergic children have a tendency toward right middle lobe atelectasis, which may be chronic or recurrent. Atopy is the most common cause of persistent right middle lobe atelectasis. Postoperative atelectasis is not uncommon, particularly when the anesthesia time is prolonged or if the surgery involves the thorax or a major abdominal operation.

Clinical Findings

A. Symptoms and Signs: The clinical findings associated with atelectasis depend on its distribution and extent. Patients may present with persistent cough or fever. Physical examination may reveal tachypnea, rales or wheezing, or a localized decrease in breath sounds. In patients with chronic atelectasis, the volume loss in the affected area may be so complete that no localized dullness to percussion or decreased breath sounds can be detected on physical examination. If there is infection in the atelectatic lung or elsewhere, there may be a temperature elevation.

B. Laboratory Findings: There may be no abnormal laboratory findings. A Mantoux test should be performed. If infection is present, there may be an elevation of the white blood count. In older patients with significant atelectasis, it may be possible to measure a decrease in lung volumes by pulmonary function testing. Most patients with significant atelectasis, particularly those with reactive airway disease (asthma), will also have decreased maximal expiratory flow rates on pulmonary function testing.

C. X-Ray Findings: Chest x-ray may show diffuse patchy, lobar, or linear infiltrates, signs of unilateral volume loss (eg, unilateral diaphragmatic elevation, mediastinal shift, hilar elevation, or elevated or lowered fissure lines), or areas of compensatory hyperinflation. When the areas of atelectasis are small, there may be difficulty in distinguishing atelectasis from pneumonia.

Treatment

Therapy should include vigorous treatment of any underlying lung disease plus vigorous chest percussion and postural drainage combined with bronchodilator administration (inhaled, oral, or both). The pulmonary physiotherapy should be directed toward the affected area. If a localized lobar or segmental atelectasis persists for 1–2 months despite optimal medical therapy, bronchoscopy may be indicated for diagnosis and treatment. Lobectomy is indicated only after failure to expand the lung with at least 1–2 years of optimal therapy. There is no evidence that intermittent positive pressure breathing is effective for atelectasis due to large airway obstruction. If foreign body aspiration is suspected, bronchoscopy should be performed after 1–2 weeks of medical therapy. Children with right middle lobe atelectasis should be evaluated for asthma and, if appropriate, treated with chronic bronchodilator therapy.

Bendixen HH & others: Impaired oxygenation in surgical patients during general anesthesia with controlled ventilation: A concept of atelectasis. N Engl J Med 269:991, 1963.

Dees SC, Spock A: Right middle lobe syndrome in children. JAMA 197:78, 1966.

Erlich R, Arnon RG: The intermittent endotracheal intubation technique for the treatment of recurrent atelectasis. Pediatrics 50:144, 1972.

Tarnay TJ: Chronic atelectasis in children. Hosp Med 6:136, May 1970.

10. BRONCHOPULMONARY DYSPLASIA

Bronchopulmonary dysplasia consists of chronic increased oxygen demand following acute clinical hyaline membrane disease. The clinical and pathologic findings are characteristic. Bronchopulmonary dysplasia occurs in approximately 20–30% of babies with clinical hyaline membrane disease who require mechanical ventilation.

Clinical Course & Manifestations

The disease has been divided into 4 stages as follows:

Stage 1 (days 1–3) is a period of acute hyaline membrane disease with a characteristic chest x-ray revealing air bronchograms and reticular granularity of the lung fields. During this period there is tachypnea, hypoxemia due to shunting through the areas of widespread alveolar atelectasis, and often hypercapnia. As a result of a deficiency of surfactant which causes diffuse microatelectasis, the lungs are stiff and the functional residual capacity low. Histologically, there is diffuse collapse of terminal air spaces, but the larger airways are entirely normal. Most patients with clinical hyaline membrane disease begin to improve after 2–3 days and are normal by 5–10 days. In contrast, those who will develop bronchopulmonary dysplasia are likely to continue to worsen over the first several days of life, requiring mechanical ventilation.

Stage 2 (days 4–10) is the period of initial regeneration. There is marked increase in oxygen requirement above normal and failure to improve clinically. The chest x-ray classically shows nearly complete bilateral opacification, although this picture may be eliminated by therapy using positive airway pressure. Histologically, there is early regeneration and metaplasia of alveolar epithelium and some necrosis of bronchiolar epithelium.

During *stage 3* (days 10–20), the period of transition to chronic disease, oxygen dependence persists, though the patient may no longer need mechanical ventilation. The chest x-ray demonstrates a "honeycomb lung," with multiple small, round radiolucent areas. On histologic examination there is regeneration and metaplasia of bronchiolar epithelium, with increased airway mucus secretion and an inflammatory cell response. There are alternating areas of emphysema and atelectasis.

Stage 4 (after 4 weeks) is the period of true chronic lung disease. There may be a requirement for increased inspired oxygen for several months although there is usually slow but progressive decrease of this requirement. There may be diffuse rales and wheezing on physical examination of the chest, with chest wall retractions, and increased chest circumference due to expiratory obstruction. The chest x-ray typically shows enlargement of the previously small radiolucent areas, beginning in the lung bases, with progression to generally radiolucent, hyperinflated lung fields with fibrous and atelectatic streaks. The histologic picture during this phase is characterized by alternating areas of atelectasis and emphysema, metaplasia of the bronchiolar epithelium, hypertrophy of medial smooth muscle in the pulmonary arterioles, and dilatation of pulmonary lymphatics. There may also be interstitial edema and eventually fibrosis.

Differential Diagnosis

The chronic lung disease following some viral pulmonary infections (especially adenovirus) or occasionally following chronic congestive heart failure due to patent ductus arteriosus may be very similar, both clinically and pathologically, to bronchopulmonary dysplasia.

Prevention

It is likely that both high positive airway pressures (barotrauma) and high inspired oxygen concentrations (oxygen toxicity) contribute to the development of this iatrogenic disease, although the relative importance of these factors has not yet been determined. Great care should be taken during the treatment of acute clinical hyaline membrane disease to minimize the patient's exposure to high airway pressure (> 30 cm water) and high oxygen concentrations (> 60% oxygen).

Treatment

Under some circumstances it is appropriate to discharge the patient from the hospital before the oxygen requirement has returned to normal. This can be done by arranging for home oxygen administration through a nasal cannula. Infants with bronchopulmonary dysplasia are likely to require several rehospitalizations for increasing respiratory distress and increased oxygen requirement, often precipitated by a mild viral infection. Some such infants, even in the absence of overt signs of heart failure, may benefit by diuretic therapy, particularly during acute exacerbations. Since excessive airway secretions and necrotic cellular debris may contribute to airway obstruction and since normal lung clearance mechanisms are not likely to be functioning properly, chest percussion and postural drainage may help these patients. It is important to maintain an adequate hemoglobin concentration in patients requiring chronic oxygen therapy in order to maximize the oxygen carrying capacity. It is helpful to follow the ECG for signs of increasing right ventricular hypertrophy, which may indicate increasing hypoxemia, and for increased serum bicarbonate which may indicate chronic hypercapnia. Adequate nutrition is also of key importance.

Prognosis

Most patients with bronchopulmonary dysplasia will demonstrate slow though progressive improvement of lung function over the first several years of life.

Bryan MH & others: Pulmonary function studies during the first years of life in infants recovering from the respiratory distress syndrome. Pediatrics 52:169, 1973.

Koch G: Neonatal respiratory distress and residual pulmonary abnormalities. Bull Euro Physiopath Resp 12:695, 1976.

Northway WH & others: Pulmonary disease following respiratory therapy of hyaline membrane disease. N Engl J Med 276:357, 1967.

Phillip AGS: Oxygen plus pressure plus time: The etiology of bronchopulmonary dysplasia. Pediatrics 55:44, 1975.

Rosan RC: Hyaline membrane disease and a related spectrum of neonatal pneumopathies. Perspect Pediatr Pathol 2:15, 1975.

Stocks J, Godfrey S: The role of artificial ventilation, oxygen, and CPAP in the pathogenesis of lung damage in neonates: Assessment by serial measurements of lung function. Pediatrics 57:352, 1976.

Taghizadh A, Reynolds EOR: Pathogenesis of bronchopulmonary dysplasia following hyaline membrane disease. Am J Pathol 82:241, 1976.

11. CYSTIC FIBROSIS

Essentials of Diagnosis

- Elevated sweat chloride (> 60 mEq/liter).
- Recurrent pulmonary infections or steatorrhea.

General Considerations

Cystic fibrosis is a genetically transmitted autosomal recessive disease characterized by widespread involvement of the exocrine glands. Approximately 5% of Caucasian population are carriers of the recessive gene, and one in 2000 infants is affected. Multiple organ systems are involved: lungs, gastrointestinal tract, sweat glands, and testes.

In the lungs there is production of abnormally viscous mucus. The respiratory cilia, which also may have a disorganized beating pattern, are unable to effectively clear this tenacious mucus. As a consequence, there is progressive obstruction of the airways, beginning with the small bronchioles, leading to air trapping and atelectasis. Secondarily acquired lung infection occurs and predisposes to destruction of the respiratory epithelium and airways, resulting in bronchiectasis. The bacteria most commonly cultured from expectorated sputum are *Pseudomonas aeruginosa,* *Staphylococcus aureus,* and *Haemophilus influenzae.* In addition, these patients are particularly vulnerable to viral respiratory tract infections.

There is wide variability in the clinical presentation and course; some patients are severely affected as infants, and others remain asymptomatic until adolescence. Any patient with malabsorption problems or repeated pulmonary infections should be suspected of having cystic fibrosis.

Clinical Findings

A. Symptoms and Signs: In severe disease, patients have foul-smelling, bulky, frequent fatty stools, failure to thrive, and frequent pulmonary infections with chronic cough productive of purulent sputum. Ten percent of newborns with cystic fibrosis present with intestinal obstruction secondary to inspissated meconium (meconium ileus). Infants with mild disease may present at an older age with symptoms resembling those of asthma. Occasional patients have no significant symptoms until early adulthood.

Physical examination may be normal or may reveal signs of pulmonary involvement and malnutrition. Manifestations of the associated lung disease include hyperexpansion of the thoracic cage with use of the auxiliary muscles of respiration, rales, rhonchi, wheezes, unevenly decreased breath sounds in different parts of the chest, cyanosis, and digital clubbing. The liver edge may be palpable well below the right costal margin, but this is probably due to a flattened diaphragm, lowering the liver, although it occasionally can be caused by cor pulmonale, and in that case would usually be associated with cardiac gallop rhythm. Patients with moderate to severe lung disease may have significant accentuation of the pulmonary component of the second heart sound. Physical signs of malabsorption include poor growth (weight gain is usually significantly more impaired than linear growth) and decreased subcutaneous tissue and muscle mass.

B. Laboratory Findings: The earliest laboratory signs of the associated pulmonary disease are a decrease in arterial oxygen tension and abnormalities of pulmonary tests of small airway patency such as the maximal midexpiratory flow rate, the flow volume loop, and the single breath oxygen test. With progression of pulmonary disease, pulmonary function testing demonstrates increasing obstructive lung disease with further decreased maximal flow rates and vital capacity and increased absolute lung volumes (first residual volume, then functional residual capacity, then total lung capacity are increased) and airway resistance. With very severe lung disease, in the preterminal period, there may be a decrease in total lung capacity.

A sweat test should be performed using the pilocarpine iontophoresis technic. A sweat chloride concentration > 60 mEq/liter is diagnostic if at least

50 mg of sweat have been collected. A concentration $<$ 50 mEq/liter is normal. Patients with sweat chloride concentrations between 50 and 60 mEq/liter present diagnostic problems.

There is likely to be increased stool fat excretion. No reliable methods are available for screening newborn stools, for intrauterine diagnosis of cystic fibrosis or for detection of the heterozygote.

With more severe lung disease, the ECG and echocardiogram may demonstrate abnormalities of the right ventricle.

Although liver involvement is histologically demonstrable at an early stage in the disease, laboratory evidence of liver involvement (increased liver enzymes and decreased liver-dependent clotting factors) does not appear until relatively late.

C. X-Ray Findings: The earliest abnormalities on chest x-ray are mild hyperinflation, best seen as loss of diaphragmatic doming on the lateral chest x-ray, and increased bronchovascular markings, particularly in the upper lobes. Later, there are diffuse infiltrates, marked hyperinflation, and areas of atelectasis interspersed with areas of "emphysema," giving an appearance of cystic lung changes. Sinus x-rays demonstrate a high incidence of sinusitis, and x-rays of the long bones may demonstrate pulmonary osteoarthropathy.

Differential Diagnosis

Cystic fibrosis must be differentiated from allergic lung diseases, immunologic deficiency diseases, chronic recurrent pneumonia, a_1-antitrypsin deficiency, anatomic airway abnormalities (eg, airway stenosis), chronic recurrent aspiration, and other causes of malabsorption.

Complications

Cardiopulmonary complications include pneumothorax, pulmonary abscess, hemoptysis, empyema, nasal polyps, sinusitis, pulmonary hypertension, cor pulmonale, respiratory failure, and pulmonary osteoarthropathy. Complications involving the intestinal tract include intussusception, impaction, rectal prolapse, recurrent abdominal pain, portal hypertension, esophageal varices, hematemesis, and failure to thrive.

Treatment

A vigorous long term multidisciplinary treatment program with good follow-up and continuity is extremely important in the treatment of patients with cystic fibrosis.

A. Pulmonary Therapy: Since all patients with cystic fibrosis probably have impaired lung clearance mechanisms and therefore accumulate viscous mucus in the airways, postural drainage and chest percussion in 9 different positions should be done at least once daily (Fig 12−2). In many patients it is helpful to precede the chest percussion by bronchodilator inhalation. All episodes of acute increases in cough, sputum production, dyspnea, or fever should be treated with oral or parenteral antibiotics depending on the severity of the acute and chronic illness as well as an increase in the frequency of pulmonary physical therapy. Antibiotics may be selected on the basis of sputum cultures, although any child with advanced cystic fibrosis will harbor *H influenzae, S aureus,* and *P aeruginosa.* The most effective oral antibiotics are trimethoprim-sulfamethoxazole (co-trimoxazole; Bactrim, Septra), 8−20 mg/kg/day of trimethoprim in 2−3 divided doses; dicloxicillin, 25−50 mg/kg/day in 3−4 divided doses; chloramphenicol, 50 mg/kg/day in 3−4 divided doses; and, for older children, tetracycline, 20−40 mg/kg/day in 3−4 divided doses. Appropriate antibiotics for intravenous administration are gentamicin, 7 mg/kg/day in 3 divided doses; carbenicillin, 400 mg/kg/day in 4 divided doses; and methicillin, 200 mg/kg/day in 4 divided doses. Some severely affected patients may have some degree of biventricular cardiac failure and may benefit by either diuretic or digitalis therapy. Oral bronchodilator therapy (theophylline, 4−6 mg/kg/dose in 3−4 daily doses) is of benefit to some patients with cystic fibrosis.

There is an increased incidence of atopy in children with cystic fibrosis, and some of these patients will benefit from intermittent antihistamine therapy.

Oxygen therapy is often indicated to maintain adequate arterial oxygen tension during acute exacerbations. In addition, severely affected children may benefit from chronic oxygen administration at home, particularly at night. Recurrent morning headaches will often disappear when nighttime oxygen therapy is initiated.

B. Intestinal Tract Therapy:

1. Meconium ileus in the newborn−Intestinal obstruction due to uncomplicated meconium ileus in the newborn can usually be relieved by diatrizoate meglumine (Gastrografin) or acetylcysteine (Mucomyst) enemas. When surgery is necessary, intestinal atresia or volvulus requiring resection may be found proximal to the meconium ileus.

2. Meconium ileus equivalent and intussusception in older children−These causes of intestinal obstruction and abdominal pain in older children can often be relieved by enema. The inspissated feces can sometimes be softened by oral acetylcysteine, liquids, or mineral oil. Intussuseption can usually be reduced by enemas, although surgery is occasionally required.

3. Pancreatic insufficiency−A number of commercial products containing lye base, trypsin, and amylase from pork pancreas (eg, Cotazym, Viokase) are available in capsule, tablet, or powder form to be taken at mealtime. The dosage of pancreatic enzyme replacement should be individualized to produce 1−2 formed stools daily. One or 2 capsules are often indicated with snacks. The enzymes may be mixed with some form of fruit (eg, applesauce). The requirement for replacement enzymes may either decrease or increase with age.

Persistence of marked diarrhea in the face of seemingly adequate replacement therapy should make one suspect other causes. Disaccharidase deficiencies and celiac disease have been reported in patients with cystic fibrosis.

The diet should be high in protein and carbohydrate, and some attempt should be made to avoid excessively fatty foods. Small infants and occasionally older children may benefit from diets containing medium-chain triglycerides (eg, Portagen). Some infants with cystic fibrosis, particularly those receiving soybase formulas, may present with hypoproteinemic edema due to difficulty in absorbing the protein. Water-soluble vitamin E preparations (approximately 100 units/day) should probably be given to all cystic fibrosis patients. Patients exposed to conditions which may cause heavy sweat loss (eg, hot weather, fever) and patients with hyponatremia should have 1 gm of salt added to the daily diet up to 2 years of age and 2 gm/day over 2 years of age.

C. Psychosocial Support: Cystic fibrosis imposes many extra psychologic, social, and financial burdens on the patient and family. Skilled counsel is an important aspect of care, particularly around the time the diagnosis is made and in the weeks before and after death.

Prognosis

Life expectancy for patients with cystic fibrosis has improved significantly in recent years, probably as a result of more aggressive therapy and more frequent diagnosis of patients with milder disease. Fifty percent of patients whose lungs can be made clear to clinical examination at the time of diagnosis will survive to 18 years of age.

Cogswell JJ & others: Chronic suppurative lung disease in sisters mimicking cystic fibrosis. Arch Dis Child 49:520, 1974.

Committee for Study for Evaluation of Testing for Cystic Fibrosis: Evaluation of testing for cystic fibrosis. J Pediatr 88:711, 1976.

Crey M & others: Five to seven year course of pulmonary function in cystic fibrosis. Am Rev Respir Dis 114:1086, 1976.

Di Sant'Agnese PA, Davis PB: Research in cystic fibrosis. N Engl J Med 295:481, 1976.

Graham DY: Enzyme replacement therapy of exocrine pancreatic insufficiency in man: Relation between in vitro enzyme activities and in vivo potency in commercial pancreatic extracts. N Engl J Med 296:1314, 1977.

Schwachman H: Gastrointestinal manifestations of cystic fibrosis. Pediatr Clin North Am 22:787, 1975.

Wood RE & others: Cystic fibrosis. Am Rev Respir Dis 113:833, 1976.

DISEASES OF THE ALVEOLI & PULMONARY INTERSTITIUM

BACTERIAL PNEUMONIA

Essentials of Diagnosis

- History of mild upper airway infection.
- Abrupt rise in temperature to 39.5–40.5° C (103.1–104.9° F).
- Tachypnea and cough.
- Chest auscultation may be normal, or there may be generalized or localized signs of rales, dullness to percussion, and increased voice transmission.
- Specific etiologic diagnosis depends upon cultures of blood and respiratory secretions.

General Considerations

The characteristic lobar involvement found in adult bacterial pneumonia is unusual in children. In infants and children, involvement is generally more diffuse and the airway is more involved (bronchial pneumonia). It is not usually possible to reliably predict the causative organism from the clinical findings. Therefore, for successful treatment, an educated guess about the causative organism is of greatest therapeutic importance.

Patients with recurrent pneumonia should be evaluated for immunologic deficiency disease, cystic fibrosis, aspirated foreign body, allergy, bronchiectasis, and other anatomic abnormalities of the airways.

Clinical Findings

A. Symptoms and Signs: The onset is usually quite rapid and is often preceded by an upper respiratory infection. Fever and tachypnea are the most important findings, especially in infants, in whom the physical examination may be otherwise normal. Any infant under 6 weeks of age with cough should be assumed to have pneumonia until this is ruled out by chest x-ray. Chest wall retractions may be seen in infants and children. Older children may also experience chills.

Physical signs may include areas of depressed breath sounds, inspiratory rales and rhonchi, wheezing, dullness to percussion, tubular breath sounds, chest wall splinting, and cyanosis. Older children may complain of chest or abdominal pain. Rales may not be heard until the disease is resolving. Abnormal physical findings in the chest may precede chest x-ray abnormalities. Friction rubs are rare.

B. Laboratory Findings: The white blood count is likely to be elevated to 18–40,000/cu mm, mostly as polymorphonuclear leukocytes. White counts under 10,000/cu mm with a shift to the left carry a poor prognosis.

Pneumococci are the most common cause of bacterial pneumonia, but other infectious agents must be considered. *Haemophilus influenzae* can cause an identical clinical picture but may not respond to penicillin alone. Pneumonia due to group A beta-hemolytic streptococci is uncommon but can be very severe. Empyema, if present, is more liquid than in pneumococcal or staphylococcal disease. Group A streptococcal infection also has a greater tendency to ulcerate the trachea than pneumococcal disease, and there may be a higher incidence of empyema. Staphylococcal infection is more apt to cause abscess formation than other organisms. Tuberculosis should be considered in any case of pneumonia that fails to respond to usual antibiotic therapy.

C. X-Ray Findings: Chest x-ray abnormalities are likely to consist of patchy infiltrates and increased bronchovascular markings (bronchopneumonia) and, occasionally, lobar consolidation.

Differential Diagnosis

Bacterial pneumonia may resemble meningitis and acute abdominal disorders. Staphylococcal pneumonia may present with ileus due to a specific toxin.

Complications

Complications of bacterial pneumonia include septicemia, lung abscess, pleural effusion, empyema, bronchiectasis, respiratory failure, pneumothorax, lung hemorrhage, septic shock, pyopneumothorax, and heart failure.

Treatment

A. Specific Measures: Any infant under 2–3 months of age with pneumonia should be admitted to the hospital for at least a brief observation. Hospitalization of older infants and children depends on the severity of their illness and the most appropriate route for antibiotics. Appropriate antibiotics should be selected on the basis of the clinical presentation, with the assistance of a Gram stain of expectorated sputum, aspirated tracheal secretions, or material taken from the lung by needle aspiration when available. Cultures of these materials and blood should be taken prior to initiating antibiotic therapy. Antibiotics may be given orally or parenterally depending on the severity of the illness but in severe cases should always be given intravenously. Penicillin is the drug of choice for pneumonia due to *S pneumoniae,* group A streptococci, and penicillin-sensitive staphylococci. Ampicillin should be used in *H influenzae* pneumonia. In resistant staphylococcal infections, intravenous sodium methicillin or nafcillin should be given. A percutaneous lung aspiration is indicated when an unusual organism is suspected or when the patient's condition is continuing to deteriorate despite usual therapy.

B. General Measures: Supportive measures such as humidified oxygen, pulmonary physiotherapy, and intravenous fluids are indicated in more severe cases. Tracheal intubation and mechanical ventilation are indicated for respiratory failure.

Prognosis

With adequate therapy, sequelae are rare; however, if staphylococcal, streptococcal, or *H influenzae* pneumonia is not adequately treated, the incidence of lung abscess and empyema may be high.

Carson AJ: Fatal *Pseudomonas aeruginosa* bronchopneumonia in a children's hospital. Arch Dis Child 46:55, 1971.

Ceruts E & others: Staphylococcal pneumonia in children. Am J Dis Child 122:386, 1971.

Jones RS, Owen-Thomas JB, Bouton MJ: Severe bronchopneu-

monia in the young child. Arch Dis Child 43:415, 1968.

Mor J & others: Inappropriate antidiuretic hormones secretion in an infant with severe pneumonia. Am J Dis Child 129:133, 1975.

Nyhan W, Rectanus D, Fausek M: *Haemophilus influenzae* type B pneumonia. Pediatrics 16:31, 1955.

Schaedler RW, Choppin RW, Zabriskie JB: Pneumonia caused by tetracycline resistant pneumococci. N Engl J Med 270:127, 1964.

Schreck KM: Observations on the epidemiology of staphylococcal infections. Am J Dis Child 105:646, 1963.

Shuttleworth DB, Charney E: Leukocyte count in childhood pneumonia. Am J Dis Child 122:393, 1971.

Thaler MM: Klebsiella-aerobacter pneumonia in infancy. Pediatrics 30:206, 1962.

CHLAMYDIAL PNEUMONIA

In 1977, Beem and Saxon described a clinical pulmonary disease associated with *Chlamydia trachomatis* infection in infants under 12 weeks of age. The symptoms and signs are those of interstitial pneumonia. The infants are afebrile and generally have symptoms confined to the respiratory tract. Tachypnea and a staccato-type cough may be associated with mucoid rhinorrhea. X-ray usually reveals only hyperinflation; in some infants, diffuse interstitial and patchy alveolar infiltrates are noted. A history of conjunctivitis in the newborn period is often obtained.

Hypoxia and rales are often noted, but wheezing has not been reported. In a second study, apneic episodes were observed in a few infants.

Eosinophilia and hyperimmunoglobulinemia (IgM, IgG) are often present. Isolation of the agent and specific serologic tests are sophisticated procedures not readily available in practice.

The course of the disease is protracted; symptoms persist for weeks, and x-ray changes and physical findings may take a month or more to resolve.

One unpublished study suggests that erythromycin or sulfonamide drugs may be useful. However, reports are available in only a few infants, and no firm conclusions can be drawn.

Beem MO, Saxon EM: Respiratory-tract colonization and a distinctive pneumonia syndrome in infants infected with *Chlamydia trachomatis.* New Engl J Med 296:306, 1977.

VIRAL PNEUMONIA

Viral pneumonia is a relatively common and potentially serious disease, particularly in infants. The viruses that most commonly cause pneumonia in the pediatric age range are respiratory syncytial virus, adenoviruses, influenza and parainfluenza viruses, and rubeola virus. Viral lung disease usually involves both the conducting airways and the alveoli.

The onset of clinical findings is often preceded by an upper respiratory infection and is generally more insidious, with slower progression than in pneumonia due to bacteria. Tachypnea, cough, chest wall retractions, rales, wheezing, decreased breath sounds, and cyanosis may be present. The white blood count and temperature may be normal or slightly elevated. Additional clinical and serologic characteristics of the infecting viruses are discussed in Chapter 25.

Complications of viral pneumonia are atelectasis, bronchiectasis, interstitial fibrosis, and hyperlucent lung (Swyer-James syndrome). The pneumonia due to respiratory syncytial or adenoviruses may resolve only very slowly over 3–12 months or may leave permanent obliterative and fibrotic changes. Respiratory syncytial virus pneumonia may first present with apnea.

Therapy is similar to that for bacterial pneumonias (humidified oxygen, vigorous pulmonary physiotherapy, and tracheal intubation and mechanical ventilation if necessary to prevent respiratory acidosis more severe than pH = 7.25, or for adequate oxygenation), although antibiotics are not indicated unless a secondary bacterial infection is suspected.

Bruhn FW & others: Apnea associated with respiratory syncytial virus infection in young infants. J Pediatr 90:382, 1977.

Becroft DMO: Bronchiolitis obliterans, bronchiectasis, and other sequelae of adenovirus type 21 infection in young children. J Clin Pathol 24:72, 1971.

Cho CT & others: Pneumonia and massive pleural effusion associated with adenovirus type 7. Am J Dis Child 126:92, 1973.

Joshi VV & others: Fatal influenza A_2 viral pneumonia in a newborn infant. Am J Dis Child 126:839, 1973.

Mactherson RI & others: Unilateral hyperlucent lung: A complication of viral pneumonia. J Can Assoc Radiol 20:225, 1969.

Simpson W & others: The radiological findings in respiratory syncytial virus infection in children. Part 2. The correlation of radiological categories with clinical and virological findings. Pediatr Radiol 2:155, 1974.

MYCOPLASMAL PNEUMONIA
(Primary Atypical Pneumonia)

The symptoms of mycoplasmal pneumonia are similar to those of pneumonias due to viruses and other bacteria. There is typically a dry, hacking cough and substernal pain. There is a wide variety of chest x-ray findings. Most typical, however, is an increase in bronchovascular markings with some areas of atelectasis. The lower lobes are more frequently involved. Occasionally there may be associated pleural effusions. Otitis media, serous otitis, pericarditis, and erythema nodosum are reported complications.

Mycoplasma pneumoniae may be differentiated from other Mycoplasma species because of its ability to lyse red blood cells. Serologic tests (cold agglutinins and specific antibody rise) confirm the diagnosis.

Culturing the organism ensures definite diagnosis.

Erythromycin and tetracycline are effective treatment. Illness may be protracted, but recovery is the rule.

Fernald GW & others: Respiratory infection due to *Mycoplasma pneumoniae* in infants and children. Pediatrics 55:327, 1975.

Stallings MW, Archer SB: Atypical *Mycoplasma pneumoniae.* Am J Dis Child 126:837, 1973.

PULMONARY TUBERCULOSIS

Essentials of Diagnosis

- Family history of tuberculosis or history of recent contact.
- Usually asymptomatic, especially in primary form.
- Miliary and progressive pulmonary disease: fever, anorexia, apathy, weight loss.
- Lymph node involvement (may cause respiratory symptoms if the airway is obstructed).
- Positive tuberculin tests and chest x-ray findings.

General Considerations

Pulmonary tuberculosis should be considered in any child who has been exposed to an adult with active disease. A recent conversion to a positive tuberculin test indicates active disease in an untreated individual. The mortality rate is higher during infancy and adolescence. Spread is by respiratory droplets, but the disease in children is usually nonprogressive and not contagious.

Clinical Findings

A. Symptoms and Signs: A history of contact with a tuberculous adult is most important. Primary tuberculosis in children is usually asymptomatic. The classic adult syndrome of chronic cough, anorexia, and loss of weight is almost never present in children. Expiratory stridor is rare. Persistent fever of 2 weeks' duration may occur with primary disease. Miliary spread and meningitis are more likely to occur in infants than in older children.

B. Laboratory Findings: Tuberculin testing (tine, Mantoux) is the most useful diagnostic tool. The tine is a good screening test, but if the diagnosis is suspected the Mantoux test (intradermal injection of Tween-stabilized PPD) should be used; it has the basic advantage that the severity of the reaction relates to the severity of the disease. The standard dose of PPD-tuberculin is 5 tuberculin units (TU) in 0.1 ml of solution, injected intracutaneously. In suspect cases, the test should be read in 48–72 hours by an experienced observer and recorded as millimeters of induration. A positive test is > 10 mm induration. Skin sensitivity develops within 2–10 weeks after infection.

Isolation of *Mycobacterium tuberculosis* is best done from gastric contents, and morning washes should be repeated 3 times. When possible, antibiotic sensitivity studies should be done on the organisms recovered.

C. X-Ray Findings: Chest x-ray in primary disease may be normal. X-ray will vary with the extent of infection from slight infiltration and hilar node invasion to atelectasis and diffuse involvement, as in miliary spread.

Differential Diagnosis

Pulmonary tuberculosis must be differentiated from atypical pneumonia, bacterial pneumonia, leukemia, malnutrition, tumors, congenital atelectasis, asthma, cystic fibrosis, and Löffler's syndrome.

Complications & Sequelae

Infants and adolescents are more likely to develop complications from pulmonary tuberculosis than people in other age groups. Complications include miliary spread, meningitis, cavitation (adolescents), atelectasis (airway obstruction), lymph node involvement outside of the chest (cervical lymph nodes), epididymitis, renal involvement, osteomyelitis of the spine, retroperitoneal and abdominal involvement, and pleurisy. Severe pleural reactions can cause the lung to become restricted or trapped.

Prevention & Treatment

See discussion in Chapter 26.

Prognosis

The prognosis with proper therapy is excellent. If the organisms are resistant to the antituberculosis drugs, the prognosis is poor.

Casteels-Van Daele M & others: Hepatotoxicity of rifampicin and isoniazid in children. J Pediatr 86:739, 1975.

Laven GT: Diagnosis of tuberculosis in children using fluorescence microscopic examination of gastric washings. Am Rev Respir Dis 115:743, 1977.

Reisinger KS & others: Congenital tuberculosis: Report of a case. Pediatrics 54:74, 1974.

Committee on Infectious Diseases: *Report*, 17th ed. American Academy of Pediatrics, 1974. [Red Book.]

Sewell EM & others: The tuberculin test. Pediatrics 54:650, 1974.

ASPIRATION PNEUMONIA

A variety of aspiration syndromes may occur in pediatric patients. These can be classified in several different categories depending on the clinical presentation and course: (1) aspiration of toxic fluids (eg, gastric acid, hydrocarbons, meconium), (2) aspiration of bacteria, and (3) aspiration of particulate matter (eg, food, meconium). Most frequent in the pediatric age range are aspiration of particulate matter (see p 287 for discussion of aspirated foreign body; p 62 for meconium aspiration syndrome of the newborn) and aspiration of toxic fluids. Aspiration of gastric acid is most common in patients with reduced levels of consciousness and in patients with disorders of the esophagus or the cardioesophageal sphincter. Hydrocarbon aspiration is a relatively common problem in pediatrics and should be suspected in any patient who has ingested hydrocarbons. Hydrocarbon aspiration typically produces a generalized chemical pneumonitis, whereas other forms of aspiration generally involve primarily the dependent portions of the lung. In the recumbent position, this would include the posterior segments of upper lobes and superior segments of lower lobes; in the upright position, the basal segments of the lower lobes are dependent.

Aspiration of Gastric Acid

The aspiration of gastric acid may be subclinical and recurrent, producing a chronic obstructive bronchitis that may progress to pulmonary fibrosis (this entity is associated with chalasia and gastroesophageal reflux), or there may be a single, larger episode of aspiration which produces the rapid onset of fever, tachypnea, diffuse rales, and severe hypoxemia. In this latter form there may also be cough, cyanosis, wheezing, apnea, and shock. The severity of this clinical syndrome is related to the acidity and volume of the aspirate as well as the general condition of the patient and probably the specific lung defense capabilities. The rapid onset of symptoms in this entity helps distinguish it from other forms of pneumonia. Radiographic abnormalities develop over the first 24–36 hours, showing diffuse or localized mottled infiltrates with or without atelectasis. A small percentage of affected patients die soon after the aspiration. The remainder show relatively rapid clinical and radiologic improvement, usually between days 2 and 5 postaspiration, but some of these will develop signs of secondary bacterial infection in the form of clinical deterioration associated with new or increasing chest x-ray infiltrates, reappearance of fever, leukocytosis, and recovery of pathogens from tracheal aspirates. This latter course is associated with a significantly worse prognosis.

Appropriate treatment for aspiration of gastric acid and other toxic fluids depends on the volume of aspirate and the clinical condition of the patient. Humidified oxygen is usually indicated to maintain adequate arterial oxygenation; and tracheal intubation, tracheal suction, and mechanical ventilation may be indicated in severely affected patients. There is no evidence to support the routine use of corticosteroids or antibiotics in such patients. Any sign of secondary bacterial infection should be treated with appropriate antibiotics. The prognosis for the majority of patients who do not develop secondary bacterial infection is excellent if there is no repeated aspiration. Patients with recurrent subclinical aspiration due to chalasia, causing chronic lung disease, may benefit by surgical correction of the incompetent cardioesophageal sphincter. The presence of gastroesophageal reflux on barium swallow in a patient with chronic lung disease does not indicate whether the lung disease or the reflux is the primary disease.

Aspiration of Hydrocarbons

Hydrocarbon aspiration may cause immediate choking, coughing, dyspnea, and transient cyanosis, with intercostal retractions and fever developing shortly thereafter. Respiratory symptoms develop usually within the first few hours if at all, although chest x-ray abnormalities may appear at any time within the first 12 hours. Chest auscultation may reveal coarse or decreased breath sounds. Initial chest x-ray abnormalities may consist of mottled perihilar densities with extension into the mid lung fields, basal pneumonitis, or atelectasis. With time, the mottled densities may coalesce into larger, patchy infiltrates. There may be peripheral obstructive emphysema and, ultimately, development of pneumatoceles and lung cysts. Clinical symptoms and x-ray abnormalities tend to begin to improve 2–5 days after aspiration. There may be high fever and an elevated white blood count.

General therapeutic measures of humidified oxygen, vigorous pulmonary physiotherapy, and mechanical ventilation, if necessary, are appropriate. There is no definite evidence to support the routine use of steroids or antibiotics in all cases of hydrocarbon aspiration; however, in debilitated patients or in patients with more significant pneumonia, antibiotics are widely used. Some patients may benefit by bronchodilator therapy. Available data suggest a good prognosis for complete recovery if the patient survives the initial aspiration.

Aspiration of Pathogenic Bacteria

Aspiration of pathogenic bacteria is differentiated from that of toxic fluids by the initial presentation with high fever and purulent sputum and a less fulminant initial process. The aspirated organisms are generally those from the oropharyngeal secretions, and the main pathogenic organisms are anaerobic streptococci, fusobacteria, and *Bacteroides melaninogenicus.* Patients who are hospitalized at the time of aspiration are at additional risk of colonization with enteric gram-negative bacilli (*Escherichia coli, klebsiella,* etc), pseudomonas, or *Staphylococcus aureus.* Antimicrobial therapy should be based on, or supported by, cultures of reliable material. While waiting for the results of such cultures, it is appropriate to start giving penicillin V for aspiration pneumonia acquired outside the hospital and gentamicin and nafcillin or some other penicillinase-resistant antibiotic for bacterial aspirations which occur in the hospital. Other supportive measures such as oxygen, pulmonary physiotherapy, circulatory support, and mechanical ventilation are appropriate when indicated.

Bartlett JG, Gorbach SL: The triple threat of aspiration pneumonia. Chest 68:560, 1975.

Bergeson PS & others: Pneumatoceles following hydrocarbon ingestion: Report of three cases and review of the literature. Am J Dis Child 129:49, 1975.

Bynum LJ, Pierce AK: Pulmonary aspiration of gastric contents. Am Rev Respir Dis 114:1129, 1976.

Cooperative kerosine poisoning study: Evaluation of gastric lavage and other factors in the treatment of accidental ingestion of petroleum distillate products. Pediatrics 29:648, 1962.

Marks MI & others: Adrenocorticosteroid treatment of hydrocarbon pneumonia in children: A cooperative study. J Pediatr 81:366, 1972.

HYPERSENSITIVITY PNEUMONITIS

Hypersensitivity pneumonitis is the result of a type 1 (immediate, IgE-mediated) or type 3 (Arthus) allergic response to an inhaled organic antigen. Examples of hypersensitivity pneumonitis are farmer's lung, bird breeder's lung, humidifier lung, and allergic bronchopulmonary aspergillosis. The antigen exposure is usually intermittent, and the disease may be acute, subacute, or chronic. The acute form is characterized by sudden onset of a nonproductive cough, chest tightness, fever, chills, malaise, and dyspnea 4–6 hours after antigen exposure. After recurrent exposures, there may be weight loss. Cyanosis, tachypnea, and basilar rales, usually without wheezing, are characteristic. Leukocytosis is common. The chest x-ray may be normal, or there may be diffuse small nodules or patchy interstitial infiltrates. Most of these findings with the acute form begin to resolve within 12–24 hours after termination of antigen exposure.

A more insidious onset of progressive dyspnea with eventual cyanosis and digital clubbing characterizes chronic hypersensitivity pneumonitis, which usually occurs after a prolonged, often intense antigen exposure. The chest x-ray shows a progressive increase in interstitial markings, and ultimately there may be a cystic appearance with decreased lung volume.

In the acute form, pulmonary function tests are initially indicative of restrictive disease, although with recurrent exposure an obstructive component may also become apparent. The signs of obstructive lung disease may predominate in the chronic form of hypersensitivity pneumonitis. Precipitants to specific molds or other offending organic antigens may be found in the patient's serum.

The optimal treatment for both acute and chronic forms is avoidance of the antigen. Both forms may be helped by cromolyn sodium and corticosteroids.

Cunningham AS & others: Childhood hypersensitivity pneumonitis due to dove antigens. Pediatrics 58:436, 1976.

Friedman PJ: Idiopathic and autoimmune type 3-like reactions: Interstitial fibrosis, vasculitis, and granulomatosis. Semin Roentgenol 10:43, 1975.

Kohler PF & others: Humidifier lung: Hypersensitivity pneumonitis related to thermotolerant bacterial aerosols. Chest 69:294, 1976.

Nicholson DT: Extrinsic allergic pneumonias. Am J Med 53:131, 1972.

Pepys J: Immunopathology of allergic lung disease. Clin Allergy 3:1, 1973.

Schlueter MP: Response of the lung to inhaled antigens. Am J Med 57:476, 1974.

IDIOPATHIC PULMONARY FIBROSIS
(Fibrosing Alveolitis)

Idiopathic pulmonary fibrosis refers to a spectrum or continuum of disease characterized by varying combinations of (1) cuboidalization of alveolar lining cells and the presence of large mononuclear cells within the alveolar spaces and (2) thickening of alveolar walls by fibrosis and inflammatory cells. The alveolar process probably represents an earlier stage of this disease, which later progresses to become primarily interstitial. Different stages of this process have previously been called desquamative interstitial pneumonitis and usual interstitial pneumonitis. The interstitial fibrosis described by Hamman and Rich in 1935 was probably a rapidly progressive and severe form of idiopathic pulmonary fibrosis. In most pediatric cases, the cause is unknown, although antecedent infections may initiate this process in some patients. In adults, drug exposure or connective tissue disorders may be causative factors. The onset of symptoms is usually after the first few weeks of life but within the first year in the reported pediatric cases.

The most common clinical findings are dyspnea, tachypnea, cough, poor weight gain, and, later, rales, digital clubbing, and cyanosis. Pulmonary hypertension and respiratory and cardiac failure develop in more severely affected patients. The ECG may demonstrate signs of right ventricular hypertrophy. Pulmonary function studies demonstrate decreased vital capacity and total lung capacity, indicating restrictive lung disease, and a diminished pulmonary diffusing capacity. In adults, the amount of hypoxemia on exercise is the best indicator of the amount of interstitial fibrosis. Lung compliance is decreased.

During the course of the disease the chest x-ray progresses from an initial diffuse ground-glass appearance with fine mottling to more coarse mottling, then to the appearance of linear markings, which are usually perihilar, and finally to the end stage chest x-ray of increased linear markings associated with hyperlucent areas, particularly at the lung bases, which may progress to a honeycomb lung pattern. The progression of this pattern generally extends over a period of 2–6 years. Cardiomegaly may be apparent on chest x-rays in severely affected patients.

There are no reported cases of spontaneous remission in children. All survivors have been treated with corticosteroids. Prednisone in a daily dose of at least 2 mg/kg should be given for 2 months. If there is improvement, steroid withdrawal should be very slow, so that at least 1 year of treatment will be completed. The mean survival of reported cases is 4–6 years.

Crystal RG & others: Idiopathic pulmonary fibrosis: Clinical histologic, radiographic, physiologic, scintigraphic, cytologic, and biochemical aspects. Ann Intern Med 85:769, 1976.

Hamman L, Rich AR: Acute diffuse interstitial fibrosis of the lungs. Bull Johns Hopkins Hosp 74:177, 1944.

Hamman L, Rich AR: Fulminating diffuse interstitial fibrosis of the lungs. Trans Am Clin Climatol Assoc 51:154, 1935.

Hewitt CJ & others: Fibrosing alveolitis in infancy and childhood. Arch Dis Child 52:22, 1977.

Scadding JG: Diffuse pulmonary alveolar fibrosis. Thorax 29:271, 1974.

EOSINOPHILIC PNEUMONIA

Eosinophilic pneumonia refers to pulmonary infiltrates on chest x-ray associated with eosinophilic infiltration in the lung seen on histologic examination, which may or may not be associated with eosinophilia of the peripheral blood. Crofton describes 5 types of pulmonary eosinophilia, most of which probably represent some form of hypersensitivity reaction.

Usually of shortest duration, and most benign, is simple pulmonary eosinophilia or Löffler's syndrome, which consists of migratory pulmonary infiltrates associated with minimal if any respiratory symptoms and fever. This entity is distinguished from prolonged pulmonary eosinophilia primarily by the duration of symptoms, which is less than 1 month with simple pulmonary eosinophilia and over 1–2 months with prolonged pulmonary eosinophilia. The prolonged variety is usually associated with high fever, malaise, productive cough, and chest pain. A third category is transient or prolonged eosinophilic infiltrations of the lung in the course of chronic asthma. This may last for 3–4 months or for years.

Tropical eosinophilia is the association of fever, expiratory obstruction, and weight loss associated with diffuse, finely nodular radiographic infiltrates. This is usually associated with a marked peripheral eosinophilia and may be due to filarial infestation. Finally, there may be pulmonary eosinophilia associated with polyarteritis nodosa and Wegener's granulomatosis, where the primary involvement is in the pulmonary blood vessels but other organs are apt to be involved also. These patients have quite severe symptoms and usually a fatal outcome.

Corticosteroids should be given if symptoms warrant treatment except in the case of tropical eosinophilia, which is best treated with the antifilarial drug diethylcarbamazine.

Carrington CB & others: Chronic eosinophilic pneumonia. N Engl J Med 280:787, 1969.

Crofton JW & others: Pulmonary eosinophilia. Thorax 7:1, 1952.

Liebow AA, Carrington CB: The eosinophilic pneumonias. Medicine 48:251, 1969.

Middleton WJ & others: Asthmatic pulmonary eosinophilia: A review of 65 cases. Br J Dis Chest 71:115, 1977.

Rogers RM & others: Eosinophilic pneumonia: Physiologic response to steroid therapy and observations on light and electron microscope findings. Chest 68:665, 1975.

PULMONARY ALVEOLAR PROTEINOSIS

This is a rare, usually fatal childhood disease of unknown cause characterized histologically by marked accumulation within the alveoli and bronchioles of an eosinophilic, granular PAS-positive material. It often presents with fever followed by dyspnea, productive cough, chest pain, and poor weight gain. There may be yellow sputum production and cyanosis in older children, and death usually several months later. Physical findings are generally sparse but may include scattered fine rales, occasional digital clubbing, and eventual cyanosis. The onset in children is usually before age 1. The chest x-ray demonstrates fine, soft, diffuse perihilar densities similar to those associated with pulmonary edema. PAS-staining material and birefringent crystals may be present in the sputum; however, most cases are diagnosed by lung biopsy or at autopsy.

No treatment has been uniformly successful. Lung lavage with heparinized saline has been beneficial in some cases.

Colon AR & others: Childhood pulmonary alveolar proteinosis (PAP). Am J Dis Child 121:481, 1971.

Costello JF: Diagnosis and management of alveolar proteinosis: The role of electron microscopy. Thorax 30:121, 1975.

Mazyck EM & others: Pulmonary lavage for childhood pulmonary alveolar proteinosis. J Pediatr 80:839, 1972.

PULMONARY ALVEOLAR MICROLITHIASIS

This often familial disease of unknown cause is characterized by extensive intra-alveolar deposits of calcium carbonate seen on x-ray. At the time of diagnosis there may be no symptoms, but dyspnea, cough, cyanosis, and eventually cor pulmonale develop subsequently. The diagnosis is most often made by chance on a routine chest x-ray which demonstrates fine, sand-like mottling distributed uniformly throughout both lung fields. In rare cases, a description of "sand" in the sputum may lead to the diagnosis.

There is no effective treatment, and the prognosis is variable.

Oka S & others: Pulmonary alveolar microlithiasis. Am Rev Respir Dis 93:612, 1966.

Viswanathan R: Pulmonary alveolar microlithiasis. Thorax 17:251, 1962.

WILSON-MIKITY SYNDROME

This is a clinical syndrome characterized by gradually progressive respiratory distress and increased inspired oxygen requirement in small premature infants who have had minimal or no previous lung disease. This clinical pattern typically begins several weeks after birth. The cause is not known, although it may be related to viral infection or immaturity of the lung. Chest x-rays show a widespread reticular pattern resembling that of stage 3 bronchopulmonary dysplasia, with small radiolucent areas (cysts) scattered throughout the lung fields. These changes become more prominent as the disease progresses.

Treatment consists of supportive care and oxygen. Mechanical ventilatory assistance is rarely needed. Antibiotics have not appeared to influence the course.

Although the course is prolonged and there is extensive lung involvement, only 10–15% of infants with this disorder die of respiratory failure or right heart failure. The others recover after several months.

The differential diagnosis includes bronchopulmonary dysplasia, viral pneumonia, patent ductus arteriosus with pulmonary congestion due to increasing left to right shunts, and chronic pulmonary insufficiency of prematurity (CPIP), which may be the direct consequence of the lung volume loss due to periodic breathing of prematurity.

Hodgman JE & others: Chronic respiratory distress in the premature infant: Wilson-Mikity syndrome. Pediatrics 44: 179, 1969.

Krauss AN & others: Chronic pulmonary insufficiency of prematurity (CPIP). Pediatrics 55:55, 1975.

Krauss AN & others: Physiologic studies on infants with Wilson-Mikity syndrome. J Pediatr 77:27, 1970.

Wilson MG, Mikity VG: A new form of respiratory distress in premature infants. J Dis Child 99:489, 1960.

EMPHYSEMA

Essentials of Diagnosis

- Dyspnea.
- Hyperexpansion of lungs.
- Distention and destruction of alveoli as shown on histologic examination.
- Progressive disease.

General Considerations

Emphysema consists of loss of the elastic properties of the lung, characterized by distention of alveoli with or without destruction of alveolar walls, resulting in air trapping. On x-ray, emphysema is seen as hyperinflation of all or part of the lung. Emphysema may be obstructive or compensatory. Compensatory emphysema occurs when normal lung expands to fill the space of collapsed lung (atelectasis) or absent lung.

Localized obstructive emphysema occurs when a bronchus is partially obstructed so that air entry past the obstruction is accomplished more easily than air exit. A whole lung, one lobe of one lung, or only one lobule may be involved. The obstruction may be intrinsic or extrinsic. In congenital or infantile lobar emphysema, severe respiratory distress may develop in the neonatal period or in early infancy as a result of compression of normal lung by the emphysematous lobe. In older children with localized emphysema, many conditions involving the airway must be considered, including asthma, foreign body, tumor, vascular ring, local inflammation due to viral or bacterial infection, and regional obstructive lung disease.

General obstructive emphysema occurs if there is widespread disease of bronchioles. It may be present in a wide range of clinical conditions including cystic fibrosis, asthma, bronchiolitis, and miliary tuberculosis.

Familial emphysema due to a_1-antitrypsin deficiency is characterized by an onset of emphysema at a relatively early age (usually early adulthood) and progressive dyspnea in the absence of clinical bronchitis in the early stages of the disease. The sex incidence is equal. Diffuse panacinar emphysema is seen microscopically on lung sections. The primary pathophysiologic mechanism is not understood, but one theory proposes that the absence of a_1-antitrypsin allows naturally occurring proteolytic enzymes as well as proteolytic enzymes released from leukocytes destroyed during infection to slowly digest the structural protein of normal lung, leading to emphysema.

Alpha$_1$-antitrypsin deficiency is inherited as an autosomal recessive trait. Although some homozygous individuals report no pulmonary symptoms, they are usually symptomatic by the third or fourth decade; isolated cases of onset in adolescence and one case involving a young girl whose symptoms began at age 18 months have been reported. Heterozygous individuals may have an increased incidence of pulmonary disease, but the data are inconclusive. It is estimated that about 5% of the population are carriers of the gene, and one in 2000 births is a homozygous recessive. Alpha$_1$-antitrypsin deficiency has also been associated with a severe form of juvenile hepatic cirrhosis.

The diagnosis may be suspected by the absence of the a_1-globulin peak in routine protein electrophoresis. Specific assay of antitrypsin activity suggests the diagnosis, although Pi (protease inhibitor) typing is most definitive.

Clinical Findings

A. Symptoms and Signs: The symptoms and signs depend upon the extent of involvement. The cardinal finding is dyspnea. In addition, cough, tachypnea, cyanosis, hyperresonant percussion sounds over the involved area, shift of cardiac impulse, and high-pitched wheezing are apt to be present. In localized or lobar involvement, the child may be asymptomatic, but careful examination of the chest will indicate poor air entry in the involved area. With increasing severity, progressive respiratory distress will be evident. In-

creased resonance on percussion, shift of the heart and trachea, wheezing, or absence of breath sounds indicates that the airway involvement is sufficient to cause air trapping.

B. X-Ray Findings: Chest x-ray or fluoroscopic examination in the generalized disease shows increased radiolucency, depressed diaphragms, and horizontal ribs. Chest x-ray is an important diagnostic procedure but does not establish the diagnosis.

Treatment

The treatment of obstructive emphysema is directed toward the underlying cause. In congenital infantile emphysema, lobectomy may be a lifesaving measure in the neonatal period. In general, only supportive measures are helpful.

Browder JA, Billingsley JG: Regional obstructive lung disease in childhood. Am J Dis Child 119:322, 1970.

Evans HE & others: Prevalence of alpha 1 antitrypsin Pi types among newborn infants of different ethnic backgrounds. J Pediatr 90:621, 1977.

Glasgow JFT & others: Alpha 1 antitrypsin deficiency in association with both cirrhosis and chronic obstructive lung disease in two sibs. Am J Med 54:181, 1973.

Talamo RC & others: Symptomatic pulmonary emphysema in childhood associated with hereditary alpha 1 antitrypsin and elastase inhibitory deficiency. J Pediatr 79:20, 1971.

DISEASES OF THE PULMONARY CIRCULATION

PULMONARY HEMORRHAGE

Acute pulmonary hemorrhage and hemoptysis may be associated with bronchiectasis (especially in patients with cystic fibrosis), lung abscess, foreign body aspiration, tuberculosis, heart disease, esophageal duplication, or coagulation disorders or may occur as idiopathic pulmonary hemosiderosis. Therapy in most cases involves treatment of the underlying disorder, and bed rest and blood transfusions may be indicated.

PULMONARY HEMOSIDEROSIS

Idiopathic pulmonary hemosiderosis refers to the accumulation of hemosiderin in the lung, particularly within alveolar macrophages, as a result of chronic or recurrent hemorrhage, usually from pulmonary capillaries. Nonidiopathic causes of a similar entity are myocarditis, polyarteritis nodosa, systemic lupus erythematosus, rheumatoid arthritis, rheumatic fever, Wegener's granulomatosis, and heart disease causing elevated pulmonary capillary or pulmonary venous pressure (especially mitral stenosis). Pulmonary hemosiderosis in association with glomerulonephritis is called *Goodpasture's syndrome*. Some infant patients with pulmonary hemosiderosis have had positive intradermal tests to cow's milk and improvement of symptoms on a milk elimination diet. This possible association between milk allergy and recurrent pulmonary hemorrhage is called *Heiner's syndrome.*

Idiopathic pulmonary hemosiderosis usually begins in the first decade of life (as early as 4 months of age) and affects males and females equally. Goodpasture's syndrome affects mostly men in the late teens or older and has a more rapid downhill course.

Clinical Findings

A. Symptoms and Signs: Idiopathic pulmonary hemosiderosis typically begins as continuous mild pulmonary bleeding with a chronic nonproductive cough, fatigue, poor weight gain, and iron deficiency anemia. There may be intermittent blood staining of the sputum and occasional heme-positive stools. The first severe pulmonary hemorrhage is likely to occur after several weeks or months and may cause substernal pain, fever, rales, and dullness to percussion over the affected area. Twenty-five percent of patients with idiopathic pulmonary hemosiderosis eventually develop digital clubbing.

The pulmonary hemorrhage of Goodpasture's syndrome is often preceded by an initial upper respiratory tract infection and is usually less severe than with idiopathic pulmonary hemosiderosis. The hemorrhage usually precedes by weeks or months the onset of acute glomerulonephritis.

During acute episodes of pulmonary hemorrhage, there may be significant dyspnea, wheezing, cyanosis, hemoptysis, tachycardia, and shock if the blood loss is extremely large. After chronic pulmonary hemorrhage, some patients may develop jaundice and hepatosplenomegaly.

B. Laboratory Findings: There is a microcytic hypochromic anemia which responds to oral administration of iron salts with an elevation of the reticulocyte count. Peripheral eosinophilia is present in 10–25% of cases. The stool guaiac test may be positive. Hemosiderin-laden macrophages are present in the gastric contents and may be found in tracheal washings. These iron-containing cells are nonspecific indications of pulmonary hemorrhage. Lung biopsy shows alveolar epithelial hypoplasia, degeneration, and shedding with large numbers of hemosiderin macrophages and variable amounts of interstitial fibrosis. Biopsy may be necessary in order to establish the diagnosis, and open biopsy is preferred.

Pulmonary function studies demonstrate a reduction of lung volumes (restrictive lung disease), decreased lung compliance, reduced oxygen saturation, and, in some patients, a decreased pulmonary diffusing capacity for carbon monoxide.

C. X-Ray Findings: The abnormalities on chest x-ray may vary from none to mild perihilar transient infiltrates to marked parenchymal involvement with infiltrates, atelectasis, emphysema, and mediastinal adenopathy.

Treatment

Any underlying disease process should be appropriately treated. Oxygen and blood transfusion may be required during acute severe bleeding episodes. Most patients benefit from oral iron therapy. Corticosteroids and immunosuppressive agents such as azathioprine have been used, but there is no convincing evidence that they are always effective in either idiopathic pulmonary hemosiderosis or Goodpasture's syndrome. In rare infants with characteristic findings of milk allergy (Heiner's syndrome), milk elimination should be tried.

Course & Prognosis

Idiopathic pulmonary hemosiderosis is characterized by intermittent episodes of acute intrapulmonary hemorrhage separated by asymptomatic intervals. After some years, there may be chronic symptoms such as exertional dyspnea and anemia in the intervals between the acute episodes of hemorrhage. The long-term course is variable, and about 50% of patients die within 5 years of the onset of the clinical disease. Most patients with Goodpasture's syndrome die of renal failure within weeks to months after the diagnosis is established. Occasional patients with Goodpasture's syndrome and idiopathic pulmonary hemosiderosis have spontaneous complete recoveries.

Aach R, Kissane J: Proliferative glomerulonephritis and pulmonary hemorrhage. Am J Med 55:199, 1973.

Goodpasture EW: The significance of certain pulmonary lesions in relation to the etiology of influenza. Am J Med Sci 158:863, 1919.

Matsaniotes N & others: Idiopathic pulmonary hemosiderosis in children. Arch Dis Child 43:307, 1968.

Soergel KH, Sommers SC: Idiopathic pulmonary hemosiderosis and related syndromes. Am J Med 32:499, 1962.

PULMONARY EMBOLISM

Pulmonary embolism is rare in children and is usually due to venous stasis or trauma. Pulmonary emboli can occasionally occur as a complication of sickle cell anemia, rheumatic fever, bacterial endocarditis, schistosomiasis, long bone fractures, dehydration, polycythemia, atrial fibrillation, or ventriculo-venous shunts for hydrocephalus. Pulmonary emboli can be single or multiple, large or small. The clinical presentation depends on the amount of the pulmonary vascular bed which is obstructed. Large pulmonary emboli may cause the acute onset of dyspnea, chest pain, chest splinting, cyanosis, tachycardia, rales with or without pleural friction rub, and occasionally hemoptysis. The chest x-ray may be normal or may show a peripheral infiltrate, small pleural effusion, or elevated diaphragm. The ECG is usually normal but may demonstrate right heart strain with very large pulmonary emboli. Pulmonary function tests usually show normal lung volumes and flow rates, with decreased pulmonary diffusing capacity for carbon monoxide and lowered arterial CO_2 and O_2 tension. Lactic dehydrogenase is usually elevated. A lung perfusion scan will show a localized perfusion defect. If either the lung scan or the arterial P_{O_2} is normal, it is extremely unlikely that the patient has had an acute pulmonary embolism.

Therapy includes the administration of oxygen and often sedation and attempts to prevent venous stasis or any extension of thrombosis by the use of anticoagulant therapy. Survival of the acute embolic period depends on the size of the embolus. The long-term prognosis in patients who survive the acute episode is related to the underlying disease.

Bell WR & others: The clinical features of submassive and massive pulmonary emboli. Am J Med 62:355, 1977.

Dalen JE & others: Pulmonary embolism, pulmonary hemorrhages and pulmonary infarction. N Engl J Med 296:1431, 1977.

Favara BE, Paul RN: Thromboembolism and cor pulmonale complicating ventriculo-venous shunt. JAMA 199:162, 1967.

Szucs MM & others: Diagnostic sensitivity of laboratory findings in acute pulmonary embolism. Ann Intern Med 74:161, 1971.

PULMONARY EDEMA

Pulmonary edema results when the rate of accumulation of extravascular lung water exceeds the capability of the pulmonary lymphatic system to remove this fluid. The edema initially accumulates in the interstitial space, first in the area surrounding small vessels and airways. The development of pulmonary edema is usually due to a change in hydrostatic or oncotic pressure gradients across the pulmonary vessel walls or increased permeability of the pulmonary capillaries. Thus it may be associated with heart disease, a wide variety of infectious and toxic lung insults, and hypoproteinemia. "Neurogenic" pulmonary edema may develop following severe CNS injury or insult. Mild pulmonary edema may cause only tachypnea, mild rales and expiratory wheezes, and slight hypoxemia. More severe pulmonary edema causes dyspnea, chest wall retraction, cyanosis, and CO_2 retention. Chest x-ray may demonstrate prominent pulmonary vascularity, often with a diffuse haziness of the lung fields. Mild pulmonary edema, especially when associated with another underlying lung disease, may be difficult to identify but may contribute to the patient's respiratory difficulty.

Appropriate therapy depends on the severity of the pulmonary edema, the underlying disease, and the age of the patient but is likely to include supplemental oxygen, diuretics, and, in some situations, restriction of fluid and salt intake, morphine, phlebotomy, rotating tourniquets on the extremities, placing the patient in a semierect position, and digitalis therapy for cardiogenic pulmonary edema. Any underlying disease should be vigorously treated.

Staub NC: Pathogenesis of pulmonary edema. Am Rev Respir Dis 109:358, 1974.

ADULT RESPIRATORY DISTRESS SYNDROME
(Shock Lung)

Essentials of Diagnosis

- Acute respiratory failure.
- Progressive severe hypoxemia.
- Markedly decreased lung compliance (stiff lung).

General Considerations

Adult respiratory distress syndrome (ARDS) is the nonspecific reaction of the lung to a variety of severe insults. It is characterized by a severe progressive hypoxemia despite inhalation of oxygen in high concentrations as a result of widespread alveolar collapse causing right-to-left intrapulmonary shunting and very stiff lungs. Some causes of ARDS are extensive viral pneumonia, widespread fat emboli, inhalation or aspiration of corrosive chemical substances, near drowning, severe shock, severe trauma, sepsis, fluid overload, and oxygen toxicity. A major consequence of the diffuse lung injury is an increase in the permeability of the capillary endothelium, causing pulmonary edema. In addition to the edema, there is histologic evidence of focal areas of thromboembolism, with multiple small pulmonary infarcts, vascular congestion, and perialveolar and interstitial hemorrhages. With longer survival, there may be more consolidation and bronchopneumonia.

Clinical Findings

A. Symptoms and Signs: ARDS usually develops in patients with no history of pulmonary disease, and its onset is usually 24–48 hours after serious trauma or illness. The onset is marked by tachypnea, chest retraction, and cyanosis. There is often relentless progression of acute respiratory failure despite all therapeutic efforts.

B. Laboratory Findings: Blood gas determinations will reveal hypoxemia and metabolic acidosis early in the course of the disease. As the process progresses, CO_2 retention develops. Calculated alveolar to arterial oxygen gradients will become progressively greater, reflecting an increasing right-to-left shunt. Because of the marked pulmonary edema and surfactant deficiency, the lungs become very stiff and the tidal volumes quite small.

C. X-Ray Findings: Initial x-rays may be normal. With the onset of symptoms of respiratory failure, bilateral patchy infiltrates will appear and alternately coalesce as lung aeration deteriorates.

Treatment

Optimal resuscitation and treatment of the underlying condition are important in minimizing the risk and severity of ARDS. General therapeutic measures should include careful monitoring of fluid intake and output in an attempt to minimize the amount of extravascular lung water, careful monitoring of intravascular pressures (a Swan-Ganz catheter is often helpful), filtering of any blood administered through a 25–40 μm filter to remove any microaggregates, vigorous chest physiotherapy and postural drainage, and attempts to maintain caloric support. Diuretics such as furosemide may be helpful. Antibiotics should be used if specific infections are suspected, but not indiscriminately or prophylactically. Early and aggressive ventilator support should be initiated when a patient requires oxygen in a concentration greater than 60% to maintain a satisfactory arterial P_{O_2}. A volume ventilator is usually desirable since very high pressures may be required for adequate ventilation. Initially, continuous positive airway pressure may be sufficient to improve oxygenation. When assist breaths are initiated, positive end-expiratory pressure, sometimes to very high levels, should be employed. Short-term treatment with corticosteroids in high doses is widely used and may be beneficial.

Extracorporeal membrane oxygenators have been used in some patients with severe respiratory failure due to ARDS. In general, the results are discouraging, while the financial burden is extreme.

Prognosis

The prognosis is generally poor because of the severity of the pulmonary insufficiency and the often severe associated precipitating insult. Skillful use of ventilators, pulmonary physiotherapy, continuous positive airway pressure, and fluid management may improve the outlook. Patients recovering from ARDS probably have persistence of some degree of interstitial lung disease, although there is progressive normalization of lung volumes and compliance.

Lamy M & others: Pathologic features and mechanism of hypoxemia in adult respiratory distress syndrome. Am Rev Respir Dis 114:267, 1976.

Murray JF: Conference report: Mechanisms of acute respiratory failure. Am Rev Respir Dis 115:1071, 1977.

Rosen AJ: Shock lung: Fact or fancy? Surg Clin North Am 55:613, 1975.

Wernault JC & others: Follow up of pulmonary function after "shock lung." Bull Europ Physiopath Respir 13:241, 1977.

CONGENITAL PULMONARY LYMPHANGIECTASIS

Congenital dilatation of the pulmonary lymphatics is a rare disease which usually causes respiratory failure and death within the first few days of life. The frequency in males is twice that in females. Lymphatic dilatation is usually secondary to a primary developmental defect of the pulmonary lymphatics, pulmonary venous obstruction, or occasionally as part of a syndrome of generalized (especially intestinal) lymphangiectasia. The onset of symptoms is usually at the time of birth, with cyanosis and severe respiratory distress. Occasionally the onset of respiratory distress may be delayed for a few days or weeks after birth. The diagnosis is definitively established by lung biopsy which demonstrates marked, irregular cystic dilatation of pulmonary lymphatic vessels and often some interstitial fibrosis. A chest x-ray demonstrates hyperaeration and diffuse nodular or reticular parenchymal lesions. If survival is prolonged, bullous changes may appear on chest x-ray. The differential diagnosis includes respiratory distress syndrome, aspiration pneumonitis, pulmonary hemorrhage, fulminant pneumonia, and, in patients who survive the newborn period, chronic lung disease, pulmonary edema, and cystic fibrosis.

There is no effective therapy for this disorder, but oxygen, digitalis, and diuretics may provide some symptomatic relief.

Felman AH, Rhatigan RM, Pierson KK: Pulmonary lymphangiectasia: Observation in 17 patients and proposed classification. Am J Roentgenol Radium Ther Nucl Med 116:548, 1972.

France NE, Brown RJK: Congenital pulmonary lymphangiectasis. Arch Dis Child 46:528, 1971.

Noonan JA & others: Congenital pulmonary lymphangiectasis. Am J Dis Child 120:314, 1970.

DISORDERS OF THE CHEST WALL

The normal function of the chest wall (rib cage and diaphragm) is essential for effective ventilation. The 2 components of the chest wall serve both a passive supportive and an active bellows function. A relatively normal chest wall configuration and size is required for normal lung growth. The diaphragm contains the major respiratory muscles in newborns and infants.

A variety of abnormalities of the rib cage and spine can interfere with normal lung function and growth. Some congenital abnormalities such as severe asphyxiating thoracic dystrophy, which may or may not be associated with other major congenital abnormalities such as achondroplasia and cerebrocostomandibular syndrome, may be incompatible with life.

Naumoff P: Thoracic dysplasia in spondyloepiphyseal dysplasia congenita. Am J Dis Child 131:653, 1977.

EVENTRATION OF THE DIAPHRAGM

Eventration of the diaphragm is abnormal elevation of one leaf of the diaphragm. It may be due to congenital maldevelopment of normal diaphragmatic muscular or tendinous structures or acquired abnormality of the phrenic nerve. In congenital eventration, the diaphragmatic abnormality may be complete or only localized and is characterized by inadequate or absent muscularization, leaving only a translucent membrane separating the thoracic and abdominal cavities.

A variety of different processes may interfere with phrenic nerve conduction, thereby causing diaphragmatic paralysis or eventration. Some causes of phrenic nerve dysfunction are neuritis, which can be on an infectious, toxic, or allergic basis; compression of the nerve roots at the level of the cervical spine; CNS diseases; or peripheral phrenic nerve damage due to surgical or other trauma, pressure, or inflammation. Phrenic nerve palsy in the newborn is usually the result of birth trauma, particularly after breech or forceps deliveries. In such cases the diaphragmatic paralysis is often associated with ipsilateral Erb's palsy. Phrenic nerve palsy is not infrequently caused by surgical trauma, particularly during correction of congenital heart lesions. Both congenital and acquired eventrations are more common on the left than on the right.

Clinical Findings

A. Symptoms and Signs: Clinical manifestations of diaphragmatic eventration are a result of decreased intrathoracic volume (decreased functional residual capacity) and of inefficient ventilation due to mediastinal mobility and paradoxic movement of the abnormal diaphragm. Typical clinical findings are tachypnea, cyanosis, sternal retraction, asymmetric chest movement and subcostal retractions. There may be decreased breath sounds and dullness to percussion at the base of the affected lung. Recurrent fevers may result from bronchopneumonia due to ineffective cough and persistent atelectasis. Most patients with diaphragmatic eventration have minimal or no symptoms after the first year or two of life. In the neonatal period and during the first year of life, the above symptoms are more common and may be associated with recurrent respiratory infections, poor feeding, and failure to thrive.

B. X-Ray Findings: The diagnosis can usually be firmly established, with regular anteroposterior and lateral chest x-rays and fluoroscopy. Complete or partial elevation of the abnormal diaphragm will be evident on regular chest x-rays. The amount of paradoxic diaphragmatic movement and mediastinal shift is best evaluated by fluoroscopy. In some cases of congenital eventration there may be no paradoxic movement of the diaphragm because of the presence of some muscle in all parts of the diaphragm. Occasionally it may be difficult to distinguish between a partial eventration and a low thoracic mass. Injection of a small amount of nonirritating radiopaque fluid into the peritoneal cavity will help outline the diaphragm and make the differential diagnosis.

Treatment

Asymptomatic eventration requires no treatment. Diaphragmatic plication significantly improves lung function and therefore is indicated for patients with significant disability (eg, prolonged increased oxygen or ventilator requirement, recurrent lower respiratory tract infections, feeding problems, or failure to thrive). Patients with acquired diaphragmatic eventration (eg, due to birth trauma or surgical injury of the phrenic nerve) may show significant improvement of diaphragmatic function over the first month or more postoperatively. If there has been no improvement at all in the first 2–4 weeks after the injury was acquired, plication is indicated if the patient has significant requirements for enriched oxygen or assisted ventilation. If the patient has milder manifestations of the eventration, a longer time for potential spontaneous recovery of diaphragmatic function should be allowed before surgical intervention. Vigorous chest physiotherapy should be administered to all patients with less than normal diaphragmatic function.

Greene W & others: Paralysis of the diaphragm. Am J Dis Child 129:1402, 1975.

Marcos JJ & others: Paralyzed diaphragm: Effect of plication on respiratory mechanics. J Surg Res 16:523, 1974.

Othersen HB, Lorenzo RL: Diaphragmatic paralysis and eventration: Newer approaches to diagnosis and operative correction. J Pediatr Surg 12:309, 1977.

Ridyard JB, Stewart RN: Regional lung function in unilateral diaphragmatic paralysis. Thorax 31:438, 1976.

Sethi G, Reed WA: Diaphragmatic malfunction in neonates and infants: Diagnosis and treatment. J Thorac Cardiovasc Surg 62:138, 1971.

SCOLIOSIS

Congenital scoliosis is likely to be severe and is often associated with other anomalies as well as with persistent respiratory failure or recurrent respiratory infections. Alveolar development is impaired. Idiopathic scoliosis is usually acquired during later childhood or adolescence and is quite common. Acquired scoliosis may also be secondary to neuromuscular disorders. Mild scoliosis has no effect on pulmonary function, but as the spinal curvature increases, patients may develop restrictive lung disease and—though usually not until adulthood—cor pulmonale and respiratory failure. Thus, surgical correction of moderately severe scoliosis is indicated to avoid these serious sequelae.

Davies G, Reid L: Effect of scoliosis on growth of alveoli and pulmonary arteries and on right ventricle. Arch Dis Child 46:623, 1971.

Hislop HJ, Sanger JO (editors). *Chest Disorders in Children: Proceedings of a Symposium.* American Physical Therapy Association, 1968.

Hull D, Barnes ND: Children with small chests. Arch Dis Child 47:12, 1972.

Miller KE & others: Rib gap defects with micrognathia: The cerebro-costomandibular syndrome: A Pierre Robin-like syndrome with rib dysplasia. Am J Roentgenol Radium Ther Nucl Med 114:253, 1972.

PECTUS EXCAVATUM
(Funnel Chest)

Minor degrees of pectus excavatum are a common and insignificant occurrence; severe deformity is rare. There is often a positive family history, and occasionally this deformity may be associated with Marfan's syndrome or homocystinuria. No abnormalities of cardiac or pulmonary function are consistently associated with pectus excavatum. The major difficulty is the psychologic impact of the cosmetic deformity, and this is most significant during the adolescent years.

Because the major indication for surgical correction is cosmetic, surgery should usually be delayed until the patient is old enough to make the decision. Careful respiratory support and vigorous chest physiotherapy are extremely important in the postoperative period in order to prevent progressive respiratory failure due to the effect of flail chest.

Holcomb GW: Surgical correction of pectus excavatum. J Pediatr Surg 12:295, 1977.

Orzalesi MM, Cook CD: Pulmonary function in children with pectus excavatum. J Pediatr 66:898, 1965.

Polgar G, Koop CE: Pulmonary function in pectus excavatum. Pediatrics 32:209, 1963.

NEUROMUSCULAR DISORDERS

A wide variety of diseases which cause weakness of the respiratory muscles can result in chronic hypoventilation and inability to effectively clear secretions and maintain normal lung volumes and may ultimately progress to respiratory failure. Such patients are particularly at risk for developing recurrent pneumonia. Examples of such causes of neuromuscular weakness are myasthenia gravis, Guillain-Barré syndrome, muscular dystrophy, Werdnig-Hoffman disease, poliomyelitis, and iatrogenic disorders such as respiratory paralysis associated with polymyxin therapy. As involvement becomes more severe, such patients will be noted to have decreased breath sounds, rhonchi, rales, wheezes, and dullness to percussion at the lung bases. Chest x-ray will demonstrate elevated diaphragms and often increased bronchovascular markings with infiltrates. Arterial blood gases will demonstrate hypoxemia and, at a later stage, CO_2 retention with respiratory acidosis which may or may not be compensated. Pulmonary function studies demonstrate a decreased functional residual capacity and decreased lung compliance. It is important to periodically measure the tidal volume and vital capacity of these patients, since a vital capacity less than twice the tidal volume indicates that the patient will be unable to produce an effective cough and may require intubation for pulmonary toilet and prevention of respiratory failure. All such patients will benefit by vigorous chest physiotherapy at regular intervals with postural drainage and chest percussion. Introduction of an artificial airway and initiation of mechanical ventilation should be considered when respiratory failure appears imminent. Correct timing of this added support is particularly important when the neuromuscular disease may be reversible, as in Guillain-Barré disease or poliomyelitis. The prognosis depends on that of the underlying cause of the muscular weakness.

Burke S & others: Respiratory aspects of muscular dystrophy. Am J Dis Child 121:230, 1971.

Gibson GJ & others: Pulmonary mechanics in patients with respiratory muscle weakness. Am Rev Respir Dis 115:389, 1977.

DISORDERS OF THE PLEURA & PLEURAL CAVITY

There is normally no gas and only a very small amount of fluid between the parietal and visceral pleural surfaces, so the pleural cavity is only a potential space. The rapid uptake of fluid and gas by the pulmonary circulation out of the pleural cavity maintains the 2 pleural surfaces in apposition under normal circumstances. Most pediatric diseases of the pleura and pleural cavity involve the abnormal accumulation of air (pneumothorax), fluid (effusion), pus (empyema), contents of the lymphatic drainage system (chylothorax), blood (hemothorax), inflammatory tissue, or some combination of these within the pleural space.

PLEURISY, PLEURAL EFFUSION, & EMPYEMA

Pleurisy may be either dry (plastic), serofibrinous (pleural effusion), or purulent (empyema). Dry pleurisy occurs most often with viral pneumonia (especially coxsackievirus pneumonia) and occasionally with upper respiratory tract infection, bacterial (especially pneumococcal) respiratory tract infection, tuberculosis, rheumatic fever, subacute infective endocarditis, systemic lupus erythematosus, pulmonary embolism, inflammatory lesions of the abdominal or chest walls, subphrenic abscess, and trauma to the chest wall. Serofibrinous pleurisy or pleural effusion most frequently accompanies infections of the lung (especially pneumococcal or tuberculous) or abdomen. In addition, pleural effusions may occur in association with metastatic lesions, rheumatic fever, polyarteritis nodosa, systemic lupus erythematosus, hypoproteinemia, congestive heart failure, ascites, pancreatitis, or pulmonary infarction. Empyema is usually secondary to bacterial pneumonia, most commonly due to staphylococci. Pneumococci and *Haemophilus influenzae* are slightly less commonly the causative agents. Empyema due to group A beta-hemolytic streptococcus is unusual but can be very severe and prolonged. Empyema may occasionally develop as a result of trauma or rupture of a lung abscess or as a complication of primary pulmonary tuberculosis. Empyema is distinguished from pleural effusion by the presence of pus in the pleural space.

Clinical Findings

A. Symptoms and Signs: Depending on the severity of the involvement, all 3 types of pleurisy may present with chest pain (especially with deep breathing or coughing), guarded and grunting respirations, diminished respiratory excursions on the affected side, dyspnea, asymmetric chest movements with respiration, and occasionally abdominal pain. The child may lie on the affected side. In addition, when there is an abnormal collection of material in the pleural cavity, as with effusion or empyema, there may be dullness to chest percussion and decreased breath sounds over the effusion, cyanosis, and mediastinal shift. A pleural friction rub is heard most often in patients with dry pleurisy. Small effusions may produce no symptoms. Patients with empyema are most likely to be severely ill, and often there has been a secondary rise in temperature or persistence of high fever during the course of pneumonia.

B. Laboratory Findings: With any of the 3 types of pleurisy, pulmonary function testing may demonstrate loss of lung volume (restrictive lung disease). Other pulmonary function abnormalities may be caused by coexistent lung disease. There are not likely to be any other laboratory abnormalities due primarily to the pleural involvement in dry pleurisy. Patients with empyema usually have an elevated white blood cell count and often a positive blood culture.

Thoracentesis is necessary to distinguish between empyema and serofibrinous effusions. The amount and mobility of pleural fluid should be evaluated before thoracentesis by a lateral decubitus chest x-ray performed with the affected side in the dependent position. Material obtained at thoracentesis should be cultured for aerobic and anaerobic organisms and tubercle bacilli and submitted for cell count and differential, Gram's and acid-fast stains, and determinations of specific gravity, glucose, protein, and lactic dehydrogenase (LDH). If appropriate, the hematocrit and the amylase content of recovered fluid should be determined and cytologic examination performed. Serum samples obtained at the same time as thoracentesis should be analyzed for protein, glucose, LDH, and, if appropriate, amylase.

Recovered fluid is considered an exudate if the pleural fluid protein to serum protein ratio is > 0.5, the pleural fluid LDH is > 200 IU, or the pleural fluid LDH to serum LDH ratio is > 0.6. An exudate results from disease (usually inflammation) of the pleural surface, as may occur with tuberculosis, pneumonia, cancer, pancreatitis, pulmonary infarction, or systemic lupus erythematosus. It may be infected or sterile. A transudate is usually a clear, sterile, yellow fluid which does not meet the above criteria for exudate and may result from a decrease in plasma oncotic pressure or increase in pulmonary or systemic hydrostatic intravascular pressures, as in congestive heart failure, renal disease, or malnutrition.

C. X-Ray Findings: In patients with dry pleurisy, the chest x-ray may be normal or there may be thickening of the pleural shadow along the thoracic wall. Pleural effusion and empyema cannot be distinguished on chest x-ray. Nonetheless, any patient in whom these diagnoses are suspected should have chest x-rays taken both in the upright position and lying on the affected side. The pleural fluid will appear as a uniform density which completely or partially obscures the underlying lung. Small collections of fluid may only blunt the costophrenic or cardiophrenic angles or may widen the interlobar septa. The fluid is apt to accumulate in the most dependent part of the pleural space, but loculated fluid will not move with changes in body position. Purulent pleural exudates are usually loculated except in the early stages of infection. Large collections of pleural fluid may cause compressive atelectasis of adjacent lung tissue and shift of the mediastinal structures toward the contralateral hemithorax. There may be radiologic abnormalities of the underlying lung due to the primary disease process.

Treatment

A tuberculosis skin test should be performed in all cases, and any underlying disease should be appropriately treated. Analgesics should be given for chest pain in patients with dry pleurisy. Thoracentesis is indicated in most patients who have significant amounts of pleural fluid, both for diagnosis and as treatment when the presence of the pleural fluid is causing respiratory distress. When an effusion reaccumulates, drainage can be performed either by repeated needle aspirations or by insertion of a chest tube for closed system drainage.

All empyemas should be treated by continuous closed system drainage using a large chest tube. Treatment should be initiated promptly after the diagnosis is established. Several chest tubes may be required simultaneously or sequentially to drain loculated areas. Chest tubes are rarely required or effective for more than 1–2 weeks. In patients with empyema, appropriate systemic antibiotics should be selected on the basis of the Gram stain and culture of the material obtained by thoracentesis. Instillation of antibiotics into the pleural cavity is indicated only in the most severe cases (if ever). Thoracotomy with open drainage is very rarely necessary to treat chronic empyema, and pleural decortication is almost never necessary in children. The prognosis for pleurisy depends upon. the extent of involvement and the underlying disease. In general, the prognosis for pleural effusion is very good, as is that for empyema if appropriate therapy is initiated promptly. Empyema can be a very serious disease, especially in young children, and the chest x-ray may not return to normal for 6–12 months.

Untreated tuberculous empyema can progress to fibrothorax with contraction scarring of the pleura and marked restriction or "trapping" of the lung.

Baum GL: Diseases of the pleura. Hosp Med 5:6, Oct 1969.

Bechamps GJ & others: Empyema in children: Review of Mayo Clinic experience. Mayo Clin Proc 45:43, 1970.

Light RW & others: Pleural effusions: The diagnostic separation of transudates and exudates. Ann Intern Med 77:507, 1972.

Vix VA: Roentgenographic recognition of pleural effusion. JAMA 229:695, 1974.

Weese WC & others: Empyema of the thorax then and now: A study of 122 cases over 4 decades. Arch Intern Med 131:516, 1973.

HEMOTHORAX

Hemothorax is defined as the accumulation of whole blood in the pleural space. It is most commonly caused by surgical or accidental trauma but can also be due to a coagulation defect or tumors of the pleura or lung. It may also be iatrogenic, associated with subclavian vein cannulation. Bleeding may be rapid or slow. Symptoms are related to blood loss or compression of pulmonary parenchyma by the pleural accumulation of blood. Hemothorax is often associated with pneumothorax in cases due to trauma. There is a significant risk of developing a hemo-empyema. For this reason, and since untreated hemothorax may result in fibrothorax, it is important to remove as much blood as possible from the pleural space by thoracotomy tube and closed system drainage.

Chetty KG, Davidson PT: A guide to the management of hemothorax. Hosp Med 11:25, June 1975.

CHYLOTHORAX

Chylothorax is accumulation of chyle in the pleural cavity, usually as a result of accidental or surgical trauma to the thoracic duct. In the newborn, chylothorax may be congenital or secondary to birth trauma. Occasionally this rare disorder may be caused by a spreading cancer or by obstruction of the thoracic duct due to enlarged lymph nodes. There may be a 2- to 10-day latent period between the injury to the thoracic duct and the appearance of chyle in the pleural cavity. The symptoms depend upon the amount of accumulated fluid. There is no associated pain, but tachypnea and dyspnea are likely with large accumulations of chyle. Other physical and radiologic findings are similar to those with pleural effusion. A white oily or milky fluid obtained at thoracentesis justifies the specific diagnosis. Chylothorax must be differentiated from the accumulation of fatty material in a chronic pleural effusion. This distinction can be made by demonstrating the appearance in the pleural fluid of a fat-soluble dye ingested by the patient. Repeated therapeutic aspirations are usually required to treat the associated respiratory distress. Continuous removal of repeated reaccumulations of chyle can frequently cause significant depletion of the patient's protein and lymphocytes.

Spontaneous closure of the defect in the thoracic duct occurs in about half of cases. Therefore, every case should be treated conservatively for about 4–6 weeks. Conservative therapy consists of continuous chest tube drainage, first discontinuing all oral feedings and then reinitiating feedings with medium chain triglyceride fats; hyperalimentation is often necessary to avoid significant protein malnutrition. If 4–6 weeks of conservative therapy are not successful in decreasing or stopping the accumulation of chyle, an attempt should be made to ligate the thoracic duct or to locate and close the site of leakage in the thoracic duct.

Brodman RF & others: Treatment of congenital chylothorax. J Pediatr 85:516, 1974.

Gershanik KJ & others: Management of neonatal chylothorax. Pediatrics 53:400, 1974.

Holm AL, Soderlund S: Experiences of postoperative chylothorax in children. Pediatr Radiol 4:10, 1974.

Kaul TK & others: Chylothorax: Report of a case complicating ductus ligation through a median sternotomy, and review. Thorax 31:610, 1976.

Kosloske AM & others: Management of chylothorax in children by thoracentesis and medium chain triglyceride feedings. J Pediatr Surg 9:365, 1964.

Seriff NS & others: Chylothorax: Diagnosis by lipoprotein electrophoresis of serum and pleural fluid. Thorax 32:98, 1977.

PNEUMOTHORAX, PNEUMOMEDIASTINUM, PNEUMOPERICARDIUM, & PULMONARY INTERSTITIAL EMPHYSEMA

Pneumothorax is not common in pediatric patients except in newborns; term infants have an incidence of 1–2%, and the incidence is higher in premature infants. Pneumothorax may be spontaneous but more commonly is associated with birth trauma, positive pressure ventilation, or continuous positive airway pressure in newborn infants or, in older children, with trauma, restrictive or obstructive lung disease such as asthma, cystic fibrosis, or pneumonia; bronchopleural fistula; or rupture of pseudocysts. It may also occur as a complication of a tracheostomy in older children. Pneumopericardium and pneumomediastinum have the same etiologic basis. In the newborn infant, pulmonary interstitial emphysema usually precedes these other manifestations of air leakage. Large accumulations of extrapulmonary air can cause significant interference with normal venous return, thus decreasing cardiac output and blood pressure.

Clinical Findings

A. Symptoms and Signs: Any type of air leak can be asymptomatic, or there may be cyanosis, tachypnea, and evidence on physical examination of gas trapping in the thorax. Tension pneumothorax presents with rapid onset of marked respiratory distress, particularly in newborns, in whom it may be associated with significant hypotension. There may be physical evidence of impaired venous return and shift of the cardiac impulse and trachea toward the unaffected side. A decrease in breath sounds is usually noted over the affected side in both newborns and older children. The older child is likely to experience sudden sharp chest pain, and there may be hyperresonance on percussion of the involved hemithorax. With pneumopericardium there may be muffled heart sounds and severe circulatory insufficiency, not infrequently causing death by cardiac tamponade. In most cases, an isolated pneumomediastinum causes no symptoms other than mild tachypnea. Rarely, severe tension pneumomediastinum may develop, causing symptoms similar to those of tension pneumothorax.

B. X-Ray Findings: The definitive diagnosis of any type of air leak is by chest x-ray. Cross-table lateral and lateral decubitus x-rays (with affected side up) are best for demonstrating pneumothorax. Pneumomediastinum usually appears as a radiolucent line following the contour of the mediastinum. Pneumopericardium is best distinguished from pneumomediastinum by the fact that the radiolucent line is continuous along the diaphragmatic cardiac border. Pulmonary interstitial emphysema appears on x-ray as a collection of small linear, reticular, or cystic radiolucencies which tend to be wider in the more peripheral lung tissue.

Differential Diagnosis

The differential diagnosis of pneumothorax on chest x-ray is usually not difficult. Occasionally there may be some difficulty distinguishing between pneumothorax and diaphragmatic hernia, lung cysts, or artifact due to overlying skin folds or clothing.

Treatment

Tension pneumothorax in a newborn or young infant requires immediate emergency needle aspiration of pleural air followed by chest tube insertion and underwater closed system drainage for several days. Needle aspiration should be performed using a needle or catheter of appropriate size for the patient, inserted into the second or third intercostal space in the midclavicular line. Pneumopericardium usually requires emergency treatment which consists of aspirating the pericardial air through a needle introduced in the subxiphoid or parasternal position. A drainage tube should be placed in the pericardial sac if there is repeated reaccumulation of pericardial air. Pneumomediastinum rarely requires aspiration. The air in the mediastinum is usually loculated into multiple cysts and therefore cannot be effectively removed by needle or mediastinal tube. There is no way to remove the abnormal air accumulations in pulmonary interstitial emphysema. Any patient with an air leak who requires resuscitation or assisted ventilation should be treated with the lowest possible inflation pressures. Small pneumothoraces (less than about 20% of the hemithorax) in stable patients of any age can be treated conservatively with bed rest. Conservative therapy would almost never be appropriate for a patient being mechanically ventilated with an air leak. In some cases, "spontaneous" resorption of pleural air can be hastened by having the patient breathe 100% oxygen. This is usually not appropriate in newborn infants because of the risk of retrolental fibroplasia. Conservative therapy while awaiting spontaneous resorption is more often indicated in older patients. A chest tube may be indicated for patients with chronic small pneumothorax in order to cause some pleural reaction to seal the air leak. Surgical procedures are occasionally indicated for a persistent air leak such as a bronchopleural fistula. Significant respiratory distress is always an indication for chest tube drainage of the pleural air.

Kirkpatrick BV & others: Complications of ventilatory therapy in respiratory distress syndrome: Recognition and management of acute air leaks. Am J Dis Child 128:496, 1974.

Mansfield PB & others: Pneumopericardium and pneumomediastinum in infants and children. J Pediatr Surg 8:691, 1973.

Ogata E & others: Pneumothorax in respiratory distress syndrome: Incidence and effect on vital signs, blood gases and pH. Pediatrics 58:177, 1976.

Reppert SM & others: The treatment of pneumopericardium in the newborn infant. J Pediatr 90:115, 1977.

Ya VYH & others: Pneumothorax in the newborn: A changing pattern. Arch Dis Child 50:449, 1975.

Zimmerman JE, Dunbar BS, Klingenmaier CH: Management of subcutaneous emphysema, pneumomediastinum and pneumothorax during respirator therapy. Crit Care Med 3:69, 1975.

DISORDERS OF
THE MEDIASTINUM

MEDIASTINITIS

Acute suppurative mediastinitis is usually secondary to esophageal perforation occurring either as a result of foreign body ingestion or iatrogenically during surgery, endoscopy, or attempted tracheal intubation. Spontaneous esophageal perforation, when it occurs, is usually due to vomiting. Nontraumatic mediastinal infection is rare.

The initial signs and symptoms of acute suppurative mediastinitis may be vague, with gradual onset of substernal pain, fever, chills, toxemia, and dysphagia. Under some circumstances there may be a brassy cough, dyspnea, and sternal tenderness. The white count is usually high. Occasionally the mediastinal process causes obstruction of venous return and venous distention. There may be a characteristic respiratory pattern of spasmodic or "halting" inspiration, sometimes accompanied by grimacing, thought to result from pain due to stretching of inflamed mediastinal structures during inspiration. The chest x-ray is characterized by widening of the upper mediastinum by a dense shadow bulging outward. The lateral x-ray may show anterior displacement of the trachea and the esophagus. There may be associated pleural effusion or pyopneumothorax and mediastinal emphysema. The key to therapy is the immediate initiation of parenteral broad-spectrum antibiotic therapy after obtaining appropriate cultures. In the absence of appropriate treatment, this disease can be rapidly progressive and death can occur. If a mediastinal abscess develops, surgical drainage may be indicated, although this is usually not necessary in the newborn if prompt antibiotic therapy is instituted. Upper airway obstruction may occur, requiring prompt creation of an artificial airway.

Engelman RM & others: Mediastinitis following open heart surgery: Review of two years' experience. Arch Surg 107:772, 1973.

Enquist RW & others: Non-traumatic mediastinitis. JAMA 236:1048, 1976.

Feldman R, Gromisch DS: Acute suppurative mediastinitis. Am J Dis Child 121:79, 1971.

MEDIASTINAL MASSES

Most mediastinal masses are asymptomatic and are discovered during routine chest x-ray. Symptoms may develop as a result of pressure on sensitive structures. Respiratory symptoms are more common in children than in adults. Most types of mediastinal masses tend to be localized to a specific mediastinal compartment, thus enhancing the accuracy of preoperative diagnosis. Some masses, however, can appear in different or several mediastinal compartments. The superior mediastinum includes the area above the pericardium and is bordered inferiorly by a line connecting the manubrium to the fourth thoracic vertebra posteriorly. The anterior mediastinum is the space between the sternum anteriorly and the pericardium posteriorly. The posterior mediastinum is bordered by the pericardium and diaphragm anteriorly and the lower 8 thoracic vertebrae posteriorly. The mid mediastinum is bounded by the other 3 compartments. The masses that are found in each compartment are listed in Table 12–5.

Mediastinal lymph nodes may be enlarged in benign or malignant disease. Benign cysts are usually abnormalities of embryologic development. An enlarged thymus is the most common mediastinal mass in children. Corticosteroids may be given to "shrink" the thymus as part of the diagnostic workup.

Clinical Findings

A. Symptoms and Signs: Respiratory symptoms result from pressure on airways, causing cough; incomplete obstruction, with wheezing or obstructive emphysema (or both); complete obstruction, with atelectasis; or compression of lung parenchyma, causing atelectasis. Pressure on the recurrent laryngeal nerve may cause hoarseness due to paralysis of the left vocal cord. Pressure on the esophagus may cause dysphagia. Dilatation of neck vessels may occur as a result of superior vena caval obstruction. Physical findings are usually absent except when a very large mass is present.

B. Laboratory Findings: Although most information is usually gained by x-ray, a variety of other tests may be helpful when certain diagnoses are being considered. Such a workup might include an ECG, fungal and mycobacterial skin tests, urinary catecholamine assay, peripheral lymph node biopsy, and mediastinoscopy.

C. X-Ray Findings: A variety of radiologic technics should be used to define the contour and location of the mediastinal mass. Regular frontal and lateral chest x-rays, tomograms, high kilovoltage x-rays to better delineate the tracheobronchial air column, esophagograms, and occasionally pulmonary angiograms and thyroid scans may be informative.

Treatment

Appropriate treatment depends on the type of mediastinal mass, although surgery is usually required either for diagnosis or treatment.

Tokorny WJ, Sherman JO: Mediastinal masses in infants and children. J Thorac Cardiovasc Surg 68:869, 1974.

Whittaker LD, Lynn HB: Mediastinal tumors and cysts in the pediatric patients. Surg Clin North Am 53:893, 1973.

CONGENITAL ABNORMALITIES OF THE LUNG

Congenital abnormalities of the respiratory tract, some of which have been discussed above, may present with clinical signs or symptoms at any time between birth and adulthood depending on the type and severity of the lesion, while others may never cause symptoms.

PULMONARY AGENESIS, APLASIA, & HYPOPLASIA

Absence or incomplete development of one or both lungs can be classified by the degree of developmental arrest. *Agenesis* refers to the complete absence of one or both lungs, *aplasia* is the absence of any pulmonary tissue beyond a rudimentary bronchus, and greater development than this but failure of the pulmonary tissue to fully develop is referred to as *hypoplasia.* Agenesis and aplasia are rare occurrences of unknown cause which are often associated with other congenital anomalies. On clinical examination there will be a shift of the cardiac impulse toward the affected side, where there is a decrease in air entry. There is likely to be decreased anteroposterior diameter of the chest on the affected side associated with decreased movement of that hemithorax with inspiration. Chest x-ray demonstrates total or partial opacification of one hemithorax, with mediastinal shift toward the affected side. Some of the contralateral lung may enter the affected hemithorax across the midline. The absence of pulmonary arteries and airways may be documented by pulmonary angiography and bronchography. Pulmonary function testing reveals decreased forced expiratory volume, decreased forced vital capacity, and small absolute lung volume as well as limited exercise tolerance. The only appropriate treatment is vigorous therapy (physiotherapy and antibiotics) for any infections in the "normal" lung. The prognosis is worse when the aplasia or agenesis occurs on the right. This may be due to the normally larger volume of the right lung or to the fact that agenesis of the right lung is more frequently associated with congenital cardiac abnormalities. Most patients with right-sided agenesis die within months. With agenesis of the left lung the chance for survival is better unless it is associated with other serious congenital abnormalities.

Pulmonary hypoplasia, or a small lung with relatively normal bronchial anatomy, may be an isolated finding or may be associated with congenital diaphragmatic hernia or eventration, renal agenesis (Potter's syndrome), abnormal chest wall development (eg, congenital scoliosis or asphyxiating thoracic dystrophy), or abnormal pulmonary arterial and venous anatomy of the right lung *(scimitar syndrome).* Unilateral pulmonary hypoplasia is apt to be associated with normal somatic growth and an increased frequency of lower respiratory tract infection in some young patients, whereas other patients may be totally free of symptoms. Physical examination may reveal decreased air entry on the affected side combined with a small hemithorax. Chest x-ray may show a small hemithorax with mediastinal shift.

A full workup is warranted before making a firm diagnosis of pulmonary underdevelopment in order to avoid misdiagnosing an acquired loss of lung volume— eg, due to airway obstruction by an aspirated foreign body or tumor.

Booth JB, Berry CL: Unilateral pulmonary agenesis. Arch Dis Child 42:361, 1967.

Jue KL & others: Anomalies of the great vessels associated with lung hypoplasia: The scimitar syndrome. Am J Dis Child 111:35, 1966.

Maltz DL, Nadas AS: Agenesis of the lung: Presentation of eight new cases and review of the literature. Pediatrics 42:175, 1968.

Punnet HH & others: Syndrome of ankylosis, facial anomalies and pulmonary hypoplasia. J Pediatr 84:375, 1974.

Thomas IT, Smith DW: Oligohydramnios, cause of the nonrenal features of Potter's syndrome including pulmonary hypoplasia. J Pediatr 84:811, 1974.

PULMONARY SEQUESTRATION

In this type of congenital malformation a small to large area of lung tissue is detached from the remaining lung. This multicystic tissue, composed of poorly developed alveoli and airways, is supplied by one or several systemic arteries arising from the thoracic or abdominal aorta. There is usually no communication— or only a deficient communication—with the rest of the bronchial tree. The venous drainage is to the pulmonary veins. Most commonly the sequestered tissue is surrounded by a pleural sac (intralobar) and located in one of the posterobasal segments of one of the lower lobes, especially the left. Occasionally, the sequestration is not surrounded by normal lung but is extralobar, with its own pleural covering. In this type there are frequently venous connections to the caval or azygos veins. The sequestration may become the site of infection or cyst formation and thus may present at any age with recurrent or chronic localized pulmonary infection. Often, however, the sequestration may be discovered as an incidental asymptomatic finding of a cystic or consolidated density on a routine chest x-ray. Extralobar sequestration may appear as a wedge-shaped radio-dense area in the retrocardiac area on the left or paravertebrally on the right. The anatomy can be defined by angiography, bronchoscopy, and bronchography. When infection occurs, there is usually some connection between the sequestration and surrounding airways.

The differential diagnosis includes foregut cysts,

congenital bronchogenic cysts, tumors, lung abscesses, eventration of the diaphragm, and adenomatoid malformation of the lung.

Sequestered lung tissue should be surgically removed in order to eliminate an actual or potential site of recurrent infection. Careful definition of the vascular supply to the sequestration should be obtained before surgery in order to avoid severing one of the related systemic arteries. The prognosis following surgery is good.

Enge I, Friestad O: Pulmonary sequestration. Scand J Thorac Cardiovasc Surg 7:181, 1973.

Iwai K & others: Intralobar pulmonary sequestration with special reference to developmental pathology. Am Rev Respir Dis 107:911, 1973.

Saegesser F, Besson A: Extralobar and intralobar pulmonary sequestration of the upper and lower lobes. Chest 63:69, 1973.

Telander RL & others: Sequestration of the lung in children. Mayo Clin Proc 51:579, 1976.

Tendse P & others: Pulmonary sequestration: Co-existing classic intralobar and extralobar types in a child. J Thorac Cardiovasc Surg 64:127, 1972.

INFANTILE LOBAR EMPHYSEMA
(Congenital Lobar Emphysema)

Infantile lobar emphysema is progressive overdistention of lung tissue, usually a single lobe, producing respiratory distress within the first 6 months of life, especially during the first 2 weeks. There is usually no indentifiable cause, although localized bronchial cartilage deficiency causing a ball valve obstruction has been reported in some cases. Other causes of a similar clinical picture include bronchogenic cysts or mucoceles, aberrant or large pulmonary arteries (especially those associated with large left-to-right shunts), mucous plugs, foreign bodies, and redundant bronchial mucosa. Sometimes the effective airway obstruction is present at birth, and early chest x-rays may demonstrate persistence of fetal lung fluid (ie, increased opacity) in the affected area. During the first week of life, this is usually replaced by air and there is gradual development of increasing hyperinflation of the affected lung. Respiratory distress classically increases within the first days or weeks of life, with tachypnea, retractions, chest asymmetry, intermittent cyanosis, expiratory wheezing, and localized decreased air entry.

The chest x-ray will demonstrate localized hyperinflation with compression of adjacent lung and mediastinal shift toward the contralateral hemithorax. With progressive hyperinflation, there may be anterior herniation of the abnormal lung into the contralateral hemithorax. Barium swallow and pulmonary angiography may be helpful in the workup to look for the presence of enlarged or aberrant vessels. Lobectomy is the treatment of choice for patients with significant respiratory symptoms. Postoperatively, many patients will have persistance of recurrent cough and wheezing episodes. Approximately 10% will develop hyperinflation of another lobe at some time in the future.

Fagan CJ, Swischuk LE: The opaque lung in lobar emphysema. Am J Roentgenol Radium Ther Nucl Med 114:300, 1972.

Lakier JB & others: Tetrology of Fallot with absent pulmonary valve: Natural history and hemodynamic considerations. Circulation 50:167, 1974.

Leape LL, Longino LA: Infantile lobar emphysema. Pediatrics 34:246, 1964.

Tsuji S & others: The syndrome of bronchial mucocele and regional hyperinflation of the lung. Chest 64:444, 1973.

CYSTIC ADENOMATOID MALFORMATION

This rare congenital anomaly of the lung is a multicystic mass of pulmonary tissue containing disordered, polypoid proliferation of respiratory epithelium and bronchiolar structures which may or may not communicate with normal airways. The cysts are lined by cuboidal or columnar epithelium. Affected infants are often born prematurely and usually begin to experience respiratory distress at birth or within the first weeks of life. The cystic mass, which may occur in any lobe of the lung and is occasionally in more than one lobe, produces symptoms of tachypnea, cyanosis, and retractions by enlargement and compression of normal lung tissue. Chest x-rays demonstrate an intrapulmonary mass which may be variably radio-dense and radiolucent, with sharp, irregular borders. There is often a shift of the mediastinum as the abnormal area becomes hyperinflated.

If the infant is symptomatic and if the abnormality appears to be localized to one lobe or lung, prompt surgical resection is indicated to avoid further compression of normal lung.

Belanger R & others: Congenital cystic adenomatoid malformation of the lung. Thorax 19:1, 1964.

Birdfell DC & others: Congenital cystic adenomatoid malformation of the lung: A report of 8 cases. Can J Surg 9:350, 1966.

Buntain WL & others: Lobar emphysema, cystic adenomatoid malformation, pulmonary sequestration, and bronchogenic cyst in infancy and childhood: A clinical group. J Pediatr Surg 9:85, 1974.

Madewell JE & others: Cystic adenomatoid malformation of the lung: Morphologic analysis. Am J Roentgenol Radium Ther Nucl Med 124:436, 1975.

PULMONARY CYSTS

Pulmonary cysts may be congenital or acquired, associated with the trachea or main bronchi (ie, extrapulmonary) or with the smaller airways or alveoli (ie, intrapulmonary), and symptomatic or asymptomatic. Distinguishing between congenital and acquired (usually postinfectious) causes may often be difficult but is of great importance since surgery is usually indicated in the former category and generally contraindicated for acquired cysts. The differential diagnosis of pulmonary cyst includes congenital cysts, cystic adenomatoid malformation, pneumatoceles, lung abscess, pulmonary sequestration, loculated pyopneumothorax, infantile lobar emphysema, a variety of mediastinal masses (see Table 12—5), and localized pulmonary interstitial emphysema.

CONGENITAL LUNG CYSTS

True congenital parenchymal lung cysts are probably very rare. Caffey states that most cysts seen in newborns and young infants are ultimately reversible and therefore likely to be acquired cysts resulting from infection. The most common forms of true congenital pulmonary cysts are bronchogenic cysts and congenital cystic adenomatoid malformation.

Caffey J: On the natural regression of pulmonary cysts during early infancy. Pediatrics 11:48, 1953.

BRONCHOGENIC CYSTS

Congenital bronchogenic cysts characteristically occur adjacent to the airway near the tracheal bifurcation. Those at the carina are usually most serious, causing obstructive respiratory symptoms, often from birth, due to tracheobronchial compression. Hilar cysts attached to one of the main or lobar bronchi are more common in older children or adults and are very likely to be asymptomatic, diagnosed only as incidental findings on chest x-ray. There is little relationship between the size of the cyst and the degree of resultant respiratory distress. The cysts are thin-walled, occasionally multilocular, white or pearly gray, and contain clear mucoid fluid. The contents of the cyst may become infected, or the airway compression by the cyst may cause the distal lung parenchyma to become hyperinflated, atelectatic, or infected. The cysts are frequently adjacent to the esophagus and may cause dysphagia. Occasionally an infected cyst may develop a communication with a bronchus, resulting in hemoptysis, purulent sputum, and associated fever. Chest x-ray may be normal or may demonstrate obstructive emphysema, atelectasis, mediastinal shift, or, in young newborns, an opacified hemithorax due to delayed clearance of fetal lung fluid. An esophagogram may demonstrate the presence of the cyst even when it is not apparent on the plain chest x-ray. The cyst is often positioned

between the esophagus and the trachea. Bronchography is rarely indicated and is a hazardous procedure in infants. Occasionally, a fluid level may be evident in a cyst, indicating communication with the tracheobronchial tree.

Appropriate treatment is surgical resection and vigorous pulmonary physiotherapy.

Bronchial cysts. (Editorial.) Br Med J 2:501, 1973.
Eraklis AJ & others: Bronchogenic cysts of the mediastinum in infancy. N Engl J Med 281:1150, 1969.

ACQUIRED PULMONARY CYSTS

Pneumatocele

Pneumatoceles are round or oval radiolucent areas with thin, well demarcated borders which appear on the chest x-ray during the course of pneumonia, usually due to staphylococcal infection or measles. Pneumonias due to infection with other viruses, tubercle bacilli, klebsiellae, group A streptococci, *Pseudomonas aeruginosa, Escherichia coli,* pneumococci, or hydrocarbon aspiration may also be associated with pneumatocele.

Pneumatocele is characterized clinically by sudden appearance, rapid changes in size and position, and potential for rapid disappearance. It typically causes no symptoms unless it is very large, and it usually regresses over a period of several weeks or months. The prognosis is excellent for eventual complete resolution with conservative therapy, which consists of chest percussion and postural drainage and appropriate antibiotic therapy for pneumonia. Bronchoscopic or surgical treatment is indicated only in the very rare case where the pneumatocele becomes infected and filled with purulent material or when it is life-threatening because of its size or location. Very rarely, rupture of a pneumatocele may cause pneumothorax and bronchopleural fistula with empyema.

Bergeson PS & others: Pneumatoceles following hydrocarbon ingestion: Report of three cases and review of the literature. Am J Dis Child 129:49, 1975.
Boisset GF: Subpleural emphysema complicating staphylococcal and other pneumonias. J Pediatr 81:259, 1972.

Lung Abscess

Lung abscesses may be multiple (especially in chronic lung disease, such as cystic fibrosis) or solitary. They may occur as a complication of bacterial pneumonia (eg, due to staphylococcus, klebsiella, pneumococcus, or group A beta-hemolytic streptococcus), secondary to aspiration of a foreign body or infected material, secondary to penetrating chest trauma, or due to infection of a pulmonary sequestration, atelectatic lung, pneumatocele, or congenital cyst. There is likely to be a rapid development of fever, dyspnea, cough, chest pain, and leukocytosis. The abscess appears on chest x-ray as a radio-dense spherical structure which may have an air-fluid level if the abscess communicates with the airway. If the abscess is in peripheral lung tissue, there may be a pleural reaction; occasionally, the abscess may rupture into the pleural space, producing empyema and a bronchopleural fistula. If the abscess develops communication with the airways, there may be production of foul-smelling purulent sputum and occasionally hemoptysis.

Optimal treatment consists of appropriate parenteral antibiotics, vigorous pulmonary physical therapy with particular attention to postural drainage, and bronchoscopy to obtain material for culture, to rule out foreign body aspiration, and to drain the abscess. If there is no significant improvement after about 1 month of optimal medical therapy (repeated bronchoscopy may be required), lobectomy should be considered. With vigorous optimal therapy, in the absence of chronic underlying disease, the prognosis is good for complete recovery.

Moore TC, Battersby JS: Pulmonary abscess in infancy and childhood. Ann Surg 151:496, 1960.
Sabiston DC & others: The surgical management of complications of staphylococcus pneumonia in infancy and childhood. J Thorac Cardiovasc Surg 38:421, 1959.

PULMONARY TUMORS

Primary tumors of the airway and parenchyma are very rare in pediatrics. Most intrathoracic tumors occur in the mediastinum. Benign pulmonary tumors which have been reported in the respiratory tract of children are hamartomas, bronchial adenomas, papillomas, angiomas, leiomyomas, lipomas, and neurogenic tumors. Although very rare, the most frequent category of malignant pulmonary tumors in children is bronchogenic carcinoma, which carries a very poor prognosis. In addition, fibrocarcinomas and leiomyosarcomas have been reported. Tumors that may metastasize to the lung are Wilms's tumor, chondrosarcoma, osteogenic sarcoma, Ewing's tumor, reticulum cell sarcoma, and soft tissue sarcoma. Tumors may be asymptomatic and detected on routine chest x-ray or may present with cough, hemoptysis, weight loss, malaise, anemia, or anorexia. Tests which may be appropriate in the workup of such problems include frontal and lateral chest x-rays, fluoroscopy, tomograms, angiography, sputum culture and cytology, tuberculin and fungal skin tests, bone marrow analysis, lymph node biopsy, mediastinoscopy, bronchoscopy, lung biopsy, and thoracotomy. Appropriate therapy depends on the type of tumor.

Brooks JW: Tumors of the chest. Page 697 in: *Disorders of the Respiratory Tract in Children,* 3rd ed. Kendig EL, Chernick V (editors). Saunders, 1977.
Hyde L, Hyde CI: Clinical manifestations of lung cancer. Chest 65:299, 1974.
Nitu Y & others: Lung cancer (squamous cell carcinoma) in adolescents. Am J Dis Child 127:108, 1974.

DROWNING

Drowning is the third most common cause of accidental death in children in the USA. Groups at particularly high risk include teenage boys, all toddlers, and patients with seizure disorders. The acute differences between salt and fresh water near drownings have little clinical significance except that hypovolemia may be a problem in the former whereas fresh water interferes much more with pulmonary surfactant and atelectasis is a more significant problem. Although electrolyte abnormalities may occur in both types of drowning, they are generally mild and do not require specific therapy.

Hypoxemia begins within seconds of submersion, and ineffective circulation begins about 2–4 minutes later. After 3–6 minutes of ineffective circulation, irreversible microscopic CNS changes begin. Laryngospasm begins early in this sequence, probably when the first water enters the posterior pharynx (Fig 12–5); aspiration of larger amounts of water generally occurs several minutes later, although 10% of victims die without ever aspirating. Thus, after 4–6 minutes of submersion, irreversible CNS changes begin. This time sequence may be delayed somewhat if the victim is submerged in very cold water or if the victim has ingested significant amounts of barbiturates.

The clinical presentation of near drowning victims varies widely. Patients with pulmonary edema will have tachypnea, rales, and often frothy sputum, cyanosis,

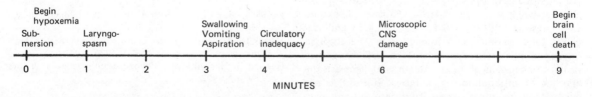

Figure 12–5. Time course of events during immersion (drowning).

and sometimes apnea. Initial chest x-rays may be normal or may demonstrate patchy, fluffy infiltrates. More severe cases will show some degree of CNS depression with or without seizures. Shock and severe metabolic acidosis may cause peripheral vasoconstriction with cool, mottled extremities.

The key to on-scene resuscitation of near drowning victims is to initiate ventilation (usually mouth-to-mouth) as early as possible. This may be in a rescue boat or when the swimming rescuer reaches shallow water. Prior to beginning mouth-to-mouth resuscitation, any foreign material should be quickly removed with the rescuer's finger from the mouth and posterior pharynx, but no time should be wasted in trying to "drain water" from the lungs. If there is no palpable heart beat, external cardiac massage should be initiated and, with mouth-to-mouth ventilation, continued in transit to the hospital. If oxygen is available, it should be given at the earliest possible moment. Upon arrival at the emergency room, cardiopulmonary resuscitation should be continued if required while an intravenous line is inserted for administration of fluid, cardiotonic drugs, and bicarbonate. In addition to the profound hypoxemia, any severely depressed near drowning victim will have a marked metabolic acidosis. Initial volume administered should be 20 ml/kg of salt-poor albumin, lactated Ringer's injection, or half normal saline. Subsequently, packed red blood cells may be more appropriate for fresh water victims, whereas plasma may be the best choice for salt water victims.

All near drowning victims should be admitted to the hospital for at least overnight observation even if they appear normal in the emergency room. Mild cases should have an initial chest x-ray and arterial blood gas determination while they breathe room air. Vital signs should be monitored frequently during the night, and arterial blood gases should be determined again prior to discharge.

The major therapeutic efforts in the hospitalized near drowning victim are directed toward the cardiopulmonary and central nervous systems. Arrhythmias, especially ventricular fibrillation, tend to occur early, and ventricular fibrillation is probably the major cause of immediate drowning deaths. Acute tubular necrosis occasionally develops, probably secondary to the period of shock and not as a result of the hemoglobinuria.

General management of the hospitalized near drowning victim includes following electrolytes, hemoglobin, fluid intake and output, and chest x-ray. Careful attention is required to maintain normal body temperature. Oxygenation is a major problem in these patients owing to the stiff, wet lungs with widespread alveolar collapse or consolidation. Positive end-expiratory pressure (PEEP), delivered by mask or endotracheal tube, should be initiated when the inspired oxygen requirement exceeds 40 or 50% oxygen in order to maintain alveolar patency and decrease the amount of intrapulmonary shunting. If PEEP is not adequate to maintain oxygenation, intermittent mandatory ventilation (IMV) should be initiated. Because

of their stiff lungs, these patients may require high ventilatory pressures. In addition, near drowning victims may require intubation for pulmonary toilet (specifically for prevention of aspiration of secretions) or for CO_2 retention or apnea in a comatose or obtunded patient. Because of the alveolar instability resulting from surfactant deficiency, it is important not to withdraw the mechanical ventilation too early. A minimum of 1–2 days is likely to be required before discontinuing the ventilator. The aspirated material may precipitate bronchospasm in some patients, necessitating bronchodilator therapy (aminophylline, corticosteroids, or isoproterenol drip). Prophylactic antibiotics are not indicated. If pulmonary infiltrates on chest x-ray persist past 24–48 hours or if the patient's pulmonary status deteriorates, there may be a secondary bacterial infection which would warrant the institution of antibiotic therapy. Some signs of secondary infection such as fever, atelectasis, leukocytosis, and tachycardia can be a direct result of the near drowning and may not indicate infection. Steroids are not indicated for the lung disease in near drowning victims.

Advances in cerebral resuscitation have lagged behind those of cardiopulmonary resuscitation, so that today one is more likely to have a successful cardiopulmonary resuscitation and be left with a patient with significant irreversible neurologic deficit. The CNS changes are probably due chiefly to the asphyxia during submersion and not to electrolyte abnormalities. Neurologic treatment consists of intravenous diazepam (Valium) for seizures, corticosteroids (eg, 1 mg/kg/day of dexamethasone) for cerebral edema in the semicomatose or comatose patient, and decreasing fluid administration to two-thirds of maintenance after initially establishing adequate circulation in order to decrease cerebral and pulmonary edema due to the shock-damaged capillaries in these organs. Any subsequent neurologic deterioration in the hospitalized patient is usually preceded by pulmonary deterioration.

Although ultimate restoration of normal pulmonary function can be expected in survivors, the prognosis for subsequent neurologic function is not as good. Patients requiring cardiopulmonary resuscitation in the emergency room have an extremely high likelihood of permanent neurologic sequelae if they survive. Vigorous, rapid cardiopulmonary resuscitation should be initiated in the emergency room, but, unless other modifying factors become apparent (eg, barbiturate overdosage), it is appropriate to stop resuscitation after 10–20 minutes if adequate cardiovascular function has not been restored.

Fandel I, Bancalari E: Near-drowning in children: Clinical aspects. Pediatrics 58:573, 1976.

Modell JH & others: Clinical course of 91 consecutive near-drowning victims. Chest 70:231, 1976.

Peterson B: Morbidity of childhood near-drowning. Pediatrics 59:364, 1977.

RESPIRATORY FAILURE

Acute, severe respiratory failure is a life-threatening situation and requires immediate therapy. There is no universally accepted definition of respiratory failure, but it can be presumed to be present when the arterial CO_2 level is elevated or when a moderate to severe degree of hypoxemia exists.

Causes of Respiratory Failure

Respiratory failure may be caused by or secondary to (1) CNS disorders, eg, head injury; (2) neuromuscular diseases, eg, myasthenia gravis, poliomyelitis, Guillain-Barré syndrome; (3) lung or airway diseases, eg, asthma, croup, peripheral lung disease such as respiratory distress syndrome, foreign body aspiration; (4) heart disease, eg, congenital heart disease; or (5) pulmonary vascular bed disorders, eg, pulmonary edema, vasoconstriction.

Principles of Treatment

Treatment is aimed at restoring arterial oxygen and CO_2 tensions to normal. Low arterial oxygen tension can be treated by increasing the concentration of inspired oxygen and application of continuous distending pressure to the lung. In the presence of severe chronic hypercapnia and hypoxia, the predominant respiratory drive may be the hypoxic stimulus; administration of oxygen under these circumstances may result in apnea, but this is a rare occurrence in the pediatric age group. It should always be borne in mind that lack of oxygen rapidly "wrecks the machinery," and severe hypoxia is not a situation that can be tolerated for long. Increased CO_2 tension is an indication that alveolar ventilation is decreased, and the only way the excess CO_2 can be eliminated is by increasing alveolar ventilation. This may require assisted ventilation.

Assisted ventilation may be administered by manual resuscitating devices or by mechanical ventilators. In general, the indications for assisted ventilation are as follows: (1) arterial oxygen tension which cannot be maintained at or near normal levels by increasing the inspired oxygen concentration; (2) elevated CO_2 tension (over 65 mm Hg); and (3) apnea. Excessive work of breathing leads to physical exhaustion, and severe respiratory failure may occur suddenly. The oxygen consumption related to excessive work of breathing may reach 40% of the total oxygen requirement.

Assisted ventilation may occasionally be indicated in the presence of normal blood gases. For example, in a patient with Guillain-Barré syndrome, when the vital capacity is reduced to twice the tidal volume, assisted ventilation may be indicated because of inability to cough and sigh effectively.

Campbell EJM: Respiratory failure. Br Med J 1:1451, 1965.
Cotton EK, Parry WH: Treatment of status asthmaticus and respiratory failure. Pediatr Clin North Am 22:163, 1974.
Downes JMB: Acute respiratory failure in infants following cardiovascular surgery. J Thorac Cardiovasc Surg 59:21, 1970.
Pontoppidan H: Acute respiratory failure in the adult. N Engl J Med 287:690, 1972.
Symposium on pathophysiology and care of respiratory failure. Crit Care Med 2:171, 1974.

SUDDEN INFANT DEATH SYNDROME
("Crib Death")

The sudden infant death syndrome (SIDS) is defined as "the sudden death of any infant or young child, which is unexpected by history, and in which a thorough postmortem examination fails to demonstrate an adequate cause for death." This entity has been known for centuries but has become of more interest recently as other causes of infant mortality are decreasing. The incidence of SIDS is 2–3/1000 live births, or approximately 7500 SIDS deaths per year in the USA. This is the largest single cause of infant death after the neonatal period. The peak incidence is at 2–4 months after birth, and 91% of SIDS deaths occur within the first 6 months of life. Less than 1% occur in the first 2 weeks.

The death characteristically occurs during sleep, particularly between midnight and 6:00 a.m. Affected infants are previously entirely healthy or may have had findings of a very mild upper respiratory infection. The incidence is increased in the winter months, in lower income groups, and in low birth weight infants. Males are affected more frequently than females in a 3:2 ratio. The death is silent.

In addition to the history, characteristic autopsy findings are necessary to establish a diagnosis of SIDS. Intrathoracic petechiae (especially on the thymus, pleura, and pericardium) are present in 87% of cases. There is usually some pulmonary edema; there may be pulmonary vascular congestion, and occasionally there may be aspirated gastric contents in the lung. Nonpolio viruses are isolated from 23–42% of SIDS victims at autopsy, but there are no consistent histologic changes to document a pathogenic role for viruses. Naeye, with special technics, has demonstrated an increase in medial smooth muscle mass in the pulmonary arterioles and prolonged retention of periadrenal brown fat in SIDS victims, both indirect evidence of previous chronic or recurrent hypoxia. The autopsy is also of great importance to rule out other specific causes of sudden death in infants such as meningitis, myocarditis, and intracranial hemorrhage.

Numerous causes have been suggested for the death of these patients, but none have been proved. It is probable that a number of causes may be responsible for the deaths in different cases. The upper airway probably plays an important role in the cause of death by one of several possible mechanisms. Subclinical gastric reflux stimulating apnea-inducing receptors in the region of the larynx is a possible cause. In animals, stimulation of such receptors can cause fatal apnea. This mechanism may combine with actual upper airway obstruction—to which the infant upper airway is particularly vulnerable—to cause a combined obstructive and central apnea in some infants. Finally, Steinschneider has documented the rare familial occurrence of prolonged sleep apneas during rapid eye movement sleep, and some of these affected infants have subsequently succumbed to apparent SIDS deaths.

Extensive psychosocial support is mandatory for families who have experienced the sudden infant death syndrome. This should be provided by trained personnel who should also work to educate both lay and professional groups about the sudden infant death syndrome.

The telephone number of the National Foundation for Sudden Infant Death, a private organization for assistance of parents, public education, and support of SIDS research, is 312-663-0650.

Beckwith JB: The sudden infant death syndrome. Department of Health, Education, and Welfare Publication # (HSA) 76-5137, 1976.

Downing SE, Lee JC: Laryngeal chemosensitivity: A possible mechanism for sudden infant death. Pediatrics 55:640, 1975.

Marx JL: Crib death: Some promising leads but no solution yet. Science 189:367, 1975.

Naeye RL: Hypoxemia and the sudden infant death syndrome. Science 186:837, 1974.

Robinson RR (editor): *SIDS 1974: The Francis E Camps International Symposium on Sudden and Unexpected Deaths in Infancy.* Canadian Foundation for the Study of Infant Deaths, 1974.

Steinschneider A: Nasopharyngitis and prolonged sleep apnea. Pediatrics 56:967, 1975.

Steinschneider A: Prolonged apnea and the sudden infant death syndrome: Clinical and laboratory observations. Pediatrics 50:646, 1972.

Tonkin S: Sudden infant death syndrome: Hypothesis of causation. Pediatrics 55:650, 1975.

Valdes-Depena M: Sudden death in infancy: A report for pathologists. Perspect Pediatr Pathol 2:1, 1975.

●   ●   ●

General References

Avery ME, Fletcher BD: *The Lung and Its Disorders in the Newborn Infant.* Saunders, 1974.

Bates DV, Macklem PT, Christie RV: *Respiratory Function in Disease,* 2nd ed. Saunders, 1971.

Comroe JH: *The Physiology of Respiration.* Year Book, 1970.

Cotes JE: *Lung Function: Assessment and Application in Medicine,* 3rd ed. Blackwell, 1975.

Crofton J, Douglas A: *Respiratory Diseases,* 2nd ed. Blackwell, 1975.

Gerbaux J, Couvreur J, Tournier G: *Pathologie Respiratoire de l'Enfant.* Flammarion Medecine—Sciences, Paris, 1975.

Kendig EL: *Disorders of the Respiratory Tract in Children,* 3rd ed. Saunders, 1972.

Kerrebijn KF & others: Chronic nonspecific respiratory disease in children, a five year follow-up study. Acta Paediatr Scand Suppl 261, 1977.

Mellins RB: Respiratory care in infants and children: Report of the Ad Hoc Committee, American Thoracic Society. Am Rev Respir Dis 105:2, 1972.

Williams HE, Phelan PD: *Respiratory Illness in Children.* Blackwell, 1975.

13...

Cardiovascular Diseases

James J. Nora, MD, & Robert R. Wolfe, MD

Cardiovascular disease is a significant cause of mortality and chronic morbidity in the pediatric population of North America even though less than 1% of children die of cardiovascular disease (as compared with over 50% of adults). Furthermore, it is becoming obvious that the prevention of adult heart disease must begin in childhood (eg, prevention of atherosclerosis by dietary modification). Preventive medicine is the most important aspect of pediatric practice, and the goal of prevention pervades all aspects of cardiovascular disease. But prevention requires an understanding of the causes of disease, and in this there are wide discrepancies ranging from significant accomplishments in the case of rheumatic fever to the very tentative steps being taken to understand the causes of congenital heart disease, atherosclerosis, and essential hypertension.

This chapter will observe the convention of dividing heart disease into congenital and acquired categories. Congenital heart disease is more common in the USA than rheumatic heart disease and other acquired forms of heart disease. About 1% of American children are born with significant congenital heart lesions, and over half of these (17,000) per year will die before 1 year of age if they are not promptly diagnosed and adequately treated.

Although it is a worthwhile exercise in deductive reasoning for the primary · physician to attempt to reach an anatomic diagnosis in a given patient with congenital heart disease on the basis of the history, physical examination, x-ray, and ECG, the fundamental question must always be, *Is this important heart disease?* The precise anatomic definition of the heart lesion is the responsibility of the personnel at the pediatric cardiac center. The responsibility of the physician outside the center is the critical one of distinguishing those patients who require the specialized care offered at the pediatric center from those who have unimportant disease.

Rheumatic fever and rheumatic heart disease, while still very common in underdeveloped countries, have been essentially eradicated in Scandinavia and continue to diminish in importance in the USA and elsewhere in areas where living standards are high. In the cardiac centers, there are 50–100 children with congenital heart lesions for every child with rheumatic heart disease. In poor areas of the USA, rheumatic fever is encountered more frequently but not to the extent that it was found 3 decades ago.

Other acquired heart diseases of significance to the pediatric patient are viral myocarditis, infective endocarditis, and pericarditis.

CLUES TO THE PRESENCE OF HEART DISEASE

Although there are traditional signs and symptoms suggesting the presence of heart disease in an infant or child, it is necessary to know how to weigh clinical findings to determine what is important disease and what is not. The presence of a heart murmur may suggest the possibility of heart disease in an infant, but all serious cardiovascular disorders are not accompanied by an easily detectable murmur.

The most important clues to the presence of heart disease requiring prompt attention are congestive heart failure and cyanosis. These clinical conditions will be discussed in more detail in subsequent sections.

DIAGNOSTIC EVALUATION

As in the diagnosis of diseases of any other organ system, an orderly sequence of evaluation is followed: (1) history, (2) physical examination, (3) electrocardiogram, (4) chest x-ray, (5) other noninvasive laboratory studies, and (6) cardiac catheterization (with angiocardiography).

HISTORY

Problem Orientation

History-taking must of course be directed to specific entities under consideration. It would be as inappropriate to discuss joint symptoms in a 3-month-old cyanotic infant as it would be to ask about hypoxemic spells in an 8-year-old girl with swollen joints and a mitral murmur. Within the bounds of these obvious extremes, there are many aspects of history-taking that should be oriented toward specific problems under consideration, and the precision of the questions is directly related to the experience and depth of knowledge of the physician asking the questions.

Family History

Cardiovascular diseases are familial. The usual sequence of concern with diagnosis and treatment is very often followed by parental questions regarding cause and chance of recurrence. Meaningful answers to these questions require a careful family history and accurate and up-to-date information regarding the cause. Etiologic factors will be considered in a subsequent section.

Poor Feeding

Not every baby who feeds poorly has something wrong with his heart, but poor feeding is apt to be one thing the mother will recognize and call to the physician's attention. It is surprising how often an infant in severe congestive heart failure will come to a pediatric cardiologist with a history of several formula changes which were made because of failure of the physician to recognize the cardiac basis of the poor feeding. The mother may say that the baby takes an hour to consume an ounce of milk and appears "too tired to eat."

Tachypnea

Another abnormality that mothers frequently notice is rapid breathing. The physician may give unwarranted reassurance by saying that all babies breathe fast. However, infants at rest rarely breathe faster than 40 respirations per minute, whereas infants in congestive heart failure usually have respiratory rates in excess of 60 (and often 80–100). Tachypnea may be considered the cardinal sign of left-sided heart failure in the pediatric patient.

Cyanosis

The physiologic basis of cyanosis and the medical and surgical approaches to the cyanotic patient will be discussed later. What should be noted here is that, curiously, many mothers do not readily recognize cyanosis—nor do inexperienced physicians. The infant with a cyanotic heart lesion may be more gray than blue (and may have no heart murmur). Cyanotic heart disease may go unrecognized because of lack of appreciation of the subtleties of diagnosing cyanosis.

Hypoxemic Spells

It is important to determine if the patient with a cyanotic heart lesion such as tetralogy of Fallot is having hypoxemic spells, because prompt surgical intervention may be required. The usual history is that—on awakening in the morning, or after a feeding or bowel movement—the infant begins breathing fast, becomes progressively more gray or blue, and cries as if having severe pain. Such a spell may progress to unconsciousness, paresis, or even death.

Other Clinical Clues

Orthopnea, dyspnea, easy fatigability, growth failure, sweating, squatting, and pneumonia are frequent clues to the presence of various forms of heart disease.

PHYSICAL EXAMINATION

Examination of an infant or child with a possible diagnosis of cardiovascular disease requires a thorough evaluation of which examination of the heart is only one part. For example, looking at the whole patient and realizing that the heart murmur under consideration is present in a child with multiple stigmas of the Ullrich-Noonan syndrome provides the physician with a great deal of assistance in reaching the diagnosis of both the cardiac and the associated noncardiac disorders of the patient, as well as providing a firm basis for discussing prognosis, etiology, and recurrence risks. Subspeciality consultants should likewise participate in the overall assessment of the patient and should not focus on one organ system to the exclusion of all else.

The physical findings most relevant to the evaluation of cardiovascular disease will be reviewed below in the sequence recommended for infants and children, which differs from the traditional general physical and cardiovascular examination of the adult. The general examination of an adult might begin with the head, including otoscopic examination of the ears; and the protocol of cardiovascular examination of the adult might specify a blood pressure determination before auscultation. Such maneuvers make infants and children cry, and the auscultatory examination is greatly compromised by crying.

The first step in the cardiovascular examination of the infant and child is observation at a distance. Does the child look ill? Is he undersized? How fast is he breathing? Is he blue? The lips and other mucous membranes and nailbeds are blue in cyanosis of central origin. Blueness of the warm body parts contrasts with the blue discoloration of the arms, legs, and face due to cold and vascular instability which characterizes peripheral cyanosis.

The physician should then approach the child more closely, play with him, give him a stethoscope to hold and examine, etc, thus winning his confidence and allaying his fear.

The next step is prompt examination of the heart: palpation first—not only for the information to be obtained, but also to provide a fear-reducing sequence—and then auscultation very early in the examination before the patient becomes uncooperative through fear or fatigue.

1. CARDIAC EXAMINATION

Evidence of cardiac enlargement may be obtained by inspection and palpation of the precordium. Asymmetric prominence of the left anterior chest wall is usually indicative of cardiac enlargement secondary to congenital heart disease.

Right ventricular hypertrophy is characterized by a heaving pulsation at the lower left sternal border or the xiphoid process. Left ventricular hypertrophy is characterized by a thrusting impulse at the apex which is displaced downward and outward. Prominent pulsations both at the apex and at the xiphoid process suggest combined ventricular hypertrophy.

A thrill is a palpable murmur consisting of a high-frequency vibration felt by the hands or fingertips. It indicates the presence of a murmur of at least grade IV/VI intensity. Thrills are localized to the area at which the murmur is most intense. The location helps to define the type of congenital or acquired heart disease (second left interspace—pulmonary stenosis; fourth left interspace—ventricular septal defect; etc).

It is at times possible to palpate one or both of the heart sounds. This is frequently referred to as a shock. It is usually an abnormal finding and is often of diagnostic significance (eg, the presence of a palpable second heart sound at the pulmonary area is suggestive of increased pulmonary arterial pressure). However, normal heart sounds may occasionally be palpated through a very thin chest wall.

Percussion

Percussion of the cardiac borders is a gross method of determining heart size but does not differentiate between right or left ventricular hypertrophy. Percussion of the cardiac borders is useful in patients with generalized cardiac dilatation or with pericardial effusion.

Auscultation

A. Heart Sounds:

1. First heart sound (S_1)—The first heart sound is related to closure of the atrioventricular valves. In most cases the first sound seems on auscultation to be single, although there are 4 components which may be detected by phonocardiography.

2. Ejection click—Early systolic ejection clicks are related to dilated great vessels. Early clicks heard at the second left interspace are pulmonary in origin and are most often due to pulmonary stenosis. Early clicks which are best localized at the lower left sternal border and apex are frequently aortic and are commonly found in aortic stenosis and truncus arteriosus. Mid and late systolic clicks best heard at the apex or widely over the thorax are usually associated with prolapse of the mitral valve. Systolic clicks are also associated with spontaneous closure of ventricular septal defects.

3. Second heart sound (S_2)— The second heart sound may be regarded as the most important auscultatory finding in the examination of the heart of the infant and child. An abnormal second heart sound (eg, single, increased pulmonary component, widely and constantly split) may be the only clue to significant cardiovascular disease in a patient with little or no heart murmur. It is due to closure of the semilunar (aortic, pulmonary) valves. The intensity and the manner of splitting of S_2 are extremely important in the diagnosis of heart disease in the pediatric age group. Physiologic splitting consists of widening of the 2 components during inspiration and narrowing (almost complete closure) during expiration. During inspiration, there is a drop in intrathoracic pressure resulting in increased filling of the right side of the heart. This results in a prolonged ejection of blood from the right ventricle and delayed pulmonic closure. The effect of respiration on the filling of the left side of the heart from the pulmonary veins is minimal since both the pulmonary veins and the left atrium are located within the thoracic cavity. Actually, there is a slight decrease in the amount of blood filling the left atrium during inspiration due to dilatation of the pulmonary veins. Accordingly, wide splitting of the second heart sound occurs during inspiration. During expiration, the reverse is true, resulting in narrowing of the 2 components. The presence of the split is detected best at the second intercostal space at the left sternal border in normal patients. The 2 components are usually of equal intensity in the pediatric age group.

4. Third heart sound (S_3)—This is due to the rapid filling of the left ventricle during early diastole. It occurs shortly (0.12–0.16 second) after S_2. It is common in infants and children and is best heard at the apex.

5. Fourth heart sound (S_4)—This sound is due to contraction of either atrium; accordingly, if present, it is heard shortly before the first heart sound. It is occasionally audible in patients with congenital heart disease associated with increased pressure within either atrium.

B. Murmurs: Every child has a heart murmur if one listens carefully under appropriate conditions. Since only one child in 100 has a congenital cardiovascular malformation and perhaps only 3 per 1000 have rheumatic heart lesions, murmurs must be put in the context that almost all are innocent. What is important is the discrimination between the innocent (or functional) murmur and the organic murmur. The "three Ps" are a convenient mnemonic device in distinguishing innocent from organic murmurs: perspective, persistence, and pigeonhole. (1) The murmur must be put into the *perspective* of the patient's overall state of health and other physical findings. (2) The innocent murmur changes or disappears much more readily with changes of position and manipulation than the organic murmur (*persistence*). (3) Each innocent murmur and each organic murmur has characteristics which make it clearly recognizable (and allows it to be placed in its appropriate *pigeonhole*).

The following characteristics of murmurs should be noted: (1) timing in relationship to the cardiac cycle (systolic, diastolic, or continuous); (2) duration;

(3) intensity, on a scale of I–VI/VI; (4) quality (blowing, harsh, rough, musical, etc); (5) area of greatest intensity; and (6) transmission (localized, widely transmitted, etc).

There are 5 types of innocent murmur:

(1) Still's murmur, a vibratory grade I–III/VI systolic murmur, best heard at the third left interspace in a line from the sternal border to the apex. This musical, groaning murmur usually disappears with the Valsalva maneuver.

(2) Functional pulmonary ejection murmur. This grade II/VI systolic murmur may be heard at the pulmonary area in the supine position. It usually disappears when the patient is upright and does not radiate to the back.

(3) Venous hum. In the sitting position, this is a grade II/VI, medium-pitched, slightly humming systolic/diastolic murmur, obliterated by digital pressure over the jugular veins or by turning the head or lying down.

(4) Carotid bruit. This ejection murmur, which should be very rarely diagnosed, originates in a carotid artery and is loudest in that location but may be referred to the base of the heart.

(5) Pericardial-pleural murmur. This is a rub-like grade III–VI/VI murmur, usually systolic, best heard at the apex or the lower left sternal border. It varies significantly with respiration and is usually secondary to a pleuro-pericardial adhesion.

Two murmurs which may be of little hemodynamic consequence to the pediatric patient are as follows:

(6) Pulmonary branch stenosis murmur of infancy. This murmur is typically heard from 2 weeks to 6 months of age and is caused by a relative and transient disparity between the size of the peripheral pulmonary arteries and the amount of blood flow they must accommodate. The grade I–II/VI systolic ejection murmurs are heard all over the chest, front, and back and in both axillas. If a murmur of this type is heard as well in the right axilla as at the base and disappears in a few months, innocent pulmonary artery branch stenosis is the likely diagnosis. In a 1-year survey of 7000 newborns, the authors found 3 times as many murmurs of innocent pulmonary artery branch stenosis as all other murmurs combined. Significant pulmonary artery branch stenosis is another disorder, and of course the murmurs persist beyond early infancy.

(7) Mitral dysfunction. The late systolic murmur at the apex initiated by a click is commonly of no hemodynamic consequence to the infant and young child, except those with connective tissue disorders such as Marfan's syndrome. It assumes greater importance in the older child and adult. Auscultatory or echocardiographic evidence of mitral valve prolapse is present in a significant proportion of preadolescent girls (up to 10%). They commonly have a slender body habitus and associated bony abnormalities of the chest. Significant problems are infrequent in such individuals, but dysrhythmias and angina may be bothersome. A click alone is not considered to be an absolute indication for subacute infective endocarditis prophylaxis. Evidence of mitral insufficiency is required.

Organic murmurs are discussed under the headings of specific cardiovascular lesions in the sections that follow.

2. NONCARDIAC EXAMINATION

Observation of the rate and depth of respiration is part of the general observation of the patient (see above). Our practice in Denver is to follow auscultation of the lungs with auscultation of the heart. Rales are of serious import in an infant with congestive heart failure and may be taken as being tantamount to pulmonary edema.

Femoral Pulse

Assessment of the femoral pulse is an essential part of the physical examination of every infant and child. The femoral pulse should be readily palpable and equal in amplitude and time of appearance with the brachial pulse. A femoral pulse that is absent or weak or one that is delayed in comparison with the brachial pulse suggests coarctation of the aorta. An absent or diminished femoral pulse may be the only clue to the etiology of a life-threatening problem.

General Comments on Arterial Pulse

A. Rate and Rhythm: Cardiac rate and rhythm are usually determined by palpation of the radial or brachial pulse. Throughout infancy and childhood, the rate is subject to great variation. Multiple determinations must be made under properly evaluated conditions before conclusions can be drawn about their significance. This is particularly important in infancy.

Marked variations in heart rate occur with activity; therefore, the resting heart rate may be most accurately determined during sleep. In older children, exercise and emotional factors have a marked effect upon the heart rate. This should be taken into account when examining the child, since many children are apprehensive and may react emotionally to the initial phases of the examination. It is possible for normal infants to have heart rates of 180 or 190 during the activity associated with a physical or electrocardiographic examination. Average resting heart rates range from 120 in infants to 80 in older children.

In the pediatric age group, the rhythm may be regular or there may be a phasic variation in the heart rate (sinus arrhythmia). Variations occasionally occur without relation to the respiratory cycle. Sinus arrhythmia is a normal finding.

B. Quality and Amplitude of Pulse: Examination of the cardiovascular system should always include a careful examination and comparison of the pulses of the upper and lower extremities. A bounding pulse is characteristic of patent ductus arteriosus or aortic regurgitation. Narrow or thready pulses are found in patients with congestive heart failure or severe aortic stenosis.

Examination of the suprasternal notch should always be included. A visible pulsation in the suprasternal notch is usually abnormal, although it may be seen in patients who are emotionally excited. A prominent pulsation is found in aortic insufficiency, patent ductus arteriosus, and coarctation of the aorta. A palpable thrill in the suprasternal notch is characteristic of aortic stenosis, valvular pulmonary stenosis, and occasionally coarctation of the aorta and patent ductus arteriosus.

Arterial Blood Pressure

Blood pressures should be obtained in the upper and lower extremities. Systolic pressure in the lower extremities determined by the auscultatory technic is usually higher than that found in the upper extremities in patients *over 1 year of age.* In normal infants, the pressure in the arms may be higher. The cuff must cover the same relative area of the arm and leg, and this usually means that a larger cuff must be used for the leg than for the arm.

A. Procedures: Because of variation of blood pressure with respiration and slower rhythmic variations (Mayer or Traube-Hering waves), pressure obtained by any method should be repeated several times.

1. Auscultatory method—The auditory recognition of Korotkoff sounds utilizing a stethoscope and sphygmomanometer is the most commonly used method of obtaining blood pressure in children and correlates well with direct intra-arterial measurements. However, despite its widespread application as the standard method of indirect blood pressure measurement, many factors grossly affect its accuracy. Among these are the dimensions of the inflatable bag within the cuff. The length of the bag should be 50–100% of the circumference of the limb, and the width should be 50% of the member circumference. A cuff that is too narrow or too short will produce a blood pressure reading that is higher than the true pressure.

2. Palpatory method—Because the application of a stethoscope head to a small limb is often awkward or impossible, palpation of the pulse characteristics distal to the occluding cuff provides an approximation of the systolic blood pressure in the infant.

3. Flush method—The flush method is also useful in small infants. Using the foot or hand, the distal extremity is blanched by manual squeezing or application of an elastic bandage and the cuff is inflated above the systolic pressure. The member is then observed as the cuff pressure is slowly reduced and the observed flush corresponds to a value approximating that of the systolic pressure. Simultaneous application of the cuffs to the upper and lower extremities and observation of flushing is a useful technic for assessing coarctation of the aorta.

4. Doppler ultrasonic method—Most recently, the combination of a small ultrasound transducer with earphones and a sphygmomanometer has proved to be especially applicable to the small infant. Considerations of cuff dimensions are still critical, however.

B. Pulse Pressure: Pulse pressure is determined by subtracting the diastolic pressure from the systolic pressure. Normally, the pulse pressure is less than 50 mm Hg or less than half the systolic pressure. A widened pulse pressure (which is associated with a bounding pulse) is present in aortico-pulmonary shunt (eg, patent ductus arteriosus), aortic insufficiency, fever, anemia, and complete heart block. A narrow pulse pressure is seen in congestive heart failure, severe aortic stenosis, and pericardial tamponade.

Venous Pressure & Pulse

The level of the distended jugular vein above the suprasternal notch when the patient is at a 45 degree angle is a determinant of venous pressure in older children and adults. Normally, one may observe the level of the transition between collapse and distention of the jugular vein approximately 1–2 cm above the notch. Because of the short, fat neck in infants and young children, this is frequently not too helpful in this age group. In addition to the level of the pulse, the wave pattern should be observed. Two waves can frequently be seen: (1) The *a* wave, due to right atrial contraction, is a rather sharply rising wave and therefore occurs immediately before or with the first heart sound or point of maximum impulse (PMI). (2) The *v* wave, caused by filling of the right atrium during ventricular systole, is a more slowly rising wave and occurs toward the end of ventricular systole.

Extremities

Cyanosis of the extremities usually indicates congenital heart disease, but severe pulmonary disease must be excluded. Cyanosis is characterized by a bluish discoloration of the nails, but the entire distal portion of the extremity may be involved.

A. Clubbing of Fingers and Toes: Clubbing implies fairly severe cyanotic congenital heart disease. It usually does not appear until approximately age 1, although occasionally, in patients with severe cyanosis, it may occur earlier. The first sign of clubbing is softening of the nail beds. This is followed by rounding of the fingernails and then by thickening and shininess of the terminal phalanx, with loss of creases.

Cyanosis is by far the most common cause, but clubbing occurs also in patients with subacute bacterial endocarditis, severe liver disease, and lung abscess.

B. Edema: Edema of the lower extremities is characteristic of right ventricular heart failure in older children and adults. However, in infants and younger children, peripheral edema is more likely to affect first the face and then the presacral region and eventually the extremities.

Abdomen

Hepatomegaly is the cardinal sign of right heart failure in the infant and child. Presystolic pulsation of the liver may occur with right atrial hypertension and systolic pulsation with tricuspid insufficiency. Congestive splenomegaly may be present in patients who have had long-standing congestive heart failure. Enlargement of the spleen is one of the characteristic features of subacute bacterial endocarditis. Ascites is occasionally present in right heart failure.

Dunkle LM, Rowe RD: Transient murmur simulating pulmonary artery stenosis in premature infants. Am J Dis Child 124:666, 1972.

Markiewicz W & others: Mitral valve prolapse in one hundred presumably healthy young females. Circulation 53:464, 1976.

Park MK, Guntheroth WG: Direct blood pressure measurement in brachial-femoral arteries in children. Circulation 41:231, 1970.

Steinfeld L, Alexander H, Cohen ML: Updating sphygmomanometry. Am J Cardiol 33:107, 1974.

Whyte RK & others: Assessment of Doppler ultrasound to measure systolic and diastolic blood pressures in infants and young children. Arch Dis Child 50:542, 1975.

The Electrocardiogram (ECG) & Vectorcardiogram (VCG)

Certainly the ECG is to be considered an essential part of the evaluation of the cardiovascular system, and frequently the information gained from this study is very useful. The ECG is the sine qua non for the diagnosis of arrhythmias and may offer the best clue to the specific diagnosis of congenital lesions (eg, left axis deviation in a blue baby suggesting tricuspid atresia). Conversely, the ECG may provide disappointingly little or no help (as in assessing right ventricular hypertrophy in the newborn or left ventricular hypertrophy in the child with congenital aortic stenosis).

It is not possible, within the limitations of this presentation, to teach the interpretation of the ECG, but a few basic facts and definitions should help to orient the student:

A. Propagation of Electrical Force: As shown in Fig 13–1, a wave of electrical force traveling toward an electrode inscribes a positive (upright) deflection; away from an electrode, a negative deflection; and perpendicular to an electrode, a low-voltage, isodipha-

sic complex. These forces are inscribed as loops on the vectorcardiogram (VCG), and abnormalities are manifested as alterations in direction and duration of force or as increased or decreased electrical force (amplitude of QRS complex on ECG or loop on VCG).

B. Age-Related Variations: The ECG and VCG evolve with the age of the patient. The rate gradually decreases and intervals generally increase with age. There is also progressive change in dominance of ventricles from right ventricular dominance in the young infant to left ventricular dominance in the older infant, child, and adult. The normal ECG of the 1-week-old would be highly abnormal for a 1-year-old, and the ECG of a 5-year-old would not be normal for an adult.

C. ECG Interpretation: Fig 13–2 defines the events recorded on the ECG. The sequence of recording the findings of the ECG is usually as follows: rate, rhythm, P wave, P–R interval, QRS complex (including axis, amplitude, and duration), Q–T interval, ST segment, T wave, and impression.

1. Rate—The paper speed at which ECGs are usually taken is 25 mm/second. Each small square is 1 mm and each large square 5 mm. Therefore, 5 large squares represent 1 second, one large square 0.2 second, and 1 small square 0.04 second. A common method of estimating the ventricular rate is to count the number of large squares between 2 QRS complexes: If QRS complexes appear at a rate of one per large square (5 per second), the ventricular rate would be 300; if QRS complexes appear every 2 squares, the ventricular rate is 150, etc. The formula is to divide the number of large squares between QRS complexes into 300 and roughly interpolate for fractions of large squares.

2. Rhythm—Cardiac rhythm is a difficult subject that does not yield easily to oversimplification. However, a working definition of normal sinus rhythm must be offered even if it is not entirely satisfactory: a normal P wave followed by a normal P–R interval and a normal QRS complex.

3. P wave—The P wave represents atrial depolarization. In the pediatric patient it is normally not taller than 2.5 mm nor more than 0.08 second in duration.

4. P–R interval—This interval is measured from the beginning of the P wave to the beginning of the QRS complex. It increases with age and with slower rates. The P–R interval ranges from a minimum of 0.11 in infants to a maximum of 0.18 in older children with slow rates. The P–R interval is commonly prolonged in rheumatic heart disease and by digitalis.

5. QRS complex—This represents ventricular depolarization, and its amplitude and direction of force (axis) reveal the relative size of (viable) ventricular mass in hypertrophy, hypoplasia, and infarction. Abnormal ventricular conduction (eg, right bundle branch block, anterior fascicular block) is also revealed. Interpretation of the QRS complex is one of the most important aspects of cardiologic diagnosis.

6. Q–T interval—This interval is measured from the beginning of the QRS complex to the end of the T wave. The Q–T duration is affected by drugs like digitalis and electrolyte imbalances such as hypocalcemia

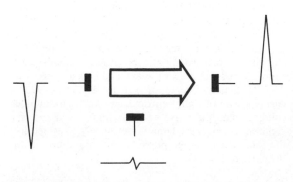

Figure 13–1. Depolarization of the myocardium. The arrow represents the wave of electrical force. As it travels toward the electrode, it inscribes a positive (upward) deflection; away from the electrode, a negative (downward) deflection; perpendicular to the electrode, a low-voltage, isodiphasic deflection.

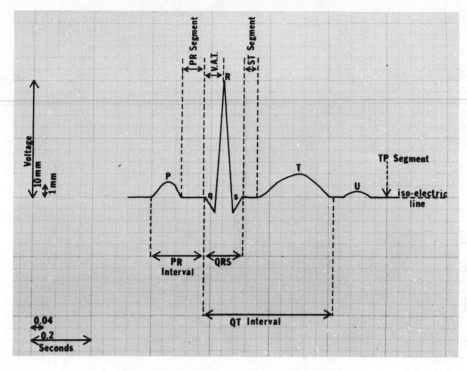

Figure 13—2. Complexes and intervals of the ECG.

and hypokalemia (really Q–U interval prolongation). The normal duration is rate-related.

7. ST segment—This short segment lying between the end of the QRS complex and the beginning of the T wave is affected by drugs and electrolyte imbalances and reflects myocardial injury.

8. T wave—The T wave represents myocardial repolarization and is altered by electrolytes, myocardial hypertrophy, and ischemia.

9. Impression—The ultimate impression of the ECG is derived from a systematic analysis of features such as those described above as compared with expected normal values for the age of the child.

D. Vectorcardiogram: The VCG reveals much of the same information as the ECG. In fact, it is possible to draw the QRS loop of the VCG with considerable accuracy from QRS complexes of the ECG. Fig 13–3 displays the ECG and VCG of the same patient. The vector interpretation of the ECG (eg, direction and shape of loop) derived by looking at the ECG is perhaps the major contribution of vectorcardiography. It is usually not necessary to obtain an actual VCG to know what the loops look like.

Ainger LE, Dixon PR: QRS spatial curves in infants. Maturational changes from birth to 4 months of age: Influence of sample size on curve contours. Am J Cardiol 29:699, 1972.

Goldman MJ: *Principles of Clinical Electrocardiography*, 9th ed. Lange, 1976.

Hastreiter AR, Abella JB: The ECG in the newborn period. (2 parts.) J Pediatr 78:146, 346, 1971.

CHEST X-RAY

Attention is directed to enlargement of the cardiac chambers and great vessels of the heart and to the vascular markings of the lungs (increased, normal, or decreased). Expert technic and interpretation are required to avoid diagnostic error. An expiratory film can make the cardiothymic silhouette look greatly enlarged in an infant, and even in a child cardiomegaly may be diagnosed where there is none because the films are not obtained on adequate inspiration. Assessment of vascular markings is subjective to begin with and also depends on technic: films that are too light may lead to overreading of vascularity, and films that are too dark may obscure increased vascularity. Some conditions—eg, tetralogy of Fallot at the stage of only mild hypoxemia—may present with chest x-rays that appear to be completely normal.

The most informative roentgenographic studies in the investigation of cardiovascular disease include posteroanterior, lateral, and right and left oblique views of the chest with barium swallow. Fig 13–4 reveals the location of the cardiovascular and adjacent structures in these 4 views.

Elliot LP, Schiebler GL: A roentgenologic-electrocardiographic approach to cyanotic forms of heart disease. Pediatr Clin North Am 18:1133, 1971.

Wesenberg RL: *The Newborn Chest.* Harper & Row, 1973.

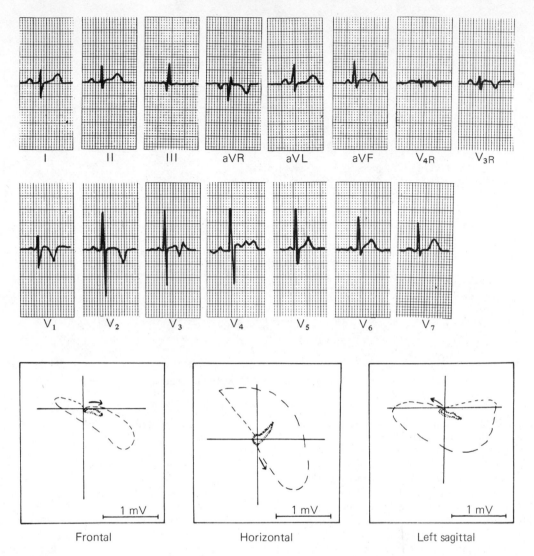

Figure 13—3. ECG and VCG of same 10-month-old infant. The direction, duration, and magnitude of electrical force are comparable in each tracing.

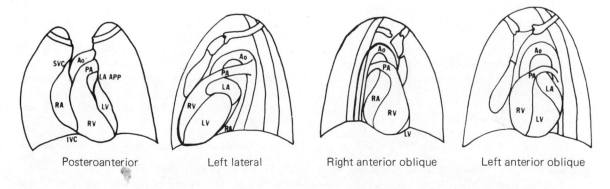

Figure 13—4. Position of cardiovascular structures in principal x-ray views. RA = right atrium; RV = right ventricle; LA = left atrium; LA APP = left atrial appendage; LV = left ventricle; AO = aorta; PA = pulmonary artery.

ECHOCARDIOGRAPHY

In recent years, echocardiography has come to play a role as essential as electrocardiography and roentgenography in the noninvasive diagnosis of pediatric cardiovascular disease. This technic reveals the sort of information regarding chamber size, anatomic relationships of great vessels and valves, valve motion, wall and septal thickness, and myocardial performance that was previously only available by cardiac catheterization. Fig 13–5 is a representative echocardiogram, but the details of interpretation exceed the limits of this presentation.

Feigenbaum H: *Echocardiography*. Lea & Febiger, 1976.

Goldberg SJ, Allen HD, Sahn DJ: *Pediatric and Adolescent Echocardiography*. Year Book, 1975.

Silverman NH: Newer noninvasive methods in pediatric cardiology: Echocardiography, isotope angiography. Adv Pediatr 23:357, 1976.

OTHER NONINVASIVE LABORATORY STUDIES

A number of other laboratory studies which provide diagnostic information will be enumerated, and 2 will be presented in a little more detail.

Complete blood count and urinalysis are routine in almost all medical evaluations. Erythrocyte sedimentation rate, C-reactive protein, and ASO titer and other evidence of streptococcal infection are important in the evaluation of rheumatic fever. Circulation time and

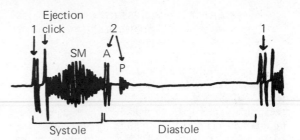

Figure 13–6. Phonocardiographic tracing showing acoustic findings in pulmonary stenosis. 1 = first heart sound; SM = systolic murmur; 2 = second heart sound; A = aortic component; P = pulmonic component.

venous pressure are now seldom performed on pediatric patients in most centers. Arterial pulse curves are of some value as a teaching aid.

Phonocardiography is also very useful as a teaching aid because it correlates visual and acoustic events. Fig 13–6 shows the acoustic findings of pulmonary stenosis: normal first sound, ejection click, "diamond-shaped" murmur, and widely split second sound with diminished pulmonary component. Terms like "diamond-shaped" murmur have entered the vocabulary by way of phonocardiography.

Arterial P_{O_2} or systemic O_2 saturation. Because cyanosis is difficult to quantitate (and sometimes to recognize) by inspection of the patient, objective laboratory determinations are required. The quantitative response of arterial P_{O_2} or O_2 saturation (eg, by earpiece oximetry) to administration of 100% oxygen is one of the most useful methods of distinguishing cyanosis produced by heart disease from cyanosis related to lung disease in sick infants. In cyanotic heart disease, Pa_{O_2} increases very little from values obtained while breathing ambient room air as compared with values during 100% oxygen administration. However, there is usually a very significant increase in Pa_{O_2} when oxygen is administered to a patient with lung disease. (An exception is noted in infants moribund with lung disease, and even in these cases administration of oxygen under intubation and assisted respiration will usually produce an increase in Pa_{O_2} significant enough to make a distinction between heart disease and lung disease.) Table 13–1 illustrates the sort of response one might expect following at least 10 minutes of 100% oxygen administration to cyanotic infants with heart disease versus lung disease.

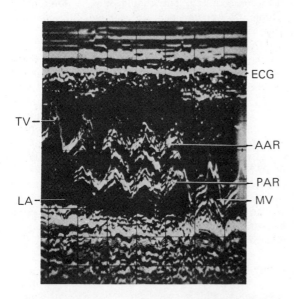

Figure 13–5. Newborn echocardiogram showing normal cardiac dimensions and anatomic relations. TV = tricuspid valve; LA = left atrium; ECG = electrocardiogram; AAR = anterior aortic root; PAR = posterior aortic root; MV = mitral valve.

Table 13–1. Examples of responses to 10 minutes of 100% oxygen in lung disease and heart disease.

	Lung Disease		**Heart Disease**	
	Room Air	100% O_2	Room Air	100% O_2
Color	Blue → Pink		Blue → Blue	
Oximetry	60% → 99%		60% → 62%	
Pa_{O_2} (mm Hg)	35 → 120		35 → 38	

CARDIAC CATHETERIZATION & ANGIOCARDIOGRAPHY

The definitive anatomic and physiologic study of infants and children with heart disease is cardiac catheterization. As stated earlier, the essential decision for the primary physician to make is to distinguish those infants and children who require the specialized diagnostic and therapeutic facilities of the pediatric cardiac center from those who may be safely managed without such facilities and consultation. The consulting pediatric cardiologist on the basis of the preceding steps of diagnostic evaluation—history, physical examination, ECG, chest x-ray, and other noninvasive laboratory studies—has a rather precise assessment of the anatomic and physiologic abnormalities in simple malformations and considerable useful information about complex malformations.

However, we personally regard it as potentially dangerous to manage sick infants and children with congenital heart diseases on the basis of physical findings and other ancillary studies rather than cardiac catheterization when this definitive study provides the requisite information for truly knowledgeable management. Cardiac catheterization in the hands of pediatric cardiologists working in laboratories fulfilling the American Heart Association standards for laboratories undertaking catheterization of infants and children is a low-risk procedure, the only significant risk being in moribund infants. Cardiac catheterization by cardiologists not having adequate training and continuing experience with infants and children and working in laboratories not completely attuned to the needs of pediatric patients is a high-risk procedure and difficult to justify.

Indications & Objectives

A. Infants:

1. Indications—

a. All infants with cyanosis presumed to be cardiovascular in origin should be catheterized as soon as a reasonably stable clinical condition can be achieved—not only for diagnosis of the anatomic and physiologic abnormality but also for possibly lifesaving procedures such as the Rashkind balloon septostomy (which takes place in the cardiac catheterization laboratory).

b. Infants in severe congestive heart failure that does not respond promptly and satisfactorily to anticongestive measures.

c. Infants in whom early operation for congenital heart disease is contemplated.

d. Infants in whom the anatomic and physiologic abnormality is sufficiently vague that appropriate medical management is not possible.

e. Infants who have evidence of complicating or potentially progressive problems, such as pulmonary hypertension and moderate to severe aortic stenosis, which will require precise longitudinal physiologic data.

2. Objectives—(In descending order of importance.)

a. To perform the study with the lowest possible morbidity and mortality. This requires pediatric cardiologists and pediatric cardiac catheterization laboratories with experience in studying infants—to gain meaningful information promptly; to care for the critically ill infant with temperature and pH control, fluid management, and all essential pediatric treatment; and to anticipate and handle life-threatening crises.

b. To gain information not available by other methods which will provide the basis for meaningful therapeutic decisions (medical or surgical).

c. Therapeutic intervention (eg, Rashkind septostomy).

d. To obtain sufficient physiologic and anatomic data so that repeat catheterization to complete the study will not be necessary.

B. Children:

1. Indications—

a. All children for whom heart surgery is contemplated (with the occasional exception of children with unequivocal patent ductus arteriosus and no evidence of an associated cardiovascular problem).

b. All children in whom there is question about the anatomic or physiologic abnormality which would significantly influence management and which cannot be completely answered by noninvasive methods.

c. Children with progressive lesions which require careful physiologic monitoring (such as aortic stenosis and pulmonary hypertension).

d. Children who have had cardiovascular surgery and require assessment of the adequacy of the repair.

e. Children with mild to moderate cardiovascular lesions when important information about the natural history is required. This should only be done in the setting of a well-designed protocol and fully informed consent.

2. Objectives—It goes without saying that conducting the study with the lowest possible risk is the most important objective of cardiac catheterization of the child as well as the infant; and the risk to the child ($< 0.2\%$) is certainly much less than to the sick infant (2%). Therapy is not an objective of catheterization of the child, as it frequently is in the infant. Complete anatomic and physiologic data are more important objectives of catheterization in children than in infants. No physician or laboratory should undertake the catheterization of a child unless prepared to obtain a completely informative study and unless physicians and surgeons are available who are capable of proceeding with whatever medical or surgical therapy may be indicated.

Contraindications

Cardiac catheterization is contraindicated in infants and children who present with no clinical urgency and none of the indications listed above. It should not be done if personnel and facilities fail to meet high standards of patient safety and clinical diagnostic and therapeutic expertise.

Cardiac Catheterization Data

Fig 13–7 shows oxygen saturation (in percent) and pressure (in mm Hg) values obtained at cardiac catheterization from the chambers and great arteries of the heart. These values would be within the normal range for a child.

A. Oxygen Content and Saturation; Pulmonary and Systemic Blood Flow (Cardiac Output): In most laboratories, evidence of left-to-right shunt is determined by changes of blood oxygen content or saturation during passage of the catheter through the right side of the heart. A significant increase in oxygen content or oxygen saturation from one chamber to another indicates the presence of a left-to-right shunt at the site of the increase. The oxygen saturation of the peripheral arterial blood should always be determined during cardiac catheterization. Normal arterial oxygen saturation is 91–97%. A decrease (at sea level) below 91% suggests the presence of a right-to-left shunt, underventilation, or pulmonary disease.

The size of a left-to-right shunt is usually expressed as a ratio of the pulmonary to systemic blood flow or as liters per minute as determined by the Fick principle:

$$\frac{\text{Cardiac output}}{\text{(liters/minute)}} = \frac{\text{Oxygen consumption (ml/minute)}}{\text{Arteriovenous difference (ml/liter)}}$$

B. Pressures: Pressures should be determined in all chambers and vessels entered. Pressures should always be recorded when a catheter is pulled back from a distal chamber or vessel into a more proximal chamber. It is not normal for systolic pressure in the ventricles to exceed systolic pressure in the great arteries or mean diastolic pressure in the atria to exceed end-diastolic pressure in the ventricles. If a "gradient" in pressure does exist, it means that there is obstruction, and the severity of the gradient is one criterion for the necessity of operative repair. A right ventricular systolic pressure of 100 mm Hg and a pulmonary artery systolic pressure of 20 mm Hg yields a gradient of 80 mm Hg. Such a patient would be classified as having severe pulmonary stenosis requiring repair.

C. Pulmonary and Systemic Vascular Resistance: The vascular resistance is calculated from the following formula and reported in units or in dynes-sec-cm^{-5}-m^2

$$\text{Resistance} = \frac{\text{Pressure}}{\text{Flow}}$$

Pulmonary vascular resistance equals mean pulmonary artery pressure divided by pulmonary blood flow per square meter of body surface area. (Pulmonary blood flow determined from the Fick principle, as noted previously.) *Systemic vascular resistance* equals mean systemic arterial pressure divided by systemic blood flow.

Normally, the pulmonary vascular resistance ranges from 1–3 units or 80–240 dynes. If pulmonary resistance is above 10 units or the pulmonary/systemic resistance ratio is above 0.7, all other diagnostic findings should be reviewed carefully to confirm the presence of pulmonary hypertension that is so severe as to render the patient inoperable.

D. Special Technics: Special technics are frequently employed during the course of cardiac catheterization. These include the following:

1. The hydrogen electrode catheter–Used to determine the presence of very small left-to-right shunts. This technic enables the operator to detect such shunts even in the absence of any increase in oxygen saturation.

2. Indicator dilution curves–This involves injection of an indicator, such as indocyanine green (Cardio-Green), at specific places in the heart and detection of the dye downstream, usually in a peripheral artery. This technic permits the detection of both right-to-left and left-to-right shunts at the specific points within the cardiovascular system. Cardiac output is frequently determined by this method.

3. Selective angiocardiography and cineangiocardiography–In this technic, contrast material is injected in a specific chamber or vessel and the course of the contrast material followed by serial large film x-rays (angiocardiography) or by motion pictures (cineangiocardiography).

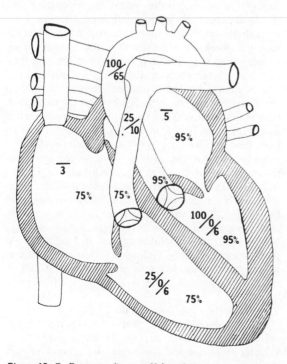

Figure 13–7. Pressures (in mm Hg) and oxygen saturation (in percent) obtained by cardiac catheterization in a normal child. $\overline{3}$ = mean pressure of 3 mm Hg in right atrium; $\overline{5}$ = mean pressure of 5 mm Hg in left atrium.

Ad Hoc Committee of the Committee on Congenital Cardiac Defects: Standards for a cardiac catheterization laboratory. A guide for cardiologists and for institutions sponsoring cardiac catheterization laboratories. America Heart Association, 1970; and Circulation 42:557, 1970.

Geypes MT, Vincent WR: *Cardiac Catheterization and Angio-cardiography in Severe Neonatal Heart Disease.* Thomas, 1974.

Stanger P & others: Complications of cardiac catheterization of neonates, infants, and children: A three year study. Circulation 50:595, 1974.

White RI: *Fundamentals of Vascular Radiology.* Lea & Febiger, 1976.

PRENATAL & NEONATAL CIRCULATION

Fetal Circulation

In the fetus, the placenta serves as the organ of respiration and for exchange of waste products for nutritive material. Oxygenated blood (80% saturated) passes from the placenta through the umbilical vein to the heart. As it flows toward the heart, it mixes with blood from the inferior vena cava and from the portal vein so that blood entering the right atrium is approximately 65% saturated. A considerable amount of this blood is shunted immediately across the foramen ovale into the left atrium. The venous blood derived from the upper part of the body is much less saturated (approximately 30%), and most of it enters the right ventricle through the tricuspid valve. Thus, the blood in the right ventricle is a mixture of both relatively highly saturated blood from the umbilical vein and desaturated blood from the venae cavae. This mixture results in a blood oxygen saturation of approximately 50% in the right ventricle.

The blood in the left atrium is derived from the blood shunting across the foramen ovale and the blood returning from the pulmonary veins. A great deal of the left ventricular output goes to the head, whereas the lower portion of the body is supplied by blood both from the right ventricle, through the patent ductus arteriosus, and from the left ventricle.

Physiologic Changes at Birth & in the Neonatal Period

At birth, 2 dramatic events occur as far as the cardiovascular-pulmonary system is concerned: (1) The umbilical cord is clamped, removing the placenta from the circulation, and (2) breathing commences. As a result, marked changes in the circulation occur. During fetal life, the placenta offers little resistance to the flow of blood so that the systemic circuit is a low-resistance one. On the other hand, the pulmonary arterioles are markedly constricted and offer strong resistance to the flow of blood into the lung. Clamping the cord causes a sudden increase in resistance to flow in the systemic circuit. As the lung becomes the organ of respiration, the oxygen tension (P_{O_2}) increases in the vicinity of the small pulmonary arterioles, resulting in a release of the constriction and thus a significant decrease in the pulmonary arteriolar resistance. Indeed,

shortly after birth the pulmonary vascular resistance is less than that of the systemic circuit.

Because of the changes in resistance, the great majority of the right ventricular outflow now passes into the lung rather than through the ductus arteriosus into the descending aorta. In fact, functional closure of the ductus arteriosus begins to develop shortly after birth. Recent studies have demonstrated that the ductus arteriosus remains patent for a variable period, usually 24–48 hours. During the first hour after birth, there is a small right-to-left shunt (as in the fetus). However, after 1 hour, bidirectional shunting occurs, with the left-to-right direction predominating. In most cases, right-to-left shunting completely disappears by 8 hours. However, in patients with severe hypoxia (in respiratory distress syndrome), the pulmonary vascular resistance remains quite elevated, resulting in a continued right-to-left shunt. The cause of the functional closure of the ductus arteriosus is not completely known. However, recent evidence indicates that the increased P_{O_2} of the arterial blood causes spasm of the ductus. Anatomically, however, the ductus arteriosus does not close until approximately 3 months of age.

In fetal life, the foramen ovale serves as a one-way valve, permitting shunting of blood from the inferior vena cava through the right atrium into the left atrium. At birth, because of the changes in the pulmonary and systemic vascular resistance and the increase in the quantity of blood returning from the pulmonary veins to the left atrium, the left atrial pressure rises above that of the right atrium. This functionally closes the flap of the one-way valve, essentially preventing flow of blood across the septum. It has been shown, however, that a small right-to-left shunt does continue for the first week of life. Although the foramen ovale remains functionally closed throughout life, the foramen ovale remains patent in about 25% of patients.

A clinical syndrome has been recognized which is characterized in term infants by onset of tachypnea, cyanosis, and clinical evidence of pulmonary hypertension during the first 8 hours after delivery. These infants have massive right to left ductal shunting for 3–7 days because of the high pulmonary vascular resistance. The clinical course is generally one of progressive cor pulmonale, hypoxemia, and acidosis, terminating in early death unless the pulmonary resistance can be lowered. The resistance can usually be reversed by instituting appropriate means to increase alveolar P_{O_2} or by intravenous administration of tolazoline. At postmortem, the only findings are increased thickness of the pulmonary arteriolar media which is felt to represent persistence of the fetal circulation (PFC).

Changes in the First Year of Life

The most significant changes occur at birth and within the neonatal period. However, pulmonary vascular resistance and the pulmonary arterial pressure continue to fall during the first year of life. This results from the involution of the pulmonary arteriole from a relatively thick-walled, small-lumen vessel to a thin-walled, large-lumen vessel. Adult levels of resistance and pressure are usually achieved by 6 months to 1 year of age.

Levin DL & others: Persistence of the fetal cardiopulmonary circulatory pathway. Pediatrics 56:58, 1975.

Rudolph AM: The changes in the circulation after birth: Their importance in congenital heart disease. Circulation 41:343, 1970.

MAJOR CLUES TO HEART DISEASE IN INFANTS & CHILDREN

1. CONGESTIVE HEART FAILURE

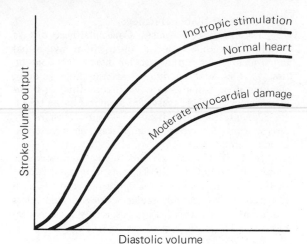

Figure 13–8. Ventricular performance curves.

There are many levels of definition of congestive heart failure. At the clinical level, a simple definition is failure of the heart to meet the circulatory and metabolic needs of the body. Congestive heart failure is one of the 2 major clues to the presence of important heart disease.* It has been estimated that congestive heart failure begins before 1 year of age in over 90% of infants and children who ever develop the disorder in the pediatric age period—and most of these patients are less than 6 months of age.

Congestive heart failure beginning in infancy may persist throughout childhood until operation relieves the underlying malformation (unless surgery is not possible). Other infants with moderately severe heart failure in the first few months of life may gradually compensate (for a variety of reasons) and not require digitalis after age 12 or 18 months even though their congenital heart lesions are still unrepaired.

Clinical Findings

The symptoms and signs of congestive heart failure have been discussed in the preceding sections on history and physical examination. Certain findings will be reviewed again here for purposes of emphasis and organization:

It may be said that the 3 cardinal signs of congestive heart failure in the pediatric patient are cardiomegaly (the sine qua non), tachypnea (left side), and hepatomegaly (right side).

Cardiomegaly represents a homeostatic (compensatory) mechanism which maintains adequate cardiac output by enlarging the capacity of the pump. This mechanism is frequently referred to as Starling's law of the heart. Up to a point, the enlarging heart can deliver a greater stroke volume output, but limits are soon reached (the descending limb of Starling's curve). Fig 13–8 shows a family of ventricular performance curves. The curve at right depicts a damaged myocar-

dium; the curve in the center, a normal myocardium; and the curve at the left, a myocardium under inotropic stimulation. One should be very cautious about the diagnosis of congestive heart failure in the absence of an enlarged heart (an exception being a condition such as total anomalous venous return below the diaphragm, which will for a short period of time be characterized by other signs of congestive heart failure without an enlarged heart). Cardiomegaly without other signs of congestive failure may well be taken as early or homeostatically compensated congestive heart failure.

Tachypnea may be considered the cardinal sign of left-sided heart failure. It may be present for a short time before hepatomegaly occurs, although pure left-sided or pure right-sided heart failure does not commonly exist independently for long.

Hepatomegaly is the cardinal sign of right-sided heart failure. The liver is capable of trapping relatively large amounts of edema fluid in the infant which would be more evident as peripheral edema in the older child and adult. It is therefore common rather than unusual for the infant in moderately severe heart failure to have an enlarged liver with no pretibial or even presacral or facial edema. Peripheral edema is found in infants only in the most severe cases of congestive heart failure.

Additional signs and symptoms of congestive heart failure are feeding difficulties, dyspnea, restlessness, easy fatigability, weak pulses, pallor, rales, peripheral edema, weight gain from fluid accumulation, tachycardia, sweating, pneumonia, orthopnea, and growth failure.

Underlying Causes of Heart Failure in the Pediatric Age Group

By far the most common cause of congestive heart failure in the pediatric patient is congenital heart disease. Causes in infancy and childhood appear in the outline below:

---

*The other being cyanosis, discussed on p 335.

A. Heart Failure in Infancy:

1. Cardiovascular causes—Congenital heart disease (producing volume overload, obstruction, myocardial impairment), congenital vascular disease (eg, coarctation of the aorta, peripheral arteriovenous shunts), acquired myocardial disease (eg, myocarditis), arrhythmias, rheumatic fever (very rare in infants in the USA).

2. Noncardiovascular causes—Acidosis, respiratory disease, central nervous system disease, anemia, sepsis, hypoglycemia.

B. Heart Failure in Childhood: Cardiovascular causes are potentially the same as in infancy except that rheumatic fever plays a more important role in childhood. Noncardiovascular causes become less important with increasing age—especially such mechanisms as acidosis and hypoglycemia.

Treatment

The physician undertaking the responsibility of caring for children must have facility with routine measures and familiarity with some emergency measures for treating congestive heart failure.

A. Routine Measures:

1. Digitalis—Digitalis is the keystone of the treatment of congestive heart failure. The major effect that is sought is improvement in myocardial performance (inotropic effect). This may be visualized as shifting the patient to a more efficient ventricular performance curve in the family of curves shown in Fig 13—8. The preparation most widely used in pediatrics is digoxin, which may be administered (in inverse order of rapidity of onset of effect) orally, intramuscularly, or intravenously. The clinical urgency of the individual case dictates how quickly digitalization should be accomplished. Although there are general guidelines, the ultimate dosage on a mg/kg basis must be individualized for each patient.

a. Protocols for digitalization—

(1) In hospital—

Age	Parenteral	Oral
Premature	0.035 mg/kg	0.04 mg/kg
2 weeks to 2 years	0.05 mg/kg	0.07 mg/kg
Under 2 weeks or over 2 years	0.04 mg/kg	0.06 mg/kg

Use of the elixir (0.05 mg/ml) is advisable even in older children because the bioavailability of the tablet preparations is unreliable.

The routine schedule consists of giving one-fourth the digitalizing dose intramuscularly or orally every 6 hours for 4 doses. For rapid digitalization, give half the digitalizing dose intravenously or intramuscularly and repeat in 4—6 hours. For very rapid digitalization, give the full digitalizing dose intravenously. For maintenance, give one-fourth to one-third the oral digitalizing dose daily (divided in morning and evening doses).

(2) Digitalization of outpatient—Give maintenance dose of digoxin (see above) divided in morning and evening doses. In less than a week, adequate digita-

lization is obtained without running the risk of a parent inadvertently failing to revert to a maintenance dosage schedule and continuing a high digitalizing dose to the point of toxicity (even death).

b. Digitalis toxicity—Slowing of the heart rate below 100 in infants, below 80 in young children, and below 60 in older children is often taken as a guide to reducing the dosage of digoxin. Any arrhythmia that occurs during digitalis therapy should be attributed to the drug until proved otherwise, although ventricular bigeminy and various degrees of atrioventricular block are characteristic of digitalis toxicity. Age-specific serum levels suggestive of toxicity during maintenance therapy are as follows: neonate, over 4 ng/ml; 1 month to 1 year, over 3 ng/ml; after 1 year, over 2 ng/ml.

c. Digitalis poisoning—This is an acute emergency which must be treated *without delay*. The sooner the stomach is emptied, the better the prognosis, but even if many hours have transpired the stomach should still be emptied. Attention must then be paid to maintaining an adequate cardiac rate and output and to controlling the arrhythmia. A useful basic intravenous solution is 10% glucose in water to which has been added 3 mEq of KCl per kg per day and 20 units of regular insulin per 1000 ml. KCl must be used with caution with electrocardiographic high-grade block. It should be given in amounts not to exceed the maintenance requirement per 24 hours for the weight or surface area of the patient. To this solution may be added isoproterenol (in the calibrated administration set) titrated in quantities appropriate to maintain adequate heart rate and output in the face of complete heart block. Phenytoin (Dilantin) may be administered through the intravenous tubing to treat arrhythmias by beginning with a 1 mg IV push followed every 5—10 minutes with doubling doses to a maximum total combined dose of 5 mg/kg. If medical management is unsuccessful, temporary transvenous pacemakers are indicated.

2. Diuretics—If digitalis alone is inadequate to achieve satisfactory compensation, diuretics may be required. For rapid inpatient diuresis, give furosemide intravenously or intramuscularly; for maintenance therapy, give thiazides orally (or, rarely, oral furosemide) by alternating every other day with oral spironolactone.

The dosages are as follows:

a. Furosemide—

(1) IV or IM, 1 mg/kg as single dose. Do not repeat more than once in a day and be cautious about using on consecutive days.

(2) Orally, 2—5 mg/kg/day.

b. Thiazides—These drugs should be given daily with spironolactone. Do not give daily for prolonged periods unless spironolactone is being given also and serum electrolytes are being monitored periodically.

(1) Chlorothiazide suspension (250 mg/tsp), 20 mg/kg/day.

(2) Hydrochlorothiazide tablets, 2 mg/kg/day.

c. Spironolactone—Give 2—4 mg/kg/day in 2 divided doses.

3. Rest and sedation—The decompensated and mildly distressed patient requires rest; the severely distressed and anxious infant or child requires sedation. Parenteral morphine, 0.1 mg/kg, is useful for sedation as well as acute pulmonary edema.

4. Oxygen—Oxygen will not make a patient with cyanotic heart disease pink but it will raise the systemic Pa_{O_2} in patients with severe congestive heart failure, overcoming the capillary-alveolar block of pulmonary edema and alleviating the hypoxemic contribution to congestive failure.

5. Salt restriction—Salt restriction must be approached with caution in infants and children. Treatment of the disease entity known as low-salt congestive heart failure is one of the more hazardous undertakings in medical management. Our feeling is that there is no place for salt-free formulas in the treatment of congestive failure in infants. Standard SMA or Similac 60/40 has about the same sodium content as human milk and about half the sodium content of cow's milk and other prepared formulas. Most cases of "low-salt failure" are largely due to overly vigorous salt restriction (sometimes combined with the other major factor, overly vigorous diuretic therapy). Clearly salty foods such as potato chips and bacon should be avoided, and no salt should be used beyond what is normally used in cooking. It is important that food be palatable enough to eat for a child, who may already be undernourished as a consequence of chronic, poorly compensated heart failure.

B. Emergency and Heroic Measures: The acute emergencies of congestive heart failure are usually related to fluid retention with pulmonary edema and low cardiac output. Some emergency therapeutic measures which may be lifesaving include the following:

1. Morphine—For acute pulmonary edema, give 0.1 mg/kg IV or subcut.

2. Diuretics—Furosemide or ethacrynic acid may be given IV in a dosage of 1 mg/kg to produce a rapid diuresis.

3. Positive pressure breathing—Pulmonary edema may sometimes be managed by intubation or mask with bag-breathing or a respirator to raise the alveolar pressure above pulmonary capillary pressure.

4. Peritoneal dialysis—Although ethacrynic acid and furosemide have largely met the need for the extremely rapid relief of fluid retention, there are 3 specific instances where peritoneal dialysis with a hypertonic solution may be indicated: (1) when fluid retention (especially pulmonary edema) is life-threatening and diuretics are unsuccessful; (2) in low-salt congestive heart failure when both the fluid retention and the electrolyte imbalance require correction; and (3) in the early postoperative care of an infant who may have an element of transient renal failure with both fluid retention and hyperkalemia.

The advantages of hypertonic peritoneal dialysis are that the procedure promptly (within minutes) draws fluid into the peritoneal cavity, where it is subject to immediate removal, while simultaneously correcting the electrolyte imbalance, whether it is low-sodium, high-potassium, or both. A suitable method is to introduce 50 ml/kg of dialyzing solution (7% glucose with balanced salt) into the peritoneal cavity, using a pediatric dialysis trocar and catheter. The fluid should be administered slowly over a 10-minute period, allowed to remain for another 10 minutes, and withdrawn by gravity drainage. More than one "run" with hypertonic solution in 12 hours should be approached with caution, but in the presence of pulmonary edema the hypertonic solution is required to withdraw fluid. If the major problem is electrolyte imbalance, such as potassium retention, a hypertonic solution is not required and the usual "isotonic" dialyzing fluid is indicated.

5. Afterload reduction—A relatively new form of therapy for "pump" failure is to effect afterload reduction by decreasing systemic vascular resistance with an intravenous infusion of vasodilators. Experience in children is limited. The procedure has been used largely in postoperative patients with reduced cardiac output and peripheral vasoconstriction. Agents such as nitroprusside have been lifesaving but must be used in a setting where central venous pressure, arterial pressure, cardiac output, etc can be carefully monitored.

Applebaum A & others: Afterload reduction and cardiac output in infants early after intracardiac surgery. Am J Cardiol 39:445, 1977.

Braunwald E: Vasodilator therapy: A physiologic approach to the treatment of heart failure. N Engl J Med 297:331, 1971.

Kim KE & others: Ethacrynic acid and furosemide: Diuretic and hemodynamic effect and clinical uses. Am J Cardiol 27:407, 1971.

Krasula R & others: Digoxin intoxication in infants and children: Correlation with serum levels. J Pediatr 84:265, 1974.

Lees MH: Heart failure in the newborn infant: Recognition and management. J Pediatr 75:139, 1970.

Levy G: Bioavailability of drugs: Focus on digoxin. Circulation 49:391, 1974.

Mason DT & others: Current concepts and treatment of digitalis toxicity. Am J Cardiol 27:546, 1971.

Nora JJ & others: Peritoneal dialysis in the treatment of intractable congestive heart failure of infancy and childhood. J Pediatr 68:693, 1966.

Schwartz A: Abnormal biochemistry in myocardial failure. Am J Cardiol 32:407, 1973.

Wedeen RP, Goldstein M, Leavitt MF: Mechanisms of edema and use of diuretics. Pediatr Clin North Am 18:561, 1971.

2. CYANOSIS

The second major clue to the presence of heart disease in the infant and child is cyanosis.* The physiologic basis of cyanosis is 4–5 gm/100 ml of reduced hemoglobin in transit through the capillaries. It becomes immediately apparent, then, that a patient with

---

*The other is congestive heart failure (see p 333).

a cyanotic heart lesion may not appear blue if he is sufficiently anemic; and a patient may look cyanotic even if his oxygen saturation is normal if his hemoglobin is very high (as in polycythemia).

Determination of the cause of cyanosis in the newborn is a frequent problem. Cyanosis may be due to CNS and blood disorders as well as to cardiac and pulmonary problems. Students often wonder why specialists in heart disease and specialists in lung disease sometimes have difficulty in determining whether a blue baby is blue because of heart disease or lung disease. The answer is that many of the clinical features and diagnostic clues are the same in cyanosis of cardiac and pulmonary origin. We find it useful to visualize this problem in terms of a Venn diagram and Boolean notation (Fig 13–9). The hatched area $H \cap \bar{L} \cap \bar{B} \cap \bar{C}$ delimits the area of tests that will reveal what is heart disease (H) and not lung ($\bar{L}$), not blood ($\bar{B}$), not CNS ($\bar{C}$). In this diagram, absence of a heart murmur, an ECG showing the usual right ventricular hypertrophy of the newborn, and a chest x-ray showing borderline heart size and vascularity could be found in an infant with cyanosis caused by heart, lung, blood, or CNS disease. These tests would fall in the unhatched overlapping areas of the Venn diagram. But the chest x-ray showing no evidence of pulmonary disease and a rise in arterial P_{O_2} from 35 mm Hg to 38 mm Hg (see Table 13–1) would be tests within the hatched area that would provide strong evidence that the cyanosis is of cardiac origin. (An excellent exposition of the use of Venn diagrams and Boolean algebra in reaching clinical decisions is provided in Feinstein AR: *Clinical Judgment.* Williams & Wilkins, 1967.)

The treatment of cyanotic heart disease is surgical correction in those patients for whom there is either a palliative or totally corrective surgical procedure. The medical management of hypoxemic spells is discussed under tetralogy of Fallot.

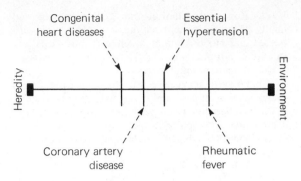

Figure 13–10. Etiologic overview.

ETIOLOGIC CONSIDERATIONS

The 4 major cardiovascular diseases are either present in or have their origins in infancy and childhood: congenital heart disease, rheumatic fever, atherosclerosis, and hypertension. Etiologic factors will be discussed in the sections devoted to these categories. An etiologic overview is presented in Fig 13–10. In all of these diseases, there is a genetic component and an important environmental interaction (with the exception of very small percentages of causes of congenital heart disease, atherosclerosis, and hypertension which have a mendelian or a chromosomal basis). Rheumatic fever is displaced toward the environmental pole and away from the other diseases, which are clustered midway between the poles. Although there appears to be an important genetic contribution to rheumatic fever, the essential etiologic factor is interaction with the group A beta-hemolytic streptococcus.

Nora JJ, Fraser FC: *Medical Genetics: Principles and Practice.* Lea & Febiger, 1974.

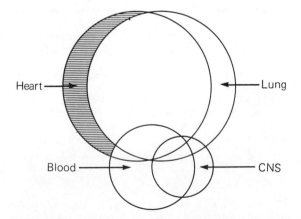

Figure 13–9. Venn diagram illustrating how much overlap may exist between the clinical and laboratory findings produced by these 4 causes of cyanosis. What is necessary is to devise special observations and tests that reveal the nonoverlapped (shaded) area of circle of heart disease. A specific test is the response of the patient's Pa_{O_2} to administered 100% O_2.

CONGENITAL HEART DISEASES

Congenital heart disease is present in about 1% of recently studied North American and British populations, making this the most common category of congenital structural malformation. Curative or palliative surgical correction is now available for over 90% of patients with congenital heart disease, but over half of all patients born with cardiovascular malformations will be dead before age 1 year if they are not promptly recognized and given the best medical and surgical care.

The customary division of congenital heart diseases into noncyanotic and cyanotic types is useful if one understands the basis for it. By convention, patients with right-to-left shunts fall into the cyanotic category whether they have readily recognizable cyanosis or not; patients who do not have right-to-left shunts—even if they are cyanotic for other reasons, such as low cardiac output—are placed in the noncyanotic category. The physiologic basis of cyanosis has been discussed above. It should be remembered that whatever brings 4–5 gm of unsaturated hemoglobin to the capillary bed produces cyanosis; if 4–5 gm of unsaturated hemoglobin are not present (as in a patient with a cyanotic heart lesion, but with anemia), cyanosis is not present.

Etiologic Considerations

On the basis of our present knowledge it can be stated that 3% of cases of congenital heart diseases are of single mutant gene origin (usually as part of a syndrome such as the Ullrich-Noonan syndrome); 5% are associated with chromosomal aberrations (such as Down's syndrome); and the remainder are best explained by multifactorial inheritance, in which there is a polygenic hereditary predisposition interacting with an environmental trigger (such as dextroamphetamine, progestogen/estrogen compounds, and probably a large number of drugs, viruses, and other environmental teratogens). Rubella virus appears not to require a hereditary predisposition to produce patent ductus arteriosus and pulmonary artery branch stenosis, but for lesions such as ventricular septal defect a positive family history is often found even when it occurs as part of the rubella syndrome. The special etiologic relationship of rubella to patent ductus arteriosus and pulmonary artery branch stenosis may be related to active proliferation of the virus in the vascular intima.

The parents' major concern in discussing the possible causes of congenital heart lesion is the chance of its recurrence in the offspring of future pregnancies. If only one first-degree relative (child or parent) is affected, the risk to the next child approximates the square root of the population frequency. For example, the population frequency of ventricular septal defect is 0.25% (25/10,000). The square root of this figure is 5% (5/100). Thus, the predicted multifactorial inheritance recurrence risk is 5%, which correlates closely with the empiric recurrence risk of 4.4%. Table 13–2 gives the risks of the 13 most common heart lesions if there is one affected first-degree relative.

The typical family that asks for counseling has one affected first-degree relative and is referred to as a type B family—ie, subject to the recurrence risks illustrated in Table 13–2. The more common the lesion, the higher the recurrence risk. Such families have a hereditary predisposition to congenital heart disease, but it is the common low-risk predisposition.

Fig 13–11 shows that there are 2 other types of families. A type A family is one with no hereditary predisposition, so that even a potent environmental trigger which moves the threshold to the left cannot move the threshold far enough to induce cardiovascular maldevelopment. A type C family is one in which the theoretical curve of polygenic hereditary predisposition is so far to the right (the family has such a strong

Table 13–2. Observed and expected recurrence risks in siblings of 1478 probands with congenital heart lesion.*

| Anomaly | Probands | Affected Siblings | | |
		No.	Percent	Exp. ($\sqrt{p}$)
Ventricular septal defect	212	24/543	4.4	5.0
Patent ductus arteriosus	204	17/505	3.4	3.5
Tetralogy of Fallot	157	9/338	2.7	3.2
Atrial septal defect	152	11/342	3.2	3.2
Pulmonary stenosis	146	10/345	2.9	2.9
Aortic stenosis	135	7/317	2.2	2.1
Coarctation of aorta	128	5/272	1.8	2.4
Transposition of great vessels	103	4/209	1.9	2.2
Atrioventricular canal	73	4/151	2.6	2.0
Tricuspid atresia	51	1/96	1.0	1.4
Ebstein's anomaly	42	1/96	1.1	0.7
Truncus arteriosus	41	1/86	1.2	0.7
Pulmonary atresia	34	1/77	1.3	1.0
Total	1478	95/3376		

*Reproduced, with permission, from Nora JJ: Etiologic factors in congenital heart disease. Pediatr Clin North Am 18:1059, 1971.

hereditary predisposition) that a high percentage of first-degree family members (often 75–100%) have some "spontaneous" congenital heart defects without the requirement of an environmental trigger. Fortunately, there are few such families, but one should assume that any family with 3 affected first-degree relatives is a type C family and that congenital heart disease is likely to recur in the majority of subsequent members of the same sibship.

Nora JJ: Etiologic factors in congenital heart diseases. Pediatr Clin North Am 18:1059, 1971.

Nora JJ: Multifactorial inheritance hypothesis for the etiology of congenital heart disease: The genetic-environmental interaction. Circulation 38:604, 1968.

I. NONCYANOTIC HEART DISEASE

ATRIAL SEPTAL DEFECT OF THE OSTIUM SECUNDUM VARIETY

Essentials of Diagnosis

- S_2 widely split and fixed.
- Grade I–III/VI ejection systolic murmur at pulmonic area.
- Diastolic flow murmur at the lower left sternal border (if shunt is significant in size).

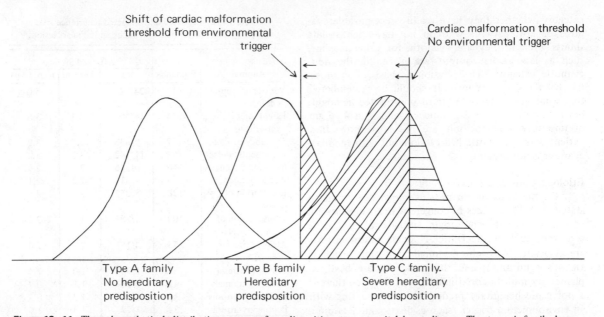

Figure 13–11. Three hypothetical distribution curves of predisposition to congenital heart disease. The type A family has no predisposition, and even the addition of an environmental trigger does not push the threshold of cardiac maldevelopment far enough to the left (or the curve of predisposition far enough to the right) to produce a congenital heart lesion. The type B family represents the usual family in which a congenital heart lesion occurs. The curve of polygenic predisposition is to the right, and the addition of an environmental trigger produces a congenital heart lesion in a portion of those predisposed. A type C family has such a strong polygenic predisposition that "spontaneous" cardiovascular malformation may occur, and the addition of environmental triggers may produce a very high frequency of malformation. (Reproduced, with permission, from Nora JJ, Fraser FC: *Medical Genetics: Principles and Practice*. Lea & Febiger, 1974.)

General Considerations

An atrial septal defect is an opening in the atrial septum permitting the shunting of blood between the 2 atria. There are 3 major types: (1) The ostium secundum type (discussed here) is the most common and is in an intermediate position. (2) The sinus venosus type is positioned high in the atrial septum, is the least common, and is frequently associated with partial anomalous venous return. (3) The ostium primum type is low in position and is a form of endocardial cushion defect; it is discussed in that section.

Atrial septal defect of the ostium secundum variety occurs in approximately 10% of patients with congenital heart disease and is twice as common in females as in males. It is uncommonly diagnosed in infancy or early childhood because of the paucity of findings. Partial anomalous pulmonary venous drainage is an infrequent associated anomaly.

Pulmonary hypertension and increased pulmonary vascular resistance are rare complications in childhood and adolescence but are significant factors after the third decade of life. As increased pulmonary vascular resistance develops, the left-to-right shunting decreases and right-to-left shunting eventually begins.

Clinical Findings

A. Symptoms and Signs: Infants may present with florid congestive heart failure often unresponsive to medical management, necessitating early total corrective surgery. However, children with atrial septal defects often have no cardiovascular symptoms. Some patients remain asymptomatic throughout life; others develop easy fatigability as older children or adults. Cyanosis does not occur until pulmonary hypertension develops. This may never occur; if it does, it is not seen until after the third decade of life. Congestive heart failure is uncommon in infants and young children.

The arterial pulses are normal and equal throughout. In the usual case, the heart is hyperactive, with a heaving impulse felt best at the lower left sternal border and over the xiphoid process. There are usually no thrills. S_2 at the pulmonary area is widely split and sometimes fixed. The pulmonary component is normal in intensity. A grade I–III/VI, blowing, ejection type systolic murmur is heard best at the left sternal border in the second intercostal space. An additional murmur of relative peripheral pulmonary artery stenosis may be heard, more commonly in infants. A mid-diastolic murmur can often be heard in the fourth intercostal space at the left sternal border. This murmur is due to increased blood flow across the tricuspid valve during diastole (tricuspid flow murmur). The presence of this murmur suggests a high flow (pulmonary to systemic blood flow ratio greater than 2:1).

B. X-Ray Findings: Chest x-rays usually demonstrate slight cardiac enlargement. The main pulmonary artery may be dilated. The pulmonary vascular markings are increased as a result of increased pulmonary blood flow.

C. Electrocardiography and Vectorcardiography: The usual ECG shows right axis deviation with a clockwise loop in the frontal plane. In the right precordial leads, there is usually an rsR' pattern. The VCG in the horizontal plane usually shows a terminal vector that is directed rightward and anteriorly.

D. Echocardiography: Two features are consistent with the diagrams: (1) paradoxic motion of the ventricular septal wall (moving in the same direction rather than the direction opposite to that of the free left ventricular wall), and (2) dilated right ventricular cavity with increased tricuspid valve excursion.

E. Cardiac Catheterization: Oximetry reveals evidence of a significant increase in oxygen saturation at the atrial level. The pulmonary artery pressure is usually normal. The right ventricular pressure is occasionally greater than the pulmonary artery pressure due to "flow." Pulmonary vascular resistance is usually normal. The pulmonary to systemic blood flow ratio may vary from 1.5:1 to 4:1. A catheter can easily be passed across the atrial septum into the left atrium if the catheterization is performed through the saphenous vein. Hydrogen electrode curves and dye dilution curves indicate a left-to-right shunt at the atrial level. The systemic arterial saturation is normal.

Treatment

It is generally recommended that ostium secundum atrial septal defects in which the pulmonary to systemic blood flow ratio is greater than 2:1 should be closed. Operation is usually performed just before the child enters school if the defect is discovered by then. The mortality rate for closure is less than 1%. Once pulmonary hypertension secondary to increased pulmonary vascular resistance has developed, closure of the defect is associated with a higher mortality rate.

Course & Prognosis

Patients with atrial septal defects usually tolerate them very well in the first 2 decades of life, and an occasional patient may live a completely normal life without symptoms. Frequently, however, pulmonary hypertension and reversal of the shunt develop by the third to fourth decade. Heart failure may also occur at this time. Subacute bacterial endocarditis is a very rare complication.

Anderson M & others: The natural history of small atrial defects. Am Heart J 92:302, 1976.

Craig RJ, Selzer A: Natural history and prognosis of atrial septal defect. Circulation 37:805, 1968.

Kumar S, Luisada AA: The second heart sound in atrial septal defect. Am J Cardiol 28:168, 1971.

Lucas RV, Hunt CF: Symptomatic atrial septal defect in infancy. Am J Cardiol 26:639, 1970.

Nora JJ, McNamara DG, Fraser FC: Hereditary factors in atrial septal defect. Circulation 35:448, 1967.

Toews WH, Nora JJ, Wolfe RR: Presentation of atrial septal defect in infancy. JAMA 234:1250, 1975.

VENTRICULAR SEPTAL DEFECTS

Essentials of Diagnosis

Small- to moderate-sized left-to-right shunt without pulmonary hypertension:
- Acyanotic, relatively asymptomatic.
- Grade II–IV/VI pansystolic murmur, maximal along the lower left sternal border.
- P_2 not accentuated.

Large left-to-right shunt:
- Acyanotic.
- Easy fatigability.
- Congestive heart failure in infancy (often).
- Hyperactive heart; biventricular enlargement.
- Grade II–V/VI pansystolic murmur, maximal at lower left sternal border.
- P_2 usually accentuated.
- Diastolic flow murmur at apex.

Insignificant left-to-right shunt or bidirectional shunt:
- Quiet precordium with right ventricular lift.
- Palpable P_2.
- Short ejection systolic murmur along left sternal border; single accentuated S_2.
- Systemic arterial oxygen desaturation may be present; pulmonary arterial pressure and systemic arterial pressures are equal; little or no oxygen saturation increase at right ventricular level by catheterization.

General Considerations

Simple ventricular septal defect (without other lesions) is the single most common congenital heart malformation, accounting for about 25% of all cases of congenital heart disease. Defects in the ventricular septum can occur both in the membranous portion of the septum (most common) and in the muscular portion. The size of the defect is more important than its position.

There are 4 different courses which patients with ventricular septal defect may follow:

(1) Spontaneous closure: Thirty to 50% of ventricular septal defects close spontaneously. These are usually small defects, and they usually close within the first few weeks or months of life. Larger defects may occasionally also close spontaneously, and there are many documented examples of spontaneous closure of ventricular septal defects in the second and third decades of life.

(2) Shunts too small to justify repair: Asymptomatic patients with hearts normal in size as seen on x-ray and without pulmonary hypertension are generally not subjected to surgical repair. Those who are studied by cardiac catheterization are usually found to have shunts of less than 2:1; and those who have had serial cardiac catheterizations have demonstrated that the shunts get progressively smaller. It is probable that many of the lesions in this category will eventually close spontaneously.

(3) Disease severe enough to require surgery: These patients may require surgery in infancy because of intractable congestive heart failure; surgery before 2 years of age because of progression of pulmonary hypertension; or surgery between 2 to 5 years of age as an elective procedure.

(4) Inoperable because of pulmonary hypertension: It is highly probable that a small percentage of patients are born inoperable—with pulmonary hypertension that does not regress. However, the majority of patients with inoperable pulmonary hypertension developed this condition progressively. On the basis of the combined data of the multicenter Natural History Study, it is becoming apparent that *most cases of irreversible pulmonary hypertension can be prevented by surgical repair of the defect before 2 years of age.*

Clinical Findings

A. Symptoms and Signs: Patients with small or moderate left-to-right shunts usually have no cardiovascular symptoms. There may be a history of frequent respiratory infections in infancy and early childhood. Patients with large left-to-right shunts frequently are sick early in infancy. Such patients have frequent respiratory infections, including bouts of pneumonitis. They grow slowly, with very poor weight gain. Dyspnea, exercise intolerance, and fatigue are quite common. Congestive heart failure may develop between 1–6 months. Patients who survive the first year usually improve, although easy fatigability may persist. With severe pulmonary hypertension (Eisenmenger's syndrome), cyanosis is present.

1. Small left-to-right shunt—There are usually no lifts, heaves, thrills, or shocks. The first sound at the apex is normal, and the second sound at the pulmonary area is split physiologically. The pulmonary component is normal. A grade II–III/VI, medium- to high-pitched, blowing pansystolic murmur is heard best at the left sternal border in the third and fourth intercostal spaces. There is slight radiation over the entire precordium. No diastolic murmurs are heard.

2. Moderate left-to-right shunt—Slight prominence of the precordium is common. There is a moderate left ventricular thrust. A systolic thrill is palpable at the lower left sternal border between the third and fourth intercostal spaces. The second sound at the pulmonary area is most often split but may be single. A grade IV/VI, harsh pansystolic murmur is heard best at the lower left sternal border in the fourth intercostal space. A diastolic flow murmur is heard and indicates that the pulmonary blood flow across the mitral valve is large and that the pulmonary to systemic blood flow ratio is at least 2:1.

3. Very large ventricular septal defects with pulmonary hypertension—The precordium is prominent and the sternum bulges. A left ventricular thrust and a right ventricular heave are palpable. A shock of the second sound can be felt at the pulmonary area. A thrill may or may not be present at the lower left sternal border. A second heart sound is usually single or narrowly split, with accentuation of the pulmonary

component. The murmur ranges from grade II–V/VI and is usually harsh and pansystolic. Occasionally, when the defect is large, very little murmur can be heard. A diastolic flow murmur may or may not be heard depending on the size of the shunt.

B. X-Ray Findings: X-rays of the chest vary depending upon the size of the shunt. In patients with small shunts, x-rays may be normal. The heart is normal in size, and the pulmonary vascular markings may be just beyond the upper limits of normal. Patients with large shunts usually show significant cardiac enlargement involving both the left and right ventricles and the left atrium. The aorta is usually small to normal in size, and the main pulmonary artery segment is dilated. The pulmonary vascular markings are significantly increased in patients with large shunts.

C. Electrocardiography: There is some correlation between the ECG and the hemodynamic findings. The ECG is normal in patients with small left-to-right shunts and normal pulmonary arterial pressures. Left ventricular hypertrophy is usually found in patients with large left-to-right shunts and normal pulmonary vascular resistance. Combined ventricular hypertrophy (both right and left) is found in patients with pulmonary hypertension due to increased flow, increased resistance, or both. Pure right ventricular hypertrophy is found in patients with pulmonary hypertension due to pulmonary vascular obstruction.

D. Echocardiography: The diagnosis of ventricular septal defect is virtually never made by means of echocardiography. Echocardiography is very useful, however, in following the hemodynamic progression as indicated by chamber size and systolic time intervals.

E. Cardiac Catheterization and Angiocardiography: Oxygen saturation is increased at the right ventricular level. The pulmonary arterial pressure may vary from normal to that in the systemic arteries. Left atrial pressure (pulmonary capillary pressure) may be normal to increased. Pulmonary vascular resistance varies from normal to markedly increased. The pulmonary to systemic blood flow ratio may vary from 1.1:1 to 4:1. Hydrogen electrode curves and dye dilution curves may indicate a shunt at the ventricular level. Angiocardiographic examination following injection of contrast material into the left ventricle reveals a left-to-right shunt at the ventricular level.

Treatment

A. Medical Management: Patients who develop congestive heart failure should be treated vigorously with anticongestive measures (see Congestive Heart Failure). If the patient responds well, he should be maintained on digitalis until surgical correction of the defect can be performed. It is often possible to discontinue digitalis after about age 2. If the patient does not respond to vigorous anticongestive measures or shows signs of developing progressive pulmonary hypertension, surgery is indicated without delay.

B. Surgical Treatment: The age for elective surgery is becoming progressively earlier in most centers (range, under 2 years to 5 years). Patients with cardiomegaly, poor growth, poor exercise tolerance, or other clinical abnormalities who have cardiac catheterization findings of significant shunt (2:1 or greater) and without significant pulmonary hypertension (greater than 10 units of resistance) are candidates for surgery. In general, patients with mean pulmonary artery pressures equal to systemic pressure who are unresponsive to oxygen administration, with little or no left-to-right shunt or bidirectional shunting, and pulmonary resistance calculated to be greater than 10 resistance units (or pulmonary/systemic resistance ratios greater than 0.7) are considered inoperable. There are patients who have pulmonary hypertension of lesser degree who remain operable, but there is a progressively greater risk with increasing pulmonary hypertension from 1% risk for patients without pulmonary hypertension to 25% for those at the upper limits of operability.

In order to prevent pulmonary hypertension from reaching inoperable levels, early surgical intervention is recommended for patients who have increased pulmonary resistance. In centers with the capability of doing total correction on infants with or without deep hypothermia, complete repair before 2 years of age is recommended. Even in these centers, patients weighing less than 10 lb may be considered for pulmonary artery banding. Pulmonary artery banding is generally being replaced by early total correction, but it may still be considered for the infant weighing less than 10 lb who is having intractable congestive heart failure and for somewhat larger infants in centers where complete correction is not feasible.

Allen HD & others: Postoperative follow-up of patients with ventricular septal defect. Circulation 50:465, 1974.

Alpert BS, Mellits ED, Rowe RD: Spontaneous closure of small ventricular septal defects: Probability rates in first five years of life. Am J Dis Child 125:194, 1973.

Clarkson PM & others: Prognosis for patients with ventricular septal defect with severe pulmonary vascular obstructive disease. Circulation 38:129, 1968.

Come P & others: Natural history of ventricular septal defect: A study involving 790 cases. Circulation 55:908, 1977.

Hoffman JI: Natural history of congenital heart disease: Problems in its assessment with special reference to ventricular septal defect. Circulation 37:97, 1968.

ENDOCARDIAL CUSHION DEFECTS

An endocardial cushion defect is a congenital cardiac abnormality which results from incomplete fusion of the embryonic endocardial cushions. The endocardial cushions help to form the lower portion of the atrial septum, the membranous portion of the ventricular septum, and the septal leaflets of the tricuspid and mitral valves. These defects are not very common. They account for about 4% of all cases of congenital heart disease. The incidence of this abnormality is 20% in patients with Down's syndrome.

Endocardial cushion defects may be divided into incomplete and complete forms. The complete form, also known as persistent common atrioventricular canal, consists of a high ventricular septal defect, a low atrial septal defect of the ostium primum variety which is continuous with the ventricular septal defect, and a cleft in both the septal leaflet of the tricuspid valve and the anterior leaflet of the mitral valve. In the incomplete form, any one of these components may be present. The most common partial form of endocardial cushion defect is the ostium primum type of atrial septal defect with a cleft in the mitral valve.

The complete form (persistent common atrioventricular canal) results in large left-to-right shunts at both the ventricular and atrial levels, tricuspid and mitral regurgitation, and marked pulmonary hypertension, usually with some increase in pulmonary vascular resistance. When the latter is present, the shunts may be bidirectional. The hemodynamics in the incomplete form are dependent upon the lesions present.

Clinical Findings

A. Symptoms and Signs: The clinical picture varies depending upon the severity of the defect. In the incomplete form, these patients may be indistinguishable from patients with the ostium secundum type of atrial septal defect. They are often asymptomatic. On the other hand, patients with atrioventricular canal usually are severely affected. Congestive heart failure often develops in infancy, and recurrent bouts of pneumonitis are common.

In the complete form, the findings are consistent with a large ventricular septal defect. The heart is significantly enlarged (both right and left), and a systolic thrill may be palpated at the lower left sternal border. The second heart sound is split, with an accentuated pulmonary component. A loud, harsh pansystolic murmur is heard at the lower left sternal border and is transmitted over the entire precordium. A pronounced diastolic flow murmur may be heard at the apex and lower left sternal borders.

When severe pulmonary vascular obstruction is present, there is evidence of dominant right ventricular enlargement. A shock of the second sound can be palpated at the pulmonary area. No thrill is felt. The second sound is markedly accentuated and single. A nonspecific short systolic murmur is heard at the lower left sternal border. No diastolic flow murmurs are heard. Cyanosis is detectable in severe cases with predominant right-to-left shunts.

The physical findings in the incomplete form depend upon the lesions. In the most common variety (ostium primum atrial septal defect with mitral regurgitation), the findings are similar to those of the ostium secundum type of atrial septal defect with or without findings of mitral regurgitation.

B. X-Ray Findings: Cardiac enlargement is present depending on the degree of specific anatomic defect and the severity. In the complete (canal) form, there is enlargement of all 4 chambers. The pulmonary vascular markings are increased. In patients with pulmonary vascular obstruction, only the main pulmonary artery segment and its branches are prominent. The peripheral markings are usually decreased.

C. Electrocardiography: In all forms of endocardial cushion defect, left axis deviation with a counterclockwise loop in the frontal plane is present. The mean axis varies from approximately −30 to −90 degrees. Since left axis deviation is present in all patients with this defect, the ECG is a very important diagnostic tool. First-degree heart block is present in over 50% of cases. Right, left, or combined ventricular hypertrophy is present depending upon the particular type of defect and the presence or absence of pulmonary vascular obstruction.

D. Echocardiography: Many suggestive patterns have been described, but excursion of the atrioventricular valve through the plane of the interventricular septal defect is characteristic. Single or multiple crystal echocardiography is highly accurate in establishing the anatomic diagnosis.

E. Cardiac Catheterization and Angiocardiography: The results of cardiac catheterization vary depending upon the type of defect present. When catheterization is performed from the leg, the catheter is easily passed across the atrial septum in its lowest portion and frequently enters the left ventricle directly. This is a result of the very low atrial septal defect and the cleft in the mitral valve. Increased oxygen saturation in the right ventricle or right atrium identifies the level of the shunt. Angiocardiography reveals a characteristic "gooseneck" deformity in the complete canal form.

Treatment

Treatment consists of anticongestive measures and eventual surgical correction. In the incomplete form, surgery is associated with a relatively low mortality rate (2−5%). The complete form is associated with a significantly higher mortality rate (about 15−25%), but complete correction in the first year of life, prior to the onset of irreversible pulmonary hypertension, is advisable.

Pulmonary artery banding procedures are contraindicated in infants with shunts predominantly at the atrial level and are less effective in predominantly ventricular level shunts than in patients with simple ventricular septal defect.

Lillehei CW & others: Persistent common A-V canal: Recatheterization results in 37 patients following intracardiac repair. J Thorac Cardiovasc Surg 57:83, 1969.

McCabe J & others: Surgical treatment of endocardial defects. Am J Cardiol 39:72, 1977.

Rastelli GC & others: Surgical repair of complete form of persistent common atrioventricular canal. J Thorac Cardiovasc Surg 55:299, 1968.

Sahn DJ & others: Multiple crystal echocardiographic evaluation of endocardial cushion defect. Circulation 50:25, 1974.

Shah CV, Patel MF, Hastreiter AR: Hemodynamics of complete atrioventricular canal and its evolution with age. Am J Cardiol 29:326, 1969.

PATENT DUCTUS ARTERIOSUS

Patent ductus arteriosus (PDA) is the persistence in extrauterine life of the normal fetal vessel which joins the pulmonary artery to the aorta. It is a common abnormality, accounting for about 12% of all cases of congenital heart disease. It is very common in children born to mothers who had rubella during the first trimester of pregnancy. There is a higher incidence of patent ductus arteriosus in infants born at high altitudes (over 10,000 feet). It is twice as common in females as in males. In intensive care premature nurseries where infants who would die with less aggressive management are salvaged, the frequency of patent ductus arteriosus may be as high as 20−60%.

The defect occurs as an isolated abnormality, but associated lesions are not infrequent. Coarctation of the aorta, patent ductus arteriosus, and ventricular septal defect are commonly associated. Even more important to recognize is the fact that patients with murmurs of patent ductus and without readily apparent findings of other associated lesions are being kept alive by their patent ducti. One would not wish to ligate a patent ductus in a patient with pulmonary atresia or merely follow with outpatient visits such a patient, who should receive immediate precise diagnosis and appropriate treatment.

Clinical Findings

A. Symptoms and Signs: The clinical findings and the clinical course depend on the size of the shunt and the degree of pulmonary hypertension.

1. Typical patent ductus arteriosus—The pulses are bounding and pulse pressure is widened (pulse pressure is greater than half of the systolic pressure). The first heart sound is normal. The second heart sound is usually narrowly split and very rarely (when the shunt is maximal) paradoxically split (ie, the second sound closes on inspiration and splits on expiration). The paradoxic splitting is due to the maximal overload of the left ventricle and the prolonged ejection of blood from this chamber.

The murmur is quite characteristic. It is a very rough "machinery" murmur which is maximal at the second intercostal space at the left sternal border and under the left clavicle. It begins shortly after the first heart sound, rises to a peak at the second heart sound, and passes through the second heart sound into diastole, where it becomes a decrescendo murmur and fades and disappears before the first heart sound. The murmur tends to radiate fairly well over the lung fields anteriorly but relatively poorly over the lung fields posteriorly. A diastolic flow murmur is often heard at the apex. Depending on the pulmonary artery pressure, the murmur may be only systolic in time. This should be fully appreciated when trying to reach a diagnosis of patent ductus arteriosus in infants. If the shunt is small, congestive failure is absent; if the shunt is large, congestive failure becomes important.

2. Patent ductus arteriosus with pulmonary hy-

pertension—The physical findings depend upon the cause of the pulmonary hypertension. If pulmonary hypertension is due primarily to a marked increase in blood flow and only a slight increase in pulmonary vascular resistance, the physical findings are similar to those listed above. The significant difference is the presence of an accentuated pulmonary component of S_2. Bounding pulses and a loud continuous heart murmur are present. In patients with pulmonary hypertension secondary to increased pulmonary vascular resistance and predominant right-to-left shunt, the findings are quite different. There may be evidence of cyanosis. The second heart sound is single and quite accentuated, and there is no significant heart murmur. The pulses are normal rather than bounding.

3. **Patent ductus arteriosus in the premature neonate with associated IRDS**—A premature during or after the clinical course of infant respiratory distress syndrome (IRDS) may have a significant associated patent ductus arteriosus which is paradoxically difficult to detect clinically but is often threatening in magnitude. A soft nonspecific systolic murmur or no murmur is more common than the classical continuous murmur. The peripheral pulse and precordium are often bounding, but typically are not characteristic for several days after the onset of a large left-to-right shunt. An early sign indicating the presence of a significant left-to-right shunt with concomitant congestive heart failure is increasing dependence on oxygen and respiratory support. In addition, increasing radiographic cardiomegaly and pulmonary edema plus increasing echocardiographic evidence of a left-to-right shunt differentiate this clinical and laboratory picture from bronchopulmonary dysplasia.

B. X-Ray Findings: In simple patent ductus arteriosus, the x-ray appearance depends upon the size of the shunt. If the shunt is relatively small or moderate in size, the heart is not enlarged. If the shunt is large, there is evidence of both left atrial and left ventricular enlargement. In both cases, the aorta is prominent, as is the main pulmonary artery segment.

C. Electrocardiography and Echocardiography: The ECG may be normal or may show left ventricular hypertrophy, depending on the size of the shunt. In patients with pulmonary hypertension due to increased blood flow, there is usually biventricular hypertrophy. In those with pulmonary vascular obstruction, there is pure right ventricular hypertrophy. Enlargement of the left atrium as measured by echocardiography is an important clue to the presence of congestive heart failure, which is especially useful in the premature with patent ductus arteriosus.

D. Cardiac Catheterization and Angiocardiography: If catheterization is performed, there is evidence of increased oxygen content or saturation at the level of the pulmonary artery. Hydrogen electrode curves are positive in the pulmonary artery and negative in the right ventricle. The catheter can often be passed through the ductus from the pulmonary artery into the descending thoracic aorta. Arteriograms taken following injection of contrast material into the aortic

arch show a shunt at the level of the ductus. If catheterization is not performed, the cardiologist must be completely satisfied that there is neither an associated lesion nor pulmonary hypertension. One should not have to tie off more than one ductus in a patient with pulmonary atresia or interrupted aortic arch to be extremely cautious about sending patients with presumptive diagnoses of patent ductus arteriosus to surgery without cardiac catheterization.

Patients with patent ductus arteriosus and pulmonary hypertension due to large left-to-right shunts show a marked increase in oxygen saturation at the pulmonary artery level and normal systemic arterial saturation. Those with marked pulmonary vascular obstruction show little or no increase in oxygen content at the pulmonary artery and a decrease in systemic arterial saturation. In both cases, a catheter may be passed through the ductus into the descending thoracic aorta.

Treatment

Treatment consists of surgical correction except in patients with pulmonary vascular obstruction. Patients with large left-to-right shunts and pulmonary hypertension should be operated on very early (even under the age of 1 year) to prevent the development of progressive pulmonary vascular obstruction. The optimal age for correction of simple patent ductus arteriosus is between ages 2–5, although the operation may be delayed until a later age without increased mortality.

Patients with nonreactive pulmonary vascular obstruction who have resistance greater than 10 units and a pulmonary/systemic resistance ratio greater than 0.7 should not be operated upon. These patients are made worse by closure of the ductus, since the ductus serves as an escape route and limits the degree of pulmonary hypertension.

Course & Prognosis

Patients with simple patent ductus arteriosus and small to moderate shunts usually do quite well even without surgery. However, in the third or fourth decade of life, symptoms of easy fatigability, dyspnea on exertion, and exercise intolerance appear, usually as a consequence of the development of pulmonary hypertension or congestive heart failure.

Spontaneous closure of a patent ductus arteriosus may occur within the first year of life. This is especially true in infants who were born prematurely. After age 1, spontaneous closure is rare. We personally prefer to follow patients with very small shunts (less than 1.5:1) and no pulmonary hypertension without surgery and with antibiotic prophylaxis of bacterial endocarditis for several more years to provide maximal opportunity for spontaneous closure. This probably represents a minority opinion, but one that we find comfortable.

Patients with large shunts or pulmonary hypertension do much less well. Poor growth and development, frequent episodes of pneumonitis, and the development of congestive heart failure are not uncommon in patients with large left-to-right shunts. If these patients do not succumb to congestive heart failure in early infancy, they frequently go on to develop pulmonary vascular obstruction in later childhood or adolescence. Life expectancy is markedly reduced, and these patients often die in their second or third decade. Those rare patients with pulmonary vascular obstruction from very early infancy are actually less symptomatic than those with pulmonary hypertension without obstruction.

Subacute infective endocarditis is a potential complication.

The problem of surgical closure of patent ductus in premature infants is not fully resolved. Indications for surgery vary widely. At some institutions it is customary to operate on virtually all prematures under 1200 gm; at others, the operation is done only rarely. Nonsurgical methods of treatment currently being assessed include 72 hours of significant fluid restriction (50–100 ml/kg/day) and administration of indomethacin to effect ductal closure.

Kitterman JA & others: Patent ductus arteriosus in premature infants. N Engl J Med 287:473, 1972.

Silverman NH & others: Echocardiographic assessment of ductus arteriosus shunt in premature infants. Circulation 50:821, 1974.

Thibeault DW & others: Patent ductus arteriosus complicating the respiratory distress syndrome in preterm infants. J Pediatr 86:120, 1975.

MALFORMATIONS ASSOCIATED WITH OBSTRUCTION TO BLOOD FLOW ON THE RIGHT SIDE OF THE HEART

1. VALVULAR PULMONARY STENOSIS WITH INTACT VENTRICULAR SEPTUM

Essentials of Diagnosis

- No symptoms with mild and moderately severe cases.
- Cyanosis and a high incidence of right-sided congestive heart failure in very severe cases.
- Right ventricular lift; systolic ejection click at the pulmonic area in mild to moderately severe cases.
- S_2 widely split with soft to inaudible P_2; grade I–VI/VI obstructive systolic murmur, maximal at the pulmonic area.

General Considerations

Obstruction of right ventricular outflow at the pulmonary valve level accounts for about 10% of all cases of congenital heart disease. In the usual case, the cusps of the pulmonary valve are fused to form a mem-

brane or diaphragm with a hole in the middle which varies from 2 mm to 1 cm in diameter. Occasionally, there may be fusion of only 2 cusps, producing a bicuspid pulmonary valve. Very frequently, especially in the more severe cases, there is secondary infundibular stenosis. The pulmonary valve ring is usually small. There is usually moderate to marked poststenotic dilatation of the main pulmonary artery and the left pulmonary artery. There is usually an inverse relationship between the severity of the obstruction and the degree of poststenotic dilatation. Patent foramen ovale is fairly common.

Obstruction to blood flow across the pulmonary valve results in an increase in pressure developed by the right ventricle to maintain an adequate output across that valve. Pressures greater than systemic are not unusual, and occasionally may range up to 200 mm Hg. As a consequence of the increased work required of the right ventricle, severe right ventricular hypertrophy and eventual right ventricular failure can occur. This is in contrast to patients with right ventricular outflow obstruction and a large ventricular septal defect (ie, tetralogy of Fallot), in whom—because of the communication between the ventricles—the maximal pressure that the right ventricle may develop is limited (equal to systemic pressure) and heart failure is extremely uncommon.

When the obstruction is severe and the ventricular septum is intact, a right-to-left shunt will often occur at the atrial level through a patent foramen ovale. Accordingly, patients with this condition may have a varying degree of cyanosis. The presence of cyanosis indicates a relatively severe degree of valvular obstruction.

Clinical Findings

A. Symptoms and Signs: The history depends upon the severity of the obstruction. Patients with a mild or even a moderate degree of valvular pulmonary stenosis are completely asymptomatic throughout infancy, childhood, and adolescence. Patients with a more severe type of valve obstruction may develop cyanosis and congestive heart failure very early—even in the neonatal period. In patients with moderately severe but not critical pulmonary stenosis, there may be progressively increasing cyanosis, easy fatigability, and dyspnea on exertion. Cyanotic spells characterized by a sudden onset of marked increase in cyanosis and dyspnea are much less uncommon than in tetralogy of Fallot. Squatting is very uncommon.

Patients with mild to moderate obstruction are acyanotic. Patients with severe or critical stenosis usually show evidence of central cyanosis. These patients are usually well developed and well nourished. They often have a round face and widely spaced eyes. The pulses are normal and equal throughout. Clubbing may occur in severe cases in which cyanosis has persisted for a long time. On examination of the heart, there may be prominence of the precordium. A heaving impulse of the right ventricle can frequently be palpated. A systolic thrill is often palpated in the pulmonic area and frequently in the suprasternal notch. The first heart sound is normal. In patients with mild to moderate stenosis, a prominent pulmonic type of ejection click is heard best at the second left intercostal space. This click varies with respiration. It is much more prominent during expiration than inspiration. In patients with severe stenosis, the click tends to merge with the, first heart sound. The second heart sound also varies with the degree of stenosis. In mild valvular stenosis, the second heart sound is normally split and the pulmonary component is normal in intensity. In moderate degrees of obstruction, the second heart sound is more widely split and the pulmonary component is softer. In severe pulmonary stenosis, the second heart sound is single since the pulmonary component cannot be heard. (On phonocardiography, the pulmonary component of the second heart sound is widely separated from the first heart sound and does not move with respiration.) An ejection type, rough, obstructive systolic murmur is best heard at the second interspace at the left sternal border. It radiates very well over the lung fields anteriorly and over the upper lung fields posteriorly. No diastolic murmurs are audible. In older children, a prominent "A" wave is seen in the jugular venous pulse. If there is congestive heart failure, the liver is enlarged.

B. X-Ray Findings: In the mild form of pulmonary stenosis, the heart may be normal in size. Poststenotic dilatation of the main pulmonary artery segment and the left pulmonary artery is often present. In moderate to severe cases, there may be a slight right ventricular enlargement and there may or may not be poststenotic dilatation of the main pulmonary artery. In patients who are cyanotic, the pulmonary vascular markings are decreased; otherwise they are normal.

C. Electrocardiography: The ECG is usually normal in patients with mild obstruction. Right ventricular hypertrophy is present in patients with moderate to severe valvular obstruction. In severe obstruction, right ventricular hypertrophy and the right ventricular strain pattern (deep inversion of the T wave) are seen in the right precordial leads. In the most severe form, right atrial hypertrophy is also present. Right axis deviation is also seen in the moderate to severe forms. Occasionally, the axis is greater than +180 degrees.

D. Echocardiography: Atrial contraction and elevated right ventricular diastolic pressure cause early opening of the pulmonary valve prior to the onset of ventricular systole.

E. Cardiac Catheterization and Angiocardiography: There is no increase in oxygen saturation or oxygen content in the right side of the heart. In the more severe cases, there is a right-to-left shunt at the atrial level. Pulmonary artery pressure is normal in milder cases and quite low in moderately to severe to severe cases. Right ventricular pressure is always higher than pulmonary artery pressure. The gradient across the pulmonary valve varies from 10–200 mm Hg. In severe cases, the right atrial pressure is often elevated, with a predominant "A" wave. Cineangiocardiography with injection of contrast material into the right ventricle

shows thickening of the pulmonary valve and the very narrow opening of the pulmonary valve. This produces a "jet" of contrast from the right ventricle into the pulmonary artery. Infundibular hypertrophy may be present. This is seen as a narrowing of the right ventricular outflow track during ventricular systole followed by a widening of this area.

Treatment

Operation is recommended immediately for all children in whom the right ventricular pressure is equal to or greater than systemic pressure or who have symptoms or cyanosis. The operative mortality rate varies from 1–10% depending upon the age and condition of the patient.

Course & Prognosis

Patients with mild pulmonary stenosis live a normal life and have a normal life span. Those with stenosis of moderate severity usually show symptoms of easy fatigability and dyspnea on exertion which may be progressive. Those with severe valvular obstruction may develop severe cyanosis and congestive heart failure in early life.

Danielson GK & others: Pulmonic stenosis with intact ventricular septum: Surgical considerations and results of operation. J Thorac Cardiovasc Surg 61:228, 1971.

Danilowitz D, Hoffman J, Rudolf A: Serial studies of pulmonary stenosis in infancy and childhood. Br Heart J 37:808, 1975.

Hultgren HN & others: The ejection click of valvular pulmonary stenosis. Circulation 40:631, 1969.

Leatham A, Weitzman D: Auscultatory and phonographic signs of pulmonary stenosis. Br Heart J 19:303, 1957.

Mustard WT, Jain S, Trusler GA: Pulmonary stenosis in first year of life. Br Heart J 30:255, 1968.

Neal WA & others: Comparison of the hemodynamic effects of exercise and isoproterenol infusion in patients with pulmonary valvar stenosis. Circulation 49:948, 1974.

2. INFUNDIBULAR PULMONARY STENOSIS WITHOUT VENTRICULAR SEPTAL DEFECT

Pure infundibular pulmonary stenosis is rare. One should suspect infundibular pulmonary stenosis where there is evidence of mild to moderate pulmonary stenosis and intact ventricular septum and (1) no pulmonic ejection click is audible and (2) the murmur is maximal in the third and fourth intercostal space rather than in the second intercostal space. Otherwise, the clinical picture may be identical.

3. DISTAL PULMONARY STENOSIS

Supravalvular Pulmonary Stenosis

This relatively rare condition is due to coarctation of the body of the main pulmonary artery or of the bifurcation of the main pulmonary artery. The clinical picture may be identical with that of valvular pulmonary stenosis, although the murmur is maximal in the first intercostal space at the left sternal border and in the suprasternal notch. No ejection click is audible. A second heart sound is usually narrowly split, and the pulmonary component is quite loud as a result of closure of the pulmonary valve under high pressure. The murmur radiates extremely well into the neck and over the lung fields.

Peripheral Pulmonary Branch Stenosis

In this condition there are multiple small coarctations of the branches of the pulmonary artery in the periphery of the lung. Systolic murmurs may be heard over both lung fields both anteriorly and posteriorly. The transient pulmonary branch stenosis murmurs of infancy (previously described under heart murmurs) are innocent. Pulmonary artery branch stenosis murmurs may be the most audible murmurs in atrial septal defects in infancy and early childhood. The most common cause of significant pulmonary artery branch stenosis is maternal rubella. In our series, pulmonary branch stenosis was found in 55% of patients with rubella syndrome and patent ductus in 43%. The hypercalcemia syndrome and the Ullrich-Noonan syndrome are also diagnostic considerations in patients with pulmonary artery branch stenosis.

Absence of a Pulmonary Artery

This condition may exist as an isolated malformation or in association with other congenital heart diseases. It is occasionally seen in patients with tetralogy of Fallot.

Dunkle LM, Rowe RD: Transient murmur simulating pulmonary artery stenosis in premature infants. Am J Dis Child 124:666, 1972.

Nihill MR, Nora JJ: Pulmonary artery coarctation. Page 759 in: *Birth Defects Atlas and Compendium.* Bergsma D (editor). Williams & Wilkins, 1973.

Ross JC & others: Congenital pulmonary artery branch stenosis. Am J Cardiol 24:318, 1969.

Rowe RD: Maternal rubella and pulmonary artery stenosis: Report of 11 cases. Pediatrics 32:180, 1963.

MALFORMATIONS ASSOCIATED WITH OBSTRUCTIONS TO BLOOD FLOW ON THE LEFT SIDE OF THE HEART

1. COARCTATION OF THE AORTA

Coarctation is a common cardiac abnormality, accounting for about 6% of all cases of congenital heart disease. Three times as many males as females are affected. In the vast majority of cases, coarctation occurs in the thoracic portion of the descending aorta.

The abdominal aorta is very rarely involved. Based on the pathologic features, coarctations are commonly classified as pre- or postductal in location. This is an oversimplification, as many are juxtaductal. The term *coarctation of aorta syndrome* is a useful concept, since most symptomatic infants will have associated patent ductus arteriosus, tubular hypoplasia of the aortic isthmus (frequently erroneously termed a coarctation), ventricular septal defect, and bicuspid aortic valve. The tubular hypoplasia of the aortic isthmus is probably related to paucity of blood flow in the fetus and often spontaneously enlarges with postnatal growth.

Clinical Findings

A. Symptoms and Signs: Patients with coarctation may or may not have cardiovascular symptoms in infancy, childhood, and adolescence. Congestive heart failure may develop in early infancy, and symptoms of decreased exercise tolerance and fatigability may appear in childhood.

The important physical finding is diminution or absence of femoral pulses. Failure to identify this diagnostic clue is due mainly to failure to look for it. Normally, the blood pressure in the upper extremities is slightly higher than in the lower extremities during the first few months of life. After 1 year of age, blood pressure higher in the arms than in the legs is suggestive of coarctation of the aorta. The actual level of blood pressure in the arms may be only moderately elevated, even in severe coarctation, or it may be significantly elevated. In the presence of severe congestive heart failure, the differences in pulses in the upper and lower extremities may not be readily apparent, but with compensation the pulses in the arms are palpably stronger than in the normal infant, whereas the pulses in the legs remain diminished or absent. The left subclavian artery is occasionally involved in the coarctation, in which case the left brachial pulse is weak. If the coarctation is uncomplicated, the heart sounds are normal. The aortic component of the second heart sound is occasionally increased in intensity. An ejection systolic murmur of grade II/VI intensity is often heard at the aortic area and the lower left sternal border. The pathognomonic murmur of coarctation is heard in the interscapular area of the back, over the area of the coarctation. This murmur is usually systolic in timing. If the coarctation is complicated by other malformations, murmurs associated with these other abnormalities will be audible.

B. X-Ray Findings: In the older child, the heart may be normal in size, although there is usually some evidence of left ventricular enlargement. The ascending aorta is usually normal in size. On barium swallow, the esophagus has a characteristic E shape. The first arc of the E is due to dilatation of the aorta just proximal to the coarctation. The second arc is due to poststenotic dilatation of the aorta. The middle bar of the E is due to the coarctation itself. In older children, notching or scalloping of the ribs caused by marked enlargement of the intercostal collaterals can be seen.

In infants in congestive heart failure, there is evidence of marked cardiac enlargement and pulmonary venous congestion.

C. Electrocardiography: ECGs in children may be normal or may show evidence of slight left ventricular hypertrophy. In infants with or without congestive heart failure, the ECG usually demonstrates right ventricular hypertrophy.

D. Echocardiography: Echocardiography reveals only secondary evidence of the coarctation. In infants with congestive heart failure, dilated right and left ventricles are noted. A striking posterior displacement of the mitral valve in the left ventricular cavity with poor excursion is common.

E. Cardiac Catheterization and Angiocardiography: These studies are useful to demonstrate the position, the anatomy, and the severity of the coarctation and to assess the adequacy of the collateral circulation. It goes without saying that coarctation of the abdominal aorta may not be approached through a thoracic incision. In fact, because of involvement of the renal arteries in some of these patients, surgery may be difficult or not possible. Surgeons generally appreciate· receiving precise anatomic and physiologic definition of the lesion.

Treatment

Infants with coarctation of the aorta and congestive heart failure require vigorous anticongestive measures. Many with isolated coarctation and no associated lesions respond well and do not require surgery in infancy. In infants with striking congestive heart failure and without associated cardiovascular abnormalities, severe systemic hypertension is often a contributing factor. Reduction of afterload with intravenous nitroprusside or propranolol followed by chronic oral propranolol is often lifesaving and allows deferral of definitive correction until a more optimal age. Infants with associated intracardiac defects sometimes need immediate surgery but frequently require revision of the recoarctation later in life. Patients who do not require surgery early in life may be corrected electively at ages 3–5 years unless significant systemic hypertension develops.

Course & Prognosis

Children who survive the neonatal period without developing congestive heart failure do quite well throughout childhood and adolescence. Fatal complications (eg, hypertensive encephalopathy, intracranial bleeding) occur uncommonly. Subacute infective endocarditis is also rare before adolescence.

Starting in the third decade of life, the patient may develop the onset of easy fatigability, dyspnea on exertion, cardiac enlargement, and left ventricular failure. Only one-fourth of these patients may be expected to live through the fourth decade. Death results from subacute infective endocarditis or hypertensive cardiovascular disease.

Infants with coarctations who develop congestive heart failure in early infancy usually succumb unless vigorously treated. If they survive this period, they may do very well without surgery and can be operated on later when the surgical risk is less.

Campbell M: Natural history of coarctation of the aorta. Br Heart J 32:633, 1970.

Maron BJ & others: Prognosis of surgically corrected coarctation of the aorta: A 20 year postoperative appraisal. Circulation 47:119, 1973.

Mathew R, Simon G, Joseph M: Collateral circulation in coarctation of aorta in infancy and childhood. Arch Dis Child 47:950, 1972.

Neches WH & others: Coarctation of the aorta with ventricular septal defect. Circulation 55:189, 1977.

Sinha SN & others: Coarctation of the aorta in infancy. Circulation 40:385, 1969.

2. AORTIC STENOSIS

Aortic stenosis may be defined from the anatomic or physiologic point of view. Anatomically, it consists of an obstruction to the outflow from the left ventricle at or near the aortic valve. Physiologically, aortic stenosis may be defined as a condition in which a systolic pressure gradient of more than 10 mm Hg exists between the left ventricle and the aorta. Aortic stenosis accounts for approximately 5% of all cases of congenital heart disease. Anatomically, congenital aortic stenosis may be divided into 4 types:

(1) Valvular aortic stenosis (75%): Critical aortic stenosis presenting in infancy usually consists of a unicuspid diaphragm-like structure without well defined commissures. Preschool and school-age children more commonly present with a bicuspid valve. Teenagers and young adults characteristically present with tricuspid but partially fused leaflets. This lesion is more common in males than females.

(2) Discrete membranous subvalvular aortic stenosis (20%): This consists of a membranous or fibrous ring 5–10 mm below the aortic valve. The ring forms a diaphragm with a hole in the middle and results in obstruction to left ventricular outflow. The aortic valve itself and the anterior leaflet of the mitral valve are often deformed.

(3) Supravalvular aortic stenosis: In this variety there is a constriction of the ascending aorta just above the coronary arteries. This condition is often associated with a family history, abnormal facies, and mental retardation (idiopathic hypercalcemia syndrome).

(4) Idiopathic hypertrophic subaortic stenosis (IHSS): In this case there is a marked hypertrophy of the entire left ventricle and, predominantly, the ventricular septum. With contraction of the ventricle, the hypertrophic portion of the septum together with the mitral valve cause obstruction of left ventricular outflow. A family history is often present.

Obstruction to outflow from the left ventricle causes the left ventricle to work harder to maintain an adequate pressure and flow in the systemic arterial circuit, resulting in hypertrophy of the left ventricle and increased oxygen requirement. If the stenosis is severe, the oxygen requirements may exceed the capacity of the coronary arteries to supply oxygen, and relative coronary insufficiency may develop. In critical aortic stenosis, left ventricular failure may occur. The left ventricle is usually able to adapt to the increased pressure load for a considerable period of time before developing heart failure or coronary insufficiency.

Clinical Findings

A. Symptoms and Signs: Most patients with aortic stenosis have no cardiovascular symptoms. Except in the most severe cases, the patient may do well up until the third to fifth decade of life, although some patients have mild exercise intolerance and easy fatigability. A small percentage of patients have significant symptoms within the first decade, ie, dizziness and syncope. Sudden death, although uncommon, may occur in all forms of aortic stenosis, with the greatest risk being IHSS.

The physical findings vary somewhat depending upon the anatomic type of lesion:

1. Valvular aortic stenosis—These patients are well developed and well nourished. The pulses are usually normal and equal throughout. If the stenosis is severe and there is a gradient of greater than 80 mm Hg, the pulses are small with a slow upstroke. Examination of the heart reveals a left ventricular thrust at the apex. A systolic thrill at the right base, the suprasternal notch, and both carotid arteries accompanies moderate disease. If only one carotid artery manifests a thrill, it is the right carotid. This is usually found in milder disease.

The first heart sound is normal. A prominent aortic type ejection click or ejection sound is best heard at the apex. Very frequently, this click can be heard at the lower left sternal border and at the aortic area. It is separated from the first heart sound by a short but appreciable interval. It does not vary with respiration. The second heart sound at the pulmonary area is physiologically split. The aortic component of the second heart sound is of good intensity. There is a grade III–V/VI, rough, medium- to high-pitched ejection type systolic murmur, loudest at the first and second intercostal spaces, which radiates well into the suprasternal notch and along the carotids. The murmur also radiates fairly well down the lower left sternal border and can be heard at the apex. The murmur transmits to the neck, and its grade correlates roughly with the severity of the stenosis.

2. Discrete membranous subvalvular aortic stenosis—The findings are essentially the same as those of valvular aortic stenosis. Absence of an aortic ejection click is an important differentiating point, and the thrill and murmur are usually somewhat more intense at the left sternal border in the third and fourth intercostal spaces than at the aortic area. Frequently, however, the murmur is equally intense at both areas. A diastolic murmur of aortic insufficiency is commonly heard after 5 years of age.

3. Supravalvular aortic stenosis—These patients often have abnormal facies and are mentally retarded. The thrill and murmur are characteristically best heard in the suprasternal notch and along the carotids, although they are well transmitted over the aortic area and near the mid left sternal border. A difference in pulses and blood pressure between the right and left arms may be found, with the more prominent pulse and pressure in the right arm.

4. IHSS—The murmur in this case is ejection in quality, grade II–III/VI, and heard from the left sternal border toward the apex and sometimes associated with a murmur of mitral insufficiency. There is often an atrial fourth heart sound and a diastolic murmur. No ejection click is audible. The arterial pulse wave has a rapid upstroke and frequently a bisferiens quality.

B. X-Ray Findings: In most cases, the heart is not enlarged. The left ventricle, however, is slightly prominent. In valvular and discrete subvalvular aortic stenosis, dilatation of the ascending aorta is frequently seen (more commonly in the former). The ascending aorta is usually normal in IHSS and supravalvular aortic stenosis.

C. Electrocardiography: There is some correlation between the severity of the obstruction and the ECG. Patients with mild aortic stenosis have normal ECGs. Patients with severe obstruction frequently demonstrate evidence of left ventricular hypertrophy and left ventricular strain, but many do not. In about 25% of severe cases, the ECG is normal. Progressive increase in left ventricular hypertrophy on serial ECGs indicates a significant degree of obstruction. Left ventricular strain is taken as a potential indication for operation.

D. Echocardiography: This has become a reliable noninvasive technic for the initial diagnosis and follow-up evaluation of IHSS. It also provides clues to the progression of other forms of aortic stenosis. Cross-sectional echocardiography holds promise for a more precise noninvasive method for assessment of severity of valvular disease.

E. Cardiac Catheterization and Angiocardiography: Left heart catheterization demonstrates the pressure differential between the left ventricle and the aorta and the level at which the gradient exists. Patients with severe aortic stenosis may be asymptomatic and have normal ECGs and chest x-rays. Serial cardiac catheterization is frequently the only reliable guide to the progression and the severity of the lesion. In the case of valvular aortic stenosis, an asymptomatic patient with a resting gradient of 80 mm Hg is considered to require surgery. In the face of symptoms, patients with lesser gradients are surgical candidates. Cineangiocardiography is helpful in demonstrating the level of the obstruction.

Treatment

The reason for requiring symptoms or a large resting gradient (60–80 mm Hg) before considering surgical repair of aortic stenosis is that the results of surgery are too frequently unsatisfactory. In many cases the gradient can only be moderately to minimally relieved without producing aortic insufficiency (which is potentially a worse disease than the lesion for which surgery was undertaken). The results of surgery in discrete subvalvular aortic stenosis are generally better than in valvular.

Patients for whom surgery is not strongly indicated should have close follow-up and limitation of exertion appropriate for the degree of severity (eg, competitive sports).

Beuren AJ & others: The syndrome of supravalvular aortic stenosis, peripheral pulmonary stenosis, mental retardation and similar facial appearance. Am J Cardiol 13:471, 1964.

Braunwald E & others: Idiopathic hypertrophic subaortic stenosis. 1. A description of the disease based upon an analysis of 64 patients. Circulation 30 (Suppl 4):213, 1964.

Champsaur G, Trusler GA, Mustard WT: Congenital discreet subvalvar aortic stenosis. Br Heart J 35:443, 1973.

Fisher RP, Mason DT, Morrow AG: Results of operative treatment in congenital aortic stenosis. J Thorac Cardiovasc Surg 59:218, 1970.

Friedman WF, Modlinger J, Morgan JR: Serial hemodynamic observation in asymptomatic children with valvular aortic stenosis. Circulation 43:91, 1971.

Nadas AS & others: Clinical course in aortic stenosis. Circulation 56(Suppl 1):47, 1977.

Weyman AE & others: Cross-sectional echocardiographic assessment of severity of aortic stenosis in children. Circulation 55:773, 1977.

3. OTHER CONGENITAL VALVULAR LESIONS

Congenital Mitral Stenosis

In this rare disorder, the valve leaflets are thickened and fused to produce a diaphragm-like or funnel-like structure with an opening in the center. Frequent associated malformations include patent ductus arteriosus, abnormality of the aortic valve, and coarctation of the aorta. Most patients develop symptoms early in life, though an occasional child may remain asymptomatic throughout childhood. Early symptoms include tachypnea and dyspnea, followed by right heart failure. Physical examination reveals a regular sinus rhythm. The first heart sound is accentuated, and the pulmonic closure sound is loud. No opening snap can be heard. In most cases, a presystolic crescendo murmur is heard at the apex. Occasionally, only a mid-diastolic murmur can be heard. Rarely, no murmur at all is heard. ECG shows right axis deviation, biatrial enlargement, and right ventricular hypertrophy. X-ray reveals evidence of left atrial enlargement and, frequently, pulmonary venous congestion. Echocardiography fails to reveal normal valve structures and shows reduced excursion. Cardiac catheterization reveals an elevated pulmonary capillary pressure and wedge pressure and pulmonary hypertension.

Cor Triatriatum

This is an extremely rare abnormality in which the pulmonary veins enter a separate chamber rather than pass directly into the left atrium. The chamber communicates with the left atrium through an opening of variable size. The physiologic consequences of this condition are very similar to those of mitral stenosis. The clinical findings depend upon the size of the opening. If the opening is extremely small, symptoms develop·very early in life. If the opening is large, patients may be asymptomatic for a considerable period of time. Echocardiography may reveal a hard shadow in the left atrium. Cardiac catheterization may be diagnostic. Finding a high pulmonary capillary pressure (high pulmonary venous pressure) and a low left atrial pressure (if the catheter can be passed through the foramen ovale into the true left atrial chamber) makes the diagnosis certain. Angiocardiographic studies may identify 2 "left atrial" chambers.

Surgical repair of cor triatriatum is usually successful only when the patient has reached an adequate size. The surgical mortality rate is very high in young children, but occasional successes are reported.

Congenital Mitral Regurgitation

This is a relatively rare abnormality which is usually associated with other congenital heart lesions, including corrected transposition of the great vessels, endocardial cushion defect, and endocardial fibroelastosis. Uncomplicated congenital mitral regurgitation is very rare. It is sometimes present in patients with Marfan's syndrome. Occasionally, there is a congenital dilatation of the valve ring with an otherwise normal valve. In other cases, the chordae tendineae are malformed, resulting in mitral regurgitation.

Congenital Aortic Regurgitation

The most common causes of this disorder include bicuspid aortic valve, either uncomplicated or with coarctation of the aorta; ventricular septal defect and aortic insufficiency; and fenestration of the aortic valve cusp (one or more holes in the cusp).

Absence of the Pulmonary Valve

This rare abnormality is usually associated with ventricular septal defect. In about 50% of cases, severe infundibular pulmonary stenosis is present (tetralogy of Fallot).

Ebstein's Malformation of the Tricuspid Valve

This uncommon abnormality consists of downward displacement of the tricuspid valve such that the greater portion of the valve is attached to the ventricular wall rather than to the fibrous ring. As a result, the upper portion of the right ventricle is within the right atrium. The portion of the ventricle below the apex of the tricuspid valve is very small and represents the true functioning right ventricle. Clinically, there is a wide spectrum of abnormalities ranging from relative absence of symptoms to death in early infancy. The severity depends upon the degree of malattachment of the valve and the associated abnormalities. Echocardiography is useful in diagnosis.

Dhanavaravibul S, Nora JJ, McNamara DG: Angiocardiographic signs in Ebstein's anomaly. Cardiovasc Center Bull 9:50, 1970.

Farooki ZQ, Henry JG, Green EW: Echocardiographic spectrum of Ebstein's anomaly of the tricuspid valve. Circulation 53:63, 1976.

Hardy KL, Roe BB: Ebstein's anomaly: Further experience with definitive repair. J Thorac Cardiovasc Surg 59:553, 1969.

Saigusa M & others: Tricuspid valve replacement with a preserved aortic valve homograft for Ebstein's malformation. J Thorac Cardiovasc Surg 62:55, 1971.

Shone JS & others: The developmental complex of "parachute mitral valve," supravalvular ring of left atrium, subaortic stenosis, and coarctation of aorta. Am J Cardiol 11:714, 1963.

Van Praagh R, Corsini I: Cor triatriatum. Am Heart J 78:379, 1969.

Vlad P: Mitral valve anomalies in children. Circulation 43:465, 1971.

Wolfe RR & others: Cor triatriatum: Total correction in an infant. J Thorac Cardiovasc Surg 56:114, 1968.

MYOCARDIAL DISEASES

This group of diseases is characterized by significant cardiac enlargement. Murmurs may or may not be present. ECG changes include left ventricular hypertrophy, ST depression, and T wave inversion.

1. GLYCOGEN STORAGE DISEASE OF THE HEART

At least 6 types of glycogen storage disease are recognized. The type that primarily involves the heart is known as Pompe's disease, or type II glycogenosis. In this disease there is a complete absence of 1,4-glucosidase activity at pH 4.0. This enzyme (acid maltase) is necessary for the hydrolysis of the outer branches of glycogen, and its absence results in marked deposition of glycogen within the myocardium. Cardiac glycogenosis is a rare heritable (autosomal recessive) disorder.

Affected infants are usually normal at birth, but onset usually begins by the sixth month of life. The findings usually include marked cardiac enlargement, a very large tongue (which causes feeding problems), and marked generalized muscular weakness. The liver is usually not enlarged unless there is congestive heart failure. These children usually have a history of retardation of growth and development, feeding problems, poor weight gain, and then the findings of heart failure. Physical examination reveals generalized muscular weakness, a large tongue, cardiomegaly, no significant heart murmurs, and occasionally evidence of congestive heart failure. Chest x-rays reveal marked cardiomegaly with or without pulmonary venous congestion.

ECG shows left ventricular hypertrophy and, usually, ST depression and T wave inversion over the left precordial leads. Echocardiography shows extremely thick ventricular wall structures.

Children with this disease usually die within the first year of life. Death may be sudden or due to progressive congestive heart failure.

Hernandez A Jr & others: Cardiac glycogenosis. J Pediatr 68:400, 1966.

Hohn AR & others: Cardiac problems in the glycogenoses with special reference to Pompe's disease. Pediatrics 35:313, 1965.

Lauer RM & others: Administration of a mixture of fungal glucosidases to a patient with type II glycogenosis (Pompe's disease). Pediatrics 42:672, 1968.

2. ANOMALOUS ORIGIN OF THE LEFT CORONARY ARTERY

In this condition, the left coronary artery arises from the pulmonary artery rather than from the aorta. In the neonatal period, while the pulmonary arterial pressure is relatively high, blood is supplied to the left ventricle from the pulmonary artery. Accordingly, during this period the child is asymptomatic and does well. However, within the first 2 months of life, the pulmonary arterial pressure decreases to normal. This results in a marked decrease of flow to the left coronary artery. Infarction of the heart usually occurs. If the patient survives, collateral channels appear which join the peripheral branches of the right with the branches of the left coronary artery. As a result, the direction of blood flow in the left coronary artery changes. Whereas previously there was some flow from the pulmonary artery into the myocardium through the left coronary, flow now occurs from the right coronary artery through the collateral into the left coronary artery and then into the pulmonary artery. In essence, then, an arteriovenous fistula is formed which further removes blood from the myocardium. This results in further myocardial infarction and fibrosis. Death occurs eventually as a result of marked dilatation of the heart and congestive heart failure. At autopsy, the left ventricle is found to be markedly fibrosed and thin.

Clinical Findings

A. Symptoms and Signs: These patients appear to be normal at birth. Growth and development are relatively normal for a few months, although detailed questioning of the parents often discloses a history of intermittent episodes of severe abdominal pain, pallor, and sweating, especially during or after feeding. These episodes are thought to be secondary to "colic" and attacks are similar to anginal attacks in adults.

On physical examination, the patients are usually well developed and well nourished. They show no evidence of congestive heart failure until terminally. The pulses are usually weak but equal throughout. The heart is enlarged but not very active. A murmur of mitral regurgitation is frequently present, although no murmur may be heard.

B. X-Ray Findings: Chest x-rays show significant cardiac enlargement with or without pulmonary venous congestion.

C. Electrocardiography: The ECG is usually diagnostic. There are T wave inversions in leads I and aVL. The precordial leads show T wave inversions from V_4-V_7. Deep, wide Q waves are often seen in leads I, aVL, and V_4-V_6. These findings of myocardial infarction are similar to those in adults.

D. Cardiac Catheterization and Angiocardiography: The diagnosis depends upon cardiac catheterization and cineangiocardiography. A small left-to-right shunt can often be detected at the pulmonary artery level as a result of the flow of blood from the right through the left coronary artery into the pulmonary artery. Frequently, however, the shunt is very small and can be detected only by the most sensitive technics such as the hydrogen electrode catheter. Cineangiocardiography following injection of contrast material into the root of the aorta shows absence of origin of the left coronary artery from the aorta. A huge right coronary artery fills directly from the aorta, and one can follow the contrast material through the right coronary system into the left coronary arteries. Occasionally, one can actually see the blood flowing into the pulmonary artery.

Treatment & Prognosis

Surgical transplantation of the coronary artery has been highly successful in some hands. Medical management until 4 years of age followed by vein graft anastomosis of the left coronary artery to the aorta gives the patient the security of a 2 coronary artery system. Other workers prefer ligation of the left coronary artery where it enters the pulmonary artery. The rationale for this procedure is that obstructing the flow from the left coronary artery into the pulmonary artery would drive coronary artery blood flow into the myocardium, thus improving myocardial oxygenation.

Implantation of the internal mammary artery into the detached left coronary artery and a 2-step procedure, ligating the left coronary artery as close to the pulmonary artery as possible in the sick infant and later anastomosing the left coronary artery to the aorta, are alternative methods of providing a 2 coronary artery system.

Koops B & others: Congenital coronary artery anomalies. JAMA 226:1425, 1973.

Nadas AS, Gamboa R, Hugenholtz PG: Anomalous left coronary artery originating from the pulmonary artery: Report of two surgically treated cases with a proposal of hemodynamic and therapeutic classification. Circulation 24:167, 1964.

Nora JJ & others: Medical and surgical management of anomalous origin of left coronary artery from pulmonary artery. Pediatrics 42:405, 1968.

Perry LW, Scott LP: Anomalous left coronary artery from pulmonary artery: Report of 11 cases; review of indications for and results of surgery. Circulation 41:1043, 1970.

3. ENDOCARDIAL FIBROELASTOSIS

This is a fairly common type of primary myocardial disease. The cause is not known, though it has been suggested that it might be due to intrauterine infection with mumps or coxsackievirus B. The entity occurs sporadically, and in general the incidence has decreased significantly during the past decade.

Pathologic examination discloses a marked milky white thickening of the endocardium, the subendocardial layers of the left ventricle, and usually the left atrium. The mitral valve is frequently involved also. The myocardial fibers themselves are fibrotic and disorganized, and associated hypervascularization is common. If sought for by serial sections, coexistent evidence of myocarditis is often found. Thus, endocardial fibroelastosis appears to be part of a continuum of primary endomyocardial diseases and may be a sequel to myocarditis.

Clinical Findings

A. Symptoms and Signs: These patients appear normal at birth, and growth and development during early infancy are normal. About half develop symptoms within the first 5 months of life, and most are symptomatic by age 1. An occasional patient may have no symptoms until age 5.

The symptoms and signs that do develop are associated with left ventricular heart failure. These include dyspnea, easy fatigability, feeding difficulties, and, eventually, findings of left and right heart failure.

On physical examination, these children are often small and undernourished. The heart is usually enlarged, and the heart tones are poor (when there is evidence of decompensation). A murmur of mitral regurgitation may be present.

B. X-Ray Findings: Chest x-rays show generalized cardiac enlargement with or without pulmonary venous congestion.

C. Electrocardiography: The ECG almost always shows evidence of left ventricular hypertrophy and, quite frequently, ST depression and T wave inversion. If there has been pulmonary hypertension secondary to left heart failure, right ventricular hypertrophy may be present. Right atrial hypertrophy is sometimes present. Complete heart block is occasionally seen.

D. Cardiac Catheterization and Angiocardiography: Catheterization reveals the absence of left-to-right shunts. Pulmonary hypertension may be present. Cineangiocardiography demonstrates diminished myocardial contractility.

Treatment & Prognosis

The treatment of this disease is medical. Early

and vigorous treatment of cardiac failure is essential. There appears to be a definite correlation between favorable outcome and early onset of treatment.

The most important part of the treatment consists of adequate and prolonged digitalis administration with the administration of chronic oral diuretics such as furosemide plus spironolactone. If the response to the usual dose is not satisfactory, the dose of both digitalis and diuretics should be increased until a satisfactory response is noted or toxicity occurs. These agents should be continued for several years.

In some cases, the child appears to improve initially but then develops recurrent bouts of heart failure. Complete recovery in such patients is very infrequent, and most eventually die with intractable congestive heart failure. The prognosis is most favorable in patients presenting between 6 months and 3 years who respond promptly to treatment.

Gersony WM, Katz SL, Nadas AS: Endocardial fibroelastosis and the mumps virus. Pediatrics 37:430, 1966.

Hastreiter AR, Miller RA: Management of primary endomyocardial disease: The myocarditis-endocardial fibroelastosis syndrome. Pediatr Clin North Am 11:401, 1964.

Hunter AS, Keay AJ: Primary endocardial fibroelastosis. Arch Dis Child 48:66, 1973.

Manning JA & others: The medical management of clinical endocardial fibroelastosis. Circulation 29:60, 1964.

MUCOCUTANEOUS LYMPH NODE SYNDROME

This syndrome was first described a decade ago in Japan and is relatively common there. Recently, small series are being reported in North America. Some of these infants have coronary artery involvement, including arteritis, aneurysms, thrombosis, occlusion, infarction, and death. The syndrome shares some features with juvenile rheumatoid arthritis, but the coronary artery disease most closely resembles infantile polyarteritis nodosa. When coronary arteritis is suspected on the basis of the ECG or coronary arteriography, steroids are recommended.

Brown JS & others: Mucocutaneous lymph node syndrome in the continental United States. J Pediatr 88:81, 1976.

Glanz S & others: Regression of coronary artery aneurysms in infantile polyarteritis nodosa. N Engl J Med 294:939, 1976.

Kawasaki T: Mucocutaneous lymph node syndrome: Clinical observation in 50 cases. Jpn J Allerg 16:178, 1967.

Kegel SM & others: Cardiac death in mucocutaneous lymph node syndrome. Am J Cardiol 40:282, 1977.

II. CYANOTIC HEART DISEASE

TETRALOGY OF FALLOT

In Fallot's tetralogy, there is a ventricular septal defect and severe obstruction to right ventricular outflow such that the intracardiac shunt is predominantly from right to left. This is the most common type of cyanotic heart lesion, accounting for 10–15% of all cases of congenital heart disease. The ventricular defect is usually located in the membranous portion of the septum but may be totally surrounded by muscular tissue and is usually quite large. Obstruction to right ventricular outflow may be solely at the infundibular level (50–75%), at the valvular level alone (rarely), or at both levels (30%). The term tetralogy has been used to describe this combination of lesions since there is always associated right ventricular hypertrophy and a varying degree of "overriding of the aorta." The overriding is present because of the position of the ventricular septal defect in relation to a dilated and often dextroposed aorta. These 2 factors (right ventricular hypertrophy and overriding aorta) plus the major lesions make up the tetralogy. A right-sided aortic arch is present in 25% of cases and an atrial septal defect in 15%.

Severe obstruction to right ventricular outflow plus a large ventricular septal defect results in a right-to-left shunt at the ventricular level and desaturation of the arterial blood. The degree of desaturation and the extent of cyanosis depend upon the size of the shunt. This in turn is dependent upon the resistance to outflow from the right ventricle, the size of the ventricular septal defect, and the systemic vascular resistance. The greater the obstruction, the larger the ventricular septal defect, and the lower the systemic vascular resistance, the greater the right-to-left shunt. Although the patient may be deeply cyanotic, the amount of pressure the right ventricle can develop is limited to that of the systemic (aortic) pressure. In other words, right ventricular pressure cannot exceed left ventricular pressure. The right ventricle is usually quite able to maintain this level of pressure without developing heart failure.

Clinical Findings

A. Symptoms and Signs: The clinical findings vary depending upon the degree of right ventricular outflow obstruction. Patients with a mild degree of obstruction are only minimally cyanotic or acyanotic; those with maximal obstruction are deeply cyanotic from birth. However, few children are asymptomatic; most have cyanosis by 4 months of age; and the cyanosis usually is progressive. Growth and development are retarded, and easy fatigability and dyspnea on exertion are common. Squatting is very common when the children become old enough to walk.

Hypoxemic spells (cyanotic spells) are characterized by the following signs and symptoms: (1) Sudden onset of cyanosis or deepening of cyanosis; (2) sudden onset of dyspnea; (3) alterations in consciousness, encompassing a spectrum from irritability to syncope; and (4) decrease in intensity or disappearance of the systolic murmur. These episodes may begin in the neonatal period and continue until nearly school age. It is unusual, however, for the initial episode to occur after 2 years of age. Acute treatment of cyanotic spells consists of giving oxygen and placing the patient in the knee-chest position. Acidosis, if present, should be corrected with intravenous sodium bicarbonate. Morphine sulfate should be administered cautiously by a parenteral route in a dosage of 0.1 mg/kg. Propranolol, 0.1−0.2 mg/kg IV, has recently been found to be useful. Chronic (daily) treatment of cyanotic spells with propranolol, 1 mg/kg orally every 4 hours while awake, remains controversial, but in a significant number of patients this regimen has prevented subsequent "spells" and made it possible to delay operation until total correction can be performed.

Patients with tetralogy are usually small and thin. The degree of cyanosis is variable. The fingers and toes show varying degrees of clubbing depending upon the age of the child and the severity of the cyanosis.

On examination of the heart, a right ventricular lift is palpable. No thrills are present. The first sound is normal; occasionally there is an ejection click at the apex which is aortic in origin. The second sound is single and best heard at the lower left sternal border between the third and fourth intercostal spaces. The second heart sound at the pulmonary area is soft; however, aortic closure is loud and heard best in the third and fourth intercostal spaces at the left sternal border. There is a grade I−III/VI, rough, ejection type systolic murmur which is maximal at the left sternal border in the third intercostal space. This murmur radiates over the anterior and posterior lung fields. Diastolic murmurs are not present.

B. X-Ray Findings: Chest x-rays reveal the overall heart size to be normal, and indeed the x-ray may sometimes be interpreted as being entirely normal. However, the right ventricle is hypertrophied, and this is often shown in the posteroanterior projection by an upturning of the apex (boot-shaped heart). The main pulmonary artery segment is usually concave, and the aorta in 25% of cases arches to the right. The pulmonary vascular markings are usually decreased.

C. Electrocardiography and Echocardiography: The cardiac axis is to the right, ranging from +90 to +180 degrees. The P waves are usually normal, although there may be evidence of slight right atrial hypertrophy. Right ventricular hypertrophy is always present, but right ventricular strain patterns are rare. An enlarged aorta overriding the septum will often be detected by echocardiography.

D. Laboratory Findings: The hemoglobin, hematocrit, and red blood count are usually mildly to markedly elevated, depending upon the degree of arterial oxygen desaturation. (But see Complications, below.)

E. Cardiac Catheterization and Angiocardiogra- phy: Cardiac catheterization reveals the absence of a significant left-to-right shunt, although the hydrogen electrode curve may be positive in the right ventricle. There is arterial blood desaturation of varying degree. The right-to-left shunt exists at the ventricular level. The right ventricular pressure is at systemic levels, and the pressure contour in the right ventricle is almost identical with that of the left ventricle. The pulmonary artery pressure is extremely low (mean ranges of 5−10 mm Hg). The gradients and pressure may be noted at the valvular level, the infundibular level, or both. The catheter frequently is passed from the right ventricle into the overriding ascending aorta.

Cineangiocardiography is diagnostic. Injection of contrast material into the right ventricle reveals the right ventricular outflow obstruction and the right-to-left shunt at the ventricular level.

Complications

A. Cerebral Infarction: Brain infarction is not uncommon. The cause varies somewhat depending upon the age of the child. Within the first 2 years of life, it is thought that the major cause of cerebral infarction is anoxia, which results from the marked arterial blood desaturation and the relative iron deficiency anemia that exists in many of these young infants.

Children with a hematocrit under 55% may be liable to the development of an anemic, anoxic infarction. This is much less common over age 2 years, when iron deficiency is less of a problem. Therefore, all children should be followed with a hemoglobin, hematocrit, and red blood count determination. If there is evidence of significant iron deficiency, these patients should be given oral iron therapy.

In older children, cerebral infarction is usually due to ischemia, making the primary therapeutic consideration one of surgically increasing pulmonary blood flow. When the hematocrit rises above 75%, the viscosity of the blood markedly increases and the possibility of thrombotic infarction also develops, making phlebotomy a second but less desirable alternative.

B. Brain Abscess: Children over 2 years of age with tetralogy of Fallot who develop CNS symptoms—especially brain damage—should be considered to have brain abscess until proved otherwise. Brain abscess is now thought to develop in areas of previous infarction which may be microscopic in size. Because of the presence of the right-to-left shunt, bacteria which usually are filtered out by the lungs can pass into the systemic circulation and hence to the area of infarction in the brain. Common presenting symptoms are those of an expanding intracranial mass. There is usually a history of a respiratory infection 1−2 weeks prior to the onset of neurologic symptoms. Treatment consists of antibiotics and, usually, surgical removal of the abscess.

Treatment

A. Palliative Treatment: Palliative treatment is recommended for very small infants who are markedly symptomatic (severely cyanotic, frequent severe anoxic spells) in whom complete correction would be difficult or impossible. It may be medical (chronic oral beta-blocking agents) or, more often, surgical (creation of a systemic arterial to pulmonary arterial anastomosis).

The earliest procedure employed for this disease (Blalock-Taussig) consisted of an anastomosis between the subclavian artery and the pulmonary artery. It is usually done on the side opposite the aortic arch. Another commonly employed anastomotic technic (Potts procedure) anastomoses the descending thoracic aorta to the left pulmonary artery. It is employed in very young infants, in whom the subclavian artery is too small for a sufficient opening. It should not be used in older infants because too large an anastomosis will result in a very large sudden increase in pulmonary blood flow and left heart failure. Furthermore, it is much more difficult to "take down" a Potts operation, which is necessary before complete correction can be undertaken.

The procedure most utilized currently is construction of an anastomosis between the ascending aorta and the right pulmonary artery (Waterston anastomosis). This procedure permits the formation of a large anastomosis and is relatively easy to take down prior to complete correction. It has the same disadvantage as the Potts procedure, ie, it is possible to create too large an opening with resultant left heart failure. Finally, an anastomosis between the ascending aorta and the main pulmonary artery may be performed.

B. Total Correction: Total correction of tetralogy of Fallot is performed under cardiopulmonary bypass. It involves opening the right ventricle, closing the ventricular septal defect, and removing the obstruction to right ventricular outflow. The surgical mortality varies from 2–15%. There seems to be a definite correlation between the severity of the disease and the mortality rate. Children who survive the operation are markedly improved. There is complete disappearance of cyanosis, and clubbing disappears shortly thereafter. Growth and development improve markedly, and these patients often become asymptomatic within a short period of time. Currently, major cardiovascular centers are performing total correction for virtually all infants with this condition, including neonates. It is somewhat discouraging to note that even with good functional result from total repair in infancy or early childhood, a significant number of patients are subject to exercise disability or sudden death due to arrhythmias.

Course & Prognosis

Infants with the most severe form of the disease are usually deeply cyanotic at birth. Anoxic spells may occur during the neonatal period. Death may occur during a severe anoxic spell. Many patients who survive the first year of life seem to improve. This may be due to the development of bronchial collateral vessels. Although anoxic spells may decrease in severity, these children remain deeply cyanotic and markedly limited in their activity. They seldom survive the second decade of life without surgical treatment.

Infants with moderate obstruction to right ventricular outflow do fairly well. Although cyanosis is present in very early life, it is usually not severe. The cyanosis may progress in severity, and anoxic spells may occur. These patients do fairly well in later childhood, but their condition progressively deteriorates during the second and third decades of life. Death occurs by the third decade as a result of cerebrovascular accidents, brain abscess, subacute bacterial endocarditis, anoxia, or pulmonary hemorrhage.

Patients with the mildest form of the disease are said to have the "acyanotic" variety. The degree of obstruction is very mild, and the right-to-left shunt is small. Very frequently, there is a predominant left-to-right shunt. However, as the patient gets older the degree of obstruction often increases. This, combined with the increased activity, results in progressively worsening cyanosis. Many of these patients live relatively normal lives without severe symptoms. Life expectancy, however, is definitely decreased, and death usually occurs by the third to fourth decade.

Bonchek LI & others: Natural history of tetralogy of Fallot in infancy: Clinical classification and therapeutic implications. Circulation 48:392, 1973.

Cole RB & others: Longer-term results following aorto-pulmonary anastomosis for tetralogy of Fallot: Morbidity and mortality. Circulation 43:263, 1971.

Eriksson BO, Thoren C, Zetterquist P: Long-term treatment with propranolol in selected cases of Fallot's tetralogy. Br Heart J 31:37, 1969.

Guntheroth WG & others: Venous return with knee-chest position and squatting in tetralogy of Fallot. Am Heart J 75:313, 1968.

James FW & others: Response to exercise in patients after total correction of tetralogy of Fallot. Circulation 54:671, 1976.

Ponce FE & others: Propranolol palliation of tetralogy of Fallot. Pediatrics 52:100, 1973.

Quattlebaum TG & others: Sudden death among postoperative patients with tetralogy of Fallot. Circulation 54:289, 1976.

Rosenquist GG & others: Ventricular septal defect in tetralogy of Fallot. Am J Cardiol 31:749, 1973.

PULMONARY ATRESIA WITH VENTRICULAR SEPTAL DEFECT

This condition consists of complete atresia of the pulmonary valve in association with ventricular septal defect. Essentially it is an extreme form of tetralogy of Fallot. Since there is no flow outward from the right ventricle into the pulmonary artery, the pulmonary blood flow must be derived either from a patent ductus arteriosus or from collateral channels.

The clinical picture depends entirely upon the size of the ductus or the collateral channels (or both). If they are large, patients may do quite well and actually do better than those with severe tetralogy of

Fallot. If effective pulmonary blood flow is small, death occurs secondary to severe anoxia early in life. This may occur suddenly with postnatal closure of a patent ductus arteriosus.

Cardiac catheterization and angiocardiography are diagnostic.

Infants who are severely hypoxemic require urgent systemic/pulmonary anastomosis in order to provide sufficient oxygenated blood to the body.

A corrective surgical procedure has been developed recently which has been successful in patients with adequate-sized pulmonary arteries. It consists of bypassing the obstructed right ventricular outflow and closing the ventricular septal defect.

Bernhard WF & others: Ascending aorta-right pulmonary artery shunt in infants and older patients with certain types of cyanotic congenital heart disease. Circulation 43:580, 1971.

Edwards JE, McGoon DC: Absence of anatomic origin from heart of pulmonary arterial supply. Circulation 47:393, 1973.

Kouchoukos NT & others: Surgical treatment of congenital pulmonary atresia with ventricular septal defects. J Thorac Cardiovasc Surg 61:70, 1971.

Mustard WT, Bedard P, Trusler GA: Cardiovascular surgery in the first year of life. J Thorac Cardiovasc Surg 59:761, 1970.

Olin CL & others: Pulmonary atresia: Surgical considerations and results in 103 patients undergoing definitive repair. Circulation 54(Suppl 3):35, 1976.

PULMONARY ATRESIA WITH INTACT VENTRICULAR SEPTUM

In this relatively rare condition, the pulmonary valve is absent and is replaced by a small diaphragm consisting of the fused cusps. The ventricular septum is intact. The main pulmonary artery segment is somewhat hypoplastic but almost always patent. In the type 1 deformity (80%), the cavity volume of the right ventricle is extremely small and the wall is thickened and fibrotic. In type 2, the right ventricular cavity is frequently of normal size.

During intrauterine life, if the tricuspid valve is intact and normal, very little blood enters the right ventricle since there is no outlet for this chamber. Almost all of the blood passes through the foramen ovale directly into the left side of the heart. In the type 2 deformity, there is usually an outlet for the right ventricle (tricuspid valve insufficiency) and the right ventricle receives a sufficient quantity of blood to permit it to develop in a relatively normal fashion.

Following birth, the pulmonary circulation is maintained primarily by a patent ductus arteriosus. Although a bronchial pulmonary collateral network is present, it is usually insufficient to maintain the pulmonary circulation. Accordingly, whether or not these patients live depends upon the patency of the ductus

arteriosus. The ductus usually remains open for only a short period of time. As it closes, hypoxia becomes progressively more severe and death eventually occurs.

Clinical Findings

A. Symptoms and Signs: These patients may be normal at birth, although they are usually cyanotic. Cyanosis becomes progressively more severe and is associated with severe dyspnea. A blowing systolic murmur may be heard at the pulmonary area and under the left clavicle due to the associated patent ductus arteriosus. In type 2 deformity, a loud pansystolic murmur due to the tricuspid insufficiency is heard at the lower left sternal border. Not infrequently, the liver is pulsating.

B. X-Ray Findings: Chest x-rays show a markedly enlarged heart with marked decrease in pulmonary vascular markings. With striking tricuspid insufficiency, right atrial enlargement may be massive and the cardiac silhouette may virtually fill the chest.

C. Electrocardiography: ECG reveals an axis which is usually normal in the frontal plane. Evidence for right atrial enlargement is usually striking. Voltage criteria for other chamber enlargement are variable.

D. Cardiac Catheterization and Angiocardiography: The diagnosis can be made on cardiac catheterization and cineangiocardiography. Right ventricular pressure is very high (greater than systemic). A cineangiocardiogram following injection of contrast material into the right ventricle reveals absence of filling of the pulmonary artery from the right ventricle. It also demonstrates the size of the right ventricular chamber and the presence or absence of tricuspid regurgitation, and right ventricular sinusoids may fill which drain into the coronary arteries.

Treatment & Prognosis

Surgery should be undertaken as soon as the diagnosis is made. Following the diagnostic aspect of the cardiac catheterization, a Rashkind atrial septostomy is performed. This opens up the communication across the atrial septum and permits adequate flow in both directions. The patient is then taken to the operating room immediately. The current procedure consists of a transventricular pulmonary valvotomy followed by an ascending aorta to right pulmonary artery anastomosis. The latter procedure is performed to ensure adequate blood flow to the lungs, since right ventricular performance (even in type 2) is poor in the immediate postoperative period. Infusion with prostaglandin E_1 to maintain patency of the ductus until surgery can be performed is currently being evaluated.

If the patient survives the surgery, the prognosis is unpredictable for type 1 or type 2 patients. The right ventricular dimensions of type 1 patients can increase significantly after the initial procedures.

Arom KV, Edwards JE: Relationship between right ventricular muscle bundles and pulmonary valve. Circulation 54(Suppl 3):79, 1976.

Dhanavaravibul S, Nora JJ, McNamara DG: Pulmonary valvular

atresia with intact ventricular septum: Problems in diagnosis and results of treatment. J Pediatr 77:1010, 1970.

Hallman GL, Cooley DA: Cardiovascular surgery in newborn infants: Results in 1050 patients less than one year old. Ann Surg 173:1007, 1971.

Miller GAH & others: Pulmonary atresia with intact septum and critical pulmonary stenosis presenting in first month of life. Br Heart J 35:9, 1973.

Neutze JM & others: Palliation of cyanotic congenital heart disease in infancy with E-type prostaglandins. Circulation 55:238, 1977.

Tousler GA, Fowler RS: The surgical management of pulmonary atresia with intact ventricular septum and hypoplastic right ventricle. J Thorac Cardiovasc Surg 59:740, 1970.

TRICUSPID ATRESIA

Essentials of Diagnosis

- Marked cyanosis from birth.
- Electrocardiogram with left axis deviation.

General Considerations

This relatively rare condition (< 1% of cases of congenital heart disease) is characterized by complete atresia of the tricuspid valve. As a result, no direct communication exists between the right atrium and right ventricle.

Tricuspid atresia may be divided into 2 types depending upon the relationship of the great vessels:

Type 1. Without transposition of the great arteries (70%): (a) No ventricular septal defect. Hypoplasia or atresia of the pulmonary artery. Patent ductus arteriosus. (b) Small ventricular septal defect. Pulmonary stenosis. Hypoplastic pulmonary artery. (c) Large ventricular septal defect and no pulmonary stenosis. Normal-sized pulmonary artery.

Type 2. With transposition of the great arteries (30%): (a) With ventricular septal defect and pulmonary stenosis. (b) With ventricular septal defect but without pulmonary stenosis.

Since there is no direct communication between the right atrium and right ventricle, the entire systemic venous return must flow through the atrial septum (either an atrial septal defect or patent foramen ovale) into the left atrium. Accordingly, the left atrium receives both the systemic venous return and the pulmonary venous return. Complete mixing occurs in the left atrium, resulting in a greater or lesser degree of arterial desaturation.

As a result of this lack of direct communication, the development of the ventricle depends upon the presence of a left-to-right shunt at the ventricular level. Therefore, severe hypoplasia of the right ventricle occurs in those forms in which there is no ventricular septal defect or in which the ventricular septal defect is very small.

Clinical Findings

A. Symptoms and Signs: In the great majority of patients with tricuspid atresia, symptoms develop very early in infancy. Except in cases in which the pulmonary blood flow is great, cyanosis is present at birth. Growth and development are very poor, and there is usually easy fatigability on feeding, tachypnea, dyspnea, anoxic spells, and evidence of right heart failure. Patients with marked increase in pulmonary blood flow (types 1c and 2b) will develop evidence of left heart failure as well.

Clubbing is present if the child is old enough. On examination of the heart, a slight bulge on the right side of the sternum may occasionally be seen. The first heart sound is normal. The second heart sound is most often single (due to aortic closure). A murmur is usually present, although it is variable. It ranges from grade I–III/VI in intensity and usually is a harsh blowing murmur heard best at the lower left sternal border.

B. X-Ray Findings: Chest x-rays are variable. The heart may be slightly to markedly enlarged. The main pulmonary artery segment is usually small or absent. The size of the right atrium varies from huge to only moderately enlarged, depending upon the size of the communication at the atrial level. The pulmonary vascular markings are usually decreased, although in types 1c and 2b they are increased.

C. Electrocardiography: The ECG is usually helpful. It often shows a left axis deviation with a counterclockwise loop in the frontal plane. The P waves are tall and peaked, indicative of right atrial hypertrophy. The size of the P wave depends upon the right atrial pressure, which in turn depends upon the size of the interatrial communication (the taller the P wave, the smaller the communication). Left ventricular hypertrophy or left ventricular preponderance is found in almost all cases. Voltage over the right precordium is usually low.

D. Cardiac Catheterization and Angiocardiography: This reveals the marked right-to-left shunt at the atrial level and desaturation of the left atrial blood. Because of the complete mixing in the left atrial chambers, oxygen saturation in the left ventricle, right ventricle, pulmonary artery, and aorta is identical to that in the left atrium. The right atrial pressure is increased. Left ventricular and systemic pressures are normal. The catheter cannot be passed through the tricuspid valve from the right atrium to the right ventricle. The course of the catheter is always from right atrium into left atrium and from there into left ventricle.

Cineangiocardiography following injection of contrast material into the right atrium is diagnostic. It reveals the lack of communication of the right atrium with the right ventricle and the right-to-left shunt at the atrial level.

Treatment

The treatment of tricuspid atresia is surgical. A new "corrective" procedure connecting the right atrium with the pulmonary arteries is currently being evaluated. Palliative procedures include: (1) systemic arterial to pulmonary arterial anastomosis (Blalock-Taussig, Potts procedure, and Waterston shunt) and (2) anastomosis of the superior vena cava to the right pulmonary artery (Glenn procedure). These procedures should be employed only in patients whose pulmonary blood flow is markedly decreased and in whom cyanosis is severe.

Course & Prognosis

The outcome depends on achieving a balance of pulmonary blood flow which permits adequate oxygenation of the tissues without producing intractable congestive heart failure.

Bargeron LM & others: Late deterioration of patients after superior vena cava to right pulmonary artery anastomosis. Am J Cardiol 30:211, 1972.

Fontan F, Baudet E: Surgical repair of tricuspid atresia. Thorax 26:240, 1971.

Hallman GL, Stasnez R, Cooley DA: Surgical treatment of tricuspid atresia. J Cardiovasc Surg 9:154, 1968.

Marcano BA & others: Tricuspid atresia with increased pulmonary blood flow: An analysis of 13 cases. Circulation 40:399, 1969.

Tatooles CJ & others: Operative repair of tricuspid atresia. Ann Thorac Surg 21:499, 1976.

HYPOPLASTIC LEFT HEART SYNDROME

This not uncommon syndrome includes a number of conditions in which there are either valvular or vascular lesions on the left side of the heart, resulting in hypoplasia of the left ventricle.

The lesions that make up this syndrome are mitral atresia, aortic atresia, or both. In all of these conditions, there is severe obstruction to either filling or emptying of the left ventricle. As a result, during intrauterine life, the quantity of blood filling the left ventricle is extremely small, resulting in hypoplasia of this chamber. Following birth, there is marked impairment of the circulation because of the very small size of the left ventricle and the obstructing lesions. Congestive heart failure develops rapidly, in most cases within several days to 3 months of life.

Patients with aortic atresia develop congestive heart failure very early, usually within the first week. Death occurs earliest in this group. Patients with mitral atresia who have large atrial and ventricular communications may live longer. Some patients have lived beyond the first decade. Patients with involvement of the aortic arch usually die within 1 month or less.

The clinical picture depends upon the type of obstructing lesion. Cyanosis is usually present early in life and is usually generalized. Patients with hypoplasia or atresia of the aortic arch may show differential cyanosis. Murmurs may or may not be present and are usually nondiagnostic. Congestive heart failure develops early.

Chest x-rays usually are relatively normal at birth. Rapid and progressive cardiac enlargement then occurs, frequently associated with pulmonary venous conges-

tion. These changes occur earliest in patients with aortic atresia.

The ECG usually demonstrates right axis deviation, right atrial hypertrophy, and right ventricular hypertrophy with relative paucity of left ventricular forces and absence of a q wave in V_6.

Echocardiography is usually diagnostic and eliminates the need for cardiac catheterization. A diminutive aorta and left ventricle with a poorly defined mitral valve in the presence of a normal and easily definable tricuspid valve is diagnostic.

Beckman CB, Miller JH, Edwards JE: Alternate pathways to pulmonary venous flow in left-sided obstructive anomalies. Circulation 52:509, 1975.

Krovetz LJ, Rowe D, Shiebler GL: Hemodynamics of aortic valve atresia. Circulation 42:953, 1970.

Meyer RA, Kaplan S: Echocardiography in the diagnosis of hypoplasia of the left or right ventricles in the neonate. Circulation 46:55, 1972.

Sared A, Folger GM: Hypoplastic left heart syndrome. Am J Cardiol 29:190, 1972.

COMPLETE TRANSPOSITION OF THE GREAT ARTERIES

Complete transposition of the great vessels is the second most common variety of cyanotic congenital heart disease, accounting for about 16% of all cases. The male/female ratio is 3:1. It is due to an embryologic abnormality in the spiral division of the truncus arteriosus.

The aorta is located anterior to the pulmonary artery—directly anterior, or to the left or right. The pulmonary artery usually ascends parallel to the aorta rather than crosses it. In most cases, associated intracardiac abnormalities are present. These include ventricular septal defect, atrial septal defect, pulmonary stenosis, and patent ductus arteriosus. Obstructive changes within the pulmonary arteriolar bed are common in patients past infancy.

Transposition of the great vessels can be classified as follows:

Group 1. Transposition with intact ventricular septum: (a) Without pulmonary stenosis and (b) with pulmonary stenosis, subvalvular or valvular (or both).

Group 2. Transposition with ventricular septal defect: (a) With pulmonary stenosis, (b) with pulmonary vascular obstruction, (c) without pulmonary vascular obstruction (normal pulmonary vascular resistance).

Since the aorta arises directly from the right ventricle, life would not be possible unless there were mixing between the systemic and pulmonary circulations; oxygenated blood from the pulmonary veins must in some way reach the systemic arterial circuit. In patients with intact ventricular septum (group 1), mixing occurs at the atrial and also at the ductal level. However, in most cases these communications are small, and the ductus arteriosus often closes shortly after birth. These patients are therefore severely cyanotic, and congestive heart failure occurs rapidly as a result of the marked increase in cardiac output. Patients with a ventricular septal defect show greater or lesser degrees of cyanosis depending upon the ratio of the pulmonary to systemic blood flow. Patients with ventricular septal defect and pulmonary stenosis (group 2b) are usually severely cyanotic because of the limited blood flow to the lungs. Patients with ventricular septal defect and pulmonary vascular obstruction (group 2b) show a moderate degree of cyanosis. Patients with ventricular septal defect and normal pulmonary vascular resistance (group 2c) show the least cyanosis but often develop heart failure very early because of the enormous pulmonary blood flow.

Congestive heart failure develops not only because of the high cardiac output but also because of the poor oxygenation of the myocardium and the presence of systemic pressure in both ventricles.

Clinical Findings

A. Symptoms and Signs: Many of the neonates are quite large, some weighing 4 kg (9 lb) at birth, and most are cyanotic at birth although cyanosis occasionally does not develop until later. Patients in groups 1 and 2a are most cyanotic; those in group 2c are least cyanotic. Retardation of growth and development after the neonatal period is common. Congestive heart failure occurs in patients in groups 1 and 2c. Patients in group 2a show no evidence of congestive heart failure but often have severe anoxic spells in early life; if they survive the first year of life, retardation of growth and development is common and cyanosis becomes progressively more severe. However, intellectual development may be unaffected.

Although these infants are usually large at birth, growth and development is retarded, so that when they reach age 6 months to 1 year they are usually below the third percentile in both height and weight. Cyanosis is marked. Clubbing is present in children over age 1. The findings on cardiovascular examination depend somewhat upon the intracardiac defects. Group 1a patients have only soft murmurs or none at all. The first heart sound is usually normal. The second heart sound is single and accentuated and is best heard at the lower left sternal border. Patients in group 1b have loud obstructive systolic murmurs which are maximal at the second and third intercostal spaces and the left sternal border, radiating well to the first and second intercostal spaces. Group 2a patients have a murmur of pulmonary stenosis (obstructive systolic murmur at the base of the heart, best heard to the right of the sternum). Those in group 2c have a systolic murmur along the lower sternal border and a mitral diastolic flow murmur at the apex.

B. X-Ray Findings: In the sick, blue newborn, at a time when any diagnostic clues are greatly appreciated, the chest x-ray in transposition is often very nonspecific. In fact, at any age, the so-called characteristic findings may be lacking.

1. Group 1a—The heart may have the characteristic appearance of an egg on a string. Pulmonary vascular markings are usually recognized as being increased.

2. Group 1b—Pulmonary vascular markings may be normal, slightly increased, or slightly decreased. The heart is moderately enlarged.

3. Group 2a—The x-ray appearance is almost identical to that seen in tetralogy of Fallot. There is a concave pulmonary artery segment. The pulmonary vascular markings are either at the lower limits of normal or decreased in size.

4. Group 2b—X-ray shows slight cardiac enlargement. The pulmonary vascular markings are prominent at the hilum and decreased in the periphery.

5. Group 2c—There is marked cardiac enlargement involving all 4 chambers. The pulmonary artery segment might be slightly larger than normal. The pulmonary vascular markings are markedly increased.

C. Electrocardiography and Echocardiography: Early in infancy, the ECG is usually of little positive help. It reveals the usual amount of right ventricular hypertrophy expected for age. The absence of positive findings of other lesions, such as left axis deviation of tricuspid atresia, provides some deductive information. Abnormal relationships of the great vessels by echo are suggestive of a lesion in the transposition group.

D. Cardiac Catheterization and Angiocardiography: Cardiac catheterization has a dual purpose in this malformation: diagnosis and therapy. The sequence is usually to enter the right ventricle and immediately record a contrast medium injection on videotape and ciné. As soon as the cardiologist has confidently demonstrated that complete transposition of the great arteries exists and that there are 2 well-developed ventricles, a Rashkind septostomy is performed.

Treatment

It has become increasingly apparent at many pediatric cardiology centers throughout the world that survival of patients with transposition of the great arteries depends on early, aggressive management.

A. Cardiac Catheterization: A catheterization routine that can be recommended for all types of transposition is as follows:

1. Newborn—Diagnostic and therapeutic cardiac catheterization should be performed as soon as the patient achieves as much stability as the clinical course indicates he will achieve. The therapeutic part of the catheterization is, of course, the Rashkind balloon septostomy, which enlarges the atrial septal communication by repeatedly pulling a dye-filled balloon across the foramen ovale, tearing the septum.

2. 4–6 months—Repeat catheterization with catheterization of the pulmonary artery (to assess progression of pulmonary vascular obstruction), determination of the presence or absence of left ventricular outflow obstruction, and repeat Rashkind septostomy if indicated.

3. 8–10 months—Repeat catheterization if definitive surgery has not taken place before this time.

B. Complete Surgical Correction:

1. Elective surgery—All patients with favorable anatomic and hemodynamic criteria for a Mustard correction should be offered such surgery before 1 year of age. The Mustard operation involves complete removal of the atrial septum with creation of a new septum that directs the systemic venous return into the pulmonary ventricle and the pulmonary venous return into the aortic ventricle.

2. Early surgery—Certain patients, especially those with rapidly rising pulmonary artery pressures (with or without ventricular septal defect) and those with rapidly progressing left ventricular outflow obstruction may require surgical intervention as early as 4–6 months of age (after the second cardiac catheterization). It is also not uncommon for a ventricular septal defect to close spontaneously and deprive the transposition patient of mixing, on which he had been relying. A patent ductus arteriosus has not proved to be an asset. Its presence accelerates rising pulmonary vascular resistance, and its spontaneous closure may disastrously disrupt the delicate balance of mixing.

3. Late surgery—Some patients, especially those in group 2b, with ventricular septal defect and pulmonary stenosis, may have had early or relatively late development of severe left ventricular-pulmonary outflow obstruction which is not ideally amenable to Mustard correction but may be more suitable for a Rastelli operation (an aortic homograft from left ventricle to pulmonary arteries).

4. Palliative surgical correction—Open atrial septectomy and aortopulmonary shunts may be used under special circumstances, but the trend is to perform early total correction whenever possible.

Azziz KU, Paul MH, Rowe RD: Bronchopulmonary circulation in *d*-transposition of the great arteries: Possible role in genesis of accelerated pulmonary vascular disease. Am J Cardiol 39:432, 1977.

Champsaur GL & others: Repair of transposition of the great arteries in 123 pediatric patients. Circulation 47:1032, 1973.

Dillon JL & others: Echocardiographic manifestations of D-transposition of the great vessels. Am J Cardiol 32:74, 1973.

Mustard WT & others: Surgical management of transposition of the great vessels. J Thorac Cardiovasc Surg 48:953, 1964.

Rashkind WJ, Miller WW: Transposition of the great arteries: Results of balloon atrio-septostomy in 31 infants. Circulation 38:453, 1968.

Rastelli GC & others: Anatomic correction of transposition of the great arteries with ventricular septal defect and subpulmonary stenosis. J Thorac Cardiovasc Surg 58:545, 1969.

ORIGIN OF BOTH GREAT VESSELS FROM THE RIGHT VENTRICLE

In this rare malformation, the aorta is completely transposed but the pulmonary artery occupies a relatively normal position. Accordingly, both great vessels arise from the right ventricle. Ventricular septal defect is present in all cases and provides the only outlet for the left ventricle.

This malformation may be divided into 2 types depending on the presence or absence of valvular pulmonary stenosis.

With Pulmonary Stenosis

Patients with double outlet right ventricle and valvular pulmonary stenosis function very much like those with severe tetralogy of Fallot. There is marked decrease in pulmonary blood flow and marked desaturation of the systemic arterial blood.

Early palliative treatment involves the construction of a systemic to pulmonary artery anastomosis in order to increase pulmonary blood flow. Definitive surgical correction is now being successfully employed in selected patients.

Without Pulmonary Stenosis

When the pulmonary valve is normal and there is no obstruction to flow into the pulmonary artery, the condition may be difficult to differentiate from a large ventricular septal defect with normal origin of the great vessels. Because of the marked increase in pulmonary blood flow, arterial blood saturation is usually around 90% and cyanosis is absent. The diagnosis is usually made by cardiac catheterization and angiocardiography. In some cases the diagnosis is made at surgery.

Treatment consists of total correction, which is moderately risky but can be done if the diagnosis is made prior to surgery.

Bharati S, Lev M: The conduction system in double outlet right ventricle with subpulmonic ventricular septal defect and related hearts (Taussig-Bing group). Circulation 54 (Suppl 3):459, 1976.

Gomes MMR & others: Double-outlet right ventricle with pulmonic stenosis: Surgical considerations and results of operation. Circulation 43:889, 1971.

Gomes MMR & others: Double-outlet right ventricle without pulmonic stenosis: Surgical considerations and results of operation. Circulation 43(Suppl 1):31, 1971.

Patrick DL, McGoon DC: Operation for double-outlet right ventricle with transposition of the great arteries. J Cardiovasc Surg 9:537, 1968.

TOTAL ANOMALOUS PULMONARY VENOUS RETURN WITH OR WITHOUT INCREASED PULMONARY VASCULAR RESISTANCE

This malformation accounts for approximately 2% of all congenital heart lesions. The pulmonary venous blood does not drain into the left atrium but either directly or indirectly (via a systemic venous connection) into the right atrium. Thus, the entire venous drainage of the body drains into the right atrium.

This malformation may be classified according to

the site of entry of the pulmonary veins into the right side of the heart.

Type 1 (55%): Entry into the left superior vena cava (persistent anterior cardinal vein) or right superior vena cava.

Type 2: Entry into the right atrium or into the coronary sinus.

Type 3: Entry below the diaphragm (usually into the portal vein).

Type 4: Multiple types of entry.

Since the entire venous drainage from the body drains into the right atrium, a right-to-left shunt is always present at the atrial level. This may take the form either of a large atrial septal defect or a patent foramen ovale. Relatively complete mixing of the systemic and pulmonary venous return occurs in the right atrium, so that the left atrial and hence the systemic arterial saturation levels approximately equal that of the right atrial saturation.

The degree of saturation of the blood (and thus the degree of cyanosis present) is determined by the ratio of the quantity of pulmonary blood flow to that of the systemic blood flow. If pulmonary vascular resistance is normal, the flow of blood into the pulmonary artery is much greater than that into the left side of the heart. In this case, there is much greater return from the pulmonary than from the systemic venous system, and the saturation within the right atrium is high. These patients function very well, with relatively normal pulmonary artery pressures, and at least physiologically are very similar to patients with very large atrial septal defects and normal pulmonary venous return.

If pulmonary vascular resistance is elevated, the ratio of pulmonary to systemic blood flow is much lower. When the pulmonary vascular resistance equals that of the systemic vascular resistance, equal amounts of blood flow in both directions. When this occurs, marked desaturation of the mixed blood develops and the patient is markedly cyanotic. Such patients do much less well and eventually develop severe right heart failure.

Clinical Findings

A. With Normal Pulmonary Vascular Resistance: The great majority of these patients have some elevation of the pulmonary artery pressure due to the marked increase in pulmonary blood flow. In most cases, the pressure does not reach systemic levels.

1. Symptoms and signs—These patients may have a history of mild cyanosis in the neonatal period and during early infancy. Thereafter, they do relatively well except for frequent respiratory infections. They are usually rather small and thin, and resemble patients with very large atrial septal defects.

Careful examination discloses duskiness of the nail beds and mucous membranes, but definite cyanosis and clubbing are usually not present. The arterial pulses are normal. The jugular venous pulses usually show a significant V wave. Examination of the heart shows left chest prominence. A right ventricular heaving impulse is palpable. On auscultation, the first heart sound is normal to moderately increased in intensity. The second sound is widely split and fixed. Frequently there is a third or fourth heart sound, producing a quadruple or quintuple rhythm. The pulmonary component of the second sound is usually normal in intensity. A grade II–IV/VI ejection type systolic murmur is heard at the pulmonary area. It radiates very well over the lung fields anteriorly and posteriorly. An early to mid diastolic flow murmur is often heard at the lower left sternal border in the third and fourth intercostal spaces (tricuspid flow murmur).

2. X-ray findings—Chest x-ray reveals evidence of cardiac enlargement primarily involving the right atrium, right ventricle, and pulmonary artery. There is a marked increase in pulmonary vascular markings. There is often a specific contour also. The most characteristic contour is the so-called snowman or figure of 8, which is seen when the anomalous veins drain into a persistent left superior vena cava. This produces marked enlargement of the superior mediastinum and results in the characteristic contour.

3. Electrocardiography—ECG reveals right axis deviation and varying degrees of right atrial and right ventricular hypertrophy. There is often a qR pattern over the right precordial leads.

4. Echocardiography—Echocardiographic demonstration of a chamber posterior to the left atrium is considered by some to be diagnostic of anomalous pulmonary venous return.

B. With Increased Pulmonary Vascular Resistance: This group includes those patients in which the pulmonary veins drain into a systemic venous structure below the diaphragm. It also includes a large number of patients in whom the venous drainage is into a systemic vein above the diaphragm.

1. Symptoms and signs—These infants are usually quite sick. Half die within the first 6 months; most are dead by age 1 unless treated surgically. Cyanosis is common at birth and is quite evident by 1 week. Another common early symptom is severe tachypnea. Congestive heart failure develops later.

Cardiac examination discloses a striking right ventricular impulse. A shock of the second sound is palpable. The first heart sound is accentuated. The second heart sound is markedly accentuated and single. A grade I–II/VI ejection type systolic murmur is frequently heard over the pulmonary area with radiation over the lung fields. Diastolic murmurs are uncommon. In many cases no murmur is heard at all.

2. X-ray findings—In the most severe and classic cases, the heart is small and pulmonary venous congestion is marked. In less severe cases, the heart may be slightly enlarged or normal in size, with only slight pulmonary venous congestion.

3. Electrocardiography—ECG shows right axis deviation, right atrial hypertrophy, and right ventricular hypertrophy.

4. Cardiac catheterization and angiocardiography—These procedures are diagnostic. Cardiac catheterization demonstrates the presence of total anomalous pulmonary venous return and (usually) the site of entry of the anomalous veins. It also demonstrates the ratio of the pulmonary to systemic blood flow and the degree of pulmonary hypertension and pulmonary vascular resistance.

Cineangiocardiography following injection of contrast material into the right ventricle or pulmonary artery demonstrates the presence of anomalous pulmonary venous return and the site of entry of the anomalous veins.

Treatment

If immediate surgical intervention is not contemplated, atrial balloon septostomy should be performed at the initial diagnostic cardiac catheterization. This procedure coupled with vigorous medical management may sustain some infants for several months. Until recently, the surgical mortality rate in infants was greater than 90%. Within the past few years, however, certain centers have reported excellent results employing either cardiopulmonary bypass or extreme hypothermia (cooling to 20° C). In such centers, the option of immediate surgical correction may be taken.

Course & Prognosis

Patients with normal pulmonary vascular resistance and only modest elevation of pulmonary artery pressures may do quite well through the second or third decade. Eventually, however, progressive increase in pulmonary vascular resistance and pulmonary hypertension does occur. Patients with increased pulmonary vascular resistance and pulmonary hypertension do poorly, and most die unless treated before age 1.

Barratt-Boyes BG, Simpson M, Neutz JM: Intracardiac surgery in neonates and infants using deep hypothermia with surface cooling and limited cardiopulmonary bypass. Circulation 43(Suppl 1):25, 1971.

El-Said G & others: Management of total anomalous pulmonary venous return. Circulation 45:1240, 1972.

Gathman GE, Nadas AS: Total anomalous pulmonary venous connection: Clinical and physiologic observation of 75 pediatric patients. Circulation 42:143, 1970.

Gersony WM & others: Management of total anomalous pulmonary venous drainage in early infancy. Circulation 43(Suppl 1):19, 1971.

Gomes MMR & others: Total anomalous pulmonary venous connection: Surgical considerations and results of operation. J Thorac Cardiovasc Surg 60:116, 1970.

Mathew R & others: Cardiac function in total anomalous pulmonary venous return before and after surgery. Circulation 55:361, 1977.

Paquet M, Guegesell H: Echocardiographic features of total anomalous pulmonary venous connection. Circulation 59:599, 1975.

PERSISTENT TRUNCUS ARTERIOSUS

Persistent truncus arteriosus probably accounts for less than 1% of all congenital heart malformations.

Only one (huge) great vessel arises from the heart and supplies both the systemic and pulmonary arterial beds. It develops embryologically as a result of complete lack of formation of the spiral ridges that divide the fetal truncus arteriosus into the aorta and pulmonary artery. A high ventricular septal defect is always present. The number of valve leaflets varies from 2–6, and the valve may be sufficient, insufficient, or stenotic.

The classification most commonly employed is into 4 types:

Type 1: One pulmonary artery which arises from the base of the trunk just above the semilunar valve and runs parallel with the ascending aorta (48%).

Type 2: Two pulmonary arteries which arise side by side from the posterior aspect of the truncus (29%).

Type 3: Two pulmonary arteries which arise independently from either side of the trunk (11%).

Type 4: No demonstrable pulmonary artery (12%). Pulmonary circulation is derived from bronchials arising from the descending thoracic aorta. (The existence of this variety of truncus is controversial. Many authorities consider it an extreme form of tetralogy of Fallot with an atretic main pulmonary artery.)

In this condition, blood leaves the heart through a single common exit. Therefore, the saturation of the blood in the pulmonary artery is the same as that in the systemic arteries. The degree of systemic arterial oxygen saturation depends upon the ratio of the pulmonary to systemic blood flow. If pulmonary vascular resistance is normal, the pulmonary blood flow is much greater than the systemic blood flow and the saturation is relatively high. If pulmonary vascular resistance is great, due either to pulmonary vascular obstruction or to very small pulmonary arteries, pulmonary blood flow is reduced and oxygen saturation is low. The systolic pressures in both ventricles are identical to that in the aorta.

Clinical Findings

A. Symptoms and Signs: The clinical picture varies depending upon the degree of pulmonary blood flow.

1. Large pulmonary blood flow—These patients do well and are usually acyanotic, though the nail beds are commonly dusky. They function similarly to patients with large ventricular septal defects and pulmonary hypertension. Examination of the heart reveals a hyperactive impulse, felt both at the apex and over the xiphoid process. A systolic thrill is common at the lower left sternal border. The first heart sound is normal. A loud early systolic ejection click is commonly heard. The second sound is single and accentuated. A grade IV/VI, completely pansystolic murmur is audible at the lower left sternal border. A diastolic flow murmur can often be heard at the apex (mitral flow murmur).

2. Decreased pulmonary blood flow—These patients have marked cyanosis early and do very poorly. The most common manifestations include retardation of growth and development, easy fatigability, dyspnea on exertion, and congestive heart failure. The heart is not unduly active. The first and second heart sounds are loud. A systolic grade II–IV/VI murmur is heard at the lower left sternal border. No diastolic flow murmur is heard. A continuous heart murmur is very uncommon except in type 4, in which the continuous murmur is due to the large bronchial collateral vessels. A very loud systolic ejection click is commonly heard.

B. X-Ray Findings: Most common are a boot-shaped heart, absence of the main pulmonary artery segment, and a large aorta which frequently arches to the right. The pulmonary vascular markings vary depending upon the degree of pulmonary blood flow.

C. Electrocardiography: The axis is usually normal, though left axis deviation occurs rarely. Evidence of right ventricular hypertrophy or combined ventricular hypertrophy is commonly present. Left ventricular hypertrophy as an isolated finding is rare.

D. Echocardiography: A characteristic tracing would exhibit override of a single great artery (similar to tetralogy of Fallot) without a demonstrable right ventricular infundibulum.

E. Angiocardiography: This procedure is usually diagnostic. Injection of contrast material into the right ventricle demonstrates the presence of a ventricular septal defect and the single vessel arising from the heart. The exact type of truncus, however, may be somewhat difficult to determine even from angiocardiograms. It may occasionally also be difficult to differentiate this condition from pulmonary atresia and ventricular septal defect (pseudo-truncus).

Treatment

Anticongestive measures and, in some cases, banding of the pulmonary artery are indicated for patients with high pulmonary blood flow and congestive failure. Aortic homografting for "total correction" of the truncus in selected patients is an exciting new therapeutic development.

Course & Prognosis

The outcome depends to a great extent upon the status of the pulmonary circulation. Patients with a low pulmonary blood flow usually do very poorly and die within 1 year. Those with increased pulmonary blood flow can survive for a variable period. A few cases of survival into the third decade have been reported. Death is usually due to congestive heart failure, hypoxia, subacute infective endocarditis, or brain abscess.

Becker AE, Becker MJ, Edwards JE: Pathology of the semilunar valve in persistent truncus arteriosus. J Thorac Cardiovasc Surg 62:16, 1971.

Gelband H, Van Meter S, Gersony WM: Truncal valve abnormalities in infants with persistent truncus arteriosus: A clinical pathologic study. Circulation 45:397, 1972.

Lee MH & others: Truncal valve stenosis. Am Heart J 85:397, 1973.

McGoon DC, Rastelli GC, Ongley PA: An operation for the correction of truncus arteriosus. JAMA 205:69, 1968.

Singh AK & others: Pulmonary artery banding for truncus arteriosus in the first year of life. Circulation 54(Suppl 3):17, 1976.

Van Praagh R, Van Praagh S: The anatomy of the common aortic-pulmonary trunk (truncus arteriosus communis) and its embryologic implications. Am J Cardiol 16:406, 1965.

Wallace RB & others: Complete repair of truncus arteriosus defects. J Thorac Cardiovasc Surg 57:95, 1969.

DEXTROCARDIA

This lesion consists of right-sided heart with or without reversal of position of other organs (situs inversus). If there is no reversal of other organs, the heart usually has other severe defects. With complete situs inversus, the heart is usually normal.

Apical pulse and sounds are heard on the right side of the chest. X-ray shows the cardiac silhouette on the right side. On ECG, the P waves are usually inverted in lead I; QRS is predominantly down in lead I; lead II resembles normal lead III and vice versa.

With situs inversus and no heart defects, the prognosis is excellent. If severe heart defects are present, definitive diagnosis is imperative since corrective surgery is frequently beneficial.

Anselm G & others: Systematization and clinical study of dextroversion, mirror-image dextrocardia, and laevoversion. Br Heart J 34:1085, 1972.

Arcilla RA, Gasul BM: Congenital dextrocardia: Clinical, angiographic, and autopsy studies on 50 patients. J Pediatr 58:39, 1961.

Cooley DA, Billig DM: Surgical repair of congenital cardiac lesions in mirror-image dextrocardia with situs inversus totalis. Am J Cardiol 11:518, 1963.

Grant RP: The syndrome of dextroversion of the heart. Circulation 18:25, 1958.

Van Praagh R & others: Anatomic types of congenital dextrocardia: Diagnostic and embryologic implications. Am J Cardiol 13:510, 1964.

Van Praagh R & others: Diagnosis of the anatomic types of congenital dextrocardia. Am J Cardiol 15:234, 1965.

• • •

ACQUIRED HEART DISEASE

RHEUMATIC FEVER

Rheumatic fever is a disease in transition. Although it is still an important disease in the USA, its frequency has diminished significantly over the past half century. Penicillin is largely responsible, but the decrease in frequency of rheumatic fever was already apparent before the antibiotic era. In the USA and other temperate zone developed countries, improvement in standards of living, general hygiene, and opportunities for medical care have reduced the incidence of this disease significantly. It is still quite common in lower socioeconomic areas within the USA and rampant in poorer nations such as India, the Philippines, and Mexico. Curiously, however, factors other than socioeconomic status may be operating in some tropical and subtropical regions, because the disease is prevalent among residents of these areas who have relatively high standards of living.

The symptomatic presentation of the disease has also changed significantly in the USA within the past 2 decades. It is unusual today for a child to present with an exsanguinating nosebleed, whereas 20 years ago the trays of nasal packs in some emergency rooms were called rheumatic fever trays. The frequency with which one encounters severe disabling carditis in children of higher socioeconomic families has also greatly diminished. One can only speculate on the reasons for these changes in the epidemiologic characteristics of the disease in different communities and on what role, if any, the liberal use of antibiotics may have played.

Group A beta-hemolytic streptococcal infection of the respiratory tract is the essential environmental trigger which acts on predisposed individuals, producing a first attack of rheumatic fever in 0.3% of untreated or inadequately treated children living in an open population in the contiguous 48 states. After a child has had an attack of rheumatic fever, the risk of recurrence following subsequent inadequately treated group A beta-hemolytic streptococcal infections is of the order of 50%—at least for the next 5 years. In other words, the mere fact that a child has had rheumatic fever once increases his risk of further attacks approximately 150 times. This is why prophylaxis with penicillin (or other appropriate antibacterial agent) is so vitally important.

The clinical presentation of an attack of rheumatic fever has a tendency to repeat itself in subsequent attacks. A patient whose first attack consists of migratory polyarthritis without carditis is likely to present the same clinical picture in subsequent attacks; and a patient with severe carditis on first attack is subject to a similar course if he has another episode of rheumatic fever. With appropriate caution, this information can be put to practical use when dealing with a patient who presents with a past history that would not support a firm diagnosis of a first episode of rheumatic fever without carditis. It should be obvious that one would not like to withhold treatment and thus permit several such "nondiagnostic episodes" to occur—because of the possibility, for example, of mitral stenosis resulting at age 35 in a patient with an equivocal history. (It is quite likely that a skilled observer could detect minimal acute mitral involvement at each of such "nondiagnostic episodes" which could eventually produce mitral stenosis.)

Further Etiologic & Epidemiologic Considerations

Like the 3 other major cardiovascular diseases presenting or having their origins in childhood, rheumatic fever is best explained on the basis of multifactorial inheritance. There is a hereditary predisposition and an environmental trigger. In Fig 13—10, rheumatic fever is seen to be much closer to the environmental pole than the other cardiovascular diseases. Respiratory infections with group A beta-hemolytic streptococci play an essential role, and the streptococcal environmental trigger is required to produce rheumatic fever no matter how strong the family history and no matter how vulnerable the patient is by virtue of his hereditary predisposition. (It should be emphasized that streptococci *not* of group A, *not* manifesting beta-hemolysis, and *not* infecting the respiratory tract are *not* associated with rheumatic fever.) How the streptococcus produces rheumatic fever in the predisposed individual is not completely clear, but some interaction with the host is assumed. The streptococcus and the myocardium have antigens in common. The body, in defending itself against streptococcal invasion, raises antibodies against antigens of this organism, but these same antibodies are also capable of attacking similar antigens present in the individual's own heart (autoimmune reaction). From this brief description, one can formulate many of the questions that require answers if autoimmunity is indeed the true mechanism.

The peak period of risk in the USA is age 5—15 years. The disease is slightly more common in girls and is now more common in blacks—perhaps reflecting socioeconomic factors. The average annual attack rate in the total American population is less than 1 per 10,000, and the presence of rheumatic heart disease in the school-age population is less than 1 per 1000. The annual death rate from rheumatic heart disease in school-age children recorded a decade ago—taking whites and nonwhites together—was less than 1 per 100,000.

Jones Criteria (Revised) for Diagnosis of Rheumatic Fever

  Major manifestations
    Carditis
    Polyarthritis
    Sydenham's chorea
    Erythema marginatum
    Subcutaneous nodules
  Minor manifestations
    Clinical
      Previous rheumatic fever or rheumatic heart disease
      Polyarthralgia
      Fever
    Laboratory
      Acute phase reaction: elevated erythrocyte sedimentation rate, C-reactive protein, leukocytosis
      Prolonged P—R interval

Plus

Supporting evidence of preceding streptococcal infection, ie, increased ASO or other streptococcal antibodies, positive throat culture for group A streptococcus, recent scarlet fever.

Two major or one major and 2 minor criteria (plus supporting evidence of streptococcal infections) justify a presumptive diagnosis of rheumatic fever. When applied in this way, the criteria are extremely useful, but the physician must know enough about the disease to be able to apply the Jones criteria intelligently. For example, Sydenham's chorea may become manifest in the absence of other major and minor criteria; or a patient may be referred with a presumptive diagnosis of rheumatic fever who has a rash that looks very much like erythema marginatum and subcutaneous nodules but no other manifestations suggestive of rheumatic fever. The clinician should know that erythema marginatum and subcutaneous nodules do not occur as isolated findings but are generally part of the presentation consisting of migratory polyarthritis, clear evidence of recent streptococcal infection, and other diagnostic clues.

Major Manifestations of Rheumatic Fever

A. Active Carditis: Any one of the following—

1. A significant *new* murmur which is clearly mitral insufficiency (with or without a transient apical diastolic Carey Coombs murmur) or aortic insufficiency. It should be remembered that mitral insufficiency, while commonly caused by rheumatic fever, has many other causes in childhood.

2. Pericarditis, manifested by a pericardial friction rub or evidence of pericardial effusion.

3. Evidence of congestive heart failure.

B. Polyarthritis: Two or more joints must be involved; involvement of one joint does not constitute a major manifestation. The joints may be involved simultaneously or (more diagnostically) in a migratory fashion. The most commonly involved joints are the ankles, knees, hips, wrists, elbows, and shoulders. Heat, redness, swelling, severe pain, and tenderness are usually all present. Arthralgia alone without the other signs of inflammation is not sufficient to meet the criterion of polyarthritis.

C. Subcutaneous Nodules: These are usually seen only in severe cases, and then most commonly over the joints, scalp, and spinal column. They vary from a few millimeters to 2 cm in diameter, and are nontender and freely movable under the skin.

D. Erythema Marginatum: While this is a specific and major manifestation of acute rheumatic fever, many physicians fail to distinguish it from other skin lesions. It usually occurs only in severe cases and is rarely an essential diagnostic clue. It consists of a macular erythematous rash with a circinate border appearing primarily on the trunk and extremities. The face is usually not involved.

E. Sydenham's Chorea: Sydenham's chorea is characterized by emotional instability and involuntary movements. These findings become progressively more severe and are often followed by the development of ataxia and slurring of speech. Muscular weakness

becomes apparent following the onset of the involuntary movements. The individual attack of chorea is self-limiting, although it may last up to 3 months. It is not uncommon to find involvement on only one side.

Minor Manifestations of Rheumatic Fever

A. Fever: The fever is usually low-grade, although occasionally it reaches 39.4–40° C (103–104° F).

B. Polyarthralgia: Pain in 2 or more joints without heat, swelling, and tenderness is a minor rather than a major manifestation.

C. ECG Changes: Prolongation of the P–R interval represents only a minor manifestation and does not qualify as active carditis.

D. Acute Phase Reactants: The sedimentation rate is accelerated and, more specifically, the C-reactive protein. Congestive heart failure does not influence the C-reactive protein and usually does not affect the sedimentation rate. Leukocytosis is the rule.

E. History: There is a prior history of acute rheumatic fever or the presence of inactive rheumatic heart disease.

Essential Manifestation

Except in cases of rheumatic fever presenting solely as Sydenham's chorea or long-standing carditis, there should be clear supporting evidence of a streptococcal infection such as scarlet fever, a positive throat culture for group A beta-hemolytic streptococcus, and increased ASO or other streptococcal antibody titers. The ASO titer is significantly higher in rheumatic fever than in uncomplicated streptococcal infections.

Other Manifestations

Associated findings may include erythema multiforme; abdominal, back, and precordial pain; and nontraumatic epistaxis, vomiting, malaise, weight loss, and anemia.

The consultant often has difficulty in reaching a retrospective diagnosis of rheumatic fever because the appropriate observations and studies were not made at the time of the acute episode. In such cases, a decision must be made which takes into account what statisticians would call type I and type II errors—the relative risk of making a diagnosis of rheumatic fever when in fact there was no episode of the disease (type II) versus failing to attribute symptoms and signs to a true episode of rheumatic fever (type I). Assuming that a murmur of mitral insufficiency is due to rheumatic fever when the cause in fact is an anomalous left coronary artery or mitral dysfunction—and not putting a ghetto child on prophylactic penicillin because the classic Jones criteria could not be elicited are examples of the diagnostic problems that can arise.

Treatment

Appropriate treatment begins with a basic understanding of the disease process. The physician must ask himself such questions as the following: How long does rheumatic fever activity generally persist with carditis and without carditis? How can the clinician be certain the disease is active? What is the goal of therapy as it relates to the disease process?

If the treatment of rheumatic fever were clearly understood, there would not be widespread dispute on many points. However, there are data in the literature—all presumably derived from well-controlled studies by reliable investigators—which are in total disagreement. It is not possible here to develop opposing arguments. The therapeutic approach presented below is intended to be generally representative of current practice.

A. Persistence of Rheumatic Activity: In the absence of carditis, the average duration of rheumatic activity is 89 ± 27 days. When carditis is present, rheumatic activity may be expected to persist for an average of 124 ± 68 days. The return of the sedimentation rate and C-reactive protein to normal (after discontinuing anti-inflammatory medication), the return of the sleeping pulse to normal, and the rise of the hemoglobin to normal levels may be taken as evidence that the rheumatic fever has become inactive. In some adolescent and preadolescent girls, the sedimentation rate does not return to normal when all other criteria for activity have disappeared. In these special cases, the physician may elect to cautiously disregard the sedimentation rate.

B. Goals of Therapy: The goals of therapy may be divided into short-term and long-term. Short-term goals range from saving the life of the patient with severe carditis to relieving joint discomfort. Long-term goals are directed toward reducing the risk of residual valvular disease and preventing recurrences.

C. Treatment of the Acute Episode:

1. Anti-infective therapy—Eradication of the streptococcal infection is essential. Depending on the weight of the patient, benzathine penicillin G in a single intramuscular injection of 0.6–1.2 million units, or 125–250 mg of penicillin orally 4 times a day for 10 days, is the preferred method. Erythromycin, 250 mg orally 4 times a day, may be substituted if the patient is allergic to penicillin.

2. Anti-inflammatory agents—

a. Aspirin—For initial relief of fever and joint symptoms (in the absence of severe carditis with congestive heart failure), give aspirin, 100 mg/kg/day orally, divided into 4 daytime doses. The maximum dose for a patient of any weight should not usually exceed 5000 mg/day (4 adult 5 gr aspirin tablets 4 times daily). Salicylate blood levels of 20–25 mg/100 ml should generally be achieved by this dosage regimen. The dosage should be reduced to 50 mg/kg/day in 1 week and maintained at this level for 1 month or until the C-reactive protein is negative and the sedimentation rate is falling. At this point, aspirin may be discontinued, but reinstituted if symptoms return.

b. Corticosteroids—There is some room for flexibility in whether or not to offer corticosteroid therapy to patients with severe carditis and congestive heart failure. Our personal preference is to withhold corticosteroids from patients with mild congestive heart failure who achieve prompt and satisfactory compensa-

tion with digitalis. The majority view would seem to favor corticosteroid therapy for all patients with congestive heart failure secondary to acute rheumatic fever. It should be realized that corticosteroids are not superior to aspirin in preventing residual valvular damage—in fact, controlled studies favor aspirin slightly (but not significantly) in this respect. Rebound phenomena are far more frequent in corticosteroid-treated patients, so that the potential for actually prolonging the acute episode managed with corticosteroids should be taken into consideration. Furthermore, one has to see only a single child with rheumatic fever develop chickenpox encephalitis while taking corticosteroids for questionable indications to insist on firm indications in the future. There is of course no question that the child with carditis and intractable or poorly compensated congestive failure requires corticosteroid treatment.

Corticosteroid therapy may be given as follows: prednisone, 2 mg/kg/day orally for 2 weeks (or comparable doses of other corticosteroids); reduce prednisone to 1 mg/kg/day the third week and begin aspirin, 50 mg/kg/day; stop prednisone at the end of 3 weeks, and continue aspirin for 8 weeks or until the C-reactive protein is negative and the sedimentation rate is falling.

3. Therapy of congestive heart failure—See p 334.

4. Bed rest and ambulation—Strict bed rest is not required for patients with arthritis and mild carditis without congestive heart failure. It is preferable to maintain a regimen of bed-to-chair with bathroom privileges and meals at the table for patients who are relatively asymptomatic while on aspirin therapy. Asymptomatic patients can be kept in bed only under duress anyway. Patients with severe carditis (congestive heart failure) have no desire to get out of bed and should be at bed rest at least as long as corticosteroid therapy is required. *Gradual* indoor ambulation followed by modified outdoor activity may be ordered when symptoms have disappeared but there is still clinical and laboratory evidence of rheumatic activity. As discussed earlier, the average duration of rheumatic fever without carditis is about 3 months (± 1 month) and with carditis 4 months (± 2 months). In neither category of patient is it likely that activity will disappear in less than 2 months.

The child should not return to school while there is clear evidence of persistence of rheumatic activity.

D. Treatment After the Acute Episode:

1. Prevention—The patient who has had rheumatic fever has a greatly increased (150 times) risk of developing rheumatic fever following the next inadequately treated group A beta-hemolytic streptococcal infection. Prevention is thus the most important therapeutic course for the physician to emphasize. The purpose of follow-up visits after the acute episode is not so much to evaluate the evolution of mitral insufficiency murmurs as to reinforce the physician's advice about the necessity for antibacterial prophylaxis. At such times the physician should stress the greater protection afforded by intramuscular benzathine penicillin

G and inform his patients that the parenteral route will be favored until they are adults, at which time their internists may elect oral medication. Failure to comply with regular oral medication programs adds an additional variable of increased recurrence risk of rheumatic fever—beyond the demonstrably lower effectiveness of oral regimens in those who follow regular regimens. At present, antibacterial prophylaxis is a lifetime undertaking, and there is currently no age at which discontinuation is advocated.

The following regimens are in current use:

a. Benzathine penicillin G, 1.2 million units IM once a month.

b. Sulfadiazine, 500 mg orally daily as single dose for patients under 60 lb; 1 gm orally daily as single dose for patients over 60 lb. Blood dyscrasias and a lesser effectiveness in reducing streptococcal infections make this a less satisfactory second choice.

c. Penicillin G (buffered), 250,000 units orally twice daily, offers approximately the same protection afforded by sulfadiazine but is much less effective than intramuscular benzathine penicillin G (5.5 vs 0.4 streptococcal infections per 100 patient years).

d. Erythromycin, 250 mg orally twice a day, may be given to those patients who may be allergic to both penicillin and sulfonamides.

2. Residual valvular damage—Chronic congestive heart failure may follow a single severe episode of acute rheumatic carditis or, more commonly, may follow repeated episodes. Methods of managing congestive heart failure have been previously discussed. It is not an easy decision to contemplate, but some children with severe valvular damage who cannot be adequately managed on medical regimens must be considered for valve replacement—and considered before the myocardium is irreversibly damaged.

The usual manifestations of residual valvular damage to children in the USA are heart murmurs of mitral and aortic insufficiency without congestive heart failure during most of the pediatric age period *as long as repeated attacks are prevented.*

Ad Hoc Committee of the Council on Rheumatic Fever and Congenital Heart Disease: Jones's criteria (revised) for guidance in the diagnosis of rheumatic fever. Circulation 32:664, 1965.

Cooperative Rheumatic Fever Study Group: The natural history of rheumatic fever and rheumatic heart disease: Ten-year report of a cooperative clinical trial of ACTH, cortisone, and aspirin. Circulation 32:457, 1965.

Kaplan EL & others: AHA committee report: Prevention of rheumatic fever. Circulation 55:1, 1977.

Markowitz M: Eradication of rheumatic fever: An unfulfilled hope. Circulation 41:1077, 1970.

Markowitz M, Gordis L: *Rheumatic Fever,* 2nd ed. Saunders, 1972.

Rheumatic Fever and Rheumatic Heart Disease Study Group: Prevention of rheumatic fever and rheumatic heart disease. Circulation 41:A-1, 1970.

Spagnuolo M & others: Risk of rheumatic recurrences after streptococcal infections. N Engl J Med 285:641, 1971.

RHEUMATIC HEART DISEASE

Mitral Insufficiency

Mitral insufficiency is the most common valvular residual of acute rheumatic carditis. It is characterized by a pansystolic murmur that localizes at the apex. In those patients who have mitral involvement, the murmur appears early in the course of rheumatic carditis, and—depending on the severity of the damage—may disappear over a period of days or months or may persist throughout the patient's lifetime. Although rheumatic fever is a common cause of mitral insufficiency in pediatric patients, the mitral insufficiency murmur cannot be taken as diagnostic of a rheumatic episode.

Among the many other causes of mitral insufficiency, the most common is the mitral dysfunction syndrome, characterized by a mid to late apical systolic murmur introduced by a click.* Other causes are myocarditis, endocardial fibroelastosis, anomalous left coronary artery, and congenital anomalies of the mitral valve, which occur as isolated lesions or as part of a complex of anomalies (eg, endocardial cushion defects). It is thus essential to define the cause of mitral insufficiency in order to provide knowledgeable management—and not to prescribe a lifetime program of rheumatic fever prophylaxis for a patient who has only mitral dysfunction or to fail to provide appropriate surgical treatment if the mitral insufficiency is secondary to an anomalous left coronary artery.

Mitral Stenosis

There are murmurs of mitral stenosis that are secondary to structural stenosis of the valve; those that are due to relative excess of flow (in large volumes of regurgitation); and those that are present during acute valvulitis (Carey Coombs murmur). Mitral stenosis due to structural stenosis is rarely encountered in the USA before 5–10 years following the first episode of acute rheumatic carditis and is much more commonly discovered in adults than in children. Early mitral stenosis murmurs, flow murmurs, and Carey Coombs murmurs are short and heard in mid-diastole. Established mitral stenosis murmurs become progressively longer in duration until they attain the classic crescendo, presystolic configuration.

Aortic Insufficiency

This early decrescendo diastolic murmur—heard maximally at the secondary aortic area—is not commonly encountered as the sole valvular involvement of rheumatic carditis, as is mitral insufficiency. It is the second most frequent valve affected in polyvalvular as well as in single valvular disease. The impression has

---

*A word of caution about diagnosing the mitral dysfunction syndrome: The echocardiographic finding of prolapse (redundancy) of the mitral valve, which characterizes mitral dysfunction, may also be found in patients with acute rheumatic fever and recently acquired rheumatic heart disease.

been offered that the aortic valve is involved more often in males and in blacks. A short aortic systolic murmur due to excess flow may accompany the aortic insufficiency murmur.

Aortic Stenosis

Dominant aortic stenosis of rheumatic origin does not occur in pediatric patients. Aortic stenosis in children is congenital. In one large series, the shortest length of time observed for a patient to develop dominant aortic stenosis secondary to rheumatic heart disease was 20 years.

Strauss AW & others: Valve replacement in acute rheumatic heart disease. J Thorac Cardiovasc Surg 67:659, 1974.

MYOCARDITIS

In the great majority of cases, the cause of myocarditis is not determined. Coxsackievirus B is the commonest infectious agent isolated. Coxsackievirus A, rubella virus, cytomegalovirus, mumps virus, herpesvirus, adenovirus, and many other viral agents have been implicated. Virtually every other infectious agent, including bacteria, fungi, rickettsiae, spirochetes, and parasites, has been suggested as a cause of myocarditis, but laboratory confirmation is seldom possible. It is important to emphasize that myocarditis is part of a spectrum of primary endomyocardial diseases and may be one of the causes of endocardial fibroelastosis.

Clinical Findings

A. Symptoms and Signs: The clinical picture usually falls into 2 separate patterns: (1) Sudden onset of congestive heart failure in a neonate who has been in relatively good health 12–24 hours previously. This is a malignant form of the disease and is felt to be solely secondary to overwhelming viremia and tissue invasion of multiple organ systems, including the heart. (2) In the older child, the onset of cardiac findings tends to be much more gradual. There is often a history of an upper respiratory infection or gastroenteritis within the month prior to the development of cardiac findings. This is a more insidious form of the disease and may have a late postinfectious or autoimmune component. Recovery from the initial infection is followed by gradual and progressive development of easy fatigability, dyspnea on exertion, and malaise.

In the newborn infant, the signs of congestive heart failure are usually quite apparent. The skin is pale and gray, and peripheral cyanosis may be present. The pulses are rapid, weak, and thready. Edema of the face and extremities may be present. Significant cardiomegaly is present, and the left and right ventricular impulses are weak. On auscultation, the heart sounds may be poor, muffled, and distant. Third and fourth heart sounds are common, resulting in a gallop rhythm. Murmurs are usually absent, though a murmur of tri-cuspid or mitral insufficiency can occasionally be heard. Moist rales are usually present at both lung bases. The liver is enlarged and frequently tender. The level of the jugular venous pulse is elevated. In the latter group, the signs of congestive heart failure are often quite subtle.

B. X-Ray Findings: Generalized cardiomegaly involving all 4 chambers of the heart can be seen on x-ray. There is evidence of moderate to marked pulmonary venous congestion. Pneumonitis is commonly present.

C. Electrocardiography: The ECG is variable. Classically, there is evidence of low voltage of the QRS throughout all frontal and precordial leads and depression of the ST segment and inversion of the T waves in leads I, III, and aVF and in the left precordial leads during the acute malignant stage. Arrhythmias are not uncommon, and atrioventricular and intraventricular conduction disturbances may be present. With the more benign form—or during the recovery phase of the malignant form—high-voltage QRS complexes are commonly seen and are indicative of left ventricular hypertrophy.

Treatment

A. Digitalis: All patients with clinical findings of myocarditis should be started immediately on digitalis. Because the inflamed myocardium is markedly sensitive to digitalis, only about two-thirds of the usual total digitalizing dose should be employed. During the initial phase of therapy, frequent ECGs should be taken. If serious arrhythmias or other evidences of digitalis intoxication develop, the drug should be stopped and not reinstituted until all evidence of digitalis toxicity has disappeared. If toxicity is not evident and there is no clinical response, digitalis doses should be increased until one or the other is noted.

B. Diuretics: Diuretics should be administered with caution since they may potentiate digitalis toxicity.

C. Corticosteroids: The administration of corticosteroids is controversial but seems more rational when used in the treatment of the more benign postinfectious autoimmune cases. If the patient continues to deteriorate despite anticongestive measures, corticosteroids are commonly employed.

Prognosis

The prognosis is related to the age at onset, the response to therapy, and the presence or absence of recurrences. If the patient is less than 6 months of age or older than 3 years, responds poorly to therapy, and manifests multiple recurrences of congestive heart failure, the prognosis is poor. Many patients recover clinically but have persistent cardiomegaly. It is possible that subclinical myocarditis in childhood is the pathophysiologic basis for some of the idiopathic myocardiopathies seen later in life.

Dominguez P, Leindrum BL, Pick A: False "coronary patterns" in the infant electrocardiogram. Circulation 19:409, 1959.

Greenwood RD, Nadas AS, Fyler DC: The clinical course of primary myocardial disease in infants and children. Am Heart J 92:549, 1976.

Hutchins GM, Vie SA: Progression of interstitial myocarditis to idiopathic endocardial fibroelastosis. Am J Pathol 66:483, 1972.

Javett SW & others: Myocarditis in the newborn infant. J Pediatr 48:1, 1956.

Woodward TE & others: Viral and rickettsial causes of cardiac disease, including the coxsackievirus etiology of pericarditis and myocarditis. Ann Intern Med 53:1130, 1960.

INFECTIVE ENDOCARDITIS

Bacterial infection of the endocardial surface of the heart or the intimal surface of certain arterial vessels (coarcted segment of aorta and ductus arteriosus) is a rare condition that usually occurs when an abnormality of the heart or great vessels exists. It may develop in a normal heart during the course of septicemia.

Essentials of Diagnosis

- Preexisting organic heart murmur.
- Persistent fever.
- Increasing symptoms of heart disease (ranging from easy fatigability to heart failure).
- Splenomegaly (70%).
- Embolic phenomena (50%).
- Leukocytosis, elevated erythrocyte sedimentation rate, positive blood culture.

1. INFECTIVE ENDOCARDITIS WITH PREEXISTING CARDIOVASCULAR DISEASE

The term subacute infective endocarditis has been inappropriately used for this category of disease. While a *Streptococcus viridans* infection superimposed on a congenital or rheumatic heart lesion may indeed be subacute, infection of the same predisposing lesion with *Staphylococcus aureus* is highly acute and runs a catastrophically rapid course. The difference between an acute and subacute course of infective endocarditis appears to reside more in the infecting organism than in the preexisting heart lesion.

The picture of infective endocarditis in the pediatric age group has changed over the past 4 decades from an invariably fatal infection in the preantibiotic era to a disease that has maintained a rather stable frequency rate (0.5% of pediatric hospital admissions) but has an altered spectrum of predisposing conditions. The most common predisposing factor is cardiovascular surgery, followed by infectious foci (including respiratory and urinary tract infections) and other types of operations (dental, ear, nose, and throat, and genitourinary). Dental procedures are less of a problem now than formerly, presumably because of the emphasis on the need for antibiotic prophylaxis before performing dental operations.

The preexisting heart lesions have, with 2 notable exceptions, remained the same as in earlier decades. Cyanotic heart lesions, most often tetralogy of Fallot, are still at highest risk, followed by aortic stenosis and ventricular septal defect. One exception is that infective endocarditis involving a patent ductus arteriosus has not been seen at the authors' institution since 1960 nor at The Children's Hospital in Boston since 1963. Preexisting rheumatic heart disease in recent studies has decreased to the point that it is found in only 5–10% of cases of infective endocarditis in children.

Clinical Findings

A. History: Almost all patients have a history of heart disease. There may or may not be a history of infection or a surgical procedure (tooth extraction, tonsillectomy).

B. Symptoms, Signs, and Laboratory Findings: In one large study, the following symptoms, signs, and laboratory findings were reported (in order of decreasing frequency): murmurs, fever, positive blood culture, weight loss, cardiomegaly, elevated sedimentation rate, splenomegaly, petechiae, embolism, and leukocytosis. Other findings include hematuria, signs of congestive heart failure, clubbing, joint pains, and hepatomegaly.

Prevention

The decreasing frequency during the past 2 decades of infective endocarditis not related to cardiovascular surgery is probably due to awareness, prompt attention to bacterial infections, and the use of prophylactic antibiotics in patients with preexisting heart disease before dental work and other operations. For this reason it is recommended that appropriate antibiotics be administered before any type of dental work (tooth extraction, cleaning) or operations within the oropharynx, gastrointestinal, and genitourinary tracts. What constitutes an appropriate antibiotic under a given condition has been specified by a committee of the American Heart Association, which has made available cards with this information for distribution to heart patients. Continuous antibiotic prophylaxis (as in the treatment of rheumatic fever) is not recommended in patients with congenital heart disease.

Treatment

In a patient with known heart disease, the presence of an otherwise unexplained fever should alert the physician to the possibility of infective endocarditis. A positive blood culture or other major findings of infective endocarditis confirm the diagnosis. If a positive blood culture is obtained and the organism is identified, specific treatment should be begun immediately. Even if blood cultures are negative after 48 hours, it is advisable to begin penicillin therapy (if there is other evidence of infective endocarditis) since most positive cultures are obtained within the first 48 hours. Penicillin is the drug of choice in most cases. Other antibiotics may be added (see Chapter 37). If congestive heart failure occurs and progresses unremittingly in the face of adequate antibiotic therapy, surgical excision of the infected area and prosthetic valve replacement should be considered.

Course & Prognosis

The prognosis depends upon how early in the course of the infectious process treatment is instituted. The prognosis is better in patients in whom blood culture is positive. If congestive heart failure develops, the prognosis is usually poor.

Even though bacteriologic cure of the infectious process is achieved, death may occur as a result of congestive heart failure secondary to severe valvular destruction. Intractable congestive heart failure may occur weeks or months following bacteriologic cure. Embolization may occur following bacteriologic cure when vegetations tear off from the involved area.

See references below.

2. INFECTIVE ENDOCARDITIS WITHOUT PREEXISTING CARDIOVASCULAR DISEASE

Infection of the endocardium in patients without preexisting heart disease may occur during the course of septicemia. These patients are extremely ill, with evidence of severe sepsis. Involvement of the heart becomes clinically manifest with the development of heart murmurs and cardiomegaly. Involvement of the heart is only part of a total systemic infection. Antibiotic treatment is the same, whether or not there is cardiac involvement.

The mortality rate is very high (approximately 50%). Even if bacteriologic cure is effected, residual cardiac damage is the rule and congestive heart failure and death may result.

Gersony WM, Hayes CJ: Bacterial endocarditis in patients with pulmonary stenosis, aortic stenosis, or ventricular septal defect. Circulation 56(Suppl 1):84, 1977.

Hurley EJ & others: Emergency replacement of valves in endocarditis. Am Heart J 73:798, 1967.

Johnson DH & others: A forty-year review of bacterial endocarditis in infancy and childhood. Circulation 51:581, 1975.

Stasen WR & others: Cardiac surgery in bacterial endocarditis. Circulation 38:514, 1968.

Taranta A, Manning JA: Committee report; prevention of bacterial endocarditis. Circulation 46:3, 1972.

Zakrzewski T, Keith JD: Bacterial endocarditis in infants and children. J Pediatr 67:1179, 1965.

PERICARDITIS

Essentials of Diagnosis

● Retrosternal pain made worse by deep in-
spiration and decreased by leaning forward.
● Fever.
● Shortness of breath and grunting respirations are common.
● Pericardial friction rub.
● Tachycardia.
● Hepatomegaly and distention of the jugular veins.

General Considerations

Involvement of the pericardium rarely occurs as an isolated event. In the great majority of cases, pericardial disease occurs in association with a more generalized process. The most common cause of pericardial involvement in children and adolescents is rheumatic pancarditis. Other important causes include viral pericarditis, purulent pericarditis, rheumatoid arthritis, uremia, and tuberculosis.

In the pediatric age group, pericardial disease usually takes the form of acute pericarditis. In most cases, there is effusion of fluid into the pericardial cavity. The consequences of such effusion depend upon the amount, type, and speed of fluid accumulation. Under certain circumstances, serious compression of the heart occurs. The direct compression and the body's attempt to correct it result in cardiac tamponade. Unless the pericardial fluid is evacuated, death occurs very rapidly.

Clinical Findings

A. Symptoms and Signs: The symptoms depend to a great extent upon the cause of the pericarditis. Pain is common. It is usually sharp and stabbing, located in the midchest and in the shoulder and neck, made worse by deep inspiration, and considerably decreased by sitting up and leaning forward. Shortness of breath and grunting respirations are common findings in all patients.

The physical findings depend upon whether or not a significant amount of effusion is present: (1) In the absence of significant accumulation of fluid, the pulses are normal and the level of the jugular venous pulse is normal. On examination of the heart, a characteristic scratchy, high-pitched friction rub may be heard. It is not restricted to any cardiac cycle and is usually located at any point between the apex and the left sternal border. The location and timing vary considerably from time to time. The heart sounds are usually normal, and the heart is not enlarged to percussion. (2) If there is a considerable accumulation of pericardial fluid, the cardiovascular findings are different. The heart is enlarged to percussion but, on inspection of the precordium, seems to be very quiet. Auscultation reveals distant and muffled heart tones. Friction rub is usually not present. In the absence of cardiac tamponade, the peripheral, venous, and arterial pulses are normal.

Cardiac tamponade is characterized by distention of the jugular veins, tachycardia, enlargement of the liver, peripheral edema, and "paradoxic pulse," in which the systolic pressure drops by more than 10 mm

Hg during inspiration. The term paradoxic pulse is a misnomer since the drop is only an accentuation of a normal event. (Normally, the systolic pressure drops by no more than 5 mm Hg.) This finding is best determined with the use of a blood pressure cuff. At this point, the patient is critically ill and has all the symptoms and signs suggestive of right-sided congestive heart failure.

Not all patients with marked cardiac compression demonstrate all the findings listed above. If the patient appears critically ill and has evidence of pericarditis and effusion, treatment should be instituted even though all the clinical signs of cardiac tamponade are not present.

B. X-Ray Findings: In pericarditis without effusion, chest x-rays are normal. With pericardial effusion, the cardiac silhouette is enlarged, often in the shape of a water bottle, with blunting of the cardiodiaphragmatic borders. When there is evidence of cardiac tamponade, the lung fields are clear. This is in contrast to patients with myocardial dilatation, who show evidence of pulmonary congestion.

Cardiac fluoroscopy usually demonstrates absence of pulsations of the cardiac borders. This is helpful in differentiating this condition from myocarditis, in which the pulsations, although feeble, are present.

C. Electrocardiography: A number of ECG abnormalities occur in patients with pericarditis. Low voltage is commonly seen in patients with significant pericardial effusion, although the voltage may be normal. The ST segment is commonly elevated during the first week of involvement. The T wave is usually upright during this time. Following this, the ST segment is normal and the T wave becomes flattened. After about 2 weeks, the T wave inverts and remains inverted for several weeks or months. In contrast to patients with myocardial infarction, there is no reciprocal relationship between the findings in lead I and lead III in the frontal plane and the right and left precordial leads.

D. Echocardiography: Echocardiography has become a most reliable form of noninvasive diagnosis of pericardial effusion. The results must be considered in the light of the clinical picture in deciding whether or not to remove the fluid.

Treatment

Treatment depends upon the cause of the pericarditis. Cardiac tamponade due to any cause must be treated by evacuation of the fluid. It is usually desirable to perform a wide resection of the pericardium through a surgical incision. However, needle insertion into the pericardial sac may be lifesaving in an emergency situation.

Prognosis

The prognosis depends to a great extent upon the cause of the pericardial disease. Cardiac tamponade due to any cause will result in death unless the fluid is evacuated.

See references below.

SPECIFIC DISEASES INVOLVING THE PERICARDIUM

Acute Rheumatic Fever

When pericarditis occurs during the course of acute rheumatic fever, it is almost always associated with involvement of the myocardium and endocardium (pancarditis). Thus, heart murmurs are almost always present. The pericarditis is usually of the serofibrinous variety and usually not associated with significant pericardial effusion.

Patients with acute rheumatic fever and pericarditis are usually very ill, with severe cardiac involvement. They respond extremely well to corticosteroid therapy. Pericarditis usually disappears rapidly (1 week) after corticosteroid therapy is started. Constrictive pericarditis almost never occurs secondary to this disease.

Viral Pericarditis

Viral pericarditis is uncommon in children and young adults. The most common cause is the coxsackievirus B4. Influenza virus has also been implicated. There is usually a history of a protracted upper respiratory infection.

The pericardial effusion usually lasts for several weeks. Cardiac tamponade is rare. Recurrences of pericardial effusion are quite common even months or years after the initial episode. Constrictive pericarditis has been reported in this disease.

Purulent Pericarditis

The most common causes of purulent pericarditis are pneumococci, streptococci, staphylococci, *Escherichia coli,* and *Haemophilus influenzae.* This is always secondary to infection elsewhere, although occasionally the primary site is not obvious. In addition to demonstrating signs of cardiac compression, these patients are quite septic and run extremely high fevers. The purulent fluid accumulating within the pericardial sac is usually quite thick and filled with polymorphonuclear leukocytes. Although antibiotics will sterilize the pericardial fluid, pericardial tamponade commonly develops and evacuation of the pericardial sac is usually necessary. Wide resection of the pericardium through a surgical incision performed in the operating room is most desirable, but pericardiocentesis is often dramatically effective and lifesaving. Drainage of the purulent fluid is followed by marked symptomatic improvement.

Allen JW & others: The role of serial echocardiography in the evaluation and differential diagnosis of pericardial disease. Am Heart J 93:560, 1977.

Bain HW, McLean DM, Walker SJ: Epidemic pleurodynia (Bornholm disease) due to coxsackie B-5 virus: Interrelationship of pleurodynia, benign pericarditis and aseptic meningitis. Pediatrics 27:889, 1961.

Benzing G III, Kaplan S: Purulent pericarditis. Am J Dis Child 106:89, 1963.

Joyner CR: Echocardiography. Circulation 46:825, 1972.

Lietman PS, Bywaters EG: Pericarditis in juvenile rheumatoid arthritis. Pediatrics 32:855, 1963.

Shabetai R & others: The hemodynamics of cardiac tamponade and constrictive pericarditis. Am J Cardiol 26:480, 1970.

Surawicz B, Lasseter KC: Electrocardiograms in pericarditis. Am J Cardiol 26:471, 1970.

* * *

HYPERTENSION*

Systemic hypertension has become more widely recognized as a pediatric problem because blood pressure determinations are being more routinely obtained in the examination of infants and children. Standards for normal blood pressure in children have been suggested, and those of Londe (see reference below) may be considered of value because they apply to the office and outpatient situation. The standards recommended by the Task Force of the National Heart, Lung, and Blood Institute are also cited.

A number of distinct pathologic conditions produce clear findings of systemic hypertension. Renal disease and coarctation of the aorta are the most common causes of elevation of arterial pressure as detected in the upper extremities in the pediatric patient. Certain disorders of the CNS and adrenal glands, certain drug effects, and some poisonings and electrolyte disturbances are responsible for systemic hypertension. Many of these conditions are curable, although some are not.

Essential hypertension is the commonest cause of pediatric hypertension. Its cause cannot be traced to a discrete lesion such as a pheochromocytoma, coarctation of the aorta, or lead poisoning. It is a familial, progressive disease, and in the USA afflicts blacks more frequently than whites. Although there may be some monogenic cases of essential hypertension, it would appear that the majority of cases are best explained by multifactorial inheritance—a polygenic hereditary predisposition interacting with environmental triggers such as obesity, sodium intake, and endogenous and exogenous vasoconstrictors. The predisposition to this disease should be identified in the pediatric patient. Early recognition should make possible early medical treatment as required.

Blumenthal S & others: Report of the task force on blood pressure control in children. Pediatrics 59:802, 1977.

Koch-Weser J: Correlation of pathophysiology and pharmacotherapy in primary hypertension. Am J Cardiol 32:499, 1973.

Loggie JM: Systemic hypertension in children and adolescents. Pediatr Clin North Am 18:1273, 1971.

*The diagnostic evaluation of renal hypertension and the treatment of hypertensive emergencies as well as the ambulatory treatment of chronic hypertension are discussed in Chapter 18.

Londe S: Blood pressure in children as determined under office conditions. Clin Pediatr (Phila) 5:71, 1966.

Moss AJ, Adams FH: *Problems of Blood Pressure in Childhood.* Thomas, 1962.

ATHEROSCLEROSIS AS A PEDIATRIC PROBLEM

It has long been appreciated that coronary artery disease tends to be familial. Risk factors have been developed which help to identify individuals and families at risk. What has only recently been recognized is that even aggressive medical treatment is relatively ineffectual if delayed until the fourth and fifth decades of life. In fact, there are data in the literature to suggest that irreversible atherosclerotic changes may become established by 20 years of age.

It is now realized that it is the pediatric patient who must be identified as being at risk in order to institute medical management at an early enough time to produce meaningful alteration of the course of atherosclerotic disease. Since many risk factors (eg, cigarette smoking) are not applicable to pediatric patients, the identification of infants and children at risk has centered on biochemical risk factors (serum cholesterol, triglycerides, and lipoprotein levels). These biochemical studies have been used to specify phenotypes, and mortality and morbidity figures have been correlated with these phenotypes.

Table 13–3 lists the Fredrickson phenotypes with their biochemical characteristics and modes of inheritance. An alternative way to describe phenotypes which is used by some investigators is to subdivide into 3 types: pure hypercholesterolemia, pure hypertriglyceridemia, and combined hyperlipidemia. In Table 13–3 it can be seen how these 3 phenotypes may be extracted from the 6 Fredrickson phenotypes.

Table 13–3. Classification of hyperlipidemias and hyperlipoproteinemias.

Type	Inheritance	Cholesterol Elevation	Triglyceride Elevation	Electrophoresis	Ultracentrifugation
I	R	+	+	Chylo	Chylo
IIa	M & D	+		Beta ↑	LDL ↑
IIb	M	+	+	Beta ↑	LDL ↑
				Prebeta ↑	VLDL ↑
III	?M ?D	+	+	Broad beta	Intermediates
IV	M		+	Prebeta ↑	VLDL ↑
V	M	+	+	Chylo	Chylo
	R			Prebeta ↑	VLDL ↑

VLDL = very low density lipoprotein
LDL = low density lipoprotein
Chylo = chylomicrons

M = multifactorial
R = autosomal recessive
D = autosomal dominant

The majority of cases of atherosclerosis are due to multifactorial inheritance factors plus environmental factors such as diet (Fig 13–10). In type I disease (? recessive) and a portion of type IIa disease (dominant), mendelian inheritance seems to prevail. The rare type IIa homozygous child is at particular risk, with myocardial infarction frequently occurring early in the second decade of life.

The pediatrician's problem is how best to identify the infant or child who will be the adult at risk of dying prematurely of atherosclerotic disease. After initial enthusiasm for identifying patients at risk through cord blood cholesterol determinations, it has become apparent that the reproducibility and reliability of this method is less than satisfactory. The ideal age at which to identify reliably the pediatric patient who will have atherosclerosis as an adult awaits the outcome of ongoing studies.

As an interim measure, recommendations regarding moderate reduction of saturated fats and cholesterol in pediatric diets would not be disputed. Severe dietary restriction or medications added to regimens for pediatric patients who cannot be confidently identified as being at risk by genetic studies and biochemical determinations may prove undesirable if not hazardous.

The unavoidable conclusion is that, although the pediatric age now appears to be the appropriate time to initiate meaningful therapy for atherosclerosis, there are many urgent questions awaiting answers before we may proceed knowledgably and effectively.

Goldstein JL & others: Hyperlipidemia in coronary heart disease. J Clin Invest 52:1544, 1973.

Kannel WB, Dawber TR: Atherosclerosis as a pediatric problem. J Pediatr 80:544, 1972.

Nora JJ, Nora AH: The pediatric roots of coronary heart disease. Chest 68:714, 1975.

DISORDERS OF RATE, RHYTHM, & ELECTROLYTE IMBALANCE

The usual or normal pacemaker of the heart is the sino-atrial (SA) node. It is located in the superior portion of the right atrium. From there the impulse spreads through the atrial fibers to the atrioventricular (AV) node. Conduction through the AV node is relatively slow and accounts for the interval in the ECG from the end of the P wave to the beginning of the Q wave. From there the impulse spreads to the common bundle of His, which divides into a right and left bundle. Impulses finally are conducted through the Purkinje fibers to the myocardium and from the endocardium to the epicardial surface.

Although the SA node is a normal pacemaker of the heart, any tissue within the heart can serve in impulse formation. As a rule, the lower the origin of the pulse, the slower the rate of discharge. However, any focus outside the SA node may take over the pacemaker function (either because of decreased irritability of the sinus node or hyperirritability of the ectopic focus) for 1–2 beats (premature contractions) or for a series of beats (ectopic tachycardia).

SINUS ARRHYTHMIA

This arrhythmia is a normal and common finding in children and adolescents. It consists of a phasic change in heart rate, usually associated with the respiratory cycle. It is characterized by acceleration of the heart rate during inspiration and a slowing of the rate with expiration. Occasionally, there may be no relationship to respirations. The P–R and the QRS intervals are normal.

PREMATURE ATRIAL CONTRACTIONS

These result from the discharge of an ectopic focus located within the atrium. Electrocardiographically, they are characterized by the premature appearance of a P wave which is different in size and shape from the normal sinus P wave. The QRS complex and the T wave are normal. The P–R interval of the premature contraction is usually less than 0.12 seconds.

The next normal sinus beat following the premature beat is slightly delayed, but the compensatory pause is incomplete—in contrast to a premature ventricular contraction. If the ectopic focus is located within the AV node, the P–R interval will be extremely short (upper node) or may appear after the QRS complex (lower node), in which case the P wave will be inverted in lead II.

Premature supraventricular contractions may be a normal finding; they occur not infrequently in patients with organic heart disease and with digitalis intoxication. Patients with organic heart disease will always demonstrate other abnormalities besides the ectopic beats (organic murmurs, abnormal x-ray, other ECG abnormalities, and symptoms referable to the cardiovascular system). Furthermore, exercise usually abolishes the ectopic beats in normal children and increases the frequency of premature contractions in patients with organic heart disease.

In normal children, infrequent supraventricular premature contractions require no treatment. The patient and the parents should be reassured that these are harmless. In patients with organic heart disease, frequent premature supraventricular contractions usually require digitalis therapy or, if this is ineffective, quinidine.

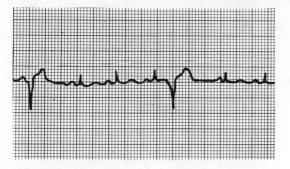

Figure 13—12. Premature ventricular contractions.

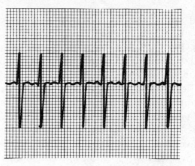

Figure 13—13. Paroxysmal atrial tachycardia.

PREMATURE VENTRICULAR CONTRACTIONS
(Fig 13—12.)

In this condition, the ectopic focus is located within the ventricle. Electrocardiographically, the premature beat is recognized by the appearance of an early, bizarre QRS complex and T wave not preceded by a P wave. There is always a complete compensatory pause (interval between 2 beats, including the premature contraction, is equal to 2 normal cardiac cycles).

Premature ventricular contractions may also occur in normal children. They are less common, however, than premature supraventricular contractions. In the normal individual, premature ventricular contractions usually are unifocal in origin and the coupling interval (interval from the end of the previous normal T wave to the beginning of the premature contraction) is exactly the same. Multifocal premature ventricular contractions and varying coupling intervals are found in patients with organic heart disease or drug intoxication. Premature contractions occasionally develop into ventricular tachycardia. Therefore, if the premature contractions are quite numerous or are associated with varying coupling intervals, treatment should be instituted. This consists primarily of the administration of quinidine.

PAROXYSMAL SUPRAVENTRICULAR TACHYCARDIA
(Fig 13—13.)

In this condition, a hyperirritable ectopic focus located below the SA node (in the atria or AV node) discharges at a very rapid rate and takes over the function of cardiac pacemaker for a period of time ranging from several seconds to several days.

Clinical Findings

A. Symptoms and Signs: The onset is usually sudden. During the early phase, older children complain of a fluttering within the chest and will be quite irritable and fearful. Infants are usually asymptomatic during this period, but if the tachycardia persists for more than 24 hours symptoms and signs indicative of impaired cardiac function will develop. In one study (see Nadas reference on p. 377), congestive heart failure developed in about 50% of patients. Three factors seem to influence the development of congestive heart failure: (1) The rate of the tachycardia: Congestive heart failure did not occur in patients who had a heart rate < 180/minute. The more rapid the rate, the more likely the development of congestive heart failure. (2) The duration of the tachycardia: The longer the tachycardia persisted, the more likely congestive heart failure was to develop. Congestive heart failure was not found in patients with tachycardia of less than 24 hours' duration; 19% had evidence of congestive heart failure after 36 hours; and 50% were in congestive heart failure after 48 hours. (3) The age of the patient: The younger the patient, the more common the incidence of congestive heart failure.

Infants in congestive heart failure secondary to paroxysmal supraventricular tachycardia are usually quite ill. They are ashen-gray and often frankly cyanotic. Pulses are difficult to count because they are very rapid and thready. The extremities are cold and clammy. The heart rate is extremely rapid and the heart tones poor. Rales are present within the lung, and the liver is enlarged.

Older children are usually not so ill when first brought to medical attention, probably because the arrhythmia is recognized early in the course.

B. X-Ray Findings: X-rays of the chest are normal during the early course of the arrhythmia. If congestive heart failure is present, the heart is enlarged and there is evidence of pulmonary venous congestion.

C. Electrocardiography: ECG is the most important tool in the diagnosis of this condition.

1. The heart rate is very rapid, ranging from 160–320/minute.

2. The rhythm is extremely regular. There is no variation in the R–R interval throughout the entire tracing.

3. P waves may or may not be present. If they are present, there is no variation in the appearance of the P wave or in the P–R interval. P waves may be difficult to find because they are superimposed upon the preceding T wave. Furthermore, if the abnormal focus is

located within the AV node, the P waves will not be seen.

4. The QRS complex is usually the same as during normal sinus rhythm. However, the QRS complex is occasionally widened. In this case, the condition may be difficult to differentiate from ventricular tachycardia (supraventricular tachycardia with aberrant ventricular conduction).

5. Termination of the tachycardia is characterized by conversion to normal sinus rhythm. Varying degrees of atrioventricular block do not develop, as is the case in atrial flutter.

Treatment

In almost all instances, paroxysmal supraventricular tachycardia can be successfully treated. However, despite conversion to normal sinus rhythm, infants who have been in severe congestive heart failure for prolonged periods with evidence of cardiovascular collapse may still succumb. This emphasizes the need for giving treatment early in the course of the tachycardia—especially in infants, in whom the onset of the arrhythmia cannot be ascertained.

A. Digitalis: Paroxysmal supraventricular tachycardia may be treated in a number of ways. In the pediatric age group, the treatment of choice is with digitalis. Conversion of the arrhythmia can almost always be achieved with this drug. Initially, however, reflex vagal stimulation may be attempted. Occasionally, maneuvers such as pressure over the eyeball may convert tachycardia of short duration. Digoxin is the preparation of choice because of its relatively rapid action. Half the calculated digitalizing dose should be administered initially. The other half should be given in 2 divided doses within the following 8 hours. If, as often happens, tachycardia is terminated before the total digitalizing dose is given, it is desirable to complete digitalization. Reflex vagal stimulation is often successful in terminating the tachycardia during the process of digitalization.

B. Other Drugs and Procedures: The use of hypertensive agents such as phenylephrine, by increasing systemic blood pressure and thus stimulating the carotid sinus, has also been successful in conversion of the arrhythmia. Phenylephrine must be given in a rapid intravenous bolus to be effective. Our method is to dilute a 1 ml (10 mg) ampule with 9 ml of normal saline to provide 1 mg/ml and to administer 0.1 mg/kg as an IV push. Oral propranolol (1 mg/kg), DC cardioversion, and, rarely, procainamide may be considered if these methods fail.

Course & Prognosis

If paroxysmal supraventricular tachycardia persists without treatment, congestive heart failure, cardiovascular collapse, and death may ensue. If the tachycardia is treated successfully, the great majority of patients do quite well. Symptoms and signs of heart failure clear up rapidly. Cardiac enlargement on x-ray, however, may persist for several days, and the ECG changes, including abnormalities of the P waves and ST

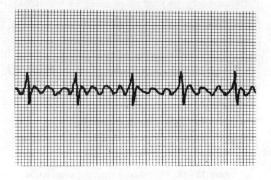

Figure 13—14. Atrial flutter.

and T wave changes, may also persist for up to 1 week.

Recurrences of paroxysmal supraventricular tachycardia are common, especially within the first year after the first attack. This is especially true in patients with Wolff-Parkinson-White syndrome (preexcitation syndrome). For this reason, all patients should remain on digitalis for at least 2 months. In case of recurrence, digitalis should be reinstituted and maintained for 6—12 months.

ATRIAL FLUTTER
(Fig 13—14.)

Although atrial flutter may occur in children with normal hearts, it is most common in patients with organic heart disease. It is characterized by an extremely rapid atrial rate (200—350/minute). In contrast to supraventricular tachycardia, however, varying degrees of atrioventricular block often exist. Whether symptoms and signs will occur or not depends upon the ventricular rate. If there is a rapid ventricular response with a heart rate greater than 200/minute, symptoms and signs of congestive heart failure frequently appear. If the ventricular response is slow (one ventricular beat for every 3—4 atrial beats), the patient's status remains essentially unchanged.

Digitalis should be given, especially if the ventricular response is rapid. Digitalization usually converts the flutter to a normal sinus rhythm, but sometimes it merely increases the AV block. In patients with organic heart disease, this may be all that can be accomplished, ie, it may be impossible to convert to normal sinus rhythm. In such a case, one should aim at maintaining the ventricular response at a relatively slow rate (80—140 beats/minute).

ATRIAL FIBRILLATION
(Fig 13—15.)

Atrial fibrillation is the most severe atrial arrhythmia. It is extremely rare in children. It is always associ-

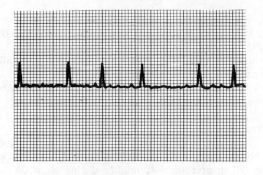

Figure 13–15. Atrial fibrillation.

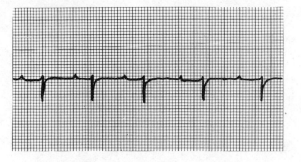

Figure 13–16. First degree heart block.

ated with organic heart disease, probably most commonly in patients with acute rheumatic fever.

Clinically, the rhythm is completely irregular and the heart sounds show a varying intensity. There is a variable pulse deficit when the rate of the heart sounds on auscultation is compared with palpation of the peripheral pulse. The ECG reveals a completely irregular rhythm without demonstrable P waves. The QRS complexes are usually normal.

All patients with atrial fibrillation should be digitalized. If the duration of fibrillation has been short, digitalization will often convert the arrhythmia to normal sinus rhythm and in any case will decrease the ventricular rate significantly. If conversion does not occur, it is desirable to maintain the cardiac rate between 70–100/minute at rest. If the ventricular rate falls below 60, digitalis should be discontinued.

If digitalis is not successful in converting the arrhythmia to normal sinus rhythm, quinidine is indicated. However, quinidine should not be administered before digitalization. If quinidine is successful, it should be continued for at least 3 months after conversion.

In refractory cases, electrical countershock may be employed. The experience in children is limited, and the results in adults have been variable.

FIRST DEGREE HEART BLOCK
(Fig 13–16.)

This is strictly an ECG abnormality, consisting of prolongation of the P–R interval. On physical examination, first degree block is associated with a soft first heart sound.

Prolongation of the P–R interval does not necessarily indicate past or present heart disease. It may occur in normal children, in which case the block is probably congenital in origin. It commonly occurs in the course of acute rheumatic carditis and in varying types of congenital heart disease, including Ebstein's anomaly of the tricuspid valve, corrected transposition of the great vessels, and endocardial cushion defect. Digitalis intoxication is frequently associated with first degree block.

Except as an indication of drug intoxication, prolongation of the P–R interval has no functional significance and requires no specific treatment.

SECOND DEGREE HEART BLOCK

In second degree heart block, an occasional P wave fails to be conducted to the ventricle. There are 2 major types.

Wenckebach Phenomenon (Mobitz Type I)

In this condition there is a progressive prolongation of the P–R interval, eventually terminating in complete block of AV conduction. The "dropped" beat usually persists for 3–5 cardiac cycles. Although this may occur in a normal heart, it is usually associated with organic heart disease. Causative factors are the same as those discussed under first degree heart block. The dropped beat usually has no functional significance. Treatment should be directed only toward the underlying heart disease or drug intoxication.

Intermittent AV Block Without Progressive Prolongation of the P–R Interval (Mobitz Type II)

This may occur haphazardly or at regular intervals every 3–4 beats. Etiologic and therapeutic considerations are the same as those of Wenckebach phenomenon.

THIRD DEGREE (COMPLETE) HEART BLOCK
(Fig 13–17.)

In third degree heart block, no atrial impulses can pass through the AV node; this results in independent contraction of the atria and ventricles. This condition should not be confused with AV dissociation, in which conduction through the AV node is intact but, because of a hyperirritable focus within the ventricle, the ventricles beat more rapidly than the atria, resulting in independent atrial and ventricular contractions. In

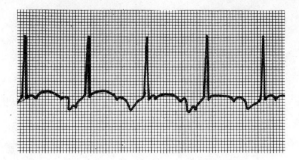

Figure 13–17. Third degree (complete) heart block.

complete heart block (with rare exceptions), the atria always beat more rapidly than the ventricles.

Complete heart block may be congenital or acquired. Congenital complete heart block may occur in the absence of any other intracardiac abnormalities or (occasionally) in association with corrected transposition of the great vessels, endocardial cushion defects, and endocardial fibroelastosis.

In the pediatric age group, almost the only cause of acquired complete heart block is open heart surgery. Transient complete heart block is not uncommon in patients undergoing correction of tetralogy of Fallot or very large ventricular septal defects. In most cases, conversion to normal sinus rhythm occurs within 1–2 weeks. Occasionally, however, complete heart block persists.

Clinical Findings

A. Symptoms and Signs:

1. Congenital complete heart block—Patients with congenital complete heart block usually do quite well. However, a number of recent reports have described Stokes-Adams attacks in these patients. The heart block is usually picked up on routine physical examination. The heart rate usually varies from 60–80/minute. In contrast to acquired heart block or complete heart block in adults, patients with congenital complete heart block can increase their heart rate 20 beats per minute during exercise. On physical examination, the heart is found to be enlarged, the heart rate slow, and loud ejection murmurs are present over the entire precordium. These murmurs are most commonly due to increased stroke volume through normal semilunar valves.

In patients with congenital heart disease and complete heart block, the history and physical findings depend upon the underlying anatomic abnormality.

2. Acquired complete heart block—Patients with heart block secondary to open heart surgery do much more poorly. The rate is usually slower than in congenital complete heart block, varying at rest from 30–50/minute. These patients cannot increase their heart rate significantly with exercise. Stokes-Adams attacks are not uncommon in this group. The mortality rate is high unless treatment is instituted.

B. Electrocardiography: The ECG is characterized by lack of any relationship between the P wave and the QRS complex. The atrial rate is always faster than the ventricular rate. The ventricular complex is usually broadened, with an abnormal T wave. In contrast to AV dissociation, no captured beats can be found on long strips of the ECG.

Treatment

Patients with congenital complete heart block who are completely asymptomatic and have a heart rate of greater than 40/minute during sleep do not require treatment. However, in many patients, when the heart rate drops below 40/minute, treatment may be necessary. This includes the oral administration of isoproterenol or ephedrine. These drugs increase the ventricular rate. If isoproterenol does not significantly increase the heart rate or decrease the number of Stokes-Adams attacks, surgical insertion of an artificial pacemaker is recommended.

Any patient with a history of a number of Stokes-Adams attacks should be started on treatment regardless of the heart rate measured at rest.

Because of the inability to significantly increase heart rate and thus cardiac output, patients with complete heart block should be restricted from participating in strenuous activities, especially competitive athletics. Except for this, they may lead normal active lives.

ELECTROLYTE IMBALANCE
(Figs 13–18 and 13–19.)

Potassium, calcium, and, to a lesser extent, magnesium imbalances are reflected in the ECG. The electrolyte disturbances of potassium are of greatest concern to the pediatrician, and some familiarity with abnormal tracings found in hyperkalemia and hypokalemia is essential. In hyperkalemia, there is gradual progression from tall peaked T waves (5–7 mEq/liter) through widening of the QRS complex (8–9 mEq/liter) to a broad, almost sine wave configuration (> 10 mEq/liter). Hypokalemia is characterized by progressive prominence of the U wave and prolongation of the Q–T (really Q–U) interval with ST segment depression.

Glenn WWL & others: Heart block in children. J Thorac Cardiovasc Surg 59:361, 1969.

Griffiths SP: Congenital complete heart block. Circulation 43:615, 1971.

Hunsaker MR, Khoury GH: Management of supraventricular tachycardia by atrial stimulation. J Pediatr 77:455, 1970.

Nadas AS & others: Paroxysmal tachycardia in infants: Study of 41 cases. Pediatrics 9:167, 1952.

Paul MH: Cardiac arrhythmias in infants and children. Prog Cardiovasc Dis 9:136, 1966.

Zoll PM: Rational use of drugs for cardiac arrest and after cardiac resuscitation. Am J Cardiol 27:645, 1971.

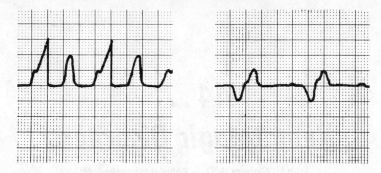

Figure 13—18. Hyperkalemia. *Left:* Serum K⁺ 8.5 mEq/liter. *Right:* Serum K⁺ 11 mEq/liter.

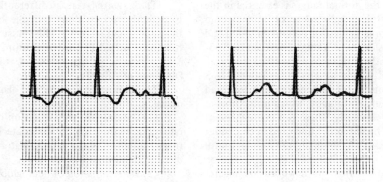

Figure 13—19. Hypokalemia. *Left:* Serum K⁺ 2.5 mEq/liter. *Right:* Serum K⁺ 3.5 mEq/liter.

●　　●　　●

General References

Cassels DE, Ziegler RF: *Electrocardiography in Infants and Children.* Grune & Stratton, 1966.

Guntheroth WG: *Pediatric Electrocardiography.* Saunders, 1965.

Nadas AS, Fyler DC: *Pediatric Cardiology.* Saunders, 1972.

Rowe RD, Mehrizi A: *The Neonate With Congenital Heart Disease.* Saunders, 1968.

Rudolph AM: *Congenital Heart Disease.* Year Book, 1974.

14 . . .
Hematologic Disorders

John H. Githens, MD, & William Hathaway, MD

Knowledge of the normal ranges is essential in the diagnosis of hematologic disorders of infancy and childhood. The normal values for peripheral blood and bone marrow are shown in Tables 14–1 and 38–3. They vary significantly with age.

The important changes shown in Table 38–3 include polycythemia in the neonatal period followed by physiologic anemia of infancy, which is maximal at 2½–3 months. Subsequently, there is a gradual rise of the hemoglobin, hematocrit, and red cell count through childhood. Adult levels are not reached until after puberty.

The red blood cells of the newborn are macrocytic (8–9 μm in diameter). There is a gradual change to microcytosis at 3 months, with return to normal diameter (7.4 μm) by 8 months.

The white blood count may normally remain higher than in the adult throughout infancy and childhood. The differential white count shows a predominance of lymphocytes, which may normally comprise as much as 80% of the white blood cells through the first 6 years of life.

I. ANEMIAS

Anemia is always a manifestation of disease or nutritional deficiency. The cause should be determined by appropriate clinical and laboratory investigations or, if necessary, by therapeutic trial with specific replacement therapy. "Shotgun" treatment with multiple drugs is never indicated.

The cell indices that are most useful are the MCHC (mean corpuscular hemoglobin concentration), the MCH (mean corpuscular hemoglobin), and the MCV (mean corpuscular volume). The normal values are shown in Table 38–3.

The primary cause of anemia in infancy is nutritional iron deficiency. Anemias due to causes other than iron deficiency fall into 2 major groups: (1) those due to impaired red cell production, maturation, or release from the marrow; and (2) those due to acute blood loss or destruction (hemolysis). The studies needed to determine the exact cause are different for these 2 groups.

The essential test in differentiating anemias due to defective production from the hemolytic group is the reticulocyte count. This must be done prior to treatment with drugs or transfusion.

Diagnosis of Anemia

The following scheme for diagnosis of anemia is useful:

(1) Careful history: Duration of symptoms, diet, rate of growth, evidence of acute or chronic hemorrhage, jaundice, and a family history of anemia, jaundice, or gallbladder disease.

(2) Determination of hemoglobin, hematocrit, red blood cell count, MCH, MCV, MCHC, and examination of the smear. •

(a) If hypochromia is shown, the cause of iron deficiency should be sought and treated. Additional studies—serum iron and iron-binding capacity, serum proteins, examination of stools for blood, and bone marrow examination—may be indicated.

(b) If normochromia (or hyperchromia) is shown, the reticulocyte count is essential. If the reticulocyte count is low (due to defect in marrow production or release), examine bone marrow; if high (due to hemolytic disease or acute hemorrhage), perform blood

Table 14–1. Normal values of cellular elements in bone marrow in older infants and children.*

	Range (%)	Mean (%)
Myeloblasts	1–5	2
Myelocytes (including pro-myelocytes)	10–25	20
Nonsegmented polymorpho-nuclear cells (including metamyelocytes)	15–30	20
Segmented polymorpho-nuclear cells	5–30	25
Lymphocytes	5–25	13
Nucleated red cells (principally normoblasts)	15–30	20
Megakaryocytes	10–35/cu mm	
Total nucleated cell count	100,000–200,000/cu mm	

*From Smith: *Blood Diseases of Infancy and Childhood*, 2nd ed. Mosby, 1966.

smear and Coombs test. If the Coombs is negative, perform red cell saline fragility test, autohemolysis test, hemoglobin electrophoresis, fetal hemoglobin determination, and Heinz body preparation. If spherocytosis or a hemoglobinopathy has not been identified, red cell enzyme studies are indicated.

ANEMIAS DUE TO DEFICIENT PRODUCTION

PHYSIOLOGIC "ANEMIA" OF THE NEWBORN & ANEMIA OF PREMATURITY

Essentials of Diagnosis

- Age 2–3 months.
- Normochromia or hyperchromia; microcytosis.

General Considerations

Physiologic "anemia" occurs in all full-term infants and reaches its low point (hemoglobin about 10–11 gm/100 ml) at about age 2½ months. The exact mechanism is not known, although it is recognized that both erythropoietin release and bone marrow production cannot keep pace with somatic growth. At this age it is not due to iron deficiency. It is associated with the transition from production of fetal hemoglobin to adult hemoglobin. The increased O_2 release capacity of adult hemoglobin provides less stimulus for erythropoietin as it replaces fetal hemoglobin. The anemia may be more severe in premature infants, in whom the hemoglobin may drop to levels of 5–6 gm/100 ml.

Clinical Findings

A. Symptoms and Signs: Slight pallor may be noted in full-term infants, but usually no other symptoms occur. If the anemia is severe in the premature infant, decreased activity and fatigue with feeding may occur.

B. Laboratory Findings:

1. Blood—Anemia is normochromic or hyperchromic, with microcytosis. Cell diameter may be as small as 5 μm. No other abnormalities are noted in the blood smear.

2. Bone marrow—The marrow appears relatively normal but shows slight erythroid hypoplasia; morphologic changes are not indicative of decreased production.

Differential Diagnosis

Iron deficiency anemia usually does not manifest itself until after the age of 2–3 months. Congenital hemolytic anemias that are associated with red cell membrane or red cell metabolic abnormalities (such as hereditary spherocytosis, pyruvate kinase deficiency, etc) are present from birth and should be considered. Congenital pure red cell hypoplastic anemia presents within the first few months of life; an extremely low reticulocyte count should suggest this diagnosis. Hemolysis associated with sepsis or following erythroblastosis fetalis should be considered. Chronic infection may increase the degree of anemia.

Treatment

Treatment should not be instituted unless the anemia is of sufficient severity to produce symptoms. Therefore, therapy is not indicated in the full-term infant. Treatment may be necessary in the premature infant if the hemoglobin drops below 7 or 8 gm/100 ml and symptoms of lethargy and fatigue are noted.

The only effective treatment is blood transfusion, which should be given in the form of packed red cells in doses of 5–10 ml/kg. The anemia will not respond at this age to iron or folic acid or other hematinics.

Prognosis

Spontaneous recovery is apparent by about 12–14 weeks of age in all infants. Anemia that persists beyond 3 months usually has another cause.

Mann DL & others: Erythropoietic stimulating activity during the first ninety days of life. Proc Soc Exp Biol Med 118:212, 1965.

O'Brien RT, Pearson HA: Physiologic anemia of the newborn infant. J Pediatr 79:132, 1971.

Stockman JA & others: The anemia of prematurity. N Engl J Med 296:647, 1977.

NUTRITIONAL ANEMIAS

Anemia is the most common manifestation of nutritional deficiency in children in the USA; it is even more frequent in other parts of the world. In the USA, iron deficiency is responsible for the majority of these nutritional anemias. Folic acid and vitamin B_{12} deficiencies are seen principally in economically underprivileged children. The need for exogenous iron is greatly increased during the first 2 years of life and again in adolescence because of the rapid growth of the child. Milk alone does not meet the iron requirements for normal growth during the first 2 years, and "solid" foods or iron supplementation is needed to prevent the development of anemia.

1. IRON DEFICIENCY ANEMIA

Essentials of Diagnosis

- Pallor, fatigue.
- Good weight gain, poor muscle tone.

- Delayed motor development.
- Poor dietary intake of iron.
- Age 6 months to 2 years.
- Hypochromic microcytic anemia.

General Considerations

The average diet contains 12–15 mg of iron (of which approximately 10% is absorbed), and the normal daily excretion of iron is less than 1 mg/day.

Iron deficiency on a nutritional basis generally occurs between 6 months and 2 years of age and is an extremely rare cause of anemia after age 3 except in adolescence. As the infant rarely outgrows his iron stores prior to the age of 4 months, iron deficiency is almost never a cause of anemia in the first 3 months of life except with severe iron deficiency in the mother or following blood loss by hemorrhage in the infant. It has been demonstrated that iron deficiency is associated with abnormalities of the intestinal mucosa that allow for loss of serum proteins as well as chronic intestinal hemorrhage. In some cases, occult gastrointestinal blood loss may be a major factor. Thus, the exudative enteropathy that may occur secondary to dietary iron deficiency further aggravates the iron depletion in the body. Other primary conditions (eg, cow's milk intolerance) may cause exudative enteropathy and initiate the iron loss.

Iron deficiency is also seen in association with chronic hemorrhage or rapid growth. Infestation with hookworm or *Trichuris trichiura* should be considered as a primary cause of chronic gastrointestinal blood loss in endemic areas.

The diagnosis depends largely on a history of a diet low in iron-containing solid foods with a high intake of milk (greater than 1 quart/day), and evidence of early rapid weight gain during the first 1–2 years of life. Hypochromia with microcytosis, decreased MCHC, and decreased serum iron with increased iron-binding capacity are characteristic.

Clinical Findings

A. Symptoms and Signs: Pallor, fatigue, irritability, and delayed motor development are common. The child is often fat and flabby, with poor muscle tone. Beeturia (red urine from the pigment of beets) occurs more frequently in iron-deficient children and may be a clue to the anemia.

B. Laboratory Findings: The hemoglobin is depressed and may be as low as 3–4 gm/100 ml. The red cell count and hematocrit are proportionately higher, producing a significantly lowered MCHC (less than 30%). The red cells on smear are microcytic and hypochromic. The reticulocyte count is normal, but it may be elevated in severe cases.

Serum iron need not be determined in childhood if the dietary and growth history readily explain the cause of the hypochromic anemia. Where there is doubt regarding the diagnosis or the cause, or if exudative enteropathy is suspected, this determination should be performed. Serum iron is low—usually below 30 μg/100 ml (normal: 90–150 μg/100 ml). Total iron-binding capacity is usually elevated to 350–500 μg/100 ml (normal: 250–350 μg/100 ml).

Bone marrow examination is usually not necessary in infants for the diagnosis of iron deficiency. Even normal children under 2 years of age deposit little or no iron in the form of hemosiderin in the marrow. In older children and adolescents, marrow examination with staining for iron may be helpful, since stainable iron should be present normally over the age of 2–3 years and will be absent in iron deficiency anemia.

The diagnosis is best confirmed by administration of an adequate dose of iron and the demonstration of a reticulocyte rise in 3–5 days and a hemoglobin rise in 7–14 days.

Differential Diagnosis

Iron deficiency anemia must be differentiated from several other hypochromic microcytic anemias caused by defective incorporation of iron into the hemoglobin molecule.

Thalassemia minor is the disorder that is most frequently confused with nutritional iron deficiency anemia, and it should be suspected in the child with an iron-resistant hypochromic anemia. Hypochromia and anemia may occur with any hemoglobinopathy involving the thalassemia gene. The serum iron will be elevated in these conditions.

Infection and inflammation interfere with erythropoiesis and utilization of iron. They produce hypochromic anemias which may be slightly microcytic. Although the serum iron and total iron-binding capacity are low, bone marrow hemosiderin will be present in the older child; search should be made for the presence of severe chronic infection or inflammatory disease. Other iron-resistant hypochromic anemias include anemia due to lead poisoning and vitamin B_6 dependent anemia.

Complications

Children with iron deficiency anemia are more susceptible than others to infection. In severe cases, heart failure may occur. Motor development is often delayed because of weakness. Anorexia and irritability cause additional feeding problems and further malnutrition. Severe iron deficiency interferes with the normal integrity of the gastrointestinal tract; exudative enteropathy associated with protein and additional iron loss may occur.

Prevention

Iron deficiency in infancy can be prevented in full-term infants if iron-containing solid foods are started by 3 months of age or if iron-fortified infant formulas are used. Small preterm infants usually require supplemental iron medication in a prophylactic dose of 0.8–1.5 mg/kg/day of elemental iron.

Treatment

A. Oral Iron: The recommended oral dose is 1.5–2 mg/kg elemental iron 3 times daily between meals (4.5–6 mg/kg/day). Although absorption is better if the medication is given between meals, it may cause gastrointestinal irritation; iron can be administered with food or even in milk. Various iron complexes and concentrates are available, but there is little evidence that any one is preferable to the others. Ferrous sulfate remains the drug of choice. Patients should be observed for a reticulocyte rise in 3–5 days and for a hemoglobin increase in 1–2 weeks.

B. Intramuscular Iron: Iron-dextran complex (Imferon) may be given intramuscularly if oral intolerance or malabsorption is present or if parental supervision is inadequate. The total dose can be calculated from the following formula:

$$\text{mg iron} = \frac{\text{Desired hemoglobin} - \text{Initial hemoglobin}}{100}$$
$$\times\ 80 \times \text{Weight in kg} \times 3.4$$

An additional 30% should be given to replace deficient iron stores. Daily doses should be limited to 1 ml (50 mg) in infants and 2 ml (100 mg) in very young children. When administering iron-dextran complex, pull the skin to one side before injecting to prevent leakage to the skin. The response of the reticulocyte count and the hemoglobin to the intramuscular product is no more rapid than to oral administration of an adequate dose of ferrous sulfate.

C. Ascorbic Acid: Large doses of ascorbic acid increase absorption of iron from food but probably do not affect the efficacy of iron medication.

D. Blood Transfusions: Transfusion therapy is reserved for children with extremely low levels of hemoglobin who are bordering on congestive failure or who have serious acute infections. Packed red cells should be used and administered slowly in a dose not to exceed 10 ml/kg. In the severely ill child with impending or frank congestive failure, a partial exchange transfusion (isovolumetric) with packed red cells should be given.

E. Diet: Ultimate management of iron deficiency anemia requires improvement in the diet, with reduction of milk intake and an increase in iron-containing foods such as meat, eggs, fortified infant cereals, and green vegetables.

Prognosis

Iron therapy will produce rapid and complete recovery within 2–4 weeks if the anemia is due to nutritional inadequacy. If the anemia persists, other causes must be found and treated.

Foman JF: *Nutritional Disorders of Children.* US Department of Health, Education, & Welfare. Publication No. (HSA) 76-5612, 1976.

Guha DK & others: Small bowel changes in iron deficiency anemia of childhood. Arch Dis Child 43:239, 1968.

Owen GM & others: Preschool children in the United States: Who has iron deficiency? J Pediatr 79:563, 1971.

Woodruff CW & others: The role of fresh cow's milk in iron deficiency. Am J Dis Child 124:26, 1972.

2. IRON-RESISTANT, HYPOCHROMIC ANEMIAS

Anemia of Infection & Inflammation

The hemoglobin usually ranges from 8–11 mg/100 ml, and the red cells may be slightly hypochromic. Serum iron and total iron-binding capacity are low. (See p 387 for details.)

Thalassemia Minor

This is one of the more common forms of iron-resistant hypochromic anemia in children of black, Mediterranean, or Southeast Asian racial origin. The hemoglobin is usually in the range of 9–11 gm/100 ml, and the red cells are significantly hypochromic. The blood smear may also show target cells and basophilic stippling. Serum iron and total iron-binding capacity are elevated. A_2 hemoglobin is elevated in beta-thalassemia minor. (See p 398 for details.)

Anemia of Lead Poisoning

The anemia associated with lead ingestion may be moderate to severe. It is hypochromic and microcytic. It can usually be suspected and differentiated from iron deficiency anemia by the presence of basophilic stippling of erythrocytes. A moderate reticulocytosis occurs. A history of pica may be found in iron deficiency anemia but is particularly characteristic of the young child with lead ingestion. The serum iron may be low, normal, or elevated depending on the nutritional status, but sideroblasts are always present in the bone marrow. Diagnostic studies for lead poisoning include long bone x-rays, serum lead levels, and urinary lead, coproporphyrin, and δ-aminolevulinic acid studies. Details of diagnosis and treatment are discussed in Chapter 30. Packed red cell transfusions may be indicated for correction of the anemia if it is severe.

Guinee VF: Lead poisoning. Am J Med 52:283, 1972.

Pyridoxine (Vitamin B$_6$) Responsive Anemia

This rare condition is usually hereditary. It is characterized by severe hypochromic, microcytic anemia. The onset may be early in infancy. Serum iron is elevated. The bone marrow shows erythroid hyperplasia with large numbers of sideroblasts (nucleated normoblasts containing iron inclusions). There is progressive hepatosplenomegaly. Abnormalities of tryptophan metabolism may be demonstrated by excessive excretion of xanthurenic acid, kynurenine, and kynurenic acid in urine after an oral loading dose of tryptophan. The diagnosis is proved by response of the anemia to parenterally administered pyridoxine. An adequate test dose is 100 mg, although most children will respond to 25 mg or less. The disorder is usually inherited as an X-linked recessive, and recovery is dependent upon continued administration of vitamin B$_6$. Phlebotomy has also been shown to be of value in older individuals in conjunction with vitamin B$_6$ therapy.

Acquired pyridoxine deficiency has been described in association with isoniazid therapy for tuberculosis. It responds readily to small oral doses of pyridoxine (2–5 mg/kg/day).

Frimpter GW & others: Vitamin B_6-dependency syndromes: New horizons in nutrition. Am J Clin Nutr 22:794, 1969.

Haden HT: Pyridoxine-responsive sideroblastic anemia due to antituberculous drugs. Arch Intern Med 120:602, 1967.

Hines JD: Effect of pyridoxine plus chronic phlebotomy on the function and morphology of bone marrow and liver in pyridoxine-responsive sideroblastic anemia. Semin Hematol 13:133, 1976.

Sideroachrestic (Sideroblastic) Anemias

The sideroachrestic anemias comprise a group characterized by iron resistance, hypochromia, large iron stores, and high serum iron levels. The anemias are all due to a disturbance in hemoglobin biosynthesis, resulting in an increased number of sideroblasts—nucleated normoblasts containing iron inclusions. The iron accumulates since the cell is unable to incorporate iron into the hemoglobin molecule. Sideroblasts occur in low concentrations in normal persons but are markedly increased in this group of iron-refractory anemias. Siderocytes, which are erythrocytes containing iron inclusions, are also markedly increased in number.

Most cases are familial, and some of them are apparently transmitted as an X-linked recessive disorder. Patients are occasionally anemic in early childhood, but the familial forms are more apt to express themselves fully in adult life.

The anemia is always hypochromic, with anisocytosis and poikilocytosis. It is refractory to parenteral iron therapy. The serum iron is increased, with almost complete saturation of the total iron-binding capacity.

Diagnostic tests (in addition to bone marrow examination) include determination of the A_2 hemoglobin level by electrophoresis studies for lead intoxication, and a therapeutic trial with vitamin B_6 in order to differentiate the other iron resistant hypochromic anemias.

Bottomley SS: Porphyrin and iron metabolism in sideroblastic anemia. Semin Hematol 14:169, 1977.

Robinson SH: Heme synthesis and hypochromic anemia. N Engl J Med 280:615, 1969.

3. MEGALOBLASTIC ANEMIAS

Megaloblastic anemias are characterized by oval macrocytes and hypersegmented PMNs in the peripheral blood and megaloblasts in the bone marrow. They are due primarily to a deficiency of folic acid or vitamin B_{12} or a combination of both. These 2 substances function as coenzymes in the synthesis of nuclear protein.

Folic acid must be converted to folinic acid with the assistance of ascorbic acid. The gastric intrinsic factor is necessary for the absorption of vitamin B_{12}. Megaloblastic anemias develop in the absence of gastric intrinsic factor or as a result of dietary deficiencies of folic acid or, rarely, vitamin B_{12}, or they may appear in the presence of ascorbic acid deficiency if the folic acid intake is low.

Folic Acid Deficiency

Dietary deficiency of folic acid occurs most frequently in infancy. It appears in an acute form within the first few months of life, and is almost always due to the combination of low folic acid intake and ascorbic acid deficiency. Whole cow's milk and human breast milk provide adequate folic acid. However, certain powdered milk products, unless supplemented, contain inadequate folate. Goat's milk is deficient in both folate and vitamin B_{12}, and its use is a major cause of nutritional megaloblastic anemia in infancy. Preterm infants and those with prolonged diarrhea are more likely to become deficient.

Folic acid deficient megaloblastic anemia also occurs in older children with severe nutritional deficiency or with serious absorption problems such as celiac disease, intestinal bypass, or blind loops of the bowel.

Megaloblastic anemia may also result from infestation with the fish tapeworm (*Diphyllobothrium latum*). The administration of certain anticonvulsant drugs (phenytoin, primidone, phenobarbital) and the use of isoniazid with cycloserine, phenylbutazone, nitrofurantoin, and methotrexate have been reported to cause megaloblastic anemia.

Folate deficiency also occurs secondary to increased utilization of folate in chronic hemolytic anemias such as sickle cell disease.

The characteristic findings are weakness, pallor, and anorexia in infancy. Glossitis and a beefy red tongue are occasionally noted, but the neurologic manifestations of pernicious anemia are not seen. The anemia is frequently severe, with hemoglobin levels below 4 gm/100 ml. The red cell count is low, and may be < 1 million/cu mm in severe cases. The blood smear shows macrocytes and significant anisocytosis and poikilocytosis. The red cells are usually normochromic or hypochromic (if iron deficiency is also present). Leukopenia with neutropenia is usually present. The PMNs are enlarged and hypersegmented. The platelets are usually moderately reduced. The reticulocyte count is low. Formiminoglutamic acid (FIGLU) is present in the urine in folic acid deficiency after histidine loading. The Schilling test (see Pernicious Anemia) will differentiate folic acid deficiency from defective vitamin B_{12} absorption. Erythrocyte transketolase activity is normal in folate deficiency but elevated in vitamin B_{12} deficiency.

The marrow examination is diagnostic. The smear is characterized by delayed maturation and the presence of the typical megaloblastic forms of the nucleated red cells. Giant metamyelocytes may be seen, and megakaryocyte nuclei may be hypersegmented.

Megaloblastic anemia due to folic acid deficiency

responds rapidly to oral or parenteral administration of folic acid in a daily dosage of 5 mg. Two to 3 weeks of treatment are usually sufficient. A significant rise in the reticulocyte count will occur within a few days after therapy is started. Ascorbic acid in a dosage of about 200 mg/day orally should be given at the same time. In generalized malnutrition, vitamin B_{12} should also be given. Dietary changes should be instituted to prevent the recurrence of megaloblastic anemia.

Complete and permanent recovery will follow the administration of folic acid and ascorbic acid. Relapses will not occur unless dietary deficiencies persist.

Kamel K & others: Folate requirements in children. Am J Clin Nutr 25:152, 1972.

Streiff RR: Folic acid deficiency anemia. Semin Hematol 7:23, 1970.

Megaloblastic Anemia of Generalized Malnutrition

Megaloblastic anemia occurs among economically underprivileged children, particularly in tropical and subtropical countries, in association with poverty and poor dietary habits. It results from a low intake of both folic acid and vitamin B_{12}, and often is associated with iron deficiency anemia. The bone marrow and other laboratory findings demonstrate the presence of megaloblastic changes in the marrow and iron deficiency. The peripheral blood usually shows both macrocytosis and hypochromia. The anemia of kwashiorkor, which occurs in severe nutritional deficiency associated with protein inadequacy, is usually normochromic and normocytic or, less commonly, macrocytic or megaloblastic.

Treatment should include folic acid, vitamin B_{12}, and iron, with dietary improvement for future prevention.

Cook JD & others: Nutritional anemia in Latin America: A collaborative study. Blood 38:591, 1971.

Congenital Megaloblastic Anemia

A few cases of megaloblastic anemia have been reported in infancy in association with a congenital metabolic block in nucleic acid formation. Large quantities of orotic acid appear in the urine because of the inborn error in pyrimidine metabolism. These patients respond well to treatment with uridine but are unresponsive to folic acid or vitamin B_{12}. Therapy must be continued probably throughout life.

Smith LH: Pyrimidine metabolism in man. N Engl J Med 288:764, 1973.

Juvenile Pernicious Anemia Syndromes
(Vitamin B_{12} Deficiency)

The pernicious anemia syndromes of childhood are all caused by impaired absorption of vitamin B_{12}. Although pernicious anemia is rare in childhood, a number of different forms have been described. A congenital deficiency of intrinsic factor has been observed, with onset of symptoms in early infancy. Several forms

of intrinsic factor defect have been differentiated with onset in the second decade—one type without antibodies, one type with antibodies to parietal cells and intrinsic factor (similar to the disease in adults), and pernicious anemia associated with various endocrinopathies.

Vitamin B_{12} malabsorption may occur in the presence of adequate intrinsic factor, with acquired intestinal lesions, with generalized intestinal malabsorption, and in a familial disease of infants characterized by selective malabsorption of vitamin B_{12}.

The clinical picture is very similar to that in the adult, with anemia resulting in pallor, fatigue, and the development of anorexia and diarrhea. The presence of a beefy, red, smooth, sore tongue and the development of neurologic manifestations differentiate this anemia from the other megaloblastic anemias of childhood. The CNS involvement includes ataxia, paresthesias of the hands and feet, impaired vibratory perception, a positive Babinski sign, and the absence of tendon reflexes.

Typical laboratory findings include a macrocytic anemia with anisocytosis and poikilocytosis. Neutropenia and thrombocytopenia are common, and the PMNs are hypersegmented. Reticulocytes are within the normal range. The bone marrow is hyperplastic and shows characteristic megaloblastic abnormalities with a delay in maturation. Giant metamyelocytes and hypersegmented megakaryocytes are found.

The serum vitamin B_{12} concentration is usually less than 100 pg/ml (normal, 300–400 pg/ml).

Treatment consists of the administration of vitamin B_{12} (cyanocobalamin) by parenteral injection. In children, a dosage of 15–30 μg IM given 3–5 times per week for 2–4 weeks (or until blood values return to normal) is usually adequate. In large children or adolescents, the dose may be increased to 100 μg given at the same intervals. A maintenance dose of 100 μg should be administered by injection each month. This therapy usually produces an excellent remission, although it must be continued throughout life. Oral administration of vitamin B_{12}, liver injections, and folic acid therapy are not recommended. Treatment with folic acid alone will allow the neurologic manifestations to progress even though the anemia may be controlled.

Katz M & others: Vitamin B_{12} malabsorption due to a biologically inert intrinsic factor. N Engl J Med 287:485, 1972.

McIntyre OR & others: Pernicious anemia in childhood. N Engl J Med 272:981, 1965.

APLASTIC & HYPOPLASTIC ANEMIAS

CONGENITAL HYPOPLASTIC ANEMIA
(Congenital Aregenerative Anemia, Congenital Pure Red Cell Anemia, Primary Erythroid Hypoplasia, Blackfan-Diamond Syndrome)

Essentials of Diagnosis
- Pallor, weakness, fatigue.
- Onset in first few months of life.
- Normochromic anemia; very low reticulocyte count (often zero).
- Normal white blood cells and platelets.

General Considerations

Congenital pure red cell anemia usually manifests itself in the first 4 months of life—often immediately after birth—and should be suspected in an infant with severe normochromic anemia and a very low reticulocyte count in the presence of normal circulating white cells and platelets. The diagnosis is made by bone marrow examination which is characterized by failure of erythropoiesis without equivalent depression of the white cells or platelets. The disorder appears to be caused by a block in the maturation of the erythroid series at the stem cell or earliest erythroblast stage. However, recent studies suggest a possible autoimmune T cell mechanism. Thymoma is not present in the congenital childhood form. Although this is sometimes observed in adults with acquired pure red cell anemia, this form is very rare in childhood.

Clinical Findings

A. Symptoms and Signs: Pallor, fatigue, and weakness becoming progressively more severe from early infancy are produced by the anemia. Short stature and growth retardation are characteristic (in untreated cases). Occasionally there are other associated anomalies, particularly of the kidneys.

B. Laboratory Findings:

1. Blood—The anemia is normocytic and normochromic, and the hemoglobin is often less than 5 gm/100 ml. The reticulocyte count is characteristically very low, and may be zero. The platelet count, white count, and differential count are normal.

2. Bone marrow—The bone marrow is characterized by a striking absence of nucleated red cell precursors without any depression of the granulocytic series or the megakaryocytes. Occasionally, very immature cells of the erythroid series may also be seen.

3. Other tests—No other studies are required for diagnosis. Levels of erythropoietin are markedly elevated, and abnormalities of tryptophan metabolites have been described in the urine following a tryptophan loading test.

Differential Diagnosis

Other conditions occurring in the neonatal period with depressed erythropoiesis in the presence of normal granulocytes and platelets include the anemia of prematurity and the anemia which often follows severe erythroblastosis fetalis. In both of these situations, reticulocytes should be present and the past history is suggestive.

Congenital pure red cell anemia may occasionally be confused with hemolytic anemia in the first few months of life when physiologic processes inhibit the normal reticulocyte response to hemolysis.

A variant of pure red cell anemia has recently been described in infants with triphalangeal thumbs and neutropenia.

Complications

The principal complications are associated with therapy. Repeated blood transfusions have resulted in widespread hemosiderosis, at. times progressing to hemochromatosis. Therapy with corticosteroids has resulted in marked impairment of physical growth and in osteoporosis.

Treatment

A. Corticosteroids: In the majority of cases the anemia responds dramatically to therapy with corticosteroids, particularly if therapy is begun before age 3. Oral prednisone is the most frequently used drug. The dosage ranges from 15 mg/day in infants up to 60 mg/day in older children. It should be given in divided doses. A significant response of the anemia will usually be seen within 3–4 weeks. Following this, the dosage should be reduced to determine the minimal level with which a remission can be obtained. Alternate day therapy is often possible and may cause less interference with growth.

Other drugs such as testosterone and cobalt have no effect in this condition.

B. Blood Transfusions: Transfusions must be given in the presence of severe anemia and as a chronic supportive measure in the child who does not respond to corticosteroid therapy. Packed cells are preferred, and, as a rule, the transfusion is not given until the hemoglobin drops to approximately 7 gm/100 ml, at which point clinical symptoms usually appear. Therapy with blood alone usually requires a transfusion every 4–8 weeks.

C. Splenectomy: Splenectomy is occasionally of value but is never curative. Its effect is probably greatest in the child who has developed splenomegaly and has an extracorpuscular hemolytic component which is presumably located in the spleen. This can be confirmed by tagging normal donor red cells with radioactive chromium (^{51}Cr) and noting their shortened survival.

D. Iron Chelation Therapy: Deferoxamine has been used as a chelating agent in patients who require repeated transfusions. Administration by intravenous or subcutaneous drip over 12–24 hours has recently been shown to be most effective. Ascorbic acid aids in mobilizing the iron stores for chelation. (See section on thalassemia.)

E. Bone Marrow Transplantation: This form of therapy has been attempted and may hold promise for the future.

Prognosis

Before the adrenocortical steroids came into use, the course of congenital pure red cell anemia in many patients was one of chronic and progressive anemia with a fatal outcome. Repeated transfusions prolong life but cause hemosiderosis and hemochromatosis by the second decade.

The results of long-term corticosteroid therapy have not yet been evaluated. Many children have been maintained in remission throughout childhood. Markedly impaired growth appears to be the primary complication of corticosteroid treatment.

Occasionally some children will have a spontaneous remission during later childhood or at adolescence. The milder cases that show a few red cell precursors in the bone marrow are more apt to have remissions.

Aase JM, Smith DW: Congenital anemia and triphalangeal thumbs: A new syndrome. J Pediatr 74:471, 1969.

August CS & others: Establishment of erythropoiesis following bone marrow transplantation in a patient with congenital hypoplastic anemia (Diamond-Blackfan syndrome). Blood 48:491, 1976.

Hoffman R & others: Diamond-Blackfan Syndrome: Lymphocyte mediated suppression of erythropoiesis. Science 193:899, 1976.

Lukens JN, Neuman LA: Excretion and distribution of iron during chronic deferoxamine therapy. Blood 38:614, 1971.

APLASTIC ANEMIA

Essentials of Diagnosis

- Weakness and pallor.
- Purpuras, petechiae, and bleeding.
- Frequent infections.
- Pancytopenia with empty bone marrow.

General Considerations

Aplastic anemia is characterized by a severe pancytopenia with an acellular marrow and normal-sized spleen.

In childhood, aplastic anemia may be of 3 general types.

(1) Fanconi's congenital pancytopenia: See below.

(2) Idiopathic aplastic anemia: In at least half of cases in childhood, no etiologic agent or specific congenital cause can be found. Recent studies suggest a possible T cell autoimmune mechanism.

(3) Secondary (acquired) aplastic anemia: Aplas-tic anemia may occur as a toxic reaction to various chemicals and drugs. Chloramphenicol accounts for the majority of cases in childhood. Other antibiotics, sulfonamides, benzene, acetone, toluene, phenylbutazone, mephenytoin, certain insecticides such as DDT, and heavy metals have all been incriminated. Glue sniffing has produced aplastic anemia and has also initiated' aplastic crises in patients with sickle cell anemia. Large amounts of radiation and high doses of cytotoxic drugs such as mechlorethamine and the folic acid antagonists will also produce severe aplasia. Aplastic anemia has been observed as a complication of severe infectious hepatitis and may be caused by other viruses also.

Clinical Findings

A. Symptoms and Signs: Weakness, fatigue, and pallor are the result of the anemia; purpura and bleeding occur because of the thrombocytopenia; and severe generalized or localized infections are frequently due to neutropenia.

B. Laboratory Findings: Severe normochromic anemia is usually present, with some microcytosis. The reticulocyte count is usually very low, but in early cases with partial marrow destruction it may be slightly elevated. The white count is usually less than 2000/cu mm, with a marked neutropenia; and the platelet count is usually below 50,000/cu mm. Thrombocytopenia is often the earliest manifestation.

The bone marrow is practically devoid of normal marrow elements and is replaced with fat. A bone marrow section is indicated for absolute diagnosis.

The fetal hemoglobin level remains elevated in congenital aplastic anemia (Fanconi type) but may or may not rise in acquired forms.

Differential Diagnosis

Other causes of pancytopenia in childhood include infiltration with leukemia, Hodgkin's disease, Niemann-Pick disease, Gaucher's disease, Letterer-Siwe disease, osteopetrosis, myelofibrosis, and various toxic agents. Most of these conditions are associated with splenomegaly.

Complications

The disease is characteristically complicated by overwhelming infection and severe hemorrhage. With long-term transfusion therapy, problems may develop in association with leukoagglutinins, erythrocyte antibodies, and hemosiderosis.

A significant complication of prolonged testosterone therapy in childhood is the development of secondary sex characteristics in boys and evidence of masculinization and hirsutism in girls. Closure of the epiphyses and stunting of growth has not been a problem in most cases, but the patient should be checked periodically with bone x-rays for epiphyseal maturation.

Treatment

A. General Measures: Severely ill children should

be protected from infection in their environment by being placed in "reverse isolation." Specific and appropriate antibiotics should be used for infection.

Transfusions are usually necessary. If bleeding is not present, packed red cells in a dose of 10–20 ml/kg should be used for treatment of the anemia when symptoms develop. For severe hemorrhage, platelet concentrates should be used. Buffy coat concentrate containing high numbers of white cells may be tried for severe antibiotic-resistant infections, although this will increase the incidence of future transfusion reactions due to the development of leukoagglutinins.

B. Drug Therapy:

1. Androgens: Androgens will produce remissions in a small proportion of both secondary and idiopathic cases of aplastic anemia in childhood. A patient who has a few residual marrow cells will respond more frequently than a patient with a totally empty bone marrow. The remission will frequently not occur until 1–2 months after treatment is started. Once a remission has been achieved, the lowest possible maintenance dose should be determined by gradual reduction of dosage. Temporary cessation of therapy may be indicated because of untoward drug side-effects. The congenital or Fanconi type of aplastic anemia is more likely to respond than the idiopathic or acquired form, although these patients usually require continued testosterone treatment and do not have spontaneous remissions. Oxymetholone given orally (2–4 mg/kg/day) has been used widely in the past. Hepatic toxicity and heptomas have been associated with long-term use. Nandrolone decanoate intramuscularly (1–1.5 mg/kg/week) has proven effective in some cases and has not been associated with hepatic complications.

2. Corticosteroid therapy–Prednisone and similar drugs are usually not effective alone in aplastic anemia, but they may enhance the effect of testosterone. Therefore, prednisone, 1–2 mg/kg orally, should be given in addition to testosterone for initial therapy: the dose is decreased if a remission occurs. Prednisone in lower doses also has a nonspecific effect which may decrease the bleeding tendency.

C. Bone Marrow Transplantation: Success has been achieved recently with the use of homologous bone marrow replacement therapy using a sibling donor with the same tissue type. Isogenic marrow grafting has been successful when an identical twin with unaffected bone marrow is the donor.

Prognosis

The prognosis in either the secondary (acquired) or the idiopathic form of aplastic anemia is extremely poor when the bone marrow is totally empty and complete pancytopenia is present. In spite of supportive measures, these patients usually die of infection or hemorrhage within a period of a few months. Very few will respond to testosterone therapy. If some marrow elements remain, however, spontaneous remissions occasionally occur, and remissions are much more common in association with testosterone therapy. In

the acquired form, a spontaneous remission may eventually occur 1–2 years after initiating treatment with testosterone or testosterone plus prednisone. In the congenital form (Fanconi type) of aplastic anemia, the mortality was at one time almost 100%. With testosterone therapy, these children often survive for many years, although relapse usually occurs when the testosterone is discontinued.

Hoffman R & others: Suppression of erythroid colony formation by lymphocytes from patients with aplastic anemia. N Engl J Med 296:10, 1977.

Meadows AT & others: Hepatoma associated with androgen therapy for aplastic anemia. J Pediatr 84:109, 1974.

Thomas ED & others: Current status of bone marrow transplantation for aplastic anemia and acute leukemia. Blood 49:671, 1977.

CONGENITAL APLASTIC ANEMIA WITH MULTIPLE CONGENITAL ANOMALIES
(Fanconi's Anemia)

This is a familial aplastic anemia in which hypoplastic or aplastic bone marrow is associated with a number of other congenital anomalies. Occasionally the pancytopenia may occur in association with a hyperplastic marrow as a result of a delay in maturation. The most common defects are skeletal and include hypoplasia or absence or anomalies of the thumb, the thenar eminence, and the radius. Other skeletal anomalies may include syndactyly, congenital dislocation of the hips, and abnormalities of the long bones. Some of these children may have patchy brown pigmentation of the skin, hypogenitalism, microcephaly, short stature, strabismus, ptosis of the eyelids, nystagmus, anomalies of the ears, and mental retardation. The condition may occur in siblings and is probably transmitted as an autosomal recessive trait. The hematologic manifestations rarely are manifested prior to age 1 and may appear at any time between ages 1–12. Thrombocytopenia is usually the first abnormality to be noted, followed later by neutropenia and anemia. Although the bone marrow in the typical patient is hypoplastic and progresses to aplasia, in rare cases it may be hyperplastic, with a delay in maturation of marrow elements.

The hematologic disorder is slowly progressive, and in most cases severe aplasia will develop. Death due to infection or bleeding will eventually occur if therapy is not instituted.

The clinical manifestations are principally those of the aplastic anemia (see above).

Fanconi's anemia is characterized by elevated fetal hemoglobin and by an increased number of chromosomal breaks. These findings are present prior to the onset of the pancytopenia and can aid in early diagnosis. The heterozygotes also have the chromosomal anomalies. Both the patients and the carriers have an increased risk of malignancy, both for leukemia and for solid tumors.

The majority of patients with aplastic anemia will respond to testosterone therapy or testosterone plus prednisone, although relapse will occur when drug therapy is discontinued. (See section on aplastic anemia for details of therapy.) Transfusion should be used in the patient who does not respond to either testosterone or a combination of testosterone and prednisone. These children are especially prone to the development of hepatomas in association with long-term oxymetholone treatment.

The prognosis is much better since testosterone therapy came into use. However, long-term experience is beginning to suggest that many of these patients may eventually become resistant to testosterone therapy and die of the aplastic anemia in early adult life. Spontaneous recovery has occurred in a few cases during adolescence.

Beard MEJ & others: Fanconi's anemia. Q J Med 42:403, 1973.

Crossen PE & others: Chromosome studies in Fanconi's anemia before and after treatment with oxymetholone. Pathology 4:27, 1972.

Krawitz S & others: Oxymetholone therapy in children with aplastic and other refractory anemias. S Afr Med J 47:1864, 1973.

Mokrohisky ST & others: Rapidly developing malignant hepatic tumor in Fanconi's aplastic anemia treated with androgenic steroids. Clin Res 25:186, 1977.

CONGENITAL HYPOPLASTIC ANEMIA WITHOUT ASSOCIATED ANOMALIES

Several families have been reported with pancytopenia and hypoplastic or aplastic marrow without associated anomalies. This is probably a recessive hereditary disorder and closely related to Fanconi's anemia. Testosterone therapy may be effective.

Zaivov R & others: Familial aplastic anemia without congenital malformations. Acta Paediatr Scand 58:151, 1969.

ANEMIA OF RENAL FAILURE
(Anemia of Uremia)

A severe normochromic anemia occurs in almost all forms of renal disease that have progressed to renal insufficiency. Although white cell production remains normal and platelet production may be normal, the bone marrow shows significant hypoplasia of the erythroid series.

The marrow hypoplasia is due to decreased circulating erythropoietin, which is normally produced principally in the kidney. Erythropoiesis is also suppressed (in vitro) by the serum of uremic patients. The only treatment available is blood transfusion, which should be given as packed cells in a dosage of 10–20 ml/kg when the hemoglobin drops below 7 gm/100 ml or when symptoms occur. Drug therapy is not effective.

The anemia of renal disease is frequently complicated by an extracorpuscular hemolytic component which occurs in the presence of significant uremia. A more severe form of hemolytic anemia that occurs occasionally in children in association with renal disease is described under the hemolytic-uremic-thrombocytopenic syndrome.

Wallner SF & others: The anemia of chronic renal failure and chronic diseases: In vitro studies of erythropoiesis. Blood 47:561, 1976.

ANEMIA OF HYPOTHYROIDISM

Certain patients with hypothyroidism develop fairly severe normochromic anemias. The red cells frequently tend to be macrocytic. However, microcytic hypochromic anemia also has been described. The bone marrow shows hypocellularity of the erythroid series, with a normoblastic pattern.

Replacement therapy with thyroid hormone is effective in treating the anemia of the hypothyroid patient. Some of the hypochromic patients also respond partially to iron.

ANEMIA OF INFECTION & INFLAMMATION

Significant anemia usually develops in serious chronic infections or inflammatory diseases such as tuberculosis, chronic osteomyelitis, rheumatic fever, and rheumatoid arthritis. The anemia usually ranges between 8 and 11 gm/100 ml of hemoglobin, and is normochromic or slightly hypochromic. The reticulocyte count is usually normal or low. The mechanism is not clearly understood. However, the primary causes are a decrease in erythropoietin and a reticuloendothelial system block in transfer of iron to nucleated red cells. In addition, there is a slight decrease in red cell survival time. The bone marrow appears normal and hemosiderin deposits are present, although the serum iron and the total iron-binding capacity are low. Evidence of underlying infection or inflammatory disease is usually obvious.

There is no effective treatment except control of the infection and transfusions if the anemia is severe.

Ward HP & others: Serum level of erythropoietin in anemias associated with chronic infection, malignancy, and primary hematopoietic disease. J Clin Invest 50:332, 1971.

ANEMIAS ASSOCIATED WITH
MARROW REPLACEMENT
(Myelophthisic Anemias)

Anemias resulting from bone marrow invasion or replacement are known as myelophthisic anemias. The most common cause in childhood is invasion with leukemic cells or lymphosarcoma. The differentiation from aplastic anemia in the hypoplastic form of leukemia can only be made by bone marrow examination. Hodgkin's disease in its advanced form may also be associated with severe marrow involvement. Other malignancies (particularly neuroblastoma) may cause diffuse involvement of the marrow. The disseminated acute form of histiocytosis or reticuloendotheliosis (Letterer-Siwe disease) may be associated with a diffuse involvement of the marrow. Certain of the lipid storage diseases such as Gaucher's disease and Niemann-Pick disease gradually invade the marrow. Osteopetrosis (Albers-Schönberg disease) in the acute infantile form is associated with severe encroachment on the marrow space by bone and usually presents initially as a myelophthisic anemia. True myelofibrosis with the development of classical agnogenic myeloid metaplasia is rarely seen in childhood.

All of these forms of myelophthisic anemia are characterized by the development of a normochromic anemia and associated thrombocytopenia. The presence of nucleated red cells and immature white cells with an elevated nucleated cell count in the peripheral blood suggests the existence of a myelophthisic process. Immature white and red cells are not always released, and they are probably related to the degree of extramedullary hematopoiesis. Splenomegaly is present in the majority of these conditions. The diagnosis is dependent upon finding the specific infiltrating process, osteopetrosis, or myelofibrosis in the bone marrow.

ANEMIAS DUE TO FAILURE OF
RELEASE FROM THE MARROW

PRIMARY REFRACTORY ANEMIA
(Refractory Normoblastic Anemia)

This condition is characterized by the paradoxic association of a hypercellular marrow and a moderate to severe chronic anemia, occasionally associated with neutropenia and thrombocytopenia. The reticulocyte count is low to normal. There are usually no other clinical findings, and the spleen is not enlarged. The marrow is markedly hypercellular, with normoblastic hyperplasia. Megaloblastic changes are usually present. Marrow hemosiderin is greatly increased.

The exact cause of this syndrome is not known, although many patients previously given this diagnosis may have had some type of dyserythropoietic anemia associated with intramedullary hemolysis (see next section). Treatment of the primary refractory anemias has been generally without success, and transfusion is the only known treatment. In rare cases, splenectomy has been of slight value; and occasional congenital cases have responded to testosterone therapy. All of these patients should be given a trial of vitamin B since the findings in pyridoxine dependent anemias may be similar.

Vilter RW & others: Refractory anemia with hyperplastic bone marrow. Blood 15:1, 1960.

DYSERYTHROPOIETIC ANEMIAS

The dyserythropoietic anemias are characterized by maturation abnormalities in the bone marrow with associated intramedullary hemolysis. The clinical manifestations include the presence of intermittent scleral jaundice and splenomegaly. Anemia may or may not be present. Some patients are well compensated, with hemoglobins and hematocrits within the normal range. The majority have a mild to moderate anemia of about 10 gm/100 ml. Occasional patients show intermittent severe anemia associated with increased jaundice. They are frequently not recognized as having a hemolytic process since the destruction takes place in the marrow and an excessive number of reticulocytes are not released. The reticulocyte count usually ranges from normal to a maximum of about 4%. In most of the reported familial cases, the mode of genetic transmission appears to be autosomal recessive.

Additional laboratory findings include the presence of marked anisocytosis and poikilocytosis on the blood smear. There is usually an elevation of the indirect serum bilirubin to approximately 2%. The haptoglobin is low or absent. Urobilin and urobilinogen are increased in the urine. The bone marrow pattern is diagnostic, with erythroid hyperplasia and characteristic erythroblasts showing several separate nuclei or with clover leaf shaped nuclei.

There is an elevated fetal hemoglobin and increased hemolysis in acidified serum (a positive Ham test) in the presence of a negative sugar water test. A high proportion of cells are agglutinated by anti-I antibody. Osmotic fragility is normal or increased. The autohemolysis test and hemoglobin electrophoresis are normal. Iron stores are increased, and iron kinetics show a rapid plasma clearance.

The exact mechanism of the ineffective erythropoiesis and the intramedullary hemolysis has not been specifically explained.

The differential diagnosis includes Gilbert's disease, since patients with little or no anemia show primarily an elevated unconjugated (indirect reacting) serum bilirubin and intermittent scleral icterus. In patients with anemia, the differential diagnosis includes the other types of mild hemolytic disease.

Treatment is symptomatic.

Crookston JH & others: Hereditary erythroblastic multinu-clearity associated with a positive acidified serum test: A type of congenital dyserythropoietic anemia. Br J Haematol 17:11, 1969.

Valentine WN & others: Dyserythropoiesis, refractory anemia, and "preleukemia": Metabolic features of the erythrocytes. Blood 41:857, 1973.

HEMOLYTIC ANEMIAS

The hemolytic anemias of childhood may be classified as hereditary or acquired. The hereditary group is of particular importance, since the manifestations usually present in infancy or childhood. They may be divided first into those associated with a defect of the red cell membrane, such as hereditary spherocytosis, and those due to abnormalities in red cell glycolysis. (This includes the majority of the non-spherocytic hemolytic anemias that are associated with specific red cell enzyme defects and the drug-induced hemolytic anemias.) Second, there is the large group of hemoglobinopathies, which includes the anemias with abnormal hemoglobin chains, those with a genetically determined decrease in production of one of the hemoglobin chains, and those with unstable hemoglobin. The majority of the acquired hemolytic anemias are on an "autoimmune" basis; are secondary to drug or chemical poisoning; or are associated with sepsis from hemolytic organisms.

DISORDERS OF RED CELL MEMBRANE

1. HEREDITARY SPHEROCYTOSIS
(Congenital Hemolytic Anemia, Congenital Hemolytic Jaundice)

Essentials of Diagnosis

- Anemia.
- Sudden weakness and jaundice.
- Splenomegaly.
- Spherocytosis, increased reticulocytes.
- Increased osmotic fragility, abnormal autohemolysis.
- Negative Coombs test.
- Positive family history of anemia, jaundice, or gallbladder disease.

General Considerations

Hereditary spherocytosis is believed to be due to

a protein abnormality mediated by a defect in phosphorylation in the red cell membrane, allowing increased sodium influx into the erythrocytes. Increased glycolysis is necessary to prevent the intracellular accumulation of sodium. Spherocytosis and decreased red cell survival occur when the cell is deprived of sufficient glucose. The cells are sequestered and destroyed in the spleen. Transfused cells from normal donors have a normal survival in the patient with spherocytosis, whereas spherocytic cells transfused into a normal recipient maintain their shortened survival rate. The disease may be mild to severe and is characterized by intermittent crises associated with rapid hemolysis and jaundice. Hypoplastic crises occasionally occur in association with decreased erythroid production in the bone marrow. In most instances, the disease is transmitted as an autosomal dominant, and abnormalities can usually be detected in one of the parents of the child even though they are asymptomatic. Occasional families have been reported in which the abnormality cannot be found in other generations, suggesting that it may sometimes be transmitted as a recessive trait or occur as a mutation. Hereditary spherocytosis may be a cause of neonatal hyperbilirubinemia and may be confused with ABO incompatibility because of the presence of spherocytes in both conditions.

Clinical Findings

A. **Symptoms and Signs:** Jaundice usually occurs in the newborn period. Splenomegaly without other symptoms characterizes many of the cases in childhood. Chronic fatigue and malaise may be present, and abdominal pain is a frequent complaint. Gallbladder pain may occur in the adolescent.

Hemolytic or aplastic crises may develop and are associated with severe weakness, fatigue, fever, abdominal pain, and jaundice.

B. **Laboratory Findings:** Mild chronic anemia is characteristic. The hemoglobin usually varies from 9–11 gm/100 ml, although a few cases may have almost normal levels of 12–13 gm/100 ml. The red cells are microcytic and hyperchromic (MCV = 70–80 fl and MCHC = 36–40%). Spherocytes characteristically are seen on the smear but may comprise no more than 10% of the cells prior to splenectomy. A persistently elevated reticulocyte count is characteristic. White cells and platelets are usually normal.

The bone marrow shows typical erythroid hyperplasia of hemolytic anemia (except during the hypoplastic crisis, when there may be marked reduction of erythropoiesis).

Osmotic fragility is increased, particularly after incubation at 37° C for 24 hours. Autohemolysis of blood incubated for 48 hours is greatly increased. Incubation with glucose or ATP will decrease the hemolysis (usually to normal levels). Serum bilirubin may show elevation of the unconjugated portion. Stool urobilinogen is usually elevated. The Coombs test is negative, and hemoglobin electrophoresis reveals a normal pattern.

Complications

Severe jaundice may occur in the newborn period with the development of kernicterus if exchange transfusion is not performed. Splenectomy in the first 2 years of life is associated with increased susceptibility to overwhelming bacterial infections (particularly pneumococcal sepsis). Gallstones (composed principally of bile pigments) occur in up to 85% of young adults with this disease, and may even develop during later childhood if splenectomy is not performed by the middle childhood years.

Treatment

There is no satisfactory medical treatment for this condition, but splenectomy is effective.

A. Exchange Transfusions: For hyperbilirubinemia in the neonatal period, exchange transfusion should be performed.

B. Surgical Treatment: Splenectomy is the treatment of choice in hereditary spherocytosis. Except in unusually severe cases, the procedure should be postponed until the child is at least 3–4 years of age because of the increased risk of infection prior to this time. The operation is indicated in all older children as soon as the diagnosis is confirmed even though the degree of hemolysis may be mild. Cholecystectomy is rarely indicated in childhood, particularly if splenectomy is performed by 10 years of age.

C. Postoperative Anti-infective Prophylaxis: Prophylactic penicillin is recommended following splenectomy in all children under 2 years of age in whom the procedure is done. It should probably be continued until at least 4–5 years of age. In older children, daily penicillin prophylaxis is recommended for at least 1 year postoperatively.

D. Treatment of Hypoplastic Crisis: The crisis is frequently precipitated by an infectious process, which should be treated with appropriate antibiotic therapy. Transfusion with packed red cells is indicated for both the hemolytic and the aplastic crisis.

Prognosis

Splenectomy will eliminate all signs and symptoms, and the red cell survival usually returns to normal following this procedure. The development of cholelithiasis will also be prevented if splenectomy is performed during childhood. The abnormal red cell morphology, increased osmotic fragility, and the abnormal autohemolysis test persist following splenectomy but are of no clinical significance.

Gomperts ED & others: A red cell protein abnormality in hereditary spherocytosis. Br J Haematol 23:363, 1972.

Greenquist AC, Shohet SB: Phosphorylation in erythrocyte membranes from abnormally shaped cells. Blood 48:877, 1976.

Zipursky A, Israels LG: Significance of erythrocyte sodium flux in the pathophysiology and genetic expression of hereditary spherocytosis. Pediatr Res 5:614, 1971.

2. OVALOCYTOSIS
(Hereditary Elliptocytosis)

Hereditary elliptocytosis is characterized primarily by the presence of large numbers of oval and elliptical cells in the peripheral blood. It is usually discovered on routine examination, and the majority of patients are asymptomatic. The morphologic abnormality of the peripheral blood is transmitted as an autosomal dominant and occurs in both sexes. Approximately 12% of the heterozygous cases demonstrate evidence of mild hemolytic disease characterized by slight splenomegaly and reticulocytosis. There may be low-grade anemia, but even in these patients the hemoglobin is frequently within normal limits. Occasionally, neonatal jaundice is sufficiently severe to require exchange transfusions.

The nucleated precursors of the elliptical cells in the bone marrow are normal in shape, with the oval appearance occurring first at the reticulocyte stage or later. The mechanism of the abnormality is not known.

A few cases have been reported of children who are homozygous for the disease. These children have severe hemolytic anemia, with splenomegaly and hematologic evidence of hemolysis.

Treatment is not usually indicated except in severe cases, for which splenectomy is usually beneficial.

Greenberg LH & others: Hereditary elliptocytosis with hemolytic anemia: A family study of 5 affected members. Calif Med 110:389, 1969.

3. STOMATOCYTOSIS

A rare form of hemolytic anemia has been described in which the red blood cells have a characteristic cup-shaped appearance. The anemia is mild, and the disease has the characteristics of a hemolytic process with elevated reticulocyte count. The red cells have increased osmotic fragility, increased autohemolysis, and reduced glutathione.

Splenectomy results in improvement.

Norman JG: Stomatocytosis in migrants of Mediterranean origin. Med J Aust 1:315, 1969.

4. ACANTHOCYTOSIS
(Abetalipoproteinemia)

This rare autosomal recessive disorder is characterized by acanthocytes (thorny cells) in the blood, progressive ataxic neurologic disease, retinitis pigmentosa, malabsorption, and abetalipoproteinemia.

Although the red cells are very abnormal, the degree of hemolysis is mild. (See also Chapter 33.)

Cooper RA, Gulbrandsen CL: The relationship between serum lipoproteins and red cell membranes in abetalipoproteinemia. J Lab Clin Med 78:323, 1971.

5. DESICCYTOSIS
(Low-Potassium Red Cells)

A severe congenital hemolytic anemia has been described that is characterized by shrunken, spiculated cells in which the hemoglobin is "puddled" on one side of the cell. Hepatosplenomegaly is also present. The defect is in the cell membrane and allows loss of potassium and water in excess of sodium gains. Splenectomy has not been of value.

Glader BE & others: Desiccytosis associated with RBC potassium loss: A new congenital hemolytic syndrome. Pediatr Res 7:350, 1973.

6. ACQUIRED CELL MEMBRANE DEFECTS ASSOCIATED WITH HEMOLYSIS

Infantile Pyknocytosis
A transient hemolytic anemia has been described in newborn infants in association with a high degree of pyknocytosis of their red cells. Pyknocytes bear a close resemblance to burr cells or acanthocytes. They occur in small numbers in all newborn and premature infants, but in infants with hemolysis as many as 50% of red cells may be pyknocytes. The exact cause remains unknown. The syndrome is characterized by hemolysis beginning during the first week of life, with jaundice, anemia, reticulocytosis, and splenomegaly. The anemia usually reaches its peak by 3 weeks of age, and recovery is spontaneous.

The diagnosis is based on the presence of large numbers of pyknocytes (> 6%) in association with a Coombs-negative hemolytic anemia.

Exchange transfusion may be necessary for the hyperbilirubinemia of pyknocytosis during the first week. Small transfusions are indicated for increasing anemia after that time.

Akerman BD: Infantile pyknocytosis in Mexican-American infants. Am J Dis Child 117:417, 1969.

Vitamin E Deficiency Hemolytic Anemia
Vitamin E deficiency may cause hemolysis and an increase in burr cells. It can be differentiated from pyknocytosis by demonstrating an increased hemolysis in hydrogen peroxide and a response to the administration of parenteral vitamin E.

The disorder occurs primarily in preterm infants after the fourth week of life and is due to poor absorption of vitamin E. It is aggravated by the oral administration of iron medication. A dosage of 25 units of vitamin E per day orally is adequate prophylaxis.

Melhorn DK, Gross S: Vitamin E-dependent anemia in the premature infant. 1. Effects of large doses of medicinal iron. J Pediatr 79:569, 1971.

Liver Disease
Red cell membrane changes may occur in liver disease and can be associated with significant hemolytic anemia. The membrane abnormality is associated with changes in serum and membrane lipid involving the cholesterol-phospholipid ratio. The most severe form (usually seen in hepatocellular disease) is characterized by "spur" cells. The more common and milder form is characterized by target cells.

Cooper RA & others: An analysis of lipoproteins, bile acids, and red cell membranes associated with target cells and spur cells in patients with liver disease. J Clin Invest 51:3182, 1972.

Renal Disease
A marked hemolytic anemia may occur secondary to the effect of elevated metabolites and urea in severe uremia. Burr cells are usually present. These changes are corrected by hemodialysis.

Hemolytic-Uremic Syndrome
Hemolytic anemia may be severe and often is the presenting complaint in this disorder. It is a microangiopathic anemia associated with destruction of red cells in small renal vessels and characterized by fragmented and burr-shaped cells. (See also Chapter 18.)

Hemolysis With Disseminated Intravascular Coagulation (DIC)
A microangiopathic hemolytic anemia with fragmented cells and burr cells is characteristic of this syndrome (see p 420).

DISORDERS OF RED CELL GLYCOLYSIS
(The Hereditary Nonspherocytic Hemolytic Anemias)

Essentials of Diagnosis
- Moderate to severe anemia.
- Elevated reticulocyte count.
- Normal osmotic fragility test with abnormal autohemolysis.
- Splenomegaly.
- Present from birth, with neonatal jaundice.
- Negative Coombs test.

General Considerations
The hereditary nonspherocytic hemolytic anemias include a number of different defects in red cell metab-

olism. A number of specific enzymes necessary for erythrocyte glycolysis have been shown to be deficient in various forms of nonspherocytic hemolytic anemia. These enzyme deficiencies include glucose-6-phosphate dehydrogenase (G6PD), 6-phosphogluconate dehydrogenase, pyruvate kinase, triosephosphate isomerase, hexokinase, hexosephosphate isomerase, phosphoglycerate kinase, adenosinetriphosphatase (ATPase), 2,3-diphosphoglycerate mutase, phosphoglucose isomerase, phosphofructokinase, glyceraldehyde-3-phosphate dehydrogenase, lactate dehydrogenase, glutathione reductase, glutathione peroxidase, glutathione synthetase, and hereditary absence of glutathione. The most frequently encountered are those associated with G6PD or pyruvate kinase deficiency. These will be discussed in more detail in succeeding sections.

Two general classes of nonspherocytic hemolytic anemia have been described by Dacie. Type I is characterized by normal red cell fragility and a normal to slightly increased autohemolysis test which is corrected by glucose. Patients with severe deficiency of G6PD fall into this type.

Type II cases are characterized by normal or slightly increased red cell fragility but a markedly increased autohemolysis that is not corrected (or only partially corrected) by glucose. Pyruvate kinase deficiency is characteristic of this group.

The hereditary pattern varies. Deficiency of G6PD is usually transmitted as an X-linked recessive trait, whereas pyruvate kinase deficiency is an autosomal recessive. Most of the other types occur as autosomal recessives, although milder forms may be transmitted as an autosomal dominant.

Clinical Findings

A. Symptoms and Signs: Moderate to severe anemia is usually present and exists from early infancy. Neonatal hyperbilirubinemia is usually marked. In severe cases, symptoms of chronic anemia and jaundice persist. The spleen is enlarged.

B. Laboratory Findings: Anemia is moderate to severe, and the hemoglobin usually ranges from 5–9 gm/100 ml. The red cells are normocytic and normochromic, although occasional microcytes are seen and, in pyruvate kinase deficiency, a few spherocytes. The reticulocyte count is markedly elevated; the white cell and platelet counts are normal. Bone marrow shows marked erythroid hyperplasia.

Red cell osmotic fragility is usually within normal limits, although in type II—and particularly in pyruvate kinase deficiency—it may be slightly increased. The autohemolysis test is usually slightly increased in type I, and partially corrected by glucose and ATP, whereas it is markedly abnormal in type II with very little correction by glucose, but complete correction with ATP. A third type (triosephosphate isomerase deficiency) is corrected by both glucose and ATP. The Coombs test is negative, and hemoglobin electrophoresis is normal.

Studies of red cell glycolysis with assays of specific enzymes are indicated in all cases that fall into this group, since the response to therapy may be dependent on the exact type of disease.

Differential Diagnosis

In the newborn period, hereditary nonspherocytic hemolytic anemia must be differentiated from erythroblastosis fetalis and ABO incompatibility by immunologic studies. It is differentiated from acquired hemolytic anemia by the early onset and the absence of a positive Coombs test. The differentiation from hereditary spherocytosis is based on the absence of spherocytes on the smear, the normal or only slightly increased red cell fragility, and the lack of complete correction with glucose in the autohemolysis test in the nonspherocytic hemolytic anemias.

Complications

The severe chronic anemia is usually associated with growth failure; hemosiderosis may occur in cases that require frequent transfusions. Cholelithiasis and cholecystitis may develop in later childhood.

Treatment

There is no specific therapy for most cases of nonspherocytic hemolytic anemia. Splenectomy is not as effective as in hereditary spherocytosis, and is of no benefit in many cases. However, many patients (including those with pyruvate kinase deficiency) do show significant improvement following splenectomy; although no patients are completely cured and many do not respond at all, the operation is probably worth a trial. The possible value of splenectomy can be estimated by determinating the red cell survival of cells from a patient with hereditary nonspherocytic hemolytic anemia after infusion into a normal individual who has undergone splenectomy for some other reason.

Prognosis

In the milder form of this disease, the prognosis is good; the patient can usually live with a mild chronic anemia. Cholelithiasis often develops in early adult life. The prognosis is similar in patients with more severe forms that show improvement following splenectomy.

In the severe types that do not respond to splenectomy, frequent transfusions are required, physical growth is stunted, and hemochromatosis may develop from the iron administered by the frequent transfusions.

Beutler E (editor): *Hereditary Disorders of Erythrocyte Metabolism.* Grune & Stratton, 1968.

Dacie JV: Recent advances in knowledge of the hereditary haemolytic anaemias. Schweiz Med Wochenschr 98:1624, 1968.

Oski FA, Naiman JL: *Hematologic Problems in the Newborn,* 2nd ed. Saunders, 1972.

1. PYRUVATE KINASE DEFICIENCY HEMOLYTIC ANEMIA

A severe chronic hemolytic anemia is associated with erythrocyte pyruvate kinase deficiency. Although this is a rare disease, it is still one of the more frequently encountered specific entities in the group of nonspherocytic hereditary hemolytic anemias. It is transmitted as an autosomal recessive condition. It presents as a moderate or severe hemolytic anemia in the immediate neonatal period, with low hemoglobin levels even in cord blood. Jaundice in the newborn is a common complication, and exchange transfusion is usually required. Splenomegaly is the only consistent clinical finding. The reticulocytes in this disorder are particularly susceptible to splenic sequestration. Leg ulcers have been described in a family with a variant type of pyruvate kinase deficiency.

The anemia is normochromic, and there is a marked elevation of the reticulocyte count. The blood smear shows some microcytes and a few spherocytes. Differentiation from hereditary spherocytosis is not easy because spherocytes may be seen in pyruvate kinase deficiency and red cell osmotic fragility may also be slightly increased; the autohemolysis test is markedly increased, as in spherocytosis. The most useful point of differentiation between the 2 diseases is the fact that the red cell fragility is only slightly increased and the autohemolysis test is only partially corrected by glucose in pyruvate kinase deficiency, whereas the latter is markedly corrected in spherocytosis.

Family studies are also helpful in differentiating the 2 conditions, since pyruvate kinase deficiency is a recessive trait whereas spherocytosis is usually a dominant.

Red cell glycolysis and specific enzyme assays for pyruvate kinase are indicated if this condition is suspected. Several different mutant forms of the enzyme have been reported, and, recently, patients have been described with a similar disorder who appear to have adequate pyruvate kinase activity by the usual assay but who are found to have a pathologic isoenzyme which can be detected only by assays using low levels of substrate.

Treatment consists of splenectomy. Significant improvement usually follows this procedure, although complete cure is not achieved. Prior to splenectomy, repeated transfusions are usually necessary every few months. No drugs or other methods of management are effective.

The prognosis following splenectomy is fairly good, although the complications of cholelithiasis should be anticipated.

Mentzer WC & others: Selective reticulocyte destruction in erythrocyte pyruvate kinase deficiency. J Clin Invest 50:688, 1971.

Müller-Soyano A & others: Pyruvate kinase deficiency and leg ulcers. Blood 47:807, 1976.

Poglia DE: An aberrant inherited molecular lesion of erythrocyte pyruvate kinase: Identification of a kinetically aberrant isoenzyme associated with premature hemolysis. J Clin Invest 47:1929, 1968.

2. GLUCOSE-6-PHOSPHATE DEHYDROGENASE DEFICIENCY (Drug-Sensitive Hemolytic Anemia, Primaquine-Sensitive Hemolytic Anemia)

Drug-induced hemolytic anemia is most commonly associated with a red cell deficiency of glucose-6-phosphate dehydrogenase (G6PD). Most persons with a G6PD defect have episodes of hemolysis only after exposure to certain drugs, although the more severe forms may be manifested by a chronic hereditary nonspherocytic hemolytic anemia of the Dacie type I.

The disease is transmitted as an X-linked trait and is of intermediate dominance. Full expression occurs in males and females who are homozygous for the gene; intermediate expression occurs in the heterozygous female carrier. About 10% of American black males manifest this enzyme deficiency, whereas only 1–2% of American black females tend to be mildly symptomatic when challenged with drugs. This disease occurs also in the Chinese and in whites (particularly Greeks, Italians, and Sephardic Jews). The exact mechanism of the enzyme defect is not quantitatively nor qualitatively identical in all of these racial groups.

Symptoms usually occur only following drug exposure, although in the neonatal period certain racial groups (Greek, Italian, and Chinese) may show increased hyperbilirubinemia, whereas full-term black babies do not. The most common offenders are the antimalarials, sulfonamides, sulfones, nitrofurans, antipyretics, analgesics, synthetic vitamin K, and uncooked fava beans. Hemolytic crises in patients with sickle cell anemia may be due in part to an associated G6PD deficiency.

The clinical picture is characterized by an acute hemolytic episode following exposure to one of these substances. The anemia is normochromic, and Heinz body formation is characteristic. An elevated reticulocyte count will appear within a few days.

Since only the older red cells are susceptible, the process becomes self-limited as a younger red cell population appears in response to the hemolytic process.

A specific laboratory diagnosis may be made by one of several tests, including the glutathione stability test, the dye reduction test using cresyl blue, the methemoglobin reduction test, or a commercially available dye reduction spot test.

Routine laboratory screening has been recommended for persons in the high-risk racial groups.

The only treatment required is discontinuing exposure to the offending agent.

Beutler E & others: Prevalence of G6PD deficiency in sickle-cell disease. N Engl J Med 290:826, 1974.

Piomelli S & others: Clinical and biochemical interactions of glucose-6-phosphate dehydrogenase deficiency and sickle cell anemia. N Engl J Med 287:213, 1972.

Yoshida A: Hemolytic anemia and G6PD deficiency. Science 179:532, 1973.

SYNTHETIC VITAMIN K-INDUCED HEMOLYTIC ANEMIA OF THE NEWBORN

Another form of drug-induced hemolytic anemia occurs following the administration of synthetic vitamin K (Synkamin, Synkayvite, Hykinone) in large doses in the newborn period. Although the level of G6PD is not decreased in the newborn infant, the drug-induced hemolysis appears to be related to instability of reduced glutathione in the newborn red cells. This may be due in part to the low blood glucose levels which are characteristic of the neonatal period.

This complication can be prevented by limiting the dose of the synthetic vitamin K product to a total of 1 mg or by the use of vitamin K_1 (Mephyton, Aqua-Mephyton, etc), which does not have the same chemical derivation.

Oski FA, Naiman JL: *Hematologic Problems in the Newborn*, 2nd ed. Saunders, 1972.

HEMOGLOBINOPATHIES—QUALITATIVE DEFECTS

1. SICKLE CELL ANEMIA

Essentials of Diagnosis

- Anemia, elevated reticulocyte count, jaundice.
- Positive sickling test, hemoglobin S and F.
- Pains in the legs and abdomen.
- Splenomegaly in early childhood, with later disappearance.
- Hemolytic crises.
- Black African ethnic origin.

General Considerations

Sickle hemoglobin is found primarily in black persons of African origin. It is seen occasionally in other racial groups in North Africa and the Middle East. Sickle cell anemia is estimated to occur in about one in 500 blacks in the USA with a much higher rate in some parts of Africa.

Sickle cell anemia occurs in individuals who are homozygous for the sickle cell gene. Sickle hemoglobin is characterized by a single amino acid substitution in the beta chain of adult type (A_1) hemoglobin. The sickling trait is transmitted as a dominant; the carrier shows a combination of hemoglobin A and sickle hemoglobin, whereas the patient with sickle cell anemia has only sickle and fetal hemoglobin. The sickling process is often initiated by low oxygen tension and low pH. The sickle cell moves slowly through capillaries, and thrombi are frequent. Thrombosis probably accounts for the abdominal pain, leg pain, and gradual decrease in the size of the spleen ("autosplenectomy").

Clinical Findings

A. Symptoms and Signs: The onset of symptoms, usually between 9 and 12 months of age, is with severe infections, splenic sequestration crises, or dactylitis (hand and foot syndrome). The anemia is moderately severe, but fatigue and weakness are minimal. Mild scleral jaundice is usually present. Crises are frequent and are characterized by pain in the bones and joints or the abdomen; severe acute hemolysis may occur. Abdominal tenderness and rigidity may occur. Fever is usually present. Severe anemia, weakness, and increased jaundice may accompany the crisis. The anemia may be hyperhemolytic or hypoplastic. Physical growth is often retarded; puberty may be delayed; and children are usually of asthenic build. Older children show enlargement of the facial and skull bones and may develop tower skull.

B. Laboratory Findings: The hemoglobin usually ranges between 7 and 10 gm/100 ml. It may drop as low as 2–3 gm/100 ml at the time of a sequestration or hypoplastic crisis. The reticulocyte count is markedly elevated. The anemia is normocytic and normochromic, but the smear shows increased numbers of target cells and abnormalities of size and shape. Sickling may be seen on the ordinary blood smear and is common at the time of crisis. The sickling phenomenon can be demonstrated by reducing the oxygen tension in the finger with a small tourniquet prior to obtaining blood, or by ringing the cover slip on a slide with petrolatum over a drop of blood. Fresh sodium metabisulfite, 2%, mixed on the slide with the drop of blood will bring out the sickling in a few minutes. Nucleated red cells are present and may equal the number of white cells. The total nucleated cell count is high. Serum bilirubin usually shows a slight elevation of unconjugated (indirect) bilirubin. The specific gravity of the urine becomes fixed at about 1.010 in later childhood, and both hemosiderinuria and hematuria may be seen.

The bone marrow shows marked erythroid hyperplasia. X-rays of the skull and spine reveal cortical thinning, enlargement of the marrow spaces, and increased trabecular markings.

Hemoglobin electrophoresis reveals sickle (S) hemoglobin and fetal (F) hemoglobin. The fetal component usually varies between 5 and 20%.

Differential Diagnosis

The most important differentiation is from the other chronic hemoglobinopathies that are also common in the black population. The differentiation from thalassemia and hemoglobin C disease is made primarily by hemoglobin electrophoresis, fetal hemoglobin determination, and the sickling test. The hematuria that occurs with sickle cell anemia must be differentiated from renal bleeding due to other causes. In crisis, the primary differentiation is from acute appendicitis in the presence of abdominal pain and tenderness and from rheumatic fever because of the frequent joint and bone pains and the systolic precordial murmur in sickle cell disease.

Hemoglobin D migrates electrophoretically on paper and starch at the same rate as S and is indistinguishable by this method. They can be differentiated by the negative sickling test in hemoglobin D disease. Study of the entire family is often of importance in determining the exact nature of the hemoglobinopathy.

Sickle cell trait associated with iron deficiency anemia can be differentiated by the presence of a low reticulocyte count, high red cell count, and hypochromia.

Complications

Increased susceptibility to overwhelming infection (especially pneumococcal) occurs in the first few years of life. Life-threatening splenic sequestration crises associated with severe anemia also may occur at this age.

The primary complications in later childhood are associated with vascular thromboses. Cerebral thrombosis and pulmonary infarcts may occur, particularly in younger children; and leg ulcers and aseptic necrosis of the femoral head are common in older children and adolescents. An increased incidence of salmonella osteomyelitis has been reported. In the adolescent, cardiac enlargement and even heart failure may occur in association with prolonged severe anemia and cardiac ischemia. Cholelithiasis is rarely seen in childhood but will be an eventual complication. Hypoplastic crises may occur and are associated with the development of a very severe and prolonged anemic state.

Treatment

Treatment is instituted primarily for the crises. There is no known effective method for reducing the rate of chronic hemolysis or preventing crises. Both the hemolytic and hypoplastic crises should be treated with transfusion. Transfusions are also helpful in terminating prolonged "painful" crises. Packed red cells are usually used. A partial exchange with packed red cells is indicated in pulmonary and other severe crises. The use of oxygen, maintenance of good hydration, and correction of acidosis are the most important measures for management of the symptoms of crisis. Rest, analgesics, and sedatives may be sufficient in mild cases. Corticosteroids have been reported to be helpful in the management of painful swelling of the hands and feet. Recent clinical trials using testosterone to stimulate marrow production have been associated with an increased incidence of thrombosis. The value of treatment with urea (to reduce sickling) must be established by further controlled studies. The use of cyanate and the alkylureas is still experimental.

Splenectomy may be of value in the child with a persistently enlarged spleen and a need for frequent transfusions. Since there is a natural tendency for the spleen to shrink in size in this disease, splenectomy is seldom indicated. Since functional hyposplenism develops as early as 6 months of age, penicillin or other prophylactic antibiotic therapy is recommended from 6 months to 5 years of age.

Prognosis

Relatively few patients with homozygous sickle cell disease die in childhood, although a fatal outcome is occasionally seen in association with overwhelming infections, cerebrovascular accidents, or cardiac failure. Many patients, however, die in early adult life. Progressive renal damage usually occurs, and death from uremia or heart failure is common.

Elbaum D & others: Molecular and cellular effects of anti-sickling concentrations of alkylureas. Blood 48:273, 1976.

Freedman ML: Treatment of crises in sickle cell anemia. Am J Med Sci 261:305, 1971.

Pearson HA & others: Functional asplenia in sickle-cell anemia. N Engl J Med 281:923, 1969.

Powars DR: Natural history of sickle cell disease. Semin Hematol 12:267, 1975.

Segel GB & others: Effects of urea and cyanate on sickling in vitro. N Engl J Med 287:59, 1972.

Smits HL & others: Hemolytic crisis of sickle cell disease: Role of glucose-6-phosphate dehydrogenase deficiency. J Pediatr 74:544, 1969.

2. SICKLE CELL TRAIT

Sickle cell trait occurs in about 8–10% of blacks in the USA and in as much as 50% of the population in certain areas of Africa. The high incidence of the carrier state in African blacks has been attributed to the increased resistance to malaria in these individuals; this tends to selectively increase their representation in the population. It is generally asymptomatic, and anemia, reticulocytosis, and morphologic red cell changes are not observed. Hematuria is the principal complication and occurs in 3–4% of cases. Progressive impairment in the ability of the kidneys to concentrate urine is sometimes noted. Infarcts (particularly in the spleen and lung) may occur in the presence of low oxygen tension at extremely high altitudes—particularly with flying in unpressurized aircraft. Except for these unusual circumstances, the prognosis is excellent and the life expectancy is normal.

Knochel JP: Hematuria in sickle cell trait. Arch Intern Med 123:160, 1969.

3. HEMOGLOBIN S-C DISEASE

Hemoglobin S-C disease is caused by the double autosomal heterozygous state for both hemoglobin S and C. The incidence in the American black population is about 1:1500. Symptoms are similar to those of homozygous sickle cell disease but are much less marked. Some patients with S-C disease are prone to vaso-occlusive crises involving the lung, kidney, retina, and femoral head. Target cells are prominent, and a mild anemia with persistent reticulocytosis is usually present. Persons with S-C disease are particularly prone to develop splenic sequestration crises at high altitudes or while flying in unpressurized aircraft. The diagnosis is confirmed by hemoglobin electrophoresis and the sickling test, along with evaluation of other members of the family. The complications and treatment are similar to those for sickle cell anemia, although most patients require no therapy. Although the severity of the disease may vary, the prognosis is much better than in homozygous sickle disease, and the life span is usually not seriously affected.

Githens JH & others: Splenic sequestration syndrome at mountain altitudes in sickle/hemoglobin C disease. J Pediatr 90:203, 1977.

Serjeant GR & others: The clinical features of haemoglobin SC disease in Jamaica. Br J Haematol 24:491, 1973.

4. SICKLE THALASSEMIA

This disease is due to the double autosomal heterozygous state for both hemoglobin S and beta-thalassemia. Symptoms are similar to those of sickle cell anemia but are less marked. Painful vaso-occlusive crises may occur. Anemia is usually mild—hemoglobin is in the range of 10—12 gm/100 ml.

Hemoglobin electrophoresis usually shows both A_1 and S hemoglobins but with S being $> 50\%$ (usually 60—80%). A_2 and fetal hemoglobins are also present and usually elevated. A few patients (with the Mediterranean beta-thalassemia gene) have only S, F, and A_2 hemoglobins, making it difficult to differentiate them from those patients with sickle cell anemia. Family studies are needed to confirm the diagnosis. Symptomatic treatment may be required for mild crises. Life expectancy is probably normal.

Pearson HA: Hemoglobin S-thalassemia syndrome in Negro children. Ann NY Acad Sci 165:83, 1969.

5. HEMOGLOBIN C TRAIT & HEMOGLOBIN C DISEASE

Hemoglobin C trait occurs in about 2% of American blacks. Individuals with the trait are heterozygous for the gene and are essentially asymptomatic; they have a normal life expectancy. The blood smear, however, reveals the presence of large numbers of target cells. Renal hematuria has occasionally been reported.

Hemoglobin C disease is rare and occurs in individuals who are homozygous for the gene. It occurs almost exclusively in blacks. The age at onset is usually about 1 year since the infant is protected by his fetal hemoglobin. Patients usually demonstrate a mild hemolytic anemia with a persistently elevated reticulocyte count. Red cell morphology is characterized by many target cells, which are usually normocytic and normochromic. Tetragonal crystals of hemoglobin can be found in the erythrocyte. Osmotic fragility is decreased. The diagnosis is made by hemoglobin electrophoresis, which usually reveals 100% hemoglobin C. Fetal hemoglobin is usually not elevated. Moderate to marked splenomegaly is the only significant clinical finding. There are usually no symptoms, although abdominal pain, arthralgia, and jaundice may occur occasionally.

Treatment is usually not required, and transfusions are rarely needed. Splenectomy is occasionally indicated if anemia is severe.

Redetski JE, Bickers JN, Samuels MS: Homozygous hemoglobin C disease: Clinical review of 15 patients. South Med J 61:238, 1968.

6. HEMOGLOBIN M DISEASE

The designation M is given to several abnormal hemoglobins which are associated with methemoglobinemia. These patients are heterozygous for the gene, and it is transmitted as an autosomal dominant. A number of different types have been described in which various abnormal amino acids are substituted in the polypeptide chain, producing a hemoglobin molecule in which the iron remains in the ferric instead of the ferrous state and cannot combine with oxygen. The defect may be on either the alpha or the beta chain. Hemoglobin electrophoresis at the usual pH will not always demonstrate the abnormal hemoglobin, and special technics are necessary to detect it by electrophoresis as well as spectroscopically.

The patient has marked and persistent cyanosis but is otherwise usually asymptomatic. Exercise tolerance may be normal, and life expectancy is not affected. When the abnormality is on the beta chain, the infant is unaffected for the first few months of life. Some persons with the M hemoglobinopathy of the beta chain may also have mild hemolysis.

This type of methemoglobinemia does not respond to any form of therapy.

Heller P: Hemoglobin M: An early chapter in the saga of molecular pathology. Ann Intern Med 70:1038, 1969.

Stavem P & others: Haemoglobin M Saskatoon with slight constant haemolysis, markedly increased by sulphonamides. Scand J Haematol 9:566, 1972.

7. OTHER ABNORMAL HEMOGLOBINS

Other hemoglobins such as D, E, G, and H are rare in the USA but occur with a higher incidence in other parts of the world. Hemoglobin D has been reported particularly from the Punjab area of India and in parts of Turkey and Africa, as well as occasionally in American blacks and American Indians. It is generally asymptomatic unless associated with another abnormal hemoglobin such as S. Hemoglobin E occurs particularly in Thailand and is usually asymptomatic except in association with other hemoglobin disorders such as thalassemia. Hemoglobin G, even in the homozygous form, has not been associated with symptoms but has been described in combination with other abnormal hemoglobins as a cause of mild anemia. Hemoglobin H has been reported primarily from Asia and, in particular, from Thailand. It is composed only of beta chains, and symptomatic disease has been described primarily in combination with alpha thalassemia. The red cells demonstrate characteristic inclusion bodies in the presence of supravital stains such as brilliant cresyl blue.

The majority of the other abnormal hemoglobins that have been described occur only in the heterozygous form and are asymptomatic.

Lehmann H: Hemoglobinopathies: Abnormal hemoglobins and thalassemias. Isr J Med Sci 4:478, 1968.

8. THERMOLABILE (UNSTABLE) HEMOGLOBINS

Since the first report in 1960, a number of families have now been described with a mild form of hemolytic anemia due to a hemoglobinopathy in which the hemoglobin is thermolabile. All of these patients with unstable hemoglobins have had mild anemia and scleral jaundice. They frequently report intermittent exacerbations of hemolysis, and in all cases a dark brown urine has been noted. Mild splenomegaly is usually present. The disorders appear to be transmitted as an autosomal dominant with symptoms occurring in the heterozygous form.

The laboratory findings reveal a typical picture of a hemolytic anemia with a mild to moderate depression of the hemoglobin and hematocrit and a significant elevation of the reticulocyte count. The unconjugated (indirect reacting) serum bilirubin is often slightly elevated and haptoglobin levels are usually zero, confirming the evidence for hemolysis. The blood smear in some patients has demonstrated marked basophilic stippling. The osmotic fragility test may show both increased fragility and increased resistance. The autohemolysis test is normal. Specific diagnostic studies include the presence of Heinz bodies, particularly after incubation at 37° C for 48 hours. Hemoglobin electrophoresis in some families has shown an abnormal hemoglobin on paper electrophoresis at pH 8.5. In all cases in which the abnormal hemoglobin was identified on electrophoresis, it has migrated more slowly than hemoglobin A_1 and frequently has been more readily identified on starch gel or agar gel. The percentage of abnormal hemoglobin identified has usually been low (in the range of 5–10%). The heat stability test is the best method for identification of the thermolabile hemoglobin. All of the reported hemoglobins precipitate with heating to 50° C for 1 hour. The dark pigment in the urine has been identified as mesobilifuscin.

At least 39 different unstable hemoglobins have been identified to date. These include Scott, Zurich, Köln, Ubi-1, Summersmith, Dacie, Seattle, St. Mary's, Galliera Genova, Sydney, King's County, and others.

The differential diagnosis includes all of the hereditary hemolytic anemias such as spherocytosis and the nonspherocytic group as well as the other hemoglobinopathies. The autosomal dominant genetic transmission tends to exclude the majority of these except for spherocytosis. The diagnostic test is a demonstration of a thermolabile hemoglobin in the blood and the presence of mesobilifuscin in the urine.

The prognosis in most patients is probably good since the anemia appears to be mild. There is no specific treatment.

White JM, Dacie JV: The unstable hemoglobins: Molecular and clinical features. Prog Hematol 7:69, 1971.

9. HEMOGLOBINOPATHIES WITH ABNORMAL OXYGEN AFFINITY

At least 13 different hemoglobinopathies have been described in which the primary clinical sign is polycythemia. The individuals have been heterozygous for the abnormal hemoglobins (eg, hemoglobins Chesapeake, Malmö, Yakima, and Rainier), and the condition is usually transmitted as an autosomal dominant. These hemoglobins have an increased oxygen affinity which results in decreased tissue oxygenation and a compensatory erythrocytosis. Most of these persons have been asymptomatic except for plethora.

At least 3 different hemoglobins have been described with low oxygen affinity. They may demonstrate cyanosis (hemoglobin Kansas) or anemia (hemoglobin Seattle).

HEMOGLOBINOPATHIES–QUANTITATIVE DEFECTS
(Thalassemia Syndromes)

1. BETA THALASSEMIA MINOR
(Thalassemia Trait, Cooley's Carrier State)

Essentials of Diagnosis

- Mild hypochromic anemia.
- Unresponsiveness to iron.
- Elevated A_2 hemoglobin.
- Usually Mediterranean, black, or Oriental racial lines.

General Considerations

Thalassemia is now known to be due to a genetic defect in the production of hemoglobin. It can affect both the alpha and the beta chains, but the majority of patients seen in the USA have beta thalassemia. The patient with thalassemia minor is heterozygous for the gene, which is transmitted as an autosomal dominant.

Clinical Findings

A. Symptoms and Signs: There are usually no symptoms, and the only physical sign may be slight enlargement of the spleen.

B. Laboratory Findings: The anemia is usually mild; the hemoglobin is rarely under 9 gm/100 ml, and may be within normal limits. The red count and hematocrit are very slightly reduced. The red cells are small and hypochromic, and the MCHC is low. Target cells are often present, and stippled cells are seen occasionally. Variations in the size and shape of the cells are often noted. The reticulocyte count may be slightly elevated but is frequently within normal limits. Osmotic fragility is markedly decreased.

The diagnosis is confirmed by finding an elevation of the A_2 hemoglobin on electrophoresis in 90% of families; fetal hemoglobin is increased in 10% of families. (In alpha thalassemia—see below—the A_2 hemoglobin is normal.) The serum iron may be normal in infancy but becomes elevated. The bone marrow may show excessive iron deposition in the older child.

Differential Diagnosis

The primary differentiation is from other mild hypochromic anemias. In childhood, nutritional iron deficiency presents the greatest problem but is readily differentiated by the finding of low serum iron levels and a response to iron therapy, as well as a normal A_2 hemoglobin level. Lead poisoning and pyridoxine responsive anemia may present with a similar hematologic picture.

Several closely related thalassemia-like carrier states have recently been described. One of these, the Lepore trait, is characterized by a mild hypochromic anemia and an abnormal hemoglobin on starch electrophoresis (but not on paper). It comprises approximately 10% of the hemoglobin.

Complications

There are no complications of thalassemia trait in childhood. In late adult life, excess accumulation of iron may lead to hemosiderosis.

Treatment

No therapy is indicated. Iron should definitely not be administered.

Weatherall DJ, Clegg JB: *The Thalassemia Syndromes,* 2nd ed. Blackwell, 1972.

2. BETA THALASSEMIA MAJOR
(Cooley's Anemia, Mediterranean Anemia)

Essentials of Diagnosis

- Very severe anemia.
- Marked erythroblastemia.
- Splenomegaly and hepatomegaly.
- Elevated fetal hemoglobin.
- Usually Mediterranean, black, or Oriental racial lines.

General Considerations

Thalassemia major appears in individuals who are homozygous for the thalassemia gene. Family studies show that both parents have thalassemia minor. Homozygous beta thalassemia is now believed to be due to a quantitative deficiency in production of beta chains of adult hemoglobin (hemoglobin A_1). This produces an intracorpuscular defect which is associated with marked hypochromia and a shortened red cell survival time. Ineffective erythropoiesis and increased intramedullary hemolysis contribute to the anemia. The gene is present in Africa, southern Europe, and Asia. It is believed that the selective increase in the gene in this area (which may reach an incidence of up to 50% in isolated communities) is due to the fact that the heterozygote has an increased resistance to malaria.

Clinical Findings

A. Symptoms and Signs: Severe anemia usually does not manifest itself clinically until about age 1 because of the protective effect of normal fetal hemoglobin. However, splenomegaly and mild anemia are often noted by 6 months. By age 2, there is usually massive splenomegaly and significant hepatomegaly, which continue until the spleen extends into the pelvis. Physical growth and sexual development are markedly impaired, and there is increased susceptibility to infections. As the child approaches the school years, the widening of the flat bones of the face and skull in association with marrow hypertrophy gives all children with thalassemia major a characteristic facies: prominence of the malar eminences, depression of the bridge of the nose, a slightly oblique appearance of the eyes, and an enlargement of the superior maxilla with upward protrusion of the lip. The anemia is severe, and after age 1 usually requires transfusions at frequent intervals. Jaundice may be present.

B. Laboratory Findings: The blood smear reveals a severe hypochromic microcytic anemia with marked anisocytosis and poikilocytosis. Target cells are prominent. Nucleated red cells are numerous and often exceed the circulating white blood cells. The hemoglobin is low (5–6 gm/100 ml). The reticulocyte count is significantly elevated. Platelet and white cell counts are frequently high. Serum bilirubin is elevated. The diagnosis is confirmed by hemoglobin electrophoresis, which reveals no abnormal hemoglobin but a marked increase in fetal hemoglobin and in A_2 hemoglobin. The exact level of fetal hemoglobin should be determined by the alkali denaturation method. Osmotic fragility is markedly decreased. The bone marrow shows marked erythroid hyperplasia with increased iron deposition.

C. X-Ray Findings: Bone x-rays are very characteristic and reveal an increase in the medullary area with thinning of the cortex. The skull has a "hair-on-end" appearance.

Differential Diagnosis

There is usually no problem in the diagnosis of homozygous thalassemia since essentially no other disease shows the characteristic peripheral blood and hemoglobin electrophoresis findings. The primary clinical differentiation is with the combinations of thalassemia and other abnormal hemoglobins such as thalassemia-hemoglobin S disease, thalassemia-hemoglobin E, etc. These have similar clinical pictures but are usually more mild. They are differentiated by the electrophoretic pattern.

Complications

Patients with thalassemia major have multiple complications. They have an increased susceptibility to infections, particularly following splenectomy. Acute benign nonspecific pericarditis is a common problem. Repeated fractures are associated with the thinning of cortical bone. The multiple transfusions which are required are ultimately associated with transfusion reactions and the development of leukocyte antibodies. Growth is impaired, and adolescent development of secondary sex characteristics is delayed. Cholelithiasis and cholecystitis are almost always present in the adolescent or young adult. The major complication, however, is the development of hemochromatosis secondary to excessive absorption and transfusion of iron in these patients. This results in cirrhosis and in heart failure. Cardiac complications are related primarily to the heavy deposition of iron in the myocardium, and death is usually due to heart failure.

Treatment

There is no specific treatment for thalassemia major. Infections should be treated promptly with antibiotics, and heart failure with digitalis and other appropriate therapy.

A. Transfusion: Blood transfusion is the primary therapeutic measure; packed red cells are indicated (in many cases, every 6–8 weeks). In the past, transfusion was given when symptoms occurred or when the hemoglobin fell below 5–6 gm/100 ml; sufficient blood was administered to raise the hemoglobin to approximately 8 gm/100 ml. Maintenance of the hemoglobin level between 10 and 12 gm/100 ml has been associated with improved vigor and well-being and fewer overall complications. There is no good evidence that more frequent transfusions increase hemochromatosis. In fact, life expectancy may be greater if the hemoglobin is maintained at the higher level.

B. Chelation: Chelating agents such as deferoxamine (Desferal) are valuable in removing some of the iron and may have the potential for increasing life expectancy. Recent studies indicate that intramuscular administration of large doses of deferoxamine (10 mg/kg IM daily) in conjunction with oral ascorbic acid (200–500 mg/day) can cause significant urinary excretion in older children who have large iron stores. Continuous intravenous or subcutaneous administration may prove to be even more effective.

C. Folic Acid: A relative folic acid deficiency may develop because of the marked overproduction of bone marrow. Folic acid, 5–10 mg daily orally, is often of value.

D. Splenectomy: Splenectomy is usually of value in the older child and is definitely indicated if the transfusion requirements become progressively greater. It is also indicated for the abdominal discomfort and distention associated with massive enlargement of the organ. Although it does not change the basic rate of homolysis, it will eliminate the hypersplenism which further shortens red cell survival. The hazard of severe and overwhelming infection following splenectomy is much greater in patients with thalassemia major than in any other group, and the use of prophylactic penicillin following this procedure is recommended.

E. Oxymetholone: Oxymetholone may stimulate bone marrow and enhance the patient's red cell production.

Prognosis

Although the prognosis has improved significantly with the use of antibiotics in the past few decades and may continue to improve with the use of chelating agents to remove iron and prevent hemosiderosis, very few patients survive into adult life although the majority reach adolescence.

Craddock PR, Hunt FA, Rozenberg MC: The effective use of oxymetholone in the therapy of thalassemia with anaemia. Med J Aust 2:199, 1972.

Graziano JH, Cerami A: Chelation therapy for the treatment of thalassemia. Semin Hematol 14:127, 1977.

Pearson HA, O'Brien RT: The management of thalassemia major. Semin Hematol 12:255, 1975.

Propper RD, Shurin SB, Nathan DG: Reassessment of desferrioxamine B in iron overload. N Engl J Med 294:1421, 1976.

3. ALPHA THALASSEMIA

Defective production of alpha chains also results in anemia. Several different forms of alpha thalassemia have been described. The disorder has been recognized chiefly in Southeast Asia (especially Thailand) and in blacks. Recent evidence suggests that 4 alpha thalassemia genes exist and that different degrees of severity of anemia are related to the number of gene deletions.

The alpha thalassemia carriers who lack one gene may be completely asymptomatic and have normal blood findings. Those with 2 deleted genes may show mild hypochromia and occasional target cells on the blood smear. No abnormal hemoglobin is demonstrated in older children, and there are no compensatory increases in hemoglobin A_2 or fetal hemoglobin. Barts hemoglobin is present in small amounts at birth.

The disorder previously called thalassemia-hemoglobin H disease is now recognized to be a form of alpha thalassemia in which 3 of the 4 genes are deleted. It has been described primarily in Southeast Asia (Philippines, southern China, and Thailand). The patient demonstrates a chronic microcytic anemia which is refractory to iron therapy and tends to resemble beta thalassemia minor. Hemoglobin electrophoresis at pH 8.5 reveals a fast hemoglobin that migrates more rapidly than A_1. This hemoglobin is composed of 4 beta chains. Characteristic red cell inclusions are demonstrated by the reticulocyte stain upon incubation. There is no satisfactory treatment. Iron should not be administered to patients with any form of alpha thalassemia.

The most severe type of alpha thalassemia is associated with deletion of all 4 genes and is incompatible with life. These severely anemic and hydropic infants have only Barts hemoglobin since they are unable to produce any alpha hemoglobin chains.

Na-Nakorn S & others: Further evidence for a genetic basis of haemoglobin H disease from newborn offspring of patients. Nature 223:59, 1969.

Orkin SH, Nathan DG: The thalassemias. N Engl J Med 295:710, 1976.

Weatherall DJ, Clegg JB: *The Thalassemia Syndromes,* 2nd ed. Blackwell, 1972.

4. THALASSEMIA VARIANTS

Double heterozygosity of thalassemia with other hemoglobinopathies such as C, S, and E are fairly common in certain parts of the world and manifest themselves clinically as milder forms of thalassemia major. The diagnosis is made by hemoglobin electrophoresis, which shows a predominance of hemoglobin F and other abnormal hemoglobin. Family studies will reveal one parent to be a thalassemia carrier and the other a carrier of C, S, or E.

5. HEREDITARY PERSISTENCE OF FETAL HEMOGLOBIN

Hereditary persistence of fetal hemoglobin has been reported in both black and Greek families. It is usually found in the heterozygous form and is associated with no symptoms. The blood counts and blood smears are normal. The fetal hemoglobin level is approximately 20% after 2 years of age and higher than normal during infancy. The homozygous form is also asymptomatic, but in combination with the sickle cell trait mild anemia may be present. The defect appears to be in the genetic mechanism that controls the switch from production of gamma to production of beta hemoglobin chains.

Conley CL & others: Hereditary persistence of fetal hemoglobin. Blood 21:261, 1963.

ACQUIRED HEMOLYTIC ANEMIAS

1. AUTOIMMUNE HEMOLYTIC ANEMIA

Essentials of Diagnosis

- Sudden pallor, fatigue, and jaundice.
- Splenomegaly.
- Positive Coombs test.
- Reticulocytosis and spherocytosis.

General Considerations

Acquired autoimmune hemolytic anemia is rare during the first 4 months of life but is one of the more common causes of acutely acquired anemia after the first year. It is caused by antibodies which coat the red cells and are responsible for the positive direct Coombs test. Circulating antibodies are demonstrated by the indirect Coombs test. The "primary" (or idiopathic) cases may be associated with an unrecognized preceding infection. The possible importance of cytomegalovirus infection has recently been emphasized. The disease may be "symptomatic" and may occur in association with a known infection such as hepatitis, viral pneumonia, or infectious mononucleosis; or it may occur as a manifestation of a generalized autoimmune disease such as disseminated lupus erythematosus or with a malignancy such as Hodgkin's disease or leukemia. The antibodies may be of the "cold-reacting" IgM type or "warm" antibodies of the IgG type.

Clinical Findings

A. Symptoms and Signs: The disease usually has an acute onset and is associated with weakness, pallor, and fatigue. Hemoglobinuria may be present. Jaundice and splenomegaly are often present. Occasional cases are chronic and insidious in onset. Clinical evidence of the underlying disease such as infection or lupus erythematosus may be present.

B. Laboratory Findings: The anemia is normochromic and normocytic and may be very severe, with hemoglobin levels as low as 3–4 gm/100 ml. Occasionally, the secondary form of acquired hemolytic anemia may be very mild and may present with evidence of a positive Coombs test but with compensated anemia. Spherocytes are usually present, and within 24 hours nucleated red cells and reticulocytes are present in the peripheral blood. There is usually a significant leukocytosis, and the platelet count may be elevated. Bone marrow shows a marked erythroid hyperplasia. Both the direct and indirect Coombs tests are usually positive. Autoagglutination may be present, and because of this the patient may be incorrectly typed as AB, Rh-positive. The indirect serum bilirubin may be elevated, and the stool and urine urobilinogen are increased.

Differential Diagnosis

The principal condition to be differentiated in childhood is hereditary spherocytic anemia in crisis, since both diseases present with acute hemolysis and spherocytosis. The Coombs test differentiates the 2 anemias since it is negative in hereditary spherocytosis. The Coombs test likewise differentiates autoimmune hemolytic anemia from essentially all other anemias except erythroblastosis.

Complications

The anemia may be very severe and result in shock, requiring emergency management. Thrombocytopenia may occur as an associated autoimmune condition. The complications of the underlying disease such as disseminated lupus erythematosus or lymphoma may be present in the symptomatic form.

Treatment

Medical management of the underlying disease is important in symptomatic cases.

A. Transfusion: Transfusion is necessary in the acute disease and may be an emergency procedure. Difficulty in cross-matching will usually be encountered. A search should be made for blood that will provide the best major cross-match. Packed, washed cells are often more compatible. The IgG antibody is often type-specific (particularly to one of the Rh antigens), and cross matching may be possible, whereas the IgM antibody is usually a panagglutinin (frequently anti-I). Transfusion occasionally must be given in spite of agglutination or a positive Coombs test in the major cross-match. Donor cells may be destroyed at a rapid rate, particularly if compatible blood cannot be found. Donor cells may be tagged with ^{51}Cr to determine their rate of survival in severe cases.

B. Immunosuppressive Therapy: Medical treatment to block the immune process is indicated. Corticosteroid therapy in the form of hydrocortisone intravenously in large doses or prednisone, 2 mg/kg/day orally, should be tried initially. If a response is observed, the dose is decreased at weekly intervals until the lowest level that will maintain the patient in remission is reached. Other immunosuppressive drugs such as cyclophosphamide, mercaptopurine, or azathioprine may be tried alone or in conjunction with corticosteroid therapy.

C. Heparin: Heparin may be useful in the IgM type (which binds complement) because of its anticomplementary effect. It may also help prevent intravascular coagulation and secondary renal disease associated with release of tissue factor from red cells.

D. Exchange Transfusion: Plasma or whole blood exchange transfusion will temporarily wash out antibody and may be a life-saving measure in severe cases.

E. Splenectomy: Splenectomy may be beneficial in cases in which all forms of medical treatment have failed. About 50% of cases may be expected to respond to this procedure.

Prognosis

In childhood the disease is self-limited in the majority of idiopathic cases, although hemolysis does not usually cease completely for months to years; the Coombs test often remains weakly positive for years. The majority of cases will show a response to corticosteroid therapy, and about 50% will improve with splenectomy. The majority of chronic cases have a basic underlying disease or immunologic disorder.

Habibi B & others: Autoimmune hemolytic anemia in children: A review of 80 cases. Am J Med 56:61, 1974.

Taft EG & others: Plasma exchange for cold agglutinin hemolytic anemia. Transfusion 17:173, 1977.

Zuelzer WW & others: Autoimmune hemolytic anemia: Natural history and viral immunologic interactions in childhood. Am J Med 49:80, 1970.

2. ACUTE ACQUIRED HEMOLYTIC ANEMIA
(Lederer's Anemia)

Severe episodes of hemolytic anemia that are not associated with a positive Coombs test are occasionally seen in children. The onset is acute and the duration short, with spontaneous recovery in a few weeks. As in autoimmune hemolytic anemia, the episode is often precipitated by an infectious process such as a urinary tract infection, but in most cases there is no evidence for red cell antibodies. The term Lederer's anemia is currently reserved for this group.

Transfusion is the treatment of choice; there is usually no problem with cross-matching the donor blood.

The prognosis is good since all cases are self-limited.

Wallerstein RO, Aggeler PM: Acute hemolytic anemia. Am J Med 37:92, 1964.

3. MISCELLANEOUS ACQUIRED (NONIMMUNE) HEMOLYTIC ANEMIAS

A wide variety of extracorpuscular mechanisms may also produce hemolysis of a nonimmune type. The role of certain drugs (eg, antimalarials, sulfonamides) and fava beans is discussed elsewhere (see p 393), since hemolysis in association with this particular group of substances occurs primarily in individuals with a deficiency of G6PD. Certain other chemicals and drugs such as arsenic and benzene may produce hemolysis by their direct effect. Exposure to physical agents such as extreme heat or cold may cause hemolysis. Hemolytic anemia is a common complication of severe burns.

Many bacterial infections with hemolytic organisms such as *Bartonella bacilliformis* and *Clostridium perfringens* produce hemolysis. In the neonatal period, hemolytic anemia may be a complication of almost any infection, but it is seen most commonly with hemolytic staphylococcal and *Escherichia coli* infections. Parasites such as malaria are characteristically associated with hemolysis. The venom of most poisonous snakes (in particular, the pit vipers of North America) contains a hemolysin, as do the venoms of certain spiders also. The management of the majority of the acquired toxic hemolytic anemias is dependent upon the removal of the offending agent or treatment of the toxic disorder. Transfusion may be important in the more severe cases.

Hemolysis in heart disease or after open heart surgery has been reported. This has usually occurred in situations in which a jet of blood was driven against a Teflon prosthesis as well as in certain congenital valvular defects and with prosthetic valve replacement. The hemolysis is on a mechanical basis.

Rodgers BM & others: Hemolytic anemia following prosthetic valve replacement. Circulation (Suppl) 39:155, 1969.

II. POLYCYTHEMIA & METHEMOGLOBINEMIA

PRIMARY ERYTHROCYTOSIS (Benign Familial Polycythemia)

This is the most common type of primary polycythemia of childhood. It differs from polycythemia vera in that it affects only the erythroid series; the white cell count and platelet count are normal. It frequently occurs on a familial basis as an autosomal dominant, although it may also occur as an autosomal recessive. There are usually no physical findings except for plethora and splenomegaly. The hemoglobin may be as high as 27 gm/100 ml, with a hematocrit of 80% and a red cell count of 10 million/cu mm. There are usually no symptoms other than headache and lethargy. Recent studies in a number of families have revealed either an abnormal hemoglobin with increased oxygen affinity, or reduced red cell diphosphoglycerate, or autonomous erythropoietin production.

Treatment is not indicated unless symptoms are marked. Phlebotomy is the treatment of choice.

Adamson JW: Familial polycythemia. Semin Hematol 12:383, 1975.

SECONDARY POLYCYTHEMIA (Compensatory Polycythemia)

Secondary polycythemia occurs in response to hypoxia in any condition that results in a lowered oxygen saturation of the blood. The most common cause of secondary polycythemia is cyanotic congenital heart disease. It also occurs in chronic pulmonary disease such as cystic fibrosis and in pulmonary arteriovenous shunts. Persons living at extremely high altitudes, as well as those with methemoglobinemia and sulfhemoglobinemia, develop polycythemia. It has on rare occasions been described without hypoxia in association with renal tumors, brain tumors, Cushing's disease, hydronephrosis, in association with cobalt therapy, and with certain unusual hemoglobinopathies.

Polycythemia occurs normally in the neonatal period; it is particularly exaggerated in premature infants, in whom it is frequently associated with other symptoms. It may occur in babies of diabetic mothers, and it has recently been described as a manifestation of Down's syndrome in the newborn and as a complication of congenital adrenal hyperplasia.

Multiple coagulation and bleeding abnormalities have been described in severely polycythemic cardiac patients. These include thrombocytopenia, mild consumption coagulopathy, and increased anticoagulants with elevated fibrinolytic activity. Bleeding at surgery may be severe.

The ideal treatment of secondary polycythemia is correction of the underlying disorder. When this cannot be done, phlebotomy is often necessary to control the symptoms. Adequate hydration of the patient and phlebotomy with plasma replacement are indicated prior to major surgical procedures to prevent the complications of thrombosis and hemorrhage. Isovolumetric exchange transfusion is the treatment of choice in severe cases.

Balcerzak SP, Bromberg PA: Secondary polycythemia. Semin Hematol 12:353, 1975.
Humbert JR & others: Polycythemia in small for gestational age infants. J Pediatr 75:812, 1969.

METHEMOGLOBINEMIA

Methemoglobin is formed when hemoglobin in a deoxygenated state is oxidized to the ferric form. Methemoglobin is being formed continuously in the red cells and is simultaneously reduced to hemoglobin by enzymes in the erythrocyte. Methemoglobin becomes unavailable for transport of oxygen and causes a shift in the dissociation curve of the residual oxyhemoglobin. Cyanosis is produced with methemoglobin levels of approximately 15% or greater. There are several mechanisms for the production of methemoglobinemia.

Congenital Methemoglobinemia Associated With Hemoglobin M

Congenital and familial methemoglobinemia associated with an abnormal hemoglobin molecule (hemoglobin M) is discussed under the hemoglobinopathies (see p 398). These patients are cyanotic but asymptomatic. They do not respond to any form of treatment.

Congenital Methemoglobinemia Due to Enzyme Deficiencies

Congenital methemoglobinemia is most frequently caused by congenital absence of a reducing factor in the erythrocyte which is responsible for the conversion of methemoglobin to hemoglobin in normal red cells. Most patients with this disease suffer from a deficiency of the reducing enzyme diaphorase I (coenzyme factor I). It is transmitted as an autosomal recessive trait. These patients may have as high as 40% methemoglobin but usually have no symptoms, although a mild compensatory polycythemia may be present.

Patients with methemoglobinemia associated with a deficiency of diaphorase I respond readily to treatment with ascorbic acid and with methylene blue (see below). However, treatment is not usually indicated.

Drug-Induced Methemoglobinemia

A number of compounds activate the oxidation of hemoglobin from the ferrous to the ferric state, forming methemoglobin. These include the nitrites and nitrates, chlorates, and quinones. Common drugs in this group are the aniline dyes, sulfonamides, acetanilid, phenacetin, bismuth subnitrate, and potassium chlorate. Poisoning with a drug or chemical containing one of these substances should be suspected in any infant or child who presents with sudden cyanosis. Methemoglobin levels in cases of poisoning may be extremely high and can produce severe anoxia and dyspnea with unconsciousness, circulatory failure, and death. Young infants and newborns are more susceptible to poisoning because their red cells have difficulty reducing hemoglobin, probably on the basis of a transient deficiency of DPNH-dependent hemoglobin reductase.

Patients with the acquired form of methemoglobinemia respond dramatically to methylene blue in a dosage of 2 mg/kg body weight given intravenously. For older children, a smaller dose (1–1.5 mg/kg) is recommended. Ascorbic acid administered orally or intravenously also reduces methemoglobin, but it acts more slowly.

Jaffé ER & others: Hereditary methemoglobinemia, toxic methemoglobinemia and the reduction of methemoglobin. Ann NY Acad Sci 151:795, 1968.

III. DISORDERS OF LEUKOCYTES

LEUKOPENIA & AGRANULOCYTOSIS

Essentials of Diagnosis

- Increased incidence of infections.
- Ulceration of the oral mucosa and throat.
- Neutropenia.
- Normal red cells and platelets.

General Considerations

The neutropenias and agranulocytosis include a wide variety of syndromes which probably have different causes. In the majority of cases the mechanism is not well understood. Many are probably secondary to exposure to drugs and chemicals, and this possibility should be investigated in all cases. In childhood, the more common drug-induced neutropenias occur with anticonvulsants, antimicrobial agents (chloramphenicol), antithyroid drugs (thiouracil), tranquilizers, antihistamines, aminopyrine, phenylbutazone, and the sulfonamides. Neutropenia is a common complication of exposure to large doses of x-ray and to cytotoxic drugs such as the antimetabolites and nitrogen mustards. There is increasing evidence that leukocyte antibodies may produce granulocytopenia on an immunologic basis. This most frequently occurs in association with repeated blood transfusions or as a result of isoagglutinins that develop during pregnancy. Autoagglutinins have also been described, particularly in association with infectious mononucleosis, lymphomas, and autoimmune diseases such as disseminated lupus erythematosus.

Viral infections characteristically produce neutropenia. Bacterial infections, particularly sepsis, are frequently associated with transient neutropenia in the newborn infant, and overwhelming bacterial infections at all ages may be indicated by neutropenia.

A significant number of neutropenic infants have hereditary disorders with deficiencies of colony-stimulating factor or defective colony-producing granulocytic precursors. Current studies of neutrophil kinetics in these congenital neutropenias may allow a more systematic reclassification.

Classifications

A number of specific leukopenias have been described in infancy and childhood:

A. Neonatal Agranulocytosis: This term has been applied to the occurrence of agranulocytosis in the neonatal period in repeated siblings. It is usually explained by transplacental iso-immunization of the mother to the leukocytes of her infant in a manner analogous to Rh immunization of the newborn. The granulocytopenia in these cases is accompanied by infection, but it is temporary and improves within 4 weeks.

B. Infantile Genetic Agranulocytosis (Kostmann type): Several families have been described in which agranulocytosis occurred from infancy in several siblings without depression of the other circulating cell elements. It has been associated with either depression of the granulocytic series in the marrow or a delay in maturation. The course has been chronic, with a high mortality rate and no response to therapy. The genetic pattern suggests an autosomal recessive transmission.

C. Chronic Benign Granulocytopenia in Childhood: Several series of cases have been described in which persistent granulocytopenia was noted throughout childhood. The bone marrow in these cases has usually shown normal cellularity but abnormal maturation of the granulocytes. In most of these cases, the neutrophils have represented about 10% of the circulating leukocytes, and infection has not been a serious problem. Spontaneous remission may occur.

D. Chronic Hypoplastic Neutropenia: A few cases have been described of chronic neutropenia associated with hypoplasia of granulocytic precursors in the marrow. The cause is not known, and complicating infections have been severe.

E. Leukopenia With Pure Red Cell Hypoplastic Anemia: A number of cases of pure red cell hypoplastic anemia have also been associated with leukopenia. This is usually mild, and an increased incidence of infection has not been observed, although oral ulceration and staphylococcal infections of the skin have been reported in a few cases.

F. Pancreatic Insufficiency and Bone Marrow Dysfunction (Schwachman's Syndrome): Neutropenia, anemia, and thrombocytopenia have been reported in association with pancreatic insufficiency in infancy and childhood. Although diarrhea, failure to thrive, short stature, and infections have been a problem, the prognosis is better than in cystic fibrosis.

G. Periodic (Cyclic) Neutropenia: This is a rare condition that may occur at any age but usually begins in infancy and childhood. It is characterized by an extreme granulocytopenia that occurs at approximately 3-week intervals, with recovery between attacks. The peripheral blood changes are reflected by a cyclic maturation arrest of the granulocytic series in the bone marrow. During the leukopenic episode, the white count is usually 2–4 thousand/cu mm, with granulocytes representing only 6–10% of the cells. The agranulocytic periods usually last about 10 days and are associated with the development of ulcers of the oral mucosa, fever, and sore throat. Various other infections may complicate the disease, and staphylococcal skin infections are common. Splenomegaly and lymphadenopathy have also been reported.

H. Neutropenia in Association With Immune Deficiency Syndromes: Neutropenia (constant or cyclic) may occur in agammaglobulinemia. It has also been observed in other forms of the immune deficiencies.

Clinical Findings

A. Symptoms and Signs: The symptoms are those of infection, with chills and fever. Sore throat and ulceration of the oral mucosa are common, and chronic or recurrent staphylococcal infection of the skin is frequent. In most cases, the spleen and liver are not enlarged.

B. Laboratory Findings: Neutrophils are absent or markedly reduced in the peripheral blood. In the purer forms of neutropenia or agranulocytosis, the monocytes and lymphocytes will be normal and the red cells and platelets not affected. The bone marrow usually shows a normal erythroid series, with adequate megakaryocytes but a marked reduction in the myeloid cells or a significant delay in maturation of this series.

Differential Diagnosis

The isolated neutropenias should be differentiated from the pancytopenias such as aplastic anemia and the hypoplastic (aleukemic) form of childhood leukemia by bone marrow examination.

Complications

The complications are essentially those of infection. Septicemia and pneumonia are the most serious. Chronic infection with antibiotic-resistant staphylococci and pseudomonas is frequent in severe cases.

Treatment

Removal of the toxic agent is essential if one can be identified. Otherwise, treatment consists of administering appropriate antibiotics. Prophylactic antimicrobial therapy is not indicated, and the patient should be managed with specific therapy directed toward the infecting organism.

Marrow stimulation with testosterone or with testosterone plus one of the corticosteroids (see Aplastic Anemia) may be tried in chronic cases, but there is little evidence that it is effective.

Fresh frozen plasma has produced remissions in a few cases with immune globulin deficiencies.

Prognosis

The prognosis varies greatly with the cause and severity of the neutropenia. In severe cases with persistent agranulocytosis, the prognosis is very poor in spite of antibiotic therapy; in mild or cyclic forms of neutropenia, symptoms may be minimal and the prognosis for normal life expectancy excellent.

Baehner RL, Johnston RB: Monocytic function in children with neutropenia and chronic infections. Blood 40:31, 1972.

Burke V & others: Association of pancreatic insufficiency and chronic neutropenia in childhood. Arch Dis Child 42:147, 1967.

Joyce RA & others: Neutrophil kinetics in hereditary and congenital neutropenias. N Engl J Med 295:1385, 1976.

Kauder E, Mauer AM: Neutropenias of childhood. J Pediatr 69:147, 1966.

PHYSIOLOGIC NEUTROPENIA

All infants and young children after the first few weeks of life have a neutropenia in comparison with adult levels. The normal white count of the infant and child may be as low as 5–6 thousand/cu mm, and the percentage of neutrophils may normally be as low as 18–20% during the first 3–4 years of life. A diagnosis of neutropenia should be considered in early infancy and childhood only if the absolute neutrophil count is below 1000/cu mm.

See Table 38–3 for normal values of leukocytes at various ages.

ACUTE INFECTIOUS LYMPHOCYTOSIS

Acute infectious lymphocytosis is a specific entity characterized hematologically by marked lymphocytosis that may range between 15–200 thousand cells/cu mm. The predominant cell is a small mature lymphocyte. The disease is apparently infectious and tends to occur in epidemic form in institutions and families. The specific agent has not been determined, although a virus is suspected. An enterovirus similar to coxsackievirus A may be the cause.

In the majority of cases the condition is asymptomatic, and the diagnosis is made on the basis of a routine blood count. Epidemics have been reported in which symptoms were noted, including fever, upper respiratory manifestations, skin rashes, abdominal pain, diarrhea, and meningoencephalitis. Lymphadenopathy and splenomegaly are not present.

The bone marrow is normal except for a slight increase in mature lymphocytes. The disease can be readily differentiated from leukemia since the lymphocytes of the peripheral blood are all mature and since chronic lymphatic leukemia does not occur in the pediatric age group. The blood smear is similar to that seen in pertussis.

There is no specific treatment. Symptomatic therapy is usually not needed.

The disease is self-limited, and the blood count usually returns to normal within a few weeks.

Horwitz MS, Moore GT: Acute infectious lymphocytosis: Etiology and epidemiologic study of outbreak. N Engl J Med 279:399, 1968.

CHRONIC NONSPECIFIC INFECTIOUS LYMPHOCYTOSIS

This syndrome is characterized by moderate leukocytosis with a predominance of lymphocytes, low-grade fever, anorexia, pallor, irritability, increased fatigability, and abdominal pain. The peripheral blood usually shows a significant lymphocytosis, with total counts reaching 25,000/cu mm with as many as 80% lymphocytes. Most of the lymphocytes are of the small, mature type, although occasional larger cells may be seen. The cause is not known, but viral infection is suspected.

The symptoms and elevated lymphocyte count often persist for several months, and therapy is not helpful. Antibiotic therapy and restriction of physical activity are not indicated.

Smith CH: Infectious lymphocytosis. Am J Dis Child 62:231, 1941.

MYELOPROLIFERATIVE SYNDROMES

1. MYELOID METAPLASIA
(Myelofibrosis, Myelosclerosis, Agnogenic Myeloid Metaplasia)

Myeloid metaplasia is a myeloproliferative condition associated with splenomegaly and a granulocytic leukemoid picture. In childhood it occurs most frequently in the secondary form and is associated with replacement of the bone marrow by tumor, storage cells, or osteosclerosis (osteopetrosis, marble bone disease). The primary form, which is associated with idiopathic myelofibrosis (agnogenic myeloid metaplasia), is extremely rare in childhood.

The peripheral blood in this condition shows not only a marked increase in granulocytes, with many immature forms at all levels of maturation, but also a significant number of nucleated red cells and large immature platelets. The presence of immature hematopoietic cells in the peripheral blood is explained by the marked extramedullary hematopoiesis that occurs in the spleen and liver in this condition.

Treatment should be directed toward the primary disease if possible. The use of testosterone (see Aplastic Anemia) may be helpful in stimulating hematopoiesis in the bone marrow.

Say B, Berkel I: Idiopathic myelofibrosis in an infant. J Pediatr 64:580, 1964.

2. FAMILIAL MYELOPROLIFERATIVE DISEASE

One family has been described with 9 children (related as first cousins) who developed a myeloproliferative disorder that appeared to be similar to either acute or subacute myelogenous leukemia. Hepatosplenomegaly, leukocytosis (with immature granulocytes), anemia, and thrombocytopenia were found. The liver and spleen showed extramedullary hematopoiesis. Six of the 9 children recovered in adolescence and 3 died in infancy.

Randell DL & others: Familial myeloproliferative disease: A new syndrome closely simulating myelogenous leukemia in childhood. Am J Dis Child 110:479, 1965.

3. MYELOPROLIFERATIVE SYNDROME WITH ABSENT C GROUP CHROMOSOME

Several observations have been made recently of myeloproliferative disorders associated with an absent chromosome of the C group. Massive hepatosplenomegaly (with extramedullary hematopoiesis), leukocytosis (with young granulocytes), anemia, and thrombocytopenia characterize this condition. The patients have usually progressed to an acute granulocytic leukemia, and the myeloproliferative phase should be considered preleukemic.

Humbert JR & others: Preleukemia in children with missing bone marrow C chromosome and a myeloproliferative disorder. Br J Haematol 21:705, 1971.

4. MYELOPROLIFERATIVE DISORDER OF DOWN'S SYNDROME

A severe myeloproliferative disorder affecting granulocytes, erythrocytes, platelets, or any combination of these cell lines may be present at birth in infants with Down's syndrome. The granulocytic hyperplasia with immature cells in the blood is the most common and has in the past been confused with acute or subacute myelogenous leukemia. It clears spontaneously and should not be treated with antileukemic therapy. There is a significant mortality rate from bleeding or infection in the first few weeks before the marrow recovers and matures.

GRANULOCYTE FUNCTION DEFECTS

1. CHRONIC GRANULOMATOUS DISEASE

The primary defect in this disorder appears to be inability to kill bacteria despite normal phagocytosis, resulting in persistent infections, frequently with bacteria of low virulence. Onset before age 1 and death before 8 years is the usual course of events. There is a marked defect in degranulation and a marked decrease in the oxidative metabolism normally associated with phagocytosis. The precise relationship of the metabolic abnormalities to the lack of bactericidal activity of the leukocyte is unclear.

The earliest manifestation is an eczematoid dermatosis occurring near a body orifice. This is followed by recurrent lymphadenopathy, suppuration, and draining granulomatous lesions. The lung parenchyma is usually involved, with enlargement of the hilar nodes on x-ray and a distinctive "encapsulating pneumonia" in some cases. Hepatosplenomegaly is characteristic but not uniformly present. Osteomyelitis occurs in about one-third of cases. Typical bacteria involved have been staphylococci (including species usually considered nonpathogenic) and enterobacteria such as enterobacter and serratia. The course of the disease is characterized by remissions and exacerbations. Remissions have lasted up to several years. Death usually results from sepsis, pulmonary infections, meningitis, and extensive visceral suppuration.

Humoral- and cell-mediated immunity is normal. Hyperimmunoglobulinemia is present, presumably because of the massive antigenic stimulation of the chronic infection. The inflammatory cycle and complement system are normal, as is the peripheral polymorphonuclear response to bacterial infection. Defective killing of intracellular bacteria is demonstrable in in vitro phagocytic systems by failure to reduce nitroblue tetrazolium to blue formazan.

Treatment is directed toward management of the infections and includes prompt antibiotic therapy with antibiotics that penetrate cell membranes well (eg, chloramphenicol), surgical drainage of suppurative lesions, and general supportive therapy.

Baehner RL, Nathan DG: Quantitative nitroblue tetrazolium test in chronic granulomatous disease. N Engl J Med 278:971, 1968.

Good RA & others: Fatal (chronic) granulomatous disease of childhood: A hereditary defect of leukocyte function. Semin Hematol 5:215, 1968.

Quie PG: Chronic granulomatous disease of childhood. Adv Pediatr 16:287, 1969.

Quie PG & others: In vitro bactericidal capacity of human polymorphonuclear leukocytes. J Clin Invest 46:668, 1967.

2. CHEDIAK-HIGASHI SYNDROME

This is a rare familial disorder that is apparently transmitted as an autosomal recessive trait. It is characterized by semialbinism, photophobia, nystagmus, excessive sweating, pale optic fundi, hepatosplenomegaly, generalized lymphadenopathy, and eventually by the development of neurologic signs and symptoms. Hematologically, there is a progressive anemia and granulocytopenia, and typical diagnostic anomalies of the leukocytes. Large granules ranging in size from 2–5 μm in diameter, which may be azurophilic or slate green, occur in the cytoplasm of the neutrophils. Extremely large red granules may also be seen in the eosinophils and are particularly prominent in the myelocytic cells of the marrow.

There is no known treatment.

The course is progressively downhill, with death occurring in childhood.

White JG: The Chediak-Higashi syndrome: A possible lysosomal disease. Blood 28:143, 1966.

3. OTHER GRANULOCYTE FUNCTION DEFECTS

Other patients have been described with defects in intracellular bacterial killing associated with genetic absence of myeloperoxidase and rarely in association with nearly total absence of leukocyte G6PD. Other persons with recurrent bacterial infections have been found to have defects in leukocyte chemotaxis ("lazy leukocyte syndrome") or defects in opsonization. The latter have most often been due to a decrease or dysfunction of the serum complement components C3 or C5. Children with recurrent or chronic bacterial infections who have normal granulocyte counts should be evaluated for these various defects in granulocyte function and for chronic granulomatous disease.

Johnston, RB, Stroud RM: Complement and host defense against infection. J Pediatr 90:169, 1977.

IV. BLEEDING DISORDERS

Bleeding disorders may be classified as (1) defects in small vessel hemostasis, which include (a) quantitative and qualitative abnormalities of platelets (thrombocytopenia, thrombasthenia, thrombopathia, and thrombocythemia) and (b) the vascular disorders; and (2) intravascular disorders (defects in blood coagulation).

The initial laboratory work-up for screening patients with bleeding disorders should include a careful history and physical examination and all of the following laboratory investigations:

(1) Bleeding time: To test small vessel integrity and platelet function.

(2) Tourniquet test: To test small vessel integrity and platelet function.

(3) Platelet count or estimation of platelet number on blood smear.

(4) Partial thromboplastin time (PTT) to measure clotting activity of factors XII, IX, XI, VIII, X, II, V, and fibrinogen.

(5) One-stage prothrombin time (PT) to screen the tissue thromboplastin system of coagulation (particularly factors II, V, VII).

(6) Thrombin time to measure antithrombin effect of fibrin split products or heparin as well as fibrinogen level (if very low).

With this battery of screening tests, it is usually possible to determine the general area of the defect and proceed with more specific tests in order to make an exact diagnosis.

ABNORMALITIES OF PLATELET NUMBER OR FUNCTION

IDIOPATHIC THROMBOCYTOPENIC PURPURA (ITP)
(Werlhof's Disease, Purpura Haemorrhagica)

Essentials of Diagnosis
- Petechiae, ecchymoses.
- Decreased platelet count.
- No splenomegaly.
- Normal bone marrow examination.

General Considerations

Acute ITP is the most common bleeding disorder of childhood. It most frequently follows infections and is particularly common after certain of the common contagious diseases (rubella, varicella, and rubeola). As a rule it is self-limited; this is particularly true of the postinfectious type, the majority of which cases recover spontaneously within a few months and approximately 90% within a year after onset. Chronic ITP is rare in childhood.

Most cases of ITP are felt to be an immunologic disorder, although platelet antibodies cannot always be demonstrated. The spleen apparently plays a major role by sequestering damaged platelets and by forming antibodies.

Clinical Findings

A. Symptoms and Signs: The onset is usually

acute, with the appearance of multiple ecchymoses, particularly over the tibias. Petechiae are often present, and epistaxis is common. There are no other physical findings, and the spleen is not palpable.

B. Laboratory Findings:

1. Blood—The platelet count is markedly reduced (usually less than 50,000/cu mm), and platelets are decreased and frequently of larger size on peripheral blood smear. The white blood count and differential count are normal. Anemia is not present unless hemorrhage has occurred.

2. Bone marrow—The bone marrow usually shows increased numbers of megakaryocytes. Eosinophils may be increased in the marrow.

3. Other laboratory tests—The bleeding time is prolonged, the tourniquet test is positive, and clot retraction is abnormal. PTT and PT are normal, although prothrombin consumption is decreased.

Differential Diagnosis

The presence of a low platelet count immediately differentiates ITP from all other bleeding disorders except those associated with thrombocytopenia. A normal white blood count and normal precursors in the bone marrow differentiate ITP from leukemia and aplastic anemia. The bone marrow is important in making the differential diagnosis. There may be a family history of hereditary or familial thrombocytopenia (see Table 14–2).

Complications

Severe exsanguinating hemorrhage and bleeding into vital organs are the primary complications of ITP. Intracranial hemorrhage is the most serious. Complications of treatment include those associated with prolonged corticosteroid therapy. Splenectomy, particularly in children under age 2, may be associated with increased incidence of infection.

Treatment

A. General Measures: Avoidance of trauma is important, and in many postinfectious cases no other therapy may be required. In the presence of hemorrhage, blood transfusions may be necessary. Platelet transfusion may be lifesaving if hemorrhage does not respond to medical therapy. The platelets (platelet concentrate or platelet pack) from 1 unit of blood per 5–10 lb of body weight are usually required to produce an observable rise in platelet count. Patients must avoid aspirin and aspirin-containing drugs.

B. Corticosteroids: Patients with a significant hemorrhagic tendency or with a platelet count less than 10,000/cu mm are treated with prednisone (2 mg/kg orally in divided daily doses) for a period of 2 weeks. The dosage is tapered and stopped during the third week. No further prednisone is given regardless of the level of the platelet count unless significant bleeding recurs, at which time the dosage of prednisone used is the smallest that will give symptomatic relief (usually 2.5–5 mg twice daily). The patient is then followed, using the general measures outlined above, until spontaneous remission occurs or until the patient is a candidate for splenectomy.

C. Plasma Transfusions: In chronic thrombocytopenic purpura, a therapeutic trial with small doses of fresh frozen plasma (5–10 ml/kg) is indicated to rule out thrombocytopenia due to a congenital deficiency of the thrombopoietic factors.

Larger doses of fresh frozen plasma (20–30 ml/kg) may occasionally produce temporary remissions in acute ITP because of the presence of this platelet-stimulating plasma factor. This form of therapy may be tried in place of corticosteroids or when they fail.

D. Splenectomy: Splenectomy produces permanent remission in the majority of cases of ITP; however, it is now usually reserved for children who have shown no evidence of spontaneous remission over a period of 6 months to 1 year, since about 90% of children with ITP will recover without surgical intervention within 1 year after onset. If symptoms are not controlled by medical management, splenectomy may be done prior to this time, and in most cases splenectomy is advised if symptoms persist beyond 1 year after onset. Fifty to 75% of chronic cases in childhood respond to the procedure, although the patient who shows a rise in platelet count with large doses of corticosteroids is most likely to have a satisfactory result.

Bleeding is rarely a complication of splenectomy, but platelet concentrates should be available during surgery. If the patient has been on corticosteroid therapy prior to surgery, the dose should be increased to the full therapeutic level during and after surgery.

Anticoagulant therapy is not indicated postoperatively even though the platelets may rise to levels of approximately 1 million.

The risk of overwhelming infection is low in the older child undergoing splenectomy. It does represent a significant risk in the young child, and the procedure should be postponed if possible until the child is older. Prophylactic penicillin for at least a year following splenectomy is indicated and is strongly recommended in the very young child.

E. Chemotherapy: In the rare child who remains thrombocytopenic after splenectomy, a trial of vincristine or cyclophosphamide may be used to stimulate a rise in platelets.

Prognosis

Spontaneous remission with permanent recovery occurs in almost 90% of cases of ITP in childhood. (The incidence of spontaneous remission is much lower in adults.)

Ahn YS & others: Vincristine therapy of idiopathic and secondary thrombocytopenias. N Engl J Med 291:376, 1974.

Baldini M: Idiopathic thrombocytopenic purpura and the ITP syndrome. Med Clin North Am 56:47, 1972.

Cohn J: Thrombocytopenia in childhood: An evaluation of 433 patients. Scand J Haematol 16:226, 1976.

Karpatkin S, Garg SK: The megathrombocyte as an index of platelet production. Br J Haematol 26:307, 1974.

Lammi AT, Lovric AV: Idiopathic thrombocytopenic purpura:

An epidemiologic study. J Pediatr 83:31, 1973.

McClure PD: Idiopathic thrombocytopenic purpura in children: Diagnosis and management. Pediatr 55:68, 1975.

THROMBOCYTOPENIA IN THE NEWBORN

Thrombocytopenia is one of the most common causes of purpura in the newborn and should be considered and investigated in any infant with petechiae or a significant bleeding tendency. A platelet count less than 150,000/cu mm establishes a diagnosis of thrombocytopenia in the neonatal period. A number of specific entities may be responsible. The most common are discussed below.

Thrombocytopenia Associated With Platelet Iso-immunization

A common cause of thrombocytopenia in the neonatal period is platelet iso-immunization, which is similar to the mechanism responsible for Rh blood group iso-immunization. Iso-immunization occurs when the platelet type of the infant differs from that of the mother and when a significant number of platelets cross from the fetal to the maternal circulation. Platelet antibodies can usually be demonstrated by complement fixation or platelet factor 3 release technics. Petechiae are usually present shortly after birth, and a male may bleed from circumcision. The bone marrow usually shows normal to increased megakaryocytes. The disease is self-limited, and severe hemorrhage usually does not occur unless surgery is performed. Platelets show a spontaneous rise within 2 weeks, with complete recovery by 4–6 weeks.

Platelet transfusions may be used in an emergency. In very severe cases, exchange transfusions with fresh whole blood is effective in removing antibody and in replacing platelets temporarily; a platelet concentrate from the mother will be more effective in raising the platelet count.

Thrombocytopenia Associated With ITP in the Mother

Infants born to mothers with ITP develop thrombocytopenia as a result of passive transfer of antibody from the mother to the infant. Evaluation of the maternal platelet count is indicated in any baby with thrombocytopenia. The persistence of antibodies in the infant's circulation is temporary, and spontaneous recovery the rule.

Congenital Amegakaryocytic Thrombocytopenia

Congenital absence of megakaryocytes is associated with severe chronic refractory thrombocytopenia beginning in the newborn period. It is frequently associated with other congenital abnormalities, particularly absence of the radius. It may be familial. This disease is considered to be the neonatal equivalent of Fanconi's syndrome, which does not usually appear in its classical form until later in childhood.

Treatment may not be necessary, although testosterone with or without corticosteroids may be tried in severe cases.

If the platelet count is extremely low, the prognosis is poor.

Thrombocytopenia Associated With Hemolytic Disease of the Newborn

Thrombocytopenia is a complication of severe erythroblastosis and may represent platelet consumption (disseminated intravascular coagulation or hypersplenism) or depressed production associated with liver disease.

Neonatal Thrombocytopenia Associated With Infections

Thrombocytopenia is commonly associated with severe generalized infections of the newborn period, and particularly with those that develop in utero. Megakaryocytes are decreased and immature, and splenomegaly is usually present. Other intrauterine infections such as syphilis, toxoplasmosis, and cytomegalic inclusion disease are almost invariably associated with thrombocytopenia, and thrombocytopenia is frequently present with bacterial sepsis and generalized infection with herpes simplex virus or other viruses.

In addition to specific treatment for the underlying disease if available, platelet transfusions may be indicated in severe cases.

Thrombocytopenia Associated With Intravascular Coagulation Syndromes

The most frequent causes of thrombocytopenia other than infection in the sick term and preterm infant are intravascular coagulation syndromes such as (1) disseminated intravascular coagulation (DIC); (2) localized large vessel thrombosis (renal artery and vein and secondary to the use of umbilical vessel catheters); (3) diffuse platelet microthrombosis, often associated with respiratory distress syndrome; and (4) organ necrosis such as necrotizing enterocolitis (NEC). Severe thrombocytopenia is frequently seen without evidence of consumption coagulopathy (low fibrinogen and other factors). If the platelet count is very low (less than 20,000/cu mm) or if bleeding is present, treatment with platelet concentrates (10 ml/kg) is often indicated.

Thrombocytopenia Associated With Giant Hemangiomas

A rare but important cause of thrombocytopenic purpura in the newborn is giant hemangioma. Platelet sequestration in the tumor results in peripheral depletion of platelets. The bone marrow usually shows marked hyperplasia of megakaryocytes. In the presence of massive hemangiomas, the thrombocytopenia may be associated with disseminated intravascular coagulation (DIC) and result in fatal hemorrhage.

X-ray treatment of hemangiomas may be indicated. Heparinization is indicated if there is evidence of DIC. Surgery is usually contraindicated because of the risk of hemorrhage. Prednisone therapy has been associated with marked regression of infantile hemangiomas.

Evans J & others: Haemangioma with coagulopathy. Sustained response to prednisone. Arch Dis Child 50:809, 1975.

Favara B.E & others: Disseminated intravascular and cardiac thrombosis of the neonate. Am J Dis Child 127:197, 1974.

Hathaway WE: The bleeding newborn. Semin Hematol 12:175, 1975.

THROMBOCYTOPENIA ASSOCIATED WITH APLASTIC ANEMIA

Thrombocytopenia is frequently the first manifestation of aplastic anemia and may be present before neutropenia and anemia develop. The child who presents with amegakaryocytic thrombocytopenia in the first few years of life—particularly if there are associated skeletal anomalies—should be considered as a possible case of congenital pancytopenia of the Fanconi type.

THROMBOCYTOPENIA IN LEUKEMIA

Thrombocytopenia is almost invariably a major finding in acute leukemia of childhood. This is discussed in Chapter 31.

THROMBOCYTOPENIA DUE TO DEFICIENCY OF THROMBOCYTOPOIETIC FACTOR

Chronic thrombocytopenia may rarely occur in association with a congenital deficiency of thrombopoietin, a plasma factor which apparently is responsible for megakaryocyte maturation and platelet production. The clinical and hematologic picture is similar to that of chronic ITP. The 2 disorders may be differentiated by the administration of fresh or freshly frozen plasma in doses of approximately 10 ml/kg; in thrombocytopoietin deficiency, this produces a dramatic and prolonged response, whereas the patient with classical ITP will respond temporarily only to large doses of plasma (about 30 ml/kg).

Patients with congenital deficiency of the thrombocytopoietic factor may be maintained in good remission with administration of freshly frozen plasma every few months.

Schulman I & others: A factor in normal human plasma required for platelet production; chronic thrombocytopenia due to its deficiency. Blood 16:943, 1960.

DRUG-INDUCED THROMBOCYTOPENIA

Drug-induced thrombocytopenia may be either amegakaryocytic or megakaryocytic. The myelosuppressive drugs and chemical toxins, as well as irradiation, tend to affect all marrow elements, including megakaryocytes. Thrombocytopenia thus is a primary presenting complication of the aplastic or hypoplastic anemias produced by these agents. They are discussed in detail in the section on aplastic anemia.

Megakaryocytic thrombocytopenia is an immune reaction resulting from sensitization of the patient by prior administration of drugs such as quinidine or quinine.

Once the cause of the purpura is understood, prevention is readily effected by removal of the sensitizing drug.

Karpatkin S: Drug-induced thrombocytopenia. Am J Med Sci 262:69, 1971.

HEREDITARY THROMBOCYTOPENIAS

At least 3 types of hereditary thrombocytopenia can be recognized based on the mode of inheritance and characteristic clinical and laboratory findings: (1) X-linked thrombocytopenia, eczema, and recurrent infections (Wiskott-Aldrich syndrome). This syndrome is characterized by low IgA and IgM immunoglobulins, impaired delayed hypersensitivity and abnormal lymphocyte function, and decreased numbers of small, poorly functioning platelets with a short life span. Variants of this disorder without the severe immunologic difficulties may be confused with chronic ITP, and patients with this disorder are at great risk of developing overwhelming infection if splenectomy is performed. (2) Bernard-Soulier giant platelet syndrome. This is a rare autosomal, incompletely recessive disorder characterized by giant, bizarre platelets of varying numbers but with normal in vitro function. (3) Thrombocytopenia with release defect (similar to the defect produced by aspirin). This heterogeneous group of thrombocytopenias with failure to release ADP may be inherited by either the recessive or the dominant mode and can also be confused with chronic ITP. Platelet function tests are usually abnormal.

Baldini MG: Nature of the platelet defect in the Wiskott-Aldrich syndrome. Ann NY Acad Sci 201:437, 1972.

Khan I, Zucker-Franklin D, Karpatkin S: Microthrombocytosis and platelet fragmentation associated with idiopathic/ autoimmune thrombocytopenic purpura. Br J Haematol 31:449, 1975.

SECONDARY HYPERSPLENISM

Thrombocytopenia is one of the earliest hematologic manifestations of secondary hypersplenism. This is discussed on p 422.

THROMBOTIC THROMBOCYTOPENIA
(Thrombohemolytic Thrombocytopenic Purpura)

Thrombotic thrombocytopenic purpura is a hemorrhagic disorder characterized by thrombocytopenia, severe purpura, fever, hemolytic anemia, transitory focal neurologic signs, and hepatic involvement. Hemolysis often precedes clinical purpura. The Coombs test may be positive (rarely), and the red blood cells show bizarre forms and fragmentation similar to that seen in the hemolytic uremic syndrome. Other clinical signs and symptoms may occur in association with widespread intracapillary and intra-arteriolar thrombi which may affect not only the brain but also the kidneys, heart, and spleen. It is believed this entity may represent a hypersensitivity syndrome closely related to diseases such as lupus erythematosus and polyarteritis nodosa. Recent evidence suggests that patients with thrombotic thrombocytopenic purpura may be undergoing disseminated intravascular coagulation and that the disease may be related to purpura fulminans.

The course is usually rapidly progressive and terminates fatally within a few weeks, although chronic cases have been described.

Treatment has not been effective, though corticosteroids and splenectomy have both been reported to be of benefit. Heparin given early in the course may be of value in preventing further development of thrombi. Trials of low molecular weight dextran or other antiplatelet agents (eg, aspirin) may be indicated.

Amorosi EL, Ultmann, JE: Thrombotic thrombocytopenic purpura: Report of 16 cases and review of the literature. Medicine 45:139, 1966.

Faguet GB & others: Thrombotic thrombocytopenic purpura: Treatment with antiplatelet agents. Am J Med Sci 268:113, 1974.

PLATELET FUNCTIONAL DEFECTS

The terms thrombasthenia, thrombopathia, and thrombocytopathy have been used to describe a variety of conditions characterized by abnormal platelet function in the presence of normal platelet counts. The tests for platelet function include clot retraction test, tourniquet test, bleeding time, platelet adhesiveness, aggregations to collagen, ADP, and thrombin, and estimation of platelet factor 3 content.

Thrombasthenia (Glanzmann's disease) is usually familial and associated with defective function of

Table 14—2. Findings in hereditary platelet diseases.*

Disease	Platelet Count	Clot Retraction	Platelet Adhesion to Glass	Platelet Aggregations	Platelet Factor 3 Release	Platelet Survival	Platelet Morphology	Genetic Transmission
Glanzmann's thrombasthenia (membrane defect)	N	↓	↓	Decreased to ADP, collagen, thrombin, epinephrine	↓	N	Decreased absorbed fibrinogen	Autosomal recessive
Thrombopathia (ADP release defect)	N or ↓	N	↓ (or N)	Decreased to collagen, epinephrine, low molar ADP	↓ (or N)	N or ↑	No abnormality except(?) small size	Variable; (?)autosomal dominant
Thrombocytopathy (platelet factor 3 defect)	N	N	N (or ↓)	N	↓	. . .	Rare increase in platelet size	(?)Autosomal dominant
Von Willebrand's disease (plasma factor defect)	N	N	↓	N	N	N	N	Autosomal dominant (occasionally recessive)
Macrothrombocytic thrombopathy (Bernard-Soulier)	↓	N	N (or ↓)	N	↓	↓	Giant platelets	Autosomal dominant
Wiskott-Aldrich syndrome	↓	N	↓	Decreased to ADP, collagen, epinephrine	N (or ↓)	↓	Reduced organelles; large number of tubules	X-linked recessive
Thrombocytopenia with intrinsic platelet defect	↓	N	. . .	N to ADP	N	↓	N	Autosomal dominant

*Modified and reproduced, with permission, from Hathaway WE: Bleeding disorders due to platelet dysfunction. Am J Dis Child 121:127, 1971.

platelets with abnormal clot retraction; a defect in platelet adhesiveness and aggregation; and inability to release platelet factor 3. The bleeding time is prolonged. Thrombasthenia has been reported both as a recessive and as a dominant, and may be either mild or severe. It should be suspected in a patient with a prolonged bleeding time and should be investigated with platelet function studies. In the presence of severe bleeding, treatment with platelet concentrates may be necessary.

Thrombopathia is characterized by an abnormality of platelet function affecting the clotting mechanism. There is a deficiency of the platelet thromboplastic factor (platelet factor 3). This abnormality is usually associated with mild bleeding. The diagnosis may only be made by investigation of platelet function in the thromboplastin generation test or by the prothrombin consumption test. Platelet concentrates are the recommended therapy. Giant platelets are frequently seen on the blood smear.

Several other hereditary (Table 14–2) and acquired diseases of platelet function have recently been described. Of practical importance are the acquired platelet function defects found in patients with uremia or after aspirin ingestion.

Roser SM, Gracia R, Guralnick WC: Portsmouth syndrome: Review of literature and clinicopathological correlation. J Oral Surg 33:668, 1975.

Stuart M: Inherited defects of platelet function. Semin Hematol 12:233, 1975.

VON WILLEBRAND'S DISEASE
(Pseudohemophilia, Vascular Hemophilia)

Essentials of Diagnosis

- History of easy bruising and epistaxis from early childhood.
- Prolonged bleeding time with normal platelet count.
- Reduced levels of AHF (AHG, factor VIII).

General Considerations

Von Willebrand's disease is a familial bleeding disorder that is usually transmitted as a dominant and occurs in both sexes. It is associated both with a prolonged bleeding time and with a reduced level of factor VIII. Although the whole blood coagulation time is usually normal, the partial thromboplastin test is abnormal.

This bleeding disorder was originally believed to be associated with an abnormality of the capillary wall since increased tortuosity of capillaries may be seen on examination of the loops in the nail bed. Recent evidence indicates that the basic defect is in the production of an antibleeding time factor (vWd factor) localized in the blood vessel endothelium and in the circulation. This factor is closely associated with factor VIII procoagulant activity and is the major part of the factor VIII molecule that can be measured immunologically (VIII antigen). Therefore, patients with von Willebrand's disease have a prolonged bleeding time due to deficiency of the vWd factor, low factor VIII procoagulant activity (3–40% of normal), and low antigenic VIII levels.

Clinical Findings

A. Symptoms and Signs: There is usually a history of increased bruising and severe prolonged epistaxis. Increased bleeding will also occur with lacerations or at surgery. Excessive menstrual flow is a problem in the adolescent female. Petechiae are usually not observed, and hemarthrosis does not occur.

B. Laboratory Findings: A prolonged bleeding time is present; platelet number and function are normal except for platelet retention in glass bead columns ("adhesiveness") and decreased platelet aggregation to the antibiotic ristocetin. These latter defects are due to the deficiency of vWd factor in the plasma. Factor VIII procoagulant activity and antigenic activity are decreased.

Treatment

The depressed levels of AHF can be easily corrected with freshly frozen lyophilized plasma or AHF concentrates (cryoprecipitates). The AHF levels increase both after transfusion of AHF and as a result of endogenous production of AHF stimulated by another plasma factor; therefore, AHF levels remain elevated longer than in classical hemophilia. In some patients, the platelet adhesiveness and bleeding time can be corrected by the use of freshly frozen, platelet-free plasma. Transfusions with cryoprecipitates may be more effective than normal plasma in correcting the bleeding time. Dosage equivalents of 10 ml/kg of freshly frozen plasma every 12 hours will correct the AHF deficiency, but more frequent transfusions may be needed to restore the bleeding time to normal.

Dental procedures involving the gums and tooth extractions should be avoided if possible. When extractions are necessary, management consists of systemic correction, local pressure, and use of aminocaproic acid (Amicar).

Prognosis

Patients with mild forms of the disease usually have a normal life expectancy, and bleeding can be controlled with the measures noted above or may cease spontaneously. In severe cases it may be difficult to control hemorrhage, although recent methods of therapy with plasma and concentrates have greatly improved the outlook. Elective surgical procedures should be avoided.

Ekert H, Firkin BG: Recent advances in haemophilia and von Willebrand's disease. Vox Sang 28:409, 1975.

Gralnick HR, Sultan Y, Coller BS: Von Willebrand's disease: Combined qualitative and quantitative abnormalities. N Engl J Med 296:1024, 1977.

THROMBASTHENIA WITH ACYANOTIC CONGENITAL HEART DISEASE

Several patients have been observed who demonstrate a history of easy bruising and bleeding from cuts or minor surgery and who have associated acyanotic congenital heart disease. Aortic stenosis is particularly apt to be associated with this problem. It is characterized by a prolonged bleeding time and by abnormal platelet function. The bleeding disorder is usually extremely mild, and some of these patients have undergone surgical correction of their heart disease without excessive hemorrhage.

Maurer HM & others: Impairment in platelet aggregation in congenital heart disease. Blood 40:207, 1972.

VASCULAR DEFECTS

ANAPHYLACTOID PURPURA
(Schönlein-Henoch Purpura, Allergic Purpura)

Essentials of Diagnosis
- Purpuric cutaneous rash.
- Urticaria.
- Migratory polyarthritis.
- Gastrointestinal pain and hemorrhage.
- Hematuria.

Clinical Findings

A. Symptoms and Signs: Migratory polyarthritis very similar to that of rheumatic fever frequently precedes the onset of the skin rash. Gastrointestinal pain, diarrhea, and gastrointestinal bleeding are common. Nephritis occurs in about 50% of cases, either with symptomless proteinuria or hematuria or with nephrotic syndrome. The skin rash is diagnostic in appearance: It is characteristically distributed on the ankles, buttocks, and elbows; purpuric areas a few millimeters in diameter are present and may progress to form larger hemorrhages. Petechial lesions occur, but the majority of skin or mucous membrane hemorrhages are slightly larger. The rash usually begins on the lower extremities, but the entire body may be involved. Erythematous and urticarial skin eruptions (which may become hemorrhagic) often accompany the hemorrhage. Cardiac involvement is rare.

B. Laboratory Findings: The platelet count, platelet function tests, bleeding time, and tourniquet test are usually negative, although the latter may be the one abnormal finding. Blood coagulation is normal. Urinalysis frequently reveals hematuria and proteinuria, but casts are unusual. Stool tests may be positive for occult blood, even though gross melena is not ob-

served. The ASO titer is frequently elevated or the throat culture positive for group A beta-hemolytic streptococci. Serum IgA globulins may be elevated.

General Considerations

Anaphylactoid purpura is characterized by a typical purpuric skin rash plus (in any combination) migratory arthritis, gastroenteritis, and nephritis. It is believed to be a vasculitis related to vessel damage by deposits of immune complexes (antigen-antibody). It is characterized by involvement of the small vessels, particularly in the skin, the gastrointestinal tract, and the kidneys. The cause of the allergic reaction is frequently not recognized, although in some parts of the world group A beta-hemolytic streptococcal infection may precede the disease in some cases. Other inciting antigens such as drugs, other infections (viruses), food allergens, insect bites, and horse serum have been implicated.

Differential Diagnosis

The hemorrhagic rash of anaphylactoid purpura can be differentiated from thrombocytopenic purpura by the presence of raised skin lesions in the former and by the platelet count. The rash of septicemia (especially meningococcemia) may be very similar, although the distribution tends to be more generalized in sepsis. Blood culture may be necessary for final diagnosis.

Complications

Intussusception of the small bowel occurs in a significant number of patients with intestinal manifestations. The most important complications derive from the renal involvement. About 8% of patients with renal involvement die as a result of advancing proliferative glomerulonephritis, and an equal number will have continuing hematuria, proteinuria, and hypertension after 2 years. About 25% have recurring hematuria, and in the remainder the renal disease clears completely. Clinical severity is proportionate to the extent of the lesion histologically; older children are more liable to severe involvement.

Treatment

There is no satisfactory treatment for anaphylactoid purpura. Corticosteroid therapy may be useful in patients with acute gastrointestinal manifestations. If the culture is positive for group A beta-hemolytic streptococci or if the ASO titer is elevated, give penicillin in full therapeutic doses for 10 days. Aspirin is useful for the arthritis, and sedatives may benefit the patient with gastrointestinal pain. Immunosuppressive drugs such as cyclophosphamide and azathioprine are now contraindicated in the treatment of the nephritis.

Prognosis

The prognosis for recovery is good, although symptoms frequently recur over a period of several months. In patients who develop renal manifestations, approximately 50% may have persistent abnormal urinary findings. This occasionally progresses to significant impairment of renal function.

Meadow SR & others: Schönlein-Henoch nephritis. Q J Med 41:241, 1972.

Trygstad CW, Stiehm ER: Elevated serum IgA globulin in anaphylactoid purpura. Pediatrics 47:1023, 1972.

INTRAVASCULAR DEFECTS; COAGULATION FACTOR DEFICIENCIES

Essentials of Diagnosis

- Generalized bleeding tendency.
- Ecchymoses (not petechiae).
- Congenital (family history) or acquired (systemic illness).

- Abnormal partial thromboplastin time or prothrombin time (or both).

General Considerations

A congenital or acquired deficiency of one or more of the coagulation factors in the blood can result in a generalized bleeding diathesis. The bleeding tendency may be mild (bleeding only at time of severe traumas or surgical procedures), moderate, or severe (frequent spontaneous hemarthroses and ecchymoses) depending on the degree of the coagulation factor deficit. Fig 14–1 depicts the interaction of these factors in producing coagulation of the blood. Hemostasis in man depends upon platelet and vascular factors as well as blood coagulation.

A specific hemorrhagic diathesis has been seen with a deficiency of each of the coagulation factors except Hageman factor (XII), calcium deficiency, and Fletcher factor. These disease entities are discussed below.

The diagnosis and classification of clinical coagu-

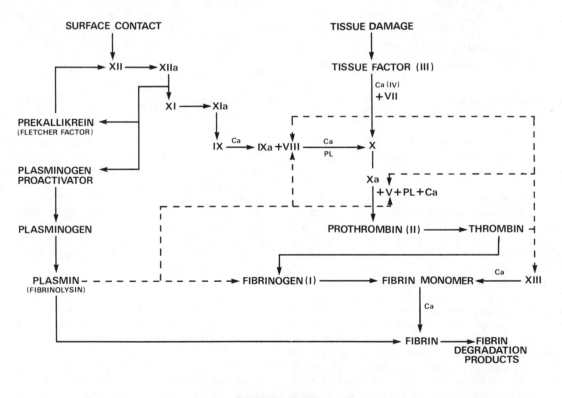

Coagulation Factors

I Fibrinogen	IX Plasma thromboplastin component (PTC)
II Prothrombin	X Stuart-Prower factor
III Thromboplastin	XI Plasma thromboplastin antecedent (PTA)
IV Calcium	XII Hageman factor
V Ac-globulin, proaccelerin, labile factor	XIII Fibrin stabilizing factor, fibrinase
VII Proconvertin, SPCA	PL Phospholipid
VIII Antihemophilic factor (AHF)	

Figure 14–1. Blood coagulation scheme and terminology of coagulation factors.

lation factor deficiencies depend upon proper performance and interpretation of specific clotting tests which are briefly reviewed below.

Coagulation Tests

A. Whole Blood Coagulation Time (Lee-White): This test is too insensitive to be of value in diagnosis or treatment of patients with mild to moderate coagulation factor deficiencies. The clotting time is influenced by heparin and can therefore be used as a rough guide to heparinization. Although simple to perform, this procedure is not an adequate screening test and should be abandoned as a "routine" test. A more useful test is the activated whole blood clotting time (ACT), which is performed by addition of an activating agent (kaolin, silica) to the clotting tube.

B. One-Stage Prothrombin Time (Quick): This procedure consists of noting the clotting time of citrated or oxalated plasma after addition of calcium and tissue thromboplastin. Normal adult values are between 11–13 seconds (100%). This is an adequate screening test for proconvertin (VII), proaccelerin (V), Stuart-Prower factor (X), prothrombin (II), and fibrinogen deficiencies. It does not measure the factors necessary for the earlier stages of coagulation.

C. Partial Thromboplastin Time (PTT): This test is performed much like the prothrombin time except that a phospholipid is added instead of tissue thromboplastin. In addition, a contact activator substance like kaolin may be added to avert the influence of glass contact. The test is very sensitive, relatively easy to perform, and inexpensive. All coagulation factors except proconvertin are measured; therefore, it is the screening test of choice. Normal adult values are as follows: with kaolin, 37–50 seconds; without contact activator, 70–100 seconds.

D. Prothrombin Consumption Test: This procedure measures all factors prior to conversion of prothrombin to thrombin (except proconvertin). The test is technically difficult to perform properly and is not as sensitive as the partial thromboplastin time.

E. Thromboplastin Generation Test (TGT): This determination is more difficult to perform than the prothrombin consumption test, but it is a reliable and sensitive estimate of plasma thromboplastin formation and is often used to confirm the diagnosis of AHF or PTC deficiency.

F. Thrombin Time: Bovine or human thrombin is added to plasma and the clotting time recorded. The normal adult range is 7–15 seconds or more, depending upon the amount of thrombin added. The test measures the conversion of fibrinogen to fibrin and is dependent upon the concentration of fibrinogen or inhibitors such as fibrin split products, antithrombins, and heparin.

G. Specific Factor Assays: Each of the coagulation factors can be assayed by an indirect clotting method using natural or synthetic factor deficient substrates and compared to the activity of normal plasma (100%). Fibrinogen is the only factor which can be measured directly by a chemical method.

H. Bleeding Time (Ivy): (Hemostasis bleeding time method.) Place a blood pressure cuff on the upper arm and inflate to 40 mm Hg. With an alcohol sponge, clean an area free of visible veins on the flexor surface of the forearm. With a sterile Bard-Parker No. 11 blade, make a puncture wound 5 mm deep and 2 mm wide. Note time of puncture; touch wound gently with sterile filter paper to absorb blood every 30 seconds until bleeding stops. Normal bleeding time is 1–7 minutes. A modification of this test using a template to make 1 mm deep and 4 mm long cut is now frequently used (template bleeding time).

I. Other Tests: Various other tests, available usually in research laboratories only, such as the thromboelastograph, thrombin generation time, euglobulin fibrinolysin time, and recalcification time, are sometimes helpful in identifying unusual circulating anticoagulants or hypercoagulability of the blood.

Hathaway WE: Easy bruising in children. Postgrad Med 61:224, March 1977.

Ratnoff OD, Bennett B: The genetics of hereditary disorders of blood coagulation. Science 179:1291, 1973.

AFIBRINOGENEMIA & DYSFIBRINOGENEMIA

Several patients have been described recently who have a bleeding tendency and delayed clotting due to an abnormal molecule of fibrinogen (congenital dysfibrinogenemia). Immunologic determinations of fibrinogen are normal, but the thrombin and prothrombin times are often prolonged. Treatment is similar to that outlined for afibrinogenemia.

Congenital absence of fibrinogen produces a definite entity which resembles hemophilia clinically. However, the condition is inherited as an autosomal recessive and affects both sexes. The patients have persistent bleeding from small injuries, hematomas, ecchymoses, and hemarthroses. Although fatal bleeding from the umbilical cord has been reported, most cases are usually much less severe than classical hemophilia.

The principal laboratory finding in afibrinogenemia is complete absence of a fibrin clot by any of the usual clotting tests attempted. Whole blood and plasma are incoagulable even upon the addition of optimal amounts of calcium, thromboplastin, and thrombin. The erythrocyte sedimentation rate is zero. There is an absence of precipitable fibrinogen upon heating of plasma to 56° C for 10 minutes. Specific assays for other coagulation factors are normal.

Transfusion with whole blood, fresh plasma, or preparations of purified fibrinogen generally control the acute bleeding episodes. The minimal hemostatic level of circulating fibrinogen is about 60 mg/100 ml (normal, 250–450 mg/100 ml). The half-life of transfused fibrinogen is about 4 days. Therefore, 10–20 ml of plasma per kg body weight or 0.05–0.1 gm of fibrinogen per kg should achieve hemostasis. This dose may need to be repeated daily depending upon the type and severity of bleeding and the rate of healing.

Menache D: Abnormal fibrinogens: A review. Thromb Diath Haemorrh 29:525, 1973.

HEMOPHILIA A
(Antihemophilic Factor [AHF],
Factor VIII Deficiency)

Classical hemophilia (hemophilia A) is a bleeding disorder characterized by decreased activity of circulating antihemophilic factor (AHF, AHG, or factor VIII). The disease occurs in males and is inherited in an X-linked recessive manner. All degrees of severity of the disease have been reported.

Clinical Findings

A. Symptoms and Signs: Patients with severe hemophilia, characterized by frequent spontaneous bleeding episodes involving skin, mucous membranes, joints, and viscera, have no circulating AHF activity. However, mild hemophilia is also recognized; these patients bleed only at times of severe trauma or surgery. They have 5–20% AHF activity. An intermediate group of patients with moderate symptoms (usually no severe joint involvement) have 1–5% AHF levels.

The most crippling aspect of hemophilia A is the tendency to develop chronic hemarthroses, especially of knees and elbows, which lead to fibrosis and joint contractures.

B. Laboratory Findings: In about 70% of families with this disease, the female carriers will have low levels of AHF (20–70%) and may occasionally be mildly symptomatic. Otherwise, low levels of AHF are not seen in a female unless the individual has von Willebrand's disease or a circulating anticoagulant or is the product of the union of a hemophiliac male and a carrier female. Carriers of hemophilia can be detected in most instances by determination of the ratio of factor VIII activity to factor VIII antigen.

Tests measuring intrinsic plasma thromboplastin formation (whole blood clotting time, plasma recalcification time, partial thromboplastin time [PTT], thromboplastin generation test [TGT], and prothrombin consumption test) are all abnormal. The bleeding time and one-stage prothrombin time are normal. The specific diagnosis is made by showing failure of "correction" in a test system (PTT or TGT) by known AHF-deficient plasma. Coagulation assays have been developed to measure the actual percentage of AHF activity in a given biologic fluid. The whole blood clotting time can be normal in the presence of as little as 1–2% AHF, and, therefore, is not a good test for diagnosis or guide to therapy. Factor VIII antigen levels are normal in classical hemophilia.

Complications

The principal complication of classical hemophilia is the development of an acquired circulating anticoagulant to AHF. Mild inhibitor or anticoagulant substances specific to AHF not uncommonly can be shown in AHF-deficient patients, but the development of a severe AHF inhibitor is a rare and dreaded complication. When this occurs, the patient is often resistant to all attempts at therapy. The inhibitor has been shown to be an antibody but is rarely amenable to immunosuppressive therapy. "Activated" prothrombin complex concentrates may be of help in stopping hemorrhage in these patients.

Another rare complication is the formation of a pseudotumor in the AHF-deficient patient. These are the result of multiple bleeding, fibrosis, serous secretion, and calcium deposition. They should be carefully evaluated and differentiated from bony or soft tissue neoplasms. Crippling due to repeated hemarthroses is the primary long-term complication.

Treatment

The basis of treatment of classical hemophilia is the administration of an AHF-containing substance in order to achieve adequate hemostasis. AHF is temperature and storage labile in biologic fluids.

The in vivo half-life of infused AHF is about 12 hours.

The following substances can be used for therapy: (1) Freshly frozen plasma or cryoprecipitates stored at −30° C for less than 12 months. (2) Lyophilized concentrates of AHF, reconstituted and given immediately.

Dosage and duration of therapy depend upon the type of bleeding seen clinically. "Open" bleeding is that which occurs from lacerations of the skin or mucous membranes, tooth extractions, surgical wounds, or severe traumatic epistaxis. Closed bleeding can be subdivided into (a) joint hemorrhage and nondissecting hematomas and (b) dissecting soft tissue hematomas.

A. "Open" Bleeding: Treat in one of the following ways: (1) Freshly frozen plasma, 10 ml/kg body weight immediately and then 5 ml/kg every 6 hours. A level of 20% (in vivo) is achieved by 10 ml/kg. Each dose must be infused as rapidly as the patient can safely tolerate it to ensure peak levels. (2) Cryoprecipitated AHF is prepared from individual blood donors and is usually supplied frozen in 20–30 ml amounts per plastic pack. The units* of AHF activity vary from 75–200 per pack. For calculations, assume 100 units per pack. To achieve a level of 40%, one pack per 5–6 kg of body weight is given. Half of this dose is given every 12 hours to maintain an in vivo level of 20%. (3) AHF concentrates (obtained commercially) supply concentrated AHF in a lyophilized form. The potency of each vial of these products is labeled in units of AHF. Dosage can be calculated as follows:

Units of AHF = Weight in kg × Desired in vivo percentage × 0.5

*A unit of AHF is the amount contained in 1 ml of fresh plasma at a 100% AHF activity level.

Treatment must be continued until adequate healing occurs, ie, 2–3 days in case of tooth extractions or epistaxis, but 7–10 days in case of lacerations and surgical wounds. The principle of therapy is to rapidly achieve a hemostatic level of AHF (at least 20%) and to maintain this level until the lesion is adequately healed. For surgical procedures, levels of 30–35% are usually necessary for hemostasis. In mucous membrane bleeding or wounds (tongue, tooth socket), the duration of AHF therapy can often be reduced to 1–2 days if a fibrinolytic inhibitor aminocaproic acid (Amicar) is given in a dosage of 100 mg/kg orally every 6 hours until healing is complete.

B. "Closed" Bleeding: Early closed bleeding in joints or soft tissue areas can often be controlled by a single infusion of freshly frozen plasma, cryoprecipitates, or AHF concentrate to reach a single peak of 20%. If bleeding is severe, this dose should be repeated in 12 hours or a higher level achieved initially (ie, 40%). However, if the lesion is a dissecting hematoma which might threaten nerve function or endanger respiration or vision, a level of 20% should be maintained for at least 48 hours.

Corticosteroids may be helpful in instances of recurrent joint bleeding. Patients with renal bleeding have also been benefited by corticosteroid therapy. Local hemostatic measures such as pressure or application of Gelfoam soaked in bovine thrombin are often helpful in case of epistaxis.

Prognosis

With prophylaxis against injury, early treatment of bleeding episodes, careful orthopedic care of joint lesions, and attention to emotional, social, and educational adjustment, the prognosis for a useful normal life is good.

Abildgaard CF: Current concepts in the management of hemophilia. Semin Hematol 12:223, 1975.
Aledort LM (editor): Recent advances in hemophilia. Ann NY Acad Sci 240:1, 1975.
Klein H & others: Detection of the carrier state of classic hemophilia. N Engl J Med 296:959, 1977.
Kurczynski EM & others: Activated prothrombin concentrate for patients with factor VIII inhibitors. N Engl J Med 291:164, 1974.

HEMOPHILIA B
(PTC [Factor IX] Deficiency)

The mode of inheritance and clinical manifestations of hemophilia B (PTC deficiency, factor IX deficiency, Christmas disease) are the same as those of AHF deficiency (hemophilia A). Congenital PTC deficiency is 20–25% as prevalent as AHF deficiency. PTC is made in the liver and is vitamin K dependent; therefore, acquired deficiencies of factor IX are fairly common.

PTC is a storage stable factor which is not consumed during coagulation and is found in the serum. The thromboplastin generation test (TGT) may be used to determine whether the first stage defect is due to PTC (serum) or AHF (plasma) deficiency. Otherwise, the diagnosis is confirmed by failure to "correct" with known PTC-deficient plasma or serum in the PTT or TGT tests. With these exceptions, the laboratory findings are the same as those noted above in the discussion of hemophilia A.

Although factor IX is storage stable and is not consumed during coagulation, the therapy of bleeding episodes is little different from that outlined above for classical hemophilia. The products that can be used include recently outdated blood bank plasma (approximately 3 weeks old) at 4° C, plus freshly frozen plasma or factor IX concentrate. Unlike factor VIII, approximately half of the administered dose of factor IX diffuses into the extravascular space. Therefore, twice the calculated factor VIII dose (see above) should be given as plasma or factor IX concentrate (Konyne) initially. Subsequently, half of the initial dose can be given to achieve the desired in vivo level. (Factor IX has a half-life of 20–22 hours in vivo.) Cryoprecipitates and AHF concentrates do not contain sufficient PTC for use in this disease. The prognosis is good if the bleeding episodes are adequately controlled.

Cederbaum AI & others: Intravascular coagulation with use of human prothrombin complex concentrates. Ann Intern Med 84:683, 1976.
Kasper CK: Surgical operation in hemophilia B: Use of factor IX concentrate. Calif Med 113:4, July 1970.

HEMOPHILIA C
(PTA [Factor XI] Deficiency)

PTA (factor XI) deficiency is a bleeding diathesis of mild to moderate severity. Inheritance is by the autosomal recessive mode. Heterozygotes rarely show a mild bleeding tendency at surgery or following severe trauma. Homozygous patients may have spontaneous hemorrhage (ecchymoses, epistaxis) in addition to bleeding due to trauma. Only rarely do patients with hemophilia C have spontaneous hemarthroses. Hemophilia C has been found mainly in Jews and comprises less than 5% of all hemophilioid diseases.

The defect may be very mild, and a sensitive coagulation test (PTT or TGT) is required to identify the deficiency. Factor XI is a stable factor found in both serum and plasma and shows increased activity on contact with glass or after storage. Therefore, differentiation from PTC deficiency may be difficult unless tests are done with fresh plasma using known PTA-deficient plasma for "correction studies." The prothrombin time and bleeding time (Ivy) are normal in PTA deficiency.

The bleeding defect is mild and requires treatment usually only at times of surgery (eg, tooth extractions) or trauma. PTA is a stable factor, and good levels are found in plasma stored for several weeks at 4° C. Therefore, the principles of treatment outlined for PTC deficiency apply equally well to PTA deficiency.

The prognosis for an average longevity is excellent.

Bick RL & others: Surgical hemostasis with a factor XI-containing concentrate. JAMA 229:163, 1974.

Rimon A & others: Factor XI activity and factor XI antigen in homozygous and heterozygous factor XI deficiency. Blood 48:165, 1976.

LIVER-DEPENDENT COAGULATION FACTORS

The following clotting factors are known to be produced in the liver: fibrinogen (I), PTC (IX), prothrombin (II), proconvertin (VII), proaccelerin (V), Stuart-Prower factor (X), PTA (XI), and factor XII. Vitamin K is necessary for the synthesis of II, VII, X, and IX. Hereditary bleeding diseases due to isolated deficiencies of prothrombin, proconvertin, proaccelerin, or Stuart-Prower factor are exceedingly rare. Congenital deficiencies of fibrinogen and PTC are discussed above.

Hereditary prothrombin deficiency, proconvertin deficiency, Stuart-Prower factor deficiency, and proaccelerin deficiency have been reported in both males and females and have a recessive mode of transmission. Mild to moderately severe bleeding manifestations can occur. The prothrombin time is uniformly prolonged in these disorders; in addition, the PTT is abnormal in all except proconvertin deficiency (formation of intrinsic thromboplastin does not require proconvertin). The diagnosis is suspected when a patient is seen with a history of bleeding manifestations, a prolonged prothrombin time without liver disease, and no response to vitamin K therapy. The diagnosis must be confirmed by specific factor assays.

Treatment consists of transfusion of whole plasma in dosages sufficient to achieve at least 20–30% correction of the prothrombin time. Fresh plasma must be used for proaccelerin (V) deficiency since this is a relatively unstable factor.

Breederveld K & others: Severe factor V deficiency with prolonged bleeding time. Thromb Diath Haemorrh 32:538, 1974.

Falter ML, Kaufman MF: Congenital factor VII deficiency. J Pediatr 79:298, 1971.

Girolami A & others: Prothrombin Padua: A "new" congenital dysprothrombinemia. J Lab Clin Med 84:654, 1974.

HAGEMAN (XII) FACTOR DEFICIENCY; FLETCHER FACTOR (PREKALLIKREIN) DEFICIENCY

Patients with factor XII deficiency constitute a medical curiosity which consists of a markedly prolonged whole blood and plasma clotting time without clinical bleeding diathesis. This phenomenon cannot be explained at present. The defect is rare and is inherited in an autosomal recessive manner. Hageman factor deficiency becomes of clinical significance in the evaluation of a markedly prolonged coagulation time. These patients have undergone major surgery without excessive bleeding. Another coagulation factor defect (designated "Fletcher factor") has similar laboratory and clinical characteristics. Recent evidence indicates that "Fletcher factor" is the same as prekallikrein. High molecular weight kininogen (Fitzgerald factor), another link to the kinin system, is also associated with a prolonged PTT when deficient in the blood. None of these "contact factors" are associated with a bleeding diathesis when absent.

Hathaway WE & others: Clinical and physiologic studies of two siblings with prekallikrein (Fletcher factor) deficiency. Am J Med 60:654, 1976.

Ratnoff OD: The biology and pathology of the initial stages of blood coagulation. Prog Hematol 5:204, 1966.

Saito H & others: Fitzgerald traits. Deficiency of a hitherto unrecognized agent, Fitzgerald factor, participating in surface-mediated reactions of clotting, fibrinolysis, generation of kinins, and the property of diluted plasma enhancing vascular permeability (PF/dil). J Clin Invest 55:1082, 1975.

Wuepper KD: Biochemistry and biology of components of the plasma kinin-forming system. Pages 93–117 in: *Inflammation, Mechanisms and Control.* Lepow IH, Ward PA (editors). Academic Press, 1972.

FIBRIN STABILIZING FACTOR (XIII) DEFICIENCY

The deficiency of a factor responsible for the stability of the fibrin clot produces a genetically transmitted hemorrhagic disorder called congenital fibrinase (fibrin stabilizing factor, factor XIII) deficiency. Cases reported to date indicate an autosomal recessive inheritance. Affected individuals have a moderately severe bleeding tendency and often present at birth with hemorrhage into the umbilical cord. The usual tests of coagulation such as PTT, prothrombin time, and TGT are all normal. Fibrinogen may be borderline to low, and increased vascular fragility has been reported. The diagnosis is made by demonstrating abnormal stability of the fibrin clot in 5 M urea solution.

Treatment consists of giving plasma transfusions to control the acute bleeding episode.

Britten AFH: Congenital deficiency of factor XIII (fibrin stabilizing factor). Am J Med 43:751, 1967.

Ikkala E: Transfusion therapy in congenital deficiencies of plasma factor XIII. Ann NY Acad Sci 202:200, 1972.

ACQUIRED COAGULATION FACTOR DEFICIENCIES

1. HEMORRHAGIC DISEASE OF NEWBORN

A generalized bleeding diathesis can occur in newborn infants who are markedly deficient in vitamin K-dependent coagulation factors (PTC, prothrombin, proconvertin, Stuart-Prower factor). This clinical syndrome is called hemorrhagic disease of the newborn. It may be present at birth or may occur any time in the first 3 days of life. All newborn infants show a moderate deficiency of these K-dependent factors at a level of 25–60% of normal adult values. However, when the levels fall below 20% in infants who are vitamin K deficient, a generalized bleeding tendency can ensue. Ecchymoses, gastrointestinal hemorrhage, hematuria, and cerebral hemorrhages may occur on the second to fourth days of life.

The prothrombin time is markedly prolonged to a level below 20% of normal. The PTT is also greatly prolonged. Platelet estimation and bleeding times are normal. In this age group, bleeding in association with a greatly prolonged prothrombin time is very suggestive of hemorrhagic disease of the newborn. The diagnosis is confirmed by the response to specific treatment.

By definition, this disorder is due to severe vitamin K deficiency. Therefore, the disease can be prevented and treated adequately by a single intramuscular injection of 1–2 mg of vitamin K_1 (phytonadione). It is also recommended that this dose be given prophylactically to all newborn infants. The prothrombin will become essentially normal within 12–24 hours, and the bleeding will stop within 6–12 hours after treatment with vitamin K. If life-threatening hemorrhage is present, a transfusion of fresh plasma (10 ml/kg) or fresh whole blood (or both) is indicated.

Since the newborn infant can usually ingest, synthesize, and utilize enough vitamin K within a few days after birth to prevent further difficulty, the prognosis is excellent.

Keenan WJ & others: Role of feeding and vitamin K in hypoprothrombinemia of the newborn. Am J Dis Child 121:271, 1971.

2. VITAMIN K DEFICIENCY IN OLDER CHILDREN

Older infants and children may develop vitamin K deficiency secondary to chronic diarrhea, malabsorption syndrome, and defective synthesis associated with prolonged antibiotic therapy. The clinical and laboratory manifestations are similar to those seen in hemorrhagic disease of the newborn. Treatment is by administration of vitamin K_1 (phytonadione) in doses of 5–10 mg IV or IM.

3. SECONDARY HEMORRHAGIC DIATHESES OF NEWBORN

Premature and full-term infants frequently develop generalized bleeding tendencies associated

Table 14–3. Coagulation factor and test values in normal pregnant women and newborn infants.*

Category	Fibrinogen (mg/100 ml)	Factors II (%)	V (%)	VII (%)	VIII (%)	IX (%)	X (%)	XI (%)	XII (%)	XIII (titer)	Platelet Count (per cu mm)	Euglobulin Lysis Time (minutes)	Partial Thromboplastin Time† (seconds)	Prothrombin Time (seconds)	Thrombin Time (seconds)
Normal adult or child	190–420	100	100	100	100	100	100	100	100	1/16	200,000–450,000	90–300	37–50	12–14	8–10
Term pregnancy	483	92	108	170	196	130	130	69	...	1/16	290,000	278	44	13	8
Premature (1500–2500 gm), cord blood	233	25	67	37	80	↓	29	...	...	1/8	220,000	214	90	17 (12–21)	14 (11–17)
Term infant, cord blood	216	41	92	56	100	27	55	36	...	1/8	190,000	84	71	16 (13–20)	12 (10–16)
Term infant, 48 hours	210	46	105	20	100	↓	45	39	25	...	200,000	105	65	17.5 (12–21)	13 (10–16)

Note: All levels expressed as means of ranges.

*Reproduced, with permission, from Hathaway WE: Coagulation problems in the newborn infant. P Clin North America 17:929, 1970.

†Kaolin PTT.

with other illness such as respiratory distress syndrome, cyanotic congenital heart disease, cerebral anoxia, and severe sepsis. Factors which are often present and possibly related to this bleeding syndrome are "physiologic" depression of coagulation factors, hypoxia, acidosis, vascular fragility, defective platelet number and function, and increased fibrinolytic activity. Laboratory tests of bleeding and coagulation parameters are difficult to interpret because of the overlap with normal infants. The values for these tests seen in "normal" full-term and premature infants are shown in Table 14–3. The pathophysiologic mechanisms of these secondary bleeding syndromes (cerebral hemorrhage, pulmonary hemorrhage, generalized bleeding tendency) are poorly understood at present.

Occasionally, these infants show the clinical and laboratory signs of disseminated intravascular coagulation (see below). Exchange transfusion or heparinization may be indicated. Otherwise, treatment is symptomatic and is mainly directed at the underlying disease or metabolic disorder. If platelets or coagulation factors are shown to be very low, specific replacement with platelet concentrates or fresh plasma can be given. Vitamin K should always be given to these infants also.

Hathaway WE: The bleeding newborn. Semin Hematol 12:175, 1975.

4. DISSEMINATED INTRAVASCULAR COAGULATION

Certain diseases occurring in children have been shown to be associated with disseminated intravascular coagulation (DIC) or consumption coagulopathy. These diseases are purpura fulminans, severe overwhelming bacterial sepsis (eg, meningococcemia, *Escherichia coli* infection), viral or rickettsial infections (eg, smallpox, Rocky Mountain spotted fever), severe thermal burns, giant hemangiomas, and the hemolytic-uremic syndrome. DIC can be triggered by a Shwartzman-like phenomenon or release of tissue thromboplastin and leads to widespread fibrin deposition (lungs, kidneys), fibrinolysis, and consumption of coagulation factors which lead to a secondary bleeding tendency.

Laboratory evaluation discloses decreased platelets, fibrinogen, proaccelerin, AHF, and prothrombin (the factors consumed during coagulation). Other factors are usually normal. Fibrinolysins are first increased and later depressed or exhausted. Degradation of fibrin leads to the accumulation of fibrin split products in the blood; these act as an anticoagulant and prolong the thrombin time.

Treatment consists of correction of the triggering event and replacement of the consumable clotting factor with fresh plasma or platelet concentrates. In the occasional patient with persistent DIC or with localized thrombotic complications (gangrene, renal cortical

necrosis), heparin may be given IV, 100 units/kg every 4–6 hours.

As shock is often associated with this disorder, early recognition and prompt treatment may be lifesaving.

Hathaway WE: Heparin therapy in acute meningococcemia. J Pediatr 82:900, 1973.

Regan DH, Lackner H: Defibrination syndrome: Changing concepts and recognition of the low grade form. Am J Med Sci 266:84, 1973.

Smith CA (editor): Chapter 22, page 307, in: *The Critically Ill Child: Diagnosis and Management,* 2nd ed. Saunders, 1977.

5. CIRCULATING ANTICOAGULANTS

Acquired anticoagulants can cause a widespread hemorrhagic diathesis. These inhibitors to coagulation are often associated with "collagen" diseases such as disseminated lupus erythematosus. Also, specific inhibitors to AHF or PTC may occur in hemophilia and may cause a severe intractable bleeding tendency. The anticoagulants appear to be antibodies and are often directed against specific coagulation factors. These inhibitors can be demonstrated using the recalcification time, prothrombin time, and PTT tests. These tests will remain prolonged rather than be corrected by addition of normal plasma in equal quantities. The most effective therapy has been with immunosuppressive agents such as prednisone or azathioprine.

Heparin and dicumarol are potent anticoagulants when administered as drugs. Heparin affects the whole blood coagulation time or PTT primarily, whereas dicumarol affects the prothrombin time by inhibiting the utilization of vitamin K.

Naturally occurring anticoagulants such as heparin, antithromboplastins, and antithrombins are rarely implicated as the cause of a bleeding diathesis, although a deficiency of antithrombin III has been associated with significant thromboembolic phenomena.

Feinstein DI, Rapaport SI: Acquired inhibitors of blood coagulation. Prog Hemostasis Thromb 1:75, 1972.

Rosenberg RD: Actions and interactions of antithrombin and heparin. N Engl J Med 292:146, 1975.

Schleider MA & others: Clinical study of lupus anticoagulant. Blood 48:499, 1976.

Shapiro SS, Hultin M: Acquired inhibitors to the blood coagulation factors. Semin Thromb 1:336, 1975.

6. FIBRINOLYSINS

Hemorrhagic tendencies due to hypofibrinogenemia secondary to increased fibrinolysins are rarely seen in children. Circumstances in which increased fibrinolytic activity may be seen include extensive surgery (especially with use of cardiopulmonary bypass procedures), liver disease, carcinomas, leukemia, and disseminated intravascular coagulation (DIC). Increased fibrinolytic activity can be diagnosed by use of the whole blood clot lysis time (normally, a formed clot lyses very slowly—48 hours or more—at 37° C), or the euglobulin lysis time, a more sensitive test. If fibrinolysins are present to a pathologic degree, ie, causing a hemorrhagic tendency, a potent fibrinolysin inhibitor, aminocaproic acid (EACA, Amicar), is available. This drug should not be used in DIC.

Nilsson IM, Isacson S: New aspects of the pathogenesis of thrombo-embolism. Prog Surg 11:46, 1973.

V. THE SPLEEN

SPLENOMEGALY

The child with a relatively isolated finding of splenomegaly frequently presents a puzzling diagnostic problem. In the diagnosis of chronic splenomegaly, the following categories of diseases should be considered: congestive splenomegaly, chronic infections, leukemia and lymphomas, hemolytic anemias, reticuloendothelioses, and storage diseases. The clinical findings and diagnostic procedures recommended with each of these entities are summarized in Table 14—4.

DEVELOPMENTAL DEFECTS OF THE SPLEEN

Simultaneous injury, at about the 25th day of embryonic life, of the splenic anlage, atrioventricular cushions of the heart, and mesentery may account for the triad of situs inversus, congenital lesions of the heart, and asplenia. Fewer than 10% of cases of congenital absence of the spleen occur without serious heart lesions. Most infants with this triad die within a few weeks. The principal evidence of asplenia in these infants consists of erythrocytic inclusions such as Howell-Jolly bodies, nucleated red cells, and Heinz bodies. A mild reticulocytosis and siderocytosis can be found. The discovery of these red cell inclusions in a patient with congenital heart disease is strong presumptive evidence for this syndrome.

No specific therapy is available.

Bisno AL: Hyposplenism and overwhelming pneumococcic infection: Reappraisal. Am J Med Sci 262:101, 1971.

Pearson HA & others: Functional hyposplenia in cyanotic heart disease. Pediatrics 48:277, 1971.

Table 14—4. Causes of chronic splenomegaly in children.

Cause	Associated Clinical Findings	Diagnostic Investigation
Congestive splenomegaly	History of umbilical vein catheter or neonatal omphalitis. Signs of portal hypertension (varices, hemorrhoids, dilated abdominal wall veins); pancytopenia, history of hepatitis or jaundice.	Complete blood count, platelet count, liver function tests, upper gastrointestinal x-rays.
Chronic infections	History of exposure to tuberculosis, histoplasmosis, coccidioidomycosis, other fungal disease; chronic sepsis (foreign body in blood stream; subacute bacterial endocarditis).	Appropriate cultures and skin tests, ie, blood cultures, PPD, histoplasmin, coccidioidin skin tests; chest film.
Infectious mononucleosis	Fever, fatigue, pharyngitis, rash, adenopathy.	Heterophil antibodies.
Leukemia, lymphoma, Hodgkin's disease	Evidence of systemic involvement with fever, bleeding tendencies, and lymphadenopathy; pancytopenia.	Blood smear, bone marrow examination, spleen biopsy.
Hemolytic anemias	Anemia, jaundice; family history of anemia, jaundice, and gallbladder disease in young adults.	Reticulocyte count, Coombs test, spherocytosis (blood smear, osmotic fragility), autohemolysis test.
Reticuloendothelioses (histiocytosis X)	Chronic otitis media, seborrheic or petechial skin rashes, anemia, infections, lymphadenopathy.	Skeletal x-rays for bone lesions; biopsy of bone, liver, bone marrow, or lymph node.
Storage diseases	Family history of similar disorders, neurologic involvement, evidence of macular degeneration.	Biopsy of rectal mucosa, liver, bone marrow, spleen, or brain in search for storage cells.
Splenic cyst	Evidence of other infections (postinfectious cyst) or congenital anomalies; peculiar shape of spleen.	Aspiration or exploration.

CONGESTIVE SPLENOMEGALY
(Banti's Syndrome)

Banti's syndrome consists of an enlarged spleen, pancytopenia, and evidences of hepatic disease such as liver enlargement, decreased liver function as shown by appropriate tests, portal hypertension, and hepatic decompensation. Three separate entities are known to produce this syndrome: (1) vascular anomalies of the splenic and portal venous system; (2) thrombophlebitis of the portal and splenic veins, often secondary to infection following neonatal catheterization of the umbilical vein; and (3) cirrhosis of the liver. The age at onset and the presenting symptoms vary according to the etiology. For further discussion of this disorder, see Chapter 16.

Infections and neoplasms of the spleen are listed in Table 14–4 and discussed elsewhere in the text.

INFECTIONS FOLLOWING SPLENECTOMY

There is good evidence that infants and children who have undergone splenectomy are subsequently more susceptible to severe bacterial infections. These infections are septicemia, meningitis, or pneumonia due to pneumococci, group A streptococci, *Haemophilus influenzae,* and enteric organisms. Children under 4 years of age and those with generalized disorders of the reticuloendothelial system are more frequently affected. The increased susceptibility to infection following splenectomy has not been explained, but it is probably related to the role of the spleen in antibody synthesis and phagocytic function. If possible, splenectomy should be delayed until after age 4, and prophylactic antibiotic therapy should be used for 1–2 years after splenectomy in susceptible patients.

Singer DB: Postsplenectomy sepsis. Perspect Pediatr Pathol 1:285, 1973.

HYPERSPLENISM

An enlarged spleen can produce varying degrees of anemia, leukopenia, or thrombocytopenia regardless of the cause of the enlargement. This pancytopenia is probably due to decreased hemic cell survival due to "trapping" of cells in the splenic pulp, but it may also be due to inhibition of release of cells from the marrow. In such instances of hypersplenism, the bone marrow is usually hyperplastic in appearance.

VI. RETICULOENDOTHELIOSES

The diseases to be discussed under this heading comprise a heterogeneous group of proliferative disorders of the reticuloendothelial system of unknown cause. Eosinophilic granuloma of bone, Hand-Schüller-Christian disease, and Letterer-Siwe disease constitute a complex of diseases of unknown cause, of histiocytic proliferation, and of unpredictable prognosis. Lichtenstein has grouped them under the term histiocytosis X. Although foam cells containing cholesterol are found in these disorders, it is currently believed that the storage cells are not the result of a primary disturbance of lipid metabolism but are secondary either to increased intracellular cholesterol synthesis or to inhibition of cholesterol from necrotic tissue.

Certain patients present primarily with signs and symptoms of lytic lesions limited to the bones—especially the skull, ribs, clavicles, and vertebrae. These lesions are well demarcated and occasionally painful. Biopsy reveals eosinophilic granuloma, which may be the only lesion the patient will develop, although further bone and even visceral lesions may occur.

Another group of patients often present with otitis media, seborrheic skin rash, and evidence of bone lesions, usually in the mastoid or skull area. They frequently also have visceral involvement, which may be indicated by lymphadenopathy and hepatosplenomegaly. This chronic disseminated form is usually known as *Hand-Schüller-Christian disease* and is associated with "foamy histiocytes" on biopsy. The classic triad of Hand-Schüller-Christian disease (bony involvement, exophthalmos, and diabetes insipidus) is rarely seen; however, diabetes insipidus is a common complication.

A third group of patients present early in life primarily with visceral involvement. They often have a petechial or macular skin rash, generalized lymphadenopathy, enlarged liver and spleen, pulmonary involvement, and hematologic abnormalities such as anemia and thrombocytopenia. Bone lesions can occur. This acute visceral form—Letterer-Siwe disease—is often fatal.

In all 3 groups there are proliferation of histiocytes; aggregations of eosinophils, lymphocytes, and plasma cells; and collection of foam cells.

The principal diseases to be differentiated from histiocytosis X are bone tumors (primary or metastatic), lymphomas or leukemias, granulomatous infections, and storage diseases. The diagnosis is established by biopsy of bone marrow, lymph node, liver, or mastoid or other bone.

Almost any system or area can become involved during the course of the disease. Rarely, these will include the heart (subendocardial infiltrates), bowel, eye, mucous membranes such as vagina or vulva, and dura mater.

Isolated bony lesions are best treated by curettage and local radiotherapy. Multiple bony involvement and visceral involvement often respond well to prednisone, vinblastine (Velban), mechlorethamine (Mustargen), or methotrexate. The current treatment of choice at the authors' institution is prednisone and vinblastine, given in repeated courses or continuously until healing of lesions occurs.

If diabetes insipidus occurs, treatment with vasopressin (Pitressin) gives good control (see Chapter 24).

In idiopathic histiocytosis, the prognosis is often unpredictable. Many patients with considerable bony and visceral involvement have shown apparent complete recovery. In general, however, the younger the patient and the more extensive the visceral involvement, the worse the prognosis.

Braunstein GD & others: Cerebellar dysfunction in Hand-Schüller-Christian disease. Arch Intern Med 132:387, 1973.

Cline MJ, Golde DW: A review and reevaluation of the histiocytic disorders. Am J Med 55:49, 1973.

Zinkham WH: Multifocal eosinophilic granuloma. Natural history, etiology, and management. Am J Med 60:457, 1976.

● ● ●

General References

Berry CL & others: Clinico-pathologic study of thymic dysplasia. Arch Dis Child 43:579, 1968.

Biggs R: *Human Blood Coagulation, Haemostasis and Thrombosis,* 2nd ed. Blackwell, 1976.

Bostrom PD & others: Splenectomy: An 11-year review. Arch Surg 98:167, 1969.

Diamond LK: The concept of functional asplenia. N Engl J Med 281:958, 1969.

Good RA, Gabrielsen AE (editors): *The Thymus in Immunobiology.* Hoeber, 1964.

Kretschmer R & others: Congenital aplasia of the thymus gland (Di George's syndrome). N Engl J Med 279:1295, 1968.

Levin JM: The thymus gland and immunity. Am Surg 35:317, 1969.

Mauer A: *Pediatric Hematology.* McGraw-Hill, 1969.

Mollison PL: *Blood Transfusion in Clinical Medicine,* 5th ed. Blackwell, 1972.

Nathan DG, Oski FA: *Hematology of Infancy and Childhood.* Saunders, 1974.

Oski FA, Naiman JL: *Hematologic Problems of the Newborn,* 2nd ed. Saunders, 1972.

Schwartz E: Therapy for blood disorders in infants and children. Pediatr Clin North Am 15:473, 1968.

Shields TW: The thymus gland. Surg Clin North Am 49:61, 1969.

Smith CH: *Blood Diseases of Infancy & Childhood,* 3rd ed. Mosby, 1972.

Stiehm ER, Fulginiti VA: *Immunologic Disorders in Infants and Children.* Saunders, 1973.

Wintrobe MM & others: *Clinical Hematology,* 7th ed. Lea & Febiger, 1974.

Wolman I: *Laboratory Applications in Clinical Pediatrics.* Blakiston, 1957.

15...
Disorders of Immune Mechanisms

Richard B. Johnston, Jr, MD, & Charles S. August, MD

INTRODUCTION

Resistance to infection is a complex phenomenon that depends upon a variety of factors, both nonspecific and specific.

NONSPECIFIC FACTORS IN RESISTANCE TO INFECTIONS

Skin & Mucous Membranes

The barrier function provided by intact skin and normal mucous membranes is one of the most important and obvious nonspecific factors in bodily defenses against infection. This function may be compromised in patients with eczema, burns, or cystic fibrosis. In this respect, inhaling irritating substances such as tobacco smoke or other environmental pollutants probably constitutes the most widespread insult to defenses against respiratory infection to which most individuals are exposed.

Phagocytes

Another important defense mechanism against infection resides in the ability of fixed and circulating phagocytic cells to clear the blood stream of infectious agents and to kill them. In addition, some phagocytes may "process" antigens and then deliver them to the lymphoid system to initiate specific immune responses. Patients with granulocytopenia, neutrophil dysfunctions, absent spleens, or "functional asplenia" (as occurs in sickle cell anemia) have diminished phagocytic function, and all are unduly susceptible to infection.

Lysozyme, Complement, & Interferon

The role played by serum lysozyme in resistance to infection is poorly understood. The complement system of serum proteins acts together with specific antibodies to enhance the phagocytosis or killing of certain microorganisms, and this appears now to be its best defined function in the body economy. Interferons—antiviral proteins which are synthesized by almost all virus-infected cells—are thought to play a critical role in the recovery of an organism from a primary viral infection.

Feigin RD, Shearer WT: Opportunistic infection in children. (2 parts.) J Pediatr 87:507, 677, 1975.

Johnston RB & others: Increased susceptibility to infection in sickle cell disease: Defects of opsonization and of splenic function. In: *Immunodeficiency in Man and Animals.* Bergsma D (editor). Birth Defects 11(1), 1975.

Lamm ME, Stetson GA: Inflammation. Page 139 in: *Clinical Immunobiology.* Vol 1. Bach FH, Good RA (editors). Academic Press, 1972.

Quie PG: Pathology of bactericidal power of neutrophils. Semin Hematol 12:143, 1975.

SPECIFIC FACTORS IN RESISTANCE TO INFECTION

Specific immunity is mediated by lymphoid cells: by plasma cells, which synthesize antibodies; and by a number of different types of lymphocytes which mediate antigen recognition, cellular immunity (delayed hypersensitivity), and immunologic memory. Both types of cells originate from stem cell precursors found in the bone marrow. Evidence suggests that such stem cells differentiate to form at least 2 major cell lines: T cells, that differentiate in the thymus; and B cells, that differentiate independently of the thymus.

Upon exposure to antigen, B lymphocytes proliferate and differentiate into plasma cells, which synthesize antibody, and into long-lived *memory cells.*

T lymphocytes perform a number of different functions. Following interaction with antigens, they divide to form an expanded population of specifically reactive cells. Some of these become cytotoxic for appropriate target cells, eg, the *killer (K) cells* involved in graft rejection. Some T lymphocytes interact and cooperate with B cells during the immune responses to certain antigens. Others may suppress or in some way regulate the proliferation and synthetic activities of both B cells and other T cells. Some T cells will become a long-lived population of memory cells.

T lymphocytes also synthesize and release a

number of soluble factors, called *lymphokines,* which serve a number of functions. These may attract, inhibit the migration of, and activate macrophages; increase vascular permeability; cause other lymphocytes to divide; or kill other cells nonspecifically.

The sequence of events that occurs when an antigen—eg, in the form of a bacterium—encounters the normal lymphoid apparatus is illustrated in Fig 15—1. This encounter establishes a population of plasma cells synthesizing specific antibody, a population of small lymphocytes capable of mediating specific delayed hypersensitivity reactions, a population of long-lived lymphocytes (so-called "memory cells") capable of responding to future challenges with the same antigen, and a population of lymphocytes capable of suppressing or regulating the immune reaction.

Since immunologic deficiency diseases may involve defects in humoral or cellular immune mechanisms (or both), it is well to consider these primary mechanisms in greater detail. Immunoglobulins are a family of structurally and functionally related glycoprotein molecules with antibody activity composed of 2 types of polypeptide chains, H (heavy) and L (light) chains according to their molecular weights. The L chains are of 2 varieties—kappa (κ) and lambda (λ)—and are the same in all immunoglobulin molecules. The H chains have regions that are distinctive for each of the immunoglobulin classes. These differences in amino acid sequences are responsible for the distinctive antigenic, physicochemical, and biologic properties of the 5 known members of the immunoglobulin family.

The immunoglobulins recognized to date are IgG, IgA, IgM, IgD, and IgE. Some properties of the immunoglobulins are shown in Table 15—1.

Cellular immunity or delayed hypersensitivity is mediated by T lymphocytes. Histologically, the reactions characteristic of cellular immunity involve infiltration of tissues by lymphocytes and macrophages as well as varying degrees of necrosis. The tuberculin reaction is the prototype of delayed hypersensitivity, and contact dermatitis is a familiar example of disease mediated by this immune mechanism. Cellular immunity is also thought to be the principal factor in allograft rejection and in graft-versus-host reactions. Ultimate containment of certain viral infections such as herpes simplex, vaccinia, varicella, and measles is thought to be mediated by a cellular immunity mechanism. The granulomatous tissue reactions to fungi and other intracellular organisms are also thought to represent cellular immune reactions.

Another population of lymphocytes exists that is capable of killing target cells coated with IgG antibody. This phenomenon is known as *antibody dependent cytotoxicity* and is mediated by lymphoid cells called killer or K cells. The role of this cytotoxic mechanism in host resistance to infection has not yet been defined.

Marchalonis JJ: Cell cooperation in immune responses. Chapter 8, pp 88—96, in: *Basic & Clinical Immunology.* Fudenberg HH & others (editors). Lange, 1976.

Rocklin RE: Products of activated lymphocytes. In: *Clinical*

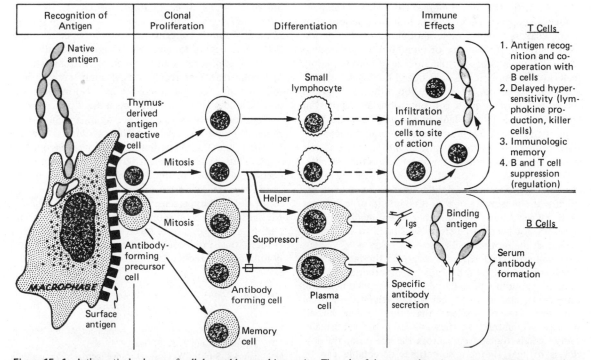

Figure 15—1. A theoretical scheme of cellular and humoral immunity. The role of the macrophage in processing antigen is not clear. (Modified and reproduced, with permission, from Meyers FH, Jawetz E, Goldfien A: *Review of Medical Pharmacology,* 5th ed. Lange, 1976.)

Table 15—1. Properties of immunoglobulins.

	IgG (γG)	IgA (γA)	IgM (γM)	IgD (γD)	IgE (γE)
Molecular weight	150,000	$(180,000)_n$	900,000	150,000	200,000
Percentage in serum	80	12	7	0.2	0.0016
Serum level (mg/ml)	12	1.8	1.0	0.03	0.00033
Half-life (days)	25	6	5	2.8	. . .
Distribution	ECF	ECF, especially secretions	Blood	. . .	ECF and fixed to target cells
Toxin neutralization	Yes	Yes	No	. . .	. . .
Bactericidal antibody activity	1	. . .	500–1000	. . .	. . .
Placental transfer	Yes	No	No	No	No
Pathologic model	IgG myeloma	IgA myeloma	IgM myeloma	IgD myeloma	IgE myeloma
Subclasses	G1, G2, G3, G4	A_1 A_2	. . .	. . .	. . .
Complement fixation	Yes	No	Yes	No	No

Immunology. Vol 3. Bach FH, Good RA (editors). Academic Press, 1976.

Wang AC: The structure of immunoglobulins. Chapter 2, pp 15–31, in: *Basic & Clinical Immunology.* Fudenberg HH & others (editors). Lange, 1976.

IMMUNITY IN THE FETUS & NEWBORN

At birth, the fetus emerges from an environment which, if normal, has protected him from serious antigenic challenge. This low level of antigenic stimulation is reflected in the paucity of lymphoid tissue throughout the body and in a virtual absence of mature plasma cells in the lymph nodes, spleen, and bone marrow.

In the serum of the newborn human, IgG is present in normal adult concentrations and is derived from the mother. IgA, IgM, IgD, and IgE are undetectable if the placenta is intact, since these immunoglobulins do not possess the specific structural sites on their heavy chains required for transport across the placenta. IgM antibodies are usually absent in the neonatal period. The absence of IgE antibodies or *reagins* explains the observation that the infant of a mother with ragweed hay fever or other reagin-mediated allergy does not become passively sensitized to substances to which the mother is allergic.

Maternal IgG antibody protects the fetus during the early months of life against diphtheria, tetanus, measles, poliomyelitis, herpes simplex, pneumococcal infections, and group A beta-hemolytic streptococcal infections to the extent that the mother herself possesses immunity to these diseases. Since normally only IgG is transported across the placenta, the low levels of IgM that are sometimes detectable can be assumed to be of fetal origin. In fact, the fetus begins to produce immunoglobulins between the second and fourth months of gestation. In congenital syphilis, toxoplasmosis, rubella, herpes simplex, and cytomegalovirus infections, cord blood and serum IgM levels are increased. Therefore, IgM levels in cord blood and shortly after birth can be used to diagnose prenatal infections. However, in most cases of infection in the neonatal period, signs of illness precede IgM elevation by several days. Thus, measurement of IgM is not as useful for diagnosing perinatal infections as it has proved to be in diagnosing intrauterine infections.

Colostrum, which contains lymphocytes, macrophages, and antibodies primarily of the IgA class, provides protection against enteric pathogens.

As maternally acquired IgG globulin (with a half-life of 25 days) is catabolized, the IgG levels in the infant fall to a nadir at about 2–3 months of age. Immunoglobulin concentrations then begin to rise as the infant begins to synthesize immunoglobulins as a result of exposure to environmental antigenic stimuli. IgM concentrations reach normal adult levels earliest, followed by IgG and then by IgA. Normal children may have low IgA concentrations until adolescence.

Although lymphocytes are abundant in the peripheral blood of newborn infants (normal mean = 5000/cu mm), cell-mediated immune reactivity is weak. Thus, newborns reject skin grafts less vigorously, become sensitized to simple chemicals such as dinitrofluorobenzene less readily, and undergo passive transfer of delayed hypersensitivity less frequently than do adults. It has been speculated that nonspecific inflammatory responses are reduced in newborn infants or perhaps that production of lymphokines by newborn lymphocytes is reduced.

Campbell AC & others: Lymphocyte subpopulations in the blood of newborn infants. Clin Exp Immunol 18:469, 1974.

Cooper MD, Lawton AR: The development of the immune system. Sci Am 230:58, Dec 1974.

Goldman AS, Smith CW: Host resistance factors in human milk. J Pediatr 82:1082, 1973.

Miller ME: Host defenses in the human neonate. Pediatr Clin

North Am 24:413, 1977.

Remington JS, Klein JO: *Infectious Diseases of the Fetus and Newborn Infant.* Saunders, 1976.

LABORATORY DIAGNOSIS OF IMMUNOLOGIC DEFICIENCY

The laboratory diagnostic approach to a suspected immunologic deficiency state includes the following procedures, most of which are well within the scope of the average hospital laboratory. (See Chapter 38.) A special list of screening procedures is given in Table 15—2.

QUANTITATIVE DETERMINATION OF IMMUNOGLOBULINS & COMPLEMENT COMPONENTS

Quantification of each of the major immunoglobulins is now a standard laboratory procedure. Kits are available from a number of manufacturers for measuring immunoglobulins by the radial diffusion method and are sufficiently reliable for clinical use. Because of the wide range of normal values at different ages (Table 15—3), a diagnosis of immunologic deficiency should not be made on the basis of insignificant deviations from the mean. Similarly, kits for estimating the concentration of the third and fourth components of complement (β_1C-globulin, β_1E-globulin) by radial diffusion are also available.

Table 15—2. Initial screening evaluation for immunodeficiency states.

Defects of phagocyte function
  White blood count and differential count (neutropenia)
  Peripheral blood smear (hyposplenia)
  Inflammatory skin window (chemotaxis defect)
  Nitroblue tetrazolium (NBT) test (chronic granulomatous disease)
Antibody deficiency
  Quantitative levels of IgM, IgG, IgA
  Isohemagglutinins, antibodies to viral and bacterial vaccine materials
  Schick test
Complement deficiency
  Hemolytic complement titer (any component deficiency)
  β_{1C} level (C3 deficiency)
Defects of cell-mediated immunity
  White blood count and differential count (lymphopenia)
  Delayed hypersensitivity skin tests
  X-ray for thymus shadow

ISOHEMAGGLUTININ DETERMINATION

Isohemagglutinins are antibodies that react with the blood group antigens A, B, M, N, P, Lewis, and Wright. These blood group substances occur widely in nature, and an individual becomes immunized presumably as a result of exposure to these antigens as they are represented on intestinal bacteria following colonization after birth. Because these antigenic determinants are common to both bacterial and red cell membranes, these antibodies agglutinate the appropriate red blood cells. Isohemagglutinin activity may be detected in cord blood but is usually maternal IgG.

There is a variable period following birth before the infant begins to produce isohemagglutinins. Therefore, during the first 2 years of life, normal infants may not have detectable isohemagglutinin activity. By the end of the second year, most normal infants have demonstrable isohemagglutinin activity in their serum (Table 15—3). These "naturally occurring" isohemagglutinins are primarily IgM but may also be IgG or IgA. Because isohemagglutinins are invariably present in all normal individuals of blood types A, B, or O after the first few years of life, their absence is strong presumptive evidence of an antibody deficiency disorder.

RESPONSE TO IMMUNIZATION

Since failure to marshal an immune response to an antigenic stimulus is characteristic of the hypogammaglobulinemic state, antibody titers should be determined before and after immunization with good immunogens. Immunizing agents used for this purpose should be of potential benefit to the patient. For this reason, only toxoids and vaccines used in conventional immunization regimens should be given. Some that have been successfully used for this purpose include diphtheria toxoid, tetanus toxoid, typhoid vaccine, and influenza vaccine. Determinations of the levels of these antibodies may be obtained from State Health Department laboratories and from the Center for Disease Control, Atlanta 30333. Administration of live viruses should be avoided in patients suspected of having immunologic deficiency disorders, since even attenuated viruses may cause prolonged and severe disease. While low titers of antibody to diphtheria, tetanus, and viral agents are commonly found in the serum of patients with immunologic deficiency disease, immunologically deficient children differ markedly from normals in response to immunization. The normal individual may show a 10-fold greater anamnestic response. The hypogammaglobulinemic individual, on the other hand, even after intensive immunization, will rarely show more than a doubling in titer and usually shows none at all.

Table 15—3. Relation of age to serum immunoglobulin (Ig) levels and isohemagglutinin activity (IHA).

	IgG (mg/100 ml) (Mean ± 1 SD and Range)	IgA (mg/100 ml) (Mean ± 1 SD and Range)	IgM (mg/100 ml) (Mean ± 1 SD and Range)	IHA Titer (Mean and Range)
Cord blood	1086 ± 290 (740–1374)	2 ± 2 (0–15)	14 ± 6 (0–22)	0*
1–3 months	512 ± 152 (280–950)	16 ± 10 (4–36)	28 ± 14 (15–86)	1:5 0–1:10†
4–6 months	520 ± 180 (240–884)	22 ± 14 (11–52)	36 ± 18 (21–74)	1:10 0–1:160†
7–12 months	742 ± 226 (281–1280)	54 ± 17 (22–112)	76 ± 27 (36–150)	1:80 0–1:640‡
13–24 months	945 ± 270 (290–1300)	67 ± 19 (9–143)	88 ± 36 (18–210)	1:80 0–1:640‡
25–36 months	1030 ± 152 (546–1562)	89 ± 34 (21–196)	94 ± 23 (43–115)	1:160 1:10–1:640§
3–5 years	1150 ± 244 (546–1760)	126 ± 31 (56–284)	87 ± 24 (26–121)	1:80 1:5–1:640
6–8 years	1187 ± 289 (596–1744)	147 ± 35 (56–330)	108 ± 37 (54–260)	1:80 1:5–1:640
9–11 years	1217 ± 261 (744–1719)	146 ± 38 (44–208)	104 ± 46 (27–215)	1:160 1:20–1:640
12–16 years	1248 ± 221 (796–1647)	168 ± 54 (64–290)	96 ± 31 (60–140)	1:160 1:10–1:320

*IHA is rarely detectable in cord blood.
†50% of normal infants have no isohemagglutinins at age 6 months.
‡10% of normal infants have no isohemagglutinins at age 1.
§Beyond age 2, all normal individuals (except those with blood type AB) have isohemagglutinins.

BONE MARROW EXAMINATION FOR PLASMA CELLS

The bone marrow is the most accessible tissue in which to look for the cells which synthesize immunoglobulins. Unfortunately, for developmental reasons, normal children may have very few mature plasma cells in the marrow for the first 2 years of life. After age 2, increasing numbers of plasma cells are seen.

If a bone marrow biopsy can be obtained, special attention should be paid to the areas around arterioles, which normally are especially rich in plasma cells. Their absence from this location is quite striking in individuals with immunologic deficiency.

LYMPH NODE BIOPSY

Biopsy of a lymph node draining the site of antigen administration can be a useful adjunct to the diagnosis of immunologic deficiency syndromes. Antigen is usually administered intramuscularly into the anterior thigh. Typhoid vaccine or DT toxoids, in the usual clinical doses and as used above to study antibody response, work well. Five to 7 days later, the ipsilateral inguinal node is removed. Cortical germinal centers and plasma cells are the morphologic counterpart of the immunoglobulin synthesizing system. The small lymphocytes of the deep cortex (paracortex) are the morphologic counterpart of the thymus-dependent cellular immunity mediating system. Deficiency of either immunologic function will usually be reflected by an abnormality in the appropriate portion of the lymph node.

EVALUATION OF DELAYED HYPERSENSITIVITY

Evaluation of the adequacy of cellular immunity or delayed hypersensitivity is considerably more difficult than evaluation of humoral immunity. This is due in part to incomplete understanding of the factors governing cellular immunity. The following tests are used both clinically and investigatively.

Skin Tests

Skin test reagents to detect evidence of delayed hypersensitivity to bacterial, viral, and fungal agents with which the patient has had natural contact include tuberculin, histoplasmin, coccidioidin, candida, mumps, vaccinia, and the group A beta-hemolytic streptococcal enzymes streptokinase and streptodornase.

For skin testing, the following materials may be

injected intradermally:

(1) Tuberculin, 0.1 ml of a 1:10,000 dilution. If negative, repeat at 1:1000. Alternatively, intermediate strength PPD may be injected in the same volume.

(2) Candida, 0.1 ml of 1:10 dilution of stock antigen (infants) or 1:1000 dilution (older children and adults).

(3) Trichophytin, as for candida.

(4) Streptococcal antigens (streptokinase-streptodornase), 0.1 ml at a concentration of 5 units of streptokinase per 0.1 ml. If negative, repeat, using 40 units/0.1 ml.

(5) Mumps antigen, 0.1 ml.

Reactions should be read immediately to assess IgE hypersensitivity, at 4 hours to assess any Arthus reactions, and at 24 and 48 hours for delayed hypersensitivity. The diameter of redness and induration should be recorded. Only reactions with induration greater than 5 mm in diameter are unequivocally positive.

While a positive delayed hypersensitivity type skin response is consistent with normal cellular immunity, a negative response may indicate only that the patient has had an inadequate sensitizing exposure to the infectious agent from which the skin test material was derived. This is especially true in infants and young children, who because of age have had little opportunity to encounter infectious agents and their products and develop delayed hypersensitivity. For this reason, certain simple chemicals which have the propensity to sensitize human skin have been used to induce delayed hypersensitivity. The agent most commonly used for this purpose is dinitrochlorobenzene (DNCB). Apply 0.05 ml of a 30% solution of DNCB in acetone (10% for infants) to the volar surface of the forearm in a ring 1 cm in diameter. Two to 3 weeks later, 0.05 ml of the sensitizing agent is reapplied in lower concentration, usually 0.1% or 0.05%. An erythematous indurated or vesicular reaction appearing at the site of the challenging dose is interpreted to mean that delayed hypersensitivity has been successfully induced and is used as presumptive evidence of normal cellular immunity. Since DNCB is a primary irritant, caution must be exercised in interpreting the results of the challenge in order to be certain that the reaction is truly one of delayed hypersensitivity and not an irritant reaction. This caution is especially pertinent in dealing with infants and small children, whose skin may react in a primary irritant manner to the low concentrations ordinarily used for challenging older children and adults.

Evaluation of Lymphocytes & Lymphocyte Function

It is now possible to determine both the numbers and functions of both B and T lymphocytes. Total lymphocytes may be counted in routine hematology laboratories and the number of small lymphocytes calculated. Most children, including newborns, have 5000–6000 lymphocytes per cu mm. Any child with fewer than 3000 lymphocytes per cu mm is suspect, and a child with fewer than 1000 lymphocytes per cu mm is definitely lymphopenic. The normal ranges for absolute lymphocyte counts in children of varying ages are given in Table 38–3.

T lymphocytes can be counted because of their unique property of binding to and forming "rosettes" with sheep erythrocytes. B lymphocytes, which possess surface-bound immunoglobulins as well as receptors for the third component of complement, can be counted by fluorescent antibody or rosetting technics. A small number of cells, called *null cells,* appear to lack both types of surface markers. While these assays are not widely available in most routine hospital laboratories, clinical immunology laboratories now commonly perform them. Normal values for B and T lymphocytes for children of varying ages are given in Table 15–4. However, because the values can vary in different laboratories, it is important to investigate any patient simultaneously with a normal control and to compare results to normal values obtained in the laboratory performing the tests.

Lymphocyte replication on exposure to the plant mitogens phytohemagglutinin (PHA), concanavalin A (ConA), or pokeweed mitogen (PWM) can be tested. PHA and ConA are chiefly mitogenic for T lymphocytes and PWM for T and B lymphocytes. Antigens to which the patient has been sensitized, eg, PPD, candida, streptokinase-streptodornase, or allogeneic leukocytes (mixed lymphocyte culture), also cause blast transformation and DNA synthesis. These responses are most accurately assessed by methods that measure lymphocyte incorporation of an isotopic precursor of DNA. Morphologic evaluation of the transformation of small lymphocytes into blasts and mitotic figures may also serve to evaluate these responses.

Aiuti F & others: Identification, enumeration and isolation of B and T lymphocytes from human peripheral blood. Clin Immunol Immunopathol 3:384, 1975.

Bellanti JA: *Immunology,* 2nd ed. Saunders, 1977.

Table 15–4. T and B lymphocytes in children and adults.*

	Percent		Absolute No. (per cu mm)	
	Mean	95% Range	Mean	95% Range
T lymphocytes				
1 week to 2 years	50	33–67	2970	1620–4320
2–10 years	57	45–69	1840	590–3090
Adults	64	51–78	1910	750–3070
B lymphocytes				
1 week to 2 years	26	14–39	1530	470–2590
2–10 years	23	16–29	720	170–1270
Adults	17	11–23	540	170–910

*Adapted, with permission, from Fleischer TA & others: Lymphocyte subpopulations (T and B) in children. Pediatrics 55: 162, 1975.

Johnston RB & others: Disorders of host defense against infection. Med Clin North Am 57:421, 1973.

IMMUNOLOGIC
DEFICIENCY DISORDERS

Immunologic deficiency disorders are characterized by increased susceptibility to bacterial infection and, in certain forms, to progressive fungal and viral disease.

Children with these disorders are subject to recurrent bacterial pneumonia, meningitis, sepsis, osteomyelitis, pyoderma, progressive vaccinia, and chronic candidal infections. Chronic otitis media, sinusitis, and bronchiectasis are frequently seen. Only very rarely does the child with recurrent "colds" turn out to have an immunologic deficiency disease definable by current diagnostic technics. An increased incidence of gastrointestinal dysfunction has been recognized, and various hematologic abnormalities, including an increased incidence of lymphoreticular malignancy, are known to occur in certain forms of the disease.

It is now apparent that the immunologic deficiency syndromes include a broad spectrum of entities with enormous variability in clinical and immunologic expression. The best defined of these syndromes are listed in Table 15–5. The nomenclature conforms to WHO recommendations. Because most of them are rare, only the more common forms will be described.

TRANSIENT HYPOGAMMAGLOBULINEMIA OF INFANCY

Essentials of Diagnosis

- Recurrent infections of skin, lungs, upper respiratory tract, or meninges, usually with pyogenic bacteria.
- Markedly diminished levels of serum IgG, IgA, and IgM.
- Normal cellular immunity.
- Lymph node biopsy which reveals absence of mature plasma cells but presence of "plasmacytoid lymphocytes."

General Considerations

Transient hypogammaglobulinemia is a syndrome which occurs in infants in whom there is a prolongation of the low levels of circulating immunoglobulins that normally occur during the first 4–8 weeks of life. If an infant fails to begin synthesizing immunoglobulins, the normal catabolism of maternal gamma globulins results in a continuing decline of the infant's immunoglobulin levels. When the level of the infant's

Table 15–5. Classification of immunodeficiency disorders.*

Antibody (B cell) immunodeficiency diseases
  X-linked hypogammaglobulinemia (congenital hypogammaglobulinemia)†
  Transient hypogammaglobulinemia of infancy†
  Common, variable, unclassifiable immunodeficiency† (acquired hypogammaglobulinemia)
  X-linked immunodeficiency with hyper-IgM
  Selective IgA deficiency
  Selective IgM deficiency
  Selective deficiency of IgG subclasses

Cellular (T cell) immunodeficiency diseases
  Congenital thymic hypoplasia (DiGeorge syndrome)†
  Chronic mucocutaneous candidiasis (with or without endocrinopathy)

Combined antibody-mediated (B cell) and cell-mediated (T cell) immunodeficiency diseases
  Severe combined immunodeficiency diseases (autosomal recessive, X-linked, sporadic)†
  Cellular immunodeficiency with abnormal immunoglobulin synthesis (Nezelof's syndrome)†
  Immunodeficiency with ataxia-telangiectasia
  Immunodeficiency with eczema and thrombocytopenia (Wiskott-Aldrich syndrome)
  Immunodeficiency with thymoma
  Immunodeficiency with short-limbed dwarfism
  Immunodeficiency with enzyme deficiency
  Episodic lymphocytopenia with lymphotoxin
  Graft-versus-host disease

*Modified and reproduced, with permission, from Ammann AJ, Fudenberg HH: Immunodeficiency diseases. In: *Basic & Clinical Immunology.* Fudenberg HH & others (editors). Lange, 1976.
†Discussed in the text that follows.

passively acquired antibody declines below those that normally protect against pyogenic bacteria and viruses, severe infections begin to appear. These infants usually begin to recover spontaneously between the ages of 9 and 15 months.

Clinical Findings

A. Symptoms and Signs: Physical signs are related to recurrent infections and the organ systems which may be involved. This particular antibody deficiency syndrome is frequently associated with episodes of bronchitis and wheezing.

B. Laboratory Findings: The principal sign is depressed serum IgG and absence of serum IgA and IgM beyond the time when these immunoglobulins normally begin to appear. This varies, of course, with the particular immunoglobulin involved, and Table 15–3 should be consulted in specific instances. Stimulation with specific antigens—eg, diphtheria and tetanus—reveals absent or markedly diminished and delayed responses. Biopsy of the regional lymph nodes carried out 4–7 days after injection of the antigen reveals absence of well formed germinal centers and plasma cells. However, plasmacytoid lymphocytes may be present which help distinguish this condition from infantile X-linked hypogammaglobulinemia.

Other laboratory findings include normal numbers of circulating small lymphocytes and normal responses of lymphocytes to stimulation in vitro with the mitogen phytohemagglutinin. Cellular immunity mechanisms are normal, as evidenced by positive skin reactions to intradermal injections of candida or streptokinase-streptodornase and normal ability to become sensitized by dinitrochlorobenzene.

Differential Diagnosis

Differential diagnosis includes virtually all the immunologic deficiency syndromes, which may be excluded by finding (1) normal cellular immune mechanisms, (2) the lymph node biopsy finding as outlined above, and (3) gradual appearance of immunoglobulins.

Treatment

The most effective treatment is a combination of vigorous specific antimicrobial therapy with monthly injections of gamma globulin (see next section).

Prognosis

The infant usually recovers from recurrent infections as he begins to achieve normal immunoglobulin levels. These children probably account for at least some of the instances in which babies with recurrent infections respond to the administration of gamma globulin and later appear to "outgrow" both their infections and the need for therapy.

Ammann AJ, Fudenberg HH: Immunodeficiency diseases. Chapter 26, pp 333–359, in: *Basic & Clinical Immunology.* Fudenberg HH & others (editors). Lange, 1976.

X-LINKED HYPOGAMMAGLOBULINEMIA
(Congenital Hypogammaglobulinemia)

Essentials of Diagnosis

- Undue susceptibility to recurrent infections with pyogenic organisms.
- Little or no difficulty with measles, chickenpox, or vaccination.
- Paucity of lymphoid tissues, particularly the tonsils.
- Profound deficiencies of all the major classes of immunoglobulins.
- Absence of cortical germinal centers and plasma cells in lymph node biopsies.

General Considerations

This disease characteristically occurs in male infants and is thought to have an X-linked pattern of inheritance. Undue susceptibility to infection usually becomes evident during the second year of life as these children contract infections with staphylococci, pneumococci, streptococci, and *Haemophilus influenzae.* Purulent sinusitis, pneumonia, sepsis, otitis, meningitis, and furunculosis are common and must be treated vigorously with specific antimicrobial agents or recurrent progressive infections will ensue. "Allergic" manifestations occur sometimes in a number of children, and some develop a condition similar to rheumatoid arthritis before the diagnosis is established. This puzzling complication usually disappears with treatment.

Clinical Findings

A. Symptoms and Signs: The symptoms and signs of X-linked hypogammaglobulinemia are those of infection and inflammation in the affected organ systems. In addition, there is an extreme paucity of lymphoid tissue. Tonsils may be absent altogether, and lateral x-rays of the nasopharynx reveal absence of adenoid tissue (Neuhauser's sign).

B. Laboratory Findings: There is marked diminution of all classes of serum immunoglobulins. The serum contains less than 200 mg of IgG per 100 ml, and serum IgA and IgM levels are usually undetectable. In addition, a failure to synthesize specific antibody may easily be demonstrated by finding absent or markedly low levels of the isohemagglutinins. A positive Schick test in the presence of a history of DTP immunization is also found. Lymphocyte counts are normal, and cellular immunity mechanisms are intact. B lymphocytes are characteristically absent. Lymph node biopsy 4–7 days after antigenic stimulation shows absence of cortical germinal center formation and plasma cells.

Differential Diagnosis

Marked diminution or absence of all classes of immunoglobulins distinguishes this disease from the selected immunoglobulin deficiencies, in which there is a disproportion between the levels of immunoglobulins. The establishment of normal cellular immunity mechanisms serves to distinguish congenital hypogammaglobulinemia from the immunologic deficiency syndromes relating to abnormalities of the thymus gland. The histology of the lymph nodes and persistence of the syndrome beyond the second year of life distinguish this from transient hypogammaglobulinemia.

Treatment

These children usually respond well to therapy with gamma globulin, available as a 16.5% solution from the American Red Cross. It is given IM in a loading dose of about 1.6 ml/kg of body weight followed by monthly injections of 0.6–0.8 ml/kg. If the amounts to be injected seem excessive, they may be given in divided doses biweekly or even weekly.

It should be remembered that available gamma globulin preparations consist largely of IgG. Even if preparations rich in IgM or IgA were available, their short biologic half-lives would require administration every 5–6 days.

At this time, gamma globulin cannot be administered intravenously because of the likelihood of producing a severe systemic reaction. Furthermore, even when given by the intramuscular route, gamma globulin administration may not be an entirely innocuous procedure. For this reason, it should only be given to children with proved deficiency of IgG and impaired ability to make specific antibody. Its indiscriminate use is to be condemned.

In selected patients, antibiotic therapy given on a continuous basis seems to be a useful adjunct.

Prognosis

The prognosis for many children with hypogammaglobulinemia, if diagnosed early and treated adequately, is quite good. However, some of these patients appear to be unusually susceptible to arthritis, leukemia, and a uniformly fatal syndrome resembling dermatomyositis.

Bruton OC: The discovery of agammaglobulinemia. In: *Immunologic Deficiency Diseases in Man.* Bergsma D (editor). Birth Defects 4(1), 1968.

Goldman AS, Goldblum RM: Primary deficiencies in humoral immunity. Pediatr Clin North Am 24:277, 1977.

Janeway CA & others: *The Gamma Globulins.* Little, Brown, 1967.

SELECTIVE IMMUNOGLOBULIN DEFICIENCY

The ability to measure quantitatively each immunoglobulin class has permitted a more precise definition of situations in which the immunoglobulin deficiency involves only one or 2 of the immunoglobulin classes, with the remainder being either normal or elevated. Patients with these disorders may have recurrent infections similar to those suffered by patients with more complete forms of the syndrome. Some have associated abnormalities of cellular immunity, and for this reason a unified description of all the syndromes is difficult. Patients with these disorders should be investigated thoroughly in all aspects of their immunologic responses, and a thorough search for underlying disease such as infection, neoplasm, or collagen disease should be made. If the immunoglobulin deficiency involves the IgG fraction, gamma globulin injections may prove therapeutically beneficial.

Ammann AJ, Hong R: Selective IgA deficiency and autoimmunity. Clin Exp Immunol 7:833, 1970.

Buckley RH: Plasma therapy in immunodeficiency diseases. Am J Dis Child 124:376, 1972.

Janeway CA & others: *The Gamma Globulins.* Little, Brown, 1967.

Schur PH & others: Gamma-G globulin deficiencies and recurrent pyogenic infections. N Engl J Med 283:631, 1970.

THYMIC HYPOPLASIA
(Pharyngeal Pouch Syndrome, DiGeorge's Syndrome)

In 1965, DiGeorge described a group of patients with congenital absence of the thymus and parathyroid glands. These patients had hypocalcemic tetany in the neonatal period and then suffered recurrent pyogenic infections. In addition, some had abnormalities of the face, palate, and ears and right-sided aortic arches.

These patients lack cellular immunity mechanisms but retain the ability to synthesize humoral antibodies. They have low normal absolute lymphocyte counts in their peripheral blood and normal levels of serum immunoglobulins. Circulating T lymphocytes are markedly reduced or absent, and B lymphocytes and null cells constitute virtually 100% of circulating lymphocytes. Plasma thymic hormone levels are very low or absent. Patients do not react with delayed hypersensitivity reactions to any of the common skin test antigens. Furthermore, they are unable to be sensitized by dinitrochlorobenzene, and skin allografts undergo markedly delayed rejections. In vitro, their lymphocytes do not undergo blast cell transformation when stimulated with phytohemagglutinin. A partial or less severe form of the syndrome has been described which is thought to be due to hypoplasia of the thymus gland rather than complete aplasia.

Immunologic function in such patients can be markedly improved by implantation of fetal thymus fragments. Beyond transplantation of fetal lymphoid tissue or the experimental administration of thymic hormone, the treatment of this syndrome is symptomatic. Because most patients hitherto described have either died in infancy or are at this time very young, the natural history and ultimate prognosis remain to be defined.

Cleveland WW: Immunologic reconstitution in the DiGeorge syndrome by fetal thymus transplant. Page 352 in: *Immunodeficiency in Man and Animals.* Bergsma D (editor). Birth Defects 11(1), 1975.

Kretschmer R & others: Congenital aplasia of the thymus gland (DiGeorge's syndrome). N Engl J Med 279:1295, 1968.

Lewis V & others: Circulating thymic hormone activity in congenital immunodeficiency. Lancet 2:471, 1977.

SEVERE COMBINED IMMUNODEFICIENCY
(Thymic Alymphoplasia, Thymic Dysplasia, Swiss Type Agammaglobulinemia)

Essentials of Diagnosis

- Recurrent severe infections with bacteria, viruses, and fungi.
- Chronic skin rashes, diarrhea, and failure to grow.
- Absent immunoglobulins in serum and fail-

- ure to synthesize specific antibody.
- Lymphopenia and absent cellular immunity mechanisms.
- Marked deficiency of thymic shadow on x-ray.
- Marked hypoplasia and disorganization of lymphoid tissue in the thymus, lymph nodes, spleen, nasopharynx, and gastrointestinal tract.

General Considerations

The essential defect in this syndrome is the embryonic failure of the thymus gland to differentiate normally. This appears to be due to absence of the lymphoid stem cell in the bone marrow. Failure of differentiation of both thymus-dependent (T cell) cellular immunity mechanisms and humoral antibody and B cell formation is the result. Patients are lymphopenic and totally lack immunologic competence. It has been found that some of these patients lack adenosine deaminase (ADA) or nucleoside phosphorylase in their red blood cells and lymphocytes. These enzyme deficiencies are transmitted as autosomal recessive traits. Children with ADA deficiency show skeletal changes and thymic involution not found in patients with the "classical" forms of this syndrome.

Clinical Findings

A. Symptoms and Signs: Infants with combined immunodeficiency become ill in the first few months of life. Persistent candida infection beyond the neonatal period may spread to the pharynx and involve the entire gastrointestinal tract. Infants then usually develop diarrhea and bronchopneumonia. They are unusually susceptible to viral infections; measles, giant cell pneumonia, hemorrhagic varicella, and fatal progressive vaccinia are common. With rare exceptions, these infants die of infection before 3 years of age.

Physical findings relate to the signs of infections in the involved organ systems. In addition, there is marked paucity of lymphoid tissue and absence of a thymic shadow on x-ray.

B. Laboratory Findings: Absence of serum IgG, IgA, and IgM is the rule, although some immunoglobulins are occasionally found. Peripheral blood lymphocyte counts are usually below 1000/cu mm. Isohemagglutinins are absent from the peripheral blood, and the Schick test is positive in spite of adequate immunization with DTP. B lymphocytes and T cell rosettes are usually absent. There is no antibody response to any administered antigen. Delayed hypersensitivity reactions are universally absent. Despite chronic candidiasis, patients with this syndrome do not respond to intradermal injections of candida antigen. They cannot be sensitized with simple chemicals such as dinitrochlorobenzene, and skin grafts are accepted indefinitely. Lymphocytes do not respond in vitro to phytohemagglutinin. Lymph node biopsies reveal totally disorganized lymph nodes with absent plasma cells and lymphocytes. At autopsy the thymuses of these patients are found to be tiny epithelial organs containing few, if any, lymphocytes, no corticomedullary differentiation, and no Hassall's corpuscles.

Differential Diagnosis

The differential diagnosis consists of distinguishing this syndrome from thymic hypoplasia (DiGeorge's syndrome) and from X-linked hypogammaglobulinemia. Patients with the former condition lack cellular immunity but are able to synthesize humoral antibodies and have normal levels of serum immunoglobulins. Patients with the latter are unable to synthesize antibodies and have reduced levels of serum immunoglobulins but intact cellular immunity mechanisms. Variants of the thymic dysplasia syndrome exist, and these are usually characterized by the presence in serum of one or all of the immunoglobulins (Nezelof type). In spite of this, it can be demonstrated that antibody synthesis in these patients is not normal, and at autopsy the thymus is identical with that of patients with the complete syndrome.

Treatment

At present the preferred treatment is transplantation of bone marrow from histocompatible donors. Successful establishment of immunologic competence has also been reported following fetal liver cell infusion, fetal thymus grafting with or without combined administration of *transfer factor,* and administration of a thymic extract called *thymosin.* This mode of therapy is experimental, and patients are best referred to treatment centers with such programs.

A high risk of inducing fatal graft-versus-host reactions in these patients with as few viable leukocytes as are contained in a single unit of transfused blood has been documented. All blood products given to these children should be irradiated (1500–3000 R) prior to administration.

Prognosis

Heretofore, all such patients have died, usually before the end of the third year. Successful transplantation of bone marrow has been achieved too recently for long-term prognosis to be accurately determined.

Good RA, Bach FH: Bone marrow and thymus transplants: Cellular engineering to correct primary immunodeficiency. Page 65 in: *Clinical Immunobiology.* Vol 2. Bach FH, Good RA (editors). Saunders, 1974.

Hoyer JR & others: Lymphopenic forms of congenital immunologic deficiency diseases. Medicine 47:201, 1968.

Meuwissen HJ & others: Combined immunodeficiency disease associated with adenosine deaminase deficiency. J Pediatr 86:169, 1975.

COMMON VARIABLE IMMUNODEFICIENCY
(Primary Acquired Hypogammaglobulinemia)

Acquired hypogammaglobulinemia is principally a disease of adults but may occur in older children.

The incidence is equal in males and females. These patients suffer undue susceptibility to pyogenic infection, particularly recurrent sinusitis and pneumonia. Some patients have been found in thoracic clinics with chronic progressive bronchiectasis. More than half of all adults are afflicted with a sprue-like syndrome consisting of diarrhea and steatorrhea. Immunoglobulins in the serum of patients with acquired hypogammaglobulinemia usually reveal levels of IgG under 500 mg/100 ml, somewhat higher than the level in children with congenital disease. However, striking immunoglobulin deficiency may be seen. IgA and IgM may also be present.

Hermans PE, Diaz-Buxo JA, Stobo JD: Idiopathic late-onset immunoglobulin deficiency: Clinical observations in 50 patients. Am J Med 61:221, 1976.

SECONDARY ACQUIRED HYPOGAMMAGLOBULINEMIA

Secondary acquired hypogammaglobulinemia occurs in patients with protein loss due to any cause or inability to synthesize serum proteins normally. Thus, patients with protein-losing enteropathies, exfoliative dermatitis, and the nephrotic syndrome—or, occasionally, severe malnutrition—may have diminished levels of serum immunoglobulins. Defective synthesis of immunoglobulins not uncommonly accompanies lymphoreticular tumors.

OTHER CONDITIONS ASSOCIATED WITH IMMUNOLOGIC DEFICIENCIES

Transient immunosuppression occurs after certain common viral diseases, the best example being measles. This is self-limited, and immunologic mechanisms usually return to normal within a few weeks. It is also clear that patients being treated with corticosteroids or other immunosuppressive agents such as azathioprine (Imuran) or antilymphocyte globulin have impaired cellular immunity mechanisms. Protein-calorie malnutrition is associated with rather specific defects in cell-mediated immunity—often coupled with elevated levels of serum immunoglobulins. Other syndromes in which impaired cellular immunity has been documented include advanced Hodgkin's disease, sarcoidosis, leprosy, Wiscott-Aldrich syndrome (see Chapter 14), ataxia-telangiectasia (see Chapter 21), and short-limbed dwarfism. Patients with protein-losing enteropathy due to intestinal lymphangiectasia have been found to lose small lymphocytes into their gastrointestinal tracts and suffer an impairment of cellular immunity functions as well as hypogammaglobulinemia.

Bergsma D (editor): *Immunodeficiency in Man and Animals.* Birth Defects 11(1), 1975. [Entire issue.]
Waldmann TA: Disorders of immunoglobulin metabolism. N Engl J Med 281:1170, 1969.
Yu DTY & others: Human lymphocyte subpopulations: Effect of corticosteroids. J Clin Invest 53:565, 1974.

●   ●   ●

General References

Bach FH, Good RA (editors): *Clinical Immunobiology.* 3 vols. Academic Press, 1972, 1974, 1976.
Bellanti JA: *Immunology,* 2nd ed. Saunders, 1977.
Bellanti JA, Dayton DH (editors): *The Phagocytic Cell in Host Resistance.* Raven, 1975.
Bergsma D (editor): *Immunodeficiency in Man and Animals.* Birth Defects 11(1), 1975. [Entire issue.]
Bergsma D (editor): *Immunologic Deficiency Diseases in Man.* Birth Defects 4(1), 1968. [Entire issue.]
Ellis EF, Henney CS: Adverse reactions following administration of human gamma globulin. J Allergy 43:45, 1969.
Fudenberg HH & others (editors): *Basic & Clinical Immunology.* Lange, 1976.
Fudenberg HH & others: Primary immunodeficiencies: Report of a World Health Organization committee. Pediatrics 47:927, 1971.

Humbert JR (editor): Neutrophil physiology and pathology. Semin Hematol 12:1, 1975.
Johnston RB, Stroud RM: Complement and host defense against infection. J Pediatr 90:169, 1977.
Medical Research Council Working Party: Hypogammaglobulinaemia in the United Kingdom. Lancet 1:163, 1969.
Merler E (editor): *Immunoglobulins: Biologic Aspects and Clinical Uses.* National Academy of Sciences, 1970.
Miescher P, Müller-Eberhard H (editors): *Textbook of Immunopathology.* Grune & Stratton, 1969.
Miller ME (editor): Symposium on the child with recurrent infection. Pediatr Clin North Am 24:275, 1977. [Entire issue.]
Ruddy S & others: The complement system of man. (3 parts.) N Engl J Med 287:489, 545, 642, 1972.
Stiehm ER, Fulginiti VA (editors): *Immunologic Disorders in Infants and Children.* Saunders, 1973.

16...
Gastrointestinal Tract *

Claude C. Roy, MD & Arnold Silverman, MD

HIATAL HERNIA

Hiatal hernias may be classified as follows:

(1) Paraesophageal hernias, where the esophagus is normal up to the esophageal hiatus but the stomach is herniated into the thorax through the hiatus. Regurgitation is not frequent, since the cardia usually maintains its competency.

(2) Sliding hernia, where the esophagogastric junction is located above the esophageal hiatus, is the most common type seen in children. It leads to regurgitation esophagitis and esophageal strictures because of incompetency of the cardiac sphincter. Inflammatory changes secondary to esophagitis lead to shortening of the esophagus and also to metaplastic changes which account for gastric mucosa lining the lower esophagus.

Clinical Findings

Paraesophageal hernias are rare and present with symptoms of complete esophageal obstruction. Symptoms of the sliding type of hiatal hernia may mimic chalasia. Attention has recently been drawn to the frequent incidence of hiatal hernia in infants with rumination. Dysphagia, failure to thrive, anemia, vomiting, aspiration pneumonia, and neck contortions (Sandifer's syndrome) are common features. Pain occurs when esophagitis is present, and bleeding may occur with hematemesis and melena. Stricture formation gives rise to the vomiting of undigested food. Large hiatal hernias often remain completely asymptomatic. There is an increased incidence of hiatal hernia and gastroesophageal reflux in children suffering from CNS disorders.

During the first few months of life, the cardiac sphincter is often incompetent and reflux can be observed. Continuous free reflux observed by cineradiography is abnormal and is almost always associated with the presence of a pouch of stomach above the diaphragm. Considerable skill and patience are needed to demonstrate small hernias. The severity of symptoms may correlate poorly with the size of the hernia. An experienced pediatric radiologist should be responsible for the cine-esophagogram. Esophagoscopy should be

*Esophageal atresia and tracheo-esophageal fistula are discussed in Chapter 3.

performed when medical measures have failed, particularly if there are x-ray changes of esophagitis and pain.

Complications

Gastroesophageal reflux is a well-known cause of disabling esophageal and respiratory complications. Since many severe recurrent respiratory problems of unexplained origin may be the result of gastroesophageal reflux and aspiration, all children with such problems should have the benefit of an esophagogram.

Treatment

In 80% of patients, conservative management is efficacious. The most important point is semi-upright positioning of the patient day and night, which should be maintained for at least 3 months after all symptoms have ceased. Infants will slip down if just propped with pillows; an infant seat is more effective. Small thickened feedings and mild sedation combined with antacids may also be of value.

Failure of medical management and the presence of strictures are indications for surgical treatment. At the time of hernia repair or of esophageal dilatation, pyloroplasty and vagotomy may be indicated—particularly if there is delayed gastric emptying.

Prognosis

Medical treatment fails in 20% of cases, and surgery becomes necessary.

Darling DB, Fisher JH, Gellis SS: Hiatal hernia and gastroesophageal reflux in infants and children: Analysis of the incidence in North American children. Pediatrics 54:450, 1974.

Randolph JG, Lilly JR, Anderson RD: Surgical treatment of gastroesophageal reflux in infants. Ann Surg 180:479, 1974.

ACHALASIA OF THE ESOPHAGUS

Esophageal achalasia is a lesion which has been associated in adults with the absence or degeneration of ganglion cells in Auerbach's plexus. It is characterized by failure of relaxation of the inferior esophageal sphincter (cardiospasm) and lack of normal peristalsis in the body of the esophagus.

Clinical Findings

A. Symptoms and Signs: Achalasia is occasionally seen in teenage children but is uncommon under the age of 5 years. The history of difficulty in swallowing solid food is intermittent at first and often goes back for many years. Affected children are described as slow eaters, consuming large amounts of fluids while eating. Familial cases have been described. Typically, the dysphagia is manifested by retrosternal pain and frequent episodes of food "sticking" in the throat or upper chest. The dysphagia is relieved by repeated swallowing movements or by vomiting. Besides dysphagia and vomiting, bouts of coughing and wheezing are reported along with recurrent pneumonitis, anemia, and weight loss.

The disease is characterized by failure of relaxation of the inferior esophageal sphincter and by lack of normal peristalsis in the body of the esophagus, leading to megaesophagus.

B. X-Ray and Manometric Studies: The barium swallow shows a grossly dilated esophagus except for a narrowing at the distal end. The narrowed segment is usually very short. Cinefluoroscopic examination may show absence of normal peristalsis and failure of relaxation of the gastroesophageal sphincter.

The esophageal motility pattern confirms the abnormal peristalsis and malfunctioning of the lower esophageal sphincter. The pressure at rest in the lower esophageal sphincter is at least twice normal and does not fall to the level of gastric pressure during swallowing. There are no true peristaltic contractions in the body of the esophagus.

Differential Diagnosis

Organic stricture of the lower end of the esophagus is the only condition which may cause diagnostic difficulties. Reflux esophagitis secondary to hiatal hernia is the most common cause of organic esophageal stricture in childhood and can be ruled out by esophagoscopy, x-rays, and manometric studies.

Treatment

Special diets and anticholinergic agents have not been successful. Dilatation is of value in a few cases and can be repeated with recurrent symptoms. More definitive results can be achieved by means of a surgical procedure (Heller) consisting of longitudinal splitting of all the muscle coats down to the mucosa.

Prognosis

Because of the shorter duration of the illness in pediatric patients and because of a proximal motility which is less disturbed, the prognosis for return of the esophagus to normal caliber after surgical treatment is very good.

Elder JB: Achalasia of the cardia in childhood. Digestion 3:90, 1970.

Vaughan WH, Williams JL. Familial achalasia with pulmonary complications in children. Radiology 107:407, 1973.

CHALASIA

Clinically, 40% of newborn infants have a tendency to regurgitate. On fluoroscopy, regurgitation can be elicited in close to 50% of normal newborns. This is due to immaturity of control over the lower esophageal sphincter.

Vomiting or excessive regurgitation after feedings (chalasia), frequently beginning shortly after birth, is common. Poor weight gain and aspiration pneumonia rarely occur. Diagnosis is based upon fluoroscopic and film demonstration of retrograde flow of barium from the stomach to the esophagus during respiration and when external pressure is applied over the abdomen.

Gastroesophageal reflux secondary to chalasia may mimic pyloric stenosis, outlet obstruction of the stomach, hiatal hernia, or esophageal stenosis.

Thickened feedings are helpful. The infant should be kept in an erect sitting position for 2–3 hours after each feeding, and it may be necessary to maintain this position 24 hours a day using an "infant seat." A low-fat diet may be helpful in some cases. Metoclopramide has been disappointing.

Chalasia is usually a mild transitory condition which normally disappears by 6 months of age. It is compatible with perfectly good health and a normal growth pattern. In rare cases, persistent vomiting, failure to thrive, esophagitis, and repeated bronchopulmonary infections may occur, in which case surgery may be required.

Cohen S: Developmental characteristics of lower esophageal sphincter function: A possible mechanism for infantile chalasia. Gastroenterology 67:252, 1974.

Ferguson CF: Esophageal dysfunction and other swallowing difficulties in early life. Ann Otol Rhinol Laryngol 80:541, 1971.

Nusslé D, Genton N, Philippe P: Clinical and radiologic course of nonoperated cardio-esophageal incompetence in the infant. Helv Paediatr Acta 24:145, 1969.

Toccalino H & others: Vomiting and regurgitation. Clin Gastroenterol 6:267, 1977.

CAUSTIC BURNS OF THE ESOPHAGUS

Stricture of the esophagus commonly follows ingestion of a caustic alkali, eg, lye, Clorox, Drano, ammonia. Lesions initially are of varying severity. Superficial esophagitis may be the only finding. On the other hand, ulceration and sometimes necrosis may lead to chemical mediastinitis and to peritonitis if the stomach is involved. The extent of burning of the mouth does not correlate well with the presence or the degree of esophageal damage.

Children who have swallowed large amounts of lye may present with oral lesions and shock. The usual clinical picture, however, is that of painful edematous lesions of the lips, mouth, and larynx. Over a period of a few hours or days, the initially extreme dysphagia subsides, and swallowing is resumed. If left untreated, the child remains asymptomatic for a few months until a stricture progressively develops. X-rays usually reveal more severe strictures in the areas of anatomic narrowing, eg, the cervical region and the point at which the left bronchus crosses the esophagus and cardia. Esophagoscopic findings are those of localized escharotic lesions. Later, the entire esophagus is twisted, shortened, and narrowed. Single, dense, fairly localized strictures may occur. Shortening of the esophagus may lead to a hiatal hernia.

The child with a history of alkali ingestion should have a careful examination of his lips and mouth, though esophageal burns are sometimes found in the absence of lip and mouth involvement. Esophagoscopy will demonstrate the lesions but cannot estimate how deeply the esophagus has been burned. Symptoms resulting from strictures may occur within 1 month following the accident, but more commonly the stricture formation does not lead to symptoms for many months or even years. Dysphagia is first manifest for solids and eventually for liquids.

The immediate home care should be familiar to all parents. Vomiting should not be induced. Hospitalization is recommended. Prednisone, 1–2 mg/kg/day (or its equivalent IV), is started immediately. Intravenous fluids may be necessary. Esophagoscopy should be done within 12–24 hours after ingestion, particularly in the young infant in whom a history of swallowing cannot be obtained. Delay in performing this procedure imposes an increased hazard of perforation. If a burn has been evidenced, corticosteroids are continued and a program of bougienage is started. In cases where x-rays show evidence of erosion into the mediastinum or peritoneum, antibiotics become mandatory.

Without early treatment, stricture formation is inevitable. Surgical replacement of the esophagus with a segment of colon may be necessary.

Chong GC, Beahrs OH, Payne WS: Management of corrosive gastritis due to ingested acid. Mayo Clin Proc 49:861, 1974.

Haller JA & others: Pathophysiology and management of acute corrosive burns of the esophagus: Results of treatment in 285 children. J Pediatr Surg 6:578, 1971.

Leape LL & others: Hazard to health: Liquid lye. N Engl J Med 284:578, 1971.

PYLORIC STENOSIS

Essentials of Diagnosis

- Vomiting, usually projectile.
- Constipation.
- Poor weight gain or weight loss.
- Dehydration.
- Palpable olive-sized tumor in the right upper quadrant.
- "String sign" and evidence of retained gastric contents on x-ray.

General Considerations

Pyloric stenosis is the second most common surgical disorder of the gastrointestinal tract in infancy (after inguinal hernia). The cause of the increase in the size of the circular muscle of the pylorus is not known. There is a coincidence of the disease in twins or fathers and sons. The disease occurs in one out of 500 births, and males are affected 3–4 times more commonly than females. The reported increased incidence in first-borns and in the spring and fall months is controversial.

Clinical Findings

A. Symptoms and Signs: Vomiting usually begins between 2–4 weeks of age and progresses to projectile vomiting after each feeding; in about 10% of cases, it may start at birth. In premature infants particularly, the onset of symptoms is often delayed. The vomitus does not contain bile but may be bloodstreaked. The infant is hungry and nurses avidly, but there is constipation and failure to gain.

Dehydration, loss of skin turgor, fretfulness, and apathy may be present. The upper abdomen is distended, and gastric peristaltic waves from left to right may be seen. An olive-sized tumor can almost always be felt to the right of the umbilicus and is readily palpable immediately after the infant has vomited.

B. Laboratory Findings: There is metabolic alkalosis with potassium depletion. Hemoconcentration is reflected by elevated hemoglobin and hematocrit values.

C. X-Ray Findings: An upper gastrointestinal series reveals delay in gastric emptying and an elongated narrowed pyloric channel ("string sign"). It is advisable for at least 2 physicians to confirm the presence of the tumor.

Differential Diagnosis

The absence of increased intracranial pressure, virilization, and hyperkalemia rules out intracranial lesions and congenital adrenal hyperplasia with adrenal insufficiency. In achalasia, the food is undigested; in annular pancreas, the vomitus contains bile. Sepsis and urinary tract infections can easily be ruled out. In simple cases of "pylorospasm," there may be a delay in gastric emptying, but the elongated narrow pyloric canal is not seen and no tumor is present.

Treatment

Pyloromyotomy is the treatment of choice and consists of incision down to the mucosa and fully across the pyloric length. Surgery for pyloric stenosis is not an emergency procedure, and the necessary time should be taken to repair dehydration and electrolyte abnormalities and to assuage any gastritis by saline gastric irrigations.

Drug therapy is not widely used or often recommended in the USA but has been used in other countries. Methscopamine nitrate, 0.1 mg dissolved in water and given orally or subcutaneously 10–15 minutes before each feeding, may be used. It is usually necessary to keep the infant in the hospital for 2–4 weeks while on therapy. It appears that medical management works best in patients whose symptoms begin late (beyond 4 weeks of age) and who suffer little dehydration despite delay in diagnosis.

Prognosis

The outlook is excellent following surgery.

Benson CD: Infantile pyloric stenosis. Prog Pediatr Surg 1:63, 1970.

Huguenard J & others: Incidence of pyloric stenosis within sibships. J Pediatr 81:45, 1972.

Pellerin D & others: Gastro-oesophageal reflux and hypertrophic pyloric stenosis. Ann Chir Infant 15:7, 1974.

NEONATAL PERFORATIONS OF THE GASTROINTESTINAL TRACT

Intrauterine perforation usually results from distal intestinal obstruction secondary to atresia, volvulus, strangulated hernia, Hirschsprung's disease, or meconium ileus. Perforation results in a sterile chemical peritonitis. Postpartum perforation gives rise to a bacterial peritonitis; it is usually secondary to an underlying intestinal obstruction but can be secondary to a gastric perforation, necrotizing enterocolitis, or even neonatal appendicitis.

Sixty percent of neonatal gastrointestinal perforations involve the stomach or the duodenum. The theory of gastric muscular defects or mechanical trauma by catheters has been largely discarded in favor of ischemic necrosis which leads to ulceration and eventually perforation of any segment of the gastrointestinal tract. Stress ulcers and necrotizing enterocolitis of the newborn are other manifestations of ischemic necrosis likely to be seen in asphyxic neonates. A high incidence of colonic perforation has been recently reported in newborn infants after exchange transfusions. Iatrogenic intestinal perforation by nasogastric intubation, enema tubes, and thermometers presents a particular threat to the newborn infant.

Prematurely born infants are more prone to develop perforation. The syndrome has been observed in identical twins. The affected newborns usually appear normal at birth; the average age at onset of symptoms is the third day of life. Refusal of feedings is followed by vomiting, sometimes bloody. The abdomen becomes rapidly distended; dyspnea and cyanosis frequently ensue and are followed by shock. X-ray findings may reveal free air under the diaphragm. The

gastric air bubble is usually absent, especially when the perforation is large.

Fluid and electrolyte balance should be corrected while the abdomen is decompressed by nasogastric suction. The perforation is then repaired.

The prognosis is poor, particularly if surgery is delayed.

Hardy JD & others: Intestinal perforation following exchange transfusion. Am J Dis Child 124:136, 1972.

Lloyd JR: The etiology of gastrointestinal perforations in the newborn. J Pediatr Surg 4:77, 1969.

Talbert JL, Felman AH, DeBusk FL: Gastrointestinal surgical emergencies in the newborn infant. J Pediatr 76:783, 1970.

PEPTIC DISEASE

The overall incidence of peptic disease in children is increasing. Peptic ulcers may occur at any age but are more frequent in the age group from 12 to 18 years. Boys are affected twice as commonly as girls, and this preponderance is even greater beyond 12 years of age. Up to age 6, most ulcers are associated with an underlying illness, a drug, or a toxic substance. A positive family history is present in 25–50% of cases of duodenal ulcers.

Gastric ulcers are as common as duodenal ulcers up to age 6. In the 6- to 18-year-old group, duodenal ulcers are 5 times as common as gastric ulcers. The pathogenesis of gastric ulcers is not understood. A number of factors favor back diffusion of hydrogen ions across the gastric mucosa and cause extensive damage to the gastric mucosa. Aspirin is the only drug that has been proved to be ulcerogenic in humans. Hypoxia, hypotension, sepsis, and increased intracranial pressure are often responsible for secondary ulcers. Excess production of pepsin or acid production is an important factor in the development of primary duodenal ulcers. The increased functional parietal mass could be inherited or acquired (islet cell adenoma, hypercalcemia). Patients with duodenal ulcers have normal fasting levels of gastrin but demonstrate increased gastrin release in response to feeding. The resultant hypersecretion of acid is neutralized by food. However, evacuation through the pylorus occurs more rapidly and is followed by a significantly higher rebound secretion of hydrochloric acid.

Clinical Findings

A. Symptoms and Signs:

1. 0–3 years—In infants past the neonatal period up to the age of 3, symptoms of primary ulcers include poor eating, vomiting, crying after meals, and melena or hematemesis. Secondary ulcers are more acute, and perforation may be the first sign.

2. 3–6 years—Vomiting related to eating is always present. Gastric outlet obstruction may give rise to protracted vomiting. Periumbilical or generalized abdominal pain is common. The typical "ulcer pain" is rarely present. Melena, hematemesis, and perforation are the rule in cases of secondary ulcers.

3. 6–18 years–Less than 50% have the typical pain leading to an early diagnosis. Melena or hematemesis (or both) is noted in over 50% of cases; occult bleeding and anemia without other symptoms are not uncommon. In addition to the acute illnesses responsible for secondary ulcers, certain chronic diseases such as chronic lung disease, Crohn's disease, cirrhosis of the liver, and rheumatoid arthritis are associated with an increased incidence of peptic disease.

B. Gastric Analysis: In children with peptic ulcers, the chief value of gastric fluid analysis is to show that there is no hypersecretion such as would occur with the Zollinger-Ellison syndrome.

C. X-Ray Findings: Radiologic signs of ulceration or a deformity should be present. The frequency with which the radiologic sign of duodenal irritability is found makes the x-ray diagnosis often unreliable. In patients with severe degrees of duodenal irritability, a niche may not be demonstrated since the barium is moved out of the bulb very rapidly.

D. Panendoscopy: Although a barium meal remains the single most widely useful diagnostic tool, the increasing availability of pediatric fiberoptic instruments is making a significant contribution to the detection of peptic ulcer disease.

Differential Diagnosis

The diagnosis of acute secondary ulcers should be suspected in any child with a severe underlying disease who suddenly presents with abdominal distention, hematemesis, or melena. A wide spectrum of symptoms is associated with primary peptic ulcers. The differential diagnosis includes chronic idiopathic recurrent abdominal pain, irritable colon syndrome, esophagitis, chronic pancreatitis, and cholelithiasis. Suspicion is warranted when abdominal pain occurs at night or in the early morning hours, when recurrent vomiting is closely related to eating, and, finally, when there is a family history of duodenal ulcers even if gastrointestinal complaints are vague.

Treatment

Bed rest is usually unnecessary unless there are signs of duodenal obstruction, active bleeding, or perforation.

With outlet obstruction, gastric suction should be maintained for a few days. Hourly feedings are necessary initially and should be continued until pain has disappeared. Foods that cause pain should be avoided. Beef broth, tea, coffee, spices, and carbonated beverages should be avoided since they enhance gastric secretion. Antacids (15–30 ml) every 1–2 hours and at bedtime are given initially and continued for some time after symptoms have disappeared in both gastric and duodenal ulcers. Anticholinergics are useful only in duodenal ulcers, where gastric hypersecretion can be present.

Surgical management is reserved for the complications, ie, perforation, hemorrhage, obstruction, or incapacitating and intractable pain.

Prognosis

Long-term studies show that 50% of children with duodenal ulcers have recurrent symptoms within a year. The prognosis for recurrence is much lower in the younger group (0–6 years). Surgery for duodenal ulcers (pyloroplasty and vagotomy) gives excellent results.

Curci MR & others: Peptic ulcer disease in childhood reexamined. J Pediatr Surg 11:329, 1976.

Deckelbaum RJ & others: Peptic ulcer disease: A clinical study in 73 children. Can Med Assoc J 111:225, 1974.

Robb JDA & others: Duodenal ulcer in children. Arch Dis Child 47:688, 1972.

Tudor RB: Gastric and duodenal ulcers in children. Gastroenterology 62:823, 1972.

CONGENITAL DIAPHRAGMATIC HERNIA

Between the eighth and tenth weeks of fetal life, the diaphragm is formed and the coelomic cavity divides into its abdominal and thoracic components. During this same stage of morphogenesis, the gastrointestinal tract undergoes its major development, elongating into the umbilical pouch and rotating on its return to the abdominal cavity. Any alteration in these 2 closely interrelated processes leads to a diaphragmatic hernia, which can be secondary to a posterolateral defect in the diaphragm (foramen of Bochdalek) or, more rarely, to a retrosternal defect (foramen of Morgagni).

All degrees of protrusion of the abdominal viscera through the diaphragmatic opening into the thoracic cavity may occur. The extent of herniation determines the severity and the timing of the symptoms. Fewer than 2% of cases are secondary to a retrosternal defect. In the posterolateral variety, more than 80% involve the left diaphragm.

Symptoms of mild to severe respiratory distress and cyanosis are usually present from birth, although some patients remain asymptomatic and the finding of a large diaphragmatic hernia with air-filled coils on x-ray is incidental to an x-ray examination. The abdomen is scaphoid. Breath sounds in the affected hemithorax are absent, with displacement of the point of maximal impulse.

Fatal cases have circulatory problems secondary to the mediastinal shift, giving rise to stretching and kinking of the great vessels. Pulmonary infections also constitute a major cause of death, along with prematurity and a high incidence of associated anomalies, mainly malrotation. The most frequent cause of death, however, is pulmonary insufficiency. The lung on the affected side is compressed and often hypoplastic. The neonate's dependence on diaphragmatic respiration and the right-to-left shunt through a lung incapable of exchanging gases precipitates anoxia and acidosis.

Eventration of the diaphragm is not, strictly speaking, a hernia. A leaf of the diaphragm, ballooned by a diminution of muscular elements, leads to identical but much milder symptoms.

Dibbins AW, Wiener ES: Mortality from neonatal diaphragmatic hernia. J Pediatr Surg 9:653, 1974.

Raphaely RC, Downes JJ: Congenital diaphragmatic hernia: Prediction of survival. J Pediatr Surg 8:815, 1973.

CONGENITAL DUODENAL OBSTRUCTION

Extrinsic duodenal obstruction is usually due to congenital peritoneal bands with or without volvulus associated with midgut malrotation, to annular pancreas, or, more rarely, to duplication of the duodenum. An intrinsic type includes atresia, where only the lumen is obliterated by a membrane or where there is a complete gap between the 2 bowel ends. Atresia and stenosis may affect the duodenum proximal or distal to the ampulla of Vater. There is often a history of polyhydramnios.

Clinical Findings

A. Atresia: Vomiting (usually bile stained) begins within a few hours after birth, with epigastric distention. Meconium may be normally passed. The association between duodenal atresia, severe congenital anomalies (30%), prematurity (25–50%), and Down's syndrome (20–30%) is striking.

B. Stenosis: Symptoms of duodenal obstruction appear later and are intermittent, being delayed for weeks, months, or years. Even though a postampullary location of the stenotic area is usual, the vomitus does not always contain bile. X-rays of the abdomen usually show gastric and duodenal gaseous distention proximal to the atretic site ("double bubble"). In cases of protracted vomiting and dehydration, there may be little air in the stomach; it is then advisable to instill 10 ml of air into the stomach to elicit the typical pattern. Total absence of gas in the intestinal tract distal to the obstruction suggests atresia or an extrinsic obstruction severe enough to completely occlude the lumen, while air scattered over the lower abdomen may indicate a partial duodenal obstruction of either the intrinsic or extrinsic variety. A barium enema may be helpful in determining the presence of a concomitant malrotation or of an area of atresia lower in the gastrointestinal tract.

Treatment

Since clinical and radiologic findings cannot do more than indicate either partial or complete duodenal obstruction, thorough exploration is necessary at operation not only to find the cause of the obstruction but to make sure that no additional pathologic anomalies are present lower in the gastrointestinal tract.

Prognosis

The mortality rate (35–40%) is significantly affected by prematurity, Down's syndrome, and associated congenital anomalies.

Fonkalsrud EW, DeLorimier AA, Hays DM: Congenital atresia and stenosis of the duodenum. Pediatrics 43:79, 1969.

Girvan DP, Stephens CA: Congenital duodenal obstruction: A 20 year review of its surgical management and consequences. J Pediatr Surg 9:833, 1974.

Wayne ER, Burrington JD: Extrinsic duodenal obstruction in children. Surg Gynecol Obstet 136:87, 1973.

CONGENITAL JEJUNAL & ILEAL OBSTRUCTION

Bile-stained or fecal vomiting usually begins in the first 48 hours of life, and distention is frequent. Meconium only is passed rectally. Prematurity and severe congenital anomalies may coexist. Atresias, stenoses, and obstructing membranes may affect multiple sites. X-ray features include dilated loops of small bowel and absence of colonic gas. Barium enema will reveal a colon of restricted caliber (microcolon) if the atresia is in the lower small bowel.

The differential diagnosis should include Hirschsprung's disease, paralytic ileus secondary to sepsis, gastroenteritis or pneumonia, midgut volvulus, and meconium ileus. This latter condition, the initial manifestation of cystic fibrosis, can be found in association with intestinal atresia.

Surgery is mandatory. The prognosis remains grave.

DeLorimier AA, Fonkalsrud EW, Hays DM: Congenital atresia and stenosis of the jejunum and ileum. Surgery 65:819, 1969.

Guttman FM & others: Multiple atresias and a new syndrome of hereditary multiple atresias involving the gastrointestinal tract from stomach to rectum. J Pediatr Surg 8:633, 1973.

Zerella JT, Martin JW: Jejunal atresia with absent mesentery and helical ileum. Surgery 80:550, 1976.

ANNULAR PANCREAS

The pancreas develops from dorsal and ventral endodermal outgrowths which fuse. The ventral pancreatic bud is bilobed; the left bud normally degenerates. If it persists and develops its own pancreatic lobe, it grows around the left side of the duodenum to join the other 2 parts of the pancreas in the dorsal mesentery.

The presence of an annular pancreas is usually associated with failure of segmental duodenal development. The symptoms are those of partial or complete duodenal obstruction. Down's syndrome and severe congenital anomalies of the gastrointestinal tract occur frequently. As with other gastrointestinal obstructive lesions of the neonate, polyhydramnios is commonly found.

Treatment consists of duodenoduodenostomy or duodenojejunostomy without operative dissection or division of the pancreatic annulus.

Merrill JR, Raftensperger JG: Pediatric annular pancreas: Twenty years' experience. J Pediatr Surg 11:921, 1976.

MIDGUT MALROTATION

Normally, the midgut, which extends from the duodenojejunal junction to the mid-transverse colon and which is supplied by the superior mesenteric artery, returns to the intra-abdominal position during the tenth week of embryonic life while the root of the mesentery rotates in a counterclockwise direction. This causes the colon to cross ventrally; the cecum moves from the left to the right lower quadrant, and the duodenum crosses dorsally to become partly retroperitoneal. When this rotation is incomplete, the posterior fixation of the mesentery is defective so that the bowel from the ligament of Treitz to the mid-transverse colon may twist, causing a volvulus around the pedicle-like mesentery. Duodenal or ileal obstruction may later result through peritoneal bands from the mobile hepatic flexure or cecum. The majority of cases are asymptomatic.

Clinical Findings

A. Symptoms and Signs: Seventy-five percent of symptomatic cases show high intestinal obstruction within the first 3 weeks of life, with bile-stained vomitus, abdominal distention, and visible peristalsis. The first signs may occur later in life, with recurring symptoms of intermittent intestinal obstruction or, more rarely, with celiac syndrome or intermittent profuse watery diarrhea. Acute gastroenteritis may be an early symptom in infants under the age of 6 months. Severe associated congenital anomalies, especially cardiac, are said to occur in over 25% of symptomatic cases.

B. X-Ray Findings: In the newborn period, complete absence of air in the small bowel suggests duodenal atresia. An upper gastrointestinal series may show partial or complete obstruction. The diagnosis of malrotation can be further confirmed by barium enema, which shows a cecum that is mobile and abnormally located.

Treatment & Prognosis

Treatment consists of surgical correction. The prognosis in the newborn period is guarded in view of the incidence of perforation with peritonitis and of extensive intestinal necrosis.

Brennom WS, Bill AH: Prophylactic fixation of the intestine for midgut nonrotation. Surg Gynecol Obstet 138:181, 1974.

Stewart DR & others: Malrotation of the bowel in infants and children: A 15 year experience. Surgery 79:716, 1976.

Venna TR, Bankhole MA: Lymphovenous obstruction in anomalous midgut rotation. Arch Dis Child 48:154, 1973.

MAJOR ABDOMINAL WALL DEVELOPMENTAL DEFECTS

Omphalocele

This is a rare condition (1:10,000 births) associated with variable herniation of intra-abdominal viscera into the base of the umbilical cord. There is no defect of the abdominal wall. It is thought to be secondary to an arrest in the intra-abdominal migration of the midgut between the fifth and ninth weeks of gestation. Primary closure of those less than 5 cm in diameter has a good prognosis. Attempts at primary repair of larger ones lead to respiratory failure, necessitating a staged enlargement of the abdominal cavity.

Gastroschisis

This consists of herniation of bowel or other viscus through an extra-umbilical defect in the anterior abdominal wall. There is no covering membrane and the eviscerated bowel loops are dark red, edematous, and adherent. They are encased in a thick matrix of fibrinous material. Gangrene may be present. All patients have associated malrotation and some degree of congenital shortening of the small bowel. Unruptured omphalocele and associated intestinal atresias are common. Closure is by stages with a prosthetic abdominal wall. Prematurity (40%), the threat of sepsis, and malnutrition remain the long-term challenges of this entity. The postoperative course is usually difficult because of protracted intestinal obstruction and intestinal dysfunction. Total parenteral nutrition is often required for extended periods of time.

Congenital Deficiency of Abdominal Musculature

This disorder is apparent from the flaccid and wrinkled appearance of the abdominal wall. Almost all of these infants are males with undescended testes; 50% present with club feet. Between 20 and 25% also have cardiac and gastrointestinal anomalies. Urinary tract anomalies consist of urethral and functional bladder neck obstructions associated with a patent urachus. Corseting counteracts the abdominal wall weakness, but 60% die in infancy as a result of renal insufficiency or respiratory failure.

Mahour GH, Weitzman JJ, Rosenkrantz JG: Omphalocele and gastroschisis. Ann Surg 177:478, 1973.

Ravitch M: The non-operative treatment of surgical conditions in children. Pediatrics 51:435, 1973.

Talbert JL & others: Surgical management of massive ventral hernias in children. J Pediatr Surg 12:63, 1977.

MECKEL'S DIVERTICULUM & OMPHALOMESENTERIC DUCT REMNANTS

The remnant of the vitelline duct known as Meckel's diverticulum is present in approximately 1.5% of the population. Complications occur 3 times more frequently in males than in females, and in 50–60% of cases within the first 2 years of life. Heterotopic tissue (gastric mucosa mostly, but also pancreatic tissue and jejunal or colonic mucosa) is 10 times as likely to be present in symptomatic cases.

Clinical Findings

A. Symptoms and Signs:

1. Hemorrhage—(40–60% of symptomatic cases.) Massive painless rectal bleeding or dark red stools is characteristic. Shock is common, with hemoglobin levels of 3–4 gm/100 ml. Gastric mucosa and an ulcer of the ileal mucosa are found in the majority of cases presenting with hemorrhage.

2. Intestinal obstruction—(25% of symptomatic cases.)

a. Intussusception—Ileocolic intussusception with early intestinal infarction. A mass is palpable.

b. Herniation or volvulus—Twisting of the bowel around a fibrous remnant of the vitelline duct extending from the tip of the diverticulum to the abdominal wall may occur with herniation around this cord or strangulation of the diverticulum in an inguinal hernia. In many cases, entrapment of a bowel loop under a band running between the diverticulum and the base of the mesentery has been associated with intestinal obstruction.

3. Diverticulitis—(10–20%.) This condition is clinically indistinguishable from acute appendicitis. Perforation and generalized peritonitis may occur in the young infant.

B. X-Ray Findings: An x-ray diagnosis is seldom made. Radionuclide imaging with 99m Tc pertechnetate may be of value to demonstrate the diverticula lined with heterotopic gastric mucosa. Angiography may be useful when bleeding is brisk.

Treatment

A. Diverticulum: Treatment is surgical. At operation, close inspection of the ileum proximal and distal to the diverticulum may reveal ulcerations and heterotopic tissue adjacent to the neck of the diverticulum.

B. Other Remnants of the Omphalomesenteric Duct: Fecal discharge from the umbilicus is evidence of a patent omphalomesenteric duct. The duct may be completely closed, leading to persistence of a fibrous cord joining ileum and umbilicus and potentially the origin of a volvulus. In other instances, a mucoid discharge may be indicative of a mucocele, which can protrude through the umbilicus and be mistaken for an umbilical granuloma since it is firm and bright red. In all cases, surgical excision of the omphalomesenteric remnant is indicated.

Prognosis

The prognosis for Meckel's diverticulum is good. Marked hemorrhage may occur but is rarely exsanguinating.

Bree RL, Reuter SR: Angiographic demonstration of a bleeding Meckel's diverticulum. Radiology 108:287, 1973.

Ho JE, Konieczny KM: The sodium pertechnetate Tc 99m scan: An aid in the evaluation of gastrointestinal bleeding. Pediatrics 56:34, 1975.

Rutherford RB, Akers DR: Meckel's diverticulum. Surgery 59:618, 1966.

Seagram CGF & others: Meckel's diverticulum: A 10-year review of 218 cases. Can J Surg 11:369, 1968.

DUPLICATIONS OF THE GASTROINTESTINAL TRACT

Duplications of the gastrointestinal tract are congenital malformations most often discovered during infancy. Duplications are spherical or tubular structures of various sizes and shapes which may occur anywhere along the gastrointestinal tract from the tongue to the anus. They usually contain fluid and sometimes blood if necrosis has taken place. Although most duplications are not communicating, they are intimately attached to the mesenteric side of the gut and share a common muscular coat. The intestinal epithelium is usually of the same type as that seen in the area of the gastrointestinal tract from which it originates. Some duplications are attached to the spinal cord and are associated with the presence of hemivertebrae (neurenteric cysts). Abdominal duplications are much more common than the thoracic ones, which are usually attached to the esophagus.

Symptoms usually become manifest in infancy and consist of vomiting, abdominal distention, colicky pain, rectal bleeding, partial or total intestinal obstruction, or an abdominal mass. Physical examination reveals a rounded, smooth, freely movable mass, and x-rays of the abdomen show a noncalcified mass displacing the intestines or compressing the stomach. Involvement of the terminal small bowel can give rise to an intussusception.

Prompt surgical treatment is indicated.

Favara B, Franciosi RA, Akers DR: Enteric duplications. Thirty-seven cases: A vascular theory of pathogenesis. Am J Dis Child 122:501, 1971.

Grosfeld JL, O'Neill JA, Clatworthy HW: Enteric duplications in infancy and childhood. Ann Surg 172:83, 1970.

Parker BC & others: Gastric duplications in infancy. J Pediatr Surg 7:294, 1972.

NECROTIZING ENTEROCOLITIS

Essentials of Diagnosis

- The patient is likely to be a small premature (< 1600 gm) and the product of an abnormal gestation and a complicated delivery.
- During the first weeks of life, regurgitation and vomiting are followed by abdominal distention, hematochezia, and signs of peritonitis.
- Lethargy, severe acidosis, sepsis, and shock rapidly supervene.
- Flat film shows intramural gas bubbles (pneumatosis intestinalis).
- Late manifestations (< 3 months) are associated with the eventual development of strictures in the ileum or colon.

General Considerations

Necrotizing enterocolitis in the newborn infant is an acute fulminating disease associated with diffuse ulceration and necrosis of the gastrointestinal tract. The ileum is the most common site of the disease. In close to three-fourths of cases, there are also lesions in the colon. The stomach and upper small bowel are rarely affected. The disease is said to affect 1–2% of all prematures, the incidence being higher in the ones weighing less than 1600 gm. Necrotizing enterocolitis may occur as a complication of a lower bowel obstruction such as meconium ileus or Hirschsprung's disease or of an exchange transfusion in full-term neonates. Risk factors in prematures include perinatal asphyxia, respiratory distress, congenital heart disease, and perhaps also hyperosmolar feedings. It is very rare in breast-fed infants.

Clinical Findings

A. Symptoms and Signs: Symptoms may occur as early as the first day and as late as the fourth week. Feedings are poorly tolerated, and regurgitation and vomiting occur. This is followed by abdominal distention and bloody stools or obstipation. Signs of perforation and peritonitis may be the initial manifestations. Severe acidosis, sepsis, and shock rapidly supervene. In others, the course is not as fulminating, and the diagnosis may be more difficult or completely missed until the baby develops signs of progressive lower small bowel or colonic obstruction, the result of acquired strictures. These late manifestations of necrotizing enterocolitis occur usually within the first 3 months after the acute phase of the illness.

B. X-Ray Findings: A plain film may show, besides small-bowel distention and evidence of obstruction, a feathered appearance indicative of ulceration and the accumulation of intramural gas bubbles (pneumatosis intestinalis). With progression of the disease and perforation, free air is seen in the peritoneum.

Treatment

When the diagnosis is entertained, oral feedings should be withheld and nasogastric suction and intravenous fluids should be started. Parenteral antibiotics are indicated. Oral antibiotics may also be given since the intestinal flora is thought to be an important pathologic factor associated with the ischemic lesion. Flat films of the abdomen are done every 6–12 hours for the first few days to detect a perforation. Feedings are resumed gradually when the nasogastric drainage is small and when the x-rays no longer demonstrate pneumatosis. Any evidence of intestinal perforation or peritonitis is an indication for immediate operation.

After discharge, neonates who have had necrotizing enterocolitis must be followed closely for signs of partial obstruction which can occur as late as a year after the initial insult.

Prognosis

Reported survival rates are quite variable, and the outcome is significantly influenced by weight and precipitating factors. It may be as low as 10% in small prematures with perinatal asphyxia. The prognosis is much better in necrotizing enterocolitis that develops in full-term neonates following an exchange transfusion.

Barlow B & others: An experimental study of acute neonatal enterocolitis: The importance of breast milk. J Pediatr Surg 9:587, 1974.

Frantz ID & others: Necrotizing enterocolitis. J Pediatr 86:259, 1975.

Lake AM, Walker WA: Neonatal necrotising enterocolitis: A disease of altered host defense. Clin Gastroenterol 6:463, 1977.

Stevenson JK & others: Aggressive treatment of neonatal necrotizing enterocolitis: 38 patients with 25 survivors. J Pediatr Surg 6:28, 1971.

Touloukian RJ, Posch JN, Spencer R: The pathogenesis of ischemic gastroenterocolitis of the neonate: Selective gut mucosal ischemia in asphyxiated neonatal piglets. J Pediatr Surg 7:194, 1972.

Virnig NL, Reynolds JW: Epidemiological aspects of neonatal necrotizing enterocolitis. Am J Dis Child 128:186, 1974.

PRIMARY PERITONITIS

The incidence of primary peritonitis has decreased remarkably with the advent of antibiotics. Most cases occur below the age of 5. In older children, the disease is 3–5 times more common in girls. The most common infecting organisms are hemolytic streptococci and pneumococci, although viruses have been implicated in a few cases. Especially at risk are infants who have undergone splenectomy for conditions such as a type of hemolytic anemia other than hereditary spherocytosis, one of the storage diseases, or histiocytosis. Peritonitis also is a potential complication of nephrosis and cirrhosis.

The onset is acute, with severe abdominal pain, fever, nausea, and vomiting. The abdomen is tender, with guarding, involuntary rigidity, and distention. Tenderness is present on rectal examination. The physical signs are identical to those associated with peritonitis secondary to, for example, a perforated appendix. However, the temperature is usually higher and the white count also higher (20,000–50,000/cu mm) than is usual in appendicitis. Diarrhea is not uncommonly seen in primary peritonitis and is much rarer in appendicitis.

Primary peritonitis must be distinguished from secondary peritonitis (see below).

A diagnostic paracentesis should be made and appropriate antibiotic therapy instituted. Surgical peritoneal drainage has been virtually abandoned save for localized abscesses.

Fogel BJ, Karpa JN, Luxemberg ER: Primary peritonitis. Clin Pediatr (Phila) 3:578, 1964.
Fowler R: Primary peritonitis: Changing aspects 1965–1970. Aust Paediatr J 7:73, 1971.

SECONDARY PERITONITIS

Secondary peritoneal infection commonly results from an abscessed or ruptured intra-abdominal viscus, usually the appendix. More rarely, peptic ulcer, cholecystitis, pancreatitis, regional enteritis, ulcerative colitis, midgut volvulus, intussusception, and strangulated hernia can cause secondary peritonitis. Abscesses may form in the pelvic, subhepatic, and subphrenic areas, but localization occurs less commonly in infants and young children than in adults.

Clinical Findings
A. Symptoms and Signs: Signs are often overshadowed by those of the underlying disorder. High fever is common except in newborn or debilitated infants, and shock may be present. Abdominal pain is diffuse and is exacerbated by movement. Vomiting is protracted, and the vomitus is greenish and eventually becomes malodorous. Constipation is marked unless there is localization, when small diarrheal stools may be passed. Restlessness, rapid pulse, and superficial grunting respirations are other common clinical features. Abdominal examination shows diffuse tenderness with muscular resistance and rebound tenderness. Peristalsis is usually absent. Irritation of the pelvic peritoneum is evidenced by pain on rectal examination.

B. Laboratory Findings: A striking polymorphonuclear response is usual; however, as the disease advances, the white blood count often drops to leukopenic levels.

Treatment
Preoperative preparation with hydration, correction of acid-base problems, antimicrobial therapy for *Escherichia coli,* gastric suction, and the relief of pain significantly improve the mortality rate.

The operative management consists of removal or repair of the affected viscus, drainage of the localized abscess, and lavage of the peritoneal cavity with saline and antibiotics.

Prognosis
The mortality rate is probably around 1% in older children and 50% in newborns.

Kiesewetter WB: Peritonitis in infancy and childhood. Am Fam Physician 5:105, March 1972.
Shandling B & others: Perforating appendicitis and antibiotics. J Pediatr Surg 9:79, 1973.

CONGENITAL AGANGLIONIC MEGACOLON
(Hirschsprung's Disease)

Essentials of Diagnosis
- Partial or complete intestinal obstruction in the newborn period.
- Vomiting, diarrhea, abdominal distention, and shock in the newborn period.
- Obstinate constipation, abdominal enlargement, ribbon-like stools, and failure to thrive in infancy or childhood.
- Absence of fecal material on rectal examination.
- Narrowed colonic segment proximal to the anus on x-ray.
- Absence of ganglion cells in the narrowed segment.

General Considerations
Hirschsprung's disease is secondary to congenital absence of parasympathetic ganglion cells in one segment of the colon (a 4–25 cm rectal or rectosigmoid segment in 90% of cases), but it may involve the entire organ in 5%. *Zonal colonic aganglionosis* has been recently described but is exceedingly rare. The aperistaltic denervated segment is narrowed, with dilatation of the proximal uninvolved colon. In long-standing cases, the portion proximal to the narrowed segment may become thinned out, and ulcerations of the mucosa occur although perforations are rare. A familial pattern has been described, particularly in total colonic aganglionosis. Hirschsprung's disease is 4 times more common in boys than in girls.

Clinical Findings
A. Symptoms and Signs: Failure to pass meconium in a newborn is rapidly followed by vomiting, abdominal distention, and reluctance to feed. The baby is irritable, and breathing may be rapid and grunting because of the abdominal distention. In other cases, symptoms appear later and are those of partial intestinal obstruction. Stools may be infrequent and loose; vomiting may be bilious initially and fecal later. Abdominal distention is invariably present. Bouts of

enterocolitis manifested by fever, explosive liquid diarrhea, and severe prostration are reported in about 50% of newborns with this disease. These episodes are serious and may lead to acute inflammatory and ischemic changes. Perforation and sepsis are not unusual. In later infancy, alternating obstipation and diarrhea predominate. The older the child, the more likely he is to present with obstinate constipation. His stools are offensive and ribbon-like, his abdomen enlarged, his veins prominent, peristaltic patterns are readily visible, and fecal masses are easily palpated. Intermittent bouts of intestinal obstruction due to fecal impaction, hypochromic anemia, hypoproteinemia, and failure to thrive are added features.

On digital rectal examination, the anal canal and rectum are devoid of fecal material and may feel narrow. If the involved segment is short, there may be a gush of flatus and of pale, liquid, offensive stool as the finger is withdrawn. The presence of fecal colonic impaction associated with an empty rectum is most suggestive of the disease. However, in cases of short segment aganglionosis, feces may be present in the rectal ampulla and soiling may be a presenting symptom.

B. Laboratory Findings: The final diagnosis rests on histologic evidence of aganglionosis. Rectal suction biopsies taken at 3, 4, and 5 cm readily establish the diagnosis, although some prefer a full-thickness rectal biopsy in order to have access to the ganglion cells between the muscular layers (Auerbach's plexus).

C. X-Ray Findings: X-ray examination of the abdomen may reveal dilated colonic loops and absence of gas from the pelvic colon on an erect lateral film. A barium enema, introducing a small amount of radiopaque material through a catheter with the tip inserted barely beyond the anal sphincter, will usually demonstrate the narrowed segment. A postevacuation film taken 12–48 hours later will show substantial residual barium. X-ray examination of the urinary tract should be done since an association between megaloureter and Hirschsprung's disease is described.

D. Special Examinations: Manometric studies are useful in establishing the diagnosis of aganglionosis, particularly in cases where the involvement is limited to a short segment, making a histologic diagnosis difficult.

Differential Diagnosis

Congenital aganglionic megacolon accounts for 15–20% of cases of neonatal intestinal obstruction. Later in life, this disease must be differentiated from psychogenic megacolon. It can also be confused with celiac disease because of the striking abdominal distention and failure to thrive.

A number of disorders are symptomatically similar to Hirschsprung's disease. Hypoganglionosis or immaturity of ganglion cells has been described, as well as some cases of achalasia of the distal rectal segment and of segmental dilatation of the colon which have a normal complement of ganglion cells. Acquired megacolon may be secondary to an anal stricture and is a frequent problem in myxedema and in children with severe mental retardation or deterioration.

Treatment

After preoperative rehydration, a colostomy should be performed in an area of the colon where ganglion cells have been demonstrated by frozen section. If the entire colon is involved, ileostomy is the procedure of choice. If enterocolitis is clinically present and radiologically demonstrated by the typical "saw tooth" appearance, saline irrigations should be repeatedly given through a rectal cannula. Plasma expanders and fluid and electrolyte homeostasis are also essential before any surgery is done. Resection of the aganglionic segment is delayed until the infant is at least 6 months of age. In healthy patients, staging is not necessary.

During operation, it is essential to ascertain from biopsies of the bowel that ganglion cells are present in the proximal portion of the resected bowel before the final anastomosis is made. Swenson's abdominoperineal pull-through procedure has been a standard procedure. The Duhamel procedure and Grob's modification of it have been said to reduce the late complications of fecal and urinary incontinence. This may relate to the fact that less pelvic dissection is necessary since the aganglionic rectum is bypassed in both these surgical technics. At present, the technic advocated by Soave is most popular. Anal myomectomy is advocated in short segment disease.

Prognosis

In the neonatal period, the mortality rate of Hirschsprung's disease reaches 25–35%. Enterocolitis before or after surgery is an ominous complication, and the mortality rate appears to be higher in infants with a long aganglionic segment.

Campbell PE, Noblet HR: Experience with rectal suction biopsy in the diagnosis of Hirschsprung's disease. J Pediatr Surg 4:410, 1969.

Davis PW, Foster DBE: Hirschsprung's disease: A clinical review. Br J Surg 59:19, 1972.

Nissan S, Bar-Maor JA: Further experience in the diagnosis and surgical treatment of short-segment Hirschsprung's disease and idiopathic megacolon. J Pediatr Surg 6:738, 1971.

Suzuki H & others: Nonoperative diagnosis of Hirschsprung's disease in neonates. Pediatrics 51:188, 1973.

Swenson O, Sherman JO, Fisher JH: Diagnosis of congenital megacolon: Analysis of 501 patients. J Pediatr Surg 8:587, 1973.

NEONATAL INTESTINAL OBSTRUCTION

Failure to pass meconium within the first 24 hours of life suggests intestinal obstruction. A diagnosis of obstruction is very likely if other symptoms such as distention or vomiting are present or if by 36 hours only a small amount of mucus or meconium has been passed. The evacuation of meconium may be quite normal in situations where the obstruction is high in the gastrointestinal tract.

The causes of neonatal intestinal obstruction can be listed as follows:

     Atresia
     Duplications, cysts, and bands
     Malrotation and midgut volvulus
     Gastrointestinal perforations
     Hirschsprung's disease
     Abnormal meconium
       Meconium ileus
       Meconium plug syndrome
     Functional obstruction
       Neurologic immaturity in prematures
       Small left colon syndrome
       Sepsis
       Respiratory distress syndrome
       Maternal drugs
     Imperforate anus

When the diagnosis is suspected, x-rays are in order. Air should reach the proximal small bowel during the first hour following delivery and the colon and rectum within 6 hours. Large amounts of air in the stomach may suggest a tracheo-esophageal fistula, while the absence of air is evidence of esophageal atresia without a fistula or with a proximal fistula. A bubble of air to the right of the spine and adjacent to the stomach bubble ("double bubble") is diagnostic of duodenal atresia. A few dilated loops beyond the stomach indicate atresia of the jejunum while many air-filled loops usually suggest a lower small bowel or colonic obstruction.

Examination of the abdomen may not show much distention if vomiting is protracted or if nasogastric drainage is being carried out. An abdominal mass suggests meconium ileus, volvulus, or duplication. If crying is brought about by light palpation, acute abdomen is a likely diagnosis. Abdominal rigidity is rarely present even in the case of peritonitis. A gray cyanotic hue with distended veins is a common finding in cases of necrotic bowel with peritonitis. If rectal examination is followed by explosive passage of stool and gas, short segment Hirschsprung's disease is likely to be present.

As soon as the diagnosis is suspected, a nasogastric tube should be inserted and intermittent suction begun. The baby should be kept in an Isolette for maintenance of central temperature and oxygenation. Systemic antibiotics, vitamin K, salt-poor human albumin, water, and electrolytes should be given immediately.

Holder TM, Leape LL: The acute surgical abdomen in the neonate. N Engl J Med 278:605, 1968.

Howat JM, Wilkinson AW: Functional intestinal obstruction in the neonate. Arch Dis Child 45:800, 1970.

Talbert JL, Felman AH, De Busk FL: Gastrointestinal surgical emergencies in the newborn infant. J Pediatr 76:783, 1970.

THE MECONIUM PLUG SYNDROME

Evidence of low intestinal obstruction becomes apparent on the second day of life. Little or no meconium is passed per rectum, and abdominal distention is usually followed by bile-stained vomiting and dehydration. On rectal examination, the anal canal may be abnormally small. Occasionally, the meconium plug may be passed and large amounts of gas and meconium follow the rectal examination.

In addition to generalized air distention seen on x-ray, fluid levels are observed in half of patients. A barium enema performed under low pressure with a soft-tipped catheter is not only diagnostic, since it reveals a change in the caliber of the colon at the site of obstruction; it can also be therapeutic in dislodging the meconium plug. The finding of a microcolon distal to the plug makes the differentiation from Hirschsprung's disease impossible, especially since the meconium plug syndrome has been reported in Hirschsprung's disease.

Surgical removal is occasionally necessary if the plug is located in the terminal ileum. Ruling out cystic fibrosis by a sweat test and Hirschsprung's disease by a rectal biopsy may be necessary if bowel function is not entirely normal after passage of the meconium.

Ellis DG, Clatworthy HW: The meconium plug syndrome revisited. J Pediatr Surg 1:54, 1966.

Swischuk LE: Meconium plug syndrome: A cause of neonatal intestinal obstruction. Am J Roentgenol 103:339, 1968.

CHYLOUS ASCITES

Congenital chylous ascites may be observed in the newborn before feeding when there is an abnormality in the lymphatic system. If the thoracic duct is involved, chylothorax may be present. Later in life, the cause may be either a congenital lymphatic abnormality or secondary to tumors or peritoneal bands.

Clinical Findings

A. Symptoms and Signs: In both forms, a rapidly enlarging abdomen, diarrhea, and failure to thrive are noted, with a fluid wave and shifting dullness. Unilateral or generalized peripheral lymphedema may be present. In older children, the history is most important in that trauma, infection, tumor, and previous surgery may play an important role.

B. Laboratory Findings: Laboratory findings include hypoalbuminemia, hypogammaglobulinemia, and lymphopenia. Ascitic fluid obtained by paracentesis will have the composition of chyle if the patient has been fed; otherwise, it is indistinguishable from ascites secondary to cirrhosis.

Differential Diagnosis

Chylous ascites must be differentiated from

ascites due to liver failure and, in the older child, from constrictive pericarditis and neoplastic or infectious agents causing lymphatic obstruction.

Complications & Sequelae

Severe chylous ascites can be fatal. Chronic loss of albumin and gamma globulin through the gastrointestinal tract may lead to edema and increase the risk of infection. Rapidly accumulating chylous ascites may cause respiratory complications.

Treatment

Specific measures are sometimes helpful when traumatic lesions or secondary obstructive phenomena can be corrected. When a congenital abnormality exists due to hypoplasia, aplasia, or ectasia of the lymphatics, little can be done for the patient. Attempts to relieve the ascites by bringing the saphenous vein into the peritoneal cavity have had partial success. A fat-free diet supplemented with medium chain triglycerides decreases the formation of chylous ascitic fluid.

The congenital form of chylous ascites may spontaneously disappear following paracentesis, exploratory laparotomy, and a medium chain triglyceride diet. Repeated paracentesis is contraindicated. Gamma globulin supplements may be needed if there is hypogammaglobulinemia.

Prognosis

The prognosis is guarded, although spontaneous cures have been reported.

Sanchez RE & others: Chylous ascites in children. Surgery 69:183, 1971.

Viswanathan U & others: Therapeutic IV alimentation in traumatic chylous ascites in a child. J Pediatr Surg 9:405, 1974.

CONGENITAL ANORECTAL ANOMALIES

Anorectal anomalies occur once in every 3000–4000 births and are more common in males. Inspection of the perianal area is essential in all newborns.

Classification

Five types are now recognized:

A. Anal Stenosis: The anal aperture is very small and filled with a dot of meconium. Defecation is difficult, and there may be ribbon-like stools, fecal impaction, and abdominal distention. This malformation accounts for perhaps 10% of cases of anorectal anomalies. It is readily corrected by digital dilatation.

B. Imperforate Anal Membrane: The infant fails to pass meconium, and a greenish bulging membrane is seen. After excision, bowel and sphincter function are normal.

C. Anal Agenesis: (90% of cases.) This results from defective development of the anus. The anal dimple is present, and stimulation of the perianal area leads to puckering indicative of the presence of the external sphincter. If there is no associated fistula, intestinal obstruction occurs. Fistulas may be perineal or vulvar in the female and perineal or urethral in the male. A perineal fistula presents as a streak of meconium buried in thickened perineal skin.

D. Rectal and Anal Agenesis: Rectal and anal agenesis accounts for 75% of total anorectal anomalies. Fistulas are almost invariably present. In the female, they may be vestibular or vaginal or may enter a urogenital sinus, which is a common passageway for the urethra and vagina. In the male, fistulas are rectovesical or rectourethral. Associated major congenital malformations are common. Sacral defects, prematurity, and hypoplastic internal and external sphincters significantly influence the prognosis for life and function.

E. Rectal Atresia: The anal canal and lower rectum form a blind pouch which is separated for a variable distance from the blind upper rectal pouch.

X-Ray Findings

X-rays taken with the infant held upside down after the first 24 hours of life and with a radiopaque object held in place at the usual location of the anus will help determine the position of the terminal end of the bowel and the surgical approach.

Treatment & Prognosis

Calibration of the stenotic anus should be undertaken in cases of anal stenosis. Excision of the membrane and dilatation is the treatment for the imperforate anal membrane. Colostomy is advocated for all cases of rectal agenesis. In patients with anal agenesis and a visible fistula of sufficient size to pass meconium, treatment can be deferred. The male without a visible fistula may have a urethral fistula; therefore, colostomy is recommended.

Of the patients with "low" defects, 80–90% are continent after surgery; with "high" defects, only 30% achieve continence. Gracilis muscle transplants may improve continence. Levatorplasty may also be used as a secondary operation following surgery for anorectal agenesis.

The overall mortality rate for anal and rectal agenesis is about 20%. The prognosis is poor in small premature infants and in infants with associated anomalies (40% of cases).

Brandesky G & others: Operations for the improvement of fecal incontinence. Prog Pediatr Surg 9:105, 1976.

Nixon HH & others: The results of treatment of anorectal anomalies: A 13 to 20 year followup. J Pediatr Surg 12:27, 1977.

Stephens FD: Embryologic and functional aspects of "imperforate anus." Surg Clin North Am 50:919, 1970.

Tank ES: Diagnosis and treatment of congenital anomalies of the anus and rectum. Dis Colon Rectum 15:135, 1972.

Taylor I & others: Anal continence following surgery for imperforate anus. J Pediatr Surg 8:497, 1973.

Wilkinson AW: Congenital anomalies of the anus and rectum. Arch Dis Child 47:960, 1972.

ACUTE APPENDICITIS

The incidence of acute appendicitis increases with age, and the disease is most frequent between the ages of 15 and 30. Luminal obstruction by fecaliths (25%) or parasites is a predisposing factor. The occurrence of appendicitis in association with enteric infections has been described.

Clinical Findings

A. Symptoms and Signs: The triad of persistent localized right lower quadrant pain, localized abdominal tenderness, and slight fever is strongly suggestive of appendicitis. Anorexia, vomiting, and constipation also occur. The clinical picture is often atypical, ie, generalized pain, tenderness around the umbilicus, and no leukocytosis. Diarrhea can substitute for constipation, and a subsiding upper respiratory tract infection may be found. Rectal examination should always be done. Since many infections give rise to symptoms mimicking appendicitis and since physical findings are often inconclusive, it is important to repeat examinations of the abdomen.

B. Laboratory Findings: Leukocytosis, seldom higher than 15,000/cu mm.

C. X-Ray Findings: A radiopaque fecalith can be detected on x-rays and is reportedly present in two-thirds of cases of ruptured appendix.

Differential Diagnosis

Since atypical cases are common, it is better to err on the side of laparotomy after ruling out the presence of intrathoracic infection (eg, pneumonia) or urinary tract infection.

Medical conditions other than pneumonia and urinary tract infections which give rise to an acute abdomen are listed below:

A. Intestinal: Salmonellosis, shigellosis, acute gastroenteritis, regional enteritis, chronic ulcerative colitis, amebiasis, ascariasis, food poisoning, megacolon, incarcerated hernia.

B. Extra-intestinal: Rheumatic fever, acute streptococcal infection, infectious lymphocytosis, porphyria, hyperlipidemia, etiocholanolone fever, familial Mediterranean fever, lead poisoning, Henoch-Schönlein purpura, pancreatitis.

Treatment

The only definitive treatment is appendectomy. When surgical facilities are not available, treat as for acute peritonitis.

Prognosis

Even when perforation occurs, the mortality rate is less than 1%.

Grosfeld JL, Weinberger M, Clatworthy HW: Acute appendicitis in the first 2 years of life. J Pediatr Surg 8:285, 1973.
Longino LA, Holder TM, Gross RE: Appendicitis in childhood. Pediatrics 22:238, 1958.
Othersen HB & others: Ruptured appendicitis in children: Continuing controversy over antibiotic combinations. J Pediatr Surg 11:405, 1976.

FOREIGN BODIES IN THE ALIMENTARY TRACT

Most foreign bodies pass through the esophagus and the rest of the gastrointestinal tract without difficulty, although anything longer than 3–5 cm may have difficulty passing the duodenal loop at the region of the ligament of Treitz. Foreign bodies lodged in the esophagus require immediate attention.

A reasonable rule is that if a foreign body remains distal to the pylorus in one location for longer than 5 days, surgical removal should be considered, especially if symptoms occur. Close observation and, preferably, hospitalization is urged for children who have swallowed open safety pins and long sharp objects.

Esophagoscopy will permit the removal of the majority of foreign bodies lodged in the esophagus. A Foley catheter introduced into the esophagus may obviate the need for endoscopy.

Brooks JW: Foreign bodies in the air and food passages. Ann Surg 175:720, 1972.
Brown EG, Hughes JP, Koenig HM: Removal of foreign bodies lodged in esophagus by a Foley catheter without endoscopy. Clin Pediatr (Phila) 11:468, 1972.
Spitz L: Management of ingested foreign bodies in childhood. Br Med J 4:469, 1971.

TRAUMATIC INJURIES OF THE GASTROINTESTINAL TRACT

Neonatal Period

Severe intra-abdominal injuries are rare in the newborn period. Listlessness, rapid respirations in conjunction with fullness of the abdomen, an abdominal mass, and rapidly developing anemia are characteristic symptoms. The incidence of trauma increases in proportion to the size of the infant and is perhaps higher in breech deliveries. A ruptured spleen usually gives rise to immediate signs. Subcapsular hematomas of the liver secondary to laceration of the liver are quite common, especially if there have been manual attempts at resuscitation. Kidney injuries give rise to retroperitoneal hematomas. Peritoneal taps are helpful in making a diagnosis and deciding whether emergency surgery is indicated. If the peritoneal fluid is bloody, immediate surgery may be required.

Childhood

Trauma is the leading cause of death and disability in children. Accidents account for 40% of the annual total of deaths of children and adolescents. Motor vehicles are responsible for 40% of the fatalities.

Abdominal trauma is found in many children brought to the hospital following serious injury. Blunt abdominal trauma gives rise to little external evidence of internal injury, and multiple injuries may distract the examiner from the abdominal injury. Solid organs are more seriously and frequently injured than hollow viscera. Contusion of the pancreas may lead to acute pancreatitis or, later, a pseudocyst. Intramural hematomas in the duodenum or at the duodenojejunal junction are frequently seen in the battered child syndrome.

Gornall P & others: Intra-abdominal injuries in battered baby syndrome. Arch Dis Child 47:211, 1974.
Hood JM, Smyth BT: Nonpenetrating intraabdominal injuries in children. J Pediatr Surg 9:69, 1974.
Sinclair MC & others: Injury to hollow abdominal viscera from blunt trauma in children and adolescents. Am J Surg 128:693, 1974.

ANAL FISSURE

Anal fissure consists of a slit-like tear in the anal canal usually secondary to the passage of large, hard, dry fecal masses (scybala). Anal stenosis and trauma can be contributory factors.

The infant or child cries with defecation and will try to hold back his stools, resulting in increasing constipation. Sparse, bright red bleeding usually follows defecation. The fissure can be seen if the patient is held in a knee-chest position and the buttocks spread apart.

When a fissure cannot be identified, it is essential to rule out other causes of rectal bleeding.

Anal fissures should be treated promptly, especially in infancy, to break the constipation-fissure-constipation cycle. Dioctyl sodium sulfosuccinate, 5–10 mg/kg/24 hours given with feedings, is usually effective against constipation. If this does not prove sufficient, 30 ml of mineral oil administered rectally with an ear syringe is advocated. The introduction of a gloved, lubricated finger twice daily lessens sphincter spasm. Hot sitz baths after defecation may be helpful. In rare cases, silver nitrate cauterization may be necessary. In protracted cases, surgery is indicated.

Arminski TC, MacLean DW: Proctologic problems in children. JAMA 194:1195, 1965.
Beck AR, Turell R: Pediatric proctology. Surg Clin North Am 52:1055, 1972.

INTUSSUSCEPTION

Essentials of Diagnosis

- Paroxysmal, episodic abdominal pain and vomiting.
- Sausage-shaped mass in upper abdomen.
- Rectal passage of bloody mucus.
- Barium enema evidence of intussusception.

General Considerations

Intussusception is the most frequent cause of intestinal obstruction in the first 2 years of life. It is 3 times more common in males than in females. In most cases the cause is not apparent, although polyps, Meckel's diverticulum, Henoch-Schönlein purpura, lymphomas, constipation, parasites, and foreign bodies are predisposing factors. Intussusception is relatively common in cystic fibrosis and usually relates to inspissated fecal material in the terminal ileum and colon.

In most instances the intussusception starts at a point immediately proximal to the ileocecal valve, so that invagination is usually ileocolic. Other forms include ileo-ileal and colo-colic. Swelling, hemorrhage, incarceration with necrosis, and eventual perforation and peritonitis occur as a result of impairment of venous return.

Clinical Findings

Characteristically, a previously thriving infant between the ages of 3 months and 1 year suddenly develops periodic abdominal pain with screaming and drawing up of the knees. Vomiting occurs soon afterward, and bloody bowel movements with mucus appear within the next 12 hours. Severe prostration and fever supervene, and the abdomen is tender and becomes distended. On palpation, a sausage-shaped tumor may be found in the early stages. In rare cases, diarrhea is an early symptom.

The intussusception can also persist for several days when obstruction is not complete, and such cases may present as separate attacks of enterocolitis. In older children, sudden attacks of abdominal pain may be related to chronic recurrent intussusception with spontaneous reduction.

Treatment

A. Conservative Measures: The use of barium enema in the treatment of intussusception is still controversial. It is a safe procedure if the following recommendations are observed.

1. No attempt should be made at hydrostatic reduction if there are clinical signs of strangulated bowel, perforation, or severe toxicity.

2. The barium solution should be allowed to drip by gravity through a Foley bag catheter inserted in the rectum from a height not more than 3½ feet above the fluoroscopy table.

3. There should be no manipulation of the abdomen during hydrostatic reduction under fluoroscopic examination for fear of increasing intraluminal pressure

and thus the risk of perforation.

4. Upon reduction, there should be free reflux of barium into the ileum; this is better elicited in a post-evacuation film, which should be repeated in 24 hours.

B. Surgical Measures: For patients with intussusception who are not suitable for hydrostatic reduction or for those in whom it is unsuccessful (25%), surgery is performed as soon as the patient has been adequately prepared. Surgery has the advantage of demonstrating any lead point (such as Meckel's diverticulum), which occurs in 5% of cases. It may be also that surgical correction is associated with a lower recurrence rate.

Prognosis

Intussusception is almost uniformly fatal if untreated. The prognosis directly relates to the duration of the intussusception before reduction. The overall mortality rate is about 1–2%.

Ein SH: Leading points in childhood intussusception. J Pediatr Surg 12:367, 1977.

Gierup J, Jorulf H, Livaditis A: Management of intussusception in infants and children: A survey based on 288 consecutive cases. Pediatrics 50:535, 1972.

Rees BI, Lari J: Chronic intussusception in children. Br J Surg 63:33, 1976.

Rosenkrantz JG & others: Intussusception in the 1970's: Indications for operation. J Pediatr Surg 12:367, 1977.

Wayne ER & others: Management of 344 children with intussusception. Radiology 107:597, 1973.

INGUINAL HERNIA

A peritoneal sac precedes the testicle as it descends from the genital ridge to the scrotum. The lower portion of this sac envelops the testis to form the tunica vaginalis, and the remainder normally atrophies by the time of birth. Persistence of the processus vaginalis presents as a mass in the inguinal region when an abdominal structure or peritoneal fluid is forced into it. The persistent sac may be very short or may extend into the scrotum. In some cases, peritoneal fluid may become trapped in the tunica vaginalis of the testis (noncommunicating hydrocele). If the processus vaginalis remains open, peritoneal fluid (hydrocele of the spermatic cord, or of the canal of Nuck in the female) or an abdominal structure may be forced into it (indirect inguinal hernia).

Most inguinal hernias are of the indirect type and occur much more frequently in boys than in girls (9:1). Hernias may be present at birth or may appear at any age thereafter.

Clinical Findings

There are no symptoms associated with an empty hernial sac. In most cases, the hernia is a painless inguinal swelling varying in size. There may be a history of inguinal fullness associated with coughing or with long periods in the standing position; or there may be a firm, globular, and tender swelling, sometimes associated with vomiting and abdominal distention.

Spontaneous reduction frequently occurs while sleeping or with mild external pressure. In some instances, a herniated loop of intestine may become partially obstructed, leading to pain, irritability, and incomplete intestinal obstruction. More rarely, the loop of bowel becomes incarcerated, and signs of complete intestinal obstruction are present. In the female, the ovary may prolapse into the hernial sac.

Inspection of the 2 inguinal areas may reveal a characteristic bulging or mass. After crying in the infant or after bearing down in the older child, the patient should be observed for evidence of swelling.

A suggestive history is often the only criterion for diagnosis, along with the "silk glove" feel of the rubbing together of the 2 walls of the empty hernia sac.

Differential Diagnosis

An inguinal mass may represent lymph nodes. They are usually multiple and more discrete. Hydrocele of the cord transilluminates. An undescended testis may be moved along the canal and is associated with absence of the testicle in the scrotum.

Treatment

Surgical treatment is indicated in all cases. There is still some controversy about the advisability of exploration of the opposite side. Herniography is helpful in determining the patency of the processus vaginalis, but patency does not necessarily lead to a hernia.

Incarcerated inguinal hernias occur most often in the first 10 months of life and are more common in girls than in boys. Manipulative reduction can be attempted after placing the sedated infant in the Trendelenburg position with an ice bag on the affected side. This conservative treatment is contraindicated if the incarcerated hernia has been present for more than 12 hours or if bloody stools are noted.

James PM: The problem of hernia in infants and children. Surg Clin North Am 51:136, 1971.

Keeley JL: Hernias and related problems in infants and children. Postgrad Med 53:169, March 1973.

Rowe MI, Clatworthy HW: The other side of the pediatric inguinal hernia. Surg Clin North Am 51:1371, 1971.

UMBILICAL HERNIA

The incidence of umbilical hernia is higher in premature than in full-term infants, in whom the frequency has been estimated to be 20%. This defect is more common in black infants.

Excessive thinning of the skin distended by the hernia and progressive enlargement of the fascial defects are reported very rarely unless there is increased intra-abdominal pressure due to organomegaly or ascites. Incarceration is the only dangerous problem and is limited to smaller hernias.

Most umbilical hernias heal spontaneously if the fascial defect has a diameter of less than 1 cm. Large defects (greater than 2 cm) may still disappear without treatment, but seldom before school age. Large defects and smaller hernias persisting up to school age should be treated surgically. Reducing the hernia and strapping the skin drawn together into a longitudinal fold over the umbilical ring does not accelerate the healing process.

Walker SH: The natural history of umbilical hernias. Clin Pediatr (Phila) 6:29, 1967.

TUMORS OF THE GASTROINTESTINAL TRACT

1. JUVENILE POLYPS

Juvenile polyps are nearly always pedunculated and solitary with a stalk covered by colonic mucosa. The chorion is hyperplastic and inflamed. The glandular portion shows branching, irregular proliferation, and cystic transformation. The polyps are always benign. Eighty percent are within reach of the sigmoidoscope and are solitary. There are a few cases of generalized gastrointestinal juvenile polyposis involving the stomach and both the small and large bowel.

Polyps are rare before age 1, but their incidence increases thereafter and reaches a maximum frequency between 4 and 5 years of age. They are uncommon after age 15 because of auto-amputation and self-destruction. They are more frequent in boys. Bright red blood in the stools, intermittent melena, and occult painless gastrointestinal bleeding with anemia are the most frequent manifestations. Abdominal pain is infrequent, but a juvenile polyp can be the lead point for an intussusception. Rectal examination, sigmoidoscopy, and barium enema are essential to a full exploration for polyps.

A polyp accessible by sigmoidoscope should be removed for biopsy. If histology confirms that it is a juvenile polyp, nothing further should be done. In the event that 3 or 4 polyps are seen above the rectosigmoid, laparotomy is recommended. Otherwise, treatment is conservative.

The prognosis is excellent, since retention polyps are never malignant and since there is a high incidence of auto-amputation.

Franklin R, McSwain B: Juvenile polyps of the colon and rectum. Ann Surg 175:887, 1972.
Toccalino H & others: Juvenile polyps of the rectum and colon. Acta Paediatr Scand 62:337, 1973.

2. FAMILIAL POLYPOSIS

This condition is characterized by the presence in the colon of large numbers of adenomatous polyps varying in size from mucosal excrescences to large stalked polyps. A family history is obtained in roughly two-thirds of cases, and the entity is transmitted genetically as a dominant with reduced penetrance. Carcinoma of the colon usually develops before age 40, or approximately 15 years after onset of symptoms.

The disease has been identified in infants but is more likely to become symptomatic in the late teens. Diarrhea is usually the first symptom. Blood loss, anemia, and abdominal pain usually supervene. The initial symptoms may be those of carcinomatosis.

Sigmoidoscopy reveals great numbers of polyps of various sizes. Barium enema reveals a normal bowel wall but a great number of filling defects.

All members of the family should be carefully examined. Subtotal colectomy has been recommended, but many authors believe that keeping the rectal stump is dangerous since carcinoma may develop despite frequent observation of the stump. Proctocolectomy with an ileostomy is the treatment of choice, since any individual with familial polyposis will eventually develop carcinoma of the colon if untreated.

Abramson DJ: Multiple polyposis in children. Surgery 61:288, 1967.
Schnug GE: Familial polyposis of the colon. Am Surg 37:449, 1971.

3. PEUTZ-JEGHERS SYNDROME

The polyps in this syndrome are classified as hamartomas. They may occur anywhere between the cardiac sphincter and the anus but occur most often in the small intestine. Mucosal pigmentation is necessary to establish the diagnosis; it usually appears at birth or in infancy and has a tendency to lessen at puberty. The lips and buccal mucosa are usually involved. The syndrome is inherited as an autosomal dominant trait.

Colicky abdominal pain, anemia, and gastrointestinal hemorrhage are common symptoms. Intussusception may occur.

Conservative treatment is advocated. Symptomatic and accessible lesions should be removed surgically. Carcinomatous change has been reported.

McKittrick JE & others: The Peutz-Jeghers syndrome. Arch Surg 103:57, 1971.
Yosowitz P & others: Sporadic Peutz-Jeghers syndrome in early childhood. Am J Dis Child 128:709, 1974.

4. GARDNER'S SYNDROME

This is a dominantly inherited condition consisting of soft tissue and bone tumors associated with multiple intestinal polyps predisposed to malignant change. The large bowel is the most common site of involvement. Management should be directed at early detection of adenocarcinoma of the bowel. All members of an affected family should be examined periodically.

Duncan BR, Dohner VA, Priest JH: Gardner syndrome: Need for early diagnosis. J Pediatr 72:497, 1968.

5. CANCER OF THE SMALL & LARGE INTESTINES

The most common small bowel malignancy in children is lymphosarcoma. Intermittent abdominal pain, an abdominal mass, evidence of intestinal obstruction, or a celiac-like picture may be present. Long-term survivals are reported in patients without lymph node involvement at surgery.

Carcinoid tumors of the small intestine and appendix are usually of low-grade malignancy and rarely show the classical syndrome of diarrhea, asthma, and flushing of the face.

Adenocarcinoma of the colon is rare in the pediatric age group. The transverse colon and rectosigmoid are the 2 most commonly affected sites. The low 5-year survival has to do with the nonspecificity of presenting complaints and the large percentage of undifferentiated types. Children with chronic ulcerative colitis or with familial polyposis are at greater risk but seldom develop cancer before age 20. Cancer of the colon usually develops in a previously intact colon.

Cain AD, Longino LA: Carcinoma of the colon in children. J Pediatr Surg 5:527, 1970.

Recalde M & others: Carcinoma of the colon, rectum, and anal canal in young patients. Surg Gynecol Obstet 139:909, 1974.

6. MESENTERIC CYSTS

These tumors are rare in infants and children. They may be small or large, and single or multiloculated. Invariably thin-walled, they contain either serous, chylous, or hemorrhagic fluid. They are commonly located in the mesentery of the small intestine but may also be seen in the mesocolon.

The majority of these cysts are asymptomatic and come to medical attention when the parents note an increase in abdominal girth. However, traction on the mesentery eventually leads to pain in a high percentage of patients. The abdominal discomfort can be mild and recurrent but may present very acutely and lead to vomiting. Volvulus is reported. A rounded mass can occasionally be palpated, and is noted on x-ray to displace adjacent intestine.

Surgical removal is indicated and often includes resection of the adjacent intestine because of a blood supply problem.

Caropreso PR: Mesenteric cysts. Arch Surg 108:242, 1974.

Hardin WJ, Hardy JD: Mesenteric cysts. Am J Surg 119:640, 1970.

THE IRRITABLE COLON SYNDROME

This is the most common cause of chronic diarrhea in the otherwise well and thriving child. The typical patient with irritable colon syndrome is a child 6–20 months of age who was a colicky baby and who starts having 3–6 loose mucoid stools per day during the waking hours. The child is active, looks healthy, has a good appetite, and is growing normally. The diarrhea is made worse by a low-residue diet and during periods of stress and infection. It clears spontaneously at about 3½ years of age. No organic disease is discoverable. The pathogenesis of the disease remains obscure. A high familial incidence of functional bowel disease is observed.

Between meal snacks and elimination of chilled fluids are helpful. Early toilet training is recommended. Dietary restriction of residues tends to increase the number of loose stools. Although bile acids are not excreted in large amounts, cholestyramine can sometimes be beneficial.

Davidson M: Nonspecific diarrhea syndrome. Page 192 in: *Current Pediatric Therapy 6.* Gellis SS, Kagan BM (editors). Saunders, 1973.

Davidson M, Wasserman R: The irritable colon of childhood. J Pediatr 69:1027, 1966.

DIARRHEAL DISEASES*

Diarrhea may be defined as water and electrolyte malabsorption leading to accelerated excretion of intestinal contents. What constitutes diarrhea is sometimes difficult to define in terms of number or consistency of stools because there are wide variations in

*Epidemic diarrhea of the newborn is discussed in Chapter 3; diarrhea due to viral infections, in Chapter 25; diarrhea due to bacterial infections, in Chapter 26; and diarrhea due to parasitic infections, in Chapter 27.

Table 16—1. Etiologic classification of diarrhea.*

Type of Disorder	Etiologic Basis
Infections	
Enteral	
Bacterial	Pathogenic *Escherichia coli,* shigellosis, salmonellosis, *Staphylococcus aureus, Clostridium perfringens, Vibrio parahaemolyticus,* yersinia, cholera.
Viral	Adenoviruses, enteroviruses, orbiviruses, Norwalk agent.
Parasitic	Amebiasis, giardiasis, ascariasis.
Parenteral	Urinary tract and upper respiratory tract infections.
Inflammatory bowel diseases	Regional enteritis, chronic ulcerative colitis, Whipple's disease, necrotizing enterocolitis of the newborn, nonspecific enterocolitis of infancy.
Anatomic and mechanical causes	Short bowel syndrome, fistula, postgastrectomy, blind loop syndrome, partial duodenal or ileojejunal obstruction, malrotation, Hirschsprung's disease, intestinal lymphangiectasis.
Pancreatic and hepatic disorders	Cirrhosis, hepatitis, biliary atresia, chronic pancreatitis, pancreatic exocrine deficiency, pancreatic hypoplasia.
Biochemical causes	Celiac disease, cystic fibrosis of the pancreas, disaccharidase deficiency, glucose-galactose malabsorption, abetalipoproteinemia, folic acid deficiency, congenital chloridorrhea with alkalosis, ·acrodermatitis enteropathica.
Neoplastic causes	Carcinoid, ganglioneuroma, Zollinger-Ellison syndrome, polyposis, lymphoma, adenocarcinoma.
Immunologic deficiencies	Ataxia-telangiectasia, Wiskott-Aldrich syndrome, agammaglobulinemia, dysgammaglobulinemia, thymic alymphoplasia and dysplasia.
Endocrinopathies	Hyperthyroidism, congenital adrenal hyperplasia.
Malnutrition	Protein malnutrition (kwashiorkor), protein-calorie malnutrition (marasmus).
Dietary factors	Overfeeding, introduction of new foods.
Food allergy	Milk colitis, allergic gastroenteropathy.
Psychogenic or functional disorders	Irritable colon syndrome.
Toxic diarrhea	Ingestion of heavy metals (eg, arsenic, lead), antibiotics, ferrous sulfate, organic phosphates.

*Slightly modified and reproduced, with permission, from Silverman A, Roy CC, Cozzetto F: *Pediatric Clinical Gastroenterology.* Mosby, 1971.

colonic function. Some infants may pass one firm stool every second to third day, whereas others may have 5—8 soft small stools daily. A gradual or sudden increase in the number of stools, a reduction in their consistency coupled with an increase in their fluid content, or a tendency for the stools to be green are more important factors.

Diarrhea may result from any of the following closely related pathogenetic mechanisms: (1) Interruption of normal cell transport processes. (2) Decrease in the surface area available for absorption by shortening of the bowel or mucosal disease. (3) Increase in intestinal motility. (4) Presence in the intestine of large amounts of unabsorbable osmotically active molecules. (5) Abnormal increase in gastric or intestinal permeability, leading to increased secretion of water and electrolytes.

The physiologic consequences of diarrhea vary with its severity and duration, the age of the patient and his state of nutrition prior to onset, and the presence or absence of associated symptoms. Acute diarrhea may lead to dehydration and acid-base disturbances (see Chapter 35). Chronic diarrhea leads to malnutrition.

Causes of Diarrhea Other Than Infectious Gastroenteritis

A. Antibiotic Therapy: Antibiotics such as ampicillin, neomycin, and tetracyclines commonly give rise to diarrhea. They lead to decreased glucose absorption and disaccharidase activity. In a clinical setting where a bacterial infection has been ruled out, they should be stopped and a lactose-free diet administered. At times, antibiotics may give rise to the overgrowth of microorganisms resistant to the antibiotic being given for acute colitis (particularly lincomycin and clindamycin) or for pseudomembranous colitis.

B. Parenteral Infections: Infections of the urinary tract and upper respiratory tract (especially otitis media) are at times associated with diarrhea, although the actual mechanism remains obscure. In the opinion of several investigators, a concomitant intestinal infection is likely.

C. Malnutrition: Malnutrition may lead to diarrhea because of an increased occurrence of enteral infections in malnourished children. Decreased disaccharidase activity, altered motility, or changes in the intestinal flora may be other factors.

D. Diet: Dietary causes of diarrhea are numerous.

Overfeeding of a colicky infant is a common example. Introduction of new foods such as fruit juices, egg yolk, vegetables, etc can cause diarrhea. Intestinal irritants (spices and foods high in roughage) are also frequent offenders.

E. Allergic Diarrhea: Diarrhea caused by gastrointestinal allergy to dietary proteins is a frequently entertained diagnosis but a poorly documented clinical entity except in cases of milk allergy, which is discussed separately.

Intractable Diarrhea of Early Infancy

A. Symptoms and Signs: The onset is within the first 3 months of life. The benign initial phase is sometimes mistaken for a feeding problem. In most cases, however, it mimics an infectious diarrhea with loose, greenish stools. The stools are rarely grossly bloody, but microscopic blood is often present. Vomiting and abdominal distention are features which suggest an underlying obstructive lesion. Dehydration, acidosis, and malnutrition rapidly supervene. After "resting the gastrointestinal tract" by means of intravenous therapy, resumption of oral feedings invariably precipitates a recurrence.

B. Diagnosis: Conditions such as enterocolitis associated with Hirschsprung's disease, cystic fibrosis, intestinal stenosis, malrotation, blind loop syndrome, short small bowel syndrome, allergic gastroenteropathy, celiac disease, disaccharidase deficiency, immunologic defects, lymphangiectasia, adrenogenital syndrome, neural crest tumors, glucose-galactose malabsorption, sepsis, urinary tract infections, and chloridorrhea may all lead to intractable diarrhea. These diagnoses and infectious gastroenteritis can be verified or ruled out by the following emergency workup:

(1) Stool cultures (3).
(2) Stool pH.
(3) Tests for fecal blood and reducing substances.
(4) Barium enema, upper gastrointestinal x-ray with small bowel follow-through.
(5) Blood count with small lymphocyte count.
(6) Blood pH and electrolytes.
(7) Sweat chloride test.
(8) Stool chymotrypsin.
(9) Protein electrophoresis and serum immunoglobulins.
(10) Rectosigmoidoscopy and rectal suction biopsy.

If these conditions are ruled out in a young infant who still has diarrhea after 3 weeks and is steadily losing weight, a primary type of intractable diarrhea (nonspecific enterocolitis) becomes the most likely diagnosis.

C. Treatment: Fasting is recommended during the first few days while blood volume, electrolyte, and acid-base disturbances are repaired. A diet free of milk, proteins, and lactose is then recommended. Reasonable success has been obtained with a medium chain triglyceride and glucose-containing formula such as Pregestimil. In most cases, either peripheral parenteral or central parenteral alimentation becomes necessary.

Hyman CJ & others: Parenteral and oral alimentation in the treatment of the nonprotracted diarrheal syndrome of infancy. J Pediatr 78:17, 1971.

Lloyd-Still JD, Shwachman H, Filler RM: Protracted diarrhea of infancy treated by intravenous alimentation. (2 parts.) Am J Dis Child 125:358, 365, 1973.

Roy CC, Silverman A, Cozzetto F: Chapter 8 in: *Pediatric Clinical Gastroenterology,* 2nd ed. Mosby, 1975.

Sunshine P & others: Intractable diarrhoea in infancy. Clin Gastroenterol 6:445, 1977.

CONSTIPATION

Constipation is the regular passage of firm or hard stools or of small, hard masses at extremely long intervals (obstipation). In its most severe form, it may be accompanied by fecal soiling or encopresis. Familial, cultural, and social factors influence the genesis, development, and course. Some children with constipation tend to absorb water from the rectum to a greater degree than control subjects. A few babies are constipated in the neonatal period and remain so despite a variety of formula changes. Psychologic factors, toilet training technics, diet (particularly excessive milk intake), overuse of laxatives, and enemas may also influence bowel habits.

Clinical Findings

Many symptoms, such as fever, convulsions, nervousness, school failure, bad breath, and the like have been improperly attributed to constipation.

A. Simple Constipation: The neonate or the infant often appears to be having difficulty passing a stool. His face may turn red, and the legs are drawn up on the abdomen even when the stool passed is quite soft. This pattern may be erroneously considered to be an indication of constipation. Similarly, the infant 6–12 months of age may become flushed, withdraw his legs, and act as though he is having a great deal of difficulty in passing a bowel movement when in fact he may be attempting to withhold a stool. Failure to appreciate this normal developmental pattern may lead to the unwise·use of laxatives or enemas. As the child becomes ambulatory, many new and exciting activities interfere with his response to the "call to stool"; he may pass enough stool to relieve the pressure while continuing to play, or may gradually develop an effective capacity to ignore the sensation of rectal fullness. In the older child, school, games, social events, and such aesthetic factors as inadequately cleaned toilets outside the home may all interfere with the development of any pattern of regularity.

B. Constipation With Encopresis: The constant or intermittent involuntary seepage of feces is characteristic of psychogenic constipation, where there is a mass of feces in the rectal ampulla and sigmoid colon. Children affected by psychogenic constipation suffer from emotional disturbances that commonly disappear

Table 16—2. Differentiation of constipation and Hirschsprung's disease.

	Constipation	Hirschsprung's Disease
Onset	2—3 years	At birth
Abdominal distention	Rarely	Present
Nutritional growth	Normal	Poor
Soiling	Intermittent or constant	Never
Rectal examination	Ampulla full	Ampulla empty

with relief of the constipation. However in certain cases, emotional problems may lead to psychogenic constipation.

Differential Diagnosis

Constipation is prevalent among mentally retarded children, particularly those with associated motor deficits. Hypothyroidism is frequently accompanied by constipation, but constipation is usually not the presenting complaint. Stenosis of the anal canal and anal fissure are among the local conditions which must be ruled out.

Distinguishing features from Hirschsprung's disease are summarized in Table 16—2. It should be remembered, however, that rare cases of short segment aganglionosis may present with symptoms and signs suggestive of chronic constipation with encopresis.

Treatment

A. Simple Constipation: A reduction of milk intake and of high-residue foods such as bran, whole wheat, fruits, and vegetables is usually curative. The use of a barley malt extract such as Maltsupex, 1—2 tsp added to feedings 2 or 3 times daily, is helpful in small infants. Stool softeners such as dioctyl sodium sulfosuccinate (Colace), 5—10 mg/kg/day, prevent excessive drying of the stool and are effective unless there is voluntary stool retention. Cathartics such as standardized extract of senna fruit (Senokot Syrup), 1—2 tsp twice daily depending on age, can be used for short periods of time.

B. Constipation With Encopresis: Remove the fecal impaction by the administration of hypertonic phosphate enemas (Fleet Enema) after overnight retention of 3—4 oz mineral oil.

Mineral oil in orange juice should be given in amounts sufficient initially (15 ml 3—5 times a day) to lead to incontinence; it should then be reduced so that 2—3 loose stools are passed daily.

The prevention of stool holding and the establishment of a regular soft bowel movement pattern is accomplished by "toileting" the child at regular times each day and by the continued administration of mineral oil over a period of several months in a reduced

dosage. A double dose of water-soluble vitamins is recommended while mineral oil is administered. After this initial phase, the use of a stool softener (Colace, 5—10 mg/kg/24 hours) should be administered on a chronic basis but not before regular toilet habits have been acquired.

Psychiatric consultation may be indicated in cases with recurrent symptoms and in those where there are overt, severe emotional disturbances.

Bently JFR: Constipation in infants and children. Gut 12:85, 1971.

Fitzgerald JF: Difficulties with defecation and elimination in children. Clin Gastroenterol 6:283, 1977.

Levine MD: Children with encopresis: A descriptive analysis. Pediatrics 56:412, 1975.

GASTROINTESTINAL BLEEDING

Vomiting or rectal evacuation of blood is an alarming symptom which will be promptly brought to the physician's attention. The history should provide detailed answers to the following questions:

(1) *Is it really blood and is it coming from the gastrointestinal tract?* A number of substances may simulate hematochezia or melena; therefore, the presence of blood should be confirmed chemically (Hematest tablet). Information concerning genitourinary problems, coughing, or epistaxis may identify a source of bleeding elsewhere than in the gastrointestinal tract.

(2) *How much blood is there and what is its color and character?* Table 16—3 lists the site of gastrointestinal bleeding in relationship to the amount and the appearance of the blood in the stools.

(3) *Is the child acutely or chronically ill?* The physical examination should be thorough no matter how ill the patient is. Alertness to signs of portal

Table 16—3. Identification of sites of gastrointestinal bleeding.

Symptom or Sign	Location of Bleeding Lesion
Effortless welling forth of bright red blood from the mouth	Esophageal varices.
Vomiting of bright red blood or of "coffee grounds"	Lesion proximal to ligament of Treitz.
Melena	Lesion proximal to ligament of Treitz. Blood loss in excess of 50—100 ml/24 hours.
Bright red or dark red blood in stools	Lesion in the ileum or colon. (Massive upper gastrointestinal bleeding may also be associated with bright red blood in stool.)
Streak of blood on outside of a stool	Lesion in the rectal ampulla or anal canal.

hypertension, intestinal obstruction, or blood dyscrasia is particularly important. The nasal passages should be inspected for signs of recent epistaxis; the vagina for menstrual blood; and the anus for fissures and hemorrhoids.

It is particularly important to assess the hemodynamic status of the patient. A systolic blood pressure below 100 mm Hg and a pulse rate above 100/minute in an older child suggest at least a 20% reduction of blood volume. A pulse rate increase of 20/minute or a drop in systolic blood pressure greater than 10 mm Hg on the patient's sitting up is a sensitive index of significant volume depletion.

(4) *Is the child still bleeding?* A determination of vital signs every 15 minutes is essential to assess ongoing bleeding. Serial hematocrits are useful—remembering, however, that plasma expansion subsequent to a loss of red cell mass may be delayed for hours and sometimes for days.

The most important maneuver for the assessment of the origin and severity of gastrointestinal bleeding is the introduction of a Levine tube in the stomach. Detection of blood in the gastric aspirate confirms a bleeding site proximal to the ligament of Treitz. However, its absence does not rule out the duodenum as the source.

Management

Blood should be drawn to rule out a hemorrhagic diathesis, and vitamin K should be given intravenously. Needs for volume replacement are best monitored by measurement of central venous pressure. In less severe cases, vital signs, serial hematocrits, and gastric aspirates are sufficient.

If blood is recovered from the gastric aspirate, gastric lavage should be performed with ice water until only a blood-tinged return is obtained. Panendoscopy is then done and is particularly useful for identifying an active bleeding site; it is superior to barium contrast study for lesions such as esophageal varices, stress ulcers, and gastritis. In cases where there has been no clinical evidence of ongoing bleeding during the 48 hours preceding admission, the upper gastrointestinal series is usually carried out as the initial diagnostic procedure. It is followed by the endoscopic procedure if the lesion is unidentified radiologically.

Except for Meckel's diverticulum, most bleeding small bowel lesions also produce intestinal obstruction. A flat film of the abdomen and a barium enema should be done in such cases prior to laparotomy. If there is no obstruction and the bleeding seemingly comes from the colon or lower ileum, rectosigmoidoscopy is done prior to barium enema. In the case of a nonobstructing small or large bowel lesion which bleeds actively and briskly (over 0.5 ml/min), angiography may be helpful. The patient with upper gastrointestinal bleeding should be maintained in a semisitting position and a calm environment. Sedation is contraindicated. Ongoing bleeding is an indication for vasopressin, 20 units per 1.73 sq m IV over a 20-minute period. Selective arterial infusion of vasopressin can also be used. It is

rarely necessary to use a pediatric Sengstaken-Blakemore tube in cases of bleeding esophageal varices.

The challenging patients are those with cirrhosis and abnormal clotting mechanisms. Emergency shunt operations are at times inevitable. Surgical treatment is also warranted in peptic disease and stress ulcers when severe ongoing bleeding continues over several days despite conservative management.

Barany F, Nilsson LHS: Diagnostic procedure in bleeding of obscure origin from the alimentary canal. Gut 11:307, 1970.

Berman WF & others: Gastrointestinal hemorrhage. Pediatr Clin North Am 23:885, 1975.

Fonkalsrud RW, Myer NA, Robinson NJ: Management of extrahepatic portal hypertension in children. Ann Surg 180:488, 1974.

Identifying the cause of gastrointestinal bleeding. (Editorial.) Lancet 2:415, 1971.

RECURRENT ABDOMINAL PAIN

In one survey, one out of 9 unselected school children had experienced at least 3 attacks of recurrent abdominal pain severe enough to affect their activities over a period longer than 3 months. An organic cause can be found in fewer than 10% of cases, and there is usually evidence that the pain is a reaction to emotional stress. The age at onset is usually between 5 and 10 years. The incidence in boys is slightly higher than in girls.

Clinical Findings

A. Symptoms and Signs: Recurrent attacks of umbilical or periumbilical pain last less than 24 hours, usually only about an hour. There may be associated pallor, nausea, vomiting, and slight fever. The pain seldom radiates. An organic cause is suggested by a change in the pattern of the attack, a negative history of colic as a baby, diarrhea, vomiting in infancy, and absence of associated emotional problems or a family history of migraine. The farther the pain is from the umbilicus, the more likely it is that an organic cause will be found. Emotional disturbances are common, with undue fears, enuresis, sleeping problems, food dislikes, and difficulties in school. It is necessary to examine the patient thoroughly both between attacks and during an attack.

The pain bears little relationship with bowel habits and activity. At times, it may occur during meals or before the child leaves for school. A definite precipitating or particularly stressful situation in the child's life at the time the pains began can sometimes be elicited. A history of functional gastrointestinal complaints and migraine headaches is found in the family members of a large number of "little bellyachers."

A thorough physical examination is essential. Abdominal tenderness, if present, is diffuse and mild,

Table 16–4. Differential diagnosis and treatment of rectal bleeding in infants and children.

Cause	Usual Age Group	Additional Complaints	Amount of Blood	Color of Blood	Blood With Movement	Treatment
Swallowed foreign body	Any age	Usually none.	Small	Dark	Yes	Surgery may be necessary.
Systemic bleeding	Any age	Other evidence of bleeding.	Variable	Dark or bright	Yes or no	As indicated.
Hemorrhagic disease of the newborn	Newborn	Other evidence of bleeding.	Variable	Dark or bright	Yes or no	Vitamin K_1, transfusion.
Allergy (milk)	Infants	Colicky abdominal pain.	Moderate to large	Dark or bright	Yes	Eliminate allergen.
Esophageal varices	>4 years	Signs of portal hypertension.	Variable	Usually dark	Yes	Medical initially; sometimes emergency surgery.
Hemangioma or familial telangiectasia	Any age	Often telangiectasia elsewhere.	Variable	Dark or bright	Yes or no	Usually none.
Peptic ulcer	Any age	Abdominal pain.	Usually small; can be massive.	Dark	Yes	Bland diet.
Duplication of bowel	Any age	Variable.	Usually small	Usually dark	Yes	Surgery.
Meckel's diverticulum	Young adult	None or anemia.	Small to large; usually large.	Dark or bright	Yes or no	Surgery.
Volvulus	Infant or young child	Abdominal pain, intestinal obstruction.	Small to large	Dark or bright	Yes or no	Surgery.
Intussusception	<18 months	Abdominal pain, mass.	Small to large	Dark or bright	Yes	Surgery.
Ulcerative colitis	>4 years	Diarrhea, cramps.	Small to large	Usually bright	Yes	Usually medical.
Bacterial enteritis	Any age	Diarrhea, cramps.	Small to large	Usually bright	Yes	Medical.
Polyp	2–8 years	None.	Small to large	Bright	No	Surgery.
Inserted foreign body	Child	Pain.	Small	Bright	No	Removal.
Anal fissure or proctitis	<2 years	Pain.	Small	Bright	No	Soften stool, anal dilatation, habit training.
Swallowed maternal blood	Newborn	None.	Variable	Dark	Yes	None.
Hiatal hernia	Any age	Dysphagia, hematemesis.	Usually small	Dark	Yes	Medical or surgical.

although discomfort over the descending colon is common.

B. Laboratory and X-Ray Findings: Complete blood count, sedimentation rate, urinalysis, stool test for occult blood, and tuberculin testing usually suffice. If the syndrome is somewhat atypical, urine cultures, intravenous urography, voiding cystography, barium enema, and upper gastrointestinal x-rays should be done.

Differential Diagnosis

Organic causes relating to the urinary and gastrointestinal tracts, as well as extra-abdominal causes, should be ruled out by appropriate studies if the clinical evidence is suggestive. Oxyuriasis, "mesenteric lymphadenitis," and "chronic appendicitis" are improbable causes of recurrent abdominal pain. Milk intolerance due to lactose intolerance usually manifests itself by both pain and diarrhea. However, abdominal discomfort may at times be the only symptom. Abdominal migraine and abdominal epilepsy are truly rare conditions.

Treatment & Prognosis

Treatment consists of reassurance based on a thorough physical appraisal and a frank and sympathetic explanation of the emotional basis. More specialized therapy for the latter is sometimes required, but drugs should be avoided. The prognosis is good.

Apley J: Psychosomatic illness in children: A modern synthesis. Br Med J 2:756, 1973.

Apley J, Hale B: Children with recurrent abdominal pain: How do they grow up? Br Med J 3:7, 1973.

Bayless TM, Huang S-S: Recurrent abdominal pain due to milk and lactose intolerance in school aged children. Pediatrics 47:1029, 1971.

Deamer WC, Sandberg DH: Recurrent abdominal pain: Recurrent controversy. Pediatrics 51:307, 1973.

Stone RT, Barbero GJ: Recurrent abdominal pain in childhood. Pediatrics 45:732, 1970.

THE MALABSORPTION SYNDROMES

The majority of diseases causing malabsorption are diseases of the small intestine or conditions which affect its normal function. Not only should the small bowel be of sufficient length, but the mucosal surface area available for absorption must not be decreased beyond a certain minimum. Anatomic abnormalities and impaired motility of the small intestine will not only interfere with normal propulsive movements and mixing of food with pancreatic and biliary secretions; it can also lead to an altered bacterial flora, which may cause malabsorption. Impairment of portal venous return, anoxia, and lymphatic abnormalities are well described causes of malabsorption. Diseases interfering with pancreatic exocrine function and with the production and flow of biliary secretions can have the same effect. Other causes include disaccharidase deficiency, glucose-galactose malabsorption, abetalipoproteinemia, malnutrition, endocrine conditions, immune deficiencies, and emotional factors (maternal deprivation). Many others are listed in the references cited at the end of this section.

Clinical Findings

The chronologic sequence of events is of great importance in determining the onset of malabsorption problems and the relationship between symptoms and the introduction of various nutrients. Gastrointestinal symptoms such as diarrhea, vomiting, anorexia, abdominal pain, and bloating are not always present, and the presenting complaints may not refer to the gastrointestinal tract. Certain physical features such as the pot belly and the wasted buttocks may indicate celiac disease. Personal observation of the stools for abnormal color, consistency, bulkiness, odor, mucus, and blood is important. In general, the investigation of this complex syndrome involves both accurate clinical appraisal and the interpretation of appropriate laboratory data.

The following are the most helpful investigations:

(1) Fat absorption: Seventy-two-hour fecal fat excretion and coefficient of fat absorption, serum carotene, cholesterol, and prothrombin time.

(2) Protein absorption: Serum protein electrophoresis, fecal nitrogen, fecal excretion of chromated Cr 51 serum albumin (Chromalbin).

(3) Carbohydrate absorption: Glucose tolerance test, D-xylose absorption test, disaccharide absorption test, stool pH and reducing substances.

(4) Absorption of folic acid and vitamin B_{12}: Schilling test, serum levels of folic acid and vitamin B_{12}.

(5) Bacteriology: Stool, duodenal juice.

(6) X-ray studies: Upper gastrointestinal series with small bowel follow-through, barium enema, and bone age.

(7) Sweat test: Chloride determination.

(8) Pancreatic exocrine function: Duodenal aspirate examined for volume, viscosity, pH, bicarbonate, trypsin, lipase, and amylase activity.

(9) Liver function tests: Bilirubin, transaminases, alkaline phosphatase, sulfobromophthalein (BSP) excretion.

(10) Miscellaneous: Peroral small bowel biopsy, rectosigmoidoscopy and rectal biopsy, immunoglobulin levels, lipoprotein electrophoresis, urine catecholamines, endocrine function tests.

Treatment & Prognosis

See specific syndromes—celiac disease, disaccharidase deficiency, etc.

Ament ME: Malabsorption syndromes in infancy and childhood. (2 parts.) J Pediatr 81:685, 867, 1972.

Anderson CM: Malabsorption in children. Clin Gastroenterol 6:355, 1977.

PROTEIN-LOSING ENTEROPATHIES

Excessive loss of plasma proteins into the gastrointestinal tract occurs in association with a number of disorders, some of which are listed below.

Disorders Associated With Protein-Losing Enteropathy

A. Cardiac: Congestive heart failure, constrictive pericarditis, atrial septal defect, primary myocardial disease.

B. Gastric: Giant hypertrophic gastritis (Menetrier's disease).

C. Small Intestine: Celiac disease, intestinal lymphangiectasia, tropical sprue, regional enteritis, Whipple's disease, lymphosarcoma, acute gastrointestinal infection, allergic gastroenteropathy, blind loop syndrome, abetalipoproteinemia, chronic volvulus.

D. Colon: Ulcerative colitis, Hirschsprung's disease.

E. Immunologic deficiency states.

Clinical Findings

The clinical signs and symptoms identified with protein-losing enteropathies are many. These include edema, chylous ascites, poor weight gain, deficiencies of fat-soluble vitamins, hypochromic anemia, or megaloblastic anemia secondary to vitamin B_{12} or folic acid malabsorption. Most patients present with severe and long-standing gastrointestinal symptomatology. Although there is nonselective "bulk loss" of a number of plasma proteins into the enteric lumen, albumin is the most depressed of the plasma proteins and is usually below 2.5 gm/100 ml. A number of methods are available for the detection of increased catabolism of plasma proteins and their quantitation in the gut, but all have certain drawbacks. Normally, the gut probably plays only a minor role in albumin catabolism, and enhanced intestinal losses of protein are solely responsible for the hypoalbuminemia that occurs in a number of conditions leading to protein-losing enteropathies. It is likely, however, that an increased rate of endogenous albumin catabolism or a decreased rate of synthesis may be operative in systemic diseases in which protein-losing enteropathies occur. The simultaneous use of iodinated I 125 serum albumin to measure overall albumin catabolism and chromated Cr 51 serum albumin (Chromalbin) to measure gastrointestinal losses appears to be most informative.

Differential Diagnosis

Malnutrition as a cause of hypoproteinemia must be excluded. Since hypoalbuminemia may be due to either a lowered production or an increased catabolic rate, it is also important to rule out hepatic disease and to make certain that no significant proteinuria is present.

Treatment

Temporary benefits can be derived from plasma or albumin infusions in the presence of severe plasma loss and anasarca. Otherwise, treatment must be directed toward the primary underlying cause.

Rothschild MA & others: Albumin synthesis. (2 parts.) N Engl J Med 286:748, 816, 1972.

CELIAC DISEASE
(Gluten Enteropathy)

Essentials of Diagnosis

- Diarrhea and steatorrhea.
- Failure to thrive; loss of weight involving mostly the limbs and buttocks.
- Abdominal distention.
- Depressed rate of D-xylose absorption.
- Villous atrophy on small bowel biopsy.
- Improvement on gluten-free diet, and histologic relapse following reintroduction of gluten into the diet within a period of 2 years.
- Normal pancreatic and biliary secretions.

General Considerations

Celiac syndrome denotes the symptom complex resulting from intestinal malabsorption. Celiac disease is a specific disease entity associated with abnormal jejunal mucosa which improves with a strict gluten-free diet.

After cystic fibrosis, celiac disease is the most frequent cause of malabsorption in infants. Most cases present during the second year of life, but the age at onset and the severity are both variable. The disease is more common in Europe and in Canada than in the USA and is uncommon in blacks and Orientals.

The exact mechanism by which gluten exerts its toxicity is unknown. Several observations suggest that the toxic effect of gliadin, the alcohol-soluble fraction of gluten, is a result of immunologic injury to the epithelial cell. Recent organ culture studies convincingly show that gliadin does not adversely affect the enterocytes directly but first triggers a local immune reaction in susceptible individuals. However, additional studies are needed before the morphologic and functional gastrointestinal changes can be attributed to an abnormal immune response.

Clinical Findings

A. Symptoms and Signs:

1. Diarrhea–Affected children often present with a history of digestive disturbances starting at 6–12 months of age–corresponding to the age at which wheat, rye, or oat glutens are first fed. Initially, the diarrhea may be intermittent and related to upper respiratory infections. Subsequently, it is continuous, with voluminous, bulky, pale, frothy, greasy, offensive floating stools. During celiac crises, dehydration, shock, and acidosis are commonly seen. Diarrhea is absent in 10% of cases. Vomiting, abdominal pain, and signs of intestinal obstruction can dominate the clinical picture.

2. Constipation, vomiting, and abdominal pain–This triad of symptoms may in a small number of cases dominate the clinical picture and suggest a diagnosis of intestinal obstruction.

3. Failure to thrive–The onset of diarrhea is usually accompanied by loss of appetite, failure to gain weight, and increased irritability.

4. Wasting and retardation of growth–In established cases, there is a loss of weight which is most marked in the limbs and buttocks. Characteristically, the face remains plump and the abdomen becomes distended secondary to a poor musculature and, more importantly, to accumulation of gas and fluid in the hypotonic intestinal tract with altered peristaltic activity.

5. Anemia and vitamin deficiencies–Anemia is usually present; it is often unresponsive to iron and may be megaloblastic. Deficiencies in fat-soluble vitamins are common. Rickets can be seen when growth has not been completely halted by the disease; however, osteomalacia is more common, and pathologic fractures may occur. Hypoprothrombinemia can be severe, and some patients are known to present with severe intestinal hemorrhages.

B. Laboratory Findings:

1. Fat content of stools–A 3-day collection of stools for fat usually reveals more than 4.5 gm/day of fecal fat. However, steatorrhea may be absent in 10–25% of cases. It is important that a nonabsorbable marker, such as charcoal or brilliant blue, be given for accurate collection. A normal child will absorb 90–98% of ingested fats. The untreated celiac patient, on the other hand, will not absorb more than 65–85% of his daily fat intake.

2. Impaired carbohydrate absorption–A low oral glucose tolerance curve is seen. Absorption of D-xylose is impaired, with blood levels lower than 20 mg/100 ml at 60 and 90 minutes.

3. Hypoproteinemia–Hypoalbuminemia can be

severe enough to lead to edema. There is evidence of increased losses of protein in the gut lumen.

C. X-Ray Findings: A small bowel series can demonstrate a typical malabsorptive pattern characterized by segmentation, clumping of the barium column, and hypersecretion. These changes can be accentuated by addition of gluten to the barium meal.

D. Biopsy Findings: Peroral intestinal biopsy provides the only reliable evidence for the diagnosis of celiac disease. It is a safe and simple procedure even in infants. Hypoprothrombinemia and severe malnutrition, however, are absolute contraindications to this procedure.

A variety of biopsy capsules are available. The Carey capsule is the least likely to cause bleeding and perforation in debilitated infants.

Under the dissecting microscope, the jejunal mucosa presents a "crazy paving" appearance rather than the slender finger-like projections which characterize normal villi. Under the light microscope, the celiac mucosa is readily recognized by amputation of the villi, by lengthening of the crypts of Lieberkühn, and by increased round cell infiltration of the lamina propria. These changes are reversible, and a normal to nearly normal appearance of the lamina propria can be expected after withdrawal of gluten from the diet.

Differential Diagnosis

The differential diagnosis must include all of the disorders that cause malabsorption. Strict adherence to 2 diagnostic criteria—ie, the characteristic small bowel microscopic changes and clinical improvement on a gluten-free diet—is essential. Since gluten enteropathy is a lifelong disease whenever the mucosal lesion is not characteristic or the response to a gluten-free diet is not as good as expected, challenge with a gluten-containing diet is indicated. Biopsy should be performed if the patient becomes symptomatic or after 2 years if the child remains healthy and is growing well on a normal diet.

Treatment

A. Diet: Treatment consists of dietary gluten restriction for life. Dietary supervision is essential. The diet should provide 25% more calories than calculated for expected weight plus 6–8 gm/kg/day of protein. Lactose is poorly tolerated in the acute stage since the extensive mucosal damage leads to acquired disaccharidase deficiency. Normal amounts of fat are advisable.

In treating a severely affected child, the diet should be tailored to the child's appetite and capacity to absorb. A full gluten-free diet can usually be given after 2–3 weeks. Clinical improvement is usually evident within a week, and histologic repair is complete after 3 months.

B. Corticosteroids: Adrenal corticosteroid therapy can produce dramatic remissions in celiac disease. Corticosteroids are particularly useful in celiac crises and in the rare patients who continue to deteriorate despite the enforcement of a strict gluten-free diet.

Gluten-Free Diet
(All possible sources of wheat, rye, and oats must be eliminated.)

Foods Allowed

Milk and cream	Fruit and fruit juices
Cheese	Cereals: Cornflakes,
Eggs	corn meal, puffed
Meat, fish, and poultry (unless breaded or creamed)	rice, or precooked gluten-free cereal
Vegetables	Soups: All clear soups
	Bread: Made from rice, corn, or gluten-free wheat flour

Foods to Be Avoided

All breads, rolls, crackers, cakes, and cookies made from wheat or rye	Commercial ice cream
	Prepared mixes and puddings
All wheat and rye cereals, spaghetti, macaroni, and noodles	Postum, Ovaltine, some instant coffees
	Beer and ale
All canned soups except clear broth	Commercial candies containing cereal products

Prognosis

Death due to celiac disease is unusual. Improvement and clinical recovery are the rule. However, disappearance of symptoms can be a protracted, intermittent process. Although good gastrointestinal tolerance for gluten may be eventually noted in a number of patients maintained on the gluten-free diet, there is evidence that they all undergo a histologic relapse on reexposure. In adults with celiac disease, the risk for development of malignant lymphoma of the small bowel or of other gastrointestinal cancer is markedly increased (10%).

Barry RE, Read AE: Celiac disease and malignancy. Q J Med 42:665, 1973.

Hamilton JR, McNeill LK: Childhood celiac disease: Response of treated patients to a small uniform daily dose of wheat gluten. J Pediatr 81:885, 1972.

Katz AJ & others: Current concepts in gluten sensitive enteropathy. Pediatr Clin North Am 22:767, 1975.

McNeish AS & others: Coeliac disease: The disorder in childhood. Clin Gastroenterol 3:127, 1974.

Rolles CJ & others: One-hour blood-xylose screening test for celiac disease in infants and young children. Lancet 2:1043, 1973.

Young WF, Pringle EM: 110 children with coeliac disease, 1950–1969. Arch Dis Child 46:421, 1971.

DISACCHARIDASE DEFICIENCY

Essentials of Diagnosis

- Watery diarrhea, explosive and frothy.
- Stool pH < 5.5.
- Reducing substances present in stools and often in urine.
- Flat glucose tolerance test following disaccharide loading.
- Quantitative decrease or complete absence of disaccharidase activity in intestinal biopsy.

General Considerations

Carbohydrates account for a substantial proportion of the human diet. The polysaccharide starch and the disaccharides sucrose and lactose are quantitatively the most important and require hydrolysis before significant absorption can take place. The accompanying scheme summarizes the digestion sequence of the common polysaccharides and disaccharides.

Disaccharidases are localized in the brush border of the intestinal epithelial cells. Absolute levels are higher in the jejunum and in the proximal ileum than in the distal ileum and in the duodenum. Some substrates can be hydrolyzed by more than one enzyme, and, conversely, some enzymes act on more than one substrate. There are 4 enzymes with maltase activity: IA, IB, II, and III. Maltase IA contributes about 50% of total maltase activity but also has some isomaltase activity. Maltase IB contributes about 25% of total maltase activity but also has some sucrase activity.

Disaccharidase deficiencies are either primary or secondary. In the primary or genetically determined form, the enzyme deficit is isolated, the disaccharide intolerance is likely to persist, intestinal histology is normal, and a family history is common.

Since disaccharidases are confined to the outer cell layer of the intestinal epithelium, they are very susceptible to mucosal damage. A number of conditions are now known to give rise to the secondary type of disaccharidase deficiency, which is transient and involves a quantitative decrease in all enzymes although lactose intolerance is by far the most common. Histologic examination reveals changes compatible with the underlying disorder. A familial incidence in these cases is uncommon.

Clinical Findings

A. Primary (Congenital):

1. Lactase—Congenital lactase deficiency is a rare condition leading to diarrhea soon after lactose is ingested. Diarrhea is the predominant symptom. The stools are frothy and acid; their pH may fall as low as 4.5 as a result of a high content of organic acids, which stimulate intestinal peristalsis. The osmotic action of unhydrolyzed lactose leads to osmotic catharsis. Vomiting is not uncommon. Severe malnutrition may occur. Reducing substances are usually present in the stools, and lactosuria may occur. Infants with lactosuria, aminoaciduria, proteinuria, acidosis, and elevated BUN have been described. It is not clear how these other abnormalities are related to lactose intolerance. An oral lactose tolerance test (2 gm/kg) in an infant suspected of the disease and from whose diet lactose has been withdrawn is likely to result in symptoms of intolerance within 8 hours, and the glucose blood levels will show no appreciable rise. If the milk does not give rise to symptoms initially, it is necessary to exclude small intestinal mucosal damage that may cause secondary lactase deficiency; this may be done by means of small bowel biopsy, which also permits direct estimation of the disaccharidase.

Patients respond to the exclusion of lactose from their diets. In most cases, congenital lactase deficiency has never been proved to be permanent since the majority of candidates for this controversial diagnosis acquire a tolerance for lactose and eventually show normal lactase levels.

2. Sucrase and isomaltase deficiency—This is a combined defect which is inherited as an autosomal recessive trait. Diarrhea usually occurs only when sucrose is fed. Abdominal distention, failure to thrive, and toilet training difficulties in association with chronic diarrhea may be the presenting symptoms. Since sucrase-isomaltase deficiencies have been found in siblings who had few or no symptoms, it is likely that a number of persons with this trait—particularly adults—remain unrecognized.

In making a diagnosis by estimating reducing substances in the stools, it is important to remember that sucrose is not a reducing sugar. The usual 5 drops of stool and 10 drops of water added to a Clinitest tablet will not give a positive reaction unless 1 N HCl is substituted for the water and the mixture allowed to boil for a few seconds before adding the tablet. A

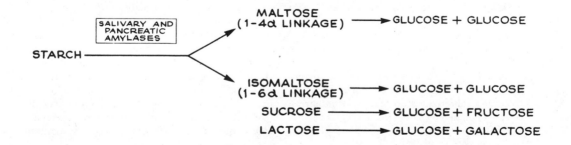

sucrose tolerance test (2 gm/kg) is likely to be flat. As with lactose, many gastric and extra-intestinal factors can account for very poor blood glucose rises. It is wise, therefore, to check the stools for the presence of sucrose and to follow the sucrose tolerance test by one for glucose. Shock may occur due to osmotic water losses in some patients with lactase or sucrase-isomaltase deficiency with a standard dose of the disaccharide for the tolerance test. In sucrase-isomaltase deficiency, exclusion of sucrose is usually sufficient. Starch intolerance is rarely a problem, since the 1–6 linkages of starch hydrolyzed by isomaltase comprise only a small proportion of the whole molecule.

B. Secondary (Acquired):

1. Secondary lactase deficiency–Diarrhea may be produced in normal individuals if a large dose of lactose is ingested. The threshold for lactose tolerance is usually much lower than that for sucrose. Lactose intolerance develops spontaneously in a certain number of children and adults. There is a high prevalence of lactose intolerance in certain racial groups (70% in American blacks) after 3–5 years of age. Disaccharidase deficiency has been described in association with many different disorders. Neomycin and kanamycin administration have been shown to reduce lactase activity in adults. The list of conditions associated with secondary lactase deficiency includes celiac disease, giardiasis, malnutrition, viral or bacterial gastroenteritis, abetalipoproteinemia, cystic fibrosis, immunoglobulin deficiencies, extensive intestinal resections, and regional enteritis.

2. Secondary sucrase deficiency–Intestinal mucosal damage tends to lower the levels of all disaccharidases. Signs of sucrose intolerance are usually masked by the more striking symptoms related to lactose. Infectious diarrhea is the most frequent cause of secondary sucrose intolerance.

Treatment

A. Lactose-Free Diet: Use a milk formula which does not contain lactose, eg, Nutramigen, Pregestimil, or soybean formulas. Exclude foods containing whey, dry milk solids, and curds. It is important to see if labels indicate any lactose content, particularly with canned puréed baby foods. Cheeses (cottage, cheddar, cream), ice cream, sherbet, and chocolate milk powders also contain variable amounts of lactose.

B. Sucrose-Restricted Diet:

1. Foods allowed–The diet described here does contain small amounts of sucrose which are usually well tolerated.

> Milk, cream, butter, cheese, salad and cooking oils
> Eggs, meat, fish
> Homemade bread and pastries containing dextrose
> Asparagus, broccoli, brussels sprouts, cucumbers, spinach, tomatoes, lettuce
> Grapes, cherries, strawberries, cranberries, blackberries
> Potatoes

> Homemade ice cream, diet carbonated beverages, diet Kool-Aid, gelatin desserts, unsweetened cocoa, vegetable juices

2. Foods to be avoided–

> Fruits and vegetables not included in the above list, especially peas, beans, and lentils
> Kool-Aid, carbonated beverages
> Jam, honey, jelly, candy, molasses, maple syrup
> Commercial ice cream, pies, cookies, cakes
> Breakfast cereals
> Medicines made up in syrup

Prognosis

In the primary type, the enzyme deficiency is theoretically a lifelong defect. However, in both lactase and sucrase deficiencies, tolerance for the offending disaccharide tends to increase with age. The prognosis in the secondary or acquired forms of disaccharidase deficiency is that of the underlying illness. It is important to remember that normal tolerance for lactose may not be regained until many months after an acute mucosal injury, eg, acute gastroenteritis.

Ament ME & others: Sucrose-isomaltase deficiency: A frequently misdiagnosed disease. J Pediatr 83:721, 1973.

Auricchio S & others: Intraluminal and mucosal starch digestion in congenital deficiency of intestinal sucrase and isomaltase activities. Pediatr Res 6:832, 1972.

Gracey M, Burke V: Sugar-induced diarrhea in children. Arch Dis Child 48:331, 1973.

Gray GM: Carbohydrate digestion and absorption: Role of small intestine. N Engl J Med 292:1225, 1975.

Lifshitz F & others: Carbohydrate intolerance in infants with diarrhea. J Pediatr 79:760, 1971.

GLUCOSE-GALACTOSE MALABSORPTION

Chronic diarrhea indistinguishable from that due to intestinal disaccharide deficiency may be due to a defect in monosaccharide absorption. The diarrhea relates to the osmotic effect of the nonabsorbed hexose. A decreased maximal rate of tubular reabsorption of glucose is often associated with the intestinal cell transport defect.

Diarrhea starting within a few days after birth constitutes the cardinal feature of the congenital form of the disease. It is usually severe and can be life-threatening. Small bowel histology is normal. Glycosuria and aminoaciduria may occur. The glucose tolerance test is flat and precipitates symptoms. Fructose is well tolerated. The diarrhea promptly subsides on withdrawal of glucose and galactose from the diet. The stool pH is not so acid as that reported in disaccharidase deficiencies; fecal reducing substances are consistently found. The clinical features associated with the acquired form of the disease are essentially the same as those seen with disaccharidase deficiency states. The acquired form is mainly seen in the perinatal period but is also described in older infants. Both disaccharides and monosaccharides, including fructose, are malabsorbed. Necrotizing enterocolitis, intractable diarrhea of early infancy, postoperative phases of neonatal gastrointestinal surgery, and protein-calorie malnutrition are acquired forms of the entity which have been described in infants with extensive small bowel resections or during the course of a bout of gastroenteritis.

In the congenital form, total exclusion from the diet of glucose and galactose is mandatory. A satisfactory formula consists of calcium caseinate, corn oil, and fructose. The prognosis is good if the disease is diagnosed early, since tolerance for glucose and galactose improves with age.

Gracey M, Burke V: Sugar-induced diarrhea in children. Arch Dis Child 48:331, 1973.

Howat JM, Aaronson I: Sugar intolerance in neonatal surgery. J Pediatr Surg 6:719, 1971.

Meeuwisse GW, Melin K: Studies in glucose-galactose malabsorption. Acta Paediatr Scand [Suppl] 188, 1969.

INTESTINAL LYMPHANGIECTASIA

This form of protein-losing enteropathy results from a congenital abnormality of the lymphatic system and is associated with lymphatic aberrations in the extremities. Obstruction to lymphatic drainage of the intestine leads to rupture of intestinal lacteals with leakage of lymph into the lumen of the bowel. Fat loss may be significant and lead to steatorrhea. Chronic loss of lymphocytes and of immunoglobulins is usual and increases the susceptibility to infections.

Clinical Findings

Peripheral edema, diarrhea, abdominal distention, lymphedematous extremities, and repeated infections are common. Laboratory findings are low serum albumin, decreased immunoglobulin levels, lymphocytopenia, and anemia. Serum calcium is frequently depressed, and stool fat may be elevated. Lymphocytes may be seen in large numbers on a stool smear. Albumin turnover studies confirm the gastrointestinal protein loss. X-ray studies reveal an edematous small bowel mucosal pattern, and biopsy reveals dilated lacteals in the villi.

Differential Diagnosis

Other causes of protein-losing enteropathy must be considered, although an associated lymphedematous extremity strongly favors this diagnosis.

Complications & Sequelae

Failure to thrive, tetany, and frequent infections are the common complications of this disease.

Lymphedema of an extremity may be disfiguring since it leads to increased bone growth and hemihypertrophy.

Treatment

Surgery is needed when the lesion is localized to a small area of the bowel or in cases of constrictive pericarditis or obstructing tumors. This may include saphenous vein-peritoneal anastomosis in intractable cases.

Medium chain triglycerides as a fat source may reduce the intestinal lymphatic pressure by eliminating long chain fats from the diet. Water-soluble vitamin and calcium supplements and gamma globulin injections may be indicated. Antibiotics are used for specific infections. Corticosteroids should be avoided.

Prognosis

The prognosis at present is not favorable, although dietary manipulations have had dramatic results in some cases.

Schussheim A: Protein-losing enteropathies in children. Am J Gastroenterol 58:124, 1972.

Shimkin PM, Waldmann TA, Krugman RL: Intestinal lymphangiectasia. Am J Roentgenol 110:827, 1970.

MILK ALLERGY

Milk allergy is more common in males and in children with a family history of allergy. Its incidence is low (0.5%) if one adopts strict clinical criteria for the diagnosis rather than the poor immunologic correlates presently available. The gastrointestinal features vary in severity and usually begin within the first 6 weeks of life. In some patients, vomiting is the predominant symptom and the diarrhea is chronic. In others, the diarrhea is very severe and may lead to the syndrome called "intractable diarrhea of early infancy." Milk protein allergy commonly leads to the presence of occult blood in the stools. Gross blood can be seen and can be associated with "milk colitis." A protein-losing enteropathy characterized by hypoalbuminemia and hypogammaglobulinemia is described in association with milk allergy. A celiac-like syndrome indistinguishable from gluten enteropathy can be secondary to milk allergy. In these cases, there may be a temporary gluten intolerance and acquired disaccharidase deficiency secondary to a severe degree of mucosal damage.

In most cases of milk allergy, milk elimination results in a rapid amelioration of symptoms. Heating reduces allergenicity of milk proteins. In evaluating the response of diarrhea suspected of being due to milk allergy, it is essential to remember that soy protein intolerance has also been reported.

Freier S, Kletter B: Milk allergy in infants and young children. Clin Pediatr (Phila) 9:449, 1970.

Kuitunen P & others: Response of the jejunal mucosa to cow's milk in the malabsorption syndrome with cow's milk intolerance. Acta Paediatr Scand 62:585, 1973.

Waldmann TA & others: Allergic gastroenteropathy. N Engl J Med 276:761, 1967.

Wilson JF, Lahey ME: Unifying concept for pathogenesis of syndrome of iron deficiency anemia, hypocupremia and hypoproteinemia in infants. J Clin Invest 44:11, 1965.

IMMUNOLOGIC DEFICIENCY STATES WITH DIARRHEA OR MALABSORPTION

It is now thought that both cellular and humoral immunity serve as a protective mechanism against invasion by pathogenic organisms and also probably prevent mucosal damage which could be caused by the normal intestinal flora.

Intermittent diarrhea is a frequent finding in immunoglobulin deficiency states, but the cause is usually obscure. It is uncommon to find pathogenic bacteria in the stools, but giardiasis is common. Fifty to 60% of idiopathic acquired hypogammaglobulinemics have steatorrhea and histologic changes consistent with the celiac syndrome. Lymphonodular hyperplasia is a common feature in this group of patients. Congenital or Bruton type agammaglobulinemics occasionally have abnormal intestinal morphology. Patients with isolated IgA deficiency have normal intestinal function but may also present with chronic diarrhea, a celiac-like picture, lymphoid nodular hyperplasia, and giardiasis. Patients with isolated cellular immunity defects or combined cellular and humoral immune incompetence all have severe chronic diarrhea leading to malnutrition. The cause of the diarrhea is unknown, and mucosal biopsies are normal. A high incidence of disaccharidase deficiency is associated with immunologic deficits in children.

Treatment must be directed at correction of the immunoglobulin defect. Gluten-free diets have been disappointing in most cases with villous atrophy. Dramatic improvement may follow the eradication of giardiasis. In patients exhibiting disaccharidase deficiencies, dietary manipulations are helpful.

Ament ME & others: Structure and function of the gastrointestinal tract in primary immunodeficiency syndromes: A study of 39 patients. Medicine 52:227, 1973.

Dubois RS & others: Disaccharidase deficiency in children with immunologic deficits. J Pediatr 76:377, 1970.

Walker WA & others: Immunology of the gastrointestinal tract. (2 parts.) J Pediatr 83:517, 711, 1973.

CHRONIC ULCERATIVE COLITIS

Essentials of Diagnosis

- Rectal bleeding, bloody diarrhea, diarrhea with mucus or pus.
- Tenesmus and crampy abdominal pain.
- Extracolonic manifestations, fever, weight loss, retardation of growth, arthralgia, arthritis, mucocutaneous lesions, erythema nodosum, jaundice.
- Ragged mucosa with loss of haustral markings on barium enema.
- Acute inflammatory changes with crypt abscesses on rectal mucosal biopsy.

General Considerations

Ulcerative colitis is an acute, intermittent or chronic, relapsing disease of the mucosa and submucosa of varying lengths of the colon and rectum characterized by bloody stools, irregularly recurring fever, and many local or extracolonic signs and symptoms. Rectal involvement is seen in more than 90% of cases. It is not a rare disorder in children and has been reported in infants. Twenty percent of cases begin before the age of 20, with a peak between ages 10–19. Impairment of physical growth, delayed appearance of secondary sex characteristics, and the risk of carcinoma make this an important disease.

An "autoimmune" basis for this disorder is suggested by the favorable response to corticosteroid treatment and by its close association with extraintestinal manifestations such as arthritis, erythema nodosum, uveitis, chronic active hepatitis, and autoimmune hemolytic anemia.

Circulating antibodies to colon tissue have been found in about 15% of patients, but it is unlikely that these antibodies play a direct role in the pathogenesis of ulcerative colitis since their attachment to colonic cells cannot be demonstrated in vivo and they are not cytotoxic to colon cells in vitro. However, lymphocytes from patients are toxic to colonic cells obtained from both normal subjects and other patients with ulcerative colitis.

Although emotional stress can exacerbate the disease, recent studies have failed to identify psychosocial factors unique to patients with ulcerative colitis.

Clinical Findings

The diagnosis of ulcerative colitis is based upon a history of an acute onset of diarrhea or nonspecific gastroenteritis, the passage of bloody stools, abdominal cramping, tenesmus, fever, malaise, and anorexia. The onset may also be insidious, with a change in bowel habits from normal to constipation or continued constipation followed by the passage of blood, mucus, or pus. Less commonly the course is fulminating, with high septic fever, extreme prostration, anorexia, vomiting, and an almost continuous bloody diarrhea. In such cases, the threat of colonic perforation is great and emergency surgery is mandatory.

The extracolonic manifestations may be the presenting symptoms and signs, especially with arthralgia or arthritis (15–20%). This is usually monarticular and involves the major joints. Joint symptoms wax and wane with the remissions and exacerbations of the primary disease. Rarely, they precede the signs of bowel involvement by months or years. Other extra-colonic findings are erythema nodosum, pyoderma gangrenosum, and liver disease, either with hepatic enlargement or with abnormalities in liver function studies for which no cause is readily apparent.

The diagnosis of ulcerative colitis is established by sigmoidoscopic examination revealing a hyperemic, friable, bleeding mucosa. Barium enema reveals the serrated edges indicating the location of the ulcers. In active or advanced colitis, there is also a loss of haustral markings and narrowing and shortening of the colon. Biopsy of the rectal mucosa reveals inflammatory cell infiltration and crypt abscesses and is particularly helpful in suggestive cases with negative sigmoidoscopic and radiologic findings.

Differential Diagnosis

Chronic ulcerative colitis must be differentiated from salmonella infections, allergic gastroenteropathy, connective tissue diseases, regional enteritis with colonic involvement (granulomatous ileocolitis), irritable colon syndrome, shigellosis, and amebiasis. The differentiation from salmonellosis, shigellosis, and amebiasis may be very difficult since these conditions also give rise to crypt abscesses.

Complications

A. Local: With progression of the disease, ulcers within the mucosa may extend to the outer layers, leading to perforations which are occasionally free but which more commonly evolve slowly, resulting in the creation of internal fistulas with other loops of bowel or with an extra-intestinal organ such as the vagina. The chronic course interspersed with acute exacerbations leads to extensive fibrosis and consequently to colonic or rectal stricture. Between areas of fibrosis, mucosa becomes "heaped up" and gives rise to pseudopolyps. Massive hemorrhage is an uncommon complication, and toxic megacolon is rare in children. Perianal fissures, abscesses, and fistulas occur.

B. Systemic: Arthritis, erythema nodosum, uveitis, and pyoderma gangrenosum may be seen. Retarded growth and chronic invalidism are almost always present. Fatty infiltration of the liver and, rarely, pericholangitis are seen in patients who have had the disease a long time. Sepsis and thromboembolic phenomena also occur.

The risk of carcinoma is about 10% after 10 years of the disease and increases to 25% after 20 years. The mortality rate from carcinoma is very high, so that prophylactic colectomy must always be considered in patients with long-standing disease.

Children with ulcerative colitis demonstrate considerably more disturbance of personality function than children suffering from other chronic diseases of the bowel. Studies have shown them to be emotionally fragile and to have increased dependency needs. Personality strength in affected children is inversely proportionate to the rapidity and severity of onset of the colitis and directly proportionate to the intensity of stress required to precipitate an exacerbation.

Treatment

No method of management has proved uniformly successful. The effectiveness of these measures must be individually determined and will further depend on the kind of relationship the physician has been able to establish with the patient, who is often apprehensive, emotionally immature, hostile, demanding, and depressed.

A. Diet: A high-protein, high-carbohydrate, high-vitamin, normal-fat diet is recommended. The main concern should be in serving attractive meals that the child will eat. Restrictive or bland diets are not necessary, although during the first year of the disease, because of a high incidence (40%) of decreased lactase activity, a trial of a milk-free diet is indicated.

B. Antibiotics and Sulfonamides:

1. Antibiotics—Appropriate antibiotics may be indicated during the initial 4—7 days of an exacerbation if stool cultures are positive.

2. Salicylazosulfapyridine—This drug is effective acutely and is useful in long-term therapy and in the prevention of relapses. It is relatively nonabsorbable and is said to have a high affinity for the submucosa. The response may be delayed for 1 week. Side-effects are common and include nausea and headaches. A serum sickness-like reaction can be a serious complication. Other side-reactions which require discontinuation of therapy include Heinz body hemolytic anemia. The dosage is as follows:

a. Children under 10 years of age—Give 2—3 gm daily as acute therapy and then reduce dosage to 1.5—2 gm daily with meals.

b. Children over 10 years of age—Give 3—4 gm daily with meals acutely, then reduce dosage to 2—3 gm daily.

C. Corticotropin and Corticosteroids: These drugs are usually restricted to life-threatening situations or to patients in whom salicylazosulfapyridine has not brought about any improvement. Complications of the chronic disease are not reduced by these agents, but emergency surgery is less often required and surgical mortality is therefore reduced.

1. Corticotropin—This drug is said to be superior to corticosteroids in the acute stage of the disease. This may relate to the poor absorption of corticosteroids when the disease is particularly acute. The usual dose of corticotropin is 40 units IV for 7—10 days, overlapping when possible with oral corticosteroids.

2. Corticosteroids—Give prednisone, 1—2 mg/kg orally daily for 2—3 weeks. The maintenance dose of prednisone is 5—20 mg daily. It can also be given on an alternate-day basis in conjunction with salicylazosulfapyridine.

Hydrocortisone retention enemas (Cortenema) are useful when the rectum is severely involved and have been effective also in the treatment of diseased areas in the transverse and descending colon.

D. Azathioprine (Imuran): Azathioprine, 1.5—2 mg/kg/day orally, can be helpful, especially in cases where a high maintenance dose of corticosteroids is necessary to keep the disease under control.

E. Symptomatic Therapy: Opiates are useful for pain but should be used with caution because they may contribute to the development of toxic megacolon. Anticholinergic agents are indicated to reduce hypermotility of the bowel. Sedatives and tranquilizers can be used as required.

F. Psychotherapy: The need for a formal psychiatric referral must be individualized. It appears, however, that every patient would benefit from a coordinated psychiatric-pediatric-surgical team approach.

G. Surgical Measures: Emergency surgery is lifesaving in the case of fulminating disease with toxic megacolon. Surgery should also be done on an emergency basis in the presence of severe hemorrhage, perforation, or obstruction. Elective colectomy should be considered in all cases where medical treatment has been unsuccessful, especially in those with 10 years of disease regardless of their degree of incapacitation because of the climbing risk of cancer. This is especially so in patients with total involvement of the colon and in those whose disease has been continuous.

Total proctocolectomy is the only acceptable surgical procedure. Recent series show that almost 30% of children require surgery within 5 years of the onset of the disease.

Prognosis

The overall prognosis for ulcerative colitis is guarded. Sixty percent survival has been reported after 20 years of the disease.

Rarely, the patient may expire during an acute fulminating attack of toxic ulcerative colitis (toxic megacolon).

Many children (30–40%) respond favorably to medical management and psychotherapy, doing well for months or years. These patients may have mild to moderate relapses, but on the whole they are able to lead a fruitful existence.

A group of patients (20–45%) whose symptoms continue despite medical therapy require early surgery.

The patient may die of carcinoma, acute exsanguinating hemorrhage, perforation of the colon, or overwhelming sepsis.

Binder V & others: Ulcerative colitis in children: Treatment, course and prognosis. Scand J Gastroenterol 8:161, 1973.

Devroede GJ & others: Cancer risk and life expectancy of children with ulcerative colitis. N Engl J Med 285:17, 1971.

Dissanayake AS, Truelove SC: A controlled therapeutic trial of long-term maintenance treatment of ulcerative colitis with sulfasalazine. Gut 14:923, 1973.

Frey CF, Weaver DK: Colectomy in children with ulcerative colitis and granulomatous colitis. Arch Surg 104:466, 1972.

REGIONAL ENTERITIS
(Crohn's Disease)

Essentials of Diagnosis

- Fever, anemia, anorexia, weight loss.
- Crampy abdominal pain, diarrhea.
- Stunting of growth.
- Anal fistulas.
- X-ray evidence of thickened circular folds, cobblestoning, rigidity of the lumen, separation and fixation of loops, "string sign."
- Histologic demonstration of submucosal inflammation with fibrosis and of granulomatous lesions.

General Considerations

The terminal ileum is most commonly involved (80–98%), but any segment or combination of segments of the intestinal tract from stomach to anus may be affected, including the regional lymph nodes. The wall is thickened and rigid, with longitudinal mucosal ulcerations and fissures, submucosal thickening, or cobblestone formation. Sinus tracts and fistulas may be present. Areas of disease may be separated by lengths of normal-appearing gut ("skip lesions"). Histologic features consist of a chronic granulomatous inflammatory reaction with edema and fibrosis involving all layers of the intestinal wall. The most useful diagnostic feature is the presence of noncaseating granulomas containing multinucleated giant cells and epithelioid cells. These focal lesions are found in 50% of cases; in another 25%, the inflammatory reaction is more diffuse. In cases where a nonspecific inflammatory process is reported, the diagnosis must be based on other criteria. The frequency of regional enteritis is equal to that of chronic ulcerative colitis in the pediatric age group, and its cause remains unknown. Occurrence of the disease in members of the same family and a significantly higher incidence among Jews suggest a genetic factor. Psychiatric studies of the disease have not disclosed any specific emotional makeup or cause.

Clinical Findings

A. Symptoms and Signs: Teenagers and young adults are most often afflicted. Cases have been described within the first few months of life. In certain instances, extra-intestinal symptoms such as arthritis, uveitis, stomatitis, erythema nodosum, unexplained fever, or failure to grow may be the presenting symptoms. Anal lesions may antedate the intestinal manifestations by a few years. Crampy abdominal pain, often triggered by food, is usually the predominant symptom. In most instances it is periumbilical, but it may localize in the right lower quadrant. Thus, in one-third of patients the symptoms may mimic an attack of acute appendicitis. Diarrhea is the presenting complaint in one-third of cases. Bloody diarrhea is less frequent than in ulcerative colitis. Anorexia, weight loss, fever, and anemia are found in the majority of patients and often precede the gastrointestinal complaints.

Sigmoidoscopy may be normal or may show diffuse involvement, with lesions indistinguishable from those of ulcerative colitis.

B. Laboratory Findings: Routine laboratory studies contribute little to the diagnosis. Some degree of anemia is usually present. Megaloblastic anemia is rare but may occur as a consequence of vitamin B_{12} or folic acid malabsorption. Evidence for a protein-losing enteropathy can be documented by a decreased serum albumin concentration. Stool examination seldom reveals the presence of blood or pus, and cultures for infectious organisms are negative.

C. X-Ray Findings: X-ray examination should include both a small bowel series and a barium enema. When both ileum and colon are involved (granulomatous ileocolitis), the disease may resemble ulcerative colitis with backwash ileitis. However, the differentiation can usually be made on clinical, radiologic, pathologic, and therapeutic grounds.

Complications

Perforation and hemorrhage are rare. Intestinal obstruction, fistulas, and abscess formation are frequent. Malabsorption syndrome may be a serious complication, manifested by protein-losing enteropathy, disaccharidase deficiency, and bile salt-induced diarrhea. Systemic complications include perianal disease, pyoderma gangrenosum, arthritis, amyloidosis, and a high incidence of severe growth retardation.

Treatment

Regional enteritis is not surgically remediable. In 33–50% of surgically treated cases, the disease will recur in previously grossly normal bowel—usually within 2 years but sometimes as late as 10 years after surgery. Recurrence at the site of anastomosis is most common; consequently, surgery is reserved for the intestinal complications of the disease such as obstruction, perforation, fistulas, and abscess formation. Recent evidence suggests that when the granulomatous process is limited to the colon (granulomatous colitis), resection may not be followed by involvement of previously intact small bowel.

Evaluation of medical regimens is made difficult by the spontaneous exacerbations and remissions so characteristic of this disease. The medical management is that of a long-term chronic illness, with goals directed toward relieving disability rather than achieving a cure.

A. Diet: Dietary management should center around providing the anorexic patient with a diet high in protein. Supplemental feedings and vitamin and iron supplementation should be encouraged. Total paren-

teral nutrition for periods of 4–6 weeks may not only improve the patient with severe malnutrition but may also induce a temporary remission.

B. Symptomatic Treatment: Rest is important when the disease is particularly active. Anxiety, depression, severe diarrhea, and pain can be treated with sedatives, tranquilizers, anticholinergic agents, and opiates or aspirin.

C. Antibiotics and Salicylazosulfapyridine: Broad spectrum antibiotics may be helpful if there is evidence that malabsorption is partly due to significant upper small bowel bacterial contamination. Salicylazosulfapyridine is not thought to be as effective in regional enteritis as in ulcerative colitis but is given to all patients with Crohn's disease in the same dosage.

D. Corticosteroids: Both short-term and chronic administration of corticosteroids are useful in the control of symptoms. Corticosteroids may alter the course of the disease and are particularly indicated in patients with systemic manifestations.

E. Immunosuppressive Therapy: Azathioprine (Imuran), 2 mg/kg/day orally, has been shown to prolong remissions, thus making it possible to maintain patients on smaller doses of corticosteroids. However, since its value is still controversial, it is reserved for a few cases where other measures have failed.

Prognosis

Although the mortality rate is low, the morbidity rate is high. The disease process is progressive in most cases, and its course is interspersed with both acute and chronic complications, leading to variable degrees of invalidism.

Ament ME: Inflammatory disease of the colon: Ulcerative colitis and Crohn's colitis. J Pediatr 86:322, 1975.

Cavell B & others: Chronic inflammatory bowel disease. Clin Gastroenterol 6:481, 1977.

Daum F, Boley SJ, Cohen MI: Inflammatory bowel disease in the adolescent patient. Pediatr Clin North Am 20:933, 1973.

Devroede GJ & others: Cancer risk and life expectancy of children with ulcerative colitis. N Engl J Med 285:17, 1971.

Guttman FM: Granulomatous enterocolitis in childhood and adolescence. J Pediatr Surg 9:115, 1974.

Homer DR & others: Growth, course, and prognosis after surgery for Crohn's disease in children and adolescents. Pediatrics 59:717, 1977.

• • •

General References

Anderson CM, Burke V: *Pediatric Gastroenterology.* Lippincott, 1975.

Davidson M (editor): Paediatric gastroenterology. Clin Gastroenterol 6:251, 1977. [Entire issue.]

Fordtran J, Sleisenger MH: *Gastrointestinal Disease,* 2nd ed. Saunders, 1977.

Grand RJ, Watkins JB (editors): Gastrointestinal and liver disease. Pediatr Clin North Am 22:719, 1975. [Entire issue.]

Gryboski J: *Gastrointestinal Problems in the Infant.* Saunders, 1975.

Roy CC, Silverman A, Cozzetto F: *Pediatric Clinical Gastroenterology,* 2nd ed. Mosby, 1975.

Walker-Smith J: *Diseases of the Small Intestine in Childhood.* Wiley, 1975.

17...
Liver & Pancreas

Arnold Silverman, MD, & Claude Roy, MD

PROLONGED CHOLESTATIC NEONATAL JAUNDICE

1. NEONATAL HEPATITIS

Essentials of Diagnosis

- Prolonged neonatal "obstructive" jaundice.
- Hepatosplenomegaly.
- Demonstration of a patent intra- and extrahepatic biliary system.
- Histologic findings on liver biopsy.
- Identification of known cause (infectious, metabolic, genetic, etc).

General Considerations

Most cases of prolonged neonatal obstructive jaundice are due to "idiopathic" neonatal hepatitis or biliary atresia, which occur with equal frequency. However, the clinical and histologic features of neonatal hepatitis may be mimicked by a variety of specific viral, bacterial, protozoal, or metabolic causes.

In particular, herpesvirus, echovirus 14 and 19, rubella virus, cytomegalovirus, and coxsackie B virus are all capable of transplacental passage to the fetus. Hepatitis B surface antigen (HB_sAg) present in the mother at the time of delivery can infect the infant either from swallowed blood products, transplacentally, or via breast milk. Susceptibility to so-called neonatal hepatitis is increased in children with cystic fibrosis and a_1-antitrypsin deficiency. An increased incidence in males, certain families, and patients with Down's syndrome supports this hypothesis of host susceptibility.

Clinical Findings

A. Symptoms and Signs: Jaundice, hepatosplenomegaly, dark urine, and pale yellow to acholic stools are the most constant physical signs. Lethargy, poor feeding, and failure to thrive frequently accompany the illness.

B. Laboratory Findings: Laboratory tests of liver function usually reflect a combination of hepatocellular injury as shown by elevated SGOT, SGPT, and bilirubin levels and obstructive features with increased serum alkaline phosphatase and acholic stools. Rose bengal sodium I 131 tests may be useful except in severely obstructive cases where results are indistinguishable from those in biliary atresia patients. The same limitations seem to apply to the peroxide hemolysis test, low-density lipoprotein (LP-X) determination, and the detection of alpha-fetoprotein. An elevated IgM value in the first 2 months of life suggests an in utero infectious cause of the jaundice.

Measurement of quantitative and qualitative serum bile acids is not helpful in differentiating biliary atresia from other causes of prolonged obstructive jaundice. However, improvement in excretion of rose bengal following cholestyramine therapy is suggestive of hepatitis.

Histologic features on liver biopsy include variable hepatocyte necrosis, lobular disorganization, cholestasis (within Kupffer's cells and hepatocytes), multinucleated giant cells, and minimal to moderate bile duct proliferation with polymorphonuclear cells, lymphocytes, and eosinophils. Portal zones show little fibrosis.

Differential Diagnosis

The major diagnostic difficulty is the differentiation of neonatal hepatitis from biliary atresia on clinical and laboratory grounds without resorting to exploratory laparotomy with liver biopsy and operative cholangiography. A conservative approach may be justified for 8–12 weeks if percutaneous liver biopsy done early in the course of the disease is primarily consistent with hepatocellular injury or if histologic examination of a biopsy specimen fails to show portal fibrosis and significant bile duct proliferation. If neither significant improvement nor resolution of the clinical and laboratory features occurs within this period, prompt operation becomes mandatory.

Infections and drugs as causes of neonatal jaundice are discussed in the next section.

Genetic, metabolic, and endocrinologic causes such as galactosemia, tyrosinosis, congenital fructose intolerance, a_1-antitrypsin deficiency, Wilson's disease, cystic fibrosis, Niemann-Pick disease, hyperalimentation, and postnecrotizing enterocolitis or other neonatal gastrointestinal insults must also be considered. Other rare causes include Zellweger's and Menkes' syndromes, which have been associated with neonatal jaundice.

Treatment

There is no specific treatment for idiopathic neonatal hepatitis. Supportive therapy includes a high-caloric formula, preferably one containing medium chain triglycerides (Pregestimil, Portagen). Supplementary vitamins A, D, E, and K in water-miscible form should be given. The bile acid binding resin cholestyramine (Questran), 4–8 gm/24 hours, and phenobarbital, 5 mg/kg, are useful in neonatal hepatitis. Beware of hyperchloremic acidosis and intestinal obstruction in the neonate treated with cholestyramine. High doses of vitamin D_3 (25–50 thousand units) may be needed also in biliary rickets. A hemolytic component may be associated with neonatal hepatitis, and blood transfusions may be needed. Bacterial infections must be treated appropriately. Where specific dietary alterations are indicated—eg, in galactosemia, tyrosinosis, and fructose intolerance—these should be instituted promptly.

Corticosteroids are of no proved value in neonatal hepatitis.

Prognosis

About 75% of infants with neonatal hepatitis will recover even after severe and prolonged illness, though most cases show improvement within 2–4 months. Of these survivors, 5–10% develop paucity of the intrahepatic bile ducts. The remainder, with continued signs of disease (jaundice, hepatosplenomegaly), eventually develop cirrhosis and die from hepatic decompensation. The prognosis appears to be worse if familial or genetic factors are present. Infants with a_1-antitrypsin deficiency are at significant risk of developing cirrhosis as a consequence of hepatitis.

Brough AJ, Bernstein J: Conjugated hyperbilirubinemia in early infancy: A reassessment of liver biopsy. Hum Pathol 5:507, 1974.

Hays DM & others: Diagnosis of biliary atresia: Relative accuracy of percutaneous liver biopsy, open liver biopsy, and operative cholangiography. J Pediatr 71:598, 1967.

Landing BH: Considerations of the pathogenesis of neonatal hepatitis, biliary atresia and choledochal cyst: The concept of infantile obstructive cholangiopathy. Prog Pediatr Surg 6:113, 1974.

Lawson EE, Boggs JD: Long-term follow-up of neonatal hepatitis: Safety and value of surgical exploration. Pediatrics 53:650, 1974.

Mathis RK, Andres JM, Walker WA: Liver disease in infants. 2. Hepatic disease states. J Pediatr 90:864, 1977.

2. NEONATAL JAUNDICE SECONDARY TO INFECTIONS & DRUGS

Specific investigative technics should be undertaken to identify the etiologic agent whenever an infectious cause is suspected in prolonged neonatal jaundice.

Bacterial Infections

The jaundice associated with sepsis may be predominantly indirect-reacting (hemolytic) or, more commonly, of the mixed type. Histologic changes attest to the inability of the liver to excrete conjugated bilirubin. Bile stasis predominates, while toxic cellular alterations and giant cell transformation occur less frequently. Cultures from all available body fluids should be obtained. A septic process involving the urinary tract is particularly common.

Escobedo MB & others: The frequency of jaundice in neonatal bacterial infections. Clin Pediatr (Phila) 13:656, 1974.

Ng SH & others: Urinary tract infections presenting with jaundice. Arch Dis Child 46:173, 1971.

Rooney JC & others: Jaundice associated with bacterial infection in the newborn. Am J Dis Child 122:39, 1971.

Viral Infections

Hepatitis virus B (HB_sAg), cytomegalovirus infection, rubella, varicella, herpes simplex, coxsackie B virus infection, echovirus infection, and adenovirus infection are specific causes of neonatal hepatitis. The transmission of HB_sAg from mother to child most often occurs during delivery, when the infant swallows maternal blood. Evidence for transplacental acquisition as well as that transmission via breast milk has recently been reported. The development of a chronic carrier state of HB_sAg in such a neonate is possible even when only minimal to mild liver disease is present. Newborns are at particular risk if the mother has had overt HB_sAg disease during the last trimester. Cross-infection may be a significant epidemiologic hazard. Hyperimmune B serum given to these neonates may prevent the carrier state from developing.

Esterley DR & others: Hepatic lesions in the congenital rubella syndrome. J Pediatr 71:676, 1967.

Gerety RJ, Schweitzer IL: Viral hepatitis type B during pregnancy, neonatal period and infancy. J Pediatr 90:368, 1977.

Hughes JR & others: Echovirus 14 infection associated with fetal neonatal hepatic necrosis. Am J Dis Child 123:61, 1972.

Merrill DA & others: Neonatal onset of the hepatitis associated antigen carrier state. N Engl J Med 287:1280, 1972.

Toxoplasmosis

Jaundice and hepatosplenomegaly are common in the congenital variety of this disease. Unless the parasite is demonstrated within the hepatic parenchyma, the liver histopathology is nonspecific. Focal to widespread necrosis, giant cells, and a generalized cellular inflammatory response have been reported.

Nahmias AJ: The TORCH complex. Hosp Pract 9:65, May 1974.

Syphilis

Syphilis is now a rare cause of neonatal jaundice. Serologic tests for syphilis on the mother and infant and prompt treatment with penicillin in positive cases are important.

Drugs

Vitamin K and the sulfonamides may cause high levels of indirect bilirubin by reducing the available binding sites of albumin or by causing hemolysis in patients with a hereditary deficiency of glucose-6-phosphate dehydrogenase. Novobiocin may impair hepatic bilirubin uptake or conjugation. Tetracyclines, especially when given intravenously, may lead to hepatic necrosis.

Stern L: Drug interactions. 2. Drugs, the newborn infant, and the binding of bilirubin to albumin. Pediatrics 49:916, 1972.

3. EXTRAHEPATIC BILIARY ATRESIA

Essentials of Diagnosis
- Prolonged neonatal obstructive jaundice.
- Hepatomegaly (splenomegaly later).
- Acholic stools (persistent).
- Laparotomy and cholangiography.
- Liver histology.

General Considerations

In Caucasians, there is no sex or familial tendency for this condition, which has an incidence of 1:8000 to 1:13,000 births. In Orientals, a female:male ratio of 2:1 is noted, as well as an increased incidence of biliary atresia. The most common abnormality found is complete atresia of all extrahepatic biliary structures, but a multitude of variations have been reported. The specific cause of biliary atresia is not known, although recent evidence supports an in utero infectious or vascular cause. Many authors now propose that neonatal hepatitis, biliary atresia, and choledochal cysts are part of a continuum representing the end product of an infantile obstructive cholangiopathy. Extrahepatic atresia has not been found in stillborn infants.

Clinical Findings

A. Symptoms and Signs: Jaundice may be noted in the newborn period but is more often delayed until 2–3 weeks of age. The urine is dark and stains the diaper, and the stools are often pale yellow, gray, or acholic. Seepage of bilirubin products across the intestinal mucosa gives some yellow coloration to the stools. Hepatomegaly is common, and the liver may feel quite firm; splenomegaly usually occurs later. Pruritus, digital clubbing, xanthomas, and a rachitic rosary may be noted in slightly older cases. Murmurs reflecting increased cardiovascular output or shunting through bronchial arteries may be heard over the entire precordium. By 2–3 months, there is poor weight gain due to fat malabsorption.

B. Laboratory Findings: No single laboratory test will consistently differentiate this entity from other causes of obstructive jaundice. Properly performed, serial rose bengal sodium I 131 tests (after a trial of cholestyramine) may be the most useful laboratory investigation. Persistent elevation of the serum alkaline phosphatase and cholesterol levels, prolongation of the prothrombin time, and elevated 5'-nucleotidase levels suggest biliary atresia, although these findings have also been reported in severe neonatal hepatitis. These tests will not differentiate the type of atresia (intrahepatic versus extrahepatic) nor indicate which cases are potentially correctable by surgery.

Histologic examination of a liver biopsy specimen obtained either by the percutaneous route or operatively is useful. Although portal tracts may be widened by fibrous tissue and bile duct proliferation, the lobule relationship to the central veins is preserved. Bile duct plugging and bile lakes are common features in extrahepatic atresia, while necrosis is rare. On occasion, giant cells may be seen. Biopsy specimens can differentiate neonatal hepatitis from biliary atresia in over 90% of cases.

Differential Diagnosis

The major diagnostic dilemma is between this entity and neonatal hepatitis. Less commonly, urinary tract infection, intrahepatic atresia, choledochal cyst, intraluminal bile duct obstruction, and extrinsic pressure on the ducts by a tumor or lymph nodes may cause prolonged obstructive jaundice.

Surgical exploration is necessary for final diagnosis. Preoperative attention to clotting studies, including partial thromboplastin time as well as prothrombin time, is mandatory. Laparotomy must always include biopsy and an operative cholangiogram if a gallbladder is present. The presence of bile in the gallbladder implies patency of the "proximal" extrahepatic duct system. Radiographic visualization of dye in the duodenum will exclude obstruction to the "distal" extrahepatic ducts. The absence of either gallbladder or bile within its lumen, or failure to visualize the duodenum on cholangiography, dictates thorough exploration of the porta hepatis.

Complications

Failure to thrive, marked pruritus, portal hypertension, hypersplenism, a bleeding diathesis, rickets, ascites, and cyanosis eventually develop. Bronchitis and pneumonia are common. Eventually, hepatic failure and death occur.

Treatment

A. Medical Treatment: With the probability that organ transplantation will provide the ultimate treatment for this disorder, medical management during the first 1–2 years is most important. All measures mentioned in the treatment of neonatal hepatitis apply here, with particular emphasis on the use of Portagen or Pregestimil (medium chain fatty acid formulas) and water-soluble vitamins. The bile acid binding resin cholestyramine is of questionable value in complete atresia, as is the use of phenobarbital. Ascites is best managed by a low-salt diet, spironolactone, and diuretics.

Potassium-depleting diuretics should be avoided. Newer potent diuretics such as triamterene (Dyrenium) and ethacrynic acid (Edecrin) may be used cautiously. Vigorous antibiotic treatment of the frequent bronchial infections will enhance early survival.

B. Surgical Measures: In extrahepatic atresia, it was hoped that liver transplantation would offer a possible solution. In some cases, actual surgical correction may be possible, but functional success is achieved in only 5%. Unfortunately, long-term survival is very rare in infants coming to liver transplantation. Greater experience with modifications of the Kasai hepatic portoenterostomy has yielded more long-term survivors with biliary atresia. Bile drainage can be expected in 60% of children operated upon before 3 months of age. A stable biliary cirrhosis may be expected in 10–20% of the survivors. This hepatic portojejunostomy procedure may be most successful in cases where the obliterative bile duct process has ceased. Ascending cholangitis is a frequent complication during the first postoperative year.

Prognosis

Uncorrected extrahepatic biliary atresia leads to biliary cirrhosis and death within the first 2 years of life in almost all cases.

Campbell DB & others: The differential diagnosis of neonatal hepatitis and biliary atresia. J Pediatr Surg 9:699, 1974.

Hays D, Synder W Jr: Untreated biliary atresia. Surgery 54:373, 1963.

Kasai M, Watanabe I, Ryoji O: Follow-up studies of long-term survivors after hepatic portoenterostomy for "non-correctable" biliary atresia. J Pediatr Surg 10:173, 1975.

Landing BH: Considerations of the pathogenesis of neonatal hepatitis, biliary atresia and choledochal cyst: The concept of infantile obstructive cholangiopathy. Prog Pediatr Surg 6:113, 1974.

Lilly JR, Altman RP: Hepatic portoenterostomy (the Kasai operation) for biliary atresia. Surgery 78:76, 1975.

Weber A, Roy CC: The malabsorption associated with chronic liver disease in children. Pediatrics 50:73, 1972.

4. INTRAHEPATIC BILE DUCT DEFICIENCY

Essentials of Diagnosis

- Obstructive jaundice.
- Absence or hypoplasia of intrahepatic bile ducts.
- Normal extrahepatic biliary system.
- Hepatosplenomegaly.
- Pruritus.
- Xanthomas.

General Considerations

Intrahepatic deficiency or agenesis accounts for less than 10% of cases of biliary "atresia." It may occur sporadically or may be part of a familial syndrome. An in utero inflammatory process (rubella), so-called neonatal hepatitis, or a hypoxic episode involving the bile ducts may be involved in the etiology, whereas the familial occurrence suggests a genetic susceptibility, perhaps due to abnormal bile. Accumulated bile acids may enhance the cirrhotic process.

Clinical Findings

A. Symptoms and Signs: Features of obstructive jaundice may be present at birth or may appear in the newborn period. Pruritus is usually striking, but the stools are seldom acholic. Hepatomegaly is slight. Splenomegaly and xanthomas are late findings. Hepatic ductular hypoplasia has been associated with a characteristic facies, vertebral malformations, cardiac murmurs, and retarded physical, mental, and sexual development.

B. Laboratory Findings: Serum bilirubin (primarily direct-reacting) is moderately elevated, as is the level of serum bile acids. Serum alkaline phosphatase and cholesterol are elevated. SGOT is normal or slightly elevated. Liver histology reveals a marked reduction in bile duct components of the intrahepatic system. This may involve primarily the major bile ducts, in which case bile plugging of the canaliculi is seen. The smaller ducts and the perilobular or interlobular ducts may be absent or hypoplastic, but large ducts can be seen in the portal triads. The degree of fibrosis may be slight or extensive, with distortion of the architectural pattern. The same variation in bile stasis has been reported.

Differential Diagnosis

Other causes of obstructive jaundice include neonatal hepatitis and extrahepatic biliary atresia. Conditions in which cellular transport of conjugated bilirubin to the canaliculi is impaired must also be considered, eg, Dubin-Johnson syndrome and Rotor's syndrome. The absence of pruritus, acholic stools, steatorrhea, elevated serum alkaline phosphatase, and bile stasis within the liver in these 2 conditions are excluding features.

A number of review reports suggest that a clinical spectrum may exist in familial cases: (1) Byler's disease, with marked obstructive jaundice, diminution in intrahepatic bile ducts, and rapid progression of liver disease to an early death, has been reported. (2) Survival with obstructive jaundice, pruritus, shortness of stature, peculiar hands, mental retardation, and ataxia were described in 4 out of 7 children in one family. Liver biopsy showed variable degrees of bile stasis, primarily in liver cells; plugging of canaliculi; and a paucity of interlobular bile ducts. (3) Hepatocyte bile stasis, jaundice, pruritus, acholic stools, steatorrhea, and early death in 2 siblings have been reported. Some of these children with hepatic ductular hypoplasia have cardiac abnormalities, and the inheritance pattern is thought to be as an autosomal dominant with variable penetrance.

Complications

Slow progressive hepatic fibrosis and biliary cirrhosis occur in most patients. Portal hypertension, hypersplenism, and ascites may develop. Pruritus early and xanthomas late in the disease are common sequelae. Depending upon the degree of obstruction, steatorrhea, failure to thrive, bleeding diathesis, and rickets may occur. Growth failure, mental retardation, ataxia, and early demise would seem to be more common in familial cases.

Treatment

Surgery has little to offer the patient with intrahepatic biliary atresia. Medical management is directed at reducing circulating bile acids by use of phenobarbital, 5–10 mg/kg/24 hours, in conjunction with the oral bile acid binding resin cholestyramine. This relieves the pruritus and lowers the serum cholesterol and bilirubin levels, which theoretically may spare the liver from the injurious effects of the primary and secondary bile acids. Dietary manipulations and water-soluble forms of vitamins A, D, K, and E are important aspects of the medical therapy.

Prognosis

The prognosis seems better in nonfamilial instances than in the familial cases. In the former, long-term survivors are not uncommonly reported. Large doses of cholestyramine started early in the disease may prolong life.

Alagille D & others: Hepatic ductular hypoplasia associated with characteristic facies, vertebral malformations, retarded physical, mental and sexual development and cardiac murmur. J Pediatr 86:63, 1975.
Heathcote J & others: Intrahepatic cholestasis in childhood. N Engl J Med 295:801, 1976.
Javitt NB & others: Cholestatic syndromes in infancy: Diagnostic value of serum bile acid pattern and cholestyramine administration. Pediatr Res 7:119, 1973.
Stiehl A: Effects of phenobarbital on bile salt metabolism in cholestasis due to intrahepatic bile duct hypoplasia. Pediatrics 51:992, 1973.

GENETIC, METABOLIC, & ENDOCRINE CAUSES OF NEONATAL JAUNDICE*

1. CYSTIC FIBROSIS

This inherited disorder must be considered in cases of prolonged obstructive jaundice in the newborn period. The findings of bile duct plugging and early fibrosis of the liver have been reported from biopsy.

*Galactosemia and tyrosinosis and congenital fructose intolerance are discussed separately in Chapter 33.

Oppenheimer EH, Esterly JR: Hepatic changes in young infants with cystic fibrosis: possible relation to focal biliary cirrhosis. J Pediatr 86:683, 1975.

2. NIEMANN-PICK DISEASE

Prolonged jaundice in the neonatal period may be the earliest manifestation of this disorder of sphingomyelin metabolism. Niemann-Pick cells seen on liver biopsy may be mistaken for the giant cells of neonatal hepatitis. Other than mild to moderate elevation of bilirubin and transaminase levels, liver function tests are within normal limits.

Crocker AC, Farber S: Niemann-Pick disease: A review of 18 patients. Medicine 37:1, 1958.
Philippart M & others: Niemann-Pick disease. Arch Neurol 20:227, 1969.

3. HYPOTHYROIDISM

Elevation of indirect-reacting bilirubin may be seen in congenital cretinism. The diagnosis should be apparent from other clinical findings.

Weldon AP, Danks DM: Congenital hypothyroidism and neonatal jaundice. Arch Dis Child 47:469, 1972.

4. BREAST MILK HYPERBILIRUBINEMIA

Persistent elevation of the indirect bilirubin fraction may be seen in breast-fed infants. The inhibitory action on glucuronyl transferase activity of pregnane-$3\alpha,20\beta$-diol in the mother's milk has been shown in vitro, but its relation to clinical jaundice is not constant. Rapid decline of bilirubin levels may be achieved by temporary discontinuation of breast feeding. Phenobarbital, 3–5 mg/kg/day, has also been employed to lower the bilirubin level.

Adlard BPF, Lathe GH: Breast milk jaundice: Effect of $3\alpha,20\beta$-pregnanediol on bilirubin conjugation by human liver. Arch Dis Child 45:186, 1970.
Ramos A & others: Pregnanediols and neonatal hyperbilirubinemia. Am J Dis Child 111:353, 1966.
Saland J & others: Navajo jaundice: A variant of neonatal hyperbilirubinemia associated with breast feeding. J Pediatr 85:271, 1974.

5. LUCEY-DRISCOLL SYNDROME

This is a rare form of transient familial neonatal hyperbilirubinemia developing during the first 48 hours of life. It is due to the presence of an as yet unidentified inhibitor of bilirubin conjugation in both maternal and infant serum.

Lucey JF & others: Transient familial neonatal hyperbilirubinemia. Am J Dis Child 100:787, 1960.

6. FAMILIAL HYPERBILIRUBINEMIA

These entities can be divided into 2 major groups depending upon whether unconjugated or conjugated hyperbilirubinemia occurs.

Unconjugated Hyperbilirubinemia
A. Crigler-Najjar Syndrome: Deficiency of the enzyme glucuronyl transferase within liver cells occurs in 2 forms. Patients with type I develop severe elevation of unconjugated bilirubin, serious neurologic defects, and, usually, kernicterus. Their bile is colorless and contains traces of unconjugated bilirubin. This defect is inherited as an autosomal recessive, and patients have no measurable glucuronyl transferase in hepatocytes. Phenobarbital is without effect, though phototherapy may keep bilirubin levels below 25 mg/100 ml. Occasional instances of this condition without neurologic complications have been found and represent the type II syndrome. Since there is some glucuronyl transferase activity, hyperbilirubinemia is less severe, and the bile is pigmented and contains bilirubin glucuronide. Inheritance here appears to be as an autosomal dominant. Such patients usually respond well to phenobarbital. Liver histology and liver function tests are normal in both types.

B. Gilbert's Disease: The most common form of the congenital hyperbilirubinemias probably represents a syndrome rather than a distinct entity. The common denominator is impaired hepatic uptake of bilirubin. The most consistent biochemical abnormality is the persistent partial reduction of hepatic bilirubin uridine diphosphate glucuronyl transferase (UDPG-T). Mild fluctuating jaundice, especially with illness, is the major clinical syndrome. A shortened red cell survival occurs in some patients. Another group has also shown some impairment of glucuronyl transferase activity. Subsidence of hyperbilirubinemia has been achieved in some patients by administration of phenobarbital.

The disease is inherited as an autosomal dominant with incomplete penetrance. Whether another illness (hepatitis) can predispose to Gilbert's disease remains controversial. Liver histology and most other liver function tests are normal except for prolonged BSP retention. An increase in the level of unconjugated bilirubin after a 2-day fast (300 kcal/day) of 1.4 mg/100 ml or greater is consistent with the diagnosis of Gilbert's disease.

Arias IM & others: Chronic non-hemolytic unconjugated hyperbilirubinemia with glucuronyl transferase deficiency. Am J Med 47:395, 1969.

Blaschke TF & others: Crigler-Najjar syndrome: An unusual course with development of neurologic damage at age eighteen. Pediatr Res 8:573, 1974.

Felsher BF, Carpio NM: Caloric intake and unconjugated hyperbilirubinemia. Gastroenterology 69:42, 1975.

Conjugated Hyperbilirubinemia (Dubin-Johnson Syndrome & Rotor's Syndrome)
These entities are rarely seen in infants, but the elevated levels of conjugated bilirubin may be confused with other causes of obstructive jaundice. Inheritance of both disorders appears to be dominant with incomplete penetrance and variable expression. The basic defect is impaired hepatocyte excretion of conjugated bilirubin, with a variable degree of impairment in uptake and conjugation complicating the picture. The early differentiation of these 2 entities on the basis of the presence or absence of pigment deposition in the liver may have been premature. In Rotor's syndrome, the liver is normal, whereas in Dubin-Johnson syndrome it is darkly pigmented on gross inspection. Microscopic examination reveals numerous dark-brown pigment granules, especially in the centrilobular regions. However, the amount of pigment varies within families, and some jaundiced members may have no demonstrable pigmentation in the liver. Other than retained pigment, the liver is histologically normal. However, excretion of BSP as well as of other dyes is also impaired.

Shani M, Seligsohn V, Ben-Ezzer J: Effect of phenobarbital on liver function in patients with Dubin-Johnson syndrome. Gastroenterology 67:303, 1974.

Shani M & others: Sulfobromophthalein tolerance test in patients with Dubin-Johnson syndrome and their relatives. Gastroenterology 59:842, 1970.

HEPATITIS A
(Short Incubation, MS-1, or Infectious Hepatitis)

Essentials of Diagnosis
- Gastrointestinal upset.
- Jaundice.
- Liver tenderness.
- Abnormal liver function tests.
- Positive liver biopsy.
- Local epidemic of the disease.

General Considerations
This disease appears to be caused by a virus or strains of related viruses (27 nm particles) and tends to occur in both epidemic and sporadic fashion. Trans-

mission by the fecal-oral route explains epidemic outbreaks from contaminated food or water supplies. Particles 27 nm in diameter have been found in stools during the acute phase of type A hepatitis. Sporadic cases usually result from contact with an affected individual. The overt form of the disease is easily recognized by the clinical manifestations, but a larger number of affected individuals have an anicteric and unrecognized form of the disease. Both forms probably confer lifelong immunity. Antibody to this virus appears within 1–4 weeks of clinical symptoms. While the great majority of children with infectious hepatitis are asymptomatic or have mild disease and recover completely, some will develop a fulminating hepatitis, chronic hepatitis, and cirrhosis. Children who die during the initial attack of the disease do so from massive hepatic necrosis secondary to overwhelming viremia, an immunologic deficiency state, or perhaps exposure to a completely different strain of virus.

Clinical Findings

A. History: A history of direct exposure to a previously jaundiced individual or of eating seafood or drinking contaminated water in the recent past should be sought. Following an incubation period of 14–50 days, the initial symptoms of fever, anorexia, and vomiting usually precede the development of obvious jaundice by 5–10 days.

B. Symptoms and Signs: Fever, anorexia, vomiting, headache, and abdominal pain are the usual symptoms. Darkening of the urine, suggesting the presence of bile, precedes jaundice. Jaundice reaches a peak in 1–2 weeks and then begins to subside. The stools may become light or clay-colored during this time. Clinical improvement can be noted during the early phase of developing jaundice. Jaundice and liver tenderness are the most consistent physical findings. Splenomegaly may be present.

C. Laboratory Findings: An elevated serum bilirubin (both direct- and indirect-reacting) is common. The SGOT and SGPT values are elevated, especially early in the course of the disease. A prolongation of BSP retention following disappearance of jaundice indicates severe residual damage. The cephalin flocculation and thymol turbidity tests are abnormal and indirectly reflect liver damage. Serum proteins are generally normal, but an elevation of the gamma globulin fraction (> 2.5 gm/100 ml) can occur and indicates a worse prognosis. As the virus disappears, the serum IgM level rises. Hypoalbuminemia, hypoglycemia, and marked reduction in prothrombin time are serious prognostic findings. Urine bile and urobilinogen will be increased. Antibody to hepatitis A virus can be detected by immune adherence test as complement fixation during the icteric phase of the disease.

If the diagnosis is in doubt, a percutaneous liver biopsy may be safely performed in most children provided the partial thromboplastin time and platelet count are normal, the prothrombin time is greater than 50%, and the serum bilirubin is less than 25 mg/100 ml. The presence of ascites may increase the risk of percutaneous liver biopsy. "Balloon cells" and acidophilic bodies are characteristic histologic findings. Liver cell necrosis may be diffuse or focal, with accompanying infiltration of inflammatory cells containing polymorphonuclear leukocytes, lymphocytes, macrophages, and plasma cells, particularly in portal areas. Some bile duct proliferation may be seen in the perilobular portal areas alongside areas of bile stasis. Regenerative liver cells and proliferation of reticuloendothelial cells are present. Occasionally, massive hepatocyte destruction is seen with scarcely a normal liver cell visible.

Differential Diagnosis

Other diseases with somewhat similar onset include infectious mononucleosis, leptospirosis, drug-induced hepatitis, Wilson's disease, and, most often, type B hepatitis.

Complications

Ninety-five percent of children recover without sequelae. In rare cases of fulminating hepatitis, the patient may die in 5 days or may survive as long as 1–2 months before death ensues. The prognosis is poor if the signs and symptoms of hepatic coma prevail, with deepening of jaundice and development of ascites. Incomplete resolution leads to subacute or chronic active hepatitis, which may have several expressions and clinical patterns. The liver disease may eventually resolve after smoldering for several years or may go on to a chronic hepatitis with cirrhosis. Rare cases of aplastic anemia following acute infectious hepatitis have also been reported.

Some attempt at isolation of the patient is indicated, although the majority of patients with type A hepatitis are noninfectious by the time the disease becomes overt. Stool, urine, and blood-contaminated objects should be handled with extreme care for 1 month after the appearance of jaundice.

Prevention

Passive immunization of exposed susceptibles can be achieved by giving 0.02–0.04 ml/kg body weight of gamma globulin IM, with casual contacts receiving approximately half this dose.

Treatment

There are no specific measures. Bed rest during the icteric phase appears to be helpful. Sedatives should be avoided whenever possible.

A. Diet: At the start of the illness, a light diet is preferable. Fruits, vegetables, and plenty of sugars are usually well tolerated. Adequate protein can be supplied by grilled meats or broiled fish with less than normal amounts of fat. B complex vitamins have been used on empiric grounds, but there is no good evidence to show that they alter the course of this disease.

B. Antibiotics: Antibiotics such as neomycin, 20 mg/kg/day orally (or kanamycin in comparable dosage), have been used to decrease the intestinal flora in anticipation of hepatic coma.

C. Corticosteroids: Corticosteroids may be detrimental to patients with hepatitis A disease.

Prognosis

See Complications, above.

Krugman S: Viral hepatitis: Recent developments and prospects for prevention. J Pediatr 87:1067, 1975.

National Research Council Symposium on Hepatitis. Am J Med Sci 266:1, 1975.

HEPATITIS B
(Long Incubation; MS-2, or Serum Hepatitis; Antigen Hepatitis)

In contrast to infectious hepatitis, serum hepatitis has a slow, insidious onset with an incubation period of 21–135 days. The disease is due to a virus (42 nm Dane particle), and until recently the parenteral route was the only known means of contracting the disease, although person-to-person spread may occur with shared razors or toothbrushes as well as venereally. The identification of hepatitis virus B antigen in 75–100% of patients with this type of hepatitis greatly assists the diagnosis of this entity. The incidence of this disease following blood transfusions varies directly with the number of units received. Recent data suggest that HB_sAg may be present in 8.7% of blood donors. The complete Dane particle (42 nm) is composed of a core (28 nm particle) which is found in the nucleus of infected liver cells and a double-shelled surface particle apparently formed in the cytoplasm. The surface antigen in blood is termed HB_sAg. These particles are found as 22 nm spherical particles in the serum but occasionally occur as filamentous structures as well. The antibody to it is HB_sAb. The core antigen is termed HB_cAg and its antibody HB_cAb. The core antigen also contains DNA polymerase, which can be measured in patients' blood during viremia.

Clinical Findings

A. Symptoms and Signs: The symptoms are nonspecific, consisting only of slight fever (which may be absent) and mild gastrointestinal upset. Visible jaundice is usually the first significant finding. It is accompanied by darkening of the urine and pale or clay-colored stools. Hepatomegaly is present. Occasionally, a symptom complex of macular rash, urticarial lesions, and arthritis antedates the appearance of icterus. The presence of HB_sAg, HB_cAb, or hepatitis B-specific DNA polymerase signifies acute hepatitis virus B disease. HB_sAb may develop much later (months to years). Carriers of HB_sAg also have detectable levels of HB_cAb, and ϵ antigen may also be present in the serum of patients with persistent antigenemia.

B. Laboratory Findings: These are similar to those discussed previously for infectious hepatitis (see above). Liver biopsy does not differentiate serum hepatitis from acute infectious hepatitis.

Differential Diagnosis

The differentiation between serum hepatitis and infectious hepatitis is made easier by a history of inoculation and an unusually long period of incubation. The history may indicate a drug-induced hepatitis.

Prevention

The best treatment is prevention. Screening of donors to eliminate individuals who may have had hepatitis is the most dependable way of preventing serum hepatitis. The use of unsterilized hypodermic equipment is a danger that must be considered. Storing plasma at room temperature for 6 months or treating it with ultraviolet rays may decrease the risk of infection. Fibrinogen is just as dangerous as plasma.

Passive immunization of individuals receiving numerous transfusions with hyperimmune gamma globulin has met with variable success. Its role in the prevention of hepatitis in neonates born of HB_sAg-positive mothers is still to be determined. Conventional immunoglobulin is potent enough to protect against hepatitis virus B disease in case of low-dose contact (nonparenteral) but provides transient passive immunity. Active immunization with both a formalin- and a heat-inactivated vaccine seems promising on the basis of early studies.

Treatment

Supportive measures such as bed rest, diet, corticosteroids, and the administration of large doses of gamma globulin have been employed with little success. Large doses of hepatitis B immune serum globulin or heat-inactivated HB_sAg-positive serum may be of therapeutic value if given at the time of exposure.

Prognosis

The prognosis is good, although fulminating hepatitis and cirrhosis may supervene. The course of the disease is variable, but jaundice in children seldom persists for more than 2 weeks. HB_sAg disappears in 95% of cases at the time of clinical recovery. Persistent asymptomatic antigenemia may occur, particularly in children with Down's syndrome or leukemia and those undergoing chronic hemodialysis. Persistence of neonatally acquired HB_sAg is common, and the presence of ϵ antigen in the HB_sAg carrier patient seems to convey a poorer prognosis.

Krugman S: Viral hepatitis: Recent developments and prospects for prevention. J Pediatr 87:1067, 1975.

Popper H, Schaffner F: Hepatitis B antigen particles and prognosis in hepatitis. N Engl J Med 288:518, 1973.

Robinson WS, Lutwick LI: The virus of hepatitis B. (2 parts.) N Engl J Med 295:1168, 1232, 1976.

Simon JB, Patel SK: Liver disease in asymptomatic carriers of hepatitis B antigen. Gastroenterology 66:1020, 1974.

Szmuness W & others: Hepatitis B immune serum globulin in prevention of non-parenterally transmitted hepatitis B. N Engl J Med 290:701, 1974.

FULMINATING HEPATITIS
(Acute Massive Hepatic Necrosis,
Acute Yellow Atrophy)

Fulminating hepatitis has a mortality rate close to 80%. Patients with immunologic deficiency diseases are particularly prone to this form of hepatitis, as are patients receiving immunosuppressive drugs.

Clinical Findings
In a number of patients the disease proceeds in a rapidly fulminant course with deepening jaundice, deterioration of laboratory indices, ascites, a rapidly shrinking liver, and progressive coma. Terminally, some laboratory values may improve at the time when the liver is getting smaller (massive necrosis and collapse). Another group of patients start off with a course typical of "benign" hepatitis and then suddenly become ill once again. Fever, anorexia, vomiting, and abdominal pain may be noted, and worsening of liver function tests parallels changes in sensorium or impending coma. A generalized bleeding tendency occurs at this time. Impairment of renal function, manifested by either oliguria or anuria, is an ominous sign. The striking laboratory findings include elevated serum bilirubin levels (usually > 20 mg/100 ml), high SGOT and SGPT (> 500 IU/liter) which may decrease terminally, low serum albumin, hypoglycemia, and prolonged prothrombin time. Blood ammonia levels may be elevated, whereas BUN is often very low initially. Hyperpnea is frequent, and a mixed respiratory alkalosis and metabolic acidosis is apparent from serum electrolyte values. A rise in the polymorphonuclear count often presages acute liver failure.

Differential Diagnosis
Other known causes of fulminating hepatitis such as drugs and other poisons may be difficult to exclude. Reye's syndrome should not be confused with fulminating hepatitis, as patients with the former are typically anicteric.

Complications
Cirrhosis of the postnecrotic type is the usual sequel in the rare pediatric survivor, with some cases of chronic active hepatitis evolving from submassive hepatic necrosis. Cerebral edema may be the cause of death in 10–15% of patients.

Treatment
Many regimens have been tried, but controlled evaluation of therapy remains difficult. Combined exchange transfusion (with fresh heparinized blood) and peritoneal dialysis—sequentially or simultaneously—temporarily repairs both the chemical and hematologic abnormalities. Response may be delayed and repeated exchange transfusions necessary. Plasmapheresis with plasma exchange, total body washout, and charcoal hemoperfusion have been used in the treatment of fulminant hepatic failure. Both cross circulation with humans and chimpanzees and organ transplantation have been tried in desperate situations.

Corticosteroids may actually be harmful. Sterilization of the colon with antibiotics such as neomycin or kanamycin to decrease ammonia formation and alteration of the intestinal flora with *Lactobacillus acidophilus* (Duphalac), 2–3 tablespoons 3 or 4 times daily, may have merit. Intravenous arginine and glutamine have been used to decrease blood ammonia levels, but their value is questionable. There is recent experimental evidence that insulin and glucagon given via the portal vein may be hepatotropic and of some help in fulminant hepatic necrosis.

Close monitoring of fluid and electrolytes is mandatory. Maintenance of normal blood glucose levels is important. Diuretics, sedatives, and tranquilizers are to be avoided or used sparingly.

Tracheostomy and mechanical support of ventilation in the comatose patient are indicated with respiratory failure. Prophylactic gamma globulin, 0.04 ml/kg IM, should be given to contacts of the patient.

Prognosis
The overall prognosis remains very grave. Exchange transfusions combined with other modes of therapy may improve survival figures, depending on the regenerative capacity of the damaged liver, but only the rare survivor escapes postnecrotic cirrhosis.

Gregory PB & others: Steroid therapy in severe viral hepatitis. N Engl J Med 294:681, 1976.

Karvountzis GG, Redeker AG, Peters RL: Long term follow-up studies of patients surviving fulminant viral hepatitis. Gastroenterology 67:870, 1974.

Rivera RA, Slaughter RL, Boyce HW: Exchange transfusion in the treatment of patients with acute hepatitis in coma. Am J Dig Dis 15:589, 1970.

Wilson RA: Acute fulminant hepatic failure: Potential therapeutic role of hemoperfusion. Gastroenterology 69:244, 1975.

CHRONIC ACTIVE HEPATITIS
(Lupoid Hepatitis, Plasma Cell Hepatitis,
Chronic Hepatitis)

Chronic active hepatitis is most common in teenage girls, though it does occur at all ages and in either sex. It may follow acute infectious hepatitis or drug-induced hepatitis or may develop in conjunction with such diseases as ulcerative colitis, Sjögren's syndrome, or autoimmune hemolytic anemia. Persistence of $HB_s Ag$ has been noted in sera of several patients. Positive LE preparations and antinuclear antibodies and systemic manifestations, such as arthralgia, acne, and amenorrhea, suggest systemic lupus erythematosus with liver involvement. However, the liver histology is consistent with that described for chronic active hepatitis and not that of systemic lupus erythematosus. A genetic susceptibility to development of this entity is suggested by the increased incidence of the histocompatibility antigens HL-A1 and HL-A8. Increased autoimmune disease in families of patients and a high prevalence of seroimmunologic abnormalities in relatives have been noted.

Clinical & Laboratory Findings

Fever, malaise, recurrent or persistent jaundice, skin rash, arthritis, amenorrhea, gynecomastia, acne, pleurisy, pericarditis, ulcerative colitis, etc may be found in the history of these patients. Cutaneous signs of chronic liver disease may be noted (eg, spider angiomas, liver palms). Digital clubbing and hepatosplenomegaly may be present.

Liver function tests reveal smoldering disease with abnormal values for bilirubin, SGOT, SGPT, BSP retention, and serum alkaline phosphatase. Serum albumin may be low. Serum gamma globulin levels are strikingly elevated (in the range 3–6 gm/100 ml), with reports of values as high as 11 gm/100 ml. Low levels of C3 complement have been seen.

Histologic examination of liver biopsy specimens shows loss of the lobular limiting plate, "piecemeal" necrosis, portal fibrosis, an inflammatory reaction of lymphocytes and plasma cells in the portal areas as well as perivascularly, and some bile duct and Kupffer cell proliferation and pseudolobule formation.

Differential Diagnosis

Laboratory findings and histology differentiate other types of chronic hepatitis (eg, Wilson's disease, persistent hepatitis, chronic pericholangitis, subacute hepatitis). Drug-induced (isoniazid, methyldopa) chronic active hepatitis should be ruled out.

Complications

Continuing disease for months to years eventually results in postnecrotic cirrhosis. Persistent malaise, fatigue, and anorexia parallel disease activity. Bleeding from esophageal varices and development of ascites usually usher in hepatic failure.

Treatment

Corticosteroids decrease the mortality rate during the early active phase of the disease. Azathioprine (Imuran) may be of value in decreasing the side-effects of long-term corticosteroid therapy but should not be used alone during the "induction" phase of treatment. Clinical and biochemical remissions occur in 75–85% of cases even though a significant number of patients are left with "inactive" cirrhosis. Treatment is continued for 1–2 years.

Prognosis

The overall prognosis for chronic active hepatitis has been significantly improved by early therapy. Some report histologic cures in 30% of cases. Survival for 10 years is common despite residual cirrhosis. The rare child with HB_sAg-positive chronic active hepatitis may respond less well to the treatment regimen.

Boyer JL: Chronic hepatitis: A perspective on classification and determinants of prognosis. Gastroenterology 70:1161, 1975.

Dubois RS, Silverman A: Treatment of chronic active hepatitis in children. Postgrad Med J 50:386, 1974.

Galbraith RM & others: High prevalence of sero-immunologic abnormalities in relatives of patients with active chronic hepatitis or primary biliary cirrhosis. N Engl J Med 290:63, 1974.

Goldstein GB & others: Drug induced active chronic hepatitis. Am J Dig Dis 18:177, 1973.

Murray-Lyon IM, Stem RB, Williams R. Controlled trial of prednisone and azathioprine in active chronic hepatitis. Lancet 1:735, 1973.

Summerskill WHJ: Chronic active liver disease reexamined: Prognosis hopeful. Gastroenterology 66:450, 1974.

Summerskill WHJ & others: Prednisone for chronic active liver disease: Dose titration standard dose and combination with azathioprine compared. Gut 16:876, 1975.

POSTNECROTIC CIRRHOSIS

Most cases of postnecrotic cirrhosis occur without a prior episode of known hepatitis, but the disease may occur as a sequel to neonatal hepatitis, viral hepatitis type A or B, chronic active hepatitis, drug hepatitis, or with certain inborn errors of metabolism. The course may be insidious, as in anicteric hepatitis, Wilson's disease, or a_1-antitrypsin deficiency, or the disease may progress with episodes of acute exacerbation of hepatitis. The underlying liver disease may be quiescent, and a stable cirrhosis may exist. The rate of development of cirrhosis may depend upon the severity of injury, persistence of the offending agent, or a self-perpetuating process of liver injury.

Clinical Findings

General malaise, loss of appetite, dyspepsia with failure to thrive, and nausea and vomiting are frequent complaints. The first indication of underlying liver disease may be ascites, gastrointestinal hemorrhage, or even hepatic coma. There is variable hepatosplenomegaly with spider angiomas and red and warm "liver" palms. A small shrunken liver may sometimes be detected by abdominal percussion. Gynecomastia may be noted in males. Digital clubbing may be present. Irregularities of menstruation and amenorrhea in adolescent girls may be early complaints.

The most significant laboratory finding is elevation of the BSP retention. Jaundice may or may not be present, and serum protein determinations often reveal a decreased level of albumin and increased level of gamma globulins. Prothrombin time is prolonged and usually unresponsive to vitamin K administration. "Burr" red cells (acanthocytes) may be noted on the peripheral blood smear.

Esophageal varices may be demonstrated by x-ray.

Liver biopsy is necessary for exact confirmation of cirrhosis.

Differential Diagnosis

The most important entity to be considered is Wilson's disease. Others might include glycogen storage disease (especially type IV), galactosemia, fructose intolerance, porphyria, and a_1-antitrypsin deficiency.

Complications

In addition to ascites and hepatic coma, complications manifested by portal hypertension (eg, bleeding esophageal varices, hypersplenism) are frequently found. On the other hand, some individuals with compensated postnecrotic cirrhosis may lead a relatively normal life.

Treatment

There is no specific treatment for postnecrotic cirrhosis except in metabolic diseases, eg, galactosemia, fructosemia, and Wilson's disease. If laboratory tests and liver biopsy reveal ongoing disease suggesting chronic active hepatitis, then corticosteroids, or a combination of corticosteroids and immunosuppressive agents, are indicated. Severe hypersplenism may be treated by splenectomy, and bleeding esophageal varices by surgical shunting procedures. Ascites may be treated with a variety of diuretic agents such as chlorothiazide (Diuril) and spironolactone (Aldactone) in combination with a low-salt diet. Newer and more potent diuretic agents (eg, ethacrynic acid) must be used with care because of their tendency to produce potassium-deficient alkalosis. Nutrition can be improved with the use of medium chain triglycerides with large doses of water-soluble vitamins.

Prognosis

The prognosis is guarded since postnecrotic cirrhosis often follows an unpredictable pattern, with death occurring in the majority of patients within 10 years of diagnosis.

Appelman HD: Cirrhosis: Morphologic dynamics for the non-morphologist. Am J Dig Dis 17:463, 1972.

Popper H & others: Hepatic fibrosis: Correlation of biochemical and morphological investigations. Am J Med 49:701, 1970.

Schaefer JW & others: Progression of acute hepatitis to postnecrotic cirrhosis. Am J Med 42:348, 1967.

ALPHA$_1$-ANTITRYPSIN DEFICIENCY LIVER DISEASE

Essentials of Diagnosis

- Serum a_1-antitrypsin level less than 100 mg/100 ml.
- Identification of specific phenotype (Pi ZZ).
- Detection of glycoprotein deposits in hepatocytes.
- Histologic evidence of cirrhosis.
- Family history of early onset pulmonary disease or liver disease.

General Considerations

A deficiency in the protease inhibitor system (Pi) predisposing patients to chronic liver disease and an early onset of pulmonary emphysema is most often associated with the Pi phenotype ZZ. Autosomal codominant inheritance seems likely, with intermediate serum levels of a_1-antitrypsin present in the heterozygote phenotype (MZ).

Table 17−1. Familial hepatic diseases associated with cirrhosis.

	Predominant Hepatic Pathology	Frequency of Hepatic Pathology	Diagnostic Procedure
Wilson's disease	Postnecrotic or macronodular cirrhosis	High	Biopsy, liver copper content, 24-hour urinary copper excretion, copper oxidase levels in serum
Cystic fibrosis	Macronodular biliary cirrhosis	Moderately high	Sweat sodium or chloride
Galactosemia	Postnecrotic cirrhosis	High	Galactose-1-phosphate, uridyl transferase levels
Glycogen storage disease (type IV)	Macronodular	High	Amylo-1,4→1,6-transglucosidase (branching enzyme)
Fructose intolerance	Postnecrotic	Rare	Absence of fructose-1-phosphate aldolase
Infantile cirrhosis of India	Postnecrotic	All	Clinical setting
Hepatic porphyrias	Postnecrotic	Rare	Porphyrin excretion, liver biopsy
Rendu-Osler-Weber syndrome	Postnecrotic	Infrequent	Skin lesion, biopsy
Tyrosinosis	Postnecrotic	Frequent	Blood and urine amino acid screening tests
a_1-Antitrypsin deficiency	Postnecrotic	Frequent	Blood a_1-antitrypsin levels

Reports of cirrhosis occurring in the heterozygote condition (SZ, FZ) have been recently published. The exact relationship between low levels of serum a_1-antitrypsin and the development of lung and liver disease is unclear. The accumulated protein in the hepatocytes can be found in most patients, but not all have features of liver disease. These inclusion bodies contain a protein component immunologically cross-reactive with serum a_1-antitrypsin, but lacking sialic acid. This structural abnormality leads to aggregation in the endoplasmic reticulum, and is resistant to sialization by sialyltransferase. The likelihood of developing severe liver disease in response to hepatic injury is definitely increased in patients homozygous for this condition. From 30–50% of adults with a_1-antitrypsin deficiency have been found to have cirrhosis. A few children will have only pulmonary or pulmonary and hepatic involvement.

Clinical Findings

A. Symptoms and Signs: a_1-Antitrypsin deficiency should be suspected in all neonates with the "idiopathic" cholestatic syndrome. Poor appetite, lethargy, slight irritability, and jaundice suggest neonatal hepatitis but are not pathognomonic of any one cause. Hepatosplenomegaly is present.

In the older child, physical findings suggestive of cirrhosis (spider angiomas, liver palms, digital clubbing, small liver size, splenomegaly) should always lead one to suspect a_1-antitrypsin deficiency. Recurrent pulmonary disease (bronchitis, pneumonia) may be present in a few children.

B. Laboratory Findings: Low levels (less than 0.2 mg/100 ml) of the a_1-globulin fraction may be noted on serum protein fractionation. Specific quantitation of a_1-antitrypsin reveals levels of over 200 mg/100 ml in normals (MM) and less than 100 mg/100 ml in homozygotes (ZZ) deficient in this glycoprotein. Heterozygotes (MZ) have levels of 100–200 mg/100 ml. Liver function tests will often reflect the underlying hepatic pathology. Bilirubin (mixed type), transaminases, and liver alkaline phosphatase are elevated in the acute stage and low albumin and prolonged BSP retention in the cirrhotic stage. Hematologic assessment may reveal evidence of hypersplenism. The esophagogram frequently shows varices in advanced cases with portal hypertension.

Pathologic evidence of a_1-antitrypsin deficiency disease is seen in liver biopsy material, where diastasefast eosinophilic intracellular granules and hyaline masses are noted, particularly in the periportal zones. This material can be definitively identified by immunofluorescent technics and electron microscopy.

Differential Diagnosis

Other specific causes of neonatal cholestatic syndrome need to be considered (giant cell hepatitis, cytomegalovirus disease, galactosemia, syphilis, fructose intolerance, choledochal cysts, biliary atresia, etc), as well as causes of insidious cirrhosis in childhood (anicteric viral hepatitis A or B, Wilson's disease, cystic fibrosis, glycogen storage disease, etc). If pulmonary symptoms predominate, then cystic fibrosis, immune deficiency disease, tracheo-esophageal anomalies, hiatal hernia, hypoplastic pulmonary artery and lung disease, etc need consideration.

Complications

The propensity of patients with a_1-antitrypsin deficiency to develop chronic liver disease as a consequence of liver injury is a striking feature of this disorder. Most, if not all, will develop cirrhosis. The infant may succumb to the liver insult. Eventually, the vagaries of chronic liver disease prevail (nutritional disturbances affecting weight and growth, bleeding from esophageal varices, ascites, and hepatic coma).

Early-onset pulmonary emphysema occurs in young adults (age 30–40 years). An increased susceptibility to hepatocarcinoma has recently been noted in cirrhosis with a_1-antitrypsin deficiency.

Treatment

There is no specific treatment for the deficiency disorder. The neonatal cholestatic condition is treated with phenobarbital, 3–5 mg/kg/day orally, cholestyramine, 4–8 gm/day orally, medium chain triglyceride-containing formula, and water-miscible vitamins. Complications of portal hypertension, esophageal bleeding, ascites, etc are treated as described elsewhere. Genetic counseling is indicated whenever the diagnosis is made.

Prognosis

With liver injury (due to viral infection, toxins, drugs, etc), 30–50% of these patients either die from progressive liver disease or develop cirrhosis. A correlation between patterns and clinical course has been documented. Liver failure can be expected 5–15 years after development of cirrhosis.

Aagenases Ø & others: Pathology and pathogenesis of liver disease in alpha-1 antitrypsin deficient individuals. Postgrad Med J 50:365, 1974.

Hadchouel M, Gautier M: Histopathologic study of the liver in the early cholestatic phase of alpha-1-antitrypsin deficiency. J Pediatr 89:211, 1976.

Odievre M & others: Alpha-1-antitrypsin deficiency and liver disease in children: Phenotypes, manifestations and prognosis. Pediatrics 57:226, 1976.

Porter CA & others: Antitrypsin-deficiency and neonatal hepatitis. Br Med J 3:435, 1972.

Talamo RC: Basic and clinical aspects of the alpha-1-antitrypsin. Pediatrics 56:91, 1975.

Talamo RC, Feingold M: Infantile cirrhosis with hereditary alpha-1-antitrypsin deficiency: Clinical improvement in two siblings. Am J Dis Child 125:845, 1973.

BILIARY CIRRHOSIS

General Considerations

Congenital abnormalities of the bile ducts and

cystic fibrosis account for all but a few cases of biliary cirrhosis. Early biliary cirrhosis may be found in cases of unsuspected cholelithiasis and in hypersensitivity reactions to certain drugs, eg, phenothiazines, hydantoins. When the extrahepatic biliary tree is atretic, the progress of disease is rapid; where hypoplasia of the intrahepatic bile ducts exists, or in cystic fibrosis, progression to cirrhosis is variable but slow. Patients who have had a hepatoportal enterostomy (Kasai procedure) often have episodes of cholangitis which contribute to the development of biliary cirrhosis.

The predominating signs and symptoms are those of persistent jaundice, marked pruritus, hepatosplenomegaly, spider nevi, palmar erythema, xanthomas, and gynecomastia in males. Failure to thrive (with height and weight retardation) and steatorrhea are frequent. Ascites may be present. Laboratory findings show the typical obstructive pattern of jaundice, with elevations of blood cholesterol, alkaline phosphatase, and bile acids. Serum albumin is often reduced, with the gamma globulin fraction elevated. Esophageal varices are common in severe biliary cirrhosis secondary to extrahepatic biliary atresia and cystic fibrosis but unusual in intrahepatic atresia.

Liver biopsy shows proliferation, dilation, and plugging of bile ducts and fibrosis. There may sometimes be confusion with congenital hepatic fibrosis.

Differential Diagnosis

In the neonatal period, extrahepatic atresia or paucity of the intrahepatic ducts must be considered as the most likely cause. Stricture or stenosis of the extrahepatic ducts may also cause biliary cirrhosis. Unrecognized choledochal cysts and chronic cholelithiasis may lead to biliary cirrhosis. Cystic fibrosis can be ruled out by the sweat test. Drug toxicity (Dilantin) should be considered. Nonobstructive dilatation of the intrahepatic biliary tree (Caroli's syndrome) can lead to biliary cirrhosis.

Complications

Progressive deterioration and loss of liver cells with marked disruption of hepatic architecture is the common course. Hepatic decompensation, ascites, and coma eventually supervene. The consequences of portal hypertension, with bleeding esophageal varices and hypersplenism, are life-threatening. Early in the disease, severe pruritus may be disabling.

Treatment

Specific treatment is available only for surgically correctable lesions involving the extrahepatic biliary system and it must be performed before the cirrhosis becomes well established. Other cases are treated by supportive measures, including medium chain triglycerides, water-soluble vitamins (A, D, E, and K), and cholestyramine (Questran) in large doses (8–15 gm/day). Antibiotic therapy is indicated in cases where ascending cholangitis or pericholangitis is suspected. Liver transplantation may be of temporary benefit. Early

(age 2–3 months) surgery using the Kasai operation is currently a popular method of treatment.

Prognosis

The prognosis is good only in surgically corrected lesions. In the remainder, this is a progressive, ultimately fatal disease.

Shier KJ, Horn RI: The pathology of liver cirrhosis in patients with cystic fibrosis of the pancreas. Can Med Assoc J 89:645, 1963.
Thaler MM, Gellis SS: Studies in neonatal hepatitis and biliary atresia. (4 parts.) Am J Dis Child 116:257, 262, 271, 280, 1968.

CHOLECYSTITIS, CHOLELITHIASIS, & ACUTE HYDROPS OF THE GALLBLADDER

Gallstones, often related to hemolytic anemias, are more common than cholecystitis in preadolescent children. Acute and chronic cholecystitis without gallstones is found in teenagers. Cholecystitis may be seen in association with a systemic disease such as typhoid fever, scarlet fever, measles, etc or secondary to anatomic obstruction, either congenital or acquired. Impairment of bile flow may be a consequence of external pressure from neoplasm, lymph node enlargement in the porta hepatis, or pancreatic pseudocyst. Bile flow is impaired by gallstones in the cystic duct, common duct, or ampulla of Vater, as well as by ductal anomalies and tumor.

Clinical Findings

A. History: Acute epigastric or right upper quadrant pain precipitated by eating fatty foods suggests biliary colic. A careful inquiry about hematologic abnormalities may elicit evidence of congenital hemolytic anemia or sickle cell disease. The incidence of cholelithiasis increases sharply in the older teenager, especially in the face of obesity and pregnancy.

B. Symptoms and Signs: Recurrent severe, steady upper abdominal pains with tenderness over the right upper quadrant is the most constant physical finding; jaundice and a palpable mass are much less frequent. Vomiting is quite common with acute hydrops.

C. Laboratory Findings: The white blood count may be normal or elevated. Serum bilirubin and alkaline phosphatase are usually variably elevated. Pancreatic amylase levels are elevated when there is obstruction at the ampulla.

D. X-Ray Findings: X-rays may visualize calculi, and an oral cholecystogram may show impairment or nonfunctioning of the gallbladder with or without calculi. Enlargement of the gallbladder and delayed or incomplete emptying following a fatty meal are definitely abnormal findings in children. Intravenous cholangiography may be necessary if oral cholecystography is nondiagnostic or if better visualization of the common duct is desired. Ultrasonography is also a useful diagnostic tool in cases of acute hydrops or cholelithiasis and should be used if the gallbladder cannot be satisfactorily visualized by the oral route.

Differential Diagnosis

The possibilities to be considered for recurrent epigastric and right upper quadrant pain include peptic disease, liver disease, pancreatic pseudocyst, intestinal or colonic inflammatory disease, and kidney disease. The association of abdominal pain in children with hematologic disorders and its postprandial occurrence after fatty foods is most helpful. The triad of pain, jaundice, and a mass should suggest choledochal cyst, but confirmation is best obtained by radiologic studies or even laparotomy. Acute hydrops is almost impossible to differentiate from other inflammatory or obstructive bowel conditions.

Complications

The major concern in long-standing cases is biliary cirrhosis. Perforation of the gallbladder is extremely rare in children but does occur in acute cholecystitis. Obstructions at the level of the ampulla can result in pancreatitis.

Treatment

Symptomatic gallbladder disease is best treated by surgical removal of the gallbladder. Common duct patency should be verified by operative cholangiography. Acute hydrops is treated by aspiration or drainage.

Prognosis

The prognosis in surgically treated patients is good. The postcholecystectomy syndrome is extremely rare in children.

Ariyan S & others: Cholecystitis and cholelithiasis masking as abdominal crises in sickle cell disease. Pediatrics 58:252, 1976.

Bartrum RJ & others: Ultrasonic and radiographic cholecystography. N Engl J Med 296:538, 1977.

Crichlow RW, Seltzer MH, Jannetta PJ: Cholecystitis in adolescents. Am J Dig Dis 17:68, 1973.

Shrand H, Ackroyd FW: Gallstones in children. Clin Pediatr (Phila) 12:191, 1973.

PYOGENIC & AMEBIC LIVER ABSCESS

Pyogenic liver abscesses are usually secondary to pyogenic seeding via the portal vein from infected viscera and occasionally from ascending cholangitis. These lesions tend to be solitary and are located in the right hepatic lobe. Bacterial seeding may also occur from infected burns, pyodermas, and osteomyelitis. Unusual causes include omphalitis, subacute infective endocarditis, pyelonephritis, and perinephric abscess.

Pyogenic liver abscesses are usually multiple, especially when associated with severe sepsis. At particular risk are children receiving anti-inflammatory and immunosuppressive agents. Likewise, children with defects in white blood cell function (chronic granulomatous disease) are more prone to pyogenic hepatic abscesses. In adults there is a male preponderance, and the abscesses are usually solitary.

Although amebic liver abscess is still rare in children, a gradual increase in frequency has been noted, presumably as a result of increased travel through endemic areas (Mexico, Southeast Asia). *Entamoeba histolytica* invasion occurs via the large bowel, though a history of diarrhea (colitis-like picture) is not always obtained.

Clinical Findings

With pyogenic liver abscess, nonspecific complaints of low-grade to septic fever, chills, malaise, and abdominal pain are frequent. Weight loss is very common, especially in delayed diagnosis. A few patients have shaking chills and jaundice. The dominant complaint is a constant dull pain over an enlarged liver which is tender to palpation. An elevated hemidiaphragm with reduced or absent respiratory excursion may be demonstrated on physical examination and confirmed by fluoroscopy. Laboratory studies show leukocytosis and at times anemia. Liver function tests reveal low-grade bilirubin elevation and an elevated alkaline phosphatase. Elevated B_{12} levels are reported. Amebic liver abscesses are usually heralded by an acute illness with high fever, chills, and leukocytosis. An occasional prodrome may also include cough, dyspnea, and shoulder pain as rupture of the abscess into the right chest occurs.

A radioisotope liver scan is the most useful diagnostic aid; its overall accuracy is around 80%. Hepatic arteriography, an ultrasonic liver scan, or portal venography has likewise had success in demonstrating liver abscesses.

The distinction between pyogenic and amebic abscesses is best made by indirect hemagglutination test.

Differential Diagnosis

Hepatitis, hepatoma, hydatid cyst, gallbladder disease, or biliary tract infections can mimic liver abscess. Subphrenic abscesses, empyema, and pneumonia may give a similar picture. Inflammatory disease of the intestines or of the biliary system may be complicated by liver abscess.

Complications

Spontaneous rupture of the abscess may occur with extension of infection into the subphrenic space, thorax, peritoneal cavity, and occasionally the pericardium. Bronchopleural fistula with large sputum production and hemoptysis can develop in severe cases. Simultaneously, the amebic liver abscess may be secondarily infected with bacteria (10–20% of cases). Metastatic hematogenous spread to the lungs and brain has been reported.

Treatment

When a solitary pyogenic liver abscess is localized, adequate surgical drainage should be performed. Both extraperitoneal and extrapleural drainage are recommended. Cultures are taken and massive specific antibiotic therapy started.

Multiple small abscesses may be impossible to drain surgically, and cultures are needed for specific antimicrobial therapy, especially anaerobic cultures.

Amebic abscesses should be treated promptly once the diagnosis is considered. Drugs of choice include either chloroquine, 20 mg/kg/day orally (up to 500 mg daily) for 10 weeks, or metronidazole (Flagyl), 250–1000 mg/day orally for 10 days.* Surgical drainage of the amebic abscess is rarely indicated except when secondary bacterial infection exists. Failure to improve after 72 hours on drug therapy indicates superimposed bacterial infection or an incorrect diagnosis. The effect of treatment is best assessed by a liver scan.

Prognosis

An unrecognized and untreated pyogenic liver abscess is universally fatal. The surgical cure rate is about 75%.

Most amebic abscesses are cured with conservative medical management.

Dehner LD, Kissane JM: Pyogenic hepatic abscesses in infancy and childhood. J Pediatr 74:763, 1969.
Reynolds TB: Amebic abscess of the liver. Gastroenterology 60:952, 1971.
Ribaudo JM, Ochsner A: Intrahepatic abscesses: Amebic and pyogenic. Am J Surg 125:570, 1973.
Rubin RH & others: Hepatic abscess: Changes in clinical, bacteriologic and therapeutic aspects. Am J Med 57:601, 1974.

EXTRAHEPATIC PORTAL HYPERTENSION

Essentials of Diagnosis

- Splenomegaly.
- Esophageal varices with hematemesis or melena.
- Elevated splenic pulp pressure.
- Normal wedged hepatic vein pressure.
- Normal liver histology.
- Impaired patency of splenic and portal veins shown by splenoportography and venous phase of superior mesenteric or splenic aortography.

General Considerations

Extrahepatic portal hypertension from acquired abnormalities of the portal and splenic veins accounts for 5–8% of cases of gastrointestinal bleeding in chil-

*See p 804 for a note of caution on the possible hazards of metronidazole.

dren. A history of neonatal omphalitis, sepsis, dehydration, and umbilical vein catheterization is present in 30–50% of cases. Symptoms may occur before 1 year of age, but in most cases the diagnosis is not made until 3–5 years of age. Splenomegaly is often the first abnormal physical finding. Massive hematemesis or melena occurs within the next few years.

A variety of portal or splenic vein malformations have been described, including valves, cavernous transformation, and atretic segments. The site of the venous obstruction may be anywhere from the hilus of the liver to the hilus of the spleen.

Clinical Findings

A. Symptoms and Signs: Splenomegaly in a well child is the most constant physical sign. Recurrent episodes of ascites may also be noted. The usual presenting symptoms are hematemesis and melena. An episode of bronchitis, tracheitis, or pneumonia with significant cough can precipitate esophageal bleeding. The presence of extrahepatic portal hypertension is suggested by the following: (1) An episode of severe infection in the newborn period or early infancy—especially omphalitis, sepsis, gastroenteritis, severe dehydration, or prolonged or difficult umbilical vein catheterizations. (2) No previous evidence of liver disease. (3) A feeling of well-being prior to onset or recognition of symptoms. (4) Transient ascites may occur following a bleeding episode.

B. Laboratory and X-Ray Findings: Most other common causes of splenomegaly may be excluded by proper laboratory tests. Cultures, heterophil titer, blood smear examination, bone marrow, and liver function tests are necessary. Mild leukopenia and thrombocytopenia are present in most cases. Esophagography will reveal varices in over 80% of these patients. In addition to normal liver function tests, confirmation of a normal liver is best obtained directly by liver biopsy or indirectly by measurement of wedged hepatic vein pressure (normal, 3–12 mm Hg). The finding of an elevated splenic pulp pressure (normal, 8–12 mm Hg) and demonstration of the block by simultaneous splenic portography confirms the diagnosis of extrahepatic portal hypertension. Filling of collateral vessels to stomach and esophagus by the dye is frequently demonstrated.

Differential Diagnosis

All causes of splenomegaly must be included in the differential diagnosis, the most common ones being infections, blood dyscrasias, lipidosis, reticuloendotheliosis, cirrhosis of the liver, and cysts or hemangiomas of the spleen. When hematemesis or melena occurs, other causes of gastrointestinal bleeding are possible, ie, gastric or duodenal ulcers, tumors, duplications, ulcerative bowel disease, and suprahepatic or hepatic venous obstructions.

Complications

The major manifestation and complication of this condition is bleeding esophageal varices. Fatal exsanguination appears to be uncommon, but hypovolemic shock or resulting anemia may require prompt treatment. Congestive splenomegaly with granulocytopenia and thrombocytopenia occurs. Rupture of the enlarged spleen due to trauma is always a threat. Leukopenia and thrombocyotopenia seldom cause major symptoms. Unexplained fluctuating episodes of ascites may develop, and retroperitoneal edema has been reported (Clatworthy's sign).

Treatment

A. Surgical Measures: The surgical treatment of this disease has been disappointing. Portacaval anastomosis would be the most satisfactory procedure, but the portal vein is often involved in the basic disease process, making it unsuitable for anastomosis except in rare cases. Most children have previously been treated by means of simultaneous splenectomy and splenorenal shunts. Sustained patency of this shunt procedure is unlikely in children under the age of 8–10 years. Thrombosis of the shunt is soon followed by recurrent and often more severe hemorrhage from esophageal varices. Splenectomy increases the risk of overwhelming sepsis. More importantly, however, it removes a "safe" group of collateral vessels running from the splenic capsule to the azygos veins, thereby bypassing the esophageal and gastric drainage system.

Other surgical decompression procedures include anastomosis of the superior mesenteric vein to the inferior vena cava (mesocaval shunt), distal splenorenal shunt (Warren procedure), or the interposition mesocaval shunt using knitted Dacron or Teflon for the graft. Esophageal and gastric resection of the varices and transthoracic ligation of the varices have been used as more desperate measures.

B. Medical Treatment: Since a few children with this disease will die as a result of esophageal bleeding, every effort should be made to control the disease medically. The chances for successful surgical shunting procedures appear to improve as the child gets older. The patient may even develop his own decompressive shunt which is adequate to prevent major bleeding from the esophageal varices.

Spontaneous cessation of hemorrhage from esophageal varices occurs frequently. Shock must be treated with blood transfusions and anemia with iron. Careful use of a pediatric Sengstaken-Blakemore tube can stop the bleeding. Freezing or cooling the varices is not recommended. A transient reduction of portal venous pressure may be achieved by the use of intravenous vasopressin (Pitressin). A dose of 0.2 units/minute in 5% dextrose in water given for 20–40 minutes often stops the bleeding. The effect of vasopressin is constriction of the splanchnic and hepatic arterioles and consequent lowering of portal venous pressure. Selective infusion of vasopressin into the superior mesenteric artery with 0.1–0.2 units/minute has also been effective in stopping esophageal bleeding. Hypertension, diminished cardiac output, and water retention may occur with this form of treatment.

Antacids, alkalies, anticholinergics, small feedings,

and positioning have been suggested to reduce gastric acidity or prevent esophageal reflux. Avoidance of contact sports in the presence of splenomegaly is advisable.

Prognosis

The prognosis depends upon the site of the block and the availability of suitable vessels for shunting procedures. Each unsuccessful surgical procedure worsens the prognosis for life. Bleeding episodes, however, seem to diminish with adolescence.

The prognosis in patients managed by medical and supportive theory may be better than in the surgically treated group, especially when surgery is performed at an early age.

Conn HO & others: Intra-arterial vasopressin in the treatment of upper gastrointestinal hemorrhage: A prospective controlled clinical trial. Gastroenterology 68:211, 1975.

Ehrlich F & others: Portal hypertension: Surgical management in infants and children. J Pediatr Surg 9:283, 1974.

Fonkalsrud EW & others: Reassessment of operative procedures for portal hypertension in infants and children. Am J Surg 118:148, 1969.

Martin LW: Changing concepts of management of portal hypertension in children. J Pediatr Surg 7:559, 1972.

Reynolds TB & others: Measurement of portal pressure and its clinical application. Am J Med 49:649, 1970.

SUPRAHEPATIC & INTRAHEPATIC (NONCIRRHOTIC) PORTAL HYPERTENSION

In the absence of cirrhosis, suprahepatic or intrahepatic causes of portal hypertension are rare in the pediatric group. Three major entities are to be considered:

(1) Hepatic vein occlusion or thrombosis (Budd-Chiari syndrome): In most instances, no cause can be demonstrated. Endothelial injury to hepatic veins by bacterial endotoxins has been shown experimentally. The occasional association of hepatic vein thrombosis in inflammatory bowel disease (ulcerative colitis, regional enteritis, infectious diarrhea) favors the presence of endogenous toxins invading the portal vein and reaching the liver. Allergic vasculitis leading to endophlebitis of the hepatic veins has been occasionally described. In addition, hepatic vein obstruction may be secondary to tumor, hyperthermia, or sepsis.

(2) Jamaican veno-occlusive disease (acute stage): This entity appears to be the result of ingestion of "bush tea" (*Crotalaria fulva*), a member of the Senecio family. It causes widespread occlusion of the small and medium-sized hepatic veins, with resultant congestion and necrosis of the neighboring parenchymal cells. The acute form of the disease generally follows a nonspecific respiratory illness. The disease may be rapidly fatal, although about 50% recover. A subacute and chronic form also exists. Increased use of herbal teas in this country has been responsible for several recently reported cases.

(3) **Congenital hepatic fibrosis:** This rare cause of portal hypertension is inherited as an autosomal recessive and requires liver biopsy for diagnosis. Splenoportography, however, is normal even though splenic pulp pressure is increased. Renal abnormalities (microcystic disease) are often associated with the hepatic lesion, so that a urogram should be routine.

Clinical Findings & Diagnostic Studies

Patients with suprahepatic causes of portal hypertension have abdominal enlargement due to ascites as the presenting complaint in all but a few cases. Abdominal pain and tender hepatosplenomegaly are frequently found. Jaundice is present in about 25% of cases. Vomiting, hematemesis, and diarrhea are less common. The presence of distended superficial veins on the anterior abdomen along with dependent edema is usually seen with inferior vena cava obstruction. Absence of the hepatojugular reflex (jugular distention when pressure is applied to the liver) is a helpful clinical sign. Liver function tests are not usually helpful. Localization is difficult. An inferior venacavogram may reveal an intrinsic filling defect from an infiltrating tumor or from extrinsic pressure and obstruction of the inferior vena cava by an adjacent tumor or nodes. Care must be taken in interpreting extrinsic pressure defects of the subdiaphragmatic inferior vena cava in the face of ascites.

Simultaneous wedge hepatic vein pressure and hepatic venography are most useful procedures. Pressures should also be taken from the right heart and supradiaphragmatic portion of the inferior vena cava. Hepatic vein pressure and splenic pulp pressure are elevated. Obstruction to major hepatic vein ostia and smaller vessels may be demonstrated by this procedure. In the absence of obstruction, reflux across the sinusoids into the portal vein branches can be accomplished. In most instances, open liver biopsy should be undertaken. Marked central venous congestion and necrosis without fibrosis are striking. Endothelial thickening of hepatic veins may also be found.

Patients with congenital hepatic fibrosis have the same mode of presentation as those with extrahepatic portal hypertension. Signs, symptoms, and results of liver function tests are similar.

Differential Diagnosis

Cirrhosis of the liver due to any cause must be ruled out. Suprahepatic (cardiac and pulmonary) or infrahepatic causes of portal hypertension must also be excluded. Although ascites may occur in extrahepatic portal hypertension, it is not common. Cutaneous signs of chronic liver disease are lacking since this entity is usually acute.

Complications

Without treatment, complete and persistent hepatic vein obstruction will lead to liver failure, coma, and death. A nonportal type of cirrhosis may develop in the chronic form of Jamaican veno-occlusive disease in which small and medium-sized hepatic veins are af-

fected. Hematemesis due to bleeding esophageal varices is frequent in the few survivors. Death from renal failure may occur in some cases of congenital hepatic fibrosis.

Treatment

Efforts to correct underlying causes must be promptly undertaken. Surgical removal of the occluding tumor or of the hepatic vein thrombi is possible when the large ostia are involved. Portacaval shunts and right atrial to inferior vena cava grafts have been attempted. Medical management with heparin, corticosteroids, and diuretics has had inconsistent results. Simple portacaval shunting is the treatment of choice in patients with congenital hepatic fibrosis.

Prognosis

Hepatic vein obstruction carries a very high mortality rate (95%). In veno-occlusive disease, the prognosis is better, with complete recovery possible in 50% of acute forms and 5–10% of subacute forms.

Murray-Lyon IM, Ockenden BG, Williams R: Congenital hepatic fibrosis: Is it a single clinical entity? Gastroenterology 64:653, 1973.

Stillman AF & others: Hepatic veno-occlusive disease due to pyrrolizidine (Senecio) poisoning in Arizona. Gastroenterology 73:349, 1977.

HEPATOMAS

Essentials of Diagnosis

- Abdominal enlargement.
- Hepatomegaly with or without a definable mass.
- Weight loss.
- Anemia.
- Laparotomy and tissue biopsy.

General Considerations

Primary epithelial neoplasms of the liver represent 0.2–5.8% of all malignant conditions in the pediatric age group. There are 2 basic morphologic types with certain clinical and prognostic differences. Hepatoblastoma predominates in male infants and children, with most cases appearing before age 3. The predominance of right-sided lesions has aroused interest since the left lobe is supplied with oxygenated blood from the umbilical vein and the right lobe with portal vein blood, which has a lower oxygen saturation.

Hepatocarcinoma is extremely rare in girls and occurs more frequently after age 3. This type of neoplasm carries a poorer prognosis than hepatoblastoma and for some reason causes more abdominal discomfort and pain. Hepatocarcinoma has been reported in children with postnecrotic cirrhosis or biliary cirrhosis, but these are the exceptions rather than the rule. The association of hepatocarcinoma with tyrosinosis and

a_1-antitrypsin deficiency cirrhosis has also been reported. An interesting aspect of primary epithelial neoplasms of the liver has been the increased incidence of associated anomalies and unusual conditions found in these children. Virilization has been reported as a consequence of gonadotropin activity of the tumor. Leydig cell hyperplasia without spermatogenesis is found on testicular biopsy. Hemihypertrophy, congenital absence of the kidney, macroglossia, and Meckel's diverticulum have been found in association with hepatocarcinoma. The late development of hepatoma in patients treated with androgens must also be kept in mind.

Clinical Findings

A. History: Noticeable increase in abdominal girth with or without pain is the most constant feature of the history. Constitutional symptoms (anorexia, fatigue, fever, chills, etc) may be present.

B. Symptoms and Signs: Weight loss, pallor, and abdominal pain associated with a large abdomen are common. Physical examination reveals hepatomegaly with or without a definite tumor mass, usually to the right of the midline. Signs of chronic liver disease are usually absent.

C. Laboratory Findings: Normal to slightly distorted liver function tests are the rule. Anemia is frequently seen, especially in cases of hepatoblastoma. Percutaneous liver biopsy can be safely performed, but final tissue diagnosis should be made at laparotomy. Cystathioninuria has been reported. Alpha$_1$ fetoglobulin may be elevated.

D. X-Ray Findings: X-ray is at times helpful in demonstrating the tumor shadow or calcified foci in the neoplasm. It is very helpful in proving the presence or absence of obvious metastases as well as in localizing the lesion to the liver. Specialized technics such as radioactive liver scans and selective celiac axis or umbilical artery angiography are generally part of the preoperative work-up.

Differential Diagnosis

In the absence of a palpable mass, the differential diagnosis is that of hepatomegaly and anemia. Hematologic and nutritional conditions should be ruled out, as well as less common entities such as lipid storage diseases, histiocytosis X, glycogen storage disease, hepatic abscess (pyogenic or amebic), cysts, and hemangiomas. Parasitic infections, toxins, and drugs can cause identical symptoms. Veno-occlusive disease and thrombosis of the hepatic veins are also rare possibilities. Tumors in the left lobe may be mistaken for pancreatic pseudocysts.

Complications

Progressive enlargement of the tumor, abdominal discomfort, ascites, respiratory difficulty, and widespread metastases are the rule. Rupture of the neoplastic liver and intraperitoneal hemorrhage have been reported. Progressive anemia and emaciation predispose to an early septic death. Metastases are most frequently to the lungs and abdominal lymph nodes.

Treatment

An energetic surgical approach has brought forth the only long-term survivors. Complete lobectomy appears to be preferred over partial resection. It appears that every isolated lung metastasis should also be surgically resected. Radiotherapy and chemotherapy have been disappointing in the treatment of primary liver neoplasms, although new combinations of drugs are continually being evaluated.

Organ transplantation has been disappointing.

Prognosis

Survival is possible only if radical surgical resection is done. In one series of cases, 15 of 37 patients were still alive without evidence of metastasis—7 of them for more than 5 years—following resection.

Alpert ME & others: Alpha-1 fetoglobulin in the diagnosis of human hepatoma. N Engl J Med 278:984, 1968.

Clatworthy HW Jr, Schiller M, Grosfeld JL: Primary liver tumors in infancy and childhood. Arch Surg 109:143, 1974.

Ishak KG, Glunz PR: Hepatoblastoma and hepatocarcinoma in infancy and childhood: Report of 47 cases. Cancer 20:396, 1967.

Meadows AT & others: Hepatoma associated with androgen therapy for aplastic anemia. J Pediatr 84:109, 1974.

WILSON'S DISEASE
(Hepatolenticular Degeneration)

Essentials of Diagnosis

- Acute or chronic liver disease.
- Deteriorating neurologic status.
- Kayser-Fleischer rings.
- Elevated liver copper.
- Abnormalities in levels of ceruloplasmin and serum and urine copper.

General Considerations

No longer considered a defect in ceruloplasmin, the increased hepatic copper may be due to an abnormal copper binding protein or to a lysosomal defect that impairs the excretion of biliary copper. Other copper-containing enzymes, notably those in the respiratory chain, may also be involved as part of a generalized disorder of copper metabolism. The disease should be considered in all children with evidence of liver disease or with suggestive neurologic signs. A family history is often present.

Clinical Findings

A. Symptoms and Signs: Hepatic involvement may be acute or may progress to postnecrotic cirrhosis in an insidious manner. Findings include jaundice, splenomegaly, Kayser-Fleischer rings, and neurologic manifestations such as tremor, dysarthria, and drooling. Deterioration in school performance is often the earliest neurologic expression of disease. The rings can sometimes be detected by unaided visual inspection as a brown band at the junction of the iris and cornea, but slitlamp examination is usually necessary.

B. Laboratory Findings: Early, liver function tests are consistent with hepatocellular damage. Late in the course, only the BSP may be useful to assess the degree of liver damage.

The laboratory diagnosis of Wilson's disease is sometimes difficult. Serum ceruloplasmin levels are usually < 20 mg/100 ml and are measured as copper oxidase rather than directly. (Normal values are 23—43 mg/100 ml.) Low values, however, are seen normally in infants under 3 months of age, and in 3—5% of homozygotes the levels may be normal. Serum copper levels are low, but the overlap with normal is too great for satisfactory discrimination. Urine copper levels in children over 3 years of age are normally < 30 μg/day; in Wilson's disease, they are > 50 μg/day. Finally, the tissue content of copper from a liver biopsy, normally < 20 μg/gm wet tissue, is > 50 μg/gm wet tissue in Wilson's disease.

Glycosuria and aminoaciduria as well as elevated serum uric acid levels have been reported. Hemolysis and, on rare occasions, gallstones may be found on routine radiography; bone lesions simulating those of osteochondritis dissecans have also been found.

The coarse nodular cirrhosis and glycogen nuclei seen on liver biopsy may distinguish Wilson's disease from other types of cirrhosis. Early in the disease, vacuolation of liver cells, fatty degeneration, and lipofuscin granules can be seen, as well as Mallory bodies. The presence of the latter in a child is strongly suggestive of Wilson's disease.

Differential Diagnosis

During the icteric phase, acute viral hepatitis type A or B, a_1-antitrypsin deficiency, chronic active hepatitis, and drug-induced hepatitis are the usual diagnostic variables. Later, other causes of cirrhosis and portal hypertension need consideration. Laboratory testing for the specific factors listed above will differentiate Wilson's disease from the others.

Complications

Progressive degenerating liver disease and hepatic coma and death are not uncommon. Recovery from the initial episode usually results in cirrhosis of the postnecrotic type. Progressive degenerating CNS disease and terminal aspiration pneumonia are common in untreated older people.

Treatment

Penicillamine (Cuprimine), 900—1200 mg/day orally, is the drug of choice in all cases, whether symptomatic or not. Dietary restriction of copper intake is not practical. The dosage of penicillamine may be reduced after urinary copper levels return to normal. Triethylenetetramine dihydrochloride (TETA) or levodopa may be helpful in cases where penicillamine is unsuccessful or results in toxicity. Liver transplantation may be curative if rejection can be controlled.

General treatment measures for acute hepatitis are as outlined for infectious hepatitis.

Prognosis

The prognosis of hepatitis due to Wilson's disease is not favorable, though reversal of the hepatic lesion following treatment has been reported in isolated cases. Eventual liver failure and coma often occur prior to brain death.

Barbeau A, Friesen H: Treatment of Wilson's disease with L-dopa after failure of penicillamine. Lancet 1:1180, 1970.
Slovis TL & others: The varied manifestations of Wilson's disease. J Pediatr 78:578, 1971.
Sternlieb I, Scheinberg IH: Chronic hepatitis as a first manifestation of Wilson's disease. Ann Intern Med 76:59, 1972.
Sternlieb I, Scheinberg IH: Prevention of Wilson's disease in asymptomatic patients. N Engl J Med 278:352, 1968.
Sternlieb I & others: Lysosomal defect of hepatic copper excretion in Wilson's disease (hepatolenticular degeneration). Gastroenterology 64:99, 1973.·

REYE'S SYNDROME
(Encephalopathy With Fatty Degeneration of the Viscera; White Liver Disease)

Essentials of Diagnosis

- Prodromal upper respiratory infection, influenza B illness, or chickenpox.
- Vomiting.
- Lethargy, drowsiness progressing to semicoma.
- Elevated SGOT, normal or slightly elevated bilirubin, prolonged prothrombin time.
- Variable hypoglycemia and hyperammonemia.
- Microvesicular steatosis of liver, kidneys, brain, etc.

General Considerations

This syndrome is being reported with increasing frequency since its recognition in 1963. Young children seem to be at greater risk. Persistent attempts to implicate a single etiologic factor have failed. Varicella, influenza A and B, echovirus 2, coxsackie A virus, rheovirus, and EB (Epstein-Barr) virus have been isolated from some patients. Epidemics of Reye's syndrome seem to cluster during influenza B epidemics. Toxic and metabolic causes, particularly salicylates, have also been incriminated. The mode of onset frequently leads to confusion with other causes of coma, particularly toxic encephalopathy and hepatic coma.

The molecular mechanisms leading to Reye's syndrome are not yet understood. Current thinking is that it reflects acute virus-induced damage to mitochondria with consequent uncoupling of oxidative phosphorylation.

Clinical Findings

A. Symptoms and Signs: Most cases give a history

of minor upper respiratory illness of short duration preceding the development of vomiting, irrational behavior, progressive stupor, and coma. Resolving chickenpox may be present in 10–20% of cases. Restlessness and convulsions may also occur. Striking physical findings are hyperpnea, irregular respirations, and dilated, sluggishly reacting pupils. Jaundice is minimal or absent. Splenomegaly is seldom present. A positive Babinski sign and hyperreflexia in association with decorticate and decerebrate posturing are consistent with severe cerebral edema.

B. Laboratory Findings: CSF is acellular and CSF glucose may be low. CSF pressure is variably elevated. The serum glucose is proportionately decreased. Moderate to severe elevations of SGOT, SGPT, and LDH are found. Serum bilirubin and alkaline phosphatase values are normal to slightly elevated. The prothrombin time is usually prolonged, and the blood ammonia is elevated in most cases. A mixed respiratory alkalosis and metabolic acidosis is seen. In a few cases, BUN has been elevated. Hyperaminoacidemia (glutamine, alanine, lysine) and hypocitrullinemia are present.

The histopathology of Reye's syndrome is most striking in the brain, liver, and kidneys; less commonly, changes in the heart and pancreas may be found. The brain shows gross cerebral edema, occasionally with evidence of herniation.

Histologically, loss of neurons and fatty vacuolation around small vessels have been noted. The liver shows diffuse microvesicular steatosis with minimal inflammatory changes. Glycogen is virtually absent from the hepatocytes in biopsies taken before giving hypertonic glucose. Ultrastructural changes are mitochondrial.

The kidney changes consist principally of swelling and fatty degeneration of the proximal lobules.

C. Electroencephalography: The EEG is diffusely abnormal, with marked slow wave activity predominating.

Differential Diagnosis

Differentiation of Reye's syndrome from acute toxic encephalopathy or from hepatic coma or fulminating hepatitis can be made on clinical and laboratory grounds. A negative history and urine screen for ingestion of poisons and drugs, absence of cells in the CSF, and absence of jaundice are significant. Fulminating hepatitis and hepatic coma in the absence of jaundice have been reported but are extremely rare. Liver biopsy is diagnostic, and the procedure is indicated in atypical cases.

Complications

Aspiration pneumonitis and respiratory failure are common, as with any comatose patient. Most patients die of cerebral complications rather than hepatic or renal failure. Herniation of the brain stem due to cerebral edema is the most serious complication. Cardiac arrhythmias may develop, and so may inappropriate ADH excretion and diabetes insipidus terminally.

Treatment

Treatment is empirical and supportive. A nasogastric tube, Foley catheter, and arterial and central venous pressure lines should be inserted immediately. Mechanical support of ventilation may become necessary if the patient reaches stage III coma (Lovejoy). Cerebral edema should be monitored directly, using either a subarachnoid transducer or intraventricular tube. Intracranial pressures (ICP) should be kept below 20–25 mm Hg. Respirator settings should keep the P_{CO_2} at 20–25 mm Hg and the arterial pH at 7.5–7.6. Mannitol infusions (1.5–2.0 gm/kg) can be given every 4 hours. At times, additional hyperosmolar agents are required to keep ICP below 25 mm Hg. Urea, 1 gm/kg intravenously, or glycerol, 1.5 gm/kg by nasogastric tube, may be tried. Maintenance fluids using 10% glucose should be given at a rate sufficient to produce a urine flow of 1–1.5 ml/kg/hour. Careful attention to central venous pressure is needed when using hyperosmolar agents. Exchange transfusions have been used with success. Peritoneal dialysis is no longer used. Vitamin K, 3–5 mg IM, should be administered. Citrulline, 100 mg/kg IV, and nicotinic acid, 500 mg IV every 30 minutes for 3 doses, have questionable value.

Prognosis

At least 70% of these patients survive. Severe neurologic residuals are not uncommon in the younger children (< 2 years) who recover from prolonged stage III–IV coma.

Aoki Y, Lombroso CT: Prognostic value of electroencephalography in Reye's syndrome. Neurology 23:333, 1973.

Aprille JR: Reye's syndrome: Patient serum alters mitochondrial function and morphology in vitro. Science 197:908, 1977.

Bobo RC & others: Reye's syndrome: Treatment by exchange transfusion with special reference to the 1974 epidemic in Cincinnati, Ohio. J Pediatr 87:881, 1975.

DeVivo DC & others: Reye's syndrome: Results of intensive supportive care. J Pediatr 87:875, 1975.

Shaywitz BA & others: Prolonged continuous monitoring of intracranial pressure in severe Reye's syndrome. Pediatrics 59:595, 1977.

ACUTE PANCREATITIS

Most cases of acute pancreatitis are due to drugs, mumps, or abdominal trauma. Less common causes resulting in acute obstruction to pancreatic flow include stones in the ampulla of Vater, choledochal cysts, tumors of the duodenum, and ascariasis. Acute pancreatitis has recently been seen as a consequence of high-dosage corticosteroid therapy and administration of sulfasalazine (salicylazosulfapyridine), thiazides, and other drugs. It may also occur in cystic fibrosis, systemic lupus erythematosus, hyperparathyroidism, and malnutrition. Alcohol-induced pancreatitis should be considered in the teenage patient.

Clinical Findings

A. Signs and Symptoms: An acute onset of severe upper abdominal pain occasionally referred to the back, with vomiting and fever, is the common presenting picture. The abdomen is tender but not rigid, and bowel sounds are diminished. Jaundice may also be noted in less than one-third of cases. In cases due to trauma, an abdominal mass may be felt that is suggestive of pseudocyst. Ascites may be noted in such cases also.

B. Laboratory Findings: Leukocytosis and an elevated serum amylase and urine diastase should be expected early. Serum lipase is likewise elevated and persists longer than serum amylase. Serum calcium may be low and signifies a poor prognosis. Hyperglycemia and slightly elevated serum bilirubin values occur.

C. X-Ray Findings: An upper gastrointestinal series may demonstrate abnormalities in the duodenum in the case of tumors, stones, pseudocyst, etc and should be ordered in cases where abdominal trauma has occurred. Plain x-rays of the abdomen may show a localized ileus (sentinel loop).

Differential Diagnosis

Other causes of acute upper abdominal pain include lesions of the stomach, duodenum, liver, and biliary system, acute gastroenteritis or atypical appendicitis, pneumonia, volvulus, and intussusception.

Complications

Complications early in the disease include fluid and electrolyte disturbances, ileus, and hypocalcemic tetany. Later, pseudocyst formation may develop and may be associated with internal fistulas. Hypervolemia is seen between the third and fifth day, at which time renal tubular necrosis may occur. Chronic pancreatitis and pancreatic lithiasis may occur as sequelae. Splenic vein thrombosis can also occur.

Treatment

Medical management includes rest, gastric suction, fluids, electrolyte replacement, and blood or plasma as needed. Pain should be controlled with meperidine. Atropine may be used intramuscularly. Recurrence of pain after oral feedings may be prevented by giving pancreatic enzymes with the meal.

Surgical treatment is reserved for stones, cysts, and anatomic obstructive lesions.

Prognosis

As most cases are due to drugs or mumps, the prognosis is excellent with conservative management. The mortality rate is 5–10% in patients treated by operation and 1% in those treated medically. The morbidity rate is also high in the surgical group as a result of fistula formation.

Jordan SC, Ament ME: Pancreatitis in children and adolescents. J Pediatr 91:211, 1977.

CHRONIC PANCREATITIS

Two general forms of chronic pancreatitis have been reported: chronic fibrosing pancreatitis and the more common hereditary chronic relapsing pancreatitis with a familial tendency. An autosomal dominant mode of inheritance has been noted.

The causes include stenotic lesions of the ampulla of Vater, strictures of the pancreatic ducts, and parasitic infestations or gallstones in the ampulla. Chronic intermittent disease may rarely follow mumps pancreatitis and may be a consequence of abdominal trauma with or without pseudocyst formation.

Pancreatitis is rarely symptomatic in cystic fibrosis.

Clinical Findings

The diagnosis of the hereditary form is usually not made in childhood unless there is a similar history in other family members. The diagnosis of chronic fibrosing pancreatitis is made by surgical exploration demonstrating a normal duct system and typical histology in the pancreatic biopsy.

A. Symptoms and Signs: There is usually a history of recurrent upper abdominal pain of variable severity but prolonged (1–6 days') duration. Radiation of the pain into the back is a frequent complaint. Fever and vomiting are not common in the chronic form. Abnormal stools and symptoms of diabetes may develop later in the course of this disease, and malnutrition due to failure of pancreatic exocrine secretions may also occur.

B. Laboratory Findings: The serum or urine amylase is usually elevated during the early acute attacks. Pancreatic insufficiency and reduced volume and bicarbonate response may be found at duodenal intubation after intravenous administration of pancreozymin (2 units/kg) (available from Kabi Diagnostica, Stockholm) and secretin (2 units/kg) (also available from Kabi Diagnostica). A 3-fold increase of normal serum amylase values is considered a positive test for obstruction.

Blood lipids and urinary amino acids are elevated in familial forms of the disease associated with hyperlipoproteinemia and should be studied in all cases. Elevated blood sugar levels and glycosuria are frequently found in protracted disease. Sweat chloride should be checked for cystic fibrosis and serum calcium for hyperparathyroidism.

C. X-Ray Findings: X-rays of the abdomen may show pancreatic or gallbladder calcifications. Contrast studies may demonstrate other obstructive lesions in the region of the duodenum. Retrograde pancreatography may become a helpful tool in the nonsurgical diagnosis. Pancreatograms show ductal dilatation rather than obvious strictures or stenotic segments.

Differential Diagnosis

Other causes of recurrent abdominal pain must be considered. Specific causes such as hyperparathyroidism, systemic lupus erythematosus, infectious disease, and ductal obstruction by tumors, stones, or helminths must be excluded by appropriate tests.

Complications

Disabling abdominal pain, steatorrhea, nutritional deprivation, and diabetes are the most frequent complications. Pancreatic carcinoma occurs more frequently in hereditary pancreatitis, especially in patients with calcifications within the gland.

Treatment

When the hereditary form of chronic pancreatitis is suspected or proved, medical management of acute attacks is indicated (see Acute Pancreatitis, above). If ductal obstruction is strongly suspected, surgical exploration should be undertaken. Pancreatography and cholangiography are usually performed at laparotomy, though sphincterotomy and biopsy are recommended when obvious obstruction is not found. Relapses seem to occur in most patients. Pseudocysts may be marsupialized to the surface or drained into the stomach or into a loop of jejunum. Prophylactic total or subtotal pancreatic resection is advocated by some workers.

Prognosis

In the absence of a correctable lesion, the prognosis is not good. Disabling episodes of pain, pancreatic insufficiency, and diabetes may ensue. Narcotic addiction and suicide are risks in teenagers with disabling disease.

Dixon JA, Englert E: Role of early surgery in chronic pancreatitis: A practical clinical approach. Gastroenterology 61:375, 1971.

Kattwinkel J & others: Hereditary pancreatitis: Three new kindreds and a critical review of the literature. Pediatrics 51:55, 1973.

ZOLLINGER-ELLISON SYNDROME

This familial syndrome, consisting of non-beta islet cell tumors of the pancreas, marked gastric hypersecretion, and severe atypical intractable peptic ulceration, is most common in males (4:1). The youngest patient so far described was 7 years old.

The ulcerogenic, gastrin-like hormone elaborated by these small pancreatic islet cell tumors and their metastases to liver or lymph nodes is responsible for the gastric hypersecretion and the intractable peptic disease. Intractable diarrhea of the secretory type may occur in the absence of peptic disease. Half of islet cell tumors in the pediatric age group have been malignant.

Clinical Findings

Severe, intermittent abdominal pain with vomiting, hematemesis, melena, diarrhea, and steatorrhea are common. X-ray findings of hypertrophied gastric rugae, duodenal dilatation, and edematous small bowel mucosa all suggest gastric hypersecretion. Gastric analysis shows a marked increase in basal volume and titratable acidity after a 12-hour overnight collection. Gastric secretion volumes of 600–2000 ml have been reported during a 12-hour period. Measurement of circulating gastrin levels in the blood is usually diagnostic (greater than 300 pg/ml). A calcium infusion test may be needed to clarify "gray zone" gastrin levels. The histamine test rarely shows more than a 2-fold increase in acid output since these patients are already secreting maximally.

Treatment

The experimental antihistamine cimetidine is expected to replace total gastrectomy as the treatment of choice. The hazard of ulcer perforation and the ineffectiveness of subtotal gastrectomy are well known. Primary and metastatic tumor tissue removal should be attempted; however, cures have been reported even when metastases have not been surgically removed and the primary tumor has not been found.

Schwartz DL & others: Gastrin response to calcium infusion: An aid to the improved diagnosis of Zollinger-Ellison syndrome in children. Pediatrics 54:599, 1974.

Wilson SD, Schulte WJ, Meade RC: Longevity studies following total gastrectomy in children with the Zollinger-Ellison syndrome. Arch Surg 103:108, 1971.

ISOLATED EXOCRINE PANCREATIC DEFECTS

Enterokinase Deficiency Disease
(Formerly Trypsinogen Deficiency Disease)

In this rare genetic defect, absence of the enzyme enterokinase leads rapidly to severe protein malnutrition and hypoproteinemia. The key step in activating the proteolytic system within the duodenum is dependent upon the enzyme.

Trypsinogen is first converted to trypsin by enterokinase. Once formed, trypsin can replace enterokinase in the activation of the proenzyme. Trypsin is also needed to activate the conversion of chymotrypsinogen to chymotrypsin as well as procarboxypeptidase to carboxypeptidase. Consequently, the absence of enterokinase results in a complete loss of pancreatic proteolytic enzyme activity. Activation studies with exogenous trypsin and homogenates of normal duodenal mucosa have shown that trypsinogen, procarboxypeptidase, and chymotrypsinogen are present in samples of the patients' pancreatic juice and are qualitatively intact. The sweat chloride test is normal, and the diagnosis is made by duodenal intubation and analysis of pancreatic enzyme activity. Anemia has been associated with this entity but not neutropenia.

Treatment consists of feeding a formula containing a casein hydrolysate such as Nutramigen or Pregestimil and adding pancreatic enzymes to the diet (Cotazym).

Polonovski D, Bier H: Pseudotrypsinogen deficiency due to a lack of intestinal enterokinase. Acta Paediatr Scand 59:458, 1970.

Tarlow MJ & others: Intestinal enterokinase deficiency. Arch Dis Child 45:651, 1970.

Isolated Pancreatic Lipase Deficiency

Deficiencies related to malabsorption of the fat-soluble vitamins are common. Neither pancreatic lipase nor a lipase inhibitor is present, while pancreatic trypsin and amylase activity are normal. The sweat chloride iontophoresis test is normal. Direct assay of pancreatic juice for enzyme activity following stimulation with pancreozymin and secretin, 2 units/kg of each IV, is required for diagnosis.

Improvement in steatorrhea occurs after the addition of pancreatic enzymes to the diet. A low-fat diet or substituting a formula containing medium chain triglycerides (Portagen) for one with long chain dietary triglycerides is helpful.

Rey J & others: L'absence congenitale de lipase pancréatique. Arch Fr Pediatr 32:5, 1966.

PANCREATIC EXOCRINE HYPOPLASIA & CHRONIC NEUTROPENIA

This uncommon disease, characterized by diarrhea and failure to thrive, is due to pancreatic exocrine insufficiency. Pathologically, there is widespread fatty replacement of the gland acinar tissue. There is no fibrosis or inflammation, and the pancreatic ducts appear to be normal. The islet cells are spared. The disease may be confused with cystic fibrosis, but the absence of elevated sweat chlorides distinguishes these entities. The association of bone marrow dysfunction is a curious but fairly constant finding. There is evidence that the disease is genetically determined.

The history of failure to thrive, diarrhea, fatty stools, and, in most cases, freedom from respiratory infections should make one suspect this entity. Important laboratory findings include normal sweat electrolytes but absent or reduced pancreatic lipase, amylase, and trypsin on duodenal intubation. Leukopenia is often present, and the thrombocyte count is sometimes depressed. Small bowel histology is normal, as are studies of absorption not dependent upon pancreatic enzymes. The bone marrow is typically hypocellular, showing a "maturation arrest" of the granulocyte series. Metaphyseal dysostosis and an elevated fetal hemoglobin may occur.

Normal sweat electrolytes and a negative history of repeated pulmonary infections differentiate this disease from cystic fibrosis. Small bowel biopsy supported by absorption tests, particularly with D-xylose, distinguishes the disorder from celiac disease. Cases of isolated lipase, trypsinogen, or enterokinase deficiency may be more difficult to distinguish. Cyclic neutropenia and neutropenia due to other causes must be considered.

The complications and sequelae of deficient pancreatic enzyme secretion are malnutrition, diarrhea, and growth failure. The major sequel seems to be short stature, although long-term follow-up studies are not available. Increased numbers of infections may be the results of chronic neutropenia.

Pancreatic enzyme replacement therapy has been fairly successful, although some patients get along without it. The prognosis appears to be good for those able to survive the increased number of bacterial infections early in life.

Schwachman H & others: The syndrome of pancreatic insufficiency and bone marrow dysfunction. J Pediatr 65:645, 1964.

Shmerling DH & others: The syndrome of exocrine pancreatic insufficiency, neutropenia, metaphyseal dysostosis and dwarfism. Helv Paediatr Acta 24:547, 1969.

● ● ●

General References

Anderson CM, Burke V: *Pediatric Gastroenterology*. Blackwell, 1975.

Andorsky M, Finley A, Davidson M: Pediatric gastroenterology. 1/1/69–12/31/75: A review. (2 parts.) Am J Dig Dis 22:56, 155, 1977.

Andres JM, Mathis RK, Walker WA: Liver disease in infants. (2 parts.) J Pediatr 90:686, 864, 1977.

Grand RJ, Watkins JB (editors): Gastrointestinal and liver disease. Pediatr Clin North Am 22:719, 1975. [Entire issue.]

Gryboski J: *Gastrointestinal Problems in the Infant*. Saunders, 1975.

Roy CC, Silverman A, Cozzetto FJ: *Pediatric Clinical Gastroenterology*, 2nd ed. Mosby, 1975.

Shiff L: *Diseases of the Liver*, 4th ed. Lippincott, 1975.

Sleisenger MH, Fordtran JS: *Gastrointestinal Disease: Pathophysiology, Diagnosis, Management*. Saunders, 1973.

18 . . .

Kidney & Urinary Tract

Rawle M. McIntosh, MD, Gary M. Lum, MD, & Donough O'Brien, MD, FRCP

EVALUATION OF THE KIDNEY & URINARY TRACT

HISTORY

Evaluation of the kidney and urinary tract begins with a careful history. The symptoms of chronic renal failure in children are protean and may be obscure. Fatigue, headaches, nausea, and anorexia are common complaints. Abdominal or flank pain may be associated with acute urinary tract infections, some forms of glomerulonephritis, or urolithiasis. The possible relationship of urinary tract symptoms to acute illnesses such as respiratory infections should be explored. Often neglected in the history is the possibility of trauma. Renal vein thrombosis, for example, may follow what was apparently a trivial episode of abdominal trauma. Symptoms relating to urination, including dysuria, polyuria, and frequency, should be sought. Excessive thirst may be present in children with renal concentrating defects. A history of unexplained fevers can often be obtained in children with chronic urinary tract infections.

The birth history, especially of oligohydramnios and birth asphyxia, is important. As with any medical history, a complete account of all medications being taken or recently taken should be obtained; along with this, the possibility of exposure to nephrotoxic agents such as heavy metals should be explored. The family history is important in the evaluation of many urinary tract symptoms. Simply inquiring about family "kidney problems" does not suffice. Specific questions should be asked about hypertension, "Bright's disease," and renal stones. The relationship of some hereditary nephropathies to hearing or visual problems must be recalled when taking the history. Construction of a formal pedigree often adds information that cannot be obtained in any other way.

PHYSICAL EXAMINATION

Although the physical examination of children with renal disease is often unrevealing, certain points deserve emphasis.

A careful measurement of blood pressure should be part of the examination of any child, especially one in whom renal disease is suspected. The cuff must be the largest one that will fit the patient; it should cover at least two-thirds of the upper arm. Accurate blood pressure measurements may be obtained in newborns with ultrasonic equipment.

An examination of the external genitalia is also important. Congenital renal anomalies, for example, are sometimes associated with obvious genital abnormalities. The urethral meatus should be examined in any child with hematuria; elaborate investigations are not needed in a child whose hematuria results from meatal excoriation. Abdominal palpation is most helpful in newborns and infants; most abdominal masses so discovered will prove to be of renal origin.

Abdominal or flank tenderness may be elicited in children with urinary tract infection. The presence of edema or ascites should also be noted. Careful ear and eye examination is important, especially when hereditary nephropathies are being considered. Ophthalmologic examination is also important in children with hypertension or those who are being treated with corticosteroids. Cardiopulmonary examination, including lower extremity blood pressures, is important in all renal patients, especially those with hypertension or nephrotic syndrome.

Kassirer JP: Clinical evaluation of kidney function: Tubular function. N Engl J Med 285:499, 1971.

Strauss J: Clinical clues to the presence of renal disease. Page 29 in: *Pediatric Nephrology.* Strauss J (editor). Stratton Intercontinental, 1974.

LABORATORY EVALUATION OF RENAL FUNCTION

Urinalysis

The urinalysis is a rapid laboratory test that should be within the competence of every physician. Commercial dipsticks (eg, Labstix) can be used to detect blood, protein, glucose, and ketones and to give an approximate measurement of pH. While useful for screening, however, dipstick urinalyses have their limitations. "Two-plus proteinuria," for example, is a meaningless result, and the detection of protein in a urine specimen requires more accurate quantitation on a timed specimen. When the kidney's acidification capability is questioned, then the use of a pH electrode rather than a pH dipstick is essential. No simple test replaces microscopic examination of the centrifuged urine sediment. The use of low illumination and a stain (Sedi-Stain) facilitates this part of the urinalysis. Casts are sought initially using a low-power objective and scanning the edges of the cover slip. Bacteria and cells are studied with a higher power objective.

A. Urine Composition: Most hospital laboratories can perform simple analyses of urine chemical composition which can provide invaluable data in assessing renal function. The urine sodium concentration reflects much about intravascular volume and renal tubular function. A low urine sodium (5 mEq/liter or less) in an oliguric patient is evidence that tubular function is intact and that renal hypoperfusion (ie, "prerenal failure") is occurring. The oliguric patient with a higher urine sodium (over 10 mEq/liter) is more likely to have impaired renal function. As will be detailed subsequently, the urine creatinine concentration, when compared to the serum creatinine, is of great value in distinguishing renal from prerenal failure.

Renal concentrating ability may be determined by measuring the urine osmolality. Infants can usually achieve a concentration of 700 mOsm/liter; after 3 months of age, this figure rises to about 1400 mOsm/liter. The urine specific gravity may be used as a rough approximation of osmolality (1.010 = 400 mOsm/liter, 1.020 = 800 mOsm/liter, 1.030 = 1200 mOsm/liter); this approximation is not valid if unusual solutes such as glucose or protein are present. Certain more specific evaluations of concentrating ability may be helpful in the diagnosis of diabetes insipidus. These are shown below.

Osmolar Clearance:

$$C_{Osm} = \frac{U_{Osm} \times V}{P_{Osm}}$$

Should rise to > 4 ml/sq m/minute in a maximally concentrating situation.

Free Water Clearance:

$$C_{H_2O} = V - C_{Osm} = V \left[1 - \frac{U_{Osm}}{P_{Osm}} \right]$$

Should be > 6 ml/sq m/minute during water diuresis.

Medullary Water Reabsorption:

$$T^c_{H_2O} = C_{Osm} - V = V \left[\frac{U_{Osm}}{P_{Osm}} - 1 \right]$$

Should be > 3 ml/sq m/minute with maximally concentrated urine during solute load.

The detection of some substances in urine is evidence of tubular dysfunction. Glucose, for example, should not be present in concentrations greater than 5 mg/100 ml; urine amino nitrogen is increased over its usual value of 2 mg/kg/day with tubular dysfunction.

Measurement of the phosphate concentration of a 24-hour urine specimen, when combined with the serum phosphate and the information from the creatinine clearance (C_{cr}). is used to calculate the tubular reabsorption of phosphate (TRP). Normal values should be ≥ 80% calculated as $(1 - C_p/C_{cr}) \times 100$.

$$TRP = 100 \left[1 - \frac{S_{cr} \times U_{PO_4}}{S_{PO_4} \times U_{cr}} \right]$$

S_{cr} = Serum creatinine in mg/100 ml
U_{PO_4} = Urine phosphate in mg/100 ml
S_{PO_4} = Serum phosphate in mg/100 ml
U_{cr} = Urine creatinine in mg/100 ml

The urinary excretion of amino acids in generalized tubular disease reflects a quantitative increase rather than a qualitative change. This can be detected by a total urinary amino nitrogen assay, the normal value being 2 mg/kg/24 hours. Glycosuria should not exceed 5 mg/100 ml; one-dimensional paper chromatography is the best test.

The ability of the proximal tubule to reabsorb bicarbonate can only be assessed by the complicated procedure of a bicarbonate infusion test to determine the threshold of HCO_3^- reabsorption. Distal tubular function is estimated by determining hydrogen ion excretion on acid loading.

Net hydrogen ion excretion is expressed as

$$UV_{H^+} = (U_{TA} + U_{NH_4^+} - U_{HCO_3^-})V$$

where U_{TA} = titratable acid, $U_{NH_4^+}$ = urine ammonium concentration, $U_{HCO_3^-}$ = urine bicarbonate concentrations, and V = volume of urine (in ml) per minute. Normal values are 45 ± 25 μEq/minute/1.73 sq m during the first year of life and 30 ± 20 μEq/minute/1.73 sq m in later childhood. In the fourth hour, after a single oral ammonium chloride challenge of 130 mEq/24 hours/1.73 sq m, values for both groups rise to 110 ± 30 μEq/minute/1.73 sq m. The hydrogen ion clearance index, H^+ excretion in mEq/minute/1.73 sq m × plasma CO_2 in mEq/liter, is 0.9 ± 0.6 in infancy and 0.6 ± 0.4 in older children. After ammonium chloride loading, this increases in both groups to 2.5 ± 1.4. Values in renal tubular acidosis are usually < 0.7 after ammonium chloride loading.

Nephrocalcinosis or urolithiasis should prompt measurement of the 24-hour excretion of calcium, oxalate, cystine, and uric acid.

B. Urine Culture: The processing of urine cultures is routine in all hospital laboratories. However, the method of urine collection by the physician varies considerably and is of great importance in the interpretation of the culture results. While culture of a "bagged" urine in an infant or a "clean catch" in a young girl may be useful if negative, a positive culture by one of these methods demands a repeat culture of a specimen collected by bladder puncture. If puncture is unsuccessful, then a catheterized specimen can be used. Although physicians are sometimes reluctant to catheterize a child, careful attention to sterile technic and a small catheter (a feeding tube in small infants) can result in an atraumatic procedure. Indeed, the importance of conclusively establishing or refuting the diagnosis of urinary tract infection justifies the procedure. These maneuvers are seldom necessary in boys.

Whereas the "colony count" was once felt to differentiate between true infection (10^5 colonies/ml) and contamination of the specimen, there is accumulating evidence that this rule does not always hold, especially in boys. Careful attention to obtaining an uncontaminated specimen is more important than following arbitrary colony count guidelines.

Brodehl J & others: Maximum tubular reabsorption of glucose in infants and children. Acta Paediatr Scand 61:413, 1972.

Brody LH, Salladay JR, Armbruster K: Urinalysis and the urinary sediment. Med Clin North Am 55:243, 1971.

Dodge WF & others: Comparison of endogenous creatinine clearance with inulin clearance. Am J Dis Child 113:683, 1967.

Edelmann CM & others: Renal bicarbonate reabsorption and hydrogen ion excretion in normal infants. J Clin Invest 46:1309, 1967.

Thalassinos NC & others: Urinary excretion of phosphate in children. Arch Dis Child 45:269, 1970.

Young JA, Freedman BS: Renal tubular transport of amino acids. Clin Chem 17:245, 1971.

Measurement of Glomerular Filtration Rate (GFR)

Most chronic (and many acute) renal diseases are associated with a decrease in the glomerular filtration rate. Measurement of GFR, then, is of use in the initial evaluation of a child with suspected renal disease and in serial follow-up of a child with established renal dysfunction.

The simplest estimate of GFR is provided by the endogenous creatinine clearance. As this test is most accurate with high urine flow rates, it is preferable to use a 12-hour daytime collection of urine with generous fluid intake unless contraindicated. To calculate the creatinine clearance, the plasma creatinine (P_{cr}) (in mg/ml), urine creatinine (U_{cr}) (in mg/ml), and urine volume (V) (in ml/min) are used in the formula shown below:

$$C_{cr} = \frac{U_{cr}V}{P_{cr}}$$

As creatinine clearance is a function of body surface area, the result must be "corrected" to a standard body surface area of 1.73 sq m:

$$\frac{\text{Patient's } C_{cr} \times 1.73 \text{ sq m}}{\text{Patient's surface area}} = \text{"Corrected" } C_{cr}$$

The normal creatinine clearance is 80–120 ml/min/1.73 sq m.

A simple and reliable substitute technic that is valid for both infants and children is to use the following formula:

$$\frac{\text{GFR}}{\text{(in ml/minute/1.73 sq m)}} = \frac{0.43 \times \text{ height in cm}}{\text{Serum creatinine in mg/100 ml}}$$

Counahan R & others: Estimation of glomerular filtration rate from plasma creatinine concentration. Arch Dis Child 51: 875, 1976.

Donckerwolcke RAMG & others: Serum creatinine values in healthy children. Acta Paediatr Scand 59:399, 1970.

Schwartz GJ & others: Plasma creatinine and urea concentration in children: Normal values for age and sex. J Pediatr 88: 828, 1976.

Blood Chemistries

The kidney's role in maintaining metabolic homeostasis is reflected in serum electrolyte concentrations. Metabolic acidosis, hyperkalemia, and abnormalities of calcium (especially the ionized fraction) and phosphorus are not uncommon in renal disease and must be sought. Abnormalities of sodium, magnesium, and uric acid are also associated with many renal diseases. The serum concentrations of urea (BUN) and creatinine are important indices of renal function. Urea appears in the urine by bulk filtration at the glomerulus; some reabsorption occurs with low urine flow rates. Creatinine, on the other hand, is excreted by filtration and tubular secretion; essentially no reabsorption of this substance occurs. The differential renal handling of these substances has diagnostic importance. In uncomplicated renal failure, the normal BUN/creatinine ratio of about 10:1 is preserved. When glomerulotubular imbalance and slow urine flow rates are present (as in the dehydrated child with "prerenal" failure), however, BUN may be disproportionately elevated. Tissue catabolism (as with starvation) may also disproportionately elevate BUN.

Chantler C: Evaluation of laboratory and other methods of measuring renal function. In: *Clinical Pediatric Nephrology.* Lieberman E (editor). Lippincott, 1976.

Evaluation of Hematuria & Proteinuria

Demonstration of proteinuria by "dipstick" on a random urine specimen should lead to quantitation of a timed specimen. A 12-hour overnight collection is preferred; this provides a concentrated specimen and minimizes the contribution of orthostatic factors. A simple turbidometric assay, using sulfosalicylic acid, will determine whether its proteinuria is significant—ie, greater than 200 mg/24 hours. Protein excretion, however, varies with age and sex. Leakage of proteins with a molecular weight < 60,000 may indicate steroid sensitivity.

Demonstration of hematuria by dipstick should lead to confirmation by microscopic urinalysis and the search for red cell casts. Especially in children with asymptomatic hematuria, the search for renal glomerular abnormalities is likely to yield the most results. It is wise to remember that the presence of red cell casts supports the diagnosis of glomerulonephritis, but the disease may be present without such casts becoming discernible in the urine.

While taking the history, pay special attention to evidence of renal disease in other family members, recent infection (especially streptococcal), and the nature of the hematuria (gross, intermittent, association with infections, especially upper respiratory). Pertinent physical findings include evidence of abdominal masses, hypertension, meatitis, or menses. These, of course, are just a few of the things one must consider in the approach to a patient with bleeding from the glomeruli. Serologic and immunologic laboratory studies are indicated to determine the extent and nature of renal disease. Some of these studies include BUN, serum creatinine and electrolytes, creatinine clearance, serum complement and protein, and quantitative protein excretion as well as the presence of antinuclear antibody factor titers, and anti-DNA antibodies. These studies are discussed later in the text in reference to particular glomerulonephritides.

Dipstick proteinuria should be followed by quantitation of protein excretion during a timed period. Significant quantitative proteinuria usually exceeds 200 mg/24 hours. In the age group under 6 years, if there are no other historical, physical, or laboratory abnormalities that suggest more serious glomerular disease, the probable diagnosis is idiopathic nephrotic syndrome of childhood. Patients in this age group often present with the full picture of nephrotic syndrome and will respond to corticosteroid therapy. Treatment is discussed more fully elsewhere in the text.

Significant proteinuria in older children suggests more serious disease, and careful attempts to document an orthostatic component to the proteinuria should be undertaken. It is therefore important in the adolescent to document the degree of proteinuria during recumbency versus the upright position. If the proteinuria is not orthostatic or if nephrotic syndrome or decreased renal function is present, further laboratory tests (see above) and renal biopsy are indicated to determine the nature of the presumed glomerular lesion.

Renal biopsy will play a role also in children who, suspected of having idiopathic nephrotic syndrome of childhood, display either a relapsing course or a dependency on or resistance to corticosteroid therapy.

McLaine PN, Drummond KN: Benign persistent asymptomatic proteinuria in childhood. Pediatrics 46:548, 1970.

Randolph MF, Greenfield M: Proteinuria. Am J Dis Child 114:631, 1967.

Rennie IBD, Keen H: Evaluation of clinical methods for detecting proteinuria. Lancet 2:489, 1967.

Robinson RR: Orthostatic proteinuria: Definition and prognosis. The Kidney. Vol 4 No. 3, National Kidney Foundation, 1971.

Wagner MG & others: Epidemiology of proteinuria: A study of 4807 school children. J Pediatr 73:825, 1968.

West CD: Asymptomatic hematuria and proteinuria in children: Causes and appropriate diagnostic studies. J Pediatr 89:173, 1976.

LABORATORY EVALUATION OF IMMUNOLOGIC FUNCTION

Much childhood renal disease is mediated by immune mechanisms. In most cases, disease is presumed to result from deposition in the kidney of circulating complexes of antigen and antibody. More rarely, antibodies may be directed at renal tissue itself.

Complete immunologic assessment of a patient requires many studies that the usual laboratory is unable to offer. Nonetheless, some basic tests are more generally available. Total serum complement (and components if possible) should be measured when immune-mediated renal injury is suspected. The serum immunoglobulins should be quantitated, and serum proteins sometimes associated with immune complex deposition should be sought (eg, antinuclear antibodies, hepatitis-associated antigen, rheumatoid factor). It has recently been reported that cold-precipitable proteins ("cryoglobulins") are associated with many immune complex diseases; these may be easily isolated from serum and characterized by standard immunochemical methods.

Berger J & others: Immunochemistry of glomerulonephritis. In: *Advances in Nephrology*. Vol 1. Hamburger J, Crosnier J, Maxwell MH (editors). Year Book, 1971.

McCluskey RT: The value of immunofluorescence in the study of human renal disease. J Exp Med 134:242, 1971.

McIntosh RM: Cryoglobulins. (Part 3.) Q J Med 44:285, 1975.

Wilson CB, Dixon FJ: Diagnosis of immunopathologic renal disease. Kidney Int 5:389, 1974.

RADIOGRAPHIC EVALUATION

Excretory urography is the initial procedure in the radiographic evaluation of the child's urinary tract. The only absolute contraindication to the procedure is dehydration; a previous reaction to the contrast material should be considered a relative contraindication. Adequate evaluation of the upper tracts is often obtained on a single 6-minute film. The multiple follow-up films routinely obtained in some centers usually constitute an unnecessary radiation exposure.

Evaluation of the lower urinary tract is indicated when vesicoureteral reflux or bladder outlet obstruction is suspected. An adequate voiding study can sometimes be obtained with the contrast media remaining in the bladder following excretory urography. If this is not possible, catheterization with instillation of contrast medium is required.

More invasive studies such as renal venography or arteriography are rarely required in children. Their main indication is in the evaluation of renal masses or in the detection of such vascular lesions as renal vein thrombosis.

Radioisotope studies provide information about renal size and function with a radiation dose much less than that provided by excretory urography. In some situations, such as the serial follow-up of children with vesicoureteral reflux, nuclear medicine technics may be the method of choice. Ultrasound and computerized axial tomography technics are beginning to be used in renal disease, particularly in the diagnosis of cysts and tumors. Only a few centers have much experience so far with children.

Johnston JH, Irving IM: Experiences with radioisotopic renography in children. Arch Dis Child 42:583, 1967.

Nogrady MB, Dunbar JS: The technic of Roentgen investigation of the urinary tract in infants and children. Progr Pediatr Radiol 3:3, 1970.

UROLOGIC STUDIES

Except for the evaluations of patients with suspected anatomic abnormalities, cystoscopy is rarely indicated in children. The yield of this procedure in children with hematuria or in girls with recurrent urinary tract infection is minimal.

Retrograde urography is rarely necessary in children. Ureteral catheterization and contrast studies may be required for the anatomic investigation of a child in severe renal failure, for the delineation of some obstructive uropathies, and for split renal function studies.

Campbell MF: *Clinical Pediatric Urology.* Saunders, 1951.

RENAL BIOPSY

The ultimate diagnostic procedure in many children with renal parenchymal disease is the renal biopsy. Satisfactory evaluation of renal tissue requires examination by light microscopy, electron microscopy, and immunofluorescence microscopy. Unless all of these methods are available, we believe it is unfair to subject a child to biopsy. When a biopsy is indicated, however, the child should be referred to a nephrologist who can perform the procedure. For example, a child with gross hematuria could have Alport's syndrome or the IgA nephropathy of Berger. The former diagnosis could not be excluded without electron microscopy; the latter diagnosis could not be made without immunofluorescence microscopy.

CONGENITAL ANOMALIES OF THE URINARY TRACT

Congenital anomalies of the genitourinary tract are present in about 10% of children. These may range in severity from asymptomatic abnormalities found only at autopsy to malformations incompatible with extrauterine or even intrauterine life.

RENAL PARENCHYMAL ANOMALIES

Kidneys may be fused in their lower poles, resulting in a so-called "horseshoe kidney." This abnormality is usually inconsequential, although some authors report a higher incidence of calculi in patients with the malformation. Unilateral renal agenesis can occur and is usually associated with compensatory hypertrophy of the contralateral kidney. Although the anomaly is usually asymptomatic, its presence should preclude participation in contact sports for fear of injury to the remaining organ. Supernumerary and ectopic kidneys can also occur and are usually of no importance.

Bilateral Renal Agenesis

Bilateral renal agenesis is a rare malformation resulting in early death. Oligohydramnios is present and probably is the cause of the pulmonary hypoplasia and peculiar (Potter) facies of these infants.

Renal Hypoplasia & Dysplasia

These represent a spectrum of anomalies. In simple hypoplasia, which may be unilateral or bilateral, renal histology is normal but the affected organs are smaller than normal. In the various forms of dysplasia, immature, undifferentiated renal tissue persists. In some of the dysplasias, the number of normal nephrons is insufficient to sustain life once the child reaches a critical body size. Thus, these lesions are usually discovered when excretory urography is performed on a child who is noted to be uremic with no history of urinary tract disease.

Simple Cysts

These are usually single and of no clinical significance, although they may be a site for development of renal stones.

Polycystic Disease

In the infantile form, this condition is associated with huge cystic kidneys, often with multiple associated cystic malformations. Some children die in the newborn period, but many survive for a few years despite hypertension and uremia. Juvenile polycystic disease occurs at a later age and is primarily manifested by liver rather than renal involvement. These diseases are inherited as autosomal recessives. An adult form of polycystic disease occurs which has an autosomal dominant hereditary pattern.

Cystic Dysplasia

Cystic dysplasias are a broad group of malformations in the hypoplasia-dysplasia group in which the renal histology is cystic.

Medullary Cystic Disease

Medullary cystic disease is characterized by varying sizes of cysts in the medulla associated with a tubulo-interstitial nephritis. Children present with renal failure and signs of tubular dysfunction (decreased concentrating ability). This lesion should not be confused with medullary sponge kidney (renal tubular ectasia), a frequently asymptomatic cystic disease.

Alexander F & others: Familial uremic medullary cystic disease. Pediatrics 45:1024, 1970.

Bernstein J: Heritable cystic disorders of the kidney: The mythology of polycystic disease. Pediatr Clin North Am 18:435, 1971.

Bernstein J: The morphogenesis of renal parenchymal maldevelopment (renal dysplasia). Pediatr Clin North Am 18:395, 1971.

Habib R: Renal dysplasia, hypoplasia and cysts. Pediatr Nephrol 1:209, 1974.

Reilly BJ, Neuhauser EBD: Renal tubular ectasia in cystic disease of the kidneys and liver. Am J Roentgenol Radium Ther Nucl Med 84:546, 1960.

Vuthibhagdee A, Singleton EB: Infantile polycystic disease of the kidney. Am J Dis Child 125:167, 1973.

DISTAL URINARY TRACT ANOMALIES

Obstruction to urine flow, infection, and stone formation, alone or in combination, are the hallmarks of most distal urinary tract anomalies. Most of these anomalies will be suggested by excretory urography and cystourethrography. Some may be managed surgically; in others, the physician has little to offer but supportive treatment and prompt recognition and management of infection.

Ureteral Anomalies

Obstruction at the ureteropelvic junction is common and may be the result of intrinsic muscle abnormalities, aberrant vessels, or fibrous bands. The lesion can cause hydronephrosis and usually presents as an abdominal mass in the newborn. Obstruction can occur throughout the rest of the length of the ureter, especially at its entrance into the bladder. Proximal hydroureter and hydronephrosis result. Obstruction or reflux may occur in ectopic ureters. Most often, these are associated with duplications of the collecting systems; the ectopic ureter generally drains the upper pole of the affected kidney. The need for repair of an ectopic ureter is related to the appearance of the kidney and the collecting system it drains.

Anomalies of Bladder & Urethra

Severe bladder malformations such as exstrophy are clinically obvious and provide an exacting surgical challenge. More subtle—but urgent in terms of diagnosis—is obstruction to urine flow from posterior urethral valves. These aberrant structures, almost invariably confined to males, usually present as anuria or a poor voiding stream in the newborn period; with severe obstruction of urine, ascites may occur. As soon as the diagnosis is suspected, confirmation by cystourethrography should be sought. Treatment consists of destruction of the valves, often by transurethral fulguration. This procedure may be preceded by a period of vesical drainage. Other distal obstructions (bladder neck obstruction, distal urethral stenosis, and meatal stenosis) were once popular diagnoses but have now fallen into disrepute as specific entities.

Complex Anomalies

The prune belly syndrome is an association of urinary tract anomalies with cryptorchidism and absent abdominal musculature. Although associated anomalies, especially renal dysplasia, usually cause early death, some patients have lived into the third decade. Early urinary diversion is essential if remaining renal function is to be preserved. At the time of this surgery, a renal biopsy should be obtained to assess the potential for future adequate renal function.

Discussion of other complex malformations, as well as such external genitalia anomalies as hypospadias, is beyond the scope of this text.

Carter TC, Tomskey GC, Ozog LS: Prune-belly syndrome: Review of 10 cases. Urology 3:279, 1974.

Poole CA: Congenital obstructive uropathies. Pediatr Nephrol 1:231, 1974.

Shopfner CE: Modern concepts of lower urinary tract obstruction in pediatric patients. Pediatrics 45:194, 1970.

GLOMERULAR DISEASE

ACUTE POSTSTREPTOCOCCAL GLOMERULONEPHRITIS

Essentials of Diagnosis

- Usually a history of group A beta-hemolytic streptococcal infection 7–14 days previously is helpful.
- General malaise, headache, vomiting, fever, loss of appetite, and sometimes abdominal pain.
- Moderate edema, especially periorbital and of the dorsa of the hands and feet.
- Hypertension, if present, is usually moderate, but it may be severe and of rapid onset

and capable of causing sudden seizures or cardiac failure.

- Proteinuria and hematuria with hyaline, granular, and red cell casts in the urine. Gross hematuria or "smoky urine" is usually present, but in subclinical cases hematuria may be minimal or absent.
- Occasionally, oliguria or even anuria and acute renal failure.
- Transient mild to moderate elevation of BUN. ASO titer may be elevated. Low C3 complement level. High erythrocyte sedimentation rate. Cryoglobulinemia, hypergammaglobulinemia.

General Considerations

Acute poststreptococcal glomerulonephritis is the most common glomerular disease in childhood. Although the cause is not established with certainty, the condition is thought to be an immune-mediated disease. An epidemiologic relationship between certain strains of streptococci and glomerulonephritis is well recognized. Presumably, antigen-antibody complexes (possibly streptococcal) are formed in the circulation and deposited in the glomeruli. These deposited complexes may incite glomerular damage through activation of the complement system.

Grossly, involved kidneys are enlarged, with punctate cortical hemorrhages. Histologically, proliferation of glomerular cells and infiltration of the glomerulus with inflammatory cells are found. Electron microscopy demonstrates characteristic subendothelial electron-dense "lumps," presumably immune deposits.

Immunofluorescence microscopy reveals deposition of complement and immunoglobulins; some workers have found glomerular deposition of streptococcal antigens.

Clinical Findings

A. **Symptoms and Signs:** One to 2 weeks following a streptococcal skin or respiratory infection, patients complain of headache, malaise, or abdominal pain. Oliguria and "coke-colored" urine may be next noted. Periorbital swelling may occur, especially in the mornings, but gross edema is unusual. Some patients may present with more severe symptoms, including hypertensive seizures, congestive heart failure, nephrotic syndrome, or acute renal failure. Hypertension, which may be severe enough to result in encephalopathy, is the major immediate complication of acute glomerulonephritis. Acute renal failure or congestive heart failure may occur in some patients.

B. **Laboratory Findings:** Urinalysis reveals hematuria of significant degree, with red blood cell casts. Proteinuria is also present. Mild elevations of BUN and creatinine may occur.

A low total serum complement or C3 is always found. The incidence of recent streptococcal infection is shown by one or more streptococcal antibodies. Circulating cryoproteins are always demonstrable.

Treatment

There is no specific treatment other than antibiotic therapy for the streptococcal infection.

Hypertension and fluid overload are managed by appropriate dietary sodium and fluid restriction. Hypotensive drugs may be required, and hemodialysis may rarely be necessary.

Prognosis

Most children with acute glomerulonephritis go on to complete recovery, although microscopic hematuria may persist for 1–2 years. An occasional patient, however, may progress rapidly to renal insufficiency. Recently, it has become evident that the long-term prognosis of acute glomerulonephritis is not as favorable as previously thought; one series reported a 50% incidence of persistent proteinuria, hypertension, or reduction in GFR.

Baldwin DS: Poststreptococcal glomerulonephritis: A progressive disease? Am J Med 62:1, 1977.

Baldwin DS & others: The long-term course of poststreptococcal glomerulonephritis. Ann Intern Med 80:342, 1974.

Gutman RA & others: The glomerulonephritis of bacterial endocarditis. Medicine 51:1, 1972.

Holland NH & others: Pathways of complement activation in human glomerulonephritis. Kidney Int 1:106, 1972.

Lewy JE & others: Clinico-pathologic correlations in acute poststreptococcal glomerulonephritis: A correlation between renal functions, morphologic and clinical course of 16 children with acute poststreptococcal glomerulonephritis. Medicine 40:453, 1971.

Vernier RL: Recurrent hematuria and focal glomerulonephritis. Kidney Int 7:224, 1975.

OTHER TYPES OF POSTINFECTIOUS GLOMERULONEPHRITIS

Glomerulonephritis has been associated with pneumococcal and staphylococcal infection as well as streptococcal infection. These glomerular diseases are also presumed to result from immune complex deposition.

Chronic infection, as occurs with infective endocarditis or ventriculoatrial shunt infections, can also result in glomerulonephritis. The treatment is that of the underlying infection with close follow-up of long-term effects on renal function.

1. RECURRENT HEMATURIA WITH FOCAL GLOMERULONEPHRITIS (IgA Nephropathy, Berger's Disease)

For many years, a syndrome characterized by asymptomatic microscopic and recurrent bouts of macroscopic hematuria, with no apparent deterioration in renal function, has been recognized in children. Histologically, patients' kidneys show changes ranging from normal morphology to segmental proliferation of a few of the glomeruli (local glomerulonephritis). Recently, many of these patients have been shown to have deposits of immunoglobulins, mainly IgA, in the mesangial regions of the glomeruli. The significance of these deposits and their role in the clinical syndrome is not clear. Association of the episodes of gross hematuria with upper respiratory infections has suggested that sequestered mesangial antigens may be the targets of the IgA. It has also been suggested that an abnormal IgA may itself be antigenic.

Between the episodes of gross hematuria, the patient's urine may either be clear or show microscopic hematuria. Proteinuria may also be present. Renal functional impairment rarely occurs, although there have been occasional reports of patients exhibiting progressive renal insufficiency. No consistent abnormalities in serum immunoglobulins have been reported. The diagnosis is made on biopsy by demonstration of the characteristic immunoglobulin pattern. Similar histologic patterns may be found in other glomerular diseases, especially systemic lupus erythematosus and anaphylactoid purpura, which must be excluded before the diagnosis is made.

In the great majority of cases, the condition is benign and nonprogressive. Since renal insufficiency has been reported, however, children should be followed with serial determinations of function as long as hematuria persists. Recurrence of IgA deposition in transplanted kidneys has been reported. No specific treatment is indicated.

Levy M & others: Idiopathic recurrent macroscopic hematuria and mesangial IgA-IgG deposits in children (Berger's disease). Clin Nephrol 1:63, 1973.

McCoy PC: IgA nephropathy. Am J Pathol 76:123, 1974.

2. MEMBRANOPROLIFERATIVE GLOMERULONEPHRITIS

The histologic findings of membranoproliferative glomerulonephritis occur in a number of glomerular diseases, including systemic lupus erythematosus and severe poststreptococcal glomerulonephritis. Membranoproliferative glomerulonephritis may also occur in the absence of other specific diseases. In one particular condition where this morphologic finding is associated with evidence of complement consumption, the condition has been designated hypocomplementemic membranoproliferative glomerulonephritis.

The development of this disease may be insidious, and it must be suspected in the course of evaluation of asymptomatic hematuria or proteinuria. Less commonly, the disease may present with gross hematuria, nephrotic syndrome, or renal insufficiency.

Urinalysis nearly always reveals hematuria, al-though it may be exclusively microscopic. Proteinuria may be slight at first but increases as the disease progresses. The serum total hemolytic complement is usually depressed, although this may fluctuate in the course of the disease. The complement profile in this disease is characterized by activation of the alternative pathway of complement metabolism. The early components (C1, C2, C4) may be normal, while C3 and C5–9 are depressed. Progressive renal insufficiency, reflected in a decreasing creatinine clearance, occurs frequently. The diagnosis is established by the characteristic histologic appearance under light microscopic examination. The findings with immunofluorescence microscopy are variable; however, the presence of C3 proactivator and properdin and the absence of the first 3 components appear to be of some diagnostic value.

Hypertension is often a severe problem. Nephrotic syndrome develops frequently.

Treatment with corticosteroids and antimetabolites has been attempted but has not been satisfactory. Hypertension should be treated if present. Close follow-up of renal function with appropriate therapy for developing chronic renal failure may be all that can be done.

Cameron JS & others: Membrano-proliferative glomerulonephritis and persistent hypo-complementaemia. Br Med J 4:7, 1970.

West CD: Membranoproliferative hypocomplementemic glomerulonephritis. Nephron 11:134, 1973.

West CD & others: Hypocomplementemic and normo-complementemic persistent (chronic) glomerulonephritis; clinical and pathologic characteristics. J Pediatr 67:1089, 1965.

ANAPHYLACTOID PURPURA NEPHRITIS

Anaphylactoid purpura (Henoch-Schönlein purpura) is a vasculitis characterized by a purpuric rash, arthritis, and gastrointestinal symptoms. Renal involvement is not infrequent.

The cutaneous manifestations and arthritis of anaphylactoid purpura are usually the first to develop, often following a respiratory infection. Hematuria is the usual presenting feature of the glomerulonephritis, which occurs in about one-third of cases.

There are no characteristic serologic features of this disease. Hematuria is constant when glomerular involvement is present; proteinuria is variable.

Most often, the glomerulonephritis of anaphylactoid purpura is mild and transient. More severe disease is suggested by deterioration of function, persistent significant proteinuria, or hypertension. The severity of the renal disease does not necessarily parallel the extrarenal manifestations. Furthermore, significant renal disease may evolve after the other manifestations have resolved.

Any child with anaphylactoid purpura should

have careful follow-up of renal status even after the acute illness has resolved. Persistent proteinuria, decreased function, or hypertension may herald the development of significant renal insufficiency. Therapy with cyclophosphamide, 1–2 mg/kg/day orally, or with prednisone, 1–2 mg/kg/day orally, and azathioprine, 3–5 mg/kg/day orally, has been advocated for progressive renal disease. Careful evaluation of renal morphology should be performed before beginning such therapy. Renal biopsy demonstrates focal glomerulonephritis, with mesangial deposition of IgA, IgG, and sometimes fibrin.

Hurley RM, Drummond KN: Anaphylactoid purpura nephritis: Clinicopathological correlations. J Pediatr 81:904, 1972.
Meadow SR & others: Schönlein-Henoch nephritis. Q J Med 41:241, 1972.

GOODPASTURE'S SYNDROME

Most immune-mediated glomerular diseases are probably caused by entrapment of circulating antigen-antibody complexes in the glomerulus. A small proportion of cases, however, are mediated by antibodies directed against the glomerular basement membrane (anti-GBM). Patients with this form of glomerulonephritis often have life-threatening pulmonary hemorrhage, presumably on the basis of antigenic similarities between the glomerular and alveolar basement membranes. While pulmonary hemorrhage is found with other forms of renal disease, its association with anti-GBM glomerulonephritis is referred to as Goodpasture's syndrome.

Goodpasture's syndrome is uncommon. The diagnosis is established by the demonstration of circulating anti-GBM antibodies in the presence of the characteristic clinical and immunohistologic picture. The mortality rate in the acute phase is high, mostly because of pulmonary hemorrhage. It has been suggested that bilateral nephrectomy may control the severe lung bleeding. Although recurrent nephritis has been reported frequently, renal transplantation has been successful in these patients after the anti-GBM antibodies have disappeared.

Wilson CB, Dixon FJ: Anti-glomerular basement membrane antibody-induced glomerulonephritis. Kidney Int 3:74, 1973.

ALPORT'S SYNDROME
(Hereditary Nephritis)

In its complete form, the hereditary nephritis of Alport is characterized by renal disease, sensorineural hearing loss, and abnormalities of the crystalline lens.

As a practical matter, the ear and eye abnormalities are much less common than the renal manifestations.

Clinically, patients generally present with hematuria, which may persist without deterioration of renal function or may progress to renal failure. Although females seem to have a higher incidence of the disease, affected males are more likely to have progressive kidney involvement.

The genetics of the disease are not established with certainty, but it appears to behave as an autosomal dominant with variable penetrance. The diagnosis is usually established by the family history. Pathologically, patients have a range of renal findings, the earliest of which appears to be focal thickening and lamination of the glomerular basement membrane at the electron microscopic level.

There is no specific treatment, although genetic counseling should be offered. Transplantation has been successful, but if a family donor is to be used it must be shown that he or she is not also affected.

Ferguson AC, Rance CP: Hereditary nephropathy with nerve deafness (Alport's syndrome). Am J Dis Child 124:84, 1972.
Kaufman DB & others: Diffuse familial nephropathy: A clinicopathological study. J Pediatr 77:37, 1970.

HEMOLYTIC-UREMIC SYNDROME

Essentials of Diagnosis

- Sudden hemolysis, fall in hemoglobin level, and burr cells in peripheral blood.
- Thrombocytopenia.
- Acute renal failure.

General Considerations

Hemolytic-uremic syndrome is the most common cause of acute renal failure in infancy. The cause is not established, but epidemiologic studies have suggested both a genetic and an infectious component. The primary lesion seems to be on the endothelium of the arterioles with formation of platelet thrombi.

Clinical Findings

A. Signs and Symptoms: Hemolytic-uremic syndrome is found most often in children under age 2 years. It usually begins with a prodromal phase characterized by gastrointestinal symptoms, including abdominal pain, diarrhea, and vomiting. Oliguria, pallor, and bleeding manifestations, principally cutaneous and gastrointestinal, occur next. Hypertension and seizures develop in a variable number of infants.

B. Laboratory Findings: The triad of anemia, thrombocytopenia, and renal failure characterizes the syndrome. The anemia is profound and is associated with burr cells and red blood cell fragments on smear. A high reticulocyte count confirms the hemolytic nature of the anemia. The platelet count is almost invariably below 100,000/μl. Other coagulation abnormalities are less constant. Serum fibrin split products are often present, but fulminant disseminated intravascular coagulation is rare. The renal failure is characterized by a high BUN and, usually, a severe oliguria. Macroscopic hematuria is often present; proteinuria and the nephrotic syndrome may also occur. Immunologic investigations are usually unrevealing. The serum complement is normal.

Complications

The complications of hemolytic-uremic syndrome are those of acute renal failure. Neurologic problems, particularly seizures, may result from electrolyte abnormalities such as hyponatremia, hypertension, or CNS vascular disease. Severe bleeding and complicating infections must be anticipated.

Treatment

As with any case of acute renal failure, meticulous attention to fluid and electrolyte status as detailed in the discussion of acute renal failure is crucial. There is evidence that early dialysis improves the prognosis; the size of the patient and the bleeding tendency will usually dictate peritoneal dialysis as the technic of choice. Seizures usually respond to control of hypertension and electrolyte abnormalities. Therapy for the metabolic manifestations is less clear. While heparinization was once employed, it has not been shown conclusively to improve prognosis and may contribute to morbidity. In view of current theories assigning a central role to platelet thrombus formation, the use of antiplatelet agents has been considered. Early reports have suggested a role for aspirin and dipyridamole in the treatment of this disease. Red cell and platelet transfusions may be necessary, but the risk of volume overload is not negligible.

Course & Prognosis

The extreme variability in the literature reports of the course of this condition makes it difficult to formulate a useful statement of prognosis. It has even been suggested that geographic factors may determine the severity of the condition. Most commonly, children recover from the acute episode within a week and follow-up examination reveals no residual renal insufficiency. A much smaller group of patients will die in the early phase from the complications of acute renal failure. Finally, some patients will recover acutely but have severe and occasionally progressive renal dysfunction. Thus, the follow-up of children recovering from hemolytic-uremic syndrome should include serial determinations of renal function for 1—2 years.

Arenson EG, August CS: Preliminary report: Treatment of the hemolytic uremic syndrome with aspirin and dipyridamole. J Pediatr 86:957, 1975.

Proesmans W, Eeckels R: Has heparin changed the prognosis of the hemolytic uremic syndrome? Clin Nephrol 2:169, 1974.

IDIOPATHIC NEPHROTIC SYNDROME OF CHILDHOOD
("Nil" Disease; Lipoid Nephrosis)

The nephrotic syndrome is characterized by proteinuria, hypoproteinemia, edema, and hyperlipidemia. It may occur in the course of virtually any glomerular disease and may be associated with a variety of extrarenal conditions. In children under age 5, the disease usually takes the form of "idiopathic nephrotic syndrome of childhood" ("nil" disease, lipoid nephrosis). This entity is characterized by certain clinical and laboratory findings outlined below. Examination of renal tissue confirms the diagnosis. Light microscopy reveals no significant glomerular changes. Most reports of immunologic investigations have been negative. The cause remains unknown; however, there have been recent suggestions of hormonal causes and of associated dysfunction of T lymphocytes.

Clinical Findings

A. Signs and Symptoms: Affected patients are generally under age 5 years at the time of their first episode. Often following a flu-like syndrome, the child is noted to have periorbital swelling and perhaps oliguria. Within a few days, increasing edema—even anasarca—becomes evident. Other than vague malaise and, occasionally, abdominal pain, complaints are few. Despite the impressive swelling and weight gain, the patient may show signs of intravascular volume depletion and may even present in shock. Hypertension is rarely present. With marked edema there may also be dyspnea due to pleural effusions.

B. Laboratory Findings: Despite heavy proteinuria, the urine sediment is usually benign. Although microscopic hematuria may rarely be found, its presence should raise the suspicion of other glomerular diseases, especially focal sclerosis. Serum chemistries reveal hypoalbuminemia and hyperlipidemia. Abnormal immunoglobulin levels such as high IgM and low IgG have also been reported. No other evidence of immunologic derangement, however, is present, eg, complement is normal and there is no cryoglobulinemia. Some azotemia may occur but is related to intravascular volume depletion rather than functional derangement. Glomerular morphology is unremarkable except for fusion of the foot processes of the visceral epithelium of the glomerular basement membrane. This finding, however, is nonspecific and is found in many proteinuria states.

Complications

Infectious complications, such as peritonitis, are seldom encountered nowadays. Hypercoagulability may be present, and thromboembolic phenomena are commonly reported.

Treatment

As soon as the diagnosis of idiopathic nephrotic syndrome is made, therapy with corticosteroids should be initiated. Prednisone (2 mg/kg/day) is the agent of choice. As soon as the urine is protein-free, the prednisone dose is reduced to 2 mg/kg every other day. Alternate-day corticosteroid therapy is continued for 6 months, after which the dosage is tapered downward over a period of 2–3 weeks and then discontinued. A similar course of corticosteroids is given if the nephrosis recurs. After 2 courses of corticosteroids, however, a course of cytotoxic therapy may be used in an attempt to achieve long-term remission. Chlorambucil is slow-acting and less toxic than the more frequently used cyclophosphamide. The dose is 0.1 mg/kg/day orally for 2 weeks and then 0.2 mg/kg/day for 6 weeks. Prednisone is given with chlorambucil at first, tapering it during the first weeks of therapy. White blood cell counts are followed weekly; if leukopenia occurs, it is mild and transient, resolving when the drug is stopped.

Renal biopsy is not essential in the child with typical idiopathic nephrotic syndrome. However, biopsy should be performed prior to institution of chlorambucil therapy or if the clinical picture is atypical. Failure of proteinuria to disappear after a month of daily corticosteroid therapy, in the absence of chronic infection, is another indication for biopsy.

Diuretics may be introduced along with corticosteroids and help to mobilize edema more rapidly. However, they are not always effective and may lead to hypoproteinemia. Intravenous albumin is useful when anasarca results in acute distress or if severe intravascular depletion occurs.

Course & Prognosis

The prognosis of the idiopathic nephrotic syndrome is often suggested by the initial response to corticosteroids. A prompt remission, lasting for 3 years, is almost always permanent. Failure to respond or early relapse usually heralds a prolonged series of relapses. Chlorambucil therapy is predictably successful only in children who respond to corticosteroids.

Grupe WE: Chlorambucil in steroid-dependent nephrotic syndrome. J Pediatr 82:598, 1973.
Siegel NJ & others: Long-term follow-up of children with steroid responsive nephrotic syndrome. J Pediatr 81:251, 1972.

FOCAL GLOMERULAR SCLEROSIS

The lesion of focal glomerular sclerosis is characterized by the presence in renal biopsy specimens of normal-appearing glomeruli as well as some partially or completely sclerosed glomeruli. At presentation the disease is often quite similar to idiopathic nephrotic syndrome; however, the response to corticosteroids is poor, and the clinical course is often one of progression to end-stage renal disease. Some of the confusion in the literature regarding this lesion stems from the varied but similar terminology applied in its description. This histologic picture has been labeled focal sclerosing glomerulonephritis, focal and segmental glomerulosclerosis, and focal and segmental hyalinosis, to name a few. Since there may be 2 forms of the disease, Habib's classification of focal and global glomerular fibrosis may be useful.

The glomerular abnormalities in this disease may be confined to the juxtamedullary glomeruli, especially early. Therefore, care must be taken to obtain biopsy tissue which includes this area of the kidney.

Because some forms of the disease (eg, global glomerular fibrosis) are believed to respond to corticosteroid therapy, histologic diagnosis is imperative. Renal biopsy is helpful in distinguishing this disorder from idiopathic nephrotic syndrome of childhood as well as indicating the prognosis.

Bohle A & others: Minimal change lesion with nephrotic syndrome and focal glomerular sclerosis. Clin Nephrol 2:52, 1974.
Habib R: Focal glomerular sclerosis. Kidney Int 4:355, 1973.
Kohaut EC & others: The significance of focal glomerular sclerosis in children who have nephrotic syndrome. Am J Clin Pathol 66:545, 1976.

RAPIDLY PROGRESSIVE GLOMERULONEPHRITIS

Glomerulonephritis characterized by rapid progression to end-stage disease is rarely seen in childhood. The cause is unknown, and association with other glomerulonephritides is obscure. Clinically, the disease cannot be readily distinguished from other glomerulonephritides that may cause rapid deterioration in renal function. Histologic analysis reveals glomerular lesions characterized by severe and extensive epithelial cell proliferation. Thus, many glomeruli will display epithelial cell crescents or fibrous scarring. In early stages, the lesions may be focal, but they rapidly extend to involve the glomeruli diffusely.

Therapy is controversial, but it has been suggested that early treatment with anticoagulants may be of help. The use of immunosuppressive agents has also been suggested. Regardless of treatment, the outcome in most cases remains discouraging.

Kincaid-Smith P: Coagulation and renal disease. Kidney Int 2:183, 1972.
Min KW & others: The morphogenesis of glomerular crescents in rapidly progressive glomerulonephritis. Kidney Int 5:47, 1974.
Suc JM & others: The use of heparin in the treatment of idiopathic rapidly progressive glomerulonephritis. Clin Nephrol 5:9, 1976.

CONGENITAL NEPHROSIS

Congenital nephrosis is a rare, uniformly fatal renal disorder which is often observed in multiple siblings in a single family. Autosomal recessive inheritance is suggested. The kidneys are pale and large and may show microcystic dilatations of the proximal tubules and glomerular changes. The latter consist of proliferation, crescent formation, and thickening of capillary walls.

The pathogenesis is unknown. A fundamental immunologic incompatibility between the mother and the infant is perhaps responsible, since mothers reject skin grafts of their nephrotic infants more rapidly than control mothers reject grafts of normal infants. Evidence of immune injury in the kidneys relates to the finding of gamma globulin and complement components on the glomerular loops.

Low birth weight with an obstetric history of large placenta, wide cranial sutures, delayed ossification, and edema are commonly noted at birth. The edema, however, may be apparent only after the first few weeks or months of life. Anasarca follows, and the abdomen is distended by ascites. Massive proteinuria associated with typical nephrotic serum protein electrophoresis and hyperlipidemia is the rule. Hematuria is not uncommon. If the patient lives long enough, progressive renal failure occurs. Most affected infants succumb to infections at the age of a few months.

Treatment has little to offer. Prevention and effective management of urinary tract infection are important. Immunosuppressives and heparin have occasionally appeared to extend renal function for a period.

Burke EC & others: Familial nephrotic syndrome. J Pediatr 82:202, 1973.
Criswold WR, McIntosh RM: Immunological studies in congenital nephrosis. J Med Genet 9:245, 1972.

FUNCTIONAL PROTEINURIA

Urine is not normally completely protein-free, but the average output is well below 100 mg/24 hours. Exertional proteinuria is now well recognized and may be accompanied by erythrocytes and casts if the exercise is violent and includes body contact. Orthostatic proteinuria is explained by hemodynamic adjustments leading to renal venous congestion. It has been suggested that lordosis may produce proteinuria by the increased convexity of the aorta compressing the left renal vein. Proteinuria is seen in about 5% of febrile illnesses and is not necessarily due to underlying renal disease.

In spite of these well recognized causes of proteinuria, the physician faced with isolated instances of proteinuria must exercise great care before making such a diagnosis (see below). Asymptomatic nonpostural proteinuria is associated in 50% of cases with histologic kidney changes which may in a small percentage of cases be due to kidney disease.

Diagnosis of Orthostatic Proteinuria
A. Procedure:
1. Have the patient empty his bladder and lie down for 1 hour. Discard urine.
2. Empty the bladder again and lie down for a second hour.
3. Empty the bladder and save the specimen, noting the exact number of minutes since previous voiding.
4. Stand quietly for 1 hour, void, and save urine in a second container, again noting the exact number of minutes since previous voiding.
5. Send both specimens to the laboratory for quantitative protein determinations and measurement of volumes.

B. Normal Values: Supine, < 0.03 mg/minute protein. Standing: < 1 mg/minute in 65%; > 1 mg/minute in 35%.

Note: Patients with true benign orthostatic proteinuria must excrete < 0.03 mg/minute proteinuria. A mere tendency to spill less protein with recumbency is an insufficient criterion.

Marks MI & others: Proteinuria in children with febrile illnesses. Arch Dis Child 5:250, 1970.
McLaine PN, Drummond KN: Benign persistent asymptomatic proteinuria in childhood. Pediatrics 46:548, 1970.
Thompson AL & others: Fixed and reproducible orthostatic proteinuria. Ann Intern Med 73:235, 1970.

URINARY TRACT INFECTIONS*

Infections of the urinary tract (UTI) can range from asymptomatic bacteriuria to severe symptomatic pyelonephritis. As in the case of many pediatric diseases, signs and symptoms are less specific in younger children. UTI is a common cause of fever of unknown origin in childhood, and even asymptomatic UTI can result in significant renal damage, especially in infants. The clinician may be misled by erroneously interpreted clinical signs and laboratory data, resulting in either overdiagnosis (antibiotic side-effects, cost, unnecessary procedures) or underdiagnosis (continued symptoms, progressive renal damage). Once the diagnosis of UTI is confirmed, an organized program of periodic follow-up should be established so that recurrences will be recognized. Most urinary tract infections can be managed by the primary physician without the need for specialized urologic procedures or surgery.

*This section is contributed by James K. Todd, MD.

Predisposing Factors

A. Age and Sex: Approximately 1% of newborns develop UTI, often associated with bacteremia. Males at this age are as likely to develop infection as females. After the newborn period, UTI is uncommon in males until later adult life, when prostatic obstruction is common. In boys with documented urinary tract infection, underlying urinary tract abnormalities should always be suspected.

The relatively high incidence of UTI in newborn and preschool girls is due to excessive perineal fecal contamination, the short urethra, and infrequent and inadequate voiding. Infection in sexually active girls is due to bacterial contamination of the bladder secondary to urethral trauma during intercourse.

B. Organisms: Although viruses are often excreted in urine, symptomatic urinary tract disease of viral origin (eg, hemorrhagic cystitis) is rare. Bacteria are by far the most common cause of urinary tract infection, the predominant organisms being *Escherichia coli,* klebsiella, enteric streptococci, and *Staphylococcus epidermidis*—all common, nonvirulent members of the normal rectal and perineal bacterial flora.

C. Route of Infection: Access of bacteria to the normally sterile bladder and kidneys appears to be retrourethral and may be enhanced by poor perineal hygiene, the short female urethra, pinworms, urethral instrumentation, or intercourse.

Once bacteria are in the bladder, the urine serves as an excellent culture medium, but infection is usually avoided by the washout effect of voiding. Foreign bodies, urinary tract obstructions or anomalies, and infrequent or inadequate voiding may allow simple transient bacterial contamination of the bladder to progress to true persistent urinary tract infection. Vesicoureteral reflux, often seen in young children with urinary tract infection, can allow bacteria to gain access to the kidneys, with resulting pyelonephritis and renal damage.

Clinical Findings

A. Symptoms and Signs: Newborns may present with fever, hypothermia, poor feeding, jaundice (late), and failure to thrive or sepsis. Infants may have fever of unknown origin, poor feeding, failure to thrive, strong-smelling urine, and irritability. Preschool children may have abdominal pain, vomiting, strong-smelling urine, fever, enuresis, increased frequency of urination, dysuria, or urgency. School-age children may develop the "classical" signs of UTI, including enuresis, increased frequency of urination, dysuria, urgency, fever, or costovertebral angle tenderness (flank pain). Occasionally, children with bacterial UTI will present with hemorrhagic cystitis.

All age groups may suffer from asymptomatic infection that nonetheless can cause renal damage, predominantly in infants and young children, who have a greater propensity to develop vesicoureteral reflux. Those children who have UTI associated with fever, flank pain, severe abdominal pain, polymorphonuclear leukocytosis, an increased sedimentation rate, or increased C-reactive protein usually prove to have pyelonephritis on more extensive urologic investigation. Asymptomatic children or those with "cystitis" symptoms (increased frequency of urination, burning on urination, dysuria, strong-smelling urine, recurrence of enuresis) may have infection of the lower tract which may asymptomatically involve the upper tract as well. It should be carefully noted that children with "classical" signs and symptoms of UTI often do not have UTI but urethral irritation due to other causes (bubble bath, feminine hygiene sprays, vaginitis, pinworms, masturbation).

B. Laboratory Tests:

1. Obtaining a proper specimen—Bag urine specimens are frequently (30–60%) contaminated and not adequate for the definitive diagnosis of UTI. Clean-catch midstream specimens (CCMS) give a more accurate estimate of the bacteriologic state of the bladder urine but give false-positive results 10–20% of the time (again due to contamination) and may (if the patient has had a recent high fluid intake) yield colony counts growing less than 10^5 colony-forming units per milliliter. Catheter-obtained urines (use a No. 5 feeding tube) are excellent for diagnosis as long as the first few milliliters are excluded from collection. The risk of introducing infection in most patients is very low. Urine specimens obtained by suprapubic needle aspiration again are excellent means of avoiding specimen contamination and confirming urinary tract infection, especially in patients with high fluid intake who have colony counts less than 10^5 colony-forming units/ml.

2. Pyuria—The microscopic finding of more than 5 white blood cells per high-power field in a urine spun sediment is termed pyuria. Approximately 50% of patients with UTI (including pyelonephritis) *do not* have pyuria, and there are many causes of increased numbers of white cells in the urine (vaginal contamination, appendicitis, viral illness) other than UTI. Thus, the presence of pyuria is a very poor basis for a diagnosis of UTI.

3. Microscopic bacteriuria—Microscopic observation of a urine spun sediment on high dry (40 X) power does allow an accurate estimation of the presence of bacteria. A count of > 100 bacteria per high-power field correlates well with actual colony counts of > 10^5 colony-forming units/ml.

4. Urine cultures—The urine culture is the mainstay of urinary tract infection diagnosis. It can be performed in the office using the streak plate method or commercial methods using agar-embedded dipslides. Colony counts > 10^5 colony-forming units/ml have in the past been considered indicative of true infection but are often associated with specimen (bag, CCMS) contamination and may miss cases of infection with lower colony counts due to diuresis.

5. Nonculture detection of UTI—Two recently evaluated tests detect the chemical alterations on urine glucose and nitrate that are due to the modifying effects of bacteria in the overnight bladder urine. These methods (nitrite test, glucose test) only work on first morning overnight urine specimens but have the advantage that they give very few false-positive results since contaminating organisms introduced during the collection process do not have time to chemically modify the urine prior to testing.

6. **Proper diagnosis of UTI**—In patients with serious symptoms of UTI, urine should be collected by catheterization or suprapubic needle aspiration to exclude contaminants which may be introduced in the CCMS or bag collection process. If bacteria are seen on the spun sediment of a catheterized or suprapubically drawn specimen or if the patient grows $> 10^3$ colony-forming units of any organism per milliliter (including *S epidermidis* or mixed organisms), the patient has a UTI.

If the patient is not severely symptomatic (or is being seen for follow-up of previous UTI), it is reasonable to postpone the visit until the next morning so that the patient can bring in a refrigerated first morning CCMS specimen. This avoids the problem of falsely low colony counts and also allows testing by chemical methods, which do not give false-positive results. If the chemical tests are positive, a urine culture should be started and therapy initiated. If the chemical test cannot be done or is negative, a spun sediment should be examined. If more than 100 bacteria are seen, a second CCMS specimen (or catheterized specimen) should be collected (to avoid the false-positive results of contaminated urine specimens) and examined. A count of > 100 bacteria per high-power field on both specimens is diagnostic of UTI.

C. X-Ray Findings: Intravenous urography should be considered with proved infection in newborns, boys, girls with symptoms of pyelonephritis, and girls with second UTIs. Voiding cystourethrograms should be performed on boys and younger girls, but it is important to note that many young children have low-grade vesicoureteral reflux which does not require urologic intervention.

Treatment

A. Initial Treatment: Once the diagnosis is confirmed, initial therapy should be based on the patient's history of antibiotic use, the location of the infection, and the cost of alternative antibiotics. Many drugs are available for treating urinary tract infection, but all of them will occasionally be ineffective because of inherent resistance of the organism.

For uncomplicated infection, a single oral antibiotic (eg, ampicillin, a sulfonamide, nitrofurantoin) which the patient has not used recently can be administered for 10 days. For the patient with recurrent infection or suspected pyelonephritis (fever, vomiting, flank pain) or whose condition is unresponsive, antibiotic susceptibilities should be determined. A patient with suspected pyelonephritis need not always be admitted to the hospital but should be treated with 2 antibiotics (ampicillin, a sulfonamide, or a cephalosporin plus gentamicin or kanamycin). This regimen assures adequate coverage until the patient improves and the results of antibiotic sensitivity tests are available, allowing selection of a single effective oral anti-

biotic. Therapy must be appropriately modified in patients with acute or chronic renal failure.

Most UTIs can be successfully treated with inexpensive drugs given orally. Success requires confirmation by negative culture 2 days after the start of therapy if symptoms persist and 3–5 days after discontinuance of therapy in all cases.

B. Treatment of Refractory Infection: Persistent bacteriuria indicates superinfection with a different organism or recurrence of infection with the same organism due to obstruction, the presence of a foreign body, or conversion of the organism to a variant form. Radiologic studies (intravenous urography, voiding cystourethrography) should be done once the first infection is controlled in boys, newborns, and girls with pyelonephritis and after the second infection in others.

Obvious structural or obstructive anomalies necessitate referral to a urologist experienced in dealing with children. Conditions frequently diagnosed and treated as abnormalities (bladder outlet obstruction, meatal stenosis, distal urethral stenosis, duplication of the ureters) are also seen in otherwise normal children who do not require therapy. Repeated urethral dilatation and cystoscopy are rarely if ever of value. Vesicoureteral reflux is common in younger children. If not severe, it will not result in renal damage and will disappear in time if repeated infections can be prevented. The presence of mild reflux does not ordinarily necessitate urologic consultation.

In patients without structural or functional urinary tract abnormalities, possible causes of recurrent infection are infrequent or incomplete voiding, poor perineal hygiene, constipation, and bubble bath use. If attempts to deal with these problems are unsuccessful, prophylaxis with agents such as nitrofurantoin, low-dose sulfonamides, or methenamine mandelate may be useful in combination with a program of frequent voiding. If methenamine mandelate is used, urine pH must be maintained at 5.5 or less.

C. Follow-Up of Patients With UTI: All patients with UTI should be checked for recurrence every 1–2 months until they have remained free of infection for 1 year. Home testing of first morning concentrated urine specimens may significantly reduce the cost of follow-up without compromising accuracy. This involves the use of nonculture detection methods, eg, nitrite and glucose.

Prognosis

As long as urinary tract infections can be confined to the lower urinary tract (bladder and below), the prognosis for life is excellent. Once an infectious process has entered the kidney, the prognosis becomes more guarded. Hence, every diagnostic and therapeutic effort should be made to prevent recurrences.

American Academy of Pediatrics Section on Urology: Screening school children for urologic disease. Pediatrics 60:239, 1977.

Kunin CM: *Detection, Prevention and Management of Urinary Tract Infections.* Lea & Febiger, 1972.

McRae CU, Shannon FT, Utley WLF: Effect on renal growth of reimplantation of refluxing ureters. Lancet 1:1310, 1974.

Slosky D, Todd JK: Diagnosis of urinary tract infection: Interpretation of colony counts. Clin Pediatr 16:698, 1977.

Stamm WE: Guidelines for prevention of catheter-associated urinary tract infections. Ann Intern Med 82:386, 1975.

Stephens FD: Urologic aspects of recurrent urinary tract infection in children. J Pediatr 80:725, 1972.

Todd JK: Home follow-up of urinary tract infection: Comparison of two nonculture techniques. Am J Dis Child 131:860, 1977.

Todd JK: Pediatrics: Urinary tract infections in children and adolescents. Postgrad Med 60:225, Nov 1976.

ACUTE HEMORRHAGIC CYSTITIS

Acute hemorrhagic cystitis affects children of any race, age, or sex. It is usually of sudden onset and is characterized by gross total or terminal hematuria, dysuria, frequency, and urgency. It is sometimes associated with suprapubic pain, fever, and enuresis. Examination of urine usually shows only red cells and microscopic pyuria.

In 20–25% of cases, a viral cause can be found; the most common offender thus far identified has been adenovirus 11. As adenovirus carriage is common, it is essential to document rises in viral neutralizing antibody titers as well as to recover the virus if it is desired to establish a viral etiology.

A small proportion of cases appear to be caused by common bacterial pathogens. These should be identified and treated by means of systemic antibiotics.

Most cases are associated with sterile urine and remain idiopathic. Sterile hemorrhagic cystitis is not uncommon in patients receiving cyclophosphamide. Diagnostic studies should exclude other causes of hematuria.

Cases of viral and idiopathic acute hemorrhagic cystitis may be expected to resolve spontaneously in 10–14 days.

Mufson MA & others: Adenovirus infection in acute hemorrhagic cystitis. Am J Dis Child 121:281, 1971.

DISEASES OF RENAL VESSELS

RENAL VEIN THROMBOSIS

Renal vein thrombosis occurs in 2 general contexts. In the newborn period, it may suddenly complicate the course of sepsis or dehydration or be observed in infants of a diabetic mother. In older children and adolescents, it may develop following trauma or without any apparent predisposing factors; in these cases, nephrotic syndrome may be associated with renal vein thrombosis.

Clinical Findings

A. Symptoms and Signs: In the newborn, renal vein thrombosis generally presents with the sudden development of an abdominal mass. If the thrombosis is bilateral, oliguria may be present; urine output may be normal with a unilateral thrombus. In older children, flank pain, sometimes with a palpable mass, is a common presentation. In other older children, however, the nephrotic syndrome may be the first sign of renal vein thrombosis.

B. Laboratory Findings: No single laboratory test is diagnostic of renal vein thrombosis. Hematuria is usually present and occasionally is gross. Proteinuria is less constant. In the newborn, thrombocytopenia may be found; this is rare in older children. Delayed opacification of the involved kidney may be seen with excretory urography; the plain abdominal film may show an enlarged renal shadow. The renal scan is helpful, but the definitive diagnostic procedure is epinephrine-assisted venacavography with renal venography.

Treatment

Anticoagulation with heparin is the treatment of choice in both newborns and in older children. No clear-cut benefit from nephrectomy has been demonstrated, although this continues to be suggested. In the newborn, a course of heparin combined with treatment of the underlying problem is usually all that is required. The management in other cases is less straightforward. The tendency for recurrence and embolization has led most workers in this field to recommend long-term anticoagulation.

Course & Prognosis

The mortality rate of renal vein thrombosis in the newborn is usually related to the underlying cause. If the child survives the acute phase, the prognosis for adequate renal function is good. The entity is much less common in older children, but they may be expected to follow the course known to occur in adults. Recurrences, in the same kidney or its mate, may occur years after the original episode of thrombus formation. Extension into the vena cava with fatal pulmonary emboli is a known complication.

The nephrotic syndrome, often with membranous glomerulonephritis, is associated with renal vein thrombosis. In some cases, thrombosis may be a complication of nephrotic syndrome. There is also evidence that the thrombus itself may result in glomerulonephritis, possibly through the release of renal tubular antigens.

Mauer SM & others: Bilateral renal vein thrombosis in infancy: Report of a survivor following surgical intervention. J Pediatr 78:509, 1971.

Moore HL & others: Unilateral renal vein thrombosis and the nephrotic syndrome. Pediatrics 50:598, 1972.

RENAL ARTERIAL DISEASE

Children are susceptible to renovascular hypertension on the basis of fibromuscular hyperplasia, congenital stenosis, or other renal arterial lesions. The proportion of hypertensive children with such demonstrable abnormalities, however, is quite small. Unfortunately, there are few clinical clues to underlying arterial lesions. They should, however, be suspected in children whose hypertension is severe, beginning at 10 years of age or under, or associated with delayed visualization on an excretory urogram. The diagnosis is established by renal arteriography with selective renal vein renin measurements. Some of these lesions may be repaired surgically, but repair may be technically impossible in many children.

ACUTE RENAL FAILURE

Essentials of Diagnosis

- History of exposure to nephrotoxic agents, sepsis, trauma, surgery, glomerulonephritis, shock, or hemorrhage.
- Severe oliguria or, more rarely, anuria.
- Progressive hyperkalemia, hyponatremia, acidosis, and rising BUN.

General Considerations

Acute renal failure is an important complication of many medical and surgical conditions. It can be defined as the sudden inability to excrete urine of sufficient quantity or adequate composition to maintain normal body fluid homeostasis. It may be due to impaired renal perfusion, as in shock (prerenal), to acute renal disease, or to obstructive uropathy.

Diminished circulating blood volume leads to lowered renal perfusion, and the decreased glomerular filtrate is further diminished by increased tubular reabsorption of sodium and water compounded by excessive amounts of circulating vasopressin (ADH) and aldosterone. Acute renal failure due to hypovolemia usually responds to volume replacement with isotonic saline solution, plasma, or blood, depending upon the cause of the deficit. If impaired renal perfusion is prolonged, however, renal cortical blood flow ceases, resulting in renal damage which may take days or weeks to resolve.

Occult postrenal obstruction must always be considered since, if the diagnosis is made early enough, relief of the obstruction will prevent the development of secondary renal failure.

It is useful to consider acute renal failure of renal origin under 2 broad headings: (1) Acute renal failure secondary to exposure of the renal parenchyma to toxic substances or reduced renal perfusion. This type is usually reversible. An initial period of oliguria is generally followed by a high-output phase. (2) Acute renal failure secondary to acute glomerulonephritis, vascular disorders with renal infarction, bilateral cortical necrosis, or necrotizing papillitis.

Clinical Findings

A reliable history of a major infection, trauma (especially crush injury), a surgical procedure, an episode of shock or hemorrhage, or exposure to a potentially nephrotoxic product is helpful in the diagnosis of acute renal failure. The hallmark of the diagnosis is oliguria (< 200–250 ml/sq m/day). Frank anuria suggests either obstructive uropathy, bilateral renal infarction, or bilateral renal cortical necrosis. Thus, the physician must be alert to inadequate urine output in any patient at risk of developing acute renal failure.

Complications

Patients with acute renal failure are unable to excrete a water load. Hence, they easily develop hyponatremia and water intoxication. Moreover, they are at great risk of rapidly developing hyperkalemia and acidemia. Hypertension, azotemia, and uremia may supervene after a few hours or days. Hemorrhage and infection may also be problems.

Treatment

A. Initial Assessment: The initial approach to an oliguric child should be aimed at classifying the problem in one of the categories outlined above and in Table 18–1. While an exact etiologic diagnosis is not

Table 18–1. Classification of causes of renal failure.

Prerenal

Dehydration due to gastroenteritis, malnutrition, or diarrhea
Hemorrhage, blood loss, aortic or renal vessel injury, trauma, surgery, cardiac surgery, renal vein thrombosis
Diabetic acidosis
Pooling of interstitial fluid into local area of injury—burns, operative site, peritonitis
Hypovolemia associated with nephrotic syndrome
Shock
Infusion of fluid with too little sodium

Renal

Hemolytic-uremic syndrome
Acute glomerulonephritis
Extension of prerenal hypoperfusion
Nephrotoxins
Renal necrosis
Intravascular coagulation—septic shock, hemorrhage
Diseases of the kidney and vessels
Iatrogenic
Severe infections
Drowning, especially fresh water
Neoplasma—hyperuricacidemia, hyperuricaciduria

Postrenal

Obstruction due to tumor, stricture, inflammation, hematoma or posterior urethral valves
Sulfonamide crystals
Uric acid crystals
Stones
Ureteroceles
Trauma to a solitary kidney or collecting system

necessary, accurate classification must be made before initiating therapy.

Postrenal failure is quite rare in children except in newborns with anatomic abnormalities and can be acutely recognized and relieved by insertion of a urethral catheter. Surgical correction follows.

The differentiation of renal failure from oliguria secondary to prenal factors is a crucial part of the diagnostic evaluation. Several factors are taken into consideration in making this decision. If the physical examination reveals dehydration and the blood pressure is low, then prenal failure should be suspected. The child with edema, however, may be either in prerenal or renal failure. A patient with nephrotic syndrome, for example, may be grossly edematous but have a severely compromised intravascular volume and thus develop prerenal oliguria.

If a central venous line is inserted and a pressure of less than 3 cm water is observed, a prerenal disturbance is likely. The presence of the central line will facilitate fluid expansion and the subsequent management of the child.

Table 18–2 lists additional factors in the differentiation of prerenal from renal failure.

B. Acute Management: An indwelling catheter should be inserted and urine output monitored hourly.

1. Prerenal factors–Exclude or rectify any prerenal factors. Oligemia should be corrected with blood, plasma, or isotonic saline solution until the blood pressure is normal. If urine output does not rise above oliguric levels within 30–60 minutes, a central venous pressure line should be inserted and additional blood, plasma, or saline should be infused until the central venous pressure has been restored to 3–6 mm Hg (or 4–8 cm water).

If diuresis does not occur in response to the above measures, begin a rapid infusion of mannitol, 0.5–1 gm/kg IV over a period of 30 minutes as a 25% solution (up to 25 gm). Also give furosemide (Lasix), 2 mg/kg as an IV push. Allow 2 hours for a response to occur. If the urine output remains low ($<$ 200–250 ml/sq m/24 hours), repeat the dose of furosemide. If no diuresis occurs, go on to the oliguric regimen given below. If diuresis does occur, continue furosemide and

mannitol if necessary to sustain it. After several hours, the patient may convert to a phase of nonoliguric renal failure which may last for several days and occasionally requires no further diuretic therapy. When this occurs, manage according to the nonoliguria regimen which follows.

2. Oliguric phase–Once it has been determined that a prolonged oliguric phase is inevitable, an oliguric renal failure regimen should be instituted without delay. It is essential that close patient monitoring be performed. The patient should be weighed at least daily; strict intake, output, and vital signs records must be kept; and laboratory determinations of hematocrit; serum sodium, potassium, chloride, calcium, phosphorus, uric acid, and creatinine; blood CO_2 content; and BUN should be done at least daily.

The principal complications of acute oliguric renal failure are (1) water intoxication and hyponatremia, (2) hyperkalemia, (3) metabolic acidosis, (4) hypertension, and (5) uremia. Therapy is directed against each of these complications.

The tendency to develop water intoxication and hyponatremia requires sharp reduction in fluid intake. This makes it difficult to provide enough calories to minimize tissue catabolism, metabolic acidosis, hyperkalemia, and uremia.

If the patient can retain oral feedings, he may be given carbohydrate- and fat-rich supplements provided they are very low in protein, potassium, and sodium (eg, Controlyte). It is usually safer, however, to administer all calories intravenously by increasing the glucose concentration in the intravenous fluids to 15–20%.

Intravenous fluids are calculated as follows: (1) Give no allotment for urine as long as oliguria persists. (2) Give only about two-thirds of the patient's estimated sensible and insensible water requirements. (The rest will be provided by water of oxidation.) In dry air, such patients usually require about 400 ml/sq m/day.

Hyperkalemia can often be controlled by administration of an ion-exchange resin such as sodium-polystyrene sulfonate (Kayexalate) given as a retention enema every 4 hours made up as an aqueous slurry containing 1 gm of resin/kg body weight. It is imperative that the cardiac effects be monitored by ECG.

Severe or persistent hyperkalemia, severe hypertension, congestive failure, severe anemia, or uremic syndrome all justify the use of peritoneal dialysis or, occasionally, hemodialysis.

3. Nonoliguric phase–Some patients with acute renal failure may initially be nonoliguric, or this phase may follow almost immediately after a renal insult or may be entered by diuretic-induced conversion from an oliguric state or during recovery after a period of prolonged oliguria. In some patients, the high-output phase is mild, lasts only a few days, and is characterized by slightly increased volumes of poorly concentrated urine. Other patients, however, may pass enormous volumes of isosthenuric, sodium-rich urine. Occasionally, this salt-wasting state may be accompanied by significant potassium wasting as well.

Management requires the provision of adequate

Table 18–2. Urine studies.

Prerenal Failure	Acute Renal Failure
Urine osmolality 50 mOsm/kg greater than plasma osmolality	Urine osmolality equal to or less than plasma osmolality
Urine sodium $<$ 10 mEq/liter	Urinary sodium $>$ 20 mEq/liter
Ratio of urine creatine to plasma creatinine $>$ 14:1	Ratio of urine creatinine to plasma creatinine $<$ 14:1
Specific gravity $>$ 1.020	Specific gravity 1.012– 1.018

quantities of water, sodium, and potassium to provide for the ongoing losses. Measurement of previous volumes coupled with determinations of urinary electrolytes (Na^+, K^+, Cl^-) provide the best guide to therapy.

C. Acute Dialysis: The indications for dialysis are based on clinical experience. There are some definite criteria, however: (1) severe hyperkalemia unresponsive to usual medical therapy; (2) unrelenting metabolic acidosis (usually in a situation where fluid overload prevents sodium bicarbonate administration); (3) fluid overload with or without severe hypertension or congestive heart failure (a situation which would seriously compromise caloric or drug administration—a definite problem in the oliguric patient); and (4) uremia symptoms, usually manifested in children by CNS depression.

The rate of rise of both BUN and serum creatinine may be helpful indicators of dialysis intervention—absolute levels as rigid criteria may not correlate with the clinical situation, but it is generally accepted that BUN should not be allowed to exceed 100 mg/100 ml.

Early dialysis, when properly performed, can simplify management and reduce the morbidity rate associated with renal failure.

The choice of peritoneal dialysis or hemodialysis depends on the availability of as well as the indications for these technics. Peritoneal dialysis is generally preferred in children because of the relative ease of performance and good results. However, when the clinical situation calls for rapid correction of systemic abnormalities or removal of toxins from the blood, hemodialysis must be instituted, as the peritoneal process is quite slow. Other contraindications to peritoneal dialysis include recent abdominal surgery or past surgery with a significant risk of adhesion formation or severe ileus.

Because of its universal availability, the technic of peritoneal dialysis will be described. However, although performance of peritoneal dialysis is a rather basic technic within the competence of many physicians, it should be done whenever possible by experienced persons. The incidence of complications is inversely related to the amount of experience the operator has had with the procedure.

1. Catheter insertion—

a. Appropriate sedative medication may be administered at the physician's discretion.

b. The bladder must be empty. The abdomen is surgically prepared (with special attention to the umbilicus, which is considered highly contaminated) and draped. Strict aseptic technic should be followed.

c. The site of insertion is approximately 2 cm below the umbilicus in the midline. The skin in this area is infiltrated with local anesthetic, and the infiltration is carried to the fascia of the rectus muscle. The site is then perforated with a 16 gauge Angiocath, and the catheter is advanced over the needle when entrance into the peritoneal cavity is assured. Fluid can then be instilled into the peritoneal cavity. Free-flowing dialysate without patient discomfort supports intraperitoneal positioning. If this is not the case, stop inflow immediately, as preperitoneal instillation of dialysate will make subsequent insertion practically impossible.

d. The abdomen is thus "primed" with enough prewarmed (37° C [98.6° F]) dialysate to distend the abdomen (see Table 18–3 for amount; the presence of ascitic fluid may reduce requirement), thus reducing the likelihood of viscus perforation and facilitating dialysis catheter insertion. After the abdomen is distended, the Angiocath is removed and the dialysis catheter is inserted.

e. The commercially available dialysis catheter is usually a stiff Teflon catheter which has a curve in the intraperitoneal perforated segment. A straight, sharpened metal stylet is provided which, when inserted into the Teflon catheter, straightens it and provides a sharp tip which eases insertion.

f. Insertion of the dialysis catheter with stylet in place may be further aided by making a small incision (2–3 mm) through the skin at the chosen site. With slow, steady pressure and some twisting motions, the catheter is pushed first through the skin and subcutaneous tissue. Sudden absence of resistance suggests entrance into the peritoneal cavity. This will be evidenced by dialysate welling up into the catheter as it is advanced (without resistance) over the stylet and into the pelvic area.

g. Exact placement depends on which position is observed to provide best function. The entire perforated segment must lie intraperitoneally (pediatric-sized catheters are small enough to be used in most infants and older children).

h. After sterile dressings are placed around the catheter, it may be held in desired place with tape. Care should be taken to prevent catheter movement once it is in place. It is especially important to avoid further insertion of the catheter once the exterior portion is contaminated.

2. Instillation of dialysate—

a. After noting the total amount of fluid used to test catheter function, begin dialysis by first making certain that at least 75% of dialysate instilled is recovered. If ascites is present at the time of dialysis, the decision whether or not ascitic fluid should be freely removed from the peritoneal cavity should be based on the patient's intravascular volume status.

Table 18–3. Volumes of dialysate in peritoneal dialysis.

Weight	Initial*	Maximum Maintenance (as Tolerated)
< 10 kg	50 ml/kg	50–100 ml/kg
10–20 kg	250–500 ml	1000–1500 ml
20–40 kg	500–1000 ml	1000–2000 ml
> 40 kg	1000 ml	2000 ml

*Initial volumes may need to be reduced to 25–35% of the amounts shown in some critically ill patients and then more fluid added slowly as tolerated.

b. Fill the peritoneal cavity with volumes as set forth in Table 18–3.

c. The dialysate is allowed to run in freely by gravity flow, and the inflow tubing is clamped when the desired inflow volume is achieved. The fluid is allowed to remain in the peritoneal cavity for 30 minutes, and the outflow tubing is then unclamped, permitting the dialysate to drain by gravity into a receptacle. An accurate record is kept of the amount instilled and the amount removed, so that it can readily be determined whether the patient is losing appropriate amounts of fluid in the process. The glucose concentration of the fluid should result in net removal of fluid from the patient. Weight should be recorded pre- and postdialysis and whenever calculations show a net fluid balance. The process is usually continued for 48 hours, performing as many cycles as possible in order to take full advantage of the time. During dialysis, vital signs should be carefully monitored, and a sample of the dialysate removed from the patient should be cultured daily, especially if the fluid becomes turbid. The catheter is removed after 48 hours, as the risk of peritonitis increases with prolonged use of this type of catheter.

3. Choosing the proper dialysate–A typical commercial peritoneal dialysate solution contains 132 mEq/liter Na^+, 102 mEq/liter Cl^-, 35 mEq/liter lactate, 3.5 mEq/liter Ca^{++}, and 1.5 mEq/liter Mg^{++}. K^+ is usually omitted unless the serum K^+ is < 4 mEq/liter. Glucose is added in varying quantities depending upon the need to withdraw fluid from the patient. Glucose solutions are available in 1.5% or 4.25% concentration. The 1.5% glucose concentration is used to maintain a slight osmotic gradient between the patient's serum and the dialysate in order to prevent fluid absorption. The higher concentration may be used to remove fluid more avidly. Higher concentrations are no longer commercially available because the removal of excessive quantities of fluid tends to result in severe hypernatremia. Lactate is used in the solutions instead of bicarbonate to provide an adequate buffer base. (The effective use of such buffers in dialysate solutions relies upon the ability to metabolize to bicarbonate.) Any other additives can be specified at the time and added to the dialysate as indicated. The only other commonly used addition is 500 units of heparin to each of the first 4–6 liters of dialysate to prevent clotting in the catheter.

4. Complications of dialysis–The complications of catheter insertion include bleeding (rarely major), bowel perforation, failure to obtain adequate return of fluid (usually requiring only repositioning of the patient or the catheter), respiratory distress (usually correctable by using smaller volumes), and infection. Infection is by far the most common and one of the more serious complications of peritoneal dialysis. However, treatment is relatively simple if infection is detected early, requiring merely the addition of appropriate antibiotics to the dialysis solution. Signs of peritonitis should be sought during the procedure but may not necessarily be present. If peritonitis is suspected, a sample of the dialysis solution from the patient should be sent for culture and sensitivity testing, and a Gram-stained smear should be examined to determine whether or not antibiotic treatment can be started while awaiting culture results.

Dysequilibrium syndrome is a complication of dialysis that usually appears early upon initiation of dialysis. The symptoms range from nausea and vomiting to severe headache and seizures. Although the cause is not completely understood, the disorder is believed to be related to rapid removal of urea with delayed removal from brain tissue resulting in cerebral edema. This complication is more commonly seen in hemodialysis and is rare with peritoneal dialysis, probably because of the slower rate of change in solute removal seen with peritoneal dialysis. In any case, this problem need not arise (or at least it will be mild if it does occur) if dialysis is initiated slowly and extreme changes are avoided.

Excessive water removal can readily be corrected by increasing intake. Mild anxiety or pain can be relieved with analgesics or sedatives providing it is not related to a true malfunction of the catheter itself. The procedure should be painless; any undue discomfort should therefore alert one to a serious intra-abdominal problem or catheter malposition.

This process of peritoneal dialysis may be repeated as necessary during the course of acute renal failure. Where the technic is available, it has been found beneficial to insert a chronic peritoneal dialysis catheter. This is especially helpful in situations where repeated dialysis may become necessary and recovery is prolonged, as this technic eliminates the need for repeated abdominal perforation. However, since this procedure is not readily performed except in specialized centers, it will not be fully discussed here.

Course & Prognosis

The period of severe oliguria, if it occurs, usually lasts about 10 days. If oliguria lasts longer than 3 weeks or if there is complete anuria, a diagnosis of acute tubular necrosis is very unlikely and a vascular accident or glomerulonephritis is more probable. The diuretic phase begins with progressive increases in urinary output followed by the passage of large volumes of isosthenuric urine containing 80–150 mEq/liter of sodium. During the recovery phase, signs and symptoms subside rapidly, although polyuria may persist for several days or weeks. Urinary abnormalities usually disappear completely within a few months.

The prognosis is excellent in acute tubular necrosis (> 90% complete recovery) but poor in other forms of acute renal failure of renal origin such as vascular accident (< 10% recovery).

Dobrin RS & others: The critically ill child: Acute renal failure. Pediatrics 48:286, 1971.

Kleinknecht D & others: Uremic and non-uremic complications in acute renal failure: Evaluation of early and frequent dialysis on prognosis. Kidney Int 1:190, 1972.

Tenchkoff H: Peritoneal dialysis today: A new look. Nephron 12:420, 1974.

CHRONIC RENAL FAILURE

Essentials of Diagnosis

- Usually a history of renal disease.
- Headache, fatigue, anorexia, pallor.
- Hypertension, anemia, acidosis, bone pains, cardiac failure.
- Elevated BUN, proteinuria; red cells and casts in urine.

General Considerations

In renal failure, kidney function is reduced to a level at which the kidneys are unable to maintain normal biochemical homeostasis. In acute renal failure, the nephrons are injured, often reversibly; in the chronic form, the nephrons are destroyed progressively, leading to gradually increasing uremia. Many kidney diseases lead to uremia, particularly chronic pyelonephritis and glomerulonephritis of various types. Renal dysplasias and cystic disease of the kidney as well as cystinosis and oxalosis are less common causes of failure.

Pathophysiology

The kidney has a remarkable ability to compensate for the persistent loss of nephrons which occurs in chronic renal failure. However, by the time the glomerular filtration rate has dropped to 15–20 ml/min/1.73 sq m, this capacity begins to be exhausted. The resulting biochemical problems can be grouped according to the major substances handled by the kidney:

A. Water: Defects in renal concentrating ability appear early in most chronic renal diseases. Thus, the patient requires a larger than normal urine volume to excrete a given solute load. Clinically, this is reflected as polyuria with a urine of low specific gravity; the patient needs an increased water intake to meet the demands of this situation. In later stages, the ability to dilute the urine may be lost, and a urine of fixed specific gravity close to that of plasma will be excreted regardless of intake.

B. Nitrogenous Products: Serum BUN, creatinine, and uric acid levels rise as the GFR falls. However, the level of BUN is affected not only by the glomerular filtration rate but also by dietary intake of protein and by urinary flow. Creatinine, on the other hand, is not reabsorbed by the tubules and is not influenced by dietary intake; for these reasons, serum creatinine has several advantages over urea as an index of renal failure.

C. Sodium and Potassium: Sodium loss is enhanced by osmotic diuresis and by a decreased capacity of the tubules to secrete hydrogen ions in exchange for sodium. Sodium retention is rare in chronic renal failure unless nephrotic syndrome is also present. Salt wasting can therefore be a serious problem and can be compounded by salt restriction or diuretics. Hyperkalemia is usually a very late problem in chronic renal failure, occurring in the oliguric phase.

D. Phosphorus and Calcium: A large percentage (85%) of the filtered phosphorus is normally reabsorbed; tubular rejection can therefore compensate for a decrease in glomerular filtration rate. However, retention of phosphorus occurs when the glomerular filtration rate drops. Serum phosphorus levels of 7–10 mg/100 ml are common, and calcium levels are correspondingly low. This phenomenon is related both to the fact that the transport of calcium across the bowel wall in uremia is unresponsive to normal amounts of vitamin D and to the reciprocal relationship of serum phosphorus and serum calcium.

E. Acid-Base Balance: Decreased ammonia production and retention of endogenous acid account for the metabolic acidosis seen in chronic renal failure.

F. Nutrition and Growth: A major problem in chronic renal failure management is the effect of dietary manipulations or restrictions plus uremia, no matter how mild, on the child's development. The clinician must be able to accept some compromise in growth and development in making the best of what remains of renal function. Dietary supplementation with essential amino acids or ketoacids may improve the nutritional status of the child with chronic renal failure. Unfortunately, the problem of unacceptability of these substances is a serious one. Early initiation of dialysis has been thought by many to be a possible solution to this problem, although nutritional status may still be a problem while on dialysis. Unfortunately, the decision is not an easy one given the extreme nature of the therapy at a time when some degree of supportive renal function still exists.

Clinical Findings

Chronic renal failure must be thought of as a total body disease, with clinical and laboratory findings relating to nearly every organ system.

Anemia is a nearly constant finding in chronic renal failure. It is usually normochromic and normocytic and results from decreased production secondary to diminished renal erythropoietin synthesis. Blood loss, hemolysis, and nutritional deficiencies also play a role. Platelet dysfunction and other abnormalities of the coagulation system are also commonly present. Clinically, bleeding phenomena, especially gastrointestinal bleeding, may be a problem.

CNS manifestations of the condition may be subtle but are usually present. Early on, confusion, apathy, and lethargy may be present; these may be unsuspected clinically until the patient is challenged with a task such as "serial sevens." With advancing uremia, stupor and coma may be present. Associated electrolyte abnormalities (eg, hyponatremia) may precipitate seizures.

Cardiovascular manifestations of chronic renal failure may be life-threatening. Uremic pericarditis may develop. Congestive heart failure is seen more often, and hypertension is quite common. The hypertension may relate to volume overload or to excessive renin excretion.

The skeleton may be severely affected. The combination of hyperparathyroidism and buffering of acids by the bone salts results in osteomalacia and rickets. Clinically, bone pain and severe deformities may result.

Anorexia is the primary gastrointestinal manifestation of this state. It is often a significant problem in that it may lead to dangerous nutritional deficiencies. Intractable vomiting may also occur with severe uremia.

Patients with chronic renal failure tend to be more susceptible to infections. Because of their generally debilitated state, they often handle infections poorly.

Treatment

A. General Measures: As with acute renal failure, the aim of treatment in chronic renal disease is the prevention of complications. The principles of management differ depending upon the degree of renal insufficiency. Thus, serial creatinine clearances (or other measurements of GFR) are essential in following these patients.

1. GFR 20–30 ml/min/1.73 sq m—With this degree of renal insufficiency, most homeostatic mechanisms are still operating effectively. The physician should be most concerned at this point with maintaining existing function. Thus, surveillance on a regular basis is essential. Blood pressure is followed carefully and hypertension treated if detected. Infections, especially those of the urinary tract, demand immediate attention. Good nutrition is important; dietary restrictions are rarely necessary at this level of function.

2. GFR 10–20 ml/min/1.73 sq m—The need for some dietary control usually becomes evident when further lowering of GFR occurs. A diet high in fats and carbohydrates and low in protein ($<$ 1 gm/kg) will provide adequate calories with some reduction in nitrogenous waste products. The need for salt restriction depends upon the urine sodium excretion. In situations where salt losses are continuing (eg, medullary cystic disease), restriction may be unnecessary or even dangerous. Generally, modest sodium restriction (1 mEq/kg/day) will be required; severe hypertension may necessitate further restriction. Patients in this category may also be hyperphosphatemic. Although dietary phosphate restriction is difficult to achieve, the use of an aluminum hydroxide antacid (Amphojel) may decrease absorption of the anion. Hypocalcemia may respond to lowering the serum phosphate, or additional measures such as vitamin D or calcium supplementation may be necessary.

3. GFR 5–10 ml/min/1.73 sq m—When GFR reaches this level, it is nearly inevitable that dialysis or transplantation will eventually be necessary. The best policy is to arrange for elective placement of an arteriovenous fistula when this stage is reached even if the child is clinically well. This early placement will allow the fistula time to mature so that it will be functioning well as soon as dialysis is required. Extremely careful follow-up is necessary at this point, with the physician's main role being early recognition of the need for dialysis. Supplemental bicarbonate may be needed for acidosis. Anemia is likely to be a problem; blood trans-

fusions, however, should be kept to a minimum because of the danger of volume overload. Where possible, deglycerated red cells should be used if transplantation is being considered. There is some evidence that the anemia of renal failure may respond to androgens.

4. GFR under 5 ml/min/1.73 sq m—With this degree of function, end-stage renal failure is well established (although it may be symptomatic at a clearance somewhere under 10 ml/min), and dialysis is necessary to maintain homeostasis. The child should have been followed carefully enough to this stage so that dialysis can be initiated electively rather than as an emergency procedure. Avoidance of such complications as pulmonary edema, hyperkalemia, or neurologic symptoms secondary to uremia is desirable. The alternative to dialysis is of course renal transplantation. Both these modes of therapy are more fully described elsewhere in this text.

B. Water and Calorie Conservation: Depending upon the degree of renal failure, strict attention must be paid to water conservation. In complete anuria, water should be supplied to replace insensible loss minus water of oxidation (about 400 ml/sq m/24 hours) plus water lost in stools, vomitus, and urine. The amount to be given should be carefully calculated at least daily and checked against body weight and, if possible, urine osmolality.

Diet is difficult to organize for any child with a fickle appetite, and especially so when water must be restricted. Flavored high-caloric solutions such as Cal-Power may be useful.

In less severe cases, restriction of protein to 1 gm/kg/24 hours or less may help to lower blood urea. However, most children in chronic severe renal failure are on dialysis. Continuing growth in this circumstance is in part dependent on a high-caloric, high-protein intake. Supplements of essential amino acids (Aminaid) may be helpful, and in time ketoacids may also come to be used extensively. Various glucose polymers are available to increase caloric intake. Sodium and potassium regulation may also be important. Water-soluble vitamins should be given in at least twice the recommended dietary allowance to children on dialysis.

C. Electrolyte Homeostasis: The principles of fluid and electrolyte therapy are discussed in Chapter 35. Meticulous medical care can often sustain children in renal failure for many weeks without dialysis.

Elevated serum phosphorus can to some extent be controlled by a low-phosphorus diet in conjunction with aluminum hydroxide gel (Amphojel), 1 tbsp 3 times a day. Calcium lactate, 4 gm 3 times a day, usually offsets urinary protein-bound calcium loss, but this is not always effective. Dihydrotachysterol, 125 μg daily or every other day, is also used and, 1a-hydroxycholecalciferol may soon be available for this purpose.

D. Blood Transfusions: Some children with renal failure become severely anemic and transfusions may be essential, but it is remarkable how little they may be affected by hemoglobin as low as 6 gm/100 ml. In general, if there is no cardiac failure and the patient is not overly fatigued, transfusions should be avoided. Since these patients may already have marginally high blood volumes, any increase may precipitate severe hypertension with convulsions or congestive failure. Packed cells should always be used and should be given very slowly and under the closest supervision. If necessary, a total or partial exchange should be used to increase the hematocrit. Vascular accidents are frequent during and immediately after improperly supervised transfusions.

E. Management of Acidosis and Osteodystrophy: A low-protein diet will be helpful in decreasing the metabolic acidosis since proteins are the largest contributors of nonvolatile acids. The acidosis can be further alleviated by the administration of an alkalinizing solution. Unless renal failure is very advanced, attempts should be made to relieve bone pain and to improve the osteodystrophy by the administration of vitamin D in doses of 25–50 thousand IU daily or more. Care must be taken to avoid metastatic calcifications. Hyperphosphatemia can be helped by aluminum hydroxide preparations administered after each meal.

F. Management of Hypertension: Hypertension in chronic renal failure is often a reflection of fluid overload. This possibility should always be considered first and treated if appropriate. Drug therapy, where needed, is described in the next section.

G. Control of Infections: Antibiotics should be given at the first sign of infection, keeping in mind that the dosage of certain antibiotics eliminated principally in the urine should be reduced in proportion to the decrease in renal function in order to prevent toxic effects.

H. Psychologic Support: As is true of most children with chronic illness, an important part of management is attention to the patient's and the family's emotional adaptation to the disease. Psychiatric counseling requires as much attention as the rather complicated medical management.

I. Dialysis and Transplantation: The best tolerated method of treatment of end-stage renal disease is a successful and uncomplicated renal transplant. The idea of transplantation in a child at first seems ideal; however, the results, despite the advances that have been made in organ transplantation procedures, are not uniformly good.

Adequate growth and well-being are directly related to acceptance of the graft, the degree of normal function, and the side-effects of medications employed. There is no guarantee that days at risk and morbidity rates will necessarily be minimized by an organ transplant. All of this depends to a large extent on what medications are required, how much difficulty is encountered with rejection of the graft, and complications in management over the long term.

Since a successful result is not always achieved, much attention has been given to improvement of technics of dialysis for children. Great advances have been made in hemodialysis, both in technic and in our understanding of the specialized approach required by this treatment. Hemodialysis now has been performed in major centers that devote their entire effort in dialysis toward the management of pediatric patients and is now being regarded as reasonable long-range method of treatment of the child with end-stage renal disease. Treatment of terminal renal failure in children may thus consist of transplantation or dialysis as the situation warrants. The demonstrated feasibility of chronic peritoneal dialysis in children is a third alternative. Peritoneal dialysis via an indwelling chronic catheter is well accepted by children. Many children can undergo dialysis at night in their homes.

Probably the best measure of the success of chronic dialysis in children is the level of physical and psychosocial rehabilitation achieved. Centers where a large experience has accumulated report substantial improvements in patient well-being. Patients continue to participate in day-to-day activities, attend school, and have even recorded reasonable growth. Although no catch-up growth has occurred, patients can grow at an acceptable rate even though they remain in the third percentile. Even associated problems such as chronic anemia and bone disease are being better controlled.

Prognosis

Severe chronic renal disease in childhood is all too often progressive and eventually fatal. The rates at which renal diseases progress are quite variable, however, and hard to predict. Intractable anemia and hypertension are bad signs, as are permanent electrolyte changes and neurologic symptoms. In the older child, there is an increasing tendency to resort to hemodialysis before a transplant, thus minimizing these complications.

Bricker NS & others: The pathophysiology of renal insufficiency. Pediatr Clin North Am 18:595, 1971.

Cameron JS: The treatment of chronic renal failure in children by regular dialysis and by transplantation. Nephron 11:221, 1973.

Fine RN & others: Hemodialysis in children. Am J Dis Child 119:498, 1970.

Grushkin CM, Korsch B, Fine RN: Hemodialysis in small children. JAMA 221:869, 1972.

Holliday MA & others: Treatment of renal failure in children. Pediatr Clin North Am 18:613, 1971.

Khan AU & others: Social and emotional adaptations of children with transplanted kidneys and chronic hemodialysis. Am J Psychol 127:1194, 1971.

Lilly JR & others: Renal homotransplantation in pediatric patients. Pediatrics 47:548, 1971.

Mauer M & others: Long term hemodialysis in the neonatal period. Am J Dis Child 125:269, 1973.

Rae A, Pendray M: Advantages of peritoneal dialysis in chronic renal failure. JAMA 225:937, 1973.

HYPERTENSION

Hypertension in children is most commonly of renal origin and is encountered usually as a looked-for complication of known renal parenchymal disease or unsuspectingly in routine physical examinations. A list of conditions which may be associated with hypertension is given in Table 18—4. Increased understanding of the respective roles of water and salt retention on the one hand and overactivity of the renin-angiotensin system on the other has done much to rationalize therapy; it is nevertheless clear that not all forms of hypertension are explicable by these 2 mechanisms.

Diagnosis

Confirmation of the diagnosis depends upon the repeated demonstration of a diastolic pressure 2 standard deviations above the mean (Table 18—5). The blood pressure cuff should be at least 20% wider than the diameter of the arm since a narrow cuff will cause falsely high readings. It is also sometimes necessary to use a "leg" cuff with overweight adolescent children. Adolescent patients may also have labile blood pressures. It is therefore important to check initial elevated readings again after a period of relaxation. It may be useful to have blood pressures recorded at home.

Evaluation of renal hypertension in children is particularly directed toward the possibility of a unilateral lesion that might be susceptible to remedy by surgery. The evaluation of nonrenal possibilities as they are indicated by the history or physical signs is detailed under these respective conditions.

Routine laboratory studies include a complete blood count, urinalysis, and urine culture and radiographic delineation of the urinary tract. A renal biopsy should always be undertaken with special care in the hypertensive patient and preferably after pressures have been controlled by therapy. Ureteric catheterization is not used now in lateralizing lesions; instead, the appropriate information is obtained from renal size, a

Table 18—5. Normal blood pressure for various ages (mm Hg).*

Ages	Mean Systolic ± 2 SD	Mean Diastolic ± 2 SD
1 month	80 ± 16	46 ± 16
6 months to 1 year	89 ± 29	60 ± 10†
1 year	96 ± 30	66 ± 25†
2 years	99 ± 25	64 ± 25†
3 years	100 ± 25	67 ± 23†
4 years	99 ± 20	65 ± 20†
5—6 years	94 ± 14	55 ± 9
6—7 years	100 ± 15	56 ± 8
7—8 years	102 ± 15	56 ± 8
8—9 years	105 ± 16	57 ± 9
9—10 years	107 ± 16	57 ± 9
10—11 years	111 ± 17	58 ± 10
11—12 years	113 ± 18	59 ± 10
12—13 years	115 ± 19	59 ± 10
13—14 years	118 ± 19	60 ± 10

*Reproduced, with permission, from Nadas A: *Pediatric Cardiology,* 2nd ed. Saunders, 1963.

†In this study the point of muffling was taken as the diastolic pressure.

rapid-sequence intravenous urogram, the renal scan, aortography with renal arteriography, and differential renal vein renin levels.

Treatment

A. Hypertensive Emergencies: A hypertensive emergency may be said to exist when CNS signs of hypertension appear, eg, papilledema or seizures. Retinal hemorrhages or exudates also indicate a need for prompt and effective control.

1. One of the most effective drugs for a true hypertensive emergency is diazoxide (Hyperstat), 5 mg/kg by a single, rapid intravenous injection.

2. A combination of intramuscular reserpine and hydralazine is often effective when rapid blood pressure control is desired. This is especially true in acute glomerulonephritis, but less so in long-standing hypertension.

a. Reserpine is given in an initial starting dose of 0.03 mg/kg IM. It may be repeated every 4—6 hours in doubled or tripled doses as necessary. Probably no more than 2—3 mg should be given at one time.

b. Hydralazine (Apresoline), 0.15 mg/kg IM, is given at the same time. The tachycardia caused by hydralazine tends to be counteracted by the bradycardia caused by reserpine.

3. A variety of other drugs are effective in the treatment of hypertensive emergencies. These include methyldopa (Aldomet), sodium nitroprusside, and minoxidil.

B. Ambulatory Treatment of Chronic Hypertension: The treatment of renoparenchymal hypertension is medical rather than surgical. In general, treatment is started with a low dose and the dose is raised at inter-

Table 18—4. Etiology of hypertension in childhood.

Renal
  Pyelonephritis
  Glomerulonephritis
  Tumor
  Hydronephrosis
  Ectopic kidney
  Renal vein abnormalities
  Renal artery abnormalities
  Cystic disease
  Trauma
  After renal transplantation
  Essential hypertension
  Blood transfusion in preexisting renal disease
Cardiovascular
  Coarctation of the aorta
  Patent ductus arteriosus
  Aortitis
  Marfan's syndrome
  Subacute bacterial endocarditis

Miscellaneous
  Lead poisoning
  Mercury poisoning
  Familial dysautonomia
  Poliomyelitis
  Radiation of the kidney
  Encephalitis
  Raised intracranial pressure
  Stevens-Johnson syndrome
  Guillain-Barré syndrome
  After genitourinary surgery
  Burns
  Reserpine overdose
  Licorice ingestion
  Acromegaly
  Hemophilia
  Acute bacterial endocarditis

vals (usually every few days) until control of blood pressure is achieved, postural hypotension becomes a problem, or undesirable side-effects occur.

Marked diurnal variations in blood pressure may occur. Hence, it is advisable to teach capable parents how to take and record blood pressures at home after arising, at mid-morning if possible, in the afternoon, and during the evening.

Table 18–6 lists the drugs commonly used to treat hypertension on an ambulatory basis. The order and combinations in which these drugs should be used are governed by the potency of the drugs, their freedom from side-effects, and the severity of the hypertension. The mildest drug is probably hydrochlorothiazide used alone, followed by reserpine and hydralazine. Propranolol and hydralazine are an effective combination. Methyldopa, guanethidine, and, as a last resort, pentolinium may also be used. Certain more recently introduced drugs promise much better control: These include minoxidil with propranolol; saralasin, an angiotensin II inhibitor; and a nonapeptide inhibitor of angiotensin I conversion to angiotensin II. Clonidine in doses of 0.2–2.4 mg daily has been favorably reported for use in adults. Studies in childhood hypertension are not yet available.

Prognosis

The long-term effects of mild hypertension with onset during childhood are not well defined. However, studies indicate that serious hypertension, if not corrected, is associated with a very poor long-term prognosis. Approximately 50% of children with diastolic blood pressures persistently above 120 mm Hg will die within 10 years of diagnosis.

Dormois JC, Young JL, Nies AS: Minoxidil in severe hypertension: Value when conventional drugs have failed. Am Heart J 90:360, 1975.

Gill DG & others: Analysis of 100 children with severe and persistent hypertension. Arch Dis Child 51:951, 1976.

Kilcoyne MM: Adolescent hypertension. 2. Characteristics and response to treatment. Circulation 50:1014, 1974.

Lieberman E: Essential hypertension in children and youth: A pediatric perspective. J Pediatr 85:1, 1974.

Loggie JMH: Hypertension in children and adolescents. Hosp Pract, June 1975.

Londe S, Goldring D: High blood pressure in children: Problems and guidelines for evaluation and treatment. Am J Cardiol 37:650, 1976.

Makker SP: Minoxidil in refractory hypertension. J Pediatr 86:621, 1975.

Malekzadeh MH & others: Hypertension after renal transplantation in children. J Pediatr 86:370, 1975.

McLaine PN, Drummond KN: Intravenous diazoxide for severe hypertension in childhood. J Pediatr 79:829, 1971.

Rance CP & others: Persistent systemic hypertension in infants and children. Pediatr Clin North Am 21:801, 1974.

•   •   •

INHERITED OR DEVELOPMENTAL DEFECTS OF THE URINARY TRACT

In recent years there has been a substantial increase in the number of renal or urinary tract diseases which have been discovered to be hereditary or developmental in origin. Many classification schemes have been proposed, although none are entirely adequate. The more important entities are listed below.

Cystic Diseases of Genetic Origin

  A. **Polycystic Disease:**

    Polycystic disease of early infancy: Neonatal polycystic disease, Meckel's syndrome

    Polycystic disease of childhood: Medullary tubular ectasia, congenital hepatic fibrosis

    Adult polycystic disease

  B. **Cortical Cysts:**

    Tuberous sclerosis complex

    Lindau's disease (cystic disease in syndromes of multiple malformations):

      Cerebrohepatorenal syndrome of Zellweger

      Autosomal trisomy syndromes D and E

      Lissencephaly and oral-facial-digital syndromes

      Schwartz-Jampel syndrome

    Asphyxiating thoracic dystrophy of Jeune

    Down's, Turner's, and Ehlers-Danlos syndromes

Table 18–6. Antihypertensive drugs for ambulatory treatment.

Drug	Oral Dose	Major Side-Effects*
Hydrochloro-thiazide (Esidrix, HydroDiuril)	2–4 mg/kg/24 hours as single dose or in 2 divided doses	Potassium depletion, hyperuricemia.
Reserpine (Serpasil, etc)	0.005–0.05 mg/kg/24 hours in 1 or 2 doses	Nasal stuffiness, depression, nausea, bradycardia, sedation.
Hydralazine (Apresoline)	0.75 mg/kg/24 hours in 4–6 divided doses	Lupus erythematosus, tachycardia, headache.
Methyldopa (Aldomet)	10–40 mg/kg/24 hours in 3 divided doses	False-positive Coombs test, hemolytic anemia, fever, leukopenia, abnormal liver function tests.
Guanethidine (Ismelin)	0.2–1 mg/kg/24 hours as single dose or in 3 divided doses	Postural hypotension, bradycardia; acute renal failure.
Propranolol (Inderal) with	0.2–1 mg/kg/24 hours in 2 doses	Syncope, cardiac failure, and hypoglycemia.
Minoxidil (a piperidine-pyrimidine)	0.15 mg/kg/24 hours in one dose	Tachycardia, angina.
Pentolinium (Ansolysen)	0.2 mg/kg/24 hours in 4 doses	Postural hypotension, urinary retention.

*Many more side-effects than those listed have been reported.

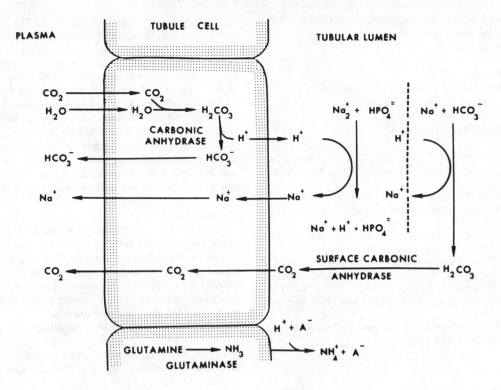

Figure 18–1. Tubular mechanisms for hydrogen ion excretion.

C. Medullary Cysts:
Medullary sponge kidney
Medullary cystic disease (nephronophthisis)
D. Hereditary and Familial Cystic Dysplasia

Dysplastic Renal Diseases
Renal aplasia (unilateral, bilateral)
Renal hypoplasia (unilateral, bilateral, total, segmental)
Multicystic renal dysplasia (unilateral, bilateral, multilocular, postobstructive, etc)
Familial and hereditary renal dysplasias
Oligomeganephronia

Hereditary Diseases Associated With Nephritis
Hereditary nephritis with deafness and ocular defects (Alport's syndrome)
Nail-patella syndrome
Familial hyperprolinemia
Hereditary nephrotic syndrome
Hereditary osteolysis with nephropathy
Hereditary nephritis with thoracic asphyxiant dystrophy syndrome

Hereditary Diseases Associated With Intrarenal Deposition of Metabolites
Angiokeratoma corporis diffusum (Fabry's disease)
Heredopathia atactica polyneuritiformis (Refsum's disease)
Various storage diseases (eg, GM_1 monosialogangliosidosis, Hurler's syndrome, Niemann-Pick disease, familial metachromatic leukodystrophy, glycogenosis type I (Von Gierke's disease), glycogenosis type II (Pompe's disease)
Hereditary amyloidosis (familial Mediterranean fever; heredofamilial urticaria with deafness and neuropathy; primary familial amyloidosis with polyneuropathy)

Hereditary Renal Diseases Associated With Tubular Transport Defects
Hartnup's disease
Immunoglycinuria
Fanconi's syndromes
Oculocerebrorenal syndrome of Lowe
Cystinosis (infantile, adolescent, adult types)
Wilson's disease
Galactosemia
Hereditary fructose intolerance
Renal tubular acidosis (many types).
Hereditary tyrosinemia
Renal glycosuria
Vitamin D resistant rickets
Pseudohypoparathyroidism
Vasopressin-resistant diabetes insipidus

Hereditary Diseases Associated With Lithiasis
Hyperoxaluria
L-Glyceric aciduria
Xanthinuria
Lesch-Nyhan syndrome, gout

Nephropathy due to familial hyperparathyroidism
Cystinuria (types I, II, III)
Glycinuria

Miscellaneous
Hereditary intestinal B_{12} malabsorption.
Total and partial lipodystrophy
Sickle cell anemia
Bartter's syndrome

Bernstein J: Heritable cystic disorders of the kidney: The mythology of polycystic disease. P Clin North America 18:435, 1971.
Bernstein J: The morphogenesis of renal parenchymal maldevelopment (renal dysplasia). Pediatr Clin North Am 18:395, 1971.
Carter JE & others: Bilateral renal hypoplasia with oligomeganephronia. Am J Dis Child 120:537, 1970.
Crocker JFS & others: Developmental defects of the kidney: A review of renal development and experimental studies of maldevelopment. Pediatr Clin North Am 18:355, 1971.
Milne MD: Genetic aspects of renal disease. Prog Med Genet 7:112, 1970.
Perkoff GT: The hereditary renal diseases. (2 parts.) N Engl J Med 277:79, 129, 1967.

DISORDERS OF THE RENAL TUBULES

The proximal renal tubule effects the reabsorption of isotonic salt from the glomerular filtrate as well as of glucose, amino acids, and phosphorus. Both the proximal and the distal renal tubules are concerned with acid-base balance through 2 mechanisms: (1) the exchange of hydrogen ion for intraluminal sodium and (2) the hydrogen ion titration of secreted ammonia into ammonium ion.

Primary tubular disorders in childhood may reflect a defect in a single transport mechanism (eg, renal tubular acidosis) or a defect in all of the major functions (eg, hypophosphatemic vitamin D resistant rickets with aminoaciduria and glycosuria).

Tubular dysfunction may also be secondary to other metabolic disorders such as galactosemia and cystinosis or part of generalized renal failure, as in advanced glomerulonephritis. Tests for these functions are described on p 491.

1. PROXIMAL RENAL TUBULAR ACIDOSIS

Essentials of Diagnosis
- Failure to thrive.
- Hyperchloremic acidosis.
- Low renal threshold for bicarbonate reabsorption.

General Considerations
The renal mechanisms for controlling acid-base

equilibrium are illustrated in Fig 18–1. The dominant process in the proximal tubule is the exchange of tubule cell hydrogen ion for intraluminal sodium. Under the influence of surface carbonic anhydrase, CO_2 is then formed, reabsorbed, and rehydrated to HCO_3^- and H^+. About 85–90% of bicarbonate reabsorption is achieved in the proximal tubules. In proximal renal tubular acidosis, the essential lesion is a lowering of the renal bicarbonate threshold, ie, the concentration of bicarbonate in the plasma above which bicarbonate appears in the urine. The exact nature of the lesion is not clear. It does not appear to involve defective function of carbonic anhydrase.

Clinical Findings
The onset is in infancy in males, with failure to thrive and hyperchloremic acidosis but without bone lesions, nephrocalcinosis, or hypokalemia. Secondary forms are seen in association with other tubular disorders, as in Fanconi's syndrome, cystinosis, Lowe's syndrome, Wilson's disease, galactosemia, hereditary fructose intolerance, and tyrosinemia.

Lightwood's syndrome, a condition characterized by failure to thrive, hyperchloremic acidosis, high urine pH, anorexia, vomiting, and constipation starting at around 6 months of age, is probably a special form of this syndrome.

Differential Diagnosis
On bicarbonate loading, these patients may be shown to have a lowered renal threshold for bicarbonate reabsorption. The actual demonstration of lowered HCO_3^- threshold is cumbersome, however, and it may be practical to make an arbitrary differentiation from distal tubular acidosis as follows: A patient who requires > 6 mEq/kg/24 hours of citrate or bicarbonate to sustain a plasma CO_2 of 22 mEq/liter and who under conditions of an acid load can acidify his urine pH below 5.4 may be said to have proximal renal tubular acidosis until proved otherwise.

The possibility that the acidosis is secondary to one of the conditions listed above should be considered.

Treatment
Treatment usually consists of giving sodium bicarbonate, 10 mEq/kg/24 hours in 3 divided doses, or whatever dose is sufficient to maintain a normal plasma HCO_3^- without causing gastrointestinal symptoms. An alternative is to give buffered citrate solution, 50 ml orally 3 times daily:

℞ Sodium citrate	50.0
Potassium citrate	50.0
Citric acid	100.0
Water, qs ad	1000.0

In addition to the above, hydrochlorothiazide (Esidrix, HydroDiuril) may be beneficial, although it may require potassium supplementation.

Prognosis
The prognosis appears to be excellent. Alkali ther-

apy can usually be discontinued after several months with no evident recurrence of symptoms or signs.

Buckalew VM & others: Hereditary renal tubular acidosis. Medicine 53:229, 1974.

Chaimontz L & others: Studies on the site of renal salt loss in a patient with Bartter's syndrome. Pediatr Res 7:89, 1973.

Donkerwolcke RA & others: Therapy of bicarbonate losing renal tubular acidosis. Arch Dis Child 45:774, 1970.

Dundon S: Treatment of osteomalacia of renal tubular acidosis. Lancet 2:1204, 1972.

Mace JW: Magnesium supplementation in Bartter's syndrome. Arch Dis Child 48:485, 1973.

McSherry E: Renal tubular acidosis in infants: The several kinds, including bicarbonate-wasting, classic renal tubular acidosis. J Clín Invest 51:499, 1972.

Modlinger RS & others: Some observations on the pathogenesis of Bartter's syndrome. N Engl J Med 289:1022, 1973.

Nash MA & others: Renal tubular acidosis. J Pediatr 80:738, 1972.

Rodriguez-Soriano J, Vallo A, Garcia-Fuentes M: Distal renal tubular acidosis in infancy: A bicarbonate wasting state. J Pediatr 86:524, 1975.

Schwartz GJ, Cornfeld D: Propranolol in Bartter's syndrome. N Engl J Med 290:966, 1974.

Simpoulos AP & others: Growth characteristics and factors influencing growth in Bartter's syndrome. J Pediatr 81:56, 1972.

Vladuti A: Renal tubular acidosis: An autoimmune disease. Lancet 1:265, 1973.

2. DISTAL RENAL TUBULAR ACIDOSIS

Acid-base regulation in the distal tubule is achieved partly by residual bicarbonate reabsorption but also by the exchange of Na^+ for hydrion against a gradient and by ammonium excretion. The defect in distal renal tubular acidosis appears to consist of inability to secrete H^+ against a gradient. It is probably transmitted as an autosomal dominant disorder.

The onset is in later childhood (after age 2) in patients with failure to grow, anorexia, vomiting, and dehydration. There is hyperchloremic acidosis, a urine pH > 6.5, and hypokalemia. Hypercalciuria may lead to rickets, and long-term complications include nephrocalcinosis, nephrolithiasis, and renal failure.

The urinary excretion of titratable acid and ammonium (U_{TA} and U_{NH_4}) is reduced, and the hydrogen ion clearance index (see p 492), which is normally ≥ 1 after an NH_4Cl load, is < 0.7. Urine pH remains above 6.5 even at plasma HCO_3^- concentrations < 13 mEq/liter.

The possibility that the tubular lesion is secondary to malnutrition, hyperparathyroidism, vitamin D intoxication, Fabry's disease, various hypergammaglobulinemic states, amphotericin B intoxication, cirrhosis, and hyperthyroidism should be considered.

In contrast to proximal renal tubular acidosis, the dose of alkali required to achieve normal plasma HCO_3^- concentration and prevent hypercalciuria sel-dom exceeds 2 mEq/kg/24 hours. Moreover, chlorothiazide may be of particular value in diminishing hypercalciuria.

Distal renal tubular acidosis is a permanent disorder which requires lifelong treatment. The prognosis is good if the diagnosis is made in time to prevent nephrocalcinosis from causing irreversible kidney damage and renal failure.

Edelmann CM Jr: The genetics of primary renal tubular acidosis. Birth Defects 6:25, 1970.

Morris RC Jr: Renal tubular acidosis: Mechanisms, classification and implications. N Engl J Med 281:1405, 1969.

Pitts RF: The role of ammonia production and excretion in regulation of acid-base balance. N Engl J Med 284:32, 1971.

Soriano JR: The renal regulation of acid-base balance and the disturbances noted in renal tubular acidosis. Pediatr Clin North Am 18:529, 1971.

CONGENITAL HYPOKALEMIC ALKALOSIS
(Bartter's Syndrome)

This syndrome is characterized by severe hypokalemic, hypochloremic metabolic alkalosis, extremely high levels of circulating renin and aldosterone, and a paradoxic absence of hypertension. The cause and pathogenesis are not known. On renal biopsy, there is striking juxtaglomerular hyperplasia. Most patients present in early infancy with severe failure to thrive. Although the prognosis is very poor, a few patients seem to have less severe forms of the disease that are compatible with longer survival.

Potassium and magnesium supplements may be beneficial in some cases, and more recently aspirin has been advocated.

Bartter's syndrome. (Editorial.) Lancet 2:721, 1976.

Mace JW: Magnesium supplementation in Bartter's syndrome. Arch Dis Child 48:485, 1973.

Norby L & others: Prostaglandins and aspirin therapy in Bartter's syndrome. Lancet 2:604, 1976.

Schwarz GJ, Cornfeld D: Propranolol in Bartter's syndrome. N Engl J Med 290:966, 1974.

RENAL GLYCOSURIA

Renal glycosuria is a disorder that apparently involves the proximal convoluted tubule of all nephrons. The basic mechanism does not seem to affect phosphorylation of glucose in the tubule but is assumed to interfere with the sodium and energy dependent steps of incorporation of glucose into the brush border. The degree to which this transport mechanism is interfered with can be quantitated by measuring the maximal tubular reabsorption of glucose (T_mG). Normal values are 260–550 mg/minute/1.73 sq m, whereas in renal glycosuria they range from 80–280 mg/minute/1.73 sq m. The test is carried out in conjunction with an inulin clearance test. The calculation is as follows:

$$T_mG \text{ in mg/minute/1.73 sq m} =$$
(Inulin clearance $\times$ Plasma glucose concentration in mg/ml) $-$
Glucose excretion in mg/minute

Structural alterations of the proximal convoluted tubules have been described; these electron microscopic changes are degenerative and correlate well with the functional insufficiency of this area of the nephron.

In most patients the total urinary glucose loss is insufficient to cause any symptoms or metabolic disturbance. Hyperglycemia does not occur. In some affected individuals, polyuria and polydipsia are present. During starvation and occasionally in pregnancy, the obligatory loss of carbohydrates may lead to acidosis.

No treatment is necessary. It is essential to rule out diabetes mellitus and renal tubular disorders, where glycosuria can be associated with aminoaciduria, phosphaturia, and acidification defects.

Horowitz L, Schwarzer S: Renal glycosuria: Occurrence in two siblings and a review of the literature. J Pediatr 47:634, 1955.
Monasterio G & others: Renal diabetes as a congenital tubular dysplasia. Am J Med 37:44, 1964.

CYSTINOSIS

Three types of cystinosis have been identified: adult, adolescent, and infantile. The adult type is a relatively benign condition characterized by corneal cystine deposition and elevated granulocyte and fibroblast cystine levels but no renal disease. The adolescent type is characterized by cystine deposition in the corneas, granulocytes, and fibroblasts and by the development of mild renal failure with Fanconi's syndrome during adolescence. Growth is normal.

The infantile type is both the most common and the most severe. Characteristically, children present in the first or second year of life with polyuria and on investigation are found to have renal rickets, generalized aminoaciduria, glycosuria, and a variable degree of renal tubular acidosis. The exact biochemical nature of the disease remains obscure. Cystine is stored in cellular lysosomes in virtually all tissues, a finding which has led to the speculation that a lysosomal cystine reductase may be absent or faulty. Eventually, cystine accumulation results in cell damage and cell death, particularly in the renal tubules. Death from renal failure between ages 6 and 12 is the rule. Whenever the diagnosis of cystinosis is suspected, a slitlamp examination of the corneas should be performed as corneal cystine crystal deposition causes an almost pathognomonic ground-glass "dazzle" appearance. Cystine crystals may also be readily observed in bone marrow aspirates, especially with phase microscopy.

Cystinosis is an autosomal recessive condition which may be diagnosed in utero by obtaining fetal cells by amniocentesis, growing them in tissue culture, and measuring the avidity with which they incorporate ^{35}S-cystine.

Dithiothreitol, vitamin C in large doses, and cysteamine are under investigation for the treatment of cystinosis. At present, the management of cystinosis is essentially that of chronic renal failure, with particular attention being paid to renal osteodystrophy. Renal homotransplantation shows significant promise in the palliation of cystinosis, although the extent of nonrenal tissue involvement with cystine remains to be defined.

Schneider JA & others: Cystinosis: A review. Metabolism 26:817, 1977.
Schneider JA & others: Prenatal diagnosis of cystinosis. N Engl J Med 290:878, 1974.

CYSTINURIA

Cystinuria, like Hartnup's disease and a number of other disorders, is primarily a disorder of amino acid transport across both the enteric and proximal renal tubular epithelium. There appear to be at least 3 biochemical types: (1) The bowel transport of basic amino acids and cystine is impaired but not that of cysteine. In the renal tubule, basic amino acids are again rejected by the tubule but cystine absorption into kidney slices in vitro seems to be normal. The reasons for the cystinuria are, therefore, still obscure. Heterozygotes have no aminoaciduria. (2) The second type is similar except that the heterozygotes excrete excess cystine and lysine in the urine and cystine transport in the bowel is normal. (3) In a third type, only the nephron is involved. The incidence of all types among institutionalized mentally retarded children is about 0.2%.

The only clinical manifestations relate to stone formation. These include ureteral colic, dysuria, hematuria, proteinuria, and secondary urinary tract infection. The urinary excretion of cystine, lysine, arginine, and ornithine is increased.

The most reliable way to prevent stone formation is to maintain a constant high free water clearance. This involves a water intake of about 400 ml/sq m every 4 hours night and day. If this is not effective, treatment with sodium bicarbonate, 6 gm/sq m/day, should also be given. Such measures will certainly prevent increases in stone formation and very often lead to dissolution.

Operative removal of the stone may occasionally be required. Penicillamine (Cuprimine) in doses of 1000–1500 mg/sq m/day will also decrease cystine excretion and bring about partial or complete dissolution of stones. It is expensive, however, and may give rise to rashes which are just as objectionable as the problem of maintaining a high water intake.

Rosenberg LE, Durant JL, Holland JM: Intestinal absorption and renal extraction of cystine and cysteine in cystinuria. N Engl J Med 273:1239, 1965.

Scriver CR & others: Cystinuria: Increased prevalence in patients with mental disease. N Engl J Med 283:783, 1970.

Segal S: Disorders of renal amino acid transport. N Engl J Med 294:1044, 1976

PHOSPHATE-LOSING RENAL TUBULAR SYNDROMES & OTHER FORMS OF RICKETS

Recent work on the metabolic products of vitamin D_3 has done much to clarify the causes of various forms of rickets. Those forms due primarily to a lack of available calcium are described elsewhere. They include deficient calcium intake or excessive urinary calcium loss, as in idiopathic hypercalciuria; lack of vitamin D_3 in the diet or from steatorrhea; and vitamin D dependency and azotemic rickets, in which there is (respectively) an inborn or acquired inability to synthesize 1,25-dihydroxycholecalciferol, the calcium transport protein stimulating factor. Treatment consists of giving supplementary calcium or vitamin D in appropriate doses.

Another group of diseases that cause rickets are those in which there is a decreased availability of phosphorus. Excessive use of aluminum hydroxide gels may be responsible, but this is very rare. Most commonly, the defect is an inherited or acquired one of tubular transport of amino acids, glucose, potassium, and hydrogen ion as well as of phosphate reabsorption. Certain generalized metabolic diseases—notably Wilson's disease, galactosemia, and cystinosis—may cause similar tubular damage. Treatment of the primary type is to give extra phosphorus. Treatment of the acquired forms is that of the basic disease.

Familial hypophosphatemic vitamin D resistant rickets is an example of a tubular nephropathy in which only phosphorus transport is affected.

Although ordinary rickets is uncommon in patients over 18 months of age, it may manifest itself for the first time in childhood. The majority of cases present during the second year of life, but some have been reported in the first 6 months.

The clinical features are variable. On the one hand the changes may be only biochemical, with a strikingly low serum phosphorus and elevated alkaline phosphatase. Muscular hypotonia may be severe; growth failure, bowing of the legs, and enlargement of wrists,

knees, and costochondral junctions are often associated with spinal deformities. Craniosynostosis has been described in infants with this disease. Pathologic fractures may be seen on x-ray, as well as certain unique findings consisting of an irregular mosaic formation of the Haversian system and trabecular "halos" of low-density bone.

In most cases the serum phosphorus is < 2mg/100 ml. Urinary calcium is low, and serum calcium may be normal or slightly low. Aminoaciduria is rare.

Treatment consists of giving 1–3 gm of phosphorus daily as a buffered monosodium and disodium hydrogen phosphate solution at pH 7.4. Magnesium oxide, 10–15 mg/kg daily by mouth, may also be of value. Supplementary vitamin D (up to 40,000 units daily) should be given if the serum calcium levels remain below normal.

Normal growth is never achieved unless every effort is made to keep the serum phosphorus level over 3 mg/100 ml throughout the 24 hours.

Fraser D & others: Pathogenesis of hereditary vitamin D dependent rickets. N Engl J Med 289:817, 1973.

Glorieux FH: Use of phosphate and vitamin D to prevent dwarfism and rickets in X-linked phosphatemia. N Engl J Med 287:481, 1972.

Haussler MR, McCain TA: Basic and clinical concepts related to vitamin D metabolism and action. N Engl J Med 297:974, 1977.

Reddy V & others: Magnesium-dependent vitamin-D-resistant rickets. Lancet 1:963, 1974.

RENAL RICKETS

Azotemic osteodystrophy appears in severe renal failure. Failure of the kidney to synthesize 1,25-dihydroxycholecalciferol, the enteric calcium transport protein stimulating factor, is thought to be an important contributing cause.

The clinical picture of uremia is usually present. In the young child, if the growth process has not been completely arrested, signs of rickets are present along with the aches and pains that reflect hyperparathyroidism. Tetany is rare despite the sporadic occurrence of a strikingly low serum calcium level since systemic acidosis sustains the level of ionized calcium. Tetany, however, may be due to low tissue Mg^{++} levels. Pathologic fractures may occur. Although the renal insufficiency may result from either acute or chronic glomerulonephritis, most cases appear to be caused by obstructive uropathies with superimposed chronic pyelonephritis.

Management should be oriented toward correction of the underlying renal disease. A low-phosphate diet with additional vitamin D is indicated.

Treatment with vitamin D, up to 40,000 IU daily orally, or equivalent amounts of dihydrotachysterol, is indicated. Serum calcium levels should be monitored for evidence of vitamin D intoxication. The use of 1α-hydroxycholecalciferol has not so far been helpful.

In certain cases of renal rickets, the secondary hyperparathyroidism may lead to the formation of a parathyroid adenoma which has autonomous function and is not under the control of calcium levels. Hypercalcemia is usually present, and surgery is indicated.

HEPATIC & CELIAC RICKETS

A lack of bile salts such as occurs in biliary atresia or hepatocellular disease causes malabsorption of virtually all lipids, including fat-soluble vitamins such as A, D, and K. The emulsifying effect of bile salts is crucial to the surface action of pancreatic lipase and to micelle formation. Severe diffuse diseases of the pancreas, such as in cystic fibrosis, will therefore also lead to malabsorption of vitamin D. Patients with disorders of the small intestine, giving rise to steatorrhea, have large amounts of fecal calcium not only secondary to the washing away of vitamin D but also due to the large amounts of calcium contained in the digestive juices.

The physical stigmas of rickets are present if the underlying hepatic or small bowel disease has not completely arrested growth. Osteomalacia is evident if growth arrest has occurred. Tetany is seldom seen. Jaundice is usually present.

Treatment of the underlying disease should include the prophylactic administration of vitamin D in water-soluble form (2000 IU daily). If rickets has developed despite the regular administration of vitamin D, it will not respond to therapeutic amounts of vitamin D (5000–10,000 IU daily) and will require 25,000–100,000 IU. Cases have been described in which the oral administration of 300,000 IU daily was ineffective and exposure to ultraviolet rays or the parenteral administration of vitamin D proved necessary.

Atkinson M, Nordin BEC, Sherlock S: Malabsorption and bone disease in obstructive jaundice. Q J Med 25:299, 1956.

Gray R & others: Vitamin D metabolism: The role of kidney tissue. Science 172:1232, 1971.

Lumb GA & others: The apparent vitamin D resistance of chronic renal failure: A study of the physiology of vitamin D in man. Am J Med 50:421, 1971.

Tougaard L & others: Controlled trial of 1α-hydroxycholecalciferol in chronic renal failure. Lancet 1:1044, 1976.

THE OCULOCEREBRORENAL SYNDROME
(Lowe's Syndrome)

This condition has been described in males only and is therefore thought to be transmitted as an X-linked recessive gene leading to anomalies involving the eyes, brain, and kidneys. The physical stigmas and the degree of mental retardation are variable. In addition to congenital cataracts and buphthalmos, the typical facies includes prominent epicanthal folds, frontal prominence, and a tendency to scaphocephaly. Muscle hypotonia is a prominent finding. The incidence of hypophosphatemic rickets is variable; it is characterized by low serum phosphorus, low to normal serum calcium, and elevated serum alkaline phosphatase. Some degree of renal tubular acidosis is usually present, characterized by hyperchloremic acidosis, an alkaline urine, and a diminution in both titratable acidity and urinary ammonia in response to an ammonium chloride challenge. The aminoaciduria is usually generalized. Mothers of affected males have punctate lens opacities.

Alkaline therapy should be given to those presenting with tubular acidosis. Vitamin D requirements range from 10,000–20,000 IU daily.

Abbassi V, Lowe CU, Calcagno PL: Oculo-cerebro-renal syndrome: A review. Am J Dis Child 115:145, 1968.

Bailey RR & others: Homozygous cystinuria in the oculocerebro-renal dystrophy of Lowe in the same family. Arch Dis Child 51:558, 1976.

DISORDERS OF THE COLLECTING DUCTS

NEPHROGENIC DIABETES INSIPIDUS

In the proximal tubule, water is reabsorbed by osmosis as solutes are being actively and passively reabsorbed. In the descending loop of Henle, water is lost against the osmotic gradient of the papillary countercurrent loop; this is not under the control of vasopressin. In the ascending part of the loop, there is no water exchange, although sodium egress dilutes the urine. Thereafter, reabsorption of water is dependent on ADH-controlled exposure to the countercurrent loop. The octapeptide hormone is fixed to the peritubular surface of the cell, where it initiates a series of reactions leading to permeability changes. An early step is the activation of adenylate cyclase, increasing tubular cyclic AMP.

Most commonly, the symptoms are limited to polyuria and polydipsia with failure to thrive. In some cases, particularly where the solute intake is unrestricted, some acclimatization to an elevated serum osmolality may develop—so-called diabetes insipidus hyperchloremicus occultus. These children are particularly liable to episodes of dehydration, fever, vomiting, and convulsions.

Clinically, the diagnosis can be made on the basis of a history of polydipsia and polyuria that is not sensitive to the administration of vasopressin or lysine-8 vasopressin. It is wise to confirm this in all cases by performing a vasopressin test. Maximal water restriction, overnight if possible, does not increase the tubular reabsorption of water (T^cH_2O) to above 2 ml/minute/sq m. Renal diabetes insipidus will show no increase in urine osmolality with the administration of active vasopressin and only a small change with hypertonic saline. Theoretically, in psychogenic diabetes insipidus, vasopressin and hypertonic saline increase urine osmolality, but constant water loading seems to diminish renal response to ADH. Urinary concentrating ability is impaired in a number of conditions—sickle cell anemia, pyelonephritis, potassium depletion, hypercalcemia, and obstructive uropathy—and as a result of nephrotoxic drugs.

In infants it is usually best to allow water as demanded and to restrict salt. Serum sodium should be estimated at intervals to ensure against hyperosmolality from inadvertent water restriction. In later childhood, sodium intake should continue to be restricted to 2–2.5 mEq/kg/24 hours. Studies have suggested that chlorothiazide, 60 mg/sq m/24 hours orally, or ethacrynic acid (Edecrin), 120 mg/sq m/24 hours orally, will decrease the C_{H_2O} significantly. When the latter drug is given, potassium chloride, 2–3 mEq/kg/24 hours orally, should also be given to prevent alkalosis due to excessive potassium loss.

Edelmann CM & others: A standardized test of renal concentrating capacity in children. Am J Dis Child 114:639, 1967.

Jamison RL, Maffly RH: The urinary concentrating mechanism. N Engl J Med 295:1059, 1976.

Kohn B & others: Hysterical polydipsia. Am J Dis Child 130:210, 1976.

Lant AF, Wilson GM: Long-term therapy of diabetes insipidus with oral benzothiadiazine and phthalmidine diuretics. Clin Sci 40:497, 1971.

PRIMARY HYPEROXALURIA

Oxalate production in man is derived from the oxidative deamination of glycine to glyoxalate (about 40%), from the serine-glycolate pathway (about 50%), and from ascorbic acid. At least 2 enzymatic blocks have been described. Type 1 is a 2-oxo-glutarate:glyoxalate carboligase deficiency which inhibits the diversion of glyoxalate to γ-hydroxy-α-ketoglutarate. Type 2 is glyoxalate reductase deficiency.

Excess oxalate combines with calcium to form insoluble deposits in the kidneys, lungs, and other tissues. The onset is in childhood. The joints are occasionally involved, but the main impact is on the kidneys, where progressive oxalate deposition leads to fibrosis and eventual renal failure.

Pyridoxine supplementation and a low-oxalate diet have been tried as therapy, but the overall prognosis is poor and most patients succumb to uremia by early adulthood. Renal transplantation is not very successful. Calcium carbimide, 1 mg/kg/24 hours, has been tried as an inhibitor of the serine-glycolate pathway of oxalate production and was shown to substantially diminish oxalate excretion in type 1 oxalosis. The use of methylene blue has also been reported. Hyperoxaluria may also occur secondary to ileal resection in some cases of chronic liver disease.

Morgan JM & others: Successful renal transplantation in hyperoxaluria. Arch Surg 109:430, 1974.

Solomons CC, Goodman SI, Riley CM: Calcium carbimide in the treatment of primary hyperoxaluria. N Engl J Med 276:207, 1967.

Vallman HB & others: Hyperoxaluria after resection of ileum in childhood. Arch Dis Child 49:171, 1974.

Watts RWE: Oxaluria. J R Coll Physicians Lond 7:161, 1973.

Williams HE, Smith LH: L-Glyceric aciduria: A new genetic variant of primary hyperoxaluria. N Engl J Med 278:233, 1968.

DISEASES OF THE RENAL PELVIS (CALCULI)

Renal calculi in children may occur as a consequence of certain inborn errors of metabolism, eg, cystine in cystinosis, glycine in hyperglycinuria, urates in Lesch-Nyhan syndrome, and oxalates in oxalosis. Stones may occur secondary to hypercalciuria in distal tubular acidosis, and large stones are quite often seen in children with spina bifida with paralyzed lower limbs. Treatment is that of the primary condition if possible. Surgical removal of stones should be considered only for obstruction, intractable severe pain, and chronic infection.

•   •   •

General References

Heptinstall RH: *Pathology of the Kidney*, 2nd ed. Little, Brown, 1974.

James JA: *Renal Disease in Childhood*, 2nd ed. Mosby, 1972.

Kincaid-Smith P (editor): *Glomerulonephritis*. Vols 1 and 2. Wiley, 1972.

Lieberman E (editor): *Clinical Pediatric Nephrology*. Lippincott, 1976.

Royer P & others: *Pediatric Nephrology*. Saunders, 1974.

Rubin MI, Barratt TM (editors): *Pediatric Nephrology*. Williams & Wilkins, 1975.

Strauss J (editor): *Pediatric Nephrology*. Vol 1. Stratton, 1974.

19 . . .
Orthopedics

Robert E. Eilert, MD

Orthopedics is the medical discipline that deals with disorders of neuromuscular and skeletal systems. Patients with orthopedic problems usually present with pain, loss of function, or deformity. Patients with such symptoms must be considered not only in terms of the bones and joints but also in a more general sense relating to the anatomy particularly of the extremities, considering the blood vessels, skin, nerves, tendons, and muscles. As is true of most medical and surgical disorders, the diagnosis of orthopedic disorders can often be made on the basis of a carefully taken history. However, the physical examination is the most important feature of orthopedic diagnosis and depends upon an intimate knowledge of human anatomy.

DISTURBANCES
OF PRENATAL ORIGIN

CONGENITAL AMPUTATIONS

Congenital amputations may be due to teratogens such as drugs or viruses, metabolic disease in the mother such as diabetes, or, in rare cases, may be hereditary defects. The history of the pregnancy must be carefully reviewed in a search for possible teratogenic factors. According to the currently accepted international classification, amputations are either terminal or longitudinal. In terminal amputation, all parts are missing distal to the level of involvement, eg, absence of the forearm, wrist, and hand in the case of a terminal below-the-elbow amputation. A longitudinal amputation consists of partial absence of structures in the extremity along one side or the other. In radial club hand, the entire radius is absent but the thumb may either be hypoplastic or completely absent, ie, the effect on structures distal to the amputation may vary. Complex tissue defects are nearly always associated with longitudinal amputations in that the associated nerves and muscles are usually not completely represented when a bone is absent. Bones within the axial skeleton likewise may be absent. Congenital absence of the sacrum is often associated with diabetes in the mother.

Terminal amputations are treated by means of a prosthesis, eg, to compensate for shortness of one leg. With longitudinal deficiencies, constructive surgery may be feasible with the objective of reducing deformity and stabilizing joints. In certain types of severe anomalies, operative treatment is indicated to remove a portion of the malformed foot so that a prosthesis can be fitted early. This applies to such anomalies as congenital absence of the fibula, which is the lower extremity bone most commonly congenitally absent. Fortunately, there is no problem with tenting of the skin by relative overgrowth of bone within the stump in congenital amputations. This problem may arise, however, in traumatic amputations unless the amputation occurs through a joint.

Lower extremity prostheses are best fitted at about the time of normal walking (12–15 months of age). Lower extremity prostheses are consistently well accepted, as they are necessary for balancing and walking. Upper extremity prostheses are not as well accepted. Fitting the child with a dummy type prosthesis as early as 6 months of age has the advantage of instilling an accustomed pattern of proper length and bimanual manipulation. Children fitted later than age 2 years nearly always reject upper extremity prostheses.

Children quickly learn how to function with their prostheses and can lead quite active lives.

Hall CB: The proposed international terminology for the classification of congenital limb deficiencies. Dev Med Child Neurol 17 (Suppl 34), 1975. [Entire issue.]

Hall CB: Recent concepts in the treatment of the limb-deficient child. Artif Limbs 10:36, 1966.

Swanson AB, Glessner JR Jr: Treatment of congenital anomalies of extremities by surgery and prosthetic replacement. J Bone Joint Surg 46A:458, 1964.

DEFORMITIES OF THE EXTREMITIES

1. METATARSUS VARUS OR METATARSUS ADDUCTUS

This disorder is characterized by adduction of the forefoot on the hindfoot, with the heel in normal position. The longitudinal arch is often creased in a vertical direction when the deformity is more rigid. The lateral border of the foot demonstrates sharp angulation at the level of the base of the fifth metatarsal, and this bone will be especially prominent. The deformity varies from flexible to rigid. Flexible deformities are usually secondary to intrauterine posture and can be reduced by manipulation by the mother.

If the deformity is rigid and cannot be corrected past the midline with passive manipulation, it is worthwhile to use a plaster cast changed at weekly intervals, with progressive loosening of the deformity obtained by manipulation and growth of the child.

"Corrective" shoes do not live up to their name. Shoes are supportive, but shoe wedges have not been effective in correcting this type of deformity and are of more use for placating the mother than for any true therapeutic value. A few minutes spent explaining what can be achieved with shoes may avoid an unnecessary expense for the family. The prognosis for this common deformity of the foot is excellent, and few long-term problems are reported.

Ponseti IV, Becker JR: Congenital metatarsus adductus: The results of treatment. J Bone Joint Surg 48A:702, 1966.

2. CLUBFOOT OR TALIPES EQUINOVARUS

This foot deformity consists of 3 elements: (1) equinus or plantar flexion of the foot at the ankle joint, (2) varus or inversion deformity of the heel, and (3) forefoot adduction. When all 3 of these deformities are present, the diagnosis of a classical talipes equinovarus or clubfoot is made. The incidence of talipes equinovarus is approximately 1:1000 live births. Any infant with a clubfoot should be carefully examined for associated anomalies, especially of the spine. Clubfeet tend to follow a hereditary pattern in some families or may be part of a generalized neuromuscular syndrome such as arthrogryposis or myelodysplasia.

Treatment consists of massage and manipulation of the foot to stretch the contracted tissues on the medial and posterior aspects, followed by splinting to hold the correction. When this is instituted in the nursery shortly after birth, correction is achieved much more rapidly. When treatment is delayed, the foot tends to become more rigid within a matter of days and weeks. Treatment in the nursery by strapping and splinting is often extremely effective. As the child gets older, casting following manipulation and stretching is necessary. The casts are applied sequentially, correcting first the forefoot adduction, then the inversion of the heel, and finally the equinus of the ankle. Treatment by means of casting requires patience and experience; if it is not done properly in sequence, secondary severe deformities of the foot may result. After full correction is obtained, braces are usually necessary for months to years to prevent recurrence of the deformity. A night brace is often prescribed for long-term maintenance of correction.

About half of children with clubfeet eventually need some operative procedure to lengthen the tightened structures about the foot.

A supple foot which is easily corrected by strapping and casting has a more favorable prognosis. If the foot is rigid and requires prolonged treatment to obtain correction, perhaps combined with surgery, the prognosis is more guarded.

Hersh A: The role of surgery in the treatment of clubfeet. J Bone Joint Surg 49A:1684, 1967.
Kite JG: Some suggestions on the treatment of clubfoot by casts. J Bone Joint Surg 45A:406, 1963.
McCanley JC Jr: Clubfoot: History of the development of the concepts of pathogenesis and treatment. Clin Orthop 44:51, 1966.
Ponseti IV, Smoley EN: Congenital clubfoot. J Bone Joint Surg 45A:261, 1963.

3. CONGENITAL DYSPLASIA OF THE HIP JOINT
(Congenital Dislocation of the Hip)

A child who has a congenital dislocation of the hip has a disturbed relationship between the femoral head and the acetabulum. The 2 structures may be in partial contact at birth, and such a condition is termed subluxation of the hip. A more severe defect is complete loss of contact between the femoral head and acetabulum, in which case there is frank dislocation of the hip with the femoral head nearly always displaced laterally and superiorly due to muscle pull. At birth there is some lack of development of both the acetabulum and the femur in cases of congenital hip dislocation. This dysplasia becomes progressive with growth unless the dislocation is corrected. If the dislocation is corrected in the first few days or weeks of life, the dysplasia is completely reversible and a normal hip will develop. As the child becomes older and the dislocation or subluxation persists, the deformity will worsen to the point where it will not be completely reversible, especially after the walking age. For this reason, it is extremely important to diagnose the deformity in the nursery.

Clinical Findings
Newborn infants display a generalized joint laxity which persists throughout early childhood. The diagnosis of congenital hip dislocation in the neonate depends upon demonstrating instability of the joint by placing the infant on its back and obtaining complete relaxation by feeding with a bottle if necessary. The examiner's long finger is then placed over the greater trochanter and the thumb over the inner side of the thigh. Both hips are flexed 90 degrees and then slowly abducted from the midline. With gentle pressure, an attempt is made to lift the greater trochanter forward. A feeling of slipping as the head goes into the acetabu-

lum is a sign of instability (as first described by Ortolani). In other infants the joint is more stable, and the
deformity must be provoked by applying slight pressure with the thumb on the medial side of the thigh as
the thigh is again adducted, thus slipping the hip posteriorly and eliciting a jerking as the hip dislocates.
This sign was first described by Barlow. The signs of
instability are the most reliable criteria for diagnosing
congenital dislocation of the hip in the newborn. X-
rays of the pelvis are notoriously unreliable until about
6 weeks of age. Asymmetric skin folds are present in
about 40% of newborns and therefore are not particularly helpful.

During the first few months of life, the signs of
instability as demonstrated by Ortolani's test or Barlow's test become less evident. Contractures begin to
develop about the hip joint, causing limitation of
abduction in the hip. Normally, the hip should abduct
fully to 90 degrees on either side during the first few
months of life. It is important that the pelvis be held
level to detect asymmetry of abduction. After the first
few weeks of life x-ray examination becomes more
valuable, with lateral displacement of the femoral head
being the most reliable sign. In mild cases, the only
abnormality may be increased steepness of acetabular
alignment, so that the acetabular angle is greater than
35 degrees. The femur is apparently shortened when
the hips are flexed, with unequal height of the knees
(Allis's sign).

If congenital dislocation of the hip has not been
diagnosed during the first year of life and the child
begins to walk, then the problem becomes more evident. There will be a painless limp and a lurch to the
affected side, as first described by Trendelenburg.
When the child stands on the affected leg, there is a dip
of the pelvis on the opposite side owing to weakness of
the gluteus medius muscle. This has been termed
Trendelenburg's sign and accounts for the unusual
swaying gait. In children with bilateral dislocations, the
loss of abduction is almost symmetric and may be
deceiving. Abduction, however, is never complete, and
x-ray of the pelvis is indicated in children with incomplete abduction in the first few months of life. As a
child with bilateral dislocation of the hips begins to
walk, the gait is waddling. The perineum is widened as
a result of lateral displacement of the hips, and there is
flexion contracture as a result of posterior displacement of the hips. This flexion contracture contributes
to marked lordosis, and the greater trochanters are
easily palpable in their elevated position. Treatment is
still possible in the first 2 years of life, but the results
are not nearly as effective as in children treated in the
nursery.

Treatment

Dislocation or dysplasia diagnosed in the first few
weeks or months of life can easily be treated by splinting, with the hip maintained in flexion and abduction.
Rigid plaster fixation is contraindicated, as this often
leads to avascular necrosis of the femoral head. Increasing the number of diapers will increase the cost of

taking care of the baby, and in any case diapers are not
adequate to obtain proper positioning of the hip. In
cases of joint laxity without true dislocation, improvement will be spontaneous and diapers are excessive
treatment. Therefore, the use of double or triple diapers is never indicated for medical reasons.

Various splints are available which do provide
proper flexion and abduction of the hip, such as the
ones designed by Pavlik, Ilfeld, or von Rosen. Treatment of these children is best supervised by an orthopedic surgeon with a special interest in the problem.

In the first 4 months of life, reduction can usually
be obtained by simply flexing and abducting the hip;
no other manipulation is usually necessary. If the dislocation persists, however, and excessive force is necessary to reduce the hip, damage to the hip joint will
occur as a result of avascular necrosis. In such cases,
preoperative traction for 2–3 weeks is important to
relax soft tissues about the hip. Following traction in
which the femur is brought down opposite the acetabulum, reduction can be easily achieved without force
under general anesthesia. It is then necessary to place
the child in a plaster cast, which is left in place for
approximately 6 months. The position in the cast
should be carefully adjusted in order to avoid stretching of the delicate blood supply to the femoral head.
The hip is flexed slightly more than 90 degrees and
abducted only 45–60 degrees. Internal rotation is
avoided as this tends to "wring out" the blood vessels
in the capsule of the joint. If the reduction is not
stable within a reasonable range following closed reduction, open reduction may be necessary combined
with plication of the lax capsule in order to maintain
reduction.

If reduction is done at an older age, operations to
correct the deformities of the acetabulum and femur
may be necessary during growth. In these complex
cases, surgery is usually done between 2 and 6 years of
age.

Barlow TG: Early diagnosis and treatment of congenital disloca-
tion of the hip. J Bone Joint Surg 44B:292, 1962.
Ponseti IV: Nonsurgical treatment of congenital dislocation of
the hip. J Bone Joint Surg 48A:1392, 1966.
Ryder CT: Congenital dislocation of the hip in the older child:
Surgical treatment. J Bone Joint Surg 48A:1404, 1966.
Salter RB: *Textbook of Disorders and Injuries of the Musculo-
skeletal System.* Williams & Wilkins, 1970.
Von Rosen S: Further experience with congenital dislocation of
the hip in the newborn. J Bone Joint Surg 50B:538, 1968.

4. TORTICOLLIS

Wryneck deformities in infancy may be due either
to injury to the sternocleidomastoid muscle during
delivery or to disease affecting the cervical spine. In
the case of muscular deformity, the chin is rotated to
the side opposite to the affected sternocleidomastoid
muscle contracture and the head is tilted toward the

side of the contracture. A mass felt in the midportion of the sternocleidomastoid muscle does not represent a true tumor but fibrous maturation of a hematoma within the muscle.

In mild cases, passive stretching is usually effective. If the deformity has not been corrected by passive stretching within the first year of life, surgical division of the muscle will correct it. It is not necessary to excise the "tumor" of the sternocleidomastoid muscle as this tends to resolve spontaneously. If the deformity is left untreated, an unsightly facial asymmetry will result.

Torticollis is occasionally associated with congenital deformities of the cervical spine, and x-rays of the spine are indicated in all cases.

Acute torticollis may follow upper respiratory infection or mild trauma in children. Rotatory subluxation of the upper cervical spine should be sought by appropriate x-ray views. Traction or a cervical collar usually results in resolution of the symptoms within 1 or 2 days.

Coventry MB, Harris LE: Congenital muscular torticollis in infancy: Some observations regarding treatment. J Bone Joint Surg 41A:815, 1959

GENERALIZED AFFECTIONS OF SKELETON OR MESODERMAL TISSUES

1. ARTHROGRYPOSIS MULTIPLEX CONGENITA
(Amyoplasia Congenita)

This congenital syndrome consists of incomplete fibrous ankylosis (usually symmetric) of many or all of the joints of the body. There may be contractures either in flexion or extension. Upper extremity deformities usually consist of adduction of the shoulders, extension of the elbows, flexion of the wrists, and stiff, straight fingers with poor muscle control of the thumbs. In the lower extremities, common deformities are dislocation of the hips, extension of the knees, and severe clubfeet. The joints are fusiform and the joint capsules are decreased in volume, producing contractures. Various investigations have attributed the basic defect to an abnormality of muscle or of the lower motor neuron. Muscular development is poor, and muscles may be represented only by fibrous bands. The joint deformities appear to be secondary to a lack of active motion during intrauterine development.

Passive mobilization of joints should be done early. Because of poor muscle control, however, joint mobility cannot be maintained by active motion. Prolonged casting for correction of deformities is contraindicated in these children, as further stiffness is often produced. Dynamic splinting combined with vigorous therapy is the most effective conservative measure. Surgical release of the affected joints is often neces-

sary. The clubfeet associated with arthrogryposis are very stiff and nearly always require surgical correction to obtain a functional position. Surgery about the knees, including capsulotomy, osteotomy, and tendon lengthening, is used to correct deformity. Dynamic correction by 2-pin skeletal traction may be effective in some knee contractures when combined with therapy to maintain motion while in traction. In the young child, a single vigorous attempt at reduction of the dislocated hip is worthwhile. Multiple operative procedures about the hip are contraindicated, as further stiffness may be produced with consequent impairment of motion. The dislocation of the hip that occurs in arthrogryposis is associated with severe dysplasia of the bones and does not respond to treatment like ordinary congenital hip dislocation. These children are often able to walk quite well with bilateral dislocation of the hips, and in cases of severe rigidity it is better to leave the hips out of joint. With lesser demands, the long-term disability is not as severe as it would be in a person with normal mobility and strength.

The long-term prognosis for physical and vocational independence is poor. These patients usually have normal intelligence, but they have such severe physical restrictions that gainful employment is hard to find.

2. MARFAN'S SYNDROME

This syndrome is characterized by unusually long fingers and toes (arachnodactyly); hypermobility of the joints; subluxation of the ocular lenses; other eye abnormalities including cataract, coloboma, megalocornea, strabismus, and nystagmus; a high-arched palate; a strong tendency to scoliosis; pectus carinatum; and thoracic aneurysms due to weakness of the media of the vessels. Serum mucoproteins may be decreased and urinary excretion of hydroxyproline increased. The condition is easily confused with homocystinuria as the phenotypic presentation is identical. The 2 diseases may be differentiated by the presence of homocystine in the urine in homocystinuria.

Treatment is usually supportive for associated problems such as flat feet. Scoliosis may involve more vigorous treatment by bracing or spine fusion. The long-term prognosis has improved for these patients as better treatment for their aortic aneurysms has been devised.

3. CLEIDOCRANIAL DYSOSTOSIS

This syndrome consists of absence of part or all of the clavicle and delay in ossification of the skull. The facial bones are often underdeveloped, with absence of the sinuses, a high-arched palate, and defective teeth. The skull is enlarged, especially in the parietal and frontal regions. Coxa vara deformity of the proximal femur is sometimes present but usually is not of sufficient magnitude to require surgery. Deficiency of ossification of the symphysis pubica may persist into adult life. The clavicular deformity allows these individuals to touch their shoulders in the midline but otherwise presents no difficulty. The pelvic deformities do not prevent normal pregnancy and childbirth. The syndrome has a strong hereditary tendency.

4. CRANIOFACIAL DYSOSTOSIS
(Crouzon's Disease)

This syndrome consists of acrocephaly, hypoplastic maxilla, beaked nose, protrusion of the lower lip, exophthalmos, exotropia, and hypertelorism. It is usually familial. No orthopedic treatment is necessary. Heroic efforts have been made by neurosurgeons and plastic surgeons to correct the grotesque deformity of these people, who generally have normal intelligence. These operative procedures are complicated and hazardous, involving multiple osteotomies of the skull and facial bones.

5. KLIPPEL-FEIL SYNDROME

This syndrome is characterized by fusion of some or all of the cervical vertebrae. Multiple spinal anomalies may be present, with hemivertebrae and scoliosis. The neck is short and stiff, the hairline is low, and the ears are often low-set. Common associated defects include congenital scoliosis, cervical rib, spina bifida, torticollis, web neck, high scapula, renal anomalies, and deafness. Examination of the urinary tract by urinalysis, blood urea nitrogen, and intravenous urograms is indicated as well as a hearing test.

Scoliotic deformities, if progressive, may require treatment. Occasionally it may be necessary to correct the high scapula, also called *Sprengel's deformity* (see below).

6. SPRENGEL'S DEFORMITY

In this congenital condition one or both scapulas are elevated and small. The child cannot raise his arm completely on the affected side, and there may be torticollis. The deformity occurs alone or may associated with Klippel-Feil syndrome.

If the deformity is functionally limiting, the scapula may be surgically relocated lower in the thorax. Excision of the upper portion of the scapula improves cosmetic appearance but has little effect on function.

Woodward J: Congenital elevation of the scapula. J Bone Joint Surg 43A:219, 1961.

7. OSTEOGENESIS IMPERFECTA

Osteogenesis imperfecta is a rare, mainly dominantly inherited connective tissue disease. The severe fetal type (osteogenesis imperfecta congenita) is characterized by multiple intrauterine or perinatal fractures. These children continue to have fractures and are dwarfed as a result of bony deformities and growth retardation. Intelligence is not affected. The shafts of the long bones are hypercellular and reduced in cortical thickness, and wormian bones are present in the skull. Other features include blue scleras, thin skin, hyperextensibility of ligaments, "otosclerosis" with significant hearing loss, and hypoplastic and deformed teeth. Recurrent epistaxis, easy bruisability, mild hyperpyrexia (which may increase significantly during anesthesia), and excessive diaphoresis are common. In the tarda type, fractures begin to occur at variable times after the perinatal period, resulting in relatively fewer fractures and deformities in these cases. These patients are sometimes suspected of having suffered induced fractures, and the condition should be ruled out in any case of nonaccidental trauma.

Metabolic defects include elevated serum pyrophosphate, increased neutrophil nitroblue tetrazolium (NBT), decreased platelet aggregation, and decreased incorporation of sulfate into acid mucopolysaccharides by skin fibroblasts. Fibroblasts are highly susceptible to infection with SV40 virus, but the transformation rates are normal. Prenatal diagnosis using amniotic fluid pyrophosphate and sulfate metabolism was accurate in a small series of patients. There is no effective treatment by medication. Surgical treatment involves correction of deformity of the long bones. Multiple intramedullary rods have been used but seldom result in improvement in long-term function.

The overall prognosis is poor, and these individuals are often confined to wheelchairs as adults.

Castells S & others: Effects of porcine calcitonin in osteogenesis imperfecta tarda. J Pediatr 80:757, 1972.
Sofield HA, Millar EA: Fragmentation, realignment and intramedullary rod fixation of deformities of long bones in children. J Bone Joint Surg 41A:1371, 1959.
Solomons CC, Millar EA: Osteogenesis imperfecta: New perspectives. Clin Orthop 96:2, 1973.
Solomons CC & others: Prenatal diagnosis of osteogenesis imperfecta. Clin Chem 21:1014, 1975.

8. IDIOPATHIC JUVENILE OSTEOPOROSIS

This is an acute disease characterized by osteoporosis and unexplained pathologic fractures of the spine and long bones. It affects boys and girls equally in the prepubertal years, and the degree of severity is variable. There is evidence of gross enteric malabsorption of calcium, which may reflect an abnormality of 1,25-dihydroxyergocalciferol synthesis.

9. OSTEOPETROSIS
(Osteitis Condensans Generalisata; Marble Bone Disease; Albers-Schönberg Disease)

The clinical manifestations of this familial and hereditary syndrome are bony deformities due to pathologic fractures, myelophthisic anemia, splenomegaly, visual and auditory disturbances, square head, facial paralysis, pigeon breast, and dwarfing. The findings may appear at any age. On x-ray examination the bones show increased density, transverse bands in the shafts, clubbing of ends, and vertical striations of long bones. There is thickening about the cranial foramens, and there may be heterotopic calcification of soft tissues. Treatment with corticosteroids to ameliorate the hematologic abnormalities should be tried.

Yu AS & others: Osteopetrosis. Arch Dis Child 46:257, 1971.

10. ACHONDROPLASIA
(Classical Chondrodystrophy)

In achondroplasia the arms and legs are short, with the upper arms and thighs proportionately shorter than the forearms and legs. Frequently there is bowing of the extremities, a waddling gait, limitation of motion of major joints, relaxation of the ligaments, short stubby fingers of almost equal length, a prominent forehead, moderate hydrocephalus, depressed nasal bridge, and lumbar lordosis. Mentality and sexual function are normal. A family history is often present. X-rays demonstrate short, thick tubular bones and irregular epiphyseal plates. The ends of the bones are thick, with broadening and cupping. Epiphyseal ossification may be delayed.

Osteotomies of the long bones are occasionally necessary if deformities are severe.

The medullary canal is narrowed, so that herniated disk in adulthood may lead to acute paraplegia.

11. OSTEOCHONDRODYSTROPHY
(Morquio's Disease)

This disorder is characterized by shortening of the spine, kyphosis, scoliosis, moderate shortening of the extremities, pectus carinatum, protuberant abdomen,

hepatosplenomegaly, and a waddling gait resulting from instability of the hips and laxity of the knee joints. The skull is minimally involved. The child may appear normal at birth but begins to develop deformities between 1 and 4 years of age as a result of abnormal deposition of mucopolysaccharides. The disorder is commonly familial. Inheritance appears to be on an autosomal recessive basis.

X-rays demonstrate wedge-shaped flattened vertebrae and irregular, malformed epiphyses. The ribs are broad and have been likened to canoe paddles. The lower extremities are more severely involved than the upper ones.

There is no treatment, and the prognosis is poor. Death may occur in childhood or adolescence. Progressive clouding of the cornea leads to increasing visual impairment.

12. CHONDROECTODERMAL DYSPLASIA
(Ellis-Van Creveld Syndrome)

Manifestations include ectodermal dysplasia, congenital heart disease, polydactyly, syndactyly, poorly formed teeth, and mental retardation. The disease is familial and inbred in certain ethnic groups such as the Amish people of Pennsylvania.

X-ray changes include chondrodystrophy; shortening and bowing of the tibias and fibulas; hyperplastic, eccentric proximal tibial metaphyses; and fusion of the carpal bones.

No treatment is available. The long-term prognosis depends on the severity of heart involvement.

Bailey JA: *Disproportionate Short Stature: Diagnosis and Treatment,* 2nd ed. Saunders, 1973.
McKusick VA: *Heritable Disorders of Connective Tissue,* 4th ed. Mosby, 1972.
Rubin P: *Dynamic Classification of Bone Dysplasias.* Year Book, 1964.

GROWTH DISTURBANCES OF THE MUSCULOSKELETAL SYSTEM

SCOLIOSIS

The term scoliosis denotes lateral curvature of the spine, which is always associated with some rotation of the involved vertebra. Scoliosis is classified by its anatomic location, in either the thoracic or lumbar spine, with rare involvement of the cervical spine. The apex of the curvature is designated right or left. Thus, a left thoracic scoliosis would denote a convex leftward curvature in the thoracic region, and this is the most common type of idiopathic curvature. Posterior curvature of the spine (kyphosis) is normal in the thoracic area, though excessive curvature may become pathologic. Anterior curvature is called lordosis and is normal in the lumbar spine. Idiopathic scoliosis generally begins at about 8 or 10 years of age and progresses during growth. In rare instances, infantile scoliosis may be seen in children 2 years of age or less.

Idiopathic scoliosis is about 4–5 times more common in girls than in boys. The disorder is usually asymptomatic in the adolescent years, but severe curvature may lead to impairment of pulmonary function or low back pain in later years. It is important to examine the back of any adolescent coming in for an incidental physical examination in order to identify scoliosis early. The examination is performed by having the patient bend forward 90 degrees with the hands joined in the midline. An abnormal finding consists of asymmetry of the height of the ribs or paravertebral muscles on one side, indicating rotation of the trunk associated with lateral curvature.

Diseases that may be associated with scoliosis include neurofibromatosis, Marfan's syndrome, cerebral palsy, muscular dystrophy, and poliomyelitis. Careful neurologic examination should be performed in all children with these disorders.

Five to 7% of cases of scoliosis are due to congenital vertebral anomalies such as a hemivertebral or unilateral vertebral bridge. These curves are more rigid than the more common idiopathic curve (see below) and will often increase with growth, especially during the rapid growth spurt during adolescence.

The most common type of scoliosis is so-called idiopathic scoliosis, which may be due to asymmetry of neuromuscular development. In 30% of cases other family members are affected also, so that a family survey is valuable for detecting the problem in siblings if one child has been found to have scoliosis.

Idiopathic infantile scoliosis, occurring in children 2–4 years of age, is quite uncommon in the USA; it is more common in Great Britain. If the curvature is less than 30 degrees, the prognosis is excellent, as 70% resolve spontaneously. If the curvature is more than 30 degrees, there may be progression, and the prognosis is therefore guarded.

Postural compensation of the spine may cause lateral curvature from such causes as unequal length of the lower extremities. Antalgic scoliosis may result from pressure on the spinal cord or roots by infectious processes or herniation of the nucleus pulposus. In such cases, the underlying cause must be sought. The curvature will resolve as the primary problem is treated.

Clinical Findings

A. Signs and Symptoms: Scoliosis in adolescents is classically asymptomatic. It is imperative to seek the underlying cause in any case where there is pain since in these instances the scoliosis is almost always secondary to some other disorder such as a bone or spinal cord tumor. Deformity of the rib cage and asymmetry of the waistline is evident with curvatures of 30 degrees or more. A lesser curvature may be detected by the forward bending test as described above, which is designed to detect early abnormalities of rotation which are not apparent when the patient is standing erect.

B. X-Ray Findings: The most valuable x-rays are those taken of the entire spine in the standing position in both the anteroposterior and lateral planes. Usually there is one primary curvature with a compensatory curvature that develops to balance the body. At times there may be 2 primary curvatures, usually in the left thoracic and right lumbar regions. Any right thoracic curvature should be suspected of being secondary to neurologic or muscular disease, prompting a more meticulous neurologic examination. If the curvatures of the spine are balanced (compensated), the head is centered over the center of the pelvis and the patient is "in balance." If the spinal alignment is uncompensated, the head will be displaced to one side, which produces an unsightly deformity. Rotation of the spine may be assessed by noting the shift of the spinous process toward the pedicle on the involved side. This rotation is associated with a marked rib hump as the lateral curvature increases in severity. Deformity of the rib cage produces a decrease in the space available for the lung and is the cause of long-term problems.

Treatment

Exercise alone will not cause permanent improvement of idiopathic scoliosis. Exercise combined with bracing is effective for curvature up to 35–40 degrees. Such treatment is indicated for any curvature that demonstrates progression on serial x-ray examination. Curvatures of less than 20 degrees usually do not require treatment unless they show progression. Curvatures greater than 40 degrees require careful monitoring and are resistant to treatment by bracing. Thoracic curvatures greater than 60 degrees have been correlated with a poor pulmonary prognosis in adult life. Curvatures of such severity are an indication for surgical correction of the deformity and posterior spinal fusion to maintain the correction. Curvatures between 40 and 60 degrees may also require spinal fusion if they appear to be progressive or are causing decompensation of the spine or are cosmetically unacceptable.

Surgical fusion involves decortication of the bone over the laminas and spinous processes, with the addition of autogenous bone graft from the iliac crest. Postoperative correction is often maintained by a Harrington rod, with cast immobilization for several months until the fusion is solid.

Treatment is prolonged and difficult and is best done in centers where full facilities are available for such treatment.

Prognosis

Compensated small curvatures that do not progress may be well tolerated throughout life with very little cosmetic concern. These patients should be counseled regarding the genetic transmission of scoliosis and cautioned that their children should be examined at regular intervals during growth. Large thoracic curvatures greater than 60 degrees are associated with shortened life span and may progress even during adult life. Large lumbar curvatures may lead to subluxation of the vertebrae and premature arthritic degeneration of the spine, producing disabling pain in adulthood. Early detection allows for simple brace treatment, at times simply using a body jacket. In patients so treated, the long-term prognosis is excellent and surgery is not necessary. For this reason, school screening programs for scoliosis have gained popular support in many sections of the country.

Goldstein LA: Surgical management of scoliosis. J Bone Joint Surg 48A:167, 1966.

James JIP: *Scoliosis.* Williams & Wilkins, 1967.

Risser JC: Treatment of scoliosis during the past 50 years. Clin Orthop 44:109, 1966.

Winter RB, Moe JH, Eilers VE: Congenital scoliosis. In: *Textbook of Disorders and Injuries of the Musculoskeletal System.* Salter RB (editor). Williams & Wilkins, 1970.

Wynne-Davies R: Infantile idiopathic scoliosis. J Bone Joint Surg 57B:138, 1975.

EPIPHYSIOLYSIS
(Slipped Capital Femoral Epiphysis)

Epiphysiolysis is the separation of the proximal femoral epiphysis through the growth plate. The head of the femur is usually displaced medially and posteriorly relative to the neck of the femur. The condition occurs in adolescence and is more common in overweight children. Slightly over 40% of the children so affected are of the obese, hypogenital body type. The cause is not clear, although some authorities have shown experimentally that the decreased strength of the perichondral ring stabilizing the epiphyseal area is sufficiently weakened by anatomic changes in adolescent years that the simple overload by excessive body weight can produce a pathologic fracture through the growth plate. Hormonal studies in these children have not demonstrated any abnormality. Anatomic study of the area of separation demonstrates a histologic picture identical to that seen with traumatic separation, and the condition occasionally occurs as an acute episode resulting from a fall or direct trauma to the hip.

More commonly, however, there are vague symptoms over a protracted period of time in an otherwise healthy child who presents with pain and limp. The pain is often referred into the thigh or the medial side of the knee. It is important to examine the hip joint in any child complaining of knee pain, particularly in adolescents. The consistent finding on physical examination is limitation of internal rotation of the hip. There usually is also an associated hip flexion contracture as well as local tenderness about the hip. X-rays should be taken in both the anteroposterior and lateral planes. These must be carefully examined in early cases in order to show an abnormality where displacement of the femoral head occurs posteriorly, which is usually most easily seen on the lateral view.

Treatment is based on the same principles that govern treatment of fracture of the femoral neck in adults in that the head of the femur is fixed to the neck of the femur and the fracture line allowed to heal. Unfortunately, the severe complication of avascular necrosis occurs in 30% of these patients. There has been a positive correlation between forceful reduction of the slip and avascular necrosis. In cases of acute slip, as evidenced by the absence of any callus formation about the growth plate, it may be possible to reduce the hip by gentle traction. In more chronic cases, a more expeditious procedure is to pin the slip in situ and perform correctional osteotomy later in order to realign the deformity. Remodeling of the fracture site often improves the position of the hip without further surgery. The pins used to maintain reduction should be removed once healing has occurred.

The long-term prognosis is guarded because most of these patients continue to be overweight and overstress their hip joints. Follow-up studies have shown a high incidence of premature degenerative arthritis in this group of patients—even those who do not develop avascular necrosis. The development of avascular necrosis almost guarantees a poor prognosis, as remodeling of the femoral head does not occur at this late stage of skeletal growth.

About 30% of patients have bilateral involvement, and patients should be followed for slipping of the opposite side, which may occur as long as 1 or 2 years after the primary episode.

Symposium: Slipped capital femoral epiphysis. Clin Orthop 48:7, 1966.

GENU VARUM & GENU VALGUM

Genu varum (bowleg) is normal from infancy through 2 years of life. The alignment then changes to genu valgum (knock-knee) until about 8 years of age, at which time adult alignment is attained. The most severely knock-kneed child seen in the orthopedist's office is 3 years of age. In questionable cases, where there is a progressive deformity that does not follow the physiologic pattern, it is worthwhile to obtain x-ray views of the knees in order to rule out any significant pathologic lesion such as rickets or proximal tibial epiphyseal dysplasia *(Blount's disease).*

No treatment is usually necessary, although an accentuated deformity may occasionally justify 3-point bracing at night.

Hugenberger PW: Leg deformities. Pediatr Clin North Am 14:589, 1967.

TIBIAL TORSION
("Toeing In")

The physician may be asked about "toeing in" in small children. The disorder is routinely asymptomatic. It is normal for the bone of the tibia to show internal rotation between its 2 ends at the knee and at the ankle. This internal rotation amounts to about 20 degrees at birth but decreases to the adult configuration of 15 degrees of external rotation by age 1. The deformity is sometimes accentuated by laxity of the knee ligaments, allowing excessive internal rotation of the leg in small children. The condition tends to correct itself during the first year of life, but in children who have a persistent internal rotation of the tibia beyond age 1 year it is worthwhile to use external rotation splinting at night to correct the rotational deformity.

FEMORAL ANTEVERSION

"Toeing in" beyond age 2 or 3 years is usually based on femoral anteversion, which produces excessive internal rotation of the femur as compared to external rotation. This femoral alignment follows a natural history of progressive decrease toward neutral up to 8 years of age, with slower change until the almost adult anteversion of 16 degrees is reached. Studies comparing the results of treatment with shoes or braces to the natural history have shown that little is gained by active treatment. Active external rotation exercises such as ballet, skating, or bicycle riding may be worthwhile. Osteotomy for rotational correction is rarely required.

Fabry G, MacEwen GD, Shands AR Jr: Torsion of the femur. J Bone Joint Surg 55A:1726, 1973.

COMMON FOOT PROBLEMS

When a child begins to stand and walk, the long arch of the foot is flat with a medial bulge over the inner border of the foot. The forefeet are mildly pronated or rotated inward, with a slight valgus alignment of the knees. As the child grows and muscle power improves, the long arch is better supported and more normal relationships occur in the lower extremities.

1. FLATFOOT

Flatfoot is a normal condition in infants. Children presenting for examination should be checked to deter-

mine that the heel cord is of normal length when the heel is aligned in the neutral position, allowing complete dorsiflexion and plantar flexion. As long as the foot is supple and the presence of a longitudinal arch is noted when the child is sitting in a non-weight-bearing position, the parents can be assured that a normal arch will probably develop. There is usually a familial incidence of relaxed flatfeet in children who have prolonged malalignment of the foot. In any child with a shortened heel cord or stiffness of the foot, other causes of flatfoot such as tarsal coalition or vertical talus should be ruled out by a complete orthopedic examination and x-ray.

In the child with an ordinary relaxed flatfoot, no active treatment is indicated unless there is calf or leg pain. In children who have leg pains attributable to flat feet, an orthopedic shoe with Thomas heel may relieve discomfort. An arch insert should not be prescribed unless passive correction of the arch is easily accomplished; otherwise, there will be irritation of the skin over the medial side of the foot.

2. TALIPES CALCANEOVALGUS

This disorder is characterized by excessive dorsiflexion at the ankle and eversion of the foot. It is often present at birth and almost always corrects spontaneously. The deformity is the reverse of classical clubfoot (talipes equinovarus) and is due to intrauterine position.

Treatment consists of passive exercises by the mother, stretching the foot into plantar flexion. In rare instances it may be necessary to use plaster casts to help with manipulation and positioning.

Complete correction is the rule.

3. CAVUS FOOT

This deformity consists of an unusually high longitudinal arch of the foot. It may be hereditary or associated with neurologic conditions such as poliomyelitis, Charcot-Marie-Tooth disease, Friedreich's ataxia, or diastematomyelia. There is usually an associated contracture of the toe extensor, producing a claw toe deformity in which the metatarsal phalangeal joints are hyperextended and the interphalangeal joints acutely flexed. Any child presenting with cavus feet should have a careful neurologic examination including x-rays of the spine.

Stretching exercises for the heel cord and arch of the foot are indicated for conservative therapy. In resistant cases that do not respond to shoe adjustments (metatarsal bars and supports), operation may be necessary to lengthen the contracted extensor and flexor tendons. Arthrodesis of the foot may be necessary later. If these feet are left untreated, they are often painful and limit walking.

The overall prognosis is much poorer than with low arch or pes planus.

4. HAMMER TOES

This is a flexion deformity, usually congenital, of either or both interphalangeal joints. It is most often asymptomatic and requires no treatment except for cosmetic reasons or if callus forms over the end of the toe.

5. BUNIONS
(Hallux Valgus)

Girls may present in adolescence with lateral deviation of the great toe associated with a prominence over the head of the first metatarsal. This deformity is painful only with shoe wear and almost always can be relieved by fitting shoes that are wide enough. Surgery should be avoided in the adolescent age group, as the results are much less successful than in adult patients with the same condition.

Funk JF Jr: Foot problems in childhood. Pediatr Clin North Am 14:571, 1967.
Kite JH: Errors and complications in treating foot conditions in children. Clin Orthop 53:31, 1967.

EPIPHYSEAL GROWTH DISTURBANCES SECONDARY TO INFECTION OR TRAUMA

In the child under 1 year of age there is direct vascular communication from the metaphysis to the epiphysis across the growth plate. For this reason, osteomyelitis occurring in the infant may produce permanent damage to the growth cartilage of the epiphysis with resulting angular deformity or decreased growth potential for the bone. Likewise, trauma, particularly of a compression variety, may damage part or all of the epiphysis. Once such damage occurs, deformity is progressive and may be severe, requiring osteotomy for angular deformity or epiphysiodesis for correction of leg length discrepancy.

ORTHOPEDIC ASPECTS OF ENDOCRINE DISEASES

Hormonal problems affecting the skeleton are discussed in Chapter 24. Only a brief orthopedic resume is presented here.

ADRENAL

Adrenocortical hyperfunction may lead to advanced skeletal age relative to chronologic age, with premature epiphyseal closure. In children receiving long-term high-dosage corticosteroid treatment, eg, in the treatment of asthma or nephrosis, there may be retardation of growth and delayed skeletal age.

THYROID

Hyperthyroidism or prolonged thyroid administration may lead to severe osteoporosis with secondary pathologic fracture.

Hypothyroidism is associated with retarded skeletal age and may result in a slipped capital femoral epiphysis in the adolescent. It is worthwhile to screen the patients with slipped capital femoral epiphysis for hypothyroidism.

PARATHYROID

1. HYPERPARATHYROIDISM

Parathyroid hormone exerts a direct effect upon bone, causing absorption of bone. Primary hyperparathyroidism is very rare in children. The skeletal effects of hyperparathyroidism in childhood are usually secondary to parathyroid stimulation by renal failure. X-ray changes associated with hyperparathyroidism are a generalized osteoporosis with cortical atrophy, which is most notable in the distal phalanges and about the necks of the metacarpals. It has been documented that slipped capital femoral epiphysis may occur as a result of the effect on the growth plate, with weakening in children with renal failure. The "brown tumors" of hyperparathyroidism are rare in childhood.

2. HYPOPARATHYROIDISM & PSEUDOHYPOPARATHYROIDISM

The signs and symptoms, laboratory findings, and x-ray findings in these 2 disorders are similar, and the distinction between them is difficult. The disease is commonly hereditary and associated with shortening of the fourth and fifth metacarpals and metatarsals. Formation of the growth plate is abnormal, and the epiphyseal ossification center may indent the metaphysis.

GONADS

In general, deficiency of gonadal hormones produces osteoporosis and delayed maturation of the skeleton. This is most commonly seen in association with Turner's syndrome in the child. Excessive amounts of estrogen such as occur in girls with Albright's syndrome produce not only sexual precocity but also premature closure of the growth centers, resulting in short stature.

DEGENERATIVE PROBLEMS
(Arthritis, Bursitis, & Tenosynovitis)

Degenerative changes may occur either in the joints or in the bursae or tendons surrounding the joints.

Degenerative arthritis may follow infection, slipped capital femoral epiphysis, avascular necrosis, or trauma or may occur in association with hemophilia. Early effective treatment of these disorders will prevent arthritis. Late treatment is often unsatisfactory.

Degenerative changes in the soft tissues around joints may occur as a result of overuse syndrome in adolescent athletes. Young boys throwing excessive numbers of pitches, especially curve balls, may develop "little leaguer's elbow," consisting of degenerative changes around the humeral condyles associated with pain, swelling, and limitation of motion. In order to enforce the rest necessary for healing, a plaster cast may be necessary. A more reasonable preventive measure is to limit the number of pitches thrown by children.

Acute bursitis is quite uncommon in childhood, and another cause should be sought when this diagnosis is made.

Tenosynovitis is most common in the region of the knees and feet. Children taking dancing lessons, particularly toe dancing, may have pain around the flexor tendon sheaths in the toes or ankles. Rest is effective treatment. At the knee level there may be irritation of the patellar ligament, with associated swelling in the infrapatellar fat pad. Synovitis in this area is usually due to overuse and is also treated by rest. Corticosteroid injections are contraindicated.

TRAUMA

SOFT TISSUE TRAUMA
(Sprains, Strains, & Contusions)

A sprain is the stretching of a ligament, and a strain is a stretch of a muscle or tendon. In either of these injuries there may be some degree of tissue tearing. Contusions are generally due to tissue compression, with damage to blood vessels within the tissue and the formation of hematoma.

A severe sprain is one in which the ligament is completely divided, resulting in instability of the joint. A mild or moderate sprain is one in which incomplete tearing of the ligament occurs but in which there is associated local pain and swelling. A severe strain may result in actual tearing of the muscle substance but more often results simply in a "pulled muscle" or "charley horse."

Mild or moderate sprains are treated by rest of the affected joint, with ice and elevation to prevent prolonged symptoms. By definition, mild or moderate sprain is not associated with instability of the joint.

If there is more severe trauma resulting in tearing of a ligament, instability of the joint may be demonstrated by gross examination or by stress testing with x-ray documentation. Such deformity of the joint may cause persistent instability resulting from inaccurate apposition of the ligament ends during healing. If instability is evident, surgical repair of the torn ligament is indicated.

The initial treatment of any sprain consists of ice, compression, and elevation. The purpose of the treatment is to decrease local edema and residual stiffness resulting from gelling of blood proteins in the interstitial space. Splinting of the affected joint protects against further injury and relieves swelling and pain.

1. ANKLE SPRAINS

The history will indicate that the injury was by either forceful inversion or eversion. The more common inversion injury results in tearing or injury to the lateral ligaments, whereas an eversion injury will injure the medial ligaments of the ankle. The injured ligaments may be identified by means of careful palpation for point tenderness around the ankle. The joint should be supported or immobilized at a right angle, which is the functional position. Adhesive taping may be effective to maintain this position but should be applied by one skilled in the use of tape and changed frequently in order to prevent the formation of blisters and skin damage. A posterior plaster splint is more easily applied and gives good joint rest if the extremity is protected by using crutches for weight-bearing. Prolonged use of a plaster cast is usually not necessary, but the sprained ankle should be rested sufficiently to allow complete healing. This may take 3–6 weeks. Because fractures usually receive more attention and adequate follow-up, the results are often better. A properly treated ankle sprain should not be the source of prolonged and repeated disability.

2. KNEE SPRAINS

Sprains of the collateral and cruciate ligaments are uncommon in children. These ligaments are so strong that it is more common to injure the epiphyseal growth plates, which are the weakest structures in the region of the knees of children. In adolescence, however, the joints and growth plates attain adult growth, and a rupture of the anterior cruciate ligament is a not uncommon result of a twisting injury and may avulse the anterior tibial spine. In such instances, the injury is apparent by physical examination and x-ray and requires anatomic reduction and immobilization for 6 weeks. In most instances, this means open operative correction.

Sprains of the collateral and cruciate ligaments, if mild, may be treated by active exercise and crutches to prevent weight-bearing. Complete separation of the ligaments should be corrected surgically to obtain secure stability of the joint. Physical therapy is important in any type of sprain to strengthen both the quadriceps and hamstring muscles around the knee. Moderate sprains should be protected for at least 6 weeks in order to prevent more serious injury from continuous sports activity.

3. INTERNAL DERANGEMENTS OF THE KNEE

Meniscal injuries are uncommon below age 12. Clicking or locking of the knee may occur in young children as a result of a discoid lateral meniscus, which is a rare type of congenital anomaly. As the child approaches adolescence, internal damage to the knee from a torsion weight-bearing injury may result in locking of the knee if tearing and displacement of the meniscus occurs. Osteochondral fractures secondary to osteochondritis dissecans may also present as internal derangements of the knee in adolescence. Posttraumatic synovitis may mimic a meniscal lesion as well. In any severe injury to the knee, epiphyseal injury should be suspected; stress films will sometimes demonstrate separation of the distal femoral epiphysis in such cases. This problem should be suspected whenever there is tenderness on both sides of the metaphysis of the femur after injury.

4. BACK SPRAINS

Sprains of the ligaments and muscles of the back are unusual in children but may occur as a result of violent trauma from automobile accidents or athletic injuries. A child with back pain should not be presumed to have had trauma to the spine unless the history warrants that conclusion. The reason for back pain should be carefully sought by x-ray and physical examination. Inflammation, infection, and tumors are more common causes of back pain in children than sprains.

5. CONTUSIONS

Contusion of muscle with hematoma formation produces the familiar "charley horse" injury. Treatment of such injuries is by application of ice, compression, and rest. Exercise should be avoided for 5–7 days. Local heat may hasten healing once the acute phase of tenderness and swelling is past.

6. MYOSITIS OSSIFICANS

Ossification within muscle occurs when there is sufficient trauma to cause a hematoma that later heals in the manner of a fracture. The injury is usually a contusion and occurs most commonly in the quadriceps of the thigh or the triceps of the arm. When such a severe injury with hematoma is recognized, it is important to splint the extremity and avoid activity. If further activity is allowed, ossification may reach spectacular proportions and resemble an osteosarcoma.

Disability is great, with local swelling and heat and extreme pain upon the slightest motion of the adjacent joint. The limb should be rested, with the knee in extension or the elbow in 90 degrees of flexion, until the local reaction has subsided. Once local heat and tenderness have decreased, gentle active exercises may be initiated. Passive stretching exercises are not indicated because they may stimulate the ossification reaction. It is occasionally necessary to excise excessive bony tissue if it interferes with muscle function once the reaction is mature. Surgery should not be attempted before 9 months to a year after injury because it may restart the process and lead to an even more severe reaction.

TRAUMATIC SUBLUXATIONS & DISLOCATIONS

Dislocation of a joint is always associated with severe damage to the ligaments and joint capsule. In contrast to fracture treatment, which may be safely postponed, dislocations must be reduced immediately. Dislocations can usually be reduced by gentle sustained traction. It often happens that no anesthetic is necessary for several hours after the injury because of the protective anesthesia produced by the injury. Following reduction, the joint should be splinted for transportation of the patient.

The dislocated joint should be treated by immobilization for at least 3 weeks, followed by graduated active exercises through a full range of motion. Physical therapy is usually not indicated for children with injuries. As a matter of fact, vigorous manipulation of the joint by a therapist may be harmful. The child should be permitted to perform his own therapy. No stretching should be permitted.

1. "PULLED ELBOW"

Infants frequently sustain subluxation of the radial head as a result of being lifted or pulled by the hand. The elbow is hyperextended and there is marked pain, with the only presenting complaint being that the child will not bend his elbow. X-rays are often normal, but there is point tenderness over the radial head. When the elbow is placed in full supination and slowly moved from full flexion to full extension, a click may be palpated at the level of the radial head. The relief of pain is remarkable, as the child usually stops crying immediately. The elbow is then immobilized in a posterior splint and sling for approximately 3 weeks.

Kempe has noted that pulled elbow may be a clue to battering. It should be remembered during examination.

2. RECURRENT DISLOCATION OF THE PATELLA

Recurrent dislocation of the patella is more common in loose-jointed individuals, especially adolescent girls. If the patella completely dislocates, it nearly always goes laterally. Pain is severe, and the patient is brought to the doctor with the knee slightly flexed and an obvious bony mass lateral to the knee joint and a flat area over the usual location of the patella anteriorly. X-rays confirm the diagnosis. The patella may be reduced by extending the knee and placing slight pressure on the patella while gentle traction is exerted on the leg. In subluxation of the patella, the symptoms may be more subtle, and the patient may say that the knee "gives out" or "jumps out of place."

In the case of complete dislocation, the knee should be immobilized for 3–4 weeks followed by a physical therapy program for strengthening the quadriceps muscle. Operation may be necessary to tighten the knee joint capsule if dislocation or subluxation is recurrent. In such instances, if the patella is not stabilized, repeated dislocation produces damage to the articular cartilage of the patellofemoral joint and premature degenerative arthritis.

EPIPHYSEAL SEPARATIONS

In children, epiphyseal separations and fractures are more common than ligamentous injuries. This finding is based on the fact that the ligaments of the joints are generally stronger than the associated growth plates. In instances where dislocation is suspected, an x-ray should be taken in order to rule out epiphyseal fracture. Films of the opposite extremity, especially around the elbow, may be valuable for comparison. Reduction of a fractured epiphysis should be done under anesthesia in order to align the growth plate with the least amount of force necessary. Fractures across the growth plate may produce bony bridges which will cause premature cessation of growth or angular deformities in the growth plate. Epiphyseal fractures around the shoulder, wrist, and fingers can usually be treated by closed reduction, but fractures of the epiphyses around the elbow often require open reduction. In the lower extremity, accurate reduction of the epiphyseal plate is necessary if a joint surface is involved in order to prevent joint deformity. Unfortunately, some of the most severe injuries to the epiphyseal plate occur from compression injuries, where the amount of force is not immediately apparent. If angular deformities result, corrective osteotomy may be necessary.

TORUS FRACTURES

Torus fractures consist of "buckling" of the cortex as a result of minimal angular trauma. They usually occur in the distal radius or ulna. Alignment is satisfactory, and simple immobilization for 3–5 weeks is sufficient.

GREENSTICK FRACTURES

With greenstick fractures there is frank disruption of the cortex on one side of the bone but no discernible cleavage plane on the opposite side. These fractures are angulated but not displaced, as the bone ends are not separated. Reduction is achieved by straightening the arm into normal alignment, and reduction is maintained by a snugly fitting plaster cast. It is necessary to x-ray these children again in a week to 10 days to make certain that the reduction has been maintained in plaster. A slight angular deformity will be corrected by remodeling of the bone. The farther the fracture is from the growing end of the bone, the longer the time required for healing. The fracture can be considered healed when there is no tenderness, no local swelling or heat, and adequate bony callus seen on x-ray.

FRACTURE OF THE CLAVICLE

Clavicular fractures are very common injuries in infants and children. They can be immobilized by a figure-of-8 dressing which retracts the shoulders and brings the clavicle to normal length. The healing callus will be apparent when the fracture has consolidated, but this unsightly lump will generally resolve over a period of months to a year.

SUPRACONDYLAR FRACTURES OF THE HUMERUS

These fractures tend to occur in the age group from 3–6 years and are potentially dangerous because of the proximity to the brachial artery in the distal arm. They are usually associated with a significant amount of trauma, so that swelling may be severe. *Volkmann's ischemic contracture* of muscle may occur as a result of vascular embarrassment. When severe swelling is present, the safest course is to place the arm in traction and carefully observe nerve function and the vascular supply to the hand. Such children should be hospitalized and followed carefully by experienced nurses. If the blood supply is compromised, exposure of the brachial artery may be necessary, although this is rarely needed when satisfactory reduction and traction are employed. Complications associated with supracondylar fractures also include a resultant cubitus valgus secondary to poor reduction. It is often difficult to ascertain adequacy of the reduction because a flexed position is necessary to maintain normal alignment. Such a "gunstock" deformity of the elbow may be somewhat unsightly but does not usually interfere with joint function.

GENERAL COMMENTS ON OTHER FRACTURES IN CHILDREN

Reduction of fractures in children is usually accomplished by simple traction and manipulation; open reduction is rarely indicated. Remodeling of the fracture callus will usually produce an almost normal appearance of the bone over a matter of months. The younger the child, the more remodeling is possible. Angular deformities remodel with ease. Rotatory deformities do not remodel, and this produces the cubitus valgus deformity sometimes seen after supracondylar fractures.

The physician should be suspicious of child battering whenever the age of a fracture does not match the history given or when the severity of the injury is more than the alleged accident would have produced. In suspected cases of battering where no fracture is present on the initial x-ray, a repeat film 10 days later is in order. Bleeding beneath the periosteum will be calcified by 7–10 days, and the x-ray appearance is almost diagnostic of severe closed trauma characteristic of a battered child.

Blount WP: *Fractures in Children.* Williams & Wilkins, 1955.

O'Donoghue DH: *Treatment of Injuries to Athletes,* 2nd ed. Saunders, 1970.

Rang M: *Children's Fractures.* Lippincott, 1974.

INFECTIONS OF THE BONES & JOINTS

OSTEOMYELITIS

Osteomyelitis is an infectious process that usually starts in the spongy or medullary bone and then extends to involve compact or cortical bone. It is more common in boys than in girls or in adults of either sex. The lower extremities are most often affected, and there is commonly a history of trauma. Osteomyelitis may occur as a result of direct invasion from the outside through a penetrating wound (nail) or open fracture, but hematogenous spread of infection from other infected areas such as pyoderma or upper respiratory infections is more common. The most common infecting organism is *Staphylococcus aureus,* which seems to have a special tendency to infect the metaphyses of growing bones. Anatomically, circulation in the long bones is such that the arterial supply to the metaphysis just below the growth plate is by end arteries, which turn sharply to end in venous sinusoids, causing a relative stasis. In the infant under 1 year of age, there is direct vascular communication with the epiphysis across the growth plate, so that direct spread may occur from the metaphysis to the epiphysis and subsequently into the joint. In the older child, the growth plate provides an effective barrier and the epiphysis is usually not involved, although the infection spreads retrograde from the metaphysis into the diaphysis and, by rupture through the cortical bone, down along the diaphysis beneath the periosteum.

1. EXOGENOUS OSTEOMYELITIS

In order to avoid osteomyelitis by direct extension, all wounds must be carefully examined and cleansed. Puncture wounds are especially liable to lead to osteomyelitis if not carefully debrided. Cultures of the wound made at the time of exploration and debridement may be useful if signs of inflammation and infection develop subsequently. Copious irrigation is necessary, and all nonviable skin, subcutaneous tissue, fascia, and muscle must be excised. In extensive or contaminated wounds, antibiotic coverage is indicated. Contaminated wounds should be left open and secondary closure performed 3–5 days later. If at the time of delayed closure further necrotic tissue is present, it should be excised. Leaving the wound open allows the infection to stay at the surface rather than extend inward to the bone.

Parenteral administration of antibiotics is satisfactory, and local irrigation is not needed. If the wound is acquired outside the hospital, penicillin is adequate for most wounds. After cultures have been read, an appropriate alternative antibiotic can be chosen if there is lingering inflammation. A tetanus toxoid booster is indicated for any questionable wound, but gas gangrene is better prevented by adequate debridement than by antitoxin.

Once exogenous osteomyelitis has become established, treatment becomes more complicated, requiring extensive surgical debridement and drainage followed by careful antibiotic management. These cases require hospitalization and the use of intravenous antibiotics.

2. HEMATOGENOUS OSTEOMYELITIS

Hematogenous osteomyelitis is usually caused by pyogenic bacteria; 85% of cases are due to staphylococci. Streptococci are rare causes of osteomyelitis today, but pseudomonas organisms have often been documented in cases of nail puncture wounds. Children with sickle cell anemia are especially prone to osteomyelitis caused by salmonellae.

Clinical Findings

A. Symptoms and Signs: In infants the manifestations of osteomyelitis may be quite subtle, presenting as irritability, diarrhea, or failure to feed properly; the temperature may be normal or slightly low, and the white blood count may be normal or only slightly elevated. In older children the manifestations are more striking, with severe local tenderness and pain, high fever, rapid pulse, and elevated white blood count and sedimentation rate. Osteomyelitis of a lower extremity often presents around the knee in a child 7–10 years of age. Tenderness is most marked over the metaphysis of the bone where the process has its origin.

B. Laboratory Findings: Blood cultures are often positive early. The most significant test in infancy is the aspiration of pus when suspicion arises because of lack of movement in a painful extremity. It is useful to insert a needle to the bone in the area of suspected infection and aspirate any fluid present. This fluid can be smeared and stained for organisms as well as cultured. Even edema fluid may be useful for determining the causative organism. The white blood cell count is usually elevated.

C. X-Ray Findings: Early in the course of the disease (during the first 3–6 days), there may be no abnormal x-ray findings. The first manifestation to appear on x-ray is nonspecific local swelling. This is followed by elevation of the periosteum, with formation of new bone from the cambium layer of the periosteum. As the infection becomes chronic, areas of cortical bone are isolated by pus spreading down the medullary canal, causing rarefaction and demineralization of the bone. Such isolated pieces of cortex become ischemic and form sequestra or dead bone fragments. These x-ray findings are late, and osteomyelitis should be diagnosed clinically before significant x-ray findings are present.

Treatment

A. Specific Measures: Antibiotics should be started intravenously, with dosage based on serum killing powers, as soon as the diagnosis of osteomyelitis is made. The recommended antibiotic is methicillin to cover penicillinase-producing *Staphylococcus aureus.* Gentamicin can also be given to combat gram-negative organisms until the results of cultures are available. Antibiotics should be continued until all signs of inflammation have ceased as judged by the absence of swelling, tenderness, and local discharge combined with laboratory findings of a normal white blood count and sedimentation rate. Serial x-rays can also be used to follow bone healing. Antibiotic therapy by the intravenous route should be continued for at least 3 weeks before it is safe to change to oral medication. Oral medication is continued for at least 1 month after the sedimentation rate has returned to normal in order to prevent resurgence of infection.

B. General Measures: Splinting of the limb minimizes pain and decreases spread of the infection by lymphatic channels through the soft tissue. The splint should be removed periodically to allow active use of adjacent joints and prevent stiffening and muscle atrophy. In chronic osteomyelitis, splinting may be necessary to guard against fracture of the weakened bone.

C. Surgical Measures: Aspiration of the metaphysis is a useful diagnostic measure in any case of suspected osteomyelitis. Osteomyelitis represents a collection of pus under pressure within the body. In the first 24–72 hours, it may be possible to abort osteomyelitis by the use of antibiotics alone. However, if frank pus is aspirated from the bone, surgical drainage is indicated. If the infection has not shown a dramatic response within 24 hours in questionable cases, surgical drainage is also indicated. It is important that all devitalized soft tissue be removed and adequate exposure of the bone obtained in order to permit free drainage. Excessive amounts of bone should not be removed when draining acute osteomyelitis since they may not be completely replaced by the normal healing process.

In questionable cases, little damage has been done bv surgical drainage, but failure to drain the pus in acute cases may lead to more severe damage.

Prognosis

When osteomyelitis is diagnosed in the early clinical stages and prompt antibiotic therapy is begun, the prognosis is excellent. If the process has been unattended for a week to 10 days, there is almost always some permanent loss of bone structure and the possibility of growth abnormality.

Clarke AM: Neonatal osteomyelitis: A disease different from osteomyelitis of older children. Med J Aust 1:237, 1958.

Waldvogel F & others: Osteomyelitis. (3 parts.) N Engl J Med 282:198, 260, 316, 1970.

PYOGENIC ARTHRITIS

The source of pyogenic arthritis varies according to the age of the child. In the infant, pyogenic arthritis often develops by spread from adjacent osteomyelitis. In the older child it presents as an isolated infection, usually without bony involvement. In teenagers with pyogenic arthritis, an underlying systemic disease is usually the cause, eg, an obvious generalized infection or an organism which has an affinity for joints, such as the gonococcus.

In infants the most common cause of pyogenic arthritis is *Staphylococcus aureus,* although gram-negative organisms may be seen. In children between 4 months and 4 years of age, *Haemophilus influenzae* is a common causative organism.

The initial effusion of the joint rapidly becomes purulent. An effusion of the joint may accompany osteomyelitis in the adjacent bone. A white blood cell count exceeding 100,000/cu mm in the joint fluid indicates a definite purulent infection. Generally, spread of infection is from the bone into the joint, but unattended pyogenic arthritis may also affect adjacent bone.

Clinical Findings

A. Symptoms and Signs: In older children the signs are striking, with fever, malaise, vomiting, and restriction of motion. In infants, paralysis of the limb may be evident due to inflammatory neuritis. Infection of the hip joint in infants can be diagnosed if suspicion is aroused by decreased abduction of the hip in an infant who is irritable or feeding poorly. A history of umbilical catheter treatment in the newborn nursery should alert the physician to the possibility of pyogenic arthritis of the hip.

B. X-Ray Findings: Early distention of the joint capsule is nonspecific and difficult to quantitate by x-ray. In the infant with unrecognized pyogenic arthritis, dislocation of the joint may follow within a few days as a result of distention of the capsule by pus. Later changes include destruction of the joint space, resorption of epiphyseal cartilage, and erosion of the adjacent bone of the metaphysis.

Treatment

Diagnosis may be made by aspiration of the joint. In the hip joint, pyogenic arthritis is most easily treated by surgical drainage because the joint is deep and difficult to aspirate as well as being inaccessible to thorough cleaning through needle aspiration. In more superficial joints, such as the knee, aspiration of the joint at least twice daily may maintain adequate drainage. If fever and clinical symptoms do not subside within 24 hours after treatment is begun, open surgical drainage is indicated. Antibiotics can be specifically selected based on cultures of the aspirated pus. Before the results of cultures are available, treatment by methicillin and gentamicin will cover the usual etiologic organisms. It is not necessary to give intra-articular antibiotics, since good levels are achieved in the synovial fluid.

Prognosis

The prognosis is excellent if the joint is drained early, before damage to the articular cartilage has occurred. If infection is present for more than 24 hours, there is dissolution of the proteoglycans in the articular cartilage with subsequent arthrosis and fibrosis of the joint. Damage to the growth plate may also occur, especially within the hip joint, where the epiphyseal plate is intracapsular.

Clawson DK, Dunn AW: Management of common bacterial infections of bones and joints. J Bone Joint Surg 49A:164, 1967.

Griffin PP: Bone and joint infections in children. Pediatr Clin North Am 14:533, 1967.

TUBERCULOUS ARTHRITIS

Tuberculous arthritis is now a rare disease in the USA. It must be considered, however, in children with resistant infections of the joints, especially if there is a history of tuberculosis in family members. Generally, the infection may be ruled out by skin testing. The joints most commonly affected in children are the intervertebral disks, resulting in gibbus or dorsal angular deformity at the site of the involvement.

Treatment is by local drainage of the "cold abscess" followed by antituberculosis therapy with isoniazid, rifampin, and ethambutol. Prolonged immobilization in a plaster bed is necessary in order to promote healing. Spinal fusion may be required to preserve stability of the vertebral column.

Kelly PJ, Karlson AG: Musculoskeletal tuberculosis. Proc Staff Meet Mayo Clin 44:73, 1969.

Seddon HJ: Fourth report of the Medical Research Council Working Party on Tuberculosis of the Spine. Br J Surg 61:69, 1974.

TRANSIENT SYNOVITIS OF THE HIP

The most common cause of limping and pain in the hip of children in the USA is transitory synovitis, an acute inflammatory reaction that often follows an upper respiratory infection and is generally self-limited. In questionable cases, aspiration of the hip yields only yellowish fluid, ruling out pyogenic arthritis. Generally, however, toxic synovitis of the hip is not associated with elevation of the white blood count or a temperature above 38.3° C (101° F). It classically affects children 3–10 years of age and is more common in boys. There is limitation of motion of the hip joint, particularly internal rotation, and x-ray changes are nonspecific, with some swelling apparent in the soft tissues around the joint.

Treatment consists of bed rest and the use of traction with slight flexion of the hip. Aspirin may shorten the course of the disease, although even with no treatment the disease usually is self-limited to a matter of days. It is important to maintain x-ray follow-up of these children, since toxic synovitis may be the precursor of avascular necrosis of the femoral head (see next section) in a small percentage of patients. X-rays can be obtained at 1 month and 3 months, or earlier if there is persistent limp or pain.

Gladhill HB: Transient synovitis and Legg-Calvé-Perthes disease. Can Med J 100:311, 1969.

Hardinge K: The etiology of transient synovitis of the hip. J Bone Joint Surg 52B:100, 1970.

VASCULAR LESIONS & AVASCULAR NECROSIS

AVASCULAR NECROSIS OF THE PROXIMAL FEMUR
(Legg-Calvé-Perthes Disease)

The vascular supply of bone is generally precarious, and when it is interrupted necrosis results. In contrast to other body tissues that undergo infarction, bone removes necrotic tissue and replaces it with living bone in a process called "creeping substitution." This replacement of necrotic bone may be so complete and so perfect that a completely normal bone results. Adequacy of replacement depends upon the age of the patient, the presence or absence of associated infection, congruity of the involved joint, and other physiologic and mechanical factors.

Because of their rapid growth in relation to their blood supply, the secondary ossification centers in the epiphyses are subject to avascular necrosis. The physicians who originally described the avascular lesions of the epiphyses and distinguished them from tuberculosis in the early 20th century were identified with the processes. Despite the number of different names referring to avascular necrosis of the epiphyses, the process is identical, ie, necrosis of bone followed by replacement.

Even though the pathologic and radiologic features of avascular necrosis of the epiphysis are well known, the cause is not generally agreed upon. Necrosis may follow known causes such as trauma or infection, but idiopathic lesions usually develop during periods of rapid growth of the epiphysis. Thus, the highest incidence of Legg-Calvé-Perthes disease is between 4 and 8 years of age.

Clinical Findings

A. Symptoms and Signs: Persistent pain is the most common symptom, and the patient may present with limp or limitation of motion.

B. Laboratory Findings: Laboratory findings, including studies of joint aspirates, are normal.

C. X-Ray Findings: X-ray findings correlate with the progression of the process and the extent of necrosis. The early finding is effusion of the joint associated with slight widening of the joint space and periarticular swelling. Decreased bone density in and around the joint is apparent after a few weeks. The necrotic ossification center appears more dense than the surrounding viable structures, and there is collapse or narrowing of the femoral head.

As replacement of the necrotic ossification center occurs, there is rarefaction of the bone in a patchwork fashion, producing alternating areas of rarefaction and relative density or "fragmentation" of the epiphysis.

In the hip there may be widening of the femoral head associated with flattening, giving rise to the term *coxa plana*. If infarction has extended across the growth plate, then there will be a radiolucent lesion within the metaphysis. If the growth center of the femoral head has been damaged so that normal growth does not occur, varus deformity of the femoral neck will occur as a result of overgrowth of the greater trochanteric apophysis.

Eventually, complete replacement of the epiphysis will become apparent as new bone replaces necrotic bone. The final shape of the head will depend upon the extent of the necrosis and collapse that has been allowed to occur.

Differential Diagnosis

Differential diagnosis must include inflammatory and infectious lesions of the joint or apophyses. Transient synovitis of the hip may be distinguished from Legg-Calvé-Perthes disease by serial x-rays.

Table 19—1. The osteochondroses.

Ossification Center	Eponym	Typical Age
Capital femoral	Legg-Calvé-Perthes disease	3—5
Tarsal navicular	Kohler's disease	6
Second metatarsal head	Freiberg's disease	12—14
Vertebral ring	Scheuermann's disease	13—16
Capitellum	Panner's disease	9—11

Treatment

Treatment consists simply of protection of the joint. If the joint is deeply seated within the acetabulum and normal joint motion is maintained, a reasonably good result can be expected. The hip is held in abduction and internal rotation in order to fulfill this purpose. Braces are generally used. Surgery may be necessary for an uncooperative patient or one whose social or geographic circumstances do not allow use of a brace (living in house trailer, in an unpaved rural area, etc).

Prognosis

The prognosis for complete replacement of the necrotic femoral head in a child is excellent, but the functional result will depend upon the amount of deformity that develops during the time the softened structure exists. In Legg-Calvé-Perthes disease, the prognosis depends upon the completeness of involvement of the epiphyseal center. In general, patients with metaphyseal defects, those in whom the disease develops late in childhood, and those who have more complete involvement of the femoral head have a poorer prognosis.

Osteochondrosis due to vascular lesions may affect various growth centers. Table 19—1 indicates the common sites and the typical ages at presentation.

Catterall A: The natural history of Perthes disease. J Bone Joint Surg 53B:37, 1971.

Goff CW: The osteochondroses, with emphasis on the Legg-Calvé-Perthes syndrome. In: *Instructional Course Lectures, The American Academy of Orthopaedic Surgeons.* Vol 13. Edwards, 1956.

Kamhi E, MacEwen GD: Treatment of Legg-Calvé-Perthes disease: Prognostic value of Catterall's classification. J Bone Joint Surg 57A:651, 1975.

OSTEOCHONDRITIS DISSECANS

This lesion is a pie-shaped necrotic area of bone and cartilage adjacent to the articular surface. The fragment of bone may be broken off from the host bone and displaced into the joint as a loose body. If it remains attached, the necrotic fragment may be completely replaced by creeping substitution.

The pathologic process is precisely the same as that described above for avascular necrosing lesions of ossification centers. However, since these lesions are adjacent to articular cartilage, there may be joint damage.

The most common sites of these lesions are the knee (medial femoral condyle), the elbow joint (capitellum), and the talus (superior lateral dome).

Joint pain is the usual presenting complaint. However, local swelling or locking may be present, particularly if there is a fragment free in the joint. Laboratory studies are normal.

Treatment consists of protection of the involved area from mechanical damage. If there is a fragment free within the joint as a loose body, it must be surgically removed. For some marginal lesions, it may be worthwhile to drill the necrotic fragment in order to encourage more rapid vascular ingrowth and replacement. If large areas of a weight-bearing joint are involved, secondary degenerative arthritis may result.

Hatcher CH: *The Fate of Aseptic Necrosis of Bone in Skeletal Diseases and Injuries. The Musculoskeletal System.* Macmillan, 1952.

NEUROLOGIC DISORDERS INVOLVING THE MUSCULOSKELETAL SYSTEM

ORTHOPEDIC ASPECTS OF POLIOMYELITIS

Muscle Recovery

In paralytic poliomyelitis it may not be possible for the complete pattern of anterior horn cell destruction to be determined in the initial stages, but some generalizations can be made:

(1) "Spotty" paralysis in a number of extremities has a good prognosis.

(2) A completely flail extremity will probably never show a significant functional recovery.

(3) Early muscle recovery is a good prognostic sign, with probable full functional recovery to be expected.

(4) Muscle recovery cannot be expected after 18 months from the time of onset.

(5) Muscle recovery must be steady and continuous. If a "plateau" is reached and maintained for 3 months, no further recovery of the muscle may be anticipated.

(6) Muscle "substitution" may produce func-

tional improvement long after the first 18 months following the acute infection. Such muscle substitution may be functionally beneficial or may produce deformity due to unbalanced muscle power.

Reconstructive Procedures

Reconstructive orthopedic procedures may be directed at dividing restricting fascial contractures, transferring musculotendinous units for better balance of motor power, corrective osteotomies for bony angulation deformities, and various procedures to equalize leg length discrepancy. Procedures used to treat such lower motor neuron paralyses cover the entire range of operative orthopedics.

ORTHOPEDIC ASPECTS OF CEREBRAL PALSY

Early physical therapy to encourage completion of the normal developmental patterns may be of benefit in patients with cerebral palsy. The greatest gains from this type of therapy are obtained during the first few years of life, and therapy should not be continued with unrealistic goals when no improvement is apparent.

Bracing and splinting are of questionable benefit, although night splints may be useful in preventing equinus deformity of the feet or adduction contractures of the hips. Orthopedic surgery can offer procedures to weaken hyperactive spastic muscles, to transfer function of deforming spastic muscles, or to stabilize joints. In general, muscle transfers are unpredictable in cerebral palsy, and most orthopedic procedures are directed at weakening deforming forces or bony stabilization by osteotomy or arthrodesis.

Flexion and adduction of the hip due to hyperactivity of the adductors and flexors may produce a progressive paralytic dislocation of the hip. Congenital dislocation of the hip is unusual in cerebral palsy, but in more severely involved children paralytic dislocation can lead to pain and dysfunction. Treatment of the dislocation once it has occurred is difficult and unsatisfactory. The principal preventive measure is abduction bracing, but this must often be supplemented by release of the adductors or hip flexors in order to prevent dislocation. In severe cases, osteotomy of the femur may also be necessary to correct the bony deformities of femoral anteversion and coxa valga that are invariably present.

Patients with predominantly an athetotic pattern are poor candidates for any surgical procedure or bracing. Neurosurgical procedures may be of some help.

Because it is difficult to predict the outcome of surgical procedures in cerebral palsy, the surgeon must examine these patients on several occasions before any operative procedure is undertaken. Follow-up care by a physical therapist to maximize the anticipated long-term gains should be arranged before the operation.

Beals RK: Cerebral palsy: Elements for decision making. In: *Instructional Course Lectures, The American Academy of Orthopaedic Surgeons.* Mosby, 1971.

Beals RK: Spastic paraplegia and diplegia: An evaluation of nonsurgical and surgical factors influencing the prognosis for ambulation. J Bone Joint Surg 48A:827, 1966.

Evans EB: The status of surgery of the lower extremities in cerebral palsy. Clin Orthop 47:127, 1966.

Phelps WM: The cerebral palsies. Clin Orthop 44:83, 1966.

Siffert RS: Children's orthopaedic surgery in the United States: Historical trends. Clin Orthop 44:89, 1966.

ORTHOPEDIC ASPECTS OF MYELODYSPLASIA

Patients born with spina bifida cystica (aperta) should be examined early by an orthopedic surgeon. The level of neurologic involvement determines the imbalance of muscular force that will be present and apt to produce deformity with growth. The involvement is often asymmetric and tends to change during the first 12–18 months of life. Early closure of the sac is the rule, although there has been some hesitancy to treat all of these patients because of the extremely poor prognosis associated with congenital hydrocephalus, high levels of paralysis, and associated congenital anomalies. Associated musculoskeletal problems may include clubfeet, congenital dislocation of the hip, arthrogryposis-type changes of the lower extremities, and congenital scoliosis, among others. The most common lesions are at the level of L3–4 and tend to affect the hip joint, with progressive dislocation occurring during growth. Foot deformities may be in any direction and are complicated by the fact that sensation is generally absent. Spinal deformities develop in a high percentage of these children, with scoliosis being present in approximately 40%. Ambulation is impossible without braces or splints, and careful urologic follow-up must be obtained to prevent complications from incontinence. A high percentage of these children have hydrocephalus, which may be evident at birth or shortly thereafter, requiring shunting. The shunts are sources of infection and may require frequent replacement.

In children who have a reasonable likelihood of walking, operative treatment consists of reduction of the hip and alignment of the feet in the weight-bearing position as well as stabilization of the vertebral scoliosis. In children who do not have extension power of the knee, ie, those who lack active quadriceps function, the likelihood of ambulation is greatly decreased. In such patients, aggressive surgery in the hip region may result in stiffening of the joints, thus preventing sitting. Multiple foot operations are also contraindicated in these children.

The overall management of the child with spina bifida should be coordinated in a multidiscipline clinic where all doctors working in cooperation with each other can work also with therapists, social workers, and teachers to provide the best possible care.

Curtis BH: *Symposium on Myelomeningocele.* Mosby, 1972.

Kilfoyle RM: Myelodysplasia. Pediatr Clin North Am 14:419, 1967.

Lorber J: Spina bifida cystica: Results of 270 consecutive cases with criteria for selection for the future. Arch Dis Child 47:854, 1972.

NEOPLASIA OF THE MUSCULOSKELETAL SYSTEM
(See Tables 19—2 to 19—6.)

Neoplastic diseases of the mesodermal tissues constitute a very serious problem because of the poor prognosis of malignant tumors in these areas. Few of the benign lesions undergo malignant transformation, and it is important to establish a proper diagnosis and thus avoid undertreatment or overtreatment. The diagnosis depends upon correlation of the clinical, x-ray, and microscopic findings.

In general, neoplasms of the mesodermal tissues are named according to the tissue produced (eg, osteosarcoma is one producing bone). However, because of the varied potentiality of mesodermal cells, several types of tissue may be present within the same tumor. This has resulted in confusion of nomenclature, with some tumors being given a bewildering combination of names. It has also resulted in a number of misdiagnoses, since a specimen from a single area may not represent tissue typical of the entire tumor. In addition, some of the tumors are so primitive that they rarely produce any recognizable type of adult tissue.

Biopsy is necessary for definitive diagnosis. Complications from biopsy are far outweighed by the advantages of correct diagnosis.

Dahlin DC: *Bone Tumors,* 2nd ed. Thomas, 1967.

Ferguson AB Jr: Benign tumors.of bone in childhood. Pediatr Clin North Am 14:683, 1967.

Jaffe HL: *Tumors and Tumorous Conditions of the Bones and Joints.* Lea & Febiger, 1958.

Lichtenstein L: *Bone Tumors.* Mosby, 1952.

Table 19—2. Differentiating features of carcinoma and sarcoma.

	Carcinoma	Sarcoma
Tissue origin	Epithelial	Mesodermal
Age incidence	Middle age	Youth
Metastases	Regional nodes	Lungs
Radiation sensitivity	Sensitive. Some cures.	Resistant
Susceptibility to chemotherapeutic agents	Some specific drug sensitivities	More resistant
Prognosis	Variable	Poor

MISCELLANEOUS DISEASES OF BONE

FIBROUS DYSPLASIA

Dysplastic fibrous tissue replacement of the medullary canal is accompanied by the formation of metaplastic bone in fibrous dysplasia. Three forms of the disease are recognized: monostotic, polyostotic, and polyostotic with endocrine disturbances (precocious puberty in females, hyperthyroidism, and hyperadrenalism, ie, Albright's syndrome).

Clinical Findings
A. Symptoms and Signs: The lesion or lesions may be asymptomatic. Pain, if present, is probably due to pathologic fractures. In females, endocrine disturbances may be present in the·polyostotic variety and associated with café-au-lait spots.

B. Laboratory Findings: Laboratory findings are normal unless endocrine disturbances are present, in which case there may be increased secretion of gonadotropic, thyroid, or adrenal hormones.

C. X-Ray Findings: The lesion begins centrally within the medullary canal, usually of a long bone, and expands slowly. Pathologic fracture may occur. If metaplastic bone predominates, the contents of the lesion will be of the density of bone. Marked deformity of the bone may result, and a shepherd's crook deformity of the upper femur is a classical feature of the disease. The disease is often asymmetric, and limb length disturbances may occur as a result of stimulation of epiphyseal cartilage growth.

Differential Diagnosis
The differential diagnosis may include other fibrous lesions of bone as well as destructive lesions such as bone cyst, eosinophilic granuloma, aneurysmal bone cyst, nonossifying fibroma, enchondroma, and chondromyxoid fibroma.

Treatment
If the lesion is small and asymptomatic, no treatment is needed. If the lesion is large and produces or threatens pathologic fracture, curettage and bone grafting are indicated.

Prognosis
Unless the lesions impair epiphyseal growth, the prognosis is good. Lesions tend to enlarge during the growth period but are stable during adult life. Malignant transformation has not been recorded.

UNICAMERAL BONE CYST

This lesion appears in the metaphyses of the long bones, usually in the femur and humerus. It begins

Table 19—3. Benign neoplasms: Osseous.

Disease	Clinical Features	X-Ray Features	Treatment	Prognosis
Osteocartilaginous exostosis (osteochondroma)	Pain-free mass. (Pain, if present, is due to superimposed bursitis.) Single or multiple. Bone mass capped with cartilage. Masses enlarge during childhood and adolescence.	Metaphyseal position. Pedunculated or sessile. Cortex of host bone "turned out" into the lesion. Cartilage cap may be calcified. Long bones predominate.	Surgical excision if symptomatic, if lesion interferes with function, or enlarging mass in adult life.	Excellent. Malignant transformation is rare.
Osteoid osteoma	Pain with point tenderness. Night pain common. Pain often relieved by aspirin.	Radiolucent central nidus (about 1 cm in diameter) surrounded by spectacular osteosclerosis. Sclerosis may obscure nidus.	Surgical excision of nidus.	Excellent. No known malignant transformation.
Osteoblastoma (giant osteoid osteoma)	Pain similar to that of osteoid osteoma.	Nidus larger than 1 cm. Osteolytic phase may predominate.	Surgical excision.	Excellent.

Table 19—4. Benign neoplasms: Cartilaginous.

Disease	Clinical Features	X-Ray Features	Treatment	Prognosis
Chondroma	Usually silent lesions. Pain may be present. Pathologic fracture may occur.	Radiolucent lesions. Long bones predominate. Most common lesion of phalanges and metacarpals or metatarsals. Calcification may be present centrally. Little or no host reaction.	Surgical excision or curettage.	Excellent. Malignant transformation of chondromas of major bones occurs rarely in childhood.
Chondroblastoma (Codman's tumor)	Pain about a joint. Pathologic fracture may occur.	Radiolucent lesion of ossification center of child or adolescent. Occasionally perforates epiphyseal cartilage. Rarely calcification. Little or no reactive bone formation.	Surgical excision or curettage.	Excellent. No known malignant transformation.
Chondromyxofibroma	Usually silent lesion. Mass may be the presenting feature. Pathologic fracture may occur.	Long bones predominate (tibia, fibula, femur, humerus). Radiolucent lesion, may enlarge the host bone. Usually metaphyseal, linearly oriented. Usually well encapsulated.	Surgical excision or curettage.	Good. Lesion may recur after local excision.

Table 19—5. Benign neoplasms: Fibrous.

Disease	Clinical Features	X-Ray Features	Treatment	Prognosis
Nonossifying fibroma (benign cortical defect; benign metaphyseal defect)	Usually silent lesion. Rarely, pathologic fracture.	Radiolucent lesion. Metaphyseal location, linearly oriented. Eccentric position. Thin sclerotic border about lesion. May be multiple lesions.	No treatment needed. Lesions heal with time and growth.	Excellent.
Giant cell tumor	Extremely rare in children.	Radiolucent lesions.	Surgical excision or curettage.	Good. Malignant transformation rare. May undergo change to fibrosarcoma.

Table 19—6. Malignant neoplasms.

Disease	Clinical Features	X-Ray Features	Treatment	Prognosis
Osteosarcoma and chondrosarcoma	Pain the most common symptom. Mass, functional loss, limp occasionally present. Pathologic fracture common.	Destructive, expanding, invasive lesion. Minimal host reaction, but, if present, usually is a triangle between tumor, elevated periosteum, and cortex. Usually radiolucent, but lesional tissue may show ossification or calcification. Metaphyseal location common. Femur, tibia, humerus, and other long bones predominate.	Surgical excision or amputation. Radiation resistant. Markedly improved prognosis (50–70%) results from use of surgery combined with doxorubicin and methotrexate in osteosarcoma. (See Chapter 31.)	Poor. Probably less than 5 or 10% cured. Metastases to lungs, occasionally to other bones. Life expectancy has been prolonged by use of chemotherapy.
Fibrosarcoma	Rare·lesions in children.	Radiolucent, destructive, expanding, invasive lesion. Little or no host reaction. Long bones predominate.	Surgical excision or amputation.	Poor. Probably 10–15% cured. Metastases to lungs.
Ewing's tumor	Pain very common. Tenderness, fever, and leukocytosis also common. Frequent pathologic fracture. Frequently multicentric.	Radiolucent, destructive lesion, frequently in diaphyseal region of the bone. May be reactive bone formation about the lesion in successive layers—"onion skin" layering.	Radiation sensitive but not curable. Surgical excision usually not desirable because of multiple areas of involvement. Chemotherapy by vincristine, doxorubicin, and cyclophosphamide.	Poor. Metastases to multiple organs.

within the medullary canal adjacent to the epiphyseal cartilage. It probably results from some fault in enchondral ossification. The cyst is "active" as long as it abuts onto the metaphyseal side of the epiphyseal cartilage and "inactive" when a border of normal bone exists between the cyst and the epiphyseal cartilage. The lesion is usually identified when a pathologic fracture occurs, producing pain. Laboratory findings are normal. On x-rays the cyst is identified centrally within the medullary canal, producing expansion of the cortex and thinning over the widest portion of the cyst.

Treatment consists of curettage of the cyst if it is producing pain. The cyst may heal after a fracture and not require treatment. Curettage should be delayed if surgery would risk damage to the adjacent growth plate.

The prognosis is excellent. Many cysts will heal following pathologic fracture.

ANEURYSMAL BONE CYST

This lesion is similar to unicameral bone cyst, but it contains blood rather than clear fluid. It usually occurs in a slightly eccentric position in the long bones, expanding the cortex of the bone but not breaking the cortex, although some extraosseous mass may be produced. On x-rays the lesion appears somewhat larger than the width of the epiphyseal cartilage, and this feature distinguishes it from unicameral bone cyst.

The aneurysmal bone cyst is filled by large vascular lakes, and the stoma of the cyst contains fibrous tissue and areas of metaplastic ossification.

The lesion may appear quite aggressive histologically, and it is important to differentiate it from osteosarcoma or hemangioma. Treatment is by curettage and bone grafting, and the prognosis is excellent.

INFANTILE CORTICAL HYPEROSTOSIS
(Caffey's Syndrome)

This is a benign disease of unknown cause that has its onset before 6 months of age and is characterized by irritability, fever, and nonsuppurating, tender, painful swellings. Swellings may involve almost any bone of the body and are frequently widespread. Classically, there are swellings of the mandible and clavicle in 50% of cases as well as of the ulna, humerus, and ribs. The disease is limited to the shafts of bones and does not involve subcutaneous tissues or joints. It is self-limited but may persist for weeks or months. Anemia, leukocytosis, an increased sedimentation rate, and elevation of the serum alkaline phosphatase are usually present. Cortical hyperostosis is demonstrable by a typical x-ray appearance and may be diagnosed on physical examination by an experienced pediatrician.

Fortunately, the disease appears to be decreasing in frequency. Corticosteroids are effective in severe cases.

The prognosis is good, and the disease usually terminates without deformity.

GANGLION

A ganglion is a smooth, small cystic mass connected by a pedicle to the joint capsule, usually on the dorsum of the wrist. It may also be seen in the tendon sheath over the flexor surfaces of the fingers. These ganglions can be excised if they interfere with function or cause persistent pain.

BAKER'S CYST

This is a herniation of the synovium in the knee joint into the popliteal region. In children the diagnosis may be made by aspiration of mucinous fluid, but the cyst nearly always disappears with time. Whereas Baker's cysts may be indicative of intra-articular disease in the adult, they usually are of no clinical significance in children and rarely require excision.

•   •   •

General References

Banks HH: Symposium on musculoskeletal disorders. (2 parts.) Pediatr Clin North Am 14:299, 533, 1967.

Bergsma D (editor): The first conference on the clinical delineation of birth defects. Parts 2, 3, & 4. The National Foundation—March of Dimes, 1969.

Caffey J: *Pediatric X-Ray Diagnosis,* 5th ed. Year Book, 1967.

Fairbank T: *Atlas of General Affections of the Skeleton.* Williams & Wilkins, 1951.

Ferguson AB Jr: *Orthopedic Surgery in Infancy and Childhood,* 3rd ed. Williams & Wilkins, 1968.

Salter RB: *Textbook of Disorders and Injuries of the Musculoskeletal System.* Williams & Wilkins, 1970.

Tachdjian MO: *Pediatric Orthopedics.* Saunders, 1972.

20...
Immune Complex Diseases

Roger Hollister, MD, & Donough O'Brien, MD, FRCP

JUVENILE RHEUMATOID ARTHRITIS
(Still's Disease)

Essentials of Diagnosis

- Nonmigratory monarticular or polyarticular arthropathy, with a tendency to involve large joints or proximal interphalangeal joints and lasting more than 3 months.
- Systemic manifestations with fever, erythematous rashes, nodules, and leukocytosis, and occasionally iridocyclitis, pleuritis, pericarditis, hepatitis, and nephritis.

General Considerations

Juvenile rheumatoid arthritis (JRA) is a common chronic disorder in the pediatric age group. Trauma, viral infections, climatic changes, and psychologic stress may act as triggering events but are not related to the fundamental cause of the disease. The course of the illness is chronic, with periods of exacerbation and remission.

The preponderance of evidence suggests an immunologic pathogenesis of the disease. Joint fluid samples frequently demonstrate immune complexes of IgG in the fluid and phagocytic cells. The concentration of complement in synovial fluid is low. The responsible antigen for this immune sequence has not been identified. Although exhaustive viral studies have failed to isolate an antigen, there remains the possibility that viral infection or alteration of normal tissues may be a cause. It remains unclear whether the host or the disease is different in adult and juvenile rheumatoid arthritis.

Clinical Findings

A. Symptoms and Signs: There are 3 patterns of presentation in juvenile rheumatoid arthritis which provide clues to the prognosis and possible sequelae of the disease. In the acute febrile form, which is most common in children under age 4, an evanescent salmon-pink macular rash, arthritis, hepatosplenomegaly, leukocytosis, and polyserositis characterize the constellation described by George Still. These patients have episodic illness, and remission of the systemic features can be expected within 1 year. They do not develop iridocyclitis.

The polyarticular pattern resembles the adult disease, with chronic pain and swelling of many joints in a symmetric fashion. Both large and small joints are usually involved. Systemic features are less prominent, though low-grade fever, fatigue, rheumatoid nodules, and anemia may be present. These patients tend to have long-standing arthritis, although the disease may wax and wane. Iridocyclitis is occasionally seen in this group.

The third pattern is the pauciarticular subset who have chronic arthritis of a few joints, often the large, weight-bearing joints in an asymmetric distribution. The synovitis is usually mild and may be painless. Systemic features are uncommon, but there is serious extra-articular involvement with inflammation in the eye. Up to 30% of children with pauciarticular juvenile rheumatoid arthritis develop insidious, asymptomatic iridocyclitis which frequently causes blindness. The activity of the eye disease does not correlate with the activity of the arthritis. Therefore, routine ophthalmologic screening with slitlamp examination must be performed every 6 months until puberty.

B. Laboratory Findings: There is no diagnostic test for juvenile rheumatoid arthritis. Rheumatoid factor tests are positive in only 10–20% of cases, more often in those with older age at onset. Antinuclear antibodies (ANA) are present in patients with iridocyclitis and may serve as an index of this complication. The acute phase reactants (ESR, CRP, a_2-globulins, and gamma globulins) are nonspecifically elevated. A normal ESR does not exclude the diagnosis. Synovial fluid examination is rarely performed in childhood but will establish the presence of inflammation or infection, especially in monarticular cases.

C. X-Ray Findings: In the early stages of the disease, only soft tissue swelling and regional osteoporosis are seen. In a few patients, late changes will include irreversible articular erosions, ankylosis, and premature epiphyseal closure. Cervical subluxation should be monitored by radiographs in patients with neck pain.

Differential Diagnosis

Monarticular arthritis is the most important differential disorder to establish. Pain in the hip or lower extremity is a frequent symptom with childhood malignancy, especially leukemia, neuroblastoma, and rhabdomyosarcoma. Infiltration of bone by tumor and actual joint effusion may be seen. X-rays of the affected site and a careful examination of the blood smear for unusual cells and thrombocytopenia are necessary. In doubtful cases, bone marrow examination is indicated.

Infectious arthritis is usually acute and monarticular except for arthritis associated with *Haemophilus influenzae* and gonorrhea, both of which are associated with a migratory pattern. Fever, leukocytosis, and increased ESR with an acute process in a single joint demand synovial fluid examination and culture to identify the pathogen. An elevated synovial fluid white count and low glucose (relative to plasma glucose) suggest sepsis.

The arthritis of rheumatic fever is migratory, transient, and often more painful than that of juvenile rheumatoid arthritis. Rheumatic fever is very rare under the age of 4 years. The murmur of rheumatic endocarditis should be carefully sought. Evidence of recent streptococcal infection is not specific for either condition. The fever pattern in rheumatic fever is low-grade and persistent in comparison to the intermittent fever in the systemic form of juvenile rheumatoid arthritis.

Articular involvement with inflammatory bowel disease, ankylosing spondylitis, psoriasis, and Reiter's syndrome most often involves the lower extremities and frequently the heel. If there are associated abdominal complaints, weight loss, etc, contrast x-rays are indicated. Arthritis is the most frequent symptom of systemic lupus erythematosus; a careful history and investigation for multisystem disease will establish the diagnosis.

Treatment

The objective of therapy is to restore function, relieve pain, and maintain joint motion. Salicylates are the treatment of choice at the outset. Aspirin, 75–100 mg/kg/day in 4 divided doses, will frequently relieve pain and inflammation and allow good physical therapy. A self-limited hepatotoxicity occurs with high-dose salicylate therapy, and most patients can continue to take aspirin. Range of motion exercises and muscle strengthening should be taught and supervised by a therapist and a home program instituted. In patients who fail to respond to aspirin, there are a number of alternatives. Prednisone in doses of less than 5 mg daily is sometimes of great value and does not seem to worsen an already poor growth pattern. Corticosteroids are also of value as a temporary measure during acute flare-ups and when there is acute systemic disease or iridocyclitis. Gold salts are of proved efficacy. The dose is 1 mg/kg/week of gold salt (eg, gold sodium thiomalate) IM. As symptoms are controlled, the frequency of injection can be gradually decreased. Regular white counts and urine testing for protein must be done. The newer nonsteroidal anti-inflammatory agents such as tolmetin, ibuprofen, and naproxen appear to offer little advantage over aspirin. Penicillamine is currently under investigation. Its potency and toxicity are similar to those of gold.

Immunosuppressive therapy with cytotoxic drugs such as cyclophosphamide remains experimental and should be reserved for patients who have failed to respond to other forms of therapy.

Iridocyclitis should be treated by an ophthalmologist. Orthopedic consultation on a regular basis is helpful, although surgery is seldom necessary.

Prognosis

In the primarily articular forms, disease activity progressively diminishes with age and ceases in about 95% of cases by puberty. In a few instances, this will persist into adult life. Problems after puberty therefore relate primarily to residual joint damage. Cases presenting in the teen years usually presage adult disease. The children most liable to be permanently handicapped are those with unremitting synovitis, hip involvement, or positive rheumatoid factor tests. Death may occur from persistent carditis or renal amyloidosis.

Calabro JJ: Management of juvenile rheumatoid arthritis. J Pediatr 77:355, 1970.

Schaller J: Juvenile rheumatoid arthritis: A review. Pediatrics 50:940, 1972.

Schaller JG & others: Histocompatibility antigens in childhood-onset arthritis. J Pediatr 88:926, 1976.

Sullivan DB & others: Pathogenic implications of age of onset in juvenile rheumatoid arthritis. Arthritis Rheum 18:251, 1975.

SYSTEMIC LUPUS ERYTHEMATOSUS

Essentials of Diagnosis

- Multisystem inflammatory disease of joints, serous linings, skin, kidneys, and CNS.
- Antinuclear antibodies (ANA) must be present in active, untreated disease.

General Considerations

Systemic lupus erythematosus (SLE) is the prototype of immune complex diseases; its pathogenesis is related to deposition in the tissue of soluble immune complexes existing in the circulation. The spectrum of symptoms in systemic lupus erythematosus appears to be due not to tissue-specific autoantibodies but rather to damage to the tissue by lymphocytes, neutrophils, and complement evoked by the deposition of antigen-antibody complexes. In systemic lupus erythematosus, many such antigen-antibody systems are present, but the best correlation exists between DNA-anti-DNA complexes and the activity of the disease. Laboratory tests of these antibodies and complement components give an objective assessment of disease pathogenesis and response to therapy. The trigger for the formation of immune complexes in systemic lupus erythematosus has not been identified. It is clear that altered cellular and humoral immunity exists from the time of onset in these patients, and data from animal models suggest that the immune aberrations antedate the disease.

A drug-related syndrome resembling systemic lupus erythematosus may be produced by procainamide, hydantoin compounds, and isoniazid, among others. These patients recover on stopping the drug and do not manifest renal disease.

Clinical Findings:

A. Symptoms and Signs: The onset is most common in females (8:1) between the ages of 9 and 15 years. The symptoms depend on what organ is involved with immune complex deposition.

1. Joint symptoms are the commonest presenting feature. Nondeforming arthritis may involve any joint, often in a symmetric manner. Myositis may also occur and is more painful than the inflammation in dermatomyositis.

2. Systemic manifestations include weakness, anorexia, fever, malaise, and loss of weight.

3. Skin lesions include butterfly erythema and induration, small ulcerations in skin and mucous membranes, purpura, alopecia, and Raynaud's phenomenon. The sun sensitivity of the dermal lesions may be striking.

4. Polyserositis may include pleurisy with effusions, peritonitis, and pericarditis. Libman-Sacks endocarditis is rarely seen since corticosteroids became available for treatment.

5. Hepatosplenomegaly and lymphadenopathy may occur.

6. Renal systemic lupus erythematosus produces few symptoms at onset but is often progressive and is the leading cause of death. Renal biopsy is indicated in all patients with evidence of renal involvement since the course of the renal disease varies with the lesion produced by immune complex deposition in the glomerular basement membrane. Late complications are nephrosis and uremia.

7. CNS involvement produces a variety of symptoms such as seizures, coma, hemiplegia, focal neuropathies, and behavior disturbances, including psychosis. The psychosis may be impossible to distinguish from corticosteroid-induced psychosis. Neurologic disease is now the second leading cause of death in systemic lupus erythematosus.

B. Laboratory Findings: Leukopenia and anemia are frequently found with a high incidence of Coombs positivity. Thrombocytopenia and purpura may be early manifestations even in the absence of other organ involvement. The ESR is elevated, and hypergammaglobulinemia is often present. Renal involvement is indicated by the presence in the urine of red cells, white cells, red cell casts, and proteinuria. Azotemia indicates severe involvement.

The antinuclear antibody (ANA) test is the most sensitive diagnostic test and has supplanted the LE preparation. The ANA test is invariably positive in patients with active untreated systemic lupus erythematosus, and a negative ANA test effectively excludes the diagnosis. Punch biopsy of involved and uninvolved skin in SLE shows deposits of immunoglobulin and complement at the dermal-epidermal junction. This rapid technic may be of aid in diagnostically difficult cases.

In managing the disease, elevated titers of anti-DNA antibody and depressed levels of serum complement (hemolytic, C3, or C4) accurately reflect active disease, especially renal, CNS, and skin disease.

Differential Diagnosis

Systemic lupus erythematosus may simulate many inflammatory diseases such as rheumatic fever, rheumatoid arthritis, and viral infections. It is essential to review all organ systems carefully to establish a clinical pattern. Renal and CNS involvement are unique to systemic lupus erythematosus. A negative ANA test excludes the diagnosis of systemic lupus erythematosus.

An overlap syndrome known as mixed connective tissue disease (MCTD), with features of several collagen-vascular diseases, has recently been described in adults and children. The symptom complex is diverse and does not readily fit previous classifications. Arthritis, fever, skin tightening, Raynaud's phenomenon, muscle weakness, and rashes are most commonly present. The importance in recognition of this disease entity is the relative infrequency of renal disease, which implies a better prognosis than SLE, and the steroid responsiveness of symptoms, which distinguishes MCTD from scleroderma. The definition of the disease includes the presence of serum antibody to an extractable nuclear antigen (ENA). Patients are initially identified by a speckled pattern of immunofluorescence in the ANA test. The specialized ENA test demonstrates very high titers of up to 1:1,000,000 of the antibody. Other laboratory findings include leukopenia and occasionally severe thrombocytopenia.

Treatment

The treatment of systemic lupus erythematosus should be tailored to the organ system involved so that toxicities may be minimized. Prednisone, 0.5–1 mg/kg/day orally, has significantly lowered the mortality rate in systemic lupus erythematosus and should be used in all cases with renal, cardiac, or CNS involvement. The dose should be varied using clinical and laboratory parameters of disease activity, and the minimum amount of corticosteroid to control the disease should be used. Alternate-day regimens of corticosteroid are frequently possible. Skin manifestations may frequently be treated with antimalarials, eg, hydroxychloroquine, 4 mg/kg/day orally. Pleuritic pain or arthritis can often be managed with salicylates alone.

If disease control is inadequate with prednisone or if the dose required produces intolerable side-effects, an immunosuppressant should be added. Either azathioprine, 2–3 mg/kg/day orally, or cyclophosphamide, 1–2 mg/kg/day orally, has been most widely used. These drugs are ineffective during acute crises such as seizures.

The toxicities of the regimens must be carefully considered. In life-threatening disease, the choices are easier. Growth failure, osteoporosis, Cushing's syndrome, adrenal suppression, and aseptic necrosis are serious side-effects of chronic use of prednisone. When high doses of corticosteroids are used (over 2 mg/kg/day), the risk of sepsis is very real. Cyclophosphamide causes bladder epithelial dysplasia, hemorrhagic cystitis, and sterility. Azathioprine has been associated with liver damage and bone marrow suppression. Immunosuppressant treatment should be withheld if the total white count falls below 3000/cu mm or the neutrophil count below 1000/cu mm. Retinal damage from chloroquine derivatives has not been observed in the recommended dosage.

Amenorrhea may result from uncontrolled systemic lupus erythematosus but may also be a consequence of prednisone, cyclophosphamide, or azathioprine administration.

Course & Prognosis

The prognosis in systemic lupus erythematosus relates to the presence of renal or CNS involvement. With improved diagnosis, milder cases of systemic lupus erythematosus are now identified. Nonetheless, the 5-year survival rate has risen from 51% in 1954 to 77% in 1974. The disease has a natural waxing and waning cycle, and periods of complete remission are not unusual. Hemodialysis and renal transplantation can be considered if medical treatment does not prevent renal insufficiency. Cessation of treatment in severe cases may lead to an unmanageable relapse.

Decker J & others: Systemic lupus erythematosus. Ann Intern Med 82:391, 1975.
Garin EH & others: Nephritis in systemic lupus erythematosus in children. J Pediatr 89:366, 1976.
Schwartz RS: Viruses and systemic lupus erythematosus. N Engl J Med 293:132, 1975.
Singsen BH & others: Mixed connective tissue disease in childhood. J Pediatr 90:893, 1977.
Singsen BH & others: Systemic lupus erythematosus in childhood: Correlations between changes in disease activity and serum complement levels. J Pediatr 89:358, 1976.

DERMATOMYOSITIS
(Polymyositis)

Essentials of Diagnosis

- Pathognomonic skin rash.
- Weakness of proximal muscles and occasionally of pharyngeal and laryngeal groups.
- Pathogenesis related to vasculitis.

General Considerations

Dermatomyositis is a rare inflammatory disease of muscle and skin in childhood which is uniquely responsive to corticosteroid treatment. The vasculitis observed in childhood dermatomyositis differs pathologically from the adult disease. Small arteries and veins are involved, with an exudate of neutrophils, lymphocytes, plasma cells, and histiocytes. The lesion progresses to intimal proliferation and thrombus formation. These vascular changes are found in the skin, muscle, kidney, retina, and gastrointestinal tract. Muscle regeneration is unusual in childhood disease. Postinflammatory calcinosis is frequent.

The autoimmune pathogenesis of dermatomyositis has been difficult to prove. Recent studies have shown that both cellular and humoral mechanisms may be involved. Lymphocytes from patients are stimulated to undergo blastogenesis in the presence of muscle tissue and will release lymphotoxin, which destroys cultured fetal muscle cells. Biopsies studied with immunofluorescent technics demonstrate immunoglobulin and complement in a perivascular distribution. The putative antigen has not been identified. Suggestive data relating adult myositis to toxoplasmosis have not been found in children, and results of viral studies have been negative.

Clinical Findings

A. Symptoms and Signs: The predominant symptom is muscular weakness in a proximal distribution affecting pelvic and shoulder girdles. Tenderness, stiffness, and swelling may be found but are not striking. Neurologic findings such as absence of tendon reflexes are not seen until late in the disease. Pharyngeal and respiratory involvement can be life-threatening. Flexion contractures and muscle atrophy produce significant residual deformities. Calcinosis may follow the inflammation in muscle and skin. Vasculitis of the intestine causing hemorrhage or perforation is less frequently seen in recent years, perhaps due to corticosteroid treatment.

The rash of dermatomyositis is very helpful in the diagnosis of unknown muscle disease. Characteristically, the rash involves the upper eyelids and extensor surfaces of the knuckles, elbows, and knees with a distinctive heliotrope color which progresses to a scaling and atrophic appearance. Periorbital edema is not uncommon. Late lesions include telangiectatic vessels on the face and extremities. None of the rashes associated with other childhood rheumatic diseases have these features of distribution. The activity of the rash frequently does not parallel the muscle disease.

B. Laboratory Findings: Elevation of muscle enzymes is the most helpful tool in diagnosis and treatment. All enzymes, including SGOT, should be screened to detect an abnormality that reflects activity of the disease. The blood count, ESR, and acute phase reactants are frequently normal. No autoantibodies are found. Electromyography is useful to distinguish myopathic from neuropathic causes of muscle weakness. Muscle biopsy is indicated in doubtful cases of myositis without the pathognomonic rash.

Treatment

Prednisone in high doses (1–2 mg/kg/day orally) has been shown to speed recovery. The dose should be maintained or increased until muscle enzymes have returned to normal. Functional recovery will lag somewhat behind laboratory improvement. With improvement, the dose may be cut to that level which maintains disease control and normal muscle enzymes. Treatment must be continued for an average of 2 years. Immunosuppressant agents are rarely required in childhood dermatomyositis. Physical therapy is critical to prevent or allay contractures.

Course & Prognosis

Most children will recover and be off medications in 1–3 years. Relapses may occur. Functional ability is very good in most patients. Myositis in childhood is not associated with an increased risk of malignancy.

Jacobs J: Methotrexate and azathioprine treatment of childhood dermatomyositis. Pediatrics 59:212, 1977.

Rose AL: Childhood polymyositis. Am J Dis Child 127:518, 1974.

Sullivan DB: Prognosis in childhood dermatomyositis. J Pediatr 80:555, 1972.

Whitaker JN: Vascular deposits of immunoglobulin and complement in idiopathic inflammatory myopathy. N Engl J Med 286:333, 1972.

POLYARTERITIS NODOSA

Polyarteritis nodosa is a rare disease, but a significant number of cases have been reported in childhood and infancy. No single cause has been found, but immune complex deposition as typified by HBAg may mediate the inflammatory events.

Pathologically, the disease is a vasculitis of medium-sized arteries with fibrinoid degeneration in the media extending to the intima and adventitia. Neutrophils and eosinophils comprise the inflammatory reaction. Aneurysms may be palpated or seen radiographically. Thrombosis of diseased arteries may cause infarction in many organs. Fibrosis of vessels and surrounding tissues accompanies the healing stages.

Symptomatology involves many tissues, and diagnosis is difficult. In childhood, unexplained fever, conjunctivitis, CNS involvement, and cardiac disease are more prominent than is the case in adult disease. Many cases appear as acute myocarditis, and the peripheral neuropathy so common in the adult is unusual. Diagnosis depends on biopsy-proved vasculitis. Testicular biopsy may be helpful if accessible tissue is not available. Mucocutaneous lymph node syndrome is a recently described entity with many pathologic similarities to polyarteritis nodosa.

The mortality rate is high, especially with cardiac involvement. Treatment consists of prednisone, 1–1.5 mg/kg/day orally, and azathioprine, 1–2 mg/kg/day orally, but controlled studies of the efficacy of therapy of this rare disease are not yet available.

Benyo RB, Perrin EB: Polyarteritis nodosa in infancy. Am J Dis Child 116:539, 1968.

Brown JS & others: Mucocutaneous lymph node syndrome in the continental United States. J Pediatr 88:81, 1976.

Gocke DJ & others: Association between polyarteritis nodosa and Australia antigen. Lancet 2:1149, 1970.

DIFFUSE SCLERODERMA
(Progressive Systemic Sclerosis)

Scleroderma is a rare disease in childhood. Both the generalized systemic type and the more localized benign form (morphea) have been described. The diagnosis is made on a clinical basis with the finding of a skin disease which progresses from an edematous phase to an atrophic, taut, immobile dermis involving some or all of the skin. Systemic involvement may include Raynaud's phenomenon, arthralgias, pulmonary fibrosis, and renal disease. Involvement of the lungs and kidneys leads to rapid demise. Histologically, the diagnosis may not be specific but includes dermal atrophy with increased fibrosis and collagen content. The pathogenesis remains obscure, but recent studies indicate an increased synthesis of immature collagen by cultured scleroderma fibroblasts.

There is no effective medical treatment of scleroderma. Physical therapy is sometimes helpful in reducing debilitation from contractures and muscle wasting.

Dobick L, Sullivan DB, Cassidy JT: Scleroderma in the child. J Pediatr 85:770, 1974.

Goel KM, Shanks RA: Scleroderma in childhood. Arch Dis Child 49:861, 1974.

MARFAN'S SYNDROME

First discovered by Marfan in 1896, this syndrome is now considered to be a diffuse abnormality of elastic tissue inherited as an autosomal dominant. The molecular defect is unknown, although the high urinary excretion of hydroxyproline indicates an increased rate of turnover of connective tissue fiber. Clinically, the impact of these changes is on the skeletal and cardiovascular systems and the eyes. Patients are characteristically tall and thin, and the upper body segment is proportionately shorter than the lower. In addition to arachnodactyly of the fingers and great toes, bony defects include pectus carinatum and excavatum, a long narrow face and pointed head, high-arched palate, and kyphoscoliosis. The attendant laxity in the ligaments leads to pes planus, winging of the scapulas, genu recurvatum, and subluxation of the patellas, hips, elbows, and other joints. Femoral and diaphragmatic hernias are noted.

Weakening of the aortic media leads to aneurysms, usually of the ascending aorta, which may involve the valve. Lax chordae may lead to mitral as well as aortic incompetence. The pulmonary artery may be dilated. Dislocation of the lens due to weakness of the suspensory ligaments is characteristic but may be confused with homocystinuria. Blue scleras, myopia, retinal detachment, and megalocornea are other abnormalities of the eye, and glaucoma, iridocyclitis, and interstitial keratitis are complications of these disorders.

There is no specific treatment, although surgical correction of the cardiovascular complications may be appropriate. Prognosis is governed by the severity of these cardiovascular lesions. Homocystinuria should be excluded.

Murdoch JL & others: Life expectancy and causes of death in the Marfan syndrome. N Engl J Med 286:804, 1972.

Siggers DC: Marfan syndrome treated with propranolol. Birth Defects 11(2):332, 1975.

EHLERS-DANLOS SYNDROME

This is a rare heritable disorder of collagen which is probably transmitted as an autosomal dominant.

Characteristically, the skin is pale, soft, and strikingly hyperextensible without being lax. Subcutaneous nodules develop over pressure points, and the skin in these areas is especially subject to trauma and the formation of shiny, parchment-like, atrophic scars. The joints are hyperextensible, and there is a tendency to dislocation of hips, patellas, elbows, clavicles, and shoulders. Blue scleras, wide epicanthal folds, and dislocation of the lens and other eye signs occur.

A number of other congenital defects have been described in association with this syndrome, notably hiatus hernia, gastrointestinal diverticula, urinary tract anomalies, and aortic aneurysm and insufficiency, the latter being conspicuously difficult to repair because of tissue friability.

There is no specific treatment.

Lichenstein JR & others: Defect in conversion of procollagen to collagen in a form of Danlos-Ehlers. Science 182:298, 1973.

McKusick VA: Multiple forms of the Ehlers-Danlos syndrome. Arch Surg 109:475, 1974.

21...
Neurologic & Muscular Disorders

Gerhard Nellhaus, MD

DISORDERS OF INFANTS & CHILDREN AFFECTING THE NERVOUS SYSTEM

ALTERED STATES OF CONSCIOUSNESS

In the patient who is comatose, stuporous, or drowsy, emergency measures must precede history.

(1) Check respiration, pulse, and color. Ensure an open airway. Consider endotracheal intubation or tracheostomy and administration of oxygen as well as respiratory assistance by mechanical means.

(2) Treat for shock if evident or imminent.

(3) Take measures to prevent or treat increased intracranial pressure. For details, see p 553.

(4) In known or suspected diabetes, consider insulin reaction and administer glucose intravenously or, if the patient can swallow, orange juice orally.

Causes of Sudden Altered States of Consciousness

(1) **Postictal state.**

(2) **Poisoning:** Common intoxicants in children include salicylates, anticonvulsants, antihistamines, tranquilizers, sedatives, or a mixture of drugs. Ethyl alcohol may cause profound hypoglycemia and coma. Inhalants such as "glue" and carbon monoxide or insecticides must be considered. Heavy metals usually produce an altered state of consciousness over a prolonged period of time.

(3) **Infections:** Bacterial, viral, mycotic, or rickettsial infections causing alterations of consciousness are usually accompanied by signs of meningitis or encephalitis, and rarely come on suddenly.

(4) **Trauma:** Brain concussion, contusion, and subdural, epidural, or intracerebral hematomas may cause states of altered consciousness. Abdominal trauma resulting in rupture of the spleen or liver may cause massive bleeding with shock and coma.

(5) **Illnesses:** Illnesses to be considered are various intracranial disturbances such as subarachnoid hemorrhage or cerebral infarction; increased intracranial pressure, as may result from obstruction of CSF pathways, tumors, or other space-occupying lesions; and "toxic encephalopathy." Primarily extracranial illnesses caus-

ing coma include diabetic coma, hyperinsulinism, liver failure, and uremia.

(6) **Combined causes:** Keep this possibility in mind, particularly with respect to an intoxicant and trauma.

Clinical Findings

The degree of alteration of the state of consciousness should be carefully noted and characterized as accurately as possible as coma, semicoma, stupor, drowsiness, or light sleep.

A. Symptoms and Signs:

1. Breathing patterns may give a clue to the underlying cause of the disorder.

a. Slow and deep breathing may be seen in heavy sleep caused by sedatives, following seizures, or in cerebral infections.

b. Slow and often shallow breathing, which may be periodic, is also seen as a result of ingestion of sedatives or narcotics.

c. Hyperventilation or irregular breathing is often associated with brain stem damage.

d. Cheyne-Stokes breathing is seen in a variety of disorders, often with symmetrical deep cerebral or diencephalic lesions.

e. Deep and rapid (Kussmaul) respirations suggest acidosis.

f. Blowing out of one cheek suggests ipsilateral facial paralysis.

g. The odor of the breath may be helpful, eg, the fruity odor of ketosis, the foul odor of uremia, or the odor of alcohol.

2. Alterations in pulse and in the color of the skin and mucous membranes will vary, as in shock, carbon monoxide poisoning, heat exhaustion, etc.

3. Inspection of the head and body should be done rapidly but carefully for evidence of injury, needle marks, petechiae, and ticks. Particularly in small children, examine the face, mouth, hands, and clothing for evidence of ingestion of toxic substances.

4. Fever suggests acute infection or heat stroke but is also seen in the postictal state and with intracranial bleeding. Hypothermia suggests ingestion of intoxicants (especially barbiturates and alcohol) or shock.

5. Nuchal rigidity suggests meningitis, subarachnoid hemorrhage, or herniation of cerebellar tonsils.

However, nuchal rigidity as a sign of the above may disappear in deep coma.

6. Eyes—(*Caution:* Do not dilate the pupils, as this obliterates critical neurologic signs.)

a. Widely dilated but reactive pupils, sometimes on one side only, are often seen in postictal states.

b. Widely dilated, fixed pupils suggest third nerve paralysis due to tentorial herniation (unless mydriatics have been used).

c. A unilateral fixed pupil usually suggests an expanding lesion on the same side but may be a false localizing sign.

d. Pinpoint pupils are commonly seen with poisonings, eg, with opiates or barbiturates, or in brain stem disorders (hemorrhage, etc).

e. Papilledema indicates increased intracranial pressure. In infants and small children, the presence of subhyaloid hemorrhages is almost always indicative of acute trauma with intracranial bleeding.

f. Visual field examination may be attempted in the lightly comatose or stuporous patient, who may blink in response to threatening movements of the hand coming in from the field of vision to be tested.

g. Check whether eye movements are conjugate or not. Disconjugate movements suggest brain stem lesions. Conjugate deviation of the eyes occurs toward the side of cerebral lesions.

7. Extremities—Asymmetric movements of the limbs or failure to move one side either spontaneously or in response to pain suggests paralysis. A hemiplegic limb will fall uncontrollably.

8. Reflexes—Testing of reflexes may be of limited value.

a. Absence of corneal reflexes usually indicates severe brain damage.

b. A positive Babinski sign may be of value if consistently present, especially if associated with other pyramidal tract signs on the same side. Fluctuating Babinski signs are often observed following seizures or in other states causing stupor.

c. Check for oculomotor paresis by performing the doll's eye maneuver (oculocephalic reflex).

d. The presence of a tonic neck reflex suggests profound brain damage.

B. Laboratory Evaluation: Best guided by the suspected cause:

1. Urinalysis—Urinalysis is generally the most helpful test. It may be necessary to catheterize the patient.

a. Glycosuria is seen in patients with diabetes, salicylism, and sometimes lead poisoning or cerebrovascular accidents.

b. Ketonuria suggests diabetes or starvation state.

c. Proteinuria is seen with renal disease, high fevers, and often lead and other poisonings.

d. A red to purple color on testing the urine with ferric chloride or Phenistix is seen in salicylism and phenothiazine ingestion.

e. Bilirubinuria suggests liver failure.

f. Coproporphyrinuria suggests lead poisoning or other heavy metal intoxication.

2. Blood—

a. Draw blood for typing and cross-matching if transfusion or surgery appears necessary.

b. Blood glucose, urea nitrogen, and pH; serum sodium, chloride, and HCO_3^-.

c. Liver function studies as indicated. High enzyme levels and ammonia, with low bilirubin, are seen in Reye's·syndrome.

d. Blood cultures if fever is present.

e. Complete blood count and differential count. Check for "stippling" in small children suspected of having lead poisoning.

f. Draw blood for toxicologic studies whenever intoxication is suspected.

3. Gastric contents—Aspirate for diagnostic and therapeutic reasons.

4. Lumbar puncture—Lumbar puncture should be performed immediately **only** when intracranial infection or toxic encephalopathy is suspected. This study can be delayed when intracranial hemorrhage is most likely and is, with rare exceptions, contraindicated in the presence of increased intracranial pressure due to a mass lesion. *Note:* The importance of obtaining CSF opening and closing pressure readings cannot be stressed enough. Papilledema is *not* a contraindication to lumbar puncture if infection is suspected; however, only a small gauge needle should be used, and only enough CSF should be withdrawn to permit cell count, protein and glucose determination, and such stains and cultures (bacterial, fungal, viral) and other studies as may be helpful. Two to 3 ml are usually adequate where microchemistry is available. (See Table 21−1.)

C. Echoencephalography: This rapid, noninvasive technic may aid in the diagnosis of cerebral edema, hydrocephalus, shift of the third ventricle or other midline structures, or large intracranial lesions such as hematomas.

D. X-Ray Evaluation: X-rays should be taken when severe head trauma, spinal cord injuries, or abdominal trauma are suspected. Nonessential x-ray studies should be deferred until the patient can cooperate or at least until he is not in an agitated or precarious state.

E. Criteria for "Brain Death"*: Legal statutes governing certification of "brain death," or, in their absence, acceptable precedents or standards, vary with governmental entities and time and must be known to the attending physician. A collaborative study in the USA recently recommended the following basic criteria for field trial:

1. Prerequisite—All appropriate diagnostic and therapeutic measures have been performed, including survey for sedative drugs, computerized tomography, radioisotope scan, or angiography, as required to rule out reversible conditions.

2. Criteria (to be present for 30 minutes at least 6

---

*Note: In contrast to "brain death," irreversible coma refers to a vegetative state in which all cerebral functions are lost but such vital functions as respiration, temperature, and blood pressure regulation may be maintained.

hours after onset of coma and apnea)—

a. Coma with cerebral unresponsiveness, ie, no purposeful responses. Spinal reflexes, usually easily differentiated, are nondiagnostic.

b. Apnea, ie, no spontaneous respirations when checked periodically over a 15-minute interval.

c. Absent cephalic reflexes, ie, those of brain stem origin.

d. Dilated fixed pupils. This is not a constant feature. Pupils may be unequal. Most sedative and narcotic drugs (except glutethimide) produce pupillary constriction.

e. Electrocerebral silence, ie, a "flat" or isoelectric EEG at maximal gains for 30 minutes. A single such recording, together with cerebral unresponsiveness and apnea, is usually diagnostic except in drug-induced coma.

3. Confirmation—Absence of cerebral blood flow. Such a demonstration by angiography or bedside brain flow study using an intravenously injected isotope is a safeguard when the diagnosis of cerebral death may be considered at a time when other criteria have not been unequivocally met. This may include patients with small amounts of sedative drugs in their blood, those with small nonreactive pupils, those undergoing therapeutic procedures making examination of brain stem function impossible, or those being considered as organ donors.

Treatment

The principle of treatment is to provide specific measures for specific problems. Emergency treatment measures are outlined at the beginning of this section.

A. General Measures:

1. Above all, maintain vital functions.

2. Observe vital signs, the state of the pupils, and levels of consciousness closely.

3. Turn the patient frequently to prevent hypostatic pneumonia.

4. Provide fluids by the intravenous route initially and by nasogastric feedings or gastrostomy if coma is prolonged.

5. Bladder care may require catheterization.

6. Avoid administration of sedatives but provide anticonvulsants when needed. Phenytoin is least likely to cloud consciousness. If the patient is very agitated and restlessness threatens to result in injuries, sedate the patient with diphenhydramine, chloral hydrate, or occasionally paraldehyde.

7. Prophylactic antibiotic therapy is rarely warranted. Where a CSF dural leak is present, antibiotics should be used as for meningitis.

B. Cerebral Edema: Treat when cerebral edema is anticipated (as after significant hypoxia or head trauma) or present (as evident by papilledema). Often a combination of approaches is necessary.

1. Physiologic program—

a. Fluid restriction to maintenance requirements, taking into consideration body temperature, tracheostomy, mist tent, and other controlling factors.

b. Hypothermia, which also reduces cerebral metabolism. Temperature should not fall below 32° C (89.6° F). It is less favored now than previously, with normothermia preferred.

c. Controlled hyperventilation, often a relatively temporary measure or instituted only in the tracheostomized patient. Arterial blood gases, especially P_{CO_2}, should be monitored carefully.

2. Corticosteroids—Used both prophylactically, especially preoperatively, and therapeutically.

a. Dexamethasone sodium phosphate, 0.15–0.25 mg/kg body weight IV initially, followed by 0.25 mg/kg/day IM in 3 or 4 doses; often tapered after 72 hours over a 3- to 4-day period.

b. Methylprednisolone sodium succinate in 4–5 times the dosage of dexamethasone (above).

3. Hypertonic solutions—These are most effective in acute cerebral edema while other therapy is being instituted. Serum electrolytes and osmolality should be monitored carefully.

a. Urea in 30% saline solution, 1–1.5 gm/kg body weight IV every 6–8 hours. This is the best established and probably the most rapidly acting agent but produces the greatest "rebound."

b. Mannitol in 20% solution, 1–3 gm (often 1.5–2 gm)/kg IV every 6 hours. Often given repeatedly in smaller doses over several days.

c. Glycerol, 10% in saline solution, 1–3 gm/kg IV every 6 hours. Also given by nasogastric tube over a longer period of time; it has the least "rebound."

4. Surgical adjuncts—Consider these when medical therapy is inadequate and *before* irreversible uncal or tonsillar herniation occurs.

a. External ventricular drainage to control CSF pressure.

b. Decompressive craniectomy, as an extreme recourse, when a bifrontal bitemporal craniotomy (Kjellberg method) should be considered.

Prognosis

The prognosis depends on the underlying cause, the severity of the brain damage, and the infections to which the patient with severe depression of consciousness is especially susceptible.

An appraisal of the criteria of cerebral death: A collaborative study. JAMA 237:982, 1977.

Ausman JI, Rogers C, Sharp HL: Decompressive craniectomy for the encephalopathy of Reye's syndrome. Surg Neurol 6:97, 1976.

Batzdorf U: The management of cerebral edema in pediatric practice. Pediatrics 58:78, 1976.

Craigmile TK, Welch K: Lumbar puncture and analysis of cerebrospinal fluid. Chapter 10 in: *Neurological Surgery.* Youmans J (editor). Saunders, 1973.

Parvey LS, Gerald B: Arteriographic diagnosis of brain death in children. Pediatr Radiol 4:79, 1976.

Plum F, Posner JB: *The Diagnosis of Stupor and Coma,* 2nd ed. Davis, 1972.

Table 21–1. Characteristics of CSF in the normal child and in some neurologic disorders.

Disease	Initial Pressure (mm H₂O)	Appearance	Cells	Protein (mg/100 ml)	Sugar (mg/100 ml)	Other Tests	Comments
Normal	< 180 mm	Clear	0–5 (some accept up to 10) mononuclear cells.	15–35 (lumbar) 5–15 (ventricular) Up to 150 (lumbar) after birth, declining rapidly.	50–80 (two-thirds of blood glucose)	Gamma globulin 8.2% or less of protein. Lactate dehydrogenase (LDH), 2–30 IU/liter.	CSF protein in first month may be up to 75 mg/100 ml, and higher in small-for-dates or premature infants; 20–50 red cells in the first days of life.
Bloody tap	Normal or low	Bloody (sometimes with clot)	One white cell for each 700 red cells.	1 mg protein for each 800 erythrocytes above "normal."	Normal		Spin down fluid; supernatant will be clear and colorless.
Acute bacterial meningitis	200–750+	Opalescent to purulent	100 to many thousands, mostly PMNs.	50 to many hundreds.	Decreased; may be none.	Smear and culture mandatory for identification. LDH > 30 IU/liter.	Blood, nose, and throat cultures; very early, sugar may be normal.
Partially treated bacterial meningitis	Usually increased	Clear or opalescent	Usually increased, PMNs usually predominate.	Elevated	Normal or decreased	LDH > 30 IU/liter.	Smear and culture often negative.
Postmeningitic hydrocephalus	Variable	Clear	0–10	Variable; may be low.	Often low	Smear and bacterial cultures negative.	Low CSF glucose may be due to disturbance in transport mechanism.
Tuberculous meningitis	150–750+	Opalescent	250–500. Monocytes predominate.	45–500	Decreased; may be none.	Smear for acid-fast organism; culture and inoculation of CSF.	Very early, PMNs may predominate; tuberculin skin test almost always positive except in fulminant cases; chest x-ray.
Fungal meningitis	Increased	Variable; often clear	10–500; early, mostly PMNs; late, mostly monocytes.	Elevated and increasing	Decreased	India ink preparations, culture, inoculations, immunofluorescence tests.	Often superimposed in patients who are debilitated or on immunosuppressive or tumor therapy.
Brain abscess	Normal or increased	Usually clear	5–500 in 80%; mostly PMNs.	Usually slightly increased	Normal; occasionally decreased.		Cell count related to proximity to meninges; findings of purulent meningitis if abscess perforates.
Acute poliomyelitis	Usually normal	Clear or slightly opalescent	10–500+, mostly monocytes; PMNs early.	Normal to 350; often progressive increase.	Normal		Stool virus and serum antibody studies.
Polyneuritis: Early	Normal and occasionally increased	Normal	Normal; occasionally slight increase.	Normal	Normal	Bacterial cultures negative; gamma globulin may be elevated.	Try to find etiology: viral infections, toxins, lupus, infectious mononucleosis, diabetes, etc.
Late		Xanthochromic if protein high		45–1500			
Aseptic meningoencephalitides	Normal or slightly increased	Clear unless cell count is above 300	0 to few hundred, mainly monocytes.	20–125	Normal; may be low in mumps.	CSF, stool, throat wash for viral cultures. LDH < 30 IU/liter.	Acute and convalescent serum antibody studies. Marked pleocytosis (up to 1000 lymphocytes) in mumps.
Neurosyphilis	Normal to 400	Clear unless protein is very high	10–100, mainly monocytes.	25–150; higher in meningitis.	Normal	Positive CSF serology. Gamma globulin may be increased.	Blood serology positive in untreated cases; *Treponema pallidum* immobilization test positive.

	Pressure	Appearance	Cells	Protein	Sugar	Serologic/Special	Comments
Parainfectious encephalomyelitis (measles, varicella, vaccinia)	80–450, usually increased	Usually clear	0–50, mainly monocytes.	15–75	Normal	CSF gamma globulin usually normal.	No organisms.
Supratentorial tumors	150–800+, usually increased	Usually clear	Usually normal	Usually normal; increased proximal to obstruction.	Normal	Radiodiagnostic studies	
Brain stem tumors	Usually normal	Clear	Usually normal	Usually normal	Normal	Radiodiagnostic studies	Increase of pressure, cells, or protein occasionally seen in late cases.
Cerebellar and fourth ventricle tumors	150–800+, usually increased	Usually clear	0–150; normal in 80%. Occasionally, cytologic identification of tumor cells.	Normal or slightly elevated	Normal	Tumor cells in CSF occasionally seen on cytologic examination. Contrast studies.	Lumbar tap contraindicated. Ventricular CSF may be normal.
Spinal cord tumors with block	Normal or low; quantitative, manometric studies.	Clear to yellow	0–100, mainly monocytes.	Normal in 15%; 45–3500 in 85%	Normal	Myelography	Color related to amount of protein; very high protein; fluid may clot.
Meningeal carcinomatosis	Often elevated	Clear to opalescent	Cytologic identification of tumor cells.	Often mildly to moderately elevated	Often depressed		Most commonly seen in childhood in leukemia; also in medulloblastoma, meningeal melanosis.
Encephalopathies (lead, anoxic, uremic, toxic)	Increased	Clear to slightly yellow	Normal, occasionally increased; mainly monocytes.	Normal or increased	Normal		Increased lead in blood and urine; increased coproporphyrins in urine; BUN high.
Cerebral concussion	Normal	Clear	Normal	Normal	Usually normal; below 50 in 15%.	Normal	The occasional reduction of sugar is probably related to the presence of blood; protein is increased in relation to admixture.
Cerebral contusion	Increased or normal	Xanthochromic or bloody	Few to several thousand red cells.			Supernatant fluid xanthochromic	
Subdural hematoma	Increased	Clear in 30%, xanthochromic in 70%	Normal (if fluid is clear).	Often normal in acute subdural hematoma if CSF is not bloody.	Normal		Blood in CSF due to co-existing other injury.
Epidural hematoma	Above 200 in two-thirds of cases	Clear	See Comments.				Lumbar tap contraindicated if this diagnosis very likely; fluid may be xanthochromic if contusion co-exists; cells, protein, and sugar assumed to be normal.
Cerebral hemorrhage	Usually high	Xanthochromic	Amount and type depend on severity of hemorrhage.	Normal to 2000; usually high.	Usually normal; occasionally high or low.	Supernatant fluid xanthochromic	
Subarachnoid hemorrhage	Usually high	Xanthochromic or grossly bloody	Presence of all cellular elements of blood.	Increase related to amount of blood	Usually high. See Comments.	Supernatant fluid xanthochromic	CSF glucose may be low 7–14 days after initial bleeding.
Demyelinating diseases	Variable; more often elevated in some leukodystrophies.	Clear	0–100, mainly monocytes.	Slightly elevated in 25%.	Normal	Gamma globulin usually increased in CSF (ie, > 8.2%).	Schilder's disease, leukodystrophies, neuromyelitis optica, multiple sclerosis, etc.

SEIZURE DISORDERS
(Epilepsies)

Essentials of Diagnosis

- Paroxysmal, usually transitory alteration of brain function of sudden onset, frequently recurrent.
- Forced movements, sensory disturbances, autonomic dysfunctions, behavioral changes, alone or in any combination, often accompanied by disturbances of consciousness.
- EEG is frequently abnormal.
- Family history of seizures in 30% of cases.

General Considerations

Four to 10% of all children will have had one or more convulsions by age 15; however, only about 2% go on to have recurrent chronic seizures or epilepsy. The causes and modifying conditions of seizures are often unclear, multiple, and additive.

Recognized causes of epilepsy include intrauterine insults, congenital malformations, and perinatal factors. After birth, systemic and CNS infections account for most seizures, with trauma, vascular disorders, metabolic and electrolyte disturbances, toxins, degenerative diseases, and physical agents responsible for only a few percent. Primary or secondary neoplastic lesions account for less than 1% of "symptomatic" seizures in children, compared with 25% in adults.

Some patients have generalized tonic-clonic or focal motor seizures chiefly during sleep—sometimes just after falling asleep and sometimes in the early morning hours. "Absence" or petit mal, akinetic, and myoclonic spells—often loosely referred to collectively as minor motor seizures—tend to occur in clusters in the morning "after breakfast" and again in the afternoon or around supper time. Lack of sleep, emotional excitement, intercurrent infections, alcohol, and some drugs may play a "triggering" role. On the other hand, some epileptics who experience difficulty in control at home may do extremely well, with no seizures and on less medication, merely when their situation changes, as when they stay with friends or relatives, go on vacation, or change schools or jobs.

Mixed seizure patterns occur frequently in children. Patterns may also change with maturation, and the treatment of one kind of seizure may unmask another.

Clinical Findings

A. Seizure Types: Based on both clinical manifestations and age at onset, the more common seizure disorders encountered in infancy, childhood, and adolescence are presented, along with pathogenetic factors, commonly encountered EEG findings, and preferred modes of treatment, in Table 21–2. It must be emphasized that there have been many diverse attempts at seizure classification, principally on the basis of clinical patterns and pathophysiology (including EEG patterns), but almost all have proved either too cumbersome or too simple. It must also be stressed that, in many of the more difficult to manage chronic epilepsies of early life, so-called partial or focal seizures or those of the "minor motor" variety (as in Lennox-Gastaut syndrome and with absences) may appear sooner or later mixed with focal seizures of the psychomotor type or with generalized (grand mal) convulsions.

B. Status Epilepticus: Any true seizure lasting an hour or more, or a series of seizures extending over such a period, constitutes status epilepticus. The term is usually applied to a prolonged generalized convulsion or a series of grand mal convulsions occurring in rapid succession without recovery of consciousness between spells. However, patients may also experience focal (motor), "psychomotor," and myoclonic status, as well as petit mal status or "spike-wave stupor" during which consciousness is impaired but not lost.

In treating status epilepticus, vigorous initial therapy is more likely to control seizures than the repeated administration of small doses of various anticonvulsants, whose cumulative effect may produce respiratory depression or marked CNS depression.

C. Breath-Holding Spells (Reflex Hypoxic Crisis): Although not a true epileptic disorder, the typical breath-holding spell is characterized by violent crying and breath-holding precipitated by slight injury, anger, frustration, fear, or the desire for attention in a young child (usually between 6 months and 4 years of age). The child becomes hypoxic and cyanotic, loses consciousness, may be opisthotonic, and may have a brief generalized seizure.

Unless the child sustains a head injury, these spells are benign. The description usually establishes the diagnosis. It is helpful to remember that cyanosis—and rarely pallor—almost always precedes loss of consciousness, whereas in grand mal epilepsy consciousness is lost first. Neurologic examination and EEG are normal, although reflex slowing produced on the EEG by ocular compression is diagnostically helpful.

Breath-holding spells almost always disappear between 4 and 6 years of age. Treatment with phenobarbital usually is of no benefit; in the spells ushered in by pallor, atropine may be useful.

D. Febrile Convulsions: Seizures occurring with fever in a child 6 months to 5 years of age that are *not* preceded at any time by a nonfebrile convulsion and *not* symptomatic of a recognized primary neurologic illness are considered separately because of their high incidence and the continuing concern over treatment.

At least 2% (perhaps as many as 5%) of young children are affected; whether to include children 1–6 months of age and up to 7 years of age is controversial. Febrile convulsions constitute about 40% of all first seizures in children. The largest number of febrile convulsions occur with temperatures above 39° C (102.2° F). Pharyngotonsillitis and otitis media are the most common associated illnesses; seizures with roseola infantum or within a week after immunization may reflect distinctive encephalopathies. Family history is positive for febrile convulsions in over 40% and for nonfebrile seizures in more than 15% of cases. Boys appear to be twice as susceptible as girls. Risk factors such as intrauterine insults, low birth weight, or perinatal complications appear to be similar to those for recurrent nonfebrile convulsions (epilepsy).

Febrile convulsions are "simple" when generalized, brief, or of less than 15 minutes' duration, and single or isolated; and "complex" when focal, prolonged, or multiple ("clustered") in a 24-hour period.

Recurrent febrile convulsions develop in 30–50% of untreated children who have had a febrile convulsion. The rate is highest within 18 months of the first episode. Young age at the initial seizure, abnormal pregnancy, low birth weight or prematurity, long or focal seizures, and abnormal developmental and neurologic status are significantly correlated with recurrences. The clustering of seizures during the first episode and an abnormal EEG recorded after a month or more show less correlation or none.

By 7 years of age, there is a 0.5% risk of a nonfebrile seizure in children with normal status and no previous febrile convulsions, a 1% risk in children with normal status who have had simple febrile convulsions, a 1.7% risk with complex initial febrile convulsions, a 30% risk when neurologic and developmental status are abnormal and the first febrile seizure was simple, and over 90% risk when a complex seizure occurs in a neurologically and developmentally abnormal child.

It is not definitely known whether the recurrence of febrile convulsions, either simple or complex, influences the incidence of subsequent febrile or nonfebrile seizures. Prophylactic treatment with phenobarbital (average initial dose 3–5 mg/kg) until age 5–6 years, maintaining serum levels at 1.5 mg/100 ml, is strongly recommended, as this reduces the recurrence rate of febrile convulsions to less than 10%. Complications with phenobarbital therapy are minimal and are outlined in Table 21–3. Most failures of phenobarbital treatment are due to noncompliance, but shigella or salmonella infections, fluid and electrolyte disorders, and other causes should be considered. The specific cause of any fever should be determined and treated appropriately.

E. Laboratory Findings: *Note:* The diagnostic work-up should be guided by the immediate condition of the child and the demands of the situation.

1. Blood—Glucose, calcium, phosphorus, and BUN or NPN; when indicated, sodium, magnesium, and phenylalanine. Check the hemogram specifically for stippling and sickling of cells. Perform serologic tests for syphilis and, in infantile spasms, for cytomegalic inclusion disease. Serologic tests for other viral diseases or for toxoplasmosis may be indicated also.

2. Urine—Reducing substances; ferric chloride or Phenistix, coproporphyrins, and chromatography for amino acids and organic acids when indicated.

3. Lumbar puncture—Although not a routine procedure, spinal tap should usually be done in infants and young children up to about 18 months of age following the first convulsion, especially if the child is febrile. *Note:* If meningitis or encephalitis is suspected as the cause of the seizure, lumbar puncture is mandatory.

Lumbar puncture is not warranted in clear-cut breath-holding spells, recurrent febrile convulsions when the cause of the fever is unequivocally extracranial, or when there is a definite risk of brain herniation (as with a posterior fossa mass). Whenever increased intracranial pressure due to a mass is suspected, skull x-rays should be examined for signs of increased pressure; if pressure is elevated, the risks of lumbar puncture should be weighed against its gains, as in infection or intracranial bleeding.

4. Subdural tap—Subdural tap should always be considered in an infant with an open anterior fontanel, particularly if there is any possibility of trauma or postmeningitic effusion.

F. X-Ray Findings: Skull films should be examined, especially for signs of increased intracranial pressure, calcifications, and lytic lesions. X-rays of long bones or a skeletal survey should be ordered when there is a suspicion of lead poisoning, trauma ("battered child"), or occult tumor.

G. Electroencephalography: Almost all children with gross structural brain disturbances have abnormal EEGs, which may be enhanced by activating technics such as light sleep, hyperventilation, and photic stimulation. However, the EEG depends upon the competence of the technician making the recording and the skill of the physician interpreting the record. Furthermore, about one-third of children with a first convulsion under 4 years of age and about 10% of epileptics later in life have normal EEGs. In 10–15% of the random "normal" population and in about 30% of nonepileptic close relatives of patients with centrencephalic epilepsy, EEG abnormalities may be observed.

1. Diagnostic value—The greatest value of the EEG in convulsive disorders is in differentiating petit mal absences and other "minor motor" seizures from "psychomotor" seizures, and "convulsive equivalents" from somatic complaints or disorders which are psychogenic in origin.

The EEG finding of mixed seizure patterns in a child who clinically demonstrates only grand mal or petit mal absences may help the physician in choosing the most appropriate anticonvulsants (Table 21–3).

The EEG may also be useful in localizing a cerebral mass (tumor, abscess, etc). In children who have persistent seizures despite adequate and prolonged anticonvulsant therapy, the EEG finding of a constant, fairly well circumscribed epileptogenic focus may lead to consideration of surgical excision.

2. Prognostic value—A normal EEG following a first convulsion suggests (but does not guarantee) a favorable prognosis. Markedly abnormal EEGs may become normal (1) immediately following intravenous injection of 50 mg vitamin B_6 in pyridoxine dependency or deficiency; (2) in infantile spasms (corticotropin or corticosteroids); (3) in petit mal absences (anticonvulsants); and (4) in petit mal and other minor motor seizures (ketogenic diet). If so, it is likely that seizure control will be achieved (although this offers

Table 21–2. Seizures by age at onset, pattern, and preferred treatment.

Age Group and Seizure Type	Age at Onset	Clinical Manifestations	Causative Factors	Electroencephalographic Pattern	Other Diagnostic Studies	Treatment and Comments*
Neonatal seizures	Birth to 2 weeks	Often "atypical": sudden limpness or tonic posturing with apnea and cyanosis; odd cry; eyes "rolling up" or nystagmus; twitchings; clonic movements—focal, multifocal, or generalized.	Neurologic insults (intracranial hemorrhage, hypoxia) tend to present more in first 3 days or after eighth day; metabolic disturbances alone between third and eighth days; hypoglycemia, hypocalcemia, hypophosphatemia, hyper- and hyponatremia, often with brain damage. Pyridoxine deficiency and other metabolic errors cause seizures after first week. Meningitis unpredictable.	Highly variable; often rhythmic slowing, independent abnormalities may shift.	Lumbar puncture; serum Ca^{++}, $PO_4^{\equiv}$, glucose, Mg^{++}; BUN, amino acid screen, blood ammonia, organic acid screen, TORCHES screen.†	Phenobarbital, 5–8 mg/kg, or phenytoin, 10 mg/kg IV (or both). Diazepam, approximately 0.2 mg/kg. Treat underlying disorder. Seizures secondary to brain damage often very resistant to anticonvulsants. When in doubt about cause, stop protein feedings until enzyme deficiencies of urea cycle or amino acid metabolism can be ruled out.
West's syndrome; "infantile spasms" (See also "Lennox-Gastaut" syndrome, below.)	3–18 months; occasionally up to 4 years	Sudden, usually symmetric adduction and flexion of limbs with concomitant flexion of head and trunk; also abduction and exterior movements—like Moro reflex. Tendency for spasms to occur in clusters, on waking or falling asleep, or when fatigued, or may be noted particularly when the infant is being handled, is ill, or is otherwise irritable. Tendency for each patient to have own stereotyped pattern.	Pre- or perinatal brain damage or malformation in approximately one-third; biochemical, infectious, degenerative causes in approximately one-third; unknown in approximately one-third. With early onset, pyridoxine deficiency, amino- or organic acidurias. Tuberous sclerosis in 5–10%. Chronic inflammatory disease and toxoplasmosis.	Hypsarrhythmia: chaotic pattern of high-voltage slow waves and random spikes in all leads in 90%; other abnormalities in rest. Rarely "normal." EEG normalization usually correlates well with reduction of seizures, but not helpful prognostically with respect to mental development.	Skull x-rays, funduscopic and skin examination; trial of pyridoxine. Amino- and organic acid screen. Chronic inflammatory disease. TORCHES screen.†	Corticotropin preferred (4–5 mg/kg/day for 10–14 days, then slow withdrawal). Some prefer oral corticosteroids. Diazepam, clonazepam. In resistant cases, ketogenic or medium chain triglyceride (MCT) diet (see text). Retardation of varying degree in approximately 90% of cases.
Febrile convulsions	6 months to 4 years	Usually generalized seizures, less than 15 minutes; rarely focal in onset. May lead to status epilepticus.	Nonneurologic febrile illness (temperature rise to 40 °C [104 °F] or higher); family history frequently positive for febrile convulsions.	Normal interictal EEG, especially when obtained 8–10 days after seizure.	In infants or whenever suspicion of meningitis exists, perform lumbar puncture.	Treat underlying illness, fever. Phenobarbital, 5 mg/kg continuously, keeping blood level about 1.5 mg/100 ml, until age 4–5 years.
"Lennox-Gastaut" syndrome; formerly "petit mal variant." Chiefly myoclonic and akinetic seizures	Any time in childhood; normally 2–7 years	Shock-like violent contractions of one or more muscle groups, singly or irregularly repetitive; may fling patient suddenly to side, forward, or backward. Usually no or only brief loss of consciousness. Half of patients or more also have generalized seizures.	Multiple causes, usually resulting in diffuse neuronal damage. History of West's syndrome; pre- or perinatal brain damage; viral meningoencephalitides; subacute sclerosing panencephalitis; CNS degenerative disorders; lead or other encephalopathies; structural cerebral abnormalities, eg, porencephaly.	Atypical slow spike-wave complexes ("petit mal variant") and frequent bursts of high-voltage generalized spikes. For "Lennox-Gastaut" syndrome, see text.	As dictated by index of suspicion. Lumbar puncture with measles antibody titer and CSF IgG. Nerve conduction studies. Urine for lead, arylsulfatase A, etc. Skin biopsy for electron microscopy and enzyme studies. Brain biopsy may be justified.	Phenobarbital; "cocktail" of phenobarbital plus methsuximide plus acetazolamide. Diazepam. Ketogenic or medium chain triglyceride (MCT) diet. Occasionally ACTH or corticosteroids. Often resistant to usual drug therapy but may respond to phenacemide or clonazepam (or both). Protect child's head with football helmet and chin padding.
Absences ("petit mal"). *Note:* Rarest seizure pattern in "pure" form. Also called "centrencephalic epilepsy."	3–15 years	Brief lapses of consciousness or vacant stares, usually in "clusters," often with blinking of eyelids or other movements. Sometimes automatisms. Often confused with "psychomotor" seizures (see below), which occur far more frequently.	Unknown. Genetic component: probably an autosomal dominant gene. Rarely may usher in childhood form of CNS lipidosis.	Three/second bilaterally synchronous, symmetric, high-voltage spikes and waves. EEG "normalization" correlates closely with control of seizures.	Hyperventilation when patient not on or on inadequate medication often provokes attacks. Studies for CNS degenerative diseases.	Ethosuximide; since many patients may also have generalized seizures, add phenobarbital if EEG suggests other abnormalities. Acetazolamide. Rarely, "diones." In resistant cases, ketogenic or MCT diet.

	Age	Clinical Features	EEG	Diagnostic Studies	Treatment
Focal seizures (motor/sensory/jacksonian). (For temporal lobe seizures, see psychomotor seizures, below).	Any age	Seizure may involve any part of body; may spread in fixed pattern (jacksonian march), becoming generalized. In children, epileptogenic focus often "shifts" and epileptic manifestations may change concomitantly.	Focal spikes or slow waves in appropriate cortical region; sometimes diffusely abnormal or even normal.	Often secondary to birth trauma, inflammatory process, vascular accidents, meningoencephalitis, etc. If seizures are coupled with new or progressive neurologic deficits, a structural lesion (eg, brain tumor) is likely.	If seizures are difficult to control or progressive deficits occur, neuroradiodiagnostic studies are imperative (see text).	Phenobarbital or phenytoin (or both). Primidone. "Cocktail" of phenobarbital plus methsuximide plus acetazolamide.
Psychomotor seizures; also called temporal lobe or limbic seizures or focal seizures of complex symptomatology	Any age‡	Aura may be a sensation of fear, epigastric discomfort, odd smell or taste (usually unpleasant), visual or auditory hallucination (either vague and "unformed" or well-formed image, words, music). Aura and seizure tend to be stereotyped for each patient. Seizure may consist of vague stare; facial, tongue, or swallowing movements; or throaty sounds; or various complex automatisms. Unlike true absences (petit mal), psychomotor seizures tend not to occur in clusters but singly and to last longer (15 seconds to minutes). History of aura (or child running to adult from "vague fear") and of *complex* automatisms establishes diagnosis. About 60% also develop generalized seizures.	As above, but occurring in temporal lobe and its connections, eg, frontotemporal, temporoparietal, temporo-occipital regions.	As above. Temporal lobes especially sensitive to hypoxia; thus, this seizure type may be sequel of birth trauma, febrile convulsions, etc. Also especially vulnerable to certain viral infections, especially herpes simplex. Remediable other causes are small cryptic tumors or vascular malformations.	Stereolateral skull films. Neuroradiodiagnostic studies, especially EMI scan or pneumoencephalogram when structural lesion suspected. Temporal lobe biopsy may be justified for immunofluorescent demonstration of herpes simplex antigen when encephalitis suspected. Carotid amobarbital injection when lateralization of speech dominance in question.	Carbamazepine, phenobarbital or primidone, or phenytoin (or all 3). Phenacemide in difficult-to-control seizures. In difficult cases and where a primary epileptogenic focus is identifiable, excision of anterior third of temporal lobe. Adjunctive psychotherapy may be justified frequently. For herpes simplex encephalitis, with its high mortality rate, a large bolus of adenosine arabinoside (AraA) may be tried. Treatment using cytarabine and idoxuridine has been abandoned.
"Convulsive equivalents"; also called "abdominal," "autonomic," "diencephalic," "thalamic-hypothalamic," epilepsy, or "vegetative" seizure disorder	Any age‡	Variety of episodic visceral or sensory disturbances for which no other cause may be found, eg, recurrent abdominal pain, cyclic vomiting, headaches, dizzy spells, episodes of profuse sweating, laughing or crying jags, other paroxysmal alterations of mood or behavior, occasionally incontinence. Unknown. The episodes may have a "migrainous" quality, and there is often a family history of epilepsy or migraine. Diagnosis depends on (1) paroxysmal, repetitive nature of attacks; (2) absence of explanatory pathologic findings; (3) positive response to therapeutic trial of phenytoin or phenobarbital.	Variety of EEG abnormalities in about 70% of cases, sometimes only during attack. One-fourth of children eventually have generalized or psychomotor seizures.		As indicated by symptomatology.	Phenytoin, about 7 mg/kg body weight (serum level 1.5 ± 0.3 mg/ 100 ml), preferred. Phenobarbital, 5 mg/kg; occasionally Donnatal in very young child.
"Benign epilepsy of childhood" (with "centrotemporal" or "rolandic" foci)	5–16 years	Partial motor or generalized seizures. Similar seizure patterns may be observed in patients with focal cortical lesions.	Seizure history or abnormal EEG findings in relatives of 40% of affected probands and 18–20% of parents and siblings, suggesting transmission by a single autosomal dominant gene, possibly with age-dependent penetrance.	Centrotemporal spikes or sharp waves ("rolandic discharges") appearing paroxysmally against a normal EEG background.	Stereolateral skull films. Serum Ca⁺⁺ and glucose, BUN, urinalysis. Neuroradiodiagnostic studies if clinical index of suspicion justifies their cost.	Phenobarbital or phenytoin (or both). Primidone. "Cocktail" of phenobarbital plus methsuximide plus acetazolamide.
Generalized seizures (grand mal)	Any age	Loss of consciousness; tonic, clonic movements, often preceded by vague aura or cry. Bladder and bowel incontinence in approximately 15%. Postictal confusion; sleep. Often mixed with or masking other seizure patterns.	Often unknown. Genetic component. May be seen with metabolic disturbances, trauma, infections, intoxications, degenerative disorders, brain tumors, etc.	Bilaterally synchronous, symmetric multiple high-voltage spikes, spikes and waves, mixed patterns. Often normal under age 4.	As above.	Phenobarbital in first 6–12 months or after 5–6 years. Phenytoin. Carbamazepine. Combinations with primidone, methsuximide, acetazolamide.

Note: When using anticonvulsants, continue treatment for at least a 2- or 3-year seizure-free period.

†TORCHES is a mnemonic formula for *toxoplasmosis, rubella, cytomegalovirus, herpes simplex,* and *syphilis.*

‡May be difficult to recognize in younger children.

Table 21–3. Guide to anticonvulsant drug therapy.

Seizure Pattern	Drug	Average Total (mg/kg/day)	in	Divided Doses	Toxicity and Precautions	Remarks
All seizures	Phenobarbital	3–6 (250–300 mg/sq m)	:	1–3	Irritability and overactivity in many children; sedative effects in others. Mild ataxia, nystagmus, skin rash. Osteomalacia may occur, especially in retarded children.	Safest overall drug. Bitter taste. Therapeutic drug level about 1.5 mg/100 ml; usually higher (up to 4 or 5 mg/ml in severe chronic epileptics). Check linear growth periodically; obtain Ca^{++} and bone films as indicated. Supplemental calcium or vit D has been suggested.
	Mephobarbital (Mebaral)	4–10	:	1–3	As above.	Tasteless. Twice the quantity of phenobarbital required for comparable effect.
	Primidone (Mysoline)	10–25	:	3–4	Drowsiness, ataxia, vertigo, anorexia, nausea, vomiting, rash.	Start slowly with 25–35% of expected maintenance dose; increase every 2 days until full dose is reached. Therapeutic blood level not fully established (about 1 mg/100 ml).
	Methsuximide (Celontin)	15–30	:	3–4	Drowsiness, ataxia, headache, diplopia, skin rash.	Effective with phenobarbital in "mixed patterns" where other drugs may be contraindicated.
	Bromides	25–75	:	3–4	Rash, drowsiness, toxic psychosis, mental dullness. Check blood bromide levels regularly.	Rarely used now. Try when usual drugs fail, especially in infantile spasms and "minor motor" seizures.
	Metharbital (Gemonil)	5–15	:	2–3	Drowsiness, irritability, rash.	Not a satisfactory drug. May be useful in seizures due to organic brain damage.
Adjuncts to above	Acetazolamide (Diamox)	5–20	:	3–4	Anorexia; numbness and tingling; increase in urinary frequency.	Supplement to other medications, especially in petit mal and other minor patterns. Also in females 4 days prior to and in the first 2–3 days of menstrual periods.
	Diazepam (Valium)	0.20 ± 0.05	:	3	Somnolence.	Most useful in minor motor seizures and infantile spasms. Often ceases to be effective after a few weeks or months.
	Carbamazepine (Tegretol)	Individualize (10–30)	: :	2–3 times a day with meals		Particularly useful in psychomotor, other focal, as well as generalized seizures. Check platelet count periodically. Therapeutic blood levels not established; possibly 0.2–1.2 mg/100 ml.
	Dextroamphetamine (Dexedrine)	0.25–0.75	:	Breakfast and noon	Nervousness, palpitations, anorexia, insomnia. Growth retardation with chronic use.	To counteract sedative effect of other drugs. Narcolepsy. In behavior disorders of younger children.
	Amphetamine (Benzedrine)	0.25–0.75	:	Breakfast and noon	As above.	As above. Less potent, but sometimes better tolerated than Dexedrine.
Any seizures except petit mal absences, akinetic, or myoclonic	Phenytoin (Dilantin)	5–9 (250 mg/sq m)	:	1–2	Gum hypertrophy, hirsutism, ataxia, nystagmus, diplopia, rash, anorexia, nausea, osteomalacia, especially in retarded children. *Warning:* Check linear growth periodically; obtain Ca^{++} and bone films as indicated. Supplemental Ca^{++} or vitamin D has been suggested. *Rare:* macro-	Generally very effective and safe. Will not cause behavior disturbances in children. Good dental hygiene reduces gum hyperplasia. May aggravate petit mal and myoclonic seizures. Severe toxicity may cause pseudodementia and liver damage. Therapeutic blood level varies with patient; usually 1.2–1.7 mg/100 ml; toxicity usually above 2 mg/100 ml but may occur at lower blood levels.

(continued from previous page) ...cytic anemia, lymph node involvement, exfoliative dermatitis, peripheral neuropathy.

Seizure Type	Drug	Dose (mg/kg)	Doses/day	Side Effects / Precautions	Remarks
	Ethotoin (Peganone)	15–30	2–3	As above.	Not very effective. Worth trying if others fail.
	Mephenytoin (Mesantoin)	4–15	2–3	Mild: Rash, drowsiness, ataxia. *Warning:* Aplastic anemia, agranulocytosis. Obtain at least monthly blood counts.	A good anticonvulsant, but fear of bone marrow depression limits use.
Psychomotor Occasionally primarily akinetic and myoclonic attacks	Phenacemide (Phenurone)	25–50	2–4	Rash, anorexia, nausea. *Warning:* Hepatitis, psychosis, blood dyscrasias. Monthly blood counts. liver function tests.	Especially effective in temporal lobe seizures when all other drugs fail.
Petit mal absences	Ethosuximide (Zarontin)	10–25	3–4	Nausea, gastric discomfort. Take with food. Rare: bone marrow depression.	Drug of choice for petit mal. Occasionally aggravates generalized seizures; may thus require phenobarbital also. Therapeutic blood level wide (4–10 mg/100 ml).
Akinetic and myoclonic attacks (Lennox-Gastaut syndrome)	Clonazepam (Clonopin)	0.1–0.2 mg/kg/day in 2–3 divided doses. Start slowly with 0.01–0.03 mg/kg in 2–3 doses per day and increase every third day to effective maintenance level or until side-effects interfere.		Drowsiness (> 50%). Behavior problems (25%). Slurred speech, ataxia, CBC, liver function tests.	Very useful with difficult to treat minor motor seizures (akinetic, myoclonic, Lennox-Gaustaut; infantile spasms; petit mal absences where Zarontin fails). As with diazepam, breakthroughs often occur after 2–3 months, but drug may be restarted after period of withdrawal. Soporific effects are greatest drawback. May aggravate generalized seizures; hence, give phenobarbital also.
	Trimethadione (Tridione)	20–50	3–4	Rash, photophobia, irritability. *Warning:* Leukopenia, agranulocytosis, nephrosis. LE phenomenon. Monthly blood counts and urinalysis.	Useful in petit mal absences if Zarontin fails. May aggravate generalized seizures; hence, give phenobarbital also.
	Paramethadione (Paradione)	20–50	3–4	As above.	As above.
	Phensuximide (Milontin)	20–40	3–4	Drowsiness, headache, slight nephrotoxicity. Monthly urinalysis.	Not very effective but may be useful when other drugs fail, or in combination.
Status epilepticus, grand mal, focal, psychomotor, and myoclonic	Diazepam (Valium)	0.2 ± 0.05 mg/kg IV initially. Repeat dose 0.1 mg/kg.		Administer slowly IV. Monitor pulse and BP. May cause respiratory depression if given to patient who has already received phenobarbital.	May need to be repeated every 3–4 hours. Follow with phenobarbital or phenytoin for long-range control.
	Phenobarbital	7–10 mg/kg IV initially. Repeat dose 5 mg/kg IV.		Less if patient has already received barbiturates.	Rule out pyridoxine deficiency, water intoxication.
	Paraldehyde	0.1–0.15 ml/kg IV; 0.2–0.3 ml/kg rectally.		Administer slowly IV mixed in saline; rectal dose in vegetable oil. Avoid in patient with pulmonary disease or in croup.	Avoid IM administration if possible: may cause fat necrosis.
	Lidocaine (Xylocaine)	2 mg/kg IV		Administer slowly.	Useful especially when reluctant to give more barbiturates or paraldehyde. Effect brief.
	General anesthesia if other measures fail.				
Infantile spasms	Use of corticotropin or corticosteroids and of ketogenic diet discussed in text. Also, clonazepam, diazepam, especially with recurrences.				

no clues to the mental status of the patient).

3. **Interpretation**—The technics of recording and interpreting the EEG constitute a separate area of specialization. The most typical patterns are mentioned in Table 21–2.

The 14 and 6 per second positive spike pattern observed most frequently in adolescents, particularly during light sleep, has been claimed to be associated with convulsive equivalents and dyssocial or asocial behavior; it is now thought to be a normal finding.

H. Special Investigations: Brain scan, computerized tomography (CT), cerebral angiography, pneumoencephalography, or ventriculography is usually indicated only when neurosurgical intervention is a distinct possibility, as in the following circumstances: (1) When there are a persistent and progressive neurologic history and findings suggestive of a focal lesion, especially in the presence of markedly localized EEG slowing. (2) When skull films show abnormal calcifications, bony rarefaction, etc, indicative of a lesion amenable to surgery. (3) In the presence of elevated CSF pressure or protein or persistently depressed CSF sugar, in cases where these findings are not explained by an infectious, toxic, hemorrhagic, or degenerative process. (4) As part of the preoperative evaluation of patients with intractable seizures who may be candidates for cortical excision, anterior temporal lobectomy, or hemispherectomy.

Differential Diagnosis

A. Fainting: In syncope, as cerebral blood flow drops, the patient usually reports that "things went black" before he "sank" to the ground. Tonic-clonic movements do not occur. As blood flow to the brain increases (when the patient lies recumbent or puts his head between his legs), consciousness returns. There are no postictal phenomena, and usually there is no retrograde amnesia.

B. Conversion Hysteria ("Hysteroepilepsy"): The differentiation from epilepsy may be extremely difficult, particularly if the patient has true seizures but also mimics his attacks. This is most often observed in immature adolescents. The character of the attacks (pseudoseizures) may be quite convincing, depending on how much the patient knows about epilepsy and whether he has had the chance to observe generalized or psychomotor seizures. If there is a strong sadomasochistic component to the conversion reaction, the patient may actually injure himself or urinate. In less sophisticated patients, the attacks tend to be "bizarre." During the attack, the patient is often resistive. Even when he mimics postictal stupor, the pupillary dilatation and Babinski responses so often seen immediately after a true seizure are usually not present. The EEG during an attack simply shows muscle artefact, but no preceding "build-up," paroxysmal activity, or postseizure slowing is seen.

C. Narcolepsy: Narcolepsy is uncommon in children. It is characterized by irresistible attacks of sleep, usually of short duration, and is frequently associated with loss of muscle tone (catalepsy) but without

sudden loss of consciousness. It is frequently precipitated by acute emotional episodes such as laughing or crying.

Complications

Emotional disturbances—notably anxiety, depression, anger, feelings of guilt and inadequacy—often occur as a reaction to the seizures in the parents of the affected child as well as in the child old enough to understand. The seizures—and particularly the hallucinatory auras and psychomotor attacks—frequently set off in the prepubescent and adolescent youngster fantasies (and sometimes obsessive ruminations) about dying and death which may become so strong as to lead to suicidal behavior and suicidal attempts. The limitations which many school systems place on epileptic children add to the problem. Commonly, the child expresses his feelings by "acting out."

Pseudoretardation may occur in poorly controlled epileptic children because their seizures—or the subclinical paroxysms sustained—may interfere with their learning ability. Anticonvulsants are less likely to "slow the child down" but may do so in toxic amounts.

True mental retardation is most commonly part of the same pathologic process that causes the seizures but may occasionally occur when seizures are frequent, prolonged, and accompanied by hypoxia.

Physical injuries, especially lacerations of the forehead and chin, are frequent in akinetic seizures. In all other seizure disorders in childhood, injuries as a direct result of an attack are impressively rare.

Treatment

The ideal treatment of seizures is the discovery and correction of specific causes. However, even when a biochemical disorder (eg, leucine hypoglycemia) or a tumor is discovered or when septic meningitis is successfully treated, anticonvulsant drugs are often still required.

A. Precautionary Management of Individual Brief Seizures: Position the patient so that he cannot injure himself nor aspirate vomitus. Beyond that, no specific therapy is necessary. The less done to the patient during a relatively brief seizure (up to 10 or 15 minutes), the better. Thrusting a spoon-handle or tongue depressor into the clenched mouth of a convulsing patient or trying to restrain tonic-clonic movements may cause worse injuries than a bitten tongue or bruised limb. Mouth-to-mouth resuscitation is rarely (if ever) necessary.

B. General Management of the Young Epileptic:
1. Education—The patient and his parents must be helped to understand the problem of seizures and their management. Many children—some even as young as 3 years of age—are capable of cooperating with the physician in problems of seizure control.

All bottles containing antiepileptic drugs should bear a contents label. The parents should know the names and dosage of the anticonvulsants being administered.

Pamphlets and books on epilepsy are available

from many sources. The local chapter of the Epilepsy Foundation of America and other community and national organizations are eager to be of service and can be a source of guidance and support as well as an outlet for the anxieties of parents and older patients.

2. Privileges and precautions in daily life— Encourage normal daily living within reasonable bounds. The child should engage in physical activities appropriate to his age and social group. After fairly secure seizure control has been established, swimming is generally permissible providing a "buddy system" or adequate lifeguard coverage is maintained. High diving and high climbing should not be permitted. After seizure control is established, physical training and sports in school, camps, community centers, etc are usually to be welcomed rather than restricted. Driving is discussed below.

Loss of sleep should be avoided.

Emotional disturbances should be treated as indicated.

Alcoholic intake, a serious problem usually beginning in adolescence, should be avoided as it may precipitate seizures.

Prompt attention should be given to infections, and evidence of further neurologic disturbances should be brought to the physician's attention.

Although every effort should be made to control seizures, this must not interfere with a child's ability to function. Sometimes it is better to let a child have an occasional mild seizure than to sedate him so heavily that he cannot function at home, in school, or at play. This often requires much art and fortitude on the part of the physician.

3. Driving—Driving becomes important to most youngsters at age 15 or 16. The restrictions vary from state to state, but in most states a learner's permit or driver's license will be issued if the patient has been under a physician's care and has been free of seizures for at least 2 years, provided the medications or basic neurologic problem do not interfere with the ability to drive.

Epilepsy and the Law, by R.L. Barrow and H.D. Fabing (Hoeber, 2nd ed, 1966), is a helpful guide to this and other legal matters as they pertain to epileptics.

C. Principles of Anticonvulsant Therapy:

1. Treat promptly with the drug most appropriate to the clinical situation as outlined in Tables 21—2 and 21—3.

2. Start with one drug—or, in some cases of mixed major and minor motor seizures, with 2—in conventional dosage and increase the dosage until seizures are controlled or to tolerated maximal dosage before adding further drugs or changing medications. The dosages given in Table 21—3 are the usual "guiding" doses, but the actual amount must be individualized.

3. Advise the parents and the patient that the prolonged use of anticonvulsant drugs will not produce "mental slowing" (although the underlying cause of the seizures might) and that prevention of seizures for about 3 years or so substantially reduces the chances of recurrence. Advise them also that anticonvulsants

are given to prevent further seizures and that they should be taken as prescribed. Changes in medications or dosages should not be done without the physician's knowledge. Unsupervised sudden withdrawal of anticonvulsant drugs may precipitate severe seizures.

Anticonvulsants must be kept where they cannot be ingested by small children or suicidal patients.

4. Check the patient at intervals, depending on the underlying cause of his seizures, the degree of control, and the toxic properties of the anticonvulsant drug or drugs used. Blood counts, urinalyses, and liver function or other biologic tests must be obtained at frequent intervals in the case of some anticonvulsants as indicated in Table 21—3.

Periodic neurologic reevaluation is important. Repeat skull films or CT scan may be indicated, eg, if there is a suspicion of a lytic lesion or intracranial calcifications. Repeat EEGs are generally not needed to achieve seizure control and need be obtained in most cases only every 1½—2 years.

5. Continue anticonvulsant treatment until the patient is free of seizures for 2—4 years or, in some cases, through adolescence. A much "improved" or normal EEG (or 2 such tracings 1½—2 years apart) is helpful in determining when anticonvulsant therapy may be discontinued.

6. In general, there is no need to withdraw anticonvulsants before taking an EEG.

7. Discontinue anticonvulsants gradually. If it becomes necessary to withdraw anticonvulsants abruptly, the patient should be under close medical surveillance. If seizures recur during or after withdrawal, anticonvulsant therapy should be reinstituted and again maintained for at least 3—4 years.

D. Side-Effects of Antiepileptic Drugs: (See also Table 21—3.)

1. Serious allergic reactions usually necessitate discontinuance of a drug. However, not every rash in a child receiving phenytoin, for example, is due to the drug. If a useful antiepileptic drug is discontinued for this reason and the rash disappears, restarting the drug in a smaller dosage is often warranted to see if the allergic reaction recurs.

2. Ataxia and other neurologic signs of drug toxicity will often disappear when the drug is reduced by 25—30% of the last daily dosage.

3. The sedative effect of many of the anticonvulsants is often easily counteracted by the judicious use of coffee or dextroamphetamine sulfate, 2.5—5 mg at breakfast and 2.5 mg at noon.

4. Gingival hyperplasia secondary to phenytoin is best minimized through good dental hygiene but occasionally requires gingivectomy. This and hypertrichosis usually disappear within 6 months after the drug is discontinued.

E. Guides to Therapy of Specific Seizure Disorders: (See also Tables 21—2 and 21—3.)

F. Status Epilepticus: Diazepam (Valium) is the drug of choice. In general, 0.2 ± 0.05 mg/kg or 6 mg/sq m administered IV over 1—3 minutes will achieve control; if necessary, half the initial amount should be given again. Pulse and blood pressure should be monitored during the injection, and if these drop markedly the injection should be temporarily halted until cardiovascular function returns to normal. In recurrent status epilepticus, diazepam may be repeated every 3–4 hours.

Once control is achieved, phenobarbital, 3–5 mg/kg, or phenytoin, 5–7 mg/kg, should be administered by IV drip, IM, or orally (depending on the particular situation) for long-term seizure control.

Phenytoin, 10 mg/kg slowly IV, is often useful in major motor and psychomotor status epilepticus, especially where it is desirable to avoid depressing the level of consciousness; lidocaine (Xylocaine) is especially useful to achieve rapid (though short-lived) control of focal motor seizures.

For further details on the use of phenobarbital and paraldehyde in status epilepticus, see Table 21.–3.

Note: General anesthesia may have to be used to control status epilepticus if the usual measures fail.

G. Corticotropin and Corticosteroids:

1. Indications–These drugs are indicated for infantile spasms not due to causes amenable to specific therapy and for akinetic and myoclonic seizures which cannot be controlled by anticonvulsant drugs.

The duration of therapy is guided by cessation of clinical seizures and EEG improvement. Corticotropin or the oral corticosteroids are usually continued in full doses for 2–4 weeks and then, if seizures have ceased, are tapered by about 25% every 2 weeks for a total treatment period of about 2 months. If seizures recur, increase the dosage to the last effective level and maintain the patient for up to 6 months on this dosage before again attempting withdrawal.

2. Dosages–

a. Corticotropin gel (Acthar Gel), starting with 4–5 units/kg/day IM in 2 divided doses. Parents can be taught to give the injections.

b. Cortisone, starting with 6–8 mg/kg/day orally in 3 divided doses.

c. Prednisone, starting with 2–4 mg/kg/day orally in 3 divided doses.

d. In akinetic and myoclonic seizures, give phenobarbital and other anticonvulsants also.

3. Precautions–Give additional potassium, guard against infections, and discuss the cushingoid appearance and its disappearance. Do not withdraw oral corticosteroids suddenly.

H. Ketogenic or Medium Chain Triglyceride Diet in Treatment of Epilepsy: A ketogenic diet should be recommended in akinetic and myoclonic seizures and petit mal absences not responsive to drug therapy, and occasionally for infantile spasms that do not respond to corticotropin or the corticosteroids. Ketosis is induced either by a diet high in fats and very limited in carbohydrates with sufficient protein for body maintenance *and* growth or by the feeding of medium chain triglycerides (MCT) or by a combination of these methods. The MCT diet induces ketosis more readily than does a high level of dietary fats and hence requires less carbohydrate restriction. The mechanism for the

anticonvulsant action of the ketogenic diet is not yet understood, although various hypotheses have been put forth. However, it is the ketosis, not the acidosis, which is effective in raising the seizure threshold. It is usually most effective in young children, ie, those under the age of 8 years, but when all other measures fail it should be tried even in adolescents.

As ketosis is achieved, a repeat EEG may be helpful; seizure control by the diet is more likely to occur if the EEG shows improvement.

The ketogenic diet is difficult, expensive, tends to be monotonous, and depends upon the ability of the mother to weigh out the foods as well as absolute adherence to the diet prescribed. Whether the ketosis is achieved by high fat meals or an MCT diet is often a matter of the physician's, the dietitian's, or the patient's preference. The result may also depend on which form of the diet is better tolerated. Full cooperation of the parents and all other family members is required, including the patient if old enough. However, when seizure control is achieved by this method, the child is alert, often is receiving no anticonvulsants or only small amounts, and parental and patient satisfaction is most gratifying.

Consult a dietitian and references on ketogenic diet (eg, Dodson & others, Keith, and Livingston & others references, below).

I. Surgery: In seizure disorders intractable to anticonvulsant therapy and primarily of focal origin, neurosurgery should be considered. Useful procedures, depending on the underlying lesion, include corticectomy, hemispherectomy, temporal lobectomy (for psychomotor seizures), and cutting of the corpus callosum. Cerebellar stimulation by chronically implanted electrodes has been advocated for ameliorating some intractable seizure disorders but is not recommended.

Aicardi J, Chevrie JJ: Convulsive status epilepticus in infants and children: A study of 239 cases. Epilepsia 11:187, 1970.

Brown JK: Convulsions in the newborn period. Dev Med Child Neurol 15:823, 1973.

Cooper IS & others: Chronic cerebellar stimulation in epilepsy. Arch Neurol 33:559, 1976.

Dodson WE & others: Management of seizure disorders: Selected aspects. (2 parts.) J Pediatr 89:527, 695, 1976.

Douglas EF, White PT: Abdominal epilepsy: A reappraisal. J Pediatr 78:59, 1971.

Huttenlocher PR: Ketonemia and seizures: Metabolic and anticonvulsant effects of two ketogenic diets in childhood epilepsy. Pediatr Res 10:536, 1976.

Juul-Jensen P: Frequency of recurrence after discontinuance of anticonvulsant therapy in patients with epileptic seizures. Epilepsia 9:11, 1968.

Keith H: *Convulsive Disorders in Children.* Little, Brown, 1963.

Lacy JR, Penry JK: *Infantile Spasms.* Raven Press, 1976.

Livingston S & others: *Comprehensive Management of Epilepsy in Infancy, Childhood and Adolescence.* Thomas, 1972.

Nellhaus G: Management of seizure disorders in infancy, childhood, and adolescence. Pages 503–520 in: *Drugs and the Developing Brain.* Vernadakis A, Weiner N (editors). Plenum, 1974.

Nelson KB: Predictors of epilepsy in children who have experienced febrile seizures. N Engl J Med 295:1029, 1976.

Wolf SM & others: The value of phenobarbital in the child who has had a single febrile seizure: A controlled prospective study. Pediatrics 59:378, 1977.

HEADACHES

Headache is not usually a psychosomatic symptom in very young children, whereas this is more often the case—even in association with vomiting—in older children and adolescents. A careful description of the headaches, associated circumstances, and other neurologic and systemic symptoms should be obtained. The family history and emotional problems should be discussed in detail. Finally, a careful systemic and neurologic examination, including blood pressure, ophthalmoscopic examination, and urinalysis, will help distinguish organic from the more common psychogenic or tension headaches.

EEG, skull and sinus x-rays, ophthalmologic evaluation, and other studies may be indicated as screening tests; even therapeutic trials of diphenylhydantoin, phenobarbital, or ergotamine are occasionally warranted.

If there is evidence of a specific intracranial cause or systemic disorder (eg, renal disease), diagnosis and treatment should be directed at the primary disorder.

Friedman AP, Harms E: *Headaches in Children.* Thomas, 1967.

Tension Headaches

Often described as "dull" or "like a tight band," of slow onset, diffuse or occipital and sometimes nuchal in location, lasting for hours, and rarely disabling, tension headaches are a frequent complaint in school-age and especially adolescent children. Home, school, social, and sexual problems are the usual underlying emotional factors. The history frequently suggests feelings of inadequacy or anxiety in the patient.

Salicylates are often successful in relieving the discomfort. Antianxiety drugs such as chlordiazepoxide (Librium), 5–10 mg 2–3 times daily, are occasionally indicated, along with supportive therapy. Primary attention, however, should be directed at the precipitating and chronic causes of the emotional strain.

Headaches Due to Refractive Error

Although rare in school-age children, more headaches are blamed on eye problems than can be substantiated by ophthalmologic examination. Attention should be directed to underlying emotional disturbances.

Waters WE: Headache and the eye. Lancet 2:1, 1970.

Migraine

Migraine attacks are usually paroxysmal, throbbing, pulsating, or pounding in character (initial vasoconstriction of intracranial vessels followed by vasodilatation of extracranial vessels); commonly unilateral; and often preceded by scintillating scotomas, slowly evolving sensory disturbances of the face and arm, and sometimes by psychic disturbances. Less frequent are transient ipsilateral visual disturbances and contralateral hemiplegia. Photophobia, nausea, gastric discomfort, and vomiting are commonly present. The child frequently seeks rest in a dark, quiet room.

Migraine of varying severity may occur in as much as 5% of the population. Onset by age 4 is not uncommon. The family history is often positive for migraine and not infrequently also for epilepsy. The EEG may be slightly abnormal. Hypoglycemia, with blood glucose levels in the range of 20 mg/100 ml, has been reported as a cause of migraine in adults but not yet in children; nevertheless, this should be ruled out by glucose tolerance tests; if the results are positive, a high-protein, low-carbohydrate, 6-feeding diet should be instituted.

Salicylates are often effective in children. The patient should be allowed to remain quiet in a darkened room. In children over 12 years of age, severe migraine may often be controlled by Fenbutal, Fiorinal, or Lanorinal,* 1 capsule every 4 hours. If these measures are ineffective, especially in the older child, and when anxiety and nausea are prominent symptoms, Cafergot P-B,† ½–1 tablet at the first sign of an attack and ½–1 additional tablet every 30 minutes for a total of 2–4 tablets, is often useful. Cafergot P-B suppositories may be used when migraine is severe and vomiting precludes oral medication.

In the prevention of severe, frequent, and disabling migraine, phenytoin (Dilantin), 5–7 mg/kg/day, may be effective, especially when the EEG is abnormal or there is a family history of epilepsy. Tranquilizers such as chlordiazepoxide (Librium) or amitriptyline (Elavil) may be useful (10–25 mg twice or 3 times daily). In children it is rarely necessary to resort to methysergide maleate (Sansert), 2–6 mg daily with meals in divided doses, depending on age and size. Methysergide is contraindicated in renal disease and vasculitis (eg, "collagen diseases"). It is reported to have caused retroperitoneal fibrosis and vascular complications.

Prensky AL: Migraine and migrainous variants in pediatric patients. Pediatr Clin North Am 23:461, 1976.

Scott DF, Moffett A, Swash M: Observations on the relation of migraine and epilepsy: An electroencephalographic, psychological, and clinical study using oral tyramine. Epilepsia 13:365, 1972.

Headache as an Epileptic Phenomenon

Headaches, when associated with epilepsy, may

---

*One capsule contains butalbital, 50 mg; aspirin, 200 mg; phenacetin, 130 mg; and caffeine, 40 mg.

†Cafergot P-B contains ergotamine tartrate, 1 mg; caffeine, 100 mg; Bellafoline (alkaloids of belladonna, as malates), 0.125 mg; and pentobarbital sodium, 30 mg.

occur as an aura (usually in psychomotor seizures) or in postictal states. Less commonly, they occur as a "convulsive equivalent." (See section on Seizure Disorders.)

Treatment consists of control of seizures. For cyclic headaches not associated with other epileptic phenomena but judged to represent a "convulsive equivalent," a therapeutic trial of an anticonvulsant is warranted. Phenytoin (Dilantin), 5–7 mg/kg/day orally, is usually more effective than phenobarbital, 3–5 mg/kg/day orally. If effective, treatment should be maintained for 2–3 years of a symptom-free period and then discontinued slowly, with reinstitution of therapy if symptoms recur.

HEAD INJURIES

Initial Evaluation

Check a child brought in because of head trauma rapidly for the following:

A. Respirations: Ensure adequate oxygenation. Hyperventilation is common in excited, irritable children. Deep, rapid, or periodic breathing is seen with brain stem involvement; intermittent gasping often precedes death.

B. State of Consciousness: (See also the section on Altered States of Consciousness.) Alterations of behavior and of consciousness may follow head trauma. In young children, it may be difficult to be certain whether there was a brief loss of consciousness immediately after the injury or whether the child had a breath-holding spell or a seizure. Following a concussion, young children are often extremely irritable.

Immediate stupor or coma suggests severe damage to the diencephalon or brain stem reticular activating system. Initial relative alertness followed by progressively deepening drowsiness, stupor, and coma within minutes, hours, or 3–4 days is observed in more extensive cerebral edema and intracranial bleeding.

C. Pulse: The pulse is often rapid shortly after head trauma. Wide fluctuations in pulse rate or marked slowing accompany direct brain stem damage or increased intracranial pressure.

D. Blood Pressure: Children often look pale and feel clammy after a head injury even though blood pressure is normal. Marked hypotension suggests bleeding into the viscera (consider splenic or hepatic rupture, particularly after an automobile or bicycle accident). Widened blood pressure or marked fluctuations often accompany direct brain stem involvement or increased intracranial pressure.

E. Ocular Signs: Note reactivity of pupils to light and their size. A 1–2 mm inequality with briskly reacting pupils may be due to congenital anisocoria but warrants continued observation. A fixed, dilated pupil in one eye may indicate ipsilateral cerebral damage or hematoma (epidural or subdural) or may be a false lateralizing sign. Bilateral fixed dilated pupils reflect

severe brain stem damage, with death often occurring in a few hours. Bilateral fixed constricted pupils may reflect brain stem damage from which the patient may recover but also suggest intoxication, eg, with barbiturates or opiates. Note voluntary and doll's eye movements.

Ophthalmoscopic examination is of paramount importance. Retinal hemorrhages occur in acute head injuries, especially with subdural hematomas. Dilated, nonpulsating retinal veins are the first sign of papilledema, which may develop within a few hours after the onset of increased intracranial pressure.

F. Inspection and Palpation:

1. Skull—Note and record signs of trauma, especially puncture wounds and deep scalp lacerations. Linear fractures, like widely separated sutures, may result in a "cracked pot sound" on percussion of the head; depressed skull fractures may be palpable. The maximum occipitofrontal head circumference should be recorded; the size and tension of the anterior fontanel, if patent, should be noted.

2. Neck—Nuchal rigidity may be due to subarachnoid hemorrhage, but cervical spine injury must be considered. Great caution is urged both in checking the neck and in moving such a patient. Prompt cervical spine films should be taken when there is the least suspicion of cervical spine fracture.

3. Ears—Bleeding from one or both ears or a hematoma over the mastoid region (Battle's sign) suggests basilar skull fracture through the petrous pyramids of the temporal bone; such bleeding may also be due to rupture of the tympanic membrane or the tearing of mucous membranes without perforation of the ear drum, and may occur without skull fracture. Note also leakage of CSF from the ears.

4. Rhinorrhea—A watery nasal discharge strongly positive for glucose (as tested with Dextrostix) suggests CSF leakage as occurs with fracture of the frontal bone and associated dural tearing. However, mucous discharges may also be glucose positive; hence, the discharge must be analyzed chemically and microscopically.

5. Skin and extremities—Rapidly inspect for signs of recent trauma, including fractures. Note also the presence of old scars.

6. Abdomen—Palpate, percuss, and auscultate the abdomen to rule out visceral bleeding, especially from the liver or spleen.

G. Motor, Reflex, and Cerebellar Examination:

1. Motor function may be difficult or impossible to evaluate in a comatose or very irritable child. Spontaneous movements and reflex withdrawal from noxious stimuli should be noted. For a short time after a concussion or convulsion, there may be transient paresis which may alternate from side to side. Consistent paresis is usually due to contusion or laceration of the brain; progressive paralysis occurs with intracranial bleeding and swelling. Paralysis may be on the same side as the injury or hematoma, due to uncal herniation (Kernohan's syndrome).

2. The reflexes (especially the plantar responses)

may vary markedly in the immediate posttraumatic period or if there has been a seizure. Pathologic reflexes are of lateralizing value when persistent and associated with motor weakness or spasticity. Transient Babinski signs and absent abdominal reflexes are common with mild head trauma in children.

3. Cerebellar testing requires that the patient be conscious and cooperative. Unsteadiness, mild intention tremor, and generalized clumsiness are common in children after head injuries. Ataxia and nystagmus, especially when associated with vertigo and vomiting, raise a suspicion of posterior fossa hematoma, a potentially curable lesion.

H. Sensory Examination: This is often difficult but should be done, especially where a spinal cord injury is suspected.

I. Temperature: Taking the child's temperature may often be delayed until the end of the examination and until the child is calmed. Never insert a thermometer into the mouth or rectum of a restless or convulsing child. If necessary, axillary temperature may be taken. Mild hypothermia immediately after the injury, followed by mild to moderate fever for 1–2 days, is observed frequently in children. Persistent moderate fever is common with subarachnoid hemorrhage.

Classification & Clinical Findings

Head injuries are usually categorized according to the more prominent clinical and pathologic findings. The clinical status, course, and prognosis of the patient depends on the nature and severity of the cerebral insult rather than on the presence and extent of superficial injuries or of skull fracture.

A. Mild: Disturbance or loss of consciousness, if it occurs at all, is transient, lasting seconds to a few minutes. There are no demonstrable residual neurologic signs. There may be no sequelae, or the posttraumatic period may be characterized by mild headache (easily controlled by salicylates), irritability, drowsiness, and occasionally vomiting in younger children. This picture is usually associated with brain concussion, but it may occur with contusion and even limited subarachnoid bleeding.

B. Moderate: Disturbance or loss of consciousness lasts several minutes to perhaps an hour. Abnormal neurologic signs are frequent (though often transient). The posttraumatic period is characterized by more severe headache, irritability, drowsiness, and confusion. Vomiting for 12–36 hours and mild to moderate fever are common. This state is usually associated with some degree of cerebral edema, contusion, or laceration.

C. Severe: Severe head injuries may result in immediate unconsciousness lasting an hour or more or in sudden or progressive deterioration of the level of consciousness after an initial lucid period. Abnormal neurologic signs may develop and persist for hours or days or may be permanent. If consciousness is preserved, the posttraumatic period may be characterized by severe unremitting headache, mental confusion,

marked fluctuations in the level of consciousness, and vomiting. This is usually associated with more extensive cerebral edema, contusion and laceration of the brain, intracranial bleeding, or brain stem damage.

The soft skulls and open cranial sutures in infants and young children may "absorb" some of the force of the head trauma and thus tend to reduce the severity of the injury or result in delayed appearance of neurologic signs.

X-Ray, Laboratory, & Other Methods of Evaluation

A. X-Ray:

1. Skull x-rays—Skull films are indicated in the following cases: (1) obvious moderate to severe and all open head injuries; (2) where a depressed or basilar fracture is suspected; (3) if a foreign body is suspected; (4) where a hypocoagulable hematologic state is present; (5) where the parent or guardian is clearly litigious; and (6) to obtain evidence, where head trauma is suspected but no history of trauma is obtained and no external signs of trauma are found, as may be the case with an abused child. X-rays should be delayed, or bedside portable views obtained, in a very restless, uncooperative child or one in danger of airway obstruction or other serious complication.

Taking skull x-rays routinely has been challenged on both medical and economic grounds. Only about 7% of skull x-rays after head trauma show fractures, but this rarely affects management. In closed head injuries, there is no correlation between fractures and complications, prognosis, or sequelae.

2. Other plain films—Whenever spinal cord injury is suspected, cervical and other spine films must be obtained (as explained above) as soon as feasible, taking care to move the patient as little as possible. X-rays of the extremities, chest, and abdomen should be taken when injury to these parts is thought likely. One common indication is suspected child abuse.

B. Echoencephalography: This rapid, innocuous procedure is employed in evaluating patients for possible intracranial hematomas, cerebral edema, or hemispheric shift.

C. Neuroradiology:

1. Brain scan—Scanning with radioactive isotopes may be useful, when the patient's status permits, in diagnosing intracranial hematomas. (Do not use ^{203}Hg in children.)

2. Computerized tomography—In CT scanning, sophisticated electronic and computer technics have been combined to "scan" the tissues in question (brain, spinal column, and other parts) at a multitude of angles by means of a slit x-ray beam. Absorption values of the sequential readings, varying with the densities of tissues and fluids, are calculated and analyzed so that a "printout" of normal and abnormal tissues and their configuration is obtained. Technical limitations are being overcome; they are relatively few, as in areas where structures and tissues of similar density are adjacent. "Enhancement" is achieved by the intravenous injection of a contrast medium for further definition of tissues. This highly accurate, safe, rapid, and basically painless method, ideal for use in children, exposes the patient to no more irradiation than the routine roentgenogram, even though it distinguishes smaller differences in tissue radiodensity.

The only significant procedural drawback is that the patient must remain motionless during the scan. Specially adapted water-rings or pillows may be fitted to the child's head to achieve this. In very young, restless, or frightened children, sedation, including use of a "cardiac cocktail" or intramuscular paraldehyde—or even general anesthesia—may be required.

3. Cerebral angiography—This may be used where CT scan is not available or for further definition of a suspected lesion. Most cerebral angiograms are now performed via the femoral route. Indications for angiography following head trauma are (1) suspected epidural hematoma, (2) suspected subdural or intracerebral hematoma, (3) suspected thrombosis, and (4) rupture of a vascular malformation or aneurysm.

4. Air studies—Ventriculography or lumbar pneumoencephalography is at times still indicated for the evaluation of posttraumatic hydrocephalus, leptomeningeal or porencephalic cysts, or cerebral atrophy.

D. Lumbar Puncture: There are few indications and many contraindications to spinal taps following head injuries. Lumbar puncture is contraindicated by increased intracranial pressure due to a suspected mass lesion, such as in epidural hematoma or intracerebral hemorrhage.

CSF examination is indicated in children when the following are likely: (1) Cerebral infection or toxic encephalopathy. (Many children will become unsteady and fall or suffer a convulsion at the beginning of these processes.) (2) Subarachnoid hemorrhage. Lumbar puncture may help differentiate concussion (CSF pressure normal or slightly elevated but cells, protein, and glucose normal) from contusion and laceration (CSF pressure often increased, with presence of red cells and xanthochromia), but this is of no help in management or prognosis.

E. Subdural Taps: These are often indicated in infants and small children following head trauma (or when there is a strong suspicion of head trauma) when the anterior fontanel is still open or the coronal sutures are sufficiently patent to allow a subdural needle (No. 20 or 22 gauge with short bevel) to pass. Subdural taps are indicated if, following the initial period, the infant continues to do poorly, has convulsions, or develops a fever; if his hemoglobin falls; or if he shows progressive neurologic signs or abnormal enlargement of head circumference. In infants up to about 18 months of age, transillumination of the head will usually be positive in chronic (but not acute) subdural hematomas.

A small amount of air (10–15 ml) may be injected after removal of an equal amount of fluid; brow-up, brow-down, and right and left lateral skull films will then disclose the extent of the subdural space and of the brain compression or atrophy.

F. Exploratory Bur Holes: Trephination of the skull may be indicated after severe closed head injuries in children whose clinical state is deteriorating rapidly, especially when neurologic signs suggest the presence of extradural or subdural hemorrhage. Bur holes for diagnostic purposes alone are no longer performed in children in whom more definitive studies, such as the CT scan, may be safely carried out first.

G. Electroencephalography: EEG is commonly abnormal in the immediate posttraumatic period, with posterior slowing in a high proportion of cases (80% or more). EEG findings are often out of proportion to clinical symptoms and are of doubtful prognostic significance. The EEG is indicated in posttraumatic epilepsy. Occasionally it is helpful in the diagnosis of subdural hematoma.

An abnormal posttraumatic EEG does not rule out functional factors and overlay. The EEG is often normal in posttraumatic and compensation neurosis.

Differential Diagnosis

Head trauma, especially when due to an accidental fall, is a common occasion for office or emergency visits. It is important to consider head trauma due to child battering or during an epileptic seizure, falls due to ataxia or other neurologic disorder, loss of consciousness due to hypoglycemia, cerebrovascular accident, intoxication, or other causes discussed in the section on Altered States of Consciousness (above).

Complications & Sequelae

A. Posttraumatic Seizures: Seizures may be focal or generalized, varying greatly with age and the site and severity of injury. Seizures in the first 24 hours occur in 6–15% of children with head injuries of all types; they are more common in younger children and following brain lacerations.

Chronic posttraumatic epilepsy in children occurs in only about 2% of the total group but in 5–10% of children who suffered brain lacerations or initial unconsciousness of an hour or more. Over 50% of these seizures occur within the first 6 months; over 80% occur within 2 years.

B. Space-Occupying Lesions: (About 1–3% of children with head injuries seen at major hospitals.)

1. Epidural hematoma—The classical picture of a hemispheric extradural (epidural) hematoma is transient disturbance or loss of consciousness followed by a symptom-free ("lucid") interval of a few hours to a day, and then progressive clouding of consciousness and evolution of a dilated fixed pupil and hemiparesis. The usual cause is bleeding from a torn middle meningeal artery or vein.

In children, this classical sequence is rare. A history of unconsciousness or impaired consciousness is frequently lacking. The symptom-free interval is often atypical because of nonspecific irritability, headache, vomiting, and other complaints; in about one-half of children, the lucid interval is longer than 48 hours' duration, and the course may be fluctuating rather than progressive, without loss of consciousness. As in adults, the site of injury is usually temporal, but fractures across the middle meningeal artery are often not present and the source of bleeding may be from its smaller branches or from torn diploic veins or bridging vessels. Extradural hematomas of clinical significance are uncommon in children under the age of 4 years.

These differences may be due to the tendency of the softer skull of infants to "give," with no fracture on impact; the escape of epidural blood through widened sutures, the fracture site, or an open fontanel; the less rapid or less massive bleeding that occurs from sources outside the middle meningeal artery; the lower systolic pressures in children, especially after blood loss; and perhaps the fact that the brain is less susceptible to pressure changes in children.

Extradural hematomas of the posterior fossa may be difficult to diagnose clinically in children. The presenting symptoms and signs may relate chiefly to the obstruction of CSF flow and consequent development of increased intracranial pressure. Cerebellar signs and cranial nerve palsies should suggest this diagnosis.

Close observation over several days is necessary to detect early signs of epidural hematoma so that neurosurgical consultation and neuroradiodiagnostic studies can be requested early.

2. Subdural hematoma—(About 4–5% of children with a history of head trauma, but the history is often lacking. The male/female incidence is 2:1.) Acute subdural hematoma may occur in association with contusion or laceration. Chronic subdural hematoma is more common. The clinical course is highly variable, depending primarily on the extent of the underlying damage to the cerebral substance and the age of the child. In infants and young children with open fontanels and sutures, there may be considerable delay before symptoms develop. The most common presenting features in children are seizures (about 75% of cases), vomiting (about 60%), drowsiness, irritability, or other personality changes (50%), developmental retardation (20%), and failure to thrive (10%). The presenting signs consist of increased head size and bulging fontanels (80%); retinal hemorrhages (40–65%); anemia (50–70%), extraocular (especially sixth nerve) palsies (40%), hemiparesis (35%), quadriplegia (10%), and fever (10%). There is a high associated incidence of scars and long bone or rib fractures due to "battering."

3. Intracerebral hematoma—(Less than 1% of children with head trauma seen at major hospitals.) Multiple small areas of hemorrhage are more common; larger hematomas may develop beneath a depressed skull fracture. The symptoms and signs vary greatly with the size and location of the hematoma. The frontal and temporal lobes are most frequently involved.

C. Subarachnoid Hemorrhage: In children, traumatic subarachnoid hemorrhage is often relatively asymptomatic and therefore infrequently diagnosed. Nuchal rigidity, disturbance or loss of consciousness, and seizures are usually the outstanding symptoms. (For further details, see Cerebrovascular Disorders.)

D. CSF Rhinorrhea and Otorrhea: (Infrequent in children.) CSF leakage from the nose occurs with fracture of the frontal bone and associated dural and arachnoid tearing. The flow of fluid is increased by erect posture, coughing, and straining. CSF otorrhea with basilar fracture may be of serious prognostic significance.

Infections, particularly meningitis, are a potential threat in CSF leakage. Most CSF leaks heal within 2 weeks in children kept at rest; chronic leaks require surgical repair of the dural tear.

E. Other Acute Paratraumatic Problems:

1. Increased intracranial pressure may be acute or subacute. Manifestations include alterations in consciousness, disturbances of behavior, vomiting, headaches, ataxia, focal weakness, and other neurologic disturbances. Findings are those of a space-occupying lesion, which must be ruled out.

2. Hyponatremia and other electrolyte disturbances are seen most commonly with cerebral edema and CSF rhinorrhea or otorrhea.

3. Infections relate to the nature and severity of the head trauma. There may be pneumonia, often due to aspiration, in children who suffered convulsions or coma. Dural tears may lead to meningitis. Infected skull fractures may result in osteomyelitis.

4. Fever, particularly in younger children, may be due to hypothalamic involvement, dehydration, subdural effusions, resorption of necrotic tissue or subarachnoid blood, and infection.

5. Retrograde amnesia for the events immediately surrounding the head injury is not uncommon, even when there was no seizure.

F. Posttraumatic CNS Structural Complications:

1. Posttraumatic hydrocephalus—The incidence of this complication is not known. It is seen most often in infants and toddlers and is most commonly due to aqueductal gliosis or basilar arachnoiditis. Congenital anomalies of the CSF passageways may play a role.

2. Posttraumatic focal deficits—Cranial nerve palsies (most commonly abducens or facial palsy), optic atrophy, anosmia, motor deficits, diabetes insipidus, or aphasia may occur, depending on the site and nature of the injury.

3. Leptomeningeal cyst—Infants and younger children (usually under age 3) with linear fracture or diastatic suture separation may develop a leptomeningeal cyst—also referred to as cephalhydrocele, spurious cranial meningocele, or "growing skull fracture." This is due to a tear of the dura and arachnoid or entrapment of the arachnoid between the separated bony parts. CSF then accumulates under the scalp, resulting in a fluctuant, often pulsatile swelling which can usually be transilluminated. It should not be aspirated because there is a risk of infection. In some cases, the continued pulsatile effect of the cerebral tissue or loculated fluid causes progressive separation of the bony parts and further damage to the underlying brain. Skull x-rays 2–3 months following the initial trauma usually establish the diagnosis. Early surgical repair of the defect is indicated.

G. Postconcussion Syndrome: The manifestations of the postconcussion syndrome in children vary markedly from those seen in adults. The symptoms also vary with age (preschool, elementary school, older child). The chief complaints usually center around disturbances of behavior (aggressiveness, regression, withdrawal, antisocial acts) and sleep, and may include enuresis, tension phenomena (irritability, emotional lability), phobias (fear of cars, fear of going out alone), and deterioration in school performance. Somatic complaints such as headache, dizziness, tinnitus, and neck pains are relatively uncommon.

Compensation neurosis in children is usually induced by the parents and may cause secondary emotional problems. Repeated questioning by adults concerning somatic symptoms and repeated physical, neurologic, or psychologic examinations may, through suggestion and arousal of anxiety, provoke multiple complaints and behavioral and emotional difficulties in the child.

H. Posttraumatic Mental Retardation: Pseudo-retardation (secondary to emotional problems) is not uncommon, but true intellectual loss usually occurs only with very severe injuries. The presence of microcephaly with a head circumference more than 2 SD below the mean for the age at which the accident occurred suggests that mental deficiency antedated the trauma. Psychologic testing may be useful.

Treatment

A. Emergency Measures:

1. Maintain airway and treat shock—See Altered States of Consciousness, above.

2. Anticonvulsants—For status epilepticus, give diazepam (Valium), phenobarbital, or paraldehyde followed by phenobarbital or phenytoin (Dilantin); the latter is less likely to raise the question of depressing consciousness. (See Seizure Disorders.)

B. General Measures:

1. Observation—Careful attention must be paid to level of consciousness, pupillary reactions, and vital signs. Children with severe injuries, loss of consciousness for more than a few minutes, or prolonged and continued seizures must be hospitalized. Most children with mild to moderate concussion need not be hospitalized and can be observed at home if their parents are reliable and live within a reasonable distance from a treatment center. The parents should check the child every few hours, especially to see if the sleeping child can be aroused normally. The parents should maintain telephone contact with the physician, and he should examine the child at least once in the first 24—48 hours after a concussion.

Since the course of epidural hematoma is quite atypical in children, with signs and symptoms often not apparent until more than 24 hours following the head injury, overnight admission of a child lucid on initial examination does not ensure early diagnosis of this serious complication.

Only continued careful observation, maintenance of contact with the parents, and prompt neurologic reevaluation when indicated will ensure early diagnosis of intracranial hematoma, hydrocephalus, posttraumatic seizures, and leptomeningeal cysts, etc.

2. Restlessness—Diphenhydramine (Benadryl) is often an effective and safe sedative in very young children. Chloral hydrate and paraldehyde may also be used. Do not use opiates or similar compounds such as pentazocine (Talwin).

3. Headache—Give aspirin as necessary in doses appropriate for the size and age of the patient.

4. Fluids—If the child is able to take fluids by mouth, maintain on clear fluids (noncarbonated soft drinks, fruit juices, etc) until it is reasonably certain that vomiting will not occur. Intravenous fluids, if indicated, should be on the low side of maintenance requirements; a slight deficit in the first 3—4 days will counteract cerebral edema and minimize the possibility of water intoxication due to inappropriate ADH secretion.

5. Tetanus prophylaxis—Tetanus toxoid (or tetanus toxoid plus diphtheria toxoid), 0.5 ml, should be given for scalp wounds, particularly if "dirty," and if the child has not had a booster within 4 years.

6. Antibiotics—These are generally best withheld until a specific need arises. With major "dirty" wounds—especially if there is dural tearing, CSF leakage, and extensive cerebral tissue damage—give antibiotics in therapeutic dosages as for purulent meningitis of unknown cause (see Chapter 37).

7. Treatment of cerebral edema—See Cerebral Edema, p 553.

8. Maintenance of normal body temperature—Hyperthermia is often best controlled by covering the child with towels soaked in alcohol and water, using a fan to aid in evaporation. The use of chlorpromazine in the immediate posttraumatic period is not recommended. Hypothermia, once favored in the treatment of severe brain injury, is no longer recommended.

9. Battering—If clinical and x-ray evidence suggests that the child has been abused, appropriate measures must be taken to ensure social service and psychiatric follow-up (see Chapter 29).

C. Surgical Measures: The chief obligation of the physician caring for the child is early recognition of complications that require prompt diagnostic studies and neurosurgical intervention, eg, extradural hemorrhage, subdural or intracerebral hematoma, posttraumatic hydrocephalus. Many subdural hematomas may be evacuated by "taps" alone.

Note: If there are compelling clinical reasons to suspect epidural hematoma, it is better to relieve pressure surgically immediately than to risk serious delay in treatment by transporting the patient a long distance to a medical center. Major lacerations are best dealt with by the surgeon.

1. Fractures—"Ping-pong ball" skull fractures in very young babies usually correct themselves within a few weeks and require no specific treatment. This is also true of very slightly depressed skull fractures. Depressed fractures involving the inner table of the skull and their accompanying dural and cerebral defects require surgical therapy.

2. Cranioplasty—Repair of major skull defects can

often be deferred in young children until the patient is of school age. It is well to remember that the skull attains about 90% of adult growth by 5–6 years of age.

Prognosis

The outlook in children who have suffered head injuries is far better than in adults. Well over 90% of those who sustain concussions and simple linear fractures are free of symptoms after the initial period. Even in severe head trauma, the mortality rate is only about 20%, as compared with 30–35% in adults; similarly, the incidence of neurologic sequelae (including seizures) in such cases is about 20%. Such sequelae are highest in cases of extensive brain laceration (about 40%) and lowest in severe contusions and cerebral edema (about 2–3%). Behavioral and emotional problems constitute the bulk of posttraumatic difficulties in children but normally disappear within a few months or a year.

DeVivo DC, Dodge PR: The critically ill child: Diagnosis and management of head injury. Pediatrics 48:129, 1971.

Dillon H, Leopold RL: Children and the post-concussion syndrome. JAMA 175:86, 1961.

Feuer H: Early management of pediatric head injury: Physiologic aspects. Pediatr Clin North Am 22:425, 1975.

Jennet B, van de Sande J: EEG prediction of post-traumatic epilepsy. Epilepsia 16:251, 1975.

McCullough DC & others: Computerized axial tomography in clinical pediatrics. Pediatrics 59:173, 1977.

Mealey J: Infantile subdural hematomas. Pediatr Clin North Am 22:433, 1975.

Roberts F, Shopfner CE: Plain skull roentgenograms in children with head trauma. Am J Roentgenol Radium Ther Nucl Med 114:230, 1972.

PERINATAL HEAD INJURIES

The incidence of head injuries during birth is not known. It has been estimated that such injuries, notably intracranial hemorrhage, account for 3–5 deaths per 1000 live births, or 10–20% of all neonatal deaths. Unlike the violent impact responsible for postnatal head trauma, perinatal injuries are produced by prolonged gradual pressure on the head. A negative pressure gradient as the head goes through the birth canal may play a role. Predisposing or contributing factors include premature birth, cephalopelvic disproportion, shoulder dystocia, breech and precipitate delivery, prolonged labor, and misapplication of forceps or vacuum extractors, complicated by hypoxia, metabolic acidosis, venous stasis, and rupture of thin-walled veins in the germinal matrix of the infant's brain.

Clinical Findings

A. Symptoms and Signs:

1. Soft tissue injuries—There may be erythema, abrasions, and necrosis of the face and scalp, caput succedaneum, scalpel injuries following cesarian sec-

tion, or cephalhematoma. The latter usually does not appear until several hours after birth and does not transilluminate; occasionally this subperiosteal hematoma grows so large as to cause symptoms due to hypovolemia.

2. Fractures—Linear skull fractures may be asymptomatic and often are not diagnosed unless accompanied by other findings. About 25% of cephalhematomas are associated with fractures. In occipital fractures with separation of the basal and squamous portions due to undue traction on the hyperextended spine while the head is still fixed in the maternal pelvis during breech delivery, there usually is massive and almost invariably fatal hemorrhage.

3. Intracranial hemorrhage—Tentorial laceration with tearing of the underlying sinuses, rupture of the great vein of Galen, or rupture of veins at the junction of the falx cerebri and tentorium usually results in massive and often fatal hemorrhage.

Rupture of more superiorly placed cerebral veins results in less extensive bleeding, producing subdural hematomas which are more readily diagnosed and treated. Acute subdural hematomas are rare in neonates and result in profound neurologic deficits and depression; subacute and chronic subdural hemorrhages are the rule. Extradural hemorrhage is exceedingly rare during birth.

The clinical manifestations of intracranial bleeding in the newborn are nonspecific, consisting principally of the triad of apneic spells, cyanosis, and convulsions. The neonate may at first be merely listless or floppy, with little spontaneous motor activity; a few hours or a day after delivery, the cry may become shrill ("cerebral cry"), the infant may be jittery or have seizures, muscle tone may become increased, or abnormal postures, including opisthotonos, may be prominent.

The fontanels may be tense and full, the sutures separated widely, the head circumference increased by 1 cm or more (due largely to cerebral edema), and the pupils irregular. Retinal hemorrhages are seen so frequently in infants who do well that no specific conclusions can be drawn from this finding. In neonates, focal neurologic signs are relatively uncommon and usually appear late; these include asymmetry of posture, tone, and reflex responses. The most dependable findings pointing to neurologic damage are persistent asymmetry or absence of the Moro response, marked absence of head control when the infant is pulled gently from the supine into the sitting position (traction response), and poor or absent sucking.

Transillumination is usually negative early since any subdural hematoma is still clotted.

B. Laboratory Findings:

1. Blood—Rapid decreases in the hematocrit or hemoglobin occur with massive bleeding, whether into the subperiosteum or intracranially. Coagulation tests may be abnormal. Hypocalcemia occurs commonly in infants following a traumatic birth, but blood glucose, phosphorus, magnesium, sodium, pH, total CO_2, and P_{CO_2} should also be determined.

2. CSF—Lumbar puncture is imperative. A moderate degree of xanthochromia, 20—50 red cells, and protein up to 150 mg/100 ml are considered by most authorities to be within the limits of normal in neonates; higher values suggest subarachnoid bleeding. A low CSF glucose in the absence of infection is most apt to be due to hypoglycemia, but it occasionally occurs 5—8 days after subarachnoid hemorrhage.

C. Subdural and Ventricular Taps: The subdural tap may yield little or no fluid early, even when there is subdural hematoma, because the blood is clotted. Later, such a tap may not only be diagnostic, but removal of subdural fluid will be therapeutic. Ventricular tap may be indicated when there appears to be intraventricular hemorrhage. It should be performed under experienced supervision.

D. Skull X-Rays: Skull x-rays should be deferred until the infant's condition is stable enough so that adequate views can be obtained; the findings, however, rarely affect management. When depressed skull fractures other than the innocuous "ping-pong ball" type are suspected, tangential views at right angles to the fracture should be obtained to indicate the extent of the depression of bone or bony fragments.

E. Computerized Tomography: CT brain scan, discussed in detail above, may be performed in infants, especially when there is unexplained cardiorespiratory or neurologic deterioration and bloody CSF. It provides information on the size and extent of intracerebral hematomas and distinguishes between subdural and intraventricular ones. Whether this will ultimately reduce morbidity and mortality rates for the neonates with intraventricular bleeding must be determined by long-range studies.

F. Electroencephalography: EEG should be deferred until the infant's condition has stabilized. A "flat" EEG or one with sharply defined paroxysmal activity is a poor prognostic sign. Other abnormalities, such as hemispheric asymmetry or high-amplitude dysrhythmic potentials, are of less prognostic value.

Treatment

Treatment is largely symptomatic. Specific treatment is directed at metabolic and electrolyte disturbances and infections. Anticonvulsants, particularly phenobarbital, 3—5 mg/kg/day IV, should be given for seizures. (See also section on Seizure Disorders.)

Repeated subdural taps are required in the presence of effusions. Shunting (subdural-peritoneal or subdural-pleural shunts may be necessary) and repeated lumbar punctures (and, rarely, ventricular punctures), particularly when the CSF is grossly bloody, are indicated to relieve irritation or pressure upon vital structures and may improve the infant's status and reduce the frequency and severity of seizures.

Vitamin K_1 (phytonadione), 1 mg IM (if not previously administered to the mother), may be given to the infant with intracranial hemorrhage to reduce the possibility of bleeding associated with vitamin K deficiency.

Significantly depressed skull fractures should be elevated surgically. Most so-called "ping-pong ball" indentations correct themselves as the brain grows.

Prognosis

The prognosis in infants with uncomplicated scalp injuries, linear fractures, "ping-pong ball" depressions, and cephalhematomas is good.

In infants with subacute and chronic subdural hematomas secondary to birth trauma, the prognosis is reasonably good if effusions are evacuated by tapping or by surgical means. However, the incidence of neurologic complications—particularly hydrocephalus, microcephaly, and seizures due to the underlying cortical damage—remains fairly high.

Neonates with major intracranial bleeding who survive frequently have focal neurologic deficits, mental retardation, and seizures. The problem may be compounded by the hypoxia which often initiates or accompanies bleeding. The overall prognosis for life of the small neonate (less than 2500 gm) with repetitive seizures due to intraventricular hemorrhage is extremely guarded.

Focal seizures, especially psychomotor (or "mesial temporal lobe") epilepsy, have been related to the squeezing of the head during the birth process even when there is no significant clinical evidence of trauma at birth. The onset of these seizures may be delayed for many years. Lesser degrees of head trauma may cause minimal cerebral dysfunction.

Abrams IF, McLennan JE, Duckett GE: Acute neonatal subdural hematoma following breech delivery. Am J Dis Child 131:192, 1977.

Anderson JM, Brown JK, Cockburn F: On the role of disseminated intravascular coagulation in the pathology of birth asphyxia. Dev Med Child Neurol 16:581, 1974.

Armstrong D, Norman MG: Periventricular leukomalacia in neonates: Complications and sequelae. Arch Dis Child 49:367, 1974.

Brown JK: Neurological aspects of perinatal asphyxia. Dev Med Child Neurol 16:567, 1974.

Davies PA, Tizard JPM: Very low birthweight and subsequent neurological defect. Dev Med Child Neurol 17:3, 1975.

Francis-Williams J, Davies PA: Very low birthweight and later intelligence. Dev Med Child Neurol 16:709, 1974.

Krishnamoorty KS & others: Evaluation of neonatal intracranial hemorrhage by computerized tomography. Pediatrics 59:165, 1977.

Leech RW, Kohnen P: Subependymal and intraventricular hemorrhages in the newborn. Am J Pathol 77:465, 1974.

Natelson SF, Sayers MP: The fate of children sustaining severe head trauma during birth. Pediatrics 51:169, 1973.

Seay AR, Bray PF: Significance of seizures in infants weighing less than 2500 grams. Arch Neurol 34:381, 1977.

Volpe JJ: Perinatal hypoxic-ischemic brain injury. Pediatr Clin North Am 23:383, 1976.

TUMORS OF THE CNS

1. INTRACRANIAL TUMORS

Essentials of Diagnosis

- Focal neurologic deficits, usually slowly progressive.
- Increased intracranial pressure with unremitting headache, vomiting, and papilledema.
- Space-occupying lesion demonstrated by neurodiagnostic studies or at operation.

General Considerations

Malignancies are (after accidents) the second most frequent cause of death in children over age 1, and CNS tumors, in two-thirds of cases infratentorial, are second only to the leukemias among neoplasms. For a variety of reasons, specific diagnosis may be delayed for 6 months or more.

The histologic types of brain tumors found in children are as follows:

(1) Gliomas (about 70%–80% of *all* brain tumors in children): (a) astrocytomas, especially of the cerebellum (25–30% of the total); (b) medulloblastomas (almost 50% of infratentorial tumors of childhood; 20% of gliomas); (c) brain stem gliomas, ependymomas, and malignant gliomas of childhood (variants of the glioblastoma multiforme of adults, each representing nearly 10% of childhood CNS tumors); and (d) gliomas of the optic nerves and chiasm (5%).

(2) Craniopharyngiomas (about 7%).

(3) Choroid plexus papillomas (about 3%).

(4) Tumors of the pineal body (3%).

(5) Other tumor types are relatively rare.

Meningiomas, acoustic neurinomas, and pituitary adenomas are rare in children. With the exception of leukemic infiltration, tumors metastatic to the brain are also uncommon; they include neuroblastoma, Wilms's tumor, and Ewing's sarcoma.

Clinical Findings (See Table 21–4.)

A. Symptoms and Signs:

1. Signs of increased intracranial pressure—These include headache, vomiting, abducens palsy, diplopia, papilledema, and, in very young children, a bulging fontanel or greater than normal increase in head circumference. These signs may be due either to obstruction of CSF flow with resulting hydrocephalus or to the tumor mass itself.

2. Focal neurologic signs—Infratentorial (especially cerebellar) tumors most commonly manifest themselves by ataxia, nystagmus, and signs and symptoms of increased intracranial pressure. Supratentorial hemispheric tumors may be manifested by progressive neurologic deficits such as contralateral hemiparesis and spasticity and by seizures; young children rarely are aware of sensory deficits. Visual difficulties, particularly hemianopsias, are rarely reported

by young children but may be demonstrated in them by opticokinetic testing or by playing with them, bringing targets into the peripheral field while having the child fix on another object in front. Progressive speech difficulties, particularly when coupled with seizures, point to involvement of the left frontotemporal or parietal lobe. Severe weight loss may occur in diencephalic, cerebellar, brain stem, and intraventricular tumors; marked obesity is sometimes seen in tumors involving the anterior third ventricle and hypothalamus.

Skin lesions may be present, eg, café au lait spots, amelanotic patches, and other stigmas of neurocutaneous dysplasia, in which there is a high incidence of brain tumor of all types.

B. Laboratory Findings: Endocrine status should be assessed if pituitary and hypothalamic involvement is suspected or evident. *Note:* Lumbar puncture for CSF examination is rarely justified—and usually contraindicated—when brain tumor is suspected. CSF obtained at the time of neuroradiologic studies or surgical intervention should be cultured and studied. Cytologic examination of CSF may reveal the presence of tumor cells, as in medulloblastoma, ependymoma, or leptomeningeal sarcoma. CSF protein may be elevated, particularly with malignant gliomas. CSF glucose may be low in the absence of infection when there is extensive meningeal infiltration by tumor, as in leukemia, medulloblastoma, pineal sarcoma, or melanosarcoma.

C. X-Ray Findings:

1. Skull x-rays may show signs of increased intracranial pressure, such as splitting of sutures in younger children and erosion of the posterior clinoids and thinning of sphenoid ridges in older children. Intracranial calcifications are found in the suprasellar region in craniopharyngiomas and also occur, usually asymmetrically, in oligodendrogliomas and other tumors. Enlargement of the optic foramens (> 8 mm) and a strikingly J-, pear-, or banana-shaped sella are seen in optic gliomas. Pineal shifts are rarely encountered on x-rays in children because of the rarity of pineal calcification at this age.

2. Computerized tomography (CT brain scan), discussed in detail on p 567, is the procedure of choice for the investigation of patients with suspected intracranial lesions and for the more accurate selection of patients for whom a further study, especially angiography, may still be indicated.

3. Isotopic scanning is both simple and useful even in the diagnosis of infratentorial tumors; however, a negative scan does not rule out the presence of tumor. It may be particularly helpful in following a patient after chemotherapy or radiation therapy.

4. Cerebral angiography via the femoral, right brachial, or carotid artery may be important in differentiating between a tumor and a vascular malformation and in demonstrating the abnormal vasculature around the tumor bed preoperatively.

5. Ventriculography is employed far less because of CT scanning. It may at times be used where midline

Table 21—4. Brain tumors.

Part Affected	Symptoms and Signs	Radiologic Findings	Tumor Type and Characteristics	Treatment and Prognosis
Cerebellum and fourth ventricle	Evidence of increased intracranial pressure.* Cerebellar signs.† Signs due to pressure on adjacent structures.‡ Personality and behavioral changes. Occasionally emaciation.	1. Signs of increased intracranial pressure on skull films.§ 2. Computerized tomography of posterior fossa; will also demonstrate hydrocephalus. 3. Brain scan of posterior fossa may be helpful. 4. Ventriculography (or positive pressure encephalography) may show tumor and hydrocephalus. 5. Angiography is a useful adjunctive study to demonstrate abnormal vascular pattern and possible herniation.	1. Astrocytoma: slow growth, frequently cystic.	Surgical removal. Follow by intensive x-ray therapy if removal is incomplete. Prognosis good if removal complete.
			2. Medulloblastoma: rapid growth, seen mostly at age 2—6 years, about 75% in boys; seeds along CSF pathways.	Surgical decompression of posterior fossa and x-ray therapy to site, cerebrum, and spinal canal. Chemotherapy. Shunt (ventriculopleural, etc) to relieve CSF obstruction. Prognosis grave: rare 5-year survivors.
			3. Less common: ependymoma, hemangioblastoma, choroid plexus papilloma.	Surgical cure possible with hemangioblastoma and choroid plexus papilloma.
Brain stem	1. Cranial nerve palsies (IX–X, VII, VI, V– chiefly sensory root), pyramidal tract signs (hemiparesis), and cerebellar ataxia. 2. Rarely, signs of increased intracranial pressure or emaciation.	Demonstration of posterior fossa and displacement of cerebral aqueduct and fourth ventricle by CT scan, pneumoencephalography, or angiography.	Astrocytoma (varying grades; polar spongioblastoma): usually rapid growth and recurrence.	X-ray therapy to site: remission rate for short periods. Prognosis grave: average survival 1 year, particularly when medulla is involved.
Midbrain and third ventricle	1. Personality and behavioral changes, often early. 2. Evidence of increased intracranial pressure.* 3. Pyramidal tract signs and cerebellar signs.† 4. Inability to rotate eyes upward. 5. Sudden loss of consciousness; seizures rare.	1. Signs of increased intracranial pressure on skull films. 2. Brain scan and echoencephalography helpful. 3. CT scan. 4. Air and contrast ventriculography in third ventricle masses. 5. Pineal rarely calcified in childhood.	Astrocytomas, teratomas including pinealoma (macrogenitosomia praecox in boys), ependymoma.	Shunt procedure (ventriculocisternal, etc) for relief of CSF obstruction and intensive x-ray therapy. Prognosis poor.
			Choroid plexus papilloma and colloid cyst (rare).	With total surgical removal, prognosis good.
Diencephalon	1. Emaciated; good intake. 2. Often very active, euphoric. 3. Few neurologic findings: occasional vertical nystagmus, tremor, ataxia. 4. Pale; without anemia. 5. Frequently: eosinophilia, decreased T_4 and pituitary reserve.	CT scan, the procedure of choice, or pneumoencephalography, showing defect in floor of third ventricle and other midline findings. Echoencephalography may be useful. EEG and angiography usually nondiagnostic.	Usually astrocytomas; less common, oligodendroglioma, glioma, ependymoma, glioblastoma.	X-ray treatment. CSF shunt for block. Prognosis variable; generally poor.

Table 21—4 (cont'd). Brain tumors.

Part Affected	Symptoms and Signs	Radiologic Findings	Tumor Type and Characteristics	Treatment and Prognosis
Suprasellar region	1. Visual disorders (visual field defects, optic atrophy). 2. Hypothalamic disorders (including diabetes insipidus, adiposity). 3. Pituitary disorders (growth arrest, hypothyroidism, delayed sexual maturation). 4. Evidence of increased intracranial pressure.*	1. Skull films: suprasellar calcification in about 90%. Deformity of sella turcica frequent. Enlarged optic foramens in optic gliomas. 2. CT scan. 3. Pneumoencephalography in absence of increased intracranial pressure; otherwise ventriculography.	Optic glioma: high incidence of café au lait spots. The feet and hands may be large in infants and young children if the diencephalon is involved.	X-ray if optic chiasm is involved. Surgical removal if only optic nerve is involved. Prognosis is fair to good. Conservative approach advised.
			Craniopharyngioma: often dormant for years.	Complete excision of craniopharyngioma with hormone replacement is now often feasible; or drainage of cyst and irradiation. Prognosis with complete removal is good.
Cerebral hemispheres and lateral ventricles	1. Evidence of increased intracranial pressure.* 2. Seizures (generalized, psychomotor, focal) in about 40%. 3. Neurologic deficits include hemiparesis (40%), visual field defects, ataxia, personality changes.	1. Signs of increased intracranial pressure. Occasionally calcifications. 2. CT scan and angiography preferred where lateralizing signs present. 3. Brain scan may be helpful, as may be echoencephalogram and EEG. 4. Air contrast studies decreasingly employed.	Gliomas; primary astrocytomas; glioblastomas in 10%. Meningiomas rare. Leptomeningeal sarcoma.	Surgical biopsy or excision where possible. X-ray treatment. Prognosis varies with tumor type. Chemotherapy gaining in trial and usage.
			Ependymoma and choroid plexus papilloma.	Surgical excision of choroid plexus papilloma; occasionally, hydrocephalus persists and requires shunt procedure.

*Evidence of increased intracranial pressure includes headache, vomiting (often without nausea, and before breakfast), diplopia, blurred vision, papilledema; personality changes, including irritability, apathy, disturbances in sleep and eating patterns, are frequent. Sudden enlargement of the head if head circumferences have been plotted is detectable when sutures are still open or after sutures have split. Alterations of consciousness. Stiff neck with tonsillar herniation.

†Cerebellar signs: ataxia, dysmetria, nystagmus. Truncal ataxia in absence of lateralizing signs most common in vermis tumors.

‡Signs due to pressure on adjacent structures: for posterior fossa, may include head tilting, cranial nerve signs, pyramidal tract signs, suboccipital tenderness, stiff neck.

§X-ray findings of increased intracranial pressure: splitting of sutures, erosion of posterior clinoids and thinning of sphenoid wings. Increased digital markings unreliable.

tumors, both infra- and supratentorial, are suspected. Contrast medium, such as Pantopaque, is instilled occasionally for better visualization of the posterior third ventricle, the cerebral aqueduct, or the fourth ventricle. This procedure will also relieve intracranial hypertension prior to attack upon (or biopsy of) the tumor.

6. Pneumoencephalography is of value in lesions not causing increased intracranial pressure, as is usually the case with brain stem glioma, optic glioma, or craniopharyngioma, and for better definition of infratentorial lesions. Its use has been greatly curtailed by CT scanning.

D. Electroencephalography may show focal slowing and is of localizing value in about 70% of supratentorial tumors. False localization may occur. In infratentorial tumors, the EEG may merely show generalized slowing in the occipital and temporal regions or bifrontal slowing.

E. Echoencephalography may be helpful in rapidly determining the presence of hydrocephalus, third ventricle shift, or subdural effusions.

Differential Diagnosis

A clinical picture similar to that of brain tumor, with a history of insidious onset and progressive, unremitting course, headache, vomiting, seizures, and focal neurologic deficits, may be produced by any of the following disorders: subdural hematoma, toxic encephalopathies (eg, lead, uremia), "pseudotumor cerebri" of varying causation, brain abscess, tuberculoma or other granuloma, encephalitides (eg, herpes simplex), degenerative CNS diseases, and slowly expanding or "leaking" cerebrovascular malformations. These can usually be differentiated by appropriate diagnostic studies.

Treatment

A. Surgical Treatment: Total extirpation is the procedure of choice if the location and type of tumor permit. Other types of surgical treatment are partial removal or biopsy, surgical decompression, and shunting procedures for relief of CSF obstruction.

B. Radiation Therapy: Radiation therapy is indicated in conjunction with surgery in many tumors. It is of particular importance to give radiation therapy along the entire neuraxis in medulloblastoma after the diagnosis has been confirmed by biopsy. Radiation therapy is given alone for intrinsic tumors of the brain stem and those around the pineal gland and quadrigeminal plate. In the latter instances, shunting for relief of obstructive hydrocephalus may first be necessary.

C. Antitumor Chemotherapy: Methotrexate, 0.5 mg/kg body weight intrathecally, about every fifth day until no cells are seen in the CSF, has been used in medulloblastoma, meningeal sarcoma, and leukemia. Intraventricular perfusion of methotrexate, with removal of perfusant from the lumbar subarachnoid space, is a recently introduced procedure. Other agents, some still in the experimental stage, are being used with increasing frequency.

D. Replacement Hormone Therapy: This is usually required in craniopharyngiomas and pituitary and hypothalamic tumors. Corticosteroids (especially dexamethasone) may be given prior to and for a few days following surgery to reduce cerebral edema. (See sections on Altered States of Consciousness and Head Injuries for details.)

E. Anticonvulsants: Anticonvulsants are given as outlined in the section on seizure disorders. In general, phenobarbital, phenytoin, and primidone (singly or in combination) are the drugs of choice for seizures due to brain tumors.

F. Emergency Medical Treatment for Increased Intracranial Pressure: See discussion on p 553.

Prognosis (See Table 21–4.)

The overall operative mortality rate is about 5%. The older the child and the less malignant the tumor, the better the outlook.

A. Benign Tumors: (About 47% of cases.) Total excision is essentially curative. In suprasellar tumors, a normal life span but with neurologic and endocrine impairment is common following surgery or irradiation (or both).

B. Malignant Tumors: (About 53% of cases.) Particularly in medulloblastoma, brain stem glioma, and most ependymomas, death within 1–5 years of diagnosis is the usual outcome. Advances in radiation and chemotherapy are improving this outlook.

Matson DD: Neoplasm, cranial and intracranial. Pages 403–642 in: *Neurosurgery of Infancy and Childhood,* 2nd ed. Thomas, 1969.

Nellhaus G: Brain tumors. Pages 91–110 in: *Clinical Management of Cancer in Children.* Pochedly C (editor). Publishing Sciences Group, 1975.

2. SPINAL CORD TUMORS

The relatively low incidence of spinal cord tumors in children often results in serious delay in diagnosis or in a misdiagnosis of "progressive cerebral palsy" or a degenerative disorder.

Such tumors may be extra- or intramedullary and include dermoid cysts, teratomas, neuroblastomas, astrocytomas, ependymomas, and other types.

Symptoms and signs usually progress more slowly than in transverse myelitis or other causes of acute flaccid paralysis (Table 21–9) and include disturbances of gait, pain in the back and legs (more common in extramedullary tumors), weakness and disturbances of sensation in the legs, and urinary incontinence of recent origin.

Neurologic findings—often symmetrical with intramedullary and asymmetrical with extramedullary tumors and varying with their site and extent—include curvature of the spine and localized tenderness; weakness, spasms, sensory deficits, and pathologic reflexes of the lower extremities; and dribbling of urine and loss of anal sphincter tone. Café au lait spots suggest neurofibromatosis. Some forms of spinal dysraphism (see below) may behave like spinal cord tumors.

The diagnosis is made roentgenographically. In 70% of patients, spine films show destructive changes of the vertebra involved; chest x-rays, which should always be obtained, show pulmonary metastases and rib erosion in almost 30% of cases.

Myelography is the procedure of choice for localization of the tumor, but it may have to be performed via a cisternal tap rather than the usual lumbar site. Where the history extends over only hours or 1–2 days, transverse myelitis is more likely; this may be aggravated by myelography. The CSF may be xanthochromic, with a high protein content, and may contain tumor cells on cytologic examination.

With benign tumors, total excision and cure is often possible. In malignant tumors, decompressive laminectomy, partial excision, irradiation, and chemotherapy are employed, but the prognosis is poor regardless of treatment.

Haslam RHA: "Progressive cerebral palsy" or spinal cord tumor? Two cases of mistaken identity. Dev Med Child Neurol 17:232, 1975.

Vogelsang H, Busse O: Neuroradiological diagnosis of intraspinal tumors in children. Neuropädiatrie 7:3, 1976.

CEREBROVASCULAR DISORDERS

General Considerations

About 1−1.5% of all admissions to teaching hospitals (or 5% of pediatric neurologic disorders) are due to cerebrovascular disorders. Intracerebral vascular disease accounts for 17% of pediatric necropsies. About half of children with leukemia have intracranial bleeding. Homocystinuria is also increasingly recognized as a cause of cerebrovascular accidents.

The deficits in children tend to be more often global or multifocal but also more difficult to demonstrate angiographically than strokes in adults.

Acute hemiplegias in childhood. The special circumstances of this syndrome—often termed acute infantile hemiplegia as if it were a single pathologic entity—require additional description. The essential feature is the relatively rapid acquisition of hemiplegia in a previously neurologically intact child. The syndrome appears most often between 1 month and 6 years of age (usually under 3 years). The onset may be sudden or may evolve over a period of minutes to 1 or 2 days, frequently with an intermittent ("stuttering") progression. Cerebral vasculitis with resultant intravascular thrombosis is considered the principal cause, but it may be difficult to demonstrate angiographically. The syndrome occurs most often in association with infections of the upper respiratory tract and, next most commonly, with head trauma and with blunt injuries to the internal carotid artery or its surrounding tissues. Almost any of the conditions underlying cerebrovascular disorders in childhood (Table 21−5) may be responsible. Frequently, however, no cause can be identified; this has led to the term idiopathic infantile hemiplegia.

Clinical Findings

A. Symptoms and Signs: These are highly variable, depending on the nature, site, and extent of the lesion. Alterations in level of consciousness, disturbances of sensorium, mood, behavior, and of cognitive and perceptual functions, the frequency of seizures, and the more widespread nature of the deficits in younger children may make it difficult to pinpoint the lesions clinically. (See Table 21−5 for a guide to the diagnosis of cerebrovascular disorders in childhood.)

Fever is observed frequently and may be part of an underlying or associated systemic disorder or may be of central origin. Vasomotor disturbances of involved extremities may be observed.

Retinal hemorrhages may occur with sudden increases in intracranial pressure, as in subarachnoid hemorrhage or from subdural hematomas, but should raise the suspicion of head trauma—especially child battering.

Seizures, which may be focal but frequently become generalized, occur in 50% or more of patients. They may precede, accompany, or follow the onset of other neurologic (especially motor) deficits.

In *acute hemiplegia,* the hemiplegia may be flaccid initially. Spasticity usually appears within a few days to 2 weeks. The right side is involved more frequently than the left. Hemianopsia and hemisensory deficits are also often present. The seizures may remain entirely confined to the involved side, resulting in the "hemiplegia-hemiepilepsy" (HHE) syndrome.

B. Laboratory Findings: Blood count, sedimentation rate, urinalysis, and electrolytes are usually normal; when grossly abnormal, they tend to reflect an underlying systemic disease rather than cerebrovascular accident.

Special studies as suggested by clinical indices may include screening for blood dyscrasias, including coagulation and cysteine screening tests, LE cell preparations, or renal function studies. Bacterial, serologic, and virologic studies should be performed in all cases associated with an inflammatory process.

Lumbar puncture should be performed in the presence of fever and meningeal signs to rule out treatable forms of intracranial infections. Except when these findings dominate the clinical picture, lumbar puncture may well be deferred until x-ray studies have shown that tentorial or tonsillar herniation is unlikely. CSF opening and closing pressures should be recorded. The color of the fluid and the distribution of erythrocytes from the initial drops to the last aliquot obtained should be carefully noted. For a differential evaluation of the findings, see Tables 21−1 and 21−5.

C. X-Ray Findings: Skull films are mandatory to rule out evidence of long-standing increased intracranial pressure, calcifications, or fractures. Chest films and a skeletal survey are often indicated—the latter especially in younger children when child abuse is suspected.

Although CT scan may be instructive, cerebral angiography remains the definitive procedure and should be performed as early as possible. It can be done percutaneously even in small infants by those skilled in the procedure. If bilateral involvement is suspected or the possibility of an arteriovenous malformation with multiple feeding vessels exists, arteriography via femoral catheterization may be most informative. In children with congenital heart disease who have had a vascular accident, cerebral angiography may be done at the time of cardiac catheterization by advancing the catheter into the aortic arch and then injecting a bolus of dye. In acute hemiplegia, carotid angiography may demonstrate occlusion of the internal carotid artery or one of the major cerebral vessels—most commonly the middle cerebral artery or one of its branches; or it may show the "beading" typical of arteritis. The pattern may be diagnostic of a space-occupying lesion such as subdural hematoma.

D. Other Neurodiagnostic Studies: EEG is helpful in assessing the effectiveness of anticonvulsant therapy but is of little help in differential diagnosis. (See Seizure Disorders, p 556.) Echoencephalography may disclose a shift of midline structures and other intracranial volume changes. Isotopic brain scan may disclose the presence and extent of the lesion or lesions and may be useful in following their resolution.

Table 21—5. Cerebrovascular disorders in childhood.

	Dural Sinus and Cerebral Venous Thrombosis	Arterial Thrombosis	Cerebral Embolism	Intracranial Hemorrhage (Primary Intracerebral and Subarachnoid)
Onset	Usually less sudden and clear-cut than in arterial occlusive disease. Usually unrelated to activity.	Sudden, but prodromal episodes may occur. Unrelated to activity.	Sudden onset; no prodrome. Unrelated to activity.	Sudden onset; severe headache, vomiting, loss of consciousness. Related to activity.
Underlying conditions	Pyogenic infections of leptomeninges and cranial structures (ear, face, sinuses). Marasmic states and severe dehydration. Congenital heart disease. Blood dyscrasias (sickle cell disease, polycythemia, thrombotic thrombocytopenia). Lead and other toxic encephalopathies. Trauma. Metastatic tumor. Sturge-Weber disease.	"Idiopathic" (hemiplegia in infancy). Cyanotic congenital heart disease. Inflammatory disease of arteries: "collagen" diseases, granulomatous (Takayasu's), acute infections, syphilis. Trauma or extrinsic compression. Dissecting aneurysm. Arteriosclerosis (progeria). Thrombotic phenomenon: homocystinuria.	Atrial fibrillation and other "arrhythmias": congenital heart disease (R→L shunt), rheumatic heart disease. Acute or subacute bacterial endocarditis. Air: complications of heart, neck, or chest surgery. Fat: complications of fractures of bone, heart surgery. Septic: pneumonia or lung abscess (especially in congenital heart disease). Newborn: infarcted necrotic placental tissue. Tumor. Coronary.	Trauma: birth (intraventricular), subdural hemorrhage, epidural hemorrhage, cavernous sinus fistula. Vascular malformations: arteriovenous, angiomas, aneurysms. Hemorrhagic disorders (leukemia, aplastic anemia, hemophilia, sickle cell anemia, thrombocytopenic/anaphylactoid purpura, liver disease, vitamin deficiencies [K, C, B_1], anticonvulsants). Hypertensive encephalopathy (renal disease, pheochromocytoma). Toxic or infectious encephalopathy. Intracranial tumors.
Neurologic findings	Altered state of consciousness. Increased intracranial pressure. Focal neurologic deficits (leg, arm). Seizures, focal and generalized.	Seizures, frequently focal. Focal neurologic deficits. Behavioral and intellectual changes. Rapid improvement at times.	Transient loss of consciousness common. Seizures, often focal. Focal neurologic deficits (sometimes multiple). Rapid improvement at times.	Consciousness commonly lost; may be regained quickly. Marked meningeal signs (**not** seen in neonate). Focal neurologic deficits. Seizures, generalized and focal.
Special clinical clues	Lateral dural sinus: mastoiditis. Superior sagittal sinus: caput medusae. Cavernous sinus: homolateral exophthalmos, periorbital edema, palsies of cranial nerves III, IV, VI, and V.	Inflammatory disease: multifocal involvement common. Takayasu's: pulseless upper limbs. Moyamoya syndrome (progressive alternating hemiplegia with basal arterial stenosis and diencephalic telangiectasia). Somatic constitution (progeria, arachnodactyly). Signs of trauma.	Emboli to other organs (spleen, kidneys, lungs). Air embolism: transient blindness. Fat embolism: respiratory distress, blood-tinged sputum in postoperative period, fat droplets in urine, retinal vessels.	Trauma (hemorrhage, subhyaloid hemorrhages, bruises, fractures on x-rays). Malformations: bruit, heart failure, hydrocephalus, cutaneous stigmas. Previous seizures/neurologic deficit. Coarctation/polycystic kidney. Hemorrhagic diathesis: skin, joints, gastrointestinal tract, newborn. Hypertensive encephalopathy: blood pressure elevated, uremia.
Skull x-rays	Signs of increased intracranial pressure within days or a few weeks, depending on age. Sinus involvement or lytic lesion.	Early: usually normal. Later: hypertrophy of skull on atrophic side of brain. Tumor. Dysplasia. Foreign body.	Normal.	Skull fractures. Characteristic calcifications. Signs of increased intracranial pressure/hydrocephalus. Deep groove in inner table from enlarged vein.
CSF	Findings vary with primary process. Protein often elevated. Sometimes bloody. If PMNs are present, suspect infection.	Early: usually normal. Later: slight monocytic pleocytosis and protein elevation.	Usually normal. Some pleocytosis and protein elevation in bacterial endocarditis.	Bloody CSF all tubes, xanthochromic supernatant. Protein elevated. Sugar may be decreased. Fluid may be clear if hemorrhage is intracerebral only.
Neuroradiologic findings	Angiogram on venous phase or sinogram may show obstruction site. Sinogram may be dangerous.	Angiography early may show occlusion or narrowing. (Later studies usually negative.)	Angiography usually normal as emboli commonly lodge in small peripheral vessels.	Angiography usually able to identify subdural and epidural hematoma, site and type of malformation, intracerebral tumor, clot.
Other studies	Echoencephalography may show midline shift. EEG may show diffuse or focal slowing. Brain scan may show increased uptake. The CT scan may show the area of infarction. None of these studies are sufficiently specific to obviate the need for other diagnostic—especially angiographic—studies.			

For subdural and (rarely justifiable) ventricular taps, see Head Injuries (p 566).

E. Electrocardiography: ECG is indicated where there is clinical evidence of heart disease, hypertension, or an arteriovenous malformation which may be causing a work overload of the heart.

Differential Diagnosis

A. Postictal (Todd's) Paralysis: Focal motor paralysis lasting 2–3 days may follow seizures which are entirely focal or of focal onset.

B. "Cerebral Palsy" with Hemiplegia: Parents sometimes become aware of the presence of hemiplegia or other neurologic deficits only when the child is ill or has his first seizure. The findings of early spasticity—and particularly of atrophy of affected limbs—favor an old deficit, often congenital or of perinatal onset.

C. Other Causes: Focal neurologic deficits, including hemiplegia, may appear suddenly with a variety of inflammatory conditions of the brain, including meningitis, encephalitis, and brain abscess. With CNS tumors, degenerative processes such as Schilder's diffuse sclerosis or multiple sclerosis, or with "slow virus" infections, the deficits are usually slower to evolve than in cerebrovascular disorders but may be apoplectic in onset. In the case of neoplasm, neurologic deficits are usually due to hemorrhage.

Complications

The complications may be those of the underlying disease process. Frequent complications include seizures (particularly generalized status epilepticus), pneumonia, coma, decubiti, contractures, and other injuries of the affected parts, and hydrocephalus.

Treatment

A. General Measures: Careful attention must be paid to airway, fluid and electrolyte balance, and infections. (See Altered States of Consciousness, p 551.) Anticonvulsant therapy should be administered from the start (even to children who do not present with seizures) because they occur in about 50% or more of cases, especially with acute hemiplegia. The preferred drug is phenobarbital, 3–5 mg/kg/day in 3 divided doses orally, by slow IV drip, or IM. Once seizures (especially status epilepticus) appear, control may be difficult and may require intravenous diazepam (Valium), paraldehyde, and phenytoin in appropriate doses. If the child has no seizures during the acute phase and none the following year, anticonvulsant therapy may then be gradually discontinued.

Corticosteroids should be given to reduce cerebral edema (see p 553). Long-term corticosteroid therapy may be indicated in children with arteritis due to lupus erythematosus, polyarteritis nodosa, pulseless disease, and other angiopathies.

Measures to lower systemic hypertension should be employed with caution. Too sudden a drop in arterial pressure may precipitate further cerebral hypoxia.

B. Specific Measures: These depend on the underlying condition and may include heparinization for multiple embolic phenomena or consumption coagulopathies, antibiotics for bacterial infections, and multiple tapping of a subdural hematoma.

C. Neurosurgical Measures: In addition to drainage of subdural hematomas (often performed by pediatricians), specific neurosurgical measures include removal of a large intracerebral clot, endarterectomy of a stenosed carotid artery and removal of thrombus; clipping, trapping, coating, or possibly "embolization" of an aneurysm; extirpation of an accessible arteriovenous malformation; excision or biopsy of a tumor; drainage of a brain abscess; or shunting for hydrocephalus.

D. Long-Term Management: In addition to anticonvulsant treatment, educational, psychologic, physical, and speech therapy are often required.

Corticectomy or hemispherectomy should be considered in children with intractable focal seizures when residual hemiparesis and hemianopsia will not be increased by surgery. In young children, even removal of the left or dominant hemisphere will not cause permanent aphasia; behavioral and functional improvement may also result.

Prognosis

The course may be brief, with complete recovery. Death may occur, depending on the precipitating cause or complications.

Residual motor and sensory deficits are common, especially with hemiplegias which occur at an early age. The upper extremity tends to be more involved than the lower. Visual field and parietal lobe defects—initially not diagnosable—often become apparent later and contribute to the learning disabilities.

Seizures—mostly focal, but also other types—persist in these children.

Impairment of mental abilities roughly parallels the frequency and severity of seizure disorders. In about three-fourths of cases there are learning disabilities, hyperactivity, disturbances of behavior, and other signs of "maturational lag."

Speech is usually least affected permanently. Even when the left hemisphere is involved, the prognosis for normal speech is good in children under age 5 or 6 except as influenced by whatever overall retardation the child may have suffered. In older children, some expressive aphasic difficulties may persist.

Amacher AL, Drake CG: Cerebral artery aneurysms in infancy, childhood, and adolescence. Child's Brain 1:72, 1975.

Falter ML, Sutton AL, Robinson MG: Massive intracranial hemorrhage in sickle cell anemia. Am J Dis Child 125:415, 1973.

Gold AP, Carter S: Acute hemiplegia of infancy and childhood. Pediatr Clin North Am 23:413, 1976.

Latchaw RE, Seager JF, Gabrielsen TO: Vertebrobasilar arterial occlusions in children. Neuroradiology 8:141, 1974.

Sedzimir CB, Robinson J: Intracranial hemorrhage in children and adolescents. J Neurosurg 38:269, 1973.

MALFORMATIONS OF THE CNS

1. SPINAL DYSRAPHISM

Essentials of Diagnosis

- Any defect of fusion in the dorsal midline.
- May be cutaneous, vertebral, meningeal, or neural.

General Considerations

Developmental anomalies involving the spinal cord and its coverings are extremely common. Damage to the embryo varies according to when such clefts occur; where they are located; whether they are single or multiple, partial or complete in dividing both the inner and outer limiting neural membranes; whether they are incipient, closed or "healing," or expanding; and how these clefts and their sequelae affect other structures in embryonic life or later.

As a matter of considerable clinical practicality, the various forms of spinal dysraphism can be grouped into (1) noncystic forms, in which there is no hernial protrusion of the meninges of the cord, and (2) cystic forms, with herniation of the meninges through a defect of the neural arch in which the hernial sac contains CSF (meningocele) and often also nervous tissue (meningomyelocele).

The incidence of those forms of neural clefts without meningeal protrusion is not known. Vestigial or primarily superficial manifestations, such as dermal dimples and sinuses, vascular nevi, and abnormal tufts of hair are extremely common. Spina bifida occulta, often an incidental x-ray finding, is estimated to occur in up to 25% of younger children in whom the posterior vertebral arches will eventually fuse, and in about 5% or more of all individuals. Spina bifida cystica occurs in about 2 per 1000 births, with one meningomyelocele per 800 births. Many environmental causes, including viral and irradiation injuries to the embryo, have been implicated epidemiologically and experimentally. Genetic factors may play a role, eg, in spina bifida cystica the family history is positive in about 8% of cases.

Clinical Findings

A. Symptoms and Signs:

1. Cutaneous manifestations—

a. Noncystic—In noncystic forms of spinal dysraphism, these may consist of a skin depression or dermal dimple, which may also mark the outlet of a fistulous or fibrous tract extending to the meninges and representing a dermal sinus. On close inspection, a tiny pore may be seen. There may be chronic or intermittent drainage of a whitish secretion from such a sinus; this may lead to cystic dilatation if the sinus is partially obliterated. Commonly seen also in the midline as evidence of dysraphism are port wine angiomatous nevi; tufts or patches or even tails of hair, which may be long and coarse, sometimes silky, and often

dark in blond children; and subcutaneous diffuse, soft lipomatous lesions. Such superficial stigmas may be absent, may appear singly or in close but variable association, or may even "split" on each side of the midline.

b. Cystic—Cystic defects are usually detected on inspection at birth, but occasionally the overlying skin is so thick that detection is delayed. A large vascular nevus, lipoma, or abnormal growth of hair may be associated superficial findings. The differentiation between meningocele and meningomyelocele is usually made by noting the absence (meningocele) or presence of neurologic deficits or the presence of neural elements on transillumination of the sac, or by eliciting reflex responses upon tapping the sac gently; but in some instances a definite diagnosis can only be established by means of surgical exploration. Pressure on the sac may cause the anterior fontanel to bulge. An exception to these statements must be made for the rare neurenteric cysts (see below), in which no superficial lesions are frequently present.

2. Orthopedic manifestations—Plainly visible or palpable anomalies of the spinal column may include scoliosis, those associated with Klippel-Feil syndrome, and occasionally bifid vertebra; in many instances, however, the abnormalities are seen only on x-ray (see below). Deformities of the feet or legs are the most common (and may be the only) evidence of noncystic spinal dysraphism. They may be highly variable in extent and kind and stationary or progressive depending upon the degree of neurologic deficit. There may be a marked difference in size between the 2 legs or feet, inversion (clubfoot) or eversion, and pes cavus or pes cavovarus. Dislocation of the hips may also be present. As would be expected from the low incidence of dysraphism involving primarily the cervical cord, the upper extremities are far less commonly involved.

3. Motor disturbances—The orthopedic manifestations are often accompanied by muscle weakness and reflex disturbances. The nature and extent depend entirely on the lesion in the spinal cord and roots and help to identify the anatomic site. Particularly in such noncystic forms as diastematomyelia—and in symptomatic spina bifida occulta and "tethering" of the cord—the first signs may appear between 2 and 8 years of age in the form of progressive leg weakness and gait disturbance. In meningomyelocele, the legs may be partially, asymmetrically, or totally paralyzed and areflexic from birth.

4. Urinary and rectal disturbances—Atonic bladder (with dribbling) and poor anal sphincter tone are commonly present at birth in lumbosacral meningomyeloceles. In noncystic forms of dysraphism, urinary incontinence usually appears after the disturbances of gait and reflects pressure on or traction of the lower cord (or both) by an adherent lipoma or other connective tissue; loss of voluntary control of the anal sphincter in these types is less common but may occur in time. When urinary incontinence is present, intravenous urography may disclose the presence of various upper genitourinary anomalies.

5. Cerebral malformations—Disturbances of brain growth with noncystic forms are relatively infrequent but may occur. With cystic forms, encephalic anomalies are far more common; hydrocephalus occurs in 65% of cases with meningomyelocele, almost invariably in association with some form of Arnold-Chiari malformation, and in 10% of meningoceles. Encephalocele, schizencephaly, cyclopia, and often microcephaly also represent aspects of dysraphism of the neuraxis; indeed, it is not unusual to find a hydrocephalic brain which, after shunting or on postmortem examination, turns out to be microcephalic. A frequent finding in such cases is mental retardation.

6. Sensory deficits—Disturbances of sensation commonly parallel the motor deficits in meningomyelocele, where the upper level of the defect may be demonstrated by pricking the infant's skin; wrinkling or corrugation denotes an intact dermatome. In noncystic forms of dysraphism, sensory disturbances are much less common; where there is pressure or traction on the cord, there may be loss of pain leading to neurogenic arthropathies (Charcot joints). Trophic disturbances of the skin may also be seen.

B. Laboratory Findings: Abnormal findings relate principally to the 2 major complications of spinal dysraphism: meningitis and urinary tract disease (see below). In meningitis, the infection is frequently mixed, with both skin *(Staphylococcus epidermidis* and others) and gram-negative organisms present. When there is dribbling or other clinical or x-ray evidence of genitourinary tract disturbance, urinalysis, urine cultures, BUN, and creatinine clearance should be obtained and followed.

C. X-Ray Findings:

1. Plain x-rays of the spine—These should be obtained in all cases of overt spinal dysraphism and will usually disclose the extent of the neural arch defect. Plain spine films obtained for other reasons usually establish the diagnosis of spina bifida occulta. In diastematomyelia, a ridge may often be protruding from the body of one or more vertebrae which splits or fixes the spinal cord or cauda equina and which may consist of bone, cartilage, and fibrous tissue; its radiopacity depends on the degree of calcification of this spur; nonvisualization on plain spine films does not rule out this diagnosis.

2. Spine tomograms—These are of particular value in cases of noncystic "tethering" of the cord and with the rarer cases of neurenteric cysts.

3. Myelography—The purpose of this procedure is usually confirmatory, and it should never be undertaken lightly. It should be performed in cases of progressively more symptomatic noncystic forms of dysraphism, particularly where diastematomyelia, tethering of the cord, or a neurenteric cyst—all of which may behave clinically like spinal cord tumors—is a possibility.

4. Skull films—These should be obtained with spina bifida cystica, macro- or microcephaly, and recurrent bacterial meningitides. In the first instances, the presence of craniolacunae (lacunar skull or lücken-

schädel) has a high correlation with hydrocephaly and the need for a shunt. In the latter instance, recurrent infection via a dermal sinus must be suspected. Its location may be cephalic, particularly near the midline occipitally or the bridge of the nose. Skull x-rays may disclose a small circular radiolucent area; tomograms may be necessary.

5. Computerized tomography—In meningomyelocele, CT scan shortly after birth should provide 2 extremely important pieces of information: (1) the presence of hydrocephalus (irrespective of occipitofrontal head circumference) and (2) the approximate thickness of the cortical mantle or pallium. Whole body scanners may be utilized to define the myelodysplastic lesion.

6. Air encephalography—Ventriculography will continue to be employed where CT scan is not available to determine the presence and extent of hydrocephalus.

7. Urologic studies—Cystometrograms and intravenous urograms are indicated in all children with obvious or suspected urinary tract involvement secondary to spinal cord involvement.

Differential Diagnosis

Meningomyelocele usually presents little diagnostic difficulty. Meningocele is not infrequently confused with a subcutaneous lipoma, and indeed the 2 may be associated. The differentiation between meningocele and meningomyelocele is sometimes only made during operation. Because of traction or pressure on the cord (or a combination of both), considerable diagnostic difficulty may be encountered in those forms of dysraphism which give rise to symptoms not unlike those of spinal cord tumors or even syringomyelia. Such may be the case (as the child grows) with fibrolipomas, tethering of the cord or cauda equina by fibrous bands to the bone or skin directly or through meningeal attachment, a tight filum terminale, or a spur which partially or completely bisects the cord (diastematomyelia). Primarily orthopedic findings such as pes cavus or Charcot joints involve consideration of Friedreich's ataxia, diabetes mellitus, congenital insensitivity to pain, familial dysautonomia, and even congenital syphilis. Lastly, the differential diagnosis must include neurenteric cyst, the remnant of an open passage between the yolk sac and neural groove present during the third week of embryonic life, which may be thoracic or lumbosacral in location and may present in infancy or not until the end of the second decade of life. Occasionally, cystic forms of dysraphism are placed anteriorly, causing symptoms of a space-occupying lesion in the thoracic, abdominal, or pelvic cavities, or of a spinal cord tumor. (See also Spinal Cord Tumors.)

Complications

Meningitis occurs in nearly 15% of cases of spina bifida cystica if the sac ruptures. It occurs far less frequently with congenital dermal sinus, but when it does it is likely to give rise to recurrent episodes of bacterial meningitis until the sinus is discovered; if it is not readily located in the back or at the nose, shaving the back of the head or a pneumoencephalogram may be required. Infections are often due to *Escherichia coli, Pseudomonas aeruginosa,* or *Staphylococcus epidermidis.*

Urinary tract infections, bladder atony, vesicoureteral reflux, hydronephrosis, and eventually renal failure are frequent complications, particularly in spina bifida cystica.

Hydrocephalus is an early and frequent problem with spina bifida cystica, and its complications, discussed on p 583, adversely affect the prognosis.

Skin problems may occur due to breakdown in the saddle area from bladder and bowel incontinence or with trophic disturbances.

Treatment

A. Neurosurgical Considerations:

1. Noncystic forms of spinal dysraphism—These may require neurosurgical intervention to relieve pressure or traction on the spinal cord, removal of a diastematomyelic spur, or excision of a dermal fistula and exploration for any connected tumor. It must be emphasized that a dermal sinus should never be probed as this may result in infection, especially of the CNS.

2. Spina bifida cystica—Approaches to this complex problem vary. Decisions about treatment must be based on the extent of neurologic and systemic involvement, the consequent morbidity, the prognosis for physical and mental function, and the emotional, social, and financial impact on the family.

a. Meningoceles—Meningoceles should be repaired early if there is danger of rupture of the sac.

b. Meningomyeloceles—The decision about immediate operation or a delay is controversial. (See Fig 21–1.)

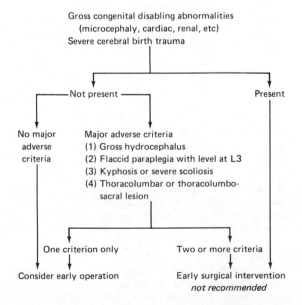

Figure 21–1. Proposed criteria for neurosurgical intervention in newborns with open meningomyeloceles. (After Stein & others.)

c. Hydrocephalus—A shunt or other measures for the relief of imminent or progressive hydrocephalus may result in collapse of the meningomyelocele, and this may be followed by epithelialization of the sac. Thus, there may be advantages to relief of hydrocephalus as a first procedure. A lacunar skull on x-ray makes the need for shunting more likely. The presence of a high (thoracic) sensory level or thin cortical mantle (< 1 cm) is a serious adverse criterion.

B. Care of the Sac When Neurosurgical Repair Is Delayed: Application of silver nitrate to the thin membrane covering a sac is advocated by some to encourage epithelialization. A "doughnut" of foam rubber or other spongy material, covered by plastic, wide enough to protect the sac and secured around the abdomen, is a useful protective appliance. It may be roofed by sterile gauze, but contact of the gauze with the sac—whether "dry" or covered with petrolatum—should be avoided.

C. Orthopedic Considerations: Surgery and braces are recommended to the extent that these measures will aid ambulation. Correction of foot deformities and dislocation of the hips should not be undertaken if there is little hope that the child will ever walk.

In a child with neurogenic arthropathy, behavioral modification to reduce the frequency of trauma to the joints as well as physically protecting the joints (as by padding) is helpful.

D. Urologic Considerations: The renal status should be assessed early and watched closely. Measures for reducing the incidence of pyuria and renal complications include suprapubic manual expression of urine from the bladder, the use of an indwelling catheter, and uretero-ileostomy.

"Prophylactic" antibiotic therapy is not advisable, but specific infections must be treated. Mandelamine (or cranberry juice) to acidify the urine to pH 5.0 or less may reduce the frequency of infections.

E. Fecal Incontinence: Constipating foods and drugs may be of help. Colostomy is sometimes advisable for social reasons in older children who are otherwise able to function.

F. Skin Care: Skin hygiene should be maintained, particularly around the anus, vulva, and pressure areas, if these are involved.

Prognosis

In noncystic forms of spinal dysraphism, the prognosis for life and function is excellent if proper treatment is carried out. The degree of residual neurologic, orthopedic, and genitourinary deficit is often minimal but depends on the extent of involvement. It is encouraging to realize that with "release" of a tethered cord urinary incontinence and gait disturbances, even when present for several years, may resolve.

In cystic spinal dysraphism, complete cures can be achieved by excision of neurenteric cysts. With meningoceles, the prognosis is that of the complications.

About two-thirds of meningomyeloceles are operable in the newborn period according to criteria proposed. The overall mortality rate at present is 15–20%; of these, about half die within the first 6 weeks of life and another third within the first year. The most common causes of early deaths are meningitis and hydrocephalus.

Among long-term survivors, 30–60% are reported as "educationally" normal (IQ > 80), although many have multiple handicaps. The features most significantly related to low intelligence are thin pallium (< 2.5 cm), high (thoracic) sensory level, and CNS infection (with or without shunt) but not a lacunar skull. Impairment of renal function with uremia is the most serious long-term threat.

In a family in which one child has been born with cystic spina bifida—and with advanced maternal age—pregnancies should be monitored between the 14th and 16th week for elevated alpha-fetoprotein and between the 19th and 20th week with serial ultrasound studies (sonography) of the fetus and amniography for the presence of a neural tube defect.

Barden GA, Meyer LC, Stelling FH: Myelodysplastics: Fate of those followed for twenty years or more. J Bone Joint Surg 57A:643, 1975.

Hunt GM, Holmes AE: Factors relating to intelligence in treated cases of spina bifida cystica. Am J Dis Child 130:823; 1976.

Lorber J: Some paediatric aspects of myelomeningocele. Acta Orthop Scand 46:350, 1975.

Nellhaus G: Neurogenic arthropathies (Charcot's joints) in children: Description of a case traced to occult spinal dysraphism. Clin Pediatr (Phila) 14:647, 1975.

Shaw JF: Diastematomyelia. Dev Med Child Neurol 17:361, 1975.

Shurtleff DB, Kronmal R, Foltz EL: Follow-up comparison of hydrocephalus with and without myelomeningocele. J Neurosurg 42:61, 1975.

Stein SC, Schut L, Ames MD: Selection for early treatment of myelomeningocele: A retrospective analysis of selection procedures. Dev Med Child Neurol 17:311, 1975.

2. HYDROCEPHALUS

Essentials of Diagnosis

- Abnormal enlargement of the cerebral ventricles due to an increased pressure gradient between the intraventricular fluid and the brain.
- In infants and children, hydrocephalus is usually accompanied by macrocephaly.

General Considerations

Most cases of hydrocephalus in infancy and childhood are due to obstruction of CSF flow, the aqueduct between the third and fourth ventricle being the most common site of blockage. Developmental causes include aqueductal stenosis or atresia; absence or atresia of the foramens of Luschka and Magendie

(Dandy-Walker syndrome); Arnold-Chiari malformation (3 types are described; myelomeningocele is frequently, but not necessarily, associated); arteriovenous malformation of the great vein of Galen, compressing the aqueduct; and other anomalies, including block of the interventricular foramens (of Monro). Intrauterine and postnatally acquired causes include principally inflammatory states, whether from infection or hemorrhage, with resulting gliosis of the aqueduct, or arachnoiditis ("communicating hydrocephalus"). Intracranial mass lesions such as tumor, abscess, and hematoma also frequently cause obstruction to CSF flow.

A nonobstructive or oversecretion type of hydrocephalus is due to choroid plexus papilloma.

Clinical Findings

A. Symptoms and Signs: Manifestations vary with age at onset, the underlying cause, and the rapidity with which hydrocephalus develops.

In infants with an open anterior fontanel and patent sutures, symptoms of increased intracranial pressure are often delayed or minimal. Instead, the head circumference enlarges too rapidly or exceeds 3 SD above the mean for age and sex as plotted on a standard head circumference graph. The anterior fontanel may be full and tense and the sutures palpably separated; there may be frontal bossing and a "setting sun" sign, in which the eyes appear to be depressed, with more sclera than normal showing above the iris. The head may transilluminate abnormally and percuss like a watermelon.

Abducens palsies with increased intracranial pressure are common in all age groups. When hydrocephalus is due to more acute obstruction, there may be vomiting, irritability and listlessness, and difficulties with vision and gait.

The findings in older infants and children may include Macewen's cracked pot sign of sprung sutures, papilledema or other eye findings, disturbances of muscle tone and reflexes, and incoordination. An unusual form of presentation is the pendular or side-to-side movement which gives rise to the "bobble-head doll syndrome." Cranial bruits are common in children, especially with increased intracranial pressure, but may suggest a vascular malformation.

B. Laboratory Findings: The composition of the ventricular or spinal fluid may offer some clues to the cause of hydrocephalus. Markedly elevated CSF protein is often seen in choroid plexus papilloma and occasionally after a CNS infection or hemorrhage. Low CSF glucose without evidence of current infection is seen in postinfectious hydrocephalus or in meningeal invasion by tumor (eg, leukemia, medulloblastoma). Increased 5-hydroxyindoleacetic acid is found in the CSF in obstructive hydrocephalus. Cytologic examination of CSF may show the presence of tumor cells.

C. X-Ray Findings: X-rays may show the cranium to be disproportionately large with respect to the face; there may be signs of increased intracranial pressure, intracranial calcifications, lytic lesions, or a large, flat occipital shelf suggestive of Dandy-Walker syndrome.

In cases of increased intracranial pressure without focal findings or in children with abnormal head enlargement without other symptoms, computerized tomography (CT scan) is recommended to determine the size of the ventricles and to rule out a choroid plexus papilloma. CT scan will often define the nature of the block even in the posterior fossa.

Air encephalography—by the lumbar route if this can be done safely or by the ventricular route (or both)—will further define the site of CSF block.

D. Special Examinations: Echoencephalography may show the ventricular dilatation. Isotope scans following the injection of radioiodinated human serum albumin into the lumbar or cisternal subarachnoid space have also been employed.

Differential Diagnosis

In the investigation of a child with a large head (macrocephaly), the following must be considered: (1) nonpathologic megalocephaly, which may be familial; (2) subdural hematoma, usually chronic or subacute and usually bilateral; (3) CNS degenerative diseases (see CNS Degenerative Disorders of Infancy & Childhood); (4) dysplasias, including cerebral gigantism and disorders of bone; (5) hydranencephaly; and (6) brain tumor.

Hydranencephaly consists of replacement of the cerebral hemispheres by a fluid-filled sac, usually due either to profound schizencephaly and bilateral porencephaly or to a massive encephalomalacic process which reduces the cerebral mantle to a thin membrane. The appearance of the neonate may be grossly normal. The head is usually not enlarged. If the diencephalon and midbrain are intact, as is usually the case, no difficulties occur with feeding, respiration, and other vegetative functions in the first months of life. Diagnosis may be delayed until the parents note slow development or defective vision. Some spasticity and persistence of primitive postural reflexes are usually evident.

Hydranencephaly may be diagnosed by transillumination of the head, air studies, or cerebral angiography.

In cases of increased intracranial pressure without hydrocephalus, the diagnosis of pseudotumor cerebri is one of exclusion. Once this diagnosis is established, its many causes (as discussed in that section) should be investigated.

Complications

In nonoperated cases, continuing increased intracranial pressure leads to neurologic deterioration. Rarely, hydrocephalus may rupture.

In "shunted" cases, complications include (1) sudden rise in intracranial pressure, due either to blockage or other malfunction of the shunt (the site varies with the type of assembly) or to displacement of the shunt mechanism, especially at the distal end as growth proceeds; (2) infections (most frequently due to coagulase-positive *Staphylococcus albus*), including septicemia, meningitis, and ventriculitis, with the shunt itself often the nidus; (3) electrolyte imbalances; and (4) subdural hematoma following abrupt collapse of enlarged ventricles.

Prevention

Early recognition of hydrocephalus is best accomplished by periodic physical and neurologic examinations, which should include head measurements.

Treatment

A. Observations and Evaluation: Careful observation over a short period is required before the decision to operate is made. It is usually best not to operate if the patient is clinically well and the rate of enlargement does not exceed that indicated on a standard head circumference chart or appears to be arresting. In moderate cases, a clinical trial of isosorbide may be warranted.

B. Surgical Treatment: The neurosurgical approach is dictated by the underlying condition as well as the surgeon's preference. Associated meningomyelocele or other anomalies must be dealt with also.

1. "Shunting technics" include a variety of ventriculovenous (ventriculojugular or ventriculoatrial) shunts, as well as ventriculoperitoneal or ventriculopleural shunts. Ventriculoureterostomy and ventriculocisternostomy are now performed rarely.

2. "Direct" nonshunting operations consist of third ventriculostomy and choroid plexectomy (imperative in choroid plexus papilloma).

3. Use of the Rickham reservoir and catheter is increasing, at least as a temporary measure.

4. Firm wrapping of the head has been recommended.

C. Prophylactic Care of Shunts: Serial head and chest x-rays should be taken to check shunt placement. Other postoperative procedures used to verify the success of surgery are manometric testing of ventricular pressure; ventriculography with CO_2; "isotopic" check with radioiodinated human serum albumin on shunt function; and echoencephalographic estimation of ventricular size.

Prophylactic periodic revision of the shunt is advocated by many neurosurgeons.

Prophylactic use of an antibiotic (eg, oxacillin) at the time a shunt is inserted to reduce infection due to *Staphylococcus albus* has been recommended.

Prognosis

In general, if progressive hydrocephalus can be arrested, the prognosis for function is improved. Even if the child is severely retarded and has other handicaps that do not threaten life, "social shunts" are justifiable since the difficulties of caring for the child are markedly eased and the cost of care, by reducing the necessity for institutionalization, is considerably lowered.

The width of the cerebral mantle may not be a reliable prognostic finding.

A. Nonoperated Group: The survival rate at 10 years is about 25%. Of the survivors, about one-fifth can function "competitively" and the remainder require supervision and maintenance. This salvage rate of competitive children is about 5% of the original group.

B. Operated Group: The survival rate at 10 years is about 60%, with over half of the surviving children able to care for themselves. (About 25% of survivors have normal or higher than normal IQs.)

C. Shunt Dependency: The question of shunt dependency is unsettled. Some data suggest that at some point in ventricular enlargement the ependymal surface may be sufficiently large to absorb the net amount of CSF not handled by the usual pathways. Such "spontaneous arrests" may occur in 40—50% of children surviving the first 1—2 years.

DeLange SA: Ventriculo-atrial shunt in progressive hydrocephalus and shunt dependency. Psychiatr Neurol Neurochir 71:65, 1968.

Halsey JH, Allen N, Chamberlin HR: The morphogenesis of hydranencephaly. J Neurol Sci 12:187, 1971.

Laurence KM: Neurological and intellectual sequelae of hydrocephalus. Arch Neurol 20:73, 1969.

Lorber J: Medical and surgical aspects in the treatment of congenital hydrocephalus. Neuropaediatrie 2:239, 1971.

Russel DS: *Observations on the Pathology of Hydrocephalus.* Medical Research Council SRS 265, Her Majesty's Stationery Office, 1966.

Tomasovic JJ, Nellhaus G, Moe P: The bobble-head doll syndrome: An early sign of hydrocephalus. Dev Med Child Neurol 17:777, 1975.

Venes JL: Control of shunt infection. J Neurosurg 45:311, 1976.

3. CRANIOSYNOSTOSIS

Primary craniosynostosis is a developmental disorder of the membranous bones of the skull that results in closure of one or more cranial sutures in utero, beginning with dysostosis of the several bones of the cranial base. Diagnosis at birth is possible by inspection and palpation confirmed by skull x-rays. The ratio of males to females is 3:1. Occasionally there is a genetic basis for the defect. Associated anomalies are found in nearly one-third of cases.

Classification

(1) Sagittal sutures only are involved in over 50% of cases, resulting in dolichocephaly (scaphocephaly) with elongation and narrowing of the skull. This deformity may occur as a dominant trait.

(2) Coronal suture involvement accounts for almost 20% of cases. When bilateral, as it is in about half of these cases, the result is brachycephaly with a broad, shortened skull.

(3) Metopic suture involvement (10%) results in a pointed, ridged forehead, or trigonocephaly.

(4) If all of the sutures are involved (about 8%), the result is a "turret" skull (oxycephaly, acrocephaly, turricephaly).

(5) Other combinations occur occasionally, such as fusion of the sagittal and coronal, lambdoidal, or metopic sutures, or of the lambdoidal and squamous sutures.

(6) Allied entities (singly or in combination) are acrocephaly with syndactyly (acrocephalosyndactyly, or Apert's disease), craniofacial dysostosis (Crouzon's disease), and hydrocephalus.

Clinical Findings

In the majority of cases there are no symptoms other than the skull deformity. Signs and symptoms of increased intracranial pressure, strabismus, visual loss, optic atrophy, mental retardation, and occasionally seizures occur with brain compression when multiple sutures are involved, or with hydrocephalus; in the latter case, the head circumference may be abnormally large.

Except where multiple sutures are involved, the normal head circumference and neurologic examination clearly differentiate primary from secondary craniosynostosis, which is usually accompanied by microcephaly.

Skull x-rays will define the suture involvement. The entire suture need not be involved. Radionuclides with a predilection for areas of osteoblastic activity will delineate the fusing—but not the fused—sutures. Decalcification of posterior clinoids and increased digital markings are present when there has been longstanding increased intracranial pressure. Symmetric involvement of sutures and craniofacial disproportion are seen in microcephaly. Suspicion of hydrocephalus justifies appropriate studies.

Treatment

If multiple sutures are involved, early neurosurgical intervention with excision of sutures in the first weeks of life is recommended. If there is a deformity of the orbits, orbital decompression is required. The principal reason for sagittal synostosis surgery is cosmetic. (See also Hydrocephalus.)

About 13% of patients, chiefly those in whom both coronal or multiple sutures are involved, require reoperation because of evidence of recurrent increased intracranial pressure or evidence of fusion after craniectomy.

The only fatalities resulting from surgery are due to failure to detect coagulation defects or to provide adequate replacement of blood loss, which is often greater than estimated. Preoperative coagulation screening and close attention to postoperative hemoglobin or hematocrit are therefore mandatory.

Prognosis

Cosmetic improvement occurs in about 75% of patients, with those operated on early and having only one or 2 sutures involved showing the best results, ie, an essentially normal-looking head (about 50% of all operated cases). It is claimed that operation also results in preservation of brain function.

Despite early surgical intervention, however (particularly in trigonocephaly), 3—5% of children with craniosynostosis exhibit varying degrees of mental retardation.

Permanent sequelae of surgical complications are infrequent.

Gates GF, Dore EK: Detection of craniosynostosis by bone scanning. Radiology 115:665, 1975.

Moss ML: Functional anatomy of cranial synostosis. Child's Brain 1:22, 1975.

NEUROCUTANEOUS DYSPLASIAS

1. RECKLINGHAUSEN'S NEUROFIBROMATOSIS

Recklinghausen's neurofibromatosis is the most common of the neurocutaneous dysplasias, a group of conditions in which nervous and skin tissues, both of ectodermal origin, are chiefly involved. However, tissues arising from meso- and endodermal embryonal layers are often affected as well. Transmitted both as a dominant trait with a highly variable degree of penetrance and as a recessive, Recklinghausen's disease may be expressed by just one of its many features or by any combination of them. Atypical forms are common.

Clinical Findings

A. Symptoms and Signs:

1. Dermatologic features—Café au lait spots on skin, freckles in axillas, hemangiomas, lymphangiomas, lipomas, and subcutaneous neurofibromas.

2. Neurologic features—Neuromas of cranial, peripheral, or autonomic nerves or of the spinal cord; optic nerve gliomas (involving either one nerve or the optic chiasm), not infrequent in childhood; acoustic (eighth nerve) neurinoma, usually bilateral in childhood; intracranial tumors, especially astrocytomas of varying degrees of malignancy; seizures (often indicative of intracranial tumors, but sometimes unrelated); nonspecifically abnormal EEGs without other neurologic deficit; and CNS malformations, including meningocele and syringomyelia.

3. Mental functioning—Moderate to severe retardation occurs in nearly 10% of individuals with neurofibromatosis. This is the case in almost all of the neurocutaneous disorders, in some of which the incidence of retardation—as well as major psychoses—is even higher.

4. Skeletal involvement—There is a high incidence of kyphoscoliosis, defects of vertebral bodies and of the skull, elephantiasic hypertrophy, and rarefaction and cyst-like destruction of bone. Recklinghausen's disease is occasionally associated with vitamin D resistant rickets.

5. Other systems—Delayed or precocious sex development, diabetes mellitus, thyroid and parathyroid disorders, pheochromocytomas, melanoblasto-sis, congenital glaucoma, and soft tissue tumors such as retroperitoneal fibrosarcomas.

B. Laboratory, X-Ray, and Other Findings: None are specific. X-rays of the skull, orbits, spine, chest, or long bones, EEGs, brain scans, and other tests such as endocrine studies must be obtained on the basis of suspected involvement.

Differential Diagnosis

The smooth-bordered café au lait spots of Recklinghausen's neurofibromatosis must be distinguished from the jagged-edged "coast of Maine" coffee-hued skin lesions seen in polyostotic fibrous dysplasia (McCune-Albright syndrome). Increased nerve growth factors have been demonstrated in blood.

Treatment

Treatment is directed toward specific problems, eg, neurosurgical removal or radiation therapy for tumors, orthopedic correction of scoliosis. The heritable nature of the disorder should be made clear.

Prognosis

The prognosis depends entirely on the manifestations: excellent where there are only skin or bone lesions, poor with malignant tumors. Most patients live normal lives.

Canale D, Bebin J, Knighton RS: Neurologic manifestations of von Recklinghausen's disease of the nervous system. Confin Neurol 24:359, 1964.

Silvers DN, Greenwood RS, Helwig EB: Café au lait spots without giant pigment granules: Occurrence in suspected neurofibromatosis. Arch Dermatol 110:87, 1974.

2. TUBEROUS SCLEROSIS

Tuberous sclerosis is a neurocutaneous dysplasia, protean in its manifestations, commonly appearing in partial form but accounting for 0.3–0.6% of institutionalized mentally retarded persons.

Clinical Findings

A. Symptoms and Signs:

1. Dermatologic features—Amelanotic spots on the skin and hair (often mistakenly called "vitiligo") may be present at birth or may appear within the first 2 years of life, and may be best demonstrated with Wood's light. Other findings include café au lait spots with smooth borders; Pringle's "adenoma sebaceum" in malar distribution, usually arising in the second to fourth year of life, of 2 types—seed-like, reddish angiofibromatous growths, and yellowish to brown, primarily fibromatous small nodules; angiomas; shagreen spots, which are grayish-green, rough, leathery patches of thickened skin; and subungual fibromas of fingers and toes found at adolescence and chiefly in girls.

2. Neurologic features—Seizures occur in a large

number of cases and may be the only manifestation in some family members. About 2–5% of cases of infantile spasms with hypsarrhythmia and mental retardation prove eventually to have tuberous sclerosis. Formation of nodules ("tubers") containing atypical large glial cells may result in the finding of cerebral calcifications on skull x-rays or irregularities of the ventricular walls on air encephalograms. The cerebellum, brain stem, and spinal cord are rarely, if ever, involved. Mass lesions include gliomas, gangliogliomas, and cystic lesions. The EEG is often nonspecifically abnormal even in asymptomatic family members.

3. Mental retardation–Mental retardation is frequent, and may be the sole manifestation in a member of an affected family.

4. Ocular involvement–Retinal phakomas or "mulberry lesions" at the edge of the optic disk are found in 7–8% of affected individuals; other eye defects include optic atrophy, nystagmus, and even blindness.

5. Skeletal involvement–Periosteal thickening and central cystic rarefactions of fingers and toes, hyperostosis of cranium, poly- and syndactyly, and vertebral defects.

6. Visceral manifestations–Renal hamartomas, rhabdomyomas of the heart, pulmonary vascular fibrosis, and various mixed tumors of other viscera.

7. Other manifestations–Endocrinopathies, cleft lip and palate, branchial cleft cysts, congenital heart disease, and genital dysplasias are occasionally present.

B. Laboratory Findings: None are specific. Diagnostic tests must be based on clinical judgment.

Differential Diagnosis

The early stages and various atypical forms of tuberous sclerosis may make the diagnosis difficult. The triad of seizures, typical skin lesions (especially of the face), and mental retardation in one individual or when present in any combination in the family supports the diagnosis. The presence of amelanotic skin or hair patches tends to differentiate this entity from Recklinghausen's disease.

Treatment

Treatment is nonspecific except as required for seizures, brain tumors, or visceral lesions. The heritable nature of the disorder should be made clear.

Prognosis

The most severely affected patients have a shortened life span, with death occurring at variable times as a result of status epilepticus, brain or visceral tumors, or intercurrent infections. In mild or atypical cases, life span may be normal

Fitz CR, Harwood-Nash DCF, Thompson JR: Neuroradiology of tuberous sclerosis in children. Radiology 110:635, 1974.

Galant SP & others: Immunological status in tuberous sclerosis. Dev Med Child Neurol 18:503, 1976.

Nevin NC, Pearce WG: Diagnostic and genetic aspects of tuberous sclerosis. J Med Genet 5:273, 1968.

3. ENCEPHALOFACIAL ANGIOMATOSIS
(Sturge-Weber Disease)

Sturge-Weber disease consists of a port wine nevus on the upper part of the face and leptomeningeal angiomatosis of the cerebral cortex on the same side, as indicated by neurologic deficits and skull x-rays. It occurs sporadically. Cutaneous port wine nevi are present at birth, but other manifestations may not become evident for a year or more.

Clinical Findings

A. Symptoms and Signs: A port wine cutaneous nevus covers at least the upper eyelid or supraorbital region of the face and scalp and may involve both sides of the face and other parts of body. Seizures, both focal and generalized, occur in up to 90% of cases, often in the first year of life. Hemiparesis on the side contralateral to the face lesion is found in about one-third of cases and is frequently associated with hemiatrophy. Mental retardation of varying degree is present in about half of cases.

Buphthalmos (congenital glaucoma) occurs in about one-third of cases; hemianopsia is common.

Angiomatous involvement of the oropharynx and viscera and hypertrophy of extremities covered by angiomatous skin may be present.

B. X-Ray Findings: Brain scan may be positive. Diagnostic double-contoured calcifications corresponding to cerebral gyri are seen on skull x-rays usually only after the second year. Skull films may also show bony enlargement with large vascular channels over the involved side. Angiography and pneumoencephalography should be reserved for children in whom complications arise or who are being considered for hemispherectomy.

C. Electroencephalography: The EEG usually shows abnormalities over the involved hemisphere early in the disease, but the findings are nonspecific.

Differential Diagnosis

The diagnosis can usually be made at birth or in the first years of life, especially when seizures and neurologic deficits appropriate to the skin lesion are present. The diagnosis is unmistakable when the typical intracranial calcifications are seen on CT scan or skull x-rays.

Complications

Intracranial bleeding may occur into the subdural or subarachnoid space, with concomitant worsening of the neurologic status.

Treatment

For the treatment of seizures, see the section on Seizure Disorders. Physical therapy may be indicated for hemiplegia. Glaucoma should be treated as outlined in Chapter 9. In cases with severe seizures, spastic hemiplegia, and hemianopsia, early hemispherectomy should be given every consideration with a view to preventing further neurologic deterioration.

Prognosis

The prognosis varies with the extent and severity of the leptomeningeal angiomatosis, the occurrence of cerebrovascular accidents, and the severity of the seizure disorder.

Nellhaus G: Sturge-Weber disease with bilateral intracranial calcifications at birth and unusual pathologic findings. Acta Neurol Scand 43:314, 1967.

4. VON HIPPEL-LINDAU DISEASE
(Retinal & Cerebellar Angiomatosis)

This unusual, dominantly transmitted disorder is characterized by angiomatosis of the retina and cerebellum. Angiomatosis of the brain stem, spinal cord, and spinal nerve roots, syringomyelia, epithelial cysts, angiomas of the liver, spleen, and kidneys, and other tumors, especially pheochromocytomas, may also be found. Cutaneous hemangiomas occur only rarely. Ocular symptoms and findings include visual difficulties, retinal hemorrhages and exudates, retinal detachment, and glaucoma; cerebellar hemangioblastoma may present as progressive ataxia, increased intracranial pressure, or subarachnoid hemorrhage. Spinal cord symptoms depend on the location and extent of the spinal angiomatosis and whether or not bleeding occurs. Visceral hemangiomas are apt to remain asymptomatic. Polycythemia is frequently present.

The diagnosis may be confirmed by family history, isotope scan of the posterior fossa and cord, and angiography.

Retinal lesions may be dealt with by photo- or diathermy coagulation. Cerebellar and spinal cord hemangioblastomas may require surgical removal.

CNS DEGENERATIVE DISORDERS OF INFANCY & CHILDHOOD

Essentials of Diagnosis

- Arrest of psychomotor development.
- Loss, usually progressive but at highly variable rates, of mental functioning, motor control, and often vision.
- Seizures of varying types are common in some disorders.
- Symptoms and signs vary with age at onset and primary sites of involvement of specific types.

General Considerations

The CNS degenerative disorders of infancy and childhood are fortunately rare. Although they may share many symptoms and signs, a careful history and clinical and laboratory evaluation frequently establish the most likely diagnosis.

Clinical Findings

A. Symptoms:

1. Where white matter is primarily involved, motor disturbances usually appear first. Hypotonia or flaccidity in infants may precede the eventual spasticity, or, if the child has begun to walk, incoordination (ataxia or dystonia) may be noted first, accompanied or followed by derangements of swallowing and of vocalization or speech. Vision is disturbed early. Convulsions usually appear late in the course if at all.

2. Where gray matter is primarily involved, convulsions often precede disturbances of mental and motor functions.

3. Where the disorder is diffuse, the clinical picture may be mixed or may present predominantly with the features of a white or gray matter disturbance.

B. Signs:

1. **Cry**—The cry is irritable and high-pitched in Krabbe's disease, Tay-Sachs disease, and Canavan's disease; diminished, weak, or absent in subacute necrotizing encephalomyelopathy (Leigh's disease); and like that of stridor or laryngospasm in infantile Gaucher's disease.

2. **Head circumference**—Often enlarged early in Canavan's disease and Alexander's disease and in the mucopolysaccharidoses; often enlarged late in metachromatic leukodystrophy and Tay-Sachs disease; and often small in Krabbe's disease and other dysmyelinogenic processes.

3. **Fundi**—"Cherry-red" maculas are seen in Tay-Sachs disease, Niemann-Pick disease, and infantile Gaucher's disease. A "salt and pepper" macula is present in late infantile and juvenile (and adult) forms of neurolipidosis (Batten-Mayou-Bielschowsky disease; Spielmeyer-Vogt disease). Optic atrophy occurs in subacute necrotizing encephalomyelopathy (Leigh's disease), Schilder's disease, and other leukodystrophies. Retinitis pigmentosa is present in abetalipoproteinemia and Refsum's disease.

4. **Hepatomegaly**—In Niemann-Pick disease, infantile Gaucher's disease, Tay-Sachs disease, generalized gangliosidosis, Wilson's disease, mucopolysaccharidoses, glycogen storage diseases, and some organic acidurias.

5. **Muscle tone and reflexes**—These are the least dependable physical clues. However, flaccidity or hypotonia coupled with areflexia may initially occur in white matter disorders in which peripheral nerve involvement is prominent, as in infantile metachromatic leukodystrophy. However, spasticity usually supervenes in time in the degenerative disorders, and deep reflexes may not be obtained because of the flexion contractures which develop.

C. Laboratory Findings: (See also Table 33–13.)

1. **Blood**—Vacuolized lymphocytes are found in many patients with neurolipidosis. Usually 10% or more of the lymphocytes are vacuolated when 300 are counted, but more than one smear may be necessary. The percentage and the size of the vacuoles depend on the duration of the disease. Vacuolized lymphocytes

are also often observed in the carriers.

Hypergranulation may be prominent in polymorphonuclear cells, and present but less marked in the mononuclear cells in some of the "storage" diseases. While not present in every patient with such a disorder, they may be observed in a high percentage of close relatives when evident in the patient. Basophilic and more focal granulations are seen in Tay-Sachs disease; azurophilic, dispersed granules are more typical of the late infantile and juvenile forms of familial amaurotic idiocy; and Alder's granulations occur in some of the mucopolysaccharidoses.

Decreased fructose-1-phosphate aldolase is found in Tay-Sachs disease and carriers. SGOT, SGPT, and LDH are often markedly increased in Tay-Sachs disease and Niemann-Pick disease. For enzyme defects in lysosomal disorders, see Chapter 33.

2. Urine—A positive screening test is found in mucopolysaccharidosis. Quantitative increases in heparitin and chondroitin sulfate determine the type. Metachromasia of shed epithelial cells and a colorimetric test showing absence of arylsulfatase A help in diagnosis of metachromatic leukodystrophy.

3. CSF—Pressure may be elevated in Schilder's diffuse sclerosis. Protein is usually markedly increased in metachromatic and globoid leukodystrophy. Gamma globulin is increased in subacute sclerosing panencephalitis (SSPE) and sometimes in Schilder's sclerosis. Measles antibody titer in CSF is increased in SSPE.

4. Nerve conduction is prolonged in metachromatic and globoid leukodystrophy and possibly in other dysmyelinogenic disorders.

D. X-Ray Findings: Skeletal alterations may suggest Gaucher's disease, GM_1 gangliosidoses, or one of the mucopolysaccharidoses. Gallbladder series shows no uptake of dye in metachromatic leukodystrophy.

E. Tissue Studies: The enzyme deficiencies may now be assayed in various tissues in a variety of the "storage" diseases.

1. White blood cell buffy coats may be examined for enzymatic activity, both in leukocytes and in lymphocytes, as well as by electron microscopy.

2. Skin punch biopsy specimens may be examined using fibroblast tissue cultures as above.

3. Nerve biopsies, when indicated by prolonged conduction time, may show typical metachromasia in metachromatic leukodystrophy. In globoid leukodystrophy, nonspecific myelin breakdown is found.

4. Liver biopsy is justified when hepatomegaly is present and is most useful in Niemann-Pick disease, the mucopolysaccharidoses, and gangliosidoses.

5. Rectal biopsy is now considered not useful.

6. Brain biopsy, if positive, is often definitive and may differentiate an acquired slow viral encephalitis (SSPE) from a biochemically determined degenerative process. In white matter diseases, the biopsy must often be deep to provide proper tissue.

Differential Diagnosis

A period of observation may be necessary before it becomes clear that one is dealing with a degenerative process. Pseudodegeneration may occur as a result of a severe seizure disorder or other illness, or a child may regress because of gross emotional neglect or stress. Retarded children with static brain damage are often thought by their parents to be regressing when in actuality a younger sibling or other child is noted to be outstripping the older one. Thus, the differential diagnosis of CNS degenerative disorders must include "cerebral palsy," seizure disorders, space-occupying lesions (including subdural hematomas or brain tumors), neurocutaneous dysplasias, chromosomal defects, disorders of glucose or protein and amino or organic acid metabolism, and chronic CNS infections.

Tables 21—6 and 21—7 summarize the important differential aspects of the clinical findings and courses of the common CNS degenerative disorders of infancy and childhood.

Complications

Pneumonia, usually due to aspiration, is the most common complication and the usual cause of death.

Prevention

The heritable nature of these disorders should be made clear. Enzymatic technics involving studies of leukocytes, skin fibroblasts, and amniotic cells are being rapidly developed to identify the carriers, affected fetuses, or presymptomatic cases.

Treatment

In most of the CNS degenerative diseases, treatment is purely symptomatic, consisting of control of seizures, maintenance of nutrition (often via feeding gastrostomy), and treatment of infections. In acute attacks of "multiple sclerosis" and optic neuritis or transverse myelitis (neuromyelitis optica, Devic's disease), corticotropin (4 mg/kg/day IM initially, with rapidly decreasing doses if there is a good response) may shorten the duration of the attack but does not alter either the frequency of exacerbations or the ultimate outcome of the disease.

Prognosis

By definition, the CNS degenerative diseases lead to progressive loss of function and premature death within months or a few years.

Antenatal detection of the sphingolipidoses. (Editorial.) N Engl J Med 288:1405, 1973.

Armstrong D, Dimitt S, VanWormer DE: Studies in Batten's disease. 1. Peroxidase deficiency in granulocytes. Arch Neurol 30:144, 1974.

Brady RO: The abnormal chemistry of inherited disorders of lipid metabolism. Fed Proc 32:1660, 1973.

Dolman CL, MacLeod PM, Chang E: Skin punch biopsies and lymphocytes in the diagnosis of the lipidoses. Can J Neurol Sci 2:67, 1975.

Horta-Barbosa L, Fucillo DA, Sever JL: Chronic viral infections of the CNS. JAMA 218:1185, 1971.

Menkes JH, Andrews JM, Cancilla PA: The cerebroretinal degenerations. J Pediatr 79:183, 1971.

Table 21–6. CNS degenerative disorders of infancy.

Disease	Enzyme Defect and Genetics	Onset	Early Manifestations	Vision and Hearing	Somatic Findings	Motor System	Seizures	Laboratory Studies	Biopsy	Course
WHITE MATTER										
Globoid (Krabbe's) leukodystrophy	Recessive. Galactocerebroside-beta-galactosidase deficiency.	First 6 months; rarely later.	Feeding difficulties. Shrill cry. Irritability. Arching of back.	Optic atrophy, mid-course to late. Hyperacusis occasionally.	Head often small. Often underweight.	Early spasticity, occasionally preceded by hypotonia. Prolonged nerve conduction.	Early. Myoclonic and generalized.	Routine blood, urine, and x-rays normal. CSF protein markedly elevated. Enzyme assay.	Sural nerve: nonspecific myelin breakdown. Brain: globoid cells.	Rapid. Death usually by 1½–2 years.
Metachromatic leukodystrophy	Recessive. Arylsulfatase A deficiency.	Second year. Less often, later in childhood.	Incoordination; especially gait disturbance.	Optic atrophy, usually late. Hearing normal.	Head enlarged late.	Combined upper and lower motor neuron signs. Ataxia. Prolonged nerve conduction.	Infrequent, usually late and generalized.	Metachromatic cells in urine; negative sulfatase A test. CSF protein elevated; occasionally normal early. "Nonfilling" of gallbladder on x-rays.	Sural nerve biopsy: metachromasia.	Moderately slow Death in infantile form by 3–5 years; in "juvenile" form, by 10–13 years.
Spongy sclerosis (Canavan's)	Recessive. Mostly Jewish. Enzyme defect not known.	First 3 months.	Arrest in development; floppiness.	Optic atrophy, usually early. Hearing normal.	Head enlarged early.	Floppy early, then rapidly very spastic with decerebrate rigidity.	Early; in about 50% of cases.	Blood, urine normal. CSF under increased pressure; protein usually normal. Cranial sutures split.	Brain: (?)nonspecific) spongiform degeneration, myelin deficiency.	Rapid. Death usually by 1½–3 years.
Pelizaeus-Merzbacher disease	X-linked recessive; rare female. (?)Disorder of glycerophosphatide metabolism.	(?) Birth to 2 years.	"Eye rolling" often shortly after birth. Head bobbing. Slow loss of intellect.	Slowly developing optic atrophy. Hearing normal.	Head and body normal.	Cerebellar signs early, hyperactive deep reflexes. Spasticity usually only very late.	Usually only late.	Blood, urine, CSF, and x-rays normal.	Brain biopsy rarely helpful; extensive demyelination; small perivascular islands of intact myelin.	Exceedingly slow, often seemingly stationary. Many survive well into adult life.
DIFFUSE, BUT PRIMARILY GRAY MATTER										
Poliodystrophy (Alpers')	Occasionally familial, possibly environmental. (?"Slow virus.")	Infancy to late childhood.	Variable: loss of intellect, seizures, incoordination.	"Cortical blindness and deafness."	Head normal initially; may fail to grow.	Variable: incoordination, spasticity.	Often initial manifestation: myoclonic, akinetic, and generalized.	Blood, urine, and x-rays normal. CSF protein normal or slightly elevated.	Extensive neuronal loss in cortex: may occur very late.	Usually rapid, with death within 1–2 years after onset.

Disease	Genetics/Enzyme	Onset	Early Symptoms	Eyes	Head/Liver/Spleen	Muscle Tone	Convulsions	Laboratory	Pathology	Course
Tay-Sachs disease and variants	93% East European Jewish. Recessive. N-Acetylhexosaminidase A deficiency. In variant forms, non-Jewish.	3–6 months. In variants, onset is usually later; deficiency of hexosaminidase A and B (Sandhoff) or partial defect of A (GM$_2$ gangliosidosis).	Variable: shrill cry, loss of vision, infantile spasms, arrest of development.	Cherry-red macula, early blindness. Hyperacusis early.	Head enlarged late. Liver occasionally enlarged.	Initially floppy. Eventual decerebrate rigidity.	Frequent, in mid-course and late. Infantile spasms and generalized.	Blood smears: vacuolated lymphocytes; basophilic hypergranulation. CSF protein normal or slightly elevated. Urine and x-rays normal. Enzyme assay.	Rectal biopsy: ballooned ganglion cells, often only late.	Moderately rapid. Death usually by 2–3 years.
Niemann-Pick disease and variants	50% Jewish. Recessive. Sphingomyelinase deficiency. In variants, later onset; enzyme defects unknown.	First 6 months. In variants, later onset; often non-Jewish.	Slow development. Protruding belly.	Cherry-red macula in 35–50%. Blindness late. Deafness occasionally.	Head usually normal. Spleen enlarged more than liver. Occasional xanthomas of skin. Emaciation early.	Initially floppy. Eventually spastic. Occasionally extrapyramidal signs.	Rare and late.	Blood: Vacuolated lymphocytes. Increased serum lipids. CSF protein normal or slightly elevated. Urine normal. X-rays: "Mottled" lungs, decalcified bones.	"Foam cells" in bone marrow, spleen, lymph nodes. Rectal biopsy occasionally positive.	Moderately slow. Death usually by 3–5 years.
Infantile Gaucher's disease (glucosyl ceramide lipidosis)	Recessive. Glucocerebrosidase deficiency.	First year; rarely, late infancy.	Stridor or hoarse cry. Retraction. Feeding difficulties.	Occasional cherry-red macula. Convergent squint. Deafness occasionally.	Head usually normal. Liver and spleen equally enlarged.	Opisthotomos early, followed rapidly by decerebrate rigidity.	Rare and late,	Peripheral blood findings variable. Increased acid phosphatase. X-rays: Thinned cortex, trabeculation of bones.	"Gaucher cells" in bone marrow, spleen. Positive rectal biopsy.	Very rapid.
Generalized gangliosidosis and juvenile type (GM$_1$ gangliosidoses)	Recessive. Beta-galactosidase deficiency.	First year; less often, second year.	Arrest of development. Protruding belly. Abnormal facies.	Occasional "cherry-red spot." Hearing usually normal.	Head enlarged early. Liver enlarged more than spleen.	Initially floppy, eventually spastic.	Usually late.	Blood: Vacuolated lymphocytes. X-rays: Dorsolumbar kyphosis, "beaking" of vertebrae.	"Foam cells" similar to those in Niemann-Pick disease.	Very rapid. Death within a few years.
Subacute necrotizing encephalomyelopathy (Leigh's)	Recessive. ?Thiamine pyrophosphate-adenosine triphosphate "inhibitor."	Infancy to late childhood.	Difficulties in feeding. Feeble or absent cry. Floppiness.	Optic atrophy, often early. Hearing normal.	Head usually normal; occasionally small.	Flaccid and immobile; may become spastic.	Rare and late.	Increased lactic acid in blood. CSF protein normal or slightly elevated. CSF, urine for "inhibitor."	Normal.	Usually rapid in infants, but more slowly progressive with death after several years in some cases.
"Steel wool" or "kinky hair" disease (Menkes')	X-linked recessive. Defect in copper absorption.	Infancy.	Peculiar facies. Secondary hair white, twisted, split. Hypothermia.	May show optic disk pallor and microcysts of pigment epithelium.	Normal to small.	Variable: Floppy to spastic.	Myoclonic, infantile spasms, status epilepticus.	Defective absorption of copper. Cerebral angiography shows elongated arteries.	Hair shows pilli torti, split shafts.	Moderately rapid. Death usually by 3–4 years.

Table 21–7. CNS degenerative disorders of childhood.*

Disease	Enzyme Defect and Genetics	Onset	Early Manifestations	Vision and Hearing	Motor System	Seizures	Laboratory Studies	Biopsy	Course
Neuroaxonal degeneration (Seitelberger)	Familial, (?) recessive. Girls more frequent than boys. Defect unknown.	1–3 years.	Arrest of development and dementia. Loss of motor functions. Occasionally loss of pain sense over trunk and legs.	Nystagmus frequent; optic atrophy and blindness. Hearing normal.	Combined upper and lower motor neuron lesions. Early, may lie in "frog" position.	Variable, but usually not a prominent feature.	Electromyography shows partial denervation, elevated serum lactate dehydrogenase and transaminase.	Brain and sural nerve: axonal swellings or "spheroids." Iron deposition in globus pallidus.	Very slowly progressive with death early in second decade or earlier.
Cerebromacular degenerations: Late infantile (Bielschowsky)	Recessive. Peroxidase deficiency in granulocytes?	2–4 years.	Ataxia. Visual difficulties. Arrested intellectual development.	Pigmentary degeneration of macula. Optic atrophy. Hearing normal.	Ataxia, spasticity progressing to decerebrate rigidity.	Often early: myoclonic and later generalized.	Blood: vacuolated lymphocytes, azurophilic dispersed hypergranulation of polymorphonuclear cells. Electroretinography helpful.	Rectal biopsy: ballooned ganglion cells.	Moderately slow. Death in 3–8 years.
Juvenile (Batten-Mayou, Spielmeyer-Vogt)	More frequent in Scandinavian and Anglo-Saxon families. Recessive. Relatively common. Peroxidase deficiency in granulocytes?	5–12 years.	Progressive visual loss. Progressive dementia. Ataxia.	Pigmentary degeneration of macula. Optic atrophy. Hearing normal.	Ataxia, slurred speech, slowly progressive spasticity.	Variable: early to mid-course, "petit mal," myoclonic, generalized.	As in late infantile form.	As in late infantile form.	Slow. Death in 7–15 years after onset.
Adult (Kufs)	Recessive. Peroxidase deficiency in granulocytes?	15–25 years.	Psychotic behavior. Dementia. Ataxia.	Normal.	Ataxia.	Myoclonic seizures, usually early.	(?) Normal.	Not known.	Very slow. May live into 60s.
Subacute sclerosing panencephalitis (Dawson's, SSPE)	None. Relatively common. Measles "slow virus" infection.	3–22 years. Rarely earlier or later.	Impaired intellect, emotional lability, incoordination.	Occasionally chorioretinitis or optic atrophy. Hearing normal.	Ataxia, slurred speech, occasionally involuntary movements, spasticity progressing to decerebrate rigidity.	Myoclonic and akinetic seizures relatively early; later, focal and generalized.	CSF protein normal to moderately elevated. High CSF gamma globulin.‡ Elevated CSF measles antibody titers. Characteristic EEG.	Brain biopsy: inclusion body encephalitis; culturing of measles virus.	Variable, from death in a few months to many years. Remissions of variable duration may occur during course of disease.

Familial sudanophilic leukodystrophy	Familial. Defect unknown.	5–10 years.	Impaired intellect, behavioral problems.	Optic atrophy common. Hearing normal.	Ataxia, spasticity.	Occasionally.	May be associated with hyperpigmentation due to adrenocortical insufficiency.‡	Brain: sudanophilia; sparing of U fibers.	Fairly rapid, death usually within 2–3 years after onset.
Schilder's diffuse sclerosis and variants†	None. Relatively common. Defect unknown.	5–10 years	Highly variable: may strike mental, motor, or visual systems first, or begin with focal seizures.	Occasionally presents with papilledema. Progressive optic atrophy. "Psychic" and organic deafness.	Ataxia, hemiparesis, or spastic diplegia.	Focal and generalized; variable in onset and frequency.	CSF protein and gamma globulin may be elevated. ‡ Occasionally increased CSF pressure.	Leukodystrophy.	Variable: death in months to years after onset with remissions of varying degree and duration possible.
Neuromyelitis optica (Devic's disease)	None. Defect unknown.	Abrupt: late infancy to late childhood. May be preceded by infection.	Optic neuritis with "painful" blindness or transverse myelitis.	Optic neuritis with loss of vision in one or both eyes. Hearing normal.	Flaccid paraplegia at first, with loss of sphincter control; later, spastic paraplegia.	None.	CSF protein may be elevated; occasionally pleocytosis. CSF gamma globulin may be elevated, usually after several attacks.‡	None.	Variable: complete remissions possible or recurrent attacks of optic neuritis or transverse myelitis.
Multiple sclerosis	None. Diagnosis difficult in childhood. Defect unknown.	2 years on.	Highly variable: may strike one or more sites of CNS. Paresthesias common.	Optic neuritis; diplopia, nystagmus at some time. Vestibulocochlear nerves occasionally affected.	Motor weakness, spasticity, ataxia, sphincter disturbances, slurred speech, mental difficulties.	Rare: focal or generalized.	CSF may show slight pleocytosis, elevation of protein and gamma globulin.‡	None.	Variable: complete remission possible. Recurrent attacks and involvement of multiple sites are prerequisites for diagnosis.

*For late infantile metachromatic leukodystrophy, Pelizaeus-Merzbacher disease, poliodystrophy, Gaucher's disease of later onset, and subacute necrotizing encephalomyelopathy, see Table 21–6.

†This includes the variants Balo's concentric sclerosis and Scholz's disease as well as transitional sclerosis, which shares features of Schilder's disease and multiple sclerosis; and the X-linked recessive form with adrenocortical atrophy.

‡CSF gamma globulin (IgG) is considered elevated in children when above 9% of total protein (possibly even > 8.3%); definitively elevated when > 14%.

Myers GJ, Hedley-Whyte ET, Fagan ME: Reevaluation of role of rectal biopsy in diagnosis of pediatric neurologic disorders. Neurology 23:27, 1973.

Poser CM: Myelinoclastic diffuse and transitional sclerosis. Pages 469–893 in: *Handbook of Clinical Neurology.* Vol 9. Vinken PJ, Bruyn GW (editors). North-Holland Publishing Co., 1970.

ATAXIAS OF CHILDHOOD

1. ACUTE CEREBELLAR ATAXIA

Acute cerebellar ataxia occurs most commonly in children 2–6 years of age. The onset is abrupt, and the evolution of symptoms is rapid. In about half of cases there is a prodromal illness with fever, respiratory or gastrointestinal symptoms, or an exanthem within 3 weeks of onset. Associated viral infections include varicella, rubeola, mumps, rubella, echovirus infections, poliomyelitis, infectious mononucleosis, and influenza. Bacterial infections such as scarlet fever and salmonellosis have also been incriminated.

Clinical Findings

A. Symptoms and Signs: The ataxia of the trunk and extremities may be quite severe, so that the child exhibits a staggering, reeling gait and inability to sit without support or to reach for objects; or there may be only mild unsteadiness. Hypotonia and tremor of the extremities may be present. Abnormal eye movements may include horizontal nystagmus. Speech may be slurred. The child frequently is irritable, and vomiting may occur.

There are no clinical signs of increased intracranial pressure. Sensory and reflex testing usually shows no abnormalities.

B. Laboratory Findings: The CSF is not under increased pressure. CSF protein and glucose are normal, although a slight lymphocytosis (up to about 30%) may be present. Attempts should be made to identify the etiologic viral agent by appropriate studies of CSF, stool, throat washings, and paired sera.

C. X-Ray and Other Findings: Skull films and long bones are normal. EEG may be normal or may show nonspecific slowing.

Differential Diagnosis

Acute cerebellar ataxia must be differentiated from acute cerebellar syndromes due to phenytoin, phenobarbital, primidone, or lead intoxication. However, with phenytoin and barbiturate intoxication, the nystagmus is usually fine, rapid, and of equal amplitude, in contrast to the coarser nystagmus of cerebellar disease. The toxic level in serum of phenytoin is usually above 20 μg/ml. Mean toxic levels of phenobarbital are reported to be above 50 μg/ml; for primidone,

above 12 μg/ml. (See section on Seizure Disorders.) With lead intoxication, papilledema, anemia, basophilic stippling of erythrocytes, proteinuria, typical x-rays, and elevated CSF protein are clinical clues, confirmed by serum, urine, or hair lead levels. The presence of an occult neuroblastoma, usually seen with the polymyoclonia-opsoclonus syndrome (see below), must also be ruled out; this may best be done by careful physical examination, x-rays of the chest and abdomen, and assays of urinary catecholamine metabolites.

In rare cases, acute cerebellar ataxia may be the presenting sign of acute bacterial meningitis or may be mimicked by corticosteroid withdrawal, vasculitides such as in polyarteritis nodosa, trauma, the first attack of ataxia in a metabolic disorder such as Hartnup's disease, or the onset of acute disseminated encephalomyelitis or of multiple sclerosis. The history and physical findings will usually differentiate these disturbances, but appropriate laboratory studies may be necessary, including gas chromatography to identify intoxicants. For ataxias with more chronic onset and course, see the sections on spinocerebellar degeneration (below) and the other degenerative disorders.

Treatment

Treatment is supportive. The use of corticosteroids has no rational justification. Chlorpromazine (Thorazine) may be useful to reduce the irritability and vomiting sometimes seen initially. Reduction of dosage or withdrawal of incriminated drugs will depend on the weight of the indications for them balanced against the severity of the side-effects.

Prognosis

Between 80–90% of children with acute cerebellar ataxia not secondary to drugs recover without sequelae within 6–8 weeks. In the remainder, neurologic disturbances, including disorders of behavior and of learning, ataxia, abnormal eye movements, and speech impairment may persist for months or years, and recovery may remain incomplete.

Roberts KB, Freeman JM: Cerebellar ataxia and "occult neuroblastoma" without opsoclonus. Pediatrics 56:464, 1975.

Weiss S, Carter S: Course and prognosis of acute cerebellar ataxia in children. Neurology 9:711, 1959.

2. POLYMYOCLONIA-OPSOCLONUS SYNDROME OF CHILDHOOD
(Infantile Myoclonic Encephalopathy, "Dancing Eyes-Dancing Feet" Syndrome)

Especially at first, the symptoms and signs of this syndrome are similar to those of "acute cerebellar ataxia," and this broad category formerly included cases of the polymyoclonia-opsoclonus syndrome. In addition to severe incoordination of the trunk and extremities, often of relatively sudden onset, there are lightning-like, violent, brief jerking or flinging movements of a group of muscles with the child in constant motion while awake. Extraocular muscle involvement results in sudden jerking, irregular eye movements, or opsoclonus. Irritability and vomiting often accompany these symptoms, but there is no depression of level of consciousness. This syndrome occurs in association with viral infections and in children with tumors of neural crest origin. Immunologic mechanisms have been postulated as responsible. Skull films usually show no evidence of increased intracranial pressure. CSF is not usually under increased pressure and may show normal or mildly increased protein. Special technics are required to show increased CSF plasmacytes and abnormal immunoglobulins. The EEG may be slightly slow, but when performed together with electromyography it shows no evidence of association between cortical discharges and the muscle movements. An assiduous search must be made to rule out tumor of neural crest origin by x-rays of the chest and abdomen, skeletal survey, and intravenous urography as well as by assays of urinary catecholamine metabolites (VMA, etc) and cystathionine. Urine evaluation should be performed only after proper dietary preparation (omission of foods rich in catecholamines) and should be performed repeatedly if normal since normal results do not rule out the presence of such tumors.

The symptoms respond (often dramatically) to large doses of corticotropin. When a neural crest (or possibly other) tumor is found, surgical excision should be followed by irradiation and chemotherapy. Life span is determined by the biologic behavior of the tumor.

The syndrome is usually self-limited but may be characterized by exacerbations and remissions. However, even after removal of a neural crest tumor and without other evidence of its recurrence, symptoms may reappear. A high incidence of mild mental retardation has also been recorded.

Moe PG, Nellhaus G: Infantile polymyoclonia-opsoclonus syndrome and neural crest tumors. Neurology 20:756, 1970.

3. SPINOCEREBELLAR DEGENERATIONS

Essentials of Diagnosis

- Cerebellar and spinal involvement in various combinations.
- Slowly progressive course.
- Family history frequently positive.
- High incidence of associated neurologic or systemic disturbances.

General Considerations

The different heredodegenerative cerebellar ataxias may represent variants of the classical form of Friedreich's ataxia and be indistinguishable from each other in the early stages. Mild and incomplete forms exist. The age at onset and rate of progression may be highly variable, though often similar in the same family or in a given variant of this group of disorders.

Clinical Findings

The following should be looked for carefully, as they appear in various combinations in the entities described briefly below: truncal and extremity ataxia, horizontal or rotatory nystagmus, slurred and staccato speech, hypotonia, kyphosis, scoliosis, high-arched feet with hammer toes, optic atrophy, retinitis pigmentosa, external ophthalmoplegia, cataracts, reflex changes, positive Babinski signs, diminished to absent vibratory and position sense, muscular atrophy, mental retardation, and cardiac disease.

Types of Heredodegenerative Cerebellar Ataxias

A. Friedreich's Spinocerebellar Ataxia: This is not only the commonest form of the hereditary ataxias but also the most variable in its manifestations. Partial forms occur frequently. Affected family members may exhibit only high-arched feet or mild scoliosis. In its complete form, with onset in childhood, findings may eventually include the typical foot deformity (in 75% or more of cases), kyphoscoliosis, ataxia; loss of 2-point discrimination, position sense, and vibratory sensation; loss of knee and ankle jerk reflexes (early) and of arm reflexes (later), positive Babinski signs, horizontal and rotatory nystagmus, staccato speech, muscular hypotonia, and impairment of mental ability. Optic atrophy and cardiac disease may also develop. Variants of peroneal muscular atrophy (Charcot-Marie-Tooth disease) and of progressive muscular dystrophy may occur in association with Friedreich's ataxia.

No specific laboratory findings are helpful. X-rays of the spine may reveal the scoliosis. ECG may show conduction defects with bundle branch block or complete heart block, or changes associated with occlusive coronary disease. Diabetes mellitus should be carefully looked for, as its association with Friedreich's ataxia is not infrequent. Muscle enzyme determinations, electrical studies, and muscle biopsy may establish the presence of muscular atrophy or dystrophy.

B. Roussy-Lévy Syndrome: Beginning usually in early childhood, there are ataxia, pes cavus, diminished or absent knee and ankle jerks, and muscular atrophy of the lower extremities and sometimes of the hands. Dysarthria and nystagmus usually are absent. The course is slowly progressive and often seems to arrest at puberty before symptoms become too severe.

C. Behr's Syndrome: Partial Friedreich's ataxia with spasticity, hyperreflexia, and optic atrophy.

D. Marinesco-Sjögren Syndrome: Partial Friedreich's ataxia with short stature, marked mental retardation, and cataracts.

E. Franchescetti's Syndrome: Partial Friedreich's ataxia combined with external ophthalmoplegia.

F. Hereditary Olivopontocerebellar Atrophy: In the juvenile form, transmitted as a dominant, there may be highly variable involvement of the cranial nerves, pyramidal tract signs, cerebellar disturbances, and striatal symptoms, including rigidity, tremor, and choreoathetosis. Mental retardation is variable.

G. Others: Among other entities to be considered are ataxia-telangiectasia of Mme Louis-Bar, abetalipoproteinemia, Refsum's syndrome, and various rare ataxic syndromes associated with neuroretinal degeneration and the also rare intermittent ataxias associated with disorders of amino acid or ammonia metabolism, such as hyperalaninemia and Hartnup's disease.

Treatment

Supportive care consists of physical therapy, the use of a walker or wheelchair when necessary, and similar measures. Orthopedic surgery may be of value when the disease appears to be only very slowly progressive or is seemingly arrested. Coronary symptoms and cardiac failure may require the use of nitrates (eg, nitroglycerin) and digitalis preparations. Diabetes mellitus should be treated.

Physostigmine is currently under investigation for the symptomatic amelioration of familial ataxias.

Prognosis

In Friedreich's ataxia, many patients are able to walk until the end of their second decade or even longer. Patients usually live for 15–20 years from the date of onset, and death is usually due to heart failure.

Many patients with Roussy-Lévy syndrome live a normal life span. In the rarer forms of spinocerebellar degeneration, the prognosis is highly variable.

Biemond A: Congenital cerebellar ataxia. Psychiatr Neurol Neurochir 74:303, 1971.
Currier RD & others: Spinocerebellar ataxia: Study of a large kindred. Neurology 22:1040, 1972.
Greenfield JG: *The Spino-cerebellar Degenerations.* Thomas, 1954.
Kark RAP, Blass JP, Spence MA: Physostigmine in familial ataxias. Neurology 27:70, 1977.

ATAXIA-TELANGIECTASIA
(Mme Louis-Bar Syndrome)

This heredodegenerative disorder is characterized by ataxia; telangiectasia of the bulbar conjunctivas, external ears, nares, and subsequently other body surfaces; and recurrent respiratory, sinus, and ear infections. The ataxia is usually noted in the second to third years of life; the telangiectatic lesions appear in the third to sixth years. Ocular dyspraxia, slurred speech, choreoathetosis, hypotonia and areflexia, and psychomotor and growth retardation may be present. In some patients, deficiencies of IgA and IgE exist. Nerve conduction velocities may be reduced. There is no treatment other than for the recurrent infections. Cases of malignancies involving the reticuloendothelial system have been reported.

DeLeon GA, Grover WD, Huff DS: Neuropathologic changes in ataxia-telangiectasia. Neurology 26:947, 1976.

THE "EXTRAPYRAMIDAL DISORDERS"

These syndromes are characterized by the presence of one or more of the following features: dyskinesias, especially the choreic syndrome, athetosis and ballismus, tremors, rigidity, and dystonias. (These terms are explained below.)

For the most part, precise pathologic and anatomic localization is not completely understood. In general, motor pathways synapsing in the striatum (putamen and caudate nucleus), globus pallidus, red nucleus, substantia nigra, and the body of Luys are involved; this "system" is markedly influenced by pathways originating in the thalamus, cerebellum, and reticular formation.

Symptoms

A. Chorea: Involuntary, purposeless, sudden jerky, irregular movements involving the face, trunk, and extremities, usually provoked and increased by voluntary activity and tension but decreased by relaxation and disappearing in sleep. Gait, in particular, is markedly disturbed; the legs are flung out or may suddenly flex, and the arms flail about. Hypotonia is frequently present. There is a waxing and waning of the grip ("milkmaid's grip"). The tongue darts in and out. Feeding, writing, and other activities requiring fine muscular coordination are impaired. There is facial grimacing. Speech is irregular and indistinct. The knee jerk may be "hung up," ie, following stimulation, the lower leg may be slow to return to the prestimulus position or even the extended position for several seconds. The arm and leg are usually affected equally; however, the 2 sides of the body may be unequally involved, so that only one side may appear to be affected (hemichorea).

B. Athetosis: A recurring series of slow, writhing movements, including vermicular movements in the fingers and waves of grimaces. Muscular hypertonia is frequently evident, and the muscles may become hypertrophied as a result of the constant movements. Speech and swallowing may be severely impaired. Tendon reflexes may be difficult to obtain.

C. Choreoathetosis: A combination of chorea and athetosis occurs rather frequently.

D. Ballismus: An involuntary movement pattern of violent flinging about of the limbs. The movements are of large amplitude and usually related to contractions of the proximal musculature. This disorder is usually unilateral (hemiballismus), of sudden onset, and may follow transient hemiplegia.

E. Dystonia: Characterized by abnormal postures and disturbed muscle tone, the movements are slow, sustained, and nonpatterned, involving chiefly the muscles of the trunk and neck and the proximal muscles of the extremities. Dystonia is made worse by voluntary activity and emotional tension. The spine is commonly twisted and the feet held in the equinus position and inverted; the hands are less affected. Occasionally, only the neck is involved (spasmodic torticollis). In addition to muscle spasm, hypertonia is common. Tendon reflexes are difficult to elicit. Initially, there are few movements, often confined to one part of the body. Eventually, however, gait and posture become bizarre, and ultimately there may be paucity of movements because of the marked rigidity and contractures.

F. Tremors: These range from fine to coarse, rhythmic oscillatory movements present at rest and often inhibited by voluntary action. Tremors are best demonstrated with the patient's arms outstretched and fingers spread.

G. Rigidity: Increased muscle tone with fairly constant contraction of the flexors and extensors, resulting in increased resistance through the full range of passive motion, and with normal or only slightly increased deep tendon reflexes.

H. "Parkinsonian" Syndrome: A combination of abnormal posture, resting tremor, and rigidity. The "pill-rolling" tremor is increased by emotional tension and inhibited by volitional actions. The rigidity is said to be of the "cogwheel" type because of a regularly jerky "give" in resistance when a flexed extremity is extended passively. Voluntary movements are slow; there is a shuffling gait, and the arms do not swing. There is often a marked paucity of movements. In children, there may be a frozen open-mouthed facies. Speech is slow and monotonous. Coordination and tendon reflexes are usually normal. In many instances, the patient can run much better than he can walk.

1. POSTNATALLY ACQUIRED EXTRAPYRAMIDAL DISORDERS

DRUG-INDUCED EXTRAPYRAMIDAL DISORDERS

Essentials of Diagnosis

- "Parkinsonian" syndrome of acute onset.
- Dystonia, dyskinesia, tetanus-like syndrome, meningismus, myoclonic jerks, or generalized seizures.
- Autonomic disturbances.
- History of administration or ingestion of phenothiazines or "tranquilizers," or presence of such drugs in the home.
- Positive urine test.

General Considerations

The diagnosis may be suspected in children who have received phenothiazine derivatives within the preceding 48 hours. Prochlorperazine (Compazine) is the most common offender. Severe bradykinesia has been reported due to anticonvulsants.

Onset is acute. The clinical picture may be greatly complicated by the signs and symptoms of the illness which led to the administration of a phenothiazine. Phenothiazine intoxication should always be suspected in the presence of extrapyramidal symptoms of acute onset.

Clinical Findings

A. Symptoms and Signs: Frequently seen are cogwheel rigidity, tremors, severe speech and swallowing disturbances, masked facies, dystonias, and dyskinesias. Constant or intermittent spasms of the neck and back muscles, jaws, face, tongue, and limbs, as well as a "sardonic smile," may suggest tetanus. Opisthotonos and spasms of the legs on straight leg raising may suggest meningismus. Oculogyric crisis may occur. Some patients have myoclonic jerks or generalized seizures, including status epilepticus. Bradykinesia may be the chief finding. Autonomic disturbances such as tachycardia, hypotension, salivation, blurred vision, and paralysis of the bladder may occur.

B. Laboratory Findings: Testing the urine with Phenistix or ferric chloride up to 18–24 hours after the last dose of phenothiazine often gives a reddish-purple reaction. Occasionally—particularly if phenothiazines have been administered over a long period of time—there may be leukopenia and disordered liver function. If antiepileptic drugs are suspected, phenobarbital and (especially) phenytoin levels should be measured. The EEG may be normal.

Differential Diagnosis

Common misdiagnoses, as may be suspected from the symptoms, are hysteria, meningitis (especially when there is an underlying febrile illness accompanied by vomiting), tetanus, and Sydenham's chorea.

Treatment

In severe cases, give one of the following: (1) diphenhydramine (Benadryl), 2 mg/kg body weight slowly IV, and repeat cautiously if necessary for a total of 5 mg/kg/day. (2) Caffeine and sodium benzoate, 10 mg/kg IV or IM (may repeat). (3) Promethazine (Phenergan), 0.5 mg/kg IM. (4) Benztropine (Cogentin), 0.5 mg IV, IM, or orally (may repeat). (5) Trihexyphenidyl (Artane), 0.5 mg orally (may repeat). (6) Phenobarbital and atropine have also been used. With bradykinesia due to phenytoin, that drug should be reduced or withdrawn.

Korczyn AD: Pathophysiology of drug-induced dyskinesias. Neuropharmacology 11:601, 1972.

SYDENHAM'S POSTRHEUMATIC CHOREA

Sydenham's chorea is characterized by an acute onset of choreiform movements and variable degrees of psychologic disturbance. It is frequently associated with endocarditis and arthritis. Although the disorder follows infections with beta-hemolytic streptococci, the interval between infection and chorea may be greatly delayed; throat cultures and ASO titers may therefore be negative. Psychic predisposition may also play a role. Chorea has also been associated with hypocalcemia and with vascular (LE), toxic, infectious and parainfectious, and degenerative encephalopathies.

Clinical Findings

A. Symptoms and Signs: See description of chorea in the introduction to this section. In addition to the jerky incoordinate movements, the following are noted: emotional lability, waxing and waning ("milkmaid's") grip, darting tongue, "spooning" of the extended hands and their tendency to pronate, and knee jerks slow to return from the extended to their prestimulus position ("hung up").

B. Laboratory Findings: Anemia, leukocytosis, and an increased erythrocyte sedimentation rate may be present. ASO titer may be elevated and C-reactive protein present. Throat culture may occasionally be positive for beta-hemolytic streptococci.

ECG may occasionally show cardiac involvement.

Differential Diagnosis

The diagnosis is usually not difficult. Tics, phenothiazine intoxication, Huntington's chorea, and hepatolenticular degeneration (Wilson's disease) as well as other rare movement disorders can usually be ruled out on historical and clinical grounds.

Treatment

There is no specific treatment. Give sedation with chlorpromazine (Thorazine), 15–25 mg 3 times daily initially and increase slowly until the involuntary movements are markedly reduced or cease or until the patient is overly drowsy; or phenobarbital, 2–3 mg/kg orally 3 times daily—with, if necessary, chloral hydrate, 250–500 mg 2–3 times daily. Haloperidol (Haldol) has recently been used, but it is not recommended for children under 12 years of age and should always be used with caution; start with 0.5–1 mg 2–3 times daily. Meprobamate may be useful in mild cases. In extreme cases, corticotropin or corticosteroids might be considered and occasionally are dramatically effective.

All patients should be given antistreptococcal prophylaxis with penicillin G (200,000 units twice daily) or sulfonamide drugs.

Prognosis

Sydenham's chorea is a self-limiting disease that may last from a few weeks to about 2 years. Two-thirds of patients relapse one or more times, but the ultimate outcome does not appear to be worse in those with recurrences. Valvular heart disease occurs in about one-third of patients, particularly if other rheumatic manifestations appear. Psychoneurotic distur-

bances, if not already present at the onset of illness, occur in a significant percentage of patients.

Aron AM, Freeman JM, Carter S: The natural history of Sydenham's chorea. Am J Med 38:83, 1965.

Shenker DM, Grossman HJ, Klawans HL: Treatment of Sydenham's chorea with haloperidol. Dev Med Child Neurol 15:19, 1973.

Shields WD, Bray PF: A danger of haloperidol therapy in children. J Pediatr 88:301, 1976.

Tierney RC, Kaplan S: Treatment of Sydenham's chorea. Am J Dis Child 109:408, 1965.

TICS OR HABIT SPASMS

Tics or habit spasms are quick repetitive movements, often stereotyped, which are alterable at will. Coordination and muscle tone are not affected. A psychogenic basis is usually readily discernible.

Tics usually represent obsessive-compulsive acts, increasing in intensity and becoming more elaborate the more attention they provoke. Unlike the child with an organic movement disorder, the child with tics is little disturbed by their presence. Tics are a common finding in children 9–13 years old.

Facial tics such as grimaces, twitches, and blinking predominate, but the trunk and extremities are often involved as well as twisting or flinging movements.

Tourette's disease is a form of tic in which extensive and varied body movements are accompanied by guttural or explosive sounds which are choked-off obscenities (coprolalia) and in which there may be abnormal neurologic and EEG findings. Familial cases and partial forms are frequent; a high percentage of afflicted persons are of eastern European Jewish ancestry. While a disturbance of catecholamine metabolism in the CNS has been suggested, plasma dopamine beta-hydroxylase and norepinephrine levels are normal.

In relatively mild cases, tics are self-limited and, when disregarded, disappear. When attention is paid to one tic, it may disappear only to be replaced by another which is often worse. If the tic and its underlying anxiety or compulsive neurosis are severe, psychiatric evaluation and treatment are needed. Drug therapy has little place in the treatment of tics except in Tourette's disease, for which haloperidol (Haldol), 10–15 mg orally daily, has been advocated in conjunction with aversive conditioning. Haloperidol should be used with caution.

Eldridge R & others: Gilles de la Tourette's syndrome: Clinical, genetic, psychologic, and biochemical aspects in 21 selected families. Neurology 27:115, 1977.

Torup E: A follow-up study of children with tics. Acta Paediatr Scand 51:261, 1962.

2. CONGENITAL CHOREOATHETOSIS & RIGIDITY

Congenital chorea, athetosis, and rigidity, in varying combinations and severity, may present in infancy or childhood or may be delayed until adolescence. The symptoms are usually not progressive, and improvement often occurs.

These patients comprise about 20% of all children with cerebral palsy (see below). Patients may be divided into those exhibiting chiefly (1) double chorea, (2) double athetosis, (3) rigidity without movement disorder, (4) atypical movement disorders, (5) transitional types between any of the aforementioned 4 groups (the majority), and (6) those in whom the disorder is complicated by paralysis, spasticity, and other symptoms. The more severe the degree of involvement, the earlier the onset. Other neurologic disorders such as seizures, visual and hearing deficits, and mental retardation may be present.

Laboratory studies often include x-rays of the skull (for microcephaly and calcification) and the hips (for dislocation); EEG, if seizures are evident clinically; amino acid chromatography (aminoacidurias are present in rare cases); tests of vision and hearing; and psychometric evaluation. There is usually little difficulty in establishing the diagnosis because of the early onset and the variety and multiplicity of the neurologic findings.

Treatment is largely confined to physical and educational therapy. In selected cases, thalamotomies have been successful. Diazepam (Valium) may reduce the rigidity, but drug therapy to date has generally been of little avail. Levodopa alone or in combination with diazepam has occasionally been effective. Orthopedic correction of deformities is indicated in some cases.

Hanson RA, Berenberg W, Byers RK: Changing motor patterns in cerebral palsy. Dev Med Child Neurol 12:309, 1970.

3. PROGRESSIVE EXTRAPYRAMIDAL DISORDERS*

HUNTINGTON'S CHOREA

Huntington's chorea is rare in the first decade of life. The childhood picture has given rise to the term "striatocortical degeneration." It varies from the adult form in several respects: (1) Dementia occurs early and progresses rapidly. (2) A "striatal" syndrome with rigidity and akinesia predominates over choreoathetoid features. (3) Cerebellar dysfunctions (tremors and

*Wilson's disease is discussed in Chapter 17.

ataxia) may be presenting features. (4) Seizures occur sooner or later in all (rare in adults). (5) Average duration of illness after onset is a little over 8 years (compared to over 13 years in adults).

The disease is transmitted in autosomal dominant fashion, but a family history is frequently denied or unobtainable.

Chromosomal analysis, dermatoglyphics, and studies of trace metals have not been helpful. A significant increase in uptake of dopamine in the blood platelets of patients with Huntington's chorea has been demonstrated. CT scan may show caudate and cortical atrophy before pneumoencephalography shows the classical "butterfly" atrophy in the region of the caudate nucleus and putamen; it may thus be most helpful in the differential diagnosis of Huntington's chorea and tardive dyskinesia. EEG is frequently but nonspecifically abnormal, showing fast, low-voltage activity as well as asymmetry and disorganization.

The initial diagnosis may include the other conditions discussed in this section as well as "cerebral palsy."

There is no treatment. The disease is fatal within a few years to about 15 years after onset. Phenothiazines, reserpine, physostigmine, and trihexyphenidyl (Artane) may afford some—if only temporary—relief. Seizures are treated in the manner discussed under Seizure Disorders. Genetic counseling to other members of the family is of paramount importance.

Buxton M: Diagnostic problems in Huntington's chorea and tardive dyskinesia. Compr Psychiatry 17:325, 1976.

Byers RK, Gilles FH, Fung C: Huntington's disease in children. Neurology 23:561, 1973.

DYSTONIA MUSCULORUM DEFORMANS

This is a rather ill-defined disorder which may be suspected when dystonia is present but encephalitis or toxic encephalopathy, hepatolenticular degeneration, and other extrapyramidal diseases have been ruled out.

In about two-thirds of cases this disorder begins with hypertonia of calf muscles, producing plantar flexion and inversion and adduction of the foot, but it may also start in the wrist or neck. The face, organs of speech, and fingers are usually spared. The disease soon progresses along the extremity to the trunk, resulting eventually in severe lordosis; slow, powerful, widespread movements, which may succeed each other in waves; and bizarre postures due to spasm of some muscle groups and relaxation of others.

This disorder is inherited (1) as an autosomal recessive, predominantly in Jewish children, with onset between 4 and 16 years of age and a rapid course; and (2) as a dominant, more variable in onset and with a slower course, with no ethnic predilection.

Symptoms and signs vary with the stage of the disease. The involuntary movements, accentuated by emotional upsets and activity (especially walking or running), are often bizarre and complex. They disappear in sleep. Strength, coordination, and reflexes are intact on examination if proper relaxation can be achieved. Intelligence is not affected, but many emotional problems develop.

Urinary dopamine levels are increased in some patients.

This condition must be differentiated from the other progressive extrapyramidal disorders discussed in this section and from hysteria.

Pallidectomy and thalamotomy have afforded relief in some patients, at least for several years. Levodopa is being tried. Sedation may be needed for sleep.

The course is usually very slowly progressive, and the disease may be arrested for several years. Children involved earliest have the most rapid course.

Zeman W, Dyken P: Dystonia musculorum deformans. Pages 517–543 in: *Handbook of Clinical Neurology.* Vol 6. Vinken PJ, Bruyn GW (editors). Wiley, 1968.

OTHER PROGRESSIVE EXTRAPYRAMIDAL DISORDERS

Hallervorden-Spatz disease and progressive pallidal degeneration are rare, slowly progressive extrapyramidal disorders whose diagnoses usually depend on the family history or autopsy findings. In familial calcification of the basal ganglia, the diagnosis is made on skull x-rays. Juvenile parkinsonism is a familial disorder due to impaired ability to synthesize dopamine; it may result in clinical symptoms first (or only) when major tranquilizers are used, but it responds to treatment with levodopa. Parkinsonism or dystonia may occur as a consequence of encephalitis.

Martin WE, Resch JA, Baker AB: Juvenile parkinsonism. Arch Neurol 25:494, 1971.
Poser CM, Huntley CJ, Polland JD: Para-encephalitic parkinsonism. Acta Neurol Scand 45:199, 1969.

INFECTIONS & INFLAMMATIONS OF THE CNS

Infections and infestations of the CNS in children, especially in neonates and infants, present with rather nonspecific symptoms. Early diagnosis depends upon a high index of suspicion, and prompt and appropriate treatment may in many instances prevent or minimize permanent CNS damage.

One of the most significant clinical attributes of any infection or infestation of the CNS is its anatomic distribution, ie, meninges, cerebrum, cerebellum, bulb,

or spinal cord. Most CNS infections in infants and young children are meningoencephalitides, although one or the other aspect (meningitis or encephalitis) may be more marked.

Laboratory Findings

A. Cerebrospinal Fluid: The diagnosis usually, though not always, depends on the CSF findings. CSF examination should include total and differential cell count, protein, and glucose with concomitant blood glucose, gamma globulin, lactic dehydrogenase, Gram's stain and cultures (including special studies for acid-fast organisms, viruses, and fungi), and tests for syphilis as indicated. (For characteristics of CSF in various neurologic conditions, see Table 21–1. See comments on lumbar puncture in Chapter 34.)

B. Other Means of Identification of Etiologic Agent: The blood, nose, throat, urine, stools, stomach, lungs, and aspirates from petechiae, vesicles, or pus pockets may all provide material for direct isolation of the responsible infective agent. When the child does not clearly have a bacterial infection, serum should be set aside at the time of admission for serologic studies about 3 weeks later with a paired convalescent serum. Heterophil studies, febrile agglutinins, and skin tests (eg, tuberculosis, trichinosis, histoplasmosis) should be performed as indicated.

C. Neurodiagnostic Studies: Special neurodiagnostic studies may occasionally be necessary to differentiate nonsurgical from specifically surgical lesions and infections, eg, encephalitis with marked focal features from brain abscess. Such studies may include echoencephalography, CT and isotope brain scans, EEG, angiography, and, rarely today, air studies.

ACUTE PURULENT MENINGITIS

The symptoms vary greatly with age (see Table 21–8). Nuchal rigidity, especially in the younger age group, may not be present; on the other hand, a stiff neck or meningismus in children is commonly due to other causes—particularly cervical adenopathy.

Clinical Findings

A. Symptoms and Signs: In addition to the symptoms and signs listed in Table 21–8, note the presence of extracranial infections, petechiae, alterations in the state of consciousness, the head circumference in the younger age group, cranial nerve palsies, and other focal neurologic deficits.

B. Laboratory Findings: CSF usually shows pleocytosis, low glucose, variable but often elevated protein, and lactate dehydrogenase values above 30 IU/ liter. Gram's stain and cultures will be positive unless the meningitis has been partially treated. Repeat lumbar punctures in suspect cases may be most helpful.

The most common etiologic agents, in order of frequency, are as follows: (1) In newborns, *Escherichia*

Table 21—8. Symptoms and signs of purulent meningitis.

Symptoms and Signs	Newborn	Up to 2 Years	Over 2 Years
Irregular respirations/ cyanosis	+		
Fever	+	+	+
Hypothermia	+		
Vomiting	+	+	+
Diarrhea	+		
Jaundice	+		
Drowsiness	+	+	+
Jitteriness	+	+	
Bulging fontanel	+	+	
Convulsions	Early	Early	Late
Stiff neck	Very late	Late	+
Headache			+
Ataxia			Early

coli and other gram-negative organisms; less commonly, *Haemophilus influenzae, Listeria monocytogenes,* hemolytic streptococci. hemolytic staphylococci, and pneumococci. (2) In older infants and children, *H influenzae* (especially in children 2—7 years of age), more prevalent in fall and early winter; pneumococci; and meningococci (epidemics every 8—10 years), more prevalent in early spring.

Complications & Sequelae

A. Seizures: There is a high incidence of convulsions in infants up to about 18 months of age. The prophylactic use of phenobarbital, 3—5 mg/kg/day, is strongly advocated during the acute phase. If a convulsion occurs, even though the child is receiving anticonvulsants, the likelihood of status epilepticus is still greatly reduced and the seizures can usually be brought under control by moderate increases in medication.

Phenytoin (Dilantin) has been found to be less helpful in the acute stage, partly because, on a maintenance dose of 5—7 mg/kg/day, it takes 7—10 days to build up therapeutic levels. (To build up the blood level of phenytoin rapidly, 10 mg/kg may be given slowly IV.)

If the patient remains free of seizures during the acute phase, anticonvulsant medication may be gradually withdrawn over a period of several days in the convalescent phase. If the patient had a seizure, it is generally advisable that anticonvulsant medication be maintained for 2—3 years since the recurrence rate of seizures following meningitis is high.

B. Water Intoxication: Cerebral edema may cause inappropriate ADH secretion. Furthermore, if the child is in a croupette, the usual water loss through insensible perspiration does not occur. Hyponatremia is therefore a frequent complication of meningitis. It is best avoided by judicious fluid administration and treated by hypertonic saline or diuretics (mannitol or urea).

C. Subdural Effusions: The incidence of subdural effusion in young infants with meningitis approaches 50%; it is less common after 18 months. Symptoms include prolongation or recurrence of fever, irritability, poor appetite, listlessness, vomiting, and, occasionally, focal or generalized seizures, and focal neurologic deficits.

Important clues to the presence of a subdural effusion are abnormal increase in head circumference, bulging or tenseness of a previously flat anterior fontanel, positive transillumination in infants up to about 18 months, and widening of sutures on x-ray. The diagnosis is made by finding 2 ml or more of subdural fluid with a high protein content on subdural tap if the fontanel is open, or through a bur hole or suture if the fontanel is closed.

Treatment is by subdural taps, if possible. If significant subdural effusion cannot be "dried up" after 4—5 weeks, neurosurgical intervention may be indicated if symptoms of increased intracranial pressure persist.

D. Hydrocephalus: Hydrocephalus is most prevalent in neonates and very young infants as a result of inflammatory obstruction of CSF pathways. An important clue to this complication is failure of the CSF glucose to return to normal levels in the face of negative bacterial cultures, most likely due to impairment of the glucose transport mechanism.

E. Other Neurologic Sequelae: Neurologic sequelae of meningitis in childhood occur in 10—20% of survivors, most often in the youngest and in those in whom diagnosis and adequate therapy were delayed. The finding of significant subdural effusions (more than 2 ml) per se has no prognostic significance. Severe seizures, prolonged depression of consciousness, and other evidence of major cerebral injury during the acute phase of meningitis, on the other hand, are the indices of major sequelae. In order of frequency, they are "minimal brain dysfunction" syndrome and mild to severe mental retardation, recurrent seizures, hearing loss, hydrocephalus (see above), and motor deficits, including hemiparesis.

Treatment

Antibiotic and fluid and electrolyte therapy are discussed in separate sections. Corticosteroids are not indicated except possibly when there is massive cerebral edema.

Treatment of complications is discussed above or in the section on tuberculous meningitis.

Prognosis

Purulent meningitis remains, despite potent specific and broad-spectrum antibiotics, a serious threat to life and neurologic competence. Among interacting factors determining outcome—and assuming good medical management once the diagnosis is made—the 3 most important are age, causative agent, and time of diagnosis. In pediatric practice, the highest mortality rate (30—50%) occurs in neonates and young infants with meningitides due to gram-negative organisms or *Staphylococcus aureus* and in those already in coma or near coma at diagnosis.

Feigin RD, Dodge PR: Bacterial meningitis: Newer concepts of pathophysiology and neurologic sequelae. Pediatr Clin North Am 23:541, 1976.

Murray JD & others: The continuing problem of purulent meningitis in infants and children. Pediatr Clin North Am 21:967, 1974.

CIRCUMSCRIBED PYOGENIC INTRACRANIAL INFECTIONS

These infections are usually secondary to a suppurative infection elsewhere; occasionally they are introduced directly, as after a compound skull fracture or penetrating foreign body (eg, pencil points). The source of infection is unknown in 5–15% of cases. Sources of direct extension are chronic otitis media and mastoiditis, the nasal cavity and accessory sinuses (frontal, sphenoid), and meningitis (via venous thrombosis). Metastatic spread occurs from the lungs and pleura or from subacute bacterial endocarditis. *Note:* Brain abscesses occur in nearly 5% of patients with cyanotic congenital heart disease, and are frequent also in patients receiving immunosuppressive agents.

The causative agents are often mixed and tend to be the same organisms responsible for middle ear and sinus infections. In metastatic abscesses, organisms may· be even more diversified and include mycotic and parasitic organisms and *Salmonella typhi.*

Clinical Findings

A. Symptoms and Signs: Manifestations often evolve rapidly and include localized severe headache, fever and malaise, drowsiness progressing to confusion and stupor, nausea and vomiting, focal and generalized seizures, and focal motor, sensory, and speech deficits varying with the site and size of the pyogenic collection, the degree of cerebral edema, and the age of the child. (*Note:* Focal neurologic signs may be obscured by depressed level of consciousness and seizures.) Meningismus is seen with meningeal involvement, cerebellar abscess, and tonsillar herniation. Point tenderness to pressure on the cranium over the abscess area may be present. Papilledema may be a late finding.

B. Laboratory Findings:

1. Blood—Leukocytosis with shift to the left and increased sedimentation rate are common.

2. Cerebrospinal fluid—Increased pressure is frequent; pleocytosis is variable, but even one polymorphonuclear cell suggests the possibility of a brain abscess. Protein may be normal to moderately elevated; the glucose is often normal. Cultures are often negative.

C. X-Ray Findings: Skull films may show signs of increased intracranial pressure. Sinus and chest films may show evidence of an inflammatory process. Brain scanning may show increased isotope uptake early in the area of an abscess. Cerebral angiography is often

the procedure of choice prior to surgical drainage in the localization of a brain abscess.

D. Electroencephalography: EEG may be most helpful. Initially there may be diffuse high-voltage, slow activity. Serial EEGs often show an abscess to be well circumscribed by the evolution of a slow wave focus.

Differential Diagnosis

The differential diagnosis between a cerebral abscess and other intracranial mass lesions may be suspected on clinical grounds but is at times difficult. In extradural abscess, the course may be protracted and relatively benign. There may be no focal findings other than meningeal signs. With subdural empyema, which is commonly a complication of frontal sinusitis and osteomyelitis, the evolution of symptoms is very rapid. The CSF is usually sterile.

Treatment

Antibiotics should be given intravenously in large amounts with broad coverage. Other medical measures include hypothermia and anticonvulsants, especially phenobarbital. Surgical evacuation of pus and excision of the abscess are indicated as soon as feasible to relieve increased intracranial pressure.

Prognosis

The mortality rate is high and is directly related to delay in diagnosis and treatment. With multiple abscesses, mortality is virtually 100%. In about 50% of cases, the duration of illness from first symptoms to death is 5–14 days. Early diagnosis and prompt treatment offer an excellent chance of complete recovery if the underlying disease process is cured.

Farmer TW, Wise GR: Subdural empyema in infants, children and adults. Neurology 23:254, 1973.

Raimondi JA, Matsumoto S, Miller RA: Brain abscess in children with congenital heart disease. J Neurosurg 23:588, 1965.

SUBACUTE MENINGOENCEPHALITIS

Subacute meningoencephalitis may occur as a complication of primary tuberculosis or may be due to fungal infection or sarcoidosis. These infections involve the meninges of the base of the brain and panarteritis of the pial vessels.

Clinical Findings

A. Symptoms and Signs: Manifestations often evolve gradually and include fever (to 39.4° C [103° F]), malaise, and irritability; headache, vomiting, and photophobia; drowsiness, stupor, and coma; focal and generalized seizures; focal motor deficits, including hemiparesis, paresis of the extraocular muscles, and Bell's palsy; and deafness. Meningeal signs may be absent or minimal, but increased intracranial pressure is common.

B. Laboratory Findings:

1. Blood—The ESR may be elevated. Salt-losing encephalopathy occurs in tuberculosis.

2. Cerebrospinal fluid—(See Table 21–1.) In both tuberculous and mycotic meningitis, cell counts may range from just above 10 to about 500/cu mm, initially mostly polymorphonuclear cells but soon predominantly lymphocytes. CSF protein is mildly to moderately elevated ("pellicle" in tuberculous meningitis). CSF glucose may initially be normal but may fall rapidly. Special stains for tubercle bacilli (acid-fast) and fungi (India ink) and appropriate cultures and inoculations should be obtained. Antibodies to cryptococcus may be demonstrated in CSF.

C. Diagnosis of Specific Types: Disorders with a similar initial clinical course and gross CSF findings include the following:

1. Tuberculous meningitis—Two-thirds of cases occur in the first decade, most between 6 and 24 months of age. A positive tuberculin skin test and chest x-ray strongly favor the diagnosis. Without treatment, the course is unremittent.

2. Mycotic meningitides—The course is usually slowly progressive, but prolonged remissions occur. Definitive diagnosis depends on cultural identification of the etiologic agent. Skin tests are often positive.

a. Cryptococcal meningitis (torulosis) is usually associated with chronic debilitating disorders such as tuberculosis, leukemia, and Hodgkin's disease or occurs in renal or liver transplant recipients.

b. Nocardiosis and aspergillosis are rare, but again are more common in patients who have undergone transplants or are receiving immunosuppressive drugs.

c. Actinomycosis may spread to the CNS from a primary site in the face, neck, or cecum.

d. Mucormycosis may produce systemic infection with orbital cellulitis or thrombosis of the internal carotid artery.

3. Central nervous system sarcoidosis—Recurrent cranial neuropathies are frequent. Eosinophilia is present in about 35% of cases and hypergammaglobulinemia in about 50%. Hypercalcemia with normal serum phosphate levels is common. Lymph node and tongue biopsies and the Kveim test may establish the diagnosis.

D. X-Ray Findings: Skull films should be examined for signs of increased intracranial pressure and calcified tuberculomas (rare). Chest films should be taken for signs of pulmonary tuberculosis or other infections.

Cerebral angiography may be indicated, especially when there is evidence of increased intracranial pressure, to rule out brain abscess or to demonstrate hydrocephalus. Note that narrowed arteries and slow cerebral circulation may be seen in encephalopathies but are particularly frequent with the panarteritis in tuberculous and mycotic meningitides.

Air studies, particularly ventriculography, may be indicated when hydrocephalus is present.

Differential Diagnosis

A. Brain Abscess: This may resemble subacute meningoencephalitis early, but focal headache and neurologic findings usually point to the diagnosis.

B. Meningeal Carcinomatosis: Leukemia, sarcoma, pinealoma, etc. The diagnosis may be made by cytologic studies of the CSF but usually requires demonstration of the tumor by other means.

Treatment

For appropriate antibiotic and anticonvulsant therapy, see under those sections. Observe carefully for toxic reactions to the anti-infective agents.

Neurosurgical evacuation of brain abscess may be required (eg, in actinomycosis) as well as neurosurgical relief of hydrocephalus by "shunting."

Prognosis

The prognosis varies with the disease process and its extent and severity. Many fungal infections, especially histoplasmosis, mucormycosis, nocardiosis, and aspergillosis, respond poorly if at all to the best available treatment.

Sodeman TM, Dock N: Laboratory diagnosis of parasitic and fungal diseases of the central nervous system. Ann Clin Lab Sci 6:47, 1976.

Symaya CV & others: Tuberculous meningitis in children during the isoniazid era. J Pediatr 87:43, 1975.

"ASEPTIC" MENINGITIS, ENCEPHALITIS, & MENINGOENCEPHALITIS*

This clinical grouping encompasses those acute and subacute inflammatory conditions of the meninges or encephalon and often, but to a variable extent, both, in which (1) no flaccid paralysis is present, ie, there is no clinical involvement of the spinal cord or peripheral nerves (see below); and (2) no bacterial or fungal organisms are found on smear or cultures of the CSF, which otherwise may show such changes as pleocytosis and increased protein. The diagnosis is often presumptive, and the diagnostic category (and even the specific entity) may be suggested by the patient's history. Clinical differentiation between entities is often difficult, since the presenting signs and symptoms overlap considerably because of the nonspecificity of pathologic involvement. Definitive diagnosis can often be established only by laboratory studies, but even this is limited by the laboratory's ability to perform viral cultures or serodiagnostic investigations.

*For consideration of specific clinical and laboratory features of the individual etiologic syndromes of aseptic meningitis, consult the chapters on viral, bacterial, and fungal diseases. Specific and supportive therapy is discussed in those chapters. Anti-infective therapy is discussed in Chapter 37.

Table 21—9. Acute flaccid paralyses in children.

	Poliomyelitis (Paralytic, Spinal, and Bulbar), With or Without Encephalitis	Landry-Guillain-Barré Syndrome	Secondary Acute Myelopathies and Polyneuropathies*	Tick-Bite Paralysis	Transverse Myelitis and Neuromyelitis Optica
Etiology	Poliovirus types I, II, and III; occasionally mimicked by mumps.	Unknown. An autosensitivity phenomenon has been postulated. Mycoplasma and viral infections (including infectious mononucleosis) and various systemic or toxic disorders may be underlying cause.	Associated with infections, especially exanthems, diphtheria, etc; vaccination, metabolic and endocrine disturbances, allergic and immune disorders, intoxicants, neoplasms, other miscellaneous conditions.	Probable interference with transmission of nerve impulse caused by toxin in tick saliva.	Unknown; immunodeficiency state (?)
History	None, or inadequate polio immunization. Upper respiratory or gastrointestinal symptoms followed by brief respite. Bulbar paralysis more frequent after tonsillectomy. Epidemic form more common in late summer and early fall.	Nonspecific respiratory or gastrointestinal symptoms in preceding 5—14 days common. Any season, though slightly lower incidence in summer.	Varies with etiology. Para-infectious paralyses may occur with or after primary illness. Paralyses due to allergic or immune disorders and neoplasms are usually of slow onset.	Exposure to ticks (dog tick in eastern USA; wood ticks). Irritability 12—24 hours before onset of a rapidly progressive ascending paralysis.	Occasionally, symptoms compatible with multiple sclerosis or optic neuritis. Progression from onset to paraplegia very rapid, usually without a history of bacterial infection.
Presenting complaints	Febrile usually. Meningeal signs, muscle tenderness, and spasm. Weakness widespread or segmental (cervical, thoracic, lumbar). Bulbar symptoms early or before extremity weakness. Anxiety. Delirium.	Symmetric weakness of lower extremities, sometimes ascending rapidly to arms, trunk, and face. Muscle tenderness and spinal root pains frequent. Verbal child may complain of paresthesias. Fever uncommon. Facial weakness early. Variant form presents chiefly as ataxia.	Symptomatology similar to Landry-Guillain-Barré syndrome, but may be masked by primary disease. In para-infectious and postvaccinal myelitides, initial complaints include low-grade fever, severe back pain, and sensory loss as well as those characteristic of encephalitis.	Rapid onset and progression of ascending flaccid paralysis; often accompanied by pain and paresthesias. Paralysis of upper extremities usually occurs on second day after onset.	Root and back pain in about one-third to one-half of cases. Sensory loss below level of lesion accompanying rapidly developing paralysis. Sphincter difficulties common.
Findings†	Flaccid weakness, usually asymmetric. Lumbar: legs, lower abdomen. Cervical: shoulder, arm, neck, diaphragm. Thoracic: intercostals, spine, upper abdomen. Bulbar: respiratory, lower cranial, upper cranial nerves. Occasionally papilledema, encephalitic syndrome, ataxia. Fever in first days. Autonomic disturbances common.	Flaccid weakness, symmetric, usually greater proximally, but may be more distal or equal in distribution. Facial diplegia in about 85%, then IX—X, XI, III—VI. Bulbar involvement may occur. Slight distal impairment of position, vibration, touch; difficult to assess in young children.	Findings similar to those in Landry-Guillain-Barré syndrome. Sensory loss may be greater. Level of spinal cord involvement may be better defined. Findings may be masked or distorted by those of the associated primary disorder or encephalitic component.	Flaccid, symmetrical paralysis. Cranial nerve and bulbar (respiratory) paralysis, ataxia, sphincter disturbances, and sensory deficits may occur. Some fever. Diagnosis rests on finding tick.	Paraplegia with areflexia below level of lesion early; later, may have hyperreflexia. Sensory loss below and hyperesthesia or normal sensation above level of lesion. Paralysis of bladder and rectum. Optic atrophy or neuritis may be present.

*See Infant Botulism on p 759.

†*Note:* In flaccid paralysis, the deep reflexes are depressed or absent.

Table 21—9 (cont'd). Acute flaccid paralyses in children.

	Poliomyelitis (Paralytic, Spinal, and Bulbar), With or Without Encephalitis	Landry-Guillain-Barré Syndrome	Secondary Acute Myelopathies and Polyneuropathies	Tick-Bite Paralysis	Transverse Myelitis and Neuromyelitis Optica
CSF	Pleocytosis (about 200 cells) with PMN predominance in first few days, followed by rapid decrease and monocytic preponderance. Glucose normal. Protein frequently elevated (50—200 mg/100 ml).	Cytoalbuminologic dissociation: 10 or fewer mononuclear cells with high protein after first week. Normal glucose. Gamma globulin may be elevated.	CSF as for Landry-Guillain-Barré syndrome. In para-infectious and post-vaccinal cases, mild pleocytosis (15—250 cells, principally monocytes) and mild protein elevation (up to 150 mg/100 ml) common.	Normal.	Usually no manometric block; CSF may show increased protein, pleocytosis with predominantly monocytes, increased gamma globulin.
EMG	Denervation after 10—21 days. Nerve conduction may be slowed slightly.	Denervation after 10—21 days. Nerve conduction velocities markedly decreased.	Denervation after 10—21 days. Nerve conduction slowed only in neuropathies.	Nerve conduction slowed; returns rapidly to normal after removal of tick.	Normal early. Denervation at level of lesion after 10—21 days.
Other studies	Initially, leukocytosis. Virus in stool and throat. Serologic titers.	Rule out specific causes such as infections, intoxications, metabolic or endocrine diseases, allergic phenomena, neoplasms. Lymphocyte transformation demonstrated. *Mycoplasma pneumoniae* implicated.	EEG diffusely slow, with focal or generalized seizure potentials when an encephalitic component is present. Appropriate studies to define associated primary disorder.	Leukocytosis, often with moderate eosinophilia.	Normal spine x-rays speak against spinal epidural abscess. Myelography is often irritative and should be very carefully considered; false positives secondary to swelling of the cord are not unknown.
Course and prognosis	Paralysis usually maximal 3—5 days after onset. Transient bladder paralysis may occur. Outlook varies with extent and severity of involvement. *Note:* Threat greatest from respiratory failure and superinfection. Early muscle atrophy common.	Course progressive over a few days to about 2 weeks. Transient bladder paralysis may occur. *Note:* Threat greatest from respiratory failure and superinfection. Majority recover completely; residual weakness in up to one-fifth of cases.	Course and prognosis vary greatly with underlying disease process, extent of the paralytic and encephalitic involvement, presence of bladder and bowel paralysis, and respiratory complications.	Total removal of tick is followed by rapid improvement and recovery. Otherwise, mortality due to respiratory paralysis is very high.	Large degree of functional recovery possible. Corticosteroids are of benefit in shortening duration of acute attack (especially the first) but not in preventing recurrences or altering the overall course.

PYOGENIC SPINAL CORD INFECTIONS

Pyogenic infections of the spinal cord, although relatively uncommon in children, must be considered in the differential diagnosis of cord lesions, as prompt treatment is required. *Staphylococcus aureus* is the most common pathogen. Infection occurs by direct extension or metastasis from a focus of infection such as a skin furuncle, osteomyelitis, empyema, perinephric abscess, infected wound, and other septic processes.

The onset of spinal cord infection, which is more rapid than that of spinal cord tumor, mimics that of noninfectious transverse myelitis. (See Table 21—9.)

Clinical Findings

A. Symptoms and Signs: The principal symptom, sometimes obscured for a while by the underlying illness, is severe localized back pain followed by root pain in the trunk or legs. Flaccid paralysis of the legs, accompanied by sensory loss, develops rapidly. Urinary retention is common. Headache, high fever, a stiff back, and vomiting are present in acute cases but often minimal in chronic ones.

Findings include rigidity of the spine, localized exquisite spine tenderness, lost tendon reflexes, and bilateral plantar extensor signs. Sensory loss, loss of urinary sphincter function, and, less commonly, fecal incontinence may occur.

B. Laboratory Findings:

1. Blood—Leukocytocis and elevated ESR are the rule. Blood cultures are often positive.

2. Cerebrospinal fluid—If epidural spinal abscess is suspected, the spinal needle is introduced only into the extradural space at the level of the lesion (region of maximal spine tenderness) to see if pus can be obtained. *Caution:* The utmost care must be exercised not to penetrate the dura and thus introduce infection into the subarachnoid space.

Lumbar puncture should be performed only after spine films have been obtained. CSF examination can be deferred and cervical puncture performed later. CSF manometrics should be performed and dye for myelography instilled while the needle is in place if a CSF block is encountered. CSF xanthochromia and pleocytosis are often present; protein is usually moderately increased; glucose is normal. CSF cultures, however, often are negative.

C. X-Ray Findings: In spinal epidural abscess, evidence of osteomyelitis or an adjacent soft tissue mass is evident on spine x-rays in about 50% of cases.

Myelography is best performed in conjunction with diagnostic lumbar puncture or via cisternal puncture.

Differential Diagnosis

The differential diagnosis involves principally 2 conditions: (1) transverse myelitis (Table 21–9) and other forms of acute flaccid paralysis, and (2) spinal cord tumors (see p 576).

Treatment

Treatment must be instituted promptly and consists'of appropriate antibiotics in massive doses, neurosurgical decompression, and evacuation of the abscess or removal of granuloma.

Prognosis

The prognosis is good if cord compression is relieved early and infection is controlled.

Bock SA, Sickler D, Chhabra OP: Spinal epidural abscess in a five-week old infant. Clin Pediatr (Phila) 15:286, 1976.
Enberg RN, Kaplan RJ: Spinal epidural abscess in children. Clin Pediatr (Phila) 13:247, 1974.

SYNDROMES PRESENTING AS ACUTE FLACCID PARALYSIS

Rapidly evolving flaccid paralysis suggests, in the early clinical stages, the following clinical possibilities: paralytic spinal poliomyelitis and encephalomyelitis, Landry-Guillain-Barré syndrome, secondary acute myelopathies and polyneuropathies, tick-bite paralysis, and transverse longitudinal myelitis. The possibility of spinal cord trauma, tumor, and epidural abscess must be considered; an adequate history will usually tend to make these conditions less likely.

Intercurrent nonspecific infections with predominantly flu-like respiratory and gastrointestinal symptoms are so common in children as to suggest the diagnosis of Landry-Guillain-Barré syndrome ("acute

idiopathic polyneuritis") almost too readily, diverting the physician's attention from the search for more specific causes.

While the sensory examination is important in these syndromes, it is often of dubious accuracy and hence of limited usefulness in the younger age group. Diagnosis, outlined in Table 21–9, is based on the clinical features of the illness as well as viral isolation and serologic studies.

Complications

A. Respiratory Paralysis: Early signs of hypoxia are increasing anxiety and a rise in diastolic and systolic blood pressures. Cyanosis is a late sign. The patient's ability to count to 20 on a single breath is a good clinical guide to still adequate vital capacity.

Early and careful attention to oxygenation is essential and may require administration of oxygen, tracheostomy, mechanical respiratory assistance, and careful suctioning of secretions.

B. Infections: Pneumonia is common, especially with respiratory paralysis. Prophylactic antibiotic administration is generally contraindicated. Specific infections are treated with appropriate antibiotics.

Bladder infections are most common when an indwelling catheter is required for bladder paralysis. Prophylactic administration of methenamine mandelate (Mandelamine), 30 mg/kg orally, is recommended, or the use of bladder irrigations with antibiotics. Recovery from myelitis may be delayed by urinary tract infection.

Treatment

There is no specific treatment except removal of ticks in tick-bite paralysis and of erythromycin in mycoplasma infection. Recognized associated disorders (eg, endocrine, neoplastic, toxic) should be treated by appropriate means. Patients may require respiratory assistance, fluids, and adequate nutrition, bladder, and bowel care.

Skin breakdown may be prevented by proper nursing care. Give antibiotics and anticonvulsants. Psychiatric support is often needed.

A. Corticosteroids: These agents are believed by some authors to be of benefit in severe and prolonged cases of Landry-Guillain-Barré syndrome, some recurrent polyneuropathies, and "idiopathic" transverse myelitis. *Caution:* They are not advised in parainfectious and postvaccinal encephalopathies.

B. Physical Therapy: Rehabilitative measures are best instituted when acute symptoms have subsided and the patient is stable. The physical therapy regimen will vary from patient to patient.

Prognosis

The prognosis varies greatly with the extent of involvement, duration of the inflammatory process, complications, and other factors. See Table 21–9.

Gamstorp I: Encephalomyelo-radiculoneuropathy: Involvement of the CNS in children with the Guillain-Barre-Strohl syndrome. Dev Med Child Neurol 16:654, 1974.

Masucci EF, Kurtzke JF: Diagnostic criteria for the Guillain-Barré syndrome. J Neurol Sci 13:483, 1971.

Sheremata W & others: Cellular hypersensitivity to basic myelin (P2) protein in the Guillain-Barré syndrome. Can J Neurol Sci 2:87, 1975.

DISORDERS OF CHILDHOOD AFFECTING MUSCLES

This section is concerned with specific muscle and neuromuscular disorders, including the muscular dystrophies, myasthenia gravis, and miscellaneous congenital neuromuscular disorders.

Certain studies commonly used in the diagnosis of muscle diseases merit special consideration.

Serum Enzymes

Certain muscle enzymes—creatine phosphokinase (CPK), aldolase, glutamic-oxaloacetic transaminase (GOT), and lactic dehydrogenase—may be helpful in establishing the diagnosis and in following the course of some muscle disorders. In practice, usually only CPK is now followed; other enzymes are now rarely used. Normal CPK values for males are 5–75 IU/liter; for females, 6–50 IU/liter. Blood should be drawn before muscle biopsy, which may lead to release of the enzyme. Corticosteroids may suppress levels despite very active muscle disease.

Electromyography

EMG is often helpful in grossly differentiating "myopathic" from "neurogenic" processes. Fibrillations occur in both. In the myopathies, very low spikes are more typical and the motor unit action potentials seen during contraction characteristically are of short duration, polyphasic, and increased in number for the strength of the contraction (increased interference pattern). "Neurogenic" findings include decreased numbers of motor units, which may be polyphasic, larger than normal, or both. The interference pattern is decreased.

In myotonic dystrophy, the EMG is characterized by prolonged discharge of electrical activity on movement of the probing needle ("dive bomber" sound), though these discharges may be found to a lesser degree also in other conditions. In myotonic dystrophy during attempted relaxation after a contraction, electrical activity persists parallel with the protracted relaxation of muscle.

Muscle Biopsy

Properly executed, this is usually most helpful. The introduction of histochemical technics, histogram analysis of muscle fiber types, and electronmicroscopy is offering new insights and hence new classifications of the myopathies. Muscle biopsy findings common to the myopathies include variation in the size and shape of muscle fibers, increase in connective tissue, interstitial infiltration of fatty tissue, degenerative changes in muscle fibers, and central location of nuclei.

Findings more characteristic of certain myopathies include the sarcoplasmic masses and striking chains of central nuclei in myotonic dystrophy; the cysts found in trichinosis or toxoplasmosis; the vacuoles found in the periodic paralyses, thyrotoxicosis, chloroquine myopathy, and lupus erythematosus; the characteristic appearances with special stains of such disorders as central core disease and nemaline myopathy; or the electronmicroscopic findings in giant mitochondrial myopathy.

Brooke MH, Kaiser KK: The use and abuse of muscle histochemistry. Ann NY Acad Sci 228:121, 1974.

Dubowitz V, Brooke MH: *Muscle Biopsy: A Modern Approach.* Saunders, 1973.

Moosa A: Muscular dystrophy in childhood. Dev Med Child Neurol 16:97, 1974.

Rosenberg RN & others: Progressive ophthalmoplegia. Arch Neurol 19:362, 1968.

THE PERIODIC PARALYSES

Primary Hypokalemic Periodic Paralysis

This condition is inherited as a dominant trait, with decreased occurrence in females, but it may appear sporadically. A family history of migraine is often present. The onset is usually about the end of the first decade of life. The proximal muscles are affected first. The muscles innervated by the cranial nerves are spared—eg, the extraocular muscles, the muscles of facial expression, mastication, and swallowing, and the tongue muscles. The diaphragm, which is usually spared, has its embryonic origin in bulbar territory. Attacks of weakness may be precipitated by rest after exercise, exposure to cold, emotional stress, high dietary intake of carbohydrate and sodium, and administration of corticosteroids.

Attacks may last for days but may be aborted by mild exercise. The disease may progress to a chronic form of weakness and atrophy, but in general attacks are less frequent after middle age.

The serum potassium is low during an attack.

Provocative tests which induce weakness and thus confirm the diagnosis include (1) exercise and (2) giving insulin, 0.25 units/kg subcut, simultaneously with glucose, 0.8 gm/kg orally.

Treatment consists of giving potassium chloride, 2–10 gm orally, to terminate an attack, and 2–10 gm at bedtime between attacks. The patient should be encouraged to eat a low-carbohydrate, low-sodium diet. Thiamine may abort the effects of carbohydrates. Unnecessary exposure to cold should be avoided.

The disorder is consistent with a normal life span.

Table 21—10. Muscular dystrophies and myotonias of childhood.

Disease	Genetic Pattern	Age at Onset	Early Manifestations	Involved Muscles
Muscular dystrophies Duchenne's muscular dystrophy (pseudo-hypertrophic, infantile)	X-linked recessive; autosomal recessive unusual. Thirty to 50% have no family history.	2–6 years; rarer in infancy or at birth.	Clumsiness and easy fatigability on walking, especially on running and climbing stairs. Walking on toes; waddling gait. Lordosis. (Climbing upon legs when rising from supine position—Gower's maneuver.)	Axial and proximal before distal. Pelvic girdle; pseudo-hypertrophy of gastrocnemius (90%), triceps brachii, and vastus lateralis. Shoulder girdle usually later. Sometimes mild articulation difficulties. Eventually, cardiac muscle (50%).
Becker's muscular dystrophy (late onset)	X-linked recessive.	Childhood (usually later than in Duchenne's).	Similar to Duchenne's.	Similar to Duchenne's.
Limb-girdle muscular dystrophy A. Pelvifemoral (Leyden-Möbius) B. Scapulohumeral (Erb's juvenile)	Autosomal recessive in 60%; high sporadic incidence. A. Relatively common. B. Rare.	Variable: early childhood to adulthood.	Weakness, with distribution according to type. Waddling gait, difficulty climbing stairs. Lordosis.	A. Pelvic girdle usually involved first and to greater extent. B. Shoulder girdle often asymmetric. Quadriceps and hamstrings may be weakest. Pseudohypertrophy of calves uncommon.
Facioscapulohumeral muscular dystrophy (Landouzy-Déjèrine). Scapuloperoneal variant	Autosomal dominant; sporadic cases not uncommon.	Usually late childhood and adolescence; rare in infancy; not uncommon in twenties.	Diminished facial movements with inability to close eyes, smile, or whistle. Face may be flat, unlined. Difficulty in raising arms over head. Lordosis. Tripping in scapuloperoneal type.	Facial muscles followed by shoulder girdle with occasional spread to hips or distal legs (scapuloperoneal variant).
Distal myopathies A. Gowers' type B. Welander's	Autosomal dominant.	A. Gowers': Some early; usually adult. B. Welander's: usually adult; occasionally adolescence.	Gowers': Wasting of cranial musculature. Welander's: weakness of hands and feet; rarely, muscles of face and tongue.	Distal muscle weakness, especially small muscles of hands and feet.
"Oculocraniosomatic syndrome" (ophthalmoplegia and "ragged reds"; progressive external ophthalmoplegia)	(?)Acquired; 80% female; other hereditary neurologic disorders may be found in patient or family.	Variable: from infancy to adult life; most at about 10 years of age.	Ptosis and limitation of eye movements; hearing and visual loss (retinitis pigmentosa); intellectual loss; cerebellar disturbances (ataxia).	Extraocular muscles, often asymmetric. Variable involvement of axial muscles; cardiac muscles with conduction defect.
Congenital myopathies: Central core	Generally, autosomal dominance with variable penetrance.	Onset generally prenatal.	Infantile hypotonia, delay in attaining motor milestones. Mild weakness.	Often diffuse and variable, mainly proximal, legs more than arms.
Nemaline (rodbody) Myotubular (centronuclear) Congenital fiber type disproportion	Autosomal recessive also reported. Genetics unclear.	Onset usually in infancy, occasionally later childhood.	Nemaline: associated dysmorphism (face, spine, feet, pigeon chest). Myotubular: may show ptosis, facial weakness.	Nemaline: some diffuse muscle wasting. May include extraocular muscles.
Myotonias Myotonia congenita (Thomsen)	Autosomal dominant (autosomal recessive cases reported).	Early infancy to late childhood.	Difficulty in relaxing muscles after contracting them, especially after sleep; aggravated by cold, excitement.	Hands especially; muscles may be diffusely enlarged, giving patient Herculean appearance.
Myotonic dystrophy (Steinert)	Autosomal dominant.	Late childhood to adolescence; neonatal and infantile forms increasingly recognized.	Myotonia of grasp, tongue; worsened by cold, emotions. "Hatchet-face." In infancy, floppiness with facial diplegia; arthrogryposis multiplex. Thin ribs on chest x-ray. Myotonic phenomena: "bunching up" of muscles of tongue, thenar eminence, finger extensors after tapping with percussion hammer. Mild to moderate MR in about 80% may precede muscular symptoms.	Wasting of facial muscles, including muscles of mastication; sternocleidomastoids, hands.

Table 21–10 (cont'd). Muscular dystrophies and myotonias of childhood.

Reflexes	Muscle Biopsy Findings	Other Diagnostic Studies	Treatment	Prognosis
Knee jerks ± or 0; ankle jerks + to ++, occasionally, extensor plantar response (Babinski sign)	Degeneration and variation in fiber size; proliferation of connective tissue. Basophilia, phagocytosis. Poor differentiation of fiber types on ATPase reaction; deficiency of type 2B fibers.	EMG myopathic. CPK (4000–5000 IU) very high with decrease toward normal over the years. ECG. Chest x-ray.	Physical therapy, braces, wheelchair eventually, weight control.	Ten percent show nonprogressive mental retardation. Death from pneumonia 10–15 years after diagnosis with 75% of patients dead by age 20.
Similar to Duchenne's	Similar to above, except type 2B fibers present.	Similar to above, although muscle enzymes may not be as elevated.	As above. Wheelchair in late childhood or early adult life.	Slower progression than Duchenne's, with death usually in adulthood.
Usually present	Variation in muscle fiber size with many very large fibers. Fiber splitting and internal nuclei common. Many "moth-eaten" whorled fibers.	EMG myopathic. CPK variable: often normal but may be elevated. ECG.	Physical therapy, weight control.	Mildly progressive: spread from lower to upper limbs may take 15–20 years. Life expectancy mid to late adulthood.
Present	Predominantly large fibers with scattered tiny atrophic fibers, "moth-eaten" and whorled fibers. Inflammatory response. Little or no fibersplitting, fibrosis, or type 1 fiber predominance.	EMG myopathic. Muscle enzymes usually normal.	Physical therapy where indicated. Wheelchair in old age.	Very slowly progressive, often with plateaus, except in infantile form where there may be difficulties in walking by adolescence. Usually normal lifespan.
Present	Nonspecifically myopathic.	EMG myopathic. Muscle enzymes may be mildly elevated.	None.	Normal life expectancy.
Depressed to ± or 0 .	Mitochondrial abnormalities. "Ragged red" fibers. Changes in fiber size, usually due to type 2 fiber atrophy.	Muscle enzymes usually normal. ECG with conduction block. Rule out myasthenia gravis, Refsum's disease. CSF protein elevated. Nerve conduction studies.	Plastic retraction of eyelids. Support of cardiac defect. Where there is evidence of denervation, corticosteroids may be helpful.	Dysphagia may develop (50%) as well as generalized muscle weakness. Prognosis fair if disease is confined to ocular muscles.
Normal to ± or 0	Specific histochemical findings determine diagnosis. Central core: amorphous areas in fiber devoid of oxidative enzymes. Nemaline: red rods with trichrome stain. Myotubular: central nuclei in areas devoid of myofibrils; type 2B fibers hypertrophy.	Muscle enzymes usually normal. CPK may be slightly elevated.	Physical therapy to prevent contractures and strengthen existing muscles. Correction of dislocated hips or other deformities.	Usually very slowly progressive or nonprogressive, with plateaus and improvements possible, depending on type. Weakness occasionally increases in adolescence.
Normal	Nonspecific and minor changes; type 2B fibers may be absent.	EMG "myotonic."	Usually none. Phenytoin, especially in cold weather, may improve muscle functioning.	Normal life expectancy, with only mild disability.
In infantile form, marked hyporeflexia	Type 1 fiber atrophy, type 2 hypertrophy, sarcoplasmic masses, internal nuclei, phagocytosis, fibrosis, and cellular reaction.	EMG markedly "myotonic." Hormonal studies, especially testosterone, glucose tolerance test, thyroid tests. ECG. Chest x-ray and pulmonary function tests. Immunoglobulins.	Procainamide, 250 mg 3 times daily orally, increased to tolerance; phenytoin, 5–7 mg/kg/day orally.	Frontal baldness, cataracts (85%), gonadal atrophy (85% of males), thyroid dysfunction, diabetes mellitus (20%). Cardiac conduction defects; impaired pulmonary function. Low IgG. Life expectancy normal to slightly decreased, though severely handicapped in late adult life.

Adynamia Episodica Hereditaria of Gamstorp (Primary Hyperkalemic Periodic Paralysis)

This form of periodic paralysis has its onset in the first decade of life and is usually detected in infancy because of "staring" eyes (myotonic form of lid lag), or the mother may note that the infant has a very feeble cry, especially on waking. It is inherited as an autosomal dominant. Pseudohypertrophy of the calves is often present. There is an increased incidence of diabetes mellitus. The attacks are relatively short, lasting 30 minutes to 2 hours, and may be precipitated by rest after exercise, cold, and fatigue. Attacks usually occur in children of school age and then abate.

The serum potassium rises during attacks. The EMG may show myotonia of the external ocular and facial muscles.

Treatment is with hydrochlorothiazide (Hydrodiuril), 50 mg orally daily, or acetazolamide (Diamox), 250 mg orally daily. Dichlorphenamide (Daranide), 50 mg orally daily, has also been recommended. The dose must be adjusted for each case.

The disorder is consistent with a normal life span.

Normokalemic Periodic Paralysis

In this disorder, the onset is in the first decade of life. It is inherited as an autosomal dominant. Attacks come on during rest after exercise, with cold, following ingestion of foods high in potassium (eg, many fruit juices), and following ingestion of alcohol. The attacks may last for days.

In normokalemic paralysis, serum electrolytes do not change during attacks. Muscle biopsy may show vacuolar myopathy.

Treatment consists of increased intake of salt; acetazolamide (Diamox), 250 mg orally daily, with dosage adjusted for each case; and fludrocortisone, 0.1 mg daily orally.

The prognosis is good.

Pearson CM: The periodic paralyses: Differential features and pathological observations in permanent myopathic weakness. Brain 87:341, 1964.

MYASTHENIA GRAVIS

Essentials of Diagnosis

- Weakness, chiefly of muscles innervated by the brain stem, usually coming on or increasing with use (fatigue).
- Positive response to neostigmine (Prostigmin) and edrophonium (Tensilon).
- The forms seen in infancy and childhood are often more difficult to distinguish clinically than the adult type.

General Considerations

Myasthenia gravis is characterized by easy fatigability of muscles, particularly the extraocular muscles, muscles of mastication, swallowing, and respiration. However, in the neonatal period or early infancy, the weakness may be constant, so that the physician merely sees another "floppy" infant. Girls are involved more frequently than boys. Siblings may be involved. The age at onset is over 10 years in 75% of cases, often shortly after menarche. If the diagnosis is made in children under age 10, congenital myasthenia should be considered in retrospect. Thyrotoxicosis is found in almost 10% of female patients. The essential abnormality, while associated with altered function of cholinesterase on the acetylcholine released at the neuromuscular junction, is still not defined; altered immunologic responses have recently been demonstrated.

Clinical Findings

A. Symptoms and Signs:

1. Neonatal (transient)—This occurs in infants born of myasthenic mothers, although sometimes the mother is not aware of nor known to have the disease. The condition is due to some, substance transmitted from the mother to the infant. Sex distribution is equal. A sibling may have died in the neonatal period with similar symptoms and nondiagnostic autopsy. The infant exhibits hypotonia and a weak Moro reflex, but the knee jerk reflexes are preserved. Most striking are ineffective sucking, difficulty in swallowing, pooling of secretions, and a weak cry despite lack of evidence of other neurologic damage. In contrast to other forms of myasthenia gravis, the eyes are usually wide open, and extraocular muscle palsies are usually not present. There is, however, obvious facial weakness.

2. Congenital (persistent)—In these infants, the mothers rarely have myasthenia gravis but other relatives may. Sex distribution is equal. Extraocular muscle palsies and ptosis are often prominent; there may be a weak cry, fatigue with sucking, and hypotonia. Symptoms are often subtle and not recognized initially. Differential diagnosis includes many other causes of the "floppy infant" syndrome (see p 617), but particularly ocular myopathy, congenital ptosis, and Möbius' syndrome (facial nuclear aplasia and other anomalies).

3. Juvenile myasthenia gravis—In this form, the symptoms and signs are more similar to those seen in adults. The patient may be first seen by an ENT specialist or psychiatrist. The more prominent signs are difficulty in chewing, dysphagia, a nasal voice, ptosis, and ophthalmoplegia. Pathologic fatigability of limbs, chiefly involving the proximal limb and neck muscles, may be more prominent than the bulbar signs and may lead to an initial diagnosis of conversion hysteria, muscular dystrophy, or polymyositis.

B. Laboratory Findings:

1. Neostigmine test—In neonates and very young infants, the neostigmine (Prostigmin) test is preferable to the edrophonium (Tensilon) test because the longer duration of its response permits better observation, especially of sucking and swallowing movements. The test dose of neostigmine is 0.02 mg/kg subcut, usually given with atropine, 0.01 mg/kg subcut. The physician should be prepared to suction the patient.

2. Edrophonium test—Testing with edrophonium (Tensilon) is used in older children who are capable of cooperating in certain tasks, such as raising and lowering their eyelids and squeezing a sphygmomanometer bulb or the examiner's hands. The test dose is 0.1–1 ml IV, depending on the size of the child. Maximum improvement occurs within 2 minutes.

3. Other laboratory tests—Thyroid function studies and LE cell preparations are indicated in older children. Where available, immunologic studies (eg, for muscle antibodies) may be useful.

C. Electrical Studies of Muscle: Repetitive stimulation of a motor nerve at slow rates (3/sec) with recording over the appropriate muscle reveals a progressive fall in amplitude of the muscle potential in myasthenic patients. A maximal stimulus must be given. At higher rates of stimulation (50/sec), there may be a transient repair of this defect before the progressive decline is seen.

In the regional curare test, tubocurarine is administered to an extremity with occluded circulation to produce a neuromuscular block. Markedly increased sensitivity of the myasthenic muscle is demonstrable.

D. X-Ray Findings: Chest x-ray and laminagraphy in older children may disclose thymus enlargement.

E. Electroencephalography: An increased incidence of seizure disorders has been reported in patients with myasthenia gravis.

Treatment

A. General and Supportive Care: In the neonate, or in a child in a myasthenic crisis or cholinergic crisis (see below), suctioning of secretions is essential. Respiratory assistance may be required. Infections should be treated promptly, usually in the hospital.

Treatment should be carried out by physicians with experience in this disorder. In older children, some of the responsibility for adjustment of drug dosage may be left to the patient.

B. Anticholinesterase Drug Therapy: *Note:* There is increasing concern that anticholinesterase drugs may eventually damage the motor end plates.

1. Pyridostigmine (Mestinon)—The dose must be adjusted for each patient. A frequent starting dose is 15–30 mg every 6 hours.

2. Neostigmine (Prostigmin)—Fifteen mg are roughly equivalent to 60 mg of pyridostigmine. It often causes gastric hypermobility with diarrhea, but it is the drug of choice in neonates, in whom prompt treatment may be lifesaving.

3. Atropine may be added on a maintenance basis to control mild cholinergic side-effects such as hypersecretion, abdominal cramps, and nausea and vomiting.

4. Immunosuppressive agents, including alternate-day therapy with prednisone, are receiving extensive clinical trials and are gaining increased favor. The advisability of their use in younger children is not definitively determined.

5. Patients who become resistant to anticholinesterase drugs may need to be taken off the drugs for a few days and be given respiratory assistance. The use of corticosteroids in such cases is sometimes beneficial.

6. Myasthenic crisis—Relatively sudden difficulties in swallowing and respiration may be observed in myasthenic patients. Edrophonium chloride (Tensilon) will result in dramatic but brief improvement and may be difficult to evaluate in the small child. Suctioning, tracheostomy, respiratory assistance, and fluid and electrolyte maintenance may be required.

7. Cholinergic crises—Cholinergic crisis may result from overdosage of anticholinesterase drugs. The resulting weakness may be similar to that of myasthenia, and the muscarinic effects (diarrhea, sweating, lacrimation, miosis, bradycardia, hypotension) are often absent or difficult to evaluate. The edrophonium (Tensilon) test may help to determine whether the patient is receiving too little of the drug or is manifesting toxic symptoms due to overdosage. Improvement after the drugs are withdrawn suggests cholinergic crisis. Respirator facilities should be available. The patient may require atropine and tracheostomy.

C. Surgical Measures: Early thymectomy is beneficial in many patients whose disease is not confined to ocular symptoms, but the effects may not be apparent for several years. Some advise irradiation prior to surgery. This requires experienced surgical and postsurgical care.

Prognosis

Neonatal (transient) myasthenia presents a great threat to life, primarily due to aspiration of secretions. With proper treatment, the symptoms usually begin to disappear within a few days to 2–3 weeks, and the child usually requires no further treatment.

In the congenital persistent form, the symptoms may initially be as acute as in the transient variety; more commonly, however, they are relatively benign and constant, with gradual worsening as the child grows older. Life span is not usually affected.

In the juvenile form, a high percentage of patients become resistant or unresponsive to anticholinesterase compounds and require treatment in a hospital where respiratory assistance can be given as needed. Spontaneous remissions in this group are infrequent, but it offers the best candidates for thymectomy.

The response to thymectomy after the first few critical days is often most gratifying, with the patient requiring no further drug therapy.

Death in myasthenic or cholinergic crisis may occur unless prompt treatment is given.

Millichap JG, Dodge PR: Diagnosis and treatment of myasthenia gravis in infancy, childhood and adolescence. Neurology 10:1007, 1960.

CONGENITAL ABSENCE OF MUSCLES*

Congenital absence (sometimes only partial) of one or more muscles, usually unilateral, and particularly of the pectoralis (sternal portion), trapezius, serratus anterior, quadratus femoris, or omohyoid, is not unusual. Heredofamilial cases have been reported. Other deformities, eg, syndactyly, microdactyly, and muscular dystrophy, may be present. Absence of muscles of the abdominal wall (prune belly) may be associated with anomalies of the gastrointestinal tract, urinary tract (Eagle's syndrome), the extremities, and cryptorchism. Treatment is determined by the specific abnormalities present.

PERIPHERAL NERVE PALSIES

1. THE ASYMMETRIC FACE

Facial asymmetry may be present at birth or develop later, either suddenly or gradually, unilaterally or bilaterally. Nuclear or peripheral involvement of the facial nerves results in sagging or drooping of the mouth and inability to close one or both eyes, particularly with crying in neonates and infants. Inability to wrinkle the forehead may be demonstrated in infants and young children by getting them to follow an object (light) moved vertically above the forehead. Loss of taste of the anterior two-thirds of the tongue on the involved side may be demonstrated in intelligent, cooperative children by age 4 or 5, though playing with a younger child and the judicious use of a tongue blade may enable the physician to note if the child's face puckers up when something sour, such as lemon juice, is applied with a swab to the anterior tongue. Ability to wrinkle the forehead is preserved, due to bilateral innervation, in supranuclear or central facial paralysis.

Injuries to the facial nerve at birth occur in 0.25–6.5% of consecutive live births. Forceps delivery is the obvious cause in some cases; in others, the side of the face affected may have abutted in utero against the sacral prominence. In many cases, no cause can be established.

Facial weakness in early life may be due to agenesis of the affected muscles, supranuclear causes (part of the Möbius syndrome), or may even be familial. Neonatal myasthenia gravis, polyneuritis, and myotonic dystrophy must be considered. Facial asymmetry due to hypoplasia of one side of the cranium associated with contralateral hemiatrophy and spastic hemiparesis

---

*Arthrogryposis multiplex, or contractures and fixation about multiple joints, is discussed briefly under the section on the floppy infant (p 617). Clubfoot, Sprengel's deformity, and torticollis are discussed in Chapter 19.

(due, in most instances, to an intrauterine cerebrovascular accident affecting one hemisphere) is usually differentiated easily, as is the hemiatrophy of one side of the body seen in Silver's syndrome.

Acquired peripheral facial weakness (Bell's palsy) of sudden onset and unknown cause is common in children. It may be a presenting sign of other disorders, such as tumor, hypertension, infectious mononucleosis, or the Landry-Guillain-Barré syndrome, but these can usually be ruled out by the history, physical examination, and appropriate laboratory tests.

In the vast majority of cases of isolated peripheral facial palsy—both those present at birth and those acquired later—improvement begins within 1–2 weeks and near or total recovery of function is observed within 2 months. Methylcellulose drops, 1%, should be instilled into the eyes to protect the cornea during the day, and the eye should be closed with cellophane tape at night. Upward massage of the face for 5–10 minutes 3–4 times a day may help maintain muscle tone. There has been renewed interest in the use of prednisone or prednisolone in Bell's palsy.

When little or no improvement occurs in 10–14 days, tests for electrical excitability of the facial nerve and electromyography by specialists are useful diagnostically and prognostically.

In the few children with permanent and cosmetically disfiguring facial weakness, plastic surgical intervention at 6 years of age or older may be of benefit. New procedures, such as attachment of facial muscles to the temporal muscle, are being developed.

Adour KK & others: Prednisone treatment for idiopathic facial paralysis (Bell's palsy). N Engl J Med 287:1268, 1972.

Manning JJ, Adour KK: Facial paralysis in children. Pediatrics 49:102, 1972.

McHugh H, Sowden KA, Levitt MN: Facial paralysis and muscle agenesis in the newborn. Arch Otolaryngol 89:131, 1969.

Salam EA, Elyahky WL: Evaluation of prognosis and treatment in Bell's palsy in children. Acta Paediatr Scand 57:468, 1968.

2. BRACHIAL PLEXUS INJURIES
(Erb's Palsy, Klumpke's Paralysis)

Traction injuries of the brachial plexus are most common in neonates, occurring in 0.1% of spontaneous, 1.2% of breech, 1.3% of forceps, and 0.25% of all deliveries. The complexity of the brachial plexus precludes any absolute classification, but injuries are usually divided into those affecting the upper plexus (Erb's palsy) and those affecting the lower plexus (Klumpke's paralysis).

Erb's palsy, involving chiefly the fifth and sixth cervical roots, is seen in 99% of cases. It is usually associated with difficult breech delivery, forceps delivery (especially in brow and face presentations), or misapplication of the vacuum extractor. The arm is maintained in adduction and internal rotation at the shoulder, with the lower arm pronated, assuming the "waiter's tip" position. Loss of sensation may be difficult to assess in neonates.

In Klumpke's paralysis, involving chiefly the lower brachial plexus (eighth cervical and first thoracic roots), the small muscles of the hand and wrist flexors are affected, causing a "claw hand." Horner's syndrome may also be present. The injury, usually manipulation during delivery, results in hyperabduction of the arm at the shoulder.

Swinging a child by one arm or jerking the arm may also cause lower plexus injuries ("nursemaid's palsy").

The palsies observed are usually due to avulsion of the plexus with contusion, edema, and some hemorrhage. X-ray studies of the shoulder will rule out fractures of the clavicle or cervical spine, or dislocations.

In most instances, recovery occurs spontaneously within a few days or weeks; however, contractures of the shoulder and especially the elbow joints and atrophy of the affected muscles are not infrequent residuals to which positioning in the so-called Statue of Liberty or airplane wing position, formerly advised, has been said to contribute. Passive range of motion exercises, which can be taught to the parents, are most helpful in preventing contractures. Electromyography can delineate the extent of injury and aid in prognosis. Surgical exploration is justified in the rare instances where residual fibrosis is compressing the roots.

Adler JB, Patterson· RL Jr: Erb's palsy: Long-term results of treatment in eighty-eight cases. J Bone Joint Surg 49A:1052, 1967.

Eng GD: Brachial plexus palsy in newborn infants. Pediatrics 48:18, 1971.

3. OTHER PERIPHERAL NERVE INJURIES

Injuries to the radial and ulnar nerves occur with fractures of the humerus; ulnar and median nerve injuries may result from deep wrist lacerations; and fracture of the fibula may cause peroneal palsy. These usually require neurosurgical attention. Femoral nerve palsies occasionally occur with diabetes mellitus in teenage youngsters.

The so-called "shoulder strap" or "pack" paralysis of the long thoracic nerve, resulting in winging of the scapula, occurs in youngsters who carry heavy rucksacks with poorly padded straps.

A most unfortunate type of paralysis is that of the sciatic nerve following injections into the buttock. Penicillin and tetracycline injected into neonates or small thin children are the most common offenders. The resulting fibrosis, chiefly around the outer portion of the sciatic nerve, comprising elements making up the common peroneal nerve, causes foot drop and adduction and inversion of the foot. Sensory loss over the outer side of the lower leg and dorsum of the foot may be demonstrated by electrical and other studies. In most cases, at least partial recovery occurs over the course of a few weeks to 6 months. Occasionally, surgical exploration of the buttock with neurolysis is justified. Postinjection sciatic neuropathy can be prevented by giving injections into the anterior lateral aspect of the thigh.

Gilles FH, Matson DD: Sciatic nerve injury following misplaced gluteal injection. J Pediatr 76:247, 1970.

Watters GV, Barlow CF: Acute and subacute neuropathies. Pediatr Clin North Am 14:997, 1967.

CHRONIC POLYNEUROPATHY

Polyneuropathy, usually insidious in onset and slowly progressive, occurs in children of any age. The presenting complaints are chiefly disturbances of gait or easy fatigability in walking or running and, slightly less often, weakness or clumsiness of the hands. Pain, tenderness, or paresthesias are infrequently mentioned. Neurologic examination discloses muscular weakness, greatest in the distal portions of the extremities, with steppage gait and depressed or absent deep tendon reflexes. Cranial nerves are sometimes affected. Sensory deficits (difficult to demonstrate in fearful children or those under 5 years of age) cover a stocking-glove distribution. The muscles may be tender, and trophic changes such as a glossy or "parchment" skin and absent sweating may occur. Thickening of the ulnar and peroneal nerves may occasionally be felt. Pure sensory neuropathies show up as chronic trauma.

The cause in children is usually not clear. Known causes include (1) toxins (eg, lead, arsenic, mercurials, vincristine, benzene); (2) metabolic disorders (diabetes mellitus, chronic uremia, recurrent hypoglycemia, porphyria, polyarteritis nodosa, lupus erythematosus); (3) hereditary, often degenerative conditions (eg, Dejerine-Sottas interstitial hypertrophic polyneuritis, some of the leukodystrophies, Refsum's disease, the spinocerebellar degenerations with neurogenic components, especially Charcot-Marie-Tooth disease, abetalipoproteinemia, and Recklinghausen's disease); and (4) "inflammatory" states such as "chronic or recurrent Landry-Guillain-Barré syndrome" and neuritis associated with mumps or diphtheria. Causes such as carcinoma, chronic alcoholism, and beriberi and other vitamin deficiencies are not reported in children.

Laboratory diagnosis is made by the marked slowing of nerve conduction. CSF protein is commonly elevated and gamma globulin is sometimes elevated. Electromyography may show a neurogenic polyphasic pattern. Nerve biopsy, with teasing of the fibers as well as staining for metachromasia, is advised to demonstrate loss of myelin and (to a lesser degree) of axons and increased connective tissue or concentric lamellas ("onion skin appearance") around the nerve fiber. Muscle biopsy may show the pattern associated with denervation. Other laboratory studies, directed toward specific causes mentioned above, include screening for heavy metals and for metabolic, renal, or vascular disorders. Chronic lead intoxication, which rarely causes neuropathy in childhood, may escape detection until the child is given calcium disodium edetate (EDTA) and lead levels are determined in timed urines. Three- and 4-fold rises then are diagnostic.

Therapy is directed at specific disorders whenever possible. Occasionally the weakness is profound and involves bulbar nerves, in which case tracheostomy and respiratory assistance are required. In most cases in which the cause is unknown or considered to be due to "chronic inflammation," corticosteroid therapy (as is not the case in acute Landry-Guillain-Barré syndrome) is often of great benefit. Prednisone, 1–2.5 mg/kg/day orally, with tapering to the least effective dose– discontinued if the process seems to be arresting and reinstituted when symptoms recur–is recommended. When treatable, symptoms regress and may disappear altogether over a period of months.

Long-term prognosis varies with the cause and the ability to offer specific therapy. In the "steroid-dependent" group, residual deficits and deaths within a few years are more frequent.

Dyck PJ & others: Severe hypomyelination and marked abnormality of conduction in Dejerine-Sottas hypertrophic neuropathy. Mayo Clin Proc 46:432, 1971.

Kasman M, Bernstein L, Schulman S: Chronic polyradiculoneuropathy of infancy. Neurology 26:565, 1976.

Matthews WB, Howell DA, Highes RC: Relapsing corticosteroid-dependent polyneuritis. J Neurol Neurosurg Psychiatry 33:330, 1970.

Schoene WC & others: Hereditary sensory neuropathy. J Neurol Sci 11:463, 1970.

Tasker W, Chutorian AM: Chronic polyneuritis of childhood. J Pediatr 74:699, 1969.

MISCELLANEOUS NEUROMUSCULAR DISORDERS

CEREBRAL PALSY

Essentials of Diagnosis

- Impairment of neurologic functions, especially voluntary motor activity.
- Nonprogressive and nonhereditary.
- Present since birth or early infancy.

General Considerations

Cerebral palsy is a term of clinical convenience for disorders of impaired brain and motor functioning with onset before or at birth or during the first year of life, basically nonprogressive, and varying widely in their causes, manifestations, and prognosis. Although the most obvious manifestation is impaired ability of voluntary muscles, the term in its broadest sense has also been applied to the minimal brain dysfunction syndrome (see below). The incidence of cerebral palsy is 1–5/1000 live births.

Classification

Classification is commonly based on the predominant motor deficit.

A. Spastic Forms: About 75% of cases. Often associated with other forms.

1. Tetraplegia–Approximately equal involvement of all 4 extremities. The main lesion is in the cortical gray matter. Cases due to perinatal damage often show symptoms earlier than those due to cortical dysplasias.

2. Hemiplegia–One side involved primarily, the right nearly twice as often as the left. Comprises nearly 40% of all cerebral palsy patients.

3. Diplegia–Legs involved more than arms.

4. Paraplegia–Legs only involved.

5. Monoplegia–One extremity only involved.

6. Triplegia–Three extremities involved.

B. Choreoathetosis: (See section on Extrapyramidal Disorders.) Often associated with rigidity or spastic tetraplegia. Comprises about 20% of all cerebral palsy patients.

C. Ataxia: Pure and in combination with other forms. Comprises about 1–2%.

Etiology

The cause is often obscure or multiple. No definite etiologic diagnosis is possible in over one-third of cases. The incidence is high among infants small for gestational age. Among known causes are intrauterine bleeding, infections, toxins, congenital malformations, birth trauma and hypoxia, neonatal infections, kernicterus, neonatal hypoglycemia, and a small number of genetic syndromes.

Associated Deficits

A. Seizures: Seizures afflict about 60% of children with cerebral palsy (chiefly children with hemi- and quadriplegia) and about one-third of children with paraplegia and movement disorders.

B. Mental Retardation: While frequent, it is present primarily in spastic tetraplegics.

C. Sensory and Speech Deficits: Impairment of speech, vision, hearing, and perceptual functions is frequently present in varying degrees and combinations.

Clinical Findings

A. Symptoms and Signs: The typical spastic child exhibits muscular hypertonicity of the clasp-knife type which may eventually end in contractures. Tendon reflexes, if sufficient muscle relaxation can be achieved, are hyperactive; clonus may be present. Plantar responses are often extensor on the involved sides. While voluntary control, especially of fine movements, is decreased, there is spread or overflow of associated movements. In extreme cases, the child may lie with his elbows flexed and fists clenched (straphanger's posture) and his legs crossed or scissored. In early infancy the child may appear floppy, although tendon jerks are abnormally increased (hypotonic, atonic, or prespastic diplegia). Rigidity often accompanies cerebral palsy.

Ataxia may be difficult to delineate due to the simultaneous presence of spasticity or hyperkinetic movements.

Microcephaly (head circumference < 2 SD from mean for age and sex and decreasing) is present in about 25% of spastic tetraplegics.

Partial atrophy of the cranium on the involved side or of involved extremities is observed frequently, but dependable statistics are not available.

A smaller hand or foot, when coupled with mild weakness on muscle testing or hyperreflexia, often justifies a diagnosis of mild cerebral palsy of which the patient or his family may not even have been aware.

B. Laboratory and Other Findings: No routine work-up can be outlined. The clinical findings, the presence or absence of seizures, and the overall outlook for the child—particularly with respect to his ability to carry on activities for daily living and his mental status—determine what studies, if any, should be performed. Hip films in abduction are indicated to rule out dislocations secondary to spasticity. EEG is indicated when seizures are present or suspected.

Pneumoencephalography or cerebral angiography is rarely indicated except when neurosurgical intervention is contemplated, as in hemiplegic children with uncontrolled seizures who may have a porencephalic cyst or may be candidates for hemispherectomy.

Urine screening tests for aminoacidurias and serum uric acid determination, where readily and inexpensively available, are sometimes indicated by the clinical findings.

Children whose motor difficulties, especially incoordination and spasticity, do not begin until the second year of life, should be checked for metachromatic leukodystrophy (Table 21–6).

Differential Diagnosis

The diagnosis is usually not difficult. When the history suggests progressive deterioration, the degenerative and metabolic disorders affecting the nervous system must be considered. In the ataxic form, cerebellar dysgenesis (sometimes familial) and other forms of spinocerebellar degenerations may have to be ruled out; in the former, skull x-rays may show a shallow posterior fossa and a hypoplastic cerebellum on pneumoencephalography.

Treatment

Realistically, a child should be helped to achieve maximum potential rather than "normality." Special educational programming depends on the physical and mental potential of the child. Not unexpectedly, the degree of improvement with physical therapy has been correlated positively with better intelligence. Treat seizures as in other children. The orthopedic aspects of cerebral palsy are discussed in Chapter 19.

Hyperactivity may be controlled to some extent with dextroamphetamine, 2.5–15 mg orally in the morning and at noon, depending on the size and age of the child. Other psychotropic drugs, such as methylphenidate (Ritalin), chlorpromazine (Thorazine), and chlordiazepoxide (Librium), may be useful.

For spasticity, diazepam (Valium), 2–5 mg orally 2–4 times a day, is often of benefit. Dantrolene (Dantrium) in amounts adequate to obtain subjective improvement in gait (0.5 mg/kg 4 times daily) may be tried in the ambulatory spastic child; however, the improvement, if any, must be weighed against such side-effects as skin eruptions, drowsiness, or paresthesias and the risk of hepatotoxicity. The safety of the drug for children under age 5 years has not been established.

At least in the USA, the role of surgery in the amelioration of spasticity or rigidity remains a matter of concern. Chronic cerebellar stimulation has been reported as a promising method for the alleviation of long-standing symptoms and improvement of functioning in patients with moderate to severe cerebral palsy.

Psychologic counseling and support of the child and his family are of paramount importance.

Prognosis

In severely involved cases, especially spastics with profound retardation and seizures which are difficult to control, death due to intercurrent infections during early childhood is not uncommon. Many children with cerebral palsy of average or near-average intelligence lead fairly normal, satisfying, and productive lives. The overall prognosis has improved.

Bleck EE: Locomotor prognosis in cerebral palsy. Dev Med Child Neurol 17:18, 1975.

Churchill JA & others: The etiology of cerebral palsy in preterm infants. Dev Med Child Neurol 16:143, 1974.

Cooper IS & others: Chronic cerebellar stimulation in cerebral palsy. Neurology 26:744, 1976.

Ford F & others: Efficacy of dantrolene sodium in the treatment of spastic cerebral palsy. Dev Med Child Neurol 18:770, 1976.

Gornal P, Hitchcock E, Kirkland IS: Stereotaxic neurosurgery in the management of cerebral palsy. Dev Med Child Neurol 17:279, 1975.

Scherzer AL, Mike V, Ilson J: Physical therapy as a determinant of change in the cerebral palsied infant. Pediatrics 58:47, 1976.

MINIMAL BRAIN DYSFUNCTION SYNDROME

This term is one of many applied to "children of near average, average, or above average general intelligence with certain learning or behavioral disabilities ranging from mild to severe, which are associated with deviations of function of the central nervous system. These deviations may manifest themselves by various combinations of impairment in perception, conceptualization, language, memory, and control of attention, impulse, or motor function."* Certain aspects of this syndrome are discussed briefly in the sections on developmental retardation and chronic brain syndromes. Neurologists are frequently requested to evaluate children whose behavior at home or in school is unacceptable to parents or teachers in order to establish the organic basis of the problem and sometimes in the hope that medical management will provide an easy solution. In terms of daily living, the children, their parents and teachers, and the professionals who become involved find the "dysfunctions" far from "minimal."

Estimates of incidence are imprecise because the syndrome is variably defined. About 3% of children of grade school age is a quasi-official estimate, with boys more frequently affected than girls. Suggested causative factors include virtually any illness or trauma occurring before, during, or after birth and affecting the brain either obviously or by implication. Multiple causes, including psychosocial factors, are usually involved.

Disturbances of feeding and sleeping patterns are often noted in early infancy, with frequent formula changes and delays in sleeping through the night. Motor milestones are usually attained at normal ages, but the child is noted to be clumsy, with troubles learning to dress himself, button his clothes, and tie his shoes. Language development is frequently reported as delayed. When the child attends preschool or school, the chief complaints are "hyperactivity," distractibility, overexcitability, short attention span, and various learning disabilities, particularly in reading and arithmetic.

On neurologic examination, the physician is apt to be less impressed by the child's "hyperactivity" than the parents or teachers. The chief findings are "maladroitness" or nonspecific incoordination; overflow "choreiform" as well as mirror movements or synkinesis (observed best by having the child wiggle the fingers of one outstretched hand and noting extraneous movements of the other hand or the feet); and difficulties in performing rapid rhythmic tasks such as hopping on one foot or clapping the hands in a rhythmic pattern. Disturbances of tone (especially mild spasticity) and hyperreflexia and occasionally Babinski responses are also found. Some clinicians accept even the most minimal of "neurologic soft signs" as evidence of brain damage. Neither eye nor hand dominance nor "mixed laterality" have proved to be related to the learning problems.

The EEG is mildly and diffusely dysrhythmic in about 40% of cases, but there is no clear correlation between the EEG findings and any of the functional disturbances; indeed, on follow-up studies, children labeled as hyperkinetic who had abnormal EEGs had normal ones later, while those with initially normal studies later had dysrhythmic EEGs.

*Clements SD: Minimal brain dysfunction in children. US Dept of Health, Education, and Welfare, NINDB Monograph No. 3, 1966, pp 9–10.

Far more useful are psychologic tests, including the WISC, Goodenough Draw-A-Man, Bender Gestalt, and Lincoln-Oseretsky Motor Development Scale. These children commonly exhibit a wide scatter on varied subtests, with marked discrepancy between verbal abilities and performances and visual-motor or audio-motor perceptual dysfunctions. Many are also found to· be mildly to moderately depressed, compulsive, and anxious because they continually fail to come up to the expectations of others.

The physician's task is not only to rule out severe and possibly progressive neurologic or emotional disorders but to act as "ombudsman" for the child and to guide his parents and teachers. He must be as accurate as possible in his diagnosis, keeping in mind that the reported complaints and disabilities, as well as the neurologic, EEG, and even psychometric findings, may be observed in children with different organic, emotional, and social problems, and that these may be present together to a greater or lesser extent. In discussing the problems, the author has often described the child as being "dyssynchronous," ie, "out of phase" in his developmental, behavioral, and educational progression and maturation. Parents quickly appreciate the term "dyssynchronous" when it is explained in terms of such analogies as the automatic shift of an automobile synchronized to changes in speed. Lack of synchronization (or letting the clutch out at the wrong time when using a standard shift) results in grinding the gears or the car's bucking like a bronco. The "dyssynchronous child" may be likened in his effect to an orchestra whose instruments are all playing slightly out of tune and off the beat or whose conductor is not in complete command, so that what is heard is somewhat chaotic and cacophonous. For the more visually oriented parent, the "dyssynchronous child" may be likened to a television image in which the horizontal and vertical alignments are out of focus or where there is a great deal of "snow," offering a recognizable but distorted picture.

The term dyssynchronous may be taken to reflect an imbalance between central excitation and inhibition, the complex· feedback mechanisms thought to produce the synchronized discharges essential to the arousal state and attentiveness, fine coordinated movements, and rhythmic electrical brain activity. The term dyssynchronous, while emphasizing the functional aspects of the disorder, also suggests something of its neurophysiologic basis as inferred from clinical findings: a disturbance, possible synaptic in character, of the timing and orderliness of neuronal interplay. This appellation avoids the implication of demonstrable and irreversible anatomic injury contained in the term brain damage; rather, it offers the hope—founded on clinical experience—of adjustment and "synchronization," with maturation aided by education. Thus, this term carries within it the challenge for investigative and therapeutic efforts.

The physician, in his role as an authority figure, can be supportive to parents, teachers, and other professionals. Behavior modification, with emphasis on and rewarding of acceptable behavior, instead of the common tendency to pay greatest attention to the child when he is misbehaving or failing, is of utmost benefit. Parents and siblings, teachers and peers can all be involved in behavior modification programs which may be best outlined by a competent clinical psychologist. Remedial tutoring is best done not by the parents but by an intelligent, calm, patient, and kind high school or college student for 20–30 minute periods several days a week. A wide variety of inexpensive methods to help a child improve his coordination and to overcome any specific learning disabilities may be devised. At present there is little rationale for "patterning" as a form of therapy.

Drug therapy is at times useful, but it is strongly recommended that it be used judiciously, sparingly, and only as an adjunct to behavior modification. Dextroamphetamine (5–20 mg in the morning and 2.5–10 mg at noon) has proved useful in diverting the nondirected "hyperkinetic" behavior into more goal-oriented activity. Methylphenidate (Ritalin) also is used widely in varying dosage. Their toxic effects (including initial suppression of growth) and their potential for abuse must be carefully considered. Pemoline (Cylert), 37.5 mg/day orally at first and increasing at 1-week intervals by 18.75 mg until the desired clinical response is obtained, has been introduced recently. Cylert is not recommended for children under age 6. The mean daily effective dose ranges from 56.25–75 mg. One of the main advantages of this drug may be its more sustained, smoother action. Side-effects, especially anorexia and insomnia, often subside with continued administration or reduction of dosage.

As he grows older, the restless hyperactive child tends to remain very active but in a more organized and less disturbing fashion. Distractibility continues to be a major handicap, resulting in significantly poorer performance in school or on jobs. Emotional immaturity continues to be characteristic of the child's behavior. Not infrequently, more serious emotional disorders, including delinquency, result from the failures and disapproval experienced by the child.

Obviously, with the large number of children involved, major educational and preventive psychologic efforts are required.

Cohen HJ, Birch HG, Taft LT: Some considerations for evaluating the Doman-Delacato "patterning" method. Pediatrics 45:302, 1970.

Council on Child Health, American Academy of Pediatrics: Medication for hyperkinetic children. Pediatrics 55:560, 1975.

Dykeman RA & others: A double-blind clinical study of pemoline in MBD children: Comments on the psychological test results. Pages 125–129 in: *Clinical Use of Stimulant Drugs in Children.* Conners CK (editor). Excerpta Medica, 1974.

Gross MD: Growth of hyperkinetic children taking methylphenidate, dextroamphetamine, or imipramine/desipramine. Pediatrics 58:423, 1976.

Kenny TJ & others: Characteristics of children referred because of hyperactivity. J Pediatr 79:618, 1971.

Touwen BC, Prechtl HFR: *The Neurologic Examination of the Child With Minor Nervous Dysfunction.* Clinics in Developmental Medicine No. 38, Heinemann, 1970.

Weiss G & others: Studies on the hyperactive child. 5. The effects of dextroamphetamine and chlorpromazine on behavior and intellectual functioning. J Child Psychol Psychiatry 9:145, 1968.

Weiss G & others: Studies on the hyperactive child. 8. Five-year follow-up. Arch Gen Psychiatry 24:409, 1971.

FLOPPY INFANT SYNDROME

Essentials of Diagnosis

- In early infancy, decreased muscular activity, both spontaneous and in response to postural reflex testing and to passive motion.
- In young infants, "frog posture" or other unusual positions at rest.
- In older infants, delay in motor milestones.

General Considerations

In the young infant, ventral suspension, ie, supporting the baby with a hand under the chest, normally results in the baby's holding his head slightly up (45 degrees or less), the back straight or nearly so, the arms flexed at the elbows and slightly abducted, and the knees partly flexed. The floppy infant droops over the hand like an inverted U. Even the normal neonate attempts to keep his head in the same plane as his body when pulled up from supine to sitting by his hands ("traction response"). Marked head lag is characteristic of the floppy infant. Hyperextensibility of the joints is not a dependable criterion.

In the older infant, delays in walking, running, or climbing stairs, or difficulties and lack of endurance in motor activities, are the usual reasons for seeking medical evaluation.

Hypotonia or decreased motor activity is a frequent presenting complaint in neuromuscular disorders but may also accompany a variety of systemic conditions or may be due to certain disorders of connective tissue.

Clinical Types

A. Paralytic Group: Significant lack of movement against gravity, such as kicking the legs, holding up arms, or attempting to stand when held or in response to stimuli such as tickling or slight pain.

B. Nonparalytic Group: Floppiness without significant paralysis.

Note: Deep tendon reflexes may be depressed or absent in both groups and thus are of no value in differentiating between them. Brisk reflexes with hypotonia, however, point to suprasegmental or generally cerebral dysfunction.

1. PARALYTIC GROUP

Hereditary Progressive Spinal Muscular Atrophies

These disorders are inherited as autosomal recessives, but rare instances of dominant transmission occur. Prevention is not possible except for genetic counseling. Treatment is supportive and consists of minimizing respiratory infections, preventing contractures, and enabling those who can do so to use crutches or a wheelchair.

A. Infantile Form (Werdnig-Hoffmann Disease): This is the commonest of the paralytic forms of floppy infant syndrome. Onset may be in utero, with loss of fetal movements, or paralysis may appear gradually or fairly abruptly in the early weeks or months of life. The infant usually lies in the frog position, breathing diaphragmatically, exhibiting sternal retraction due to paralysis of intercostal muscles, and moving the legs only slightly if at all. The facies is alert. Cry may be weak, and secretions tend to pool in the pharynx due to bulbar involvement. Fasciculation of the tongue is seen frequently. Fasciculations of the muscles of the extremities are usually hidden by baby fat. Tremor of the fingers may be seen, usually in slightly older and less severely involved children. Deep tendon reflexes are lost early—first in the lower extremities—as the paralysis proceeds cephalad. Sensation is normal.

The diagnosis is based on a "neurogenic" EMG pattern and muscle biopsy, which shows a neuropathic pattern of large bundles of atrophied fibers interspersed with bundles of normal or hypertrophied fibers. Soft tissue x-rays show marked muscle atrophy, and this may help in gauging needed depth for muscle biopsy. Muscle enzymes are usually normal but may be slightly elevated late in the disease.

Pneumonia, often due to aspiration, is the commonest complication, and most of the afflicted infants die within 2–3 years.

B. Variants: Less rapidly progressive forms may represent a continuum of the disorder, but—pending biochemical definition—not specific entities.

1. Weakness appearing late—Muscle weakness, chiefly of the legs, may not be recognized until the time when infants might be expected to sit up by themselves or to be walking; there may be other signs of retarded motor development as well. Intelligence is not affected. Muscles of respiration may be relatively spared, and the upper extremities may be strong enough so that the child can learn to walk with crutches, the legs and lower trunk being braced, or to use a wheelchair. Hence, maximum physical rehabilitation is indicated. In general, the more insidious and the later the onset of weakness and the more limited its extent, the better the prognosis. Some patients may live a normal life span.

2. Juvenile spinal muscular atrophy of Kugelberg-Welander—Onset is between 2 years of age and the late teens. The larger proximal muscles, especially of the pelvic girdle, are affected first; the lower legs and arms are involved relatively late. The muscles of the trunk and those supplied by the cranial nerves are usually spared. Muscle enzymes are usually normal, the EMG is "neurogenic," and muscle biopsy is similar to that seen in Werdnig-Hoffmann disease. Progression is usually slow. Males may be affected more severely. Every effort should be made to permit the patient to lead as independent a life as possible.

Myopathies

The congenital, relatively nonprogressive myopathies, muscular dystrophy, myotonic dystrophy, polymyositis, and periodic paralysis are discussed elsewhere. Most cases of congenital or early infantile muscular dystrophy reported in the past probably belong in the group of congenital myopathies.

Glycogenosis With Muscle Involvement

These are described under Glycogen Storage Disease in Chapter 33. Patients with type II (Pompe's disease, due to a deficiency of acid maltase) are most likely to present as floppy infants. The weakness in type III (limit dextrinosis) is less marked than in type II, while the rare instances of type IV (amylopectinosis) are severely hypotonic. Muscle cramps on exertion or easy fatigability, rather than floppiness in infancy, is the presenting complaint in type V (McArdle's phosphorylase deficiency) or the glycogenosis due to phosphofructokinase deficiency or phosphohexose isomerase inhibition.

Myasthenia Gravis

Neonatal transient and congenital persistent myasthenia gravis, presenting as "paralytic" floppy infants, is described elsewhere in this chapter.

Infant Botulism

A syndrome of severe generalized weakness of acute onset in previously well and active young infants has been related to the presence in the stool of *Clostridium botulinum* organisms and either toxin type A or B. These infants, 2 weeks to a few months of age, develop over the course of hours to several days increasing irritability, lethargy, constipation, poor feeding, and weakness of cranial and skeletal musculature. There is weak cry, difficulty with sucking and swallowing, pooling of saliva, ptosis and loss of facial movements, often striking loss of head control, and generalized hypotonia, with corresponding diminution or loss of sucking, gag, and stretch reflexes. While cranial nerves VII, IX, X, and XI have been constantly involved, III, IV, and VI involvement may also be present with internal and external ophthalmoplegia. *Respiratory arrest may occur.* On electromyography, brief, low-amplitude motor unit action potentials overly abundant for the amount of power exerted or stimulus used are found. It is important to note that all of these infants received foods additional to their breast or formula feedings, yet none of the foods contained toxin. None of the other family members were ill. In none of the infants was toxin found in the serum. Botulinus toxin appears to be formed in the infant gut.

Treatment requires supportive care, including gavage feeding and mechanical ventilation. Botulinus antitoxin has not been required. The illness may persist for several weeks, but complete recovery has occurred in all children.

The differential diagnosis includes myasthenia gravis, in which there is a response to neostigmine, and infantile polyneuritis, especially of the "steroid-responsive" type. In that condition, there is (1) prolonged nerve conduction time and denervation on EMG examination; (2) usually marked elevation of CSF protein for age; and (3) lack of progressive cerebral involvement, as in metachromatic and globoid leukodystrophies. Nerve biopsy may be justified. Diagnosis of this polyneuropathy may require a therapeutic trial of corticosteroids, resulting in improvement.

Arthrogryposis Multiplex, or Congenital Deformities About Multiple Joints

This symptom complex, sometimes associated with hypotonia, may be of "neurogenic" or "myopathic" origin (or both) and may be associated with a wide variety of other anomalies. Orthopedic aspects are discussed in Chapter 19.

Spinal Cord Lesions

Exceedingly limp newborns, usually the product of breech extraction with stretching or actual tearing of the lower cervical to upper thoracic spinal cord, are still occasionally seen. Klumpke's lower brachial plexus paralysis may be present; the abdomen is usually exceedingly soft, and the lower extremities are flaccid. Urinary retention is present initially, but later the bladder may function autonomously. Spine films are usually not helpful, although myelography may define the lesion. After a few weeks, spasticity of the lower limbs becomes obvious. Treatment is symptomatic, being directed at bladder and skin care, and eventual mobilization on crutches or in a wheelchair. The problem can be prevented by careful obstetric delivery.

2. NONPARALYTIC GROUP

In the "floppy" state without paralysis, tendon reflexes, though depressed, may be elicited. Muscle enzymes and EMG are usually normal. Prolonged nerve conduction velocities point to polyneuritis or leukodystrophy. Muscle biopsies, utilizing special staining technics and histographic analysis, often show a remarkable reduction in size of type II fibers associated with decreased voluntary motor activity.

CNS Lesions (Above Spinal Cord)

Limpness in the neonatal period and early infancy and subsequent delay in achieving motor milestones are the presenting features in a large number of children with a variety of CNS disorders. In many, but not all, the reduction in spontaneous motor activity accompanies mental retardation; in these cases, there may be a history of delayed development or regression suggesting brain damage. Close observation and scoring of motor patterns and adaptive behavior, as by the Denver Developmental Screening Test, usually confirms this. Several categories deserve specific attention.

A. "Prespastic Diplegia": This group includes neonates who have had various forms of pre- or perinatal encephalopathy, eg, encephalopathy due to hypoxia, toxins, and intracranial hemorrhage or infection. Findings include profound limpness at or shortly after birth, depressed or absent deep tendon reflexes initially, other signs of CNS difficulties such as poor sucking and feeding, weak or shrill cry, poor Moro responses, weak or absent grasp responses, and visual and auditory inattention. Tendon reflexes usually become hyperactive within a few weeks. When the infant is held up, supported under the armpits by the examiner's hands, his legs are flexed at the hips and knees and, instead of going limp, the infant exhibits increased tone (Foerster's sign). Because of their floppy state, these infants have been referred to in the past as hypotonic—or even atonic—diplegics; however, most, if not all, eventually exhibit hypertonicity, thus meriting the diagnosis of "prespastic diplegia."

B. Hypotonic, Hypokinetic Forms of "Minimal Brain Dysfunction" Syndrome: Floppiness may occur in children with normal or nearly normal intelligence who eventually exhibit aberrant behavior, maturational lag, and learning disabilities. The diagnosis in early life may be difficult, and close follow-up is indicated.

C. Hypotonia With Various Forms of Mental Deficit: Children with chromosomal defects, particularly trisomy 21, may exhibit floppiness without paralysis. However, in most children with mental retardation who are floppy, presumably because of deficient higher nervous activity, there is no specific diagnosis.

D. Degenerative CNS Disorders: Degenerative diseases of infancy presenting with hypotonia include globoid and metachromatic leukodystrophy, subacute necrotizing encephalomyelopathy, infantile amaurotic idiocy, and generalized gangliosidosis. Though relatively rare, the impact of such a diagnosis on the family, the dire prognosis for the child, and the importance of genetic counseling justify the often exhaustive investigations necessary in these disorders (Table 21–7).

E. Others: Congenital choreoathetosis, discussed earlier, often presents as hypotonia; involuntary movements of the limbs and facial grimacing are not noted until the second half of the first year or even later. Delays in the attainment of motor milestones are the rule.

Children with congenital cerebellar ataxia and, even more rarely, those with exceedingly early forms of Friedreich's ataxia show hypotonia and subsequent incoordination when they begin to reach, sit, stand, or walk. Pneumoencephalography, sometimes justified by the lack of clear clinical definition and the severity of symptoms, may disclose cerebellar dysplasia.

"Systemic" Causes

Limpness without motor paralysis is a presenting or accompanying feature of many other disorders seen in children. These include the following:

A. Malnutrition: *Examples:* Nutritional deprivation, cystic fibrosis, celiac disease, scurvy, rickets.

B. Debilitating Diseases: *Examples:* Severe infections; congenital heart, lung, and renal diseases.

C. Metabolic Disorders: *Examples:* Infantile hypercalcemia, hypophosphatasia.

D. Endocrinopathies: *Examples:* Hypothyroidism, adrenocortical hyperfunction, gonadal dysgenesis (Turner's syndrome), hypotonia-hypogonadal-obesity (HHO) syndrome of Prader-Willi.

E. Familial dysautonomia (of Riley-Day).

Heritable Disorders of Connective Tissue

Children with osteogenesis imperfecta, Marfan's syndrome, Ehlers-Danlos syndrome, and congenital laxity of ligaments, besides being floppy, are often "double-jointed" or "rubber-jointed." The first 3 disorders present characteristic pictures discussed elsewhere. The last condition is entirely benign.

Essential Hypotonia

Floppy infants who do not fall into the previously mentioned categories are often classified as having "essential" or, less properly, "benign congenital" hypotonia. This is, perforce, a diagnosis of exclusion, made less and less frequently as diagnostic acumen and technics improve. In essential hypotonia, the family history is usually negative. The muscles show no atrophy or fasciculations; tendon reflexes may be present, diminished, or absent. Respiratory difficulties are encountered occasionally. "Immaturity" of the motor end plates has been offered as a possible cause of the condition. Muscle biopsy, which should include special stains and electron microscopy, may show either no pathologic features or universally small fibers without histochemical or connective tissue changes. The outlook is for partial to full recovery in well over 50% of children so reported.

Abroms IF & others: Cervical cord injuries secondary to hyperextension of the head in breech presentations. Obstet Gynecol 41:369, 1973.

Clay SA & others: Acute infantile motor unit disorder: Infantile botulism? Arch Neurol 34:246, 1977.

Dubowitz V: *The Floppy Infant.* Clinics in Developmental Medicine No. 31. Heinemann, 1969.

Paunier L & others: Spinal muscular dystrophy with various clinical manifestations in a family. Helv Paediatr Acta 28:19, 1973.

PSEUDOTUMOR CEREBRI
(Benign Intracranial Hypertension, Serous Meningitis, Meningeal Hydrops, Otitic Hydrocephalus, Toxic Hydrocephalus)

Essentials of Diagnosis

- Symptoms and signs of increased intracranial pressure.
- Normal or small ventricular system.

General Considerations

By definition, the diagnosis of pseudotumor cerebri can be made only by excluding intracranial disorders which result in significant distortion, displacement, or enlargement of the ventricular system.

Pseudotumor cerebri, as reflected in its many synonyms, may be due to or associated with any of the following: (1) Inflammatory processes such as mastoiditis and lateral sinus obstruction (more often on the right than the left), poliomyelitis, Landry-Guillain-Barré syndrome, head trauma, Schilder's diffuse sclerosis, and other demyelinating disorders. (2) Encephalopathies such as lead poisoning, hypo- or hypervitaminosis A, or toxicity due to tetracyclines or nalidixic acid, cystic fibrosis and other chronic lung disorders. (3) Endocrinopathies such as hypocalcemia, Addison's disease, functional hyperpituitarism (perhaps); menstrual dysfunctions, including menarche, pregnancy, and galactorrhea. (4) Prolonged corticosteroid therapy, especially with triamcinolone, usually during withdrawal. (5) Enzyme deficiency such as galactokinase.

Clinical Findings

A. Symptoms and Signs: The presenting symptoms are nonspecific and nonlocalizing: headache, vomiting, blurred vision, photophobia, diplopia, dizziness, tinnitus, incoordination, drowsiness and stupor, and, rarely, convulsions.

On physical examination, signs of the causative or associated disorder may be present. Neurologic findings, in order of frequency, are papilledema, abducens nerve palsies, nystagmus, ataxia, pyramidal tract signs, and central or peripheral facial weakness. Visual acuity and visual fields should be evaluated in any child whose cooperation can be gained and whose intelligence and age (often as early as 3–4 years) permit reliable testing.

B. Laboratory Findings: Studies should be guided by the clinical suspicion of the causes previously mentioned. Lumbar puncture may be performed if the ventricles are normal or small, both to measure and to reduce the elevated CSF pressure. The CSF is acellular, and protein and glucose are normal.

C. X-Ray Findings: X-rays of the mastoid sinuses, chest, and abdomen and a skeletal survey may provide diagnostic information.

D. Neurodiagnostic Studies: As discussed in the section on tumors of the CNS, tests to rule out a space-occupying intracranial lesion include skull x-rays, computerized tomography (CT) scan, and EEG before proceeding to definitive contrast studies. The EEG is normal or slightly slow. In nonlocalized increased intracranial pressure, the CT scan is the procedure of choice to demonstrate the presence or absence of hydrocephalus. Especially when the ventricles are small, as is often the case in pseudotumor cerebri, ventriculography may be difficult to perform; hence, if contrast studies are deemed necessary to supplement the CT scan, right retrograde brachial angiography and fractional pneumoencephalography may be considered.

Treatment

Specific associated conditions are treated appropriately.

In patients receiving corticosteroids, a temporary increase in dosage may succeed in alleviating symptoms, after which very gradual withdrawal may be initiated.

Measures aimed at reducing CSF pressure generally are of transient value. In a child with intractable headache, vomiting, and other somatic complaints, lumbar puncture with removal of sufficient CSF to lower initial pressure by 50% may be of benefit. Acetazolamide and hyperosmolar diuretics have offered no benefit, but glycerol and furosemide have been said to be of value.

Visual acuity should be determined at frequent intervals. If there is loss of acuity or if the disorder is present in a young child (in whom visual acuity is difficult to measure) with long-standing increased intracranial pressure, subtemporal decompression should be considered.

Prognosis

Pseudotumor cerebri is usually a self-limited condition with no residua. Careful follow-up is recommended since some cases recur or a brain tumor eventually becomes manifest.

Greer M: Benign intracranial hypertension (pseudotumor cerebri). Pediatr Clin North Am 14:819, 1967.

HYPOXIC ENCEPHALOPATHY

Essentials of Diagnosis

- Disturbance of neurologic status.
- Any situation resulting in decreased oxygen to brain.

General Considerations

Hypoxic encephalopathy may be due to any one of the 4 types of hypoxia, given here in order of frequency: (1) *hypoxic,* due to reduction in the availability of oxygen to tissues due to a decrease in the partial pressure of oxygen (P_{O_2}) in the arterial blood, as in respiratory difficulties (eg, asphyxiation), interference

with gas exchange in the lungs, or arteriovenous shunting; (2) *stagnant,* with reduction of available oxygen due to slowed circulation, as in local brain edema or circulatory failure (cardiac arrest); (3) *anemia,* with reduced oxygen-carrying capacity of the blood, as in anemic hemorrhage or carbon monoxide poisoning; and (4) *histotoxic,* with a reduction of oxygen utilization by tissues due to interference with cellular metabolism, as in certain poisonings (eg, glutethimide [Doriden], propoxyphene [Darvon], or cyanide) or in connection with certain metabolic disorders.

The clinical spectrum of hypoxic encephalopathy and sequelae involves 3 major factors: (1) the nature of the hypoxic process, (2) the neurologic status of the patient prior to the hypoxic episode, and (3) the rapidity of onset, severity, and duration of hypoxia.

Clinical Findings

A. Symptoms and Signs: Mild hypoxia causes headache, troubles in mentation, drowsiness, confusion, listlessness or restlessness, apathy or hyperirritability, and, rarely, delirium.

Moderate hypoxia of gradual onset, allowing cerebral blood flow or the hemoglobin to increase, allows the manifestations just mentioned to be mild and soon to disappear; the symptoms are common when one first moves to a higher altitude.

Severe hypoxia of sudden onset and lasting 1–3 minutes manifests itself by profound disturbance of cerebral function, including loss of consciousness, convulsions, decorticate and decerebrate posturing, often high fever, and rapid evolution of papilledema. If the patient recovers from the immediate episode, he may exhibit true or psychic blindness, aphasia, spasticity, rigidity, choreo-athetotic or pill-rolling movements, and abnormal reflexes such as snouting, sucking, and forced grasp. Seizures are often a continuous problem.

Hypoxia of abrupt onset, marked severity, and lasting 3 or more minutes may result in failure to regain consciousness as well as severe cerebral edema. If the patient survives, he may progress from hypotonic and hyporeflexic to spastic. Such an episode often leads to irreversible brain damage, with medullary compression and accompanying cardiac and respiratory failure.

B. Laboratory Findings: Blood gases and serum electrolytes should be obtained as soon as possible. Blood levels for toxins should be examined as indicated. A chest x-ray and ECG should be obtained as soon as feasible. EEGs can be delayed.

The CSF may be under increased pressure and, with sufficient tissue damage, show an increase in protein.

Differential Diagnosis

The history of a hypoxic episode establishes the diagnosis. In the absence of such history, hypoglycemic and toxic encephalopathies must be considered. Aspiration of foreign bodies by young children, causing respiratory obstruction, is frequently missed.

Complications

As in any comatose patient, aspiration pneumonitis, infections, electrolyte and fluid imbalances, decubitus ulcers, and contractures may occur. Stress ulcers occur infrequently in children.

Treatment

A. Specific Measures: Prompt reversal of specific causes, eg, removal of a patient from a source of carbon monoxide or extraction of a foreign body, is obviously of urgent importance. Blood gases, fluids, and electrolytes must be monitored closely. Emergency care, treatment of cerebral edema, and antibiotic therapy are discussed in the sections on altered states of consciousness and head trauma.

B. Anticonvulsants: (For treatment of status epilepticus, see Seizure Disorders.) Prophylactic phenytoin (Dilantin), 10 mg/kg IV immediately, followed 6—8 hours later by the maintenance dose of 7 mg/kg IV, IM, or orally daily, is advised because of the frequency of seizures as a sequel to hypoxic encephalopathy. Seizures may cause further brain damage. If the patient recovers neurologically intact, without seizures and with a normal EEG, anticonvulsant therapy may be gradually discontinued. *Note:* Exercise caution in using paraldehyde in cases of severe pulmonary involvement or pneumonias. Barbiturates should be avoided because they involve a risk of further depression of the CNS.

C. Chronic Care: Respiratory toilet, maintenance of nutrition via a nasogastric or gastrostomy tube if necessary, proper skin, bladder, and bowel care, and early physical therapy are often required.

Prognosis

Mild hypoxia usually ends in rapid recovery without sequelae. However, the so-called "minimal brain dysfunction syndrome" has been ascribed to milder hypoxic episodes, especially when these occurred during birth or in early infancy.

Moderately severe hypoxia, particularly if it developed relatively slowly, may result in good recovery, especially in the neonate. The effects of severe hypoxia, however, are often not appreciated in infants for a few weeks or months, after which delayed psychomotor development, microcephaly, spasticity, sometimes choreo-athetosis and ataxia, and frequently seizures become manifest.

Moderately severe hypoxia of acute onset after the neonatal period may be followed by a period of apparent improvement for 1—10 days. The patient may then deteriorate and be permanently impaired mentally and neurologically.

Once there is evidence of medullary compression, with slow irregular respirations, irregular cardiac activity, loss of doll's eye movements and ciliospinal reflexes, fixed pupils, and often flaccidity with absence of deep reflexes but bilateral extensor responses, the prognosis for recovery is extremely poor.

Schneck SA: *Cerebral Anoxia in Clinical Neurology.* Baker AB (editor). Hoeber, 1972.

CONGENITAL NYSTAGMUS & SPASMUS NUTANS

Two benign types of spontaneous pendular horizontal nystagmus are congenital (familial) nystagmus and spasmus nutans. They are similar initially. Intermittent lateral nodding or tilting of the head is seen in both types; strong light inhibits the nystagmus. Strabismus, neurologic and EEG abnormalities, and a family history of nystagmus, more frequent than in controls, suggest organic causes.

Congenital nystagmus, usually of both eyes, is noted—often as an isolated finding—at or shortly after birth. The family history is often positive, and the disorder may be transmitted as a dominant or an X-linked recessive (hence more common in boys).

Spasmus nutans tends to appear in the third or fourth month as the triad of nystagmus affecting predominantly (or only) one eye (more often the left), head nodding, and head tilting. Sex distribution is equal. Although familial cases are reported, the mode of transmission is not known. Disturbances of the mother-child relationship, nutrition, illumination (room darkness), teething, illness, and trauma are no longer considered to be causative or contributing factors.

The differential diagnosis includes serious causes of nystagmus (often "searching" in type) due to impaired vision as from chorioretinitis, optic atrophy, or optic nerve or cerebellar tumors. Irregular jerking of both eyes may be the principal manifestation of a seizure disorder or part of the polymyoclonia-opsoclonus syndrome.

The passage of time defines congenital nystagmus as permanent. Spasmus nutans is self-limiting, ceasing between the second and fifth year in three-fourths of infants without and in one-third of those with associated strabismus or other neurologic abnormalities.

Therapy is directed at any treatable neurologic disorder and correction of strabismus. Congenital nystagmus and spasmus nutans, being benign, require—in addition to diagnosis—reassurance of the parents. Epileptic nystagmus responds to phenobarbital or phenytoin.

Jayalakshmi P & others: Infantile nystagmus: A prospective study of spasmus nutans, congenital nystagmus, and unclassified nystagmus of infancy. J Pediatr 77:177, 1970.

Kelley TW: Optic glioma presenting as spasmus nutans. Pediatrics 45:295, 1970.

White JC: Epileptic nystagmus. Epilepsia 12:157, 1971.

● ● ● ●

General References

Chusid JG: *Correlative Neuroanatomy & Functional Neurology*, 16th ed. Lange, 1976.

Ford FR: *Diseases of the Nervous System in Infancy, Childhood and Adolescence*, 5th ed. Thomas, 1966.

Matson DD: *Neurosurgery of Infancy and Childhood*, 2nd ed. Thomas, 1969.

Menkes JH: *Textbook of Child Neurology*. Lea & Febiger, 1974.

Swaiman KF, Wright FS (editors): *The Practice of Pediatric Neurology*. Mosby, 1975.

22...
Developmental Problems of Childhood

Harold P. Martin, MD

This chapter deals with the common developmental problems of childhood that may confront the practicing physician. It thus includes not only the child with apparent neurologic dysfunction but also the child who may not be able to do things that other children of the same age do—eg, walk, talk, endure separation from the mother at school age. The child may just "seem different," eg, may be less active, even apathetic, with "strange" ways of relating to the examiner or to parents or age-mates. There may or may not be physical findings of note. The following list of disorders that must be included in the differential diagnosis should account for well over 95%·of such children the physician who takes pediatric patients may encounter in daily practice.

(1) Mental retardation of primary biologic origin.

(2) Mental retardation of primary environmental origin.

(3) Motor disability ranging in degree from minimal neurologic dysfunction to cerebral palsy.

(4) Sensory or perceptual disability.

(5) Language delay or deviation.

(6) Learning disability; in older children, school learning problems.

(7) Personality deviation or impaired parent-child interaction.

(8) Normal child; not truly "deviant."

IDENTIFICATION OF PATIENTS WITH DEVELOPMENTAL PROBLEMS

In most cases the child's deviation from the norm comes to the attention of the alert clinician during routine well child visits. The first clues are derived from historical data and a physical examination that includes assessment of developmental skills. The parents may come to the office expressing specific concern about the child's development. The increasing use of routine developmental screening devices such as the Denver Developmental Screening Test (DDST) (see Chapter 2) has resulted in the early identification of many children at risk. Screening tests are also now increasingly administered by nonclinicians such as welfare workers and personnel at day care centers and preschool nurseries. Children who "fail" such tests should be brought to the family physician or pediatrician for further evaluation.

A fourth means of identifying children who may be developmentally handicapped is the close scrutiny of children at high biologic or social risk of developmental disability.

Children identified as having or suspected of having developmental problems should first be given an appropriate screening test by the physician whether or not such a test has already been performed by someone else. It may be clear from the history or the physical examination that the child's development is significantly delayed in some area. Nonetheless, a developmental screening test or battery of tests is necessary to give the clinician information about other areas of development. For example, the infant may be slow in motor milestones, and that may be the parents' only concern, but the clinician must assess that child's level of achievement in the interrelated areas of language, problem-solving, personality functioning, and sensory skills. Developmental screening must of course always be accompanied by a meticulous history and physical examination.

EVALUATION FOR DEVELOPMENTAL DISABILITIES

History

A. Past Medical History: The history of the pregnancy, labor, and delivery should include such factors as excessive or minimal weight gain, exposure to radiation, infections, medications, threatened or attempted abortion, preeclampsia-eclampsia, inadequate prenatal care, excessively rapid or prolonged labor, heavy sedation, and abnormal fetal presentation. The history of the newborn baby's sleep pattern, feeding history, and energy level may provide clues to early CNS damage. Significant events after the newborn period include unexplained high fevers, trauma, severe infections, inadequate nutrition, and other serious medical problems.

B. Family History: The physician must determine by skillful and considerate questioning whether there is any family history of mental disability or any condition or disease associated with retardation. For the purpose of assessing the child's genetic endowment, it is helpful to know of siblings, uncles, aunts, or cousins of the parents who were stillborn or died in infancy before a diagnosis of retardation could be made. Complete obstetric information about the mother is essential, including questions about abortions, relative infertility, and difficulties with previous pregnancies, all of which may have a bearing upon biologic ability to support a pregnancy.

C. Developmental History: A record of prior developmental milestones helps to clarify the degree of disability. A change in the rate of development may provide a clue to the time of postnatal neurologic damage. The baby book, if available, is a useful means of objectively assessing early developmental landmarks such as smiling, reaching, and turning over.

D. Records: Prenatal and nursery records on mother and child often suggest causative factors not elicited in the history taken from the parents. Apgar scores, length of gestation, newborn head circumference, and nurses' observations of the newborn are important facts that parents are rarely able to recall. In older children, school records should be requested and should include reports of teachers' observations and any testing done by school personnel. Evaluations by other professionals should be reviewed.

Physical Examination

The emphasis in physical examination is on neurologic function, including head circumference, transillumination of the skull, ophthalmoscopic examination through dilated pupils, strabismus, and amblyopia. Subtle signs not historically considered as part of a classical neurologic examination are helpful, eg, grasping patterns, quality of motor performance, and development of early reflex behavior such as equilibrium and balance. Hearing and vision must be assessed more carefully than in a child who is developing normally. If there are any doubts about hearing and vision, appropriate consultation should be obtained. Auditory disorders are often confused with retardation. Audiograms and complete ophthalmologic examinations should be routinely performed on all children with suspected developmental or learning disabilities. The complete examination should include special attention to minor congenital anomalies such as abnormal palmar creases, syndactyly, malformations of the ears, and other facial abnormalities. Although any one specific minor congenital anomaly may occur in the normal population, the risk of CNS maldevelopment or damage during the prenatal period is quite high in any child who has more than 2 or 3 minor congenital anomalies.

The physical examination also provides an opportunity for the clinician to assess the behavior of the child, both with the examiner and with the parent. Unusual anxiety or an indifference to people or aberrations of the child's investment and attachment to the parents are usually spotted easily.

Laboratory Examination

Laboratory examination of the child (other than routine blood and urine studies if not done recently) should only be ordered on the basis of clinical indications.

Family Assessment

The physician should determine how the family views the child—what their questions are—how they perceive the difficulty—and how the family functions in relation to the child, especially if the family sees the child as completely normal or "just lazy." There are many misconceptions about retardation, eg, that all retarded children should be institutionalized or that they will sexually act out, be delinquent, or stop learning at some specific age. Unspoken concerns about heritable diseases, the part either parent may have played in causing the problem, and the effect on the siblings are often present. The physician must determine whether the parents need more extensive counseling to assist them in accepting their defective child and planning constructively for care of the child.

The family assessment should include a conclusion about why the family is bringing the child to the physician at this time for this complaint. The physician should be alert for "hidden agendas," ie, the "real" reason for the parents' visit to the doctor at this time may actually be marital discord, breakdown of parent-child interaction, guilt over one's role as a parent, pressure from relatives, or unhappiness in one or both parents. If the physician is oblivious to these factors, the parent may be unsatisfied with the physician's procedures and recommendations. In practice, parents may or may not be immediately aware of these underlying problems. Frequently, however, they may reveal the actual nature of the difficulty when they talk with more intensity or feeling about their most immediate pressing concerns than about the developmental history of the child. The physician may also elicit information about any underlying reasons for the visit by inquiring how the parents' concern about the child's developmental problems has affected them.

Evaluation in a Natural Setting

There are several important reasons why an evaluation should include observation of the child at home or in school. Anxiety or fear of the office setting may preclude adequate developmental screening or a satisfactory physical examination. The child may simply refuse to do many tasks, especially those involving gross motor skills or language. The physician then does not know whether the child is incapable of performing the task or is simply refusing to comply. Before further diagnostic testing is undertaken, a nurse, nurse practitioner, or child health associate from the medical office should spend time in the home observing the child. In some instances, a visit to a preschool nursery may be better than a home visit. Such observation can usually provide information about language skills, problem-solving tasks, relations with age-mates, and gross motor function. At these visits a developmental screening test or neurologic examination can often be completed where this was not possible in the physician's office.

Developmental Consultation With Other Professionals

In some patients, development is clearly abnormal but the exact nature of the developmental problem is not clear. In such cases, appropriate consultation should be obtained. If the child's behavior seems unusual or bizarre, consultation with a child psychologist or psychiatrist should help determine whether or not a psychic disturbance may be responsible for aberrant development. A speech pathologist can contribute to the diagnosis of problems leading to abnormal speech and language. Social workers are particularly helpful in assessing complex family relationships and in locating sources of assistance and treatment available in the community. Physical and occupational therapists, public health nurses, and specialists in neurology, orthopedics, ophthalmology, and developmental pediatrics can also help the primary physician in evaluating and managing the developmentally disabled child. It is helpful to compile a listing of these sources of assistance.

Perhaps the most common type of consultation required lies in the field of developmental or intelligence testing. Few primary care physicians have either the training or the inclination to administer detailed intelligence or developmental tests and should therefore depend on a child psychologist or specialist in developmental pediatrics for the administration and interpretation of such tests.

Consultation with an interdisciplinary child development clinic is sometimes indicated, particularly when the abnormality has many causes, thus making it necessary to obtain the help of several professionals.

DIFFERENTIAL DIAGNOSIS

Mental Retardation Having a Primary Biologic Basis

A. Evaluation: Mental retardation has been defined by the American Association on Mental Deficiency as "significantly subaverage general intellectual functioning existing concurrently with deficits in adaptive behavior and manifested during the developmental period." This definition includes both those children whose intellectual deficits are a result of biologic damage and those whose function is handicapped by adverse social circumstances. It should be noted that the definition also includes any handicap in "adaptive function," eg, in personal independence, social responsibility, and ability to cope in society. Thus, a child may have normal intelligence despite the presence of a disability such as blindness or cerebral palsy that impedes adaptive behavior. Conversely, mental retardation cannot be diagnosed exclusively on the basis of an IQ test, especially if the child is coping quite normally in the areas of personal skills and social interaction. It

should also be stressed that some deficits influence a wide range of intellectual functions.

Mental retardation cannot be established on the basis of a screening test alone but will require a complete developmental history, physical examination, and full testing of intellectual abilities. As noted above, detailed developmental and intelligence testing will usually require examination by a clinical specialist in child psychology or developmental pediatrics, who must interpret the test results for the referring physician.

A low score on an IQ test may have any number of explanations: the child may be having seizures; may not see or hear well; may be ill or feverish; may be frightened and anxious; may be mute; or may be handicapped by cultural orientation of the test that is different from that of the child. Mental retardation is but one of several hypothetical explanations for poor performance on any intelligence test, although mental retardation may indeed be the most common reason for a low IQ score. The consultant and the referring primary physician together must then decide on a reason for the child's subaverage performance. The history, physical examination, and data about the child's performance in other settings and situations must all be evaluated in formulating the diagnosis.

A diagnosis of biologically based retardation rests on exclusion of other physiologic causes of retarded function such as sensory deficit or frequent seizures; exclusion of nonbiologic causes of retardation such as emotional deprivation or emotional disorder; and a careful search for biologic origin of the retardation. Biologic bases might include one of the following categories:

(1) Following infection or intoxication: Includes prenatal infections such as rubella, toxoplasmosis, and cytomegalic inclusion disease; postnatal infections, especially encephalitis and meningitis. Intoxication includes preeclampsia and hyperbilirubinemia.

(2) Following trauma or physical agent: Prenatal, perinatal or postnatal injuries, including child abuse; anoxia.

(3) Metabolic and nutritional disorders: Undernutrition; various metabolic disorders such as aminoacidopathies, mucopolysaccharidoses, glycogen storage diseases, and endocrine disorders.

(4) Gross brain disease of postnatal period: Neoplasms and heredodegenerative disorders, eg, tuberous sclerosis, leukodystrophy.

(5) Prenatal influence: Cerebral malformations of unknown cause, hydrocephalus, primary microcephaly, and other malformations.

(6) Chromosomal abnormality: New staining technics and automated karyotyping are greatly increasing the specificity and ease of detecting chromosomal lesions.

(7) Gestational disorders: Prematurity, small-for-gestational-age babies, and postmature babies.

A specific cause can be cited in probably only 60% of cases of mental retardation. There are many children with mental retardation in whom the clinician will only be able to pinpoint the timing and not the cause of the brain damage. Nonetheless, this pinpointing of the timing of brain damage may be quite helpful to the parents in eliminating other fantasized causes of damage and may also be helpful in genetic counseling.

Extensive laboratory testing is not necessary in the evaluation of the retarded child. In addition to a current urinalysis and blood count, the only other routine examinations recommended are urine and serum amino acid assays. In children under age 18 months whose retardation is of unexplained origin, blood studies for rubella, cytomegalovirus disease, and toxoplasmosis should be performed. Other laboratory tests are performed if findings in the history and physical examination suggest a specific disease. Some of these tests and the indications for them are as follows:

1. EEG—An EEG will not help in determining whether or not the child is retarded. However, it should be considered when there is a possibility of a seizure disorder or of a focal or structural abnormality of the brain.

2. Skull films—Skull films should be obtained in microcephalic children, in cases of an abnormally shaped skull, or in cases of suspected prenatal infections. Evidence of calcification should be sought.

3. Thyroid studies—Thyroid studies should be performed in the presence of retardation of unknown cause accompanying any other symptom associated with hypothyroidism, such as hypotonia or failure to thrive. Serum TSH determination is the best test but is not always as readily available as the T_4.

4. Chromosomal analysis—Chromosomal analysis is indicated if the child has an unusual appearance, if there is a family history of a disorder which could be chromosomal, if there are 2 or more minor anomalies in the retarded child, or if the clinical picture fits known chromosomal syndromes such as Down's syndrome. As improved laboratory identification of subtle abnormalities such as small translocations becomes easier, parents and siblings of the affected child should also be offered chromosomal analysis for the purpose of genetic counseling.

B. Causes: In assessing the causes of mental retardation, the following priorities should be considered:

(1) Causes which are treatable, eg, hypothyroidism, phenylketonuria, subdural hematoma.

(2) Causes which have significance in genetic counseling, eg, chromosomal abnormality.

(3) Syndromes, or disease entities in which the prognosis is known. A specific syndrome may suggest associated defects, eg, cardiac disease in children with a history of congenital rubella.

(4) Degenerative diseases such as leukodystrophy or glycogen storage disease.

It is easier for parents to accept a diagnosis of retardation when a cause can be identified. This knowledge should help in overcoming the defense of denial, in relieving feelings of guilt, and in expunging the parents' fantasies about what might have gone wrong to damage the child's brain.

C. Management:

1. Specific causes, if any, should be treated (eg, phenylketonuria).

2. The child's condition, prognosis, and needs should be explained to the parents so that they will understand what they can do to help, what they should refrain from doing, what they can hope for, and what they need not fear.

3. Routine medical care is essential because many mentally retarded children are especially susceptible to infection, accidents, and other medical and surgical disorders.

4. Counsel the parents. It is essential that the physician or an appointed delegate meet with the parents on a regular basis (every few months during the child's infancy and once or twice a year thereafter) without the child present, to discuss the child's progress and problems, the effect of the child on the family, and future concerns. The family will need much help from the physician in the first few weeks of working through their grief and pain at having a handicapped child.

5. Stimulate the intellectual abilities of the retarded child. Most retarded children are capable of functioning better than they do. They require more cognitive stimulation than the average child as they are usually less curious and venturesome, and they need more repetition and practice to master skills. This stimulation can be provided by the parents but should be supplemented quite early by enrollment in an organized day care center or preschool or homebound infant stimulation program for the developmentally disabled. The local Association for Retarded Citizens (ARC) or appropriate state health and education agencies will be able to provide information about special programs for handicapped children.

6. The Association for Retarded Citizens (ARC) is composed principally of parents of mentally retarded children. These men and women can offer emotional support, can suggest or provide useful reading materials, and can share practical solutions to common problems such as getting baby-sitters, using local resources, etc.

7. Consider institutionalization only when it is absolutely necessary. Fewer than 1% of mentally retarded children belong in institutions for the retarded. Very few communities fail to offer the medical and educational resources the retarded child needs. If the presence of the retarded child in the family is causing significant hardship, foster home placement rather than institutionalization is preferable unless there are specific services the institution offers that are not available to a child living with a family. State institutions may perform special services such as taking the child for limited periods to give the family a respite from the stress of everyday care of the child, or they may help in modifying some types of behavior problems, eg, toilet training or dealing with temper tantrums.

8. The physician should continue to be available to the family over a protracted period. As the child

grows older, new problems will emerge relating to schooling, sexuality, reactions of siblings, etc. A physician who is available to the family for both medical and family problems will be able to anticipate difficulties and help the family deal with the acute and chronic stresses placed upon them by a handicapped child.

Mental Retardation Having an Environmental Basis

A child's intellect can be affected by environmental factors. Social and economic conditions affecting health and function are increasingly being recognized as a legitimate concern of physicians who treat children.

Environmental conditions that can result in retardation may be divided into 3 categories. The first is inadequate parenting, as shown in the deprived, neglected, or abused child. In the second category, parenting is good, but crowding, large family size, poor housing, and social stress do not allow adequate stimulation of the child. The third category is genetic susceptibility.

A. Inadequate Parenting: Spitz and others showed in the 1930s and 1940s that children in hospitals and foundling homes who were deprived of their mothers suffered death, marasmus, or mental retardation. Later, it was shown that children of mothers who were depressed, ill, or emotionally unavailable to their babies failed to show normal intellectual development. Silver in the mid 1960s pointed out the retardation and growth failure occurring in *deprivation dwarfism.* Since that time, numerous studies of deprivation and neglect have shown that mental retardation may result. More recently, studies have emphasized the psychologic and developmental wounds of the abused child.

The diagnosis of inadequate parenting requires the assistance of a professional in the mental health field except where deprivation is accompanied by obvious neglect of basic nutritional and medical care. It is usually the physician who first identifies or suspects this condition, and it is the physician's responsibility to raise this diagnostic possibility.

Management is difficult. The first priority is to try to improve parenting abilities and instill positive parental attitudes toward the child. If this is successful, the child can remain with the biologic parents. If not, social agencies and the judicial apparatus will participate with the physician in deciding whether the risk of retarded development is so great that the child must be removed from the biologic parents and be cared for by someone else.

B. Social and Economic Disadvantage: Eighty percent of mildly retarded children in the USA are members of the lowest socioeconomic classes. Biologic high-risk factors such as prematurity, difficult delivery, high-risk pregnancy, or low Apgar scores are significantly more liable to affect development in economically disadvantaged children. In fact, the income and educational level of the parents provide a better general prediction of the eventual IQ of infants than any presently known tests of development or intelligence

in young children. There are obvious exceptions: Children with Down's syndrome will have intellectual handicaps regardless of their home environment; conversely, a few children raised in adverse social conditions will escape the anticipated blunting of intellectual capacity. Nonetheless, most children who grow up with the stigma of retardation and learning disabilities are found in families with the lowest incomes and lowest level of parental education. It should be stressed that this disadvantage is not irrevocably foreordained, not genetic, and not irremediable.

A young retarded child with poor and uneducated parents confronts the physician with a dilemma. Biologic causes must be sought as noted above. The physician must exercise caution in assuming that the functional retardation can be explained solely on the basis of some high-risk event such as prematurity, because it has been shown that in another socioeconomic class the retardation would not result. A number of stimulation programs show that such children will often develop normally if they receive additional cognitive stimulation.

The relationship between poverty and retardation is obviously complex. Nutrition and medical care of children in poverty-stricken areas may be so inadequate that the risk of biologic causes of brain damage is increased. Schools geared to serve the middle class and intelligence tests that measure culturally acquired attributes which are then scored as "intelligence" often mislabel poor children as mentally retarded who have the potential for normal or above-normal achievement. It can be argued that genetically inferior adults tend to be less competitive in the job market and thus may be overrepresented in the lowest economic classes. However, when young infants from the lowest socioeconomic class are given the benefit of stimulation programs or are adopted into families in better circumstances, their intellectual abilities and learning skills frequently are found to be within the normal range.

Treatment consists of enrolling the child in a Head Start or other cognitive stimulation program.

C. Genetic Disorders: What has been called genetically based mental retardation does not usually have a truly genetic foundation. There are numerous recent studies showing normal or superior abilities in children who, according to the family history, could be assumed to be genetically inferior. Twin studies and adoption studies also point out the dangers inherent in overemphasizing genetic endowment. The often limited intellectual abilities of parents of mentally retarded children are usually not a *genetic* deficit but rather are part of a whole matrix of suboptimal family and social conditions. Recognition of this fact led to the establishment of Head Start centers a decade ago. Early assessment of the results of such programs showed that the gains of children in the programs tended to disappear during the early years at public school. More recent studies show that this need not occur and may be prevented by reaching the children earlier, ie, before age 3–4 years.

The physician should not automatically assume

that there is a genetic basis for impaired intelligence in infants and children whose parents have been shown to be limited in intelligence by the results of traditional middle-class intelligence tests. Such parents can provide excellent parenting. Assistance that tries to improve cognitive stimulation for the child both at home and at alternative sites such as preschool and day care centers will result in normal intellectual development by a majority of such children.

Sensory Deficits

Vision and hearing deficits in infancy still go undiagnosed, and most of these children are thus erroneously thought to be mentally retarded, whereas the real cause of developmental delays and problems is sensory loss rather than intellectual impairment. As more newborns survive, child development clinics are treating increasing numbers of infants with visual loss due to retrolental fibroplasia, which results from high concentrations of oxygen used in the treatment of premature infants. Nonetheless, screening for hearing and vision is still overlooked in many nurseries and at many well baby examinations.

A baby in the first month of life should be able to focus on a bright object or light and follow a moving object at least 90 degrees. By age 3–4 months, the child can see and focus for extended periods on objects as small as a raisin. Babies in the first month of life will react to a moderately loud sound by a quieting reaction, a Moro reflex (startle reaction), or a change in facial expression. Well before age 6 months, the baby will turn toward a voice and localize other sounds. Chapter 11 discusses detection and management of children with auditory loss.

One type of auditory loss that deserves emphasis is a mild (20–40 dB) loss, chiefly of high-frequency sounds. The parents will usually not suspect that the child has a hearing loss, and such a child will frequently perform well enough to pass the screening test performed by the physician. This mild handicap frequently results in articulation disorders or in speech and language delays of mild to moderate degree. Hence, any child with a significant articulation disorder or one whose speech and language are delayed in the presence of normal development in other areas should be referred to an audiologist for thorough hearing assessment.

There has not been adequate emphasis on the urgent need for special stimulation and early special educational help for children with severe visual and auditory deficits. In most states of the USA, state agencies sponsor special programs for the deaf and blind, which should be started in infancy. These handicapped children need above-average parenting to ensure sufficient cognitive and personality development.

Especially for the blind child, early developmental or intellectual testing by an experienced clinical psychologist or developmental pediatrician is indicated because blind children reach developmental milestones later than sighted children. They are slower in turning toward sounds, walking, and talking. In order to avoid an unjustified diagnosis of mental retardation, the physician must be aware of the differing patterns of development of children with sensory deficits.

Some children whose sensory end organs for sight, hearing, and somatosensory stimuli (touch, kinesthesia, proprioception) are intact can receive and transmit stimuli received by those end organs but cannot appreciate and understand what is seen, heard, or felt. The degree of such "perceptual handicaps" may vary enormously.

Motor Delays & Deviations

Most parents know when a baby should roll over, sit, stand, and walk. However, they usually do not know when a child might be expected to transfer objects from hand to hand, develop consonant sounds, know colors, or understand prepositions. The development of the infant will therefore be assessed by parents and physician primarily on the basis of motor development.

There are 2 facets of motor development to be assessed by the physician. The first is motor skill acquisition: When does the child accomplish a particular skill, eg, rolling over, walking, running, negotiating stairs, riding a tricycle? The second aspect of motor development is the *quality* of the child's motor acts: Is the child as coordinated in motor movements as other children of the same age? An illustration of this aspect would be the recognition that although a child may be walking unaided by age 12–16 months, the gait may be abnormal (eg, wide-based or unsteady) or asymmetric.

The most obvious neuromotor disability is *cerebral palsy*. This is an anatomically nonprogressive motor disability present at birth or appearing shortly thereafter. The hallmark of cerebral palsy is abnormality of muscle tone. Although the most common type (spasticity) involves hypertonicity, almost as common is the child who has erratic or fluctuating tone. The physician should also look carefully for signs of abnormal reflex development. There are 2 types of reflexive behavior that require assessment.

First are automatisms of the infant: the Moro, grasp, tonic, and labyrinthine reflexes and the asymmetric tonic neck, symmetric tonic neck, trunk incurvation, and crossed extension responses. Although each of these reflex behaviors has a slightly different time course, it is reasonable to expect all of these infantile reflexes to have disappeared by age 4–6 months. When they are retained, there is a delay in maturation of the CNS or outright damage to the brain. These reflexes are frequently present in the child with cerebral palsy and may interfere with normal function as much as or more than the abnormality of tone or the tremors, athetosis, or choreiform movements.

The second group of automatisms that must be assessed are those that should start to develop by age 8 months and be easily elicited by age 12 months. These include such reflexive behaviors as protective and righting responses, the Landau reflex, and the parachute reflex. When these are delayed, absent, or asymmetric,

CNS damage or maldevelopment should be suspected.

The role of the physical therapist is chiefly to help parents learn how to handle and position the child with cerebral palsy more easily. There remains a place for passive exercises to prevent contractures; however, it must be stressed that exercises alone are inadequate treatment. Various approaches to treatment have been developed to deal with different types of cerebral palsy, but in no case has the superiority of one method over another been documented. The child with cerebral palsy can be helped to learn to develop equilibrium and balance. Reflexes that interfere with motor function (such as an asymmetric tonic neck) can be eliminated, or the child can learn alternative ways of performing motor acts so that the reflex will not interfere. As well as the real assistance in motor function provided by good physical therapy, there is the additional benefit to the parents in having something concrete to do that may help their child. If the physician fails to provide positive programs for handicapped children, the parents may seek out practitioners of discredited or unevaluated treatment regimens at great expense for essentially no result.

Infants with abnormalities or minor deviations from the norm in motor function and reflexive behavior are increasingly being identified early in the first year of life. The infant with a poorly organized or immature CNS may be irritable, difficult to hold, unable to mold well to the shoulder, and difficult to diaper, feed, and soothe. Early diagnosis with appropriate advice on special ways of soothing, feeding, and handling the baby can be most supportive.

The disorder of function in a child with cerebral palsy may be uneven and often progresses with age. The 6-month-old infant with cerebral palsy may be quite hypotonic and only later, between 12–24 months of age, develop spasticity or choreoathetosis. When the primary disability of the child is impaired equilibrium and balance, the disability in function will be noted most dramatically after the child attempts to walk. Motor disability that interferes with lucid speech will only be noted after the child has reached the age when clear speech is expected. Some children with many neurologic signs of neuromotor disability in infancy will appear almost normal in 1–2 years. The converse is also true.

The child with neuromotor dysfunction may have handicaps in other developmental areas, eg, intellect, sensory awareness, or language. The assessment of these other areas of development requires professionals who are experienced in the difficult task of evaluating the intelligence and learning abilities of physically handicapped children. All too often the child with a motor handicap is thought to be retarded in infancy because so few developmental landmarks are available for assessment, especially when the child's speech is handicapped by motor disability.

The need for a comprehensive educational setting for children with cerebral palsy and other motor disabilities deserves mention. Such educational programs, often sponsored by the Cerebral Palsy Association, provide necessary specific therapies and consultation with specialists in neurology and orthopedics and also offer an educational setting that directs attention toward cognitive development, socialization, and personality development.

Speech & Language Delays & Deviations

Delay in language development (see Chapter 2) is often the most striking symptom of almost any type of developmental deviation. Absence of language is one of the most prominent symptoms of autism and has been used as a prognostic sign, ie, if the autistic child has not developed language adequate for communication by age 5, the prognosis for recovery is very poor. In many types of brain damage, language is the most severely affected function. For example, in Down's syndrome, language is typically more delayed than any other area of development with the exception of gross motor skills, which are inversely related to the degree of hypotonia. Communication disorders are commonly delayed in older children with learning disabilities. There is also a remarkably high incidence of language disorders in children who have been abused and neglected. Thought disorders are manifested by bizarre and idiosyncratic communication patterns. A complete evaluation will necessarily screen for evidence of biologic, emotional, and social problems and for dysfunction in the parent-child relationship. A speech pathologist should assist the physician in establishing diagnosis and treatment.

One of the most common problems facing the private practitioner is the 3- to 5-year-old who has a mild delay in expressive speech or a mild-to-moderate articulation problem. Most commonly, there are no signs of retardation, sensory loss, emotional problems, or aberrant parent-child interactions. Most such children, if they are enrolled in preschool, will show a surge in language development within 6–8 months. It is often not clear why such a course of action results in acceleration in speech and language development; it may be modeling of age-mates, or it could be that other children and teachers will not understand or not tolerate nonverbal communications and poorly articulated speech. If there has been no acceleration in speech or language development in this time period, the child should be referred to a speech pathologist for therapy.

Learning Disabilities

The term learning disability denotes difficulty in learning academic subjects in a school setting when intelligence is normal and there are no gross signs of emotional disturbance, sensory deficit, emotional disadvantage, or motor handicap. Only children with serious emotional disturbance, mental retardation, or sensory handicap, especially of vision or hearing, should be excluded from this diagnostic category. Children with normal intelligence may have learning disabilities resulting from minimal brain dysfunction, mild emotional problems, social disadvantage, family dysfunction, or inappropriate and inadequate instruction. When parents present with a child and a complaint of inadequate learning, the first task is to assess the child's intelligence, vision, and hearing and to rule out serious emotional disturbances as the cause of failure to learn.

The physician's next responsibility is to diagnose or rule out a variety of physical, psychologic, and social causes of the disability. The educational system, however, and not the physician is responsible for the development of an appropriate educational program for the child.

A. Evaluation: In evaluating a child with school learning problems, physicians must be ready to vary their routine in order to achieve an understanding of the whole child. Office personnel should first obtain a signed release of information from the parents, and all pertinent data should be solicited from the school. This should include records of all testing that has been done, data from the school nurse and social worker or school psychologist, and the impressions and observations of the child's teachers. Most teachers will be reluctant to share sensitive information about the child or family in writing. It is therefore essential that the physician or someone in the office have a telephone conversation or interview with the teacher to elicit information that the physician might not be able to acquire in any other way. All pertinent records, including prenatal and newborn data as well as previous medical or developmental evaluations, should also be obtained.

The second step is to procure a careful neurologic, psychiatric, and social history. It is essential to obtain a developmental and family history from the parents when the child is not present. Both parents should be interviewed, and there are many occasions when it would be wise to see each one individually as well. They should be asked what they think might be the cause of the child's learning difficulty. Patterns of child rearing, parents' expectations of the child, and attitudes toward the child must be explored because deviations are commonly discovered that are either causing or exacerbating the child's problems at school. It is important to remember that most children with learning problems also have behavior problems. Frustrations over failure may lead to anger, overactivity, impulsiveness, confusion, and more failure. Not infrequently, learning disabilities are associated with marital strife, indifference, or overconcern on the part of the parents. These family and emotional reactions may be the cause of the learning disability or they may be the result, but identification and treatment are needed in either case.

In examining the child in the absence of the parents, it is possible to make an assessment of the child's intelligence and emotional status. The presence of any possible handicaps, chronic illnesses, or deviations of function which have been suggested by the history can now be confirmed by the physical examination.

CNS dysfunction or immaturity must be carefully investigated by the physician, who is the only profes-sional person able to confirm this diagnosis. In addition to the history, at least 30 minutes should be devoted to performing a detailed neurologic examination. The most common signs of CNS dysfunction associated with learning disabilities are as follows:

(1) Poor coordination of gross or fine motor skills.

(2) Delay in acquisition of motor skills.

(3) Poor ability to plan and execute a motor task (dyspraxia).

(4) Impaired ability to inhibit movement, as shown by associated movements, mirror movements, and fidgeting.

(5) Signs of neurologic immaturity, such as persistent tonic neck reflex, poor equilibrium, and righting reactions.

(6) Impaired somatosensory perception, as shown by tests of proprioception, stereognosis, 2-point tactile discrimination, graphesthesia (drawing on the skin of the child), or finger identification when touched (ie, the examiner touches a finger on the child's hand, and the child, with a finger of the other hand, indicates which finger was originally touched).

(7) Poor visual-motor integrative skills, which are assessed by having the child draw geometric forms, play catch with a ball, and imitate gestures of the examiner.

(8) Poor understanding and processing of auditory input, which are assessed informally or by having the child repeat digits or nonsense sounds.

(9) A driven hyperactivity, not related to stress or situation, which the child is unable to control.

(10) Mild hemiparesis (easily overlooked), suggested by differences in skills performed with the left and right sides or when there is lack of lateral preference by age 5 or lack of lateral dominance by age 7.

(11) Hyperactive deep tendon reflexes, tight heel cords, and ankle clonus.

(12) Poor eye tracking and poor control of tongue or oropharyngeal musculature.

(13) Symptoms or signs not specific to CNS dysfunction and which must therefore be differentiated from emotional instability, poor attention span, and a history of delayed language development.

The physician should undertake a careful screening for emotional problems that may be causing the learning disability or may be secondary to it. Some children in this category will actually be learning normally, ie, will have normal achievement test scores but poor grades. Another possible indication of an emotional basis for learning disabilities is a great deal of scatter on the child's performance in a spectrum of tests and subtests such as the Illinois Test of Psycholinguistic Abilities (ITPA), McCarthy's Scales of Children's Abilities, and the Wechsler Intelligence Scale for Children (WISC). It is especially important to assess the child's self-concept; self-deprecation may be shown by the things that the child says, by picture drawings, or by the child's daydreams, fantasies, or expectations of the future. Some children may mask their feelings of poor self-worth with a facade of bravado.

B. Management: The management of retardation, sensory handicap, and significant neuromusculature handicap is described elsewhere in this book. When these are responsible for the learning disability, their appropriate management should help alleviate the chief complaint. When the child's difficulty is due to inappropriate or inadequate school experiences or is based upon social or cultural differences arising from economic disadvantage, the physician must undertake the sensitive task of communicating this opinion to the school system. An overworked school staff may label such a child as "dumb," predelinquent, or unmotivated. School personnel may prefer to blame the child or each other for poor performance, even though everyone concerned is doing the best that can be done in difficult circumstances. The physician may be able to discern a pattern of isolated areas of normal or even superior adaptive behavior by the child outside the school, such as at home or in the neighborhood, and then use these perceptions in helping the child to build a foundation for better performance. Or the child's teachers may be urged to take the view that since poor prior schooling, low family income, minority status, or a disorganized family structure has caused the child to lag behind, the child consequently deserves special attention and a greater effort on the part of the school staff to find and capitalize on individual learning abilities and make certain that performance does not lag behind capacity.

The most important part of the treatment of children with CNS dysfunction is communication of the physician's findings to parents, teachers, and the children themselves. Parents and teachers must abandon their diagnoses of laziness, poor motivation, bad attitude, or emotional disorder. Above all, parents and children must not be allowed to view the problem as "brain damage" or defect. It should be explained to these children that some tasks and activities are simply more difficult for them than for other children but that they are not retarded, brain-damaged, lazy, or unworthy and that their nervous system functions in such a way that they find it difficult to perform certain tasks such as rapidly receiving and processing sensory information, screening out distracting visual, auditory, and tactile data, and performing motor tasks smoothly and effortlessly. These children will need special understanding and individual instructional approaches from their educators in order to acquire the knowledge and skills they need. The educators in the schools must then take up the challenge of finding how best to enable these children to learn.

If these children are hyperactive and other methods of controlling this symptom have failed, medications such as dextroamphetamine (Dexedrine) or methylphenidate (Ritalin) may help. When these medications are given to control hyperactivity, it is essential that the physician have the help of the teacher in monitoring any changes in behavior. A monthly checklist filled out by the teacher will be most helpful in making this assessment as regularly and as objectively as possible.

Children with minimal cerebral dysfunction, whether or not associated with learning disabilities, may require and benefit from specific help with their motor coordination through occupational or physical therapy. Speech and language therapy is also frequently needed. It is essential to note, however, that learning in school may not improve when children receive these therapies. Articulation, motor coordination, and perceptual-motor disabilities may improve, but academic performance may not. In many cases, disabilities in these areas are not the cause of the learning disability but are associated with it. Attempts to change handedness are of no value in the treatment of learning disabilities. Treatment of reading disabilities by eye exercises has not been shown to be beneficial. It is up to the physician and the educator to assess the symptoms, determine whether or not each symptom constitutes an impediment to learning, and decide whether that symptom needs treatment regardless of whether or not it is a direct cause of the learning disability.

Tactful discussion of the findings with these children can serve a therapeutic purpose. Children with school learning problems have a basis in reality for their poor self-concept. Teachers, parents, siblings, and age-mates may have reinforced such children's feelings of personal inadequacy. They must be helped to discard their fantasies about mental retardation, brain damage, babyishness, or basic unworthiness. Children of school age can be helped to understand the nature of their learning problems.

C. Educational Programs: The knowledge the physician has gained about the child's personality, neurologic status, and family—perhaps reinforced by consultation with other professionals—is invaluable when transmitted to an aware and competent educational staff. The physician's data and interpretations need to be shared with experts at the school so that they can be incorporated into the professional field of educational theory to build an educational program for the child. The physician may continue to function as a champion or ombudsman for the child in the school setting. The parents, however, may not be regarded with similar respect. The physician must also be prepared to offer continuing support to the family and child just as in the case of children with other chronic disabilities.

Personality Deviations

There are several helpful ways to consider personality deviations in children. The first relates to normal personality development. Specific milestones can be associated with norms for a given age just as has been done with motor and language milestones, eg, smiling, recognition of strangers, anxiety with strangers, separation anxiety, parallel play with age-mates, cooperative play with age-mates, temper tantrums, fantasy play, use of a transitional object (security blanket), imaginary playmates, etc. The physician can then see if the child's behavior corresponds to what can be expected for the child's age.

An alternative method of looking at normal development is to consider the tasks of differing age periods. For the first year, the tasks of the infant are to develop trust in parenting figures, to develop attachment to them, and to begin the process of individuating from the parents. From age 1–3, the child is developing autonomy. This is seen in increasing mastery over body functions (feeding, toileting, dressing, mobility) and in the use of "no" and tantrums to assert the child's autonomous choices. From the third to fifth years, the child shows increasing development of mastery and initiative. During this time, the child is developing a clearer sense of self and learning a great deal about the world, whereas earlier the knowledge gained was about himself or herself. Play with age-mates, dramatic play, and the word "why" predominate. With the start of public school, the child enters a stage of tremendous learning, when rules, logical thinking, and "facts" such as state capitals are assimilated at a rapid rate. Tabletop games become popular, as well as reading and rather complex gross motor play. Skipping rope, organized sports, jacks, and skateboards enter the child's play patterns. The physician who is familiar with normal developmental tasks can identify the child who is deviating from the usual pattern of development, and evaluation and treatment can follow.

A third view of personality development is that intellectual handicap may be due to emotional disorders. A child's learning may be impeded by excessive shyness, fear of failure, fear of growing up, anxiety, and similar problems. In any list of differential diagnoses for delays in language acquisition, learning disorders, or retarded mental function, emotional factors must rank high. Usually there will be behavioral symptoms in addition to the delay in development, but these symptoms may be difficult to elicit by the physician and may not be bothersome or visible to the parents. Quietness and shyness may be pleasing to the parents even though these attributes are hindering normal development. A child's fear of growing up, anxiety, or fear of trying something and failing may not be noted by the parents.

Ideally, the physician should have known the child since infancy and have a good understanding of the parents, siblings, and family function. If this is the case, the physician is in a good position to evaluate and understand the personality of the child.

Individual personality evaluation requires a comprehensive history from the parents and observations of the child. It usually takes about 30 minutes to obtain a history from the parents without the child being present. It is essential to adopt the position of wanting to know what kind of person the child is rather than taking the stance of a medical detective who is looking for clues to pathologic processes. It is helpful, regardless of the child's age, to begin by inquiring what the child was like during the neonatal period and during early infancy. This will give information about the temperament of the baby and about the ease or difficulty presented by this child from the very beginning. The history should cover the following points:

(1) Temperament of the child from infancy.

(2) Response of the child to stress.

(3) Personality milestones: Eg, smiling, anxiety with strangers, separation anxiety, mastery of body functions, play with age-mates, tantrums, masturbation, night terrors, desire for privacy, etc.

(4) Affects of the child: Under what conditions is the child sad, frustrated, happy, or afraid, and how does the child deal with those feelings?

(5) Interaction and play patterns with other children.

(6) Any unusual symptoms or behaviors of the child.

(7) Feelings of the parents about the child and how they deal with problems presented by the child.

(8) Important events in the child's life: Eg, hospitalizations, losses, illnesses, birth of siblings, changes in baby-sitters, etc, and reaction to those important events.

The other important source of data is observation of the child. The most important and convenient time to do this is during the physical examination and especially during developmental screening. The advantages of this observation period are squandered if a technician or other assistant performs the developmental screening examination. The physician who elects to personally perform the physical examination and developmental screening can observe such factors as reactions to praise, reactions to setting of limits, tolerance of frustration, ability to imitate, affect of child (sad, shy, happy, etc), perseverance, investigativeness, reaction to strange adult, and the child's need for the mother when under stress.

A second readily accessible source of information is the child's behavior in the waiting room. This is a time when play with age-mates and more natural behavior of the child and parent can be observed. The receptionist can easily be trained to observe children in the waiting room and make written comments about the child and the parents while they are waiting.

A member of the physician's staff should visit the child and parents at home and should go to the preschool nursery or day care facility. Information gathered from these sources is much less expensive than consultation with a mental health professional. At home, the child is less frightened, spontaneous play can be observed, and parent-child interaction is apt to be less stilted and artificial than in the doctor's office.

Of course, emotional and biologic problems are not mutually exclusive, and children with chronic handicaps are at much greater risk of psychologic maladaptation than children in the general population. This should be of special concern to the child's physician, because children with chronic handicaps are rarely evaluated for emotional health despite the obvious stress their handicap places on their self-concept and their relations with their age-mates. A further problem is that mental health professionals have had little experience or inclination to offer help to such children. Recently, attention has been paid to the emotional stress of such chronic handicaps as diabetes, cystic fibrosis, asthma, and hemophilia. However, much less attention has been paid to the mental health needs of children with retardation, cerebral palsy, delays in language acquisition, and other developmental disabilities. Because of the heightened risk of emotional disorder in such handicapped children, the primary physician must periodically assess the emotional and social life of the developmentally disabled children under treatment and must become an active advocate for those children when disturbances in emotional development become apparent.

Emotional disorders of the child and dysfunction of the family may be treated by the physician or by a mental health professional. Most physicians find it helpful to seek corroboration of a tentative diagnosis in the psychosocial area in consultation with a child psychiatrist, clinical psychologist, or psychiatric social worker. Counseling or psychotherapy may then be carried out by the consulting professional or by the physician when it is within the scope of that doctor's interest and expertise. The physician is in a unique position to help identify the problem and offer solutions, particularly when the child's problems stem from deviations in parental attitudes toward the child, child-rearing practices, or messages of indifference or overconcern by parents. The physician's knowledge of the family over the years should assist in identification of such factors. As a nonjudgmental counselor, the doctor is in a position to help the family understand that such situations are not pathologic or signs of mental illness but are nonetheless playing an important role in the child's problems.

Normal Child

There are 2 circumstances in which a child brought to the clinician with suspected mental retardation or other developmental disability will be found to be perfectly normal.

The first situation occurs when a child has done poorly on some developmental screening test. The child may perform normally on the repeat screening, which must be done before further evaluation is indicated. Some children who do poorly on tests in the doctor's office will perform normally when the test is performed in the home. For the most part, such children are normal. Poor performance on a screening test may have many explanations, all of which are obvious to the reader. A child may be fearful or shy. This is not a pathologic sign but must be viewed as a personality trait which the physician would do well to note and discuss with the parents because this same child may find it difficult to adapt to other frightening situations, such as starting school. Well child visits provide an excellent opportunity to identify such traits and characteristics, which may result in unnecessary stress to the child and family.

A more complex situation occurs when parents feel that the child is delayed in development, retarded, or handicapped but the physician finds no signs of deficiency in the child. There are 2 possible explanations in such cases:

(1) The parents have unusually high expectations of this child or of children in general. This attitude has been described in abusive parents, who may expect precocious or unusually good behavior of a child. The parent may be distressed that the child is not toilet-trained by age 12 months or may feel there is something pathologic about the normal ("terrible 2") behavior of a 2-year-old. They may describe a child as hyperactive when the activity level of the child is within normal limits. This is not only true of abusive parents but is also commonly noted in people who are otherwise excellent parents. It is possible that this particular child is disappointing to the parents and that a complaint of developmental delay is their way of expressing their concern and disappointment.

(2) The parents have some legitimate concern about the child but either do not know exactly what it is or cannot bring themselves to say it. It helps to inquire of the parents what things the child does especially well, what things the child does poorly, what things they enjoy about their child, what things they do not enjoy, what things they worry about. Such information can be gathered before the office visit. Many parents will be more forthright about their child when they fill out answers to such questions in private rather than when they are asked such things in the physician's office. Although the child's learning and language and motor skills are normal, the parents may be identifying some subtle signs of emotional disorder or may be subliminally aware of an unhealthy parent-child interaction. It is the physician's difficult job to uncover the real reasons for the parents' concern about developmental disability when none exists.

HELPING PARENTS

One of the most difficult but critically important roles of the primary physician is conveying bad news to parents and helping them understand and deal with a diagnosis of chronic disability.

Typically, the first reaction is denial. This may take the form of outright rejection of the diagnosis and a search for another opinion. It is helpful if the physician understands and tolerates the parents' skepticism and offers to be both their guide in the continued evaluation of the child and the coordinator of treatment and education programs if these should be needed.

The parents may next become angry, or sad and depressed. Both emotions may occur in sequence. Having an "imperfect," chronically handicapped child is a cruel disappointment. Unable to find a legitimate object of their anger and resentment, the parents may try to blame the physician who first told them the bad news, but it may be the obstetrician, the delivery room nurse, or some other medical staff person. Parents may become angry with relatives, neighbors, or friends they feel are not accepting the child.

Depression and sadness are especially difficult to

deal with if the physician too is distressed by these tragic episodes of medical practice. A parent whose depression is severe and unrelenting may need help from a mental health professional. More often, however, the family physician or pediatrician can help parents through this phase by acknowledging and sharing their sadness and gently pointing out the child's strengths and the brighter aspects of the child's future. The parents of a handicapped child usually feel they must accept the child's disability as a cross they are called upon to bear. It may be only in the presence of the physician that they can express their sadness and despair. One of the key elements in depression and despair is hopelessness, which can be combated in a number of ways. Stimulation of cognitive or motor skills, for example, can be presented as a prescription or planned program which, while not curative, will help the child. Referral of the child to such stimulation programs or specific therapies as indicated will also help the parents gain a sense of purpose and direction in providing help for their child. It is essential at this point to realize that most adults have a much gloomier picture of developmental problems than is indicated. They may believe that their child's outlook necessarily means institutionalization, an end to learning after a certain period, social ostracism, etc. When these fantasies are unjustified, as they usually are, it will be helpful to correct them and describe a more realistic picture of the prognosis.

Many parents of handicapped children have difficulty dealing with guilt feelings. This is especially true when no cause of the handicap can be identified. The mother will think of every break in her diet during pregnancy and all of the things she might have done to cause the problem. It is necessary to deal directly with the parent's sense of guilt, which is usually grounded in the belief that if one's offspring is defective there must be something wrong with the parent also. When genetic or chromosomal causes are operative, this guilt will be fueled by the realistic knowledge that the condition has been transmitted through hereditary mechanisms. It may be necessary to consult with a mental health professional if this guilt persists or interferes with the ability of the parents to adequately care for their child.

It is important to note that all parents do not follow the same pathway of adapting themselves to a child's handicap. Some parents intellectualize the problem and hold themselves at a distance (emotionally) from the child. Many fathers find a second job and thus avoid having to endure much contact with the child. Some adults find solace in working for the "cause" of handicapped children—sometimes even asking the physician to use their child for any research that might help handicapped children.

The role of the primary physician in dealing with parents is that of education and of counseling. To fill either role and ignore the other would be a disservice to the child. Parents need to know how their child is functioning, what is wrong with the child's development, what the future holds, and what can be done to help. The parents also must be allowed to feel that the physician understands and accepts their reactions to the child's problem, even though these may be illogical and disturbing. Having a child with developmental problems is stressful for the parents and for the marriage. Divorce, suicide, and emotional problems are more frequent in parents of handicapped children than in the general population. Since having stable and relatively healthy parents is an important need of the developmentally disabled child, the child's physician should do everything possible to help the patient have a family in which he or she can grow and develop maximally.

●　　●　　●

General References

Grossman HJ (editor): *Learning Disorders.* Saunders, 1973.

Haslam RHA (editor): Habilitation of the handicapped child. Pediatr Clin North Am 20:1, 1973. [Entire issue.]

Kenny TJ, Clemmens RL: *Behavioral Pediatrics and Child Development.* Williams & Wilkins, 1975.

Kimsbourne M: Disorders of mental development. Pages 488–515 in: *Textbook of Child Neurology.* Menkes JH (editor). Lea & Febiger, 1974.

Knobloch H, Pasamanick B: *Developmental Diagnosis,* 3rd ed. Harper, 1974.

Martin HP & others: The development of abused children. Pages 25–73 in: *Advances in Pediatrics.* Schulman I (editor). Year Book, 1974.

Meier JH: *Developmental and Learning Disabilities.* University Park Press, 1975.

Meier JH: Early intervention in the prevention of mental retardation. Pages 305–409 in: *The Prevention of Genetic Disease and Mental Retardation.* Milunsky A (editor). Saunders, 1975.

Schain RJ: *Neurology of Childhood Learning Disorders.* Williams & Wilkins, 1972.

Schmitt BO & others: The hyperactive child. Clin Pediatr (Phila) 12:154, 1973.

23...

Psychosocial Aspects of Pediatrics & Psychiatric Disorders

Dane G. Prugh, MD, & Anthony J. Kisley, MD

GENERAL PRINCIPLES OF PSYCHIATRIC EXAMINATION & TREATMENT

THE APPROACH TO INTERVIEWING

Most physicians find that the traditional question and answer or "check list" method of taking a history is not flexible enough to ferret out significant psychosocial material. The "open-ended question" allows the parent or patient to take the lead and to respond with material that he is most concerned about. The physician·should feel comfortable with his own interviewing technics and not attempt to imitate too closely those of someone else.

In addition to what the patient says, the physician can learn much from observation of the patient and from noting how the emotional relationship between himself and the patient is developing. The quality of this relationship will influence both the accuracy of the data obtained and the response to recommended therapeutic measures. A warm, friendly, and nonjudgmental attitude will make it easier for the patient and his parents to talk freely. The doctor's skill in "listening actively" will enable him to discover the multiple determinants in what the patient says. Quick advice should be avoided, as well as premature promises about the success of treatment; both can promote overdependency or lead to disappointment.

Adequate time should be permitted for interviews. A good deal can be learned in 20–30 minutes, and longer interviews can be scheduled if necessary. Appointments should be promptly kept.

Interviewing the Parents

At the initial contact with the family, both parents should be seen together. Valuable impressions can be gained about the marital relationship, attitudes about parenthood, and attitudes toward the child and his illness or adjustment problem.

In most cases, the physician can simply begin by asking what seems to be the matter. The parents should be encouraged to tell the story in their own way, guided as necessary by comments and questions.

The ostensible chief complaint may turn out not to be the parents' greatest concern. Considerable patience may be required, and intrusive (or leading) questioning early in the interview only delays the flow of significant material.

Observing the parents' attitudes and feelings will help direct the physician's inquiries to fill in gaps in the history. Repeating an emotion-laden word or phrase may enable a parent who temporarily blocks to continue. A note to oneself about things the parent does not say may give important clues later. The physician should be alert to what the parents' feelings toward him are and what they seem to expect of him. A sympathetic, tolerant, and respectful attitude will help convince them that he is interested in helping them with their problem.

The physician must respect the dignity of the people he deals with in his professional role. He should learn his patients' names and not call all women "mother" to save himself the trouble. If he often encounters "troublesome" parents with whom he cannot seem to get along, he should examine his own attitudes and behavior even to the extent of obtaining psychiatric consultation. Occasionally he may have to suggest that the parents might feel more comfortable with or better served by another physician.

Parental demands for quick advice and easy solutions are usually symptoms of their own anxieties. They soon lose confidence in a physician who jumps to conclusions based on insufficient facts. No parent loses respect for a physician who says he doesn't yet know what is wrong or what to do and that further investigation and thought are necessary.

Certain historical data carry an emotional charge, and some revelations are painful and difficult. This is particularly true of familial or hereditary illnesses and of emotional disturbances in children and parents. For example, parents of children having seizures may at first withhold information about epilepsy in close relatives. Parents also recognize that their feelings about their child may be partly responsible for his behavioral disturbances. In asking questions about behavior problems, it is important not to adopt an approach which the anxious parent may misinterpret as a critical attack. Questions such as, "Did you want this child?" "Does your son masturbate?" "Was she jealous of the new baby?"—all are too frequently doomed, in the initial interview, to provoke conventional and socially acceptable replies or defensive indignation. Such information must be gathered by inference or by the use of indirect questioning. Nonverbal behavior such as blushing, nailbiting, or neuromuscular tension may give important clues.

The history should elicit relevant details about the family's circumstances—eg, their position as members of a minority group, the father's depression about unsatisfying work experiences, the mother's part-time employment which takes her out of the home at the child's bedtime. It is important to determine whether there are or have been family illnesses which may be relevant to the child's problem, but the experienced physician will avoid the monotonous listing of all possible illnesses.

In securing details of the child's birth, growth and development, and past illnesses and of the parents' child-rearing practices, it must be remembered that parents have difficulty in recalling many items with accuracy. Confirmation from other sources may be required.

The most significant emotional data often do not emerge during the first interview. Parents can rarely discuss their deep feelings until a basic sense of trust in their doctor has been allowed to develop. The parents must be allowed to talk at their own pace. The act of talking helps to discharge initial tensions and overcome anxiety. Expectant waiting is vital even if the mother appears to be on the verge of tears. The physician can, with practice, curb his natural impulse to interrupt the expression of strong emotions, and might better encourage crying by a tense and troubled mother. The release of such feeling in a sympathetic atmosphere may be of help to the parent and may strengthen the relationship with the physician.

In terminating the initial interview, it is wise to return to the area of the parents' major concern. The physician can then ask questions prompted by the leads he has gained up to this point. This indicates to the parents that he has fully comprehended their concern and will endeavor to deal constructively with it.

Interviewing the Child

Infants and young children of preschool age are usually seen with the mother. The physician may give the child a toy, tongue depressor, or other object to play with. If the parent talks too freely in the child's presence, the child may play in the waiting room while the pediatrician and the parent talk alone.

The physician may learn a good deal by observing the child at play during the interview. Impressions of the child's level of development can be gained from the degree of complexity and organization of his play, his attention span, and other clues. The child's attitude toward the physician, often reflecting parental anxiety, may also be apparent in his drawings, his play with dolls, and his general demeanor.

With older children and adolescents, the initial interview may be handled in different ways under differing circumstances. If the parents are concerned about what they think is an emotional problem, it may be wise to see them together first without the child so that they can talk freely. If information taken while the appointment is being made reveals a bitter struggle between an adolescent and his parents, it may be best to see the adolescent first so that he may feel sure he has a chance to tell his story even though he should be told that the doctor cannot take sides. With anxious, suspicious children, it is advisable to see one or both parents and the child together at the first interview since the child may fear that the parent is imparting secret information about him; later, the parents and the child can be seen separately.

At the end of an evaluation, it may help to see the parents and the child together.

At some point, the physician should see the child alone. This is best done in an office rather than an examining room. The parents should tell the child that he is going to see a doctor who is interested in the problems that make boys and girls worried or unhappy.

With an older child, verbal data may be more accurate and voluminous after a positive relationship has been established. At the first contact, school age children or adolescents may be inhibited and withdrawn. The physician should avoid making premature judgments of the child's mental status under these circumstances.

If the physician is unaggressive and friendly and keeps his conversation at the child's level (without talking down to him), he can easily secure the child's cooperation and confidence. He may show the child some toys, suggesting that they talk while he plays. Once engrossed, the child may begin talking spontaneously, or the physician may comment on his activities.

Through observation of the child's play, the physician may learn a great deal about his conflicts or anxieties. The 4-year-old who has a smaller boy doll "beat up" a larger boy doll before "throwing it off a cliff" reveals much about his feelings toward his 6-year-old brother. It is wise not to make immediate interpretations of the child's feelings, however, as he may become too anxious. Later, the physician may bring up the child's feelings about his siblings, referring to the play incident and suggesting that maybe he feels "like that boy." Firm but kindly limits should be set on aggressive or destructive play.

With the child who can talk fairly freely, one can gain impressions of the meaning to him of his symptoms or disability in terms of its effect upon his adjustment at school, within his peer group, and in the home. With frightened or withdrawn children, data of this sort may have to be sought indirectly by asking what they want to do when they grow up. If a school age child cannot offer at least one possibility, it can be inferred that he has some fears about "growing up." The child can be asked to make 3 wishes; a significantly depressed child may not be able to think of one. If an ill child does not include "getting well" as at least one of his wishes, he usually has conflicts about returning to school or other (perhaps unconscious) fears.

A sick child can be asked what he would do if he were well, or a child who cannot talk easily about himself can be asked what a hypothetical child ("Let's pretend we know a boy who . . .") would wish for or do in a particular situation. Most children cannot talk easily at first about their feelings toward their parents. With such an approach, most children from late preschool age onward can be helped to understand their symptoms or behavior as a problem or a worry which can be remedied.

The preadolescent and adolescent child is usually capable of understanding the reason for the interview and, if adequately prepared by the parents, may openly express his desire for help with his problems. If the parents have used the visit to the physician as a threat or punishment, or if the child is present at the recommendation of school or judicial authorities, the physician should quickly clarify the situation with the youngster so that a therapeutic alliance can be established. Authoritarianism, lectures, and unsought advice are detrimental to such a relationship. Frightened adolescents should be put at ease. Hostile or defensive youngsters usually have reasons for their behavior, and a physician who can accept these attitudes nonjudgmentally is likely to discover the reasons. An open and neutral position and an evident desire to help will in time convince even the most resistant adolescent that the physician is sincere.

A formal mental status examination is difficult in children and often insulting to adolescents. Clinical observations, questions about school, and asking the child to write his name or to draw a picture will usually provide sufficiently accurate impressions of his attention span, orientation in time and place, and perceptual and motor functions. School age children, when asked to draw a picture of a person, will usually draw a person of the same sex.

Some estimate of the child's intelligence may be obtained in a rough fashion through similar methods. Pediatricians have demonstrated their capacity, in a controlled study, to make a surprisingly accurate evaluation of the Developmental Quotient of infants and young children. Their main errors lie in underestimating the capacities of sick children and overestimating the abilities of mentally retarded ones.

Most available tests of reading ability are complicated and lengthy. The physician should familiarize himself with first, second, and third grade readers and should have one of each available in case a reading problem is suspected. For adequate evaluation in the cognitive area, referral to a clinical psychologist is indicated.

Observation of Child & Parent

From the moment the parent enters the office, valuable clinical impressions are available to the physician or to an alert nurse or secretary. Some parents cannot permit the child to answer a question independently, manifesting a need to dominate the child or the situation. Other parents constantly correct the child or

require him to sit impossibly still, disclosing unrealistically high standards of behavior and conformity.

If the father and mother are interviewed together, they may disclose disagreements in child-rearing practices. Some parents pay little attention to their children, such as the mother who does not stand close to her infant to prevent him from falling off the examining table. Disturbed parents, with unconscious needs to deny the extent or seriousness of the child's obvious illness, may belittle him or urge him to act as if he were well.

The physician should record such observations and test them against later impressions. Observations of this sort are most readily available to the physician who visits the home and enjoys continuity of contact with the parents and child. On a home visit, the standards of parental care and the patterns of family living are often more evident than in the office. Valuable observations of this nature can also be gathered in a clinic waiting room by the receptionist or nurse.

Gardner RA: *Therapeutic Communication with Children: The Mutual Storytelling Technique.* Jason Aronson (New York), 1971.

Korsch BM: Pediatrician-patient relations. In: *Ambulatory Pediatrics.* Green M, Haggerty R (editors). Saunders, 1968.

THE APPROACH TO PHYSICAL EXAMINATION OF THE CHILD

Preparation for the Examination

The physician can anticipate active participation by the child in the physical examination, but he must be prepared for resigned submission, passive resistance, or even active refusal and violent battle. The degree of rapport already established with the parent and child may determine the diagnostic success of the examination. If the child is seriously ill, the physical examination may be done while the latter portion of the history is being taken to save time and to decrease the suspense of the anxious child and the parent.

Refusal by preschool children to remove certain items of clothing may indicate anxiety over being so completely exposed rather than sexual modesty. This initial apprehension should be respected, and it is soon overcome. Older children may retain their underpants, which can be dropped for genital examination when they are more at ease.

A relaxed and unhurried approach is vital. A few moments spent in conversation, using the child's first name or nickname, may save time and struggle. Some explanation of each step, as in examining the throat or darkening the room for ophthalmoscopic examination, can be given quietly, using terms the child can understand.

Permitting a young child to handle certain instruments such as the stethoscope before they are used (eg, listening to their own heartbeat) may overcome tension. "Blowing out" the light of the otoscope is a time-honored pediatric method of distracting toddlers from their apprehension about the examination.

Variations in Handling of Different Ages

A. Very Young Infants: With the very young infant, little difficulty is encountered if the mother is relaxed and trusting. Pacifiers may be used if the baby is crying or restless. Much of the examination may be performed while the mother holds and feeds the infant, affording the physician an opportunity to observe her feeding approach and the mother a chance to talk about any fears she may have about the infant's physical status or developmental progress.

B. Older Infants Up to Age 1½: In the second half of the first year, stranger or separation anxiety causes most infants to show some fear of the physician even if they have seen him regularly for health examinations. The physician may hand the mother a tongue depressor or similar object to give to the infant while he sits in her lap during the interview, permitting him to appraise the physician from a safe vantage point. If he is crawling or toddling, the infant may later move toward the physician and make friendly overtures.

The infant often resists being examined on his back or on the examining table, and it may be best to examine him on his mother's lap, permitting her to hold his head against her shoulder for examination of the ears and throat. The nurse may be able to obtain a more positive initial response from the older infant than the physician.

C. Ages 1½–3: During the normal period of negativism in the latter part of the second and early part of the third year, the child may refuse to cooperate with some parts of the examination such as opening his mouth to permit examination of the throat. Patience is required. A stubbornly negativistic child, diverted at this point to some other activity, may later abandon his rebellious stand. Physical battles inevitably result in the child's loss of trust in the physician.

D. Preschool Children: The preschool child can usually be examined on a table. Most children at this age are frightened when they are compelled to lie down and feel less anxious when they are sitting.

E. School Age Children: With children of school age, as with older preschool children, much can be learned during the physical examination about the child's attitudes toward his own development; his feelings about himself as a developing individual; his feelings about his body and its adequacy; his fears or misconceptions about parts of his body and how they are working; and his concern about minor blemishes. If the child feels secure with the physician, he may himself bring up his fears or concerns. The parent may verbalize similar concerns during an unhurried examination.

F. Adolescents: With adolescents, feelings of modesty may become apparent during the examination. Such feelings should be respected, and these young people should be handled in the same way as adults. Fears may emerge in boys concerning growth lags or other real or imaginary deviations; in girls, about the onset of menses and the development of secondary sex characteristics. During the examination of girls of this age, a nurse should always be present.

Parent Attendance

Some physicians prefer to exclude an anxious mother from the physical examination, recognizing that the child often submits more passively in her absence. This approach carries with it not only the pain of separation but also the implication of punishment by the physician. The parent may react with feelings of guilt or resentment, surmising that the physician thinks she is a poor parent. It is almost always best to permit the parent to remain with the infant or young child.

An apprehensive parent who asks to leave during the examination should usually be permitted to do so, but it is better that she leave before rather than during the examination. If the mother leaves the room, the child should be told where she will be and when she will return. If restraint is indicated, it should be carried out promptly, with a brief explanation of its need.

Precautions in Examination

The physician's hands and the instruments he uses should be warm, since any coldness to the touch may add to the child's fear or resistance. With younger children, examination of the ears and throat should be done last. Rectal temperatures may be resisted, in which case an axillary temperature reading will suffice. For children beyond infancy, rectal examinations should be performed with great care and gentleness and with adequate explanation. A "blowing" game may aid in securing cooperation during examination of the chest. Time spent in putting the child at ease will provide sufficient relaxation of the abdominal musculature for an accurate examination of the abdomen. Caution should be observed in the vaginal inspection of preadolescent or adolescent girls.

After the examination, the child should be given time to ask questions about procedures or instruments used or about any other phase of the examination. Plans for preparation of the child for further laboratory procedures, other medical or surgical experiences, or hospitalization should be considered.

The physician should always terminate the interview with a friendly and personal farewell to the child.

SPECIAL TESTS

Psychologic Tests

When properly administered by trained personnel, psychologic tests can be of great diagnostic assistance. Like laboratory tests, they must be interpreted in the light of the clinical findings. A single psychologic test, like a single laboratory test, may not be accurate, especially if the child is tired, sick, or anxious.

Intelligence testing is discussed in Chapter 22.

Electroencephalography

Although the older literature indicates that a large percentage of patients with emotional illnesses have abnormal EEGs, recent investigators have found a strikingly high incidence of so-called abnormal waves in normally developing children. For example, it was once thought that 14- and 6-per-second spikes were associated with behavioral disorders, but these wave patterns have also been found in normal children and adolescents. In one large study, well over one-half of children without symptoms showed these abnormalities, especially children between 4–9 years of age. Many so-called abnormal waves may be better described as transient phenomena occurring during critical periods of integrative development in the CNS.

The EEG should be interpreted only as one of many factors in the clinical evaluation of the patient.

Preparation of the child for EEG testing is important, as the wires and machine may arouse fears of "electricity." The child may also need to be told that the machine cannot read his mind.

Metcalf DR, Jordan K: EEG ontogenesis in normal children. In: *Drugs, Development, and Cerebral Function.* Smith WL (editor). Thomas, 1971.

Osselton JW, Kiloh LG: *Clinical Electroencephalography.* Butterworth, 1961.

IMPLEMENTATION OF RESULTS OF THE CLINICAL EXAMINATION

Once the physician has achieved a balanced appraisal of the child and his family, his plan of therapy or his approach to well child care must be communicated effectively to parents and patient. He should be confident and at times authoritative in his recommendations, but humility, patience, and understanding are the most appropriate and useful attitudes. The physician must bear in mind the apprehension with which the parents await his diagnosis and recommendations. He should use simple language and write out detailed or complicated instructions for care.

In discussing with parents a child's emotional problem, the physician should not imply that they have "caused" it. The parents may suspect that the problem is an emotional one. If they initially thought the problem was a physical one, the physician can begin by saying that he is happy to reassure them that there are no serious physical abnormalities. He can add that he feels the symptoms can be caused or aggravated by "emotional tension," and then ask the parents whether they have noticed evidence of any such tension. He can indicate that such problems are "nobody's fault" and can suggest that there are ways of helping the child to overcome his difficulties. He can further

indicate that, with help, they might think of things that should be done or things that they might, in hindsight, want to change about their ways of handling the child. Most parents will respond positively, after some initial defensiveness, to such an approach.

The physician should also give the child, in the presence of his parents or alone, a brief explanation of his illness and the plan for treatment, in age-appropriate terms.

INDICATIONS FOR PSYCHIATRIC REFERRAL

The decision about what kind of cases a pediatrician can treat and which he should refer to a child psychiatrist or child guidance clinic depends to a large extent on the pediatrician's interests and training. Of all health professionals, the pediatrician is in the best position to educate parents about the nature of childhood and to help them handle ordinary behavior problems. However, every pediatrician has cases in his practice that he cannot be expected to handle. When doubt exists, consultation with a child psychiatrist is useful.

Criteria for Referral

The following criteria should be considered as guidelines for referral.

A. Home Environment: A severely handicapping home environment or seriously disturbed parents will generally warrant a prolonged relationship with mental health professionals.

B. Age Discrepancy: At certain ages, most children have outgrown particular habits or behavior. If they do not, psychiatric study may be indicated.

C. Intensity or Frequency of Symptoms: Under emotional or physical stress, most children may regress, but persistent regressive behavior may indicate psychologic fixations.

D. Degree of Social Disadvantage or Impairment: Certain modes of behavior tend to be self-perpetuating, eg, the aggressive child who makes many enemies has no choice but to continue to fight.

E. The Child's Inner Suffering: This is frequently overlooked by parents, teachers, and physicians, as with the well behaved student who is not achieving.

F. Intractable Behavior: The persistence of symptoms, despite the efforts of the child and others to change them, is a cardinal clue to intrapsychic conflicts.

Preparation for Referral

When the pediatrician has decided that referral is necessary, his preparation of the child and parents can help to ensure a successful outcome. Parents may be afraid of the word psychiatry; may feel that they have failed as parents; or may fear that they will be lectured or condemned.

The physician must explain to the parents why the child needs help. It is best to discuss the symptoms in terms of the child's discomfort, as indications of "lack of confidence" or of being "mixed up" about himself.

The second step involves dealing with the parents' possible objections to psychiatric aid. Some parents need to be told that normal children can have emotional problems and that they need not fear that the child will be stigmatized. Parents need reassurance about the confidentiality of such matters. A sense of guilt may prevent them from accepting help or recognizing their own involvement. The physician must not argue with the parents and should explain that there are undoubtedly many important reasons for their child's difficulties.

The last step involves conveying a realistic understanding of what psychiatric therapy can accomplish. The physician should not make extravagant promises or concrete predictions but should convince the parents that help is both needed and available.

In talking with the child, openness and honesty are essential. He should be told where he is going and why, and he should know what his basic problem is.

Freud A: Assessment of childhood disturbances. Psychoanal Study Child 17:149, 1962.
Moskowitz JA: The pediatrician calls for psychiatric referral. Notes on achieving a successful consultation. Clin Pediatr (Phila) 7:733, 1968.
Schwab JJ, Brown J: Uses and abuses of psychiatric consultation. JAMA 205:65, 1968.

PSYCHOTHERAPY

There are several different schools of psychotherapy based on different frames of references, but the aims and methods of treatment tend to be similar in all. In some types of emotional problems, a supportive or directive approach is indicated; in others, exploration of the patient's defenses and life experiences; in still others, the therapeutic effect of allowing the patient to talk about (ventilate) his feelings is of dominant importance. Psychotherapy may also be classified as interpretive, suggestive, persuasive, or educative; or in terms of its depth, duration, and intensity. Isolating a single therapeutic element as a basis for classification is an artificial approach since each of the factors listed is present in some degree in every psychotherapeutic relationship. The dimensions of psychotherapy are best described as a continuum extending from the supportive end, where little uncovering of deeper conflicts occurs, to the insight-promoting end, in which "operative" or interpretative activity is predominant.

Adams PL: *A Primer of Child Psychotherapy.* Little, Brown, 1974.

Hammer M, Kaplan AH: *The Practice of Psychotherapy with Children.* Dorsey, 1967.
Harrison SI, Carek DJ: *A Guide to Psychotherapy.* Little, Brown, 1966.
Swanson FL: *Psychotherapists and Children: A Procedural Guide.* Pitman, 1970.
Zick GH: *Family Therapy.* Behavioral Publications, 1972.

PSYCHOPHARMACOLOGIC AGENTS

Psychoactive drugs have achieved a significant place in the treatment of emotional disorders of childhood. They cannot replace the interpersonal relationship which is the main tool of the physician, but they can be effective in reducing anxiety and overactivity. Reduction of impulsiveness and irritability is usually accompanied by less anxiety and improved attention span. On occasion, drug therapy can increase spontaneous activity and responsiveness in states of apathy and depression. The effects upon complex behavior patterns, on the other hand, are much more difficult to predict during drug therapy.

There is no evidence that psychoactive drugs can improve intellectual functioning directly. Although it is possible to modify a child's responses to current experiences with drugs, they cannot undo previously learned behavior or alter neurotic patterns. Much information is still needed on the effects of specific drugs and their mode of action, as our knowledge remains largely empiric.

Principles of Drug Treatment

A. Drug and Diagnosis Must Be Matched: The condition of a disturbed child must be accurately diagnosed if he is to receive the most effective treatment. An appropriate drug—eg, an antipsychotic tranquilizer—can help control behavior even in severe psychoses. With appropriate drug administration, some severely disturbed children may become amenable to psychotherapy. Although neurotic disorders rarely respond lastingly to drugs, some children with intrapsychic conflicts suffering from persistent anxiety, inhibitions, and phobias become more spontaneous and increase their adaptive functioning when given tranquilizing drugs.

Personality disorders and mental retardation are generally not benefited by drugs. Hyperkinesia may benefit from stimulant drugs. Reactive disorders rarely justify drug use except as sedation is necessary for cases of acute anxiety.

B. Benefit Should Exceed Toxicity: The physician who uses drugs should have a thorough knowledge of their pharmacologic properties, including their side-effects and potential toxicity. The severity of the child's disorder and the potential for improvement must justify the possible impact of side-effects and toxicity.

C. Special Precautions in Young Patients: Data

cannot always be extrapolated from adult medicine to pediatrics. A child's response to a psychoactive drug may be quite different from that of an adult.

Special clinical testing of drugs potentially valuable for disturbed children is essential, as a drug's action may be other than predicted because of the immature and developing qualities of the child.

Dosage must be individualized for each patient, since undertreatment as well as overtreatment may result from metabolic differences at different ages. Dosage must be carefully regulated so as not to impair a child's intellectual acuity and maturation.

D. Use Familiar Drugs: A well tested and familiar drug should be employed until a newer or unfamiliar one establishes its superiority. Unexpected toxicity from a less well known agent may not become apparent until it has been in general use for a long period.

E. Use Drugs Sparingly: Drugs should not be used any longer than necessary. Lowering the dosage periodically will permit the observation of improvement or worsening of the symptoms being treated.

F. Seek Other Forms of Therapy: Since pharmacotherapy of emotional disorders affects symptoms rather than the underlying disease, the physician must continue his attempts to identify and eliminate the physical, psychologic, and social etiologic factors in the emotional disturbance.

MAJOR TRANQUILIZERS

The major ("antipsychotic") tranquilizers have been of greatest use in treating hospitalized, severely disturbed, or psychotic children because they exert a calmative effect on agitated, impulsive, or excited states without causing paradoxical excitement or anesthesia. They can also reduce or eliminate delusions, hallucinations, and some schizophrenic ideation and thus make these children more communicative.

The dosage is increased at intervals of several days until a satisfactory response is obtained or until side-effects limit further increases in dosage or force discontinuance of therapy. In acute situations, an initial parenteral dose may be given.

These agents should not be used to alleviate neurotic anxiety.

The antipsychotic tranquilizers can be classified according to their chemical structure or pharmacologic properties.

Phenothiazine Derivatives & Similar Potent Drugs

The tranquilizers most commonly used are phenothiazine derivatives. Chlorprothixene (Taractan) is chemically and pharmacologically similar. Haloperidol (Haldol) is a butyrophenone comparable to the stimulant tranquilizers listed below but is not approved for use in patients under 12.

The phenothiazines can be further classified according to the degree of sedation induced and the likelihood of extrapyramidal side-effects.

A. Sedation Prominent: The only important example is promethazine (Phenergan).

B. Standard Agents: Included are chlorpromazine (Thorazine) and thioridazine (Mellaril).

C. Stimulant Tranquilizers: These agents cause comparatively less sedation for the same therapeutic effect but are also more likely to cause extrapyramidal side-effects. Trifluoperazine (Stelazine) and prochlorperazine (Compazine) are the important drugs in this group. Children are especially susceptible to side-effects and may manifest violent dystonias or choreiform movements as well as tremors, rigidity, and akathisia. Parenteral administration should be avoided.

Other side-effects are atropine-like or anticholinergic responses (constipation, blurred vision, dryness of the mouth, difficult micturition), postural hypotension, and lethargy or drowsiness. Endocrine abnormalities, skin changes (dermatitis, photosensitivity), and lowered body temperature are less common.

Rare cases of aplastic anemia and agranulocytosis have been reported. Cholangiolitic jaundice (intrahepatic obstruction) was once a common side-effect of chlorpromazine administration but is now rare. Convulsions may occur when very high dosages are used or when epilepsy or other predisposition to convulsions is present. The "seizures" that are seen after accidental ingestion of stimulant tranquilizers are usually actually dystonias.

Toxicity or troublesome side-effects can be managed by decreasing the dosage or changing to another drug. Extrapyramidal signs can usually be relieved by antiparkinsonism drugs.

Antihistamines & Other Less Potent Tranquilizers

Diphenhydramine (Benadryl) and other antihistamines and hydroxyzine (Atarax, Vistaril) are tranquilizers of limited potency. The dosage cannot be increased because of atropine-like side-effects.

The antihistamines were used to induce sleep even before the concept of tranquilizing drugs was introduced. Children often become disinhibited when given barbiturates or the antipsychotic tranquilizers. The sedation caused by these agents is not as subjectively unpleasant at bedtime as it is during the day.

Rauwolfia Alkaloids (Reserpine)

Reserpine has been replaced as an antipsychotic tranquilizer by the phenothiazines, and its use is now limited to the treatment of hypertension. In addition to the side-effects mentioned above, it causes nasal congestion, gastric hypersecretion, and diarrhea.

MINOR TRANQUILIZERS

In contrast to the antipsychotic tranquilizers, minor tranquilizers are basically antianxiety agents. Some are also used as anticonvulsants and as sedatives. The 3 main classes are the benzodiazepines, ie, diazepam (Valium), chlordiazepoxide (Librium), and flurazepam (Dalmane); the propanediols, ie, meprobamate (Equanil, Miltown); and the barbiturates.

Barbiturates mimic the effects of alcohol. They suppress the higher control centers and may have a mild euphoriant or depressant effect as well as adversely affecting psychomotor coordination. The barbiturates are addicting and are often used as a means of suicide. Tolerance develops easily, so that increasing doses are required to procure equivalent effects.

In terms of drug management, compared to the propanediol family of drugs and the barbiturates, the benzodiazepines are less depressing to the CNS vital center and therefore have less suicidal potential. An additional advantage of the benzodiazepines over the barbiturates is that the margin between the therapeutic and sedative doses is wider, allowing greater latitude in establishing optimal therapeutic doses.

Any antianxiety agents should be used with great sensitivity and thoughtfulness, since these drugs are not specific for target symptoms but are directed at "anticipatory anxiety," which has specific inherent dynamic constellations.

SEDATIVE-HYPNOTICS

In contrast to the antipsychotic tranquilizers, the sedatives are antianxiety agents. They are, of course, also anticonvulsants and used to induce sleep.

The drugs listed below have a number of effects in common. The first 4 properties listed are the stages of anesthesia produced by increasingly larger doses.

(1) Sedation, relief of anxiety, encouragement of normal sleep.

(2) Disinhibition, excitement, drunkenness: Paradoxical excitement is common in children, especially when the continued stimulation of pain, restraint, or anxiety is present.

(3) General anesthesia.

(4) Medullary depression and death.

(5) Anticonvulsant effect.

(6) Habituation and withdrawal: Rare in children, although misuse of secobarbital and other sedatives involves younger age groups each year.

(7) Spinal cord depressant action: These drugs are theoretically but not practically useful as voluntary muscle relaxants.

Classification

The sedatives can be classified according to their chemical structure as barbiturates, piperidinediones (glutethimide [Doriden]), dicarbamates (meprobamate), alcohols (chloral hydrate), ethers (paraldehyde), or benzodiazepines (chlordiazepoxide [Librium]). However, it is more useful to classify them according to their rapidity of action and duration of effect. Those with a rapid onset of action have short

duration of action, and those with a prolonged effect have a longer latent period.

A. Short-Acting: Pentobarbital, secobarbital, chloral hydrate.

B. Intermediate-Acting: Amobarbital, meprobamate, diazepam (Valium), chlordiazepoxide (Librium), flurazepam (Dalmane).

C. Long-Acting: Phenobarbital, mephobarbital (Mebaral), oxazepam (Serax).

STIMULANTS

Stimulants have been found to be effective in the treatment of children who are hyperactive, eg, children with *minimal brain dysfunction (MBD)*, which is characterized by a chronic history of short attention span, emotional lability, impulsiveness, and moderate to severe hyperactivity. Minor neurologic signs, abnormal EEG, and learning problems may also be present. Drugs are not indicated for all children with MBD, and least of all for those whose symptoms are related to environmental factors. Although some hyperactive children with chronic or acute anxiety may respond to stimulants, care should be taken not to regard drug therapy as the only resource that can be offered the child and his family. The decision to prescribe medication will depend upon an assessment of the chronicity and severity of the symptoms.

Treatment for school-age children with either dextroamphetamine or methylphenidate (Ritalin) is initiated with 5 mg at breakfast and lunch, increasing by 5 mg increments every several days until improvement occurs or side-effects (anorexia or insomnia) appear. Dosages of up to 30 mg/day of dextroamphetamine and 40 mg/day of methylphenidate may be needed. Frequent consultations with the classroom teacher will help determine the drug's effectiveness and permit dosage adjustments. If after 2 weeks no noticeable change in symptomatology has occurred, the drug should be discontinued.

Caution should be exercised in the use of stimulants with children under 6 years of age.

If effective, these drugs can be continued until puberty, when they are usually no longer necessary and when abuse can more readily occur.

Alexandris A, Lundell F: Effect of thioridazine, amphetamine, and placebo on hyperkinetic syndrome and cognitive area in mentally deficient children. Can Med Assoc J 98:92, 1968.

Charlton MH: Use of Ritalin in hyperactive children. NY State J Med 2:2058, 1972.

Connors CK, Eisenberg L, Barcai A: Effect of dextroamphetamine on children: Studies on subjects with learning disabilities and school behavior problems. Arch Gen Psychiatry 17:478, 1967.

ANTIDEPRESSANTS & LITHIUM

Whether the antidepressant drugs (tricyclics, monoamine oxidase inhibitors) will find a place in pediatric practice has not been established. The types of depression treated successfully with these drugs in adults do not occur as clearly in children and adolescents. Imipramine and other drugs in this group can have serious toxic effects.

On the other hand, there is mounting evidence in the literature that lithium has been effective in the treatment of bipolar type (manic-depressive) disorders, which do occur, though rarely, in adolescence. Lithium is useful for the acute manic phase as well as serving as a modulator for the highs and lows characteristic of the bipolar patient. Lithium can be lethal if given without careful patient selection, adequate clinical control, and frequent determination of serum lithium levels.

Herreno FA: Lithium carbonate toxicity. JAMA 266:1109, 1973.

Stallone F & others: The use of lithium in affective disorders. 3. A double-blind study of prophylaxis in bipolar illness. Am J Psychiatry 130:1006, 1973.

THE PEDIATRICIAN & OTHER SERVICES IN THE COMMUNITY

The pediatrician can contribute to the early treatment and in some cases prevention of some major current social issues. Such problems as adoption, disturbed families, delinquency, child battering, illegitimate pregnancies, and homicide can be partially solved or prevented by the kind of early intervention the pediatrician is in a position to offer. Physicians responsible for the care of children should be familiar with the mental health, family service, and other agencies in their communities and should use them when necessary.

PSYCHOTHERAPEUTIC ASPECTS OF THE ROLE OF THE PEDIATRICIAN

Various aspects of the psychotherapeutic role of the pediatrician in dealing with children and their parents include, among others, emotionally supportive contacts during the prenatal period; later, helping the parents to promote the child's healthy personality development; and preparation of the child and parents for potentially stressful experiences such as hospitalization or surgery.

Some aspects of supportive psychotherapy which the pediatrician can use in dealing with parents and with older children and adolescents have already been mentioned. In working with parents of children with mild psychologic disorders or with chronic illnesses or handicaps, he can provide emotional support. He can help them to ventilate their feelings and to develop spontaneous insights by helping to clarify conflicting feelings or by offering gentle confrontation of inconsistencies in their attitudes.

The pediatrician may reflect feelings back to the parents by repeating emotion-laden words, offering them an opportunity to explore conflicts further. At times he can verbalize for them certain feelings or thoughts. He may offer advice or counseling and can help them work through feelings already recognized, particularly in the case of serious illness. By suggestion, persuasion, and other means, he can facilitate constructive changes in the parents' attitudes and behavior.

The use of toys and play interviews can help younger children to clarify their fears, confusion, or conflicts, offering them a chance to discharge tension or master anxieties through "playing out" their feelings.

Verbal discussion and counseling can be helpful for older children and adolescents if they can talk easily, but improvement may often occur on a nonverbal level as a result of the young person's perception of the pediatrician's attitudes toward him and his parents.

Confidentiality of the older child's or adolescent's intimate revelations should be maintained and explained to the parents. Exceptions should be made only with the young person's knowledge and only when obviously necessary, such as a potential suicide attempt or serious delinquency.

Attention should be paid to attitudes or feelings which are transferred from past experiences with key figures onto the pediatrician. Awareness of the origin of these transferences will help the pediatrician to avoid reacting to the situation as if the attitudes were directed personally toward him. It may at times be wise to confront the parent or child with the fact that such attitudes or feelings derive from other experiences. If certain types of behavior often make him angry or frustrated, the pediatrician must examine his own responses. Such feelings may be influenced by his own past experiences, representing a type of countertransference which may not be appropriate to the circumstances.

The pediatrician may sometimes employ family interviews, especially if communication between parents and child or adolescent seems blocked. He must take an active, directive approach in such situations, helping the family to maintain control and to avoid explosive releases of hostile feelings. Group discussions, often with the aid of a social worker or other mental health professional, may be of value for parents of chronically ill children or for adolescents with hemophilia, diabetes, or other chronic disorders. They may be employed with groups of parents of well children also in a kind of "child study" approach.

The pediatrician may act as a coordinator of the contributions of other professionals in the health team, as in a comprehensive approach to the management of children in a hospital ward. In the community, he may act as a consultant to nursery schools, public schools, courts, camps, social agencies, or child guidance clinics. He can also use his influence to promote the development of needed mental health resources, which may aid him and other health professionals in preventing emotional disorders and further unhealthy adaptation and personality development.

Bolian GC: Diagnosis and treatment: Psychosocial aspects of well child care. Pediatrics 39:280, 1967.
Shulman JL: The management of the irate parent. J Pediatr 77:338, 1970.

SPECIFIC CLINICAL DISORDERS

Although the definition of normality in development and behavior has a certain relativity because of individual variations and different cultural settings, an assessment of healthy behavioral responses can be made.

Appropriateness of behavior to the age of the child or stage of development is a basic consideration, and the same is true of the balance of progressive versus·regressive forces and the general "smoothness" of development. The latter includes the clinician's assessment of the child's adaptation in the present as well as his mastery of stresses in the past. Such considerations may be modified in accordance with the child's endowment, his current developmental level, the nature of the stresses to which he is subjected in his particular family and social setting, and other factors. The following classification is adapted from that offered by the Committee on Child Psychiatry of the Group for the Advancement of Psychiatry (see reference on p 668).

HEALTHY RESPONSES

1. DEVELOPMENTAL CRISES

Developmental crises are brief and transient upheavals which are definitely related to a particular developmental stage and involve attempts to resolve appropriate psychosocial tasks. The child appears normal except for the manifestations of the developmental crisis.

Examples include "stranger" and "separation" anxieties of the second half of the first year, related to the capacity of the infant to distinguish between the mother and others. Anxiety, oppositional behavior, and other manifestations are most marked when developmental tasks are normally most demanding, as when the young child is first separated from the parent.

Treatment consists of a supportive counseling approach to help the child master the crisis and move on to the next stage of development. Anticipatory counseling of the parents is helpful so that they will not handle the child too permissively or too punitively at such times. Inappropriately handled, a developmental crisis may become a reactive disorder (see below) or may crystallize into a psychoneurotic or personality disorder. If a developmental crisis comes too early or too late, it may represent a developmental deviation.

2. SITUATIONAL CRISES

Situational crises are usually transient and brief and are related to situations in the family or environment which represent acutely stressful circumstances for a particular child. The resulting behavioral problems appear to be normal adaptive responses to crisis situations and not deeply disturbed behavior. The child appears normal on examination except for his behavioral response to the crisis situation.

Examples of situational crises include the death of a parent or other serious family crisis and the mild regression that may occur upon return from the hospital after a tonsillectomy. Depression may be apparent in grief reactions. Depressive equivalents may be manifested by temporary loss of appetite, sleep disturbances, or change in activity level. Regression is often characterized by a transient refusal to speak in infants or loss of bowel and bladder control in toddlers.

Treatment is primarily supportive, since the crises are self-limited. Anticipatory guidance of the parents and preventive measures such as preparation of the child and parents for hospitalization can be vital.

Prolonged stressful circumstances with inadequate parental response can lead to reactive disorders or more structured psychopathology.

Erickson E: Growth and crises of the healthy personality. In: *Symposium on the Healthy Personality.* Supplement II. Josiah Macy Jr Foundation, 1950.
Friedman SB: Management of death in a parent or sibling. In: *Ambulatory Pediatrics.* Green M, Haggerty R (editors). Saunders, 1968.
Sugar M: Children of divorce. Pediatrics 46:588, 1970.

REACTIVE DISORDERS

Pathologic behavior or symptoms may occur in response to·disturbing events or situations. They are usually transient but may develop into more severe and chronic psychopathology. Such responses are most common in preschool and early school age children.

The child is usually normal on examination but may have had previous adaptive difficulties.

The reactive disorders differ from situational crises in the matter of degree. A disturbing situation arising acutely may have a profound effect. Examples include illness and hospitalization, accidents, loss of a parent, school pressures, and parental behavior problems. The important consideration is not the strength of the stimulus but the intensity of the child's reaction, which is a function of his ego development, his adaptive capacity, his past experience, and his original endowment. Physiologic concomitants such as peptic ulcer or ulcerative colitis may be precipitated in the predisposed youngster. Depression or regressive behavior may include withdrawal, thumbsucking, wetting or soiling, or excessive daydreaming and preoccupation with fantasy.

Treatment is similar to that of situational crisis: supportive counseling for the parents, with anticipatory guidance and clarification of misconceptions, and emotional support for the child. "Replacement" therapy in the hospital, with the use of parent substitutes or liberalized visiting hours, will help to compensate for emotional deprivation. In some cases, a reactive disorder may be superimposed upon a psychoneurosis, a personality disorder, or even a chronic psychosis of moderate severity. A reactive disorder involving temporary arrest in development may evolve into a developmental deviation or psychoneurosis, and formal intensive psychotherapy may be necessary.

DEVELOPMENTAL DEVIATIONS

Developmental deviations become manifest over a period of months or years as characteristics of the child's development. A single parameter of development may be involved (eg, motor or sensory), or the deviation may be characterized by lags, unevenness, or precocities in maturational steps.

Included in this diagnosis are deviations in maturational patterns such as capacity for control or rhythmic integration in such bodily functions as sleeping, eating, speech, or bowel and bladder functions. Specific types of deviations involved are described briefly below.

Types of Developmental Deviations

A. Motor Development: Eg, hyperactivity, hypoactivity, incoordination, and handedness, along with other predominantly motor capacities, where brain damage is not involved.

B. Sensory Development: Difficulty in monitoring stimuli from tactile to social in nature. Such children may overreact or be apathetic to stimuli.

C. Speech Development: Significant delays other than those due to deafness, oppositional behavior, elective mutism, brain damage, or early childhood psychosis. Disorders of articulation, rhythm, or phonation, or

an infantile type of speech comprehension, may be evident. Normal word repetition by a healthy child in the preschool phase and stuttering as a conversion symptom are not included in this group.

D. Cognitive Function: Problems of symbolic or abstract thinking such as reading, writing, and arithmetic. "Pseudoretarded" and significantly precocious youngsters are in this category.

E. Social Development: Eg, children with delayed capacities for parental separation, marked shyness, dependence, inhibitions, and immaturely aggressive behavior.

F. Psychosexual Development: Eg, timing of sexual curiosity, persistence of infantile auto-erotic patterns, or markedly precocious or delayed heterosexual interests.

G. Affective (Emotional) Development: Eg, moderate anxiety, emotional lability not appropriate to the child's age, marked overcontrol of emotions, mild depression or apathy, and cyclothymic behavior.

H. Integrative Development: Lack of impulse control or frustration tolerance and uneven use or overuse of defense mechanisms (eg, projection or denial).

Treatment

In many cases, no formal treatment is necessary. Explanation to the parents of the nature of the deviation may suffice, and counseling about management of the child is often helpful.

Psychotherapy is necessary in cases involving sweeping lags in maturational patterns or developing personality disturbances.

The amphetamines may be useful for the hyperactive child; speech therapy when there is a lag in speech development; and remedial tutoring for the youngster with a cognitive lag.

Chess S: Individuality in children: Its importance to the pediatrician. J Pediatr 69:676, 1966.
Thomas A, Chess S: *Temperament and Development.* Bruner/Mazel, 1977.

PSYCHONEUROTIC DISORDERS

Psychoneurotic disorders are ordinarily chronic and structured in nature, pervading the whole personality. They are characterized by psychologic symptoms (free-floating anxiety, obsessive thoughts, and phobias) which can be crippling. They arise from the child's internalized unconscious conflicts, often with apparent reference to current family situations.

Psychoneuroses in flagrant form are not common before early school age. No gross disturbances in reality testing are observed in spite of the apparent irrationality of the child's fears or other symptoms.

Types of Psychoneuroses in the Pediatric Age Group

A. Anxiety Type: The conflict breaks into awareness as an intense and diffuse feeling of apprehension or impending diaster—in contrast to normal apprehensions, conscious fears, or content-specific phobias. The physiologic concomitants of anxiety, in contrast to psychophysiologic disorders, do not lead to structural changes in involved organ systems.

B. Phobic Type: There is unconscious displacement onto an object or situation in the external environment that has symbolic significance for the child. For example, there may be a conscious fear of animals, school, dirt, disease, elevators, etc. Phobias, with their internalized and structured character, should be distinguished from developmental crises involving separation anxiety and the mild fears and transient phobias of the stressful experiences in reactive disorders. School phobias are discussed below.

C. Conversion Type: The original conflict is expressed as a somatic dysfunction of organs supplied by the voluntary portion of the CNS—usually the striated musculature or somatosensory apparatus. Included are disturbances of motor function, as in paralysis or motor tics; alterations in sensory perception, as in cases of blindness or deafness; disturbances in awareness, as in conversion syncope or convulsive-like phenomena; and disturbances in the total body image, as in psychologic invalidism associated with extreme weakness or bizarre paralyses. Dysfunctions of the upper and lower ends of the gastrointestinal tract, as in certain types of vomiting or encopresis; of the voluntary components of respiration, as in hyperventilation and respiration (coughing or barking); and of the genitourinary organs, as in certain types of enuresis or bladder atony, may also be conversion expressions. EEG changes are nonspecific, and local structural abnormalities have not been demonstrated except those secondary to long-standing conversions. Personality disorders and borderline psychoses may be associated and may justify multiple diagnoses.

D. Dissociative Type: Includes fugue states, cataplexy, transient catatonic states without underlying psychosis, and conditions with aimless motor discharge or "freezing." Disturbances in consciousness may occur with hypnagogic or hypnopompic or so-called twilight states, marked somnambulism, and pseudodelirious and stuporous states. Depersonalization, dissociated personality, amnesia, Ganser's syndrome (in adolescents), and pseudopsychotic states or "hysterical psychoses" may be present episodically. Although a hysterical personality may be involved, other psychopathologic disorders may be present also. Panic states (usually reactive disorders), acute brain syndromes, psychotic conditions, and epileptic equivalents must be differentiated.

E. Obsessive-Compulsive Type: The countless rituals (eg, excessive orderliness and washing compulsions) with marked anxiety resulting from interference by the parents or others. This disorder must be distinguished from the normal ritualism in early childhood associated with bedtime or toilet training or the pseudocompulsive rituals in the early school age.

F. Depressive Type: Often expressed differently in children than in adults. Symptoms include eating and sleeping disturbances and hyperactivity. Chronic depressive disorders are modified by the child's stage of development and must be distinguished from the more acute reactive disorders in which depression may be involved (eg, the anaclitic type). Depression may be a component of any clinical problem from developmental crisis to psychosis.

Treatment

Treatment may be minimal, eg, supportive counseling, since some mild psychoneurotic disorders resolve spontaneously. However, intensive psychotherapy for parents and child is often required and is usually successful, especially in the anxiety, phobic, conversion, and depressive types. Severe obsessive-compulsive and dissociative types often require child analysis.

Tranquilizing agents are of limited value but may be used to control free-floating anxiety.

Enger NB, Walker PA: Hyperventilation syndrome in childhood. J Pediatr 70:521, 1967.

Goodwin DW & others: Follow-up studies in obsessional neurosis. Arch Gen Psychiatry 20:182, 1969.

Judd LL: Obsessive-compulsive neurosis in children. Arch Gen Psychiatry 12:136, 1965.

Poznanski EO, Krahenbuhl V, Zrull JP: Childhood depression: A longitudinal perspective. J Am Acad Child Psychiatry 15:491, 1976.

Rock NL: Conversion reactions in childhood. J Am Acad Child Psychiatry 10:1, 1971.

Sandler J, Joffee WG: Notes on childhood depression. Int J Psychoanal 46:88, 1965.

Toolan JM: Depression in children and adolescents. Am J Orthopsychiatry 32:404, 1962.

PERSONALITY DISORDERS

Personality disorders in childhood (not commonly seen in flagrant form before late school age) are usually chronic and structured in nature, pervading the child's entire personality. They are manifested as chronic or fixed pathologic behavioral characteristics derived from responses to earlier conflicts which have become ingrained in the personality structure rather than psychologic symptom formation. No gross distortion in reality testing is observed in spite of the apparent irrationality of the child's behavior.

In discussing these disorders, the concept of a continuum is useful. At one end are the relatively well organized personalities with, for example, constructively compulsive traits or somewhat overdependent features, representing mild to moderate exaggerations of healthy personality trends. These may blend into the environment and may almost pass unnoticed unless the interpersonal network of relationships suddenly or radically changes. At the other end are markedly impulsive, sometimes poorly organized personalities which dramatically come into conflict with society as a result of their sexual or social patterns of behavior.

Symptom formation of a psychoneurotic nature is rarely seen, and in most cases the traits are not perceived by the child as a source of anxiety. Premonitory patterns are often seen during infancy and early childhood as fixations in early psychosexual and psychosocial development.

The clinical picture dictates the subcategories, which include compulsive, hysterical, anxious, overly dependent, oppositional, overly inhibited, isolated, mistrustful, tension discharge, sociosyntonic, and sexual deviation.

Treatment & Prognosis

Treatment and prognosis vary according to severity. In its milder forms, the disorder may offer sublimatory outlets (eg, compulsiveness may make for good work habits). More severe forms are more crippling and interfere with effective academic or social functions (eg, delinquency, poor impulse control) or conflict with a new social setting such as the military service when a sociosyntonic personality moves out of his subculture and into the army.

While counseling of children and parents may be sufficient in cases of mild disorders of the obsessive, hysterical, anxious, overly dependent, oppositional, or overly inhibited types, intensive psychotherapy on an outpatient basis is usually necessary for more severe disorders, including the true sexual deviations. Day hospitalization programs with a psychoeducational approach or special classes are indicated if associated learning difficulties are present.

Children with moderate to severe isolated, mistrustful, tension discharge, or impulse-ridden personality types generally require intensive treatment on a residential basis. This is particularly the case when delinquency and drug or alcohol problems are involved. A residential setting, whether it be a hospital, cottage type group living setting, group foster home, or treatment-oriented correctional institution, should provide warmth, structure, consistent limits, and positive relationships with a well trained staff who have adequate mental health consultation.

Cloward RA, Ohlon LE: Some current theories on delinquent subcultures. Pages 540–564 in: *Childhood Psychopathology.* Harrison S, McDermott J (editors). Internat Univ Press, 1972.

Zuger B: Effeminate behavior present in boys from early childhood. 1. The clinical syndrome and follow-up studies. J Pediatr 69:1098, 1966.

PSYCHOTIC DISORDERS

Psychoses may be of sudden or gradual onset in infancy, childhood, or adolescence, with differences in the clinical picture in relation to developmental level. The essential features are failure to develop awareness of or withdrawal from reality, with preoccupation with inner fantasy life; failure to develop emotional relationships with human figures, or retreat from established relationships; inability to express emotions appropriately or to use speech communicatively; and bizarre, stereotyped, or otherwise seriously inappropriate behavior.

Hallucinations and delusions, as well as other classic characteristics of adult psychoses, are rarely encountered until late school age or early adolescence.

Obsessions, compulsions, phobias, and other psychologic or behavioral symptoms may occur in psychotic children. They are markedly intense and tenacious, and the child usually has no awareness of their lack of logic or appropriateness.

Type of Psychoses in the Pediatric Age Group
A. Psychoses of Early Childhood:

1. **Early infantile autism**—Must be distinguished from autism secondary to brain damage or mental retardation. The onset is within the first year of life, and the child remains aloof from all human contact, being preoccupied with inanimate objects. The child resists any change with outbursts of temper or anxiety when routines are altered. Speech is delayed or absent, and sleep and feeding problems are severe. Intellectual functioning is restricted or uneven, probably related to perceptual and communication problems.

2. **Interactional psychotic disorders**—These disorders of infancy and early childhood include the so-called "symbiotic psychoses." The problem revolves around the failure of the youngster to master the step of separation and individuation, often because of the mother's inability to allow the child to separate from her. The psychotic disorder is often precipitated in the second to fifth year by some shift in the mother-child relationship such as the birth of a sibling or a family crisis. The overdependent child then shows intense separation anxiety and clinging, with regressive manifestations. The picture is one of gradual withdrawal, emotional aloofness, autistic behavior, and distorted perception of reality.

3. **Other psychotic disorders**—Other psychoses of early childhood include "atypical" or fragmented ego development in children who exhibit some autistic behavior and emotional aloofness.

B. Psychoses of Later Childhood: Schizophreniform psychotic disorders occur in the school age period and are characterized by a gradual onset of neurotic symptoms followed by concrete thinking, loose associations, hypochondriacal tendencies, and intense temper outbursts. Later developments may include a breakdown in reality testing, autism, anxiety, and uncontrollable phobias. Bizarre behavior and stereotyped motor patterns, such as whirling, are often observed. Other children may have sudden and wild outbursts of aggressive or self-mutilating behavior, inappropriate mood swings, and suicidal threats or attempts. The range of other psychotic behavior seen in adults may occur, usually in older children. Organic brain syndromes and severe panic states with a tempo-

rary thought disorder due to anxiety require careful differential assessment.

C. Psychoses of Adolescence:

1. Acute confusional state—This is a "psychosis" of adolescence with an abrupt onset of acute and intense anxiety, depressive trends, confusion in thinking, and feelings of depersonalization. The crisis of identity is very common, but evidence of a true thought disorder or marked breakdown in reality testing is usually lacking. While rapid recovery is the rule, a deep-seated personality disorder may underlie the psychotic picture. Differential considerations include neurotic panic states and the severe upsets seen in normal adolescents.

2. Adult types of schizophrenia—These occur in late adolescence, with minor differences related to the developmental level. Manifestations include the myriad symptoms seen in adults.

Treatment & Prognosis

Treatment and prognosis vary considerably. The psychotic disorders of early childhood have a more guarded prognosis.

A. Young Children: Patients with early infantile autism have a guarded prognosis and often require long-term hospital care. Interactional psychotic disorders fare somewhat better and may respond to outpatient treatment of the child and the parents. Such treatment can often clarify the child's basic intellectual endowment and help the parents to accept, when necessary, later placement for treatment. In the management of these young children, play therapy as a restitutional experience for emotional deprivation—and simultaneous therapy for the parents—may be usefully combined with the contributions of a therapeutic nursery school. Operant conditioning (positive reinforcement by praise, affection, or reward for healthy behavior) has been helpful in teaching these youngsters speech and socialization. Placement in a nursery school requires preceding treatment to alleviate the separation anxiety of the child and the parents.

Family conjoint therapy and tranquilizing agents have limited value, the latter being useful when the child is very anxious, hyperactive, or destructive.

B. School Age Children: For the school age child with a schizophreniform psychosis, short-term psychiatric hospitalization with several weeks to several months of milieu therapy and individual psychotherapy for the child and parents often assists the youngster with an acute onset to recompensate so that further therapy can be continued on an outpatient basis. This may include family conjoint therapy (wherein the family is treated together and separately). The chronically psychotic child may require long-term residential treatment or long-term placement in small cottage type group living quarters or professional group foster homes.

The psychoactive drugs are useful mainly in controlling outbursts of panic or aggressive behavior.

C. Older Children: The adolescent or postadolescent psychotic disorders often respond well to brief psychiatric hospitalization of only a few days or weeks. This is particularly true of the acute confusional state. Patients with sweeping regressive states may require several months of hospitalization. Very few adolescents, even with adult type schizophrenic disorders, require long-term hospitalization, and only a small proportion have further episodes or become chronically schizophrenic.

Psychoactive drugs are more effective in adolescents than in children and are used adjunctively with psychotherapeutic measures.

Campbell M: Biological intervention in psychoses of childhood. J Autism Child Schizo 3:347, 1973.

Gittelman M, Birch HG: Childhood schizophrenia. Arch Gen Psychiatry 17:16, 1967.

Jordan K, Prugh D: Schizophreniform psychosis in childhood. Am J Psychiatry 128:323, 1971.

Kanner L: Early infantile autism. J Pediatr 25:211, 1944.

PSYCHOPHYSIOLOGIC DISORDERS

The psychophysiologic disorders involve organs or organ systems which are innervated by the autonomic nervous system—in contrast to conversion disorders, which involve the striated musculature and somatosensory apparatus. Biologic predisposing factors appear to be involved, with probable latent biochemical defects. Psychologic and social factors act as additional predisposing, precipitating, and perpetuating influences. More than one organ system may be involved.

Anxiety is not alleviated by these disorders—in contrast to conversion disorders, where anxiety is repressed and "bound" in the symbolic symptom.

No type-specific personality profile, parent-child relationship, or family pattern has as yet been associated with individual psychophysiologic disorders, although some may occur in conjunction with personality disorders.

These disorders may be mild or severe and transient or chronic. A continuum probably exists ranging from cases with milder biologic predisposition and greater psychologic involvement to those which are more heavily "loaded" biologically, requiring less psychologic influence for their appearance and perpetuation.

A brief summary of the various organ systems affected and the clinical manifestations follows. For treatment and prognosis, see p 653.

Skin

Psychophysiologic skin disorders include certain cases of neurodermatitis, seborrheic dermatitis, psoriasis, pruritus, alopecia, eczema, urticaria, angioneurotic edema, and acne. Atopic eczema may persist into childhood or may disappear and recur in late childhood and adolescence, with patches of dermatitis becoming widespread and severe during early adolescence. Affected children are generally rigid, tense, and at times compulsive, with a tendency to repress strong emotions, particularly toward an overcontrolling mother. Exacerbations during adolescence are usually related to increased conflicts over independence and sexuality. The latter considerations are also involved in urticaria patients, who are often shy, passive, and immature, with feelings of inadequacy, unconscious exhibitionistic trends, and overdependency upon the mother.

Kremer MM: Psychological impact of acne in adolescents. J Am Med Wom Assoc 24:309, 1969.

Musculoskeletal System

Psychophysiologic musculoskeletal disorders include certain cases of low back pain, rheumatoid arthritis, "tension" headaches and other myalgias, muscle cramps, bruxism, and specific types of malocclusion (the latter may involve some conversion components). Children with rheumatoid arthritis often exhibit conflicts over the handling of aggression and dependency, and exacerbations are often related to shifts in family balance.

Cleveland SE, Reitmann EE, Brewer EJ: Psychological factors in juvenile rheumatoid arthritis. Arthritis Rheum 8:1152, 1965.

Respiratory System

Psychophysiologic respiratory disorders may include certain cases of bronchial asthma, allergic rhinitis, chronic sinusitis, hiccup, breathholding spells, and hyperventilation. Psychologic factors contributing to asthmatic attacks include threatened separation from the parents and parental marital conflicts.

Enger NB, Walker PA: Hyperventilation syndrome in childhood. J Pediatr 70:521, 1967.
Purcell K: Distinctions between subgroups of asthmatic children. Pediatrics 31:486, 1963.

Cardiovascular System

Psychophysiologic cardiovascular disorders may overlap with respiratory disorders and include some cases of paroxysmal tachycardia, peripheral vascular spasm (eg, Raynaud's disease and central angiospastic retinopathy), migraine, erythromelalgia, causalgia, vasodepressor syncope, epistaxis, essential hypertension, hypotension, and eclampsia in adolescents. Intense autonomic responses to emotional trauma can trigger paroxysmal tachycardia which may lead to syncope. Children with orthostatic hypotension often appear to be tense, anxious, emotionally restricted, and "not sure where they stand" in their families. Similar characteristics occur in children or adolescents with vasodepressor syncope, often precipitated by sudden fright or pain anticipation. This syncope should be distinguished from conversion syncope which often occurs in hysterical girls who have other conversion phenomena but no vascular changes. Migraine presents during the school age period (headache is rare in pre-

school children) and is often triggered by emotional crises. The patients tend to be rather rigid, sometimes compulsive individuals in tense families.

Falstein EI, Rosenblum AH: Juvenile paroxysmal supraventricular tachycardia: Psychosomatic and psychodynamic aspects. J Am Acad Child Psychiatry 1:246, 1962.
Green M: Fainting. In: *Ambulatory Pediatrics*. Green M, Haggerty R (editors). Saunders, 1968.
Holguin J, Fenichel E: Migraine. J Pediatr 70:290, 1967.
Katcher AL: Hypertension in adolescent children. Med Clin North Am 48:1467, 1964.

Gastrointestinal System

The psychophysiologic gastrointestinal disorders comprise a large category of varied clinical disorders. Since the gastrointestinal tract is so responsive to emotional factors, it is unusual to find gastrointestinal disorders which are not affected by the psychic adjustment of the individual. Some of the more common problems include pylorospasm, gastric hyperacidity, pseudo-peptic ulcer syndrome, idiopathic celiac disease, nontropical sprue in adolescents, megacolon (aganglionic type), constipation, diarrhea, and cyclic vomiting in tense, overprotected children in families with these tendencies.

A. Peptic Ulcer: Peptic ulcers in school age children and adolescents are different from those in adults and probably more common. Abdominal pain is not well localized, nausea and vomiting are common, and symptoms are not closely related to meals. Individuals who develop peptic ulcer have high blood pepsinogen levels from infancy, reflecting tendencies toward gastric hypersecretion. In children who have difficulty in handling hostile feelings, are demanding of affection, and are passive and dependent, peptic ulcers are apt to develop in stressful situations.

B. Ulcerative Colitis: Children with ulcerative colitis are often overdependent, passive, inhibited, and compulsive, and frequently manipulate the parents. Precipitation of fulminant cases usually takes place in a situation with actual or threatened loss of emotional support from a key figure. Exacerbations are frequently related to family crises. Other psychologic factors include familial patterns of autonomic response to stress, involving the lower gastrointestinal tract in "bowel oriented" families, conditioning of the defecation reflex to emotional conflict in coercive toilet training, and maternal overprotection and overdominance in early childhood. These factors lead to overdependence and resentment by the child.

C. Regional Ileitis: Patients with regional ileitis have psychosocial similarities to those with ulcerative colitis and mucous colitis, the latter being generally less disturbed.

D. Obesity: Obesity results basically from an excess of intake over output of calories as a result of hyperphagia, usually in families with a tendency toward overeating and obesity. From a psychosocial view, there are 2 major groups: the *reactive* type, responding to an emotionally traumatic experience (eg, the death of a parent or a school failure); and the *developmental* type, where the origins are principally in the disturbed family's tendencies toward overeating, with probably some biologic predisposition also involved. The child is often overvalued by the family, sometimes because of the loss of a previous child. He becomes obese as a result of overfeeding and continues to be obese from infancy on. The mother usually dominates and protects the child, and, after an early period of demanding behavior, the child goes on to become passive, overdependent, and immature. In such children, feelings of helplessness, despair, and withdrawal from social interaction are associated with more overeating, and food is used as a solace to ward off depression or feelings of hostility. The "wall of weight" is a way of hiding from social problems and is often used to ward off sexual conflicts with feelings of ugliness or unattractiveness.

E. Anorexia Nervosa: This syndrome occurs in late school age to postadolescence, usually in females. It consists of loss of appetite, denial of physical hunger, aversion to food, severe weight loss, emaciation and pallor, amenorrhea, lowered body temperature; decreased metabolism, pulse rate, and blood pressure; flat or occasionally diabetic blood sugar curves, dry skin, brittle nails, cold intolerance, and, in severe and protracted cases, other symptoms and signs such as gastric hypoacidity and diarrhea. Activity levels remain high even with marked emaciation. Patients are often preoccupied or irritable and have difficulty in verbalizing their feelings. The onset is often related to menarche or traumatic incidents with serious dieting which continues out of control. The parents are frequently in the food business. The mother and daughter often have an ambivalent (hostile-dependent) relationship, and the involvement with the father often has had a seductive quality. During preadolescence, such patients are often overconscientious, energetic, high achievers, but they remain strongly dependent upon the parents.

Three main groups of patients are seen: (1) those with psychoneurotic disorders (mixed hysterical and phobic trends) with sexual implications and symbolic meanings attributed to eating and body weight; (2) those with obsessive-compulsive personality disorders; and (3) schizophrenic or near-psychotic individuals with massive projection tendencies and fears of poisoning. A few show the syndrome as a severe reactive disorder, at times with strongly depressive trends.

F. Recurrent Abdominal Pain: This common syndrome occurs in 10–13% of children, but over 90% show no physical basis for the pain. In most cases, symptoms are epigastric or periumbilical and are usually related to some emotional crisis in tense, apprehensive, timid, and often overly conscientious children who have experienced parental overprotection. Fourteen- and 6-per-second EEG spikes are not diagnostic; they occur in many normal children in the early school age period. School phobia or identification with a family member with abdominal pain is sometimes reported.

Apley J: The child with recurrent abdominal pain. Pediatr Clin North Am 14:63, 1967.

Bruch H: *Eating Disorders.* Basic Books, 1973.

Davidson M: The irritable colon of children (chronic nonspecific diarrhea syndrome). J Pediatr 69:1027, 1966.

Finch SM, Hess JH: Ulcerative colitis in children. Am J Psychiatry 118:819, 1962.

Green M: Psychogenic recurrent abdominal pain: Diagnosis and treatment. Pediatrics 40:84, 1967.

Heald F: Obesity in the adolescent. In: *Symposium on Adolescence.* Meiks LT, Green M (editors). Saunders, 1960.

Illingworth RS: Practical observations and reflections. 2. Vomiting without organic cause. Clin Pediatr (Phila) 4:685, 1965.

Leiken SJ, Caplan H: Psychogenic polydipsia. Am J Psychiatry 123:1563, 1967.

Lesser LI & others: Anorexia nervosa in children. Am J Orthopsychiatry 30:572, 1960.

Lowe CU, Coursin DB, Heald FP: Obesity in childhood. Pediatrics 40:455, 1967.

Menking M & others: Rumination: A near-fatal psychiatric disease of infancy. N Engl J Med 280:802, 1969.

Prugh DG, Jordan K: The management of ulcerative colitis in childhood. In: *Modern Perspectives in International Child Psychiatry.* Howells J (editor). Oliver & Boyd, 1969.

Reinhart JB, Succop RA: Regional enteritis in pediatric patients: Psychiatric aspects. J Am Acad Child Psychiatry 7:252, 1968.

Genital & Urinary Systems

Psychophysiologic genitourinary disorders include certain cases of menstrual disturbances, functional uterine bleeding, leukorrhea, polyuria and dysuria, vesical paralysis, urethral and vaginal discharges, and persistent glycosuria without diabetes. Disturbances of sexual function (eg, vaginismus, frigidity, frequent erections, dyspareunia, and priapism) are often conversion reactions but may include psychophysiologic components. Menstrual problems are the rule in early adolescence, but they may be intensified or perpetuated by emotional conflicts. Dysmenorrhea has an incidence of up to 12% of high school girls and may be influenced by attitudes of inconvenience or disgust, particularly in middle class girls. Persistence of the symptom indicates difficulty in accepting the feminine role and the responsibilities of womanhood. Premenstrual tension is often intensified by sexual or identity conflicts. Habitual abortion occurs with significant conflicts over sexuality and motherhood. Impotence in adolescent boys is rare, but it may cause problems in teenage marriages—as may frigidity in girls.

Heald FP, Masland RP, Sturgis SH: Dysmenorrhea in adolescence. Pediatrics 20:121, 1957.

Heiman M: The role of stress situations and psychological factors in functional uterine bleeding. J Mt Sinai Hosp 23:755, 1956.

Endocrine System

Psychophysiologic endocrine disorders include certain cases of hyperinsulinism, growth disturbance, diabetes, hyperthyroidism, and, in adolescents, pseudocyesis and disorders of lactation. Emotional conflicts about "growing up" are related to some cases of delayed puberty or delayed onset of menarche. In pseudocyesis, enlargement of the abdomen is a conversion phenomenon, but the physiologic changes of pregnancy derive from obscure psychologic influences on endocrine function. It usually occurs in hysterical personalities with underlying conflicts over feminine identity and motherhood. In more seriously disturbed adolescents, it may occur after the first experience of kissing or petting. Diabetes is significantly influenced by psychologic mechanisms. It is often precipitated or exacerbated in a setting of increased conflict, most often involving a real or threatened loss of a key relationship. Although most juvenile diabetics show increased symptoms in adolescence, those more disturbed may have an exceptionally "stormy course," with coma precipitated by emotional conflict, rebellious overeating, or inattention to insulin requirements. Children and adolescents with thyrotoxicosis often experience the onset in gradually intensifying stressful situations, particularly those involving emotional relationships.

Glaser HH: Physical and psychological development of children with early failure to thrive. J Pediatr 73:690, 1968.

Greaves D, Green PE, West LJ: Psychodynamic and psychophysiological aspects of pseudocyesis. Psychosom Med 22:24, 1960.

Silver HK, Finkelstein M: Deprivation dwarfism. J Pediatr 70:317, 1967.

Nervous System

Psychophysiologic nervous system disorders include idiopathic epilepsy (grand mal, petit mal, psychomotor epilepsy, and epileptic equivalents), narcolepsy, certain types of sleep disturbance, dizziness, vertigo, hyperactivity, motion sickness, and some recurrent fevers of psychologic origin.

A. Epilepsy: Epilepsy, with its unfortunate stigma, frequently produces psychic trauma, although a personality disorder, may antedate its onset. The youngster may have feelings of inferiority, shyness, and feel different from others. Irritability, temper outbursts, or aggressive behavior may be exhibited prior to a seizure. These children tend to experience fears of death before a seizure and may fear they have said or done something "bad" during the interval of postictal amnesia. The anxious parents are frequently overly restrictive about activity. They often blame themselves for the hereditary factor and often equate the seizures with death or "craziness."

Few children deteriorate, intellectually or otherwise, if adequate seizure control is achieved. Seizures often are more frequent or precipitated initially during periods of emotional conflict or family crises. Some children learn ways of inhibiting or touching off seizures, the latter skill sometimes being used in a manipulative way.

The diagnosis of "epileptic equivalent" on the basis of exaggerated fears, repeated tantrums, aggressive behavior, marked withdrawal, or sleepwalking in association with an abnormal EEG is often inappropriate. Most of the children suspected of such equivalents show disturbances in behavior related to conflicts within the family.

A variety of conditions which were formerly thought to bear some relationship to idiopathic epilepsy include migraine, recurrent abdominal pain, cyclic vomiting, and narcolepsy.

B. Narcolepsy: Narcolepsy is uncommon in childhood and more frequent in boys. It is characterized by paroxysmal and recurrent attacks of irresistible sleep, often precipitated by a sudden alteration in emotional state related to conflictual situations. Attacks may come on suddenly from 1−2 times a day to many times a day. They may be associated with cataplexy and hypnagogic hallucinations. The sleep during attacks is light, and the patient is easily awakened. Nocturnal sleep is usually normal, although an earlier appearance of REM sleep has been reported. The major factors are usually psychopathologic, often related to conflicts over competition or the expression of unacceptable aggressive influences. The EEG is normal between attacks, and there is no significant relationship to epilepsy. Narcolepsy is to be differentiated from the Pickwickian syndrome, in which sudden attacks of somnolence occur in markedly obese children.

C. Motion Sickness: Motion sickness in cars, trains, elevators, swings, etc is more common in children than in adults; seasickness and airplane sickness are less frequent in children. Psychologic factors are involved to varying degrees in different children. Tense, apprehensive, or phobic children are most often affected, and family arguments during driving are frequent precipitating factors. Most children improve markedly by adolescence.

D. Hyperactivity: This picture occurs in many children without signs of brain damage. Anxious children who are active from birth may show this symptom, with impulsiveness and distractibility in response to parental overrestrictiveness or other family tensions.

Barbero GJ: Cyclic vomiting. Pediatrics 25:740, 1960.

Berlin I, Yaeger CL: Correlation of epileptic seizures, electroencephalograms and emotional state. Am J Dis Child 81:664, 1951.

Friedman AP, Harms E: *Headaches in Children.* Thomas, 1967.

Laybourne PC: Psychogenic vomiting in children. Am J Dis Child 86:726, 1953.

Yoss RE, Daly DD: Narcolepsy in children. Pediatrics 25:1025, 1960.

Fever

Fever of psychophysiologic origin may occur in children who show excitement or continued emotional tension in the absence of physical overactivity. Chronic low-grade fever may occur in infants with "hospitalism" or in school age children who are anxious or tense. In the latter case, the mother is often overanxious and continues to take the child's temperature every day long after the subsidence of a mild infection. The fever usually disappears upon discontinuation of the daily measurements. Discussion of the parents' apprehension related to guilt or other feelings rather than simple reassurance may be helpful.

Renbourn ET: Body temperature and pulse rate in boys and young men prior to sporting contests: A study of emotional hyperthermia with a review of the literature. J Psychosom Res 4:149, 1960.

Organs of Special Sense

Psychophysiologic disorders of organs of special sense include certain cases of glaucoma, blepharospasm, amblyopia, Ménière's syndrome, and certain types of tinnitus and hyperacusis.

Fowler EP, Zeckel A: Psychosomatic aspects of Ménière's disease. JAMA 148:1265, 1952.

General Principles of Treatment & Prognosis in Pediatric Psychophysiologic Disorders

Treatment and prognosis are related to the multiple interactive factors involved in these disorders. Included are the nature of the biologic predisposition, the degree of personality disturbance and family disruption, the extent of the contribution of psychosocial factors to the perpetuation of the disorder, and the likelihood of its response to psychotherapeutic treatment and medical measures.

The basic approach to treatment should be founded upon an adequate diagnostic evaluation with due consideration to the relative importance of somatic and psychologic factors.

In some disorders, only treatment of the basic emotional deprivation, with "replacement measures" offered by parent substitutes, together with parental treatment, offers any chance of amelioration. In others with mild psychologic components, as in some cases of asthma, medical measures alone will suffice. In some mildly disturbed children—eg, in cases of obesity, menstrual problems, and recurrent abdominal pain—the pediatrician may use a supportive psychotherapeutic approach to the child and parents, with psychiatric consultation initially and as needed. If the patient is hospitalized, seeing him for brief periods at the beginning or end of each day may be more effective than 1–2 hours a week, with the encouragement of an initially dependent relationship upon the pediatrician and, later, gradual "weaning." Long-term follow-up may be indicated, particularly for children with ulcerative colitis (even those treated surgically), who may have later exacerbations at times of emotional trauma.

In more seriously disturbed children with severe conditions of tension headache, asthma, menstrual problems, narcolepsy, quiescent ulcerative colitis, and management problems of diabetes, intensive psychotherapy for the child and parents may have to be carried out by a child psychiatrist or other mental health professional. In most such disorders, supportive psychotherapeutic measures should be undertaken at the beginning, with later use of more intensive measures if necessary. In potentially serious and life-threatening disorders such as acute ulcerative colitis or diabe-

tes, psychotherapeutic treatment should never be undertaken without concomitant medical treatment and follow-up.

In some instances, notably anorexia nervosa, psychiatric hospitalization may be required. Under these circumstances, the psychiatrist may act as a coordinator, drawing upon the contribution of the pediatrician and other consultants regarding the medical or surgical aspects of treatment.

Certain basic principles in the handling of children with psychophysiologic (and many other) illnesses can be listed briefly as follows: *continuity* of the relationship with the child and parents by a single physician (usually the pediatrician); *communication* among professionals, in order to bring about true and respectful *collaboration* among disciplines and *consistency* in management; *consultation* with child psychiatrists and other specialists; and *coordination* of all such activities into a unified plan of therapy with the most appropriate balance of physical, psychologic, and social measures.

Mirsky IA: Physiologic, psychologic, and social determinants of psychosomatic disorders. Dis Nerv Syst 21:50, 1960.
See also General References at end of chapter.

BRAIN SYNDROMES

Essentials of Diagnosis

- Impairment of orientation, judgment, discrimination, learning, memory, other cognitive functions; emotional lability.
- Evidence of cerebral dysfunction, including (1) abnormal neurologic findings, (2) definitively abnormal EEG, (3) perceptual-motor disturbances on psychologic testing, and (4) a history of insult to the CNS. (Three out of 4 should be present to establish the diagnosis.)
- Psychologic disturbances, either preexisting or secondary to brain damage. There is no "pure" cerebral dysfunction without accompanying psychologic reactions.

General Considerations

Brain syndromes result from localized or diffuse damage to brain tissue, particularly the cerebral cortex, due to any cause. The severity of the associated psychotic, neurotic, or behavioral disorders is not necessarily proportionate to the degree of brain damage. The psychologic accompaniment of brain damage is determined by predisposing personality patterns, current emotional conflicts, the child's level of development, family interpersonal relationships, and the nature of the brain disorder and its meaning to the child and his parents. As in adults, such associated disorders are often regarded as having been released by the brain disorder or superimposed on or intertwined with it. In infants and young children, however, later personality development may be influenced by such disorders, whose manifestations may be quite different from those in older children and adults. The young child appears to be able to a great extent to compensate for insults to the CNS as he matures. Functions most recently developed may be most vulnerable to such insults, whereas those developed earlier may be less affected. On the other hand, functions not yet developed may be interfered with, particularly those relating to the cognitive aspects of learning and impulse control. It is thus much harder in children than in adults to correlate the severity of cognitive impairment with the severity of the brain pathology.

Children affected by localized rather than diffuse brain lesions may react in various ways depending only in part upon the brain functions which are interfered with.

Brain syndromes of diffuse nature are classified as acute (reversible) or chronic (permanent). The emphasis in the following paragraphs is on the psychologic and social consequences of brain damage in children.

Clinical Findings

A. Acute Brain Syndromes: Acute brain disorders may be due to intracranial infection, systemic infection, drug or poison (including alcohol) intoxication, trauma, circulatory disturbances, certain types of convulsive disorders, metabolic disturbances such as chronic renal problems, and certain disorders of unknown etiology (eg, multiple sclerosis).

The principal manifestation in children (as in adults) is delirium, a disturbance in awareness resulting from alterations of cerebral metabolism. The clinical picture may be gross and easily identifiable, characterized by wildly agitated or confused behavior and hallucinatory experiences arising from distorted perception or interpretation of stimuli. A subclinical form, however, may present with subtle disturbances in awareness or mildly stuporous states, withdrawn or "difficult" behavior, or irrational fears. In such cases, a rough mental status examination adapted to the child's level of development will often reveal disorientation and misinterpretation of external stimuli. An EEG may aid in diagnosis, revealing large, slow waves and disorganization which disappear upon correction of the disturbance in cerebral metabolism. Perceptual-motor difficulties may persist for some time and may lead to learning difficulties upon return to school even though the brain lesion has completely healed.

Recognition of subclinical forms may be difficult, and the clinician must keep the possibility in mind to avoid overlooking the delirium or to prevent misdiagnosis as psychotic behavior on a psychosocial basis.

Preexisting or underlying psychotic, psychoneurotic, or personality disorders may become more manifest after such insults to the CNS, and reactive disorders or later developmental deviations in cognitive or other areas may result.

B. Chronic Brain Syndromes: These disorders result from relatively permanent, more or less irreversible, diffuse impairment of cerebral tissue function. They may be due to congenital cranial anomalies, cerebral palsy, and other disorders arising from prenatal or perinatal damage to the brain, CNS syphilis, intoxications of various types, brain trauma, convulsive disorders, disturbances of metabolism, growth, or nutrition, intracranial neoplasm, or heredodegenerative factors such as Schilder's encephalopathy, Heller's infantile dementia, etc. Some disturbances in memory, judgment, orientation, comprehension, affect, and learning capacity may persist permanently, accompanied by remarkable compensations at times in individual children during the course of development.

There appears to be no specific type of personality disorder in children with chronic brain syndromes. Many children become overly dependent, with frequent developmental lags in personality organization and other developmental deviations. These psychologic factors appear in varying admixtures with the effects upon behavior of the underlying brain damage, and some of the psychologic features may be the child's reactions to his perceptions of his own limitations.

One particular syndrome frequently seen in young children with diffuse cerebrocortical damage is frequently but not invariably characterized by hyperactivity, distractibility, impulsiveness, and EEG and EMG abnormalities. Difficulties in perceptual-motor functions, spatial orientation, and cerebral integration lead to problems in employing symbols (eg, reading and writing) and in abstract concept formation. Specific neurologic lesions are rarely demonstrable, and the diagnosis must be based on the history and clinical findings. However, children with significant psychologic disturbances may also exhibit difficulties in impulse control, distractibility, and hyperactivity; together with delayed perceptual-motor development and dysrhythmic EEG patterns. Signs of cerebral dysfunction are not always due to organic lesions alone; therefore, diagnoses of "organicity" or "minimal brain damage" based principally on behavioral manifestations seem open to much question.

Many children with chronic brain syndrome are not significantly retarded in intellectual development. They often show significant learning difficulties, however, due to perceptual-motor handicaps, and may function at a mentally retarded level with psychologic and social factors playing a contributory role. If mental retardation is present, this should be specified by means of appropriate tests. In each instance, the predominant personality picture associated with the brain syndrome should be noted, eg, developmental deviations of affective nature, or personality, psychoneurotic, or psychotic disorders.

Cerebral palsy. (See also Chapter 21.) Children with cerebral palsy exhibit motor disabilities of a predominantly extrapyramidal type characterized by choreiform and athetoid movements and frequent sensory and perceptual defects, all of which predispose to learning difficulties and poor achievement on intelligence tests. Speech problems are often present. The physical defects, combined with the child's inability to discharge tensions through physical activity and play, produce anxiety, emotional conflicts, and feelings of difference from others and a negative self-image. Some parents feel guilty and handle the child overprotectively, whereas others may feel ashamed, resentful, or hopeless. Insufficient stimulation or a pessimistic appraisal of the child's prospects by parents, physicians, and teachers may lead to inadequate education in addition to the inherent learning problems.

Children with cerebral palsy are often emotionally immature, introverted, overly dependent, fearful, irritable, and egocentric. Emotional conflicts are commonly most severe during adolescence, although children with athetosis or ataxia may be surprisingly cheerful and outgoing (often with lack of insight into their limitations).

An important and encouraging characteristic of cerebral palsy is its stationary, nonprogressive course.

Treatment

A. Acute Brain Syndrome: The essential problem in the psychologic management of acute brain syndrome is the control of delirium while the underlying cause is being sought and treated. The child must be helped to deal with misperceptions of stimuli in his environment. He may misinterpret shadows as "witches" or "ghosts," or may see medical instruments as the weapons of "killers"—the doctors and nurses. When his parents are not present, a school age child may fear that they are dead or have abandoned him. Instead of darkening the room to cut down on stimuli, it is important to keep the room adequately lighted, especially at night, when such misperceptions are most severe and frightening. A special nurse, relative, or foster grandmother should be in the room at all times during the day and should be available at night in order to serve as an external "auxiliary ego" who can help the child correct his misperceptions and misinterpretations.

Chloral hydrate is probably the best tolerated sedative in childhood delirium, and large doses may be required. Paraldehyde given orally or rectally is the ideal sedative in adolescents, although the odor may be offensive. Barbiturates tend to cause confusion and should be avoided.

It is essential to maintain the tie with the parents, the only truly familiar figures in the delirious child's confused world, through daily visiting or overnight stay by the mother, even for school age children. If a parent is ill or far·away and cannot visit regularly, substitute mothering becomes all the more vital. A familiar blanket or toy from home, or postcards which can be read to the child, will be of some help.

The anxieties and guilt of the parents must also be dealt with, especially in cases involving accidents or poisonings.

B. Chronic Brain Syndrome: Treatment measures, in addition to those directed toward the basic cause of brain dysfunction, include remedial education in small "ungraded" classes from which the child should move to normal classes as soon as possible. Individual tutor-

ing may help to retain the child in his age-appropriate classroom. Special remedial teaching technics using auditory, tactile, and kinesthetic stimuli may be of value.

Children with brain damage and significant emotional problems, including anxiety over performance, problems in impulse control, a negative self-image, and resistance to learning, often respond to psychotherapy for themselves and their parents. Such therapy may at first be largely supportive. Educational components, including some tutoring, may be included.

Cerebral palsy. (See also Chapter 21.) Whereas some parents of cerebral palsied children may simply give up, others go to great lengths to push the child toward normality with "gimmicks" or cure-alls such as the Doman-Delacato approach, which involves a great deal of effort and money. This has been shown by a controlled study to be of no more value than other training methods and may cause emotional problems as a result of the pressure it exerts on the child.

In addition to physical therapy, speech therapy, and drug therapy (including tranquilizers) as indicated, special educational measures, sheltered workshops, and group therapy or discussions for the parents of such children may be helpful, as may individual psychotherapy for the more seriously disturbed. There is no substitute for the physician's continuing supportive relationship with the child and his parents, working with representatives of other disciplines. Children with cerebral palsy, many of whom are not inherently retarded, may make surprisingly adequate emotional and vocational adjustments in spite of continuing problems.

Psychoactive drugs may be of some value. Hyperactivity, impulsiveness, and distractibility may be controlled by the judicious use of amphetamines. The phenothiazines may be of help in the control of anxiety or destructive behavior. Residential treatment may be necessary for children with·severe emotional disturbances.

Prognosis

A. Acute Brain Syndrome: The prognosis for children with acute brain syndrome depends upon the degree of structural brain damage and upon host resistance factors. With appropriate antibiotic therapy, the various types of bacterial meningitis may resolve with little residual damage. The viral encephalitides cannot be controlled so well, but children who have been in coma even for several months may regain complete function, gradually "relearning" lost skills from walking to reading. In all of these disorders—particularly head trauma—the response of the child is influenced by parental reactions. A minor concussion may provoke overprotective patterns of parental behavior with psychologic difficulties during convalescence in spite of complete recovery.

If the child recovers completely, the possibility of persistence of perceptual-motor deficits for some weeks should be explained to the parents and teachers in order to permit gradual return to optimal academic performance.

B. Chronic Brain Syndrome: Infants and children show a remarkable tendency to compensate for diffuse damage to the cerebral cortex, especially if attention is paid to the psychosocial needs of the child and his parents.

Birch HG (editor): *Brain Damage in Children.* Williams & Wilkins, 1964.

Green M: Delirium. In: *Ambulatory Pediatrics.* Green M, Haggerty R (editors). Saunders, 1968.

COMMON PROBLEMS IN PEDIATRIC PRACTICE

COLIC

Colic or paroxysmal fussing is a common problem in young infants. It is most common in the evening. It may build up in a crescendo, with the baby drawing his legs up onto the abdomen, and is frequently relieved by the passage of flatus. This period usually begins at age 2–3 weeks and disappears by 10–12 weeks— so-called "3-months colic." The course is not clear, but "developmental colic" may be related to overready response to stimulation, irregular gastrointestinal peristalsis, and other as yet unintegrated autonomic functions characteristic of the first 2–3 months. The evening hours in the home often involve more stimulation from the father, anxiety about the infant's sleep on the part of a tired young mother, and perhaps concerns about the reactions of relatives or neighbors to continued crying.

Observations suggest that prolonged and severe colic, often persisting until the latter part of the first year, occurs most commonly in infants who are overactive and tense from birth (the so-called hypertonic infant, with a "lean and hungry look"). There may be some relationship to greater activity of the infant in utero and higher levels of maternal anxiety during pregnancy. Maternal and family tension, as well as possible allergic tendencies, have also been implicated.

Management of Colic

Anticipatory guidance about avoiding overstimulation (particularly of more active infants) during the first 3 months may be helpful in minimizing developmental colic, and so is the knowledge that it ordinarily disappears by 3 months. A pacifier can be soothing and does no harm unless used too freely by an overly anxious parent to prevent any crying or unless employed as a substitute for tactile, rhythmic, and other forms of soothing. If colic is prolonged and severe, more sucking time during feeding may be required for emotional satisfaction.

Counseling is important, giving the parent an opportunity to "think out loud," with the nonjudgmental help of the physician, about family tensions centering around living arrangements, overstimulation of the infant by the father on his return home in the evening, arguments over handling the infant, criticisms of in-laws in the home, or other matters.

Brazelton TB: Crying in infancy. Pediatrics 29:579, 1962.

Harley LM: Fussing and crying in young infants: Clinical considerations and practical management. Clin Pediatr (Phila) 8:138, 1969.

Paradise JL: Maternal and other factors in the etiology of infantile colic. JAMA 197:191, 1966.

SCHOOL PHOBIA

A special type of inability to attend school called school phobia is a syndrome involving a morbid or irrational dread or fear of some aspect of the school situation. Somatic complaints include abdominal pain, nausea, vomiting, diarrhea, headache, pallor, faintness, feelings of weakness, and low-grade fever. These symptoms appear in the morning before school, usually disappear by the time school is out or before, and do not appear on weekends or school holidays.

The basic fear is not of going to school but of leaving home or of separation from the family. Such fears occur in mild form, often with abdominal pain, in many normal children going off to full day school for the first time. With reassurance and firm support from the parents, they usually disappear within a few days, although they may recur during the first several years of school attendance, after vacations, or during convalescence from illness. Some young school age children with more intense fears are undergoing prolonged separation anxiety or experiencing a developmental crisis.

The classical school phobic picture of psychoneurotic nature usually occurs in an overly dependent, shy, and anxious child who has an overly solicitous or too controlling mother and a passive father. The mother often has a strong need for closeness with the child, fears that he is growing away from her, and communicates her anxiety about his welfare during the process of separation. There is usually a precipitating factor such as an unpleasant experience at school, illness or a new baby at home, or an increase in marital friction. The child's fear of separation is displaced onto the school as a "dangerous" place; his unconscious feelings of resentment over parental domination are projected onto the school as fears of punishment or attack. The mother takes the child's fears too seriously and becomes concerned about his safety.

The child becomes more guilty and socially isolated the longer he is permitted to remain at home and clings more closely to the mother even as she becomes increasingly frustrated and angry at his inability to go to school.

In young children in the early grades, the school phobia syndrome usually involves marked separation anxiety, a developmental crisis, or a mild form of phobic neurosis. In junior and senior high school students, it is usually a manifestation of a more severe personality disorder or occasionally a borderline psychosis.

Management of School Phobia

The pediatrician plays an important role in the management of this pediatric-psychiatric emergency. The emergency situation represents the first phase of treatment, which may be handled by the pediatrician if he understands the background of the difficulty and is willing to work with the parents, the child, and the school authorities.

Early return to school is the immediate goal. The pediatrician should first do a thorough physical appraisal; if abdominal pain or other gastrointestinal symptoms have been present for weeks or months, he should do a barium x-ray series in order to rule out peptic ulcer (often of the acute type), which occasionally coexists with school phobia. If the physical findings are within normal limits, the pediatrician should reassure the parents that no physical abnormalities are present and explain that "emotional tension" can be responsible for all the symptoms. He should further explain, in a noncritical, nonjudgmental way, that the child seems to be easily frightened by "new experiences," of which school is the most typical. Rather than interpreting their role in the problem, he should ask the parents what they feel might be involved.

With this approach, many parents can begin to recognize, without too much defensiveness or guilt, that they have kept the child "too close" to them. The pediatrician can suggest that they "think out loud" with him about ways to help the child become more independent. He should emphasize the importance of the child's early return to school—pointing out, if necessary, that every day at home will only make it harder for the child to have a successful school experience.

The pediatrician should talk with the principal or, with his permission, with the teacher, school social worker, or psychologist in order to learn how they interpret the problem. If the school authorities agree, he should suggest to the mother that she take the child to school and, if necessary, to the classroom, even remaining there briefly. If the mother is too anxious, the father may accompany her or may take the child to school himself. If neither parent feels able to accompany the child, it may be possible for an adult relative, another adult (such as the school nurse), or even an older child to pick up the child and see that he gets to school. Once in the classroom, the younger school age child usually settles in and does well academically. In some cases, it may be necessary to arrange for return to school at first on a part-time basis or to one class only. It may sometimes by necessary to change teachers or even arrange a transfer to another school.

Certain children may be unable to remain for long in the classroom and may ask to go home because of abdominal pain or other symptoms. The teacher should send the child to the school nurse, who can let him lie down briefly and then return him, with reassurance and encouragement, to the classroom. If he is permitted to call his parents, they may not be able to resist his appeals to come and take him home. No matter how worried the parents are, the physician should not give a medical certificate for home teaching since psychologic invalidism and other psychopathology may result.

If these emergency measures are not effective, early referral to a psychiatric clinic is warranted. In a few cases, a threat of legal intervention may be necessary to galvanize helpless parents into action.

Even if early return to school is achieved, referral for psychotherapy is usually indicated to work out underlying conflicts and prevent return of symptoms. If the parents are reluctant to take this step, the pediatrician can take comfort from follow-up studies which show that most such children are able to remain in school and to perform adequately without crippling neurotic symptoms.

With children in junior high or high school, who are usually more severely disturbed, the "first aid" approach should be tried and may be successful. Often it is not, however, and many adolescents with the school phobia syndrome require long-term intensive psychotherapy and even psychiatric hospitalization. With some mildly disturbed adolescents, brief pediatric hospitalization, drawing upon psychiatric consultation, may be all that is required.

Schmitt B: School phobia, the great imitator: A pediatric viewpoint. Pediatrics 48:433, 1971.

Williams HR, Prugh DG: School phobia. In: *Ambulatory Pediatrics*. Green M, Haggerty R (editors). Saunders, 1968.

Wolden S: School phobia and other childhood neuroses: A systematic study of the children and their families. Am J Psychiatry 132:8, 1975.

ENURESIS & ENCOPRESIS

Two major challenges for the pediatrician are offered by enuresis and encopresis. These symptoms are not necessarily associated with any specific personality picture. Both represent normal patterns until the expected age of training. Thereafter, they may represent a regressive component of a reactive disorder (in late preschool children), a developmental deviation in control mechanisms, a conversion symptom as part of a psychoneurotic disorder, or one of a constellation of symptoms in a chronic personality disorder or psychosis.

1. ENURESIS

Continuing enuresis (beyond about age 4) may be diurnal or nocturnal. Both types are often associated with coercive toilet training in infancy, except for an occasional child whose overpermissive parents have not attempted to train him, the child who has been seriously neglected, or the child with an apparent developmental lag in bladder control mechanisms, without other disturbance, whose parents handle him supportively and continue to pick him up at night. Some family tendencies toward enuresis are seen.

Diurnal enuresis is constant dribbling during the day beyond the point of occasional accidents caused by anxiety or momentary "forgetting" to empty a full bladder, as often happens in late preschool children. It may become a problem if the child enters nursery school, or it may remain mild and relatively unnoticed until kindergarten. It may or may not be associated with nocturnal enuresis, and is associated with a higher incidence of encopresis.

Diurnal wetting may be influenced by shyness about asking to go to the toilet, fear of strange toilets, negativistic tendencies, or chronic anxiety. In older school age children, it is most often encountered in chronically anxious children, those with personality disorders of the anxiety type, and those with oppositional personality traits. In general, it is more difficult to treat with the usual methods (described below) than the nocturnal type. A supportive relationship with the pediatrician and counseling for the child and the parents may be of help. Psychiatric consultation should usually be obtained, however, and many of these children require referral for intensive psychotherapy.

Children with *nocturnal enuresis* seem to experience greater than normal urgency in response to bladder distention during sleep. Their bladder capacity is not strikingly diminished, however, and, at least as measured by EEG studies, their sleep is not deeper. There appears to be no association with epilepsy (most epileptic children do not have enuresis). Most have no neurologic disorders related to true incontinence or structural abnormalities of the bladder or proximal urethra. The problem seems to be one of external sphincter control, and abnormalities higher in the urinary tract appear to play no significant role.

Diagnostic studies should ordinarily go no further than a urinalysis to rule out cystitis (which might cause urinary urgency) or, at most, an intravenous urogram if abnormalities are suspected. Retrograde cystoscopy in children with normal urine specimens should be avoided as it can provoke severe anxiety in young school age children, who still have fears of bodily (especially genital) mutilation. If done without general anesthesia in neurotic adolescents, the experience can become paradoxically pleasurable, particularly in girls with hysterical trends and masochistic needs.

Classification of Causes

Children with nocturnal enuresis fall into several groups from a psychosocial point of view, which may account for the conflicting findings in the literature regarding personality pictures and parent-child relationships.

A. Developmental Lag: One group shows a continuing struggle for control with the parents in this area, often arising from an apparent developmental lag in control mechanisms which upsets the parents. These are not usually seriously disturbed children, although they may be timid, somewhat anxious, and show some immature behavior. The symptom is more or less "encapsulated," and may represent a failure to achieve conditioned nighttime control.

B. Psychoneurotic Disorders: Boys with nocturnal enuresis are usually passive, somewhat inhibited, and often overly dependent or with phobic trends. They may identify with a dominant mother or be fearful of a punitive father. The symptoms appear to be of a conversion nature, involving relaxation of the external sphincter in relation to unconscious sexual conflicts, often expressed in terrifying nightmares during which loss of control occurs.

Girls with this symptom seem to be more active, sometimes overly independent, and competitive toward boys, with a tendency toward more masculine identification in an attempt to handle sexual fears. The content of the conversion symptom seems to carry an unconsciously hostile component toward their mothers or toward men who could injure them.

C. Tension Discharge Disorders: Children (usually boys) with tension discharge disorders, frequently of the impulse-ridden type, show problems in control in a number of areas. They often have dysrhythmic EEGs, although these seem to be related to immaturity in CNS development rather than to other causes. In some children with previously repressed neurotic conflicts, fire-setting is encountered, together with dreams of firemen or of firehoses putting out fires. In many cases the fathers have been overly punitive and the mothers unaffectionate. Broken homes are a frequent historical component, and most of these children have experienced considerable emotional deprivation.

D. Other Disorders: A few disturbed children, with much resentment underlying passive-aggressive behavior, demonstrate a "revenge" type of enuresis, ie, bedwetting represents a conscious, volitional act, usually carried out secretly. Psychotic children may have enuresis because of negativism or due to an inability to comprehend the significance of toilet training.

Treatment

Treatment should be related to the type of personality and family picture. For children whose enuresis represents a developmental lag in bladder control mechanisms, often with a related struggle for control, various methods can be employed successfully, eg, the gold star chart, drugs such as atropine or imipramine (Tofranil), and conditioning approaches such as the Eneurtone apparatus. Probably the most important ingredient in all these approaches is a positive doctor-parent relationship.

In the context of such a relationship, the physician should explain to the parents that the child cannot help the enuresis. They should be assured that the problem is not "their fault" and encouraged to stop pressuring or punishing the child in favor of his prescription, whatever it may be. By developing a positive relationship with the child, the pediatrician can help him with feelings of guilt, shame, or resentment and develop motivation for independent control with the help of the prescribed method. In some instances, control has been achieved during the evaluation process even before the prescription has been written.

Maxwell MD, Seldrup J: Imipramine in the treatment of childhood enuresis. Practitioner 207:809, 1971.

Oppel WC, Harper PA, Rider RV: Social, psychological, and neurological factors associated with nocturnal enuresis. Pediatrics 42:627, 1968.

Silberstein RM, Blackman S: Differential diagnosis and treatment of enuresis. Am J Psychiatry 121:1204, 1965.

Stanfield B: Enuresis: Its pathogenesis and management. Clin Pediatr (Phila) 11:343, 1972.

Werry JS, Cohrssen J: Enuresis: An etiologic and therapeutic study. J Pediatr 67:423, 1965.

2. ENCOPRESIS

Children with encopresis fall into 3 different groups. In many cases, the symptom begins as stool withholding in late infancy, and the majority of these children have experienced coercive toilet training.

Classification of Causes

A. Developmental Failure: In one group, failure to develop conditioned control of the external anal sphincter results in continuous soiling from infancy. These children generally have a relaxed anal sphincter. "Paradoxic diarrhea" often occurs, with a flow of mucoid material around a central fecal mass. These children frequently show strong oppositional behavior tendencies, with negativism in response to parental pressure or restrictions. Nonaganglionic megacolon of psychophysiologic origin may be present.

B. Inhibited, Dependent Children: Another group of children with encopresis often exhibit inhibited, dependent, compulsive tendencies and may show much concern about cleanliness in other areas. The symptom, often of regressive onset, seems to be a type of conversion reaction, representing the expression of unconscious hostility and resistance toward the parents—usually a dominating, overcontrolling, compulsive mother with strong unconscious interests in bowel functions and a passive, retiring, uninterested father. Soiling occurs rarely at school but is common on the way home, as the child returns to the area of conflict. "Hiding" the stool, wrapped in underwear, in a bureau drawer where the mother will find it frequently underlines the hostile significance of the soiling. In these children, the stool is often soft and formed, without paradoxic diarrhea.

C. Seriously Disturbed Children: Still another group of children with encopresis are much more seriously disturbed. They may manifest deep personality disorders, of mistrustful or isolated nature, with defects in reality testing of near-psychotic proportions, and some have shown "revenge" encopresis. Some may have been frankly psychotic since infancy, failing to comprehend control, whereas in others encopresis may have developed as one of a group of bizarre symptoms involved in a schizophreniform psychotic disorder. Paradoxic diarrhea may or may not be present. A few children have psychotic parents who have made no attempt to offer training. The parents of most are themselves disturbed, and they may occasionally interfere with treatment because of their fears or suspicions.

Treatment

Treatment should be geared to the personality and family patterns. If fecal impaction is present, hypertonic phosphate or oil retention enemas can be used in the hospital. Later, a mild laxative can be prescribed. Mineral oil is effective, but many children and parents are upset by the "leaking" that occurs. A regular evacuation each day may help reestablish bowel habits.

The support of the pediatrician, helping the parents to understand that the symptom is not their fault nor the child's and encouraging them not to use pressure or punishment in controlling it, is fundamental to any therapeutic approach. The child is usually embarrassed and guilty and can rarely talk about it easily, but he can be encouraged to participate in the reestablishment of bowel routines and control.

The above approach is surprisingly effective in the group who have resisted control by overly rigid parents and to some extent in school age children who develop the regressive type with conversion mechanisms. The doctor can offer the child a "way out," as it were.

Psychiatric consultation may be necessary, and some children and parents may require intensive long-term psychotherapy.

"Cleaning out" procedures and establishment of bowel routines may be resisted by the child or the parents out of fear of harm.

Silver D: Encopresis: Discussion of etiology and management. Clin Pediatr (Phila) 8:225, 1969.

SUICIDAL ATTEMPTS

Depression in adolescents, as in younger children, often takes different forms from depression in adults. Overt depression, with feelings of worthlessness, psychomotor retardation, and other physical changes, is much less common than in adults. Withdrawal, excessive daydreaming, anorexia, mood swings, sleep disturbances (inability to fall asleep or inability to get up in the morning), hyperactivity or hypoactivity, feelings of helplessness or hopelessness, or even hostility, temper outbursts, or aggressive behavior (warding off a depression) are common depressive equivalents of which the adolescent may not be consciously aware.

Suicidal threats are common in children and often represent attempts to punish the parents. ("You'll be sorry if I die.") Children are unable to comprehend the reality of death until age 9 or 10 years. Suicidal attempts are rare and usually do not reflect serious wishes to die but rather a desire for self-punishment or retaliation against the parents; however, they may accidentally be successful or may be carried out more efficiently than intended. The incidence of attempts rises rapidly after age 14. Although accurate reporting is rare, suicide is the fourth most frequent cause of death in late adolescence and the second most frequent cause in college students of high economic status.

Adolescent suicide rates vary from country to country (highest in Japan, Switzerland, and Finland) and from region to region (highest in the Rocky Mountain and Pacific Coast states in the USA). They appear to be higher in middle class groups and in urban areas, and show some seasonal incidence in temperate countries (highest in the spring) and some variation in relation to historical epochs and social crises. The adolescent suicide rate has increased significantly in the USA in the recent past (from 2.8 per 100,000 in 1954 to 3.8 in 1962, a 36% increase). This increase may be due in part to more honest reporting of suicides previously recorded as accidental. The rate among boys, particularly, may be even higher if automobile accidents are considered, since self-destructive or suicidal motives may be involved in deaths due to vehicle accidents.

In the USA, the suicide rate was formerly higher among adolescent girls than boys. The rate of successful suicide in boys is now at least double that of girls, although girls make more attempts. Boys most commonly employ firearms and explosives, with hanging or strangulation next; girls most frequently have employed poison or drugs, although firearms and explosives have recently become more common.

In addition to social, economic, or historical factors and a greater acceptance of suicide as a method of protest or problem-solving, it may be that child-rearing attitudes related to shame, guilt, or achievement and individual and family or situational factors are involved in most specific suicidal attempts. A small proportion of adolescents who attempt suicide are psychotic, and these episodes may be bizarre attempts at self-mutilation rather than actual suicide. Some have chronic personality disorders (hysterical and others), and their attempts may be clearly manipulative of parents or peers. Immature, sensitive, shy, anxious, emotionally labile adolescents with low self-esteem who come from disorganized or disturbed families are vulnerable to stressful events and may regard suicide as a solution. Others are reasonably healthy adolescents reacting to some specific situation such as chronic illness, pressure for school achievement, or sudden loss of another person or of self-esteem, as with a broken love affair or a bitter fight with a parent. Depression, feelings of

unworthiness, internalized anger at another (with guilt and depression), boredom, attempts to gain affection and esteem or to punish a parent or a boy or girl friend, a desire to join a dead relative, or even the acting out of an unconscious wish of a parent or identification with a parent who has committed suicide may be involved in the attempt, with more than one factor usually involved. Many adolescents do not really wish to die, and the attempt is a "cry for help." Even a true wish to die is more short-lived in adolescents than in adults. The adolescent often tells the parents about the attempt or leaves a note or a bottle where it may easily be found. He may change his mind in the middle of the act (sometimes too late); he may feel backed into a corner by his own threats of suicide if his "bluff is called," and may feel that he has to make the attempt to maintain his integrity.

Many parents are ashamed and guilty when their adolescent son or daughter attempts suicide, and the doctor may unconsciously conspire with them to forget it or "sweep it under the rug." Even suicidal threats should always be taken seriously. If an attempt is made which produces no response from the parents, the adolescent may try again with tragic results.

Signs of depression or depressive equivalents are a serious indication that suicide may be attempted. Although emotional lability is one of the characteristics of adolescence, true depression should never be dealt with by a "pat on the back" or a "buck up" approach. An opportunity to ventilate feelings to an understanding adult may be of great help, or more formal therapy may be necessary.

If an adolescent asks for a chance to talk with a physician or other adult, an interview should be arranged promptly. It is hard enough to encourage teenagers to talk to adults at most times; if a request for an opportunity to talk is made, granting it may help to prevent impulsive suicide attempts.

If a suicidal attempt has been made, pediatric hospitalization can provide the time, with the help of a psychiatrist and social worker, to convince the parents of the seriousness of the adolescent's plea for help. Supportive counseling or environmental rearrangement may suffice, or more intensive psychotherapy can be started at once if indicated.

It is unwise to send home from the emergency room an adolescent who has made even a patently superficial and manipulative suicidal attempt such as the ingestion of a small amount of an innocuous drug or a quantity of barbiturates which can easily be dealt with by gastric lavage. The family will often not return for follow-up therapy, and more serious attempts may occur. If the adolescent appears seriously disturbed, emergency psychiatric hospitalization is necessary.

Barter JT, Swaback DO, Todd D: Adolescent suicide attempts. Arch Gen Psychiatry 19:523, 1968.

Faigel HC: Suicide among young persons: A review of its incidence and causes, and methods. Clin Pediatr (Phila) 5:187, 1966.

Lewis M, Solnit A: The adolescent in a suicidal crisis: Collaborative care on a pediatric ward. In: *Modern Perspectives in Child Development.* Solnit A, Provence S (editors). Internat Univ Press, 1963.

DRUG ABUSE

Drug addiction and the use of drugs by adolescents are some of the most controversial topics of our times. Physicians should keep informed about what drugs are being abused in their geographic areas and be prepared to give appropriate counseling to parents and teenagers as well as to treat overdoses and side-effects.

LSD & Other Hallucinogens

The biologic effects of LSD and related compounds have been carefully studied; they resemble sympathomimetic agents and produce such changes as increased pulse and heart rate, rise in blood pressure, mydriasis, tremors of extremities, cold sweaty palms, flushing, chills and shivering, increased salivation, nausea, and anorexia. The psychologic effects may last for periods of 1–2 hours to more than a day. The LSD effect usually lasts 4–8 hours.

The effects depend on the person taking the drug, his expectation of what will happen, the setting in which it is taken, the other people in the setting, previous experiences with the drug, the physiologic and psychologic states of the subject, and other variables.

Changes in perception (especially visual) are often experienced by nonpsychotic subjects who take oral doses of LSD as small as 30 μg. They include enhancement of colors, alterations in the perception of one's own body, vivid hallucinations, and synesthesias. Mood changes include depression, euphoria, or lability of mood; anxiety is frequent, sometimes to the point of panic. Feelings of depersonalization and estrangement are often reported. Changes in thinking may include flights of ideas, perseveration, a feeling of insight into universal and transcendental phenomena (the "psychedelic experience"), and intense preoccupation with one's own thought and bodily processes. Other cognitive changes consist of difficulty in concentration on reality-oriented tasks, distractibility, abandonment of logical and causal thinking, and changes in time sense.

Untoward psychologic effects ("bad trips") include the appearance of a serious schizophreniform psychotic illness (usually precipitated by the drug experience in borderline psychotic individuals); prolonged depressive reaction (including a number of reported suicides); continuing anxiety (panic), depersonalization, and recurrent catatonia, with intermittent return ("flashback") of hallucinatory experiences; and serious injury or death in a few cases.

Some reports have indicated that persons who take LSD have an increased number of "breaks" in chromosomes, lasting at least 6 months, and that the offspring of women who have taken LSD early in pregnancy also exhibit such chromosomal alterations (continuing up to 5 years of age). Similar findings have been reported in animals. These results need to be carefully validated, but caution in the use of LSD, especially by pregnant women, seems justified on this basis.

Because the manufacture and sale of many of the compounds used as hallucinogens is a federal offense, the extent of their abuse is difficult to determine. Statements regarding large numbers of young people who have experimented with or used these drugs are often exaggerated and inflammatory. Various surveys report that up to 15% of college students in selected colleges have admitted trying LSD. Undoubtedly, a number have tried the experience once only for "kicks" or out of curiosity; some anxious persons with conflicts have continued the practice; and others with "an empty feeling," alienated and isolated (anomie), may continue to seek stimulation of any kind by the use of these drugs. Some report the experience openly as frightening; others describe it in rapturous terms.

Although feelings of universal insight seem to occur in some individuals, there is no evidence that LSD changes personality for the better. In addition, those who experience such insights rarely can describe them clearly to others, and there is little evidence that the experiences have resulted in any personal or social benefit. The use of LSD as an adjunct to psychotherapy in chronic alcoholism and chronic neurosis has been reported, but no carefully controlled studies are available.

LSD is relatively easy to manufacture and easily available from illegal sources, and there is no way to detect its presence in the body. Thus, in spite of realistic concerns about adverse psychologic and biologic effects of LSD (and presumably other psychedelic drugs also), there is no easy way to control its distribution. The largest group of users appears to be teenagers and young adults who characteristically are "looking for answers" and are only too ready to rebel against the established order and break its rules. To make laws against use or possession of these drugs is more likely to encourage experimentation with them than the reverse. Such legislation also means that large numbers of young people who will soon outgrow their rebelliousness in the course of development will be socially hampered by a police record.

At present, the incidence of experimentation with these drugs seems to be decreasing. Young people are aware of the information about chromosomal damage and appear to respect that type of data even more than rules or laws.

Marihuana

Marihuana is more widely used today than the psychedelic (hallucinogenic, psychotomimetic) drugs, with estimates of up to 20% or more in college students. Its effects are not well studied because of its illegal status; they appear to involve relaxation of inhibitions in some individuals, although most users describe an introspective attitude under the influence of marihuana even in a group setting. The drug does not appear to be significantly involved in episodes of antisocial, destructive, or criminal behavior. It is not addictive and does not predispose to other addictions. The furor among adults over its use seems unjustified, as most young people control its use or eventually give it up.

Heroin

Heroin does seem to have some addictive qualities, although physical dependence on it or other "addictive" drugs (with great desire and increasing tolerance) involves also certain psychologic needs for escape from reality conflicts, fear of withdrawal symptoms, or a conditioning process. Deaths have occurred from overdosage, and tetanus, malaria, hepatitis, syphilis, and other infections have resulted from the use of unsterile needles.

The Hydrocarbons

Inhalation of hydrocarbons (glue or plastic cement, lighter fluid, or gasoline fumes) seems to produce a state somewhat resembling alcoholic intoxication, ie, an initial "jag" with pleasant exhilaration, euphoria, and excitement. Ataxia, slurred speech, and at times diplopia and tinnitus follow, with drowsiness, stupor, and brief coma appearing later. As tolerance develops, large amounts of inhalant become necessary to produce a reaction. Nausea, anorexia, weight loss, irritability, inattentiveness, somnolence, excessive salivation, and fetor oris may result from glue-sniffing, but serious physiologic effects do not occur. Gasoline sniffing, which has been reported in children as young as 18 months of age, has caused occasional accidental deaths.

Although not addictive, the hydrocarbons offer easy habituation. They are used—particularly glue—principally by boys who usually have significant psychosocial problems which lead to the habituation. The same is true of individuals who become habituated to the amphetamines, barbiturates, alcohol, or tobacco in childhood or early adolescence.

Management of Drug Abuse

The approach to the use of drugs should be medical, psychologic, and social rather than restrictive or punitive. This is true of serious addictive problems as well; even alcoholism has been recognized recently by the courts as an illness requiring treatment and not primarily an offense against society. Indeed, recent indications are that alcohol is becoming the agent most widely used by young people.

An understanding approach by the parents to guidance and discipline, with some limits but with some flexibility, will prevent many young people from resorting to the habitual use of drugs of any kind.

For those who have experienced "bad trips" or other untoward effects of drug abuse, or those in higher-income families who engage in chronic drug abuse because of emotional disturbance or rebellion, psychiatric treatment is usually indicated. Younger adolescents who have indulged in glue-sniffing because of psychologic problems may often be successfully treated by the pediatrician with the help of psychiatric

consultation and therapy for the parents by a social worker or other mental health professional. Other social and economic measures are necessary to deal with the fundamental problems of poverty and discrimination which favor the use of drugs by adolescents in disadvantaged neighborhoods.

Deisher RW & others: Drug abuse in adolescence: The use of harmful drugs—a pediatric concern. Pediatrics 44:131, 1969.

Freedman A, Wilson E: Childhood and adolescent addictive disorders. (2 parts.) Pediatrics 34:254, 283, 1964.

Litt IF, Cohen MI: The drug-using adolescent and pediatric patient. J Pediatr 77:195, 1970.

MANAGEMENT OF PSYCHOLOGIC ASPECTS OF ILLNESS & INJURY

ACUTE ILLNESS OR INJURY

The child's response to acute illness or injury depends upon the particular organ system affected, his level of psychosocial development, the meaning of the illness to the child and his family, the nature of necessary treatment, and other factors. In general, there are broad patterns of responses characteristic of children at different developmental levels, with variations due to individual differences.

The direct effects of acute illness on behavior may include listlessness, prostration, irritability, or disturbances in sleep and appetite. Restlessness and hyperactivity often complicate the management of milder illnesses, especially in preschool children. In biologically predisposed youngsters, physiologic concomitants of anxiety may appear, including tachycardia, palpitation, hyperventilation, and diarrhea—at times leading to diagnostic confusion with hyperthyroidism, rheumatic fever, etc. Struggles for control between a young child and his parents may cause eating and sleeping problems which may persist long after recovery.

Emotional and behavioral regression in response to illness is common in older infants and young children and occurs to some degree in school age children and adolescents as well. Depression may also occur with return of primitive fears and feelings of helplessness and hopelessness. In more severe reactions, compulsive or ritualized, stereotyped behavior may occur and may subside rapidly or continue as a reactive disorder.

Misinterpretations of the meaning of the illness or accident as punishment are common in preschool children and may occur in school age children as well. Late preschool and early school age children may have fears of bodily mutilation, especially when sensitive areas such as the genitals, eyes, or mouth are involved. In older school age children, conversion and dissociative reactions may be encountered, often associated with subclinical delirium in response to drug administration or high fever or during convalescence.

The potentially deleterious effects of bed rest too strenuously enforced must be borne in mind and balanced against the sometimes doubtful advantages.

CHRONIC ILLNESS & SERIOUS INJURY

Chronic illness or handicapping injuries may have serious consequences for the child's personality development and family functioning. The child's previous adaptive capacity and the parent-child family balance appear to be the most important prognostic factors. These children's personalities appear to fall along a continuum ranging from overdependent, overanxious, and passive or withdrawn to overly independent, with strong tendencies to deny illness. A number of these youngsters become realistically dependent and accept their limitations, developing adequate social roles and methods and sublimating their energies in constructive ways. Parental patterns range from overanxiousness, overprotectiveness, and overindulgence, often with difficulties in setting limits on the child's demands, to refusal to accept the severity of the child's disability, projection of personal guilt onto others (including the doctor), reluctance to cooperate with treatment programs, and, occasionally, rejection or isolation of the child.

Most parents ultimately learn to accept the child's limitations without discomfort, permit an appropriate degree of dependency, and help him explore constructively his capacities and strengths.

Child's Reaction

Many children with chronic illnesses or handicaps have difficulties in maintaining a sound body image. Adolescents especially may show marked reactions to disfigurement or physical handicap.

In reaction to catastrophic illness or injury, school age children and adolescents show a phasic response consisting initially of an *impact phase* involving realistic fears of death, soon followed by marked regression, strong denial of long-term damage, and the use of primitive fantasy (eg, daydreams of being a great athlete). After some days or weeks, the *phase of recoil* is characterized by dawning recognition of the seriousness of the situation and by grief, or "mourning for the loss of the self"; this represents a constructive process, but it may be masked by demanding behavior. Severe depression may be present during this phase. The *phase of restitution* is characterized by the reemergence of premorbid personality traits such as overdependence or unrealistic overindependence. Management must be geared to the patient's progress through these phases.

Parents' Reaction

Parents show a parallel phasic response. A phase of "denial and disbelief" may persist for days, weeks, or months, sometimes accompanied by "shopping" for other opinions. During the succeeding phase of "fear and frustration," the parents may be depressed and guilty and may project blame onto each other or onto other persons. Marital crises may occur during this time. After weeks or months, the parents usually arrive at the phase of "intelligent inquiry and planning," in which they are able to handle their feelings and to live fairly comfortably although with some ambiguity.

Attempts to force either the parents or the child to face the reality of the situation before they are ready only increase the denial. Indeed, some denial— within limits—may be necessary for the maintenance of hope.

Management of Initial Reactions

During the management of chronic illness or handicap, the child and parents can be helped to focus on small, day-to-day steps as well as to ventilate feelings of frustration, anxiety, or guilt. Other supportive measures include suggestions for occupational therapy in the home, encouragement of gradual resumption of activity, and redirecting the child's interests so that he can compensate for activities denied to him by excelling in others. Parents often need to be restrained from overprotecting or overindulging such children.

Home teachers may make it possible for the child to keep up with his schooling. The child should attend school, even on a part-time basis, either in a special class or, ideally, in a regular class. Vocational training compatible with the adolescent's intellectual and physical capacities can be arranged with the help of community resources. For the child who is so seriously handicapped that he cannot leave home, service agencies can often build a social club around him in the home. Group discussions among parents of children with similar problems may be of value in offering emotional support, as may similar approaches with handicapped adolescents.

Paradoxic Responses to Treatment

Children with deep-seated emotional conflicts who have adapted to the role of an invalid in families with unhealthy interpersonal relationships may find it difficult to respond to treatment in a positive way and may instead decompensate or develop a variety of symptomatic reactions. A gradual rehabilitative approach is necessary for such children and parents, and psychiatric consultation or formal psychotherapy is often required.

Prognosis

Emotional factors such as depression over actual or symbolic loss of key figures or lack of motivation to recover may adversely influence the course of serious illnesses such as carcinoma, leukemia, lymphoma, and especially infectious hepatitis, which seems to exert a specific depressive effect upon the psyche. Supportive psychologic measures should be part of the total treatment plan for children and adolescents with many of these disorders. Psychiatric consultation is often helpful and should be sought whenever the physician feels that an emotional component he cannot deal with is menacing his patient's total mental and physical well-being.

Downey JA, Low NL: *The Child With Disabling Illness: Principles of Rehabilitation.* Saunders, 1974.

Green M, Solnit AJ: Reactions to the threatened loss of a child: A vulnerable child syndrome. Pediatrics 34:58, 1964.

Korsch B, Barnett HL: The physician, the child, and the family. J Pediatr 58:707, 1961.

Lief HI, Lief VF, Lief NR (editors): *The Psychological Basis of Medical Practice.* Harper, 1963.

Mattsson A: Long-term physical illness in children: A challenge to psychosocial adaptation. Pediatrics 50:801, 1972.

Prugh DG: Toward an understanding of psychosomatic concepts in relation to illness in children. In: *Modern Perspectives in Child Development.* Solnit AJ, Provence S (editors). Internat Univ Press, 1963.

Prugh DG, Eckhardt LO: Children's reactions to illness, hospitalization, and surgery. In: *Comprehensive Textbook of Psychiatry,* 2nd ed. Freedman AM, Kaplan HI, Sadock BJ (editors). Williams & Wilkins, 1975.

HOSPITALIZATION

The management of children before, during, and after hospitalization is an important part of pediatric treatment, since most children have this experience at some time or other (3.5 million a year under age 15). Hospitalization, with its separation from home and the various treatment procedures encountered, may cause a variety of reactions depending upon the child's level of psychosocial development, the family's response, the meaning of the illness and hospitalization, the type of treatment required, and other factors. The older the child, the more he will understand the realistic meaning of this experience and the less likely he will be to misinterpret its significance.

Child's Reaction to Hospitalization

A. Infants Under Age 6 Months: Young infants usually show temporary "global responses" to unfamiliar methods of feeding and handling, which may confuse mothers on return home.

B. Older Infants: Beginning in the second half of the first year, infants experience stranger anxiety and fears of separation, with regression and depression.

C. Young Children: Children up to age 4 appear most vulnerable to separation from the mother. Children of this age often experience a sequence of protest, despair, and detachment, the latter often associated with withdrawal and depression if separation without adequate mother-substitute relationships continues beyond a few days or 1–2 weeks.

D. Age 4 to Early School Age: The child from age 4 through the early school age period, although he may experience separation anxiety, is usually more preoccupied with fears of bodily mutilation.

E. Older School Age Children: Older children are usually able to comprehend the reality of the hospital experience more objectively but may still show signs of mild regression and anxiety over bodily functioning, etc. Fears of genital inadequacy, muscular weakness, and of loss of body control or of helplessness during anesthesia may enhance the feelings of anxiety and inferiority that are characteristic of this stage of development. The same trends may be seen in adolescents but in a muted form. They may have difficulty in accepting the authority of the medical staff.

Parents' Reaction

Parental reactions to a child's illness may be compounded by hospitalization. Some parents may fear criticism from the hospital staff regarding their role in the illness itself or their effectiveness as parents. Consequently, some may adopt a strongly rival attitude toward nurses or physicians in an attempt to disarm the implied criticism of their own parental abilities. Feeling left out or unwanted is also common among parents. A few parents project their own guilt onto the hospital staff and blame them for the child's difficulties. Some parents with excessive anxiety are themselves unable to separate comfortably from the child; a few, with intense guilt, may be unable to visit.

Preparation for Hospitalization

All children should be told simply and truthfully why they are going to the hospital. They should be given a general impression of what being in a hospital is like and what will be done to make them comfortable. They must be assured that their parents will remain in contact with them. When the physician decides that hospitalization is necessary, he should inform the parents what to tell the child and deal as necessary with their apprehension, guilt feelings, or conflicts.

Preschool children should not be prepared for elective hospitalization more than a week or so in advance—enough time for questions but not too much for anxiety to build up. In some instances, a group session with the physician, parents, and child may be helpful in order to support anxious parents or to give the child the feeling of being involved in the planning.

Thorough exposition of the medical or surgical implications and procedures is not necessary for most children, although adolescents may wish to know more details. Practical discussions about mealtimes, use of a bedpan, etc may be of value for older preschool children. "Playing out" situations in the hospital with a toy doctor's or nurse's kit may help to prevent anxiety. Visits to the hospital may be useful for school age children. Booklets about "going to the hospital" may be of value if an opportunity for questions is offered, but they should not convey the impression that being in hospital is like "being at a party," with all sorts of entertainment, etc.

Reactions to Painful Procedures

Procedures such as venipunctures, injections, and lumbar punctures are frightening to young children, and very young children cannot be expected to cooperate unassisted. An older child can sometimes be made interested in the doctor's instruments and their purpose, so that he can cooperate to some extent in controlling his response to pain. The doctor should always explain that some pain will occur, without minimizing or exaggerating it. He should tell the child when and where it will hurt and encourage him to cry if he feels like it. Firm but kindly restraint should be used as necessary, with the explanation that it is being done to help the child hold still so that "it won't hurt so much." The main thought to be conveyed is that the young patient, the doctor, and the nurse have an alliance which will help get the task done with as little hurt as possible.

Post-Hospitalization

Most children manifest at least mildly disturbed behavior for a few days or several weeks after returning home. This post-hospitalization reaction may persist if reinforced by parental anxiety or guilt. Anticipatory guidance and support for the parents in gradually "weaning" the child from regressive behavior can be of valuable preventive significance.

During convalescence, some children do not want to relinquish the greater dependency involved in the acute phase of the illness and may dread the imminent return to competitive school responsibilities. Flexibility in matters of bed rest, meals, and treatment routines may be appropriate, eg, rest on the living room couch, in contact with others, may be more therapeutic than in the bedroom, where the relative isolation can lead to further regression.

The child should return to an integrated family life and to school as soon as possible and should resume his responsibilities gradually as his capacities return to normal.

The Child in the Hospital

Hospitalization is not necessarily a traumatic experience for a child, although it should be used as sparingly as possible. Preschool or previously disturbed children are most vulnerable to adverse reactions. In addition to improvement in physical health as a result of hospitalization, some older children benefit from the opportunity to relate to other children and adults outside the home, especially if the family has been disturbed or isolated.

Previously unrecognized psychologic problems in a child with physical illness may become obvious as a result of a comprehensive evaluation in a hospital setting, where one may observe at greater length the behavior of the child and the interaction with his parents.

During hospitalization, the child's "life space" and his ties with reality should be maintained. The teacher is a familiar nonmedical figure, and schooling should be available even during brief periods of hospitalization. Recreational therapists ("play ladies"), social group workers, and occupational therapists can provide valuable emotional support and opportunities for "playing out" feelings about the hospital staff and procedures while at the same time offering age-appropriate recreational outlets.

Early ambulation (in carts if necessary) and family style eating arrangements offer social experiences which may facilitate convalescence and improve appetite.

It is sometimes difficult to coordinate the activities of physicians, consultants, nurses, social workers, teachers, recreational staff, "foster grandmothers," and other persons involved. A weekly or biweekly ward management conference chaired by a senior pediatrician or clinical director will facilitate communication and increase the effectiveness of the total effort.

The most vital mental health need while the child is in the hospital is maintenance of the tie between the child and his family. The "therapeutic alliance" between the parents and the hospital staff is a concept of great importance. Hospital organization should provide a balance between the advantages of the parents' presence and the treatment obligations of the staff, with separate visiting and treatment areas if possible. Flexible daily visiting schedules are directly correlated with less disturbed behavior on the part of the older preschool and school age child, and cross-infection has been shown to be minimal. Some facilities permit unrestricted visiting and overnight stay by parents. For preschool children, who are more anxious over separation and whose understanding is limited, overnight stay or "living in" by the mother is the most effective preventive measure. Individualized planning about visiting is necessary, since some parents will not be able to take advantage of such opportunities for a variety of reasons.

Alternative plans to hospitalization should be considered whenever possible. For example, motel facilities adjacent to a children's hospital have been developed where the parents of a child who is being studied diagnostically may stay. Day care can be planned for children with chronic illnesses or diagnostic problems who do not require hospitalization. Greater use can be made of home care if a "family team" can be organized for this purpose.

Glaser MD: Group discussions with mothers and hospitalized children. Pediatrics 26:132, 1960.

Mason EA: The hospitalized child: His emotional needs. N Engl J Med 272:406, 1965.

Robertson J: *Young Children in Hospitals.* Basic Books, 1958.

Shore MF (editor): *Red is the Color of Hurting: Planning for Children in the Hospital.* US Department of Health, Education, & Welfare, 1966.

Solnit AJ: Hospitalization: An aid to physical and psychological health in childhood. Am J Dis Child 99:155, 1960.

SURGERY

The child who requires an operation usually needs special preparation if psychologic problems are to be avoided. For school age children, the explanation should be simple and brief, without many details, and the child should be permitted to ask as many questions as he wishes both before and after surgery. Most children can talk more freely and understand more fully if a simple drawing is used to explain the procedure. Even early adolescent boys may fear, for example, that a colectomy for ulcerative colitis may somehow interfere with their capacity for "becoming a man." The pediatrician should make sure that preparation takes place, no matter whether he or the surgeon does it. Preparation of the parents is equally important, as they too may have significant misconceptions. If possible, elective operations should be avoided in children age 4–6 since fears of bodily mutilation are greatest at this time.

Anesthesia

Anesthesia may evoke fears of death or of loss of self-control in school age children. They may have fears they will say or do "something bad" and may also be concerned about what might be done to their bodily organs while they are helpless. Induction and recovery states should be explained in appropriate terms. Some children need to be reassured they will not awaken before the operation is over. Others may mistake the onset of unconsciousness as impending death and need to be told that "forced sleep" is temporary and will be followed by complete awakening and survival. Preliminary "playing out" of the induction process by the anesthetist or other personnel aids in the child's mastery of the situation. If possible, the child should be spared the experience of seeing instruments, the operating room, etc.

Since oral barbiturates may have a stimulant effect on preschool children unless given in large doses, administration of a basal anesthetic (eg, thiopental) in the child's room (with the mother present) may help relax an overly anxious child and prevent resistance on the way to the operating room. When the child awakes, the mother should be there to greet him; this is especially important in young children. School age children can be helped to adjust to the ward setting and staff by being admitted a day in advance of an operation. (This is not ordinarily helpful for preschool children.)

Principles of this kind have also been shown to be effective in cutting down on the amount of anesthetic necessary and in reducing the incidence and severity of postoperative reactions.

Mutilating Operations

Special problems may arise in regard to operations with unavoidably mutilating results, such as amputations. If the child misinterprets the procedure as a punishment for a past misdeed, he may become aggressive (in fantasied self-defense) or withdrawn (feeling helpless and hopeless).

Occasionally, persistent denial of loss of a body part, such as a limb, can lead to difficulties in planning for prosthetic devices. Psychiatric consultation should be freely used.

Burns

If a severely burned child is guilty about the accident and fearful of the loss of his parents' love, he may become seriously depressed, respond poorly to surgical procedures, and fail to heal adequately. The presence of a mother substitute such as a foster grandmother may be lifesaving for a regressed and depressed preschool child whose parents cannot hold him because of his burns. Hypnosis may be helpful in stimulating trust and minimizing pain during dressing changes; drugs are not as helpful in children as in adults. Most children with extensive burns have significant emotional problems following even successful surgical treatment. Psychotherapy has been shown to ameliorate or prevent such problems.

Bernstein NR: Observations on the use of hypnosis with burned children on a pediatric ward. Internat J Clin Exper Hypnosis 13:1, 1965.

Cytryn L, Cytryn E: Psychological implications of cryptorchidism. J Am Acad Child Psychiatry 6:131, 1967.

Fine RN & others: Renal homotransplantation in children. J Pediatr 76:347, 1970.

Fineman L, Blom GE, Waldfogel S: Emotional implications of tonsillectomy and adenoidectomy in children. Psychoanal Study Child 7:126, 1952.

Loomis E: The child's emotions and surgery. In: *Pre- and Post-Operative Care in the Pediatric Surgical Patient.* Kieswelter WB (editor). Year Book, 1956.

TERMINAL ILLNESS

Recent advances in medical and surgical care have brought about a change in the composition of the patient population in many children's hospitals. The pediatric practitioner is spending more and more of his time in caring for children with chronic and sometimes fatal illnesses. The physician must be able to deal constructively with parents and children in these tragic circumstances. The management of dying children is perhaps one of the most difficult tasks the pediatrician faces today.

Explaining a fatal illness is a complicated task often attended by some risk. However, not to interpret the fatal illness at some level is a disservice to the patient and his family. Knowing the individual child and family and understanding the child's concept of death may provide the physician with some guide to individual answers in specific situations.

The Young Child

The young child who is dying expresses mainly his fear of separation from his parents and his wish to avoid pain. When death comes acutely, the child's awareness is often blunted by delirium, stupor, or coma. In a more gradual terminal experience, there is often evidence of depression, withdrawal, fearfulness, and apprehension. Although most children with a fatal illness do not directly ask if they are going to die, this question may be raised by some children over the age of 4 or 5. Parents, physicians, and nurses may have preferences about how to respond. When such questions are raised, the physician can ask why the child thinks he might die and may find that the child is worried about whether he will be alone or whether the doctor will make him feel "all right."

It is better not to tell the child that he might die without first discussing it with the parents and obtaining their permission. They may wish to answer the question themselves or they may wish to have help, either from the physician or from their religious counselors, in answering such questions.

The Older Child

Older children and adolescents have more understanding about impending death than the parents or hospital staff may realize.

Staff members often maintain an unconscious "conspiracy of silence," and may even stay away from the child to avoid the topic. In some cases, everyone involved may feel more comfortable if the topic is brought into the open. The young person can be told that he might die but that everything possible will be done to help him get well. He should be assured that relief from pain will be available and that he will not be left alone if he becomes seriously ill.

When a child dies, other children on the ward inevitably sense that something serious has happened and may need to be reassured that their condition is different.

Reactions of Parents

Parental reactions include the entire continuum from complete withdrawal from the child, through "mourning in advance" and an early detachment, to the extreme of denial and unrealistic expectations accompanied by poor reality testing. The reaction of the parents also depends on the circumstances of the illness or injury, the degree of their guilt, and the nature of the prior family relationship.

The physician must keep in mind the nature of the disease, the age of the child, and the family concept of death. Once he is certain of the diagnosis and prognosis, the parents should be told, frankly but gently, even though they may be overwhelmed and may want to go elsewhere for further medical care. The possibility of a fatal illness should never be mentioned to parents as part of a differential diagnosis, since some disturbed parents may continue to handle the child as if he were going to die even if that possibility is ruled out.

If the parents are able to help care for the child in the hospital during the terminal phase, they should be encouraged to do so. Some parents cannot bring themselves to help, however, and they should not be made to feel guilty if this is so. The physician must be ready to accept whatever feelings the parents display, even permitting them to bring other family members in to mourn with the child or to take the child home to die if that is their cultural tradition. Parents should be allowed to vent their feelings and perhaps even be encouraged to engage in the normal mourning process if there is an obvious lack of expression in an overly inhibited family. In the hospital, parents may gain much emotional support from other parents or social workers. Other community resources may be available also, so that the parents can have someone to whom they can express their feelings outside the hospital. Ministers, other family members, or psychiatric consultants may be helpful in understanding such situations and in working out a plan for some sort of help.

Parents frequently require a continuing supportive relationship with the pediatrician after the child's death. An appointment should be made to see them within several weeks, as their guilt and anxiety may lead them to repeat questions already asked. Such an opportunity for "working through" their feelings may help them to avoid immediately conceiving another child to take the place of the lost one, with obvious difficulties ahead.

Easson WM: *The Dying Child: Management of the Child or Adolescent Who Is Dying.* Thomas, 1970.

Friedman SB: Management of fatal illness in children. In: *Ambulatory Pediatrics.* Green M, Haggerty R (editors). Saunders, 1968.

Toch R: Management of the child with a fatal disease. Clin Pediatr (Phila) 3:418, 1964.

• • •

General References

Ackerman N: *Treating the Troubled Family*. Basic Books, 1966.

Alt H: *Residential Treatment for the Disturbed Child*. Internat Univ Press, 1960.

Apley J, McKeith R: *The Child and His Symptoms*. Davis, 1968.

Bakwin H, Bakwin RM: *Clinical Management of Behavior Disorders in Children*, rev ed. Saunders, 1967.

Berlin IN: *Bibliography of Child Psychiatry: With a Selected List of Films*. American Psychiatric Association, 1963.

Berlin IN (editor): *Bibliography of Child Psychiatry and Child Mental Health*, 2nd ed. Human Sciences Press, 1976.

Caplan G (editor): *Emotional Problems of Early Childhood*. Basic Books, 1955.

Committee on Child Psychiatry: *The Diagnostic Process in Child Psychiatry*. GAP Report No. 38. Group for the Advancement of Psychiatry, 1957.

Committee on Child Psychiatry: *Psychopathological Disorders in Childhood: Theoretical Considerations and a Proposed Classification*. GAP Report No. 62. Group for the Advancement of Psychiatry, 1968.

Erikson EH: *Childhood and Society*. Norton, 1950.

Finch SM: *Fundamentals of Child Psychiatry*. Norton, 1960.

Freedman AM, Kaplan H: *Comprehensive Textbook of Psychiatry*, 2nd ed. Williams & Wilkins, 1974.

Freud A: *Normality and Pathology in Childhood: Assessment of Development*. Internat Univ Press, 1965.

Green M, Haggerty RJ (editors): *Ambulatory Pediatrics*. Saunders, 1968.

Harrison SI, Carek DJ: *A Guide to Psychotherapy*. Little, Brown, 1966.

Helfer RE, Kempe CH: *The Battered Child*. Univ of Chicago Press, 1968.

Hoch P: *Depression*. Grune & Stratton, 1954.

Hoch P, Zubin J (editors): *Psychopathology of Childhood*. Grune & Stratton, 1955.

Hoffman L, Hoffman M (editors): *Review of Child Development Research*. Russell Sage Foundation, 1966.

Hollender M (editor): *The Psychology of Medical Practice*. Saunders, 1958.

Howells JO (editor): *Modern Perspectives in International Child Psychiatry*. Oliver & Boyd, 1968.

Kanner L: *Child Psychiatry*. Thomas, 1962.

Kliman G: *Psychological Emergencies of Childhood*. Grune & Stratton, 1968.

Patton RG, Gardner LI: *Growth Failure and Maternal Deprivation*. Thomas, 1963.

Pearson GHJ (editor): *A Handbook of Child Psychoanalysis*. Basic Books, 1968.

Psychoanalytic Study of the Child. Internat Univ Press, 1945–present. [Annual. Various editors.]

Schulman JI: *Management of Emotional Disorders in Pediatric Practice: With a Focus on Techniques of Interviewing*. Year Book, 1967.

Sex and the College Student. GAP Report No. 60. Group for the Advancement of Psychiatry, 1965.

Shaw CR (editor): *The Psychiatric Disorders of Childhood*. Appleton-Century-Crofts, 1966.

Shirley HF: *Pediatric Psychiatry*. Harvard Univ Press, 1963.

Slavson SR: *Analytic Group Psychotherapy With Children, Adolescents, and Adults*. Columbia Univ Press, 1950.

Solnit AJ, Provence S (editors): *Modern Perspectives in Child Development*. Internat Univ Press, 1963.

Verville E: *Behavior Problems of Children*. Saunders, 1967.

24...
Endocrine Disorders

Henry K. Silver, MD, & Ronald W. Gotlin, MD
With Revisions by Georgeanna J. Klingensmith, MD

Endocrine disorders are relatively infrequent in childhood, but a knowledge of the endocrine system is essential in order to differentiate its disorders from congenital malformations and from normal variations in the timing and pattern of development (ie, "constitutional" deviations from average). One should attempt to understand the pathogenesis of endocrine abnormalities so that the physiologic and chemical evidences of specific hormonal dysfunctions can be correlated with structural abnormalities, particularly as they affect growth and development.

DISTURBANCES OF GROWTH & DEVELOPMENT

Disturbances of growth and development are the most common presenting complaints in the pediatric endocrine clinic. It is estimated that over 1 million children in the USA have abnormally short stature and that there are at least 10 million children whose growth is potentially abnormal.

Failure to thrive is a term usually reserved for infants who fail to gain weight and is most often due to undernutrition (see p 672).

Tall stature is a much less frequent presenting complaint than short stature and is usually a matter of concern to adolescent girls. The recent trend toward acceptance of tall stature in women has decreased the number of young people evaluated and treated for tall stature in our clinics.

SHORT STATURE

Abnormally short stature in relation to age is a common finding in childhood. In most instances it is due to a normal variation from the usual pattern of growth. The possible roles of such factors as sex, race, size of parents and other family members, nutrition, pubertal maturation, and emotional status must all be evaluated in the total assessment of the child.

The causes of unusually short stature are listed in Table 24–1. In most instances, the causes can be differentiated on the basis of significant findings in the history and physical examination or by laboratory tests.

1. CONSTITUTIONAL SHORT STATURE

Many children have a constitutional delay in growth and skeletal maturation. Puberty is delayed. In all other respects, they appear entirely normal. There is often a history of a similar pattern of growth in one of the parents or other members of the family. Normal puberty eventually occurs, and these children usually reach normal adult height although at a later than average age.

In the majority of children with constitutional short stature, the rate of growth is decreased either in the second year of life or just prior to puberty. At other times the growth curve parallels the third percentile.

No treatment for the short stature is indicated. The child and the parents should be helped to understand the normality of the situation.

2. PITUITARY DWARFISM
(Growth Hormone Deficiency)

Growth hormone (GH) deficiency is an uncommon cause of short stature; approximately half of cases are idiopathic (rarely familial); the remainder are secondary to pituitary or hypothalamic disease (craniopharyngioma, infections, tuberculosis, sarcoidosis, toxoplasmosis, syphilis, trauma, reticuloendotheliosis, vascular anomalies, and other tumors such as gliomas). GH deficiency may be an isolated defect or may occur in combination with other pituitary hormone deficiencies. Idiopathic growth hormone deficiency affects both sexes equally. The idiopathic form associated with multiple hormone deficiencies is more common in males.

Table 24—1. Causes of short stature.

Familial, racial, or genetic

Constitutional retarded growth and delayed adolescence

Endocrine disturbances
  Hypopituitarism
    Isolated somatotropin deficiency
    Somatotropin deficiency with other pituitary hormone deficiencies
  Hypothyroidism
  Adrenal insufficiency
  Cushing's disease and Cushing's syndrome (including iatrogenic causes)
  Sexual precocity (androgen or estrogen excess)
  Diabetes mellitus (poorly controlled)
  Diabetes insipidus
  Hyperaldosteronism

Primordial short stature
  Intrauterine growth retardation
    Placental insufficiency
    Intrauterine infection
  Primordial dwarfism with premature aging
    Progeria (Hutchinson-Gilford syndrome)
    Progeroid syndrome
      Werner's syndrome
      Cachectic (Cockayne's syndrome)
  Short stature without associated anomalies
  Short stature with associated anomalies (eg, Seckel's bird-headed dwarfism, leprechaunism, Silver's syndrome, Bloom's syndrome, Cornelia de Lange syndrome, Hallerman-Streiff syndrome)

Inborn errors of metabolism
  Altered metabolism of calcium or phosphorus (eg, hypophosphatemic rickets, hypophosphatasia, infantile hypercalcemia, pseudohypoparathyroidism)
  Storage diseases
    Mucopolysaccharidoses (eg, Hurler's syndrome, Hunter's syndrome)
    Mucolipidoses (eg, generalized gangliosidosis, fucosidosis, mannosidosis)
    Sphingolipidoses (eg, Tay-Sachs disease, Niemann-Pick disease, Gaucher's disease)
    Miscellaneous (eg, cystinosis)
  Aminoacidemias and aminoacidurias

  Epithelial transport disorders (eg, renal tubular acidosis, cystic fibrosis, Bartter's syndrome, vasopressin resistant diabetes insipidus, pseudohypoparathyroidism)
  Organic acidemias and acidurias (eg, methylmalonic aciduria, orotic aciduria, maple syrup urine disease, isovaleric acidemia)
  Metabolic anemias (eg, sickle cell disease, thalassemia, pyruvate kinase deficiency)
  Disorders of mineral metabolism (eg, Wilson's disease, magnesium malabsorption syndrome)
  Body defense disorders (eg, Bruton's agammaglobulinemia, thymic aplasia, chronic granulomatous disease)

Constitutional (intrinsic) diseases of bone
  Defects of growth of tubular bones or spine (eg, achondroplasia, metatropic dwarfism, diastrophic dwarfism, metaphyseal chondrodysplasia)
  Disorganized development of cartilage and fibrous components of the skeleton (eg, multiple cartilaginous exostoses, fibrous dysplasia with skin pigmentation, precocious puberty of McCune-Albright)
  Abnormalities of density of cortical diaphyseal structure or metaphyseal modeling (eg, osteogenesis imperfecta congenita, osteopetrosis, tubular stenosis)

Short stature associated with chromosomal defects
  Autosomal (eg, Down's syndrome, cri du chat syndrome, trisomy 18)
  Sex chromosomal (eg, Turner's syndrome-XO, penta X, XXXY)

Chronic systemic diseases, congenital defects, and malignancies (eg, chronic infection and infestation, inflammatory bowel disease, hepatic disease, cardiovascular disease, hematologic disease, CNS disease, pulmonary disease, renal disease, malnutrition, malignancies, collagen vascular disease)

Psychosocial dwarfism (maternal deprivation)

Miscellaneous syndromes (eg, arthrogryposis multiplex congenita, cerebrohepatorenal syndrome, Noonan's syndrome, Prader-Willi syndrome, Riley-Day syndrome)

At birth, affected subjects are of normal weight but length may be reduced. Growth retardation is evident during infancy, and there may be infantile fat distribution, youthful facial features, small hands and feet, and delayed sexual maturation. Excessive wrinkling of the skin is present in older individuals. Dental development and epiphyseal maturation ("bone age") are delayed to a greater degree than height age (median age for patient's height). In cases resulting from CNS disease, headaches, visual field defects, abnormal skull x-rays, and symptoms of posterior pituitary insufficiency (polyuria and polydipsia) may precede or accompany the growth hormone deficiency.

Growth hormone deficiency is associated with low levels of GH in the serum and a failure of GH rise in response to arginine, insulin-induced hypoglycemia, or during normal physiologic sleep. Glucose-6-phosphate dehydrogenase deficiency, spontaneous hypoglycemia, augmented insulin sensitivity, and decreased gonadotropin levels may be present, as well as other pituitary hormone deficiencies.

The treatment of choice is human pituitary growth hormone. Protein anabolic agents (testosterone, fluoxymesterone, oxandrolone, norethandrolone, etc) may be effective in promoting linear growth, but these drugs may cause undue acceleration of epiphyseal closure with resultant limitation of growth potential and short stature in adult life.

3. HYPOTHYROIDISM

Hypothyroidism in childhood (see p 676) is invariably associated with poor growth and delayed osseous maturation. In occasional cases, short stature may be the principal finding.

4. PRIMORDIAL SHORT STATURE
(Intrauterine Growth Retardation)

Primordial short stature may occur in a number of disorders, including craniofacial disproportion (eg, Seckel's bird-headed dwarfism), Silver's syndrome, some cases of progeric and cachectic dwarfism (eg, Hutchinson-Gilford dwarfism), or may occur in individuals with no accompanying significant physical abnormalities. Children with these conditions are small at birth; both birth weight and length are below normal for gestational age. They grow parallel to but below the third percentile. Plasma growth hormone levels are usually normal but may be elevated. In most instances, skeletal maturation ("bone age") corresponds to chronologic age or is only mildly retarded, in contrast to the striking delay often present in children with GH and thyroid deficiency.

There is no satisfactory treatment for primordial short stature.

5. SHORT STATURE DUE TO EMOTIONAL FACTORS
(Psychosocial Short Stature)

Psychologic deprivation with disturbances in motor and personality development may be associated with short stature. Although the growth retardation in some of these subjects is the result of undernutrition, in others undernutrition does not seem to be a factor. In some instances, in addition to being small, the child may have increased (often voracious) appetite and a marked delay in skeletal maturation. These children are of normal size at birth and grow normally for a variable period of time before growth stops. A history of feeding problems in early infancy is common. Emotional disturbances in the family are the rule. Plasma growth hormone levels are variable; the normal sleep-related circadian rise may be absent as a consequence of restless sleep. Treatment with growth hormone is not associated with increase in growth velocity. Polydipsia and polyuria are sometimes present.

Foster home placement or a significant change in the psychologic and emotional environment at home usually results in significantly improved growth, a decrease of appetite and dietary intake to more normal levels, and personality improvement.

DIFFERENTIAL DIAGNOSIS OF SHORT STATURE

Short stature may accompany or be caused by a large number of conditions (Table 24–1). When the etiologic diagnosis is not apparent from the history and physical examination, the following laboratory studies, in addition to bone age, are useful in detecting or categorizing the common causes of short stature:

(1) Complete blood count (to detect chronic anemia, infection, malignancies).

(2) Erythrocyte sedimentation rate (elevated in collagen vascular disease, malignancy, chronic infection, inflammatory bowel disease).

(3) Urinalysis and microscopic examination (occult pyelonephritis, glomerulonephritis, renal tubular disease, etc).

(4) Stool examination for occult blood, parasites, and parasite ova (inflammatory bowel disease, overwhelming parasitism).

(5) Serum electrolytes and phosphorus (mild adrenal insufficiency, renal tubular diseases, parathyroid disease, rickets, etc).

(6) Blood urea nitrogen (occult renal insufficiency).

(7) Buccal smear and karyotyping (should be performed in all short girls with delayed sexual maturation with or without clinical features of Turner's syndrome).

(8) Thyroid "function" assessment: T_4 and TSH

assay (short stature may be the only sign of hypothyroidism).

(9) Growth hormone evaluation. Blood samples for growth hormone determination should be obtained following 20 minutes of exercise, during normal sleep, or after administration of one of the conventional provocative agents (arginine, glucagon, levodopa, and insulin-induced hypoglycemia). Samples obtained during the first 90 minutes of sleep are preferable since they demonstrate both the presence and the physiologic release of growth hormone.

Goodman HG, Grumbach MM, Kaplan SL: Growth and growth hormone. 2. A comparison of isolated growth hormone deficiency and multiple pituitary-hormone deficiency in 35 patients with idiopathic hypopituitary dwarfism. N Engl J Med 278:57, 1968.

Gotlin RW, Mace JW: Diagnosis and management of short stature in childhood and adolescence. (2 parts.) Curr Probl Pediatr 2:3, Feb 1972, and 2:3, March 1972.

Gotlin RW, Mace JW, Silver HK: Raised nyctohemeral (night and day) growth-hormone levels in conditions with primordial short stature. Lancet 1:626, 1971.

Hall K, Filipsson R: Correlation between somatomedin A in serum and body height development. Acta Endocrinol (Kbh) 78:239, 1975.

Mace JW, Gotlin RW, Beck P: Sleep related human growth hormone release: A test of physiologic growth hormone secretion in children. J Clin Endocrinol 34:339, 1972.

Marti-Henneberg C, Niirianen AK, Rappaport R: Oxandrolone treatment of constitutional short stature in boys during adolescence: Effect on linear growth, bone age, pubic hair, and testicular development. J Pediatr 86:783, 1975.

Root AW, Bongiovanni AM, Eberlein WR: Diagnosis and management of growth retardation with special reference to the problem of hypopituitarism. Pediatrics 78:737, 1971.

Silver HK, Finkelstein M: Deprivation dwarfism. J Pediatr 70:317, 1967.

Tanner JM & others: Clinical longitudinal standards for height, weight, height velocity, and stages of puberty. Arch Dis Child 51:170, 1976.

FAILURE TO THRIVE (FTT)

Failure to thrive is present when there is a perceptible declination of growth from an established pattern or when the patient's height and weight plot consistently below the third percentile. (The term is usually reserved for infants who for various reasons fail to gain weight.) Linear growth and head circumference may also be affected; when this occurs, the underlying condition is generally more severe. There are many reasons for failure to thrive (see below and Table 24–1), although a specific cause often cannot be established.

Classification & Etiologic Diagnosis

The diagnosis of failure to thrive is usually apparent on the basis of the history and physical examination. When it is not, it is helpful to compare the patient's chronologic age with the height age (median age for the patient's height), weight age, and head circumference. On the basis of these measurements, 3 principal patterns can be defined which provide a starting point in the diagnostic approach.

> **Group 1.** (Most common type.) Normal head circumference; weight reduced out of proportion to height: In the majority of cases of failure to thrive, malnutrition is present as a result of either deficient caloric intake or malabsorption.
>
> **Group 2.** Normal or enlarged head circumference for age; weight only moderately reduced, usually in proportion to height: Structural dystrophies, constitutional dwarfism, endocrinopathies.
>
> **Group 3.** Subnormal head circumference; weight reduced in proportion to height: Primary CNS deficit; intrauterine growth retardation.

An initial period of observed nutritional rehabilitation, usually in a hospital setting, is often helpful in the diagnosis. The child should be placed on a regular diet for age and his intake and weight carefully plotted for 1–2 weeks. During this period, the presence of lactose intolerance is determined by checking pH and the presence of reducing substances in the stools. If stools are abnormal, the child should be further observed on a lactose-free diet. Caloric intake should be increased if weight gain does not occur but intake is well tolerated. The following 3 patterns are often noted during the rehabilitation period. Pattern 1 is by far the most common.

> **Pattern 1.** (Most common type.) Intake adequate; weight gain satisfactory: Feeding technic at fault. Disturbed infant-mother relationship leading to decreased caloric intake.
>
> **Pattern 2.** Intake adequate; no weight gain: If weight gain is unsatisfactory after increasing the calories to an adequate level (based on the infant's ideal weight for his height), malabsorption is a likely diagnosis.
>
> If malabsorption is present, it is usually necessary to differentiate pancreatic exocrine insufficiency (cystic fibrosis) from abnormalities of intestinal mucosa (celiac disease). In cystic fibrosis, growth velocity commonly declines from the time of birth and appetite usually is voracious. In celiac disease, growth velocity is usually not reduced until 6–12 months of age and inadequate caloric intake may be a prominent feature.
>
> **Pattern 3.** Intake inadequate:
>
> (1) Sucking or swallowing difficulties: CNS or neuromuscular disease; esophageal or oropharyngeal malformations.
>
> (2) Inability to eat large amounts is common in patients with cardiopulmonary disease

or in anorexic children suffering from chronic infections, inflammatory bowel disease, and endocrine problems (eg, hypothyroidism). Patients with celiac disease often have inadequate caloric intake in addition to malabsorption.

    (3) Vomiting, spitting up, or rumination: Upper intestinal obstruction (eg, pyloric stenosis, hiatal hernia, chalasia), chronic metabolic aberrations and acidosis (eg, renal insufficiency, diabetes mellitus and insipidus, methylmalonic acidemia), aldosterone insufficiency, increased intracranial pressure, psychosocial abnormalities.

Laboratory Aids to Diagnosis

The laboratory may provide adjunctive information helpful in the differential.

A. Initial: Initial laboratory investigations at the time of admission might be limited to the following:

1. Blood—Complete blood count, sedimentation rate.

2. Urine—Urinalysis (including microscopic examination of sediment) and culture and colony count.

3. Stool—Culture, pH, reducing substances, and Hematest.

4. Tuberculin test.

5. Other tests as specifically indicated.

B. Definitive: The following laboratory investigations are recommended after the period of nutritional rehabilitation, when the patient has been classified in one of the 3 categories listed above.

1. Pattern 1—No further diagnostic laboratory tests are indicated. Maternal (and family) psychologic evaluation may be indicated.

2. Pattern 2—Evaluation of malabsorption.

a. Stool fat (72-hour specimen) on a diet with normal fat content.

b. Stool trypsin on *fresh* specimen.

c. Sweat chloride test.

d. Peroral small bowel biopsy with histology, analysis of intestinal disaccharidase activity, duodenal aspiration for pancreatic enzyme activity, culture and examination for *Giardia lamblia.*

e. Liver function tests (eg, serum alkaline phosphatase, bilirubin).

3. Pattern 3—

a. With vomiting—

(1) Serum electrolytes, pH, total CO_2, glucose, BUN, serum and urine osmolarities, serum and urine organic and amino acids.

(2) Upper gastrointestinal series and cineesophagography.

(3) Skull x-rays for increased intracranial pressure.

b. Without vomiting—

(1) Sigmoidoscopy, rectal biopsy (ulcerative or granulomatous colitis).

(2) Barium enema (ulcerative colitis or Hirschsprung's disease).

(3) Upper gastrointestinal series and follow-through (regional enteritis, malrotations).

(4) Thyroid function test (eg, T_4, PBI).

C. Other Tests: Further testing (adrenal function tests, intravenous urograms, etc) may be indicated.

Treatment

Treatment will vary according to the underlying disorder. Most patients will gain weight and thrive on an adequate caloric intake. Maternal counseling and support are often required over a prolonged period. In some cases, foster home placement may be required.

Prognosis

The outcome is dependent on the underlying disorder. In general, infants whose length and, particularly, head circumference are affected along with weight have a less favorable prognosis.

Hannaway PJ: Failure to thrive: A study of 100 infants and children. Clin Pediatr (Phila) 9:96, 1970.

Hufton IW, Oates RK: Nonorganic failure to thrive: A long-term follow-up. Pediatrics 59:73, 1977.

Kempe CH, Helfer R: *Helping the Battered Child and His Family.* Lippincott, 1972.

Newberger EH, Howard RB: A conceptual approach to the child with exceptional nutritional requirements. Clin Pediatr (Phila) 12:456, 1973.

TALL STATURE

Tall stature is usually of concern only to adolescent and preadolescent girls. The upper limit of acceptable height of both sexes appears to be increasing, but there are occasions when the patient and her parents desire to influence the pattern of growth.

On the basis of family history, previous pattern of growth, stage of physiologic development, assessment of epiphyseal development ("bone age"), and standard growth data, the physician should make a tentative estimate of the patient's eventual height. Although there are several conditions (Table 24—2) which may produce tall stature, by far the most common cause is a constitutional variation from normal.

Reassurance and counseling should be tried first and are usually the only forms of therapy required. If the predicted height appears to be excessive, hormonal therapy with estrogen (eg, ethinyl estradiol), 0.2—0.3 mg daily, cycled with a progestational agent 7 days out of 28 days, has been suggested. Estrogens are of less value when the physiologic age (as determined by stage of sexual maturity and epiphyseal development) has reached the 12-year-old level and may be of little value even when administered at earlier ages. Estrogens act to accelerate epiphyseal closure and may be continued until fusion occurs.

Because of the unknown long-term effects of hormone administration to children, these agents should be used with great caution.

Table 24—2. Causes of tall stature.

Constitutional (familial, genetic)

Endocrine causes
    Somatotropin excess (pituitary gigantism)
    Androgen excess (tall as children, short as adults)
        True sexual precocity
        Pseudosexual precocity
    Androgen deficiency (normal height as children, tall as adults)
        Klinefelter's syndrome
        Anorchia (infection, trauma, idiopathic)
    Hyperthyroidism

Genetic causes
    Klinefelter's syndrome
    Syndromes of XYY, XXYY (tall as adults)

Miscellaneous syndromes and entities
    Marfan's syndrome
    Cerebral gigantism (Soto's syndrome)
    Total lipodystrophy
    Diencephalic syndrome
    Homocystinuria

Carrington ER: Relationship of stilbestrol exposure in utero to vaginal lesions in adolescence. J Pediatr 85:295, 1974.

Haigler ED Jr, Hershman JM, Meador CK: Pituitary gigantism. Arch Intern Med 132:588, 1973.

Mace JW, Gotlin RW: Cerebral gigantism: Triad of findings helpful in the diagnosis. Clin Pediatr (Phila) 9:662, 1970.

Wettenhall HNB, Cahill C, Roche AF: Tall girls: A survey of 15 years of management and treatment. J Pediatr 86:602, 1975.

THYROID

FETAL DEVELOPMENT OF THE THYROID

By the seventh week of intrauterine development, the thyroid gland has migrated to its definitive location and the thyroglossal duct has atrophied. Cell differentiation and function progress over the next 7 weeks, and by the 14th week the thyroid is capable of hormone synthesis. At this stage, thyroid-stimulating hormone (TSH; thyrotropin) is detectable in the fetal serum and pituitary gland.

Under normal conditions, neither TSH nor thyroid hormone crosses the placenta in appreciable amounts, and the fetal pituitary-thyroid axis functions independently of, though in parallel with, the maternal pituitary-thyroid axis.

Trace amounts of free thyroxine (T_4) and triiodothyronine (T_3) are capable of transplacental passage, and administration of the latter in large doses has been recommended in pregnant women when a hypothyroid offspring is anticipated. Antithyroid drugs, including radioactive iodine, freely cross the placenta, and goitrous hypothyroid newborns may be born to hyperthyroid mothers who undergo treatment during pregnancy.

Although maternal TSH does not reach the fetus, pregnant hyperthyroid mothers may transmit long-acting human-specific thyroid stimulator* transplacentally, resulting in thyrotoxic newborns who may exhibit exophthalmos. Since human-specific thyroid stimulator may be present in the serum of "controlled," previously hyperthyroid mothers, the possible transmission of human-specific thyroid stimulator should be considered in all mothers in whom hyperthyroidism is or has been present.

Physiology

Under the stimulation of pituitary TSH, the thyroid gland traps, concentrates, and organifies iodine, synthesizes and couples mono- and diiodotyrosine, and releases active thyroid hormones into the circulation (Fig 24—1).

The quantity released is proportionate to the needs of the organism and is maintained by a negative feedback mechanism involving pituitary TSH and "free" thyroid hormone (Fig 24—2).

Active hormone produced in excess of physiologic needs is stored within the thyroid follicles as colloid. Upon release into the circulation, T_4 and T_3 are bound to thyroxine-binding globulin (TBG), albumin, and prealbumin. The binding affinity of TBG for T_4 is approximately 20 times greater than for T_3. A small percentage ($< 1\%$) of T_3 and T_4 is not bound but is "free" and exists in equilibrium with the "bound" form. The physiologic activity of thyroid hormone depends on the amount of free T_3 and T_4. The level of free hormone is measured directly or determined by the total amount and binding affinity of the thyroid-binding proteins.

Causes of Thyroid Disturbances

Physiologic disturbances of the thyroid gland may be due to the following causes:†

(1) Decreased thyroid tissue: Hypofunction may result from congenital aplasia or hypoplasia, destruction due to inflammatory disease (thyroiditis), neoplasm, antithyroid antibodies, thyroidectomy, or irradiation.

(2) Inborn errors in the synthesis of thyroid hormone: Defects may occur in any of the metabolic steps shown in Fig 24—1 as well as in the binding and release of T_4 and T_3 from thyroglobulin.

(3) Iodine deficiency.

(4) Inhibition of thyroidal iodide uptake and concentration by drugs (eg, thiocyanates, perchlorates, nitrates).

---

*Formerly called LATS or LATS protector, which is now known to be of physiologic significance only in rodents.
†Adapted from Wilkins.

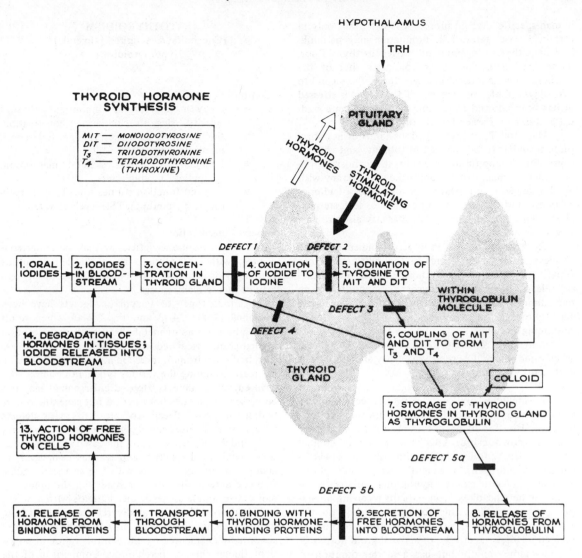

Figure 24–1. Synthesis of thyroxine (T_4) and triiodothyronine (T_3). (Adapted, with permission, from: Current Concepts of Thyroid Disease. [Programmed instruction course in *Spectrum*.] Pfizer Laboratories Division, Chas Pfizer & Co, Inc, 1965.) (See Table 24–3 for causes of defects.)

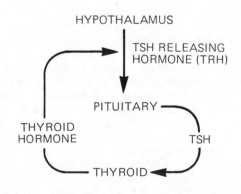

Figure 24–2. Pituitary-thyroid control.

(5) Interference with thyroid enzyme activity by antithyroid compounds. Antithyroid compounds include thiourea, thiouracil and its derivatives, cobalt, large doses of iodides, and certain foods such as cabbage, turnips, and soybeans. Iodides also interfere with the release of thyroid hormone.

(6) Disorders of the hypothalamus and pituitary gland which result in impairment of either thyrotropin-releasing hormone or thyrotropin secretion.

(7) Nervous stresses.

Release of Thyroid Hormone & Its Function

The principal functions of the thyroid gland are to synthesize and store T_4 and T_3 and to release them in response to bodily need. A number of chemical reactions are involved in thyroid hormone formation. The thyroid gland is regulated and stimulated by TSH;

human-specific thyroid protector is important only in certain disease states. TSH production may be inhibited by either endogenous or exogenous thyroid hormone. At birth, the T_4 approximates that of the mother. There is a rapid increase during the second to fifth days of life—particularly if the infant is stressed or has been allowed to become cool—and then a gradual decrease over several weeks or months.

The total T_4 is low in various forms of hypothyroidism and may be reduced in subacute and chronic thyroiditis, hypopituitarism, nephrosis, cirrhosis, hypoproteinemia, malnutrition, and following therapy with T_3. Prolonged administration of high doses of adrenocorticosteroids as well as sulfonamides, testosterone, phenytoin (Dilantin), and salicylates may also produce a decrease in T_4.

The total T_4 is high in hyperthyroidism and may be elevated in various forms of thyroiditis and acute hepatitis; in some types of inborn errors in the synthesis, release, or binding of thyroid hormone; following the administration of estrogens or during pregnancy; and following the administration of various iodine-containing globulins.

Individuals receiving T_4 therapeutically may have an elevated serum T_4 even though they are maintained in the euthyroid state.

TBG is increased in pregnancy, after estrogen therapy (including oral contraceptives), occasionally as a genetic variation, in certain hepatic disorders, following administration of phenothiazines, and occasionally from unknown cause. TBG is decreased in familial TBG deficiency; following the administration of glucocorticoids, androgens, or anabolic steroids; in nephrotic syndrome with marked hypoproteinemia; in some forms of hepatic disease; in patients receiving phenytoin; and as an idiopathic finding. T_4 and T_3 are the active components of the thyroid gland, comprising 90% and 10%, respectively, of active thyroid hormone. T_3 acts more rapidly but has a shorter duration of action; there is no marked qualitative difference in its metabolic effect. The thyroid hormones accelerate various oxidative systems, thus increasing the consumption of oxygen.

Fisher DA: Advances in the laboratory diagnosis of thyroid disease. (2 parts.) J Pediatr 82:1, 187, 1973.

Inada M & others: Estimation of thyroxine and triiodothyronine distribution and of the conversion rate of thyroxine to triiodothyronine in man. J Clin Invest 55:1337, 1975.

Rosenberg IN: Evaluation of thyroid function. N Engl J Med 286:924, 1972.

Vigneri R: Triiodothyronine and thyrotropin-releasing hormone interaction on TSH release in man. Hormones 3:250, 1972.

HYPOTHYROIDISM
(Congenital & Acquired [Juvenile] Hypothyroidism)

Essentials of Diagnosis

- Growth retardation, diminished physical activity, sluggish circulation, constipation, thick tongue, poor muscle tone, hoarseness, intellectual retardation.
- Delayed dental and skeletal maturation. "Stippling" of epiphyses.
- Thyroid function studies low (T_4 and erythrocyte T_3 binding); TSH levels elevated.

General Considerations

Thyroid hormone deficiency may be either congenital (with or without the physical features of cretinism) or acquired (juvenile hypothyroidism) and may be due to many causes.

Various types of enzymatic defects have been described (Table 24–3 and Fig 24–1) which result from inborn errors of metabolism. With the exception of that group associated with congenital nerve deafness (Pendred's syndrome), there are no distinguishing clinical features among the various types. In children who have enzymatic defects, thyroid enlargement may not be present in the newborn period but generally occurs within the first 2 decades of life. Enzymatic defects have a familial autosomal recessive inheritance pattern.

Under the influence of increased TSH stimulation, rapid uptake occurs and reaches peak levels in about 2 hours. In patients with the very rare iodide trapping defect, the goiter is small and the uptake of radioactive iodine is negligible. Patients with a defect in iodide organification rapidly release labeled iodine from the gland; this release may be significantly and abnormally augmented by the administration of potassium thiocyanate or perchlorate. Comparison of the PBI and T_4 may be helpful in coupling and deiodinase defects, revealing a greater than normal discrepancy in the blood levels of these substances which reflects impaired thyroglobulin proteolysis, abnormal plasma binding, or the presence of abnormal circulating iodoproteins. Further clarification of the defect generally requires chromatographic fractionation of iodinated compounds in the serum, urine, and thyroid tissue.

A number of drugs and goitrogens taken during pregnancy (eg, cabbage, soybeans, aminosalicylic acid, thiourea derivatives, resorcinol, phenylbutazone, cobalt, and iodides in therapeutic doses for asthma—particularly in individuals who have also received adrenocortical steroids) have been reported to cause goiter and in some instances hypothyroidism also. Since many of these agents cross the placental barrier freely, they should be used with great caution during pregnancy. If taken by the pregnant woman, the goiter and decreased thyroid function that is produced in the newborn are generally transient and seldom a problem.

Many cases of acquired hypothyroidism, particularly in the presence of a history of goiter, appear to be

Table 24—3. Causes of hypothyroidism.*

A. Congenital (Cretinism):	4. Iodide deficiency (endemic cretinism).
1. Aplasia, hypoplasia, or associated with maldescent of thyroid—	5. Idiopathic.

A. Congenital (Cretinism):
1. Aplasia, hypoplasia, or associated with maldescent of thyroid—
   a. Embryonic defect of development.
   b. Autoimmune disease (?).
2. Familial iodine-induced goiter secondary to metabolic inborn errors—
   a. Iodide transport defect (defect 1).
   b. Organification defect (defect 2)—
      (1) Lack of iodine peroxidase.
      (2) Lack of iodine transferase; Pendred's syndrome associated with congenital nerve deafness.
   c. Coupling defect (defect 3).
   d. Iodotyrosine deiodinase defect (defect 4).
   e. Abnormal iodinated polypeptide (defects 5a and 5b)—
      (1) Resulting from defect in intrathyroidal proteolysis of thyroglobulin.
      (2) Abnormal plasma binding preventing use of T_4 by peripheral cells.
   f. Possible inability of tissues to convert T_4 to T_3.
3. Maternal ingestion of medications during pregnancy—
   a. Maternal radioiodine.
   b. Goitrogens (propylthiouracil, methimazole).
   c. Iodides.
4. Iodide deficiency (endemic cretinism).
5. Idiopathic.

B. Acquired (Juvenile Hypothyroidism):
1. Thyroidectomy or radioiodine therapy for—
   a. Thyrotoxicosis.
   b. Cancer.
   c. Lingual thyroid.
   d. Isolated midline thyroid.
2. Destruction by x-ray.
3. Thyrotropin deficiency—
   a. Isolated.
   b. Associated with other pituitary tropic hormone deficiencies.
4. TRH deficiency due to hypothalamic injury or disease.
5. Autoimmune disease (lymphocytic thyroiditis).
6. Chronic infections.
7. Medications—
   a. Iodides—
      (1) Prolonged, excessive ingestion.
      (2) Deficiency.
   b. Cobalt.
8. Idiopathic.

*"Defect 1" etc refers to specific defects in Fig 24—1.

the result of previously unsuspected lymphocytic thyroiditis.

Clinical Findings

The severity of the findings in cases of thyroid deficiency depends on the age at onset and the degree of interference with production of thyroid hormone. Congenital hypothyroidism may be recognized during the first month of life but may be so mild as to go unrecognized for months. Every effort should be made to establish the diagnosis of hypothyroidism as early as possible since untreated hypothyroidism may be associated with irreversible damage to the CNS. Newborn screening programs are becoming available to facilitate prompt diagnosis and therapy of congenital hypothyroidism. Screening programs utilize either T_4 or TSH. TSH may be a more sensitive index of thyroid hypofunction.

A. Symptoms and Signs:

1. Functional changes—Even with congenital absence of the thyroid gland, the first finding may not appear for several days or weeks. Findings include physical and mental sluggishness; pale, gray, cool or mottled skin; nonpitting myxedema, decreased intestinal activity (constipation); large tongue, poor muscle tone, giving rise to a protuberant abdomen, umbilical hernia, and lumbar lordosis; hypothermia; bradycardia, diminished sweating (variable); decreased pulse pressure; hoarse voice or cry; delayed transient deafness; and slow relaxation after elicitation of tendon reflexes. Nasal obstruction and discharge and persistent jaundice may be present in the neonatal period.

The skin may be dry, thick, scaly, and coarse, with a yellowish tinge due to excessive deposition of carotene. The hair is dry, coarse, brittle (variable), and may be excessive. Lateral thinning of the eyebrows may occur. The axillary and supraclavicular fat pads may be prominent in infants. Muscular hypertrophy (Debré-Sémélaigne syndrome) occasionally is present.

2. Retardation of growth and development—Findings include shortness of stature, infantile skeletal proportions with relatively short extremities, infantile naso-orbital configuration (bridge of nose flat, broad, and underdeveloped; eyes seem to be widely spaced); delayed osseous development (retarded "bone age"); delayed closure of the fontanels, and retarded dental development. Slowing of mental responsiveness and retardation of development of the brain may occur, and in many cases a coincidental congenital malformation of the brain is present also.

3. Alterations in sexual development (usually retardation, sometimes precocity)—Menometrorrhagia in older girls; galactorrhea occasionally.

B. X-Ray Findings: Epiphyseal development ("bone age") is delayed. Centers of ossification, especially of the hip, may show multiple small centers or a single, stippled, porous or fragmented center (epiphyseal dysgenesis). Vertebrae may show anterior beaking. The cardiac shadow is increased. Coxa vara and coxa plana may occur.

C. **Laboratory Findings:** T_4 is decreased. Radioiodine uptake is below 10% (normal: 10–50%).* (Both may be normal or elevated in goitrous cretinism and in some cases of thyroiditis.) The binding of T_3 by erythrocytes or resin in vitro (T_3 test) is lowered. Serum cholesterol and carotene are usually elevated but often low or normal in infants and rarely low in older children; cessation of therapy in previously treated hypothyroid patients produces a marked rise in serum cholesterol levels in 6–8 weeks. The basal metabolic rate is low, but the test is difficult to perform and unreliable in children. With primary hypothyroidism, the plasma TSH is elevated. Urinary creatine excretion is decreased and creatinine increased. Serum alkaline phosphatase is occasionally reduced, and urinary hydroxyproline is low. Circulating autoantibodies to thyroid constituents may be present. Erythrocyte glucose-6-phosphate dehydrogenase activity is decreased. Plasma growth hormone may be decreased, with subnormal response to insulin-induced hypoglycemia and arginine stimulation.

Differential Diagnosis

The various causes of primary hypothyroidism due to intrinsic defects of the thyroid gland must be differentiated from pituitary and hypothalamic failure with secondary thyroid insufficiency as a result of deficiency of TSH. TSH measurements before and after TRH and T_4 and radioactive iodide uptake studies before and after exogenous TSH administration (5–10 units daily for 3 days) are useful in differentiation. Since pituitary insufficiency may be associated with both secondary hypoadrenocorticism and secondary hypothyroidism, treatment of the latter alone may precipitate an adrenal crisis.

Down's syndrome, chondrodystrophy, generalized gangliosidosis, I-cell disease, Hurler's and Hunter's syndromes, and certain other causes of short stature as well as macroglossia due to abnormalities of the lymphatics of the tongue can all be readily distinguished by the clinical manifestations and by appropriate laboratory studies. Although other individual findings of the hypothyroid child may suggest exogenous obesity, congenital heart disease, or some type of anemia as the primary diagnosis, a careful appraisal of the entire clinical and laboratory picture should permit establishment of the proper diagnosis.

Treatment

A. **Medical Treatment:** Levothyroxine or desiccated thyroid is the drug of choice. Begin therapy with 0.05 mg levothyroxine for 1–2 weeks. Use 0.025 mg levothyroxine initially for myxedematous infants. In-

*The presence of iodides in bread in recent years has resulted in significant decrease in normal values of radioiodine uptake. The normal levels for any particular area should be ascertained.

crease dosage by 0.025–0.05 mg every 1–2 weeks until the required level is reached. Children will usually require 0.10–0.11 mg/sq m, or 0.0038 mg/kg/day, with a minimum requirement of 0.05 mg. Serum T_4 and TSH should be used as a guide to adequate therapy.

The hypothyroid patient is quite responsive to thyroid, usually shows improvement 7–21 days after starting therapy, and is very sensitive to slight excesses of thyroid hormone. The normal individual can take comparatively large doses of thyroid with very little effect. If a patient can tolerate significantly more than the usual therapeutic doses of thyroid hormone (> 130 mg in the young child, > 220 mg in the older child), the diagnosis of hypothyroidism should be questioned.

Triiodothyronine (sodium liothyronine, Cytomel) may be employed when a more rapid and short-lived effect is desired (eg, in the TSH suppression test) but probably is not as effective for maintenance therapy as desiccated thyroid or levothyroxine. When levothyroxine or triiodothyronine is administered, the T_4 should be lower when the patient is euthyroid. In the treatment of neonatal goiter with or without hypothyroidism resulting from drugs and goitrogens taken by the pregnant woman, temporary treatment with triiodothyronine or levothyroxine is sufficient to bring about rapid disappearance of the enlargement.

B. **Surgical Measures:** Rarely, respiratory obstruction may occur, requiring surgical excision of the thyroid isthmus (rather than tracheostomy).

Barnes ND: Thyroid stimulator hormone measurement in children with thyroid disorders. Arch Dis Child 54:497, 1975.

Hayek A & others: Pertechnetate for detection of cryptic thyroid tissue in childhood hypothyroidism. Pediatrics 79:466, 1971.

Homoki J & others: Thyroid function in term newborn infants with congenital goiter. J Pediatr 86:753, 1975.

Klein AH & others: Improved prognosis in congenital hypothyroidism treated before age three months. J Pediatr 81:912, 1972.

Klein AH & others: Neonatal thyroid function in congenital hypothyroidism. J Pediatr 89:545, 1976.

Medreios-Neto GA & others: Partial defect of iodide trapping mechanism in two siblings with congenital goiter and hypothyroidism. J Clin Endocrinol 35:370, 1972.

Rezvani I, DiGeorge AM: Reassessment of the daily dose of oral thyroxine for replacement therapy in hypothyroid children. J Pediatr 90:291, 1977.

Schalch DS & others: Abnormalities in release of TSH in response to TRH in patients with disorders of the pituitary hypothalamus and basal ganglia. J Clin Endocrinol 35:609, 1972.

Turks MI & others: New radioimmunoassay for plasma T_3: Measurements in thyroid disease and in patients maintained on hormonal replacement. J Clin Invest 51:3104, 1972.

HYPERTHYROIDISM

Essentials of Diagnosis

- Nervousness, irritability, emotional lability, tremor, excessive appetite, weight loss, per-

spiration, and heat intolerance.
- Goiter, exophthalmos, tachycardia, increased pulse pressure.
- Thyroid function studies elevated (eg, T_4, T_3, T_3R).

General Considerations

The cause of hyperthyroidism has not been determined, but an immunologic basis is likely. In addition, psychic trauma, psychologic maladjustments, disturbances in pituitary function, infectious disease, and heredity have all been incriminated. Regardless of the inciting event or agent, mediation of the disease process may result from long-acting human-specific thyroid stimulator, an antibody produced by the lymphocytes. Transient congenital hyperthyroidism may occur in infants of thyrotoxic mothers, usually as a consequence of the transplacental passage of human-specific thyroid stimulator. However, infantile hyperthyroidism—or hyperthyroidism at any age—may occur in the absence of serum human-specific thyroid stimulator. Hyperthyroidism may be found with tumors of the thyroid, with other tumors producing thyrotropin-like substances, and with exogenous thyroid hormone excess.

Clinical Findings

A. Symptoms and Signs: Hyperthyroidism is 5 times as common in females as in males. The disease is most likely to appear in childhood at age 12–14 years, with only 20% of cases present before 10 years of age. The course of hyperthyroidism tends to be cyclic, with spontaneous remissions and exacerbations, but it tends to progress rapidly. Findings include weakness, dyspnea, emotional instability, "nervousness" (inability to sit still), marked variability in mood, tremors and movements which may simulate chorea, personality disturbances, warm and moist skin, flushed face, palpitation, tachycardia (even during sleep), systolic hypertension with increased pulse pressure, and dysphagia. Proptosis and exophthalmos are common in hyperthyroid children. Goiter is present in more than 80% of cases and is characteristically diffuse and usually firm. A bruit and thrill may be present. Variable degrees of accelerated growth and development occur, and loss of weight is common in spite of polyphagia. (An occasional adolescent may gain weight.) Amenorrhea may occur in adolescent girls. There is an increased incidence of diabetes mellitus in thyrotoxicosis.

B. Laboratory Findings: The T_4 and free T_4 are elevated except in rare cases in which only the blood triiodothyronine is elevated ("T_3 thyrotoxicosis").* There is increased binding of radioactive T_3 to shed blood or resin in the T_3 test. Radioiodine uptake is above 35–40% at 24 hours and suppressed less than 40% after administration of T_3 (25 μg 3–4 times daily

---

*Certain organic iodine compounds, eg, iophenoxic acid (Teridax) may cause prolonged elevation of the PBI. If administered to the mother, they may cross the placenta in significant amounts and will affect the infant's PBI for months to years.

for 7 days). The basal metabolic rate is elevated, but testing for BMR is frequently unreliable and is seldom used. Serum cholesterol is low; glycosuria may occur. Agglutinating antibodies to thyroglobulin are found in most patients. Circulating TSH is usually depressed, and human-specific thyroid stimulator is often present in plasma (particularly in the newborn infant). Erythrocyte glucose-6-phosphate dehydrogenase activity is increased. Urinary hydroxyproline is increased, and urinary creatine may be elevated.

C. X-Ray Findings: Rarely, abnormal skull x-rays are found in some patients with primary pituitary disease. Skeletal maturation may be accelerated; in the newborn, it may be associated with subsequent premature closure of the cranial sutures.

Differential Diagnosis

Although the well established case of hyperthyroidism seldom presents a problem in diagnosis, the findings in the early stage of the disease may be confused with chorea, or, more commonly, with the euthyroid child with a goiter (usually an adolescent girl) who is nervous, emotionally labile, and manifests a rapid pulse and increased perspiration. Careful and sometimes repeated clinical and laboratory evaluation may be required before the proper diagnosis can be established. Moreover, it should be recognized that thyrotoxic symptoms may occur with thyroiditis and rarely with thyroid cancer.

Various states with signs of hypermetabolism (severe anemia, leukemia, chronic infections, pheochromocytoma, as well as muscle wasting disease) may occasionally be confused with hyperthyroidism, but differentiation can usually be readily made by the clinical manifestations and by appropriate laboratory studies.

Treatment

The course of hyperthyroidism may exhibit fluctuations of improvement and remission. In some mild cases therapy may not be required.

Both surgical and medical methods are available for treating the manifestations of hyperthyroidism.

A. General Measures: Rest in bed is advisable only in severe cases, in preparation for surgery, or at the beginning of a medical regimen. The diet should be high in calories, carbohydrates, and vitamins (particularly vitamin B_1).

Propranolol (Inderal), a beta-adrenergic blocking agent, may be necessary to control symptoms of nervous instability and tachycardia. Propranolol will not alter thyroid function. Propranolol may also be helpful in controlling life-threatening cardiac complications which may occur in thyroid storm (severe thyrotoxicosis, fever, and altered consciousness).

B. Medical Treatment: With medical treatment, clinical response may be noted in 2–3 weeks and adequate control in 1–3 months. The thyroid frequently increases in size after initiation of treatment but usually will decrease in size within several months.

1. Propylthiouracil—This drug interferes with the intrathyroidal hormonogenesis and the peripheral conversion of T_4 to T_3; with the binding of iodine to thyroid protein; and with hormone synthesis. The correct dose must always be individually assessed. Propylthiouracil may be used in the initial treatment of the patient with hyperthyroidism, but if the T_4 fails to return to a normal range—or if it rises rapidly with reduction in drug dosage after 18–24 months of therapy—continued or alternative therapy may be necessary. Relapses occur in 10–30% of cases, and severe cases may not respond. Therapy should be continued for at least 2–3 years with the smallest drug dosage that will produce a euthyroid state. The safety of prolonged treatment has not been evaluated.

    a. Initial dosage—75–300 mg/day in 3–4 divided doses 6–8 hours apart until tests of thyroid function are normal and all signs and symptoms have subsided. Larger doses may be necessary.

    b. Maintenance—50–100 mg/day in 2–3 divided doses. Some authors recommend continuing the drug at higher levels until the euthyroid state is approached or reached and then giving oral thyroid. Thyroid may also be given if the gland enlarges significantly or remains enlarged after 2–3 months with propylthiouracil therapy.

    c. Toxicity—Granulocytopenia, fever, and rash may occur. Discontinue the drug and consider giving antibiotics and a short course of one of the adrenocortical steroids.

    2. Methimazole (Tapazole)—This drug may be used in 1/10–1/15 the dosage of propylthiouracil. However, toxic reactions may be more common with methimazole than with propylthiouracil.

    3. Iodide—Medical treatment with continuous iodide administration alone usually produces a rapid response but is generally recommended only for acute management since the effectiveness of iodide is short-lived; a progressive increase in dosage is often required for satisfactory control; and toxic reactions to iodide are not uncommon.

    C. Surgical Measures: Subtotal thyroidectomy is considered by many to be the treatment of choice, especially when a close follow-up of the patient is difficult or impossible. In childhood, surgery should be employed in patients when medical treatment is impossible or has been unsuccessful. The patient should be prepared first with bed rest, diet, and propranolol (as above), and with iodide and propylthiouracil as follows: Propylthiouracil (as above) should be given for 2–4 weeks. Iodide (as saturated solution of potassium iodide) is added 10–21 days before surgery is scheduled. Iodides act by blocking the effect of TSH on the thyroid, with resultant decrease in iodine trapping (with reduction of vascularity), and by inhibiting the release of hormone, thus reducing the possibility of thyroid storm. Give 1–10 drops daily for 10–21 days. Continue the drug for 1 week after surgery.

    Progressive exophthalmos following surgery is uncommon in childhood.

    D. Radiation Therapy: X-ray and radioactive iodine (^{131}I) generally are not recommended in children because of the possibility of an ultimate increased incidence of cancer, but the significance of this relationship remains to be proved.

    E. Congenital (Transient) Hyperthyroidism: Temporary treatment of congenital hyperthyroidism may be necessary, in which case iodides appear to be the drugs of choice. Reserpine or propranolol may be necessary to control cardiac arrhythmias. Transection of an enlarged thyroid isthmus may be of value if respiratory distress is present.

Course & Prognosis

    Improvement may occur without therapy in as many as one-third of cases, but partial remissions and exacerbations may continue for several years. With medical treatment alone, prolonged remissions may be expected in one-half to two-thirds of cases. Surgical therapy probably yields about the same number of satisfactory results. Postoperative hypothyroidism is not uncommon, and hypoparathyroidism and other complications may occur after surgery. Because of the comparatively high incidence of carcinoma in nodular goiters of childhood, such glands should be removed routinely once the thyrotoxicosis is in remission.

    Congenital hyperthyroidism has a significant mortality in the neonatal period, but the eventual prognosis in surviving infants is excellent.

Brewsher PD & others: Propranolol in the surgical management of thyrotoxicosis. Ann Surg 180:787, 1974.

Hayek A & others: Long-term results of treatment of thyrotoxicosis in children and adolescents with radioactive iodine. N Engl J Med 283:949, 1970.

Hayles A: Problems of childhood Graves' disease. Mayo Clin Proc 47:850, 1972.

Henneman G & others: Dissociation of serum LATS activity and hyperfunction and autonomy of the thyroid gland in Graves' disease. J Clin Endocrinol 40:935, 1975.

Hollingsworth DR, Mabry CC, Eckerd JM: Hereditary aspects of Graves' disease in infancy and childhood. J Pediatr 81:446, 1972.

Marsden P & others: Hormonal pattern of relapse in hyperthyroidism. Lancet 1:944, 1975.

Mitsuma T & others: T_3 toxicosis in childhood: Hyperthyroidism due to isolated hypersecretion of triiodothyronine. J Pediatr 81:982, 1972.

GOITER

    Goiter or struma is any enlargement of the thyroid gland. It has recently been noted with increasing frequency in children and adolescents. Enlargement of the thyroid may result from inflammation, infiltrative processes, or neoplasms, but in most instances the goiter is produced by the action of a relative excess of TSH or human-specific thyroid stimulator. These may develop autonomously or in response to an increased need for thyroid hormone. When the level of circulating hormone is inadequate, the normal pituitary produces more TSH in an attempt to stimulate the thyroid gland to increased activity.

The enlarged gland may vary greatly in size, shape, and consistency; regardless of these characteristics, the functional activity of the gland may be normal (euthyroid), decreased (hypothyroid), or increased (hyperthyroid). If augmented production is sufficient to produce physiologic quantities of hormone, the individual will be euthyroid; but if maximum stimulation of the thyroid is still associated with deficient production, hypothyroidism results.

Goiters resulting from deficient production of thyroid hormone are seen in children with inborn enzymatic defects, those with both iodine deficiency and excess, and when ingestion of antithyroid drugs or naturally occurring goitrogens has interfered with normal hormonogenesis.

Goiters may also be found in hyperthyroidism, various forms of thyroiditis, tumors, hemorrhage, infiltration with amyloid, and in an idiopathic form, particularly during adolescence. The administration of various drugs (aminosalicylic acid, thiourea derivatives, resorcinol, phenylbutazone, iodides, and cobalt) may be associated with the development of goiter.

Other causes of goiter are discussed above (see pp 676–679) and in the following sections.

Classification

A. Neonatal Goiter: Infants whose mothers are deficient in iodine or have been receiving iodides or antithyroid hormones may be born with goiters or may develop them during the first few days of life. The goiter is diffuse and relatively soft but may be large enough to compress the trachea, esophagus, and adjacent blood vessels.

Regression usually occurs in a few weeks. It may be hastened by the administration of small doses of thyroid. If evidence of hyperthyroidism appears, therapy with iodine or thiouracil drugs (or both) for a few weeks may be necessary.

B. Nodular Goiter: Nodular goiter in childhood occurs most commonly in chronic lymphocytic thyroiditis (see below). The presence of one or more nodules in the thyroid gland of a child raises the possibility of malignancy, as a thyroid nodule is more likely to be malignant in a child than in an adult. Nodules may also be the result of cyst formation, hemangiomas, or lymphangiomas.

The likelihood that a nodule is malignant increases when the nodule is single, hard, associated with paratracheal lymph node enlargement, or does not concentrate radioactive iodine. In the absence of these characteristics, nodular goiter in childhood should be treated with full replacement doses of desiccated thyroid or levothyroxine for a period of 1–2 months. If the nodule fails to decrease in size, it should be removed. Nodules occurring in chronic thyroiditis and hyperthyroidism should also be followed carefully because they too may be associated with an increased risk of malignancy.

Clinical Findings

There is usually no associated disturbance of function, although TSH levels may be elevated and in some instances mild hypothyroidism may occur. Symptoms of pressure due to goiter are very uncommon in childhood.

Prevention

Prevention in endemic areas consists of the use of iodized salt containing 1 mg of iodine per 100 gm of salt, or the administration of an iodide-containing drug. Routine iodinization of the water supply is also a satisfactory preventive measure.

Treatment

Remove or avoid precipitating factors if possible. Desiccated thyroid, 65–195 mg daily orally, is of value when treatment is necessary. Iodine therapy alone is effective when the goiter is due to iodide deficiency.

Surgery is occasionally necessary if significant pressure symptoms persist or for possible malignancy if a nodular lesion fails to regress despite therapy with thyroid hormone.

Course & Prognosis

Adolescent goiter may subside without treatment, but thyroid therapy may be necessary. Recent evidence suggests that most cases of adolescent goiter are the result of chronic lymphocytic thyroiditis.

Gillie RB: Endemic goiter. Sci Am 224:93, June 1971.

Hopwood NJ & others: Functioning thyroid masses in childhood and adolescence. J Pediatr 89:710, 1976.

Hung W & others: Goiters in euthyroid children. J Pediatr 82:10, 1973.

Kusakabe T: A goitrous subject with structural abnormality of thyroglobulin. J Clin Invest 35:784, 1972.

Silver HK, Gotlin RW: Goiter in infancy and childhood. Postgrad Med 42:A-133, Nov 1967.

See also Fisher & others reference, below.

ACUTE THYROIDITIS

Acute thyroiditis is uncommon but may occur after various infections, including those of the skin, pharynx, or larynx. At present, acute thyroiditis is apt to be the result of viral infections (mumps, adenovirus, measles, cat scratch fever, etc) or may be caused by bacteria (streptococci, pneumococci, staphylococci). There is usually no associated endocrine disturbance. Specific antibiotic therapy, if available, should be administered. Adrenocortical steroids may be of value.

SUBACUTE THYROIDITIS

Subacute thyroiditis (DeQuervain's giant cell thyroiditis, granulomatous thyroiditis, giant cell thyroiditis) is rare in this country. In most cases the cause

cannot be identified. Subacute thyroiditis is characterized by an insidious onset, fever, malaise, sore throat,
dysphagia, pain in the thyroid gland that may radiate
to the ears, and mild and transient manifestations of
hypermetabolism. The thyroid gland is firm, and the
enlargement may be confined to one lobe. Radioiodine
uptake is usually reduced.

The disease is usually self-limited and of short
duration, but it may persist for years. Thyroid hormone preparations and adrenocorticosteroids have
been employed with variable success in the treatment
of serious cases.

Greene JN: Subacute thyroiditis. Am J Med 51:97, 1971.

CHRONIC LYMPHOCYTIC THYROIDITIS
(Chronic Autoimmune Thyroiditis, Hashimoto's Thyroiditis, Lymphadenoid Goiter)

Essentials of Diagnosis
- Firm, freely movable, and diffusely enlarged goiter.
- T_4 normal, elevated, or decreased depending on stage of disease.
- Antibodies to various thyroid gland fractions.

General Considerations
Chronic lymphocytic thyroiditis is being seen
with increasing frequency in all age groups and currently is the most common cause of goiter and hypothyroidism in childhood. In children and adolescents, it
has a peak incidence between the ages of 8–15 years
and occurs most commonly in females. The exact
cause is not known, but many authors believe chronic
thyroiditis to be associated with an "autoimmune
phenomenon" since antibodies to various thyroid
gland fractions have been reported in many cases. Antibody formation is believed to be stimulated by the
release of abnormal thyroid gland proteins which then
act as antigens. At present there is no conclusive evidence that antithyroid antibodies actually initiate the
changes involving normal thyroid tissue, and the finding of "autoantibodies" has been neither consistent
nor unique to chronic thyroiditis.

Clinical Findings
A. Symptoms and Signs: The goiter is characteristically firm, freely movable, nontender, "pebbly" in
consistency, and diffusely enlarged, although it may be
asymmetric. In long-standing cases, nodules and, rarely, malignant changes have been described. The onset is
usually insidious. Most cases occur without clinical
manifestations and are completely painless. The
symptoms consist mainly of moderate tracheal compression with a sense of fullness, hoarseness, and
dysphagia. There are no local signs of inflammation
and no evidence of systemic infection.

B. Laboratory Findings: Laboratory findings are
variable. The T_3R and T_4 levels may be normal, elevated (10%), or depressed. TSH levels may be high.
Radioactive iodine uptake is elevated at 4–6 hours,
but the iodine is not bound normally to thyroglobulin
and is subsequently released at an abnormally rapid
rate. Enhanced release is reflected by a low 24-hour
radioiodine uptake value. The rate of release may be
increased after the administration of perchlorate or
thiocyanate. At least low titers of antithyroid antibodies are usually present.

Treatment
The treatment of choice for autoimmune thyroiditis is thyroid hormone in full therapeutic doses.
Approximately one-third to one-half of patients will
have a good response. Adrenocorticosteroids have been
used and do produce a reduction in the size of the
gland, but the gland usually enlarges again when corticosteroids are discontinued. Subtotal thyroidectomy is
occasionally necessary when the gland is particularly
large and fails to respond adequately to medical therapy. Regardless of the type of treatment employed,
hypothyroidism is a common end result of autoimmune thyroiditis.

Allison AC: Self-tolerance and autoimmunity in the thyroid. N
    Engl J Med 295:821, 1976.
Fisher DA & others: The diagnosis of Hashimoto's thyroiditis. J
    Clin Endocrinol 40:795, 1975.
Loeb PB & others: Prevalence of low titer and negative anti-
    thyroglobulin antibodies in biopsy-proved juvenile
    Hashimoto's thyroiditis. J Pediatr 82:17, 1973.
Papapetrou RD: Long-term treatment of Hashimoto's thyroid-
    itis with thyroxine. Lancet 2:1045, 1972.
Rallison ML & others: Occurrence and natural history of
    chronic lymphocytic thyroiditis in childhood. J Pediatr
    86:675, 1975.

RIEDEL'S STRUMA
(Chronic Fibrous Thyroiditis, Woody Thyroiditis, Invasive Thyroiditis)

Riedel's struma is rare in this country, particularly in children. The cause is not known, but the disease may represent a late stage of chronic lymphocytic
thyroiditis. The disease is characterized by marked and
invasive fibrosis which extends beyond the thyroid
gland to involve the trachea, esophagus, blood vessels,
nerves, and muscles of the neck, so that the gland
becomes fixed to these tissues. Since differentiation
from carcinoma of the thyroid is usually impossible by
clinical means alone, the diagnosis is usually made by
surgical biopsy.

Adrenocorticosteroids may be helpful, but
surgery is frequently necessary to relieve fibrotic
obstruction or constriction of neighboring structures.

Greene JN: Subacute thyroiditis. Am J Med 51:97, 1971.

CARCINOMA OF THE THYROID

Carcinoma of the thyroid is uncommon in childhood, but there is evidence that its incidence is increasing. In a significant number of cases, a history of irradiation, particularly to the neck and chest, can be obtained. In others, the gland has most likely been under excessive stimulation (ie, TSH or LATS protector). The most prominent findings are localized thyroid enlargement, neck discomfort, dysphagia, and voice changes of recent onset. The thyroid gland may be fixed to surrounding tissues. Thyroid function studies are normal.

Papillary carcinoma is the most common form in childhood, and the prognosis with treatment is relatively good, with a survival rate greater than 80% after 10–20 years. Surgical extirpation of the entire gland and removal of all involved lymph nodes is the treatment of choice. Radical neck dissection is seldom necessary. About 1–2 months following surgery, when the patient has become definitely hypothyroid, a diagnostic scan should be carried out with radioactive iodine; if metastases are found, they should be removed or treated with therapeutic doses of radioactive iodine. Replacement therapy with thyroid hormone is initiated and continued· for about 6–12 months, at which time thyroid therapy is temporarily withdrawn and the patient rescanned after becoming mildly hypothyroid. Follow-up scanning and skeletal survey by x-ray is recommended at yearly intervals.

Other less common malignant tumors of the thyroid include follicular, medullary, and undifferentiated carcinomas, lymphomas, and sarcomas. Medullary carcinoma of the thyroid may be familial (autosomal dominant) and has been associated with excessive elaboration of gastrin, calcitonin, pheochromocytoma, parathyroid hyperplasia, and mucosal neuromas. The treatment and prognosis depend upon the cell type present.

Dobyns BM & others: Malignant and benign neoplasms of the thyroid in patients treated for hyperthyroidism: A report of the Cooperative Thyrotoxicosis Therapy Follow-up Study. J Clin Endocrinol Metab 38:976, 1974.

Fisher JM: Cancer in the irradiated thyroid. N Engl J Med 292:975, 1975.

Keiser HR & others: Sipple's syndrome: Medullary thyroid carcinoma, pheochromocytoma, and parathyroid disease. Ann Intern Med 78:561, 1973.

Pilch BZ & others: Thyroid cancer after radioactive iodine diagnostic procedures in childhood. Pediatrics 51:898, 1973.

Roeher HD & others: Juvenile thyroid carcinoma. J Pediatr Surg 7:27, 1972.

Scott MD, Crawford JD: Solitary thyroid nodules in childhood: Is the incidence of thyroid carcinoma declining? Pediatrics 58:521, 1976.

THE PARATHYROIDS

HYPOPARATHYROIDISM

Essentials of Diagnosis

- Tetany with numbness, tingling, cramps, carpopedal spasm, positive Trousseau and Chvostek signs, loss of consciousness, convulsions (usually focal), photophobia, diarrhea, and laryngospasm.
- Candidal infections, defective nails and teeth, cataracts, and calcific bodies in the subcutaneous tissues and basal ganglia.
- Serum and urine calcium low; serum phosphorus high; urine phosphorus low; alkaline phosphatase normal or low; azotemia absent. Low parathyroid levels.

General Considerations

Hypoparathyroidism may be idiopathic (possibly as the result of an autoimmune phenomenon) or may result from parathyroidectomy. Hypoparathyroidism may develop following thyroidectomy, when it may appear acutely (with variable severity of symptoms) or insidiously over several years and may be transient or permanent. Parathyroid deficiency has been reported following x-ray radiation of the neck or the administration of therapeutic doses of radioactive iodine for carcinoma of the thyroid. Transient hypoparathyroidism may occur in the neonate in hypomagnesemic states; in the offspring of hyperparathyroid or diabetic mothers; or as a physiologic variation in some infants, particularly those who have received a milk formula with a high phosphate/calcium ratio.

Idiopathic, apparently autoimmune hypoparathyroidism with demonstrable antibodies to parathyroid tissue, is frequently associated with candidal infection, Addison's disease, pernicious anemia, thyroiditis, and steatorrhea. Congenital absence of the parathyroids may occur in association with congenital absence of the thymus (with resultant thymic dependent immunologic deficiency) and cardiovascular, cerebral, and ocular defects (eg, DiGeorge's syndrome).

Clinical Findings

A. Symptoms and Signs: Prolonged hypocalcemia causes tetany (see below), photophobia, blepharospasm, diarrhea, chronic conjunctivitis, cataracts, numbness of the extremities, poor dentition, skin rashes, alopecia, ectodermal dysplasias, candidal infections, "idiopathic" epilepsy, or symmetrical punctate calcifications of basal ganglia. In early infancy, respiratory distress may be the presenting finding.

Tetany is manifested by numbness, cramps, and twitchings of the extremities; carpopedal spasm and laryngospasm; positive Chvostek sign (tapping of the face in front of the ear produces spasm of the facial muscles), positive peroneal sign (tapping the fibular

Table 24–4. Rickets and disorders of calcium metabolism.

Disease Condition	Synonym	Inheritance Pattern	Major Clinical Features	Serum Concentration				Urinary Excretion			
								Basal Conditions		Response to Parathyroid Hormone	
				Ca⁺⁺	P	Alk Ptase	PTH	Ca⁺⁺	P	P	Cyclic AMP
"Idiopathic" (spontaneous), surgical, or "autoimmune" hypoparathyroidism	Autoimmune polyendocrinopathy with thyroiditis and hypoparathyroidism (Schmidt's syndrome). Absence of parathyroid glands and thymic aplasia (DiGeorge's syndrome)	X-linked or autosomal recessive in autoimmune type	Tetany, seizures, photophobia, diarrhea, positive Chvostek and Trousseau signs, candidiasis. In autoimmune type, other autoimmune diseases (eg, adrenal insufficiency, thyroiditis, pernicious anemia, diabetes mellitus).	↓(N)	↑(N)	↓	↓	↓(N)	↓	N	N
Pseudohypoparathyroidism and pseudopseudohypoparathyroidism	Albright's syndrome type I and type II	X-linked dominant	Brachymetacarpal and metatarsal short stature; mental subnormality; ectopic calcification of lenses, basal ganglia, and subcutaneous tissue.	↓(N)	↑(N)	↓↑(N)	↑	↓(N)	↓	↓	↓
Pseudohypoparathyroidism type II	PTH unresponsiveness	Unknown	Seizures. Phenotype normal.	↓	↑		↑	↓	↓	↓	N
Pseudohypohyperparathyroidism with osteitis fibrosa	Renal resistance to parathyroid hormone with osteitis fibrosa	Probably familial	Clinical features of hypocalcemia. Phenotype normal.	↓	↑	↑	↑	N(↑)	↓(N)	↑	↓
Pseudoidiopathic hypoparathyroidism			Clinical features of hypoparathyroidism. Phenotype normal.	↓	↓		↑*	↓	↓	N	N

*Molecular anomaly of PTH proposed.

Table 24–5. Rickets and disorders of calcium metabolism.*

Disease Condition	Synonym	Inheritance Pattern	Clinical Features	Metabolic Features						Treatment
				Serum Concentration				Urinary Excretion		
				Ca⁺⁺	P	Alk Ptase	PTH	Ca⁺⁺	P	
Hypoparathyroid states	See Table 24–4.									Vitamin D and calcium
Transient tetany of the newborn			Tetany, focal seizures. More common in prematures and infants of diabetic mothers. Rarely described in association with maternal hyperparathyroidism.	↓	↑ (N)	↓ (N)	↓ (N)	↓ (N)	↓ (N)	Diet high in calcium, low in phosphate. Vitamin D may be necessary.
Malabsorption syndrome	Disease entities associated with malabsorption include cystic fibrosis, celiac disease, sprue, Schwachmann's disease; hypoplasia of cartilage and hair.	Generally familial with mode of inheritance related to specific disease	Steatorrhea, failure to thrive. Some forms associated with neutropenia, skeletal anomalies, immunologic deficiencies, and abnormalities of cartilage and hair.	↓ (N)	(N) ↓	↑ (N)	↑ (N)	↓	N (↑↓)	Vitamin D, calcium, and magnesium (hypomagnesemic states)
Chronic renal insufficiency			Growth failure, undernutrition, skeletal changes.	↓ (N)	↑	↑ (N)	↑	↓ (N)	↑	Diet high in calcium, low in phosphorus; vitamin D
Vitamin D–deficient rickets	Infantile rickets		Rickets.	↓ (N)	↓	↑	↑	↓	↓	Vitamin D
Familial hypophosphatemic vitamin D–resistant rickets	(1) Hereditary vitamin D–resistant rickets (2) Phosphate diabetes (3) X-linked hypophosphatemia	X-linked dominant (occasionally autosomal dominant or sporadic)	Skeletal deformities, growth retardation.	N (↓)	↓	N	N (↑)	N	↑	Oral phosphate
Hereditary vitamin D–refractory rickets	(1) Hypophosphatemic vitamin D–refractory rickets (2) Pseudo-vitamin D–deficiency rickets	Autosomal recessive	Severe rachitic bone changes; generalized aminoaciduria.	↓	↓ (N)	↑	↑		↑	Vitamin D in large doses

*Tubular reabsorption of phosphate (TRP) normally is 83–98%; the lower values are associated with higher serum levels of phosphorus. In hypoparathyroidism, TRP varies from 40–70%. Low values for TRP are also found in some forms of inherited renal tubular disease, eg, vitamin D–resistant rickets.

side of the leg over the peroneal nerve produces abduction and dorsiflexion of the foot), positive Trousseau sign (prolonged compression of the upper arm produces carpopedal spasm), and positive Erb sign (use of a galvanic current to determine hyperexcitability); unexplained bizarre behavior, irritability, loss of consciousness, convulsions, and retarded physical and mental development. Headache, vomiting, diarrhea, increased intracranial pressure, papilledema, and pseudopapilledema may occur. The symptoms of hypocalcemic tetany may be confused with respiratory or metabolic alkalosis or primary hyperaldosteronism.

B. Laboratory Findings: (Table 24—4.) Serum calcium is decreased, serum phosphorus increased, and serum alkaline phosphatase usually normal. Urinary excretion of calcium and phosphorus is decreased. The Ellsworth-Howard test is positive, ie, there is a markedly increased excretion of urinary phosphorus and cyclic AMP following a single intravenous injection (200—500 units) of parathyroid extract. False-negative results are common. There is a rise in serum calcium, a fall in serum phosphorus, and an increase in urine phosphorus following the intramuscular injection of parathyroid extract, 400—1000 units in divided doses daily for 3—4 days. Renal clearance of phosphorus is decreased, and the maximum tubular reabsorption of phosphate falls by 12—30%.

C. X-Ray Findings: Soft tissue and cerebral (basal ganglia) calcification may occur in idiopathic hypoparathyroidism.

Differential Diagnosis

The differential diagnosis of hypoparathyroidism includes pseudohypoparathyroidism as well as several very uncommon disorders (Table 24—4) and the other causes of hypocalcemia listed in Table 24—5. The presence of convulsions may suggest epilepsy and other chronic disorders of the CNS, while the combination of findings referable to the CNS (headache, vomiting, increased intracranial pressure, and convulsions) may make the differentiation from brain tumor difficult.

Other causes of cataracts and basal ganglia calcification as well as malabsorption syndrome and chronic diarrhea also enter into the differential diagnosis.

Treatment

The objective of treatment is to increase and maintain the serum calcium at an approximately normal level. A simple, practical method of regulating therapy is with the Sulkowitch urine test, but this test may not always accurately reflect hypercalciuria, particularly in infants.

A. Acute or Severe Tetany: Correct hypocalcemia immediately with calcium intravenously and orally. Dihydrotachysterol may be of value. Parathyroid hormone is seldom employed in the treatment of hypoparathyroidism because of its erratic action, unpredictable potency, and the potential danger of impure parenterally administered commercially available preparations.

Because calcium chloride may cause necrosis and abscess formation at the site of injection, calcium gluconate, 0.1—0.2 gm/kg as a 10% solution injected slowly IV, is generally preferred. Injection should be made slowly, with careful monitoring of the heart. Subsequent control may be obtained with calcium orally, although intravenous calcium may be repeated. For short-term therapy, calcium chloride as a dilute solution orally is useful because it produces systemic acidosis and an increase of ionized calcium; calcium lactate is preferred for prolonged oral therapy.

B. Maintenance Management of Hypoparathyroidism and Chronic Hypocalcemia:

1. Drugs—Give calciferol or dihydrotachysterol. Calciferol may not reach its peak effect for 3—7 days, but activity persists for weeks or months. Careful control of dosage with frequent determinations of serum calcium and urine concentrating ability is essential to avoid hypercalcemia, with resultant nephrocalcinosis and renal damage.

2. Diet—Give a high-calcium diet, with added calcium gluconate or lactate. The latter is preferable since it appears to possess a vitamin D-like effect at the intestinal level, lowering the dosage requirement of vitamin D. The dose is 300—1200 mg of calcium lactate 3—4 times daily with meals. The diet should be low in phosphorus (omit milk, cheese, and egg yolk).

Course & Prognosis

The initial manifestations of the idiopathic form of hypoparathyroidism may appear in the neonatal period, thus suggesting tetany of the newborn. More often, they appear at a later age in a previously well child. Some of the less dramatic manifestations (diarrhea, dullness, unhappiness, irritability, apprehension) may be present for a prolonged period before the presence of convulsions brings the patients to the attention of a physician.

With adequate treatment, many of the findings may be reversed and normal progress expected.

Blizzard RM, Gibbs JH: Candidiasis: Studies pertaining to its association with endocrinopathies and pernicious anemia. Pediatrics 42:231, 1968.

Fanconi A & others: Serum parathyroid hormone concentrations in hypophosphatemic vitamin D–resistant rickets. Helv Paediatr Acta 29:187, 1974.

Fraser D & others: Pathogenesis of hereditary vitamin D–dependent rickets: An inborn error of vitamin D metabolism involving defective conversion of 25-hydroxyvitamin D to 1α,25-dihydroxyvitamin D. N Engl J Med 289:817, 1973.

Kooh SW & others: Treatment of hypoparathyroidism and pseudohypoparathyroidism with metabolites of vitamin D: Evidence for impaired conversion of 25-hydroxy-vitamin D to 1α,25-dihydroxyvitamin D. N Engl J Med 293:840, 1975.

Linarelli LG & others: Renal cyclic AMP response to parathyroid hormone in premature hypocalcemic infants. J Pediatr 84:914, 1974.

Root A & others: Serum concentrations of parathyroid hormone in infants, children and adolescents. J Pediatr 85:329, 1974.

Root AW, Harrison HE: Recent advances in calcium and metabolism. 1. Mechanisms of calcium homeostasis. 2. Disorders of calcium homeostasis. J Pediatr 88:1, 177, 1976.

Schneider AB, Sherwood LM: Pathogenesis and management of hypoparathyroidism and other hypocalcemic disorders. Metabolism 24:871, 1975.

Tsang RC & others: Parathyroid function in infants of diabetic mothers. J Pediatr 86:399, 1975.

PSEUDOHYPOPARATHYROIDISM
(Albright's Syndrome & Pseudopseudohypoparathyroidism)

Pseudohypoparathyroidism is a familial hereditary X-linked disease with a female to male ratio of approximately 2:1 in which there is adequate parathyroid hormone but a failure of response of the end organ, the renal tubule (and perhaps bone), to the hormone. It may have the same symptomatology, physical signs, and chemical findings as idiopathic hypoparathyroidism (Table 24–4). In addition, these patients have round, full faces, irregularly shortened fingers (with the index finger often longer than the middle finger), a short, thick-set body, delayed and defective dentition, and mental retardation. The hair is dry and coarse and nails and skin are thickened, but candidiasis has not been reported. X-rays may show thickness of the long bones with limitation of growth at the metaphyseal ends. There may be chondrodysplastic changes in the bones of the hands, demineralization of the bones, thickening of the cortices, and exostoses. The first, fourth, and fifth metacarpals and metatarsals may be relatively more shortened than the second or third, so that there may be "dimples" in place of some of the knuckles when the hand is clenched into a fist. Ectopic calcification of the basal ganglia and subcutaneous tissues may occur, and corneal and lenticular opacities may be present.

Treatment is the same as for hypoparathyroidism.

Similar phenotypic findings may be found in *pseudopseudohypoparathyroidism,* which is probably a variant of pseudohypoparathyroidism in which the blood chemistry findings are normal. No treatment is necessary. Lenticular and intracranial calcifications may occur in the presence of normal serum calcium.

In both pseudo- and pseudopseudohypoparathyroidism, the parathyroid glands are hyperplastic, serum levels of parathyroid hormone are elevated, and the kidneys are relatively unresponsive to parathyroid hormone. Elevated calcitonin concentration is the consequence rather than the cause of hypocalcemia.

Frame B & others: Renal resistance to parathyroid hormone with osteitis fibrosa: "Pseudohypohyperparathyroidism." Am J Med 52:311, 1972.

Greenberg SR & others: Pseudohypoparathyroidism: A disease of the second messenger. Arch Intern Med 129:633, 1972.

Schneider AB, Sherwood LM: Pathogenesis and management of hypoparathyroidism and other hypocalcemic disorders. Metabolism 24:871, 1975.

HYPERPARATHYROIDISM

Essentials of Diagnosis

- Elevated blood levels of parathyroid hormone.
- Serum (and urine) ionized calcium elevated; urine phosphate high with low or normal serum phosphate; alkaline phosphatase normal or elevated.
- Polyuria, polydipsia, hypertension, nephrocalcinosis, uremia, intractable peptic ulcer, constipation, renal stones.
- Bone pain and, rarely, pathologic fractures. X-ray shows subperiosteal resorption, loss of lamina dura of teeth, renal parenchymal calcification or stones, and bone cysts.

General Considerations

Hyperparathyroidism may be primary or secondary. The most common causes of primary hyperparathyroidism are adenoma of the gland (rare in childhood) and diffuse parathyroid hyperplasia or hypertrophy. The most common causes of the secondary form are chronic renal disease (glomerulonephritis, pyelonephritis) and congenital anomalies of the genitourinary tract. Rarely, hyperparathyroidism may be found in osteogenesis imperfecta, malignancies with bony metastases, and rickets. Familial hyperparathyroidism may be associated with multiple adenoma of the parathyroid, anterior pituitary, and pancreas, and peptic ulcer in adult life.

Clinical Findings

A. Symptoms and Signs:

1. Due to hypercalcemia—Hypotonicity and weakness of muscles; apathy, nausea, vomiting, and poor tone of the gastrointestinal tract with constipation; loss of weight, hyperextensibility of joints, hypertension, cardiac irregularities, bradycardia, and shortening of the Q–T interval. Calcium deposits may occur in the cornea or conjunctivas ("band kerotopathy"). Detection of this important finding may require slit-lamp examination of the eye. Coma occurs rarely. Intractable peptic ulcer occurs in adults and rarely in children.

2. Due to increased calcium and phosphorus excretion—Loss of renal concentrating ability with resultant polyuria, polydipsia, precipitation of calcium phosphate in the renal parenchyma or as urinary calculi, and progressive renal damage.

3. Related to changes in the skeleton—Osteitis fibrosa, subperiosteal absorption of phalanges, absence of lamina dura around the teeth, spontaneous fractures, "moth-eaten" appearance of skull, and bone pain. If the patient drinks adequate quantities of milk, renal stones will occur but bone disease will not.

B. Laboratory Findings: See Table 24–6.

C. X-Ray Findings: Bone changes may not occur in children, although nephrocalcinosis may be observed radiographically. When bone changes occur, the distal

Table 24—6. Laboratory findings in hypercalcemia.*

	Serum Concentration			Urinary Excretion		
	Ca^{++}†	P	Ptase	Ca^{++}	P	Bone Pathology
Hyperparathyroidism	↑	↓ or N	N or ↑	N or ↑	↑	Generalized osteitis fibrosa cystica
Hyperparathyroidism with impaired renal function	↑	N or ↑	↑	↑	↑	Generalized osteitis fibrosa cystica
Excessive vitamin D	↑	↑	N or ↑	↑	N or ↑	
Excessive dihydro-tachysterol	↑	↓		↑	↑	
Neoplasms of bone	N or ↑	N	N or ↑	↑	N or ↑	Bone destruction
Hyperproteinemia	Total, ↑ Ionized, N	N	N	N	N	
Idiopathic hypercalcemia	↑	N or ↑	N	N or ↑	N	See text below.

*Modified and reproduced, with permission, from Silver, Kempe, & Bruyn: *Handbook of Pediatrics,* 12th ed. Lange, 1977.
†Repeated determinations of ionized calcium are advisable; total serum calcium levels may be within normal limits in some cases of hyperparathyroidism.

clavicle is initially affected. Later, one finds a generalized demineralization with a predilection for subperiosteal cortical bone.

Treatment

Treatment consists of complete removal of the tumor or subtotal removal of hyperplastic parathyroid glands. Preoperatively, fluids should be forced and the intake of milk restricted. The administration of phosphate and sulfate salts has been reported to be successful in reducing the hypercalcemia in primary hyperparathyroidism without renal damage. Postoperatively, observe carefully for evidence of hypocalcemic tetany; this may occur with total serum calcium within normal limits if a precipitous drop in calcium has occurred. The diet should be high in calcium and vitamin D.

Treatment of secondary hyperparathyroidism is directed at the underlying disease. Diminish the intake of phosphate with aluminum hydroxide orally and by reducing the intake of milk. It has recently become apparent that the hypocalcemia of renal disease results from impaired renal activation of vitamin D. Administration of 1,25-dihydrotachysterol should prove therapeutically efficacious in the near future.

Course & Prognosis

Although the condition may recur, the prognosis following subtotal parathyroidectomy or removal of an adenoma is usually good. Renal function may remain abnormal. The prognosis of the secondary forms depends on correcting the underlying defect.

Bergman L & others: Primary hyperparathyroidism in a child investigated by determination of ultrafiltrable calcium. Am J Dis Child 123:174, 1972.
Bjernulf A & others: Primary hyperparathyroidism in children. Acta Paediatr Scand 59:249, 1970.
Landing BH, Kamoshita S: Congenital hyperparathyroidism secondary to maternal hypoparathyroidism. J Pediatr 77:842, 1970.
Schrott HG & others: Calcium infusion with phosphate deprivation tests in patients with primary hyperparathyroidism and with normocalcemia and nephrolithiasis. Metabolism 21:205, 1972.

OTHER RELATED DISEASES

1. IDIOPATHIC HYPERCALCEMIA

Idiopathic hypercalcemia is an uncommon disorder characterized in its severe form by peculiar ("elfin") facies (receding mandible, depressed bridge of nose, relatively large mouth, prominent lips, hanging jowls, large low-set ears, prominent eyes, occasional esotropia, and hypertelorism), failure to thrive, mental and motor retardation, irritability, purposeless movements, constipation, hypotonia, polyuria, polydipsia, hypertension, and cardiac defects (ie, supravalvular aortic stenosis). Generalized osteosclerosis is common, and there may be premature craniosynostosis and nephrocalcinosis with evidence of urinary tract disease. In addition to the hypercalcemia, there may be hypercholesterolemia, azotemia, and elevation of serum carotene and vitamin A.

Clinical manifestations may not appear for several months. The disease may be due to the increased intake of vitamin D during pregnancy, a defect in the metabolism of or responsiveness to vitamin D, abnormal sterol synthesis, or some as yet unrecognized mechanism.

Treatment is by rigid restriction of dietary calcium and vitamin D.

2. IMMOBILIZATION HYPERCALCEMIA

Abrupt immobilization of a rapidly growing adolescent following an injury may lead to a rapid decrease in bone deposition with continued bone resorption and calcium mobilization. This may result in hypercalcemia.

Friedman WF, Mills LF: The relationship between vitamin D and the craniofacial and dental anomalies of the supravalvular aortic stenosis syndrome. Pediatrics 43:12, 1969.

Hyman LR & others: Immobilization hypercalcemia. Am J Dis Child 124:723, 1972.

3. HYPOPHOSPHATASIA & PSEUDOHYPOPHOSPHATASIA

Hypophosphatasia is an uncommon inherited (autosomal recessive) condition characterized by a specific deficiency of alkaline phosphatase activity in serum, bone, and tissues. Inadequate calcification of bone matrix, with localized areas of radiolucency, is radiographically and histologically similar to the bone lesions of other types of rickets, although in hypophosphatasia the lesions are not limited to sites of rapid growth. The earlier the age at onset, the more severe the condition. Failure to thrive, feeding problems, dwarfing, hyperpyrexia, premature loss of teeth, widening of the sutures, bulging fontanels, convulsions, bony deformities, hyperpigmentation, conjunctival calcification, band keratopathy, and renal lesions have been reported in some cases. Premature closure of cranial sutures may occur. Signs and symptoms may be similar to those of idiopathic hypercalcemia; late features include osteoporosis, pseudofractures, and rachitic deformities. Serum calcium is frequently elevated. The plasma and urine of patients and heterozygote carriers contain phosphoethanolamine in excessive amounts. In some cases, marked metaphyseal irregularities may occur. Recently, a condition has been described in which the clinical features of hypophosphatasia are seen in association with normal levels of alkaline phosphatase (thus the term pseudohypophosphatasia).

No specific treatment is available, but adrenocorticosteroids may be of value. The mortality is high in severe cases, particularly in infancy, but improvement may occur in children who survive early childhood. Adults are usually asymptomatic.

Condon JR: Pathogenesis of rickets and osteomalacia in familial hypophosphatemia. Arch Dis Child 46:269, 1971.

Russell RGG & others: Inorganic pyrophosphate in plasma in normal persons and in patients with hypophosphatasia, osteogenesis imperfecta, and other disorders of bone. J Clin Invest 50:961, 1971.

Scriver CR & others: Pseudohypophosphatasia. N Engl J Med 281:604, 1969.

ADRENAL CORTEX

ADRENOCORTICAL INSUFFICIENCY
(Adrenal Crisis, Addison's Disease)

Essentials of Diagnosis

Acute form (adrenal crisis):

- Vomiting, dehydration, hypotension, circulatory collapse.
- Serum sodium low; serum potassium high.
- Eosinophilia; blood and urine adrenocorticosteroids low.
- A definite precipitating factor usually present (eg, acute illness, trauma).

Chronic form (Addison's disease):

- Weakness, fatigue, pallor; episodes of nausea, vomiting, and diarrhea; increased appetite for salt.
- Increased pigmentation, hypotension; small heart.
- Serum sodium low, serum potassium high; blood and urine adrenocorticosteroids decreased; eosinophilia.

General Considerations

Adrenocortical hypofunction may be due to congenital absence; atrophy (toxic factors, autoimmune phenomena); an enzymatic defect leading to decreased production of cortisol; infection (eg, tuberculosis); destruction of the gland by tumor or hemorrhage (Waterhouse-Friderichsen syndrome) and calcification; or may occur as a consequence of inadequate secretion of corticotropin (ACTH) due to anterior pituitary or hypothalamic disease. In the latter condition, hyperpigmentation does not occur. Any acute illness, surgery, trauma, or exposure to excessive heat may precipitate an adrenal crisis. A temporary salt-losing disorder, possibly due to either mineralocorticoid deficiency or renal tubular insensitivity to mineralocorticoid, may occur during infancy.

Fractional adrenocortical types of insufficiency, including forms with deficiency of glucocorticoid, aldosterone, or other mineral-regulating steroids but normal production of other hormones of the adrenal have been described.

Clinical Findings

A. Symptoms and Signs:

1. Acute form (adrenal crisis)—Manifestations include nausea and vomiting, diarrhea, abdominal pain, dehydration; fever, which may be followed by hypothermia; hypotension, circulatory collapse, and confusion or coma.

2. Chronic form (Addison's disease)—Tuberculous destruction of the adrenals was formerly the most common cause of Addison's disease. The leading causes of adrenal insufficiency today are hereditary enzy-

matic defects with congenital adrenal hyperplasia and idiopathic loss of adrenal function, the latter thought to be due to autoimmune mechanisms. Adrenal destruction may also occur secondary to infectious processes and neoplasms. A rare form of familial Addison's disease may be seen in association with cerebral sclerosis and spastic paraplegia. Idiopathic Addison's disease may be familial and has been described in association with hypoparathyroidism, candidiasis, hypothyroidism, pernicious anemia, and diabetes mellitus. The finding of circulating antibodies to adrenal tissue and other tissues involved in these conditions suggests that some autoimmune mechanism may be the cause; however, the pathogenesis is not understood.

Signs and symptoms include fatigue, hypotension, weakness, failure to gain or loss of weight, increased appetite for salt, diarrhea; vomiting, which may become forceful and sometimes projectile; and dehydration. Diffuse tanning with increased pigmentation over pressure points, scars, and mucous membranes may be present. A small heart may be seen on x-ray.

B. Laboratory Findings:

1. Suggestive of adrenal insufficiency—Serum sodium, chloride, and bicarbonate, P_{CO_2}, and blood pH and blood volume are decreased. Serum potassium and blood urea nitrogen are increased. Urinary sodium is elevated, and the sodium:potassium ratio is high despite low serum sodium.

Eosinophilia* and moderate neutropenia may be present.

2. Confirmatory tests—The following tests measure the functional capacity of the adrenal cortex:

a. Corticotropin (ACTH) stimulation test—See p 1051. This is the most definitive test.

b. Plasma ACTH levels are elevated while cortisol and urinary 17-hydroxycorticosteroid levels are low and fail to rise with ACTH stimulation.

c. Urinary 17-hydroxycorticosteroid excretion is decreased.

d. Urinary 17-ketosteroid output is decreased except in cases due to congenital adrenal hyperplasia or tumor of the adrenal cortex. This test is of little value in younger children, who normally excrete less than 1 mg/day.

e. The metyrapone (Metopirone) test (see p 1051) is useful in demonstrating normal pituitary function and in the diagnosis of adrenal insufficiency secondary to pituitary insufficiency. This test may provoke acute adrenal insufficiency in an individual with compromised adrenal function.

Differential Diagnosis

Acute adrenal insufficiency must be differentiated from severe acute infections, diabetic coma, various disturbances of the CNS, and acute poisoning. In the neonatal period, adrenal insufficiency may be

clinically indistinguishable from respiratory distress or intracranial hemorrhage.

Chronic adrenocortical insufficiency must be differentiated from anorexia nervosa, certain muscular disorders (myasthenia gravis, etc), salt-losing nephritis, chronic debilitating infections (tuberculosis, etc), and recurrent spontaneous hypoglycemia.

Treatment

A. Acute Form (Adrenal Crisis):

1. Replacement therapy—

a. Give hydrocortisone sodium succinate (Solu-Cortef), 1–2 mg/kg diluted in 2–10 ml of water IV over 2–5 minutes. Follow with an infusion of normal saline and 5–10% glucose, 100 ml/kg/24 hours IV, containing 50–250 mg of hydrocortisone sodium hemisuccinate. Cortisone acetate, 1 mg/kg IM, may be used after initial replacement therapy; the onset of action of this preparation given intramuscularly is delayed, and its effect may continue for several days.

b. Repeat intramuscular medication every 24 hours until stabilization is achieved and then reduce gradually.

c. Give desoxycorticosterone acetate, 1–2 mg/day IM, as part of initial therapy and regulate dose depending on state of hydration, electrolyte status, weight, and heart size.

d. Ten percent glucose in saline, 20 ml/kg IV in the first 2 hours, may be of value, particularly in infants with adrenal crisis who have congenital adrenal hyperplasia. Avoid overtreatment.

2. Hypotension—Specific treatment includes volume expansion (eg, hydrocortisone sodium succinate, normal saline solution, albumin). Rarely, one of the following additions is necessary:

a. Isoproterenol (Isuprel), 2.5–5 mg in 500 ml of 5% dextrose and 0.45% saline solution infused over a period of 2–8 hours to maintain blood pressure. Plasma or blood transfusion, 22 ml/kg, should be used also as necessary to maintain blood pressure.

b. Levarterenol bitartrate (Levophed), 4 ml (1 mg/ml) added to 1000 ml of electrolyte solution for use by IV drip. Determine response to an initial dose of 0.25–0.5 ml of dilute solution per 10 kg and then stabilize flow at a rate sufficient to maintain blood pressure (usual rate: 0.5–1 ml/minute). This drug is very potent, and great care must be employed in its use.

c. Phenylephrine (Neo-Synephrine)—See Chapter 36 for dosage.

3. Infections—Treat infections with large doses of appropriate antibiotic or chemotherapeutic agents.

4. Waterhouse-Friderichsen syndrome with fulminant infections—The use of adrenal corticosteroids and levarterenol in the treatment or "prophylaxis" of fulminant infections is felt by some not to be justified since it may augment the generalized Shwartzman reaction seen in the renal cortices of fatal cases of meningococcemia. However, corticosteroids should be used in the presence of adrenal insufficiency, particu-

---

*A normal number of eosinophils during stress (eg, the day after operation or in the presence of a severe infection) is also suggestive of insufficiency.

larly with hypotension and circulatory collapse.

5. Fluids and electrolytes—Give 10% glucose in saline, 20 ml/kg IV. *Caution:* Avoid overtreatment. Total parenteral fluid in the first 8 hours should not exceed the maintenance fluid requirement of the normal child (see Chapter 35). Fruit juices, ginger ale, milk, and soft foods should be given as soon as possible.

B. Maintenance Therapy of Chronic Form (Addison's Disease): Following initial stabilization, the most effective substitution therapy generally consists of giving hydrocortisone or cortisone together with supplementary desoxycorticosterone or fludrocortisone.

Additional hydrocortisone, desoxycorticosterone, or sodium chloride, singly or in combination, may be necessary with acute illness, surgery, trauma, exposure to sudden change in temperature, or other stress reactions.

Supportive adrenocortical therapy should be given whenever surgical operations are performed on patients who have at some time received prolonged therapy with adrenocortical steroids. (See below.)

1. Glucocorticoid (hydrocortisone or equivalent)—Increase the dosage of all glucocorticoids to 2–4 times the usual dosage during intercurrent illness or times of stress.

a. **Hydrocortisone**—Give 20–25 mg/sq m/day orally in 3–4 divided doses. Give 50% in the morning, 25% in the afternoon, and 25% at bedtime.

b. **Cortisone acetate**—25–30 mg/sq m/day orally divided in 3 daily doses as hydrocortisone, or 12.5 mg/sq m/day IM given as 37.5 mg/sq m IM every 3 days.

c. **Prednisone**—5–6 mg/sq m/day orally in 2–3 doses. Its potency may preclude necessary minor modulations in dosage. More potent glucocorticoids should not be used.

2. Mineralocorticoid (desoxycorticosterone acetate [DOCA] and related drugs)—Dose should be gradually increased or decreased to maintain normal serum sodium levels and avoid increased blood volume with hypertension. Increases with stress are not necessary.

a. **Fludrocortisone (Florinef)**—0.05–0.2 mg orally once a day.

b. **DOCA in oil**—1 mg/day IM.

c. **Pellets** containing DOCA may be implanted subcutaneously in the subscapular area. In general, two 125 mg pellets provide adequate therapy. Reimplantation is necessary every 6–9 months.

d. **Desoxycorticosterone pivalate**—May be given following prolonged stabilization; 25 mg/ml IM of this long-acting macrocrystalline suspension every 3–4 weeks corresponds to 1 mg of DOCA in oil IM daily. Hypertension (without hypernatremia) may occur following DOCA administration and may persist for months following its discontinuation. A waxing and waning effect may be seen during therapy.

3. Salt—The child should be given ready access to table salt; an infant should be offered salted food or formula once a day. Rarely, sodium chloride (enteric-coated tablets), 1–2 gm/day, may be needed in addition to mineralocorticoid therapy.

C. Corticosteroids in Patients With Adrenocortical Insufficiency Who Undergo Surgery:

1. Preoperatively—Give cortisone acetate IM as follows (single dose):

a. 48 hours before surgery, 100% of maintenance.
b. 24 hours before surgery, 100% of maintenance.
c. 12 hours before surgery, 100% of maintenance.
d. 1 hour before surgery, 100% of maintenance.

2. During operation—Give cortisone acetate intramuscularly, 100–200% of maintenance daily, for 1–2 days. Begin oral preparation as soon as possible and give full maintenance doses daily. If significant stress occurs postoperatively, give 3–5 times the maintenance dose.

Course & Prognosis

A. Acute: The course of acute adrenal insufficiency is rapid, and death may occur within a few hours unless adequate treatment is given. Spontaneous recovery is unlikely. Newborn infants with severe adrenal hemorrhages seldom respond even to vigorous therapy. Patients who have received treatment with adrenal corticosteroids may exhibit adrenal collapse if they undergo surgery or other acute stress for as long as 6–24 months after corticosteroids are discontinued.

In all forms of acute adrenal insufficiency, once the crisis has passed, the patient should be observed carefully and evaluated with appropriate laboratory tests to assess the degree of permanent adrenal insufficiency.

B. Chronic: Adequately treated chronic adrenocortical insufficiency is consistent with a relatively normal life. Since these patients may become dehydrated quickly during minor infections, they must be observed carefully and receive prompt treatment under such circumstances.

Bottazzo GF, Florin-Christensen A, Doniach D: Islet-cell antibodies in diabetes mellitus with autoimmune polyendocrine deficiencies. Lancet 2:1279, 1974.

Franks RC: Urinary 17-hydroxycorticosteroid and cortisol excretion in childhood. J Clin Endocrinol 36:702, 1973.

Gutai JP, Migeon CJ: Adrenal insufficiency during the neonatal period. Clin Perinatol 2:163, 1975.

Pakravan P & others: Familial congenital absence of adrenal glands: Evaluation of glucocorticoid, mineralocorticoid, and estrogen metabolism in the perinatal period. J Pediatr 84:74, 1974.

ADRENOCORTICAL HYPERFUNCTION

1. CUSHING'S SYNDROME

Essentials of Diagnosis

- "Truncal type" adiposity with thin extremities, moon face, weakness, plethora, easy bruisability, purplish striae, growth retardation.

- Hypertension, osteoporosis, glycosuria.
- Elevated serum and urine adrenocorticosteroids with loss of normal diurnal variation; low serum potassium; eosinopenia.
- Early in the disease process, few of the classical features may be present.

General Considerations

The principal findings in Cushing's syndrome in childhood result from excessive secretion of glucocorticoids and androgens. Depletion of body protein stores and abnormal carbohydrate and fat metabolism are typical. There may also be lesser degrees of overproduction of the mineralocorticoids. It has been suggested that in Cushing's syndrome with bilateral adrenal hyperplasia there is decreased responsiveness of the hypothalamic-pituitary "feedback" mechanism which regulates the release or production of ACTH. This may then result in a constant but only slightly excessive elevation in the secretion of ACTH or lead to qualitative or quantitative change in the diurnal variation.

Cushing's syndrome is more common in females. In children under 12, it is usually iatrogenic (secondary to therapeutic doses of corticotropin or one of the corticosteroids). It may rarely be due to an adrenal tumor or associated with a basophilic adenoma of the pituitary gland, adrenocortical hyperplasia, or an extrapituitary ACTH-producing tumor.

Clinical Findings

A. Symptoms and Signs:

1. Due to excessive secretion of the glucocorticoid hormones—"Buffalo type" adiposity, most marked on the face, neck, and trunk (a fat pad in the interscapular area is characteristic); easy fatigability and weakness, plethoric facies, purplish striae, easy bruisability, ecchymoses, hirsutism, osteoporosis, hypertension, diabetes mellitus (usually latent), pain in the back, muscle wasting and weakness, and marked retardation of growth.

2. Due to excessive secretion of mineralocorticoids—Hypernatremia, increased blood volume, edema, and hypertension.

3. Due to excessive secretion of androgens—Hirsutism, acne, and varying degrees of excessive masculinization.

4. Menstrual irregularities occur during puberty in older girls.

B. Laboratory Findings:

1. Blood—

a. Serum cortisol levels are elevated. There may be a loss of the normal diurnal variation.

b. Serum chloride and potassium may be lowered.

c. Serum sodium and HCO_3^- content may be elevated (metabolic alkalosis).

d. Plasma ACTH concentrations are slightly elevated with adrenal hyperplasia; decreased in cases of

adrenal tumor; and greatly increased with ACTH-producing pituitary or extrapituitary tumors. The white count shows polymorphonuclear leukocytosis with lymphopenia, and the eosinophil count is low (below 50/cu mm). The red cell count may be elevated.

2. Urine—

a. Urinary free cortisol excretion is elevated. This may be the most diagnostic test.

b. Urinary 17-hydroxycorticosteroid levels are elevated.

c. Urinary 17-ketosteroids may be normal but are usually elevated in association with adrenal tumor.

d. Glycosuria may be present.

3. Response to corticotropin (ACTH) and corticosteroids—The response to corticotropin (ACTH) stimulation is excessive in patients with adrenal hyperplasia; a poor response is usually found in those with tumor. There is a diminished adrenal response to small doses (0.5 mg) of dexamethasone in the dexamethasone suppression test; larger doses will cause suppression of adrenal activity when the disease is due to adrenal hyperplasia. Adenomas and adrenal carcinomas may rarely be suppressed by large doses of dexamethasone (4–16 mg daily in 4 divided doses).

C. X-Ray Findings: Urograms may be abnormal. Adrenal calcification may be present. Osteoporosis (evident first in the spine and pelvis) with compression fractures may be seen in advanced cases.

Differential Diagnosis

Children with obesity, particularly in the presence of striae and hypertension, are frequently suspected of having Cushing's syndrome. The growth rate may be helpful in differentiating the two. Children with Cushing's syndrome have a poor growth rate, while those with exogenous obesity usually have a normal or slightly increased growth rate. In addition, the color of the striae (purplish in Cushing's syndrome, pink in obesity) and the distribution of the obesity assist in the differentiation. The urinary free cortisol excretion is always normal in obesity. The urinary excretion of corticosteroids may not be helpful since they may be elevated in obesity (usually in proportion to the weight and surface area).

Treatment

In all cases of primary adrenal hyperfunction due to tumor, surgical removal, if possible, is indicated. Corticotropin (ACTH) should be given preoperatively and postoperatively to stimulate the nontumorous adrenal cortex, which is generally atrophied. Adrenocortical steroids should be administered for 1–2 days before surgery and continued during and after operation. Supplemental potassium, salt, and mineralocorticoids may be necessary. (See above outline of corticosteroid administration in surgical patients.)

For adrenal hyperplasia, total adrenalectomy is usually necessary although pituitary irradiation, radioactive implantation, electrocoagulation, or ablation has sometimes been of value in adults. Substitution therapy may be necessary after these measures.

The use of mitotane (Lysodren; o,p'DDD), a DDT derivative toxic to the adrenal cortex, has been suggested, but the drug's usefulness in children with adrenal tumors has not been determined.

Prognosis

If the tumor is malignant, the prognosis is poor; if benign, cure is to be expected following proper preparation and surgery.

Pituitary enlargement has been reported in some cases of Cushing's syndrome following both partial and complete adrenalectomy.

Cushing's syndrome (perhaps due to adrenal hyperplasia) may occasionally undergo spontaneous remission.

Although most of the changes resulting from adrenocorticosteroid excess disappear, hypertension, diabetes mellitus, and osteoporosis may persist, and the rate of growth may continue to be poor.

Eddy RL & others: Cushing's syndrome: A prospective study of diagnostic methods. Am J Med 55:621, 1973.

Krieger D & others: Cyproheptadine-induced remission of Cushing's disease. N Engl J Med 293:893, 1975.

Lee PA, Weldon VV, Migeon CJ: Short stature as the only clinical sign of Cushing's syndrome. J Pediatr 86:89, 1975.

McArthur RG & others: Cushing's disease in children: Findings in 13 cases. Mayo Clin Proc 47:318, 1972.

Orth DN, Liddle GW: Results of treatment in 108 patients with Cushing's syndrome. N Engl J Med 285:243, 1971.

2. ADRENOGENITAL SYNDROME

Essentials of Diagnosis

- Pseudohermaphroditism in females, with urogenital sinus, enlargement of clitoris, and other evidence of virilization.
- Isosexual precocity in males with infantile testes.
- Excessive (isosexual) masculinization in males.
- Excessive growth; early development of sexual hair.
- Urinary 17-ketosteroids elevated; urinary pregnanetriol increased in commonest form.
- May be associated with water and electrolyte disturbances, particularly in the neonatal period.

General Considerations

The congenital familial (autosomal recessive) form of adrenogenital syndrome is due to an inborn error of metabolism with a deficiency of an adrenocortical enzyme. Various types are recognized, including the following:

(1) Deficiency of 21-hydroxylase (approximately 80% of cases), resulting in inability to convert 17-hydroxyprogesterone into compound S (11-desoxy-

cortisol). Mild forms result in androgenic changes (virilization) alone, but severe cases are associated with salt loss and electrolyte imbalance.

(2) Deficiency in 11β-hydroxylation and a failure to convert compound S to compound F (cortisol). Associated with virilization and usually with hypertension but no disturbance of electrolytes. Deoxycorticosterone and its metabolites are present.

(3) A defect in 17-hydroxylase, with the enzyme deficiency in both the adrenals and the gonads. Hypertension, virilization, and eunuchoidism may be present. Serum aldosterone levels may be low.

(4) A defect in 3β-hydroxysteroid dehydrogenase activity and a failure to convert Δ^5-pregnolone to progesterone. Associated with incomplete masculinization, with hypospadias and cryptorchidism in the male. Some degree of masculinization may occur in the female. Severe sodium loss occurs, and the infant mortality rate is high.

(5) Cholesterol desmolase deficiency with congenital lipoid adrenal hyperplasia. Clinical features are similar to those of 3β-hydroxysteroid dehydrogenase deficiency (above). Urinary corticosteroid excretion does not occur.

Over 90% of cases manifest a deficiency of either the 21- or 11β-hydroxylase enzyme.

In some forms the infant may appear normal at birth, with onset occurring later. In all forms there is excessive secretion of ACTH, causing adrenal hyperplasia and increased urinary excretion of metabolites of various precursors but decreased production of hydrocortisone. Increased pigmentation, especially of the scrotum, labia majora, and nipples, frequently results from excessive ACTH secretion.

Pseudohermaphroditism in the female may also occur as a result of virilizing maternal tumors or the administration of androgens, synthetic progestins, diethylstilbestrol, and related hormones to the mother during the first trimester of pregnancy. In these cases the condition does not progress after birth, and cortisol deficiency and abnormal steroidogenesis are not present. Pseudohermaphroditism may occur with gonadal dysgenesis.

Adrenogenital syndrome may also result from tumors of the adrenal, ovary (rare in childhood), or testes or from idiopathic adrenal hyperplasia later in life.

Clinical Findings

A. Symptoms and Signs:

1. Adrenogenital syndrome in females—In females with potentially normal ovaries, masculinization occurs and sexual development is along heterosexual lines.

a. Congenital bilateral hyperplasia of the adrenal cortex (pseudohermaphroditism)—The abnormality of the external genitalia may vary from mild enlargement of the clitoris to complete fusion of the labioscrotal folds, forming a penile urethra, and enlargement of the clitoris to form a normal-sized phallus. If left untreated, growth in height and skeletal maturation are excessive, and patients become muscular. Pubic hair appears early (often before the second birthday); acne may be excessive; and the voice may be deep. Excessive pigmentation may develop. Dentition is normal or only slightly advanced for the chronologic age. Similar abnormalities may be present in siblings and cousins. Signs of associated adrenal insufficiency may be present during the first days of life or later.

b. Postnatal adrenogenital syndrome (virilism)— This disorder may be due to adrenal hyperplasia or tumor or to arrhenoblastoma (extremely rare). Enlargement of the clitoris occurs, but other changes of the genitalia are not found. The family history is negative for similar abnormalities. If a tumor is present, it may be palpably enlarged. Other findings are similar to those of pseudohermaphroditism.

2. Adrenogenital syndrome in males (macrogenitosomia praecox)—In males, sexual development is along isosexual lines.

a. Congenital bilateral hyperplasia of the adrenal cortex—The infant may appear normal at birth, but during the first few months of life enlargement of the penis will be noted. There may be increased pigmentation resulting from excessive secretion of ACTH. Other symptoms and signs are similar to those of the congenital form in females. The testes are soft and not enlarged except in the rare male in whom aberrant adrenal cells may be present in the testes and produce unilateral or bilateral symmetric or asymmetric enlargement. Males with the 3β-hydroxysteroid dehydrogenase defect usually show incomplete masculinization with cryptorchidism and hypospadias, whereas females show a mild degree of masculinization. Signs of adrenal glucocorticoid insufficiency may be present. In the complete form of the 21-hydroxylase deficiency, mineralocorticoid deficiency may lead to hyponatremia, hyperkalemia, anorexia, vomiting, decreased blood volume, circulatory collapse, and death.

b. Tumor—The findings may be identical with those of congenital bilateral hyperplasia of the adrenal cortex except that they appear at a later age. The tumor may be palpably enlarged. Rarely, an adrenal tumor in a male may produce feminization with gynecomastia.

B. Laboratory Findings:

1. Blood—

a. 21-Hydroxylase deficiency—17-Hydroxyprogesterone levels are markedly elevated.

b. 11β-Hydroxylase deficiency—Plasma 11-deoxycortisol (compound S) is elevated.

c. Serum sodium will fall and potassium will rise in the complete 21-hydroxylase deficiency. The peak time for hyponatremia to occur is 7–10 days of age.

d. Plasma renin activity may be elevated in the complete form of the 21-hydroxylase deficiency.

2. Urine—

a. 21-Hydroxylase deficiency—17-Ketosteroids, pregnanetriol, and testosterone levels are elevated. (*Note:* Urinary pregnanetriol levels are sometimes normal in the neonatal period. During the first 3 weeks of life, normal infants may excrete up to 2.5 mg/day.) Aldosterone may be reduced, and excessive sodium

loss occurs in salt-losing forms.

b. 11β-Hydroxylase deficiency—11-Deoxycortisol (compound S), tetrahydro-compound S, deoxycorticosterone, and 17-ketosteroids and testosterone levels elevated.

c. 17-Hydroxylase deficiency—17-Ketosteroid and aldosterone levels decreased; corticosterone and deoxycorticosterone levels increased.

d. 3β-Hydroxysteroid dehydrogenase deficiency—17-Ketosteroid levels moderately elevated.

e. Cholesterol desmolase deficiency—All steroid excretion is markedly decreased.

f. Tumor—Excretion of dehydroepiandrosterone may be greatly elevated.

3. Buccal smear—In any newborn with ambiguous genitalia, a buccal smear interpreted by an experienced individual should be done as soon as possible. Ideally, fluorescent staining for the Y chromosome should be performed if the buccal smear is interpreted as chromatin-negative. In female pseudohermaphrodites, the nuclear chromatin pattern is positive.

4. Dexamethasone suppression test—If the administration of dexamethasone, 2–4 mg/day in 4 doses for 7 days, reduces 17-ketosteroids to normal, hyperplasia rather than adenoma is the probable diagnosis.

C. X-Ray Findings: Vaginograms using contrast media may indicate the presence of a urogenital sinus. Defects in the urogram, displacement of the kidney, and calcification in the area of the adrenal may be seen on x-rays of patients with tumors. Bone age is advanced with 21- and 11β-hydroxylase defects but may not be evident in the first year. The adrenal may be radiologically enlarged on plain films of the abdomen, but extraperitoneal pneumography *(caution)* may be required to demonstrate the increased size.

Treatment

A. Congenital Hyperplasia of the Cortex:

1. Initially, cortisone acetate, 10–25 mg/day orally or 10–25 mg IM every 3 days to infants and 25–100 mg/day orally to older children, will suppress abnormal adrenal steroidogenesis within 2 weeks. The maintenance dose is the same as that given on p 690. In congenital hyperplasia, if oral medication is given, 50% of the daily dose should be given in the late evening to suppress the early morning ACTH rise. Dosage is regulated to maintain a normal growth rate, a normal rate of osseous maturation, and the normal range of urinary 17-ketosteroid excretion; in cases of 21-hydroxylase deficiency, the urinary pregnanetriol level should also be kept within the normal range. In adolescent females, menses are a sensitive index of adequacy of therapy. Therapy should be continued throughout life in both males and females because of the possibility of malignant degeneration of the hyperplastic adrenal.

2. Other aspects of treatment are as for Addison's disease (eg, mineralocorticoid therapy and glucocorticoid increases with stress; see p 690). Occasionally, inadequate mineralocorticoid therapy will lead to inadequate ACTH suppression and elevated 17-ketoste-

roid production in the face of adequate or excessive glucocorticoid therapy.

3. Clitororecession is often indicated in the first year of life. Vaginoplasty for labial fusion should be performed in early childhood. The latter may be indicated during infancy if vaginal-urinary reflux and genitourinary tract infections occur. Partial clitoridectomy is occasionally indicated in a girl with an abnormally large or sensitive clitoris.

B. Tumor: Because the malignant lesions cannot be distinguished clinically from the benign ones, surgical removal is indicated whenever a tumor has been diagnosed. Preoperative and postoperative treatment is as for Cushing's syndrome due to tumor.

Course & Prognosis

When therapy is started in early infancy, abnormal metabolic effects are not observed and masculinization does not progress.

Unless adequately controlled, uncomplicated congenital adrenal hyperplasia causes sexual precocity and masculinization throughout childhood. Affected individuals will be tall as children but short as adults. Treatment with the corticosteroids permits normal growth, development, and sexual maturation. If started when somatic development is over 12–14 years (as determined by bone age), true sexual precocity may supervene, with thelarche and often menses in females and testicular androgen production in males.

Patient education stressing lifelong therapy is important for compliance in adolescence and later life.

Female pseudohermaphrodites mistakenly raised as males for more than 3 years may have serious psychologic disturbances if their sex is "changed" after that time. If the condition is not recognized for several years and the child is raised as a male, removal of the ovaries and uterus is indicated.

When adrenogenital syndrome is caused by a tumor, progression of signs and symptoms will cease after surgical removal; however, evidences of masculinization, particularly deepening of the voice, may persist.

Bongiovanni AM: Disorders of adrenocortical steroid biogenesis. Page 857 in: *The Metabolic Basis of Inherited Disease,* 3rd ed. Stanbury JB, Wyngaarden JB, Fredrickson DS (editors). McGraw-Hill, 1972.

Federman DD: Disorders of sexual development. N Engl J Med 277:351, 1967.

Gutai J & others: The detection of the heterozygous carrier for congenital virilizing adrenal hyperplasia. J Pediatr 90:924, 1977.

Hughes IA, Winter JSD: Serum 17 OH-progesterone in the diagnosis and management of congenital adrenal hyperplasia. J Pediatr 88:766, 1976.

Klingensmith GJ & others: Glucocorticoid treatment of girls with congenital adrenal hyperplasia: Effects on height, sexual maturation and fertility. J Pediatr 90:996, 1977.

Lovas B, Hasur F, Bertrand J: Exchangeable sodium and aldosterone secretion in children with congenital adrenal hyperplasia due to 21-hydroxylase deficiency. Pediatr Res 4:145, 1970.

Milunsky A, Tulchinsky D: Prenatal diagnosis of congenital adrenal hyperplasia due to 21-hydroxylase deficiency. Pediatrics 59:768, 1977.

Shaekleton CH & others: Difficulties in diagnosis of adrenogenital syndrome. Pediatrics 49:198, 1972.

Wentz A & others: Gonadotropin output and response to LRH administration in congenital virilizing adrenal hyperplasia. J Clin Endocrinol Metab 42:239, 1976.

3. PRIMARY HYPERALDOSTERONISM

Primary hyperaldosteronism may be caused by a benign adrenal tumor or by adrenal hyperplasia. It is characterized by paresthesias, tetany, weakness, periodic "paralysis," low serum potassium, elevated serum sodium, hypertension, metabolic alkalosis, and production of a large volume of alkaline urine with elevated protein content and low fixed specific gravity; the latter does not respond to vasopressin (Pitressin). The glucose tolerance test is frequently abnormal. Plasma and urinary aldosterone are elevated, but other steroid levels are variable. Edema is absent. Plasma renin levels are decreased (in contrast to increased levels in secondary hyperaldosteronism, eg, that due to renal vascular disease and Bartter's syndrome). In patients with tumor, the administration of ACTH may further increase the excretion of aldosterone. Marked decrease of aldosterone-induced hypokalemia, alkalosis, hypochloremia, or hypernatremia after the administration of a glucocorticoid or an aldosterone antagonist such as spironolactone (Aldactone), which blocks the action of aldosterone upon the renal tubule, may be of diagnostic value.

Treatment is with glucocorticoid administration, surgical removal of the tumor, or subtotal or total adrenalectomy for hyperplasia.

Conn JW: Primary aldosteronism and primary reninism. Hosp Pract 9:131, Oct 1974.

Giebink GS & others: A kindred with familial glucocorticoid-suppressible aldosteronism. J Clin Endocrinol 36:715, 1973.

Kowarski A, Katz H, Migeon CJ: Plasma aldosterone concentration in normal subjects from infancy to adulthood. J Clin Endocrinol 38:489, 1974.

Mace JW & others: Magnesium supplementation in Bartter's syndrome. Arch Dis Child 48:485, 1973.

ADRENOCORTICOSTEROIDS & CORTICOTROPIN (ACTH)

Under the regulation of adrenocorticotropin hormone (ACTH, corticotropin), the intact adrenal elaborates adrenocorticosteroids having glucocorticoid activity and a minimal but significant amount of mineralocorticoid effect. The latter is complemented by adrenocorticosteroids which possess primarily mineralocorticoid activity and are under the regulatory control of vascular compartment volume and electrolyte concentration (ie, sodium). Adrenal androgens are also elaborated, but in the normal subject the quantity is insignificant before puberty.

Numerous synthetic preparations possessing variable ratios of glucocorticoid and mineralocorticoid activity are available (Table 24—7), and are employed widely in a variety of clinical conditions. These agents are not curative and may have many undesirable side-effects. Moreover, prolonged use of these agents orally, parenterally, or topically may result in suppression of ACTH with ultimate adrenal atrophy and insufficiency.

Actions

The adrenocorticosteroids exert an effect on virtually every tissue of the body, but the exact mechanism of their action is not known.

(1) Glyconeogenesis and glycogen synthesis in the liver.

(2) Stimulation of fat synthesis and redistribution of body fat.

(3) Catabolism of protein with an increase in nitrogen and phosphorus excretion.

(4) Decrease in lymphoid and thymic tissue, resulting in a decreased cellular response to inflammation and hypersensitivity.

(5) Alteration of CNS excitation.

(6) Retardation of connective tissue mitosis and migration, decreasing wound healing.

(7) Improved capillary tone and increased vascular compartment volume and pressure.

(8) In the case of mineralocorticoids, control of cation flux across membranes, with sodium retention and potassium excretion.

Uses

The adrenocorticosteroids and corticotropin are commonly employed in the following conditions in childhood:

(1) Adrenogenital syndrome, adrenal insufficiency. (Corticotropin is not effective in these disorders.)

(2) Nephrotic syndrome.

(3) Ulcerative colitis and ileitis.

(4) Allergic disorders: Bronchial asthma (including status asthmaticus), intractable hay fever (pollinosis), urticaria, angioneurotic edema, serum sickness, atopic dermatitis, atopic eczema, exfoliative dermatitis.

(5) Inflammatory eye disease: Uveitis, chorioretinitis, sympathetic ophthalmia, iritis, iridocyclitis, retinitis centralis, herpes zoster (not herpes simplex) ophthalmicus, optic neuritis, retrobulbar neuritis.

(6) Collagen diseases: Rheumatoid arthritis, acute rheumatic fever, disseminated lupus erythematosus, scleroderma, dermatomyositis.

(7) Neoplastic diseases (temporary remission): Pulmonary granulomatosis, lymphoma, Hodgkin's disease, acute leukemia.

Table 24—7. Adrenocorticosteroids.

	Trade Names	Potency/mg Compared to Cortisol* (Glucocorticoid Effect)	Potency/mg Compared to Cortisol (Sodium-Retaining Effect)
Glucocorticoids			
Hydrocortisone (cortisol)†	Cortef, Cortril, Hydrocortone, Solu-Cortef	1	1
Cortisone	Cortone	4/5	1
Prednisone	Deltasone, Meticorten, Paracort	4—5	2/5
Prednisolone	Delta-Cortef, Hydeltra, Meticortelone, Prednis, Sterane	4	2/5
Methylprednisolone† ‡	Medrol	5 6	Minimal effect
Triamcinolone† ‡	Aristocort, Kenacort, Kenalog	5—6	Minimal effect
Paramethasone	Haldrone	10—12	
Fluprednisolone	Alphadrol	13	
Dexamethasone†	Decadron, Deronil, Dexameth, Gamma-corten, Hexadrol	25—30	Minimal effect
Betamethasone† ‡	Celestone	25	
Mineralocorticoids			
9a-Fluorocortisol	Florinef	15—20	300—400
Desoxycorticosterone acetate	Doca, Percorten	No effect	15
Desoxycorticosterone pivalate (trimethylacetate)	Percorten pivalate	No effect	
Aldosterone		30	500

*To convert hydrocortisone dosage to equivalent dosage in any of the other preparations listed in this table, divide by the potency factors shown.

†Available for topical use in dermatologic disorders.

‡There is no indication that these preparations offer any advantage over prednisone and prednisolone.

(8) Blood dyscrasias: Idiopathic thrombocytopenic purpura, allergic purpura, aplastic anemia, acquired hemolytic anemia.

(9) Miscellaneous conditions: Idiopathic hypoglycemia, infantile cortical hyperostosis, reticuloendotheliosis, thymic enlargement, sarcoidosis, pulmonary fibrosis, transfusion reactions, contact dermatitis (including poison oak), drug reactions, neurodermatitis.

Contraindications

A. Absolute Contraindications: Active, questionably healed or suspected tuberculosis (unless treated concomitantly with specific antituberculosis agents).

B. Relative Contraindications: These drugs should be used with extreme caution in herpes simplex of the eye, osteoporosis, peptic ulcer and other active diseases of the gastrointestinal tract (except ileitis and ulcerative colitis), active infections, marked emotional instability, and thrombophlebitis.

Untoward Reactions of Therapy

With high dosage or prolonged use, adrenocorticosteroids may lead to any or all of the clinical manifestations of Cushing's syndrome. These side-effects may result from either synthetic and exogenous agents (by any route, including topical) or from the use of corticotropin, which stimulates excess production of endogenous adrenocorticosteroids. Use of a large single dose given once every 48 hours (alternate day therapy) lessens the incidence and severity of side-effects.

A. Endocrine Disorders:

1. Hyperglycemia and glycosuria (of particular significance in early chemical diabetes).

2. Production of Cushing's syndrome.

3. Persistent suppression of pituitary-adrenal responsiveness to stress with danger of hypoadrenocorticism or pituitary insufficiency.

B. Electrolyte and Mineral Disorders:

1. Marked retention of sodium and water, producing edema, increased blood volume, and hypertension.

2. Potassium loss with symptoms of hypokalemia.

3. Hypocalcemia, tetany.

C. Protein and Skeletal Disorders:

1. Negative nitrogen balance, with loss of body protein and bone protein, resulting in osteoporosis and pathologic fractures and aseptic bone necrosis.

2. Suppression of growth, retarded skeletal maturation.

3. Muscular weakness.

D. Effect on Gastrointestinal Tract:

1. Excessive appetite and intake of food.

2. Activation or production of peptic ulcer.

3. Gastrointestinal bleeding from ulceration or from unknown cause (particularly in children with hepatic disease).

4. Fatty liver with embolism, pancreatitis, nodular panniculitis.

E. Lowering of Resistance to Infectious Agents; Silent Infection; Decreased Inflammatory Reaction:

1. Susceptibility to acute pulmonary or disseminated fungal infections; intestinal parasitic infections.

2. Activation of tuberculosis; false-negative tuberculin reaction.

3. Stimulation of activity of herpes simplex virus.

F. Neuropsychiatric Disorders:

1. Euphoria, excitability, psychotic behavior, and status epilepticus with EEG changes.

2. Increased intracranial pressure with "pseudotumor cerebri" syndrome.

G. Hemorrhagic Disorders:

1. Bleeding into the skin as a result of increased capillary fragility.

2. Thrombosis, thrombophlebitis, cerebral hemorrhage.

H. Miscellaneous:

1. Myocarditis, pleuritis, and arteritis following abrupt cessation of therapy.

2. Cardiomegaly.

3. Nephrosclerosis proteinuria.

4. Acne (in older children), hirsutism, amenorrhea.

5. Posterior subcapsular cataracts; glaucoma.

Controls to Minimize Dangers of Corticosteroid Therapy

A. Laboratory Controls: During therapy with corticosteroids the following determinations should be obtained at periodic intervals: blood pressure, weight, hematocrit and erythrocyte sedimentation rate, fasting blood glucose, serum potassium and CO_2 content (if prolonged therapy with large doses is necessary), stool examination for occult blood.

B. Other Recommendations:

1. Always reduce the dosage as soon as therapeutic objectives are achieved. Intermittent use is a preferable, safer method of treatment.

2. Terminate administration gradually. Abrupt withdrawal of corticotropin or the corticosteroids may cause a severe "rebound" of the disease; abrupt withdrawal of corticosteroids may cause symptoms of adrenal insufficiency. When discontinuing therapy, withdraw the evening dose first.

3. When treating less severe disorders, give corticosteroids during the daytime only, since this causes less suppression of endogenous ACTH.

4. When prolonged therapy with adrenocortical steroids is necessary, alternate-day therapy will lessen the growth-suppressive influence of corticosteroids.

5. Give therapeutic doses of adrenocortical steroids to any child undergoing surgery, any child with a severe infection, or any child under other significant types of stress who has previously received daily corticosteroid therapy for longer than 4 months during the past 6 months to 2 years.

6. If a child receiving steroids develops chickenpox, the dosage of the steroid should not be reduced but increased (unless it is already at a high level). Steroid withdrawal in these circumstances may have a fatal outcome.

7. If edema develops, place the patient on a low-

sodium diet or administer thiazide diuretics.

8. Give potassium in divided doses if prolonged therapy or high dosage is employed.

9. Sodium fluoride has been reported to stimulate calcium retention in some patients with corticosteroid-induced osteoporosis.

10. Liberal intake of protein may decrease the risk of developing osteoporosis.

11. Continuous therapy with antacids is of value in minimizing the risk of peptic ulcer formation.

Dosage

Precise dosage of these drugs in various diseases has not been determined. The recommended dosages listed below may be used as a guide for the therapy of most diseases. (See specific diseases for further guidance.) Maintenance dosage should be adjusted depending upon the clinical response and the effect desired; if possible, it should be no higher than the minimum dosage required for adequate control of the disease (as shown by symptoms, signs, and laboratory evidence of activity).

A great many topical corticosteroids are available in various strengths for the treatment of inflammatory skin conditions. A significant amount of percutaneous absorption of corticosteroids may occur through both intact and inflamed skin. Corticosteroids are frequently prescribed in the form of aerosols and enemas for the treatment of respiratory and gastrointestinal disorders (eg, asthma, ulcerative colitis). Absorption and systemic steroid effects may occur by these routes.

See Table 24-7 for conversion of other adrenocortical steroids to hydrocortisone equivalents.

A. Corticotropin Gel: 0.5 unit/kg or 15 units/sq m IM daily in 2 equal doses 12 hours apart.

B. Hydrocortisone:

1. Physiologic maintenance–

a. IM–0.44 mg/kg (13 mg/sq m) once daily.

b. Orally*–0.66 mg/kg (20 mg/sq m) per day.

2. Early pharmacologic therapy–

a. IM–4.4 mg/kg (130 mg/sq m) once daily.

b. Orally*–6.6 mg/kg (200 mg/sq m) per day.

3. Therapeutic maintenance–

a. IM–1.3–2.2 mg/kg (40–66 mg/sq m) once daily.

b. Orally*–2–3.3 mg/kg (60–100 mg/sq m) per day.

Gaddie J & others: Aerosol beclomethasone dipropionate in chronic bronchial asthma. Lancet 1:691, 1973.

Kenny FM: Clinical observations on the use of adrenal steroids: Comments on side effects and approaches to avoiding them. Clin Pediatr (Phila) 11:395, 1972.

*In 4 equal doses 6 hours apart (preferred) or 3 equal doses every 8 hours.

ADRENAL MEDULLA

PHEOCHROMOCYTOMA
(Chromaffinoma)

Pheochromocytoma is an uncommon tumor which may be located wherever there is any chromaffin tissue (adrenal medulla, sympathetic ganglia, carotid body, etc). It may be multiple, familial (autosomal recessive), recurrent, and sometimes malignant.

Clinical manifestations of pheochromocytoma are due to excessive secretion of epinephrine or norepinephrine. Attacks of anxiety and headaches should arouse suspicion. Other findings are palpitation and tachycardia, dizziness, weakness, nausea and vomiting, diarrhea, dilated pupils with blurring of vision, abdominal and precordial pain, hypertension (usually persistent), discomfort from heat, and vasomotor and sweating episodes. The symptoms may be sustained, producing all of the above findings plus papilledema, retinopathy, and enlargement of the heart. There is an increased incidence of pheochromocytomas in patients and families with the pheochromatoses (neurofibromatosis and medullary carcinoma of the thyroid; see p 683). Neuroblastomas, neurogangliomas, and other neural tumors may cause increased secretion of pressor amines and occasionally simulate the findings of a pheochromocytoma. Carcinoid tumors may produce cardiovascular changes similar to those associated with pheochromocytoma.

Laboratory diagnosis is possible in over 90% of cases. Serum catecholamines are elevated, particularly while the patient is symptomatic, and urinary excretion of catecholamines parallels this elevation. (Elevated levels may be limited to the period of a paroxysm.) The 24-hour urine collection shows increased excretion of metanephrines and vanillylmandelic acid (VMA, 3-methoxy-4-hydroxymandelic acid). Attacks may be provoked by mechanical stimulation of the tumor or by administration of histamine, tyramine, or glucagon. The phentolamine (Regitine) test is abnormal but usually is not necessary for diagnosis. Displacement of the kidney may be shown by routine x-ray or after presacral insufflation of air. Angiocatheterization and measurement of blood levels of catecholamines are particularly helpful in localizing the tumor prior to surgery.

Surgical removal of the tumor is the treatment of choice; this is a dangerous procedure and may produce sudden paroxysm and death. The oral administration of phentolamine (Regitine) preoperatively has been recommended to prevent the extreme fluctuations of blood pressure which sometimes occur during surgery. Profound hypotension may occur as the tumor is removed; this may be controlled with an infusion of levarterenol, which may have to be continued for 1–2 days.

Complete relief of symptoms is to be expected

after recovery from removal of the nonmalignant tumor unless irreversible secondary vascular changes have occurred. If untreated, severe cardiac, renal, and cerebral damage may result.

Axelrod J, Weinshilboum R: Catecholamines. N Engl J Med 287:237, 1972.

Robinson AT: Pheochromocytoma in childhood. Arch Dis Child 48:137, 1973.

Saxena KM: Endocrine manifestations of neurofibromatosis in children. Am J Dis Child 120:265, 1970.

PITUITARY

DIABETES INSIPIDUS

Essentials of Diagnosis

- Polydipsia (4–40 liters/day); excessive polyuria.
- Urine sp gr < 1.006.
- Inability to concentrate urine on fluid restriction. Hyperosmolality of plasma.
- Responsive to vasopressin.

General Considerations

Diabetes insipidus with inability to elaborate a concentrated urine may result from deficient secretion of vasopressin (ADH), lack of response of the kidney to ADH, or failure of osmoreceptors to respond to elevations of osmolality.

Hypofunction of the hypothalamus or posterior pituitary with deficiency of vasopressin (neurogenic diabetes insipidus) may be idiopathic or may be associated with lesions of the posterior pituitary or hypothalamus (trauma, infections, suprasellar cysts, tumors, reticuloendotheliosis, or some developmental abnormality). Familial ADH deficiency may be transmitted as an autosomal dominant or X-linked recessive trait. In nephrogenic diabetes insipidus, the renal tubules fail to respond to physiologic or pharmacologic doses of vasopressin, and no lesion of the pituitary or hypothalamus can be demonstrated; this disease is believed to be X-linked with variable degrees of penetrance, with a milder variant in carrier females (see Chapter 18). When no specific cause for neurogenic diabetes insipidus can be determined, the search for an underlying lesion should be continued for many years.

Clinical Findings

The onset is often sudden, with polyuria, intense thirst, constipation, and evidences of dehydration. When the child awakens at night to urinate, he is very thirsty and drinks copiously. In young infants on an ordinary feeding regimen, polyuria may not be obvious and the infant may present with severe dehydration manifested by a high fever, circulatory collapse, and convulsions. In long-standing cases, growth retardation, lack of sexual maturation, and CNS damage may occur. The inability to concentrate urine is reflected by serum osmolalities that may be elevated to 305 mOsm/kg (occasionally higher), but urine osmolality remains below this level. Familial diabetes insipidus may have an insidious onset and a progressive course.

In cases of ADH deficiency and associated damage to the hypothalamic thirst center or hypothalamic-pituitary centers controlling ACTH production, the clinical features may be "masked" and polydipsia may not occur. The administration of corticotropin (ACTH) or adrenocorticosteroids may "unmask" the ADH deficiency by increasing the glomerular filtration rate and distal tubule perfusion.

Differential Diagnosis

Diabetes insipidus may be differentiated from psychogenic polydipsia (compulsive water drinking, potomania) and polyuria by permitting the usual intake of fluid and then withholding water for 7 hours. The test should be terminated if distress is clinically notable and associated with a weight loss exceeding 3% of body weight. Patients with long-standing psychogenic polydipsia may be unable to concentrate urine initially, and the test may have to be repeated on several successive days. Eventually, in these patients, dehydration will increase urine osmolality well above plasma osmolality. With neurogenic and nephrogenic diabetes insipidus, the urine osmolality usually does not increase above 280 (sp gr 1.010) even after the period of dehydration. Normal children and those with psychogenic polydipsia will respond to the dehydration with a urinary osmolality above 450 mOsm/kg (sp gr > 1.020). The vasopressin (Pitressin) and hypertonic saline tests may be employed to distinguish between the various forms of diabetes insipidus. The subcutaneous injection of nicotine, which is a direct stimulus of vasopressin release, may be of value in identifying cases due to primary osmoreceptor failure but has had limited clinical trial in children.

Decreased urinary concentrating ability may also occur in various forms of hypercalcemia, with hypokalemia, and in various forms of renal tubular abnormalities (eg, Fanconi's syndrome).

Treatment

A. Medical Treatment: Replacement with lypressin (lysine-8-vasopressin, Syntopressin Spray, lysine-8-vasopressin drops [Diapid]), vasopressin tannate (Pitressin Tannate), or posterior pituitary powder for nasal insufflation is of value for cases with a deficiency of pitressin.

The use of one of the thiazide diuretics, ethacrynic acid, or even salt restriction may be of value for short periods in both the neurogenic and nephrogenic types. Moreover, the treatment of nephrogenic diabetes insipidus appears to be enhanced by the administration of abundant quantities of water at short intervals, low-sodium diet, and minimum but nutritionally adequate amounts of protein.

Chlorpropamide (Diabinese) has been found to have an antidiuretic effect through its augmentation of endogenous ADH. It may be tried in cases with a partial deficiency in doses of 100–250 mg once or twice a day. Maximal effects may take 1–2 weeks. Hypotension and hypoglycemia are uncommon side-effects.

B. Other Therapy: X-ray therapy, surgery, antitumor chemotherapy, or a combination of these may be used for some cases of tumor (eg, reticuloendotheliosis).

Prognosis

In the absence of associated defects, life expectancy should be normal (if severe dehydration in infancy is avoided). Hydronephrosis and hydroureter are not uncommon sequelae of prolonged polyuria; patients should also be observed carefully for urinary tract infection.

Andersson B: Thirst and brain control of H_2O balance. Am Sci 59:408, 1971.

Aronson AS & others: Treatment of diabetes insipidus in children with DDAVP (1-deamino-8D-arginine vasopressin), a synthetic analogue of vasopressin. Acta Paediatr Scand 62:133, 1973.

Bode HH, Crawford JD: Nephrogenic diabetes insipidus in North America: The Hopewell hypothesis. N Engl J Med 280:750, 1969.

Malone JI, Vallet L, Bongiovanni AM: A partial defect in antidiuretic hormone secretion: Chlorpropamide response. J Pediatr 81:92, 1972.

Nash FD & others: Symposium on control of anti-diuretic hormone secretion. Fed Proc 30:1376, 1971.

PINEAL

The pineal gland is made up of parenchymal cells (pinealocytes) and is often assigned an endocrine function. The pineal may be involved in regulation of somatic growth, sexual maturation, body pigmentation, blood sugar regulation, and a day/night-sensitive neuroendocrine regulatory function. Tumors destroying the pineal may be associated with sexual precocity in males, possibly either through loss of an inhibitor hormone produced by the pineal or by tumor extension into the hypothalamus. Cases of gonadotropin-secreting choriocarcinomas of the pineal with secondary Leydig cell activation and resultant sexual precocity have been reported. Inasmuch as other space-occupying lesions in the same region (eg, cysts, teratomas, and hamartomas) have been associated with sexual precocity (and, at times, retarded sexual maturation), probably as a result of pressure changes upon the hypothalamus and without associated destruction of the pineal gland, a definite endocrine effect cannot be assigned to the pineal at present. Intracranial calcifi-

cation may be associated with disturbances of the pineal but may be of questionable significance in the older individual since calcification is noted in 70% of normal persons by the sixth decade.

The pineal. (Editorial.) Lancet 2:1235, 1974.

Quay WB: Diagnosis of destructive lesions of the pineal. Lancet 2:42, 1970.

Relkin R: Relative efficacy of pinealectomy: Hypothalamic and amygdaloid lesions in advancing puberty. Endocrinology 88:415, 1971.

OVARY

The ovary produces 2 types of hormones: estrogens and progesterone. At least 3 natural estrogens have been isolated: estrone, estriol, and estradiol-17β (most potent). Estrogens stimulate the growth of the uterus, vagina, and breasts. Small amounts of estrogens are elaborated throughout childhood, with a marked increase at puberty, but it is not clear whether the prepubertal production is derived from the ovary or from the adrenal cortex.

OVARIAN TUMORS

Ovarian tumors are not rare in children and account for approximately 1% of cases of female sexual precocity. They may occur at any age; are usually large, benign, and unilateral; and may be estrogen-producing. The most common estrogen-producing tumor is the granulosa cell tumor (see below), but thecomas, luteomas, mixed types, and theca-lutein and follicular cysts have all been described in association with sexual precocity. Sexual development may be complete, with advanced skeletal development, sexual hair, nipple pigmentation, and menstrual bleeding; in other cases, sexual hair may be conspicuously absent. In most instances, an ovarian tumor is palpable abdominally or rectally by the time sexual development has occurred, but there are notable exceptions to this rule.

Urinary estrogens are elevated, and the vaginal smear is positive for estrogen effect. Urinary gonadotropins are usually normal or decreased for the age.

Other ovarian tumors (teratomas, chorioepitheliomas, and dysgerminomas) have been reported in association with sexual precocity.

Treatment is surgical removal, and recurrences are uncommon.

Barber HR: Ovarian cancer in children: Guide for a difficult decision. CA 25:334, 1975.

Edwards RG: Steroid assays and preovulatory follicular development in human ovaries primed with gonadotrophins. Lancet 2:611, 1972.

Gerald PS: Origin of teratomas. N Engl J Med 292:103, 1975.

Harris BH, Boles ET Jr: Rational surgery for tumors of the ovary in children. J Pediatr Surg 9:289, 1974.

Kobayashi M: Use of diagnostic ultrasound in trophoblastic neoplasms and ovarian tumors. Cancer 38 (Suppl):441, 1976.

Lippe BM & others: Pelvic pneumography in the diagnosis of endocrine and gynecologic disorders in children. J Pediatr 78:779, 1971.

Peters H, Himelstein-Braw R, Faber M: The normal development of the ovary in childhood. Acta Endocrinol (Kbh) 82:617, 1976.

Teilum G: *Special Tumors of Ovary and Testis and Related Extragonadal Lesions: Comparative Pathology and Histological Identification.* Munksgaard, 1971.

Wollner N & others: Malignant ovarian tumors in childhood: Prognosis in relation to initial therapy. Cancer 37:1953, 1976.

TESTIS

The testes contain 3 types of cells: interstitial (Leydig) cells, germinal epithelium of the seminiferous tubules, and Sertoli cells. The Leydig cells produce the testicular androgens androstenedione and testosterone, both of which contribute to the urinary ketosteroid pattern. Testosterone is far more potent, and changes in its secretory rate may produce obvious masculinization without contributing significantly to the total urinary 17-ketosteroid fraction. (The other major ketosteroid precursors are produced by the adrenal cortex.) Testicular androgens, produced under the stimulation of anterior pituitary luteinizing hormone (LH, ICSH), appear in boys in appreciable amounts at about 11–12 years of age and are responsible, wholly or in part, for the growth of the penis and the development of secondary sexual characteristics, including pubic, axillary, and facial hair. FSH stimulates the development of germinal epithelium. The production of testicular androgens contributes to the maturation of testicular germinal epithelium and thus promotes spermatogenesis. Androgens induce nitrogen retention, accelerate bone growth, and determine the closure of epiphyseal junctions.

The Sertoli cells activate the germinal epithelium and may produce a hormone that depresses the formation of follicle-stimulating hormone (FSH) of the anterior pituitary. In addition, the Sertoli cells have the function of affording mechanical support for the germinal epithelium.

It is improbable that the testes have any major significant endocrine function before puberty.

Gonadal deficiency may be primary, eg, from absence or destruction of testicular tissue, or secondary, eg, following pituitary insufficiency. It may be due to either disturbed tubular or disturbed Leydig cell function but usually involves both.

Primary testicular failure may be due to an embryologic defect, a genetic defect (enzyme defect or hormone receptor defect), inflammation and destruction following infection (mumps, syphilis, tuberculosis), trauma, tumor, irradiation, or surgical castration. Secondary hypogonadism may result from pituitary insufficiency (destructive lesions in or near the anterior pituitary, irradiation of the pituitary, or starvation) or occasionally from dysfunction of either the thyroid or adrenal glands.

Forest MG, Cathiard AM, Bertrand JA: Total and unbound testosterone levels in the newborn and in normal and hypogonadal children: Use of a sensitive radioimmunoassay for testosterone. J Clin Endocrinol 36:1132, 1973.

Guthrie RD, Smith DW, Graham CB: Testosterone treatment for micropenis during early childhood. J Pediatr 83:247, 1973.

Johnsen SG, Bennett EP, Jensen VG: Therapeutic effectiveness of oral testosterone. Lancet 2:1473, 1974.

Paulsen CA: Recognition and management of testicular failure. Hosp Pract 7:133, Nov 1972.

Teilum G: *Special Tumors of Ovary and Testis and Related Extragonadal Lesions: Comparative Pathology and Histological Identification.* Munksgaard, 1971.

CRYPTORCHIDISM

Cryptorchidism (undescended testes) is a common disorder in children. It may be unilateral or bilateral and may be classified as ectopic, total, or incomplete.

Approximately 3% of term male newborns and 20% of premature males have undescended testes at birth. In over half of these cases, the testes will descend by the second month; by age 1 year, 80% of all undescended testes are in the scrotum. Further descent may occur through puberty, the latter perhaps stimulated by endogenous gonadotropin. If cryptorchidism persists into adult life, failure of spermatogenesis may occur but testicular androgen production usually remains intact.

The incidence of malignancy (usually seminoma) is appreciably greater in those testes which remain in the abdomen after puberty.

Cryptorchidism may merely represent delayed descent of the testes or may be due to prevention of normal descent by some mechanical lesion such as adhesions, short spermatic cord, fibrous bands, or endocrine disorders causing hypogonadism (uncommon). It is probable that many abdominal testes are congenitally abnormal and that this abnormality in itself prevents descent.

A causal relationship between failure of spermatogenesis and an abdominal location after puberty is assumed, but this relationship has not been established. The normally descended testis of a male with unilateral cryptorchidism may not have normal spermatogenesis; unusual cases have been described in which persistent intra-abdominal testes have been associated with normal spermatogenesis. The apparent abnormality of an abdominal testis may be reversible (even if the testes are histologically abnormal at the time they are placed in the scrotum) since they may later manifest normal histology and function.

Treatment

The best age for medical or surgical treatment has not been determined, but there is a recent trend toward operation in early childhood. Although there is a difference of opinion about whether lack of descent until puberty will cause damage to the testes, in general, delaying treatment for 5–10 years (or even longer) appears to involve no greater risk of sterility than early surgical correction (with the hazard of surgical injury to the testis). Surgical repair is indicated for cryptorchidism persisting beyond puberty since the incidence of malignancy is appreciably greater in those glands which remain in the abdomen beyond the second decade of life.

A. Unilateral: Most cases are due to local mechanical lesions or a defective testis on the involved side. If pseudocryptorchidism (see below) has been ruled out and if descent has not occurred by mid-puberty, surgical exploration and relocation should be attempted by a surgeon skilled in this procedure. Surgical intervention may be delayed until serum or urine gonadotropin have been at pubescent levels for 6–12 months.

Testes with short spermatic cords should be relocated at the abdominal wall and later to a scrotal site (if possible) after "stretching" has increased spermatic cord length.

Gonadotropin therapy (chorionic gonadotropins, 500 units IM 2–3 times a week for 5–8 weeks, or 3000 units/sq m 3 times a week for 2 weeks) is recommended by some before surgery and may be of value if surgery is carried out prior to puberty. When surgery is postponed until mid puberty, it is doubtful that exogenous gonadotropins are more effective than the gonadotropin produced endogenously.

B. Bilateral: The timing for surgery in the male child in whom pseudocryptorchidism has been ruled out is still controversial. Histologic changes may be seen in the intra-abdominal testes by 3–4 years of age, but the relationship of these changes to fertility is unproved. Some suggest that surgery should be done prior to age 5; others recommend waiting until early in puberty. Treatment with chorionic gonadotropin may be tried prior to surgery (see above).

The child with bilaterally undescended testes should be evaluated for sex chromosome abnormalities and genetic sex determined by buccal smear or chromosome analysis in the newborn period (see p 694).

Androgen treatment (ie, testosterone enanthate) is indicated only as replacement therapy in the male beyond the normal age of puberty who has been shown to lack functional testes.

C. Pseudocryptorchidism: This disorder consists of retractile testes that are normally located extra-abdominally but not found in the scrotum at the time of examination.

In palpating the scrotum for the testes, the cremasteric reflex may be elicited, with a resultant ascent of the testes into the inguinal canal or abdomen. To prevent this, the fingers first should be placed across the upper portion of the inguinal canal, obstructing ascent. Examination while the child is in a warm bath is also helpful.

No treatment is necessary, and the prognosis for testicular competence is excellent.

Bramble FJ: Reproductive and endocrine function after surgical treatment of bilateral cryptorchidism. Lancet 2:311, 1974.

Dougall AJ, Maclean N, Wilkinson AW: Histology of the maldescended testis at operation. Lancet 1:771, 1974.

Lattimer JK & others: The optimum time to operate for cryptorchidism. Pediatrics 53:96, 1974.

Samenow SE: Cryptorchidism and character. Med Arts Sci 25:9, 1971.

Santestebam A: Cryptorchidism in the newborn. Pediatrics 51:310, 1973.

PRECOCIOUS SEXUAL DEVELOPMENT

Sexual development may be considered precocious if it develops before the age of 10 years in boys or 8 years in girls. The causes are outlined in Table 24–8. True (complete) precocious puberty refers to sexual maturation in which the hypothalamic-pituitary mechanism initiates sexual development; in pseudoprecocity, the process is initiated elsewhere. True precocious puberty is always isosexual and may be associated with the production of mature sperm or ova. In pseudoprecocity, sex characteristics may be isosexual or heterosexual; secondary sexual characteristics develop, but the gonads do not mature and the patient is infertile. In the pseudosexual variety, gonadal development and fertility may occur at the normal time.

Precocious puberty is 9 times more common in girls than in boys. It may have its onset at any age. In constitutional precocious puberty, no etiologic factor can be found. Sexual and genital maturation and body growth tend to proceed along the normal pattern but are accelerated. (The earliest recorded pregnancy occurred at age 5 years 7 months.) In males, a positive family history is often present. Breast development is usually the first sign in females, but the pattern of development may be variable; the interval between breast development and menstruation may be less than 1 year or more than 8 years. Psychologic development tends to be consistent with chronologic age. In male pseudoprecocious puberty (eg, adrenogenital syndrome), the penis enlarges but the testes do not; in the constitutional form, boys manifest enlargement of testes as well as the penis. However, enlargement of the testes may not be commensurate with that of the penis

Table 24—8. Causes of isosexual precocious development.

True (complete) precocious puberty
Constitutional (functional, idiopathic)
Tumors producing destruction of the pineal (principally in males)
Polyostotic fibrous dysplasia (McCune-Albright syndrome) (principally in females; often incomplete; usually infertile)
Hypothalamic lesions (hamartomas, hyperplasia, congenital malformations, tumors)
Tumors in vicinity of the third ventricle
Internal hydrocephalus
Cerebral and meningocerebral infections (postencephalitis, postmeningitis)
Degenerative, possibly congenital encephalopathy
Tuberous sclerosis
Von Recklinghausen's disease
Cystic arachnoiditis
Therapeutic administration of gonadotropin
Exogenous obesity
 	
Pseudoprecocious (incomplete) puberty
Adrenal abnormalities
  Adrenocortical hyperplasia (males)
  Adrenocortical tumors
  Hyperplastic ectopic adrenal tissue
  Cushing's syndrome (males)
	Gonadal tumors
	  Tumors of the ovary—Granulosa cell tumor (most common), theca cell tumor, teratoma, choriocarcinoma, dysgerminoma, luteoma
	  Tumors of the testes—Interstitial (Leydig) cell tumor, teratoma
	Premature pubarche (premature adrenarche) (both sexes)
	  Without cerebral disease (constitutional?)
	  With cerebral disease
	Premature thelarche (premature gynarche) (females)
	  Without cerebral disease (constitutional?)
	  With cerebral disease
	Drug-induced
	
	Unclassified causes
	With elevated gonadotropins
	  Associated with hypothyroidism
	  Presacral teratoma
	  Primary liver cell tumors (hepatoma) (males only)
	  Choriocarcinoma and seminoma of the testes
	Others
	  Hyperinsulinism
	  Primordial dwarfism
	  Silver's syndrome (short stature, congenital asymmetry, and variations in the pattern of sexual development)
	  Thyrotropin-releasing hormone excess

since tubular elements may not be stimulated to the same extent as in normal puberty. Children grow rapidly in childhood but may be short as adults since osseous maturation ("bone age") advances at a more rapid pace than linear growth ("height age").

When radioimmunoassays for pituitary gonadotropins are employed, pubertal elevations are demonstrable; however, bioassay methods may not detect elevations since they lack sufficient sensitivity. 17-Ketosteroids may be elevated to the pubertal range. Luteal cysts of the ovaries are frequently found and probably reflect only gonadotropin activity, although an etiologic role has been inferred by some.

Treatment is seldom helpful. In girls, the administration of medroxyprogesterone acetate (Depo-Provera), 400 mg IM every 4 weeks, may arrest and reverse the condition either by inhibiting gonadotropin production or by a direct effect on the ovary, but treatment may have no effect on the acceleration of bone age and may be associated with hypertension and glucose intolerance. Psychologic management of the patient and family is important.

Early menarche may be associated with late menopause.

During the first 2 years after onset, females with sexual precocity should have a thorough abdominal and rectal examination every 4—6 months for the presence of a possible ovarian neoplasm since evidence of precocious sexual development may precede the finding of a palpable abdominal mass by several months. Physical examination may be augmented by abdominal-pelvic ultrasound or by pneumogynogram

performed by a skilled radiologist. In females, 75—85% of cases of precocious puberty are constitutional or idiopathic; about half of cases in males are due to congenital adrenal hyperplasia (pseudoprecocious puberty); many cases of central (true) precocious puberty in males are due to intracranial mass lesions.

In males, observe carefully for tumors of the testes and adrenals.

Since certain cases of precocious puberty resulting from organic brain lesions may produce no clinical manifestations for prolonged periods, children should be examined periodically for evidence of increased intracranial pressure or other CNS disturbances (skull x-ray, eye examination, visual fields, EEG).

Escobar ME & others: Plasma concentration of oestradiol in premature thelarche and in different types of sexual precocity. Acta Endocrinol (Kbh) 81:351, 1976.

Forbes GB: Relation of lean body mass to height in children and adolescents. Pediatr Res 6:32, 1972.

Hall R, Warrick C: Hypersecretion of hypothalamic releasing hormones: A possible explanation of the endocrine manifestation of polyostotic fibrous dysplasia (Albright's syndrome). Lancet 1:1313, 1972.

Kulin HE & others: Gonadotropins during childhood and adolescence: A review. Pediatrics 51:260, 1973.

Reiter EO & others: Responsivity of pituitary gonadotropes to luteinizing hormone-releasing factor in idiopathic precocious puberty, precocious thelarche, precocious adrenarche, and in patients treated with medroxyprogesterone acetate. Pediatr Res 9:111, 1975.

Richman RA & others: Adverse effects of large doses of medroxyprogesterone in idiopathic isosexual precocity. J

Pediatr 79:963, 1971.

Root AW: Endocrinology of puberty. (2 parts.) J Pediatr 83:1, 187, 1973.

Root A & others: Isosexual pseudoprecocity in a 6-year-old boy with a testicular interstitial cell adenoma. J Pediatr 80:264, 1972.

DIABETES MELLITUS*

Essentials of Diagnosis

- Hyperglycemia and glycosuria, with or without ketonuria.
- Weight loss, polyuria, polydipsia, and abdominal or leg cramps.
- Enuresis, mild appetite loss, emotional disturbances, lassitude.
- 20% of cases present in coma or precoma.
- Diminished glucose tolerance.

General Considerations

Diabetes mellitus is a common disease in childhood. Its incidence in a clinically overt form may be as high as 0.4%. It was regarded primarily as an expression of insulin deficiency until technical advances in the ability to measure plasma insulin levels showed that this was not always the case.

In most cases of juvenile diabetes—if observed early—there is insulin in the circulating blood, and some investigators have observed hypertrophy of the islet tissue. However, this hypertrophic stage is short-lived, and early and progressive degenerative changes of the B cells lead to the complete disappearance of insulin from the pancreases of young juvenile diabetics within 2 years after onset. These pancreatic changes are in striking contrast with the absent or mild ones noted in the maturity onset type of diabetes. Juvenile diabetics, with rare exceptions, are insulin-dependent, since endogenous insulin is insufficient and rapidly disappears completely.

When juvenile diabetes is finally explained in molecular terms, it seems probable that it will be found to be due to many causes. Even now it is difficult to be satisfied with the concept that the conventional form of the disease develops in the same way as some of its related syndromes such as Prader-Willi syndrome, lipoatrophic diabetes, myotonic dystrophy, or Friedreich's ataxia.

The influence of heredity in juvenile diabetes is still far from clear. Certainly there is an increased incidence of the HLA antigens HLA-B8 and HLA-Bw15. There is some evidence also that the underlying genetic defect is production of an abnormal insulin. Current thinking, however, favors direct or autoimmune damage to the B cell by viruses such as mumps virus,

*This section is contributed by Donough O'Brien, MD, FRCP.

coxsackievirus B4, and perhaps other coxsackieviruses of the B series.

The basic biochemical lesion is that insulin no longer stimulates protein synthesis at the ribosomal level or effectively binds hexokinase to the electron transport chain on the mitochondrial surface. The latter leads to diminished availability of oxaloacetate. To replace these lessened energy resources from glucose, increased breakdown of fat and protein to acetylcoenzyme A occurs. Peripheral utilization of fatty acids and amino acids, however, is incomplete, and both are converted to ketone bodies in the liver.

Present evidence is that proinsulin, the single-chain precursor molecule of insulin, constitutes up to 15% of circulating insulin but that it is not of importance in the causation of diabetes.

Clinical Findings

A. Symptoms and Signs:

1. Severe diabetes—In most affected children, diabetes is first recognized during the initial rapid deterioration in carbohydrate metabolism, with about 20% of patients being actually in or near coma when first seen. The characteristic symptoms of loss of weight, polyuria, polydipsia, and abdominal or leg cramps are recognized largely in retrospect.

Evanescent diabetic states may occur with severe infections such as pneumonia, meningitis, or encephalitis or as a complication of corticosteroid therapy.

2. Mild diabetes—With increasing frequency, the disease may present in a more benign fashion. A few will be detected before overt symptoms appear, being accidentally discovered on urinalysis; others are the ketosis-resistant cases, with enuresis as evidence of polyuria, with moderate weight loss, or with mild problems of poor appetite and lassitude or emotional disturbances. Very rarely, diabetes may present as a delayed overcompensation to a glucose load, with hypoglycemia 3 hours or so after a glucose load, or as nonketotic (hyperosmolar) coma. In children, there are usually no specific signs suggestive of diabetes other than dehydration, exhaled acetone, or coma. "Adult onset" diabetes is occasionally seen in an obese teenager. This can be managed by diet restriction with or without sulfonylureas. By extending screening programs to young people, more such cases might be identified.

Well controlled diabetics show no abnormal physical signs.

3. Prediabetes and pseudodiabetes—*Prediabetes* is a condition in which there is an abnormal response to a glucose load but no clinical evidence of diabetes mellitus. Criteria for diagnosis are as follows: (1) Two values above the 97th percentile at 60 and 120 minutes and one below the 50th percentile at 180 minutes, or one value at or above the 97th percentile at 60 or 120 minutes and one below the 10th percentile at 180 minutes. These reflect a delayed insulin response to the glucose load. (2) Three values above the 97th percentile at 60, 120, and 180 minutes. Either criterion must be met in 2 tests. (3) Two fasting levels > 110 mg/100 ml or one value at 30 minutes > 200 mg/100 ml. (See p 1047.) There is much argument about whether these children should be treated. The author's view is that treatment should not be given.

Pseudodiabetes is a transient diabetic state occurring in the newborn or occasionally in older children with infections. It may require a short course of treatment with regular insulin.

4. Hyperosmolar nonketotic coma—This is characterized by severe hyperglycemia, hyperosmolality, and dehydration without ketoacidosis. It is usually seen in adult onset diabetes; it is uncommon in children. Restoration of extracellular water is a primary goal of treatment.

B. Laboratory Findings:

1. Glycosuria—Glycosuria may be identified by glucose oxidase tapes, eg, Tes-Tape and Clinistix, which are very sensitive tests and thus not always suitable for routine urine testing in treatment despite their convenience. Clinitest tablets are less sensitive; placing 2 drops of urine and 10 drops of water on a tablet yields a colored precipitate which can be compared to a color chart to indicate glucose concentrations between 0 and 5%. Placing 8 drops of urine in 5 ml of Benedict's solution and bringing it to a boil will give comparable changes from translucent blue to a brown-red precipitate according to the degree of reduction.

2. Hyperglycemia—A fasting blood sugar of over 120 mg/100 ml is almost certainly indicative of diabetes mellitus; the upper limit of normal is usually regarded as 100 mg/100 ml, using a true glucose determination.

3. Glucose tolerance tests—Glucose tolerance tests, although a traditional confirmatory test for diabetes, are not usually necessary in childhood. The oral test is to take fasting 30, 60, 90, and 120 minute blood samples for serum glucose determination following an oral dose of glucose of 70 gm/sq m. (See surface area nomograms, Figs 36—1 and 36—2.) The glucose should be given as flavored corn syrup (Glucola; glucose solutions may be used instead but may produce nausea and vomiting). A level of over 120 mg/100 ml at 2 hours is considered evidence of diabetes.

4. Serum insulin levels—Serum insulin levels may be normal or moderately elevated at the onset of juvenile diabetes. A delayed insulin response to glucose is indicative of prediabetes.

5. Other laboratory measurements—A number of additional laboratory parameters are coming to be used in the appraisal of long-term control. Red cell sorbitol levels are normally 5.3 ± 2.1 (1 SD) nmol/ml packed red cells and in diabetics rise to 33 ± 14. Hemoglobin A_{Ic} levels are 14 ± 2.5% of total hemoglobin in childhood diabetics and 6.5 ± 1.5% in normal children. The utility of these determinations is not yet fully established, however.

Differential Diagnosis

The differential diagnosis of diabetes mellitus is not difficult since this is virtually the only condition which gives rise to glycosuria and hyperglycemia with ketosis.

Abnormal glucose tolerance tests with glycosuria may be encountered in a variety of conditions in which there is an increased production of glucocorticoids or catecholamines. These include certain hypothalamic and pituitary tumors, adrenal tumors or hyperplasia, and pheochromocytomas. Since the hyperglycemia in these states is a reflection of increased gluconeogenesis and glycogenolysis and not of insulin insufficiency, there is no ketosis. Renal glycosuria is not associated with hyperglycemia.

Treatment

A. Management of Ketosis and Coma:

1. General management—The treatment of severe diabetic acidosis must be based on fundamental principles. Insulin must be given to restore normal carbohydrate utilization and triglyceride synthesis. Extracellular fluid volume must be restored to compensate for losses due to vomiting and to the osmotic diuresis caused by unmetabolized glucose in the urine. Serum hyperosmolality must be gradually normalized and intracellular stores of potassium replenished. The serum phosphorus level must be raised in some cases in order to maintain normal erythrocyte 2,3-diphosphoglycerate levels and tissue oxygenation. Severe acid-base distortions may have to be corrected both for homeostatic reasons and to ensure optimal insulin action. Over the long term, nutritional balance should be brought into the normal range for age and sex.

2. Initial laboratory studies—The laboratory routine should include a complete blood count, examination of the urine for blood cells, protein, ketone bodies, and sugar; and appropriate cultures as required for the investigation of suspected infectious disease.

The acid-base status should be estimated by measuring blood pH and P_{CO_2} or serum bicarbonate. Baseline serum (or plasma) ketones, glucose, sodium, potassium, and chloride levels should be recorded, as well as BUN, serum phosphate, and serum osmolality in severe cases. Serum acetoacetic acid should be measured by Acetest tablet dilution. (More specific tests are too time-consuming for routine use.)

3. Initial management—The following protocol is for children with diabetic ketoacidosis who have been hospitalized because they are new diabetics; because they have severe acidosis, CNS symptoms, or repeated vomiting; because they are unable to take oral fluids; or because they have not responded to home or outpatient management. It does not apply to diabetes complicated by lactic acidosis, renal failure, or hyperosmolar coma.

a. General clinical management—

(1) Take a routine history and perform a physical examination, with special attention to the possibility of infection as a precipitating cause.

(2) Reassure the patient and keep him warm. Antiemetics (eg, promethazine, 0.5 mg/kg IM) may be helpful if the child is vomiting but not comatose.

(3) If there is vomiting or abdominal distention

with a risk of aspiration due to coma or precoma, start gentle continuous gastric suction. Unconscious patients must be catheterized.

(4) Start a flow sheet for medications, fluids, insulin, and laboratory values. Record all intake and output meticulously. Keep all records in a format that anyone can easily and accurately grasp.

(5) In severe cases, assess the degree of shock and the need for blood or other volume expanders. Also attach an ECG monitoring line for K^+ changes.

b. Insulin—No insulin should be given until a baseline serum glucose level has been determined. There are a variety of acceptable ways of replenishing insulin in diabetic acidosis using combinations of intravenous, intramuscular, and subcutaneous administration. The regimen advocated here consists of giving small doses of insulin by continuous intravenous infusion. This achieves a relatively constant serum insulin level without the hazard of hypoglycemia and a smoother and more predictable fall in serum glucose and ketones. The normal initial dose is 0.2–0.3 unit/kg IM, which in severe cases with profound acidosis and neurologic signs can be increased up to 0.5–1 unit/kg. Albumin need not be added to the solution.

In general, insulin should be repeated in a dosage of 0.1–0.15 unit/kg IV hourly until the serum acetoacetic acid is only moderately elevated when tested by Acetest tablet in 1:2 dilution. During this period, serum acetoacetic acid by Acetest tablet should be measured every 2 hours before the insulin dose. Blood glucose by Dextrostix should be measured hourly as a screening measure to detect hypoglycemia early if it occurs. If the serum glucose has fallen below 250 mg/100 ml and serum acetoacetic acid is still elevated, the intravenous insulin regimen should be continued until serum ketones are normal and glucose should be administered intravenously. In the interval before serum acetone levels (at 1:2 Acetest dilution) fall, regular insulin should be given subcutaneously in a dosage of 0.1–0.15 unit/kg every 4–6 hours.

The first dose of long-acting insulin (equal parts of semilente and ultralente or 1 part of regular to 3 or 4 of NPH) should be started on the first or second morning after admission provided vomiting has stopped. A tentative starting total dose of 0.5–1 unit/kg/24 hours is advised in new patients.

c. Fluid and electrolyte management—

(1) **Initial volume expansion**—If the patient is in a severely dehydrated or borderline shock state, give 20 ml/kg (600 ml/sq m) or more of physiologic solution (isotonic saline or lactated Ringer's injection) over the first hour. If the serum glucose is high (> 250 mg/100 ml), there is no reason to add glucose until the serum glucose falls below this level. Blood glucose levels should be determined at hourly intervals to be certain that hypoglycemia does not occur—or the Dextrostix method can be used. If the patient is severely acidotic or has not voided, it may be desirable to wait to add potassium until after the initial fluid volume reexpansion in the first hour of therapy. Patients with severe circulatory failure may need plasma or whole blood as well as extracellular water volume expansion.

(2) **Twenty-four-hour fluid volume**—

(a) **Replacement**—If weight loss over a short time has occurred, replace this acute weight loss with physiologic salt solution. If the body weight before onset is unknown, treatment must be guided by estimation of hydration status based on physical examination; losses vary from 5–15% of body weight for mild to severe losses. (If in doubt, replace 10% of body weight.) Deficits can usually be replaced at a rate of 50% in the first 8 hours and 25% in each of the second and third 8-hour periods. Remember to subtract the quantities given in the first hour of reexpansion from the 24-hour totals. Measure and record urine or emesis (gastric drainage if tube is in place) output at intervals of 4–8 hours to be certain that initial estimates are adequate.

(b) **Maintenance**—The maintenance requirement is 60–80 ml/kg (the lower quantity for an adolescent and the higher for a 1-year-old), or 1500–2500 ml/sq m. Maintenance sodium requirements are 3–5 mEq/kg/24 hours. Divide maintenance fluids evenly over the first three 8-hour periods.

(c) **Special additional losses**—Additional replacement fluids may be required if there has been severe vomiting or other fluid losses.

(d) **Potassium**—Potassium is a special problem because high urinary losses occur in association with normal serum levels due to the inability of K^+ to be retained intracellularly in the presence of acidosis. As acidosis is corrected, it is not unusual to see serum potassium levels fall in spite of large potassium replacements. In general, all intravenous fluids should contain 20–30 mEq K^+/liter once voiding is established. ECG strips (lead II) may give the best indication of total body potassium deficit or change. Supplements may be in the form of potassium chloride or phosphate.

(e) **Phosphorus**—Serum phosphorus, like potassium, may be initially elevated in diabetic acidosis only to fall rapidly during therapy. It is still not clear that low serum phosphorus causes clinical problems, but there is some evidence that neurologic disturbances may respond to raising the serum phosphorus. On theoretic grounds, a low serum phosphorus may be reflected in a low red cell 2,3-diphosphoglycerate, causing a leftward shift of the O_2 dissociation curve. This in turn may cause peripheral anoxia, especially with restoration of normal blood pH. In replacing phosphate, either give all potassium requirements as potassium, checking serum phosphate levels, or use the following formula:

$$\frac{\text{Dose (in ml) of Travenol potassium phosphate solution (3 mEq } K^+ \text{ and 66 mg P per ml)}} = (3.5 - \text{Serum phosphorus in mg/100 ml}) \times (\text{Body weight in kg} \times 0.1)$$

The dose may be repeated every 3 hours until serum phosphorus levels reach 3 mg/100 ml.

(f) **Osmolarity**—Measurement of serum osmolarity may be helpful in severely comatose patients. If the serum osmolality is very high (> 350), the blood sugar and dehydration should be corrected less rapidly. Osmolarity should not be rapidly decreased because CNS damage may result. The treatment of hyperosmolar nonketotic coma is different from the treatment outlined here.

d. Acid-base management—Specific acid-base correction with alkali is usually not necessary unless the blood pH is under 7.15. If acidosis is severe enough to warrant therapy, correction should be slow. When bicarbonate is given, the following formula can be used and the bicarbonate infused over a period of 4–8 hours:

$$\text{mEq bicarbonate required} = \text{Base excess in mEq/liter} \times 0.3 \times \text{Body weight in kg}$$

If the base excess is unknown, the formula $(22 - HCO_3{}^-) \times 0.3 \times$ body weight in kg will also give an approximation of the mEq/liter of bicarbonate needed. Because bicarbonate crosses the blood-brain barrier and other cells slowly, the CO_2 formed from $HCO_3{}^- + H^+ \leftrightharpoons H_2CO_3 \leftrightharpoons H_2O + CO_2$ crosses rapidly (forming intracellular H_2CO_3), and accentuation of intracellular acidosis can occur. Acidosis, however, will usually correct itself with volume expansion and stopping of organic anion formation.

4. Continuing management of the ketotic patient —After the first period of adjustment, there is seldom any need to give insulin more than once a day. On the first convenient morning after admission, the patient should be started on a mixture of equal parts of ultra- and semilente insulin in a single dose consisting of one-fourth of the total required during the resuscitation period. One part of regular insulin to 3 or 4 of lente is also satisfactory. Other mixtures of soluble, NPH, protamine zinc, and lente insulins can be devised; the duration of action of these preparations is shown in Table 24–9. In general, the ultralente/semilente mixture is best, offering greater stability of insulin release and a smaller chance of subcutaneous fat necrosis and injection tumors. Most children seem to require a more nearly 50:50 proportion of the relatively short-acting

Table 24–9. Duration of action of various insulins.

Insulin	Duration of Maximum Effect (hours)	Total Duration of Effect (hours)
Regular	4–6	6–8
Actrapid pork	2–7	8–9
Globin	6–10	12–18
NPH	8–12	12–18
Crystal II beef	5–18	13–23
Protamine zinc (PZI)	14–20	24–36
Semilente	4–6	12–16
Lente (30% semi, 70% ultra)	8–12	18–24
Ultralente	16–18	24–36

semilente and ultralente than exists in the lente preparation (30:70 ratio of semi to ultra). Protamine zinc insulin is seldom used in children.

In the following days, the patient should be encouraged to return to full activity and a normal diet, while the insulin dosage is adjusted on the basis of serum and urine glucose levels and urine acetone along the lines suggested below for long-term management. At this stage, education of the patient and family must begin. After the nature and prospects of the disease have been explained, they must be shown the technics of giving insulin and of testing the urine for acetone and sugar. It is important to go over these routines repeatedly, especially in the early months of the disease. A good clinic nurse, especially one who can make home visits, can be invaluable in helping families to understand and manage diabetes in a child.

B. Management Without Acidosis: Most cases of juvenile diabetes now present without severe acidosis. The initial phase of treatment can usually be conducted on an outpatient basis if the family and physician can assign sufficient time for the purpose. However, it still may be better to confirm the diagnosis, establish insulin treatment, and start patient education, both generally (about the disease) and specifically (in terms of insulin administration, diet management, and urine testing), while the child is an inpatient.

Patients without acidosis should be started on 0.5 units/kg/day of a mixture of equal parts of semi- and ultralente insulin given once a day 30 minutes before breakfast. A preliminary regimen involving 2 or more doses of regular insulin should not be necessary. The insulin is gradually increased until hyperglycemia and glycosuria are controlled. The patient should be ambulatory and active even in the hospital.

It is probably not necessary to contrive an episode of hypoglycemia, even under controlled conditions. However, patients or their parents must be warned of the characteristic symptoms of headache, abdominal pain, and shakiness and instructed to control it with a snack, orange juice, lump of sugar, etc.

C. Long-Term Management of All Patients: The objective of long-term management is to achieve "control." In children, this can be defined as a high level of physical and emotional health, continuing normal growth with freedom from hypoglycemic reactions, no acetone in the urine, and glycosuria that seldom exceeds 1000 mg/100 ml in early morning, pre-lunch, pre-supper, or late evening urine specimens. Since routine urine testing is a measure of concentration, it is useful also from time to time to check a 24-hour urine glucose, which should be less than 20 gm/sq m/24 hours. The following are important in achieving this:

1. Patient follow-up and continuing education— Continued observation of the child with diabetes is most important. Initially, this should be weekly or at any time the need should arise; telephone contacts should be encouraged. During this period, if patients will keep careful records of urine glucose and acetone, it is usually possible to anticipate the fluctuations in insulin need which are characteristic of the early years of juvenile onset diabetes. Later on, supervision can be much less close and will depend primarily on the patient's and the family's confidence in managing diet and insulin dosage. Puberty is often a period of instability in carbohydrate metabolism, but more frequently the problems at this age are, again, the emotional ones which may stem from feelings of being different or apart from the group as a result of the diabetes. The patient must be encouraged to participate in all activities, even the strenuous ones, care being taken to avoid hypoglycemia. It is important, particularly in the early months, constantly to renew and augment the patient's and family's understanding of diabetes in both general terms and in the specific practical matters of giving the injections, diet management, activity, and immediate treatment of infections. Many families need emotional support and counseling.

2. Insulin—Mixtures of equal parts of semilente and ultralente insulin, or regular and NPH or lente insulin in the proportion of 1:2, are most often given for routine once a day use. Cases that are difficult to control can occasionally be improved by 2 doses of regular insulin, one each before breakfast and before supper. Insulin resistance is rare in children, but patients requiring over 2 units/kg/day may be helped by using pure pork insulin, sulfated insulin, or dalanated insulin. U-100 insulin is purer and less likely to cause resistance. Insulin should normally be administered, if possible by the patient, 30 minutes before breakfast. The anterior and lateral aspects of the thighs are easiest for self-administration, and the exact site should be changed daily so that a given site is used no oftener than once or twice a month. Some children are helped by "body maps," but in general it is very desirable to handle the disease with minimum attention to being different from the normal.

Initially, insulin requirements will increase to around 1 unit/kg/day, but in most new diabetics, after 1–2 months, the requirement will be reduced to the point at which the total dose may be < 5 units a day. (See oral hypoglycemic agents, below.)

Insulin dosage should be readjusted from time to time on the basis of glycosuria. Parents and patients should be encouraged to acquire confidence in making small adjustments in insulin dosage in response to gradual changes with growth and short-term increases with infection. Ready access to the pediatrician for advice is important. Ideally, daily physical exercise should be kept constant, but this is often difficult. Physical exertion diminishes insulin requirements.

3. Oral hypoglycemic agents—These drugs play a minimal role in the management of juvenile diabetes. They are helpful in the occasional case of maturity onset diabetes in young persons. It may also be possible to manage juvenile diabetics on oral hypoglycemic agents during the period 2–4 months after onset, when insulin requirements may be minimal. The sulfonylureas, which have an initial primary effect as stimulators of insulin secretion, are at least therapeutically warrantable. In any case, all but a few young diabetics eventually have to return to a regimen of injected insulin. It is poor management to raise false hopes of continued oral control at a time when the physician should be concentrating on educating the family about the care of the child.

4. Diet—Effective control can nearly always be achieved without a strict dietary regimen. The rather equivocal advantage, in terms of cardiovascular complications, that is claimed for rigid dietary control is offset in young children by the practical and emotional problems that accompany the restrictions required.

In most cases it is sufficient to establish, with the help of a dietitian, that the family diet offers a conventional assembly of calories (100 kcal × age in years + 1000), about 15–20% from proteins, 35–40% from fat, and 45–55% from carbohydrates, as well as other nutrients. Thereafter, control can be sustained on an unweighed diet but with a similar distribution of food groups from day to day.

There is increasing evidence, however, that in the adolescent it is important to strive for optimal control. Weighing diets is seldom necessary, but understanding the exchange system may be helpful in achieving control. A brief summary of the system is given here. A more complete reference is the pamphlet *Exchange Lists for Meal Planning,* published by the American Diabetes Association, 1 West 48th Street, New York, NY 10020. In general, the idea of the exchange diet is to develop "equivalents" in each food group that are similar to each other in quantities of sugar and in calories. Instructions concerning the diet should be given by a dietitian or nutritionist. The food groups, with examples of foods having similar values in each of the groups, are as follows:

a. Milk exchanges—One exchange is the quantity required to equal about 8 gm of protein or 32 kcal.

Skimmed or nonfat milk	1 cup
1% milk (also includes ½ fat exchange)	1 cup
2% milk (also includes 1 fat exchange)	1 cup
Yogurt made from skimmed milk	1 cup
Yogurt from 2% milk (includes 1 fat exchange)	1 cup

b. Vegetable exchange—One-half cup of most vegetables (cooked or raw) has about 5 gm of carbohydrate and 2 gm of protein (25 kcal) and is considered one exchange. Raw lettuce may be taken in larger quantities, but salad dressing usually equals fat exchange. Some vegetables are higher in carbohydrate, equal to 15 gm carbohydrate and 2 gm protein, and should be considered equivalent to one bread exchange in quantity. These include: corn (1/3 cup or 1 ear), white potato (one baked or ½ cup mashed), yam or sweet potato (¼ cup), green peas (½ cup), squash (½ cup), and lima beans (½ cup).

c. Fruit exchange—One fruit exchange contains about 20 gm of carbohydrate (40 kcal) and essentially no fat or protein.

Juices	Grape juice	1/4 cup
	Apple or pineapple	1/3 cup
	Orange and grapefruit	1/2 cup

1 small apple, orange, pear, or peach; ½ banana, ½ cup berries, ¼ of a small canteloupe, 1 cup watermelon.

d. Bread exchange—One bread exchange contains about 15 gm of carbohydrate and 2 gm of protein (70 kcal). Examples are as follows:

One slice of bread, ½ hamburger or hot dog bun, ¾ cup of unsweetened cereal (the box may state the grams of carbohydrate per cup), ½ cup noodles, 3 cups popcorn; crackers (6 small saltines, 2 squares of graham cracker, 3 of most other crackers), one pancake or waffle (5″), 15 potato or corn chips.

e. Meat exchanges are wisely divided by the ADA into *lean meats, medium fat meats,* and *high fat meats.* One oz of the lean meats contains 7 gm of protein and 3 gm of fat (55 kcal). The best of the lean meats are poultry (chicken and turkey without the skin) and fish, although many roasts (beef, lamb, veal) and cottage cheese have also been placed in this group. The *medium fat* group equals one meat and ½ fat exchange and includes 1 oz of corned beef, most cuts of pork, liver and other organ meats, 1 oz of most cheeses, one egg, or 2 tbsp of peanut butter. The *high fat* meat group includes 1 oz of hamburger, most steak, spare ribs, cold cuts (one slice), hot dogs (one small), and cheddar cheese (1 oz).

f. Fat exchange—Fat is necessary for the body and is particularly important during periods of fasting (eg, overnight), when it is slowly converted to sugar. One fat exchange contains 5 gm of fat (45 kcal). The polyunsaturated fats are currently believed best for use, with one exchange equaling 1 tsp margarine or 1 tsp of any vegetable oil (except coconut). One exchange of saturated fat includes 1 tsp butter, 1 strip bacon, or 2 tbsp cream.

5. Managing hypoglycemia—It is wise for the patient to carry hard candy in case hypoglycemic symptoms are experienced. This is especially likely following unanticipated strenuous physical exertion. In certain cases, it is also advisable for the parents to be instructed in the use of glucagon to counteract hypoglycemia by giving 1 mg IM. If glucagon is used, the child must be given some easily absorbed carbohydrate as soon as possible to restore the liver glycogen. "Instant glucose" is a very viscous glucose solution obtainable in tubes from the local Diabetes Association. It can be squeezed into the cheeks of a semiconscious child and absorbed without danger of aspiration.

6. Urine testing—Patients should be told to use the early morning urine as it is voided when making estimations of urine sugar. With other specimens, the bladder should first be emptied and a second specimen, voided 15–30 minutes later, used for the actual test. In cases where control is poor, it may be helpful to take serial blood sugars over a single day as a guide to insulin adjustment and to collect a number of 24-hour urine specimens for total sugar output. Urine sugar may be estimated with sufficient accuracy for clinical purposes with Clinitest tablets and should not exceed 20 gm/sq m/24 hours. (Use 2 drops of urine and 10 drops of water and compare the color of the precipi-

tate to the chart graduated on a scale of 0–5%.) Twenty-four-hour collections should not be asked for on a school day unless this can be arranged unobtrusively with the aid of the school nurse. Glucose oxidase tapes such as Tes-Tape or Clinistix are less reliable although convenient in juvenile diabetes.

Urine samples should also be tested for acetone using Acetest papers. It is usually sufficient to do this during periods of poor control, with glycosuria.

7. Blood sugar estimations—Isolated blood sugar estimations are of limited value. However, in cases that are difficult to control, it may be very helpful to obtain blood glucose samples every 3 hours—1 hour before and 2 hours after each meal (6 hours between meals)—as well as overnight for a single 24-hour period.

Complications

Complications during the course of diabetes in children are not common. During presenting coma, extensive neurologic signs may develop, but the outlook is good. Hypoglycemia, which is also rarely a presenting symptom, may be frequent and severe enough to cause brain damage. Urinary tract infections and tuberculosis are modest special risks. Degenerative vascular disease, peripheral neuritis, and exudative retinopathy may occasionally be seen in childhood. Poorly controlled diabetes in young children over a long period may lead to a syndrome of hepatomegaly, delayed puberty, and dwarfism (Mauriac's syndrome). Emotional disturbances are common, especially in the early teen years. Vaginal candidiasis is seen occasionally.

Some children become very readily ketotic during episodes of stress. In some instances they may be helped by small doses of propranolol.

One of the commonest causes of poor control is the Somogyi phenomenon, which occurs as a result of sequential overdosage of insulin in response to occult hypoglycemia, followed by pressor amine-induced hyperglycemia spuriously interpreted as due to insufficient insulin. Treatment in this instance consists of reduction of the insulin dosage.

Both atrophy and hypertrophy of subcutaneous fat occur around injection sites. In the former the patient is instructed to use U-100 insulin or pork or single peak insulins and to inject around the site. With hypertrophy, the area should be spared for a few weeks and insulin shots widely dispersed.

Prognosis

Parents will want to know in what ways the overall life expectancy may be altered for their diabetic children. In this respect, there is now a mean expectancy of some 20 years after the onset of the disease before the onset of major complications. However, the prepubertal years do not contribute to the anticipated time of onset of these complications.

Baum JD & others: Immediate response to a low dose of insulin in children presenting with diabetes. Arch Dis Child 50:373, 1975.

Bruck E: Posthypoglycemic hyperglycemia in diabetic children.

J Pediatr 84:672, 1974.

Chase HP & others: *Understanding Juvenile Diabetes,* 3rd ed. Univ of Colo Med Ctr Press, 1977.

Drash A: The control of diabetes mellitus: Is it achievable? Is it desirable? J Pediatr 88:1074, 1976.

Drash A: Diabetes mellitus in childhood. J Pediatr 78:919, 1971.

Lee RG & others: Stunted growth and hepatomegaly. J Pediatr 91:82, 1977.

Rosenbloom AL & others: Advances in commercial insulin preparations. Am J Dis Child 128:631, 1974.

Schwarz R: Diabetic acidosis and coma. Pediatrics 47:902, 1971.

PRADER-WILLI SYNDROME

These children show obesity, short stature, and mental retardation with amyotonia in the newborn period. The males show hypogonadism. There is a tendency to develop diabetes in later childhood.

Dunn MG: The Prader-Labhart-Willi syndrome. Acta Paediatr Scand, Suppl 186, 1968.

Hall BD, Smith DW: Prader-Willi syndrome. J Pediatr 81:286, 1972.

• • •

General References

Alsever RN, Gotlin RW: *Handbook of Endocrine Tests in Adults and Children.* Year Book, 1975.

Bacon GE: *A Practical Approach to Pediatric Endocrinology.* Year Book, 1975.

Gardner LI: *Endocrine and Genetic Diseases of Childhood and Adolescence,* 2nd ed. Saunders, 1975.

Stanbury JB, Wyngaarden JB, Fredrickson DS (editors): *The Metabolic Basis of Inherited Disease,* 3rd ed. McGraw-Hill, 1972.

Vilee DB: *Human Endocrinology: A Developmental Approach.* Saunders, 1975.

Wilkins L: *The Diagnosis and Treatment of Endocrine Disorders in Childhood and Adolescence,* 3rd ed. Thomas, 1965.

Williams RH: *Textbook of Endocrinology,* 5th ed. Saunders, 1974.

25 . . .

Infections: Viral & Rickettsial

Vincent A. Fulginiti, MD

I. VIRAL INFECTIONS*

Laboratory Diagnosis

The specific etiologic diagnosis of viral infections is seldom possible on clinical grounds alone. Apart from exanthems such as measles and chickenpox and certain CNS infections (paralytic poliomyelitis and rabies), the clinical syndromes caused by different viruses frequently resemble one another. Therefore, laboratory tests are required for specific diagnosis.

The proper collection, shipping, and identification of specimens are essential to adequate diagnosis. In the discussions of specific viral diseases which follow are listed the specimens to be submitted, special procedures in handling and shipping such specimens (where applicable), and what information the physician can expect from the viral diagnostic laboratory.

General considerations which apply to the diagnosis of viral diseases are as follows:

(1) Viral diagnosis usually depends upon isolation of the offending agent or demonstration of the host response on the basis of a rising titer of specific serum antibody (or both).

(2) Specimens for isolation of viruses consist of appropriate body fluids, secretions, or tissue. An adequate sample can usually be obtained by swabbing the appropriate orifice or mucous membrane and immersing the swab immediately in media designed to protect the agent during shipping and handling—usually a mixture of salts and protein which can be supplied by the laboratory. (Veal infusion broth with 0.5% albumin or Hank's balanced salt solution is adequate.) It is almost always necessary to freeze the specimen immediately and keep it frozen until it reaches the laboratory. (Respiratory syncytial virus and cytomegalovirus may be destroyed by freezing and must be kept on ordinary ice during transport.)

(3) Viral antibody titration depends upon the collection of paired sera—a first ("acute") specimen collected as early as possible in the course of the illness and a second ("convalescent") serum collected usually 2–4 weeks later. Accurate serologic diagnosis depends upon aseptic direct venipuncture, careful separation of

*For prevention, see Chapter 5.

serum to avoid hemolysis, and maintenance in the frozen state until receipt in the laboratory.

(4) "Quick" diagnostic technics are available for some viral infections, eg, fluorescent antibody diagnosis of rabies, inclusion body identification in herpetic, vaccinial, and varicella infections. In general, these are presumptive tests which require confirmation by means of more elaborate technics.

Lennette EH, Schmidt NJ: *Diagnostic Procedures for Viral and Rickettsial Diseases,* 5th ed. American Public Health Association, Inc, 1974.

POXVIRUSES

VARIOLA*
(Smallpox)

Essentials of Diagnosis

- History of contact with smallpox patient within past 2 weeks (Ethiopia or Somalia).
- Severe prodrome with high fever, severe backache, and prostration.
- Occasionally a "swimming trunk" rash, centrifugal in distribution, that lasts 3 days.
- Secondary rise in temperature.
- Typical rash appears on third to fifth days, beginning on the face and distal extremities and spreading centrally. Macules progress rapidly to papules, vesicles, umbilication, pustules, and crusts in 3 weeks.
- Early hemorrhagic form may only have prodrome and purpura (no rash).

General Considerations

All ages are susceptible. Immunity following vaccination varies with the interval from last successful

*Smallpox has now been virtually eliminated, occurring only in Ethiopia and Somalia. This description is included until the disease is totally eradicated.

vaccination. Vaccination confers virtually complete protection for 1 year, but protection diminishes progressively to nil by 20 years.

A minor form of the disease with lessened mortality rate has been noted in some parts of the world in the past (variola minor, alastrim), although the virus causing this type is indistinguishable from that of smallpox.

Clinical Findings

A. History: A history of prior contact and vaccination status is essential. The incubation period is usually 11–12 days, but it can vary from 7–21 days. No illness is usually apparent until the prodrome, but a nonspecific flu-like "illness of contact" is occasionally noted shortly after exposure. Reported "successful" vaccination should be corroborated by observation of a scar.

B. Symptoms and Signs:

1. Prodrome–The onset of the illness is abrupt, with a sudden rise in temperature to 40–40.6° C (104–105° F), severe backache, and extreme prostration. This prodromal period lasts 2–4 days. A morbilliform eruption may occur in the groin and lower abdomen (swimming trunk rash) during the prodrome.

2. Rash–The typical rash heralding the disease appears on the third to fifth day. It begins on the face, wrists, and ankles and spreads over the extremities. At first, erythematous macules appear, each of which becomes a papule, then a vesicle, and finally a pustule, often with umbilication. The course in a given patient may vary, but the rash usually progresses for 7–14 days after its first appearance. Encrustation and a scar result, particularly with secondary bacterial infection. Mucosal lesions are seen at the time of appearance of the skin rash. Corneal infection may occur.

The more fulminant forms of the disease are associated with a confluent rash; the less severe forms with discrete or even minimal rash.

3. Hemorrhagic smallpox–Hemorrhage may appear in the prodrome in "early" hemorrhagic disease, and death occurs before the pocks appear. A "late" hemorrhagic form is recognized in which hemorrhage occurs into established typical smallpox lesions.

C. Laboratory Findings: Leukopenia occurs early, but leukocytosis is more common by the time the disease is recognizable. Other hematologic abnormalities may be expected, with bleeding, bacterial superinfection, and electrolyte imbalance.

Hemorrhagic disease (early) is associated with accelerator globulin deficiency, depression of prothrombin, and marked thrombocytopenia. Late hemorrhagic disease is accompanied by thrombocytopenia.

Virus may be isolated in relatively high titer from the blood and papules early in the disease. In hemorrhagic forms, viremia is persistent until death.

Rapid diagnosis may be accomplished by light microscopic identification of elementary bodies (Gutstein stain), electron microscopic visualization of virus, fluorescent antibody staining of virus antigen in infected cells, and by identification of virus by precipi-

tation with antisera in agar or by fixation of complement. The best source of material for all of these tests is scrapings from the base of a papule collected with a sharp No. 11 scalpel blade after light cleansing with alcohol. The scrapings and swabs (collected simultaneously) may be shipped dry to the laboratory or, where available, in appropriate virologic material (veal infusion broth or Hank's balanced salt solution with added antibiotics). Freezing during transit is desirable but not essential. Bacterial cultures should be obtained.

The diagnosis of smallpox has taken on added significance since compulsory routine vaccination has been abolished. Many physicians in practice today are unfamiliar with the disease and with the requisite laboratory diagnostic tests. Introduction of smallpox from the 2 remaining endemic areas in the world (Ethiopia and Somalia) could result in small epidemics unless the first cases were diagnosed promptly and effective therapeutic measures taken. For these reasons, the Center for Disease Control (CDC) in Atlanta maintains a constantly available team to provide diagnostic assistance and therapeutic advice. Physicians familiar with the disease can be dispatched rapidly to any part of the country. The physician who encounters a suspected case should not postpone seeking this expert help. Even if doubtful, any case in which smallpox is considered in the differential diagnosis warrants notification by phone call to the CDC.

D. X-Ray Findings: X-rays may help in the diagnosis of pneumonia and osteomyelitis.

Differential Diagnosis

The prodrome is frequently confused with dengue, enterovirus infections, and almost any febrile illness. The prodromal rash may be confused with that of measles. A history of contact and isolation of virus from the blood establish the diagnosis.

Hemorrhagic smallpox must be distinguished from meningococcemia, coagulation disorders, typhus, and other acute hemorrhagic exanthems.

Eruptive smallpox is often mistaken for varicella. In smallpox, the rash has a centrifugal distribution, all lesions are in the same stage of development, and there is a history of a febrile prodrome and of contact with a case of smallpox within the past 3 weeks.

Complications & Sequelae

Virus multiplication in tissues other than skin results in keratitis and blindness, laryngeal ulceration and edema, encephalitis, pneumonia, and osteomyelitis. Acute psychoses and orchitis have been reported also. Secondary bacterial infection of the skin, abscess formation, and septicemia are common. Bronchial pneumonia is common later in the course.

Prevention

Routine smallpox vaccination is no longer recommended. Prevention of the disease in exposed susceptibles can be achieved with methisazone (Marboran) given during the incubation period (see p 1043) and with vaccinia immune gamma globulin.

Treatment & Prognosis

Give supportive care, with attention to shock, blood replacement, and fluid and electrolyte balance. Appropriate antibacterial therapy should be employed when bacterial superinfection occurs.

The overall mortality rate in smallpox is 25%, but this is because fulminating and hemorrhagic diseases are almost universally fatal, whereas discrete smallpox is rarely fatal (1% or less). Recovery is usually complete in survivors, although postencephalitic symptoms and osteomyelitis may prolong convalescence.

Kempe CH: Smallpox. In: *The Biologic Basis of Pediatric Practice.* Cooke R (editor). McGraw-Hill, 1969.
Mack TM: Smallpox in Europe, 1950–1971. J Infect Dis 125:161, 1972.

COMPLICATIONS OF SMALLPOX VACCINATION

Essentials of Diagnosis

- History of recent vaccination.
- Typical vaccinial vesicles in sites other than vaccination area.
- Lack of healing of primary vaccination site after 15 days.
- Rash, corneal ulceration, and CNS symptoms following vaccination.
- Personal or family history of serious infections or hematologic or immunologic disease.

General Considerations

In most individuals, dermal vaccination results in a predictable, benign, local skin infection beginning on the third postinoculation day as a papule, progressing to vesiculation, forming a pustule, scabbing, and ultimately scarring during the next 3 weeks. In a few patients, untoward reactions occur which can be classified as shown in Table 25–1. As can be seen, most complications are infections, and many occur because of poor selection of vaccinees (immunologic deficiency states, malignancies, eczema, etc) or poor or ill-advised local care of the vaccination site.

Clinical Findings

Findings vary with specific complications. Important elements are the history of recent vaccination, excessive trauma in the preparation of the vaccination site, bathing during the "take," manipulation or irritation of the site, the prior presence of a bacterial respiratory or skin infection, allergic conjunctivitis, and prior or concurrent inflammatory skin lesions (eczema, burns, pyoderma, exanthems, etc).

A. Symptoms and Signs of Specific Complications:

1. Noninfectious rashes—Macular, maculopapular, or vesicular rashes of presumed "allergic" or "hypersensitivity" origin have been noted at the height of the primary take (7–14 days). The rash may be localized or generalized, and is usually intensely erythematous and associated with a marked degree of erythema and induration surrounding the normal-appearing primary site. Pruritus and excoriation may be present. This is not an infective complication, and virus is not recoverable from the rash. No complications are observed.

2. Bacterial superinfection—This usually occurs in a child with recurrent or concurrent streptococcal respiratory infection. It may also be associated with skin infections (streptococcal or staphylococcal) elsewhere on the body. Manipulation of the primary vaccination causes seeding of the bacteria. Examination reveals an impetiginous vaccination site, and lifting a corner of the scab allows a thin, serous exudate to escape which on bacteriologic examination with

Table 25–1. Complications of vaccination.

Major Category	Specific Syndromes
Noninfectious rashes	"Erythema multiforme," macular ("toxic eruption"), maculopapular
	Vesicular, urticarial (cf generalized)
Bacterial superinfection	Streptococcal, staphylococcal, mixed
	Tetanus, syphilis
Vaccination by abnormal route	Intramuscular, oral, etc
Accidental inoculation (may occur in vaccinated individual or be acquired by contact with vaccinated individual)	Into normal skin, but more often into abnormal skin—eg, burns, pyoderma, exanthem, eczema; other dermatitides—eg, varicella, herpes
	Mucosal (usually oral or conjunctival)
	Corneal (keratitis)
Congenital vaccinia	Disseminated infection
Generalized vaccinia	Benign or progressive ("malignant")
Progressive vaccinia	In hypogammaglobulinemic (congenital X-linked, thymic alymphoplasia)
	In dysgammaglobulinemia
	With malignancies (chronic lymphatic leukemia, Hodgkin's lymphoma, etc)
Encephalitis	Postvaccinial
Unusual	Hemolytic anemia, arthritis and osteomyelitis, laboratory infections, pericarditis and myocarditis

Gram's stain is seen to contain many cocci and which on culture yields a profuse growth of streptococci or staphylococci (or both). Secondary lesions may be noted near the primary site or elsewhere.

3. Accidental inoculation—"Secondary" lesions may occur anywhere on the body at the time of or shortly after the vesiculopustular stage of vaccination, but are most frequent on exposed surfaces (nares, face, periorbital regions, extremities). If the child has been bathed, the diaper area may be involved. The individual lesions resemble a primary vaccination, and virus may be recovered from them.

Significant areas may become involved if the skin was previously abnormal. Thus, life-threatening vaccinia virus spread occurs in eczema (eczema vaccinatum), severe burns, and extensive dermatitides. The secondary lesions resemble primary vaccinations, but they are modified by the underlying disease and their atypical appearance may cause a delay in diagnosis. A history of contact with a recently vaccinated individual may lead to rapid diagnosis. Fever may be marked, and secondary bacterial infection with purulent drainage may occur. Virus is recoverable from the skin, and failure to detect serum antibody 1 week or more after onset is a grave prognostic sign.

Accidental inoculation of the conjunctivas is manifest by intense inflammation characterized by increased vascularity, pannus formation, and occasionally by a purulent exudate. If keratitis occurs, cloudiness of the cornea, severe photophobia and pain, and a fluorescein-stainable ulcer are noted.

4. Congenital vaccinia—This rare complication may occur following vaccination of a pregnant woman or contact of a pregnant woman with a vaccinated individual. Death in utero or massive, generalized infection of the infant with multiple cutaneous lesions may occur and may be fatal.

5. Generalized vaccinia—Blood-borne spread of vaccinia virus results in typical "pocks" on normal skin in an individual with a normal-appearing primary "take." The vaccination response is generally at its height (6–8 days). Virus can be recovered from the secondary lesions, and serum antibody, although it may be delayed, is produced in normal amounts.

6. Progressive vaccinia (vaccinia necrosa or gangrenosa)—Failure of the primary vaccination site to heal after 2 weeks establishes the diagnosis of progressive vaccinia. Bacterial infection must be ruled out, but the diagnosis should not be unduly delayed. The primary lesion fails to resolve normally, and slow progression at the margin with a "soft" vesicular border is observed. Central necrosis may be pronounced. Small "satellite" lesions may appear in uninoculated skin surrounding the primary site or at a distance from it. They resemble a primary take at first, but each progresses as does the primary. With delayed diagnosis, large areas of skin become involved and extensive peripheral spread is noted. The child usually remains well, with little fever or systemic signs. Secondary bacterial infection, usually due to gram-negative organisms, occurs late.

Virus is recovered in high titer from all skin lesions. Serum antibody is usually absent. No skin reaction at 24–48 hours is noted following intradermal injection of killed vaccinia virus. Other findings include those of the underlying disease (decreased serum globulins in hypogammaglobulinemia, abnormal peripheral blood and bone marrow in leukemia, etc).

7. Postvaccinial encephalitis—Following primary vaccination by 10–13 days, headache, vomiting, and drowsiness may herald encephalitis. Physical findings include cranial nerve palsies, coma, spastic paralysis, and occasionally nuchal rigidity. CSF pleocytosis (lymphocytic) and increased CSF protein are usually observed. Virus is usually not recoverable from CSF or autopsy material.

B. Laboratory Findings: Definitive diagnosis of the infectious complications depends upon isolation or other identification of vaccinia virus (complement-fixing, hemagglutinating, precipitating antigens) from skin lesions. This is best accomplished by scrapings or swab specimens from the base of a scalpel-denuded papular or vesicular lesion. Identification of virus in blood can be accomplished in progressive vaccinia.

Determination of the immune response of the host is also important in the diagnosis. Intradermal injection of 0.1 ml of heat-inactivated vaccinia virus produces a delayed type skin response in normal vaccinees. This reaction is absent in patients with progressive vaccinia.

Serum neutralizing antibody can almost never be detected in progressive vaccinia or in overwhelming eczema vaccinatum.

Underlying diseases such as hypogammaglobulinemia, leukemia, etc should be investigated by appropriate laboratory tests. Bacterial infections are identified by standard bacteriologic technics utilizing material from pustules, blood specimens, or other appropriate materials.

Prevention

Smallpox vaccination is no longer recommended for children. (See Chapter 5.)

Treatment

Vaccinia immune globulin (VIG) is now available both from the Center for Disease Control (CDC) in Atlanta and from a commercial source. In serious complications, the physician is advised to obtain the free consultation available from the CDC panel of experts *before* instituting therapy, especially the administration of VIG. Diagnostic and therapeutic errors can be avoided by such consultation. Often the disease is masked without being cured by VIG and diagnosis is thus made much more difficult. On occasion, VIG is contraindicated or another therapy is preferred. The very infrequency of complications in any single physician's practice is a strong indication for expert consultation in any severe condition suspected of being secondary or related to smallpox vaccination.

A. Hypersensitivity Reactions: Use of antihistamines, starch baths, and sedation aid in control of severe pruritus.

B. Bacterial Superinfection: Appropriate antibiotic therapy based upon bacteriologic findings is indicated.

C. Accidental Inoculation: Most cases require no therapy. With lesions around the eyes or in areas exposed to trauma and moisture, the use of vaccinia immune globulin (VIG), 0.3–0.6 ml/kg body weight, may result in more rapid healing.

Eczema vaccinatum or any extensive infection of skin in patients with no immunologic defect may respond to VIG, 0.6–1 ml/kg. With lack of serum antibody and overwhelming infection, higher doses of VIG (up to 10 ml/kg), methisazone (see Progressive Vaccinia, below), or exchange transfusion may be helpful.

D. Congenital Vaccinia: If the pregnant woman has been vaccinated, VIG is indicated to help prevent viremic spread to the fetus.

E. Generalized Vaccinia: No therapy is usually necessary.

F. Progressive Vaccinia: Because of the slowly progressive nature of this illness and because the mortality rate without treatment is 100%, all patients should be treated in centers experienced with this complication. Massive amounts of VIG may be necessary. Experiments have shown that methisazone (Marboran) in a dosage of 200 mg/kg orally immediately followed by 200 mg/kg/day in 4 divided doses for 3 days is of value in 50% of cases. Repeated exchange transfusions with blood from a recently vaccinated donor may be beneficial.

Prognosis

If recovery occurs, it is usually complete. This is especially true of those complications that do not constitute a threat to life. In progressive vaccinia, the mortality rate is 100% without therapy and 30% or less with current therapy. Eczema vaccinatum is occasionally fatal despite therapy.

The mortality rate in postvaccinial encephalitis is 30–40%; residual neurologic damage is frequent in survivors.

Sequelae include blindness (keratitis), neurologic handicap (encephalitis), scarring (bacterial infection), and osteomyelitis (progressive vaccinia).

Douglas RG & others: Treatment of progressive vaccinia. Arch Intern Med 129:980, 1972.
Fulginiti VA, Kempe CH: Poxvirus diseases. Chap 25 in: *Practice of Pediatrics.* Vol 2. Brennemann-Kelley, Prior, 1970.
Kempe CH: The end of smallpox vaccination in the United States. Pediatrics 49:489, 1972.
Neff JM & others: Complications of smallpox vaccination, U.S., 1963. Pediatrics 39:916, 1967.

MOLLUSCUM CONTAGIOSUM

The typical lesions of this uncommon viral infection are white to pink, pearly, hard, rapidly maturing asymptomatic papules which umbilicate and extrude a central core of friable exudate. The most common sites are the face, back, arms, and buttocks. The incubation period is believed to be 2 weeks.

A history of contact is not usually present in sporadic cases, but outbreaks have been observed in schools or institutions. The histologic picture is diagnostic. Prickle cells of the epithelium undergo degeneration, and round hyaline cytoplasmic masses are seen (molluscum bodies, or Henderson-Paterson inclusions). Virus isolation is possible but not readily available.

Molluscum contagiosum is rarely confused with other lesions. Solitary lesions must be distinguished from malignancies.

Surgical excision is rarely necessary. Incision or cautery, usually chemical–or both incision and cautery–is successful in eradicating lesions. Podophyllum resin, silver nitrate, trichloroacetic acid, and phenol have all been used successfully.

Molluscum contagiosum is usually a self-limited, benign disease. Autoinoculation (rare) results in hundreds of lesions and a chronic course.

Overfield TK, Brody JA: An epidemiological study of molluscum contagiosum. J Pediatr 69:640, 1966.
Rosenberg EW, Yusk JW: Molluscum contagiosum: Eruption following treatment with prednisone and methotrexate. Arch Dermatol 101:439, 1970.

MYXOVIRUSES

INFLUENZA

Except in major epidemics, clinical identification of influenzal infection may be impossible. Influenza is mimicked by other respiratory viral infections. "Flu" syndrome seen in adults is uncommon in children.

Virus isolation is both possible and desirable. Increase in serum antibody is valuable in identifying epidemics.

Influenza viruses cause sporadic clinical illness in infants and children in nonepidemic infections which account for 5–10% of all serious respiratory infections. Most frequent is the upper respiratory infection (URI) syndrome, although croup, bronchiolitis, and pneumonia also occur. During epidemics, a sudden onset of fever and "toxic" symptoms may accompany respiratory manifestations.

In 1976, an influenza isolate with the antigenic characteristics of the swine influenza type A variant was responsible for a localized outbreak of disease in Fort Dix, New Jersey. In the following year, extensive surveillance failed to detect another focus. Since the swine variant is believed to be the cause of the 1917–1918 pandemic, a massive campaign was undertaken to immunize the entire American public. Plagued by technical production problems, by problems in determining liability, and by the unexpected occurrence of Guillain-Barré syndrome in vaccinees, the effort was finally abandoned.

It is not known if swine influenza will recur; current vaccines do not contain this type of A antigen. USPHS, WHO, and others will continue their surveillance efforts through the 1978–1979 seasons.

Reye's syndrome (encephalopathy with fatty degeneration of the viscera) has recently occurred in epidemic fashion closely paralleling influenza type B epidemics. Other viral agents—notably varicella—had previously been implicated in the etiology of this syndrome. The exact relationship between influenza virus and Reye's syndrome is unclear. If an upper respiratory infection is followed by excessive vomiting and convulsions, one should consider this diagnosis. Coma, hypoglycemia, and liver dysfunction are later confirmatory findings. (See Chapter 17 for details of the diagnosis and treatment of Reye's syndrome.)

Clinical Findings

A. History: The history is compatible with various types of respiratory infections of "viral" nature. A history of the same illness in other members of the family or school group, or more severe illness in younger siblings, can often be obtained.

B. Symptoms and Signs: There are no distinguishing clinical characteristics except the abrupt onset of high fever and "toxic" symptoms which are in contrast to most other respiratory viruses. Influenza C virus has been associated with the croup syndrome in infants.

C. Laboratory Findings: The usual laboratory tests are of little help. Specific diagnosis depends upon isolation of virus from respiratory secretions. A swab of nasopharyngeal or throat secretions should be sent in appropriate media to the laboratory. Paired sera obtained early in the course of the illness and after 2–3 weeks are of value in retrospective diagnosis. Early identification of virus type is important in control of epidemics by immunization.

D. X-Ray Findings: Chest x-rays may reveal extensive bronchial pneumonia or simply hyperaeration.

Differential Diagnosis

This is primarily an etiologic differential diagnosis since many viruses produce the same syndrome. With croup, it is important to differentiate from *Haemophilus influenzae* epiglottitis (cherry-red epiglottis, severe systemic illness, positive throat and blood cultures) and spasmodic or allergic croup (history of early respiratory symptoms or fever), obstructive croup (history of choking or gagging on food, x-ray demonstration of foreign body or its effects).

Complications & Sequelae

Pneumonia may be followed by bacterial superinfections (particularly staphylococcal), with empyema, pyopneumothorax, etc. Croup may be associated with drying of the tracheal mucous membranes (with subsequent encrustation and obstruction), cardiac arrest, subcutaneous or mediastinal emphysema, and pneumothorax.

Prevention

Amantadine (Symmetrel), may reduce the risk of influenza due to type A_2 if administered prior to infection. The dosage is as follows: 1–9 years: 4–9 mg/kg/day (do not exceed 150 mg/day) in 2 or 3 doses; 9–12 years: 200 mg/day in 2 doses (total dose).

Influenza vaccine is discussed in Chapter 5.

Treatment

Supportive measures are critical, especially in croup. Support of the airway, judicial tracheostomy, and attention to hydration and nutrition and to peripheral cardiovascular integrity may be lifesaving. (Croup is discussed further in Chapter 12.)

Prognosis

In general, complete recovery is the rule. Children—particularly young infants with croup—may die from cardiac arrest or other complications. Tracheostomy may prolong convalescence and require care beyond the period of acute infection.

Brocklebank JT & others: Influenza A infection in children. Lancet 2:497, 1972.

Douglas RG Jr: Influenza: The disease and its complications. Hosp Pract 11:43, Dec 1976.

Glezen WP: Influenza prophylaxis for children. Am J Dis Child 131:628, 1977.

Hall CE & others: The Seattle virus watch. 4. Comparative epidemiologic observations of infections with influenza A and B viruses, 1965–1969, in families with young children. Am J Epidemiol 98:365, 1973.

Lindsay MI & others: Hong Kong influenza. JAMA 214:1825, 1970.

Linnemann CC & others: Reye's syndrome: Epidemiologic and viral studies, 1963–1974. Am J Epidemiol 101:517, 1975.

Wright PF & others: Influenza A infections in young children. N Engl J Med 296:829, 1977.

PARAINFLUENZA

The parainfluenza viruses are among the more important respiratory viruses in childhood because they cause croup and upper respiratory illness. Parainfluenza type 3 is most important very early in life, as most 1-year-old infants have been infected. The history, differential diagnosis, complications, and treatment are as for influenza (see above).

Although it is difficult to distinguish parainfluenza infections from other respiratory viral illness, the presence of hoarseness suggests this etiology. This is particularly true if one member of the family has croup and the others upper respiratory infection with hoarseness. Viral diagnosis is feasible, and identification of group and type is possible by laboratory examination of secretions and by antibody titration.

Recovery is the rule. Reinfection is common, but second infections tend to be less severe and with less fever.

Cooney MK & others: The Seattle virus watch. 6. Infections with parainfluenza, mumps, and respiratory syncytial viruses and *Mycoplasma pneumoniae*. Am J Epidemiol 101:532, 1975.

MUMPS

Essentials of Diagnosis

- History of exposure 14–21 days previously.
- Unilateral or bilateral parotid gland swelling.
- Aseptic meningitis with or without parotitis.
- Pancreatitis, orchitis, oophoritis (or combination).

General Considerations

Mumps is a common childhood infection which is asymptomatic in 30–40% of cases. Most children are infected, and lifetime immunity results. A few remain susceptible throughout adolescence and adult life, when parotitis with orchitis may occur.

Clinical Findings

A. History: Contact results in infection 14–21 days later. Only 60–70% of cases develop symptoms, and bilateral (or unilateral) painful swelling of the parotid glands is usually the only manifestation of the disease. Parotitis may be accompanied by mild respiratory symptoms. Occasionally, CNS symptoms appear prior to or in the absence of parotid gland involvement. Abdominal pain is a frequent complaint and may represent pancreatic involvement.

Recently, mumps virus pancreatitis has been suggested as a precursor of juvenile diabetes mellitus. Most of the evidence is epidemiologic, ie, a correlation between the incidence of mumps and of diabetes in children within 2–4 years. Specific data linking mumps virus infection of the pancreas and subsequent diabetes mellitus are lacking.

B. Symptoms and Signs:

1. Parotitis or salivary gland form—Smooth, tender enlargement of the affected salivary gland or glands is the most common finding. Lymphedema of the face is frequently present also and makes the swelling indistinct at its margins. Obliteration of the angle of the mandible is a useful diagnostic sign, as is the alignment of the fusiform swelling with the line formed by the long axis of the ear and the ramus of the mandible. Upward and lateral displacement of the earlobe is noted. The opening of Stensen's duct may be pointed and reddened.

Submaxillary or sublingual gland involvement produces swelling in the lateral and anterior aspects of the neck, respectively. Both are palpated just beneath the mandible and may appear to be fused with it as a result of surrounding lymphedema.

Systemic symptoms may consist of high fever and headache or mild respiratory symptoms or may be absent.

2. Meningoencephalitis—Mumps virus is the most common cause of aseptic meningitis in childhood. CSF pleocytosis is said to occur in 10–50% of all cases of mumps, although overt clinical symptoms are less common.

Aseptic meningitis may be accompanied by, may precede, or may occur in the absence of parotitis. Fever and headache increase, nuchal rigidity is noted, and gastrointestinal symptoms (nausea and vomiting) may occur. CNS irritability is uncommon, and convulsions are rare. Recovery is rapid, with symptoms subsiding in 3–10 days, almost always without sequelae.

3. Pancreatitis—Mild to moderate abdominal pain may be present in the parotitic form of mumps. When severe epigastric pain occurs in association with nausea, persistent vomiting, high fever, chills, and severe prostration, pancreatitis should be suspected.

4. Orchitis or oophoritis—The gonads may be involved in postpubertal individuals with sudden onset of fever, chills, systemic symptoms, and testicular (males) or lower abdominal pain (females). Testicular swelling and extreme pain occur. Symptoms subside in 3–14 days, with abdominal tenderness being most persistent.

5. Other glandular involvement—Rarely, overt inflammation of the thyroid, Bartholin's glands, and breasts may be seen.

6. Endocardial fibroelastosis and subacute thyroiditis have recently been said to be due to mumps virus infection, but the association has not been proved.

C. Laboratory Findings: In almost 75% of patients, serum amylase levels rise in proportion to the glandular swelling. Return to normal values occurs in 2–3 weeks. CSF pleocytosis with lymphocytosis (often 500–1000 cells/cu mm) is associated with elevated CSF protein and normal CSF glucose values.

Mumps virus may be isolated from saliva, the pharynx, or urine and, in cases of aseptic meningitis, from the CSF. A 4-fold rise in serum antibody titer is diagnostic and is particularly useful in the diagnosis of nonsalivary gland forms of the disease. Serum should be collected as early as possible in the clinical course and again in 2 weeks.

The mumps virus skin test is an unreliable indicator of prior mumps virus infection and should not be relied upon in the diagnosis or differential diagnosis of mumps.

Differential Diagnosis

The glandular forms of the disease must be distinguished from other acute causes of swelling in the neck: cervical lymphadenitis (location; coexistence of pharyngeal, tonsillar, or skin infection; leukocytosis with shift to the left; discreteness, absence of serum amylase elevation), acute suppurative parotitis (local inflammation, unilateral involvement, leukocytosis, purulent secretion from salivary duct), acute obstructive parotitis (visualization of calculus in the duct, history of previous episodes), other viral parotitides (coxsackievirus and lymphocytic choriomeningitis virus infections, distinguishable by virologic methods), acute lymphoma or lymphosarcoma (painless enlargement, involvement of lymph nodes, bone marrow findings), and acute episodes of recurrent parotitis (history of previous episodes; sialography reveals sialectasia).

Pancreatitis and oophoritis may be confused with other causes of acute abdominal pain such as a ruptured viscus, acute appendicitis (especially in females with right-sided oophoritis), peptic ulcer, etc. A history of exposure to mumps, a high degree of suspicion, and serum amylase elevation all contribute to accurate diagnosis.

Meningoencephalitis occurring in the absence of parotitis must be distinguished from all other causes. This can usually be done by means of laboratory evaluation.

Complications

Rare sequelae of meningoencephalitis include deafness (auditory nerve damage), postinfectious encephalitis syndrome or myelitis, and facial neuritis.

Contrary to common belief, mumps orchitis and oophoritis do not result in sterility. Most often it is unilateral, and even with bilateral infection total atrophy of the gonads is unlikely.

Mumps myocarditis, arthritis, and hepatitis are rare.

Treatment

Control of fever, pain, and discomfort is occasionally necessary. Orchitis is best treated by conservative management, with rest, testicular support, and analgesics, although some physicians favor systemic corticosteroid therapy, which may result in more rapid subsidence of testicular swelling. Surgical intervention and hormonal therapy appear to offer no advantages. To prevent orchitis, administration of mumps hyperimmune gamma globulin appears to be effective in reducing the incidence by 75%. Several commercial preparations are available.

Prognosis

Mumps is usually a self-limited infection lasting approximately 1 week in all forms. Recovery is spontaneous and complete, and sequelae are rare. Immunity is lifelong. Episodes of parotitis after mumps infection are due to other causes.

Azimi PH & others: Mumps meningoencephalitis in children. JAMA 207:509, 1969.

Dufour FD & others: Correlation between the potency of mumps virus skin test antigen and cutaneous delayed hypersensitivity. J Pediatr 81:742, 1972.

Johnstone JA & others: Meningitis and encephalitis associated with mumps infection: A 10-year survey. Arch Dis Child 47:647, 1972.

Levitt LP & others: Mumps in a general population. Am J Dis Child 120:134, 1970.

Modlin JF & others: Current status of mumps in the United States. J Infect Dis 132:106, 1975.

St. Geme JW & others: Immunologic significance of the mumps virus skin test in infants, children, and adults. Am J Epidemiol 101:253, 1975.

Shultz HA & others: Is mumps virus an etiologic factor in juvenile diabetes mellitus? J Pediatr 86:654, 1975.

RESPIRATORY SYNCYTIAL VIRUS (RSV) DISEASE

Essentials of Diagnosis

- Bronchiolitis in very young infants is probably due to RSV.
- Illnesses are indistinguishable from other respiratory viral diseases (see Influenza).

General Considerations

RSV is the single most important cause of viral respiratory disease in infants and children, accounting for nearly 40% of all serious respiratory illnesses and for almost 70% of all cases of bronchiolitis. Children are infected early in life, and by age 1 most have acquired antibody. RSV infection appears to occur even when serum neutralizing antibody is present, and reinfection is common.

Clinical Findings

A. **History:** (See also Influenza.) A history of preceding upper respiratory symptoms is frequent in RSV infections, which then progress to lower tract disease. Fever is a more frequent finding in RSV infection than in other myxovirus diseases. Apneic episodes have been described in the course of RSV infections in premature and young infants.

B. **Symptoms and Signs:**

1. **Upper respiratory infections**—Nonspecific symptoms of rhinitis, nasal stuffiness, and bronchitis. Cough and fever may be more frequent with RSV infections.

2. **Bronchiolitis**—Dyspnea and, frequently, severe respiratory distress, usually associated with copious, occasionally thick nasal and pharyngeal secretions, are the principal manifestations. Hyperaeration of lungs occurs, with fine rales and marked expiratory wheezing. Fever may be high. Retractions may be evident, and severe respiratory effort is a frequent finding.

3. **Bronchial pneumonia**—Dyspnea and tachypnea are evident. Rales may or may not be present. Expiratory wheezing is not part of the picture of bronchial pneumonia.

C. **Laboratory Findings:** Virologic diagnosis depends upon isolation of RSV or demonstration of 4-fold antibody rise in paired sera. Throat or nasopharyngeal swabs placed in appropriate media and kept cold but not frozen are essential. Freezing may destroy the virus.

D. X-Ray Findings: In bronchiolitis, generalized hyperaeration is often quite marked, with depression of the diaphragm, precardiac and retrosternal hyper-aerated lungs, and diminished respiratory excursion on fluoroscopy. Pneumonia results in a similar pattern to a less marked degree. Patchy, diffuse peripheral infiltrates may be seen with both but are more prominent in pneumonia.

Differential Diagnosis

The differentiation between RSV and other respiratory viral infections can only be made by laboratory identification of the virus. Clues to RSV infection include wheezing, fever, and cough, which are prominent in RSV infection but may occur with other types of infection also. Bronchiolitis must be distinguished from pneumonia (lack of expiratory wheezing, prominence of pulmonary infiltrates) and allergic asthma (history of recurrence, family history, other signs or symptoms of atopy). Aspiration of a foreign body is characterized by a history of unilateral emphysema and endoscopic visualization; cystic fibrosis is diagnosed on the basis of sweat chloride determination, family history, and a history of meconium ileus or gastrointestinal symptoms.

Complications

Secondary bacterial infection may occur. Cardiac failure is a rare complication.

Treatment

Maintenance of airway and oxygenation is critical, and may be lifesaving in bronchiolitis. Cold vapor produced by bubbling oxygen through water should be administered by means of a croup tent. Hydration—usually by administration of intravenous fluids, since patients handle feedings poorly and may aspirate oral liquids—is essential. Expectorants have been used but seem less satisfactory than moist oxygen. If cardiac failure develops, administer digitalis.

Less well documented therapeutic attempts include administration of epinephrine (0.1 ml of 1:1000 solution subcut) or aminophylline (5 mg/kg IV every 6 hours), intravenous administration of hydrocortisone (25 mg every 6 hours), tracheostomy, and intermittent positive pressure breathing. Controlled trials have not shown these methods of therapy to be superior to good nursing care with attention to oxygenation and moist air.

Antibiotics have also been advocated, but there is no rationale for their use.

Prognosis

Bronchiolitis is rarely fatal, and recovery is usually complete. Respiratory symptoms and signs, cough, and wheezing may persist or may recur with subsequent respiratory infections whether or not they are due to RSV. There is some evidence linking RSV bronchiolitis to subsequent asthma.

Beem M: Repeated infections with respiratory syncytial virus. J Immunol 98:1115, 1967.

Bruhn F, Mokrohisky ST, McIntosh K: Apnea associated with respiratory syncytial virus infection in young infants. J Pediatr 90:382, 1977.

Bruhn F, Yeager AS: Respiratory syncytial virus in early infancy. Am J Dis Child 131:145, 1977.

Glezen WP & others: Epidemiologic patterns of acute lower respiratory disease of children in a pediatric group practice. J Pediatr 78:397, 1971.

Hall CB, Douglas RG: Clinically useful method for the isolation of respiratory syncytial virus. J Infect Dis 131:1, 1975.

Kim HW & others: Clinical and immunological response of infants and children to administration of low temperature adapted respiratory syncytial virus. Pediatrics 48:745, 1971.

MEASLES
(Rubeola)

Essentials of Diagnosis

- History of exposure 9–14 days previously.
- Three-day prodrome consisting of fever, conjunctivitis, coryza, and cough.
- Koplik's spots—pathognomonic small whitish specks on a red base on buccal mucous membranes—appear 1–2 days before rash.
- Maculopapular, confluent rash begins at hairline and spreads downward over the face and body in 3 days.
- Leukopenia. Multinucleated giant cells (Warthin-Finkeldey cells) in oral and nasal scrapings.

General Considerations

Measles is an acute, highly contagious disease usually affecting preschool children. Over 95% of persons are infected prior to age 15. Immunity is solid and lifelong.

Clinical Findings

A. History: A history of contact can usually be elicited and is particularly important in sporadic episodes. During epidemics, contact may be frequent and usually is with another member of the family.

B. Symptoms and Signs: After an incubation period of 9–14 days, the illness begins with high fever and lassitude, which persist and are accompanied in the next 3 days by increasing cough, coryza, and conjunctivitis. The cough is barking and harsh, and more noticeable at night. Severe conjunctival inflammation may be present, and photophobia is common. Preceding or accompanying the rash, Koplik's spots appear as small white specks on an intensely red base. Koplik's spots may be absent, but when present are pathognomonic of measles. They may be few in number or may involve the entire buccal mucous membrane, and occasionally are seen on the nasal mucous membranes also. The rash begins near the hairline as faint macules and papules and rapidly progresses to involve the face, trunk, and arms. When the rash appears on the lower extremities, it begins to fade on the face, and then gradually disappears over a 3–6 day interval. The lesions begin as discrete macules and papules and rapidly coalesce, involving large areas of skin. Fine desquamation may accompany healing. The coryzal symptoms reach their peak during the first 4–5 days and are accompanied by a harsh "barking" cough which persists throughout the illness, which lasts 9–10 days, and may be manifest after all other symptoms have subsided.

The general appearance (the "measly" look) of a child with florid measles is characteristic. The patient is red-eyed, with puffy eyelids and a swollen bridge of the nose, a distressed look, and copious, thin nasal secretions. The child with measles sits listlessly in bed, his apathy punctuated by violent harsh coughing. Combined with a confluent red rash, the clinical picture is one of extreme (though temporary) distress.

C. Laboratory Findings: Marked leukopenia is present early in the course. White counts as low as 1500–3000/cu mm are not uncommon, and lymphocytosis is marked. If bacterial superinfection occurs, abrupt leukocytosis with a shift to the left may be evident.

In doubtful prodromal cases, examination of nasal secretions or oral scrapings may reveal the characteristic Warthin-Finkeldey giant cells (large multinucleated cells).

Measles virus can be recovered from the blood or nasal and oropharyngeal secretions during the prodrome and early part of the rash. However, this is seldom necessary to establish the diagnosis. A 4-fold rise in serum antibody can be demonstrated in paired sera.

D. X-Ray Findings: In typical, uncomplicated measles, chest x-rays may reveal patchy pneumonic infiltrates or the typical "hilar pneumonia" pattern. Overaeration is frequent, and in the presence of bacterial pneumonia the x-ray may reveal lobular or lobar consolidation. With staphylococcal or, less commonly, pneumococcal pneumonia, empyema or pyopneumothorax may be evident.

Differential Diagnosis

Measles must be differentiated from other common exanthematous diseases of childhood. Table 25–2 lists the principal distinguishing features.

Abdominal pain (see below) in measles may be due to appendicitis or may result from gastrointestinal infection without appendicitis.

Acute prodromal measles with CNS manifesta-

Table 25–2. Differential diagnosis of exanthematous diseases.

Disease	Incubation Period	Prodrome	Exanthem	Enanthem	Other Diagnostic Features
Measles	9–14 days	3 days. Cough, coryza, conjunctivitis.	Red, maculopapular, confluent, face to feet, lasts 7–10 days, may desquamate.	Koplik's spots	Cough prominent.
Rubella	16–18 days	Usually none	Pink, maculopapular, discrete, spreads rapidly, lasts 3–5 days.	None or faint	Lymphadenopathy may be prominent.
Roseola infantum	10–14 days	3 days fever; "well" child.	Rose, macular, discrete, fleeting.	None	Child remains well. Occasional febrile convulsion with first rise in temperature.
Fifth disease (erythema infectiosum)	About 7–14 days	None	"Slapped cheek," lace-like rash on extremities, may reappear, lasts 7–14 days.	Variable	Rash is characteristic. May appear when extremity is warmed (bathing, clothing, etc).
Scarlet fever	2–5 days	1–2 days. Fever, vomiting, sore throat.	Red, punctate, sandpaper feel, confluent blush, lasts 7 days, desquamation.	Red pharynx, tonsillitis, palatal petechiae, strawberry tongue.	Circumoral pallor, increased rash in skin folds, "toxic" child.
Enterovirus infection	Variable (usually short)	Variable	May resemble any of above. Echo, petechial; coxsackie, vesicular.	Variable	Concurrent familial illness, gastroenteritis, epidemic locally.

tions must be differentiated from other causes of fever and convulsions. The presence of conjunctivitis and cough is helpful, as is the finding of giant cells in nasal scrapings or the presence of Koplik's spots.

Complications & Sequelae

A. Upper and Lower Respiratory Tract: Bacterial infection occurs in 5–15% of all cases of measles; otitis media and pneumonia are the most common forms. Sinusitis, mastoiditis, tonsillopharyngitis, and cervical adenitis also occur.

Viral complications include severe bronchial pneumonia and a peculiar viral pneumonia known as Hecht's giant cell pneumonia. The latter occurs frequently without rash and may be fatal.

B. Encephalitis: Occurring in 1:1000 instances of measles, this illness begins with fever, CNS signs (coma, convulsions, bizarre behavior, etc), and vomiting 3–8 days after the onset of rash. Sixty percent of patients recover completely; 25% have severe sequelae; and the remainder die.

Diagnosis can be suspected clinically and confirmed by the finding of CSF pleocytosis (lymphocytosis) and an elevated CSF protein, with normal or slightly elevated CSF glucose content.

C. Hemorrhagic Measles: Rarely, a fulminating form of measles is seen, with hemorrhage into the gastrointestinal tract, mucous membranes, and CNS. Fever and toxicity are pronounced, and the rash is purpuric and typically morbilliform. CNS symptoms (coma, convulsions, etc) may be prominent.

D. Thrombocytopenia: Following the onset of the rash, or days later, bleeding may occur into the rash. This is usually associated with a decrease in the platelet count.

E. Gastrointestinal Complications: These are uncommon in the USA but are a leading cause of death elsewhere. True appendicitis, diarrhea, and vomiting may be observed, often with a progressive course and fatal outcome.

F. Eyes: Secondary bacterial conjunctivitis is common. Corneal ulceration, gangrenous meibomianitis, membranous conjunctivitis, and optic nerve damage are rare complications of measles.

G. Cardiac Complications: Myocarditis and cardiac failure occur occasionally.

H. Effect on Other Diseases and Conditions: Measles during pregnancy may result in stillbirth, abortion, or premature delivery. Tuberculosis is exacerbated by intercurrent measles, and transient anergy to tuberculin is frequent. Nephrosis, asthma, and eczema may temporarily abate during measles virus infection.

Treatment

Good nursing care is essential, with attention to relief of cough, maintenance of clear nasal passages, reduction of fever, and cleansing of the conjunctivas.

Bacterial complications should be specifically diagnosed and effective antimicrobial therapy employed. Streptococcal infections are common.

Antimicrobial prophylaxis should not be used since it may result in bacterial infections with resistant organisms.

Prognosis

Measles is usually a self-limited disease lasting 7–10 days. Most often it is without permanent sequelae, although it is a severe infection.

The most serious complication, encephalitis, may result in permanent disability or death in 40% of cases.

Rarely, a progressive degenerative CNS disease, ending in death, occurs as a late sequel (years after infection) of measles. This disease has had various eponyms attached to it but is currently termed subacute sclerosing panencephalitis (SSPE). Specimens of brain from patients with SSPE have been co-cultured with measles virus-susceptible cells in tissue culture. Whole measles virus has been isolated by this method, providing direct evidence for its role in SSPE. It is believed that measles virus remains latent in the neural cells of infected infants and children and produces the slowly progressive SSPE at some time in the future. Some authorities maintain that latent or "slow" measles virus infections are also operative in multiple sclerosis and Jakob-Creutzfeldt disease, both chronic degenerative CNS diseases.

Barkin RM: Measles mortality: Analysis of the primary cause of death. Am J Dis Child 129:307, 1975.

Hinman AR: Resurgence of measles in New York. Am J Public Health 62:498, 1972.

Krugman S: Present status of measles and rubella immunization in the United States. J Pediatr 90:1, 1977.

Landrigan PJ: Epidemic measles in a divided city. JAMA 221:567, 1972.

Lobes LA, Cherry JD: Fatal measles pneumonia in a child with chickenpox pneumonia. JAMA 223:1143, 1973.

Meuden V & others: Subacute sclerosing panencephalitis: A review. Curr Top Microbiol Immunol 57:1, 1972.

Murphey JU, Yumis EJ: Encephalopathy following measles infection in children. J Pediatr 88:937, 1976.

Olson RW, Hodges GR: Measles pneumonia. JAMA 232:363, 1975.

PICORNAVIRUS INFECTIONS

The picornaviruses include the enteroviruses (poliovirus, echovirus, and coxsackievirus) and the rhinoviruses.

ENTEROVIRAL INFECTIONS

The enteroviruses resemble one another in size, morphology, biochemical and biophysical characteristics, and in the illnesses they cause. Since a large majority of the types of enteroviral infections can be produced by more than one type of virus, we will present the common clinical categories and then refer to specific syndromes peculiar to each of the groups.

Types of Infection Common to All Enteroviruses

A. Fever Alone: Infection may be accompanied solely by fever of variable height and duration.

B. Respiratory Illness: Undifferentiated upper respiratory infection may occur.

C. Gastrointestinal Illness: Nausea, vomiting, and diarrhea have been associated with enteroviral infection.

D. Exanthematous Illnesses: A variety of rashes have been reported, including scarlatiniform, morbilliform, rubelliform, petechial, and vesicular varieties.

E. Combinations of Above: Illnesses in which all or some of the above symptoms occur together have been recorded. This is particularly true for the echovirus group.

F. CNS Infections:

1. Aseptic meningitis—Fever, gastrointestinal symptoms associated with nuchal rigidity, headache, lethargy, and CSF pleocytosis can result from infection with any of the enteroviruses.

2. Encephalitis—Cortical symptoms, including disturbances of sensorium, convulsions, and coma, have been noted.

3. Paralytic illness—Although occasionally due to the echoviruses or coxsackieviruses, this syndrome is almost exclusively produced by polioviruses and will be considered separately below.

G. Isolated Myocarditis: Inflammation of the myocardium with attendant precordial chest pain, dyspnea, cough, tachycardia, cyanosis, and fulminant congestive heart failure has been attributed to poliovirus and coxsackievirus infection.

Horstmann DM & others: Enterovirus surveillance following a community-wide oral poliovirus vaccination program: A seven year study. Am J Epidemiol 97:173, 1973.

Lake AM & others: Enterovirus infections in neonates. J Pediatr 89:787, 1976.

Sells CJ, Carpenter RL, Ray CG: Sequelae of central nervous system enterovirus infections. N Engl J Med 293:1, 1975.

1. PARALYTIC POLIOMYELITIS

Essentials of Diagnosis

- Muscle weakness, headache, stiff neck, fever, nausea, vomiting, sore throat.
- Lower motor neuron lesion (flaccid paralysis) with decreased deep tendon reflexes and muscle wasting.
- CSF shows excess cells. Lymphocytes predominate; rarely more than 500/cu mm.
- No history of immunization.

Clinical Findings

A. Symptoms and Signs: Following (or blending with) an undifferentiated illness (fever, lassitude, gastrointestinal symptoms), the onset of paralysis is heralded by nuchal rigidity and stiffness of the back. Varying degrees of CNS depression or excitability may be observed, followed by pain and tenderness in the affected muscles, a brief period of hypertonicity and spasm with transient hyperactive reflexes, asymmetric flaccid paralysis, and loss of superficial and deep reflexes but maintenance of sensation. Deviations from the above pattern are common, especially in very young infants.

Involvement of the cervical spinal cord segments and the brain stem may lead to respiratory muscle paralysis and cranial nerve involvement with palatal, facial, and laryngeal paralysis. Severe involvement results in loss of function of the respiratory and circulatory centers with irregular respirations, apnea, and peripheral vascular collapse.

Paralysis generally extends during the first week, reaching its limits as the fever subsides. No change is noted for days or weeks; if spontaneous recovery is to occur, muscle strength and function and reflexes begin to improve at this time. The ultimate extent of paralysis should not be judged until 12–18 months have passed without continuing improvement. In recent years, paralytic poliomyelitis has been observed in the following groups: (1) those infected outside the USA; (2) normal children following OPV; (3) contacts of immunized children; and (4) immunodeficient or immunosuppressed individuals.

B. Laboratory Findings: Poliovirus may be isolated from the throat or the stools. Fecal excretion may persist for weeks beyond the acute phase. Specific viral etiology can be detected by serum antibody increase in paired sera.

CSF findings are those of aseptic meningitis. There may be mild early pleocytosis with polymorphonuclear leukocytosis rapidly shifting to lymphocytosis. Protein concentration is normal initially, but during the second to third weeks of illness it rises roughly in parallel with the paralysis.

Differential Diagnosis

Most cases of paralytic polio occurring in the USA in recent years are either (1) due to other enteroviruses, (2) due to infrequent epidemics with wild strains in unimmunized individuals, or (3) secondary to oral poliovirus vaccine. With the dramatic reduction in wild virus, the few cases of nonepidemic paralytic disease are of types (1) and (3). Therefore, the clinician should make every effort both to report paralytic disease and to obtain appropriate viral cultures and paired sera for etiologic identification. Local health departments with liaison with the Center for Disease Control (CDC) in Atlanta can provide the necessary consultation and laboratory assistance.

Aseptic meningitis due to any cause may be confused with poliovirus infection. However, paralysis is usually due to poliovirus infection and must be differentiated from Guillain-Barré syndrome or infective polyneuritis (sensory loss frequently present, symmetric paralysis, CSF shows albuminocytologic dissociation, ie, high protein concentration, little or no increase in leukocytes), other infective polyneuritides (history of preceding illness, mumps, diphtheria, etc), and paralysis or pseudoparalysis due to other causes (signs of scurvy, syphilis, fractures, arthritides, infection of bone, etc).

Complications & Sequelae

Bulbar poliomyelitis may result in respiratory arrest, muscular or central in origin, requiring assisted ventilation and tracheostomy.

Paralysis may remain and result in loss of function necessitating relearning, bracing, wheelchair ambulation, etc.

Hypertension is usually brief in duration but may persist.

Immobilization in a respirator may result in stasis pneumonia, decubitus ulcers, renal calculi, and disuse atrophy of nonparalyzed muscles. Careful attention to skin care, exercising, and coughing will help to prevent these complications.

Treatment

Complete bed rest is essential. The immediate disability must be accurately assessed so that difficulties can be anticipated and treated promptly rather than as an emergency. Special attention must be given to neurologic evaluation to detect beginning respiratory paralysis.

The Kenny method (heat packs) reduces spasm and tenderness and makes possible early rehabilitation to avoid disease atrophy and reeducate involved muscle groups.

A clear airway should be maintained, preferably without the use of intubation, either endotracheal or transtracheal. If necessary, tracheostomy should be anticipated and performed electively in an operating suite with experts in attendance under optimal conditions. The use of oxygen, assisted ventilation, and humid respirators may be necessary.

Prognosis

The mortality rate in paralytic disease varies from 5–10%, and permanent incapacitating paralysis occurs in 15% of cases. Mild paralysis may occur in as many as 30% of cases. In general, pregnant women and other adults are more severely affected than infants and children.

Abramson H, Greenberg M: Acute poliomyelitis in infants under one year of age. Pediatrics 16:478, 1955.

Poliomyelitis today. (Editorial.) Br Med J 1:415, 1975.

Schonberger LB & others: Vaccine-associated poliomyelitis in the United States. Am J Epidemiol 104:202, 1976.

Weinstein L: Poliomyelitis: A persistent problem. N Engl J Med 288:370, 1973.

WHO Expert Committee on Poliomyelitis: *First, Second, and Third Reports.* WHO Technical Report Series Nos. 81, 145, 203. World Health Organization, 1954, 1958, 1960.

Wilfert CM & others: An epidemic of echovirus 18 meningitis. J Infect Dis 131:75, 1975.

2. HERPANGINA
(Coxsackie Group A, Types 2–6, 8, and 10)

There are usually no prodromal symptoms. Similar illnesses may be observed in the community, or other forms of coxsackievirus infection may be noted.

Herpangina is characterized by fever, sore throat and painful swallowing, anorexia, and vomiting, which occur with abrupt onset in association with tiny vesicles (which rapidly ulcerate) on the anterior fauces and elsewhere in the posterior pharynx. The ulcers are often arrayed linearly on the anterior fauces, lending a characteristic (diagnostic) appearance to the throat. Fever may be prominent, particularly in the young. Convulsions may occur with the first rise in temperature. Symptoms and signs persist for 2–6 days.

Virus can be isolated from throat swab and stool specimens. Serologic diagnosis is of aid only in epidemics, where the specific virus type has been isolated.

Herpangina in its classic form is seldom confused with other illnesses. Oral ulceration associated with fever is seen in primary herpetic gingivostomatitis (ulcers over most of the oral mucosa, lack of epidemic pattern). Distinguish also from aphthous ulceration (usually no fever; lesions may be anterior), ulcerative pharyngitis associated with leukemia or its treatment (lymphadenopathy, splenomegaly, etc; characteristic peripheral blood and bone marrow changes), and other viral exanthems (history of contact, exanthem, course of disease).

Parotitis or vaginal ulceration may occur, but recovery is complete.

The disease is self-limited, and only symptomatic therapy is required.

Parrott RH: The clinical importance of group A coxsackieviruses. Ann NY Acad Sci 67:230, 1957.

3. PLEURODYNIA
(Coxsackie B Viruses; Epidemic Myalgia; Bornholm Disease)

Pleurodynia may begin with vague prodromal symptoms of malaise, anorexia, headache, and muscle aches, but the onset is usually unheralded and abrupt. Other coxsackievirus infections may be observed in the community. Pleurodynia may be epidemic.

Pleurodynia characteristically begins with severe, usually unilateral chest pain which frequently is paroxysmal and pleuritic and therefore is aggravated by respiratory movements. The patient is asymptomatic between episodes. The pain is severe and dramatically described by the patient as crushing or vise-like (hence the name "devil's grip"). Headache, fever, malaise, apprehension, abdominal pain, hiccups, vomiting, diarrhea, and stiff neck have all been noted. The illness may last as long as a week but is quite variable. Mild forms are also seen. Physical signs include apprehension, fever, limitation of respiratory excursions, muscle tenderness, normal breath sounds, and an ipsilateral pleural friction rub in one-fourth of cases. Mild to moderate nuchal rigidity may be present.

Virus can be recovered from the stools or from throat swabs. Serologic diagnosis may be possible since coxsackievirus B3 and B5 are the most common offenders, but any of the group B coxsackieviruses can produce the disease.

Any cause of sudden pleurisy must be distinguished from pleurodynia. Thus, bacterial pneumonia (leukocytosis, empyema, productive cough, bacteriologic findings), tuberculosis (history of exposure, positive tuberculin test, identification of mycobacteria), and other infectious and noninfectious causes of pleuritis must be differentiated. Abdominal or muscular pain may suggest acute surgical conditions (appendicitis, ulcer, perforation, etc). The superficial nature of the tenderness, the associated fever and pulmonary findings, and epidemiologic evidence may suggest the diagnosis of pleurodynia.

Almost all patients recover completely without complications. A few cases have been reported associated with aseptic meningitis, orchitis, pericarditis, and pneumonia.

Analgesics, splinting of the chest, and other supportive measures are indicated.

Hierholzer JC & others: Prospective study of a mixed coxsackievirus B3 and B4 outbreak of upper respiratory illness in a children's home. Pediatrics 49:744, 1972.

4. GENERALIZED NEONATAL INFECTION
(Coxsackie B Viruses)

Sudden onset of fever associated with acute heart failure occurring in more than one infant should arouse the suspicion of generalized neonatal infection. Sick infants are usually in nurseries or recently discharged. Case-finding is important and may lead to the correct diagnosis. A history of mild gastrointestinal symptoms 1–2 days before the major illness is common. The mother may have had an upper respiratory tract infection just prior to delivery. Cyanosis, tachycardia, and increasing size of the liver and heart are all observed. Pneumonic symptoms may predominate early, and cough, dyspnea, and vomiting are prominent manifestations. In more than half of cases, the disease progresses rapidly to death in circulatory collapse. Cardiac murmurs are not heard. Despite the preponderance of cardiac signs and symptoms, the infection is a generalized one, and encephalitis, pancreatitis, focal hepatitis,

and myositis are all observed at autopsy. ECG changes are those of severe myocardial damage. Chest x-ray reveals a large heart.

In general, the illness is produced by coxsackievirus groups B3 and B4. Virus can be recovered from the feces before death and from the myocardium and other tissues postmortem. Serologic confirmation is possible in surviving infants.

Other causes of acute congestive heart failure in neonates must be considered, but the epidemic nature and findings of coxsackievirus infection should be diagnostic.

Intensive supportive measures, including oxygenation, support of ventilation and circulation, and digitalization, are mandatory.

Reported mortality rates are variable but approach or exceed 50%. If the patient survives, recovery is rapid and complete.

Hanson LA & others: Clinical and serological observations in cases of coxsackie B3 infections in early infancy. Acta Paediatr Scand 55:577, 1966.

5. ISOLATED MYOCARDITIS & PERICARDITIS
(Coxsackie B Viruses)

Myocardial or pericardial infection with coxsackieviruses occurs in humans and in several other animal species. The clinical findings are similar to those observed in myocarditis or pericarditis due to other causes. Severity ranges from very mild clinical disease to fulminant fatal infections. The diagnosis is suggested by the clinical findings and substantiated by virus isolation from the stools or pericardial fluid during life, from the myocardium postmortem, or by a rise in serum antibody in paired sera in survivors.

Myocarditis is treated as outlined above for generalized neonatal infection. Pericardial aspiration is indicated for pericarditis.

Bharucha PE, Nair KG: Coxsackie B1 endocarditis. Clin Pediatr (Phila) 14:186, 1975.
Burch GE & others: Interstitial and coxsackie B myocarditis in infants and children. JAMA 203:55, 1968.

6. ACUTE LYMPHONODULAR PHARYNGITIS
(Coxsackie A10)

Papular whitish-yellow lesions of the uvula, anterior pillars, and pharynx in association with sore throat, fever, and headache have been observed in a single outbreak of coxsackievirus A10 infection. The illness lasted for 1–2 weeks and was uncomplicated. The papules did not vesiculate, which differentiates this disease from herpangina.

Treatment is symptomatic.

7. VESICULAR EXANTHEM
(Hand-Foot-Mouth Disease; Coxsackie A5, A10, & A16)

Several epidemics of a vesicular exanthem which in its complete form involves the oral mucosa, tongue, and interdigital and digital surfaces of both the upper and lower extremities (hence the term hand-foot-mouth disease) have occurred due to infection with coxsackievirus A16. Incomplete forms are also seen, and coxsackievirus A16 may cause nonvesicular disease in the community at the same time.

Diagnosis is by virologic isolation and serology. Treatment is symptomatic.

Adler JA & others: Epidemiologic investigation of hand, foot, and mouth disease. Am J Dis Child 120:309, 1970.
Tindall JP, Callaway JL: Hand, foot and mouth disease: It's more common than you think. Am J Dis Child 124:372, 1972.

8. ECHOVIRUS EXANTHEMATOUS DISEASE

Echovirus types 4, 9, and 16 have been definitely associated with epidemics of exanthematous illness; 10 other echovirus types have also been related to such illnesses. Other clinical findings have also been noted, including the aseptic meningitis syndrome.

Echovirus types 4 and 9 cause a usually maculopapular but sometimes petechial rash, and vesicular rashes, even with crusting, have occasionally been noted. Association with aseptic meningitis and lymphadenitis has been observed. The rash is usually present for just a few days but may persist for 10 days.

In echovirus type 16 disease (Boston exanthem), the rash appears during or shortly after defervescence, thus simulating roseola infantum. A punched-out ulcerative exanthem may be seen. Aseptic meningitis due to echovirus 16 usually occurs without rash. The rash lasts 1–5 days and may be associated with pharyngitis and cervical, suboccipital, and postauricular lymphadenopathy, but there are no appreciable respiratory symptoms.

Cherry J: Newer viral exanthems. Adv Pediatr 16:233, 1969.
Hall C & others: The return of Boston exanthem. Am J Dis Child 131:323, 1977.

RHINOVIRUSES

A large group of viruses with properties similar to those of the enteroviruses have recently been shown to cause the common cold in adults. Their role in the production of disease in infants and children is not completely understood at present. They have been isolated from the nose and throat in a wide range of upper respiratory illnesses in children and less frequently in lower tract diseases.

Fox JP & others: The Seattle virus watch. 5. Epidemiologic observations of rhinovirus infections, 1965–1969, in families with young children. Am J Epidemiol 101:122, 1975.

HERPESVIRUSES

HERPES SIMPLEX

Essentials of Diagnosis

- Recurrent small grouped vesicles on an erythematous base, especially around oral and genital areas.
- May follow minor infections, trauma, stress, or sun exposure.
- Regional lymph nodes may be swollen and tender.

General Considerations

Primary herpesvirus infection is asymptomatic in most individuals. When manifestations occur, they usually take the form of gingivostomatitis in children under 4 or 5 years of age. Secondary or recurrent herpes occurs far more frequently even in the absence of a history of primary infection; thus, the virus is felt to remain hidden or "latent" following first infection. Various excitants (fever, menses, trauma, severe infections, sunshine, etc) result in uncovering of the virus with a resulting "fever blister" or "cold sore" type of infection. Thus, immunity is imperfect despite demonstrable levels of circulating antibody.

Two types of herpesvirus have been identified. Type 1 is involved in lesions of the oral cavity, CNS, and skin. Type 2 is responsible for genital disease and probably accounts for all cases of congenital herpes infection. Type 2 has also been linked with carcinoma of the cervix.

Clinical Findings

A. History: In primary infections, no history of previous disease is elicited; in recurrent disease, a history of severe gingivostomatitis or vulvovaginitis in early childhood can sometimes be elicited. In recurrent herpes, a history of similar episodes following exposure to the same excitants is usually present.

B. Symptoms and Signs:

1. Herpetic gingivostomatitis—Fever, irritability, pain in the mouth and throat and upon attempted swallowing, and lassitude with disinterest in surroundings are seen in varying degrees. Examination reveals extensive shallow, yellowish ulcers of the buccal, gingival, tonsillar, and pharyngeal mucosa, frequently with crusting of the lips, a half-open mouth with drooling, foul breath odor, and cervical lymphadenopathy. The disease lasts 7–14 days.

2. Herpetic vulvovaginitis or urethritis–Manifestations are similar to those of gingivostomatitis (both may occur) except that they appear on the vulva and vagina. Urination may be painful or withheld, especially in males. Inguinal lymphadenopathy is frequently present.

3. Recurrent herpetic lesions–Sensory symptoms varying from vague discomfort to neuralgic pain may precede or accompany the appearance of erythematous papules on the mucocutaneous junction of the lips. Rapid vesiculation, pustulation, and crusting occur. Fever is usually absent unless it is the inciting factor. Regional lymphadenopathy and lymphadenitis occur infrequently. Lesions appear in groups and tend to involve the same area in recurrences. Severity is variable, and the illness often causes discomfort without being incapacitating.

4. Herpetic keratoconjunctivitis–A variety of forms of herpetic corneal infection have been described according to the depth and extent of the infection. Almost all forms are accompanied by conjunctival inflammation, often purulent in appearance. Cloudiness and ulceration of the cornea may be noted. Ulceration may be diagnosed by application of fluorescein to the eye, whereupon a dendritic (branched) pattern may be seen. Deeper forms include stromal edema and hypopyon with rupture of the globe. Ophthalmologic consultation is indicated for accurate diagnosis and treatment.

5. Herpetic encephalitis–This rare disease may take the form of aseptic meningitis or may begin with cortical symptoms and cranial nerve palsies. Convulsions and coma are frequent, and death occurs in the second to third weeks of illness.

6. Neonatal herpetic infection–This form of infection occurs in infants of nonimmune parents, and a history of recent herpes infection in either parent may be obtained. The illness may be present at birth but usually manifests itself in the first week of life with generalized vesiculation of the skin, high or low temperature, jaundice, progressive hepatosplenomegaly, dyspnea, signs of cardiac failure, hemorrhage, and CNS manifestations. Death occurs following a 2–4 day course of illness. "Mild" neonatal herpes infections result in vesicular rash usually unassociated with overt CNS disease. The rash may recur repeatedly in the first months of life, and CNS function may ultimately be impaired.

7. Eczema herpeticum (Kaposi's varicelliform eruption)–The appearance of fever, prostration, and vesicular lesions in a patient with eczema should lead to a diagnosis of intercurrent herpesvirus or vaccinia virus infection. Although varying in severity, eczema herpeticum is frequently fulminant and fatal, especially when large areas of skin are involved.

C. Laboratory Findings: CSF pleocytosis (lymphocytosis) is present in aseptic meningitis. Virus can be recovered from vesicular fluid, skin and corneal scrapings, throat swabs, blood, CSF, and appropriate tissue specimens. Enrichment of collection media with protein enhances virus stability if a delay in handling specimens is unavoidable.

A 4-fold or greater rise in serum antibody is detectable in paired sera from patients with primary infection. This is of little aid in recurrent infection, since titer rises do not occur. A negative titer may help to rule out herpes in vesicular lesions.

Smears taken from the bases of vesicles or ulcers suspected of being herpetic can be stained with hematoxylin and eosin to reveal the typical Cowdry type A intranuclear inclusion bodies. These consist of eosinophilic oval masses within the nucleus, which has marginal chromatin. Fixation produces a distinct halo around the inclusion. Giemsa stains of tissue best visualize the giant cells with their multinucleate or syncytial structure.

Electronmicroscopic examination of vesicular fluid may result in rapid identification of herpes simplex virus, as can fluorescent antibody staining.

Differential Diagnosis

Herpetic gingivostomatitis must be differentiated from herpangina (posterior pharyngeal ulcers only, linear array on anterior pillars, isolation of coxsackie A viruses); aphthous ulceration (one or only a few ulcers, previous history, lack of systemic symptoms); ulcerative pharyngitis of agranulocytic disease (history, other physical findings, blood and bone marrow findings), and Stevens-Johnson syndrome (multiple mucosal involvement, "iris" lesions of skin, history of sulfonamide or other drug ingestion).

Recurrent herpes labialis can easily be differentiated from impetigo by the characteristic history and course of the former and bacterial isolation and response to treatment of the latter.

Herpetic keratoconjunctivitis must be differentiated from vaccinial keratoconjunctivitis (history or presence of recent vaccination or contact, isolation of virus) and from adenovirus keratoconjunctivitis (pain in adenovirus infection of cornea, epidemic nature, isolation of virus).

Meningoencephalitis can only be differentiated from other causes by laboratory studies.

Generalized neonatal infection is differentiated from similar illness due to coxsackie B viruses by lack of skin involvement, epidemic nature in nursery, and isolation of virus.

Eczema vaccinatum can be differentiated from eczema herpeticum by the history of exposure to smallpox vaccination, typical vacciniform lesions, and the fact that eczema vaccinatum lesions tend to be in the same stage. In some cases, differentiation is difficult and laboratory diagnosis is necessary.

Complications, Sequelae, & Prognosis

Primary skin and mucosal infections are usually self-limited, with complete and prompt recovery, although limited recurrences occur.

Herpetic keratoconjunctivitis can lead to blindness or perforation of the cornea with loss of the eye.

Encephalitis or neonatal generalized infection is frequently fatal.

Treatment

A. Specific Measures: Idoxuridine (IDU, Herplex, Stoxil, Dendrid) has been used successfully in superficial mucosal, corneal, and skin infections. It is of proved curative effect if used promptly in superficial ulcerative keratitis and possibly of ameliorative effect in skin infections. One to 2 drops are instilled onto the cornea every 1–2 hours around the clock for maximum effect. (Follow manufacturer's directions, as new formulations may appear.)

Some experience has been gained with the use of systemic antiviral agents in the treatment of herpes encephalitis and generalized neonatal infection. Idoxuridine and both cytarabine and vidarabine have been utilized, though idoxuridine and cytarabine have been abandoned and the best hope seems to lie with vidarabine (Ara-A). Such agents work by inhibiting the enzymes necessary for viral synthesis and by substituting for essential nucleotides in the viral DNA molecule. Unfortunately, they also affect normal DNA and thus possess a high degree of toxicity. Some investigators have reported promising results with these compounds; others report lack of success.

Vidarabine appears to have a dramatic effect upon the mortality rate (reduction from 70% in controls to 28% in treated) but did not influence morbidity in survivors. No toxicity was observed. In encephalitic syndromes not due to herpesvirus infections, no effect was shown. This collaborative study suggests that early diagnosis by means of brain biopsy and early treatment in the stage of lethargy before coma has occurred will yield optimal results.

In anecdotal reports, human immune globulin has been claimed to be beneficial in neonatal herpetic infections. The doses have been large, and, because of the variability of the disease, these reports cannot be validated. This must be regarded as a questionable use of gamma globulin (see p 131).

B. General Measures: In gingivostomatitis, considerable discomfort is experienced, with resultant lack of fluid and caloric intake. Since this is a 7–14 day illness, maintenance of fluid intake is vital. Dehydration can be avoided by hospitalization and intravenous administration of fluids and electrolytes. In less severe instances, discovering the optimal temperature of fluids tolerated (cool is usually best) can ensure intake. It is rarely necessary to use topical "caine" anesthetics, thus avoiding potential sensitization. Mild antiseptic mouthwashes are occasionally of benefit. There is no rationale to the use of local antibiotics. Systemic administration of analgesics occasionally is necessary and facilitates intake of food and fluids.

The treatment of encephalitis and neonatal infection is symptomatic and supportive (see above).

Herpetic keratoconjunctivitis is best treated with idoxuridine (see above). The use of topical corticosteroids in the acute ulcerative disease is contraindicated. In instances of stromal edema or of persistent deep lesions, topical corticosteroids may be of aid but should be combined with idoxuridine and given only under an ophthalmologist's direction.

Eczema herpeticum is best treated as an extensive "burn" so that appropriate attention is directed to replacement of fluid and electrolytes and to protein nutrition. Prevention of secondary bacterial infection is accomplished by continuous bacteriologic guidance and antibacterial therapy.

In severe complications, the use of systemic corticosteroids is often advocated. There are theoretical objections to the use of such agents, since experimental evidence indicates that they enhance viral spread. Pooled adult gamma globulin has been advocated, but there is no evidence that it has a beneficial effect.

Recurrent herpes labialis has been treated in a variety of ways, including injections of vitamin B_{12}, the use of reticulose (a supposed antiviral substance), and repeat smallpox vaccination. No evidence of a controlled nature is available to indicate that any of these or other forms of therapy are uniformly beneficial. Saline injections and no other treatment can result in "cure" of recurrent herpes. Smallpox vaccination has resulted in untoward effects in some patients and should be avoided.

In pregnancies complicated by herpes cervicitis or infection of the external genitalia, cesarian section has been advocated to prevent contamination of the infant during passage through the birth canal. This advice still holds, although it has been reported that herpetic infection of the newborn is not necessarily prevented in all instances.

In both the labial and genital forms of recurrent herpes infection, the application of a vital dye (eg, proflavine, neutral red) to the lesions with subsequent exposure to light has been reported to be of some benefit. The carcinogenic hazards of this form of therapy are not definitely proved, but some experts feel it should not be utilized.

Barr RJ & others: Rapid method for Tzanck preparations. JAMA 237:1119, 1977.

Francis DP & others: Nosocomial and maternally acquired *Herpesvirus hominis* infections. Am J Dis Child 129:889, 1975.

Gershon AA & others: Herpes simplex infection of the newborn. Am J Dis Child 124:739, 1972.

Illis LS & others: Treatment of herpes simplex encephalitis. J R Coll Physicians Lond 7:34, 1972.

Juel-Jensen BE, MacCallum FO: *Herpes Simplex, Varicella, and Zoster.* Lippincott, 1972.

Nahmias AJ, Dowdle WR: Antigenic and biologic differences in *Herpesvirus hominis.* Prog Med Virol 10:110, 1968.

Nahmias AJ, Roizman B: Infection with herpes simplex viruses 1 and 2. (3 parts.) N Engl J Med 289:667, 719, 781, 1973.

Smith JB & others: Multicystic cerebral degeneration in neonatal herpes simplex virus encephalitis. Am J Dis Child 131:568, 1977.

Whitley RJ & others: Adenine arabinoside therapy of biopsy proved herpes simplex encephalitis. N Engl J Med 297:289; 1977.

Wolontis S, Jeansson S: Correlation of herpes simplex virus types 1 and 2 with clinical features of infection. J Infect Dis 135:28, 1977.

VARICELLA (Chickenpox) & HERPES ZOSTER (Shingles)

Essentials of Diagnosis

Varicella:

- History of exposure within 2–3 weeks; appearance of characteristic vesicles over a 2–5 day period, usually without prodrome.
- Lesions rapidly evolve from macules to papules to "dewdrop" superficial vesicles to encrustation in centripetal distribution. Macules, papules, vesicles, and crusts are all observable at any one time (pleomorphic).

Herpes zoster:

- History of chickenpox.
- Preeruptive pain (infrequent in children) in region of rash.
- Clusters of confluent vesicles in unilateral dermatomal distribution. Successive crops may appear.
- Examination of early vesicular scrapings reveals Tzank giant cells or characteristic intranuclear inclusions (see Herpes Simplex, above).

General Considerations

Varicella and herpes zoster are caused by the same virus. Varicella is the primary infection and herpes zoster appears to be a recurrent infection. In the USA, varicella is primarily a disease of childhood; in large areas of the tropics, it is principally a disease of adults. No known animal reservoir exists, and the disease is transmitted from person to person in epidemics with a high degree of contagiousness (80–90% of exposed susceptibles are infected). Herpes zoster is sporadic and considerably less infectious, resulting in varicella in 15% of exposed susceptibles.

Clinical Findings

A. History: A history of contact 10–20 days (average, 12–13 days) prior to onset is typically obtained. There is usually no prodrome, but a mild febrile illness with rhinitis is occasionally noted for 1–3 days before the rash appears. A history of contact may be lacking in zoster, but the disease has occurred (in adults) following exposure to varicella. Severe pain along the nerve root distribution of the rash may precede the rash by several days.

B. Symptoms and Signs:

1. Varicella—In typical varicella, the onset is abrupt with the appearance of the rash. Systemic symptoms, if any, are mild. The rash appears in crops, with faint erythematous macules rapidly developing into papules and vesicles. The vesicles are characteristic; they are thin-walled, and superficially located on the skin with a distinct areola (dewdrop on a red base). They rupture easily, rapidly encrust, and frequently become impetiginized. Successive crops (usually 3) appear in the next 2–5 days, giving rise to the pleomorphic appearance of the rash: lesions in all stages can be seen at one time. The rash is heaviest on the trunk and sparse on the extremities. Barring bacterial infection, the crust falls off in 1–3 weeks, leaving no scars.

Deviations from the above pattern vary from very mild disease with just a few vesicles to as many as 5 successive crops with involvement of most of the skin. Rarely, hemorrhagic lesions occur and are associated with thrombocytopenia, particularly in children with leukemia receiving antimetabolites. Infrequently, a zoster-like cluster of lesions appears during the course of primary varicella. Bullous and gangrenous forms are recognized.

Systemic symptoms are usually absent or mild but may be severe, and generally parallel the extent of skin involvement.

An enanthem is recognizable which consists of shallow mucosal ulceration (the vesicle is rarely seen). When it involves the posterior pharynx or esophagus, swallowing may be painful and difficult.

2. Zoster—Herpes zoster is usually unilateral and limited to one or more adjacent dermatomes. Thoracic and lumbar forms are most common, although the ophthalmic division of the trigeminal nerve, cervical roots, and other divisions may be affected. Maculopapules appear in closely arrayed patches, rapidly vesiculate, and frequently coalesce; they follow the dermal distribution of the nerve root, and often end abruptly at the midline of the body. Concomitant or preceding pain, often very severe, occurs less frequently in children than in adults.

C. Laboratory Findings: The usual laboratory tests are of little aid. Sepsis may be accompanied by an abrupt increase in the white blood count with neutrophilia.

Although virus isolation and serologic tests are available, they are seldom necessary. Etiologic identification may be important in distinguishing varicella from smallpox or in the diagnosis of unusual and atypical forms of the disease.

Giant cells with multinucleate or syncytial structure may be found in vesicular scrapings, as may inclusion bodies of the eosinophilic intranuclear type (Cowdry type A) also.

D. X-Ray Findings: Chest films may reveal diffuse nodular pneumonia ("viral") and emphysema in varicella pneumonia.

Differential Diagnosis

Typical chickenpox is seldom confused with other illnesses. Severe forms must, in rare cases, be differentiated from smallpox (history of exposure, typical 3-day severe prodrome, lesions all in same stage of development, centrifugal distribution, hard, pearly, nodular, deep-seated lesions, absence of giant cells and intranuclear inclusions, isolation of the virus) and mild forms from the vesicular exanthem due to coxsackievirus infection (sparseness of rash, history of chickenpox, failure to form crusts, isolation of specific virus). Also to be distinguished are impetigo (lack of exposure history, response to therapy), multiple insect bites or papular urticaria (history of bites, papular and excoriated but no vesicles), rickettsialpox (primary eschar, smaller lesions, lack of crusting, serologic diagnosis), and dermatitis herpetiformis (chronic course, symmetry of eruption, urticaria, residual pigmentation).

Complications & Sequelae

Complications are uncommon. Secondary bacterial infection may occur if the lesions are manipulated. Septic sequelae may then ensue, including local abscesses, lymphangitis, septicemia, osteomyelitis, and others.

Varicella pneumonia is rare in children except in severe generalized forms of the disease such as occur in neonatal disease and disseminated forms associated with malignancy or immunosuppressive drug therapy. Its onset is in the first week of rash with fulminant pulmonary manifestations (cough, dyspnea and tachypnea, pain, cyanosis, rales, splinting). Chest films show characteristic diffuse pulmonary nodular infiltrates throughout both lung fields. The disease may be fatal, especially in adults and in disseminated forms.

Varicella in the neonate is often mild but may be fulminant, with extensive visceral infection and death.

Varicella occurring in patients with malignancies or receiving immunosuppressive therapy can be very severe and often fatal. Hemorrhagic forms of the disease and disseminated visceral lesions, including pneumonia, are common. The role of corticosteroid therapy is controversial, but most authorities feel that the underlying disease is more important in the development of severe infections than is administration of corticosteroids alone.

Patients receiving corticosteroids for illnesses not associated with immunologic suppression (eg, asthma, juvenile rheumatoid arthritis) require no adjustment in dose upon exposure. Those patients whose underlying illness predisposes to disseminated disease should have the dose of corticosteroids reduced as much as possible and zoster immune globulin administered.

Varicella encephalitis occurs infrequently and is milder than measles encephalitis. Eighty percent fully recover; 15% have sequelae; and 5% die. The onset is insidious, usually in the first week of rash, and is followed by varying CNS signs and symptoms.

Fatal hypoglycemia has been reported in infants with varicella and is believed to be associated with decreased carbohydrate intake and concomitant salicylate therapy.

Rare complications include transverse myelitis, optic neuritis, hepatitis, and orchitis.

Treatment

Symptomatic measures include fluids, control of itching (sedative antihistamines, colloidal baths), attention to cleanliness (trimming of nails, handwashing, bathing), and antipyretics where indicated (avoid high or repeated doses of aspirin, especially in young infants). Antimicrobial agents should not be administered prophylactically, but infections should be treated as they occur. Topical therapy is often sufficient for mild skin infection, but systemic administration may be necessary.

Supportive and symptomatic treatment for the complications of varicella are indicated. In the disseminated forms of infection, massive amounts of passive antibody in the form of zoster immune globulin or convalescent plasma from adults recently ill with zoster may be of aid.

The effects of antiviral chemotherapy in varicellazoster infections are confused and controversial. Advocates of vidarabine or cytarabine imply benefit in uncontrolled observations. A large-scale controlled study of cytarabine not only failed to demonstrate a favorable effect but reported increased morbidity and mortality rates.

However, a recent trial with vidarabine given by intravenous infusion suggested that there was accelerated clearing of varicella-zoster virus from vesicles and cessation of new vesicle formation with no drug toxicity. These early favorable results resulted in a recommendation that vidarabine be further studied in young individuals with lymphoreticular malignancies and early in the course of their disease.

Prognosis

Varicella is usually benign and self-limited. Complications in children are infrequent and fatalities rare.

Asano Y & others: Protection against varicella in family contacts by immediate inoculation with live varicella vaccine. Pediatrics 59:3, 1977.

Brunell PA, Gershon AA: Passive immunization against varicella-zoster infections and other modes of therapy. J Infect Dis 127:415, 1973.

Brunell PA & others: Zoster in children. Am J Dis Child 115:432, 1968.

Gordon JE: Chickenpox. Am J Med Sci 244:362, 1962.

Johnson MT: Treatment of varicella-zoster infections with adenosine arabinoside. J Infect Dis 131:225, 1975.

Norris FH & others: Herpes zoster meningoencephalitis. J Infect Dis 122:335, 1970.

Stevens DA & others: Adverse effect of cytosine arabinoside on disseminated zoster in a controlled trial. N Engl J Med 289:873, 1973.

Whitley RJ & others: Adenine arabinoside therapy of herpes zoster in the immunosuppressed. N Engl J Med 294:1193, 1976.

ARBOVIRUSES

Four clinical syndromes of importance in children are associated with arbovirus infection: encephalitis, dengue, yellow fever, and febrile illnesses such as Colorado tick fever. In general, a cycle of infection between an arthropod and nonhuman vertebrates is established in nature, and humans are infected as a secondary host. Dengue and urban yellow fever are exceptions, as the mosquito transmits the viruses directly from human to human.

ENCEPHALITIS SYNDROMES

Essentials of Diagnosis

- High fever, severe headache, nuchal rigidity, stupor, coma, convulsions, and other CNS symptoms predominate.
- CSF pleocytosis and slight protein elevation (normal in St Louis encephalitis).
- Isolation of virus from blood, CSF, or postmortem specimens (brain, blood).
- Identification of serum antibody rise in paired specimens obtained 3–4 weeks apart.

General Considerations

The major types of arbovirus encephalitis occurring in the USA are St Louis (SLE), California group, and eastern and western equine (EEE and WEE). In recent years, Venezuelan equine encephalitis has been introduced into the USA from its usual endemic areas in Central and South America. A minor cause of arbovirus encephalitis is Powassan, which occurs in the northern USA and Canada.

Clinical Findings

A. History: A history of encephalitic death in horses may precede human cases of EEE and WEE. The epidemic nature of the illness may alert the physician to new cases.

B. Symptoms and Signs: After an incubation period of 5–10 days (as long as 3 weeks in SLE), a sudden onset of high fever and headache heralds the illness. Signs of CNS irritability (convulsions, nausea and vomiting) and depression (coma, stupor, lethargy) appear in association with a stiff neck or back, increased deep tendon reflexes, tremors, muscle weakness, and occasionally paralysis. Mild or asymptomatic infections are observed in WEE and SLE but are uncommon with EEE.

The illness may be abortive, with rapid recovery, or may progress to severe illness and even death. In general, EEE tends to be the most severe.

C. Laboratory Findings: In EEE and WEE, CSF pleocytosis of moderate degree is noted (50–1000 cells/cu mm) and protein concentration may be slightly elevated. CSF glucose concentration remains normal.

Attempts at virus isolation should be made early in the course of an epidemic in order to alert physicians and to inform public health officials. Heparinized blood, CSF, and CNS tissue from fatal cases should be submitted to appropriate diagnostic laboratories. The USPHS maintains diagnostic facilities for this purpose. Serologic diagnosis can be accomplished by demonstration of a 4-fold or greater antibody rise between acute and convalescent sera (7–21 days apart).

Differential Diagnosis

Arbovirus encephalitis must be differentiated from other causes of encephalitis by appropriate laboratory means. Brain tumor, lead and other poisonings, and CNS injuries occurring during an epidemic of arbovirus encephalitis must also be differentiated. The history, appropriate neurologic and neurosurgical diagnostic procedures, and negative virologic studies aid in the differentiation.

The abortive forms must be distinguished from aseptic meningitis due to any cause and from enteroviral infections, particularly since the peak incidence of both illnesses often coincides. Only laboratory study can make the distinction, as the clinical syndromes may be identical. For this reason, throat and stool specimens as well as blood and CSF should be submitted to the virus diagnostic laboratory.

Complications & Sequelae

Infants may develop convulsions, hydrocephalus, mental retardation, and severe CNS damage.

Treatment

Control of convulsions by barbiturates is indicated. The unconscious patient requires continuous care, with attention to the airway, oxygenation, and support of the circulation.

Prognosis

Mortality from encephalitis is greatest with EEE and may exceed 50%, whereas the mortality rate in WEE and SLE is usually less than 25% (often 5–7%).

Barrett FF & others: St. Louis encephalitis in children during the 1964 epidemic. JAMA 193:381, 1965.

Gunderman JR, Stamler R: Neurophysiological residuals seven years after acute encephalitis. Clin Pediatr (Phila) 12:228, 1973.

Powell KE, Blakey DL: St. Louis encephalitis, the 1975 epidemic in Mississippi. JAMA 237:2294, 1977.

Sudia WD, Newhouse VF: Epidemic Venezuelan equine encephalitis in North America: A summary of virus-vector-host relationships. Am J Epidemiol 101:1, 1975.

DENGUE
(Group B Arboviruses)

Dengue in children usually occurs during the preschool or early school years. It is characterized by a sudden onset of fever, severe headache, and retro-ocular pain; severe pain in the extremities and back (thus the term breakbone fever), lymphadenopathy, and a maculopapular or petechial (hemorrhagic) rash.

The fever and course are often diphasic, with an "exacerbation" following temporary improvement. CNS and pneumonic symptoms may occur. Shock and peripheral vascular collapse may result in death in the first week of illness.

Leukopenia and thrombocytopenia may be marked. Hemorrhagic disease may be associated with prolonged bleeding time and maturation arrest of megakaryocytes. Virus may be recovered from the blood. Complications include hemorrhage, shock, and postinfectious asthenia.

Treatment consists of supportive measures for shock, blood replacement for severe hemorrhage, and, in severe cases, corticosteroids. Antipyretics and analgesics suffice for uncomplicated cases.

Fatality rates vary from epidemic to epidemic but are usually low. No sequelae have been observed in survivors.

Dengue. (Editorial.) Lancet 2:239, 1976.

Ehrenkranz NJ: Pandemic dengue in Caribbean countries and the southern United States: Past, present and potential problems. N Engl J Med 285:1460, 1971.

Ventura AK & others: Placental passage of antibodies to dengue virus in persons living in a region of hyperendemic dengue virus infection. J Infect Dis 131(Suppl):62, 1975.

YELLOW FEVER

The severity of yellow fever varies, and mild and inapparent infections occur. In the classic illness, 3 phases are seen following an incubation period of 3–7 days. The first is nonspecific, with abrupt onset, fever, headache, lassitude, nausea and vomiting, and vague muscle aching. A short period of remission is followed by the severe "toxic" phase with high fever associated with bradycardia (Faget's sign), severe jaundice, and gastrointestinal hemorrhage often progressing to shock and death. The disease may be fulminant, with no remissive period; or may be abortive, with only mild nonspecific symptoms. The disease is usually less severe in children.

Leukopenia is the rule. Proteinuria, azotemia, hyperbilirubinemia, elevated BUN, and disturbed liver function tests are observed. Virus can be isolated from the blood in the first 3–4 days of illness and irregularly thereafter. Serologic diagnosis is possible by examination of paired sera obtained 2–4 weeks apart.

Midzonal hepatic cell necrosis with eosinophilic inclusions (Councilman bodies) and relative absence of inflammation are seen at postmortem examination and can be diagnostic.

Treatment is symptomatic and supportive, including fluid and blood replacement, antipyretics, and support of peripheral circulation.

Despite prolonged convalescence in some severely affected patients, no permanent sequelae are noted in survivors. Mortality rates vary, and may be conditioned by age, race, and the status of other arbovirus immunity.

Cahill KM: Yellow fever. NY State J Med 63:2990, 1963.

COLORADO TICK FEVER

Three to 6 days after the bite of an infected tick (*Dermacentor andersoni*), a sudden onset of high fever occurs with retro-ocular, back, and muscular pain. This phase lasts 2–3 days, and a remission of 2–3 days may follow, whereupon a second, usually more severe episode of fever, severe headache, and muscular pain occurs. Rarely, several such episodes occur. In 10–15% of patients, a generalized maculopapular or petechial rash may be present. Symptoms subside slowly, and recovery is usually complete within 10–14 days.

Marked leukopenia (often 1500–2000/cu mm), with a shift to the left occurring on the third to sixth day, is characteristic. In the hemorrhagic forms, thrombocytopenia may be present. Virus may be regularly isolated from the blood during the illness and occasionally from CSF. Serologic testing reveals an increase in antibody 4–6 weeks after onset.

Any cause of fever must be considered in the early phases, but the typical clinical course, leukopenia, and virus isolation serve to distinguish Colorado tick fever. The appearance of a rash may lead to confusion with other viral exanthems, meningococcemia, and various thrombocytopenic states. Bacteriologic and hematologic studies may be of aid in diagnosis.

Encephalitis and severe hemorrhages have been reported. Nuchal rigidity, stupor, headache, or signs of CNS irritability suggest meningoencephalitis and should prompt a lumbar puncture.

Hemorrhage (frequently severe) involving the skin, mucous membranes, gastrointestinal tract, and genitourinary tract may occur.

Treatment is symptomatic and supportive. Transfusion of whole blood may be necessary if hemorrhage occurs.

Most cases are uncomplicated and self-limiting.

Silver HK, Meiklejohn G, Kempe CH: Colorado tick fever. Am J Dis Child 101:30, 1961.

Spruance SL, Bailey A: Colorado tick fever: A review of 115 laboratory confirmed cases. Arch Intern Med 131:288, 1973.

ADENOVIRUSES

There are more than 24 human types of adenoviruses, but relatively few produce illness in children. A carrier state involving one or more adenoviruses is common in young children. Immunity is type-specific.

Many forms of adenovirus disease are recognized:

(1) Pharyngoconjunctival fever: Fever, exudative pharyngitis, and follicular conjunctivitis.

(2) Follicular conjunctivitis: Sporadic illness with preauricular adenopathy and occasional corneal opacification.

(3) Epidemic keratoconjunctivitis: Epidemics of severe conjunctivitis and corneal infiltration traceable to some common source, eg, ophthalmologic examination.

(4) Others: Adenoviruses have been linked with a pertussis-like syndrome, with intussusception, and with a form of obliteration pneumonitis in immunodeficient individuals.

In most of the respiratory infections caused by adenoviruses, the signs and symptoms are not unlike those produced by any of the respiratory viruses. Conjunctivitis and exudative pharyngitis are more commonly due to adenoviral infection than to other viruses and may provide an etiologic clue in local outbreaks.

Specific diagnosis can be made by virus isolation from stools, respiratory secretions, or conjunctival specimens and by identification of antibody responses. A 4-fold antibody rise in paired sera is essential to the diagnosis. Since these viruses may be "carried" in the pharynges of normal children, serologic evidence of infection should be sought; lack of evidence of other respiratory viral etiology supports the diagnosis.

Azizirad H & others: Bronchiolitis obliterans. Clin Pediatr (Phila) 14:572, 1975.

Fox JP, Hall CE, Cooney MK: Observations of adenovirus infections. Am J Epidemiol 105:362, 1977.

Fox JP & others: Observations of adenovirus infections: Virus excretion patterns, antibody response, efficiency of surveillance, patterns of infection, and relation to illness. Am J Epidemiol 89:25, 1969.

Guyer B & others: Epidemic keratoconjunctivitis: A community outbreak of mixed adenovirus type 8 and type 19 infection. J Infect Dis 132:142, 1975.

Nelson KE & others: The role of adenoviruses in the pertussis syndrome. J Pediatr 86:335, 1975.

MISCELLANEOUS VIRUSES

RUBELLA

Essentials of Diagnosis

- Variable clinical expression in childhood.

"Typical case":

- Maculopapular, discrete, rash with rapid caudal progression (3 days).
- Lymphadenopathy preceding and outlasting rash.
- Minimal respiratory and systemic symptoms.

In congenital rubella (usually in combination):

- Thrombocytopenic purpura.
- Deafness.
- Cataract, glaucoma, retinopathy.
- Congenital heart defect.
- Psychomotor retardation.
- Growth retardation.
- Evidence for specific organ infection (hepatitis, osteomyelitis, etc).

General Considerations

It is now appreciated that rubella may be an asymptomatic illness or one associated solely with lymphadenopathy, although the typical illness in children consists principally of a 3-day exanthem. This virus is of major importance because of its proved teratogenic effects on the unborn fetus of a susceptible woman.

Clinical Findings

A. History: The incubation period is 14–21 days (usually 17 days), and in children there is no prodrome. (In adults and adolescents, fever, mild respiratory and constitutional symptoms, and lymphadenopathy may precede the eruption by 1–5 days.)

Maternal exposure to rubella, particularly during the first 12 weeks of gestation, may be associated with fetal disease whether or not a history of illness is elicited in the mother.

B. Symptoms and Signs: Lymphadenopathy may be the first sign of the illness, and is often present for several days prior to rash. Any nodes may be involved, but the suboccipital and postauricular groups are most frequently enlarged. (Lymph node enlargement is not pathognomonic of rubella.) The rash appears first about the face as a pinkish, discrete, macular eruption and rapidly spreads to the trunk and proximal extremities. Within 2 days it fades from the face and trunk and involves the distal extremities. Thereafter, it rapidly disappears and only rarely desquamates. In children, the rash may be the first sign of rubella.

Fever and systemic symptoms are usually absent or are very mild. Rarely, in infancy, a severe rash and constitutional symptoms occur. In the epidemic form in 1964, many children were observed with systemic symptoms, some so severe as to suggest rubeola.

Purpura and petechiae may occur in a small percentage of patients during an epidemic. Arthritis is not uncommon, particularly among adolescent girls and young women. The involved joints may be normal in appearance or may simulate acute rheumatoid arthritis.

Rubella infection during pregnancy may result in fetal infection with varied manifestations. Maternal viremia may produce placental infection and may result in infection of fetal tissues. The critical factor is the exact timing of these events in relation to fetal growth and development. Although estimates vary, most data support the concept that teratogenesis is largely confined to rubella infections occurring in the first 16 weeks of pregnancy. There are reports of isolated deafness in association with infections after this time. Chronic infection, persistent for years after birth, also is related to early fetal infection. Depending upon the exact developmental events taking place at the time of infection, the following manifestations may appear in the fetus and newborn:

1. Growth retardation—This is related to inhibition of cellular multiplication by rubella virus and is manifested as low birth weight ("small for gestational age") and postnatal growth failure.

2. Cardiac anomalies—Among the more common defects are branch stenosis of the pulmonary arteries, patent ductus arteriosus, and ventricular septal defect, although a variety of defects, some very complex, have been described.

3. Eye defects—Congenital glaucoma, cataracts, cloudy corneas, and a distinctive retinopathy (diffuse, sharply demarcated areas of black pigmentation scattered about the retina) are common. Microphthalmia may be noted, particularly in infants with other features of growth retardation.

4. Developmental ear defects—These are usually bilateral and due to maldevelopment of the organ of Corti or the cochlea. The deficit may be so subtle that it is not detected until abnormal speech development calls attention to deafness.

5. Hematologic defects—Thrombocytopenia is the most common defect, ranging from mild to severe, resulting in petechial skin eruption or frank purpura, often at birth or shortly thereafter. The so-called "blueberry muffin" skin rash is due to petechial and purpuric bleeding. Lymphocytopenia may occur with an associated immunologic defect. Hemolytic anemia has also been described.

6. CNS defects—Chronic and persistent viral encephalitis begins in the fetus and results in varying degrees of mental retardation. Syndromes noted have included minimal brain dysfunction (MBD), behavioral disorders, movement disorders, and a slowly progressive degenerative CNS disease resembling subacute sclerosing panencephalitis (SSPE). The decrease in brain growth may be manifest as microcephaly.

7. Immunologic defects—A variety of immunodeficiencies have been attributed to fetal rubella, including cell-mediated immune disorders, hypoimmunoglobulinemias, and complex deficiencies. The usual immunologic response in congenital rubella uncomplicated by immunodeficiency is high levels of fetal IgM rubella antibody admixed with maternally derived IgG rubella antibody. As maternal antibody wanes, the IgM persists, eventually being replaced with IgG rubella antibody actively synthesized by the child.

8. Gastrointestinal disease—The following have been described, usually in association with chronic rubella: hepatitis, pancreatitis, splenitis, diabetes, and malabsorption syndromes.

9. Bone infection—A characteristic rubella osteomyelitis has been described, with circular metaphyseal radiolucent areas associated with metaphysitis.

10. Miscellaneous—A variety of defects have been described whose association with rubella is less certain than those listed above.

C. Laboratory Findings: Leukopenia or thrombocytopenia is seen in some patients. Virus may be recovered prior to the rash (up to 7 days) and as late as 2 weeks after onset. Throat specimens and urine are good sources, but blood must be examined before the onset of rash. Fecal specimens may also yield the virus.

A rise in rubella antibody may be detected between paired sera collected 2 or more weeks apart. Since antibody may be present early in the rash stage of rubella, it is important to collect specimens as early as possible.

In congenital rubella, the following may be detected:

1. Thrombocytopenia, frequently < 10,000 platelets/cu mm.

2. Hemolytic anemia, neuroblastemia, reticulocytosis, an erythroid hyperplastic marrow, and eventual decrease in hemoglobin.

3. Increased levels of direct-reacting bilirubin and evidence of hepatocellular dysfunction.

4. Virus may be recovered from peripheral leukocytes, throat, stool, and urine for months or years after birth. Recovery of virus from the lens has occurred after many years.

5. High and persistent rubella antibody titer in the serum.

6. Abnormalities in immunoglobulin concentration (variable, but includes depression of IgA and IgG levels with increased IgM levels).

7. A defect in cellular immunity.

8. CSF pleocytosis and increase in protein.

D. X-Ray Findings: Signs of pneumonia may be present in congenital rubella. Radiographic evidence of rubella osteomyelitis consists of alternating linear densities and translucent streaks in the metaphyses of the long bones.

Differential Diagnosis

Rubella must be differentiated from other acute viral exanthematous diseases (Table 25–2). In general, the 3-day course of the pinkish rash, prior lymphadenopathy, and minimal or absent prodromal symptoms serve as useful clinical criteria for diagnosis. However, in cases where the distinction is important (as in the pregnant female), virus isolation and serology are essential.

Arthritis or arthralgia raises the possibility of rheumatoid arthritis (fever, splenomegaly, history, multiple joint involvement), and the distinction may be blurred by a positive latex fixation test. The transient nature of rubella arthritis may aid in the differentiation.

Congenital rubella must be differentiated from other infections acquired in utero, including toxoplasmosis (by specific antibody studies), cytomegalovirus infection (by virus recovery and specific antibody studies), and congenital syphilis (by serologic study).

Complications & Sequelae

A. Encephalitis: Encephalitis occurs in no more than one out of 6000 cases of rubella. The manifestations are those of postinfectious encephalitis due to any cause, although rubella encephalitis tends to be mild, with less frequent sequelae and few fatalities. A severe encephalitis, much like measles-associated subacute sclerosing panencephalitis, has been described after congenital rubella.

B. Rubella During Pregnancy: Rubella in pregnant women is not unusually severe, but the potential risk to the fetus is great. The following generalizations may be made in the light of currently available evidence:

The risk to infants following maternal rubella is greatest in the first 3–4 months of pregnancy. In Cooper's study, only one out of 16 infants born to mothers infected after the fourth month were abnormal, whereas 243 out of 291 were abnormal when infection occurred before the end of the fourth month. The risk in this series was greatest in the first 2 months, when 157 out of 166 infants were abnormal; next highest in the third month, with 64 of 82 infants affected; and lowest in the fourth month, with 22 out of 43 infants involved.

Gamma globulin administered to the exposed pregnant female has no effect in preventing fetal infection.

Treatment

A. Specific Measures: Despite the demonstration of antiviral activity of amantadine in vitro, no specific therapy for rubella is available.

B. General Measures: The usual case requires no therapy. Purpura is usually confined to the skin, and no treatment is necessary. It is conceivable that severe hemorrhage might occur, requiring transfusion of whole blood or platelets. Arthritis is controlled with aspirin and limitation of motion.

C. In Pregnancy: Therapeutic abortion is recommended in some pregnancies. This practice is tempered by local standards, religious beliefs, and law.

Prognosis

Rubella is almost always a self-limited, uncomplicated disease with complete recovery. Congenital rubella can result in death or prolonged handicap.

Cooper LZ & others: Rubella: Clinical manifestations and management. Am J Dis Child 118:18, 1969.

Donowitz M, Gryboski JD: Pancreatic insufficiency and the congenital rubella syndrome. J Pediatr 87:241, 1975.

Hambling MH: Effect of a vaccination programme on the distribution of rubella antibodies in women of childbearing age. Lancet 1:1130, 1975.

Hattis RR & others: Rubella in an immunized island population. JAMA 223:1019, 1973.

Heggie AD, Robbins FC: Natural rubella acquired after birth. Am J Dis Child 118:12, 1969.

Horstmann DM: Rubella and the rubella syndrome: New epidemiologic virologic observations. Calif Med 102:397, 1965.

Lebon P, Lyon F: Non-congenital rubella encephalitis. Lancet 2:468, 1974.

Stoffman J, Wolfish MG: The susceptibility of adolescent girls to rubella. Clin Pediatr (Phila) 15:625, 1976.

Weil ML & others: Chronic progressive panencephalitis due to rubella virus simulating subacute sclerosing panencephalitis. N Engl J Med 292:994, 1975.

CYTOMEGALIC INCLUSION DISEASE
(Cytomegaloviruses)

Essentials of Diagnosis

- The syndrome of hepatosplenomegaly, microcephaly, and chorioretinitis occurring in a jaundiced infant with a petechial rash is classical.
- Variants occur with only part of the syndrome.
- Periventricular intracranial calcification.
- Inclusion bodies (owl's eye) in cells sedimented from freshly voided urine or in liver biopsy.
- Detection of virus in urine or saliva. (*Note:* Do not freeze specimens. Keep at 0–4° C.)

General Considerations

It was originally thought that the cytomegaloviruses produce only a characteristic fulminant, generalized neonatal infection, but it has recently been shown that in older children and adults they may cause pulmonary or gastrointestinal infections also. Patients receiving immunosuppressive therapy may develop clinical disease by unmasking of latent virus infection, usually in the lungs.

Many investigators believe that additional illnesses will be attributable to the cytomegaloviruses, since they are ubiquitous and most individuals are infected (as shown by the finding of serum antibody and, occasionally, asymptomatic virus excretion).

Cytomegalovirus infection may result from infusion of blood containing the virus. An appreciable risk occurs in a susceptible patient receiving large quantities of whole blood (cardiac surgery, etc).

Clinical Findings

A. History: Since the maternal disease is asymptomatic, the history is of little value. A history of prior cytomegalovirus infection in an infant virtually assures that subsequent siblings will be unaffected despite chronic shedding of the virus by the mother.

B. Symptoms and Signs: In full-blown neonatal disease, jaundice, massive hepatosplenomegaly associated with CNS signs (lethargy, convulsions, etc), and a petechial-purpuric rash are present. Milder forms of the disease are seen. Fewer infants have chorioretinitis and cerebral calcification, but almost all have some degree of microcephaly, occasionally striking. Surviving infants are usually severely mentally and physically handicapped, and hepatosplenomegaly and jaundice may persist. A syndrome resembling infectious mononucleosis may occur without accompanying heterophil antibody rise. Isolated hepatitis has been described.

Pulmonary disease has been observed in cytomegalovirus-infected children. Interstitial pneumonitis is the most common lesion, but wheezing or tachypnea with positive x-rays is also observed. The illness may be prolonged and intractable and most often occurs in immunodeficient or immunosuppressed individuals.

C. Laboratory Findings: Anemia, thrombocytopenia, and hyperbilirubinemia are usually present. CSF pleocytosis and elevated protein with normal glucose concentration are found. Typical owl's eye intranuclear basophilic inclusions can be found in cells in freshly voided urine. Delay in examination may result in lack of visualization of the inclusions. Tissue from other organs can also be utilized; examination of liver biopsy material can establish the diagnosis.

Virus can regularly be isolated from the urine for many months and even years after birth. Salivary and fecal excretion of virus is also detectable, but for shorter periods.

Diagnosis by antibody determination is clouded by the widespread incidence of infection; more than 70% of all infants have antibody in their cord sera. Therefore, serologic diagnosis is less helpful than isolation of virus and histologic technics.

D. X-Ray Findings: Skull films may show typical periventricular calcification.

Differential Diagnosis

Cytomegalic inclusion disease must be differentiated from other causes of jaundice, hepatosplenomegaly, and petechial rash in the newborn, principally toxoplasmosis (diagnosed by elevated Feldman-Sabin dye test antibody titer and suggested by generalized instead of periventricular cerebral calcification); generalized herpetic neonatal infection (presence of vesicular skin lesions, lack of cerebral calcification, specific virologic tests); generalized coxsackievirus infection (myocarditis predominates, epidemic nature, isolation of virus); hemolytic disease of newborn (no microcephaly, positive Coombs tests, demonstration of incompatibility for rhesus or ABO antigens); bacterial sepsis, including syphilis (positive blood culture or serology, osseous changes, lack of microcephaly); and galactosemia (galactosuria and galactosemia, proteinuria, aminoaciduria, and absence of other signs of cytomegalovirus infection).

Pneumonia in older individuals must be differentiated from *Pneumocystis carinii* infection, which is usually accomplished by identification of the parasite.

Complications & Sequelae

Residual cerebral damage frequently results in mental and physical retardation of marked degree. Institutionalization may be necessary for total care of the patient.

Treatment

There is no specific treatment. Symptomatic therapy may reduce immediate morbidity but usually does not influence the final outcome.

Floxuridine may be of benefit in severe cytomegalovirus infections in children with leukemia or other diseases associated with immunosuppression.

Prognosis

The exact mortality rate is difficult to estimate because of a broad base of asymptomatic infections. Fulminant forms of the disease are almost universally fatal in the neonatal period.

Sensorineural hearing loss occurs frequently in both symptomatic and asymptomatic infants with congenital cytomegalovirus infection. Symptomatic cytomegalovirus infection may also result in impaired vision.

Cox F, Hughes WT: Cytomegaloviremia in children with acute lymphocytic leukemia. J Pediatr 87:190, 1975.

Hanshaw JB: Congenital cytomegalovirus infection: A fifteen year perspective. J Infect Dis 123:555, 1971.

Henson D & others: Cytomegalovirus infections during acute childhood leukemia. J Infect Dis 126:469, 1972.

Reynolds DW & others: Maternal cytomegalovirus excretion and perinatal infection. N Engl J Med 289:1, 1973.

Smith SD & others: Pulmonary involvement with cytomegalovirus infections in children. Arch Dis Child 52:441, 1977.

Stagno S & others: Auditory and visual defects resulting from symptomatic and subclinical congenital cytomegaloviral and toxoplasma infections. Pediatrics 59:669, 1977.

Weller TH: The cytomegaloviruses: Ubiquitous agents with protean clinical manifestations. (2 parts.) N Engl J Med 285:203, 267, 1971.

Yeager A & others: Congenital cytomegalovirus infection outcome for the subsequent sibling. Clin Pediatr (Phila) 16:455, 1977.

ROSEOLA INFANTUM
(Exanthem Subitum)

Roseola infantum is a usually benign, self-limited infection which has been transmitted by filtrates of blood. No specific virus has been isolated.

Clinical Findings

A. History: The typical clinical picture is 3 days of sustained high fever, often with a febrile convulsion at onset, in a child who otherwise appears well. Roseola occasionally occurs in epidemics, even in young adults.

B. Symptoms and Signs: A discrete pink rash is the most characteristic finding. It is often evanescent, and typically appears as the fever decreases or shortly thereafter. The rash is occasionally generalized and may coalesce. Any sustained fever in an infant or child under 3 years of age should therefore alert the physician and parents to look for a rash, which may be mild or transient. The temperature falls to lower than normal after defervescence. Edema of the eyelids has been said to be diagnostic, but this is not regularly observed and may not be specific.

C. Laboratory Findings: Leukocytosis with a shift to the left may be present at onset, but leukopenia is more common and may be marked at the time of rash.

Differential Diagnosis

The presence of high fever and the frequency of initial convulsions may suggest other causes of this combination, including bacterial meningitis and encephalitis. The age of the child, well-being following recovery from the seizure, and the typical course plus a normal CSF are helpful in the differentiation.

Complications & Sequelae

Some workers claim that encephalitis is common, but sequelae occur infrequently if at all.

Treatment

Fever can be controlled with supplemental fluids, gentle tepid water sponge baths, and aspirin. Convulsions are usually self-limited and single, requiring no therapy. Barbiturates are rarely required. With a history of prior "febrile" convulsions, administration of elixir of phenobarbital, 15 mg 3 times daily, should be considered. Antimicrobial agents are not indicated and are of no benefit.

Prognosis

Roseola is almost universally benign, and complete recovery is the rule.

Juretić M: Exanthem subitum: A review of 243 cases. Helv Paediatr Acta 18:80, 1963.

ERYTHEMA INFECTIOSUM
(Fifth Disease)

This disease (of presumed viral origin) is characterized by an intensely erythematous, slightly raised, hot eruption of the cheeks ("slapped face") followed after 1 day by a maculopapular eruption on the extensor surfaces of the proximal extremities. With spread and continued evolution, the rash assumes a striking reticular or lacy pattern. The rash is frequently enhanced by a warm bath or by wrapping the arm in a towel. It lasts for a few days to several weeks, often clearing and reappearing. There are usually no other symptoms, and resolution is eventually complete.

Complications or sequelae are rare. No treatment is necessary.

Balfour HH & others: A study of erythema infectiosum: Recovery of rubella virus and echovirus 12. Pediatrics 50:285, 1972.

Hall C, Horner F: Encephalopathy with erythema infectiosum. Am J Dis Child 131:65, 1977.

INFECTIOUS MONONUCLEOSIS

Essentials of Diagnosis

- Fever, pharyngitis, lymphadenopathy, and splenomegaly.
- Lymphocytosis with atypical lymphocytes.
- Positive heterophil test.

General Considerations

Infectious mononucleosis is an acute, self-limiting infectious disease characterized by increased numbers of atypical lymphocytes and monocytes in the peripheral blood. The disease is presumed to be due to a virus (EB virus). The disorder can occur at any age but is seen most frequently in children and young adults. In the majority of patients the serum reveals an increased titer of agglutinins for sheep red cells (heterophil antibody test). However, in children under 5 years of age, the heterophil test is often negative.

Clinical Findings

A. Symptoms and Signs: Children with infectious mononucleosis often present with fever, sore throat, exudative tonsillitis, malaise, generalized lymphadenopathy, and splenomegaly. Other clinical features may be headache, epistaxis, jaundice, and abdominal pain. A morbilliform or maculopapular exanthem is not unusual. Almost any system may be involved; hepatitis, encephalitis, meningitis, polyradiculoneuritis, pneumonitis, and carditis have all been reported. There is an increased susceptibility to rupture of the spleen. Recently, spatial and visual distortion have been reported in adolescents.

B. Laboratory Findings:

1. Peripheral blood—The leukocyte count varies greatly; although the usual white count is 10–20 thousand/cu mm, a normal or low count may be present. A rather constant feature is the appearance of increased numbers of atypical lymphocytes and monocytes in the peripheral blood smear, ranging from 50–90% of the total differential count. The hemoglobin, hematocrit, and platelets are usually normal. Thrombocytopenia and autoimmune hemolytic anemia occasionally may be complicating factors.

2. Screening test for mononucleosis—A rapid screening test (Monospot) has been developed for the diagnosis of mononucleosis. This slide test relies upon the differential reactivity of patients' sera with guinea pig kidney and beef red blood cells in the presence of a reactor system, horse erythrocytes. The test is rapid, sensitive, easy to perform, and inexpensive. False-negative reactions are rare; false-positive reactions have been reported in 5–14% of sera containing other heterophil antibodies in such diseases as hepatitis, cytomegalovirus infection, adenovirus infection, leukemia, and rubella. One advantage of this test is its ability to detect patients with low levels of sheep red cell agglutinins (20–40), thus enabling diagnosis to be made where other technics fail.

3. Serology—The heterophil antibody (Paul-Bunnell) test is often positive in a titer above 1:112. Early in the course of the disease or in young children, this test may be negative. An attempt to make the heterophil test more reliable uses differential agglutination after absorption as follows:

Serum Source	Heterophil Agglutinins Present After Absorption By	
	Guinea Pig Kidney	Beef Cells
Infectious mononucleosis	+	–
Normal sera	–	+
Serum sickness	–	–

Differential Diagnosis

Differential diagnosis includes leukemia (usually with pancytopenia or circulating "blast" cells), acute infectious lymphocytosis (increase in small mature lymphocytes), viral exanthems (clinical course differs), infectious hepatitis (fewer atypical lymphocytes and absence of lymphadenopathy), and aseptic meningoencephalitis (absence of splenomegaly and lymphadenopathy). In addition, many young infants and children have a few atypical lymphocytes without evidence of illness.

Treatment

Treatment is symptomatic. Emphasis is on supportive care when the major systems (liver, heart, nervous system) are involved. In older children and adolescents the symptoms may be quite severe, and hospitalization and bed rest are often necessary. In severe disease, some success has been noted in controlled trials with corticosteroids or chloroquine.

Prognosis

The prognosis is good for complete recovery after a period of illness of 3–6 weeks or, with major system involvement, longer. Rupture of the spleen and secondary infection are the major complications.

Balfour HH & others: Penicillin associated exanthems in infectious mononucleosis identical to those associated with ampicillin. Clin Pediatr (Phila) 11:417, 1972.

Brodsky AL, Heath CW: Infectious mononucleosis epidemiologic patterns at United States colleges and universities. Am J Epidemiol 96:87, 1972.

Copperman SM: "Alice in Wonderland" syndrome as a presenting symptom of infectious mononucleosis in children. Clin Pediatr (Phila) 16:143, 1977.

Fermaglich DR: Pulmonary involvement in infectious mononucleosis. J Pediatr 86:93, 1975.

Fernbach DJ & others: Infectious mononucleosis. Pediatr Clin North Am 19:957, 1972.

Niederman JC & others: Infectious mononucleosis: Epstein-Barr virus shedding in saliva and the oropharynx. N Engl J Med 294:1355, 1976.

Ragab AH, Vietti TJ: Infectious mononucleosis, lymphoblastic leukemia, and the EB virus. Cancer 24:261, 1969.

RABIES

Essentials of Diagnosis

- History of animal bite (wild, sick, or unidentified).
- Early hypesthesia or paresthesia in area of bite.
- Increasing irritability with clear sensorium.
- Hydrophobia—initially to drinking, later to sight of water.
- Progressive symptoms to death.
- Isolation of rabies virus from animal brain confirming Negri body visualization or fluorescent antibody identification.
- CSF may be normal, or there may be pleocytosis and slightly elevated protein.
- Mild to moderate peripheral leukocytosis.

General Considerations

Rabies is an almost unexceptionally fatal disease which is transmitted to humans by the bite of a rabid animal. The variable results following such bites are due to the presence or absence of virus in the animal's saliva, the extent and location of the wound, the promptness with which preventive measures are instituted, and the immune status of the bitten individual. Accurate diagnosis and correct therapy depend upon determination of the presence or absence of rabies. This requires knowledge about the prevalence of rabies in the community, the immunization status of the animal, and observation of the living animal for at least 10 days following the bite.

Clinical Findings

A. History:

1. The animal bite—In most instances, a clear-cut history of animal bite is obtained. The animal is usually a dog, but may be a wild skunk, fox, wolf, etc or unknown to the patient. Multiple bites may have occurred. If the animal was a pet, unusual behavior and an unprovoked bite should suggest rabies. Death of the animal complicates the history. With prolonged incubation periods, the history of animal bite, particularly in a young child or if the wound was slight, may be lacking.

Rabies may also be transmitted by bats; rarely, the bat's environment, particularly in caves, may serve as a means of transmission where no bite is involved.

2. The animal—Peculiar behavior of an animal during observation is noted. The dog, the usual offender, may become hyperirritable and begin to bite anything in its environment. Conversely, progressive lethargy and paralysis may be seen ("dumb" rabies). If the animal remains healthy for 10 days or more after the bite, the possibility of rabies is remote.

3. The patient—Following the bite, no symptoms occur for 10 days to many months. The duration of the incubation period is related to the site of the bite in relation to the brain and to the severity of the bite (and therefore to the amount of rabies virus inoculated). Very short incubation periods have been associated with direct intracranial bites and prolonged ones with slight trauma to the distal extremities.

B. Symptoms and Signs: The first symptom in the typical form of the disease relates to the region of the bite. Tingling or loss of sensation is reported. The patient then experiences increasing apprehension, anxiety, and hyperexcitability despite a clear sensorium. Episodes of convulsive movements, irrational behavior, or frank delirium may alternate with lethargy. Progressive aversion to water or the act of swallowing ensues, and drooling and spasmodic contraction of the muscles of deglutition follow.

The course is progressive and culminates in death. Increasing CNS depression, cardiovascular and respiratory instability, and fever end in death 5–7 days after onset.

C. Laboratory Findings: Rabies virus may be recovered from saliva during life or from CNS tissue or salivary glands after death. Virus identification rarely leads to premortem diagnosis because death occurs before laboratory studies can be completed. A presumptive diagnosis can be made on the basis of examination of the animal's brain, if available, for rabies virus content. Fluorescent antibody or Negri body identification should always be confirmed by virus isolation.

Examination of CSF is of little aid. Most often it is normal, although elevation of the white cell count and protein may occur. The presence of peripheral leukocytosis is of little diagnostic significance.

Differential Diagnosis

Differentiation from other forms of encephalitis is usually not difficult. The history of animal bite, an appropriate incubation period, and the characteristic clinical course should be sufficient. Adequate virologic diagnosis of other forms of encephalitis should be attempted.

Prevention*

Despite adequate support, almost all patients die. Therefore, treatment at the time of the animal bite is directed at preventing the clinical disease.

The World Health Organization has outlined its recommendations for the use of rabies hyperimmune serum and vaccines in the prophylactic treatment of animal bites. However, local conditions should modify these recommendations, particularly because the risk of bites by domestic animals in many areas is almost negligible as a result of absence of a convenient reservoir in the wild animal population or insufficient opportunities for contact between domestic and wild animals. The guidelines laid down by the California State Department of Public Health (see below and Chapter 5) can be made applicable to local conditions. Early and adequate local treatment of the wound, local epidemiologic factors, veterinary consultation, adequate field investigation, and the facts and circum-

*See also Chapter 5.

stances associated with the bite may modify the physician's judgment with regard to the systemic treatment indicated in individual cases. The following is intended only as a guide.

A. Local Treatment of the Wound: If the animal is not overtly rabid and has been impounded, cleanse the wound carefully with bland soap and water and irrigate copiously with saline solution. Debride devitalized tissues. Give tetanus prophylaxis. If the animal is known to be rabid, or if the attack was unprovoked and the animal has been killed or has escaped, cauterize the wound with fuming nitric acid, irrigate copiously with saline, and cleanse with soap and water.

B. Antirabies Immunization:*

1. No lesion (indirect contact; licks of unabraded skin)—No treatment even if animal is overtly rabid.

2. Licks of abraded or scratched skin or mucosa—No treatment if animal remains healthy. Start vaccine at first sign of rabies in animal.

3. Bites other than multiple bites or face, head, or neck bites—

a. Start vaccine at first sign of rabies in animal.

b. Stop treatment on fifth day after exposure if the animal at first showed signs suggestive of rabies but is normal after 5 days.

c. Start vaccine immediately (see Chapter 5) if the animal is overtly rabid or it has escaped, was killed, or cannot be identified.

4. Multiple bites or face, head, or neck bites—

a. Start human rabies immune globulin immediately. Give no vaccine as long as the animal remains normal.

b. Start vaccine at first sign of rabies in animal.

c. Stop vaccine if animal is normal on fifth day after exposure.

d. Give human immune globulin immediately, followed by vaccine, if the animal is rabid, escaped, killed, or unknown; or for bites by a wild animal (especially a skunk, raccoon, fox, or bat, although all warmblooded animals except birds or rodents are suspect).

Treatment

Experience with 3 recent cases of rabies suggests that prolonged survival and, in one case, apparent recovery may occur if vigorous early supportive therapy is utilized. Early tracheostomy, careful attention to maintaining oxygenation, circulatory support, and ventilation are suggested.

Prognosis

Although rare instances of survival in suspected rabies have been reported, the disease is almost always fatal. Whether application of vigorous early supportive therapy will alter this prognosis cannot be stated at present.

*Modified from recommendations of the California State Department of Public Health, May, 1960. Physicians in rabies-enzootic areas are advised to consult WHO Technical Report Series No. 321, 1966, prepared by the Expert Committee on Rabies of the World Health Organization.

Gode GR & others: Intensive care in rabies. Lancet 2:6, 1976.

Hattwick MAW & others: Recovery from rabies. Ann Intern Med 76:931, 1972.

Hattwick MAW & others: Skunk-associated human rabies. JAMA 222:44, 1972.

Kappus KD: Canine rabies in the US, 1971−73: Study of reported cases with reference to vaccination history. Am J Epidemiol 103:242, 1976.

Loofbourow JC & others: Rabies immune globulin (human). JAMA 217:1825, 1971.

U.S. Public Health Advisory Committee on Immunization Practices: Rabies. Morbid Mortal Wkly Rep, Suppl 21, p 17, June 24, 1972.

II. RICKETTSIAL INFECTIONS (RICKETTSIOSES)

The rickettsiae are pleomorphic coccobacillary organisms which are intracellular parasites. They are now classified as true bacteria.

Characteristically, human infections occur as a result of arthropod contact. Only those diseases encountered in pediatrics will be considered here.

Common characteristics of rickettsiae and the infections they produce may be listed as follows:

(1) Asymptomatic multiplication in the arthropod host.

(2) Intracellular replication.

(3) Limited geographic and seasonal occurrence related to arthropod ecology.

(4) Local primary lesions (rickettsialpox, scrub typhus, tick typhus).

(5) Fever, rash, and respiratory symptoms predominate.

(6) Nonspecific (Weil-Felix reaction, H proteus agglutinins) and specific antibodies develop following human infection.

(7) Infections respond to the tetracyclines and chloramphenicol.

RICKETTSIALPOX

Rickettsialpox is an acute, self-limited disease caused by infection with *Rickettsia akari.* It is transmitted by mites from the common house mouse. Following an incubation period of 2 weeks, fever, chills, myalgia, headache and photophobia appear abruptly. At the site of the mite bite, a primary firm, red papule appears which vesiculates and becomes crusted with a black eschar. Two to 4 days after onset, a generalized papulovesicular eruption appears which evolves to crusting within 2 days. The crusts are shed in 1−2 weeks. The differential diagnosis includes varicella, variola, flea typhus, Rocky Mountain spotted fever,

and scrub typhus. Leukopenia is frequent early in the illness, and complement-fixing antibodies appear during or after the second week of illness. The drug of choice is tetracycline (see Chapter 37).

TICK TYPHUS
(Rocky Mountain Spotted Fever, Boutonneuse Fever, North Queensland Tick Typhus, Spotted Fevers, Etc)

The tick-borne rickettsioses have many features in common, and are all produced by rickettsiae which may be considered subspecies of *R rickettsii.* They differ in the locale of infection and bear regional names for the illnesses. All are transmitted by the hard ticks, including the genera Dermacentor, Haemaphysalis, Amblyomma, and Rhipicephalus. Animal hosts vary and include rodents, rabbits, and dogs.

1. ROCKY MOUNTAIN SPOTTED FEVER

The name of this disease is a misnomer since it is seen throughout the USA and is found with greater frequency in some eastern and southeastern states than in the Rocky Mountain region. The ixodid ticks serve as the vector for *Rickettsia rickettsii.* Most cases are seen in the late spring and early summer in children who frequent wooded and rural areas.

There has been a recent increase in the number of cases of Rocky Mountain spotted fever throughout endemic areas in the USA. Most cases occurred in the East (from Massachusetts to Florida), the Southeast, and the Midwest. Very few have been reported in the Rockies or Far West.

Following an incubation period of 3−7 days, chills, fever, and influenza-like symptoms appear suddenly. There may be associated headache, sore throat, retro-orbital pain, photophobia, nosebleed, myalgias, arthralgias, gastrointestinal symptoms, and abdominal pain. Severe CNS manifestations may occur, ie, coma, delirium, stupor, and profound lethargy. Physical findings initially include conjunctivitis, fever, splenomegaly (in 50% of cases), and, occasionally, cyanosis, hepatomegaly, and jaundice. Within 2−11 days (usually 3−5 days), a tiny red macular eruption appears on the wrists and ankles and spreads to involve the entire extremities and the trunk, usually sparing the face. The macules grow larger and become petechial within 2−3 days.

Laboratory findings may include proteinuria, bilirubinuria, and hematuria. The diagnosis may be established by culture or complement fixation tests. Proteus OX-19 and OX-2 agglutinins become detectable during the second week (Weil-Felix reaction). The illness may be complicated by myocarditis, pneumonia, and cerebral infarction.

Before the availability of antimicrobial agents, the mortality rate was 25—75%. Specific therapy includes the tetracyclines or chloramphenicol (see Chapter 37). For persons at high risk, a vaccine is available.

Annual Summary 1976. Morbid Mortal Wkly Rep 25:53, Aug 1977.

DeShazo RD & others: Early diagnosis of Rocky Mountain spotted fever. JAMA 235:1353, 1976.

Kahn LI: Rocky Mountain spotted fever (Clinical Conference, St. Louis Children's Hospital). Clin Pediatr (Phila) 8:331, 1969.

Lee RV: Keeping the rickettsioses in check. Drug Ther 5:37, July 1975.

Peters AH: Tick-borne typhus (Rocky Mountain spotted fever). JAMA 216:1003, 1971.

2. OTHER FORMS OF TICK TYPHUS

African tick typhus is generally mild, usually terminating by rapid lysis in the second week. An abrupt onset is usual, with severe headache, constipation, insomnia, photophobia, myalgia, and arthralgia. Mental disturbances may occur but are not severe. In a varying proportion of cases, an eschar is already developed at onset, with painful enlargement of regional lymph nodes. The eschar may be anywhere on the body, at the site of the tick bite, but is usually on covered parts. The rash is similar to that of the American type, but is less often petechial and may be transitory or absent, especially outside the Mediterranean region. In the mildest cases, there may be no more than a few days of fever with headache, with or without an eschar and lymphadenopathy.

North Queensland tick typhus has been little studied. Fever lasts less than a week and may be intermittent. The rash is variable in character.

EPIDEMIC TYPHUS
(Louse Typhus)

This disease is produced by infection with *R prowazekii* and is transmitted in the feces of the body louse. Following an incubation period of 8—12 days, during which malaise, cough, nausea, coryza, headache, and chest pain may occur, the disease begins with an abrupt rise in temperature accompanied by chills and severe prostration. Headache, nausea and vomiting, gastrointestinal symptoms, cough, nonpleuritic chest pain, stupor and delirium, and severe muscle aching may occur. Conjunctivitis, flushing, splenomegaly (one-third of cases), rales, low blood pressure, and a rash may be seen. The rash is characteristic, beginning on the third to eighth day of illness with pink maculopapules that appear on the trunk and spread to the extremities. The rash usually spares the face, scalp, palms, and soles, and may become hemorrhagic.

Leukopenia may be present during the first week, and leukocytosis during the second. Proteinuria is common, and hematuria may occur. Although rickettsiae can be isolated, the diagnosis is usually made by the appearance of proteus OX-19 (and occasionally OX-2) agglutinins and specific complement-fixing antibody titers during or after the second week of illness.

The illness usually lasts 2—3 weeks, and convalescence may be prolonged. A recrudescent form of the disease is seen in adults (Brill's disease).

Therapy consists of tetracyclines or chloramphenicol (see Chapter 37.)

ENDEMIC TYPHUS
(Murine Typhus)

Endemic typhus is caused by *R mooseri* and is usually transmitted by fleas from a rodent (house rat) reservoir. Body lice may become infected and transmit the agent in their feces.

The illness is gradual in onset. Although the symptoms resemble those of epidemic typhus, they are milder and shorter in duration. The prognosis is also better, and fatalities and complications are rarely seen. Proteus OX-19 agglutinins and specific complement-fixing antibody titers appear in the second week.

Adams WH & others: The changing ecology of murine (endemic) typhus in Southern California. Am J Trop Med Hyg 19:311, 1970.

• • •

FEVER OF UNDETERMINED ORIGIN
(FUO)*

It is virtually impossible to be certain of the cause of fever in the first week of illness unless a specific and localizing diagnosis can be made on the basis of the history, clinical findings, or laboratory findings, including the results of viral and bacterial cultures, x-rays, etc. In the first 5 days of illness, a fever is most apt to be due to acute infection. Viral infections are rarely febrile beyond 10 days, though untreated or inadequately treated bacterial infections can last for weeks or months.

In the second week of fever, if no clinical or laboratory findings point to an infectious cause, consideration must be given to silent encapsulated infections (most commonly abscesses of the brain, kidney, bone, liver, lung, etc). Noninvasive radiologic scanning technics are now available for the investigation of these possibilities.

*Contributed by C. Henry Kempe, MD.

At the end of 2 weeks, one should consider the 2 other common major groups of diseases causing fevers of a chronic nature: autoimmune disorders and neoplasms. The most common autoimmune disorder causing chronic fever in childhood is acute juvenile rheumatoid arthritis; in older children, lupus erythematosus and other autoimmune diseases should be considered. The most common neoplasm of childhood is acute lymphatic leukemia. In the preleukemic state, fever may be the only symptom, although the platelet count in peripheral blood may be low.

In summary, the first week of fever can reasonably be thought to be due to acute infection; in the second week, chronic bacterial infection should be considered; and after 2 weeks one must entertain the possibilities of the 2 most common other causes: autoimmune disease, especially juvenile rheumatoid arthritis, and neoplasia, principally leukemia.

The lists that follow are by no means complete.

Infectious Diseases

Bacterial, mycotic, parasitic, spirochetal, and viral infections of various tissues, organs, and systems, including abscesses in the following locations: alveolar, appendiceal, intracranial, intraspinal, perinephric, pulmonary, retropharyngeal, and subphrenic

Acute infectious lymphocytosis
Acute yellow atrophy
Amebiasis
Appendicitis
Ascariasis
Bronchiectasis
Brucellosis
Cat scratch disease
Cholangitis
Coccidioidomycosis
Empyema
Encephalitis
Exanthems
Haverhill fever
Hepatitis
Histoplasmosis
Infectious mononucleosis
Influenza
Leptospirosis
Lymphocytosis, acute
Malaria
Mastoiditis
Mediastinitis
Meningitis
Myalgia, epidemic
Myocarditis
Osteomyelitis
Otitis media
Pancreatitis
Poliomyelitis
Psittacosis
Salmonellosis
Septicemia
Shigellosis
Sinusitis
Spinal epidural infections
Spirillum fever
Streptococcal disease
Syphilis
Torulosis
Toxoplasmosis
Trichinosis
Tuberculosis
Tularemia
Urinary tract infections

Diseases of "hypersensitization"

Dermatomyositis
Lupus erythematosus
Polyarteritis nodosa
Rheumatic fever
Rheumatoid arthritis
Serum sickness

Blood Diseases & Neoplastic Diseases

Agranulocytosis
Cervical cord tumors
Ewing's tumor
Hemolytic anemia
Hodgkin's disease
Leukemia
Sickle cell anemia
Transfusion reaction
Other tumors

Central Nervous System Disorders

Brain tumors
Convulsive states
Hemorrhage, intracranial
Hypothalamic lesions
Medullary lesions
Third ventricle lesions

Dehydration

● ● ●

General References

Blanic H, Rake C: *Rickettsial Disease of the Skin, Eye and Mucous Membranes of Man.* Little, Brown, 1955.

Committee on Infectious Diseases: *Report,* 18th ed. American Academy of Pediatrics, 1974.

Hoeprich PD: *Infectious Diseases.* Harper & Row, 1972.

Horsfall FL, Tamm I: *Viral and Rickettsial Infections of Man,* 4th ed. Lippincott, 1965.

Jawetz E, Melnick JL, Adelberg EA: *Review of Medical Microbiology,* 12th ed. Lange, 1976.

Krugman S, Ward R: *Infectious Diseases of Children,* 5th ed. Mosby, 1973.

Lennette EH, Schmidt NJ: *Diagnostic Procedures for Viral and Rickettsial Diseases,* 5th ed. American Public Health Association, Inc, 1974.

Melnick JL (editor): *Progress in Medical Virology.* Karger, 1973.

26 ...
Infections: Bacterial & Spirochetal

Jerry J. Eller, MD

BACTERIAL INFECTIONS

GROUP A BETA-HEMOLYTIC
STREPTOCOCCAL INFECTIONS

Distinct clinical entities are seen in specific age groups.

(1) In early childhood, the disease is mild, with low-grade fever, serous nasal discharge, pallor, and failure to thrive.

(2) In middle childhood, an abrupt onset of fever, sore throat with exudate, and vomiting may be prominent symptoms. The eruption of scarlet fever is finely papular, erythematous, and in appearance much like a mild sunburn. The diagnosis is confirmed by a positive culture of group A beta-hemolytic streptococci from a throat swab.

(3) The adult type (after 10 years of age) has a more insidious onset with fewer toxic symptoms.

Streptococcal respiratory infections are caused by group A beta-hemolytic streptococci. Transmission is by inhalation of droplets from an infected individual. The average incubation period is 1–3 days. Outbreaks of group A streptococcal infections on maternity and newborn services have occurred. Raw and processed powdered milk and contaminated eggs are sources of organisms in food-borne epidemics, which are occasionally reported.

Streptococcal infections of the lungs, brain, and endocardium are life-threatening unless promptly treated.

Vaginal, skin, and respiratory tract infections are of concern principally because they may lead to the development of sensitizing antibodies which predispose to the later development of rheumatic fever or acute glomerulonephritis.

In scarlet fever, the host responds to the erythrogenic toxin of the streptococcus by development of an erythematous eruption, strawberry tongue, Pastia's lines, and other manifestations. Strain differences between streptococci causing infection without eruption and those causing scarlet fever have been demonstrated, and the difference in clinical response relates to the presence in the host of specific antibodies against the erythrogenic toxin.

Clinical Findings

A. Symptoms and Signs:

1. Respiratory infections—

a. Infancy and early types—The onset is insidious, with very mild constitutional symptoms, ie, failure to thrive, low-grade fever, chronic serous nasal discharge, chronic cervical adenitis, and pallor. Otitis media is common. Pharyngitis and exudate are rare in this age group.

b. Childhood type—Onset is sudden, with high fever—at least 39–40° C (102–104° F)—marked malaise, and usually repeated vomiting. The pharynx is sore and edematous and the tonsillar area generally shows exudate. Anterior cervical lymph nodes are tender and enlarged. Small petechiae are frequently seen on the soft palate. Fine discrete petechiae on the upper abdomen and trunk may suggest meningococcemia, leukemia, idiopathic thrombocytopenic purpura, and subacute infective endocarditis. In scarlet fever, the skin is diffusely erythematous and appears like a sunburn. The rash is most intense in the axillas and groin and on the abdomen and trunk. It blanches on pressure except in the skin folds, which do not blanch and are pigmented (Pastia's sign). The rash usually appears 24 hours after the onset of fever and rapidly spreads over the next 1–2 days. Desquamation begins on the face at the end of the first week and becomes generalized by the third week. A retrospective diagnosis of scarlet fever may be made by observing desquamation of the fingers several weeks after a febrile disease. Early, the surface of the tongue is coated white, with the papillae enlarged and bright red ("white strawberry tongue"). Subsequently, desquamation occurs and the tongue appears beefy red ("red strawberry tongue"). The face generally shows circumoral pallor. Petechiae may be seen on all mucosal surfaces.

c. Adult type—The adult type is characterized by exudative or nonexudative tonsillitis with fewer systemic manifestations, lower fever, and no vomiting. Complications due to sensitization do occur. Scarlet fever is not common in this age group.

2. Impetigo—Streptococcal impetigo begins as a papule that vesiculates, leaving a denuded area covered by a honey-colored crust. A mixture of *Staphylococcus aureus* along with streptococci is isolated in about 66% of cases. The lesions spread readily and diffusely. Local lymph nodes often become swollen and inflamed. Such a child may develop high fever and be acutely ill.

3. Cellulitis—The portal of entry is often an insect bite or superficial abrasion on an extremity. There is a diffuse and rapidly spreading cellulitis which involves the subcutaneous tissues and extends along the lymphatic pathways with only minimal local suppuration. Local acute lymphadenitis occurs. The child is usually acutely ill, with fever and malaise. The involved area is swollen, warm, tender, and painful. The infection may extend rapidly from the lymphatics to the blood stream.

4. Necrotizing fasciitis—*(This is a medical and surgical emergency.)* Formerly called streptococcal gangrene, this is an uncommon but dangerous entity. Infection with group A beta-hemolytic streptococci after trauma to an extremity causes extensive necrosis of superficial fascia with undermining of surrounding tissue and extreme systemic toxicity. Initially, the skin overlying the infection is pale red without distinct borders, resembling subcutaneous cellulitis. Blisters or bullae may appear. The pale red skin progresses to a distinct purple color. The involved area may develop mild to massive edema.

5. Group A streptococcal infections in newborn nurseries—Group A beta-hemolytic streptococcal nursery epidemics are still of importance. The organism may be introduced into the nursery from the vaginal tract of a mother or from the throat or nose of a mother or a member of the staff. The organism then spreads from infant to infant. The umbilical stump is colonized while the infant is in the nursery. As is true also in staphylococcal infections, there may be no or few clinical manifestations while infants are still in the nursery; most often, a colonized infant develops a chronic, oozing omphalitis days later at home. The organism may spread from the infant to other family members. More serious and even fatal infections may develop, including sepsis, meningitis, empyema, septic arthritis, and peritonitis.

B. Laboratory Findings: Leukocytosis with a marked shift to the left is seen early. Eosinophilia regularly appears during convalescence and is a useful retrospective diagnostic sign.

Beta-hemolytic streptococci are cultured with ease from the throat. The organism may be cultured from the skin—and by needle aspiration from subcutaneous tissues and other involved sites—and from infected nodes. Occasionally, with overwhelming infections, blood cultures are positive. Group A streptococci may be identified most easily by demonstrable sensitivity on disks containing standardized concentrations of bacitracin. Few false-negatives are reported by this method. Grouping by fluorescent antibody technics is preferred and correlates best with the original precipitin reactions described by Lancefield. Grouping is dependent upon the presence of a specific "C carbohydrate substance" in the cell wall. Typing is dependent upon the presence of specific M precipitins or T agglutinins in the cell wall and is cumbersome enough to be reserved for epidemiologic surveys.

Antistreptolysin (ASO) titers rise above 150 units within 2 weeks after an acute infection. Elevated ASO and anti-DNase B titers are useful in documenting prior throat infections in cases of acute rheumatic fever. On the other hand, elevated anti-DNase B and antihyaluronidase titers are most useful in associating pyoderma and acute glomerulonephritis. Elevation of 2 or more of these antibody titers in children 5–18 years of age with isolated Sydenham's chorea suggests a streptococcal etiology. Streptozyme is a useful 2-minute slide test which detects antibodies to streptolysin O, hyaluronidase, streptokinase, DNase B, and NADase.

The presence of erythrogenic toxin in scarlet fever may be demonstrated during the first hours of the rash by a blanching reaction following the local intradermal injection of 0.1 ml of human gamma globulin. Blanching is best seen 8–14 hours after injection. This is best done on the lateral chest or abdominal wall.

The urine may show proteinuria, cylindruria, and minimal hematuria early. More commonly, true sensitizing poststreptococcal nephritis is seen 2–4 weeks after the respiratory infection.

Differential Diagnosis

Streptococcosis of the early childhood type must be differentiated from pneumococcosis and from adenovirus and other respiratory virus infections. Streptococcal pharyngitis must be differentiated from such virus infections as herpangina (coxsackievirus A), acute lymphonodular pharyngitis (coxsackievirus A10), nonbacterial exudative pharyngitis (adenoviruses), herpes simplex stomatitis, and pharyngeal erythema associated with respiratory syncytial and parainfluenza viruses.

In diphtheria, systemic symptoms, vomiting, and fever are all less marked; the pseudomembrane is confluent and adherent; and the throat is less red.

Infectious mononucleosis causes more marked generalized adenopathy and splenomegaly and shows a typical blood picture and a positive heterophil test.

Pharyngeal tularemia causes white rather than yellow exudate. There is little erythema, and cultures for beta-hemolytic streptococci are negative. Response to specific antibiotic therapy is prompt. Leukemia and agranulocytosis may be diagnosed by bone marrow examination.

Scarlet fever must be differentiated from other exanthematous diseases, principally rubella. Erythema due to sunburn, drug reactions, fever, and the prodromal rashes of chickenpox and smallpox must at times be considered.

Complications

The most common complications of group A beta-hemolytic streptococcal infections are chronic purulent or serous rhinitis, sinusitis, otitis, mastoiditis, cervical lymphadenitis (which may be suppurative), pneumonia and empyema, septic arthritis, and meningitis. Spread of streptococcal infection from the throat to other sites, principally the skin (impetigo) and vagina, is common also and should be considered in every instance of chronic vaginal discharge or chronic skin infection such as that complicating childhood eczema.

Both acute rheumatic fever and acute glomerulonephritis are nonsuppurative complications of group A streptococcal infections.

A. Acute Rheumatic Fever: The infecting group A streptococcus must be present in the pharynx for at least 8 days before rheumatic fever can develop. Only a small percentage of the general population is susceptible to rheumatic fever. "Target organs" bearing the brunt of inflammation, eg, heart, nervous system, and joints, vary among susceptible individuals. Rheumatic fever is rare in infancy, possibly because streptococcal sensitization is unusual before age 4. The disease has a familial tendency. Infection with any pharyngeal M type group A streptococcus may lead to rheumatic fever. The communicability of streptococcal infections is greatest during the acute phase of respiratory illness and in the first 2 weeks of the carrier state. An important factor in the incidence of rheumatic fever is the severity of the preceding pharyngitis, which reflects on the virulence of the streptococcal strain infecting the upper respiratory tract. The incidence of first attacks of rheumatic fever is proportionate to the degree of antistreptolysin O (ASO) titer increase. Second attacks of rheumatic fever are common in the absence of prophylaxis.

B. Acute Glomerulonephritis: Acute glomerulonephritis is uniformly distributed geographically. Streptococcal skin infections, which are more prevalent in warmer climates, are not rheumatogenic. Acute nephritis, however, can follow streptococcal infections of either the pharynx or the skin. Thus, the higher prevalence of skin infections in the southern and tropical latitudes compensates for the lower prevalence of pharyngitis and results in a more even geographic distribution of acute glomerulonephritis as compared to acute rheumatic fever. Glomerulonephritis may occur at any age, including infancy. Acute glomerulonephritis in infants may be related to the fact that infants commonly develop streptococcal skin infections. In most reported series of acute glomerulonephritis, males predominate by a ratio of 2:1, whereas acute rheumatic fever occurs with equal frequency in both sexes. The male predominance may result from epidemiologic factors or from some unknown host factors. The preceding infection may be either of the pharynx or of the skin. However, the M types of the pathogenic group A hemolytic streptococcus differ depending upon the site of infection. Pharyngeal infections leading to glomerulonephritis include M types 1, 4, 12, and 18, with limited evidence for 3, 6, and 25. Skin M types leading to nephritis include 2, 31, 49, 52–55, 57, and 60. It is not clear why acute glomerulonephritis but not rheumatic fever follows streptococcal skin infections.

The incidence of acute glomerulonephritis after streptococcal infection is variable and has ranged from 0–28%. Several outbreaks of acute glomerulonephritis in families have involved 50–75% of siblings of affected patients in 1- to 7-week periods. Second attacks of glomerulonephritis are rare. Infection with a particular M type streptococcus results in persistent protective immunity against homologous organisms. Acute glomerulonephritis is caused by only a relatively small number of M types. The average latent period between infection and the first attack of glomerulonephritis is 10 days. This contrasts with acute rheumatic fever, which has a longer latent period lasting 18 days. The latent period between infection and exacerbation in acute rheumatic fever is shorter than that in the first attack of glomerulonephritis. This is thought to be evidence that poststreptococcal glomerulonephritis is related to an antigen-antibody reaction reflecting an anamnestic response. One of the most striking differences between acute glomerulonephritis and acute rheumatic fever is the behavior of serum complement. Whole serum complement and C3 are increased in acute rheumatic fever, as they are in other inflammatory conditions. In acute glomerulonephritis, however, whole serum complement, C3, and properdin are reduced for the first 2–6 weeks of the disease, presumably reflecting some aspect of the immunologic pathogenesis. General and local activation of the complement system by circulating antigen-antibody complexes appears to play a role in the pathogenesis of acute glomerulonephritis but not of acute rheumatic fever.

Prevention of Complications

Penicillin G, 200,000 units orally twice daily, or benzathine penicillin G, 1.2 million units IM once a month (usually for life), prevents reinfection with the group A beta-hemolytic streptococcus in individuals with proved rheumatic fever and thus prevents recurrences. A similar approach to the prevention of recurrences of acute glomerulonephritis is debatable but probably worthwhile in childhood when there is any suspicion that repeated streptococcal infections coincide with flare-ups of acute glomerulonephritis. Mass prophylaxis with benzathine penicillin may be required to abort an epidemic of acute glomerulonephritis.

Treatment

A. Specific Measures: Treatment is directed not only toward eradication of acute infection but also to the prevention of rheumatic fever and nephritis. Sibling contacts of patients with pyoderma-associated nephritis should be treated as early in the course of skin infection as possible. This is best accomplished with penicillin. The use of sulfonamides in the treatment of streptococcal disease is to be discouraged because they do not prevent the development of sensitizing antibodies and therefore do not lower the incidence of rheumatic fever or nephritis.

1. Penicillin—In children, oral penicillin is adequate for most infections. Give penicillin G, 200–400 thousand units, or penicillin V, 125–250 mg every 6 hours between meals for 10 days. Parenteral therapy is indicated if there is vomiting or sepsis and other serious infections.

A single dose of benzathine penicillin G (Bicillin), 0.6–1.2 million units IM, is preferred for treatment of pharyngitis and impetigo. Mild cellulitis may be similarly treated. Cellulitis requiring hospitalization should be treated with aqueous penicillin G, 150,000 units/kg/day IV or IM in 4 divided doses until there is marked improvement. Procaine penicillin G, 25,000 units/kg/day IM in 2 doses, may then be given to complete a 7- to 10-day course. Acute cervical lymphadenitis may require incision and drainage. Treatment of necrotizing fasciitis requires emergency surgical debridement. Aqueous penicillin G should be given as 300,000 units/kg/day IV in 6 divided doses for 7 days after surgery. Smaller doses may then be given intramuscularly until the patient is completely healed.

Ampicillin, nafcillin, cloxacillin, and dicloxacillin are also effective in the treatment of streptococcal infections. Penicillinase-producing staphylococci play a controversial role in penicillin treatment failures.

2. Other antibiotics–For serious, life-threatening infections in patients with known penicillin allergy, give cephalothin, 100–200 mg/kg/day in 4–6 divided doses. For milder infections, give erythromycin, 40 mg/kg/day orally in 4 divided doses for 10 days.

Clindamycin and cephalexin are effective oral antibiotics. The dosage of clindamycin is 75 or 150 mg 3 times daily; for cephalexin, 25–50 mg/kg/day in 3 divided doses. Each of these drugs should be given for 10 days. Lincomycin may be effective. Tetracycline-resistant strains have been reported.

3. Reasons for treatment failure include the following:

a. Failure to take or absorb full course of antibiotics as prescribed.

b. Streptococci found after adequate treatment frequently are other than beta-hemolytic group A.

(1) Reported falsely as beta-hemolytic if human blood agar rather than sheep blood agar plate is used.

(2) Reported falsely as group A if the wrong concentration of bacitracin disk is used. (The laboratory should use 0.02 unit–not 0.1 unit–bacitracin disks.)

c. Reinfection by another family member–A sick child will spread organisms to about 40% of childhood siblings and to about 20% of adult members of the household. These family members then may reinfect the originally sick and treated child.

d. The creation in vivo of protoplasts no longer sensitive to penicillin, with later reversion to the parent pathogenic form, is another interesting but presently speculative cause of penicillin treatment failures.

e. Failure to eradicate organisms from tonsillar tissues. A larger dose of antibiotic than usually recommended may be required to penetrate into the tonsils.

4. Control of nursery epidemics–

a. Treat all infants with positive cultures with aqueous penicillin G, 100,000 units/kg/day IM in 2 doses for 10 days.

b. Apply bacitracin ointment every 8 hours to the umbilical stump of each infant until discharge from the nursery.

c. Treat all other infants prophylactically with a single IM dose of 150,000 units of benzathine penicillin G.

d. Continue prophylactic bacitracin ointment and benzathine penicillin G for 15 days or until the outbreak is controlled.

B. General Measures: Analgesic lozenges or gargles with 30% glucose or hot saline solution may be used for relief of sore throat. A soft, bland diet, including noncarbonated high-glucose drinks such as apple juice, grape juice, and pear juice, and iced milk or sherbet is helpful. Aspirin may be useful for fever.

With impetigo, crusts should first be soaked off; areas beneath the crusts should then be washed with 3% hexachlorophene 3 times daily.

C. Treatment of Complications: Acute complications are best treated with penicillin. Prevention of rheumatic fever and glomerulonephritis is best accomplished by early adequate penicillin treatment of the streptococcal infection (see above).

D. Treatment of Carriers: Carriers of group A beta-hemolytic streptococci are much less likely to spread the disease to contacts than acutely infected individuals. Carrier states are difficult to abolish, and it may be well to be certain that a group A hemolytic strain is involved before it is attempted.

Contacts should be cultured 2 days after initiating treatment in the index case, and all contacts with positive cultures should be treated. As an alternative plan, all family contacts may be treated. Treatment consists of a single dose of benzathine penicillin G, 1.2 million units IM, or therapeutic doses of oral penicillin G or V. Hemolytic streptococci found after adequate treatment frequently are other than group A.

E. Streptococcal Vaccine: Since immunity to group A streptococcal infection appears to depend on immune responses against the M protein, considerable interest is directed toward developing vaccines containing the M proteins of the serotypes most often implicated in rheumatic fever.

Prognosis

Death is rare except in sepsis or pneumonia in infancy or early childhood. The febrile course is shortened and complications eliminated by early and adequate penicillin treatment.

Anthony BF & others: The dynamics of streptococcal infections in a defined population of children: Serotypes associated with skin and respiratory infections. Am J Epidemiol 104:652, 1976.

Bell SM, Smith DD: Quantitative throat-swab culture in the diagnosis of streptococcal pharyngitis in children. Lancet 2:61, 1976.

Bergner-Rabinowitz S & others: The new streptozyme test for streptococcal antibodies. Clin Pediatr (Phila) 14:804, 1975.

Breese BB & others: The treatment of beta hemolytic streptococcal pharyngitis: Comparison of amoxicillin, erythromycin estolate and penicillin V. Clin Pediatr (Phila) 16:460, 1977.

Burech DL, Koranyi KI, Haynes RE: Serious group A streptococcal diseases in children. J Pediatr 88:972, 1976.

Derrick CW, Dillon HC: Erythromycin therapy for streptococcal pharyngitis. Am J Dis Child 130:175, 1976.

Kaplan EL, Wannamaker LW: C-reactive protein in streptococcal pharyngitis. Pediatrics 60:28, 1977.

Krause RM: Prevention of streptococcal sequelae by penicillin prophylaxis: A reassessment. J Infect Dis 131:592, 1975.

Peter G, Hazard J: Neonatal group A streptococcal disease. J Pediatr 87:454, 1975.

Smith EWP & others: Varicella gangrenosa due to group A beta hemolytic streptococcus. Pediatrics 57:306, 1976.

Wannamaker LW: A penicillin shot without culturing the child's throat. JAMA 235:913, 1976.

STREPTOCOCCAL INFECTIONS OTHER THAN GROUP A

Most patients with group B streptococcal disease are infants less than age 3 months. However, serious and often life-threatening infection has been reported occasionally in women with puerperal sepsis, in immunocompromised patients, in patients with cirrhosis and spontaneous peritonitis, and in diabetics with cellulitis. The importance of group B streptococci as a cause of infection among newborns and infants is now well established. Two distinct clinical syndromes distinguished by differing perinatal events, age at onset, and serotype of the infecting strain have been described in these infants.

The first syndrome, early onset illness, is observed in the newborn less than 5 days old. The onset of symptoms in the majority of these infants occurs in the first 48 hours of life. Apnea is often the first sign. There is a high incidence of associated maternal obstetric complications, especially premature labor and prolonged rupture of the membranes. Newborns with early onset disease are severely ill at the time of diagnosis and have a case-fatality ratio of more than 50%. Although the majority of infants with early onset type infections have low birth weights, term infants may also develop fatal infection. Newborns with early onset type infection acquire the group B streptococcal organism from the maternal genital tract in utero or during passage through the birth canal. When early onset infection is complicated by meningitis, as occurs in approximately 30% of cases, more than 80% of the bacterial isolates belong to serotype III. Postmortem examination of babies with early onset disease almost always reveals pulmonary inflammatory infiltrates and hyaline membrane formation. These hyaline membranes have been shown by both routine and fluorescent antibody staining to contain large numbers of group B streptococci.

The late onset meningitis type infection occurs in infants after the first week of life (between 10 days and 4 months of age); the mean age at onset is about 4 weeks. Maternal obstetric complications are infrequently associated with the late onset type infection. These infants are usually not as severely ill at the time of diagnosis as those with early onset disease, and the mortality rate is significantly lower (approximately 20%). However, up to 50% of infants with late onset type meningitis have neurologic sequelae following recovery. Although the majority of infants with late onset disease have meningitis, other clinical manifestations have recently been described. These signs include asymptomatic bacteremia, otitis media, ethmoiditis, conjunctivitis, cellulitis, breast abscess, pleural empyema, septic arthritis, impetigo, and osteomyelitis. Strains of group B streptococci possessing the capsular type III polysaccharide antigen are isolated from more than 95% of infants with late onset disease, irrespective of clinical manifestations. The exact mode of transmission of the organisms is not well defined. It is clear that, unlike newborns with early onset type infection, those with disease occurring after the first week of life have no apparent predisposition to invasive infection other than colonization of the mucous membranes with type III strains of group B streptococci.

An absolute increase in the number of symptomatic group B streptococcal infections among newborns and young infants has occurred throughout the USA.

Current data suggest that chemoprophylaxis is not an effective means of eradicating the asymptomatic colonization state in either the pregnant woman or the newborn. Penicillin G is a highly effective antibiotic for the treatment of group B streptococcal disease. In vitro and clinical data on susceptibility of group B streptococci to penicillin G with reference to concentration of organisms in CSF and peak levels of penicillin G in CSF suggest that doses of penicillin of more than 250,000 units/kg/day may be necessary to eradicate the organism from the CSF. The combination of a penicillin with an aminoglycoside may be more effective against group B streptococci than penicillin G alone. For this reason, initial therapy with both drugs may be beneficial. Treatment of group B streptococcal meningitis is with penicillin G for 10 days: under 1 week of age, 200,000–250,000 units/kg/day IM or, preferably, IV, divided into 3 doses given every 8 hours; over 1 week of age, 250,000–350,000 units/kg/day IV or IM, divided into 4 doses given every 6 hours. Gentamicin in the recommended dosage for the newborn of 5–7.5 mg/kg/day IM or IV may be beneficial. For sepsis without meningitis, treatment for 5–7 days is adequate.

Many women of childbearing age possess circulating antibody to the neutral buffer polysaccharide antigen of type III group B streptococci. This antibody seems to be transferred to the newborn via the placental circulation. It seems that pregnant women delivering healthy infants have significant levels of IgG antibody to this antigen in their sera. In contrast, sera obtained from women delivering infants with proved type III group B streptococcal disease of either the early or late onset type rarely have detectable antibody in their sera. If deficiency of maternal antibody directed against type III or other type-specific polysaccharide antigens is a major determinant in the pathogenesis of group B streptococcal infection, immunization using a purified protein polysaccharide preparation may be a reasonable means of prevention in women who are antibody-deficient.

Group D (enterococcus) hemolytic streptococcus is a less frequent cause of neonatal sepsis. Treatment is for 5—7 days with ampicillin: under 1 week, 100 mg/kg/day IV or IM in divided doses every 8—12 hours; over 1 week of age, 150 mg/kg/day IV or IM in divided doses every 6—8 hours, *and* kanamycin, 20 mg/kg/day IM in divided doses every 12 hours. Enterococcus is a common cause of urinary tract infections and can be treated with ampicillin. Viridans streptococci are the commonest cause of subacute infective endocarditis, and enterococci cause about 10% of cases.

Treatment of Subacute Infective Endocarditis

(See Chapter 13 for cardiovascular management.)

Subacute infective endocarditis is best treated with both penicillin and streptomycin. Endocarditis caused by a viridans streptococcus sensitive to 0.2 μg/ml or less of penicillin G may be successfully treated with penicillin V, 125 mg/kg/day orally in 6 divided doses every 4 hours for 3—4 weeks. An average serum killing level of 1:16 or higher should be maintained. Strains resistant to 0.2 μg/ml of penicillin G should be treated with aqueous penicillin G given intravenously. Streptomycin is also given in a dosage of 30 mg/kg/day IM in 2 divided doses.

For enterococcal endocarditis, give 300,000 units/kg/day of aqueous penicillin G by continuous IV infusion or in 6 divided doses IV for 6 weeks. Concurrently, streptomycin is given for 2 weeks in a dosage of 30 mg/kg/day IM in 2 divided doses and then 15 mg/kg/day for an additional 4 weeks. The maximum dose of streptomycin for adolescents is 2 gm/day. Two hours after an intramuscular injection of streptomycin, the serum killing level should be 1:8 or higher.

In case of penicillin allergy, treatment may be given after desensitization. Otherwise, vancomycin is given in a dosage of 40 mg/kg/day IV in 4 divided doses every 6 hours for 6 weeks, along with streptomycin. The maximum dose of vancomycin for adolescents is 2—3 gm/day.

Ablow RC & others: A comparison of early-onset group B streptococcal neonatal infection and the respiratory-distress syndrome of the newborn. N Engl J Med 294:65, 1976.

Baker CJ, Kasper DL: Correlation of maternal antibody deficiency with susceptibility to neonatal group B streptococcal infection. N Engl J Med 294:753, 1976.

Feigin RD: The perinatal group B streptococcal problem: More questions and answers. N Engl J Med 294:106, 1976.

Hall RT & others: Antibiotic treatment of parturient women colonized with group B streptococci. Am J Obstet Gynecol 124:630, 1976.

Kenny JF: Recurrent group B streptococcal disease in an infant associated with the ingestion of infected mother's milk. J Pediatr 91:158, 1977.

McCracken GH Jr, Feldman WE: Editorial comment. J Pediatr 89:203, 1976. [Comment on Vollman JH & others: Early onset group B streptococcal disease: Clinical, roentgeno-

graphic, and pathologic features. J Pediatr 89:199, 1976.]

Paredes A, Wong P, Yow MD: Failure of penicillin to eradicate the carrier state of group B streptococcus in infants. J Pediatr 89:191, 1976.

Paredes A & others: Nosocomial transmission of group B streptococci in a newborn nursery. Pediatrics 59:679, 1977.

Roe MH, Todd JK, Favara BE: Nonhemolytic group B streptococcal infections. J Pediatr 89:75, 1976.

Stewardson-Krieger P, Gotoff SP: Neonatal meningitis due to group C beta-hemolytic streptococcus. J Pediatr 90:103, 1977.

PNEUMOCOCCAL INFECTIONS

Essentials of Diagnosis

- Very high fever, with few other signs of illness in the early childhood form.
- Marked leukocytosis.
- Cough and diffuse rales (pneumonia).
- Bulging fontanels and neck stiffness (meningitis).
- Diagnosis confirmed by blood, sputum, or CSF culture.

General Considerations

Pneumococcal fever (with bacteremia), pneumococcal pharyngitis, sinusitis, otitis, pneumonitis, and occasionally pneumococcal meningitis, vaginitis, and peritonitis are all part of a spectrum of "pneumococcosis" that may occur at any time during childhood. Recently, several reports of children with bacteremia who were well enough to be evaluated in walk-in clinics suggest that blood cultures may also be a necessary procedure for febrile patients who are not hospitalized. Many patients with *Streptococcus pneumoniae* bacteremia have no clinical evidence of an infectious process at the time of evaluation. Clinical findings which correlate with bacteremia in ambulatory patients include age (under 24 months), degree of temperature elevation (above 39.4° C), and leukocytosis (above 15,000/cu mm). Although each of these findings is in itself nonspecific, a combination of them should prompt a high index of suspicion. This constellation of findings in a child who has no focus of infection and who is not "toxic" is not an indication for antibiotic therapy, but it should call for blood cultures. Although several children in the studies apparently eliminated the pneumococci without antimicrobial therapy (presumably accomplished from an extravascular infectious focus that disseminated the disease in the blood), others developed severe pneumococcal disease, including meningitis. Patients of any age with pneumococcal bacteremia are at risk of developing life-threatening infectious processes.

Eighty-two types of pneumococci have been identified. In patients of all age groups, types 1—8, 14, 18, and 19 occur most frequently.

In recent years, the incidence of pneumococcal pneumonia in children has dropped sharply. This may be due to the widespread use of antibiotics, but it may also be that viral studies are now available which establish a viral etiology for serious lower respiratory tract infections previously misdiagnosed as due to pneumococci.

The highest incidence of pneumococcal meningitis is during the first year of life, but the disease may occur at any age. The child with sickle cell disease appears unusually susceptible.

Disseminated intravascular coagulation with or without Waterhouse-Friderichsen syndrome has been observed with pneumococcal bacteremia. In the reported cases, there is a high incidence of asplenia. The spleen seems to be important in the control of pneumococcal infection by clearing organisms from the blood and producing an opsonin which enhances phagocytosis. Autosplenectomy may explain why the older child with sickle cell disease is at increased risk of developing serious pneumococcal infections.

For more than 30 years, penicillin has been the agent of choice for pneumococcal infections. During this time, the majority of strains of *S pneumoniae* have been highly susceptible to penicillin. However, during the last 10 years there have been sporadic reports of pneumococci with increased resistance to penicillin.

Clinical Findings

A. Symptoms and Signs: Fever usually appears abruptly, often accompanied by chills, in an otherwise well appearing child. There may be no respiratory symptoms, and in a child under 2 years of age a diagnosis of roseola infantum may be suspected because the child appears well otherwise. There may be some irritability; mild pharyngitis may be present, but exudate is not seen. Cervical adenopathy is uncommon. In pneumococcal sinusitis, mucopurulent discharge may occur. In infants and young children, cough and diffuse rales are found more often than the lobar distribution characteristic of adult forms of pneumococcal pneumonia. Respiratory distress is manifest by flaring of the alae nasi, chest retractions, and tachypnea. In older children, the adult form of pneumococcal pneumonia with signs of lobar consolidation may be found, but sputum is rarely bloody. Thoracic pain resulting from pleural involvement is sometimes present. With involvement of the right hemidiaphragm, pain may be referred to the right lower quadrant.

Vomiting is common at onset but seldom persists. Convulsions are relatively common at onset in infants. It is not unusual for the infant to have meningismus manifested by nuchal rigidity.

Meningitis. In infants, fever, irritability, and convulsions are common. Some neck stiffness may be detected. The most important sign is a tense, bulging anterior fontanel. In older children, fever, chills, headache, and vomiting are common symptoms. Classical signs are nuchal rigidity associated with positive Brudzinski and Kernig signs. With progression of untreated disease, the child may develop opisthotonos, stupor, and coma.

B. Laboratory Findings: Leukocytosis is pronounced (20,000–45,000/cu mm), with 80–90% polymorphonuclear neutrophils. Bacteremia is more likely to be detected in infections with types 1, 3, and 14. The presence of pneumococci in the nasopharynx is not diagnostic, whereas large numbers in endotracheal aspirates are much more confirmatory. Needle aspiration of the lung rarely is indicated. The quellung test can be used for identification on clinical specimens in which the Gram stain suggests pneumococci. An omniserum containing antibodies to all 83 known pneumococcal capsular polysaccharide type antigens is available from the Statens Seruminstitut in Copenhagen. CSF usually shows an elevated white count of several thousand, chiefly PMNs, with decreased glucose and elevated protein levels. Gram-positive diplococci are often seen on stained smears of CSF sediment. Counterimmunoelectrophoresis is a definite adjunct for rapid and specific diagnosis of pneumococcal meningitis.

Differential Diagnosis

In roseola infantum, the diagnostic rash coincides with the disappearance of symptoms 3–4 days after onset. Leukopenia is present instead of leukocytosis.

Children with signs of upper respiratory tract infection who develop moderate respiratory distress and signs of lower respiratory disease are most likely to be infected with respiratory syncytial virus or parainfluenza virus types 1, 2, or 3. Hoarseness is often present, and there may be a marked bronchiolitic component. X-ray of the chest shows perihilar infiltrates and increased bronchovascular markings.

Staphylococcal pneumonia causes early cavity formation and empyema.

In primary pulmonary tuberculosis, x-rays show a primary focus associated with hilar adenopathy and often signs of pleurisy. Miliary tuberculosis presents a classical x-ray appearance.

The child with cystic fibrosis has patchy infiltrates, areas of emphysema and atelectasis, and a positive sweat test.

Pneumonia caused by *Mycoplasma pneumoniae* is most common in the age group 8–12 years and older. Onset is insidious, with infrequent chills, low-grade fever, prominent headache and malaise, and cough which is hacking, irritating, and productive of small amounts of mucoid sputum. Physical findings are scanty in comparison with x-ray changes.

Pneumococcal meningitis is excluded or diagnosed by lumbar puncture.

Complications

Complications include otitis media, mastoiditis, and occasionally meningitis and sinusitis secondary to pneumococcal fever or pneumococcal pharyngitis, and empyema accompanying pneumonia. Peritonitis is often a complication of chronic glomerulonephritis and nephrosis. Both pneumococcal meningitis and peritonitis are more likely to occur independently without coexisting pneumonia.

Treatment

A. Specific Measures: Penicillin is the drug of choice, but erythromycin is also effective. In recent years there have been several reports of occasional pneumococcal strains (including type 14) resistant to tetracyclines. For several reasons, tetracyclines are not the drugs of choice for children under 5 years of age (see Chapter 36).

1. Pneumonia—For infants, give aqueous penicillin G, 50—100 thousand units/kg/day IM in 2 or 3 divided doses. Aqueous procaine penicillin G, 600,000 units IM daily for 7 days, is recommended for children. Pneumonia which is not severe may be treated with oral penicillin G, 400,000 units 4 times daily for 7—10 days. In case of penicillin allergy, give erythromycin, 40—50 mg/kg/day orally in 4 divided doses. Oral cephalexin or clindamycin may be used.

2. Otitis media—Treat with oral penicillin or ampicillin or a substitute as described above for 7—14 days.

3. Meningitis—Until pneumococcal meningitis is confirmed by culture, give ampicillin, 300 mg/kg/day IV in 6 divided doses. After bacteriologic confirmation, give aqueous penicillin G, 300,000 units/kg/day IV in 6 divided doses. Intrathecal penicillin is occasionally given at onset in small children and infants. Treatment must be continued until the patient has been afebrile for 5 days, the CSF white cell count is 30/cu mm or less, and CSF glucose and protein have returned to normal. This usually requires 10—14 days.

4. All children with blood cultures that are positive for pneumococcus must be reexamined as soon as possible. The child with a focal infection such as pneumonia or meningitis should receive a course of antimicrobial therapy. The child with persisting and unexplained fever who appears to be septic should be hospitalized and treated with parenterally administered penicillin G. Therapy should be continued for 5 days after the fever has abated. Only if the child is afebrile, bright, and alert should management on an ambulatory basis be considered. The physician must be confident that close contact will be maintained with the family and that medications will be administered appropriately. If the physician is assured of these considerations, a second blood culture is performed (a lumbar puncture is not done); oral penicillin V, 100 mg/kg/day, is prescribed and the initial dose given at once; and the family is instructed to call at least once a day or at any time if an untoward sign develops. If the child remains well and the second blood culture is negative, oral therapy is given for a total of 5 days. Some children may be afebrile at times in the course of the disease and yet still have continuous bacteremia that progresses to meningitis.

B. General Measures: Supportive and symptomatic care is required.

Prognosis

Case fatality rates of less than 1% should be achieved in pneumococcal disease other than meningitis, in which rates of 5—20% still prevail.

Bratton L, Teele DW, Klein JO: Outcome of unsuspected pneumococcemia in children not initially admitted to the hospital. J Pediatr 90:703, 1977.

Coonrod JD: CIE detection of bacterial antigens in meningitis. J Pediatr 90:676, 1977.

Feigin RD & others: Countercurrent immunoelectrophoresis of urine as well as of CSF and blood for diagnosis of bacterial meningitis. J Pediatr 89:773, 1976.

Klein JO: Pneumococcal bacteremia in young child. Am J Dis Child 129:1266, 1975.

McCarthy PL & others: Bacteremia in children: An outpatient clinical review. Pediatrics 57:861, 1976.

Myers MG & others: Complications of occult pneumococcal bacteremia in children. J Pediatr 84:656, 1974.

Quie PG: "Walk-in" bacteremia. Pediatrics 57:827, 1976.

Waldman JD & others: Sepsis and congenital asplenia. J Pediatr 90:555, 1977.

STAPHYLOCOCCAL INFECTIONS

General Considerations

Staphylococcal infections are an important cause of serious neonatal infections and lung diseases in early childhood. There are marked strain differences in pathogenicity. Penicillin has revolutionized the specific therapy of diseases caused by strains of staphylococci which are not penicillinase producers. More than 80% of strains causing hospital-acquired staphylococcal disease are resistant to penicillin.

The first form of bacterial resistance to penicillins identified was that caused by penicillinase (β-lactamase). Penicillinases have been identified in almost all bacteria that are highly resistant to benzylpenicillin, and they are probably the most common mechanism of resistance to penicillins. A second form of resistance to penicillins is "intrinsic" resistance, ie, not caused by drug inactivation. Its clinical importance was first noted in gram-negative bacilli when it became apparent that β-lactamase alone could not account for the resistance observed. The purest form of intrinsic resistance to β-lactam antibiotics is that of penicillinase-negative segregants of methicillin-resistant *Staphylococcus aureus;* these organisms are highly resistant to methicillin (and other penicillins and cephalosporins) but produce no β-lactamase. Penicillin tolerance, a third form of penicillin resistance, differs in that the minimum inhibitory concentration (MIC) of penicillins for the tolerant organisms is low (sensitive range), but the minimum bacterial concentration (MBC) is high, often more than 100 times the MIC. Although one of the many desirable attributes of penicillin is that it kills bacteria at almost the same concentration at which they are inhibited, identification of penicillin-tolerant staphylococci in patients who have staphylococcal bacteremia, osteomyelitis, or pneumonia and who have failed to respond adequately to antibiotic treatment indicates that the slow rates of killing may well be a critical factor in each clinical course.

Brain abscess occurs by extension or metastatically from such infected peripheral sites as chronic otitis media, sinusitis, infected skin lesions, and infected myelomeningoceles. Brain abscess also occurs in association with cyanotic congenital heart disease and pulmonary arteriovenous fistulas and after penetrating head wounds, including those inflicted by lead pencil points.

Cultures from brain abscesses most often reveal aerobic and anaerobic streptococci. *S aureus* is the second most frequently isolated pathogen. Isolates include a great variety of aerobic and anaerobic gram-positive and gram-negative bacteria and fungi.

The staphylococcal scalded-skin syndrome has been expanded to include several different dermatologic reactions all of which are probably produced by a toxin elaborated by infection with phage group II staphylococcus. Reactions in the skin include, in infants, generalized exfoliative (Ritter's) disease; in children, toxic epidermal necrolysis, generalized scarlatiniform erythema without exfoliation (staphylococcal scarlet fever), and localized bullous impetigo.

Septic (purulent) pericarditis without antecedent infection is rare. *S aureus* is the most common primary etiologic agent and is found in 40–50% of cases. The primary sites of infection in purulent pericarditis due to *S aureus* are the lungs and pleura in 20% of cases and the skin and wound and soft tissue abscesses in 30% of cases. Less commonly, the pericardium may become infected by *S aureus* from the upper respiratory tract, osteomyelitis, or meningitis. After *S aureus*, the most common organisms causing purulent pericarditis are the pneumococci, *Haemophilus influenzae*, and meningococci, followed by gram-negative coliforms. Bacteroides and anaerobic streptococci have only rarely been reported as causes of purulent pericarditis.

Severe staphylococcal sepsis has been reported in normal adolescents. Organisms isolated are generally methicillin-sensitive. Lack of clinical response is often related to delay in adequate surgical drainage of infected material.

Acute suppurative cervical adenitis is a common problem occurring most frequently between age 1–2 years. The presence of a probable bacterial source of infection (tonsillitis, pharyngitis, otitis media, facial or scalp impetigo, or dental disease) may establish the cause. The frequent absence of a focus of infection makes identification of the bacterial organism difficult. Infants under age 4 months may have significant cervical adenitis (2 × 2 cm) caused by *S aureus* and yet have no obvious source of infection. Suppurative adenitis in infants less than age 4 months is unusual. Needle aspiration and biopsy of acutely inflamed lymph nodes larger than 2 × 2 cm in a patient without a focus of infection is advisable, with incision and drainage when fluctuation is present. A penicillinase-resistant penicillin is the preferred therapy.

Clinical Findings

A. Symptoms and Signs:

1. Pyoderma is seen as impetigo, primarily in the neonatal period; in older children, acute and chronic skin infections are often seen as part of a family infection. Impetigo caused purely by *S aureus* begins as a papule that becomes and remains bullous.

2. Osteomyelitis frequently follows trauma, primarily to the head or to the long bones, and is regularly accompanied by septicemia.

3. Staphylococcal pneumonia in infancy is characterized by abdominal distention, high fever, respiratory distress, and toxemia. It often occurs without predisposing factors or after minor skin infections. The organism is necrotizing, producing broncho-alveolar destruction. Pneumatoceles, pyopneumothorax, and empyema are frequently encountered. Rapid progression of disease is characteristic. Presenting symptoms may be typical of paralytic ileus, suggestive of an abdominal catastrophe. When this is suspected, the abdominal films should always be accompanied by a chest film to rule out the staphylococcal pneumonitis.

Staphylococcal pneumonia usually is peribronchial and diffuse and begins with a focal infiltrative lesion progressing to patchy consolidation. Most often only one lung is involved (80%), more often the right. Purulent pericarditis occurs by direct extension in about 10% of cases, with or without empyema.

4. Staphylococcal food poisoning is produced by enterotoxin. The most common source is poorly refrigerated and contaminated food. The disease is characterized by vomiting, prostration, and diarrhea occurring within 2–6 hours after ingestion of contaminated foods.

5. Brain abscess is characterized by fever, headache, irritability, focal neurologic signs, and signs of increased intracranial pressure. Percussion tenderness over the abscess is an important localizing sign. Skull films, serial EEGs, brain scans, and echoencephalograms are helpful in diagnosis. A definitive diagnosis prior to surgery is most frequently made by carotid arteriography or ventriculography.

6. Septic pericarditis is characterized by symptoms and signs of the primary infection and high spiking fever. A pericardial friction rub is audible in about 20% of cases. Clinical, x-ray, and ECG evidence of a pericardial effusion develops. Pus is commonly aspirated from the pericardial sac. On occasion, a large effusion will be coagulum-free but grow the organism.

B. Laboratory Findings: Moderate leukocytosis, (15,000–20,000/cu mm) with a shift to the left is usually found. The sedimentation rate is elevated. Cultures of pus from sites of infection prove the diagnosis. Cultures of tracheal aspirates and material from pleural taps are positive in pneumonia. Blood cultures are often sterile in pneumonia but positive in osteomyelitis. CSF culture is usually negative with brain abscess, but CSF pressure is usually elevated, with mild pleocytosis and elevated protein. Culturing large numbers of *S aureus* in suspected food suggests that the organism is responsible in cases of food poisoning.

Bacteriophage typing is extensively utilized for epidemiologic studies.

Differential Diagnosis

Klebsiella pneumoniae (Friedländer's) pneumonia is rare but tends to cause lobar consolidation with bulging fissures seen on x-ray. Rare nursery outbreaks have been reported. The organism is a secondary invader associated with antibiotic usage, debilitating states, and chronic respiratory conditions and rapidly forms abscesses or empyema.

Primary pneumonias caused by group A hemolytic streptococci and *H influenzae* may also cause pneumatoceles and empyema.

See Pneumococcal Infections for further differential diagnosis of bacterial pneumonia.

Tracheo-esophageal fistulas in infancy may be demonstrated by careful x-ray examination. Such infants may develop aspiration pneumonia involving the upper lobes.

Staphylococcal osteomyelitis may be confused with conditions causing pain and limitation of motion of an extremity, including rheumatic fever, septic arthritis, cellulitis, and fractures and sprains.

Staphylococcal enterocolitis is associated with the suppression of normal intestinal flora and the presence of large numbers of the organisms on smears and cultures of the stool. Staphylococcal food poisoning as a separate entity is usually epidemic in nature and usually is not associated with fever. Shigellosis and salmonellosis must be distinguished. Brain abscess must be distinguished from viral encephalitis, meningitis, generalized sepsis, lead poisoning, brain tumors and other encephalopathies, and space-occupying lesions.

Purulent pericarditis must be distinguished from pericarditis with acute rheumatic fever, in which there are usually murmurs and manifestations of endocarditis. Collagen diseases (especially rheumatoid arthritis) with pericarditis must also be differentiated. Tuberculous pericarditis is usually painless and is associated with a friction rub lasting for weeks or months. The child usually has pulmonary tuberculosis. Viral pericarditis is associated with chest pain, a prominent friction rub, and pericardial effusion which is either serous, containing fibrin and a few lymphocytes, or serosanguineous. There is usually evidence of other infections in the community due to coxsackievirus B1–6, including pleurodynia, aseptic meningitis, or perhaps a nursery outbreak of encephalomyocarditis. Pericarditis associated with hemolytic anemia or uremia occasionally must be distinguished from purulent pericarditis.

Complications

Various infections of the skin (particularly in newborns and infants), including impetigo, paronychia, and cellulitis, may be followed by mastitis, omphalitis, pneumonia, meningitis, and brain abscess. Ritter's disease is a generalized bullous exfoliative dermatitis associated with phage types 3B/55/71. Epidemic strains in nurseries have included phage types 52A/79/80/81/71 and 77. Extension of the osteomyelitic process may lead to septic arthritis and subcutaneous abscesses. Chronic osteomyelitis still occurs in inadequately treated acute cases. Septic pericarditis leads to heart failure and fatal tamponade.

Treatment

A. Specific Measures:

1. Pneumonia–Prompt administration of a penicillinase-resistant penicillin, eg, methicillin, oxacillin, or nafcillin, is indicated until the sensitivity of the etiologic agent to penicillin G has been determined. The dosage of methicillin is 200–300 mg/kg/day IV in 6 divided doses. The dosage of oxacillin is 100–200 mg/kg/day in 6 divided doses; of nafcillin, 50–100 mg/kg/day IV in 4 divided doses. Cephalothin may be given in a dosage of 100–200 mg/kg/day IV in 6 divided doses.

A few methicillin-resistant strains associated with serious illness have been reported in the USA, and more such reports have come from Europe. If the organism is penicillin-sensitive, penicillin G is preferred. Give 300,000 units/kg/day IV in 4 or 6 divided doses. Parenteral therapy is continued for 3 weeks or until there has been marked clinical improvement. Pyopneumothorax and empyema should be treated by placement of one or more chest tubes into the pleural space accompanied by massive systemic antibiotic therapy.

2. Newborn infections–(See also Chapter 3.) Methods available to stop a nursery epidemic include the following:

a. Prompt and adequate management of known infections.

b. Prevention of colonization of newborns with epidemic strains by the following means:

(1) Routine hexachlorophene bathing of newborns has been discontinued for the past 3 years because of evidence of absorption causing CNS damage. Local application of bacitracin is a safe and effective method of controlling staphylococcal colonization and disease in infants in nurseries.

(2) Removal and treatment of personnel carrying the epidemic strain.

(3) Segregation of infants according to age, and early discharge (within 3 days after birth).

(4) Complete cleansing and disinfection of nurseries after discharge of colonized and infected infants.

(5) Restriction of visitors to the nursery area.

(6) Elimination of breast feeding.

(7) Consideration of prophylactic antibiotics.

(8) Elective colonization of infants with a relatively nonvirulent strain of *S aureus* such as 502A. This procedure is still in the investigational stage but shows promise provided strict methodology is adhered to.

c. "Rooming-in" has definite psychologic benefits but probably is not so important in stopping an epidemic as once thought.

3. Skin infection–See Chapter 8.

4. Brain abscess–(See Chapter 21 for neurosurgical management.) An established abscess must be treated surgically. Some neurosurgeons prefer repeated aspirations; others prefer total excision of the abscess as an initial surgical maneuver. Broad spectrum anti-

---

Prevention of Cross-Infection in Hospitalized Patients

(1) Avoid unnecessary treatment with antibiotics.

(2) Observe strict aseptic technic in operating rooms. (Heart-lung machines have been found to be contaminated with staphylococci.)

(3) Observe strict isolation precautions for patients with infectious diseases.

(4) Maintain scrupulous cleanliness in the hospital to reduce dust-borne and other types of contamination from fomites.

(5) Care of patients with purulent discharges:

(a) Observe strict isolation, especially from patients with burns, eczema, etc.

(b) Use masks and gloves.

(c) Dispose of infectious material promptly in impermeable bags.

(d) Disinfect unit after patient is discharged.

(6) Choose antibiotics carefully by means of sensitivity tests. Monitor "serum killing powers" at intervals.

(7) Prevent contact between patients and staphylococcal infections or carrier states.

(8) Establish an infection committee to review nosocomial infections continuously and make recommendations.

---

biotic coverage should begin before the first surgical procedure, using penicillin G, 300,000 units/kg/day IV in 4 or 6 divided doses, and chloramphenicol, 100 mg/kg/day IV in 4 divided doses. In cases where the organism is identified by culture, drugs shown to be appropriate by sensitivity tests should be used. Although the value of topical antibiotics has not been determined, the abscess cavity may be irrigated with bacitracin solution, 500 units/ml, prior to surgical closure and for 1 or 2 days postoperatively. Systemic antibiotics should be continued for 3–4 weeks or until the abscess has healed.

5. Osteomyelitis—(See Chapter 19 for surgical management.) Some orthopedists believe that immediate surgical drainage of the metaphysis is the local treatment of choice in the early stage of metaphysitis. Antibiotic treatment should be started immediately with methicillin, 200–300 mg/kg/day IV in 6 divided doses. Penicillin G, 300,000 units/kg/day IV in 4–6 divided doses, should be given if the organism is penicillin-sensitive. It is mandatory that a serum killing power be determined at the time of the expected peak blood level of the antibiotic (about 30 minutes after an intravenous dose). The level of the drug should be maintained at a serum killing power of 1:32 or higher. The assay of antibiotics that are more than 50% protein-bound (eg, cephalothin, cefazolin, nafcillin, oxacillin) should be done in serum, or an adjustment should be made for protein binding. For example, if a 1:32 broth dilution of serum containing cefazolin is bactericidal for a staphylococcal strain, it could be anticipated that the bactericidal dilution in serum would only be about 1:5. For cephalothin, a 1:32 dilution in broth would be about 1:11 in serum. Nafcillin and oxacillin, which have higher protein binding, would be even more affected. If there is metaphysitis without x-ray changes, parenteral antibiotic therapy should be continued for 3 weeks. With x-ray changes of osteomyelitis, parenteral therapy should be continued in the hospital for 4–5 weeks. The serum killing power should be determined every other day for the first week and then weekly for the next 4 weeks. During the fifth week of hospitalization, a transition from

parenteral to oral therapy may be made, maintaining a peak serum killing power of 1:32. Oral therapy should be continued for an additional 2 or 3 weeks. Dicloxacillin, 25–100 mg/kg/day orally in 4 divided doses, or penicillin V, 250–500 mg orally 4 times daily, may be used. Probenecid (Benemid), 10 mg/kg/dose given 4 times daily, with penicillin V may be required to achieve adequate penicillin blood levels. Cephalexin may be given orally in a dosage of 100–200 mg/kg/day in 4 divided doses.

Persistence of fever is due to (1) inadequate drainage, (2) multiple lesions, (3) metastatic lesions, (4) phlebitis (drug-induced), and (5) drug fever. Drug fever associated with methicillin most commonly occurs during the second or third week of treatment. In association with an elevated temperature, leukopenia, eosinophilia, and micro- or macroscopic hematuria are seen. These signs subside usually within 24 hours after the drug is stopped. Eosinophilia usually persists for a while.

6. Septic pericarditis—When pus is present in the pericardial sac, optimum treatment consists of maximim intravenous doses of antistaphylococcal antibiotics for 4 weeks plus surgical pericardiostomy, which permits constant drainage and prevents reaccumulation of fluid. The child should be digitalized preoperatively or immediately after surgical drainage.

B. General Measures: Moist heat applied to local infections will hasten localization and drainage. Oxygen, intravenous fluids, and other supportive care are indicated in staphylococcal pneumonia and other systemic infections. Blood transfusion may be indicated if the patient is severely anemic.

Prognosis

Septicemia, brain abscess, and widespread pneumonitis in infancy all have a serious prognosis. Infants who recover from serious staphylococcal pneumonia appear to have a good long-term prognosis without development of chronic respiratory disease. Osteomyelitis is now never fatal if promptly treated.

Even with optimal treatment, the mortality rate of septic pericarditis remains about 20%.

Compton AB & others: Nephropathy caused by methicillin therapy for staphylococcal septicemia. South Med J 69:872, 1976.

Hill HR & others: Recurrent staphylococcal abscesses associated with defective neutrophil chemotaxis and allergic rhinitis. Ann Intern Med 85:39, 1976.

Johnson JD & others: A sequential study of various modes of skin and umbilical care and the incidence of staphylococcal colonization and infection in the neonate. Pediatrics 58:354, 1976.

Koblenzer PJ: Toxic epidermal necrolysis (TEN; Ritter's disease) and staphylococcal scalded skin syndrome (SSSS): A description and review. Clin Pediatr (Phila) 15:724, 1976.

Kunin CM: Erythromycin in staphylococcal infections. JAMA 232:1217, 1975.

Nolan CM, Beaty HN: *Staphylococcus aureus* bacteremia: Current clinical patterns. Am J Med 60:495, 1976.

Sabath LD & others: A new type of penicillin resistance of *Staphylococcus aureus.* Lancet 1:443, 1977.

Shanson DC, Kensit JG, Duke R: Outbreak of hospital infection with a strain of *Staphylococcus aureus* resistant to gentamicin and methicillin. Lancet 2:1347, 1976.

Shulman ST, Ayoub EM: Severe staphylococcal sepsis in adolescents. Pediatrics 58:59, 1976.

MENINGOCOCCAL INFECTIONS

Essentials of Diagnosis

- Fever, headache, vomiting, convulsions.
- Petechial rash of skin and mucous membranes.
- Signs of meningitis.

General Considerations

Infection with *Neisseria meningitidis* is most commonly a subclinical nasopharyngitis or upper respiratory carrier state. Fewer than 1% of carriers develop serious illness via the blood stream with involvement of the meninges, joints, or other sites or with fulminating sepsis followed by rapid circulatory collapse and death.

The meningococci have classically been divided into 4 serologic groups (A, B, C, and D). Additional groups known as X, Y, Z, and A4317 have now been described. The serologic subgroups serve as specific markers for studying outbreaks and transmission of disease; they are also important in the development of specific meningococcal vaccines. Major epidemics of meningococcal disease prior to 1963 were caused by group A strains. In the past several years, however, group A organisms have accounted for only 2% of meningococcal isolates in the USA. Group B, the most common serogroup, accounts for 45%; group C for 32%; group Y, 18%; group A, 2%; and other serogroups, 3%. About 25% of all isolates are resistant to sulfadiazine. Resistance is found in 75% of group C strains. Two out of 6 group A strains are resistant to sulfonamides. In contrast, less than 5% of group B and Y isolates are resistant. None of the isolates are resistant to rifampin. Group B is encountered more often in children younger than 5 years of age and also in persons 30 years of age and older. Serogroup C predominates in children 5–14 years of age, and serogroup Y is the most common group isolated from persons between 15 and 29 years of age.

Children from ages 2–4 to age 12 develop progressive immunity by virtue of an asymptomatic carrier state. These children usually carry nontypeable, nonpathogenic strains of *N meningitidis* or other bacteria which nevertheless produce cross-reacting protective antibodies. Young adults carry a higher percentage of typeable and pathogenic organisms. The meningococci are second only to *Haemophilus influenzae* type B as a cause of meningitis in children. The highest attack rate occurs within the first year of life.

Pathogenic strains differ in their virulence. Endotoxins may damage the walls of blood vessels directly and cause hemorrhage. Endotoxins may also induce disseminated intravascular coagulation, resulting in the production of damaging fibrin thrombi. Myocarditis is a significant factor in the fatal outcome of acute meningococcal infections. Pulmonary edema may result from the direct action of endotoxins on the CNS.

Vaccines prepared from purified meningococcal polysaccharides (groups A and C) appear to be nontoxic. Unfortunately, as immunizing agents they appear to be least effective in infants who are under age 1 year.

Changing sexual habits and social attitudes have been responsible for a greater incidence of *N meningitidis* in the flora of the female and male urogenital tract and anus.

Clinical Findings

A. Symptoms and Signs: Disseminated meningococcal infection is generally one of 3 types: meningococcemia, meningitis, or fulminating sepsis.

1. Meningococcemia—There often is a prodrome of upper respiratory infection followed within 2 days by high fever, headache, nausea, and often diarrhea. A petechial rash on the skin and mucous membranes and occasionally bright pink tender macules or papules over the extremities and trunk are seen and may have hemorrhagic centers. Chronic meningococcemia is characterized by periodic bouts of fever, arthralgia or arthritis, and recurrent petechial lesions. Splenomegaly is often present. The patient may be fairly free of symptoms between bouts.

2. Meningitis—In most children, meningococcemia is followed within a few hours by the onset of a typical acute purulent meningitis with severe headache, stiff neck, nausea, vomiting, and stupor. The Kernig and Brudzinski signs are positive.

3. Fulminating sepsis—A most virulent and rapidly progressing form of meningococcemia (Waterhouse-Friderichsen syndrome) is seen in which massive skin and mucosal hemorrhages and shock occur. This syndrome may occur in other generalized bacterial infections, particularly those due to *H influenzae* or pneumococcosis. Characteristically, the blood pressure falls rapidly as massive bleeding into the skin and mucosal membranes occurs. Death occurs generally within 12 hours. In those who survive, marked renal impairment, extensive skin necrosis, and prolonged convalescence are usual. Meningitis may or may not be present.

B. Laboratory Findings: Leukocytosis is marked. If petechial or hemorrhagic lesions are present, meningococci can readily be demonstrated on smear by puncturing the lesions and expressing a drop of tissue fluid. Meningococci are also readily found in smears of buffy coat. The spinal fluid is generally cloudy and contains more than 1000 white cells per cu mm, with many polymorphonuclear cells containing gram-negative intracellular diplococci. A gram-stained smear of the CSF sediment may fail to show the organisms, however, even in the absence of previous antibiotic therapy. Meningococci can usually be cultured from the nasopharynx or blood by the use of chocolate agar incubated in an atmosphere of 5–10% CO_2. In the case of partially treated meningitis, nonviable organisms from the CSF may be identified as meningococci, using an immunofluorescent antibody technic.

Serogrouping is routinely accomplished by the agglutination technic. The precipitation technic is easy to perform. Meningococcal capsular polysaccharide has been detected by counterimmunoelectrophoresis (CIE) in the serum, CSF, synovial fluid, and pericardial fluid of patients with meningococcal infections. CIE provides rapid, specific confirmation of the diagnosis when it is important to identify the causative organism in order to initiate proper management with the appropriate antibiotics. The Limulus lysate assay, which detects endotoxin, also helps to support the diagnosis. It may not be until later that *N meningitidis* grows on blood cultures, thus confirming hematogenous infection.

Examination of a stained blood smear for the presence of platelets will show whether significant thrombocytopenia is present. The combined findings of severe thrombocytopenia, markedly abnormal prothrombin time and partial thromboplastin time (PTT), increase in fibrin split products, and significant depletion of prothrombin, factor V, factor VIII, and fibrinogen indicate intravascular coagulation.

Differential Diagnosis

The petechial lesions of meningococcemia may be mistaken for the skin lesions seen in other disseminating infections due to *H influenzae* or pneumococci or caused by enteroviruses (echovirus types 6, 9, 16; cox-sackievirus types A2, 4, 9, and 16 and type B4).

Eruptions seen in bacterial endocarditis, leptospirosis, Rocky Mountain spotted fever, and other rickettsial diseases as well as the prodrome of smallpox must also be differentiated.

Blood dyscrasias as a cause of petechial eruptions may be excluded by bone marrow examination.

Complications

Blood-borne infections may lead to arthritis, osteomyelitis, endocarditis, pericarditis, pneumonia, unilateral ophthalmia, and bilateral deafness. Menin-

gitis may lead to chronic CNS damage manifested by convulsions, paralysis, and impairment of intellectual functions. Subdural collections of fluid and hydrocephalus are important complications.

Prevention

Household contacts are at risk. Less intimate contact (eg, with hospital personnel or school classmates) is not clearly associated with increased risk. Secondary cases of meningococcal disease have been reported in several day care centers. It would therefore seem prudent to regard nursery school contacts in the same light as intimate household contacts and employ chemoprophylaxis. Sulfadiazine, 0.5 gm every 12 hours for 4 doses, will reduce the carrier rate and limit spread of the disease if the strains of the organism causing the disease are sulfonamide-sensitive. If the strain is resistant to sulfonamides, rifampin, 10 mg/kg twice daily for 2 days for children 1–12 years of age, is the drug of choice. If the initial case of infection is due to serogroup A or C meningococci, vaccinating contacts of the patient with the appropriate meningococcal polysaccharide vaccine will provide additional protection. Such contacts must be identified, and the physician must make certain that they comply with recommendations about prophylaxis. Countercurrent immunoelectrophoresis has played an important diagnostic role in helping to establish appropriate chemoprophylaxis.

Treatment

A. Specific Measures: Give aqueous penicillin G, 400,000 units/kg/day IV in 6 divided doses. Treatment is continued until the patient has been afebrile for 5 days, the CSF count shows fewer than 30 white cells, and the CSF glucose and protein levels are normal. Patients allergic to penicillin should probably be treated with chloramphenicol or with penicillin G after rapid desensitization and concomitant corticosteroid administration.

B. General Measures: Treatment uses the VIP approach to physiologic support (**V**, ventilation; **I**, infusion; **P**, pump [heart]).

1. Ventilation—The airway and adequate alveolar ventilation must be maintained; this may require a tracheostomy. Arterial blood gases should be monitored. Humidified oxygen by nasal catheter is usually required.

2. Infusion—A central venous pressure catheter should be inserted and the CVP monitored carefully (normal CVP: 3–10 cm water). Hourly urine output should also be monitored (normal: 2–4 ml/kg/hour).

a. Fluid management—Isotonic electrolyte solution, plasma, or blood, 1–2 ml/kg, is infused over a 10-minute period with constant monitoring in order to treat hypovolemic shock. Wait 10 minutes before infusing more fluids. A rise in CVP of 2 cm water is acceptable. In the presence of hypovolemic shock, intermittent infusions should be continued until the CVP remains constant in a range of 5–10 cm water and an adequate urine volume of 2 ml/kg/hour is obtained.

b. Acid-base and electrolyte status (pH, electrolytes, BUN, creatinine)—As noted above, profound metabolic acidosis occurs in advanced septicemic shock. This should be monitored. An infusion of 1 mEq/kg of sodium bicarbonate may be given in an attempt to temporarily correct the acidosis and improve cardiac function, but the primary effort should be directed toward restoring tissue perfusion and aerobic metabolism.

3. Pump (heart) failure—In some patients, particularly those with meningococcemia, there may be decreased cardiac output associated with an increased CVP. Myocarditis is a significant factor in the fatal outcome of acute meningococcal infections. The patient should be treated for heart failure if the CVP increases by more than 5 cm water during the 10-minute waiting period after an infusion or if the CVP exceeds 16 cm water at any time. In the presence of heart failure, the intravenous administration of a rapidly acting digitalis preparation with constant ECG monitoring is recommended. If poor perfusion of vital tissues (decreased renal output) continues, a beta-adrenergic stimulator should be used.

a. Isoproterenol—As a beta-adrenergic stimulator, isoproterenol has the desirable effect of decreasing peripheral vascular resistance as well as exercising an inotropic effect on the heart. A continuous infusion of 0.2–0.4 mg in 100 ml of isotonic solution given at a rate of 1 ml/minute will often result in increased urine output and a decline in CVP.

b. Dopamine (Intropin)—As an endogenous catecholamine, dopamine exercises a direct effect on both beta and alpha receptors. It has been effective in some cases where isoproterenol has failed. Dopamine is administered beginning at a rate of 5 μg/kg/minute IV. The rate of infusion is gradually increased every 15–20 minutes until blood pressure and urine output are satisfactory.

c. Corticosteroids—Evidence indicates that very large doses of hydrocortisone produce an increase in blood pressure and decreased peripheral resistance through the mechanism of arteriolar vasodilation. Nonhemodynamic effects of corticosteroids which may contribute to increased survival include a positive inotropic effect on the heart, stabilization of lysosomes, and binding of endotoxin. Hydrocortisone (Solu-Cortef) is given in a dose of 50 mg/kg as a bolus injection IV followed by 50 mg/kg as a continued infusion over the next 12 hours.

d. Phenoxybenzamine (Dibenzyline)—This alpha-adrenergic blocking agent has been shown to be of value in humans with septic shock. Lowering of the CVP when this drug is being used indicates the need for more fluid volume correction. Its use requires experience and close monitoring. When administered IV, phenoxybenzamine must be well diluted and infused slowly. The usual dosage is 1 mg/kg diluted in 250–500 ml of 5% glucose in 0.9% sodium chloride solution and infused over a period of at least 1 hour.

C. Treatment of Disseminated Intravascular Coagulation (DIC): As noted above, DIC often accompanies septic shock. Usually DIC improves when other measures to restore blood volume and tissue perfusion are instituted. However, in the case of frank bleeding, rising BUN or creatinine, or "shock" lung known to be associated with fibrin deposits, heparinization is indicated. The initial dose is 50 units/kg IV. Every 4 hours, 100 units/kg are added to the infusion. The dosage should be titrated to give a clotting time of 20–30 minutes.

Prognosis

With prompt treatment, the prognosis is excellent, except in the fulminating form of the disease. Convalescence may require several weeks, especially if skin involvement is pronounced.

Eickhoff TC: Meningococcal prophylaxis. JAMA 234:150, 1975.

Jacobson JA, Filice GA, Holloway JT: Meningococcal disease in day-care centers. Pediatrics 59:299, 1977.

Lauer BA, Fisher CE: *Neisseria lactamica* meningitis. Am J Dis Child 130:198, 1976.

McCormick JB, Bennett JV: Public health considerations in the management of meningococcal disease. Ann Intern Med 83:883, 1975.

Meningococcal disease: Prevention and control. Clin Pediatr (Phila) 16:311, 1977.

The Meningococcal Disease Surveillance Group: Meningococcal disease: Secondary attack rate and chemoprophylaxis in the United States, 1974. JAMA 235:261, 1976.

Pickering LK: Chemoprophylaxis against *Neisseria meningitidis:* The role of countercurrent immunoelectrophoresis. JAMA 236:1882, 1976.

GONOCOCCAL INFECTIONS

General Considerations

Gonorrhea remains the world's most commonly reported communicable disease. *Neisseria gonorrhoeae,* a member of the aerobically growing genus Neisseria, is a gram-negative diplococcus. Although morphologically similar to other neisseriae, it differs in its ability to grow on selective media and to ferment glucose. The organism can be subdivided according to colony variation into 4 types; types 1 and 2 are capable of producing disease in man. Colony types 1 and 2 have pili when observed with the electron microscope, and colony types 3 and 4 do not. These pili are hair-like protein structures which extend from the cell wall and are known to be related to the cell's capacity for adherence. The pili may be responsible for antiphagocytic properties of the cell and may protect the gonococcus from the action of complement and antibody. The existence of a capsule on *N gonorrhoeae* has recently been demonstrated. The cell wall of *N gonorrhoeae* acts as a powerful endotoxin which is liberated when the organism dies and is responsible for the production of a cellular exudate. The incubation period of infection is short, averaging 3–5 days.

Until very recently, penicillin resistance was relative, not absolute. Gonococci are now being encountered that elaborate penicillinase and are therefore totally resistant to penicillin. Initially, most isolates of these gonococci in the USA were related to travelers who had returned from the Philippines, but more recent local outbreaks have occurred that have no demonstrable epidemiologic connection to travelers returning from the Far East.

Penicillinase-resistant penicillins are relatively resistant to the penicillinase produced by the gonococcus but show too little intrinsic activity against gonococci to be clinically useful. Among the cephalosporins, the most active drugs on the basis of weight appear to be cefamandole, cefoxitin, and especially cefuroxime. All isolates to date are sensitive to spectinomycin. Many of the penicillinase-producing gonococci show low-level resistance to tetracycline, but none has an MIC for tetracycline of more than 4 μg/ml. Treatment with spectinomycin has been very effective to date. Only limited clinical experience in treatment of infections caused by penicillinase-producing gonococci has been obtained using other drugs. Since infection with penicillinase-producing gonococci is still very uncommon in the USA (less than 5% of cases), it has been recommended that the present treatment policies remain unchanged. However, spectinomycin should be given as initial therapy for infections acquired in areas where the disease is highly prevalent.

Gonococcal disease in the pediatric patient is not rare and may be transmitted venereally or nonvenereally. Prepubertal girls usually manifest gonococcal vulvovaginitis because of the anterior placement of the vulva, neutral-alkaline pH of the vagina, thin vaginal mucosa, and lack of protecting hair and soft tissue. Progression of vulvovaginitis to salpingitis and peritonitis in the prepubertal girl has been reported but is unusual because of the complete absence of endocervical glandular structures that harbor the organism. The triad of fever, abdominal pain, and vaginal discharge should alert the physician to the possibility of salpingitis and periappendicitis.

Clinical Findings

A. Symptoms and Signs:

1. Asymptomatic gonorrhea—Most cases of gonorrhea are apparently asymptomatic, with genital carriage in up to 80% of women, rectal carriage in up to 50% of women and a high percentage of homosexual males, urethral carriage in up to 40% of men, and pharyngeal carriage in either sex. The incidence of asymptomatic gonorrhea in children and adolescents cannot be ascertained because most pediatricians do not include screening for gonorrhea in routine evaluations.

2. Uncomplicated genital gonorrhea—

a. Male with urethritis—Frequency and urgency on urination with urethral discharge and erythema and, rarely, balanitis. The patient is usually afebrile, and inguinal lymphadenopathy is rarely present.

b. The young female child with diffuse vaginitis—The only evidence at this stage may be dysuria and polymorphonuclear neutrophils in the urine. Vulvitis characterized by erythema, edema, and excoriation accompanied by a purulent discharge may follow.

c. Postpubertal female with symptomatic cervicitis—Characterized by a purulent discharge, dysuria, and occasionally dyspareunia. Lower abdominal pain is absent. Physical examination reveals an afebrile patient with positive findings limited to the cervix, which is frequently hyperemic and tender when touched by the examining finger. This tenderness is not worsened by moving the cervix, nor are the adnexa tender to palpation.

3. Tonsillopharyngitis—Presents as an acute exudative pharyngitis with bilateral cervical lymphadenopathy and fever. It often constitutes a variant of child abuse.

4. Conjunctivitis and iridocyclitis—Probably spread from infected genital secretions by the fingers.*

5. Progressive local infection (salpingitis)—The interval between initiation of genital infection and the onset of ascent of infection is variable and may range from days to months, with menses frequently the initiating factor. With the onset of a menstrual period, gonococci invade the endometrium, causing transient endometritis. Subsequently, salpingitis may occur, resulting in pyosalpinx or hydrosalpinx, or it may lead to the escape of gonococci into the peritoneum, causing peritonitis or perihepatitis. Gonococcal salpingitis occurs in an acute, subacute, or chronic form depending in part on the duration of infection, the quality of antibiotic treatment for cervicitis, and possibly on the virulence of the organism. All 3 forms have in common tenderness on gentle movement of the cervix and bilateral tubal tenderness during pelvic examination.

a. Gonococcal perihepatitis—(Often referred to as Fitz-Hugh and Curtis syndrome.) In the typical clinical pattern, there is right upper quadrant tenderness in association with signs of acute or subacute salpingitis. Pain may be pleuritic and referred to the shoulder. Hepatic friction rub is a valuable but inconstant sign.

b. Prostatitis—The most frequent complication of gonococcal urethritis in the male is local extension to the prostate. This gland may become enlarged, causing symptoms of urinary obstruction, or may be tender to palpation.

c. Gonococcal epididymitis—Should be considered in the differential diagnosis of a mass in the scrotum of an adolescent male. The mass is commonly tender, erythematous, and warm but may rarely be indurated and nontender.

6. Disseminated gonorrhea—Dissemination follows asymptomatic more often than symptomatic genital infection and often results from gonococcal pharyngitis and anorectal gonorrhea.

a. Arthritis—This is the form of disseminated disease most commonly encountered in children and adolescents. It is more common in females, who may have

---

*Gonococcal ophthalmia neonatorum is discussed in Chapter 9. Infants may also develop anogenital colonization during birth with subsequent gonococcal sepsis and arthritis.

been asymptomatic until development of arthritis. Initially, there is polyarthralgia or polyarthritis. This is followed by arthritis involving virtually any joint, especially the knees, ankles, and wrists. Tenosynovitis is an especially important clue. This is most common about the ankles and wrists. Frank sheath abscesses may occur.

b. Dermatitis—There may be vesiculopustules on an erythematous base, hemorrhagic papules, or hemorrhagic bullae, most commonly over the distal portions of the extremities and around the joints. The rash begins as tender, pointing erythematous macules. Vasculitis is present histologically. The gonococcus seldom can be isolated from the lesions. However, a Gram stain may be helpful.

c. Carditis—A rare but frequently fatal manifestation of disseminated gonococcal infection is endocarditis. Acute in its onset, it is typically preceded by transient polyarthritis or arthralgias. The aortic valve is most frequently involved.

d. Meningitis—Because of the morphologic similarities of *N gonorrhoeae* and *N meningitidis,* it is not surprising that the former may cause meningitis and that the latter may be found in pelvic disease. The clinical manifestations are similar to those of meningitis due to *N meningitidis,* both in the neonate and in the adolescent. The differentiation can be made only by carbohydrate fermentation testing.

B. Laboratory Findings: Demonstration of gram-negative kidney bean–shaped diplococci on smears of urethral exudate in males is presumptive evidence of gonorrhea. Negative smears do not rule out gonorrhea; cultures are needed. In girls with suspected gonorrhea, both the cervical os and the anus should be cultured. Gonococcal pharyngitis requires culture to substantiate the etiologic diagnosis. In patients with peripheral manifestations of gonococcal sepsis (skin lesions, arthritis), there is a less than 15% chance of isolating gonococci from the blood. There is a 25% chance of isolating gonococci from a joint, and little chance of isolating gonococci from skin lesions. Bacteriologic documentation of genital infection strongly supports a diagnosis of extragenital gonorrhea and is the usual means of establishing the diagnosis of gonococcal sepsis. Thayer-Martin medium suppresses nearly everything except oxidase-positive *N gonorrhoeae* and *N meningitidis* and is especially useful when gonococci must be isolated from an area colonized by multiple bacterial strains such as are present in the cervical os, anus, and pharynx. Culture on Thayer-Martin medium is presently considered to suffice for the diagnosis of gonorrhea. If bacteriologic diagnosis is critical, suspected material should be cultured on chocolate agar as well. Thayer-Martin medium is not necessary for culturing blood or synovial fluid. In circumstances where transportation is necessary, material should be directly inoculated into Transgrow medium prior to shipment to an appropriate laboratory.

Repeat cultures should be obtained from patients who fail to respond to penicillin, and the isolates should be tested for production of penicillinase by screening with a 10-μg disk of penicillin G. All isolates of penicillinase-producing gonococci should be reported. Patients known to have acquired infections with penicillinase-producing gonococci should have a rescreening culture performed a few weeks after successful therapy, and maximal efforts should be made to trace and treat their infected sexual contacts. In performing rectal cultures, the physician should insert a cotton sterile swab 1 inch into the anal canal, avoiding feces. The direct fluorescent antibody (FA) test on a smear directly obtained from the patient probably is not much better than a Gram-stained smear alone. No serologic tests are available. A new antipilar antibody test is promising.

Differential Diagnosis

Urethritis, alone or in association with prostatitis, proctitis, and epididymitis, may be caused by other bacteria or may represent only nonspecific urethritis.

Vulvovaginitis in a prepubertal female may be due to infection caused by miscellaneous bacteria, candida, and herpesvirus; discharges may be caused by trichomonads, oxyuris, and other parasites; and inflammation may be secondary to foreign bodies. Symptom-free discharge (leukorrhea) normally accompanies rising estrogen levels.

Cervicitis in a postpubertal female, alone or in association with urethritis and involvement of Skene's and Bartholin's glands, may be due to infection caused by other bacteria, candida, herpesvirus, trichomonas, discharge resulting from inflammation caused by foreign bodies (usually some form of contraceptive device), or leukorrhea associated with birth control pills.

Salpingitis may be due to infection with other organisms or may be associated with appendicitis, urinary tract infection, or ectopic pregnancy.

Extragenital infections (arthritis, pharyngitis, endocarditis, meningitis, ophthalmitis, skin lesions) may be caused by other organisms besides gonococci.

Complications

Other manifestations of gonococcal infection such as liver abscesses, osteomyelitis, and pericarditis are now all rare. Postgonococcal urethritis syndrome is not rare; the cause is uncertain.

Prevention

Prevention of gonorrhea is principally a problem of sex education.

Treatment*

A. Uncomplicated Gonococcal Infections in Adolescents: The drug regimen of choice is aqueous procaine penicillin G, 4.8 million units IM, divided into at least 2 doses and injected at different sites at one visit,

---

*These dosages must be modified for use in infants and children. Spectinomycin has not been approved for use in children. Tetracycline should not be used for children under 8 years of age. For penicillin-allergic patients, erythromycin or tetracycline may be used.

together with 1 gm of probenecid orally just before the injections. The following alternative regimens can be used: (1) ampicillin, 3.5 gm orally, together with 1 gm probenecid orally administered at the same time; (2) tetracycline, 1.5 gm immediately by mouth followed by 0.5 gm by mouth 4 times a day for 4 doses (total dosage, 9.5 gm); or (3) spectinomycin, 2 gm IM, recommended only for patients who do not respond to treatment with other antibiotics or who are likely to be infected with penicillinase-producing *N gonorrhoeae* (PPNG). Nonpenicillinase-producing gonococci with absolute resistance to spectinomycin have been detected, and if the drug is used indiscriminately, the probability that PPNG will acquire spectinomycin resistance will increase. These strains are also relatively resistant to tetracycline. Pharyngeal infection commonly fails to respond to spectinomycin. Prophylactic treatment of sexual partners employs these same dosages. Follow-up urethral and other appropriate cultures should be obtained from males and cervical, anal, and other appropriate cultures from females 7–14 days after completion of treatment.

B. Postgonococcal Urethritis: This syndrome is best treated with tetracycline, 0.5 gm orally 4 times daily, for at least 7 days.

C. Gonococcal Sepsis: Give aqueous penicillin G, 7–10 million units IV daily by continuous drip for 3 days; then ampicillin, 2 gm orally daily for 7 days. Treat for 10 days. Metastatic disease may require at least 10 million units IV daily for at least 10 days for meningitis and for at least 3–4 weeks for endocarditis.

D. Arthritis: Gonococcal arthritis is ordinarily quite responsive to penicillin given IM, and massive IV therapy is unnecessary.

Dans PE: Treatment of gonorrhea and syphilis: Part 1. Gonorrhea. South Med J 68:1287, 1975.

Elliott WC & others: Treatment of gonorrhea with trimethoprim-sulfamethoxazole. J Infect Dis 135:939, 1977.

Faigel HC: Asymptomatic gonorrhea. (Commentary.) Clin Pediatr (Phila) 15:673, 1976.

Hein K, Marks A, Cohen MI: Asymptomatic gonorrhea: Prevalence in a population of urban adolescents. J Pediatr 90:634, 1977.

Karney WW & others: Spectinomycin versus tetracycline for the treatment of gonorrhea. N Engl J Med 296:889, 1977.

Kaufman RE & others: National gonorrhea therapy monitoring study: Treatment results. N Engl J Med 294:1, 1976.

McCormack WM: Treatment of gonorrhea: Is penicillin passé? (Editorial.) N Engl J Med 296:934, 1977.

Nelson JD & others: Gonorrhea in preschool and school-aged children: Report of the Prepubertal Gonorrhea Cooperative Study Group. JAMA 236:1359, 1976.

Penicillinase-producing gonococci. (Editorial.) Lancet 2:725, 1976.

Sparling PF & others: Summary of the conference on the problem of penicillin-resistant gonococci. J Infect Dis 135:865, 1977.

Thornsberry C & others: Spectinomycin-resistant *Neisseria gonorrhoeae*. JAMA 237:2405, 1977.

ANTHRAX

General Considerations

Anthrax is a disease caused by *Bacillis anthracis* and is transmitted to humans through broken skin or mucosa or by inhalation or ingestion from a variety of domestic animals. The characteristic lesion of human anthrax is a necrotic cutaneous ulcer, the "malignant pustule." A degree of suspicion is necessary in making the diagnosis, especially if a potential source of contamination is present. Cases have occurred among children of industrial workers. A specific toxin affecting capillary permeability and leading to fluid loss has been identified.

Clinical Findings

A. Symptoms and Signs:

1. Cutaneous anthrax ("malignant pustule")—This form of the disease usually begins on an exposed body surface as a painless, mildly pruritic, erythematous papule which soon vesiculates. Within 1 day, ulceration leads to the formation of a black eschar. The ulcer may be surrounded by marked edema and swelling which is nontender and nonpitting. Mild tenderness and enlargement of regional lymph nodes are seen. Constitutional symptoms may be very mild despite extensive local changes. Septicemic spread may occur with extensive systemic manifestations, but this is uncommon.

2. Pulmonary anthrax (woolsorter's disease)—The pneumonic form of the disease is characterized by high fever, malaise, headache, cough, and evidence of widespread pneumonitis by auscultation and x-ray. Widening of the mediastinum is suggestive of the disease.

3. Gastrointestinal anthrax—A central necrotic ulcer of the stomach surrounded by edema may be accompanied by massive ascites.

B. Laboratory Findings: The exudate from a "malignant pustule" usually shows little cellular reaction, and the causative gram-positive bacilli are present in small numbers. The smear may also show contamination with staphylococci. Cultures of the skin exudate, blood, and sputum may be positive for *B anthracis.* A serologic test exists with which a diagnosis can be made in patients who have been given antibiotics prior to collection of specimens for culture.

Differential Diagnosis

In scrub typhus, a cutaneous black eschar is associated with a generalized maculopapular eruption.

Pneumonitis associated with Q fever may need to be distinguished from pulmonary anthrax. Infection occurs by inhalation of contaminated products of infected sheep and cattle.

The pulmonary lesions may resemble those of tuberculosis, neoplasms, sarcoidosis, and fungal infections.

The cutaneous lesion occasionally may be mistaken for tuberculosis, pyoderma, carcinoma, and granulomas.

Treatment

Treatment consists of procaine penicillin G, 50,000 units/kg/day IM in 4 divided doses for 10–14 days. Streptomycin may be added if there is no clinical response within 24 hours. One of the tetracyclines may be given as an alternative to penicillin in a dosage of 25–50 mg/kg/day orally in 4 divided doses. Erythromycin or streptomycin may also be used.

Prognosis

The mortality rate approaches 20% in the untreated cutaneous form of the disease. Prognosis with early treatment is excellent. Pulmonary anthrax has a serious prognosis.

Brachman PS: Anthrax. Ann NY Acad Sci 174:577, 1970.

Christie AB: The clinical aspects of anthrax. Postgrad Med J 49:565, 1973.

Davies DG, Harvey RWS: Anthrax infection in bone meal from various countries of origin. J Hyg (Camb) 70:455, 1972.

Dutz W, Saidi F, Kohout E: Gastric anthrax with massive ascites. Gut 11:352, 1970.

Lamb R: Anthrax. Br Med J 1:157, 1973.

McSwiggan DA, Hussain KK, Taylor IO: A fatal case of cutaneous anthrax. J Hyg (Camb) 73:151, 1974.

BOTULISM

Essentials of Diagnosis

- Nausea and vomiting.
- Diplopia.
- Difficulty in swallowing and speech occurring within 12–36 hours after ingestion of home-canned food.

General Considerations

Botulism is a serious food poisoning caused by *Clostridium botulinum,* which produces 6 type-specific neurotoxins. Humans are affected by types A, B, E, and F. Toxin is absorbed from the gut and reaches motor nerves, where it acts at synapses and neuromuscular junctions.

C botulinum organisms and toxin have been identified in the feces of infants age 5–20 weeks who had illnesses clinically consistent with botulism. Clinical findings included constipation, weak sucking and crying ability, pooled oral secretions, cranial nerve deficits, generalized weakness, and, on occasion, sudden apnea. A characteristic electromyographic pattern termed "brief, small, abundant motor-unit action potentials" (BSAP) was observed. The source of *C botulinum* toxin for infants is thought to be in vivo (gastrointestinal) production following ingestion of *C botulinum* organisms. Studies are under way to determine the full clinical spectrum, incidence, and potential public health importance of this infectious disease in view of its newly recognized incidence in infants.

Food contamination is a well-recognized source of botulism. Wound contamination with *C botulinum* is uncommon. It should be considered in any patient who, soon after trauma, develops symmetric cranial nerve paralysis and progressive descending motor weakness without sensory impairment. The most frequent presenting symptoms are diplopia, dysarthria, and dysphagia. Progressive motor paralysis with respiratory failure is common. Fever may be present. Gastrointestinal symptoms and changes in sensorium are absent. Confirmation of the diagnosis is established by isolating *C botulinum* from the wound or by demonstrating botulinum toxin in the patient's serum.

Most cases of botulism follow ingestion of improperly prepared home-canned foods, the remnants of which are often fed to domestic animals such as chickens, causing their death and confirming the diagnosis. The immunologically distinct strain designated as type F was recognized in an outbreak caused by the ingestion of homemade liver paste on the Dutch island of Langeland in 1960. Type F subsequently was recovered from marine samples taken off the coasts of California and Oregon and from salmon in the Columbia River. An outbreak caused by type F occurred in California in 1966.

Clinical Findings

A. Symptoms and Signs: An abrupt onset occurs 12–36 hours after ingestion of food which may have had a rancid or putrid odor or taste. There is lassitude or fatigue, generally with headache. Double vision followed by photophobia and nystagmus occurs, and within a few hours, difficulty in swallowing and in speech. Pharyngeal paralysis occurs in serious cases, and food may be regurgitated through the nose and mouth. The sensorium is clear and the temperature normal. Death usually results from respiratory failure.

B. Laboratory Findings: Suspected food should be recovered and examined for the presence of toxin by injection into mice. Laboratory findings in the patient are usually normal. With the use of electrophysiologic technics, electrical abnormalities can be found. Early in the course, when the patient has marked clinical weakness, the rested muscle shows a depressed response to a single supramaximal stimulus applied to the nerve (normal, 6–12 mV). Later in the course, a marked augmentation of muscle action potential is seen after rapid repetitive stimulation (50/second) of the nerve. This finding is characteristic of neuromuscular block.

Differential Diagnosis

Spinonuchal rigidity and CSF pleocytosis distinguish bulbar poliomyelitis from botulism.

A symmetrical ascending motor paralysis associated with sensory findings and albumino-cytologic dissociation are seen in Guillain-Barré syndrome (infectious neuritis).

The history and related findings characterize postdiphtheritic polyneuritis.

In methyl chloride poisoning, pulmonary edema is associated with CNS depression.

In sodium fluoride poisoning, there is severe

nausea, vomiting, and diarrhea in addition to CNS depression. Poisoning with methyl alcohol, organic phosphorus compounds, or atropine may have to be ruled out.

Tick paralysis is characterized by a flaccid ascending motor paralysis which begins in the legs.

Myasthenia gravis usually occurs in adolescent girls and is characterized by ocular and bulbar symptoms with normal pupils, fluctuating weakness, and the absence of other neurologic signs.

Complications

Difficulty in swallowing leads to aspiration pneumonia. Serious respiratory paralysis may be fatal.

Prevention

Proper sterilization of all canned foods is indicated. Energetic boiling for 10 minutes before eating home-canned food would prevent the disease. Cans with bulging lids or jars with leaking rings should be destroyed. Prophylactic antitoxin should be given to asymptomatic persons within 72 hours of ingesting an incriminated food. Vomiting should be induced, and purgatives and high enemas should be administered.

Treatment

A. Specific Measures: Botulinus antitoxin, trivalent (types A, B, and E), should be given intravenously as soon as the diagnosis is made or suspected after skin testing for horse serum sensitivity. The antitoxin as well as 24-hour diagnostic consultation, epidemic assistance, and laboratory testing services are available from the Center for Disease Control. The trivalent antitoxin contains 7500 IU of type A, 5500 IU of type B, and 8500 IU of type E per vial. It is recommended that 2 vials be given as initial therapy. This dose may be repeated within 2–4 hours. A small supply of quadrivalent antitoxin (types A, B, E, and F) is stored at the Center for Disease Control. Guanidine hydrochloride, 15–35 mg/kg/day orally in 3 doses, reverses the neuromuscular block and is a useful adjunct in the treatment of botulism.

B. General Measures: General and supportive therapy consists of absolute rest in bed, aspiration of the respiratory tract through a tracheostomy (if necessary), oxygen and assisted respiration for respiratory paralysis, fluid therapy, and administration of purgatives and high enemas. Treatment with penicillin will eliminate viable organisms continuing to produce toxin.

Prognosis

The mortality rate is 65% in the USA but much lower in Europe. In nonfatal cases, symptoms subside over 2–3 months and recovery is eventually complete.

Arnon SS & others: Infant botulism: Epidemiological, clinical and laboratory aspects. JAMA 237:1946, 1977.

Barker WH Jr & others: Type B botulism outbreak caused by a commercial food product, West Virginia and Pennsylvania, 1973. JAMA 237:456, 1977.

Berg BO: Syndrome of infant botulism. Pediatrics 59:321, 1977.

Merson MH & others: Current trends in botulism in the United States. JAMA 229:1305, 1974.

Midura TF, Arnon SS: Infant botulism: Identification of *Clostridium botulinum* and its toxins in faeces. Lancet 2:934, 1976.

Paust JC: Respiratory care in acute botulism: A report of 4 cases. Anesth Analg (Cleve) 50:1003, 1971.

Pickett J & others: Syndrome of botulism in infancy: Clinical and electrophysiologic study. N Engl J Med 295:770, 1976.

TETANUS

Essentials of Diagnosis

- History of skin wound.
- Spasms of jaw muscles (trismus).
- Stiffness of neck, back, and abdominal muscles, with hyperirritability and hyperreflexia leading to fatal convulsions.

General Considerations

Tetanus is caused by *Clostridium tetani,* an anaerobic, gram-positive organism that produces a potent toxin. The toxin reaches the CNS by retrograde axon transport, is bound to gangliosides, increases reflex excitability in neurons of the spinal cord by blocking function of inhibitory synapses, and affects synaptic transmission at the myoneural junction by accumulation of acetylcholine. Intense muscle spasms result. The organism enters the body by contamination of a wound which may be very minor. In many cases, no history of wound contamination can be obtained. In the newborn, infection frequently occurs through the umbilical cord. It may also occur after smallpox vaccination if an infected poultice is used. The incubation period ranges from 1–54 days (in nearly 90% of cases, within 14 days). In the USA there is an increased incidence of tetanus in the lower Mississippi Valley and in the Southeast. Wounds leading to tetanus usually have 2 things in common: (1) they have not been washed and kept clean, and (2) they often have scabbed over to allow a little pus to form beneath.

Clinical Findings

A. Symptoms and Signs: The first symptom is often minimal pain at the site of inoculation followed by hypertonicity and spasm of the regional muscles. Characteristically, difficulty in opening the mouth (trismus) is evident within 48 hours. The disease may then progress to extensive stiffness of the jaw and neck, increasing dysphagia and irritability, and generalized hyperreflexia with extreme rigidity and spasms of all muscles of the abdomen and back. There is no involvement of the sensorium, and the patient is conscious and lucid. Difficulty in swallowing and convulsions triggered by minimal stimuli such as sound, light, or movement may occur. Recurrent spasms are seen, as well as opisthotonos, clenching of the fists, and pain lasting 10–20 seconds. In most cases the temperature is only mildly elevated. A high or subnormal temperature is a bad prognostic sign. A profound circulatory disturbance associated with sympathetic overactivity may occur on the second to fourth day, which may contribute to the mortality. This is characterized by elevated blood pressure, increased cardiac output, tachycardia (> 120 beats/minute), and dysrhythmia. Reduction of effective circulatory volume with leakage of fluid and solute to the interstitium has been recently documented.

B. Laboratory Findings: The diagnosis is made on clinical grounds. There is a mild polymorphonuclear leukocytosis. The CSF is normal with the exception of some elevation of pressure.

Differential Diagnosis

Poliomyelitis is characterized by asymmetric paralysis in an incompletely immunized child.

The history of a bite, absence of trismus, and pleocytosis of the spinal fluid distinguish rabies.

Local infections of the throat and jaw should be easily recognized.

In strychnine poisoning, spasms of the jaw muscles are not common, and periods of relaxation between spasms are more obvious.

Tetany is confirmed by finding hypocalcemia.

Complications

Malnutrition, pneumonitis, and respiratory obstruction are complications which can be prevented by skilled nursing care.

Prevention

A. Tetanus Toxoid: Active immunization with tetanus toxoid is routinely advised. Primary immunization of infants is completed after 4 injections. A booster is given upon entry into school. A diphtheria and tetanus (DT) booster is then required every 10 years. A serum antitoxin content of 0.01 unit/ml indicates that protection is adequate. A booster at the time of injury is practical if none has been given in the past 3 years, or if none has been given within 1 year in case of a heavily contaminated wound.

An attack does not confer immunity, and every patient who recovers from an attack should be given a complete course of active immunizations without delay.

B. Tetanus Antitoxin: Horse serum antitoxin was formerly used in nonimmunized individuals with soil-contaminated wounds, compound fractures, gunshot wounds, etc. Tetanus immune gamma globulin (human) should now be employed instead. Much lower doses are required than with horse serum, and the child does not require prior sensitivity testing or observation following its administration. For children under 5 years of age, give 125 units IM; for children 10 years of age or older, 250 units IM. After severe exposure or delayed therapy, 500 units may be required. Tetanus toxoid should be administered at the same time since

there is no apparent evidence for significant interference with immune response by the concomitantly administered immune globulin.

C. Treatment of Wounds: Proper surgical cleansing and debridement of possibly contaminated wounds will decrease the likelihood of tetanus.

Treatment

A. Specific Measures: Human tetanus antitoxin, 3000–6000 units IM, is preferred to horse serum (50,000–100,000 units IV) because it causes no sensitivity reactions and has a much longer half-life. Surgical exploration of wounds with excision of all necrotic tissue is indicated after effective relaxant therapy has been initiated. Local therapy with antitoxin is contraindicated. Penicillin G is given in a dosage of 150,000 units/kg/day IV for 14 days.

B. General Measures: The patient is kept in a quiet dark room with minimal stimulation. Diazepam (Valium) is given in a dosage of 0.6–1.2 mg/kg/day IV in 6 divided doses. In the newborn, the drug may be given in 2 or 3 divided doses. Large doses (up to 25 mg/kg/day) may occasionally be required for older children. Diazepam is given intravenously until muscular spasms become infrequent and the generalized muscular rigidity much less prominent. The drug may then be given in the same total daily dose orally in 3 divided doses. With continued improvement, the daily oral dose may be reduced after physical therapy is started and then finally discontinued.

A synthetic corticosteroid has been tried and has been associated with decreased mortality. The optimal dose of dexamethasone for children is 20–40 mg daily IM. The drug should be started as soon as the diagnosis is made and continued until there is marked clinical improvement.

Tracheostomy is generally desirable early in the course of the disease. Hyperbaric oxygen therapy is said to be of value but requires specialized equipment not generally available. Intravenous fluids are used as required to minimize the need for oral feeding.

Cardiovascular instability may be treated with propranolol (Inderal), beginning with 0.2 mg IV and guided by continuous monitoring of the ECG, heart-rate, and intra-atrial pressure. Further increments of 0.2 mg are given at 2–3 minute intervals until a normal sinus rhythm at a rate of 100/minute or less is reached. The total intravenous dose should not exceed 3 mg. The drug may then be given in a maintenance dosage of 0.5–0.8 mg/kg/day intragastrically in 4 divided doses until the patient has recovered sufficiently to reduce the oral dose of sedative. In some cases, hypertension associated with elevated systemic resistance may persist after the heart rate has been stabilized with propranolol. In such a case, bethanidine (Esbatal) or other hypotensive agent may be efficacious; bethanidine is given intragastrically every 2 hours for a total dose of 0.6–0.8 mg/kg/day.

Prognosis

The fatality rate in newborns is high (70–90%). A

fatality rate of 20–40% can be expected in pediatric practice. Many deaths are due to pneumonia or respiratory embarrassment. If the patient lives, recovery is complete.

Mortality rates tend to increase when (1) the incubation time is short, (2) the site of infection is less accessible and closer to the CNS, (3) there is no acquired immunity, (4) spasms are more frequent and severe and associated with apnea, and (5) the temperature is under 36.7° C (98° F) or over 38.9° C (102° F).

Edsall G: Passive immunity to diphtheria and tetanus in the newborn. J Infect Dis 134:314, 1976.

Human antitoxin for tetanus prophylaxis. (Editorial.) Lancet 1:51, 1974.

Illis LS, Taylor FM: Neurological and electroencephalographic sequelae of tetanus. Lancet 1:826, 1971.

Meira AR: Duration of immunity after tetanus vaccination. Lancet 2:659, 1973.

Nathenson G, Zakaewski B: Current status of passive immunity to diphtheria and tetanus in the newborn. J Infect Dis 133:199, 1976.

Stanfield JP, Gall D, Bracken PM: Single dose antenatal tetanus immunization. Lancet 1:215, 1973.

Weinstein L: Tetanus. N Engl J Med 289:1293, 1973.

GAS GANGRENE

Essentials of Diagnosis

- Massive edema, skin discoloration, bleb formation, and pain in an area of trauma with contamination.
- Serosanguineous exudate from wound.
- Crepitation of subcutaneous tissue.
- Clostridia cultured or smeared from exudate.

General Considerations

Gas gangrene (clostridial myositis) is an infection caused by one or more of several anaerobic gram-positive bacilli of the genus Clostridium *(Cl perfringens [Cl welchii], Cl novyi, and Cl septicum)*. These are soil and fecal organisms usually placed in traumatized devitalized tissue. *Cl perfringens,* the principal causative agent of gas gangrene, produces at least 12 toxins. Alpha toxin is a lecithinase and damages cell membranes by splitting lecithin into phosphocholine and diglyceride. Beta toxin has a necrotizing effect; other toxins are necrotizing, hemolytic, and proteolytic. Multiple toxins are necrotizing and hemolytic, and, together with distention of tissue caused by interference with blood supply and by gas formed from carbohydrates, favor the spread of gangrene. The spread of alpha toxin, in particular, is responsible for the clinical features. Alpha toxin production can be suppressed in broth cultures of *Cl perfringens* by increasing the partial pressure of oxygen in the broth to 250 mm Hg by exposure of cultures to a pressure of 3 atmospheres.

The pathophysiology of necrotizing enterocolitis (NEC) of the newborn is not understood. It is thought to be caused by ischemia of the bowel. This would favor the conversion of clostridial spores—which can occur very early in the intestinal tract of newborns—to toxin-producing, invading bacilli. The histology of resected gut specimens from a small number of patients with NEC who had undergone operation was similar to that in cases of gas gangrene of the bowel and in experimentally provoked cases of pneumatosis cystoides intestinalis. In one case, *Cl perfringens* type A was cultured in great numbers with the use of anaerobic technics. The clostridia in these cases may play an important role in the development of NEC.

Nonclostridial infection can mimic clostridial infections. The former is usually associated with a mixed flora consisting of 2 or more of the following: *E coli,* klebsiella, pseudomonas, enterococcus, anaerobic streptococci, and bacteroides. Such cases have previously been reported to have a poor prognosis and high mortality rate similar to that found in clostridium-induced infection. Nonclostridial organisms are the usual causative organisms of distal gangrene in diabetic patients who have crepitation or x-ray evidence of subcutaneous gas.

Clinical Findings

A. Symptoms and Signs: The onset is sudden, usually 1–5 days after a traumatic injury with an open wound which has been inadequately debrided or has been closed by suture after fairly heavy contamination. The skin around the wound becomes discolored, there is a serosanguineous exudate, and crepitation may be felt in the subcutaneous tissues. Pain and swelling are usually intense. If clostridial septicemia occurs, intravascular hemolysis and jaundice are the rule. Shock and renal failure are ominous signs of far-advanced disease.

B. Laboratory Findings: Isolation of the organism is accomplished by anaerobic culture. Smears may demonstrate morphologically characteristic clostridia.

C. X-Ray Findings: Although the diagnosis is generally made on clinical grounds, x-ray may demonstrate subcutaneous gas.

Differential Diagnosis

Gangrene caused by streptococci is associated with massive bullae. Crepitus in the subcutaneous tissues or x-ray evidence of gas is diagnostic of gas gangrene.

Treatment

A. Specific Measures: Give penicillin G, 150,000 units/kg/day IV in 4 divided doses, and continue until clinical remission occurs. Treatment may be supplemented with tetracyclines.

Polyvalent gas gangrene antitoxin is now rarely employed in pediatric practice because of the danger of horse serum sensitivity and the adequacy of other specific measures.

Tetanus toxoid with or without antitoxin should be given.

B. Surgical Measures: Where hyperbaric oxygen is

used, surgery should be limited to incisions into the phlegmonous area in cases with massive necrosis; removal of necrotic tissue after clinical resolution; and reconstructive measures as necessary.

C. Hyperbaric Oxygen: Hyperbaric oxygen therapy has been shown to be dramatically effective. An environmental oxygen pressure of 2 atmospheres (30 psi) will produce a partial pressure of oxygen in gangrenous tissue of 250 mm Hg at a depth of 5 cm. A patient may be exposed to 2 atmospheres absolute (30 psi) in pure oxygen in a small "one-man chamber" for 2-hour periods for as many sessions as necessary until there is clinical remission of disease. Hyperbaric oxygen therapy is usually continued for 2 or 3 sessions after clinical remission has occurred. Large chambers that can accommodate medical staff as well as the patient may be used in the treatment of gas gangrene. Care must be taken to eliminate risks from pressure, 100% oxygen, and spark production.

Prognosis

Without adequate and early therapy, the prognosis is extremely poor. With a combination of antibiotics, hyperbaric oxygen therapy, and surgery, the mortality rate is about 20%.

Alexander CS, Sako Y, Mekulic E: Pedal gangrene associated with the use of dopamine. N Engl J Med 293:591, 1975.

Bessman AN, Wagner W: Nonclostridial gas gangrene: Report of 48 cases and review of the literature. JAMA 233:958, 1975.

Gorbach SL, Thadepalli H: Isolation of clostridium in human infections: Evaluation of 114 cases. J Infect Dis 131 (Suppl):S81, 1975.

Pedersen PV & others: Necrotising enterocolitis of the newborn: Is it gas-gangrene of the bowel? Lancet 2:715, 1976.

Thomas M & others: Hospital outbreak of *Clostridium perfringens* food-poisoning. Lancet 1:1046, 1977.

DIPHTHERIA

Essentials of Diagnosis

- A gray, adherent pseudomembrane, most often in the pharynx but also in the nasopharynx or trachea.
- Sore throat, serosanguineous nasal discharge, hoarseness, and fever in a nonimmunized child.
- Peripheral neuritis or myocarditis.
- Positive culture.

General Considerations

Diphtheria is an acute infection, usually of the throat or nose but also of the mucous membranes or skin, caused by a gram-positive pleomorphic rod, *Corynebacterium diphtheriae,* which produces a powerful exotoxin. Corynebacteria are 0.5–1 μm in diameter and several μm long. Characteristically, they possess irregular swellings at one end that give them a

"club-shaped" appearance. Irregularly distributed within the rod, often near the poles, are granules staining deeply with aniline dyes (metachromatic granules), which give the rod a beaded appearance.

There are 3 colony types that grow on McLeod's blood agar containing potassium tellurite: (1) var *gravis,* (2) var *mitis,* and (3) var *intermedius.* Variants of toxigenic strains are often nontoxigenic. When some nontoxigenic (avirulent) diphtheria organisms are infected with bacteriophage from certain toxigenic (virulent) diphtheria bacilli, the offspring of the exposed bacteria are lysogenic and toxigenic, and this trait is subsequently hereditary. Thus, acquisition of phage leads to toxigenicity. Whereas toxigenicity is under control of the phage gene, virulence (invasiveness) is under control of the bacterial gene.

The toxin is absorbed into the mucous membranes and causes destruction of epithelium and a superficial inflammatory response. The necrotic epithelium becomes embedded in the exuding fibrin and red and white cells along with normal mouth and throat flora, so that a grayish "pseudomembrane" is formed, commonly over the tonsils, pharynx, or larynx. Any attempt to remove the membrane exposes and tears the capillaries and results in bleeding. The regional lymph nodes in the neck enlarge, and there may be marked edema of the entire neck. The diphtheria bacilli within the membrane continue to produce toxin actively. This is absorbed and results in distant toxic damage, particularly degeneration and necrosis in heart muscle, liver, kidneys, and adrenals, and is sometimes accompanied by hemorrhage. The toxin also produces nerve damage, resulting in paralysis of the soft palate, eye muscles, or extremities. The incubation period is 1–6 days. More serious damage by exotoxin involves the heart, causing early myocarditis. A late manifestation is polyneuritis. Death may occur as a result of respiratory obstruction or acute toxemia and circulatory collapse. The patient may succumb after a somewhat longer time as a result of cardiac damage or may recover after perhaps showing evidence of neurotoxic injury. The clinical course depends on (1) the location and extent of the membrane, (2) the amount of toxin absorbed, (3) the patient's immunity status, and (4) early institution of treatment. In the USA, the disease most commonly affects nonwhite unimmunized children in the Southwest and South.

Clinical Findings

A. Symptoms and Signs:

1. Pharyngeal diphtheria—Early manifestations of diphtheritic pharyngitis are a mild sore throat, moderate fever, and malaise, followed fairly rapidly by severe prostration and circulatory collapse. The pulse is more rapid than the fever would seem to justify. A membrane forms in the throat and may spread into the nasopharynx or the trachea, producing respiratory obstruction. The membrane is tenacious and gray and is surrounded by a narrow zone of erythema and a broader zone of edema. Difficulty in swallowing is present, and noisy breathing becomes evident even without laryngeal obstruction. High fever and prostration are characteristic. Palatal paralysis may occur. A disturbed sensorium is seen. Hemorrhages from the mouth and nose are common. Petechiae may appear on the skin and mucous membranes. The cervical lymph nodes become swollen, and swelling is associated with brawny edema of the neck ("bull neck").

2. Nasal diphtheria—Primary nasal diphtheria occurs in about 2% of cases and is characterized by a serosanguineous nasal discharge and excoriation of the upper lip. Fever and constitutional manifestations may be absent.

3. Laryngeal diphtheria—In about 25% of cases, the larynx is invaded. Occasionally, it may be the only manifestation of the disease. Stridor is apparent. Progressive laryngeal obstruction can lead to cyanosis and suffocation.

4. Other forms—Cutaneous or vaginal diphtheria and wound diphtheria comprise fewer than 2% of cases and are characterized by ulcerative lesions with membrane formation. These may be particularly difficult to identify in the presence of burns or wounds thought to be necrotic on a nonspecific basis. Prompt diagnosis and treatment are essential.

B. Laboratory Findings: Diagnosis is a clinical judgment based on available data. Once a presumptive diagnosis is made, immediate specific treatment should be given. Direct smears are unreliable. Identification by the fluorescent antibody technic is reliable only when done by experienced personnel. Material is first obtained from the nose and throat and from skin lesions, if present, for culture on Löffler's blood agar or other media. From 16–48 hours are required before identification of the organism is possible. A toxigenicity test is then performed. The white blood count is usually normal, but there may be a slight leukocytosis. The red cell count may show evidence of rapid destruction of erythrocytes and hemoglobin. Urinalysis frequently shows proteinuria of a transient nature.

Differential Diagnosis

A foreign body in the nose can be seen with a nasal speculum.

Infants with "snuffles" have other signs of congenital syphilis.

Nasal discharge associated with respiratory viral infections is usually clear and not blood-tinged. Other family members often have symptoms.

The child with acute streptococcal pharyngitis has a sudden onset of high fever, sore throat, and appears acutely ill. Exudate is usually confined to the tonsils.

Exudative pharyngitis may be associated with adenovirus infections. Normal flora is obtained on throat culture. There is no clinical response to penicillin.

Infectious mononucleosis is differentiated by generalized lymphadenopathy, a characteristic blood picture, and a positive heterophil agglutination test.

Agranulocytosis and leukemia are diagnosed by bone marrow examination. (See Streptococcal Infections for differential diagnosis of pharyngitis.)

Acute epiglottitis caused by *Haemophilus influenzae* type B is identified by physical examination and culture.

Acute spasmodic croup is recurrent, worse at night, and may be of allergic origin.

Croup caused by the parainfluenza viruses is associated with symptoms of the common cold with or without fever. Many children in the community will have colds, with some degree of hoarseness. Unpredictably, the occasional child with a mild "croupy cough" will develop stridor and upper airway obstruction rapidly and require a tracheostomy.

Complications

A. Myocarditis: Diphtheritic myocarditis is characterized by a rapid, thready pulse, indistinct and poor heart sounds, cardiac arrhythmias, cardiac failure, hepatomegaly, and fluid retention. Myocarditis can occur 2–27 days after onset of pharyngitis. Cardiac failure most commonly occurs during the second week. ECG changes are characteristic of myocarditis. Conduction system disturbances are not uncommon. Left anterior hemiblock is frequent. Complete heart block signifies a poor prognosis.

B. Toxic Polyneuritis: This complication involves principally the nerves innervating the palate and pharyngeal muscles during the first or second week. Nasal speech and regurgitation of food through the nose are seen. Diplopia and strabismus associated with ocular palsy occur during the third week or later. Neuritis may also involve peripheral motor nerves supplying the intercostal muscles and diaphragm and other muscle groups. Generalized paralysis usually occurs after the fourth week.

C. Bronchopneumonia: Secondary pneumonia is common in fatal cases, especially in association with the laryngeal form.

D. Nephritis: Mild generalized edema, proteinuria, and hyaline casts associated with a decreased urine output are seen in 10–15% of cases.

Prevention

Immunizations with diphtheria toxoid combined with pertussis and tetanus toxoids (DTP) should be employed routinely for infants for a total of 4 injections. A booster is given at 4–6 years, and then an adult type of diphtheria and tetanus (Td) toxoids at 12–14 years. Thereafter, a Td booster is indicated every 10 years.

Care of exposed susceptibles. Children exposed to diphtheria should be examined for signs and symptoms of early diphtheria. If any are found, treat as for diphtheria. Asymptomatic individuals should receive diphtheria toxoid and either erythromycin orally or benzathine penicillin G intramuscularly and be observed daily.

1. Benzathine penicillin G—Age 1–5 years, 600,000 units IM as single dose; over 5 years, 1.2 million units IM as single dose.

2. Erythromycin—Up to 50 lb, 250 mg as estolate (syrup) twice daily for 7 days; 50–100 lb, 250 mg (capsule) 3 times daily for 7 days; over 100 lb, 250 mg (capsule) 4 times daily for 7 days. Failure to take the full course of prescribed drug means that the carrier state will not be eradicated. In epidemic situations where there are many exposed contacts, treatment with benzathine penicillin G is effective and assures that the person is treated. A previously unimmunized, asymptomatic individual who cannot be observed daily should receive, in addition to the above, 10,000 units of diphtheria antitoxin IM.

Treatment

A. Specific Measures:

1. Antitoxin—Every effort must be made to administer diphtheria antitoxin as early as possible. Delay beyond 48 hours must be avoided, if possible, because administration of large doses of antitoxin beyond that point may have little effect in altering the incidence or severity of complications. A syringe containing 1 ml of epinephrine chloride (1:1000) dilution should always be available when antitoxin is being injected. The dose is 0.01 ml/kg/dose of a 1:1000 aqueous solution, with a maximum dose of 0.5 ml. Preliminary sensitivity testing of the patient to horse serum should always be made before antitoxin is administered. Both a skin test and an eye test should be done. For the skin test, 0.1 ml of a 1:1000 dilution of antitoxin in isotonic saline should be injected intradermally. A positive skin test consists of the appearance of a significant wheal and flare occurring at the injection site after a period of 15–20 minutes. For the eye test, one drop of a 1:10 dilution of antitoxin in isotonic saline is instilled into the conjunctival sac. A positive reaction consists of conjunctivitis occurring 15–20 minutes after instillation. If either of these tests is positive, the patient is considered to be sensitive to horse serum and desensitization should be accomplished. Diphtheria antitoxin is administered on the basis of the following schedule: mild pharyngeal diphtheria, or when careful examination indicates that the membrane is small or confined to the anterior nares or tonsils, 40,000 units; moderate pharyngeal diphtheria, 80,000 units; severe pharyngeal or laryngeal diphtheria, combined types, or late cases, 120,000 units. Diphtheria antitoxin is infused in 200 ml of isotonic saline over a 30-minute period.

2. Antibiotics—Antibiotics eliminate the organism from the respiratory tract and skin, terminate the carrier state, stop exotoxin production, and eliminate secondary bacterial infections, particularly those caused by a beta-hemolytic streptococcus. Penicillin is the drug of choice. If the patient can swallow, 250 mg of phenoxymethyl penicillin are given by mouth 3 times a day. Patients unable to swallow may receive procaine penicillin G, 600,000 units twice daily IM. The duration of therapy is 10 days. For the patient allergic to penicillin, erythromycin, 25–50 mg/kg body weight daily, is given, preferably by the oral route, for 10 days.

B. General Measures: Bed rest in the hospital for 10–14 days is usually required. No special food restrictions or additions are needed. Food of a consistency that can be swallowed comfortably in a diet that is adequate in all the nutritional elements is sufficient. Parenteral therapy is indicated only for those patients who cannot swallow, generally because of dysphagia, palatal paralysis, or airway obstruction. Patients may have considerable pharyngeal discomfort during the first few days of illness, and irrigation of the pharynx with warm isotonic saline solution may be helpful. Codeine phosphate, 3 mg/kg/day divided into 6 doses, may be helpful.

All patients must be isolated from other persons until antibiotic treatment has made respiratory secretions noninfectious. A private room is preferable. Because antibiotic administration is effective in eliminating the carrier state, many patients may be free of organisms early in the course of the disease (1–7 days). Isolation may usually be discontinued after 5 days of administration of specific antibiotics. The staff should wear gowns and masks and should wash their hands thoroughly after attending patients with diphtheria. Discharge from the hospital is delayed in uncomplicated cases until 2 or 3 consecutive daily throat and nose cultures contain no *C diphtheriae*. These cultures should not be taken until at least 48 hours have elapsed since the cessation of antibiotic treatment.

C. Treatment of Complications:

1. Myocarditis—Consultation with a cardiologist is usually indicated. From 40 to 65% of patients will show minor ST and T wave changes in the ECG. Patients are generally routinely kept in the hospital for 2 weeks. It is advisable, at least in children, to restrict strenuous exercise for 4 weeks after discharge from the hospital. More serious diphtheritic myocarditis is characterized by a rapid, thready pulse, indistinctive and poor heart sounds, cardiac arrhythmias, cardiac failure, hepatomegaly, and fluid retention. Myocarditis can occur from 2–27 days after the onset of pharyngitis. Cardiac failure most commonly occurs during the second week. ECG changes are characteristic of myocarditis. Conduction system disturbances are common. Left anterior hemiblock is frequent. Complete heart block signifies a poor prognosis. Strict bed rest must be enforced in an attempt to prevent sudden death from slight physical activity. The patient should remain supine in bed and should not attempt self-care. An attendant should be present at the bedside. Digitalis is not well tolerated and should be reserved for therapy of congestive heart failure and arrhythmias with a rapid ventricular response. The value of adrenocorticosteroid therapy is difficult to assess. However, prednisone, 1–2 mg/kg/day for approximately 2 weeks, is advised to lessen the severity of myocarditis. Bed rest is continued for at least 1 month, with graduated activity allowed if there is no occurrence of myocarditis or development of peripheral neuritis.

2. Laryngeal obstruction—Consultation with an ear, nose, and throat specialist is usually required. Bronchoscopy may be used to remove dislodged membrane from larger bronchi, where it may cause death by asphyxia. Tracheostomy may be required early in the course of severely ill patients. The physician should be alert for the development of secondary bronchopneumonia caused by hospital-acquired gram-negative bacilli. Corticosteroids may be of use in acute laryngeal diphtheria. Hydrocortisone sodium succinate (Solu-Cortef), 5 mg/kg/day IM or IV, is given in 3 divided doses for 1 or 2 days or longer. An equivalent dose of prednisone is then given orally when possible and gradually reduced over a 5- to 8-day period.

3. Neurologic complications—Neurologic consultation may be indicated for more severe complications. Palatal paralysis, the most common and often the only paralysis, usually appears early during the course of diphtheria. Intravenous therapy or nasogastric feeding may be required. Paralysis of respiratory muscles usually appears from 6—8 weeks after the onset of pharyngitis. Assisted or controlled ventilation by mechanical means is indicated until the patient can resume spontaneous respiration with satisfactory alveolar inhalation.

4. Shock—In the absence of either myocarditis or peripheral neuritis, severe shock may rarely appear suddenly during the course of diphtheria. This is usually associated with overwhelming toxemia. Under these circumstances, it is best to manage the patient with the measures used for gram-negative septic shock.

D. Treatment of Carriers: All carriers should be treated. Erythromycin or clindamycin is the drug of choice. The dose for erythromycin is 20—50 mg/kg/day divided into 3 or 4 oral doses; for clindamycin, 20 mg/kg/day orally divided into 4 doses. Treatment is continued for 10 days. All carriers must be confined at home. Before they can be released, carriers must have 2 negative cultures of both the nose and the throat taken 24 hours apart and obtained at least 24 hours after the cessation of antibiotic therapy. Cultures are generally taken on days 11 and 12 after treatment.

Prognosis

Mortality rates vary from 3—25% and are particularly high in the presence of early myocarditis. Neuritis is fatal only if an intact airway and adequate respiration cannot be maintained. Permanent damage due to myocarditis occurs rarely.

Death may occur as a result of respiratory obstruction or acute toxemia and circulatory collapse. The patient may succumb after a somewhat longer time as a result of cardiac damage or may recover after perhaps showing evidence of neurotoxic injury.

Edsall G: Passive immunity to diphtheria and tetanus in the newborn. J Infect Dis 134:314, 1976.

Franz ML, Carella JA, Galant SP: Cutaneous delayed hypersensitivity in a healthy pediatric population: Diagnostic value of diphtheria-tetanus toxoids. J Pediatr 88:974, 1976.

Gerry JL, Greenough WB III: Diphtheroid endocarditis: Report of nine cases and review of the literature. Johns Hopkins Med J 139:61, 1976.

Nathenson G, Zakzewski B: Current status of passive immunity to diphtheria and tetanus in the newborn. J Infect Dis 133:199, 1976.

ESCHERICHIA COLI INFECTIONS

Essentials of Diagnosis

- Sudden onset of explosive watery stools with fever and vomiting in newborns or gradual onset of foul-smelling, green diarrheal stools in children under 2 years of age.
- Sick newborn with labile temperature, poor feeding, irritability, jaundice, irregular respirations.
- Child with symptoms of acute urinary tract infection.

General Considerations

Institutional epidemics of gastroenteritis are caused by *Escherichia coli,* including serotypes O26, O55, O86, O91, O111, O112, O119, O124, O128, and O142, which are spread to the infant from hospital personnel, mothers, or infected infants (who may be asymptomatic). Early diagnosis and treatment, including that of carriers in institutions, is essential to prevent widespread disease. Strains of *E coli* not necessarily associated with gastroenteritis can cause neonatal sepsis, the diagnosis of which must be made on clinical grounds and prompt therapy started while awaiting results of blood cultures. Most acute urinary tract infections in children are due to *E coli* infection.

Routine serum grouping of *E coli* in sporadic cases of diarrhea using commercial sera currently available in the USA is for practical purposes useless.

Of major importance is a newly discovered virus which closely resembles the reoviruses. It has been shown to belong to a group of viruses (rotaviruses) which have the appearance on electron microscopy of a double-rimmed wheel. Rotavirus is associated with more than 50% of cases of diarrhea occurring in young children during the months of November through April and 78% of infants with diarrhea in December and January. Infants 6—24 months of age are most susceptible to infection.

Eighty percent of *E coli* strains causing neonatal meningitis possess specific capsular polysaccharide (K1 antigen), which, alone or in association with specific somatic antigens, confers virulence. K1 antigen is associated with approximately 40% of strains causing neonatal septicemia. *E coli* strains are common inhabitants of the gastrointestinal tract of healthy babies, children, and adults. The *E coli* K1 organisms do not appear to cause gastrointestinal disease.

Investigators have studied the somatic (O) and capsular (K) antigens of *E coli* found in the urine of children with acute pyelonephritis, acute cystitis, and asymptomatic bacteriuria and in the feces of healthy school children. Typing antisera for 16 capsular polysaccharide K antigens were used, and 5 antigens (1, 2, 3, 12, and 13) accounted for 70% of isolates from patients with acute pyelonephritis. These 5 K antigens were found to a lesser extent in 3 other study groups. Thus, only a few K polysaccharides are associated with virulent *E coli* infections of the upper urinary tract.

Strains of *E coli* isolated from cases of gastroenteritis in humans and animals have little or no tendency to grow in the kidney. Estrogen may predispose to the development of kidney infection in females and may have an important link with the virulence of the *E coli* organism causing infection.

Clinical Findings

A. Symptoms and Signs:

1. Enteropathic *E coli* gastroenteritis—Usually there is a gradual onset of diarrhea which is not associated with high fever or vomiting in a child under 2 years of age. The stools are loose, slimy, foul-smelling, and green. In a nursery outbreak, the newborn may have fever and associated vomiting and rapidly develops dehydration and metabolic acidosis. In the latter case, weight loss may be spectacular. Within a period of 6–8 hours, 10% dehydration may occur.

2. Neonatal sepsis—Overt signs include jaundice, hepatosplenomegaly, fever, and anemia; subtle signs include listlessness, labile temperature control, apneic spells or irregular respiration, irritability, and failure to suck vigorously. Meningitis is associated with sepsis in 25–40% of cases. Other metastatic foci of infection may be present, including pneumonia and pyelonephritis. Sepsis may also lead to congestive heart failure, hyponatremia, tissue hypoxia, lactic acidemia, severe metabolic acidosis, circulatory collapse, disseminated intravascular coagulation, and death.

3. Neonatal meningitis—High fever, full or bulging fontanels, vomiting, coma, twitching or frank convulsions, pareses or paralyses (ocular, facial, limb), poor or absent Moro reflex, and opisthotonos; occasionally, hyper- or hypotonia and stiff neck. Sepsis coexists or precedes meningitis in a large number of cases. Thus, signs of sepsis often accompany those of meningitis. CSF shows a cell count of over 10/cu mm, usually several hundred or thousands, mostly PMNs. (More than a few PMNs almost always indicate meningitis.) Gram-stained smear of CSF may show organisms. CSF glucose concentration is low, usually less than half that of blood. CSF protein is elevated to 100 mg/100 ml in full-term newborns. CSF protein is normally elevated in prematures (mean, 180 mg/100 ml) even in the absence of meningitis. The diagnosis is established by a positive culture of CSF.

4. Acute urinary tract infection—Classical symptoms include dysuria, increased urinary frequency, and fever in the older child. Such nonspecific symptoms as anorexia, vomiting, irritability, failure to thrive, and unexplained fever are seen in children under 2 years of age. As many as 1% of girls of school age and 0.05% of boys have undiagnosed and asymptomatic but significant urinary tract infections.

B. Laboratory Findings: Culture of enteropathogenic *E coli* by repeated anal swab is routine, but for rapid diagnosis fluorescent antibody studies give an almost immediate answer which permits control measures to prevent epidemic spread in nurseries. Blood cultures are positive in neonatal sepsis. Cultures of spinal fluid, urine, and the umbilicus should also be obtained. A positive culture with a significant colony count (100,000 colonies per ml) from a clean catch, midstream urine sample—or any growth from a bladder tap—confirms the diagnosis of acute urinary tract infection. Recently, a method for distinguishing pyelonephritis from cystitis has been reported. Bacteria in the urinary sediment are stained with fluorescein-tagged antihuman globulin. Positive fluorescence indicates that the bacteria are coated with human antibodies and correlates well with the presence of pyelonephritis.

Differential Diagnosis

The clinical picture of enteropathogenic *E coli* infection may resemble salmonellosis or shigellosis or certain enterovirus (echovirus 18, 9) and adenovirus infections. The diagnosis depends upon stool cultures.

Neonatal sepsis can be clearly differentiated only by blood culture identification.

Complications

Gastroenteritis frequently results in metabolic acidosis and dehydration, requiring vigorous corrective therapy. (See Chapter 35.) Neonatal sepsis may result in seeding of meninges, brain, bone, etc and the development of hemolytic anemia. Recurrent urinary tract infections associated with vesicoureteral reflux may lead to irreversible kidney damage and early death from uremia.

Treatment

A. Specific Measures:

1. *E coli* gastroenteritis—The drug of choice is neomycin, 100 mg/kg/day orally in 3 divided doses for 3–5 days. If the organism is neomycin-resistant, give colistin, 5–10 mg/kg/day orally in 2–3 doses. Good results have also been obtained with gentamicin, 25 mg/kg/day orally in 2 divided doses.

2. *E coli* sepsis, pneumonia, pyelonephritis—In the first week of life, give ampicillin, 100 mg/kg/day IV or IM in divided doses every 8–12 hours; over 1 week of age, give 150–200 mg/kg/day IV or IM in divided doses every 4–6 hours *and* gentamicin in the following dosages: under 1 week of age, 5 mg/kg/day IM in divided doses every 12 hours; over 1 week of age, 7.5 mg/kg/day IM in divided doses every 8 hours. Gentamicin may be given intravenously as an infusion over 1–2 hours in the same dosages as for intramuscular use. Treatment is for 7–10 days. Kanamycin may be used instead of gentamicin if the strain is susceptible. The dosage of kanamycin is 20 mg/kg/day IM in 2 divided doses every 12 hours.

3. *E coli* meningitis—Give ampicillin, 100–300 mg/kg/day IV or IM in 3 divided doses, and gentamicin, 5–7.5 mg/kg/day IM in 3 doses. In addition, give gentamicin intrathecally daily for 5 days. The intrathecal dose for a full-term infant is 2 mg; for a small premature infant, 1 mg. Continue with parenteral antibiotics for 3 weeks, then stop treatment and then reevaluate sterility of CSF after 2–4 days of observation. Do not perform subdural taps unless a symptomatic subdural collection is suspected on the basis of bulging fontanels, enlarged head circumference, seizures, focal neurologic signs, or persistent or recurrent fever. In such a case, perform daily subdural taps with caution, removing a maximum of 10–15 ml daily from each side of the coronal suture for 2 weeks. In case of subdural empyema, continue parenteral antibiotics and introduce 0.5–1 mg of gentamicin into the infected subdural space at the time subdural taps are performed. In infants not responding to treatment, a diagnostic ventricular tap is indicated and 2 mg of gentamicin instilled into the ventricular space. If the ventricular fluid shows evidence of infection with the presence of PMNs or organisms by Gram stain or culture, 2 mg gentamicin should be instilled daily until the fluid is sterile.

4. Acute urinary tract infection—Particularly in girls, the first urinary tract infection is most often a cystitis, commonly caused by *Escherichia coli.* Treatment for 10–14 days is indicated. Several different agents are equally efficacious: sulfisoxazole or trisulfapyrimidines, 120–150 mg/kg/day orally in 4 divided doses; ampicillin, 125–250 mg orally 3 times daily; or nitrofurantoin, 5–7 mg/kg/day orally in 4 divided doses. A follow-up culture should be obtained after 36–48 hours of treatment. If the culture is positive, change treatment according to culture and sensitivities. With recurrent or chronic infection, it should be routine to distinguish pyelonephritis from lower tract infection by direct or indirect technics. Especially promising is the testing for antibodies coating bacteria found in urinary sediment with fluorescein-tagged antihuman globulin, positive fluorescence indicating pyelonephritis. Therapy should be continued for 6 weeks in such cases. Long-term suppressive therapy may be given when indicated with the following drugs: (1) nitrofurantoin, 1–2 mg/kg orally in a single daily dose at bedtime; (2) trimethoprim-sulfamethoxazole (Bactrim, Septra), 2 mg of the former component and 10 mg of the latter per kg orally once daily; or (3) methenamine mandelate (Mandelamine), 250 mg/30 lb/day orally in 4 doses. If methenamine mandelate is used, acidification of the urine to a pH below 5.5 with ascorbic acid is recommended.

B. General Measures: In gastroenteritis, early correction of metabolic acidosis and dehydration is indicated. The jaundice encountered in hemolytic *E coli* sepsis of the newborn often requires blood transfusion. Principles of importance in the management of urinary tract infection, in addition to specific treatment, include the following general measures: (1) diagnosis of existing mechanical defects by intravenous urography, voiding cystourethrography, cinefluoroscopy, and cystoscopy; (2) surgical correction of defects; (3) frequent culture after an initial infection to detect significant asymptomatic bacteriuria before the onset of repeated clinical illness (every 3 months for the first year, then every 6–12 months for an indefinite period); and (4) long-term suppressive therapy (for years) in cases not controlled by the means outlined above.

Prognosis

Gastroenteritis should no longer be of serious import provided general and specific therapy is given early. On the other hand, neonatal sepsis still carries a mortality rate of over 50%. As many as 20% of children with recurrent urinary tract infections may eventually succumb to the effects of the disease.

Donta ST & others: Enterotoxigenic *Escherichia coli* and diarrheal disease in Mexican children. J Infect Dis 135:482, 1977.

Echeverria P, Lew MA, Smith AL: Apparent emergence of aminoglycoside-resistant *Escherichia coli* during neonatal meningitis. N Engl J Med 293:913, 1975.

E. coli enteritis. (Editorial.) Lancet 2:1131, 1975.

Gangarosa EJ, Merson MH: Epidemiologic assessment of the relevance of the so-called enteropathogenic serogroups of *Escherichia coli* in diarrhea. N Engl J Med 296:1210, 1977.

Guerrant RL & others: Toxigenic bacterial diarrhea: Nursery outbreak involving multiple bacterial strains. J Pediatr 89:885, 1976.

Harle EMJ, Bullen JJ, Thomson DA: Influence of estrogen on experimental pyelonephritis caused by *Escherichia coli.* Lancet 2:283, 1975.

Jelliffe EFP, Overall JC Jr: Breast feeding and incidence of *E. coli* infections in newborn nurseries. J Pediatr 90:1038, 1977.

Marker SC, Blazevic DJ: Enteropathogenic serotypes of *E. coli.* J Pediatr 90:1037, 1977.

Merson MH & others: Travelers' diarrhea in Mexico: A prospective study of physicians and family members attending a congress. N Engl J Med 294:1299, 1976.

Neter E: Enteropathogenicity of *Escherichia coli.* (Editorial.) Am J Dis Child 129:666, 1975.

Rowe B, Scotland SM, Gross RJ: Enterotoxigenic *Escherichia coli* causing infantile enteritis in Britain. Lancet 1:90, 1977.

Sach DA & others: Diarrhea associated with heat-stable enterotoxin-producing strains of *Escherichia coli.* Lancet 2:239, 1975.

Sach RB: Enterotoxigenic *Escherichia coli:* An emerging pathogen. (Editorial.) N Engl J Med 295:893, 1976.

Speer ME & others: Fulminant neonatal sepsis and necrotizing enterocolitis associated with a "nonenteropathogenic" strain of *Escherichia coli.* J Pediatr 89:91, 1976.

PROTEUS & PSEUDOMONAS INFECTIONS

Essentials of Diagnosis

- Organisms tend to lodge in damaged or infected tissues in debilitated children.
- Occurs as a "superinfection" in patients treated for some other infection or receiving prophylactic chemotherapy.
- Positive cultures.

General Considerations

Members of the proteus and pseudomonas groups, although not hardily invasive, are becoming increasingly important as causes of infection in debilitated individuals or those receiving antibiotic therapy. Spread from local sites can occur in many locations, including the urinary and respiratory tracts, ears, mastoids, paranasal sinuses, eyes, and skin. Invasion of the meninges is occasionally seen. There is a tendency for infection to occur in debilitated patients or those with neoplastic disease or extensive burns. Pseudomonas can be isolated from the respiratory tract of a majority of patients with cystic fibrosis of the pancreas as the disease progresses. Pseudomonas produces a vasculitis affecting the media of small blood vessels which leads to infarction and gangrene. *Pseudomonas aeruginosa* sepsis may be accompanied by characteristic peripheral lesions called ecthyma gangrenosum. Previously thought rare, childhood osteomyelitis caused by *P aeruginosa* has resulted from puncture wounds of the feet. Difficulties in diagnosis and treatment are due mainly to the chronic nature of the infection and to the resistance of the organism to many antibiotics. Children with acute hematogenous osteomyelitis are typically quite ill. In contrast, osteomyelitis caused by pseudomonas presents insidiously, with few systemic effects. Melioidosis is an uncommon but serious infectious disease of tropical areas caused by *P pseudomallei*. Although many cases have been recognized in adults, the disease is not well recognized in children.

Nosocomial infections with *P aeruginosa* and *Proteus vulgaris* are spread by a variety of hospital equipment and solutions. Proteus is second only to *Escherichia coli* as a gram-negative rod associated with urinary tract infection.

Clinical Findings

The diagnosis is made by specific culture. Pseudomonas infection is frequently associated with a low white count and agranulocytosis.

Prevention

A. Debilitated Patients: Colonization of extensive second and third degree burns by pseudomonas can lead to fatal septicemias. Topical treatment with 0.5% silver nitrate solution, 10% mafenide (Sulfamylon) cream, or gentamicin ointment will greatly inhibit pseudomonas contamination of burns. Silver nitrate can lead to serious systemic depletion of sodium and chloride, so that children on silver nitrate therapy must have their serum electrolytes checked frequently. Mafenide (Sulfamylon) may cause pain, sensitization, and acidosis. Gentamicin is an excellent topical agent, but many centers discourage its topical use because of its potential for selecting out resistant organisms. Silver sulfadiazine is a drug that is as effective as any of the above. No matter what topical agents are used, the burns must be debrided frequently and kept clean or pseudomonas will colonize dead tissue beneath the eschar and invade the dermal vessels and lymphatics.

Pseudomonas vaccines show some potential for preventing infection in patients with severe burns, immunodeficiency, and cystic fibrosis and in those who are particularly susceptible to invasion by these bacteria as a result of the kinds of treatment methods used. Multivalent vaccines are needed for effective protection against a full range of serotypes found in hospitals. Such vaccines have been developed in the USA and in Great Britain, and some evidence of their clinical value in the treatment of severely burned patients has been reported. Patients with cystic fibrosis show good antibody response to vaccination. Leukemic patients show a smaller antibody response and more toxic effects of the vaccine. However, the toxic effects are reduced if vaccine is injected together with an adrenal corticosteroid.

B. Nosocomial Infections: Faucet aerators, communal dispensers of green soap, improperly cleaned inhalation therapy equipment, infant isolettes, and numerous back rub solutions and lotions have all been associated with pseudomonas epidemics. Constant vigilance and frequent cultures are essential in order to minimize spread of pseudomonas between patients.

Treatment

Susceptibility of clinical isolates of *P aeruginosa* and enteric gram-negative bacilli to amikacin and other aminoglycosides has been reported. At a concentration of 8 μg/ml, gentamicin inhibited 50% and tobramycin inhibited 67% of 200 isolates. At 16 μg/ml, amikacin inhibited 96.5% of 200 isolates; the respective figures for kanamycin and streptomycin were 28.5% and 24%. The virtual absence of cross-resistance between amikacin and gentamicin and between amikacin and the other 4 aminoglycosides was confirmed.

A. Proteus: Some strains of *Proteus mirabilis* are relatively susceptible to penicillin V or to ampicillin, 100—300 mg/kg/day orally in 4 divided doses. Other strains are susceptible to the cephalosporins and kanamycin. Gentamicin, 5—7.5 mg/kg/day IM in 3 divided doses, is quite effective. Carbenicillin is a semisynthetic penicillin which is active against indolepositive proteus and appears to be quite useful clinically, especially for urinary tract infections. The dose is 50—200 mg/kg/day IV or IM in 4 divided doses. Carbenicillin indanyl sodium is a new oral form useful for urinary tract infections.

B. Pseudomonas: Gentamicin, 5—7.5 mg/kg/day in 3 divided doses IM or IV (1-hour infusion), and carbenicillin, 250—400 mg/kg/day in 6 divided doses IV, singly or together (with synergy), have become the standard agents for use in serious pseudomonas infections. Treatment should be continued for 10—14 days.

With pseudomonas meningitis, parenteral therapy should be supplemented by daily intrathecal or intraventricular administrations of 1—2 mg gentamicin for 5 days. Parenteral treatment should be continued for 3 weeks.

The greatest chances for cure of pseudomonas osteomyelitis are with combined surgical and antibiotic treatment. The erythrocyte sedimentation rate is the best clinical indication of an effective cure. Antibiotic therapy must be continued until the sedimentation rate has returned to normal; this usually takes about 4 weeks. A 6-week course of antibiotics would seem to provide an ample safety margin and ensure a successful outcome.

Solutions for nebulizer inhalation should contain 2–10 mg of polymyxin B per ml. The dose for inhalation is 2 ml 4 or more times per day. For local therapy, polymyxin B, 0.1% solution or ointment, may be useful. Gentamicin may also be used as an ointment.

The treatment of melioidosis is often difficult; fatality rates as high as 95% are not uncommon with the acute fulminant form of the disease. The current antibiotics of choice are tetracycline and chloramphenicol, but antibiotic sensitivity tests should be performed on all isolates.

Prognosis

Because debilitated patients are most frequently affected, the mortality rate is high. The disease may, however, have a protracted course.

Amirak ID & others: Amikacin resistance developing in patient with *Pseudomonas aeruginosa* bronchopneumonia. Lancet 1:537, 1977.

Brown DA, Calcaterra TC: Pseudomonas meningitis complicating head and neck surgery. Laryngoscope 86:1386, 1976.

Laraya-Cuasay LR, Cundy KR, Huang NN: Pseudomonas carrier rates of patients with cystic fibrosis and of members of their families. J Pediatr 89:23, 1976.

Meyer RD & others: Gentamicin-resistant *Pseudomonas aeruginosa* and *Serratia marcescens* in a general hospital. Lancet 1:580, 1976.

Pattamasukon P, Pichyangkura C, Fischer GW: Melioidosis in childhood. J Pediatr 87:133, 1975.

Pseudomonas vaccines. (Editorial.) Lancet 2:168, 1975.

Rapkin RH: *Pseudomonas cepacia* in an intensive care nursery. Pediatrics 57:239, 1976.

Reed RK & others: Peripheral nodular lesions in pseudomonas sepsis: The importance of incision and drainage. J Pediatr 88:977, 1976.

Reynolds HY, Di Sant'Agnese PA, Zierdt CH: Mucoid *Pseudomonas aeruginosa:* A sign of cystic fibrosis in young adults with chronic pulmonary disease? JAMA 236:2190, 1976.

KLEBSIELLA-ENTEROBACTER INFECTIONS

General Considerations

The klebsiella-enterobacter organisms are encapsulated gram-negative bacilli found among the normal flora of the mouth, respiratory tract, and intestines. For historical reasons, organisms isolated from the respiratory tract have been called klebsiella and those from the genitourinary tract aerobacter (enterobacter). One-fourth to one-third of children with acute urinary tract infections have a recurrence of the infection within a year. Enterobacter is a common urinary tract pathogen and is more likely to be a cause of recurrent or chronic infections. Klebsiella causes a progressive, serious (sometimes fatal) bronchopneumonia which may lead to cavity formation. The organism is a

secondary invader associated with antibiotic usage, debilitating states, and chronic respiratory conditions. Rare nursery outbreaks have occurred. Nosocomial colonization with kanamycin-resistant *Klebsiella pneumoniae* in nurseries is becoming an increasing problem.

Necrotizing enterocolitis (NEC) in newborns is suspected on the basis of abdominal distention and ileus. Guaiac-positive or bloody stools are common. Other clinical findings, such as peritonitis or perforation, shock, and disseminated intravascular coagulation, are present in patients with extensive involvement. The diagnosis of NEC is confirmed radiologically on the basis of pneumatosis intestinalis and adynamic ileus. When NEC occurs, stool cultures reveal a significantly increased frequency of klebsiella as compared to findings in control patients. Other data suggest that the combined presence of certain intestinal bacteria and enteric feedings, perhaps requiring a background of mucosal ischemia, may be significant in causing the development of NEC and its radiologic hallmark, pneumatosis intestinalis.

Clinical Findings

A. Symptoms and Signs: *K pneumoniae* rapidly forms abscesses or empyema. The onset is usually sudden, with chills, fever, dyspnea, cyanosis, and profound toxicity. The sputum is often red ("currant jelly"), mucoid, sticky, and difficult to expectorate. Physical findings and white counts are variable. The disease may be fulminating and progress rapidly to a fatal outcome. In subacute forms, there is a tendency to necrosis of lung tissue and abscess formation. Lobar consolidation with bulging fissures is seen on x-ray.

B. Laboratory Findings: The diagnosis is established by culture of the sputum, pleural fluid, or blood and urine.

Differential Diagnosis

Staphylococcal pneumonia in the first 2 years of life is many times more common as a cause of pneumatoceles, cavity formation, and empyema.

Treatment

A. Specific Measures: Many of these infections are difficult to treat, and antibiotic sensitivity tests are desirable. At present, cephalothin, 75–100 mg/kg/day IV or IM in 4 divided doses, is the drug of choice for a *K pneumoniae* superinfection in the newborn. Treatment should be continued for 7–10 days. In older children, doses of 100–200 mg/kg/day IV may be used for serious infections. Other effective antibiotics include gentamicin, polymyxin B, colistin, kanamycin, cephaloridine, and cephalexin (oral preparation). Despite the historical aspects of nomenclature, the majority of isolates from the urinary tract are nonmotile and belong to the Klebsiella genus. These latter organisms causing acute infections are susceptible to oral cephalexin given as 25 mg/kg/day in 3 divided doses for 14–21 days. However, isolates classed as Enterobacter species are usually motile and are resistant to cephalexin.

Recurrent urinary tract infections should be treated for 6 weeks to 3 months before stopping an effective antibiotic. (See under *E coli* infections for management of urinary tract infections.) Combinations of chloramphenicol or streptomycin and tetracyclines have also been used successfully.

B. General Measures: Causes of urinary tract obstruction should be investigated and surgically corrected. Oxygen and supportive therapy are required for klebsiella pneumonia. Intercostal tube drainage connected to a water seal is needed to manage empyema.

Prognosis

Klebsiella is usually a secondary invader, and, in the respiratory tract, progresses rapidly, causing abscesses, empyema, and necrosis. The mortality rate in untreated cases is upward of 80%. With vigorous, adequate treatment, this may be reduced to 40%.

Frants ID III & others: Necrotizing enterocolitis. J Pediatr 86:259, 1975.

Guerrant RL & others: Toxigenic bacterial diarrhea: Nursery outbreak involving multiple bacterial strains. J Pediatr 89:885, 1976.

Hamory B, Ignatiadis P, Sande MA: Intrathecal amikacin administration: Use in the treatment of gentamicin-resistant *Klebsiella pneumoniae* meningitis. JAMA 236:1973, 1976.

SALMONELLA & GASTROENTERITIS & MENINGITIS

Essentials of Diagnosis

- Nausea, vomiting, headache.
- Fever and diarrhea.
- Abdominal pain.
- Meningismus.
- Culture of organism from stool, blood, or other specimens.

General Considerations

The genus Salmonella comprises more than 1400 serotypes. The more important serotypes in human disease—exclusive of *Salmonella typhi* and *S cholerae-suis*—are *S enteritidis* bioserotypes: *S typhimurium, S montevideo, S newport, S oranienburg, S schottmül-leri, S bareilly,* and *S derby. S typhimurium* has been the most frequently isolated serotype in most parts of the world.

Salmonella organisms are motile and are therefore able to penetrate the mucin layer of the small bowel and attach to epithelial cells. Some plasmid-containing salmonella organisms can produce a toxigenic component of the diarrhea. Organisms penetrate beneath the epithelial surface and localize there, causing fever, vomiting, watery diarrhea, and occasionally mucus with some polymorphonuclear leukocytes in the stool. Although the small intestine is generally regarded as the principal site of human salmonella infection of the food poisoning type, studies have demonstrated the presence of active colitis. *S typhimurium* frequently involves the large bowel. It has been suggested that colonic involvement is common in human salmonellosis and probably plays an important role in causing the diarrhea.

Salmonella enteral infections in childhood occur in 2 major forms: (1) gastroenteritis (including food poisoning), which may be very mild or severe and complicated by sepsis with or without focal suppurative complications; and (2) enteric fever (typhoid fever and paratyphoid fever). (See next section.) While the incidence of typhoid fever has decreased, the incidence of salmonella gastroenteritis caused by a variety of strains has greatly increased in the past 15 years in the USA. The highest attack rates occur in children under 6 years of age, with a peak in the age group from 6 months to 2 years old. Nursery epidemics have occurred, and infants under 6 months of age are susceptible.

The organisms are widespread in nature, infecting domestic animals (pets, including pet turtles, and fowl), rodents, and arthropods. Most nonhuman isolations of salmonellae are from poultry. Contaminated egg powder and frozen whole egg preparations used to make ice cream, custards, and mayonnaise are often responsible for outbreaks. Animal-to-human transmission occurs by ingestion of animal excreta, infected animal meat, and animal products. Transmission from human to human occurs by the fecal-oral route via contaminated food, water, and fomites.

Most cases of salmonella meningitis (80%) have occurred in infancy. About 25% of cases have occurred in nursery epidemics. In newborns, meningitis tends to run a rapid course, with diarrhea as a prominent manifestation.

Clinical Findings

A. Symptoms and Signs: The infant develops fever, vomiting, and diarrhea. The older child may complain of headache, nausea, and abdominal pain. Stools may be watery or may contain mucus and in some instances blood. Diarrhea may be mild to moderate, or profuse, suggestive of shigellosis. Drowsiness and disorientation may be associated with striking meningismus. Splenomegaly is occasionally noted. In the usual case, diarrhea is moderate and subsides after 4–5 days, but it may be protracted.

B. Laboratory Diagnosis: Diagnosis is made by isolation of the organism from the stools and blood and in some cases from the urine, CSF, or pus from a suppurative lesion. The white count usually shows a polymorphonuclear leukocytosis. Typing of the isolate is done with specific antisera.

Differential Diagnosis

In staphylococcal food poisoning, the incubation period is shorter (2–4 hours) than in salmonella food poisoning (12–24 hours). In shigellosis, pus cells are likely to be seen on a Wright-stained smear of stool, and there is more likely to be a shift to the left in the peripheral white count. In shigellosis as well as in enteropathogenic *E coli* enteritis and other diarrheal diseases, culture of the stools or other appropriate diagnostic laboratory tests will establish the diagnosis. Meningitis may need to be excluded by lumbar puncture.

Complications

Bacteremia can occur. Septicemia with focal manifestations occurs most commonly with *S choleraesuis* but also with *S enteritidis, S typhimurium,* and *S paratyphi* B and C. The organism may localize in any tissue, producing abscesses and causing arthritis, osteomyelitis, cholecystitis, endocarditis, meningitis, pericarditis, pneumonia, and pyelonephritis. In sickle cell anemia and other hemoglobinopathies, there is an unusual predilection for osteomyelitis to develop. Severe dehydration and shock are more likely to occur with bacillary dysentery but may occur with salmonella gastroenteritis.

Prevention

Measures for the prevention of salmonella infections include thorough cooking of foodstuffs derived from potentially infected sources; proper refrigeration during storage; and recognition and control of infection among domestic animals, combined with proper meat and poultry inspections. Adults with occupations involving care of young children should have negative stool cultures for 3 successive days.

Patients traveling to an endemic area should be vaccinated.

Treatment

A. Specific Measures: In the usual case of uncomplicated salmonella gastroenteritis not associated with sepsis, there is no evidence that antibiotic treatment shortens the course of the clinical illness or the length of time the organism is present in the gastrointestinal tract. In fact, there is evidence that antibiotic treatment prolongs the carrier state.

However, in order to prevent sepsis and focal disease, antibiotic treatment is indicated for newborns, for moderately or severely ill young infants, and for children with sickle cell disease, liver disease, recent gastrointestinal surgery, cancer, depressed immunity, and chronic renal and cardiac disease. Ampicillin, 100–150 mg/kg/day IM in 4 divided doses for 4–5 days, is recommended. Amoxicillin, 50 mg/kg/day orally in 3 divided doses, may also be effective. Patients developing bacteremia during the course of gastroenteritis should be given parenteral ampicillin for 7–10 days. Longer treatment is indicated for specific complications. If clinical improvement does not follow and in vitro sensitivity tests indicate resistance to ampicillin, chloramphenicol should be given, 100 mg/kg/day IV or orally in 4 divided doses.

Salmonella meningitis is best treated with both chloramphenicol, 100 mg/kg/day IV, and ampicillin, 200–300 mg/kg/day IV, each given in 4 divided doses.

Chloramphenicol should be given for 2–3 weeks; ampicillin for 4–6 weeks. An average CSF killing level of 1:4–1:8 should be maintained. Selection of a multiple antibiotic-resistant strain is less likely to occur if both antibiotics are used to treat this serious disease.

Nursery or hospital epidemics. An outbreak may be stopped by treating hospitalized asymptomatic contacts with colistin, 10 mg/kg/day orally in 3 divided doses, until they can be discharged. Excretion of the organism in the stools will stop while the infants are taking oral colistin. The carrier state will occur as soon as the colistin is stopped. Sick infants should be treated with ampicillin as outlined above to prevent bacteremia and suppurative complications. They should then be treated with oral colistin until discharge from the hospital.

B. Treatment of the Carrier States: About half of patients are still infectious after 4 weeks. During the first year of life, particularly under 6 months, there is a greater tendency to remain a convalescent carrier. Antibiotic treatment of carriers is not indicated.

C. General: Careful attention must be given to maintaining fluid and electrolyte balance, especially in infants. Severe dehydration must be vigorously treated as outlined in the section on bacillary dysentery.

Prognosis

In gastroenteritis, the prognosis is good if adequate measures are used to control diarrhea. In sepsis with focal suppurative complications, the prognosis is more guarded.

The case fatality rate for salmonella meningitis is about 85% in infants. There is a strong tendency for relapse to occur if treatment is not prolonged.

Anderson ES: The problem and implications of chloramphenicol resistance in the typhoid bacillus. J Hyg (Camb) 74:289, 1975.

Appelbaum PC, Scragg J: Salmonella meningitis in infants. Lancet 1:1052, 1977.

Cherubin CE & others: Emergence of resistance to chloramphenicol in salmonella. J Infect Dis 135:807, 1977.

Gilman RH & others: Relative efficacy of blood, urine, rectal swab, bone-marrow, and rose-spot cultures for recovery of *Salmonella typhi* in typhoid fever. Lancet 1:1211, 1975.

Grant RB, Bannatyne RM, Shapley AJ: Resistance to chloramphenicol and ampicillin of *Salmonella typhimurium* in Ontario, Canada. J Infect Dis 134:354, 1976.

Ryder RW & others: Salmonellosis in the United States, 1968–1974. J Infect Dis 133:483, 1976.

Vaisrub S: Tracking down *Salmonella typhi.* (Editorial.) JAMA 233:1196, 1975.

TYPHOID FEVER & PARATYPHOID FEVER

Essentials of Diagnosis

- Acute onset of headache, anorexia, vomiting, constipation or diarrhea, dehydration, and fairly high fever.

- Meningismus, splenomegaly, and rose spots with abdominal distention and tenderness.
- Leukopenia; positive blood, stool, and urine cultures.
- Elevated Widal agglutination titers.

General Considerations

Typhoid fever is caused by the gram-negative rod *Salmonella typhi;* paratyphoid fevers, which may be clinically indistinguishable, may be caused by a variety of strains but most frequently by *S paratyphi* A, B, and C. Children have a shorter incubation period than do adults (usually 5–8 days instead of 8–14 days). Symptoms of typhoid fever in children may vary from the mildest to the most severe, but in general, except for the very young, the disease is milder than in adults. The organism enters the body through the walls of the intestinal tract and multiplies in the reticuloendothelial cells of the liver and spleen. Reinfection of the intestinal tract occurs as organisms are excreted from the biliary tract. The onset of disease depends upon when a sufficient number of *S typhi* reach the blood stream and mesenteric lymph nodes. Symptoms appear to be due to the systemic effects of endotoxin and other bacterial products. Bacterial emboli in the capillaries of the skin produce the characteristic skin lesions.

In 1972 and 1973, a nationwide outbreak of typhoid fever occurred in Mexico. Isolates of *S typhi* resistant to chloramphenicol in vitro were common in the Mexican epidemic, and this antibiotic was clinically ineffective against typhoid fever caused by the resistant strain. Recently, resistance to chloramphenicol in *S typhi* has also been reported in Chile, France, India, Indonesia, Thailand, and Vietnam. The appearance in Mexico of strains of *S typhi* resistant to both chloramphenicol and ampicillin was also documented.

Clinical trials with amoxicillin have revealed a greater efficacy for this drug than for ampicillin when the isolate is ampicillin-sensitive. Oral administration of trimethoprim-sulfamethoxazole is effective therapy for chloramphenicol-resistant strains and probably for ampicillin-resistant and amoxicillin-resistant strains as well.

An association between glucose-6-phosphate dehydrogenase deficiency and typhoid fever has been observed.

Clinical Findings

A. Symptoms and Signs: In children, the onset is apt to be sudden rather than insidious, with malaise, headache, crampy abdominal pains and distention, and sometimes constipation followed within 48 hours by diarrhea, high fever, and considerable toxemia. Disturbances of the sensorium may be seen with irritability, confusion, delirium, and stupor. Vomiting and meningismus may be prominent in the young. The classic 3-stage disease seen in adult patients seems to be shortened in children. Thus, the prodrome may be shortened to only 2–4 days, whereas the fastigium, which is characterized by fever, diarrhea, and abdominal distention and mild to marked toxemia,

may last only 2–3 days. The defervescence stage generally lasts 1–2 weeks. Relapse may occur 1–2 weeks after the temperature returns to normal.

During the prodromal stage, physical findings may be absent or there may merely be some abdominal distention and tenderness, meningismus, and minimal splenomegaly. The typical typhoidal rash (rose spots) tends to appear during the second week of the disease, and may erupt in crops for the succeeding 10–14 days. Rose spots are pink papules 2–3 mm in diameter which fade on pressure, are found principally on the trunk and chest, and generally disappear within 3–4 days.

B. Laboratory Findings: During active clinical infections, typhoid organisms can be isolated from many sites, including blood, stool, and urine. Organisms are also present in the spleen, bone marrow, gallbladder, and lymphatics. Organisms are also frequently isolated from blood during the initial 7–10 days of the clinical syndrome. Later, cultures of urine and stool become positive. The majority of patients will have negative stool cultures by the end of a 6-week period. Two antigens (Widal test) are used for the diagnosis of typhoid fever: the H (flagellar) antigen and the O (somatic) antigen. A low H antigen titer and a rise in titer against O antigen in serum samples drawn 1 week apart or a single specimen showing an O titer of 1:160 usually represents acute infection with *S typhi* or occasionally with another member of this salmonella group. A third antigen, Vi, is present almost exclusively in the blood of typhoid carriers; the O and particularly the H antibodies are frequently low in titer or absent in such patients.

Leukopenia is commonly encountered in the second week of the disease. However, total leukocyte counts above 10,000 are not unusual. Urinalysis generally reveals 1+ or 2+ protein. Mild anemia may be present unless massive bleeding occurs (see Complications, below). Disseminated intravascular coagulation has been reported in association with typhoid fever.

Elevated sedimentation rates and the presence of C-reactive proteins are seen during the febrile period.

Differential Diagnosis

Typhoid and paratyphoid fevers must be distinguished from other serious prolonged fevers associated with normal or low white counts. These include typhus, primary atypical pneumonia, brucellosis, tularemia, miliary tuberculosis, psittacosis, and lymphomas.

A positive diagnosis of typhoid fever is made by laboratory means.

Complications

The most important complication of typhoid fever is hemorrhage from the gastrointestinal tract. This generally occurs toward the end of the second week or during the third week of the disease. The clinical signs and symptoms are those of acute blood loss, including the appearance of gross blood in the stools and early evidence of shock. Epistaxis is the most common type of hemorrhage.

Intestinal perforation is a dangerous complication and one of the principal causes of death. The sites of perforation generally are the terminal ileum or the proximal part of the colon. The clinical manifestations are indistinguishable from those of acute appendicitis, with pain, tenderness, and rigidity in the right lower quadrant. The x-ray finding of free air in the peritoneal cavity is diagnostic.

Bacterial pneumonia, meningitis, septic arthritis, and osteomyelitis are uncommon complications, particularly if specific treatment is given promptly. Cardiovascular collapse and electrolyte disturbances may lead to death. Occasionally there are metastatic abscesses. Hepatic involvement with jaundice occurs occasionally. Acute cholecystitis associated with gallstones is rare. Infection of the urinary tract occurs in about 25% of cases.

Prevention

Paratyphoid A and B vaccines or triple vaccines should no longer be employed. Routine typhoid immunization is not recommended in the USA. Selective typhoid fever immunization is indicated in the following circumstances: (1) Intimate exposure to a known typhoid carrier, as would occur with continued household contact. (2) Community or institutional outbreaks of typhoid fever. (3) Foreign travel to areas where typhoid fever is endemic. There are no data to warrant continuing the practice of typhoid vaccination for persons attending summer camps or where flooding has occurred.

A. Primary Immunization: Children 6 months to 10 years, 0.25 ml subcutaneously on 2 occasions separated by 4 or more weeks; adults and children over 10 years, 0.5 ml subcut on 2 occasions separated by 4 or more weeks.

B. Booster: Under conditions of continued or repeated exposure, a booster dose should be given every 3 years. Even if more than 3 years have elapsed, a single booster injection should be sufficient. The booster dose, regardless of age, is 0.1 ml intradermally.

Treatment

A. Specific Measures: Chloramphenicol is the drug of choice in typhoid fever. Ampicillin is much less effective. The dosage of chloramphenicol is 50–100 mg/kg/day orally in 4 divided doses. For infants under 1 month of age, the daily dose should not exceed 25 mg/kg. Oral therapy is preferable to systemic therapy. Where vomiting is a problem, it is well to supplement parenteral therapy with oral medication as soon as possible. Occasionally, drug administration through a gastric tube is required. Chloramphenicol palmitate, while well tolerated, is not advised because of the irregular absorption of this lipase-dependent compound. A suspension of the crystalline form from the capsule is preferred. In patients unable to take oral medication, the succinate ester may be given intravenously as a 10% solution; it is given slowly over at least 1 minute or incorporated into intravenous fluids such as isotonic saline or 5% dextrose.

If chloramphenicol therapy is contraindicated (hematologic disorders, anemia, etc), give parenteral ampicillin in doses of 150 mg/kg stat followed by 150 mg/kg/day in 4 divided doses. Treatment should be continued for 14–21 days. Fever usually returns to normal within 3–5 days.

Amoxicillin, 100 mg/kg/day orally in 3 divided doses, has been shown to be effective. As noted above, strains of *S typhi* resistant to both chloramphenicol and ampicillin have been introduced into the USA; trimethoprim-sulfamethoxazole (Bactrim, Septra) can be effective in the treatment of these resistant strains. The dosage is 10 mg of the former and 50 mg of the latter per kg per day orally in 2 divided doses.

B. General Measures: If toxicity is marked, a short course of corticosteroids may be indicated when antibiotics are begun. Prednisone, 1 mg/kg/day orally during the first 4 days of chloramphenicol therapy, generally results in marked improvement of the patient's condition.

General support of the patient is exceedingly important and includes rest, good oral hygiene, and careful observation with particular regard to evidence of internal bleeding or perforation. A high-caloric liquid diet should provide ample calories and at least 2 gm of protein per kg body weight. Potassium depletion should be corrected. Small transfusions with whole blood may be needed in the anemic patient even in the absence of frank hemorrhage.

Prognosis

A convalescent carrier stage in children often continues for 3–6 months after the acute infection. This does not require retreatment with antibiotics nor exclusion from school or other activities.

With specific antibiotic therapy, the prognosis is excellent.

Anderson ES: The problem and implications of chloramphenicol resistance in the typhoid bacillus. J Hyg (Camb) 74:289, 1975.

Baine WB & others: Typhoid fever in the United States associated with the 1972–1973 epidemic in Mexico. J Infect Dis 135:649, 1977.

Clarke PD, Geddes AM: Drugs for typhoid fever. Lancet 1:545, 1977.

Colon AR, Gross DR, Tamer MA: Typhoid fever in children. Pediatrics 56:606, 1975.

Scragg JN, Rubidge CJ: Amoxicillin in treatment of typhoid fever in children. Am J Trop Med Hyg 24:860, 1975.

BACILLARY (SHIGELLA) DYSENTERY

Essentials of Diagnosis

- Cramps and bloody diarrhea.
- High fever, malaise, clouded sensorium, convulsions.
- Pus and mucus in diarrheal stools; isolation of shigella strain.

General Considerations

Shigellosis is a serious disease of children under 2 years of age with an appreciable mortality rate. Because of the variability of antibiotic sensitivity for strains of shigella now encountered, it remains an important therapeutic problem. In older children, the disease tends to be self-limited and milder.

The genus Shigella is divided into 4 major groups: *Shigella dysenteriae, S flexneri, S boydii,* and *S sonnei.* In turn, the *S dysenteriae* group comprises 7 members, the *S flexneri* group, 12 members, and the *S boydii,* 7 members. A sharp upswing in isolations of *S sonnei* has occurred nationwide, with a shift to predominance of *S sonnei* over *S flexneri.*

Although shigellosis occurs in individuals of all ages, for unexplained reasons it is rare in infants under 3 months of age. However, on rare occasions, shigellae may be transmitted from the mother to the newborn infant during delivery. Shigellosis during the neonatal period often differs from the disease in older children. Diarrhea and refusal to take feedings are the most common symptoms. Bloody diarrhea and fever occur less frequently. Vomiting, convulsions, or high fever is almost never encountered. Shigellosis can be contracted by swimming in polluted water.

S dysenteriae accounts for less than 1% of all shigella infections in the United States. It causes the most severe diarrhea of all species and the greatest number of extraintestinal complications.

Clinical Findings

A. Symptoms and Signs: Onset is abrupt, with abdominal cramps, tenesmus, chills and fever, malaise, diarrhea, and often a cloudy sensorium suggesting encephalitis. In the most severe forms, blood and mucus are seen in the watery stool and convulsions may occur. In older children, the disease may be mild and the diagnosis therefore missed. In young children, a fever of 39.4–40° C (103–104° F) is common.

Respiratory symptoms of bronchitis are common. The anal sphincter shows lax tone. Rarely, there is rectal prolapse. In over 50% of cases, other family members will also have diarrhea.

B. Laboratory Findings: The white count is high, with a shift to the left. The appearance of more band forms than segmented neutrophils in the differential smear may be an important diagnostic clue. The stool shows blood, mucus, and pus and a positive culture for shigella. Hemoconcentration with a marked elevation in hematocrit is common shortly after onset.

Differential Diagnosis

Diarrhea due to echovirus infections tends to be seen in the summer months in outbreaks. Intestinal infections caused by salmonellae and enteropathogenic *Escherichia coli* are differentiated by culture. Amebic dysentery is diagnosed by microscopic examination of fresh stools; intussusception by an abdominal mass, currant jelly stools, and absence of fever. Epidemic outbreak and an incubation period of 6 hours or less characterize staphylococcal food poisoning.

Complications

Dehydration, acidosis, and shock occur in infancy. In some cases, a chronic form of dysentery occurs, characterized by mucoid stools and poor nutrition. Otitis media, pneumonia, and nonsuppurative arthritis are occasional complications.

Treatment

A. Specific Measures: Ampicillin is the antibiotic of choice and is given IV, IM, or orally in a dosage of 100 mg/kg/day in 4 divided doses for 5 days. With this drug there will be a 50% reduction in duration of fever and diarrhea and in fecal excretion of shigella. Therapeutic failure with ampicillin correlates closely with in vitro resistance. Tetracycline, 25 mg/kg/day orally in 4 divided doses, may be effective. If the strain is sensitive in vitro, chloramphenicol may be used in a dosage of 100 mg/kg/day orally in 4 divided doses. Sulfonamides are as effective as ampicillin if the organism is susceptible, but most strains are resistant. For multiply resistant strains, give nalidixic acid, 55 mg/kg/day orally in 4 divided doses, or trimethoprim-sulfamethoxazole (Bactrim, Septra), 10 mg of the former and 50 mg of the latter per kg per day orally in 2 divided doses.

B. General Measures: In severe cases, immediate rehydration by means of saline, glucose, and potassium is an emergency procedure, generally requiring a cutdown in a suitable vein. To combat circulatory collapse and shock, special nursing observation is required.

In milder cases, after initial rehydration with parenteral fluids, clear liquids may be required for 2 or 3 days followed by glucose-containing liquids such as grape juice, apple juice, liquid Jell-O, or ginger ale. Subsequently, boiled skimmed milk or any 12 kcal/oz formula may be introduced, followed by return to a regular light diet somewhat low in fat.

A mild form of chronic malabsorption syndrome may supervene and require prolonged dietary control.

Prognosis

Except in the very young patient with septicemia, the prognosis is excellent if ampicillin is given early and vascular collapse is treated promptly by adequate fluid therapy.

Caceres A, Mata LJ: Serologic response of patients with Shiga dysentery. J Infect Dis 129:439, 1974.

Chang MJ & others: Trimethoprim-sulfamethoxazole compared to ampicillin in the treatment of shigellosis. Pediatrics 59:726, 1977.

Davis TC: Chronic vulvovaginitis in children due to *Shigella flexneri.* Pediatrics 56:41, 1975.

Farrar WE Jr, Eidson M, Wells JG: Extensive urban outbreak caused by antibiotic-sensitive *Shigella sonnei.* JAMA 235:1026, 1976.

Keusch GT, Jacewicz M: The pathogenesis of shigella diarrhea. 5. Relationship of Shiga enterotoxin, neurotoxin, and cytotoxin. J Infect Dis 131 (Suppl):S33, 1975.

Levine MM & others: Shigellosis in custodial institutions. 4. In vivo stability and transmissibility of oral attenuated streptomycin-dependent shigella vaccines. J Infect Dis 131:704, 1975.

Nelson JD, Haltalin KC: Amoxicillin less effective than ampicillin against shigella in vitro and in vivo: Relationship of efficacy to activity in serum. J Infect Dis 129 (Suppl):S222, 1974.

Nelson JD & others: Trimethoprim-sulfamethoxazole therapy for shigellosis. JAMA 235:1239, 1976.

Panaranda ME, Mata LJ: Transfer of ampicillin resistance from *Shigella dysenteriae* type 1 to *Escherichia coli.* Lancet 2:154, 1976.

Rahaman MM, Huq I, Dey CR: Superiority of MacConkey's agar over salmonella-shigella agar for isolation of *Shigella dysenteriae* type 1. J Infect Dis 131:700, 1975.

Torrence MB & others: Ampicillin-resistant shigella. JAMA 226:1359, 1973.

Weissman JB & others: Impact in the United States of the Shiga dysentery pandemic of Central America and Mexico: A review of surveillance data through 1972. J Infect Dis 129:218, 1974.

Weissman JB & others: Shigellosis in day-care centres. Lancet 1:88, 1975.

Weissman JB & others: The role of preschool children and day-care centers in the spread of shigellosis in urban communities. J Pediatr 84:797, 1974.

CHOLERA

Essentials of Diagnosis

- Sudden onset of very severe diarrhea.
- Persistent vomiting without nausea.
- Extreme and rapid dehydration and electrolyte loss, with rapid development of vascular collapse.
- Contact with a case of cholera and the presence of a cholera epidemic in the community.
- Positive smears and culture.

General Considerations

Cholera is an acute diarrheal disease caused by *Vibrio cholerae* and transmitted by contaminated water or food in the endemic areas of the world. The incubation period is very short, 1–3 days, and the disease is generally so dramatic that in a frank case the diagnosis is obvious. Chronic carriers of *V cholerae* are rare. Mild cases are important causes of infection in others. Young children may play an important role in transmission of the infection. Higher titers of vibriocidal antibody are seen with increasing age. Infection occurs in individuals with low titers. The age-specific attack rate is highest in the age group under 5 years and declines with age. Sanitation and personal hygiene may prevent cholera in areas where the vibrios persist in the environment. A protein enterotoxin produced by *V cholerae* has been shown to be highly active in inducing experimental cholera in animals. The toxin is only active in the small bowel. The motility of *V cholerae* enables the organism to penetrate the mucosa of the small bowel.

Nutritional status is a determining factor in the severity of the diarrhea in patients with cholera. Duration of diarrhea, but not volume of stool per hour, has been prolonged by 30–70% in those adults and children suffering from severe malnutrition.

Clinical Findings

A. Symptoms and Signs: Sudden onset of massive, frequent, watery stools, generally light gray in color ("rice water") and containing some mucus but no pus. Vomiting may be projectile and is not accompanied by nausea. Within 2–3 hours, the tremendous loss of fluids has resulted in severe and life-threatening dehydration, hypochloremia, and loss of cellular potassium, with marked weakness and collapse. This is a medical emergency. Renal failure with uremia and irreversible peripheral vascular collapse will occur if fluid therapy is not administered.

B. Laboratory Findings: Markedly elevated hemoglobin (20 gm/100 ml), marked acidosis, hypochloremia, and hyponatremia are seen.

Using darkfield microscopy and Ogawa/Inaba specific antisera, a presumptive diagnosis can be made within a matter of minutes. This is based on the immobilization by specific antisera of the highly motile cholera vibrios. In the absence of such facilities, confirmation of a clinical diagnosis will take 16–18 hours for a presumptive diagnosis and 36–48 hours for a definitive bacteriologic diagnosis after the arrival of a specimen of stool or rectal swab at the laboratory.

Prevention

Cholera vaccine is given as 2 injections, 0.5 ml subcut, not less than 4 weeks apart, with boosters of 0.5 ml every 6 months while at risk. In endemic areas, all water and milk must be boiled, food protected from flies, and rigid sanitary precautions observed. All patients with cholera should be strictly isolated and their surroundings carefully decontaminated.

Chemoprophylaxis is indicated for household and other close contacts of cholera patients. Drug administration should be initiated as soon as possible after the onset of the disease in the index patient. One of the tetracyclines given as a single daily dose of 500 mg for 5 days is effective in preventing subsequent infection in children.

Treatment

Physiologic saline must be administered at once in large amounts to restore blood volume and urine output and to prevent irreversible shock. Potassium supplements are required. Sodium bicarbonate, 2–4% solution given intravenously, may also be needed initially to overcome profound acidosis. In general, children need more potassium and less sodium replacement than adults. Some hypotonic fluids should also be given intravenously in order to replace water lost in excess of electrolytes.

Recent reports indicate that moderate dehydration and severe acidosis can be corrected in 3–6 hours by oral therapy alone. Give 1000 ml/hour of warmed (45°C) oral solution during a 6-hour period. The composition of the solution (in mEq/liter) is as follows:

Na$^+$, 120, HCO$_3^-$, 48, Cl$^-$, 87, and K$^+$, 25—together with 110 mM glucose per liter. Intravenous fluids should be given initially in cases with frank shock.

Treatment of children with one of the tetracyclines, 25 mg/kg/day orally in 4 divided doses for 5 days, modifies the clinical course of the disease and prevents clinical relapse.

Prognosis

With early and rapid replacement of fluids and electrolytes lost through the massive diarrhea, the case fatality rate should be less than 1%. If significant symptoms appear and no treatment is given, the mortality rate is over 50%.

Berkenbile F, Delaney R: Stimulation of adenylate cyclase by *Vibrio cholerae* toxin and its active subunit. J Infect Dis 133 (Suppl):S82, 1976.

Cholera worldwide. Morbid Mortal Wkly Rep 26:201, June 24, 1977.

Holmgren J, Lonnroth I: Cholera toxin and the adenylate cyclase-activating signal. J Infect Dis 133 (Suppl):S64, 1976.

Levine RJ & others: Cholera transmission near a cholera hospital. Lancet 2:84, 1976.

Levine RJ & others: Failure of sanitary wells to protect against cholera and other diarrheas in Bangladesh. Lancet 2:86, 1976.

Mekalanos JJ, Collier RJ, Romig WR: Simple method for purifying choleragenoid, the natural toxoid of *Vibrio cholerae*. Infect Immun 16:789, 1977.

Minneman KP, Iversen LL: Cholera toxin induces pineal enzymes in culture. Science 192:803, 1976.

Nalin DR: Failure of aspirin to reverse intestinal secretion after cholera toxin in dogs. Lancet 2:576, 1976.

Palmer DL & others: Nutritional status: A determinant of severity of diarrhea in patients with cholera. J Infect Dis 134:8, 1976.

Pierce NG, Sack RB, Sircar BK: Immunity to experimental cholera. 3. Enhanced duration of protection after sequential parenteral-oral administration of toxoid to dogs. J Infect Dis 135:888, 1977.

Wishnow RM, Lifrak E, Chen CC: Mode of action of *Vibrio cholerae* enterotoxin in cultural adrenal tumor cells. J Infect Dis 133 (Suppl):S108, 1976.

BRUCELLOSIS

Essentials of Diagnosis

- Intermittent fevers, primarily in the evenings or at night.
- Easy fatigability, arthralgia, anorexia, sweating, and irritability.
- Relative lymphocytosis, positive blood culture, agglutination titer of 1:160 or greater.

General Considerations

Brucella infections in humans are caused by 3 species: *B abortus* (cattle), *B suis* (hogs), and *B meli-*

tensis (goats). Infection usually occurs through ingestion of contaminated milk or milk products or by contact through minor skin or mucosal abrasions. The incubation period is 8–30 days.

Clinical Findings

A. Symptoms and Signs: The onset is insidious, with vague symptoms of weakness and exhaustion, intermittent night fevers, and sweating. In children, physical findings are generally absent, although splenomegaly is occasionally seen. Slight lymphadenopathy may be present.

B. Laboratory Findings: The white count is normal, with absolute lymphocytosis. The organism can be recovered from the blood and urine and, though rarely, from the CSF and other tissues. There is little difficulty in obtaining positive blood cultures from patients infected with *B melitensis* or *B suis*. However in *B abortus* infections there are fewer organisms circulating in the blood. In case of suspected *B abortus* infections, it is well to obtain about 0.5 ml/kg of venous blood and distribute it among a series of blood culture bottles. All blood cultures should be subcultured twice a week for at least 8 weeks before a negative result is reported. An elevated brucella agglutinin titer (1:160 or above) confirms the diagnosis.

Where there is a questionable or doubtful positive agglutination test, 2 additional serologic tests may be helpful. An agglutination test may be repeated after treating the serum with mercaptoethanol. A titer of 1:40 or higher is considered positive. If the serum fixes complement using brucella antigen at a titer of 1:10 or higher, it is considered positive. The results of conventional serologic tests (direct and indirect agglutination tests and complement fixation tests) allow identification of 2 groups of infected individuals: (1) acutely infected persons who have IgM (and IgG) antibody to *B abortus* somatic antigen, and (2) individuals who have either chronic brucellosis or a subclinical infection in which immunity is being repeatedly stimulated by contact with brucella organisms. Both types in the second category have IgG and IgA (but not IgM) antibody to *B abortus* in their serum, which is usually detectable by positive agglutination and positive complement fixation reactions but is sometimes undetectable by these tests. Recently, a radioimmunoassay (RIA) has been devised to measure the serum antibody against *B abortus* in each of the immunoglobulin classes IgM, IgG, and IgA. This test was applied to 46 sera from individuals with various clinical types of brucellosis, and the results were compared with the results of conventional tests. The RIA provided a highly sensitive primary type assay which avoided the difficulties with blocking or nonagglutinating antibody. It thus has many advantages in the diagnosis of acute and chronic stages of brucella infection in humans. The RIA successfully detected antibody in many instances in which conventional serologic tests were negative. IgM antibodies are associated with acute cases and IgG or IgA with chronic cases of brucellosis. One case in which *B abortus* was isolated by blood culture but which failed to yield antibody by conventional tests showed substantial levels of IgM and IgG antibody by RIA. In other cases, the RIA helped to eliminate the diagnosis of brucellosis by revealing absent or low antibody levels.

In case of involvement of the CNS, the CSF may rarely show a growth of brucella in culture or be positive for agglutinins.

An intracutaneous test with brucella antigens may be performed and read at 48–72 hours. A positive test indicates prior exposure to the antigenic components of the organism. It does not indicate the current status of infection.

Four-fold rises in serum antibody may occur after performing a skin test. The skin test should not be used in routine diagnosis when serologic tests are available.

Differential Diagnosis

A variety of causes of fever without localization, including neoplastic and granulomatous diseases which may cause lymphadenopathy and hepatosplenomegaly, have to be distinguished. It is desirable to look for evidence of brucellosis in patients with arachnoiditis or meningomyelitis of obscure origin.

Complications

Following hematogenous spread, secondary foci of infection may lead to endocarditis, pyelonephritis, meningoencephalitis, and osteomyelitis. In older children, infection of the bile ducts results in jaundice. In the malignant form, hepatic necrosis may occur. Neurologic complications may appear at the onset of the illness or at any time during the clinical course, including convalescence, or long after acute symptoms have subsided. Leptomeningitis is an early feature and may lead to adhesive arachnoiditis in the cranium or in the spinal cord.

A psychiatric form of the disease is well known which is likely to be associated with a mild encephalitis.

Treatment

A. Specific Measures: Tetracycline, 50 mg/kg/day orally in divided doses every 6 hours, is given for 21 days. In case of a relapse, treatment is repeated. Only in very severe cases of acute brucellosis or in suppurative brucellosis due to *B suis,* simultaneous administration of streptomycin, 20–40 mg/kg IM as a single daily dose for 1 week, is advised. During the second week, streptomycin is continued at the level of 15 mg/kg while tetracycline is continued orally for the full 21 days.

B. General Measures: Limited physical activity and bed rest are indicated while there is fever. Aspirin will relieve headache and somatic pains. Codeine sulfate, 30 mg orally every 12 hours, is occasionally required early in the course of antibiotic therapy.

Prognosis

With specific therapy, the prognosis is now excellent and the chance for prolonged invalidism markedly reduced.

Bigler WJ & others: Trends of brucellosis in Florida: An epidemiologic review. Am J Epidemiol 105:245, 1977.

Brucellosis. (Editorial.) Lancet 1:436, 1975.

Busch LA, Parker RL: Brucellosis in the United States. J Infect Dis 125:289, 1972.

Daikos GK & others: Trimethoprim-sulfamethoxazole in brucellosis. J Infect Dis 128 (Suppl):S731, 1973.

Street L, Grant WW, Alva JD: Brucellosis in childhood. Pediatrics 55:416, 1975.

TULAREMIA

Essentials of Diagnosis

- A cutaneous or mucous membrane lesion at the site of inoculation and regional lymph node enlargement.
- Sudden onset of fever, chills, and prostration.
- History of contact with infected animals, principally wild rabbits.
- Culture of mucocutaneous ulcer or regional lymph nodes confirms the diagnosis.

General Considerations

Tularemia is caused by *Francisella tularensis,* a gram-negative organism usually acquired from infected animals, principally wild rabbits, by ingestion of contaminated meat or infected water; by contamination of the skin or mucous membranes; by inhalation of infected material; and by bites of ticks or fleas or deerflies which have been in contact with infected animals. Strains of high virulence for humans are usually associated with tick-borne tularemia of rabbits; those of lowered virulence are linked with the water-borne disease of rodents. The incubation period is short, usually 3–7 days, but may vary from 2–25 days.

Rabbits are the classic vectors of tularemia. It is appropriate to seek a history of rabbit hunting, skinning, or food preparation in any patient who has a febrile illness with tender lymphadenopathy, often in the region of a draining skin ulcer. However, a history of exposure to ticks may be equally helpful in the prompt initiation of appropriate therapy.

All the reservoirs of *F tularensis* in nature are not known. The rabbit tick *Haemaphysalis leporis-palustris* may maintain tularemia infection in rabbits that succumb to the disease. This tick has been shown to be infected in nature and to transmit the bacteria to its eggs and larvae but does not appear to attack humans. Rabbits thus infected may transmit the disease directly to humans or to ticks that attack humans, such as the eastern dog tick *(Dermacentor variabilis),* the Lone Star tick *(Amblyomma americanum),* or the western wood tick *(D andersoni).*

Oropharyngeal tularemia is a common type of tularemia found in the pediatric age group and can progress to septicemia or tracheal obstruction with a fatal outcome. It is caused by the ingestion of food or water contaminated with *F tularensis* or by manual-oral contact after handling an infected host. Frequently, more than one member of the family is infected. This form of tularemia is very severe. It must be distinguished from more common causes of exudative pharyngitis such as streptococcal infection or infectious mononucleosis. In addition, the frequently observed necrotic gray membrane can mimic that of diphtheria.

Clinical Findings

A. Symptoms and Signs: Several clinical types are seen in children. Most infections start as a reddened papule which may be pruritic, quickly ulcerates, and is not very painful (ulceroglandular form). Shortly thereafter, there may be marked systemic manifestations, including high fever, chills, weakness, vomiting, and enlargement of the regional lymph nodes which are usually very tender and quickly become fluctuant. Drainage may occur. Pneumonitis occasionally is found clinically or by x-ray (pneumonic form). A detectable skin lesion is occasionally absent, and localized lymphoid enlargement exists alone (glandular form). Oculoglandular and oropharyngeal forms also occur in children. In the absence of any primary ulcer or localized lymphadenitis, a prolonged febrile disease reminiscent of typhoid fever can be seen (typhoidal form). Splenomegaly is common, and an evanescent maculopapular rash may be seen on the trunk and extremities.

B. Laboratory Findings: *F tularensis* can be recovered from ulcers or regional lymph nodes as well as from sputum in patients with the pneumonic form. An intradermal skin test is positive early in the disease; it resembles the tuberculin skin tests. The skin test does not result in a significant serologic response and may therefore be used in addition to serologic tests for diagnosis. The white blood count is not remarkable, and the ESR is usually normal. Agglutinins are present after the second week of illness, and in the absence of a positive culture their development confirms the diagnosis. An agglutination titer of 1:160 or higher is considered positive.

Differential Diagnosis

The typhoidal form of tularemia may mimic typhoid, brucellosis, miliary tuberculosis, Rocky Mountain spotted fever, and infectious mononucleosis. Pneumonic tularemia resembles atypical and mycotic pneumonitis and bacterial pneumonia. The ulceroglandular type of tularemia resembles pyoderma caused by staphylococci or streptococci, rat-bite fever, plague, anthrax, cat scratch fever, and rickettsialpox as well as accidental vaccinia inoculation. The oropharyngeal type must be distinguished from herpetic gingivostomatitis, herpangina, and lymphonodular pharyngitis due to coxsackievirus type A, nonspecific tonsillopharyngitis due to adenovirus, infectious mononucleosis, and blood dyscrasias.

Prevention

Reasonable attempts should be made to protect children from bites of insects, principally ticks, fleas, and deerflies, by the use of proper clothing and repellents. Drinking water from streams in endemic areas should be avoided. Children should be cautioned to stay away from wild game. If contact occurs, thorough washing with soap and water is indicated.

Treatment

A. Specific Measures: Give streptomycin, 30–40 mg/kg/day IM in 2 divided doses for 8–10 days. The maximum daily dose is 1 gm. The tetracyclines and chloramphenicol are also effective but are not advised as sole medication.

B. General Measures: Antipyretics and analgesics may be given as necessary. Skin lesions are best left open. Glandular lesions occasionally require incision and drainage.

Prognosis

With streptomycin treatment, the prognosis is excellent.

Alford RH, John JT, Bryant RE: Tularemia treated successfully with gentamicin. Am Rev Respir Dis 106:265, 1972.

Bloom ME, Shearer WT, Barton LL: Oculoglandular tularemia in an inner city child. Pediatrics 51:564, 1973.

Boyce JM: Recent trends in the epidemiology of tularemia in the United States. J Infect Dis 131:197, 1975.

Guerrant RL & others: Tickborn oculoglandular tularemia: Case report and review of seasonal and vectorial associations in 106 cases. Arch Intern Med 136:811, 1976.

Szalay GC: Tularemia in an inner city child. Clin Pediatr (Phila) 13:375, 1974.

Tyson HK: Tularemia: An unappreciated cause of exudative pharyngitis. Pediatrics 58:864, 1976.

PLAGUE

Essentials of Diagnosis

- Sudden onset of fever, chills, and prostration.
- Regional lymphangitis and lymphadenitis with suppuration of nodes (bubonic form).
- Hemorrhages into skin and mucous membranes and shock (septicemia).
- Cough, dyspnea, cyanosis, and hemoptysis (pneumonic form).
- History of exposure to infected animals.

General Considerations

Plague is an extremely serious, acute infection caused by a gram-negative bacillus, *Yersinia pestis*. It is a disease of rodents which is transmitted to humans by the bites of fleas. Rodent plague in animals of the field and forest is called sylvatic plague; plague in rodents associated with humans is called murine plague. Plague bacilli have been isolated from rodents in 15 of the western states in the USA. Cases associated with wild rodents occur sporadically.

Human plague in the USA appears to exhibit a definite cycle: peak years occur approximately every 5 years. This periodicity is thought to reflect a comparable cycle in wild animal reservoirs of infection.

Yersinia enterocolitica is a gram-negative bacillus which has been associated with a variety of human clinical disorders, including diarrhea, acute mesenteric adenitis, abscesses, septicemia, arthritis, and skin rash. It has been isolated from many animal species, including pigs, cats, and dogs. Only rarely, however, has it been isolated from animals epidemiologically associated with human disease.

Clinical Findings

A. Symptoms and Signs: The disease assumes several different clinical forms, the 2 most common being bubonic and pneumonic.

1. Bubonic plague—Bubonic plague begins with a sudden onset of high fever, chills, headache, vomiting, and marked delirium or clouding of consciousness. Although the flea bite is rarely seen, the regional lymph node is painful and tender, 1–5 cm in diameter, and usually suppurates and drains spontaneously after 1 week. The plague bacillus is known to produce an endotoxin which causes vascular necrosis. Bacilli may overwhelm regional lymph nodes and enter the circulation to produce septicemia. Severe vascular necrosis results in widely disseminated hemorrhages in skin, mucous membranes, liver, and spleen. The term "black death" was used during the Middle Ages because of the large, discolored hemorrhagic skin areas. Myocarditis and circulatory collapse may result from damage by the endotoxin.

Plague meningitis may occur secondarily following bacteremic spread from an infected lymph node, and suboptimal antibiotic therapy employing penicillin may permit multiplication of organisms in a protected site in the meninges.

2. Pneumonic plague—The pneumonic form occurs primarily during epidemics as a result of man-to-man airborne transmission. Lung necrosis results in abundant sputum that is initially watery but rapidly becomes bloody and loaded with organisms. Patients are toxic, cyanotic, and dyspneic.

B. Laboratory Findings: Aspiration of a bubo leads to visualization of bacilli on a stained smear. Pus, sputum, and blood all yield the organism, although laboratory infections are common enough to make isolation dangerous. Blood-agar cultures yield positive results in 24–48 hours. The white count is markedly elevated, with a shift to the left.

Difficulty in isolating *Y enterocolitica* using routine stool isolation technics may be a major reason why many clinical laboratories fail to identify this pathogen more frequently in sick patients. A cold enrichment isolation technic is required.

Differential Diagnosis

The febrile phase of the disease may be confused with such illnesses as typhoid fever and typhus. The bubonic form resembles tularemia, anthrax, cat scratch fever, streptococcal adenitis, and cellulitis. Skin lesions may suggest a rickettsial infection. Buboes in the groin need to be differentiated from chancroid, lymphogranuloma venereum, and incarcerated hernia. Primary gastroenteritis and appendicitis may have to be distinguished.

Prevention

Proper disposal of household and commercial wastes and chemical control of rats are basic measures for control of the reservoir of murine plague. Flea control is instituted and maintained with the liberal use of DDT and other insecticides. Children of vacationing parents in remote camping areas should be cautioned not to handle dead or dying animals. Travelers to wilderness areas in the enzootic western states are considered to be at low risk of infection, and immunization of visitors to these areas is not recommended.

Vaccination is recommended for those traveling or living in areas of high incidence. (See Chapter 5.)

Treatment

A. Specific Measures: Streptomycin and tetracyclines should both be used. The dose of streptomycin is 20–40 mg/kg IM in 2 divided doses for 5 days followed by one of the tetracyclines, 50 mg/kg/day IM in 3 divided doses. The total daily dose of streptomycin should not exceed 1 gm. Treatment should be continued until the patient has been afebrile for 4 or 5 days. In simple bubonic plague, sulfonamides are also effective.

In septicemia and pneumonic plague, treatment must be started in the first 15–24 hours of the disease if survival is to be expected. Treatment with streptomycin started 36–48 hours after onset of the disease may result in death due to liberation of plague toxin. The mechanism may be analogous to the Jarisch-Herxheimer reaction, with release of toxin from dead plague bacilli. Any case of painful bubo should be treated without delay.

Bubonic plague is not highly contagious. Every effort is made to effect resolution of buboes without resorting to surgery. Pus from draining lymph nodes should be handled with rubber gloves.

B. General Measures: Pneumonic plague is highly infectious, and rigid isolation is required. All contacts should receive prophylaxis with sulfadiazine, 100–200 mg/kg/day orally in 4 divided doses for 7 days.

Prognosis

The mortality rate in untreated bubonic plague is about 50%; it is 90% in the septicemic form, and nearly 100% in the pneumonic form. The mortality rate of the septicemic form is reduced to 10% or less with early streptomycin treatment.

Bartelloni PJ, Marshall JD, Cavanaugh DC: Clinical and serological responses to plague vaccine U.S.P. Milit Med 138:720, 1973.

Butler T & others: *Yersinia pestis* infection in Vietnam. 1. Clinical and hematologic aspects. J Infect Dis 129 (Suppl):S78, 1974.

Isaacson M & others: Unusual cases of human plague in southern Africa. S Afr Med J 47:2109, 1973.

Meyer KF & others: Plague immunization. 1. Past and present trends. J Infect Dis 129 (Suppl):S13, 1974.

HAEMOPHILUS INFLUENZAE TYPE B INFECTIONS

Essentials of Diagnosis

- Purulent meningitis in children under age 2 years with direct smears of CSF showing long filamentous forms as well as gram-negative pleomorphic rods.

- Acute epiglottitis: High fever, dysphagia, and croup. White blood count > 20,000/cu mm.

- Otitis media: Low-grade fever, chronic nasal discharge, and bilaterally inflamed tympanic membranes with little pain.

- Septic arthritis: Fever, circumferential redness, swelling, local heat, and pain with active or passive motion of the involved joint.

- Cellulitis in infants: Sudden onset of fever and distinctive cellulitis in an infant, often involving the cheek, and starting as a mild swelling with central erythema that rapidly progresses to a lesion without a distinct border with central reddish discoloration, surrounded by and merging into purplish areas that fade peripherally.

- Orbital cellulitis: Sudden onset of pain, swelling of the orbital area, purple discoloration of involved skin, and bilateral haziness of maxillary and ethmoid sinuses.

- Insidious onset of pneumonia in an infant, with x-ray picture of lobar consolidation or patchy bronchopneumonia; empyema.

- High, spiking fever in an infant with meningitis or pneumonia, transient pericardial friction rub, ST segment and T wave ECG changes, clinical and x-ray evidence of pericardial effusion, and aspiration of pus from the pericardial sac.

- In all cases, a positive culture from the blood or from aspirated pus confirms the diagnosis.

General Considerations

Haemophilus influenzae type B is perhaps the most important bacterial pathogen in childhood. It causes meningitis, acute epiglottitis (supraglottic croup), acute septic arthritis, orbital and facial cellulitis, pneumonia, and septic pericarditis. *H influenzae* type B infections occur most frequently in the age group from 6 months to 4 years (epiglottitis: 2–5

years). With the exception of pneumonia and septic pericarditis, this organism is the leading cause of all these infections in this age range. Ninety percent of blood samples from newborns show bactericidal antibody, presumably reflecting passive transfer of antibody from protected mothers. The age distribution of infection is explained by the loss of passive protection by 4–6 months of age, the progressive infection of susceptible individuals, and acquisition of protective antibodies in early childhood. The chief virulence factor for *H influenzae* type B organisms appears to be the polyribose phosphate (PRP) capsule, which is antiphagocytic. Many children 4 months to 3 years of age have low or nondetectable levels of anticapsular antibodies. In the period from 3½–8 years of age, anticapsular antibodies appear in the serum and reach adult levels. Although many infants and children are colonized early with *H influenzae* species, most of the strains are nonencapsulated. The very low nasopharyngeal colonization rate of *H influenzae* type B in infants and children suggests that the homologous organism is not the usual stimulus for the development of anticapsular antibodies. The type B capsule is immunologically cross-reactive with the capsules of certain species of bacilli, diphtheroids, lactobacilli, *Staphylococcus aureus, S epidermidis,* streptococci, *Escherichia coli,* and pseudomonas. Thus, it appears that natural immunity is acquired from encapsulated bacteria which share antigenic determinants with *H influenzae* type B PRP. In the past 3 decades, the prevalence and incidence of *H influenzae* type B infections serious enough to require hospitalization have been increasing. There is no clear explanation for this increase. Recently, reports of systemic disease in newborns and adults have increased. However, the number of systemic infections has increased in all age groups, and the highest age-specific attack rate still occurs in children from 6 months to 4 years of age.

In 1974, the first 2 cases of illnesses due to ampicillin-resistant *H influenzae* type B were reported. The mechanism of resistance appears to be a plasmid-mediated elaboration of β-lactamase (penicillinase) by the resistant organisms. At the end of 1975, ampicillin-resistant strains comprised 5–10% of all type B strains isolated in certain regions of the USA. Associated clinical illnesses have included meningitis, pneumonia, epiglottitis, sepsis, and otitis media. Isolates have been made from cultures of CSF, blood, sputum, and throat and ear aspirates. Most *H influenzae* type B isolates are highly sensitive to ampicillin. *H influenzae* type B resistant to chloramphenicol has been observed. These strains carry plasmids mediating resistance to chloramphenicol or tetracycline.

Tympanocentesis performed in children with acute otitis media has demonstrated that a pneumococcus can be isolated from about 50% of cases and *H influenzae* from about 20%. However, most of the *H influenzae* strains are nonencapsulated and nontypable. Type B accounts for about 10% of the *H influenzae* strains. A recent report indicates that the incidence of ampicillin resistance in nonencapsulated strains causing otitis media increased from 0.6% in 1973 to 2.4% in 1976. All isolated resistant strains produced β-lactamase. Patients infected with such ampicillin-resistant organisms require therapy with antimicrobial agents which are not susceptible to degradation by penicillinase. Also, ampicillin-resistant *H influenzae* should be suspected in situations where ampicillin therapy of otitis media is unsuccessful.

There is epidemiologic evidence that *H influenzae* type B meningitis occurs more frequently in urban and rural areas of low socioeconomic status. Children with sickle cell disease also appear to have increased susceptibility. Acutely ill children 6–36 months of age, with temperatures higher than 39° C (102.2° F) and nonspecific symptoms associated with an elevated white blood count, may have *H influenzae* type B bacteremia. Type B bacteremia is second only to pneumococcal bacteremia in incidence. Experimental evidence suggests that if the bacteremia has a concentration of 1000 or more cells per ml of blood, metastatic foci such as meningitis or septic arthritis will occur. If the cell count per ml of blood is substantially lower, these serious infections do not occur.

The initial therapy for infants over 2 months of age and for children with meningitis, arthritis, cellulitis, epiglottitis, or sepsis thought to be due to *H influenzae* type B should include both chloramphenicol and ampicillin. In many hospitals, tube dilution sensitivity tests for both ampicillin and chloramphenicol are routinely performed on isolates obtained from CSF, joint fluid, and blood. The full course of therapy should be continued with the single most appropriate antibiotic, ie, ampicillin or chloramphenicol. In this age group, meningitis of undetermined origin may be treated with a combination of ampicillin and chloramphenicol without fear of antibiotic antagonism.

Clinical Findings

A. Symptoms and Signs:

1. Meningitis—Findings may be very minimal. Nothing clinically distinguishes it from other forms, although petechiae are less common than in meningococcal meningitis, and fever and generalized toxemia are apt to be very high. Characteristically, there is a history of upper respiratory infection in a young infant who subsequently frowns a good deal, becomes increasingly stuporous, and may show nuchal rigidity. If the fontanel is open, evidence of increased intracranial pressure may be seen.

2. Acute epiglottitis—The most characteristic clinical aid in the early diagnosis of *H influenzae* croup is evidence of dysphagia characterized by a refusal to eat or swallow saliva even by very young children. This finding, plus the presence of a high fever in a toxic child—even in the absence of direct examination of the epiglottis (cherry-red epiglottis)—should strongly suggest the diagnosis and lead to prompt intubation. (See Chapter 12 for details.)

3. Otitis media, septic arthritis, cellulitis in infants, orbital cellulitis, pneumonia, septic pericarditis—See Essentials of Diagnosis, above.

B. Laboratory Findings: Very high leukocytosis (> 20 thousand/cu mm) with a marked shift to the left is characteristic of *H influenzae* infections. Blood culture is almost always positive. Positive culture of aspirated pus or fluid from or near the involved site proves the diagnosis.

In meningitis (before treatment), spinal fluid smear reveals, in addition to the characteristic pleomorphic gram-negative rods, pathognomonic long filamentous forms.

Countercurrent immunoelectrophoresis (CIE) can be used to detect polyribose phosphate (PRP), the capsular antigen of *H influenzae* type B, in CSF, joint fluid, urine, and serum, using a high titer, type-specific rabbit antiserum. The test is useful in the specific diagnosis of patients with meningitis who have received antibiotic therapy. Up to 20% of treated children with meningitis have detectable antigen in sterile serum or spinal fluid. Recent evidence indicates that both the concentration of PRP in serum or spinal fluid at onset of therapy for meningitis and the duration of antigenemia provide prognostic information concerning the clinical course. Antigenemia may last from days to weeks in certain infants.

C. X-Ray Findings: A lateral view of the neck should be taken in suspected acute epiglottitis. Haziness of maxillary and ethmoid sinuses occurs with orbital cellulitis; lung consolidation and pleural fluid with pneumonia; and a characteristically enlarged heart shadow with purulent pericarditis.

D. Electrocardiography: Elevated ST segments and flattened T waves and low voltage occur with purulent pericarditis.

Differential Diagnosis

A. Meningitis: Differentiate from head injury, brain abscess, tumor, lead encephalopathy, and other forms of meningoencephalitis due to viral, fungal, and bacterial agents, including tuberculous meningitis.

B. Acute Epiglottitis: In croup caused by viral agents (parainfluenza 1, 2, and 3, respiratory syncytial virus, influenza A, adenovirus), the child has more definite upper respiratory symptoms, slower progression of obstructive signs, and only low-grade fever. Spasmodic croup occurs typically at night in a child with a history of previous attacks; these attacks may be of allergic origin. A history of sudden onset of choking and paroxysmal coughing suggests aspiration of a foreign body. Occasionally, retropharyngeal abscess or laryngeal diphtheria may have to be differentiated from epiglottitis.

C. Septic Arthritis: Acute osteomyelitis, prepatellar bursitis, cellulitis, rheumatic fever, and fractures and sprains.

D. Cellulitis in Infants: Erysipelas, streptococcal cellulitis, insect bites, and trauma.

E. Orbital Cellulitis: Erysipelas, paranasal sinus disease without orbital cellulitis, allergic inflammatory disease of the lids, vaccinial or herpes simplex conjunctivitis, herpes zoster infection, metastatic neuroblastoma, and primary orbital tumors.

F. Pneumonia: See p 297.

G. Septic Pericarditis: See p 369.

Complications

A. Meningitis: Subdural effusion, subdural empyema, involvement of cranial nerves, hydrocephalus; late intellectual sequelae include handicaps of perceptual and motor functioning and abstract thinking ability.

B. Acute Epiglottitis: Mediastinal emphysema, pneumothorax; rarely, bacteremic spread to meninges or joints.

C. Otitis Media: Sinusitis, mastoiditis, and occasionally bacteremic spread to other sites.

D. Septic Arthritis: May result in rapid destruction of cartilage and ankylosis if diagnosis and treatment are delayed.

E. Cellulitis in Infants: Bacteremia may lead to metastatic meningitis, osteomyelitis, or pyarthrosis.

F. Orbital Cellulitis: Cavernous sinus thrombosis is a rare sequel. With the onset of this complication, the child develops severe pain and general toxicity, papilledema, and decreased vision.

G. Pneumonia: Empyema; rarely, pneumatocele and pneumothorax.

H. Septic Pericarditis: Myocardial abscesses and heart failure; cardiac tamponade.

Prevention

Evaluation of *H influenzae* type B purified polysaccharide vaccine has shown that injection of a wide range of dosages does not provoke untoward reactions and elicits a serum antibody response in at least 95% of adults. Response is maximal in 2–3 weeks and is sustained for at least 5 years. Reinjection of the purified antigen does not elicit an anamnestic response. The antibody response of infants and children differs from that of adults and is age-dependent. Infants up to 6 months of age respond poorly, both with respect to the percentage responding with more than a 2-fold increase in antibodies and with respect to the average postinjection level of antibodies. Since any successful immunization program for *H influenzae* type B must be completed by 4–6 months of age, it is apparent that the administration of purified polysaccharide antigen would not protect the most vulnerable young infants and children. Children 2 years of age and older who are able to respond to the polysaccharide vaccine have a significant decrease in the attack rate of *H influenzae* type B meningitis compared to that of control children in the same age group. The *E coli* K100 antigen cross-reacts with *H influenzae* type B. Colonization with the cross-reacting K100 strain in adults gives a significant boost to anticapsular type B antibodies as measured in sera. Under study is a less purified vaccine containing the outer cell membrane complex of lipopolysaccharide-protein PRP of *H influenzae* type B.

Individuals with X-linked antibody synthesis deficiency are highly susceptible to repeated and severe *H influenzae* type B infections, including meningitis. Passive immunization of these individuals with pooled immunoglobulin shown to contain anti-type B antibody confers a high degree of protection.

It has been a common observation that multiple cases of *H influenzae* type B meningitis occur in up to 3% of affected families. Since there is no chemoprophylaxis available for *H influenzae* type B meningitis, it would seem advisable to hospitalize any ill siblings of the patient, perform a diagnostic workup, including examination of CSF, and begin full therapeutic doses of ampicillin and chloramphenicol.

Treatment

Refer to the comments made above under General Considerations concerning the problem of ampicillin-resistant strains of *H influenzae* type B. With the exception of acute otitis media, all of these diseases are potentially fatal and require immediate hospitalization and treatment. Each disease should be treated with ampicillin, 200–400 mg/kg/day IV in 6 divided doses until there is marked improvement; in some cases, the treatment course may then be completed with ampicillin given intramuscularly in 4 divided doses. Chloramphenicol, 100 mg/kg/day IV in 4 divided doses, is the drug of choice if there is a known allergy to ampicillin.

A. Meningitis: A repeat lumbar tap should be performed after 24–36 hours of treatment. The CSF should then be sterile. Treatment should be continued until the patient has been afebrile for 5 days, the CSF cell count is 30 cells or less, and the sugar and protein have returned to normal; this usually requires 10–14 days. It is preferable to give the entire course of antibiotic intravenously in 6 divided doses per day. No treatment failures need be expected using a dosage of 300 mg/kg/day. The intravenous site should be rotated every 48–72 hours.

Most common causes for exacerbation of fever or persistence of fever beyond 6 days are the following: chemical phlebitis at injection site, drug fever, subdural effusions, acquisition of hospital-acquired viral or bacterial superinfection, and metastatic disease requiring drainage (eg, subdural empyema, septic pericarditis, arthritis).

In case of subdural effusion, a maximum of 15 ml are allowed to drip freely from each side of the anterior fontanel daily. If fluid is still present after 2 weeks neurosurgical consultation is advised.

Supportive therapy with intravenous fluids, oxygen, sedation, and tube feeding should be given as required.

B. Acute Epiglottitis: An immediate intravenous dose of 200 mg/kg of ampicillin is given, followed by 200 mg/kg/day IV in 6 divided doses. In most cases, establishment and maintenance of a free airway are most important considerations. Signs of increasing airway obstruction are a clear indication for tracheostomy, which should be done electively with the assistance of a skilled bronchoscopist. Antibiotic treatment should be continued for 10 days. In case of penicillin sensitivity, give chloramphenicol as an alternative drug.

High humidification and intravenous fluids are required. Improvement of cyanosis by placing the child in an oxygen atmosphere gives a false sense of security to the physician. The basic problem is upper airway obstruction, which may require tracheostomy.

C. Otitis Media: Give ampicillin orally in a dosage of 100 mg/kg/day in 4 divided doses for 7–14 days *or* amoxicillin, 50 mg/kg/day orally in divided doses every 8 hours. Some physicians prefer to use an oral penicillin-sulfonamide combination such as phenoxymethyl penicillin, 25–50 mg (40,000–80,000 units)/kg/day, *plus* trisulfapyrimidines, 120 mg/kg/day orally in 4 divided doses.

Oral decongestants may be used but are now considered less important than once thought. Careful follow-up is indicated for the secondary occurrence of serous otitis and hearing loss.

D. Septic Arthritis: Ampicillin is given in a dosage of 200–300 mg/kg/day IV in 6 divided doses until there is marked improvement. The same dose may then be given intramuscularly in 4 divided doses to complete a 3-week course of treatment. On admission, surgical incision and drainage are required whenever there is a significant collection of pus in the joint.

The joint should be immobilized. Give antipyretics and analgesics as required and maintain adequate hydration.

E. Cellulitis and Orbital Cellulitis: Give ampicillin as for septic arthritis and supportive and symptomatic treatment as required. There is usually marked improvement after 72 hours of treatment. Antibiotics should be given for 7–10 days.

F. Pneumonia: Give ampicillin as for septic arthritis and oxygen, intravenous fluids, and other supportive care as required. Treat for 3 weeks. Empyema should be treated by placement of one or more chest tubes into the pleural space. When possible, a chest tube should be removed after 4 or 5 days.

G. Septic Pericarditis: Give ampicillin as for septic arthritis. Continue treatment for 4 weeks. Pericardiocentesis may be lifesaving to prevent fatal tamponade. Open pericardiostomy should be performed to allow for continuous drainage of pus and to prevent reaccumulation.

Digitalis, oxygen, and intravenous fluids should be given as required.

Prognosis

The case fatality rate for *H influenzae* meningitis is 5–10%. Young infants have the highest mortality rate. Nuerologic sequelae should be watched for but are appreciably reduced with prompt antibiotic treatment.

The case fatality rate in acute epiglottitis is 15–20%; deaths are associated with bacteremia and the rapid development of airway obstruction.

With optimal medical and surgical drainage, the case fatality rate for septic pericarditis in infants still is 20%.

The prognosis for the other diseases requiring hospitalization is good with the institution of early and adequate antibiotic therapy.

Committee on Infectious Diseases: Current status of ampicillin-resistant *Haemophilus influenzae* type B. Pediatrics 57:417, 1976.

Delage G & others: *Haemophilus influenzae* type B infections: Recurrent disease due to ampicillin-resistant strains. J Pediatr 90:319, 1977.

Echeverria P & others: *Haemophilus influenzae* B pericarditis in children. Pediatrics 56:808, 1975.

Feigin RD & others: Prospective evaluation of treatment of *Haemophilus influenzae* meningitis. J Pediatr 88:542, 1976.

Granoff DM: *Haemophilus influenzae* type B and epiglottitis. J Pediatr 88:1068, 1976.

Granoff DM, Nankervis GA: Cellulitis due to *Haemophilus influenzae* type B: Antigenemia and antibody responses. Am J Dis Child 130:1211, 1976.

Harlow M, Chung SMK, Plotkin SA: *Haemophilus influenzae* septic arthritis in infants and children. Clin Pediatr (Phila) 14:1146, 1975.

Herson VC, Todd JK: Prediction of morbidity in *Haemophilus influenzae* meningitis. Pediatrics 59:35, 1977.

Khuri-Bulos N, McIntosh K: Neonatal *Haemophilus influenzae* infection. Am J Dis Child 129:57, 1975.

Lindberg J & others: Long-term outcome of *Haemophilus influenzae* meningitis related to antibiotic treatment. Pediatrics 60:1, 1977.

Long SS, Phillips SE: Chloramphenicol-resistant *Haemophilus influenzae.* J Pediatr 90:1030, 1977.

Manten A, van Klingeren B, Dessens-Kroon M: Chloramphenicol resistance in *Haemophilus influenzae.* Lancet 1:702, 1976.

Marston G, Wald ER: *Haemophilus influenzae* type B sepsis in infant and mother. Pediatrics 58:863, 1976.

Molteni RA: Epiglottitis. Incidence of extraepiglottic infection: Report of 72 cases and review of the literature. Pediatrics 58:526, 1976.

Schwartz R: Resistance of *H influenzae* to ampicillin. J Pediatr 89:1041, 1976.

Smith AL: Antibiotics and invasive *Haemophilus influenzae:* Current concepts. N Engl J Med 294:1329, 1976.

Smith EWP, Ingram DL: Counterimmunoelectrophoresis in *Haemophilus influenzae* type B epiglottitis and pericarditis. J Pediatr 86:571, 1975.

Syriopoulou V & others: Incidence of ampicillin-resistant *Haemophilus influenzae* in otitis media. J Pediatr 89:839, 1976.

Todd JK, Bruhn FW: Severe *Haemophilus influenzae* infections: Spectrum of disease. Am J Dis Child 129:607, 1975.

Wald ER, Levine MM: Frequency of detection of *Haemophilus influenzae* type B capsular polysaccharide in infants and children with pneumonia. Pediatrics 57:266, 1976.

Waldman LS, Kosloske AM, Parsons DW: Acute epididymoorchitis as the presenting manifestation of *Haemophilus influenzae* septicemia. J Pediatr 90:87, 1977.

Ward J, Smith AL: *Haemophilus influenzae* bacteremia in children with sickle cell disease. J Pediatr 88:261, 1976.

Whisnant JK & others: Host factors and antibody response in *Haemophilus influenzae* type B meningitis and epiglottitis. J Infect Dis 133:448, 1976.

PERTUSSIS
(Whooping Cough)

Essentials of Diagnosis

- Staccato, paroxysmal expiratory cough ending with a high-pitched inspiratory "whoop."
- Prodromal catarrhal stage (1–3 weeks) characterized by cough, coryza, and occasionally vomiting.
- Leukocytosis with absolute lymphocytosis.
- Diagnosis confirmed by fluorescent stain or culture.

General Considerations

Pertussis is an acute communicable infection of the respiratory tract caused by *Bordetella pertussis.* The disease has the most serious impact on children under 2 years of age. Transmission is through infected individuals, generally a family contact. The incubation period is 7–14 days, and infectivity is greatest during the catarrhal and early paroxysmal cough stage (for about 4 weeks after onset). Of all reported deaths in the USA due to pertussis from 1960–1967, 72% were infants 1 year of age or younger. The highest fatality rate is noted in infants 2–3 months of age.

Active immunity following pertussis is not permanent. Repeated subclinical or mild infections probably act as boosters to maintain immunity, thus making it appear that immunity is lifelong. Most women of childbearing age lack sufficient protective antibody to ensure passive transfer of IgG antibody to the fetus during the later months of pregnancy. Although passive immunity in newborn infants due to maternal antibody is comparatively weak, it apparently attenuates the disease in young infants when present. Immunity may wane to a low level with increasing age; consequently, the disease may recur in a severe form later in life.

Clinical Findings

A. Symptoms and Signs: In children over 2 years of age, mild cases lasting 5–14 days occur, and symptoms may consist only of low-grade fever and irritating cough with mild paroxysms. In the younger child, symptoms of pertussis last about 8 weeks. The onset is insidious, with mild catarrhal upper respiratory tract symptoms (rhinitis, sneezing, and an irritating cough). Slight fever may be present. After about 2 weeks, cough becomes paroxysmal, with each cough followed by a sudden inspiratory whoop. Vomiting commonly occurs, and coughing through tenacious mucus may result in large bubbles at the nose and mouth. Coughing is accompanied by sweating, prostration, and exhaustion. This stage lasts for 2–4 weeks, with gradual improvement. Cough suggestive of chronic bronchitis lasts for another 2–3 weeks and then usually fades away. Paroxysmal coughing may continue in the absence of any active infection for some months.

B. Laboratory Findings: White blood cell counts of 20–30 thousand/cu mm with 70–80% lymphocytes appear near the end of the catarrhal stage. The blood picture may resemble lymphocytic leukemia. Identification of *B pertussis* by fluorescent antibody technic or culture from nasopharyngeal swabs proves the diagnosis. The organism may be found in the respiratory tract in diminishing titers beginning in the catarrhal stage and ending about 2 weeks after the beginning of the paroxysmal stage. A Bradford wire swab specimen is obtained from the nasopharynx. Culture of the specimen is done on special media. The combination of culture and fluorescent antibody staining is the diagnostic method of choice. Sterilized Bordet-Gengou agar base should be stored in the refrigerator and liquefied just prior to use. Freshly withdrawn defibrinated sheep's blood is added to make a final concentration of 20% in pour plates. Plates used for culture should have been prepared within 72 hours. Serum agglutinins appear late in the infection and are of little value in diagnosis.

Differential Diagnosis

Cough in acute bacterial pneumonias in infants is usually associated with high fever, tachypnea, and chest retractions, often out of proportion to auscultatory findings. In viral respiratory infections, several members of a family usually have symptoms. The infant may develop stridor, wheezing, or signs of pneumonia. Pertussis is differentiated by the progressive course and characteristic "whoop." Children with cystic fibrosis of the pancreas have a positive sweat test, steatorrhea, and often a positive family history. A positive chest x-ray and tuberculin test distinguish the young child with tuberculosis. A foreign body aspirated into the tracheobronchial tree may be identified by proper x-ray and endoscopic technics. Parapertussis resembles mild pertussis and can be distinguished only by culture. Adenoviruses (types 1, 2, 3, or 5) and respiratory syncytial virus have been reported in association with the pertussis syndrome. From available data it appears that adenoviruses may be reactivated from a latent state during pertussis and may enhance the lymphocytosis.

Complications

Pneumonia may be widespread and may be the direct cause of death, particularly in an infant. Asphyxia in children having serious paroxysmal attacks may lead to brain damage with or without convulsions. Cerebral edema is a common postmortem finding. Cerebral hemorrhage and bleeding into the conjunctivas or from the nose may occur. Increased intrapulmonary pressure may also lead to interstitial or subcutaneous emphysema and pneumothorax.

Pertussis probably has been an important primary respiratory disease, leading to chronic bronchiectasis.

Diagnostic lumbar puncture is occasionally desirable in order to ascertain the presence of blood when subarachnoid hemorrhage is suspected on clinical grounds.

Prevention (See Chapter 5.)

Active immunization should be routinely administered, with pertussis vaccine given in combination with diphtheria and tetanus toxoids (DTP). Little or no maternal immunity is passively transferred to the newborn.

Chemoprophylaxis with erythromycin should be administered to exposed susceptible contacts in the family, particularly those under 2 years of age, for 10 days after contact with an infected person is terminated or, if it is not possible to end the contact, for the duration of cough in the infected individual.

In exposed immunized children under 4 years of age, a booster injection of pertussis vaccine should be given. Erythromycin chemoprophylaxis is also indicated.

Treatment

A. Specific Measures: Antibiotics have no effect on the clinical course of pertussis when administered in the paroxysmal stage of the disease. Erythromycin regularly eliminates pertussis organisms from patients with the disease within a few days and makes them noninfectious. Patients should be treated with erythromycin, 35–50 mg/kg/24 hours orally in 4 divided doses for a period of 14 days. Treatment for less than 14 days is frequently complicated by bacteriologic relapse. Although ampicillin is known to be effective against *B pertussis* in vitro, it is ineffective in producing bacteriologic cures in vivo. This discrepancy has been explained by its poor penetration into respiratory tract secretions. Erythromycin penetrates into the secretions in effective concentrations.

In controlled studies, pertussis immune globulin has not been shown to be of benefit in the treatment of pertussis. Therefore, its use is no longer recommended.

B. General Measures: Nursing care to permit adequate nutritional support during the period of most exhausting paroxysms is one of the most important therapeutic considerations. Frequent small feedings, and refeeding if vomiting occurs, are recommended. Gavage tube feeding and parenteral fluid supplementation may be essential in serious cases in which the nutritional state is poor and continued weight loss cannot be prevented by other means. Gastrostomy feedings may be required.

Minimizing stimuli which trigger paroxysms is probably the best way of controlling cough. In general, cough mixtures are of little benefit.

C. Treatment of Complications: Respiratory insufficiency due to pneumonia or other pulmonary complications should be treated with oxygen and with high humidity. Control convulsions by means of oxygen and parenteral sodium phenobarbital.

Prognosis

The prognosis of pertussis is much improved in recent years because of adequate attention to nursing care. However, the disease is still of serious importance in infants under 1 year of age; about 70% of

deaths due to pertussis occur in this age group. For unknown reasons, the mortality rate is higher among females.

Altemeier WA III, Ayoub EM: Erythromycin prophylaxis for pertussis. Pediatrics 59:623, 1977.

Buck C, Mortimer EA: Whooping-cough vaccination. Lancet 1:746, 1977.

Kendrick PL: Can whooping cough be eradicated? J Infect Dis 132:707, 1975.

Linnemann CC Jr, Perry EB: *Bordetella parapertussis:* Recent experience and a review of the literature. Am J Dis Child 131:560, 1977.

Linnemann CC Jr & others: Use of pertussis vaccine in an epidemic involving hospital staff. Lancet 2:540, 1975.

Nelson KE & others: The role of adenoviruses in the pertussis syndrome. J Pediatr 86:335, 1975.

TUBERCULOSIS

Essentials of Diagnosis

- All types: Positive tuberculin test, chest x-ray, history of contact, and demonstration of organism by stain and culture.
- Pulmonary: Fatigue, irritability, and undernutrition, with or without fever and cough.
- Glandular: Chronic cervical adenitis.
- Miliary: Classical "snowstorm" appearance of chest x-ray; choroidal tubercles.
- Meningitis: Fever and manifestations of meningeal irritation and increased intracranial pressure.

General Considerations

Tuberculosis is a chronic granulomatous disease caused by *Mycobacterium tuberculosis.* It remains a leading cause of death throughout the world, although in the USA human disease caused by the bovine type has been virtually eliminated by pasteurization of milk and control of disease in cattle. The case rate in children under 15 years of age showing a demonstrable lesion is 7 per 100,000 population. For every case of diagnosed disease there are about 80 asymptomatic infections manifested only by tuberculin skin test conversion. Children under 3 years of age are most susceptible, and lymphohematogenous dissemination through the lungs and spread to extrapulmonary sites, including the brain and meninges, eyes, bones and joints, lymph nodes, kidneys, intestines, larynx, and skin are more likely to occur in infants. Increased susceptibility occurs again in adolescence, particularly in girls within 2 years of menarche. Prolonged household contact with an active adolescent or adult case usually leads to infection of infants and children. This is a particularly serious problem among crowded urban populations. The case rate and death rate in nonwhite children are 2–5 times those in white children. The primary complex in infancy and childhood consists of a small parenchymal lesion in any area of the lung with caseation of regional nodes and healing by calcification. There is a strong tendency for lymphohematogenous spread early in primary infection, but chronic pulmonary disease is not common (see Chapter 12). Postprimary tuberculosis in adolescents and adults occurs in the apexes of the lungs and is likely to cause chronic, progressive cavitary pulmonary disease with less tendency for hematogenous dissemination.

Clinical Findings

A. Symptoms and Signs:

1. Pulmonary—See Chapter 12.

2. Miliary—Diagnosis is made on the basis of a classical snowstorm appearance of lung fields on x-ray. The majority also have a fresh primary complex and pleural effusion. Choroidal tubercles are seen in as many as 60% of cases. Other lesions may be present and may be associated with osteomyelitis, arthritis, meningitis, tuberculomas of the brain, enteritis, and infection of the kidneys.

3. Meningitis—Symptoms include fever, vomiting, headache, lethargy, and irritability, with signs of meningeal irritation and increased intracranial pressure, including cranial nerve palsies, convulsions, and coma. Choroidal tubercles are pathognomonic when associated with these signs and symptoms. Otorrhea or acute otitis media may be seen.

4. Glandular—The primary complex may be associated with a skin lesion drained by regional nodes or chronic cervical node enlargement and infection of the tonsils. Involved nodes may become tender, fixed to the overlying skin, and suppurative and may drain.

5. Enteritis—Chronic diarrhea, tenesmus, anemia, fever, and wasting are seen.

B. Laboratory Findings: The Mantoux test using intermediate strength PPD, 0.0001 mg (5 TU) or 0.0002 mg (10 TU), is read as positive at 48–72 hours if there are over 10 mm of induration. The PPD now used should be stabilized with polysorbate 80 (Tween-80) and is identified as PPD-T. The tine test or Heaf test may be used in surveys, but positive responses should be verified by Mantoux testing. The ESR is usually elevated. The CSF in tuberculous meningitis shows slight to moderate pleocytosis (50–300 white cells), decreased glucose, and increased protein.

The detection of mycobacteria in body fluids or discharges is now best done by examination of auramine O stained preparations with blue light (incandescent lamp) fluorescence microscopy, which is superior to the Ziehl-Neelsen method. Specimens are plated for isolation and direct susceptibility to primary drugs (INH, streptomycin, ethambutol, PAS) without reference to microscopic findings on specific culture media. A tentative bacteriologic diagnosis can usually be made within 6 weeks. Sensitivities of the organism should be checked at regular intervals.

C. X-Ray Findings: Chest x-ray shows a fresh primary complex or pleural effusion.

Differential Diagnosis

Pulmonary tuberculosis must be differentiated from sarcoidosis, fungal, parasitic, and bacterial pneumonias, lung abscess, foreign body aspiration, lipoid pneumonia, and mediastinal malignancy. Cervical lymphadenitis is most apt to be due to streptococcal, staphylococcal, or recurrent viral infections. Cat scratch fever and infection with atypical mycobacteria may need to be distinguished from tuberculosis also. Viral meningoencephalitis, head trauma (battered child), lead poisoning, brain abscess, acute bacterial meningitis, brain tumor, and disseminated fungal infections must be excluded in tuberculous meningitis.

Prevention

A. BCG Vaccine: BCG vaccination confers definite but only partial protection and is advised for tuberculin-negative children known to be exposed (limited contact) to adults with active or recently arrested disease. It is advisable to give BCG to newborn infants of tuberculous mothers. BCG is administered intracutaneously over the deltoid or triceps muscle. The dosage is 0.05 ml for newborns and 0.1 ml for older infants and children. The child should not remain in contact with the infected member of the family for at least 2 months afterwards. BCG should never be given to a tuberculin-positive individual; to one with definite or suspected agammaglobulinemia, thymic alymphoplasia, or dysplasia; or to one with skin infection or burns or a recent smallpox vaccination. Some authorities feel that BCG vaccination should be made compulsory for tuberculin-negative school children in slums (urban and rural) before they are admitted to school.

B. Isoniazid (INH) Chemoprophylaxis: Daily administration of INH in therapeutic doses is advised for children who cannot avoid intimate household contact with adolescents or adults with active disease. The dose of isoniazid is 10 mg/kg orally, not to exceed 300 mg daily. Isoniazid is continued throughout the period of exposure and for 6 months after the contact has been broken. BCG is not given during the period of isoniazid chemoprophylaxis.

C. Other Measures: The source contact (index case) should be identified, isolated, and treated to prevent other secondary cases. Exposed tuberculin-negative children should be skin tested every 2 months for 6 months after contact has been terminated. Routine tuberculin skin testing is advised at 12 months of age before live viral vaccines are administered. Routine testing of school children should be done in the first grade and again in the seventh grade. Only when the prevalence of tuberculin sensitivity exceeds approximately 1% (or 10 per 1000) in the schoolage population do the benefits of routine periodic testing appear to outweigh its cost.

Among very malnourished and very ill children with overwhelming infection with bacteriologically proved tuberculosis, it is very common (30%) to find no reaction to intermediate strength PPD. Usually (but not always) the second strength test will be positive. About 20% of patients with recently acquired active disease which is not an overwhelming infection will have negative intermediate strength PPD reactions shortly after admission to a diagnostic ward. After a few weeks, about 98% of these latter cases will have positive intermediate tuberculin reactions.

Certain viral infections, including measles, influenza, varicella, mumps, and probably others; some viral vaccines (measles, influenza, rubella); and administration of corticosteroids and other immunosuppressants may depress or suppress tuberculin reactivity for 2–6 weeks. Malnutrition may have a similar effect.

Treatment

A. Specific Measures: Most patients in the USA are hospitalized at the beginning of treatment but receive most of the prolonged drug course as outpatients. Treatment failure is usually due to the inability of patients (and parents) to cooperate in the long program of therapy.

1. Isoniazid (INH)–INH is given alone to any child without a demonstrable lesion who is tuberculin-positive (with Mantoux reaction measuring less than 18 mm) and is (1) under 6 years of age, (2) adolescent, (3) known to have converted within 1 year, or (4) receiving corticosteroids, antimetabolites, or ionizing irradiation. The dosage is 20 mg/kg orally once a day (or intravenously or intramuscularly if the drug causes vomiting) for 12 months.

2. Aminosalicylic acid (PAS)–Since children have a better tolerance for PAS than do adults, there is still a role for PAS as a primary drug in the treatment of tuberculosis in children. PAS-C, 150 mg/kg/day orally in 2 divided doses, is given in addition to INH for 18–24 months in the following conditions: cervical or hilar lymphadenitis; segmental lung shadow or pleural effusion; tuberculin conversion within the year if there is a demonstrable or "suspicious" lesion; tuberculin-positive reaction measuring 18 mm or more; or a tuberculin-positive girl with a reaction measuring 12 mm or more whose menarche has occurred or will occur within 2 years.

3. Ethambutol (Myambutol)–Ethambutol has not yet been recommended for children under 13 years of age because there is a lack of studies in the USA demonstrating the safety of this drug in children. However, the experience with children in European countries is encouraging. Ethambutol as a second oral drug is used in cases of PAS intolerance and is both effective and well tolerated. In children, the dosage is 15 mg/kg/day orally in 2 divided doses. Retrobulbar neuritis is an uncommon complication of ethambutol treatment in adults, but monthly visual acuity testing is recommended when the drug is being given. Visual acuity can be tested in a 3-year-old child using pictures. The Snellen chart can be used by 5 years of age. Green color vision can also be checked at 5 years of age.

4. Streptomycin or kanamycin–In serious or progressive forms, including meningeal, miliary, renal, osseous, cavitary, and chronic pulmonary tuberculosis, give streptomycin, 20–30 mg/kg/day IM in 1 or 2 doses for 2–4 months in addition to 2 oral drugs. In case of streptomycin resistance, kanamycin, 15 mg/kg/day IM, is given for 1–3 months. Periodic audiometric tests are advisable when either drug is used.

5. Rifampin–Rifampin has been shown in studies conducted in the USA and abroad to be as effective as INH alone. In the USA it is available only for oral use. The dosage is 10–20 mg/kg/day, not to exceed 600 mg/day. It is taken as a single daily dose, either 1 hour before or 2 hours after a meal. It may be used as the third drug, when indicated, to replace streptomycin. At the National Jewish Hospital, Denver, rifampin–not streptomycin–is used as the third drug for treatment of patients with tuberculous meningitis. However, there are now scattered case reports in the European literature of serious–sometimes fatal–hypersensitivity reactions, primarily involving the kidneys. These reactions have been reported where therapy has been intermittent. The patient should be cautioned against intentional or accidental interruption of the daily dosage regimen.

6. Retreatment–Retreating drug-resistant tuberculosis requires giving the patient 3 drugs which he has never had before and to which his organisms are fully susceptible. In vitro sensitivities are mandatory.

B. General Measures:

1. Corticosteroids–These drugs are useful for suppressing inflammatory reactions in meningeal, pleural, and pericardial tuberculosis and for the relief of bronchial obstruction due to hilar adenopathy. Prednisone is given orally, 1 mg/kg/day for 6–8 weeks, with gradual withdrawal at the end of that time.

2. Bed rest–Rest in bed is only indicated while the child feels ill. Isolation is necessary only for children with draining lesions or renal disease and those with chronic pulmonary tuberculosis. Otherwise, children receiving INH–or INH plus ethambutol or PAS– are noninfectious and may attend school.

Prognosis

If bacteria are sensitive and treatment is completed, most patients make lasting recovery. Retreatment is more difficult and less successful. With antituberculosis chemotherapy (especially isoniazid), there should now be nearly 100% recovery in miliary tuberculosis. Without treatment, the mortality rate in both miliary tuberculosis and tuberculous meningitis is almost 100%. In the latter form, about two-thirds of treated patients survive. There may be a high incidence of neurologic abnormalities among survivors if treatment is started late.

Brasfield DM, Goodloe TB, Tiller RE: Isoniazid hepatotoxicity in childhood. Pediatrics 58:291, 1976.

Greenberg HB, Trachtman L, Thompson DH: Finding recent tuberculous infection in New Orleans: Results of tuberculin skin tests on New Orleans children from the inner city and contact investigation program. JAMA 235:931, 1976.

Harris VJ & others: Cavitary tuberculosis in children. J Pediatr 90:660, 1977.

Idriss ZH, Sinno AA, Kronfol NM: Tuberculous meningitis in

childhood: Forty-three cases. Am J Dis Child 130:364, 1976.

Podgore JK: Simultaneous administration of isoniazid and BCG to the infant of a tuberculous mother. J Pediatr 89:679, 1976.

Steigman AJ, Kendig EL Jr: Frequency of tuberculin testing. Pediatrics 56:160, 1975.

INFECTIONS
WITH ATYPICAL MYCOBACTERIA

Essentials of Diagnosis

- Chronic unilateral cervical lymphadenitis.
- Granulomas of the skin.
- Chronic bone lesion with draining sinus (chronic osteomyelitis).
- Reaction to PPD-S (standard) of 5–8 mm, negative chest x-ray, and history of contact with tuberculosis.
- Positive skin reaction to a specific atypical antigen.

General Considerations

Various species of acid-fast mycobacteria other than *Mycobacterium tuberculosis* are now known to cause asymptomatic subclinical infections in wide segments of the population with occasional manifest clinical disease closely simulating tuberculosis. Strain cross-reactivity with *M tuberculosis* can be demonstrated by simultaneous skin testing (Mantoux) with PPD-S (standard) and PPD prepared from one of the atypical antigens. The larger skin reaction represents infection with the homologous strain.

The Runyon classification of mycobacteria now used includes the following:

Group I—Photochromogens (PPD-Y): Yellow color develops upon exposure to light in previously white colony grown 2–4 weeks in the dark. Group includes *M kansasii* and *M balnei* and tends to be more prevalent in the midwestern USA.

Group II—Scotochromogens (PPD-G): Colony is definitely yellow-orange after incubation in the dark. Organisms may be found in small numbers in the normal flora of some human saliva and gastric contents. Subclinical infection is widespread in the USA, but clinical disease appears rarely. Group includes *M scrofulaceum.*

Group III—Nonphotochromogens (PPD-B): "Battey-avian-swine group" grows as small white colonies after incubation in the dark with no significant development of pigment upon exposure to light. Infection with *M intracellulare* ("Battey bacillus") is prevalent in the south and southeastern USA and probably in the New England states. Infection with avian strains is prevalent in Great Britain.

Group IV—"Rapid growers": *M fortuitum* is the recognized pathogen. Within 1 week after inoculation, forms a colony closely resembling *M tuberculosis* morphologically.

Clinical Findings

A. Symptoms and Signs:

1. Pulmonary disease—*M kansasii* accounts for 60% and *M intracellulare* for 30% of pulmonary tuberculosis due to organisms other than *M tuberculosis.* Clinical features and x-ray appearance can be identical to disease caused by *M tuberculosis.*

2. Cervical lymphadenitis—Due to *M intracellulare, M kansasii,* and *M scrofulaceum.* The submandibular or anterior cervical (tonsillar) node is enlarged on one side and persists as a troublesome lump which is discovered fortuitously. There is no response to treatment with penicillin. Such a child might show evidence of pulmonary infection on x-ray (uncommonly) or evidence of disseminated disease (rarely).

3. Swimming pool granuloma—Due to *M marinum.* This is a solitary chronic granulomatous lesion, usually on the elbow, which develops after minor trauma in infected swimming pools.

4. Chronic osteomyelitis—Due to *M kansasii* and *M scrofulaceum.* The child has swelling and pain over a distal extremity, radiolucent defects in bone, fever, and clinical and x-ray evidence of bronchopneumonia. Such cases are rare.

5. Meningitis—Due to *M kansasii.* Disease may be indistinguishable from tuberculous meningitis.

6. Disseminated infection—Rarely, a clinical syndrome resembling an acute hematopoietic malignancy has been reported in association with isolation of *M kansasii,* scotochromogens, *M fortuitum,* or *M intracellulare* from bone marrow, lymph nodes, or liver. Chest x-rays are usually normal.

B. Laboratory Findings: In most cases there is a small reaction (< 10 mm) when Mantoux testing is done with PPD-S. The chest x-ray is negative, and there is no history of contact with tuberculosis. Biopsy of the lesion shows a granulomatous reaction with caseation. Acid-fast bacilli are demonstrated in stained biopsy material. Tuberculosis may be suspected and treatment started with antituberculosis drugs. With these findings, including a Mantoux reaction of < 10 mm, disease due to one of the atypical mycobacteria should be suspected. Simultaneous tuberculin testing with the infecting atypical antigen (PPD-Y, G, or B) will usually give a reaction 2–5 mm greater than the reaction to PPD-S.

Definitive diagnosis is made by isolating the causative agent from clinical material on a medium as described for the isolation of *M tuberculosis.*

Differential Diagnosis

See section on differential diagnosis in the discussion of tuberculosis above and in Chapter 12.

Treatment

A. Specific Measures: Treatment should be individualized and based on in vitro drug sensitivity studies. Recent data indicate that INH, ethambutol, and streptomycin will result in bacteriologic conversion of response in 85% of patients with *M kansasii* infection regardless of in vitro sensitivity. Rifampin is a highly effective drug in this infection and can be used early in therapy or may be reserved for the 15% who fail to respond to other drugs or for the group who later relapse. Chemotherapeutic treatment of *M intracellulare* is much less satisfactory. Rifampin has not markedly altered these responses. Response of *M fortuitum* infections to chemotherapy alone is poor, and drainage procedures are usually required. Swimming pool granuloma due to *M marinum* is treated either with drugs or by surgical excision, with good results. In case of pulmonary and disseminated disease where in vitro resistance appears to be complete, an oral 3-drug regimen of isoniazid, rifampin, and ethambutol plus daily administration of streptomycin or kanamycin IM may be used.

B. General Measures: Isolation of the patient is usually not necessary. General supportive care is indicated for the child with disseminated disease.

Prognosis

The prognosis is good for localized disease, though fatalities occur in immunocompromised children with disseminated disease.

Chang MJ, Barton LL: *Mycobacterium fortuitum* osteomyelitis of the calcaneus secondary to a puncture wound. J Pediatr 85:517, 1974.

Dusty mycobacteria. (Editorial.) Lancet 1:524, 1976.

Herndon JH, Dantzker DR, Lanoue AM: *Mycobacterium fortuitum* infections involving the extremities: Report of three cases. J Bone Joint Surg 54A:1279, 1972.

Kubala E: Some aspects of disease caused by atypical mycobacteria. Scand J Respir Dis (Suppl) 80:11, 1972.

Mandell F, Wright PF: Treatment of atypical mycobacterial cervical adenitis with rifampin. Pediatrics 55:39, 1975.

Pergament M, Gonzalez R, Fraley EE: Atypical mycobacteriosis of the urinary tract. JAMA 229:816, 1974.

LEPROSY

Essentials of Diagnosis

- Pale, anesthetic macular—or nodular and erythematous—skin lesions.
- Superficial nerve thickening with associated sensory changes.
- History of residence in endemic area.
- Acid-fast bacilli in skin lesions or nasal scrapings, or characteristic histologic nerve changes.

General Considerations

Leprosy is a chronic intracellular infectious disease unique to humans. It is usually not fatal. The estimated incubation period of leprosy is 3–5 years.

Thirteen percent of reported cases occur from infancy through 19 years of age.

Clinical Findings

The onset of leprosy is insidious. The lesions involve the cooler tissues of the body: skin, superficial nerves, nose, pharynx, larynx, eyes, and testicles. The skin lesions may occur as pale, anesthetic macular lesions 1–10 cm in diameter; diffuse or discrete erythematous, infiltrated nodules 1–5 cm in diameter; or as a diffuse skin infiltration. Neurologic disturbances are manifested by nerve infiltration and thickening, with resultant anesthesia, neuritis, paresthesia, trophic ulcers, and bone resorption and shortening of digits. The disfiguration due to the skin infiltration and nerve involvement in untreated cases may be extreme.

The disease is divided clinically and by laboratory tests into 2 distinct types: lepromatous and tuberculoid. In the lepromatous type the course is progressive and malign, with nodular skin lesions; slow, symmetric nerve involvement; abundant acid-fast bacilli in the skin lesions, and a negative lepromin skin test. In the tuberculoid type, the course is benign and nonprogressive, with macular skin lesions, severe asymmetric nerve involvement of sudden onset with no bacilli present in the lesions, and a positive lepromin skin test. In the lepromatous type an acute febrile episode with evanescent skin lesions may occur and may last for weeks. Eye involvement (keratitis and iridocyclitis), nasal ulcers, and epistaxis may occur in both types but are most common in the lepromatous type.

Systemic manifestations of anemia and lymphadenopathy may also occur.

Histologic nerve changes are usually characteristic.

Differential Diagnosis

The skin lesions of leprosy must often be distinguished from those of lupus erythematosus, sarcoidosis, syphilis, erythema nodosum, erythema multiforme, and vitiligo; nerve involvement, sensory dissociation, and resulting deformity may require differentiation from syringomyelia and scleroderma.

Complications

Intercurrent tuberculosis is common in the lepromatous type. Amyloidosis may occur with longstanding disease.

Treatment

Drug therapy must be given during periods of exacerbation of the disease. Drugs should be given cautiously, with slowly increasing doses, and must be withheld when they show signs of producing an induced exacerbation with leprotic fever; progressive anemia with or without leukopenia; severe gastrointestinal symptoms, allergic dermatitis, hepatitis, or mental disturbances; or erythema nodosum. It is important, therefore, to observe temperature, blood counts, and biopsy changes in lesions at regular intervals. The duration of treatment must be guided by progress, preferably as judged by biopsy. Treatment must be continued for several years but often indefinitely because recrudescence may occur after cessation of therapy.

Emergence of drug resistance is a recognized problem with sulfone therapy. Inadequate dosage and irregular treatment appear to be contributing factors. Prevention of drug resistance is by adequate and continuous therapy. When sulfone resistance does emerge, clofazimine or rifampin may be considered as substitutes for the sulfones.

A. Dapsone (Avlosulfon, DDS) is given orally to a maximum of 300 mg a week (occasionally up to 600 mg/week, the full adult dose). Start with 25 mg twice weekly and increase to the maximum by 25 mg increments every week, by which time the dose of 300 mg weekly may be spread in daily or other fractions. Selected cases may be treated as outpatients. Children tolerate all the sulfones well in doses proportionate to age (eg, 300 mg/week for a child of 12). If the lepra reaction occurs, stop treatment until recovery is complete and then start again at the beginning or change to another sulfone. (Although all sulfones apparently act in the body in the same way as DDS, some produce fewer reactions.)

B. Solapsone (Sulphetrone), a complex substituted derivative of DDS, may be given orally or parenterally. The adult oral dose is 0.5 gm 3 times daily initially, increasing gradually until a total daily dose of 6–10 gm is being given. The parenteral preparation (50% aqueous solution) is given deeply subcutaneously or intramuscularly in doses beginning with 0.1 ml twice a week and doubling each 2 weeks to a maximum of 3 ml/week in divided doses.

C. Sulfoxone sodium (Diasone) is given orally, 300 mg daily Monday through Friday for 1 week and 600 mg daily Monday through Friday thereafter.

D. Clofazimine (B663; Lamprene), a phenazine dye, is the treatment of choice for patients with DDS-resistant leprosy. The usual dose is 100 mg orally twice weekly. The major side-effect is yellow-red discoloration of the skin, which deepens to brown and blue black. Although pigmentation disappears slowly after withdrawal of the drug, this side-effect is unacceptable to some patients.

E. Surgical care of the extremities (hands and feet) requires careful consideration.

F. BCG vaccination is being studied and shows promise as a means of immunizing children. Both dapsone and BCG are being tested for their prophylactic value for family contacts of patients with lepromatous leprosy.

G. Rifampin is unlike other drugs which are bacteriostatic against *M leprae* in that it is bactericidal. The recommended dose is 600 mg daily. Because the drug is currently so expensive, its principal role is that of an adjunct in the treatment of lepromatous leprosy.

Prognosis

Untreated lepromatous leprosy is progressive and fatal in 10–20 years. In the tuberculoid type, spontaneous recovery usually occurs in 1–3 years; it may, however, produce crippling deformities.

With treatment, the lepromatous type regresses slowly (over a period of 3–8 years), and recovery from the tuberculoid type is more rapid. Recrudescences are always possible and it may be safe to assume that the bacilli are never eradicated. Deformities persist, however, after complete recovery, and may markedly interfere with function and appearance.

Golden GS, McCormick JB, Fraser DW: Leprosy in the United States, 1971–1973. J Infect Dis 135:120, 1977.

Jacobson RR, Hastings RC: Rifampin-resistant leprosy. Lancet 2:1304, 1976.

Pearson JMH, Rees RJ, Waters MFR: Sulphone resistance in leprosy: A review of one hundred proven clinical cases. Lancet 2:69, 1975.

Russell DA & others: Prevention of leprosy by azedapsone. Lancet 2:771, 1975.

BARTONELLOSIS
(Oroya Fever, Carrión's Disease)

Bartonellosis is an acute or chronic infection caused by *Bartonella bacilliformis,* a gram-negative, pleomorphic microorganism occurring in certain mountainous areas of South America. It is transmitted to humans by the sandfly *Phlebotomus verrucarum.* The acute and noneruptive phase (Oroya fever) is characterized by mild or severe fever occurring 2–6 weeks after infection. There may be malaise, headaches, bone and joint pains, and moderate to severe anemia which is of the macrocytic, hypochromic type. Hepatosplenomegaly and lymphadenopathy are common. Superinfection with bacterial pathogens, especially salmonellae, is common at this stage. The acute phase lasts 2–6 weeks. In the severe form of the acute disease, mortality has been 90–95%. In those who survive, the eruptive phase (verruga peruana) begins 2–6 weeks later and lasts from a few weeks to 2 years. Hemangioma-like lesions (verrugas) 1–3 mm in size appear in the skin. There are also subcutaneous lesions, but the miliary skin lesions are more widespread and may become secondarily infected. No scars form unless infections are not treated. In Oroya fever the organisms are seen in the peripheral blood smear by Giemsa stain or by blood culture. Skin lesions may also reveal the organisms. Leukocytosis is rare, but hyperbilirubinemia, reticulocytosis, and megaloblasts and normoblasts are commonly seen.

Chloramphenicol is the drug of choice because of its effect on salmonella superinfection. Penicillin, streptomycin, and tetracyclines in large doses have been used effectively. Blood transfusion is often required.

Recavarren S, Lumbrera H: Pathogenesis of verruga of Carrión's disease: Ultrastructural studies. Am J Pathol 66:461, 1972.

Reyes del Pozo E: Bartonellosis or Peruvian verruca. J Am Med Wom Assoc 24:422, 1969.

Schultz MG: A history of bartonellosis (Carrión's disease). Am J Trop Med Hyg 17:503, 1968.

Wernsdoyer G: Possible human bartonellosis in the Sudan: Clinical and microbiological observations. Acta Trop (Basel) 26:216, 1969.

PSITTACOSIS
(Ornithosis)

Essentials of Diagnosis

- Fever, cough, malaise, chills.
- Rales all over chest; no consolidation.
- Long-lasting x-ray findings of bronchopneumonia.
- Isolation of chlamydia or rising titer of complement-fixing antibodies.
- Exposure to infected birds.

General Considerations

Psittacosis is caused by *Chlamydia psittaci,* a member of the psittacosis-LGV-trachoma group. When the agent is transmitted to humans from psittacine birds (parrots, parakeets, cockatoos, and budgerigars), the disease is often called psittacosis or parrot fever. However, other avian genera (pigeons, turkeys) are common sources of infection in the USA, and the general term ornithosis is often used. The agent is an obligatory intracellular parasite. Human-to-human spread occasionally occurs. The incubation period is 7–15 days.

Clinical Findings

A. Symptoms and Signs: The onset is usually rapid, with fever, chills, headache, backache, malaise, myalgia, epistaxis, dry cough, and prostration. Signs include those of pneumonitis, alteration of percussion note and breath sounds, and rales. Pulmonary findings may be absent early. Rose spots, splenomegaly, and meningismus are occasionally seen. Delirium, constipation or diarrhea, and abdominal distress may occur. Dyspnea and cyanosis may occur later.

B. Laboratory Findings: The white count is normal or decreased, often with a shift to the left. Proteinuria is frequently present. The ornithosis agent is present in the blood and sputum during the first 2 weeks of illness and can be isolated by inoculation of clinical specimens into mice or embryonated hens' eggs. Tissue culture cells, such as HeLa or monkey kidney, can also be used for isolation. Complement-fixing antibodies appear during or after the second week. The rise in titer may be minimized or delayed by early chemotherapy.

C. X-Ray Findings: The x-ray findings in psittacosis are those of central pneumonia which later becomes widespread or migratory. Psittacosis is indistinguishable from viral pneumonias by x-ray.

Differential Diagnosis

This disease can be differentiated from acute viral pneumonias only by the history of contact with potentially infected birds. Rose spots and leukopenia suggest typhoid fever.

Complications

Myocarditis, pericarditis, hepatitis, and secondary bacterial pneumonia.

Treatment

Give tetracyclines in full doses for 14 days. Supportive oxygen is often needed. The patient should be kept in strict isolation.

Durfee PT: Psittacosis in humans in the United States, 1974. J Infect Dis 132:604, 1975.

CAT SCRATCH DISEASE

Essentials of Diagnosis

- History of a cat scratch or contact (95%).
- Healing primary lesion (papule, pustule, conjunctivitis) at site of inoculation.
- Regional lymphadenopathy.
- Aspiration of sterile pus from a node.
- Negative laboratory studies excluding other causes.
- Positive skin test.
- Biopsy of enlarged node showing histopathology consistent with cat scratch disease.

General Considerations

Cat scratch disease is a nonfatal infectious disease of uncertain cause, although the agent is now believed to belong to the chlamydia group, which includes also the agents of psittacosis, lymphogranuloma venereum, and trachoma. Stained sections of primary skin lesions and involved lymph nodes show large numbers of intracellular and extracellular granule-like elementary bodies similar to those seen in psittacosis. Herpes-like virus particles have been seen in cell cytoplasm in tissue taken from infected people. These viruses may be passengers and not etiologic agents. It is possible that more than one agent produces cat scratch disease.

The cat or kitten is merely the healthy carrier of the agent. Also implicated as the source of the scratch or bite are dogs, monkeys, thorns, codfish bones, and wooden splinters. The clinical picture is that of a regional lymphadenitis associated with a distal skin lesion without intervening lymphangitis. The disease occurs worldwide and is more common in the fall and winter.

Clinical Findings

A. Symptoms and Signs: About 50% of patients develop a primary lesion at the site of the scratch or inoculation. The lesion usually is a papule or pustule and is located most often on the arm or hand (50%), head or leg (30%), or trunk or neck (10%). The lesion may be conjunctival (10%). Symptoms are usually not manifest until regional lymphadenopathy accompanied by malaise, lassitude, headache, and fever develop, 10–30 days after the original inoculation. At that time there is some exacerbation of redness and swelling of the primary lesion, which is healing. Axillary, cervical, submental, preauricular, epitrochlear, inguinal, and femoral nodes are commonly involved. Multiple site involvement is seen in about 10% of cases. Involved nodes may be hard or soft and 1–6 cm in diameter. They are usually tender. About 25% of involved nodes suppurate. Overlying skin may or may not be inflamed. Lymphadenopathy may persist for 2 weeks to 8 months but usually lasts about 2 months.

Unusual manifestations include exanthem with nonpruritic maculopapular rash, erythema multiforme or nodosum, or purpura; conjunctivitis with Parinaud's syndrome, parotid swelling, pneumonia, chronic sinus drainage, osteolytic lesions, mesenteric and mediastinal adenitis, and compression peripheral neuritis.

Encephalopathy, believed to represent a delayed hypersensitivity reaction, is unusual but may occur within 1–6 weeks of the onset of adenopathy. Manifestations include coma or convulsions, involvement of cord and nerve roots, lethargy or confusion, choreoathetosis, behavior disorders, and optic neuritis.

B. Laboratory Findings: Skin test antigens are prepared from materials aspirated from nodes of infected individuals although such crude products should be used with extreme caution. Lack of chemical standardization and antigenic variation among different lots of test material are obvious disadvantages. The test is performed by the intracutaneous injection of 0.1 ml of antigen. A positive reaction consists of 5 mm or more of induration or any degree of erythema at the injection site 48–72 hours later. A positive reaction indicates prior contact with the etiologic agent and is not necessarily diagnostic of the present illness. The skin test should be repeated in 1 month in a case where cat scratch disease is clinically suspected but the initial skin test is negative.

Histopathologic examination shows characteristic changes. The lymph node architecture is displaced by multiple areas of central necrosis showing acidophilic staining and surrounded by foci of epithelioid cells and scattered giant cells of the Langhans type. There is usually some elevation in the sedimentation rate. In cases with CNS involvement, the CSF is usually normal but may show a slight pleocytosis and modest elevation of protein.

Differential Diagnosis

Cat scratch disease must be distinguished from pyogenic adenitis, tuberculosis (typical and atypical), tularemia, plague, brucellosis, Hodgkin's disease, lymphoma, rat-bite fever, acquired toxoplasmosis, infectious mononucleosis, lymphogranuloma venereum, and fungal infections.

In the atypical forms of cat scratch disease such as encephalitis, rash, Parinaud's syndrome, parotid swelling, or purpura, the differential diagnosis includes the common causes of these manifestations.

Treatment

The best therapy is reassurance that the adenopathy is benign and will subside spontaneously within 4–8 weeks in most cases. Aspirin may be given for pain. In case of suppuration, node aspiration under local anesthesia with an 18 or 19 gauge needle relieves painful adenopathy within 24–48 hours. In the rare instance of compression peripheral neuritis, excision of the involved node is indicated. In encephalitis, corticotropin gel, 0.8 units/kg/day IM in divided doses every 12 hours for 2–3 weeks, is recommended in addition to supportive therapy.

Prognosis

The prognosis is uniformly good.

Bradstreet CMP, Dighero MW: Cat-scratch fever skin-test antigen. Lancet 1:913, 1977.

Quillian WW II, Quillian WW, Lancaster JW: Non-thrombocytopenic purpura associated with cat-scratch disease. Pediatrics 53:279, 1974.

Schulkind ML, Ayoub EM: Cell-mediated immunity in cat-scratch disease. J Pediatr 85:199, 1974.

SPIROCHETAL INFECTIONS

SYPHILIS

Essentials of Diagnosis

- *Congenital:* In all types, there will be a history of untreated maternal syphilis, a positive serologic test, and positive darkfield examination.
- *Newborn:* Hepatosplenomegaly, characteristic x-ray bone changes, anemia, increased nucleated red cells, thrombocytopenia, abnormal spinal fluid, jaundice, edema.
- *Young infant (3–12 weeks):* Snuffles, maculopapular skin rash, mucocutaneous lesions, pseudoparalysis (in addition to x-ray bone changes).
- *Childhood:* Stigmas of early congenital syphilis (saddle nose, Hutchinson's teeth, etc), interstitial keratitis, saber shins, gummas of nose and palate.
- *Acquired:* Chancre of genitalia, lip, or anus in child or adolescent. History of sexual contact.

General Considerations

Syphilis is a chronic, generalized infectious disease caused by a slender spirochete, *Treponema pallidum.* In the acquired form, the disease is transmitted by sexual contact. Primary syphilis is characterized by the presence of an indurated chancre. A secondary eruption involving the skin and mucous membranes appears in 4–6 weeks. After a long latency period, late lesions of tertiary syphilis involve the eye, skin, bone, viscera, CNS, and cardiovascular system.

After a precipitous decline in incidence between 1947 and 1957, a great increase has been reported in adults, adolescents, and even young children.

Congenital syphilis usually results from transplacental infection after the fourth month of gestation and may result in stillbirth or manifest illness in the newborn, in early infancy, or later in childhood. First trimester fetal syphilis has been found in the products of conception in therapeutic abortions. Syphilis occurring in the newborn and young infant is comparable to secondary disease in the adult but is more severe and life-threatening. Late congenital syphilis (developing in childhood) is comparable to tertiary disease.

Clinical Findings
 A. Symptoms and Signs:
  1. Congenital syphilis—
  a. Newborn—Jaundice, anemia with or without thrombocytopenia, increase in nucleated red blood cells, hepatosplenomegaly, and edema are seen. There may be overt signs of meningitis (bulging fontanel, opisthotonos), but CSF is more likely to be abnormal (increased protein, modest increase in cells). The majority of affected newborns show x-ray changes in the long bones.
  b. Young infant (3–12 weeks)—The infant may appear normal for the first few weeks of life only to develop "snuffles," a syphilitic skin eruption, mucocutaneous lesions, and pseudoparalysis of the arms or legs. Shotty lymphadenopathy may sometimes be felt in addition to organomegaly. Other signs of disease seen in the newborn may be present. Anemia has been reported as the only presenting manifestation of congenital syphilis in this age group. "Snuffles" (rhinitis) almost always appears and is characterized by a profuse mucopurulent discharge which excoriates the upper lip. A syphilitic rash is common on the palms and soles but may occur anywhere on the body; it consists of bright red, raised maculopapular lesions which gradually fade. Moist lesions occur at mucocutaneous junctions (nose, mouth, anus, genitalia) and lead to fissuring and bleeding.

Syphilis in the young infant may lead to stigmas recognizable in later childhood. Thus, such a child may have rhagades or scars around the mouth or nose, a "saddle" nose, and a high forehead (secondary to mild hydrocephalus associated with low-grade meningitis and frontal periostitis). The permanent upper central incisors may be peg-shaped with a central notch (Hutchinson's teeth), and the cusps of the sixth-year molars may have a lobulated mulberry appearance.
  c. Childhood—Bilateral interstitial keratitis (6–12 years) is characterized by photophobia, increased

lacrimation, and vascularization of the cornea associated with exudation. Chorioretinitis and optic atrophy may also be seen. Meningovascular syphilis (2–10 years) is usually slowly progressive, with mental retardation, spasticity, abnormal pupil response, speech defects, and abnormal spinal fluid. Deafness sometimes occurs. Thickening of the periosteum of the anterior tibias produces saber shins. A bilateral effusion into the knee joints (Clutton's joints) may occur but is not associated with sequelae. Gummas may develop in the nasal septum, palate, long bones, and subcutaneous tissues.
  2. Acquired syphilis—The primary chancre of the genitals, mouth, or anus may occur as a result of intimate sexual contact. If the chancre is missed, signs of secondary syphilis may be the first manifestation of the disease.
 B. Laboratory Diagnosis:
  1. Darkfield microscopy—Treponemes can be seen in scrapings from a chancre and from moist lesions.
  2. Serologic tests for syphilis (STS)—All nontreponemal tests currently used are flocculation tests. The most widely used is the Venereal Disease Research Laboratory (VDRL) slide flocculation test. The rapid plasma reagin (RPR) teardrop card test is used for screening only. Specimens showing any degree of reactivity should be subjected to further serologic testing, including quantitation by another nontreponemal test such as the VDRL slide test. Infected newborns may have negative or low titers at birth. High cord blood titers may reflect passive transfer of antibodies. Elevated IgM (> 20 mg/100 ml) or IgA (> 10 mg/100 ml) strongly suggests prenatal infection. Rising titers usually occur within 4 months in infected infants. The VDRL or FTA-ABS test should be employed to screen umbilical cord or neonatal serum for serologic evidence of congenital syphilis, and the IgM FTA-ABS test is especially useful when production of intrauterine IgM antibody has already begun but VDRL and routine FTA-ABS antibody levels have not reached a sufficient magnitude in relation to maternal values to be of diagnostic significance. Since false-positive IgM FTA-ABS reactions occur in less than 10% of cases, the FTA-ABS test is a useful confirmatory procedure. Unfortunately, the false-negative rate can exceed 35%. Since this test for congenital syphilis is insensitive, it cannot be used as a screening procedure, and it cannot replace serial quantitative testing with a nontreponemal test such as the VDRL.
 C. X-Ray Findings: Osteochondritis and periostitis involve the long bones. Occasionally the phalanges and metatarsals are involved. Periostitis of the skull is seen. Bilateral symmetrical osteomyelitis with pathologic fractures of the medial tibial metaphyses (Wimberger's sign) is almost pathognomonic.

Differential Diagnosis
 A. Newborn: Sepsis, congestive heart failure, congenital nephrosis, toxoplasmosis, disseminated herpes simplex, cytomegalovirus infection, and, particularly, hemolytic disease of the newborn have to be differen-

tiated. Positive Coombs test and blood group incompatibility distinguish hemolytic disease.

B. Young Infant: Pseudoparalysis—a flaccid paralysis occurs in poliomyelitis, and signs of scurvy do not appear until the latter half of the first year of life. Injury to the brachial plexus, acute osteomyelitis, and septic arthritis must be excluded. "Snuffles"—coryza due to viral infection—will often respond to symptomatic treatment. Rash—ammoniacal diaper rash—and scabies may be confused with a syphilitic eruption.

C. Childhood: Interstitial keratitis and bone lesions of tuberculosis are distinguished by positive tuberculin reaction and chest x-ray. Arthritis associated with syphilis is unaccompanied by systemic signs, and joints are not tender. Mental retardation, spasticity, and hyperactivity are shown to be of syphilitic origin by strongly positive serologic tests.

D. Acquired Syphilis: Herpes genitalis, traumatic lesions, and other venereal diseases must be differentiated.

Prevention

A serologic test for syphilis should be performed at the initiation of prenatal care and repeated once during pregnancy. Adequate treatment of mothers with secondary syphilis before the last month of the pregnancy will reduce the incidence of congenital syphilis from 90% to less than 2%. The serology of the father and siblings should also be checked.

Treatment

A. Specific Measures: Penicillin is the drug of choice against *T pallidum.* If the patient is allergic to penicillin, erythromycin or one of the tetracyclines may be used.

1. Congenital—Prompt treatment of the infant with penicillin is indicated if there is clinical or x-ray evidence of disease or the cord blood serology is positive and the mother has not been adequately treated. With equivocal findings, the infant may be given protective treatment or followed at monthly intervals with quantitative serologic tests and physical examinations. Rising titers or clinical signs usually occur within 4 months in infants with infection.

Infants with congenital syphilis should have a CSF examination before treatment. Infants with abnormal CSF should receive either of the following: (1) aqueous crystalline penicillin G, 50,000 units/kg IM or IV daily in 2 divided doses for 14—21 days, or (2) aqueous procaine penicillin G, 50,000 units/kg IM daily for 14—21 days. Infants with normal CSF should be given benzathine penicillin G, 50,000 units/kg IM in a single dose. If neurosyphilis cannot be excluded, the procaine or aqueous penicillin regimens are recommended for a minimum of 10 days. Penicillin therapy for congenital syphilis after the neonatal period should use the same dosages recommended for neonatal congenital syphilis. For larger children, the total dose of penicillin need not exceed the dosage used in adult syphilis of more than 1 year's duration.

For interstitial keratitis, a topical corticosteroid

(drops or ointment) should be applied to the affected eye at 2-hour intervals. Herpetic keratitis must be excluded before using topical corticosteroids. The pupil should be kept dilated with a mydriatic.

2. Acquired—1.2 million units of benzathine penicillin G is given IM in each buttock (total dose of 2.4 million units).

B. General Measures: Care should be given to the maintenance of adequate nutrition. Treatment of anemia with transfusion may be necessary before penicillin treatment to prevent a severe Herxheimer reaction.

Prognosis

Severe disease, if unexpected, may be fatal in the newborn. Complete cure can be expected if the young infant is treated with penicillin. Serologic reversal will usually occur within 1 year. Treatment of primary syphilis with penicillin is curative. Permanent neurologic sequelae may be seen with meningovascular syphilis.

Fiumara NJ: Syphilis in newborn children. Clin Obstet Gynecol 18:183, 1975.

Harter CA, Benirschke K: Fetal syphilis in the first trimester. Am J Obstet Gynecol 124:705, 1976.

Kaplan B & others: The glomerulopathy of congenital syphilis: An immune deposit disease. J Pediatr 81:1154, 1972.

Kaplan JM, McCracken GH: Clinical pharmacology of benzathine penicillin G in neonates with regard to its recommended use in congenital syphilis. J Pediatr 82:1069, 1973.

Primary and secondary syphilis—United States, April 1977. Morbid Mortal Wkly Rep 26:207, June 24, 1977.

ENDEMIC SYPHILIS
(Bejel, Skerljevo, Etc)

Endemic syphilis is an acute and chronic infection caused by an organism morphologically indistinguishable from *Treponema pallidum;* it is distinguished from sporadic syphilis by its occurrence in children in crowded, poor households in particular localities, by virtual absence of primary lesions, and the predilection of secondary lesions for oral and nasopharyngeal mucosa as well (in places) as the soles (plantar hyperkeratosis). It is distinguished from yaws by its occurrence in areas in which yaws is not endemic and by the absence of primary lesions and the presence of buccal lesions. It may be confused with angular stomatitis due to vitamin deficiency. It has been reported in a number of countries, including Latin America, often with local names: bejel in Syria and Iraq; skerljevo in Bosnia; dichuchwa, njovera, and siti in Africa. Each has local distinctive characteristics.

Secondary oral lesions are the most common manifestations. Generalized lymphadenopathy and secondary and tertiary bone lesions are common in bejel. Secondary lesions tend to heal in about a year.

Laboratory findings and treatment are the same as for primary syphilis.

Guthe T, Luger A: The control of endemic syphilis of childhood. Int J Dermatol 5:179, 1966.

Hasselmann CM: On endemic, "non-venereal" syphilis. Int J Dermatol 11:57, 1972.

Luger A: Non-venereally transmitted "endemic" syphilis in Vienna. Br J Vener Dis 48:356, 1972.

PINTA
(Carate)

Pinta is a nonvenereal spirochetal infection caused by *Treponema carateum*. It occurs endemically in rural areas of Latin America, especially in Mexico, Colombia, and Cuba; the Philippines; and some areas of the Pacific. A nonulcerative, erythematous primary papule spreads slowly into a papulosquamous plaque showing a variety of color changes (slate, lilac, black). Secondary lesions resemble the primary one and appear within a year after it. These appear successively, new lesions together with older ones. They are commonest on the extremities, but may cover most of the body. Mild local lymphadenopathy is common. Atrophy and depigmentation occur later. Some cases show pigment changes and atrophic patches on the soles and palms, with or without hyperkeratosis, which are indistinguishable from "crab yaws."

Diagnosis and treatment are the same as for primary syphilis.

Mikhail GR, Tanay A: Pinta or pinta-like syphiloderm? Dermatol Trop 3:131, 1964.

Padillia-Goncalves A: Immunologic aspects of pinta. Dermatologica 135:199, 1967.

Pardo-Castello V: Dermatoses of the Americas. Dermatol Trop 2:232, 1963.

Smith JL, Israel CW: A neuro-ophthalmologic study of late yaws and pinta. Trans Am Ophthalmol Soc 68:292, 1970.

YAWS
(Pian, Frambesia)

Yaws is a contagious disease largely limited to tropical regions which is produced by *Treponema pertenue*. It is characterized by granulomatous lesions of the skin, mucous membranes, and bone. Yaws is rarely fatal, although if untreated it may lead to chronic disability and disfigurement. Yaws is acquired by direct nonvenereal contact. The disease is usually acquired in childhood, although it may occur at any age. The "mother yaw," a painless papule which later ulcerates, appears 3–4 weeks after exposure. There is usually associated regional lymphadenopathy. Six to

12 weeks later, similar secondary lesions appear and last for several months or years. Late gummatous lesions may follow, with associated tissue destruction and alterations involving large areas of skin and subcutaneous tissues. The late effects of yaws, with bone change, shortening of digits, and contractions, may be confused with similar changes occurring in leprosy. CNS, cardiac, or other visceral involvement is rare. The Wassermann and flocculation tests are positive, and the spirochetes may be demonstrated by darkfield examination.

Cleanliness of lesions is very important in treatment. Specific measures consist of giving one of the following: (1) procaine penicillin G, 300,000 units IM daily for 7–10 days; (2) one of the tetracyclines, 0.5 gm orally every 6 hours for 10 days; or (3) dichlorophenarsine (Clorarsen), 40 mg IV weekly for 3–6 weeks.

Cahill KM: Tropical medicine for temperate climates: Treponematosis and rickettsiosis. NY State J Med 64:647, 1964.

Lees RE: A selective approach to yaws control. Can J Public Health 64:52, 1973.

Wilson J: Syphilis and yaws: Diagnostic difficulties and case report. NZ Med J 78:18, 1973.

RELAPSING FEVER

Relapsing fever is the name of a group of clinically similar acute infectious diseases caused by several different species of spirochetes of the genus Borrelia. The disease is transmitted to humans by insect vectors (head and body lice and ticks). The insect is infected by feeding on human acute cases (lice) or the animal reservoir (ticks), and transmits the disease to humans when insect feces or crushed insects are rubbed into the bite puncture wound, excoriated areas of skin, or the eyes. The disease is endemic in various parts of the world, including the western USA. The incubation period is 2–15 days (average, about 7 days).

Clinical Findings

A. Symptoms and Signs: The disease is characterized by relapses occurring at intervals of 1–2 weeks after the preceding episode with an interim asymptomatic period. The relapses duplicate the initial attack but become progressively less severe. Recovery occurs after 2–10 relapses.

The attack is of sudden onset with fever, chills, tachycardia, nausea and vomiting, myalgia, arthralgia, bronchitis, and a dry, nonproductive cough. Hepatomegaly and splenomegaly appear later. Jaundice may be present. An erythematous rash appears early in the course of the disease over the trunk and extremities, followed later by rose-colored spots in the same area. Petechiae may also be present. In severe cases, neurologic and psychic manifestations are present. After 3–10 days, the fever falls by crisis. Jaundice, iritis, conjunctivitis, cranial nerve lesions, and uterine hemorrhage are more common in the relapses.

B. Laboratory Findings: During the acute episodes, the urine shows protein, casts, and occasionally erythrocytes; the blood shows a marked polymorphonuclear leukocytosis and, in about one-fourth of cases, a false-positive serologic test for syphilis. During the paroxysm, spirochetes may be found in the patient's blood on darkfield examination or on a blood smear stained with Wright's or Giemsa's stain; or the blood may be injected into a rat and the spirochetes found 3–5 days later in the tail blood. The Weil-Felix test may be positive in a titer of 1:80 or more.

Differential Diagnosis

The late manifestations of relapsing fever may be confused with those of malaria, leptospirosis, dengue, yellow fever, and typhus.

Complications

Facial paralysis, eye diseases such as iridocyclitis, vitreous opacities, and optic atrophy, and possibly hypochromic anemia.

Treatment

Treatment either with (1) tetracycline drugs, 0.5 gm orally every 6 hours for 7 days; or (2) aqueous penicillin, 50,000 units IM every 3 hours, or procaine penicillin G, 300,000 units IM daily for 10 days. Chloramphenicol is often of value.

The more severely ill patients should be hospitalized and should receive intensive care during and after reaction to treatment. Antibiotic treatment should be started at the beginning of a paroxysm or after the fever has dropped in order to avoid a "Jarisch-Herxheimer" reaction, which can be dramatic and even fatal. This reaction is probably due to released endogenous pyrogen. Some severely ill patients have died within hours of an intravenous dose of tetracycline or penicillin.

Prognosis

The overall mortality rate is usually about 5%. Fatalities are most common in debilitated or very young children. With treatment, the initial attack is shortened and relapses largely prevented.

Bryceson ADM & others: Louse-borne relapsing fever: A clinical and laboratory study of 62 cases in Ethiopia and a reconsideration of the literature. Q J Med 39:129, 1970.

DeZulueta J & others: Finding of tick-borne relapsing fever in Jordan by the malaria eradication service. Ann Trop Med Parasitol 65:491, 1971.

Goodman RL, Arndt KA, Steigbigel NH: Borrelia in Boston. JAMA 210:722, 1969.

Smith L, Brown TG: Relapsing fever: A case history. Calif Med 110:322, 1969.

Thompson RS & others: Outbreak of tick-borne relapsing fever in Spokane County, Washington. JAMA 210:1045, 1969.

RAT-BITE FEVER

Rat-bite fever (sodoku) is caused by *Spirillum minus* and transmitted to humans by the bite of a rat. The incubation period is 5–28 days.

Clinical Findings

A. Symptoms and Signs: The original rat bite, unless infected by other organisms, heals promptly, only to be followed after the incubation period by a flare-up at the original site. The area of the rat bite then becomes swollen, indurated, and painful, assumes a dusky purplish hue, and may ulcerate. Regional lymphangitis and lymphadenitis, fever, chills, malaise, myalgia, arthralgia, and headache are present. Splenomegaly may occur. A dusky red, sparse maculopapular rash appears on the trunk and extremities.

After a few days, both the local and systemic symptoms subside, only to reappear again in a few days. This relapsing pattern of fever of 24–48 hours alternating with an equal afebrile period becomes established and may persist for weeks. The local and systemic findings, however—including the rash—usually recur only during the first few relapses.

B. Laboratory Findings: Leukocytosis is often present, and a blood STS may be falsely positive. The organism may be identified by darkfield examination of the ulcer exudate or aspirated lymph node material or by animal inoculation of exudate or blood. The organism cannot be cultured in artificial media.

Differential Diagnosis

In case of a rat bite, the chief problem is distinguishing between infection with *S minus* and *Streptobacillus moniliformis*. *S moniliformis* is characterized by a short incubation period (usually less than 10 days), lack of flare-up of the primary lesion at the onset of systemic symptoms, a high incidence of arthritis (50%), and a low incidence of false-positive STS (15%). This organism can usually be isolated from blood, joint fluid, or pus. Agglutinins against the organism develop during the second or third week of illness. A prolonged incubation period, relapsing instead of sustained fever, and few or no manifestations of arthritis suggest *S minus* infection.

Rat-bite fever may also need to be distinguished from tularemia, relapsing fever, malaria, and chronic meningococcemia.

Treatment

Treat with aqueous penicillin, 100,000 units every 3 hours IM; procaine penicillin G, 300,000 units IM every 12 hours; or tetracycline drugs, 0.5 gm orally every 6 hours for 7 days. Give supportive and symptomatic measures as indicated.

Prognosis

The reported mortality rate is about 10%, but this should be markedly reduced by prompt diagnosis and treatment.

Bradford WL: Rat-bite fever. Pages 461–462 in: *Pediatrics,* 16th ed. Rudolph AM (editor). Appleton-Century-Crofts, 1977.

Farquahar JW, Edmunds PN, Tilley JB: Sodoku in a child. Lancet 2:1211, 1958.

Holmgren EB, Tunevall G: Rat-bite fever. Scand J Infect Dis 2:71, 1970.

LEPTOSPIROSIS

Essentials of Diagnosis

- Biphasic course lasting 2 or 3 weeks.
- Initial phase: high fever, headache, myalgia, and conjunctival injection.
- Apparent recovery for a few days.
- Return of fever associated with meningitis.
- Jaundice, hemorrhages, and renal insufficiency (severe cases).
- Culture of organism from blood and CSF (early) and from urine (later).
- Positive leptospiral agglutination test during convalescence.

General Considerations

Leptospirosis is a zoonotic disease caused by many antigenically distinct but morphologically similar bacteria called leptospires. Humans acquire leptospirosis through accidental contact with infected animals. Classically, the severe form—Weil's disease, with jaundice and a high mortality rate—was associated with infection with *Leptospira icterohaemorrhagiae* following immersion in water contaminated with rat urine. It is now well known that a particular host species (dog, rat, cattle, etc) may serve as a reservoir for one or more serotypes of leptospires, and, conversely, that a given serotype may have multiple animal species as hosts.

Leptospirosis now occurs more commonly in children, students, and housewives than in persons with constant occupational exposure. Urban and suburban cases are now more prevalent than cases from rural areas. Cases acquired from contact with dogs are more than twice as prevalent as those acquired from cattle, swine, or rodents.

The incubation period is 7–12 days. Cases occur in all age groups.

Clinical Findings

A. Symptoms and Signs:

1. Initial phase—Chills, fever, headache, myalgia, conjunctivitis (episcleral injection), photophobia, cervical lymphadenopathy, and pharyngitis occur commonly. This phase lasts for 3 to 4 days up to 1 week.

2. Phase of apparent recovery—Symptoms typically (but not always) subside for 2–3 days.

3. Systemic phase—Fever reappears, completing the "saddleback" temperature curve, and is associated with muscular pain and tenderness in the abdomen and back, nausea and vomiting, and headache. Lung, heart, and joint involvement occasionally occurs. These manifestations are due to extensive vasculitis.

a. CNS—The CNS is most commonly involved. Mild nuchal rigidity is usual, but delirium, coma, and focal neurologic signs may be seen.

b. Renal and hepatic—In about 50% of cases, either or both organs become involved early in the illness. Gross hematuria and oliguria or anuria are sometimes seen. Dysuria is not prominent. Jaundice may be associated with an enlarged and tender liver.

c. Gallbladder—Leptospirosis is a rather common cause of acalculous cholecystitis in children. Such patients may have elevated bilirubin and alkaline phosphatase levels without primary hepatitis. A cholecystogram may demonstrate a nonfunctioning gallbladder. Cholecystotomy or cholecystectomy is required. Pancreatitis is an unusual manifestation.

d. Hemorrhage—Petechiae, ecchymoses, and gastrointestinal bleeding may be severe.

e. Rash—The rash of leptospirosis may be maculopapular and generalized, or petechial or purpuric. Occasionally, erythema nodosum occurs.

Peripheral desquamation of the rash may occur. Gangrenous areas are sometimes noted over the distal extremities. In such cases, skin biopsy demonstrates the presence of severe vasculitis involving both the arterial and the venous circulations.

B. Laboratory Findings: Leptospires may be seen in the blood and CSF only during the first 10 days of illness. They appear in the urine during the second week and may persist for 30 days or longer. Small amounts of blood inoculated into Fletcher's semisolid medium or EMJH semisolid medium will permit isolation of the organism. Multiple cultures should be taken. Identification by dark-field examination is not reliable. Fluorescent antibody technics have been used to demonstrate leptospires in urine and tissues.

The white count may be normal but is more likely to show leukocytosis with liver involvement. Serum bilirubin levels, when elevated, usually remain below 20 mg/100 ml but may go higher. Other liver function tests may be abnormal, although the SGOT usually shows only slight elevation. An elevated serum creatinine phosphokinase is frequently found. CSF shows a moderate elevation of cells ($<$ 500) and protein (50–100 mg/100 ml), but CSF glucose is normal. Urine often shows microscopic pyuria, hematuria, and, less often, proteinuria (++ or greater). BUN is usually below 100 mg/100 ml. The ESR is usually markedly elevated. With lung involvement, chest x-ray may show pneumonitis. EEG and ECG occasionally show abnormal tracings.

The most widely used but least specific rapid screening test for leptospiral disease in human sera is the macroscopic slide agglutination test. The antigen is available commercially, and the test can be performed easily by small hospital laboratories. If positive results are obtained, the titer and specific serotype are determined by microscopic agglutination procedures using live organisms (performed at the Center for Disease Control, Atlanta). Leptospiral agglutinins generally do not reach detectable levels until the first or second week of disease and increase to peak levels by the third to fourth week. A 1:100 titer is considered significant. A 4-fold or greater rise in microagglutinins is usually sought.

Differential Diagnosis

Fever and myalgia associated with the characteristic conjunctival (episcleral) injection should suggest leptospirosis early in the illness. During the prodrome, causes of fever and general myalgia such as malaria, typhoid fever, typhus, rheumatoid arthritis, brucellosis, and influenza may be suspected. Depending upon the organ systems involved, a variety of other diseases need to be distinguished, including aseptic meningitis of viral or tuberculous origin, encephalitis, poliomyelitis, polyneuritis, viral hepatitis, glomerulonephritis, viral or bacterial pneumonia, rheumatic fever, and acute surgical abdomen.

Prevention

Preventive measures include avoidance and treatment of contaminated water and soil, rodent control, vaccination of dogs and other domestic animals, and good sanitation.

With known exposure, give procaine penicillin G, 50,000 units/kg/day IM for 7 days.

Treatment

A. Specific Measures: The efficacy of specific antibiotic treatment has not been clearly established. Treatment within the first 4 days of illness (prodrome) reduces the severity of the disease but has little effect if started later. Give procaine penicillin G, 50,000 units/kg/day IM in 4 divided doses. Continue treatment for 7–10 days. A predictable increase in fever and other signs and symptoms occurs in the majority of patients after the initiation of penicillin treatment.

Tetracyclines may be used as an alternative to penicillin. Give 20 mg/kg/day orally in 4 divided doses.

B. General Measures: Symptomatic and supportive care is indicated, particularly for renal and hepatic failure and hemorrhage.

Prognosis

In the vast majority of cases, leptospirosis is anicteric and recovery is complete. The disease usually lasts 1–3 weeks, but the course may be prolonged. Relapse may occur.

There are usually no permanent sequelae associated with CNS infection. The mortality rate may reach 20% or more in patients who have severe kidney and hepatic involvement.

Barton LL & others: Leptospirosis with acalculous cholecystitis. Am J Dis Child 126:350, 1973.

Buckler JMH: Leptospirosis presenting with erythema nodosum. Arch Dis Child 52:418, 1977.

Geistfeld JG: Leptospirosis in the United States, 1971–1973. J Infect Dis 131:743, 1975.

Pierce JF, Jabbari B, Shraberg D: Leptospirosis: A neglected cause of nonbacterial meningoencephalitis. South Med J 70:150, 1977.

Poh SC, Soh CS: Lung manifestations in leptospirosis. Thorax 25:751, 1970.

Wong ML & others: Leptospirosis: A childhood disease. J Pediatr 90:532, 1977.

• • •

General References

Committee on Infectious Diseases: *Report,* 17th ed. American Academy of Pediatrics, 1974.

Eickhoff TC: Surveillance of nosocomial infections in community hospitals. J Infect Dis 120:305, 1969.

Jawetz E, Melnick JL, Adelberg EA: *Review of Medical Microbiology,* 13th ed. Lange, 1978.

Krugman S, Ward R, Katz S: *Infectious Diseases of Children and Adults,* 6th ed. Mosby, 1977.

27...
Infections: Parasitic

LTC Richard O. Proctor, MD, MPH&TM, FAAP, & T. Jacob John, MBBS, MRCP, DCH

PROTOZOAN INFECTIONS

MALARIA

Essentials of Diagnosis

- Fever, frequently paroxysmal, with shaking chills and marked diaphoresis.
- Splenomegaly and anemia.
- Severe headache, delirium, coma, and convulsions (in cerebral malaria), vomiting, diarrhea, and jaundice.
- Malarial parasites in blood smears.

General Considerations

Despite all attempts at eradication, malaria continues to cause an estimated 30 million new cases and a million deaths annually. In some areas previously cleared (notably South Asia), malaria is now resurgent.

Four species of parasites infect man: *Plasmodium vivax, P falciparum, P malariae,* and *P ovale* (in declining order of frequency). Various species of female anopheline mosquitoes act as vectors. Male and female gametocytes ingested by the mosquito fertilize and develop into sporozoites which are injected into fresh hosts. They develop in parenchymal cells of the liver (pre-erythrocytic cycle), resulting in the release of merozoites into the circulation. Those that escape phagocytization infect red blood cells, mature, and divide into merozoites that are released when the erythrocytes rupture (erythrocytic cycle, schizogony). Others may continue to develop in liver cells (exo-erythrocytic cycle). Merozoites sustain the infection in fresh red cells and repeat the erythrocytic cycle according to a synchronous pattern of 48 or 72 hours, depending on the species of Plasmodium. A few merozoites develop into gametocytes. In time, the erythrocytic cycles dwindle and disappear, and the exo-erythrocytic cycle forms the source for new erythrocytic cycles, causing relapses, except for falciparum malaria, which has no exoerythrocytic cycle, so that relapses after long intervals do not occur.

Malarial infections constitute an intense form of antigenic stimulation leading to the production of antimalarial antibodies detectable by various technics.

Susceptibility to malarial infection varies in different populations, and some individual genes confer some degree of natural immunity (eg, hemoglobin S, hemoglobin F, G6PD deficiency, thalassemia). Natural immunity appears not to prevent infection by the sporozoites, but the clinical manifestation of the disease is reduced or absent, either because of acquired immunity or a sustained premunition.

Repeated infection results in partial immunity, chiefly due to increased cellular rather than humoral defenses. Passive immunity appears to be acquired by the newborn via placental antibody transfer. Congenital malaria is relatively common in babies born to nonimmune but infected mothers but is rare in babies of immune mothers despite heavy placental infections with *P falciparum.*

Malaria must be considered even in nonmalarial areas when the clinical syndrome with fever occurs in a patient who has received blood transfusions or shared a syringe or needle during illicit drug use. An exoerythrocytic cycle does not develop in such cases.

Clinical Findings

A. Symptoms and Signs: The clinical manifestations vary to some degree according to the species of parasite. Minor variations also occur between strains of the same species. In children, the initial clinical picture can be flu-like. In infants, it may be limited at first to fever, vomiting, and diarrhea. On first exposure, the incubation period is 2 weeks for vivax, falciparum, and ovale malaria and about 3–5 weeks for quartan (malariae) malaria. Initially, intermittent or continuous fever occurs and lasts for a variable period. The fever may disappear, only to appear in further episodes. Periodicity characteristic of the species may become established in first or subsequent attacks. In vivax (benign tertian), falciparum (malignant tertian), or ovale malaria, fever occurs on alternate days. In the quartan type, the day of fever is followed by 2 afebrile days. Fever that occurs every day is called quotidian. Considerable variation in the above periodicities occurs as a result of "broods" of the same species or mixed infection. Each paroxysm consists of chills lasting up to 1 hour accompanied by headache, back and muscle pains, and nausea and vomiting; rapid elevation of temperature lasting for several hours accompanied by prostration; and then remission with intense perspiration. These parox-

---

Antiparasitic Drugs & Synonyms

Amodiaquine dihydrochloride (Camoquin, Flavoquine)	Mebendazole (methyl-5-benzoylbenzimidazole-2-carbamate, Vermox)
Amphotericin B (Fungizone)	Melarsoprol (Mel B)
Antimony potassium tartrate (tartar emetic)	Metronidazole (Flagyl)
Antimony sodium dimercaptosuccinate (stibocaptate, Astiban)	Niclosamide (Yomesan)
Antimony sodium gluconate, pentavalent (Pentostam)	Niridazole (Ambilhar)
Bephenium hydroxynaphthoate (Alcopara)	Paromomycin sulfate (Humatin)
Bithionol (Bithin)	Pentamidine isethionate (Lomidine)
Carbarsone	Piperazine citrate (Antepar)
Chloroguanide (Paludrine, Proguanil)	Primaquine phosphate (Neo-Quipenyl, Primaquine)
Chloroquine hydrochloride or diphosphate (Aralen, Avloclor, Nivaquine, Resochin)	Pyrantel pamoate (Combantrin)
Dapsone (Avlosulfon)	Pyrimethamine (Daraprim)
Dehydroemetine dihydrochloride	Pyrimethamine-sulfadoxine (Fansidar)
Dichlorvos (Dichlorman)	Pyrvinium pamoate (Povan)
Diethylcarbamazine citrate (Hetrazan)	Quinacrine hydrochloride (mepacrine, Atabrine)
Diiodohydroxyquin (Diodoquin)	Quinine dihydrochloride and quinine sulfate
Diloxanide (Entamide)	Sodium suramin (Antrypol, Germanin)
Diloxanide furoate (Furamide)	Stibophen (Fuadin)
Emetine hydrochloride	Stilbazium iodide (Monopar)
Ethylstibamine (Neostibosan)	Sulfonamides
Furazolidone (Furoxone)	Tetrachlorethylene
Glycobiarsol (Milibis)	Tetracyclines
Hexylresorcinol (Crystoids Anthelmintic)	L-Tetramisole (Decaris)
Hycanthone methanesulfonate (Etrenol)	Thiabendazole (Mintezol, Thibenzole)
Jonit (phenylene-diisothiocyanate-1,4)	Trimethoprim-sulfamethoxazole (co-trimoxazole)
Lucanthone hydrochloride (Miracil D, Nilodin)	Tryparsamide

---

ysms coincide with the periodicity of the erythrocytic cycle of the parasites, which for unknown reasons develops a curious synchrony. Thus, in its classic form, malaria is manifested by remissions and relapses of paroxysmal fever.

Between attacks, the child may feel well or ill. The spleen gradually becomes palpable and continues to enlarge. Rapid splenic enlargement may cause pain. Herpetic lesions may appear on the lips. Anemia and slight jaundice may become manifest. In the absence of reinfections and complications, the relapses die down in less than a year for falciparum malaria and in a few years for vivax malaria. Quartan malaria may remain dormant or "cryptic" for years or decades and then reappear.

B. Laboratory Findings: The most important part of the investigation is thick and thin blood smears (stained with Giemsa's or Wright's stain), the former for screening and the latter for detailed study. The parasites seen in blood smears are trophozoites, schizonts, and gametocytes—except for falciparum malaria, in which only gametocytes and ring stage trophozoites are ordinarily found in peripheral blood.

Currently available serologic methods of diagnosis include indirect immunofluorescence, passive hemagglutination, and enzyme-linked immunosorbent assay. The latter 2 do not always detect early infection, and the former is the present method of choice. Serologic tests are useful in the detection of carriers among blood donors and also where diagnosis cannot be made by blood smears.

Other laboratory findings include low red and white cell counts, increased unconjugated blood bilirubin, increased serum gamma globulin, and a lowered C3 level. The serologic test for syphilis may be falsely positive.

Differential Diagnosis

Malaria must often be differentiated from tuberculosis, typhoid, and other febrile illnesses, especially recurrent ones such as brucellosis, rat-bite fever, relapsing fever, febrile episodes of lymphoreticular diseases, urinary tract infections, and periodic fevers. Malaria may coexist with other diseases or may be present in unusual circumstances such as undiagnosed postoperative fever. The various complications of *P falciparum* infection are a diagnostic challenge.

Complications & Sequelae

Apart from malignant tertian malaria, the other forms of malaria are relatively free from complications. Chronic malaria may result in anemia and debility. An enlarged spleen may rupture on trivial trauma. Red cells infected with *P falciparum* trophozoites have a tendency to adhere to blood vessels, and in certain viscera, infected red cells and the population of parasites increase in a vicious cycle, causing obstruction and anoxic necrosis which may result in enteritis with gastrointestinal bleeding, interstitial pneumonia, and "encephalitis" (commonly called cerebral malaria).

Severe intravascular hemolysis resulting in hemoglobinuria and shock (blackwater fever) occurs rarely in falciparum malaria. The mortality rate is very high in cerebral malaria and in blackwater fever. Blackwater fever was very common in the past when quinine was widely used as a therapeutic agent.

Severe hemolytic reactions, which may be fatal, occur in black patients who have erythrocyte deficiency of G6PD and are given full doses of primaquine. Where the condition is suspected, one-eighth of the recommended dose is given to start and very gradually increased.

The nephrotic syndrome is seen as a complication of chronic *P malariae*. Massive splenomegaly may lead to hypersplenism with anemia.

Heavy placental infection with the malarial parasite in the pregnant woman interferes with the growth of the fetus and is a common cause of low birth weight. Though rare, infection across the placenta to the fetus occurs.

Prevention

Widespread prophylaxis may not be justified in malarial areas with immune populations of children because later withdrawal of prophylaxis leaves the child highly susceptible to severe disease. However, for nonimmune children living in endemic areas and therefore constantly at risk of infection or reinfection, the best procedure is prophylaxis. Since true prophylaxis (prevention of infection by the destruction of sporozoites) is unavailable, a drug is given that suppresses schizogony and clinical symptoms. It should be started 1 or 2 weeks prior to arrival in any endemic area. The most commonly used suppressive drug is chloroquine, given as follows (dosage expressed as portions of a 250 mg tablet): up to age 1 year, ¼ tablet per week; age 1–3 years, ½ tablet per week; age 7–10 years, ¾ tablet per week; age 11–16 years, 1 tablet per week; over age 16 years, 2 tablets per week. Other suppressive drugs include chloroguanide, 2–3 mg/kg/day; amodiaquin, 7.5 mg/kg/week; and pyrimethamine, 0.5 mg/kg/week. If the suppressive drug is taken for about 4–6 weeks after a person leaves the endemic area, falciparum malaria usually does not become manifest but the other forms of malaria may because of the uncontrolled exoerythrocytic cycle. To avoid this, a course of primaquine may be given as described below.

Because falciparum malaria resistant to chloroquine is widespread in Southeast Asia and South America, chloroquine prophylaxis is not always effective in these areas. The combination of pyrimethamine (25 mg) and sulfadoxine (500 mg), called Fansidar, has been found to be effective in preventing falciparum malaria. The dose is 3 tablets for adults, 2 tablets for teenagers, 1 tablet for children age 5–9, ½ tablet for children age 2–4, and ¼ tablet for children under age 2. Weekly, biweekly, and even monthly doses are effective. Although weekly chloroquine-primaquine plus daily dapsone are recommended as prophylaxis against chloroquine-resistant falciparum malaria, both primaquine and dapsone may cause hematologic disorders.

Since most malarial vectors are night biters, mosquito nets to sleep in and mosquito repellents are important preventive measures. While chemoprophylaxis and the environment engineering or chemical control of mosquito populations currently represent the most feasible mass preventive measures, biologic control of mosquitoes and malarial vaccines are under study for future use.

Treatment

Any child with unexplained fever or coma who has a history of travel in a zone of malarial transmission, blood transfusion or illicit drug injection must be regarded as having malaria until an alternative diagnosis has been established.

A. Specific Measures: In a child with malaria, the first aim of treatment is to terminate the paroxysms with drugs that act on the erythrocytic cycle, ie, chloroquine or quinine. Primaquine may also be used in conjunction with chloroquine to prevent relapses in vivax infections by destroying the exoerythrocytic reservoir of infection.

1. Chloroquine diphosphate–Given once daily orally for 2 days, this is the drug of choice for *P vivax* and nonresistant *P falciparum* infections, which it completely eradicates. Toxic symptoms include nausea, vomiting, and diarrhea. The dosage is as follows:

a. Give 10 mg/kg (maximum, 600 mg) as initial dose. Follow with 5 mg/kg in 6 hours and then 5 mg/kg 18 hours after the second dose and 5 mg/kg 24 hours after the third dose.

b. If oral therapy is not possible, give chloroquine hydrochloride, 2 mg/kg IM or IV immediately and the same dosage once each day for 2 more days. *Caution:* 5 mg/kg or more of injected chloroquine may cause convulsions or even death.

2. Quinine–In chloroquine-resistant falciparum infection, fever persists over 48 hours. Change treatment to quinine.

a. Quinine sulfate, 0.6 gm 3 times daily orally for 5–7 days.

b. Quinine dihydrochloride, 0.5 gm IV diluted in 100 ml or more of physiologic saline solution. *Give very slowly (over 30 min or more).* Use only for patients unable to take oral medication. Follow with oral medication. *Caution:* A very dangerous drug.

3. Primaquine phosphate–A drug used in combination with chloroquine in *P vivax* infections only. It is reported to eradicate the infection and prevent relapses. *Caution:* Primaquine is a toxic drug and must be used with careful laboratory follow-up. Never use in blacks without first testing for G6PD deficiency. If anemia, leukopenia, or methemoglobinemia appears, discontinue use of the drug immediately. Never use with quinacrine or within 5 days of quinacrine therapy.

Give orally once daily for 14 days as follows: up to 15 lb, 2 mg; 15–40 lb, 4 mg; 40–80 lb, 6 mg; 80–120 lb, 10 mg; over 120 lb, 20 mg.

Falciparum malaria contracted in an area reporting strains resistant to chloroquine must be treated with other drugs from the beginning to prevent the rapid build-up of a potentially fatal parasitemia.

4. Newer drugs—Among the drugs that have been tried for chloroquine-resistant falciparum malaria, 2 are very promising. They are pyrimethamine-sulfadoxine (Fansidar) and mefloquine. After 1 or 2 days of quinine therapy (see above), a single dose of Fansidar (see under Prevention) or of mefloquine (not commercially available) has been found to be curative in 96–100% of cases.

B. General Measures: Fluid therapy is most important. Urge oral intake and, if not satisfactory, give parenteral fluids. Control high fever and treat anemia with iron.

Prognosis

In the majority of cases, the prognosis with proper therapy is excellent. In small infants and in the presence of malnutrition or chronic debilitating disease, the prognosis is more guarded.

Asch AJ: Malaria at the Hospital for Sick Children, Toronto. Can Med Assoc J 115:405, 1976.

Butler T & others: Algorithms in the diagnosis and management of exotic diseases. XIII. Malaria. J Infect Dis 133:721, 1976.

Chin N & others: A comparative evaluation of sulfalenetrimethoprim and sulfamethoxine-pyrimethamine against falciparum malaria in Thailand. Am J Trop Med Hyg 22:308, 1973.

Clyde DF: The problem of drug resistant malaria. Am J Trop Med Hyg 21:736, 1972.

Clyde DF & others: Prophylactic and sporontocidal treatment of chloroquine-resistant *Plasmodium falciparum* from Vietnam. Am J Trop Med Hyg 20:1, 1971.

Donno L: Antifolic combinations in the treatment of malaria. Bull WHO 50:223, 1974.

Hall AP: The treatment of malaria. Br Med J 1:323, 1976.

Heyneman D: Medical staff conference: Malaria. Calif Med 118:38, Feb 1973.

Kean BH: Malaria—the mime. Am J Med 61:159, 1976.

Kuti OR: Malaria in childhood. Adv Pediatr 19:319, 1972.

Lewis AN, Ponnampalam TJ: Suppression of malaria with monthly administration of combined sulfadoxine and pyrimethamine. Ann Trop Med Parasitol 69:1, 1975.

Miller LH: Current prospects and problems for a malaria vaccine. J Infect Dis 135:855, 1977.

Powell RD: Development of new antimalarial drugs. Am J Trop Med Hyg 21:744, 1972.

Powell RD, Brewer GJ: Glucose-6-phosphate dehydrogenase deficiency and falciparum malaria. Am J Trop Med Hyg 14:358, 1965.

Powell RD, Tigertt WD: Drug resistance of parasites causing human malaria. Annu Rev Med 19:81, 1968.

Ree GH: Complement and malaria. Ann Trop Med Parasitol 70:247, 1976.

Scholtens RG, Nájera JA (editors): Proceedings of the Inter-American Malaria Research Symposium. Am J Trop Med Hyg 21:607, 1972.

Simpson B & others: Sulphadoxine and pyrimethamine as treatment for acute *Plasmodium falciparum* malaria. Trans R Soc Trop Med Hyg 66:222, 1972.

Sodeman TM: The use of fluorochromes for the detection of malaria parasites. Am J Trop Med Hyg 19:40, 1970.

Thompson PE: The challenge of drug-resistant malaria. Am J Trop Med Hyg 22:139, 1973.

Thompson PE, Werbel LM: *Antimalarial Agents. Chemistry and Pharmacology.* Academic Press, 1972.

Trager W, Jensen JB: Human malaria parasites in continuous culture. Science 193:673, 1976.

Voller A, Bartlett A, Bidwell DE: Enzyme immunoassays for parasitic diseases. Trans R Soc Trop Med Hyg 70:98, 1976.

WHO: Information on malaria risk for international travellers. WHO Weekly Epidemiological Record 3:25, 1973.

Woods WG & others: Neonatal malaria due to *Plasmodium vivax.* J Pediatr 84:669, 1974.

Ziai M & others: Malaria prophylaxis and treatment in G-6-PD deficiency: An observation on the toxicity of primaquine and chloroquine. Clin Pediatr (Phila) 6:243, 1967.

AMEBIASIS

Essentials of Diagnosis

- Acute dysentery: Evidence of colitis, ie, diarrhea with blood and mucus, pain, and tenderness.
- Chronic dysentery: Recurrent symptoms of diarrhea and abdominal pain.
- Hepatic amebiasis: Enlarged and tender liver.
- Amebic abscess: Reddish-brown pus.
- Amebas or cysts in stools or abscesses.

General Considerations

Amebiasis in children is a common and serious problem in some tropical countries but is rare where sanitation is good. Infants and children of all ages may be infected, and the younger the patient the greater the chance that infection has been acquired within the family.

Only the trophozoites (vegetative forms of *Entamoeba histolytica*) invade tissues, and only the cysts can survive outside the host and infect others. Infection occurs by ingestion of the cysts. The question of pathogenicity of strain variants and other species of amebas is controversial. The so-called small race is now considered a separate nonpathogenic species, *Entamoeba hartmanni. E coli* is nonpathogenic.

Infection by *E histolytica* causes disease only in a minority (10–25%) of cases. Asymptomatic carriers often pass cysts and, rarely, vegetative forms.

Clinical Findings

A. Symptoms and Signs: The symptoms of amebic dysentery vary greatly in severity. Typically there is diarrhea with several small stools, not too foul-smelling, with clear mucus and a variable amount of blood. The onset may or may not be sudden. Fever is variable and not usually high. Older children may complain of abdominal pain, either localized over the cecum or sigmoid or generalized. In severe cases, dehydration and prostration may supervene.

Symptoms in chronic intestinal amebiasis also vary greatly in severity. Recurrent complaints of changing bowel habits, abdominal pain, and tenderness over the colon are usual. Chronic dysentery may or may not be preceded by an acute attack. Amebomas are rare in children.

B. Laboratory Findings: The most important investigation is that of satisfactory stool specimens. In acute dysentery, a fresh fecal sample is mounted in warm saline on a warm slide and examined under the microscope. The trophozoites are distinguished by unidirectional movement, size (50–60 μm), a clear ectoplasm, and ingested red cells. In acute dysentery in children, sigmoidoscopy is not usually recommended. It may be done, however, for obtaining ulcer scrapings to look for amebas. Characteristically, the mucosa looks inflamed, with shallow ulcers scattered over otherwise intact mucosa.

In suspected chronic amebiasis, a series of stools should be examined for cysts, preferably on alternate days. Cysts are round or oval, with a diameter 1–2½ times that of a red cell. Immature cysts contain 1–2 nuclei and often 2 chromatoid bodies. More mature cysts contain 4 nuclei and no chromatoid bodies. Staining with Lugol's iodine brings the above features into prominence. If necessary, the stools may be collected after a saline purge. Cysts under 10 μm in diameter are considered to be nonpathogenic *E hartmanni*.

Serologic procedures, such as complement fixation, indirect hemagglutination, counterelectrophoresis, and latex agglutination tests, are of value in extraintestinal amebiasis. Barium enema helps in the differentiation of chronic dysentery from other colonic lesions, but it cannot be used before a search for parasites.

Moderate leukocytosis may be present.

Differential Diagnosis

Acute bacillary dysentery has a more explosive onset and foul-smelling diarrhea, often with blood and mucus. Fever and leukocytosis are often high. A smear of feces reveals the presence of large numbers of neutrophilic leukocytes and bacteria. The final proof is the cultural demonstration of pathogenic bacteria and the absence of amebas.

Other causes of bloody stools such as polyps, anaphylactoid purpura, and nonspecific ulcerative colitis must be differentiated from amebiasis. Schistosomiasis, balantidiasis, regional enteritis, and tuberculous enteritis must be distinguished from acute or chronic amebiasis.

Other causes of chronic and recurrent diarrhea also need to be considered, eg, sprue and malabsorption syndromes.

Complications & Sequelae

Complications may be generally classified as alimentary or extra-alimentary. Acute dysentery may result in perforation of the bowel and peritonitis. Granulomatous proliferations (ameboma) are extremely rare in children.

Amebic hepatitis following amebic colitis consists of hepatic enlargement and tenderness in the absence of demonstrable abscesses. Liver function tests may be only slightly abnormal.

Amebic liver abscess is usually solitary and in the right lobe. Fever, chills, hepatic enlargement, and tenderness are usually present but may be absent in debilitated children. Diagnosis may be readily made with radioisotope (technetium) uptake studies. Rarely, such abscesses rupture into the peritoneum, pleura, lungs, or pericardium. Metastatic abscesses may occur in the lungs, brain, or spleen. Cutaneous and genital lesions are extremely rare.

Treatment

A. Medical Treatment: Several antiamebic drugs are available, but no drug is consistently effective in eradicating infection in 100% of cases. Moreover, drugs vary in their effect against trophozoites or cysts in the intestinal lumen, in the tissues of the intestinal wall, and in the liver and other organs.

1. Amebic dysentery—Several drugs are available for relief of symptoms and eradication of infection. From among the regimens suggested below, any one may be chosen.

a. Metronidazole, given orally in the following dosage, for 10 days: 40–50 mg/kg/day in 3 divided doses, up to a maximum of 2250 mg/day. *Caution:* Metronidazole has recently been shown to be carcinogenic in rodents and mutagenic in bacteria.

b. Oral tetracycline for 5–7 days along with or followed by oral diiodohydroxyquin. The dosage of tetracycline is 15–25 mg/kg/day in 4 divided doses. *Caution:* Tetracyclines are not recommended in children below 7 years of age. The dosage of diiodohydroxyquin is 40 mg/kg/day in 3 divided doses, up to a maximum of 2 gm/day, for 20 days. *Caution:* To avoid toxicity resulting in optic neuritis, do not exceed dosage or duration of therapy. Contraindication: iodine intolerance.

c. Diloxanide furoate, 20–25 mg/kg/day in 3 divided oral doses for 10 days, especially in mild cases. This drug is not available in the USA.

d. Emetine hydrochloride or the less toxic dehydroemetine should be used only in life-threatening dysentery. The dosage is 1 mg (emetine) or 1.5 mg (dehydroemetine)/kg/day IM for 5–8 days. *Caution:* Toxicity may result in peripheral neuritis or myocarditis.

e. Paromomycin, a nonabsorbable antibiotic, given orally in doses of 10–20 mg/kg/day in 3 divided portions for 5 days, is also usually effective.

2. Hepatic amebiasis—Metronidazole, chloroquine phosphate, and dehydroemetine (or emetine) are effective against hepatic amebiasis. In amebic hepatitis, suspected liver abscess, and in proved abscess in a patient who is not very sick, metronidazole, given as described under amebic dysentery, may effect a cure. Failure of treatment, severity of illness, and life-threatening hepatic amebiasis are indications for combination treatment with dehydroemetine (or emetine) plus metronidazole or chloroquine phosphate. The dosage of chloroquine is 10 mg/kg orally twice daily for 2 days and then once daily for 19 days. Opinions vary regarding indications for aspiration of amebic liver abscess. The author recommends aspiration of large and accessible abscesses.

In cases of extra-abdominal amebiasis with pus, treatment should be started as above and pus drained surgically.

3. Chronic amebiasis—Chronic intestinal infection with continued excretion of cysts should be treated to prevent hepatic amebiasis. Effective drugs are dehydroemetine (or emetine), metronidazole, diloxanide furoate, diiodohydroxyquin, chiniofon, iodochlorhydroxyquin, carbarsone, and glycobiarsol. Glycobiarsol, an arsenical, is given in the following dosages: children under 6 years, 250 mg orally once daily for 10 days; older children, 500 mg orally once daily for 10 days. If metronidazole or diloxanide furoate fails to eradicate infection, one of the iodine compounds and one arsenical may be given either together or sequentially.

B. Follow-Up Care: A diligent examination of a series of at least 3 samples of feces should be done on alternate days to make sure that infection has been eradicated in all treated cases.

Prognosis

With prompt diagnosis and adequate treatment, if complications can be avoided, the prognosis is good. In ruptured liver abscesses and in brain abscesses, the prognosis is poor.

Behrens MM: Optic atrophy in children after diiodohydroxyquin therapy. JAMA 228:693, 1974.

Biagi F, Beltran F: The challenge of amoebiasis: Understanding pathogenic mechanisms. Int Rev Trop Med 3:219, 1969.

Cahill KM & others: Symposium on amoebiasis. Bull NY Acad Sci 47:435, 1971.

Gilman RH, Prathap K: Acute intestinal amoebiasis: Proctoscopic appearances with histopathological correlation. Ann Trop Med Parasitol 65:359, 1971.

Maddison SE & others: Comparison of intradermal and serologic tests for diagnosis of amebiasis. Am J Trop Med Hyg 17:540, 1968.

Neal RA: The pathogenesis of amoebiasis. Gut 12:483, 1971.

Nnochiri E: Observations on childhood amoebiasis in urban family units in Nigeria. J Trop Med Hyg 68:231, 1965.

Pittman FE, Pittman JC: Amebic liver abscess following metronidazole therapy for amebic colitis. Am J Trop Med Hyg 23:146, 1974.

Powell SJ: New developments in the therapy of amoebiasis. Gut 11:967, 1970.

Powell SJ: Therapy of amebiasis. Bull NY Acad Med 47:469, 1971.

Powell SJ, Wilmot AJ, Elsdon-Dew R: Single and low dosage regimens of metronidazole in amoebic dysentery and amoebic liver abscess. Ann Trop Med Parasitol 63:139, 1969.

Scragg J: Amoebic liver abscess in African children. Arch Dis Child 35:171, 1960.

Tharavanij S: Immunity in amoebiasis. Pages 22–38 in: *Proceedings of Seminar on Filariasis and Immunology of Parasitic Infections, Singapore.* Sandosham AA, Taman V (editors). Singapore and Bangkok, 1969.

WHO Expert Committee: *Amoebiasis Report.* Pages 1–52.

Technical Report Series No. 421. World Health Organization, 1969.

Wilmot AJ: *Clinical Amoebiasis.* Blackwell, 1962.

Wolfe MS: Nondysenteric intestinal amebiasis: Treatment with diloxanide furoate. JAMA 224:1601, 1973.

Woodruff AW, Bell JS: Amoebiasis: The evaluation of amoebicides. Trans R Soc Trop Med Hyg 61:435, 1967.

PRIMARY AMEBIC MENINGOENCEPHALITIS (PAM)

Essentials of Diagnosis

Naegleria:

- Upper respiratory syndrome followed by rapidly progressing, usually fatal meningoencephalitis.
- Generally healthy young persons with a history of swimming in soil-contaminated water 3–7 days prior to onset.
- Amebas with large central karyosome in fresh wet mount slide of uncentrifuged CSF. Can be cultured in Stamm's medium.

Hartmannella-Acanthamoeba (H-A):

- Variable clinical picture, sometimes with multiple organ involvement.
- More insidious onset of severe meningoencephalitis.
- History of preexisting debilitating disease (metabolic, infectious, or malignant), an immunosuppressed state, or trauma to skin, mucous membranes, and eye.

General Considerations

Beginning in 1965, two distinct genera of free-living, soil- and water-inhabiting amebas were recognized as capable of producing fatal purulent meningoencephalitis. The smaller of the 2, Naegleria (8–15 μm), appears to penetrate the posterior nasopharynx, entering the cranium via the cribriform plate. Its higher incidence in children and young adults may reflect their increased exposure through fresh water swimming and possibly an immunity in older persons based on prior undiagnosed infections. The cysts of Naegleria are not destroyed even by 10 ppm of residual chlorine in water but are susceptible to an 0.7% concentration of NaCl. Naegleria may, under adverse environmental conditions, develop 4–6 flagella transiently.

Acanthamoeba (15–45 μm) does not produce flagella but does possess tapered hyaline projections from its ovoid surface. Both genera are uninucleate, with a large distinguishing central nucleolus. The mechanism by which Acanthamoeba enters the CNS is unclear. Infection has followed skin or mucous membrane trauma in which initial induration disappeared only to be replaced by multiple organ granulomas and eventual meningoencephalitis. The epidemiology of both organisms is far from complete.

Clinical Findings

A. Symptoms and Signs: Naegleria infection has been almost invariably fatal within a week from the appearance of CNS signs. Presentation is frequently with high fever, severe frontal headache, and nausea and vomiting, although the history may include a prior episode of upper respiratory tract infection. Mental signs include stupor, coma, and convulsions followed by death. Patients with Acanthamoeba infections have presented with a variety of clinical pictures including chronic nodular, granulomatous disease of the skin, kidneys, adrenals, pancreas, and brain. Abscesses and hydrocephalus have also been found in cases of Acanthamoeba infection. The amebas themselves produce little exudate in the immediate vicinity but leave behind as they progress a trail of severely lysed and necrotic tissue.

B. Laboratory Findings: Laboratory identification can be made by direct wet mounts of CSF or nasal smears, antiserum staining of fixed tissue or CSF, and cultures on special media.

Differential Diagnosis

Primary amebic meningoencephalitis caused by Naegleria has been likened to meningococcal meningitis in its rapid progression and initial upper respiratory symptoms. Acanthamoeba, on the other hand, more closely resembles chronic mycotic disease of the brain.

Prevention

Amebic meningoencephalitis appears to be a relatively rare disease, and, although it has occurred in time-place clusters of more than one case, its appearance is erratic. Prevention at present would seem to depend upon maintenance of clean swimming pools and education of young people about the danger of swimming anywhere in warm stagnant water. Persons with a history of trauma to the skin, mouth, or eye and those with debilitating disease or who are immunosuppressed for any reason should be suspect if suggestive peripheral lesions or CNS signs appear.

Treatment

Animal experiments and the outcome of treated cases suggest that the best chance of success in treatment of Naegleria rests in early use of intravenous amphotericin B (1 mg/kg/day), with consideration of intrathecal and/or intraventricular use (0.1 mg on alternate days) if improvement does not occur within 48 hours. Acanthamoeba appears to be sensitive to sulfadiazine given intravenously, although in vitro tests have been less encouraging. There are 3.65 mEq of sodium per gram of sulfadiazine, and this should be borne in mind in planning electrolyte management. Corticosteroids, while theoretically of value in the patient with cerebral edema, appear to bind amphotericin B and may result in a critical reduction of the drug in vivo. Chloroquine was credited with the survival of one patient but has failed to produce amelioration in others. Penicillin and other antibiotics have been used without apparent benefit in the treatment of amebic meningoencephalitis. Since treatment must be instituted at the earliest possible time, it is well to use both amphotericin B and sulfadiazine pending positive identification of the organism. Attention must be given to supportive care and the prevention of complicating nosocomial infection. Rehabilitation may be indicated in survivors.

Prognosis

In spite of early successes, the general outlook, especially in infections with Naegleria, is grave. The patient must present early and the diagnosis must be suspected and treatment started before the process becomes irreversible. With Acanthamoeba infection of the CNS, the time factor may still be critical and the history more difficult to interpret.

Carter RF: Primary amoebic meningoencephalitis: An appraisal of present knowledge. Trans R Soc Trop Med Hyg 67:193, 1972.

Duma RJ: Primary amoebic meningoencephalitis. CRC Crit Rev Clin Lab Sci 3:163, 1972.

Duma RJ & others: Primary amoebic meningoencephalitis caused by Naegleria: Two new cases, response to amphotericin B, and a review. Ann Intern Med 74:923, 1971.

Marino JT: Amplification of primary amebic meningoencephalitis. J Pediatr 86:160, 1975.

Nagington J, Richards JE: Chemotherapeutic compounds and acanthamoebae from eye infections. J Clin Pathol 29:648, 1976.

Ringsted J & others: Probable Acanthamoeba meningoencephalitis in a Korean child. Am J Clin Pathol 66:723, 1976.

Willaert E: Primary amoebic meningoencephalitis: A selected bibliography and tabular survey of cases. Ann Soc Belg Med Trop 54:429, 1974.

GIARDIASIS

Most infections with *Giardia lamblia* are asymptomatic or cause only mild symptoms. Diarrhea of insidious onset is the most common manifestation. In some children, steatorrhea with large frothy stools may occur. Vague abdominal pain and tenderness occasionally occur, with few constitutional symptoms.

The organisms usually reside in the duodenum and jejunum. The diagnostic feature is the presence of the organisms in duodenal aspirate or in fresh stools; vegetative forms in diarrheic stools and cysts in formed stools. The frequency and consistency of stools appears to have no relation to the number of organisms seen in the stool specimen. The most sensitive method of diagnosis is to examine smears and sections of upper small intestinal biopsy for trophozoites which are pear-shaped, with 4–5 pairs of notable flagella. There are 2 nuclei with central karyosomes and 2 parabasal bodies, altogether resembling the caricature of a face. They are 12–15 μm in diameter. The cysts are elliptical, with a clear wall and 4 nuclei with karyosomes. Excretion of the cysts is responsible for spread of infection.

Giardiasis must be differentiated from tuberculous enteritis, steatorrhea due to other causes, and chronic amebiasis. Giardiasis may coexist with any of these diseases, and a therapeutic trial may help to clarify the role of Giardia in the total clinical picture.

Metronidazole is the drug of choice.* The dosage is 250 mg orally 3 times daily for 10 days. Alternatively, quinacrine, 8 mg/kg/day in 3 doses for 5 days, will usually clear the infection. Furazolidone (Furoxone) is another drug that has been found to be highly effective in the therapy of giardiasis. The dosage is 6–10 mg/kg/day orally in 4 divided doses orally for 1 week. It is very popular in India because of its low cost.

Ament ME: Diagnosis and treatment of giardiasis. J Pediatr 80:633, 1972.

Ananthasubramanian P & others: Drug trial in giardiasis with furazolidine. Indian Pediatr 13:779, 1976.

Bassily S & others: The treatment of *Giardia lamblia* infection with mepacrine, metronidazole and furazolidone. J Trop Med Hyg 73:15, 1970.

Danciger M, Lopez M: Numbers of Giardia in the feces of infected children. Am J Trop Med Hyg 24:237, 1975.

Kamath KR, Murugasu R: A comparative study of four methods for detecting *Giardia lamblia* in children with diarrheal disease and malabsorption. Gastroenterology 66:16, 1974.

Khambatta RB: Metronidazole in giardiasis. Ann Trop Med Parasitol 65:487, 1971.

Knight R & others: Progress report: Intestinal parasites. Gut 14:145, 1973.

Madanagopalan N & others: A correlative study of duodenal aspirate and faeces examination in giardiasis before and after treatment with metronidazole. Curr Med Res Opin 3:99, 1975.

Walzer PD & others: Giardiasis in travelers. J Infect Dis 124:235, 1971.

Yardley JH, Takano J, Hendrix TR: Epithelial and other mucosal lesions of the jejunum in giardiasis: Jejunal biopsy studies. Bull Johns Hopkins Hosp 115:389, 1965.

BALANTIDIASIS

Dysentery due to *Balantidium coli* infection is far less common than amebiasis. The clinical picture may mimic that of amebic dysentery. It is believed that pigs are the main source of infection. Ingested cysts result in colonic infection by trophozoites. *B coli* usually will live free in the lumen of the intestine; rarely, it may cause ulceration in the colon. In severe infection, the entire lower bowel may be affected.

There may be no symptoms, or symptoms essentially similar to those of acute amebiasis may occur, ie, diarrhea with or without blood and mucus. Slight

leukocytosis may be present, and some degree of eosinophilia is not uncommon.

Examination of fresh feces reveals motile trophozoites, ciliated ovoid bodies approximately $100 \times 50 \mu m$ with a reniform macronucleus, a micronucleus, and several vacuoles. The cysts are about $40 \times 60 \mu m$, containing most of the internal features of the trophozoite.

Intestinal perforation is the major complication. Liver lesions do not occur.

Treatment is with tetracyclines, 20–50 mg/kg/day orally in divided doses for a week; carbarsone in gelatin capsules with 0.25 gm twice a day for 10 days or a 1% enema in a 2% sodium bicarbonate solution (adult dosages); or paromomycin, 1–2 gm daily for 5–10 days.

Marsden PD, Schultze MG: Intestinal parasites. Gastroenterology 57:724, 1969.

Powell SJ: Drug trials in amoebiasis. Bull WHO 40:956, 1969.

Woody NC, Woody HB: Balantidiasis in infancy. J Pediatr 56:485, 1960.

TOXOPLASMOSIS

Essentials of Diagnosis

- Congenital toxoplasmosis: Fever, rash, hepatosplenomegaly, chorioretinitis, hydrocephalus or microcephalus, and mental retardation (in various combinations).

- Acquired toxoplasmosis: Fever, rash, lymphadenopathy, chorioretinitis, encephalitis, and myocarditis (in various combinations). Chronic infection may be afebrile and associated only with lymphocytosis.

- In both cases, the demonstration of *Toxoplasma gondii* or serologic evidence of infection is required for confirmation.

General Considerations

Toxoplasma gondii is a protozoan parasite of various animals and man whose life cycle has been shown to be very similar to that of the coccidian parasite Isospora. Widespread occurrence of asymptomatic infection in man has been demonstrated by seroepidemiology. The vegetative organism is crescentic and 4–7 μm long. It has a single nucleus. In tissues, the parasites appear intracellularly, often in small clusters. True cysts with large numbers of spore-like inclusions form in various tissues but are particularly common in the brain. These are thought to be the stages infective to cats in the brains of mice or possibly to man eating infected meat.

Toxoplasmosis may be congenital or acquired. Congenital toxoplasmosis is acquired in utero from the mother. Most acquired infections, including those of gravid women, remain clinically unrecognized.

The mode of transmission to man remains unclear, though it is thought to be from undercooked

*For *Caution,* see p 804 under Amebiasis.

meat, especially lamb or mutton. Recent work has established that the cat and other felines are probably the normal final hosts and the only ones in which an intestinal Isospora-like stage is found, with infective oocysts being passed in the feces. The organisms may persist in tissues for long periods.

Clinical Findings

A. Congenital Toxoplasmosis: The infected newborn may manifest skin rash (hemorrhagic or otherwise), hepatosplenomegaly, and jaundice. Thrombocytopenia is common. Some infants exhibit CNS disease during the first several weeks of life. Hydrocephalus, microcephalus, CSF pleocytosis and elevated protein, intracranial calcifications, and mental retardation occur in various combinations. Chorioretinitis is common. The systemic manifestations may occur alone or be accompanied or followed by encephalitic features depending upon the stage in utero when the transplacental infection took place.

The organisms may be visualized in or isolated (usually in mice) from infected tissues or CSF. High levels of antibodies (demonstrated by the Sabin-Feldman dye test or hemagglutination test) are present both in the mother and the baby. The demonstration of IgM (19S) antibodies in the baby is further proof of infection.

B. Acquired Toxoplasmosis: Symptomatic acquired infection, though rare, may occur at any age. The clinical manifestations include fever and the following features in varying combinations: generalized lymphadenopathy, muscular pain, maculopapular rash, hepatosplenomegaly, encephalitis, usually unilateral chorioretinitis, pneumonia, and myocarditis. The course may be short or may extend over several weeks. The diagnosis may be confirmed by the demonstration of the organisms or by serology.

The toxoplasmin skin test is of limited diagnostic value. Some clinicians feel that the skin test may aggravate acquired toxoplasmic chorioretinitis.

Differential Diagnosis

Congenital toxoplasmosis may be mistaken for hepatitis due to other causes, septicemia, cytomegalovirus infection, and maternal rubella syndrome. The acquired form must be differentiated from viral encephalitis, viral myocarditis, infectious mononucleosis, and lymphoreticular and lymphoproliferative diseases. Because of the lymphoid proliferation, it may be difficult to differentiate lymphoid toxoplasmosis from lymphosarcoma even on biopsy.

Complications

Nephritis and nephrotic syndrome have recently been recognized as complications of both acquired and congenital toxoplasmosis.

Treatment

A combination of pyrimethamine and a sulfonamide (sulfadiazine or trisulfapyrimidines) is recommended for 3–4 weeks in suspected or proved cases.

Pyrimethamine is given orally in doses of 0.5 mg/kg twice daily in infants and once daily in older children. Sulfadiazine or trisulfapyrimidines are given orally in a dosage of 100 mg/kg daily in 4 divided doses. Both of these drugs may cause gastrointestinal upsets which may necessitate interruption of treatment. Pyrimethamine may cause leukopenia, thrombocytopenia, and, very rarely, agranulocytosis; frequent blood counts should be performed and the drug stopped if the counts fall very low. Folinic acid, 1–3 mg IM once a week, may be given to combat the drug's toxicity.

The neurologic damage that occurs in congenital toxoplasmosis does not subside after treatment. In acquired toxoplasmosis, in the absence of encephalitis and myocarditis, one must use discretion in instituting potentially dangerous therapy. The infection is usually self-limited.

In chorioretinitis, especially in the acquired form, a course of corticosteroids should be given along with antitoxoplasmosis drugs, eg, prednisone, 1 mg/kg orally initially and then reduced gradually. The corticosteroid may be stopped in 3–4 weeks and anti-infective therapy continued until the activity of the eye lesion abates. For recurrence of eye lesions, corticosteroids may be given alone.

The antibiotic spiramycin has been used to treat acquired and congenital toxoplasmosis, especially in Europe. Information on its efficacy is limited, and it is not licensed in the USA.

Boughton CR: Toxoplasmosis. Med J Aust 2:418, 1970.

Desmonts G, Couvreur J: Congenital toxoplasmosis: A prospective study of 378 pregnancies. N Engl J Med 290:1110, 1974.

Feldman HA: Toxoplasmosis. (2 parts.) N Engl J Med 279:1370, 1431, 1968.

Guignard JP, Torrado A: Interstitial nephritis and toxoplasmosis in a 10-year-old child. J Pediatr 85:381, 1974.

Hoare CA: The developmental stages of Toxoplasma. J Trop Med Hyg 75:56, 1972.

Hogan MJ, Kimura SJ, O'Connor GR: Ocular toxoplasmosis. Arch Ophthalmol 72:592, 1964.

Hutchison WM & others: The life cycle of the coccidian parasite *Toxoplasma gondii* in the domestic cat. Trans R Soc Trop Med Hyg 65:380, 1971.

Jones TC: Acquired toxoplasmosis. NY State J Med 69:2237, 1969.

Remington JS: Toxoplasmosis. Page 27 in: *Obstetric and Perinatal Infections*. Charles D, Finland M (editors). Lea & Febiger, 1973.

Shahin B, Papadopoulou ZL, Jenis EH: Congenital nephrotic syndrome associated with congenital toxoplasmosis. J Pediatr 85:366, 1974.

LEISHMANIASIS

1. VISCERAL LEISHMANIASIS
(Kala-Azar)

Essentials of Diagnosis

- High fever, remittent or intermittent—occasionally hectic.
- Splenomegaly and hepatomegaly; often lymphadenitis.
- Progressive anemia, leukopenia, and wasting.
- Demonstration of *Leishmania donovani* in smears of bone marrow or in splenic, hepatic, or lymph node aspirate.
- Positive formol-gel test, complement fixation test, or immunofluorescence test.

General Considerations

Leishmania donovani is a protozoan parasite transmitted by the sandfly (species of Phlebotomus) from man to man (India), from dogs to man (Mediterranean region), or from various carnivores or rodents to man (Sudan). Infantile kala-azar is common in the Mediterranean area; in India, older children are more susceptible; and in other parts of the world, leishmaniasis is primarily an adult disease, probably varying with the timing and intensity of exposure.

The parasites infect and multiply in the reticuloendothelial cells of the spleen, liver, bone marrow, and lymph nodes. In the human body they exist as ovoid bodies 2–4 μm in diameter. With Leishman's or Giemsa's stain, they exhibit a round nucleus and a rod-shaped rhizoplast enclosed in faintly bluish cytoplasm. Appropriate touch-preparation smears show these organisms intracellularly or extracellularly, though the normal site of infection is the macrophage. In the sandfly as well as in artificial (NNN) medium, the parasites exist in a flagellated form, the promastigote.

Clinical Findings

A. Symptoms and Signs: In infants and children, the onset is usually acute, with high fever and gastrointestinal upsets. The spleen enlarges rapidly. There may also be enlargement of the liver (though to a lesser degree) and lymphadenopathy.

In older children, the illness is usually less severe and more prolonged. They remain febrile over long periods, develop hyperpigmentation, lose weight, and become progressively anemic and wasted.

Hypopigmented patches and nodular lesions of varying severity may occur on the face, forearms, and thighs in patients a year or longer after treatment for visceral leishmaniasis. This condition, called dermal leishmanoid or post-kala-azar dermal leishmaniasis, has been reported in India and Africa. The nodular lesions harbor numerous parasites.

B. Laboratory Findings: The diagnosis is confirmed by the presence of *L donovani* in smears of bone marrow or splenic or lymph node aspirate. Rarely, blood smears may reveal the organisms. Blood or bone marrow may be cultured on NNN medium to prove the diagnosis. In chronic cases, a drop of commercial formalin coagulates about 1 ml of serum at room temperature (aldehyde or formol-gel test). Complement fixation and immunofluorescence tests are also available, and an indirect hemagglutination test is under development.

Leukopenia is common, and often quite marked. Thrombocytopenia (with skin hemorrhages) also is common. Anemia and markedly elevated serum gamma globulins are also characteristic.

Differential Diagnosis

Febrile illnesses associated with splenomegaly, such as infective endocarditis, typhoid fever, brucellosis, lymphoproliferative and lymphoreticular diseases, trypanosomiasis, schistosomiasis, and malaria, must be differentiated from kala-azar. Dermal leishmanoid simulates leprosy, yaws, or lupus vulgaris.

Treatment

Correction of nutritional deficiencies (including anemia) and treatment of complicating infections should be done along with specific therapy.

The drugs used in kala-azar are pentavalent antimony compounds (ethylstibamine, urea stibamine, and antimony sodium gluconate) and pentamidine isethionate.

Indian leishmaniasis is easily controlled by treatment, but in Africa the response to specific treatment has been less satisfactory.

The antimony compounds may be given intramuscularly or by slow intravenous injection. Ethylstibamine is given on alternate days in doses of 25 mg in infants less than age 1 and 50 mg in older children for 5 or 6 injections. If parasitism persists after about 2 months, treatment should be repeated. Urea stibamine is given in doses of 10–50 mg on alternate days for a total of 150–750 mg. Antimony sodium gluconate is given in doses of 0.1 ml/kg (20 mg antimony per ml) for 6 injections on alternate days. Antimony compounds may cause vomiting, diarrhea, and muscle cramps; temporary interruption of therapy may be necessary.

Pentamidine may be given intramuscularly in doses of 3 mg/kg of the base daily for 10 days. This drug is useful where the disease is resistant to antimony compounds.

For the nodular type of dermal leishmanoid, a course of a pentavalent antimony compound must be given.

In the USA, antimony sodium gluconate and pentamidine are available through the Parasitic Disease Drug Service, Center for Disease Control, Atlanta (Telephone: 404-633-3311).

Prognosis

In untreated cases, death usually occurs as a result of bacterial complications such as pneumonia.

Adler S: Leishmania. Adv Parasitol 2:35, 1964.

Beveridge E: Chemotherapy of leishmaniasis. Exp Chemother 1:257, 1963.

Hicsönmez G, Ozsoylu S: Kala-azar in childhood: A survey of clinical and laboratory findings and prognosis in 44 childhood cases. Clin Pediatr (Phila) 11:465, 1972.

Hoogstraal H, Heyneman D: Leishmaniasis in the Sudan Republic. 30. Final epidemiologic report. Am Soc Trop Med Hyg 18:1091, 1969.

Leishmaniasis. Bull WHO 44:471, 1971. [Special number; various authors.]

2. CUTANEOUS LEISHMANIASIS
(Oriental Sore)

Leishmania tropica is morphologically identical with *L donovani*. The vector is also the sandfly, but of a different species from the vectors of kala-azar. Cutaneous leishmaniasis has been reported from all inhabited continents. Endemic foci are mostly in India, the Asian countries west of India, and North Africa. Russian investigators recognize 2 forms: the dry type, in urban areas, spread from man to man; and the moist type, in rural areas, transmitted from rodents to man. An area of autochthonous transmission has been identified in south central Texas.

The lesions develop at the sites of sandfly bites after an incubation period of weeks to months. They begin as itchy papules and develop into granulomatous ulcers with scabs. The ulcers gradually extend, and satellite lesions occasionally appear. These lesions occur mostly on the face and limbs, especially in children. The lesions occasionally remain atypical with no ulceration. The onset may or may not be accompanied by fever. After several months, the lesions heal slowly, leaving behind depressed and deforming scars.

In endemic areas the diagnosis is suspected on clinical grounds and confirmed by demonstration of the causative organisms in smears or fluid aspirated from the margins of the lesions. Such specimens may also be cultured on NNN medium.

The leishmanin skin test is positive in all cases except in anergic individuals.

Discrete ulcers may be cleaned and treated with local or systemic antibacterial therapy and allowed to heal, assuring immunity and avoiding potentially toxic drugs. Mild chemical cauterization is recommended by some investigators. In instances of multiple or extensive ulceration and lesions on the face, antibacterial therapy should be accompanied by specific therapy with pentavalent antimony compounds as for visceral leishmaniasis. Stibophen, supplied in 5 ml ampules of 6.3% solution, is an alternative drug. It is given intramuscularly as follows: 0.5 ml on the first day; 1 ml on the second day; third day onward, 1 ml for children weighing less than 15 kg, or 1 ml/15 kg on alternate days for 9 injections.

Prognosis

The prognosis is good except for deforming scars which can be minimized by early treatment.

Bray RS: Leishmaniasis in the Old World. Br Med Bull 28:39, 1972.

Fraser WM & others: Cutaneous leishmaniasis. JAMA 194:1142, 1963.

Johnson CM: Cycloguanil pamoate in the treatment of cutaneous leishmaniasis. Am J Trop Med Hyg 17:819, 1968.

Lainson R, Shaw JJ: Epidemiological considerations of the leishmanias with particular reference to the New World. In: *Ecology and Physiology of Parasites.* Fallis AM (editor). Univ of Toronto Press, 1971.

Shaw PK & others: Autochthonous dermal leishmaniasis in Texas. Am J Trop Med Hyg 25:788, 1976.

Vegas FK: Leishmaniasis tegumentaria americana. Biblioteca Academia Ciencias Fisicas, Matematicas y Naturales 11:1, 1972.

3. MUCOCUTANEOUS LEISHMANIASIS

Except for a few reports, most cases of mucocutaneous leishmania infection are reported from South America. Several different species are now recognized and cause widely varying clinical manifestations. *L braziliensis* causes espundia, the most destructive form of the disease; *L mexicana* causes chiclero's ulcer in Mexico, Guatemala, and Honduras; *L peruviana* causes uta in British and French Guiana and Peru; and several other forms have recently been described. *L braziliensis* is morphologically identical with *L donovani* and is also transmitted by sandflies. The chronic ulcerative lesions may be indistinguishable from those of oriental sore, or they may develop into destructive mucocutaneous lesions over the naso-oral regions. Healing is slow, and in untreated cases heavy scarring occurs. Lesions similar to oriental sore or punched-out ulcers may occur on the face or limbs.

The diagnosis is confirmed by demonstration of *L braziliensis* at the margins of the ulcer. The leishmanin test is usually positive.

Treatment is similar to that of oriental sore, with pentavalent antimonials and antibacterial therapy. Pyrimethamine given orally has been found useful. It is given in 3 ten-day courses of 50 mg/day orally with a rest period of 1 week between courses.

Amphotericin B has been used successfully recently in the treatment of mucocutaneous leishmaniasis.

Crofts MAJ: Use of amphotericin B in mucocutaneous leishmaniasis. J Trop Med Hyg 79:111, 1976.

AFRICAN TRYPANOSOMIASIS
(Sleeping Sickness)

Essentials of Diagnosis
- Trypanosome chancre and erythematous

- nodule at the site of fly bite.
- Fever, progressive anemia and debility, splenomegaly, lymphadenitis, skin rash.
- Changes in personality, disturbances of speech and gait, progressive apathy and somnolence, involuntary movements, and coma.
- Detection of trypanosomes in a wet blood film in rhodesiense infections and by lymph node puncture in gambiense infections.

General Considerations

Trypanosomiasis occurs in parts of tropical Africa. The more virulent Rhodesian form, caused by *Trypanosoma rhodesiense,* occurs chiefly in East Africa, but the Gambian form, caused by *T gambiense,* is more widespread. Both species are transmitted by the bites of tsetse flies (various species of Glossina). In human blood the 2 are morphologically similar—actively motile, slender, wavy, spindle-like bodies with a central nucleus and a prominent flagellum, the trypomastigote stage. Variation in size and body form occurs, with both elongated and "stumpy" forms. This is apparently related to antigenic variation by the parasite and infectivity for the vector.

Gambian trypanosomiasis occurs more commonly in children than the Rhodesian form, except in epidemics of the latter.

Clinical Findings

A. Signs and Symptoms:

1. Rhodesian trypanosomiasis—During the first week, an erythematous, pruritic, and occasionally painful nodule appears at the site of the fly bite, which subsides in a few days. Some patients do not develop this reaction. Fever appears by the second week. It varies in intensity but occurs intermittently or continuously, accompanied by headache, muscular pain, tenderness, and transient skin rashes. Progressive splenomegaly and, to a lesser degree, hepatomegaly are common. Cervical, femoral, or axillary lymph nodes may become palpable. In a few months, weakness, lassitude, emaciation, personality changes, disturbances of speech and gait, and involuntary movements appear. Death may occur before the onset of the classic somnolence.

2. Gambian trypanosomiasis—The early and intermediate stages are similar to those of the Rhodesian form but the progression is slower. Lymphadenitis is more prominent, especially of the posterior cervical glands (Winterbottom's sign). CNS involvement sets in after several months to years. The child becomes very lethargic and sleeps most of the time. Severe emaciation and edema are common. Terminally, coma is followed by death.

B. Laboratory Findings: A wet or stained thick blood smear should be examined for trypanosomes. Repeated examinations are sometimes necessary. Bone marrow aspirate or, preferably, a lymph node aspirate is more likely to be positive in the early and intermediate stages. In the late stages, CSF, especially after

centrifugation, may exhibit the organisms. CSF pleocytosis and elevated protein are usually found. Even in the absence of gross CNS symptoms and signs, pleocytosis and elevated protein are evidences of CNS invasion.

Anemia, elevated erythrocyte sedimentation rate and serum gamma globulins, and hypoproteinemia are some of the accompanying nonspecific features.

Differential Diagnosis

Malaria is not usually difficult to distinguish, but kala-azar may at times be mistaken for trypanosomiasis. Fever, splenomegaly, and lymphadenitis may occur also in lymphoreticular and lymphoproliferative diseases and should be differentiated from trypanosomiasis in endemic areas. Meningitis, especially tuberculous and cryptococcal, and intracranial neoplasms may mimic the CNS manifestations of this disease.

Treatment

A. Specific Measures:

1. Suramin, an organic urea compound, is the drug of choice in the early and intermediate stages without CNS involvement in both the Rhodesian and Gambian forms. It should be given as fresh 10% aqueous solution intravenously in the following dosage: Give a test dose of 20–50 mg with facilities for resuscitation in the event of severe reaction. Continue with 5 doses of 20 mg/kg on days 1, 3, 7, 14, and 21. The appearance of heavy and persistent proteinuria or dermatitis is an indication for discontinuing therapy.

2. Pentamidine isethionate is an alternative drug which may be given in doses of 3–4 mg/kg IM daily for 10 days. It may induce hypotension or hypoglycemia. It is less effective in the Rhodesian form than the Gambian form.

Suramin and pentamidine do not penetrate the CNS, so that treatment with arsenicals is necessary when the brain is involved.

3. Melarsoprol, an arsenical, is the drug of choice in stages with CNS involvement, especially in patients with average nutrition and little renal or hepatic damage. It is given IV as 3.6% solution in propylene glycol, 3.6 mg/kg on alternate days for 3 injections. In severe CNS disease, the course may be repeated after 3 weeks. Any evidence of arsenical toxicity such as mental confusion, encephalopathy, or peripheral neuritis should immediately be treated with dimercaprol (BAL). Headache, vomiting, and proteinuria are indications for discontinuing therapy.

A closely related drug, Mel W, is water-soluble and may be given intramuscularly or subcutaneously. Give fresh 5% aqueous solution in doses of 1, 2, 2, and 4 mg/kg on successive days. In advanced late cases, repeat after 2 weeks. It is less toxic than melarsoprol but is also less effective in Rhodesian trypanosomiasis.

4. Tryparsamide, another arsenical, is less toxic than melarsoprol but may cause optic atrophy. It is more effective against *T gambiense* in CNS than against *T rhodesiense.* The dose is 20–40 mg/kg IV given at weekly intervals for 10 injections. Treatment should be stopped at the appearance of the slightest symptom related to the eyes. In severe and late cases, the course may be repeated after a month.

During the treatment of CNS disease, suramin or pentamidine also should be given to eradicate parasites from the blood and reticuloendothelial system.

B. General Measures: When facilities are available, patients should be hospitalized for therapy. Concurrent infections and nutritional deficiencies should be adequately treated.

Prognosis

Spontaneous recovery occurs occasionally in early cases, and early and intermediate cases do well with treatment. After the CNS has been invaded, the prognosis is less favorable. Untreated cases have an extremely high mortality rate, ie, death occurs within 1 year in Rhodesian and within 10 years in Gambian forms.

Hoare CA: *The Trypanosomes of Mammals. A Zoological Monograph.* Blackwell, 1972.

Mulligan HW (editor): *The African Trypanosomiases.* Wiley-Interscience, 1970.

Robertson DHH: Chemotherapy of African trypanosomiasis. Practitioner 188:80, 1962.

Weinman D: Problems of diagnosis of trypanosomiasis. Bull WHO 28:731, 1963.

AMERICAN TRYPANOSOMIASIS
(Chagas' Disease)

Essentials of Diagnosis

- Chagoma—an erythematous, painful nodule at the site of primary cutaneous infection.
- Unilateral conjunctivitis and palpebral and facial edema—"Romaña's sign."
- Fever, lymphadenitis, myocarditis, occasionally meningoencephalitis.
- Mega-esophagus, megacolon.
- *Trypanosoma cruzi* in blood, bone marrow, or aspirates of lymph nodes or spleen.

General Considerations

Chagas' disease is confined to South and Central America, with the highest incidence in Brazil and Argentina. The causative agent, *Trypanosoma cruzi,* infects man and various animals. It is transmitted through the feces of reduviid bugs—by rubbing feces in skin abrasions or the eye. The organisms multiply locally and invade blood and other tissues.

Clinical Findings

A. Symptoms and Signs: Infants and children are frequently infected in endemic areas. In most cases, a transient lesion (chagoma) develops at the site of primary infection, characterized by an erythematous painful nodule. It is soon followed by local lymph-adenitis, unilateral palpebral and facial edema, conjunctivitis, intermittent or continuous fever, generalized lymphadenitis, hepatosplenomegaly, and myocarditis (tachycardia, cardiomegaly, arrhythmias, and cardiac failure). Occasionally, meningoencephalitis may occur.

In chronic cases, especially in older children and young children who survive the early stages, the main abnormality is myocardial damage. Damage to the myenteric nerve plexuses may result in mega-esophagus and megacolon.

B. Laboratory Findings: In acute Chagas' disease, wet and stained thick blood smears should be examined for *T cruzi.* If they are negative, bone marrow and lymph node or splenic aspirate should be examined. Blood or other specimens may be inoculated into mice, rats, or guinea pigs or cultured in NNN medium. Another method, suitable only during the early, blood-borne phase of the disease, is to feed clean laboratory-grown bugs on patients and to look for the organisms in the bugs' feces after 3–8 weeks. A complement fixation test is also available.

In the acute phase, there is often high leukocytosis, mostly due to mononuclear cells. Cases with myocarditis have x-ray and ECG abnormalities.

Differential Diagnosis

Trichinosis, kala-azar, and bacterial sepsis should be differentiated. In endemic areas, nonpathogenic trypanosomes (*T rangeli*) may be found in blood.

Treatment

Recent experimental trials of metronidazole do not offer much promise that this drug will be of use in trypanosomiasis. However, a new drug, Bayer 2502 (Lampit), has been tried in Brazil and has shown promise. Information regarding Bayer 2502 may be obtained from the Center for Disease Control in Atlanta.

Prognosis

Acute infection may prove fatal to infants and children. Mortality is particularly high in meningoencephalitis. Chronic disease with myocardial damage carries a poor prognosis.

Earlam RJ: Gastrointestinal aspects of Chagas' disease. Am J Dig Dis 17:559, 1972.

Laranja FS & others: Chagas' disease: A clinical, epidemiologic and pathologic study. Circulation 14:1035, 1956.

Olivier MC, Olivier LJ, Segal DB (editors): *A Bibliography on Chagas' Disease (1909–1969).* Index-Catalogue of Medical and Veterinary Zoology. Special Publication No. 2. US Government Printing Office, Washington DC, 1972.

METAZOAN INFECTIONS

NEMATODE INFECTIONS

1. HOOKWORM DISEASE

Essentials of Diagnosis

- Weakness and pallor, with a hypochromic, microcytic anemia.
- Abdominal discomfort, weight loss.
- Occult blood in stool.
- Ova in fecal smears.

General Considerations

The hookworms that commonly infect man are *Ancylostoma duodenale* and *Necator americanus.* Their life cycles are identical, and both occur widely in the tropical and subtropical regions of the world, with Necator the predominant form in the Americas and elsewhere in tropical areas. The larger Ancylostoma is the predominant form in temperate regions, especially North Africa, Europe, Asia, and Japan. It is considerably more pathogenic since it can withdraw substantially more blood per worm.

The adult worms reside mostly in the jejunum. They feed on blood; blood loss from one Ancylostoma may be 0.1–0.5 ml/day, and that from Necator somewhat less. Ova are deposited in the bowel and expelled in feces. In suitable damp, shaded soil, the eggs hatch and develop after about 2 weeks into infective larvae. On contact with human skin (walking bare-footed or handling soil), they penetrate and enter the blood stream, reach the lungs, exit into the alveoli, migrate toward the pharynx, and are swallowed. In the upper intestine, they develop into adults.

In some communities where no organized drainage and sanitation are available, over 90% of individuals may be infected.

Another species, *A braziliense,* a dog or cat hookworm, is a rare human parasite. The infective larvae cause cutaneous larva migrans. This condition has been reported mainly from the American continents.

Clinical Findings

A. Symptoms and Signs: At the skin sites where large numbers of larvae penetrate, especially on and between the toes, intense itching ("ground itch") may occur, particularly in rainy seasons. In cutaneous larva migrans, the larvae penetrate the skin and wander under it, causing irritation, redness, and a slowly creeping eruption.

Small numbers of worms cause no symptoms, and symptoms directly related to the presence of these parasites are never notable. Abdominal pain, discomfort, and distention and changes in bowel habits occasionally occur with heavy infection.

B. Laboratory Findings: Diagnosis is made by identification of ova in fecal smears. They are oval, about 60 × 40 µm, with a segmented egg of 4–16 cells visible through the thin eggshell. Eggs of the 2 species, *Necator americanus* and *Ancylostoma duodenale,* are identical, but identification by means of geographic distribution usually is possible. Moderate to severe anemia of the microcytic hypochromic type is usually present in patients who are chronically ill with hookworm disease. Hypoalbuminemia is an integral part of the disease in these patients and is related to the worm load.

Tests for occult blood in feces are usually positive if there are a sufficient number of worms. Mild to moderate eosinophilia is common.

Complications & Sequelae

By causing a continuous loss of blood, hookworm aggravates nutritional deficiencies. Thus, a progressive iron deficiency anemia is produced in people who are on a low iron intake. Supplemental iron usually prevents hookworm anemia. In patients with borderline folic acid intake, megaloblastic anemia may be produced. The anemia is so insidious that patients may seek medical attention only after cardiac decompensation has occurred. In addition to cardiac failure, hypoalbuminemia may also exist and contribute to anasarca.

Prevention

Prevention of hookworm infection is achieved by avoiding fecal contamination of soil and skin contact with contaminated soil.

Treatment

A. Specific Measures:

1. Bephenium hydroxynaphthoate is the drug of choice, particularly for *A duodenale* infection. It is also effective against roundworms (Ascaris) and can be administered in mixed infections. It is given in a single dose, on an empty stomach, 2.5 gm for children under 20 kg and 5 gm for those above 20 kg. Food should be withheld for 2 hours after administration, but no purgation is necessary. Because of its bitter taste, it is best mixed with fruit juice, flavored liquid, or milk. It may provoke nausea and vomiting, but other side-effects are few. Treatment may be repeated after an interval of 3–4 weeks.

2. Tetrachlorethylene is equally effective and widely used, especially for *N americanus.* It is given orally in a single dose of 0.1–0.12 ml/kg to a maximum of 5 ml on an empty stomach. No purgation is necessary, but a light supper with no fat on the previous night is recommended to prevent absorption of the fat-soluble drug. In severely anemic or debilitated children, treatment for anemia should precede the above therapy. Since it may stimulate roundworms into activity and migration, tetrachlorethylene is better avoided in mixed infection or only given after piperazine therapy. The drug may cause abdominal discomfort and nausea and vomiting. It deteriorates unless kept in a cool place in dark air-tight containers.

3. Newer drugs—A new broad-spectrum anthelmintic of considerable promise against hookworms and other intestinal roundworms is mebendazole (see under Ascariasis). If early reports of its high efficacy and low toxicity are confirmed, mebendazole may become the drug of choice for hookworm infections. Another highly effective drug with low toxicity is pyrantel pamoate (see under Enterobiasis). Jonit is as effective as bephenium and tetrachlorethylene (especially against Necator), with comparable safety. The dosage is three 100 mg tablets at 12-hour intervals after meals.

4. Cutaneous larva migrans may be arrested by topical preparation of 15% thiabendazole powder in a water-soluble base. Oral thiabendazole is effective and the drug of choice. The adult dose is 25 mg/kg twice daily for 2 days.

B. General Measures: In many anemic children, oral iron therapy is of greater value than anthelmintics. Exchange blood transfusions may be lifesaving in severely anemic children in cardiac failure. In less severe cases, parenteral iron therapy is of value.

Prognosis

Except in severely anemic children, the prognosis is good.

Ball PAJ, Bartlett A: Serological reactions to infection with *Necator americanus*. Trans R Soc Trop Med Hyg 63:362, 1969.

Botero D, Castano A: Comparative study of pyrantel pamoate, bephenium hydroxynaphthoate and tetrachlorethylene in the treatment of *Necator americanus* infections. Am J Trop Med Hyg 22:45, 1973.

Burman NN & others: Morphological and absorption studies of small intestine in hookworm infestation (ankylostomiasis). Indian J Med Res 58:317, 1970.

CCTA-WHO: *African Conference on Ancylostomiasis.* Brazzaville, 1961. WHO Technical Report Series No. 255. World Health Organization, 1963.

Rowland HAK: A comparison of tetrachloroethylene and bephenium hydroxynaphthoate in ancylostomiasis. Trans R Soc Trop Med Hyg 60:313, 1966.

2. ASCARIASIS

Essentials of Diagnosis

- Abdominal discomfort and colic.
- The passage of roundworms in feces or the demonstration of ascaris ova.

General Considerations

The roundworm, *Ascaris lumbricoides,* is a cosmopolitan human parasite. Where indiscriminate defecation by children is allowed, the ova are spread widely in the soil where they remain viable for long periods. The ova contaminate food, fingers, toys, etc and are swallowed, to hatch in the upper small intestine. The escaping larvae penetrate the gut wall and, through the portal circulation and the right side of the heart, reach the pulmonary capillaries. They penetrate into the alveoli, are coughed up and swallowed, and mature in the small intestine. Males and females mate, and the female lays thousands of eggs each day.

Clinical Findings

A. Symptoms and Signs: In the great majority of instances, the infection remains silent. However, abdominal pain, anorexia, gastrointestinal upsets, loss of weight, irritability, and short febrile episodes have been attributed to the presence of these worms. Occasionally the worms are excreted in feces or ascend to the stomach and are vomited out.

Large numbers of the larvae migrating through the lungs may cause an acute and often transient "pneumonia" accompanied by eosinophilia (Löffler's syndrome). This syndrome seems to be rare in India. In pediatric practice, large numbers of worms in the gut lumen can cause symptoms of intestinal obstruction.

B. Laboratory Findings: Except when a history of passing roundworms is obtained, the diagnosis is made by the detection of ova in fecal smears. They are approximately 45×60 μm with a brown (bile-stained), heavily mamillated outer coat, a thick middle, and a delicate inner coat covering a densely granular egg cell.

Complications

Large numbers of worms occasionally cause intestinal obstruction, which may be precipitated by treatment in cases of massive infection.

Worms may penetrate the gut wall and cause peritonitis; block the appendiceal lumen, causing acute appendicitis; or block the common bile duct and cause acute obstructive jaundice.

Treatment

In asymptomatic infections, especially in older children, there is no urgency for treatment. The infection is self-limited within a year unless reinfection occurs.

Pyrantel pamoate and mebendazole are the currently recommended drugs of choice. The dosage of pyrantel pamoate is 11 mg/kg as a single oral dose, up to a maximum of 1 gm. The dosage of mebendazole is 100 mg twice daily for 3 days. If follow-up stool examination is positive for ova, treatment should be repeated. For caution regarding mebendazole, see under Enterobiasis.

Piperazine compounds (citrate, adipate, hydrate, or phosphate) are also highly effective and are available as tablets or syrup. Dosage is usually calculated in terms of the hydrous base, piperazine hexahydrate. Piperazine citrate is widely used as a single dose of 75–100 mg/kg, up to a maximum of 3 gm, taken orally after breakfast, either once or, preferably, on 2 consecutive days. No purge is required, and treatment can be repeated after a week in heavy infections. Little or no toxicity is encountered.

Other suitable drugs include thiabendazole (25

mg twice a day for 2 days), hexylresorcinol (dosage as in trichuriasis), and L-tetramisole, 5 mg/kg for 1–2 days.

In massive infection, treatment may result in intestinal obstruction by masses of paralyzed worms.

In the presence of surgical complications, enterotomy with evacuation is perhaps the safest procedure. The administration of a piperazine drug is recommended after about 2 weeks.

Prognosis

The prognosis is good except when massive infection results in bowel gangrene or perforation and peritonitis; in these instances, death may result.

Castro L de P & others: Treatment of ascariasis by tetramisole: Analysis of 1000 cases. Rev Assoc Med Bras 16:43, 1970.

Fernando N: Surgical ascariasis in children (a review of 50 cases). J Trop Pediatr 4:61, 1958.

Franz KH, Schneider WJ, Pohlman MH: Clinical trials with thiabendazole against intestinal nematodes infecting humans. Am J Trop Med Hyg 14:383, 1965.

Goodwin LG, Standen OD: Treatment of ascariasis with various salts of piperazine. Br Med J 1:131, 1958.

Myalvaganam C & others: Extra-intestinal ascaris granuloma. J Trop Med Hyg 72:98, 1969.

Piggott J & others: Human ascariasis. Am J Clin Pathol 53:223, 1970.

Seftel HC, Heinz HJ: Comparison of piperazine and tetramisole in treatment of ascariasis. Br Med J 2:93, 1968.

Tripathy K & others: Effects of Ascaris infection on human nutrition. Am J Trop Med Hyg 20:212, 1971.

Warren KS, Mahmoud AAF: Algorithms in the diagnosis and management of exotic diseases. XXII. Ascariasis and toxocariasis. J Infect Dis 135:868, 1977.

Wolfe MS, Wershing JM: Mebendazole: Treatment of trichuriasis and ascariasis in Bahamian children. JAMA 230:1408, 1974.

3. ENTEROBIASIS
(Oxyuriasis; Pinworm or Seatworm Infection)

Essentials of Diagnosis

- Pruritus ani, especially at night.
- Worms in stool; ova on perianal skin.

General Considerations

Enterobiasis occurs all over the world. Infection is caused by the pinworm or seatworm, *Enterobius vermicularis.* The adult worms reside in the cecum and colon. The gravid females crawl out and deposit thousands of eggs in the skin folds of the anus, especially at night, causing intense itching. When the child scratches, the ova stick to the fingertips and under the nails and eventually get to the mouth and are swallowed, resulting in autoinfection. Contamination of clothes and the environment leads to the infection of fresh hosts; it is not unusual for several members of the same household to harbor pinworms.

Clinical Findings

A. Symptoms and Signs: Pinworms have been blamed for a multitude of minor ills for which proof is difficult to find (eg, bruxism, insomnia, short attention span). A cause and effect relationship can be observed, however, for pruritus ani and pruritus vulvae. Pinworms can induce tiny mucosal ulcers and have been identified in the submucosa and the deeper layers of the bowel wall. They are rarely a cause of appendiceal inflammation. The parasite's ability to penetrate the intact mucosa is controversial, but there seems to be little doubt that they can exploit any breach that is already present. The female worm may become disoriented in her normal migration to deposit eggs, reaching instead the peritoneal cavity via the human female genital tract. Migration into the female urethra has been suggested as one cause of urinary tract infection. In any of these ectopic sites, the parasite may produce a granuloma. Often they produce no symptoms.

B. Laboratory Findings: The diagnosis is confirmed by the detection of ova on the perianal skin. A transparent adhesive tape held tight over the bottom of a test tube with the sticky surface outward is applied to the anus and perianal skin; this is preferably done in the morning, before defecation or washing. The tape is then mounted over a drop of toluene on a glass slide and examined under the microscope. Occasionally, ova and even adult worms may be seen in stools.

The ova measure about 50–60 × 20–30 μm and are oval with one flat surface. The coiled larva is usually visible through the translucent shell.

Differential Diagnosis

All instances of pruritus ani or vulvae are not caused by enterobiasis, though in the absence of other demonstrable causes a therapeutic trial is justifiable.

Treatment

A. Specific Measures: To prevent intrafamilial cross-infection, it is worthwhile treating all individuals in a household simultaneously. Treatment should be repeated after 2 weeks to eradicate infection.

1. Pyrantel pamoate is a highly effective drug active against Ascaris and hookworm as well as pinworm. It is given in a single dose (11 mg/kg), is tasteless, and has minimal side-effects (maximum 1 gm).

2. Mebendazole is a highly effective new drug which is active against pinworm as well as whipworm, Ascaris, and hookworm. It is given in a single dose of 100 mg irrespective of age. *Caution:* Avoid in pregnant women. Experience is scanty in children under 2 years of age.

3. Pyrvinium pamoate in syrup, single dose of 5 mg/kg body weight (maximum of 0.25 gm). It may cause nausea and vomiting, and it turns the stools red.

4. Piperazine compounds (citrate, adipate, hydrate, or phosphate) are nontoxic in therapeutic dosage and are widely used in syrup form. The dosage is 50 mg/kg to a maximum of 2 gm daily in the evenings for 7 days.

B. General Measures: Strict personal hygiene helps prevent autoinfection. Infected children should wear undergarments even while sleeping so that direct contact of fingers with perianal skin can be avoided. The nails should be kept short and clean. Bedclothes and undergarments of infected children should be removed without shaking (to prevent dispersal of ova) and laundered frequently. Since treatment is satisfactory and clinical complications minor, it is often necessary to reassure concerned parents and to prevent their undertaking extreme measures at household sanitation ("pinworm psychosis").

Chandrasoma PT, Mendis KN: *Enterobius vermicularis* in ectopic sites. Am J Trop Med Hyg 26:644, 1977.

Fierlafijn E, Vanparijs OF: Mebendazole in enterobiasis: A placebo-controlled trial in a pediatric community. Trop Geogr Med 25:242, 1973.

Leuin MB: Night cries in little girls. Pediatrics 44:125, 1969.

Mathias AW Jr: *Enterobius vermicularis* infection: Certain effects of host-parasite relationships. Am J Dis Child 101:174, 1961.

Miller MJ & others: Mebendazole: An effective anthelmintic for trichuriasis and enterobiasis. JAMA 230:1412, 1974.

Simon RD: Pinworm infestation and urinary tract infection in young girls. Am J Dis Child 128:21, 1974.

Yokogawa M & others: Mass treatment of *Enterobius vermicularis* infections with pyrantel pamoate. Jpn J Parasitol 19:593, 1970. [In Japanese.]

4. TRICHURIASIS
(Trichocephaliasis, Whipworm)

The whipworm, *Trichuris trichiura*, is a worldwide human and animal parasite. It is still found with regularity in southern USA and was the most common intestinal parasite found among a sample of students of Latin background as far North as Connecticut. The adult worms reside in the cecum and colon, and ova are passed in feces, where they develop to the infective stage in 3–4 weeks. Infective (larvated) eggs then reach the human alimentary canal in contaminated soil, vegetables, toys, etc and hatch in the upper small intestine. There are usually no symptoms except when infection is heavy, causing abdominal pain especially in the right iliac fossa, abdominal distention, and diarrhea. Massive colonic infection may cause dysentery clinically similar to amebic dysentery. The diagnosis is based on demonstrations of ova in fecal smears. They are about 50 × 20 μm, brown, and oval, with 2 polar plugs in the shell. Proctoscopy may reveal grayish-white worms with narrow anterior and broad posterior portions attached to hyperemic mucosa. The whole worm measures 3–5 cm. Mild to moderate eosinophilia may occasionally be present.

The treatment of choice is mebendazole, a new drug that has recently been shown to be highly effective against trichuriasis as well as roundworm, pinworm, and hookworm. The dosage is 100 mg twice daily for 3 days for children of all ages. For caution see under Enterobiasis.

Alternative drugs include thiabendazole (25 mg/kg twice a day for 2 days), stilbazium iodide (20 mg/kg daily for 3 days), and hexylresorcinol, either orally as enteric-coated tablets (100 mg per year of age, once, before breakfast), or rectally as a 0.1% retention enema. *Caution:* Hexylresorcinol is a local irritant to oral mucosa and perianal skin.

Hargus EP & others: Intestinal parasitosis in childhood populations of Latin origin. Clin Pediatr (Phila) 15:927, 1976.

Hutchison JGP: Clinical trial of mebendazole: A broad spectrum antihelminthic. Br Med J 2:309, 1975.

Jung RC, Beaver PC: Clinical observations on *Trichocephalus trichiuris* (whipworm) infestation in children. Pediatrics 8:548, 1951.

Knight R & others: Progress report: Intestinal parasites. Gut 14:145, 1973.

Lynch DM & others: *Trichuris trichiura* infestations in the United Kingdom and treatment with difetarsone. Br Med J 4:73, 1972.

Muqbool S, Lawrence D, Katz M: Treatment of trichuriasis with a new drug, mebendazole. J Pediatr 86:463, 1975.

Wolfe MS, Wershing JM: Mebendazole: Treatment of trichuriasis and ascariasis in Bahamian children. JAMA 230:1408, 1974.

5. STRONGYLOIDIASIS

Essentials of Diagnosis

- Productive cough, blood-streaked sputum.
- Abdominal pain, distention, diarrhea.
- Progressive nutritional deficiencies, eosinophilia.
- Larvae in stool or duodenal aspirate.

General Considerations

Unlike the other helminths considered in this chapter, *Strongyloides stercoralis* has parasitic and free-living forms, which can survive and multiply for a few generations as free-living soil dwellers. As a human parasite, it has been found in most tropical and subtropical regions of the world. The adult worms live in the submucous tissue and the mucosal folds of the duodenum and occasionally occupy the entire length of the intestines. Eggs are deposited in the intestinal mucosa and hatch rapidly. Therefore, both in feces and in duodenal aspirates, the larvae are found commonly but the eggs rarely. However, larvae can occasionally change to the infective stage before leaving the anus, penetrate the bowel wall, enter the blood stream, and initiate an internal autoinfection.

In suitable soil and moisture, the larvae develop rapidly into the skin-penetrating infective stage. Under less suitable conditions, free-living adult worms may develop and reproduce for several nonparasitic generations. Contact with human skin (walking bare-footed or handling soil) facilitates the penetration of skin by the infective larvae, which follow a course much like that of the hookworms and reach the pulmonary capillaries through the blood stream. They escape into alveoli, travel up the bronchial tree, and enter the alimentary canal. In the duodenum, they mature into adults.

Older children and adults are more often affected than young children. Even in areas where the general incidence of strongyloidiasis is low, an occasional patient presents with massive parasitization, chiefly due to internal autoinfection.

Clinical Findings

A. Symptoms and Signs: The site of skin penetration may go unnoticed, or a transient pruritic papular eruption may occur. After heavy exposure, respiratory signs and symptoms may be caused by the migrating larvae. Cough, often productive, with streaks of blood in the sputum, may occur. Abdominal pain, distention, vomiting, and diarrhea with large and pale stools, often with mucus, are the common features.

B. Laboratory Findings: The diagnosis is confirmed by the presence of larvae in feces and duodenal aspirates. They are about 225 μm long, with a double-bulb esophagus which is almost half the length of the larva.

Larvae can sometimes be seen in sputum. A mild to moderate eosinophilia may be present.

C. X-Ray Findings: There may be patchy areas of infiltration on chest x-ray. A barium meal may reveal evidence of duodenitis, including coarse mucosal folds, a widened lumen, and clumping of barium. In severe cases, a pipe-like appearance may occur in the duodenum and elsewhere. These findings simulate those of sprue, regional enteritis, and occasionally ulcerative colitis.

Differential Diagnosis

Symptomatic strongyloidiasis must be differentiated from sprue, other causes of malabsorption, regional enteritis, tuberculous enteritis, and hookworm disease.

Complications & Sequelae

In heavy infection with Strongyloides, chronic diarrhea and malabsorption eventually lead to severe nutritional deficiencies and debility. Paralytic ileus has been known to occur. Several workers have reported fatal strongyloidiasis, nearly all of which were cases of internal reinfection, with massive infection levels and larval worms found throughout the viscera.

Treatment

A. Specific Measures: The treatment of choice is with thiabendazole, 25 mg/kg orally twice daily or 50 mg/kg once daily for 2 days. Close follow-up of treated patients is recommended, as relapses are common. In such instances, specific therapy should be repeated.

B. General Measures: In serious infections, attention to the nutritional and fluid and electrolyte needs is urgent. In many fatal cases, death appears to be due to the severe nutritional defects or to paralytic ileus.

Prognosis

The prognosis is good in mild infection but poor in symptomatic heavy infections with complications.

Beal CB & others: A new technique for sampling duodenal contents. Am J Trop Med Hyg 19:349, 1970.

Bras G & others: Infection with *Strongyloides stercoralis* in Jamaica. Lancet 2:1257, 1964.

Huchton P, Horn R: Strongyloidiasis. J Pediatr 55:602, 1959.

Most H & others: The treatment of Strongyloides and Enterobius infections with thiabendazole. Am J Trop Med Hyg 14:379, 1965.

Purtillo DT, Meyers WM, Connor DH: Fatal strongyloidiasis in immunosuppressed patients. Am J Med 56:488, 1974.

Rivera E & others: Hyperinfection syndrome with *Strongyloides stercoralis*. Ann Intern Med 72:199, 1970.

Walker-Smith JA & others: Strongyloidiasis causing small-bowel obstruction in an aboriginal infant. Med J Aust 2:1263, 1969.

6. TRICHINOSIS

Essentials of Diagnosis

- Vomiting, diarrhea, and abdominal pain within 48 hours of ingesting infected meat.
- Fever, periorbital edema (84% of patients), myalgia, and eosinophilia (97% of patients) about 1 week later.
- Encysted *Trichinella spiralis* larvae in muscle (biopsy).

General Considerations

T spiralis is a small roundworm (1.5 mm male, 4 mm female) which inhabits the intestines of hogs and several other flesh-eating animals. The larvae are ingested in the muscle meats of pork, bear, walrus, etc. They are liberated by digestion of their capsule and immediately enter the mucosa of the upper small intestine, where they develop into adult worms before emerging. The fertilized female burrows again into the mucosa, where she may release more than 1000 larvae within the next few weeks to months. The larvae enter the blood stream and reach the striated musculature before becoming encysted. They may cause significant damage to many tissues as they migrate. Man is thereby a dead end for the parasite. Trichinosis is largely a disease of North America, parts of Europe, and the Soviet Union. In 1975, the number of cases reported in the USA was 284, with one death. Most of these occurred in single-source outbreaks of 2–28 persons each. Only 36 patients (13%) were under 19 years old. Ground beef may be contaminated with pork left in the grinding machine.

Clinical Findings

Illness begins when excysted larvae from infected meat penetrate the small bowel mucosa, producing nausea, vomiting, diarrhea (occasionally with some bleeding), and abdominal cramps. This occurs 1–2 days after ingestion. Most patients are without symptoms or experience only the gastrointestinal phase in a mild form. In some cases, the migration of larvae is heralded by fever, edema (especially face and eyelids), and moderate to severe myalgia. Muscles with a low glycogen content (eg, diaphragm) are more apt to be heavily invaded. Larval migrations are extensive, however, and symptoms may indicate involvement of the heart, lungs, kidneys, and brain. The patient may become progressively more neurotoxic and die at 4–6 weeks. Although recuperation may begin about the fifth week, the continued release of larvae can result in symptoms for several months. A rash can occur. Splenomegaly is not uncommon.

Differential Diagnosis

At times, a typhoidal picture may be seen in trichinosis. The triad of periorbital edema, eosinophilia, and myalgia is so characteristic that it is only necessary to be aware of its meaning (ie, trichinosis) to make the presumptive diagnosis.

Complications & Sequelae

Marked inflammation of virtually any tissue can occur. If the mass of larvae is sufficiently large, the toxicity can threaten life.

Prevention

The United States Department of Agriculture does not inspect meat in the USA for trichinosis. There are, however, laws in all 50 states requiring the cooking of swill fed to hogs. Since hog-to-hog or hog-rat cycles of transmission are still possible, it is necessary to educate the public about personal prevention. All pork should be heated to at least 65° C (149° F) at the center of the cut. The same applies to all sylvatic meats (bear, walrus, etc). It is thought that freezing meat at −15° C (5° F) for 3 weeks prevents transmission, but there is some recent question about this.

No animal that is used for food should be allowed access to carrion. Hog farms in particular should be cleared of rats.

Treatment

Although thiabendazole (50 mg/kg/day for 1 week) has been successful in some cases in treating the larval phase of trichinosis, its use is sometimes limited by side-effects. Mebendazole has recently shown promise in its larvicidal effects (including the encysted form) as well as some effect against the mature worm. It has been used at a dosage of 50 mg/kg/day up to 14 days in mice. Considering its relative lack of toxicity, it deserves a trial in humans. Insufficient data exist to justify a recommendation for the use of thiabendazole in pregnant women or children under 2 years of age. Corticosteroids have proved useful in decreasing the severity of symptoms, but their use may aid survival of the mature female worm and thus the total numbers of larvae liberated. General supportive measures are indicated. Where exposure has been recognized before the onset of initial gastrointestinal symptoms, saline purga-

tives may help eliminate some developing larvae. No therapy to date is considered truly specific.

Prognosis

The vast majority of symptomatic cases can be managed without significant threat to life or fear of residual disability. Death, when it occurs, generally occurs at about the fifth week. Survivors of this critical period usually recover.

Despommier D & others: Immunodiagnosis of human trichinosis using counterelectrophoresis and agar gel diffusion techniques. Am J Trop Med Hyg 23:41, 1974.

Fernando SSE, Denham DA: The effect of mebendazole and fenbendazole on *Trichinella spiralis* in mice. J Parasitol 62:874, 1976.

Gould SE & others: Diagnostic patterns: *Trichinella spiralis*. Am J Clin Pathol 40:197, 1963.

Maynard JE, Kagan IG: Trichinosis. Practitioner 191:622, 1963.

7. DRACUNCULOSIS
(Dracontiasis, Guinea Worm Infection)

Dracunculus medinensis (guinea worm) is a common parasite of man in some parts of India, West Asia, and Africa. Infection results from drinking water containing small copepod crustaceans (Cyclops) harboring mature larvae. The larvae penetrate the intestinal mucosa, develop in the abdominal cavity for about a year, and then the mated female worms migrate to the subcutaneous tissues of the lower extremities or back. They may also reach various other tissues and die, causing few or no symptoms. The female lies under the skin, from which larvae are discharged through a skin blister near the head of the female adult worm, when the skin is in contact with water. Thus, farm workers and water carriers who wade into step-in wells both suffer from and perpetuate dracontiasis.

There have been few reports on the infection in children, though pediatric infection is known to occur in India.

The symptoms mostly refer to the blister or ulcer caused by the worm. The lesion is usually on the lower limb and discharges a milky fluid that shows the white worm. Fever and urticaria may occur prior to or during the blister formation. In cryptic infection, eosinophilia may be the sole evidence, although intense pruritus occasionally occurs. Calcified worms can be seen on x-rays and may be palpable. The ulcer may become bacterially infected. Premature death of worms in the subcutaneous tissues may result in inflammatory lesions and sometimes in a sterile abscess. A filarial skin test is available which is seldom needed for diagnosis.

In ulcerated dracontiasis, a moist antiseptic dressing (eg, acriflavine) accelerates the discharge of larvae and the death of the worm. Afterward, the worm can be pulled out gradually, about 2–3 cm a day, using a suitable instrument such as a clean match stick on which it can be wound. If more rapid withdrawal is attempted, the worm might rupture and cause a severe cellulitis.

A neomycin-bacitracin cream or systemic antibiotics should be given when bacterial infection is evident.

Diethylcarbamazine has been reported to be effective against immature forms and in maximal doses even against adult forms. Niridazole, 25 mg/kg daily for 7 days, may be effective, but direct worm removal is preferred.

Hodgson C, Barrett DF: Chronic dracunculosis. Br J Dermatol 76:211, 1964.

8. VISCERAL LARVA MIGRANS
(Toxocariasis)

Essentials of Diagnosis
- Marked eosinophilia and hepatomegaly in children with pica.
- The demonstration of larvae in liver biopsy.

General Considerations
Visceral larva migrans occurs in young children infected with the larvae of the dog or cat roundworm, *Toxocara canis* or *T cati.* Most of the reported cases are from North America and the British Isles. A history of pica is helpful in diagnosis. The presence of worm-infested dogs in the environment leads to the ingestion of eggs.

The life cycle and transmission of dog and cat roundworms are quite similar to those of Ascaris in man. When the eggs are ingested in large numbers by children via feces-contaminated soil, the larvae hatch out in the intestines, migrate through the blood stream, and are caught up in granulomatous inflammatory lesions in the liver, occasionally in the lungs, and rarely in other tissues, where they may remain, or wander about, for months to several years.

A similar syndrome can also be caused by the rodent whipworm, *Capillaria hepatica.*

Clinical Findings
A. Symptoms and Signs: The common presenting symptoms are anorexia, fever, and pallor. Abdominal distention and cough occur occasionally. Hepatomegaly is common, and splenomegaly is not unusual. Cutaneous hemorrhagic lesions have been reported in a few instances. Blindness and epileptiform convulsions may be atypical forms of presentation.

B. Laboratory Findings: Anemia is usually present and may be the reason for the pica. High leukocytosis, mainly due to eosinophilia (30–90%), is almost a constant feature. Hypergammaglobulinemia and high titers of blood group isoagglutinins are commonly found. The diagnosis may be confirmed by finding nematode larvae in a liver biopsy specimen, preferably performed by the open method. The larvae may be seen in secretions in granulomatous lesions or in crushed or papain-digested specimens. In fatal cases, larvae have been found in muscle and brain also.

C. X-Ray Findings: Infiltrations can often be seen on chest x-ray.

Differential Diagnosis
Pallor and pica in children with other symptoms may be associated with lead poisoning. These 2 conditions have been reported to occur simultaneously. Transient eosinophilia (less than 3 weeks) may occur during the migration of Ascaris larvae. More prolonged eosinophilia may occur in strongyloidiasis and trichinosis. Other helminths do not usually cause eosinophilia to a comparable degree.

Tropical eosinophilia, probably due to filariasis, may occur in infants and toddlers, especially in India. Pulmonary signs and symptoms are common, and hepatomegaly and fever may occur. Pica is not a feature.

Eosinophilia may be prominent in schistosomiasis and hydatid disease in association with hepatomegaly. Collagen diseases with eosinophilia and eosinophilic leukemia also should be differentiated.

Complications & Sequelae
Myocarditis, convulsive disorders, encephalitis, and ocular involvement such as retinal mass and endophthalmitis may occur due to the presence of larvae in these tissues. The ocular complications may be mistaken for retinoblastoma.

Treatment
A. Specific Measures: Thiabendazole is considered the best available drug for systemic helminth infections (25 mg/kg twice a day until symptoms subside or toxic effects occur). Diethylcarbamazine is also active against the larvae. The dosage is 10–30 mg/kg/day orally in 3 divided doses for 2 weeks. Medical treatment is especially indicated when pulmonary symptoms are prominent.

B. General Measures: In most cases, the prevention of reinfection is all that is required since the condition disappears without treatment. Removal of the source of Toxocara ova is important. The treatment of anemia with iron may be of value in stopping pica.

For endophthalmitis or for severe cases, especially with massive pulmonary infiltrates, corticosteroids have been recommended. These appear to reduce hepatocyte necrosis and cellular infiltration without changing the fibrous lesions. Antihistamines have not altered the pathologic features significantly in mouse studies.

Prognosis
Some severe cases have been fatal. Endophthalmitis leads to blindness. The majority of patients recover if continued infection is avoided.

Beaver PC: The nature of visceral larva migrans. J Parasitol 53:3, 1969.

Campbell WC, Cuckler AC: Thiabendazole in the treatment and control of parasitic infections in man. Tex Rep Biol Med 27:665, 1969.

Shrand H: Visceral larva migrans: *Toxocara canis* infection. Lancet 1:1357, 1964.

Snyder CH: Visceral larva migrans: Ten years' experience. Pediatrics 28:85, 1961.

Woodruff AW: Toxocariasis. Br Med J 3:663, 1970.

Zyngier FR, Santa Rosa G: Multiple infection with *Toxocara canis:* Influence of antihistamines and corticosteroids on the histopathologic response. Ann Trop Med Parasitol 70:445, 1976.

9. ONCHOCERCIASIS

Essentials of Diagnosis

- Localized or generalized pruritus.
- Subcutaneous nodules (adult worms).
- Superficial punctate keratitis.
- Late iridocyclitis.
- Eosinophilia.
- Biopsy evidence of *Onchocerca volvulus.*

General Considerations

Onchocerca volvulus is a filarial nematode found across central Africa and in Central America and southern Mexico. It is transmitted by species of Simulium (black flies). The infective larvae deposited after the bite of an infected Simulium will slowly develop in the subcutaneous tissues, which form an enclosing tumor, encapsulating the large female and possibly several smaller male worms. Microfilariae are developed in the female and shed in large numbers. These minute pre-larvae wander in subcutaneous tissue fluids and the eyes but do not enter the blood stream, as do the other pathogenic filariae of man.

Clinical Findings

A. Symptoms and Signs: About half of infected patients develop localized areas of nodularity or skin tumors associated with itching and resulting in excoriation and chronic pigmentary and morphologic skin changes. Common sites include the bony prominences of the trunk, extremities, and head.

Ocular infestation results in an early superficial punctate keratitis. Iridocyclitis may ultimately occur and is a serious complication which may lead to glaucoma, cataracts, and blindness.

B. Laboratory Findings: Eosinophilia of 15–50% is common. Aspiration of nodules will usually reveal microfilariae, and adult worms may be demonstrated in excised nodules. Microfilariae are not found in the blood but can be identified in skin or conjunctival snips or in skin shavings. The snip is performed by tenting the skin with a needle and cutting off a bit of skin above the needle tip. A blood-free shaving may be cut with a razor blade from the top of a ridge of skin firmly pressed between thumb and forefinger. The snip or shaving is examined in a drop of saline under a coverslip on a slide. Shavings or snips should be taken from several sites over bony prominences of the scapular region, hips, and thighs. In ocular onchocerciasis, slit lamp examination will usually reveal many microfilariae in the anterior chamber. Complement fixation and skin tests are of doubtful value because of high false-positive reaction rates.

Treatment

A. Specific Measures:

1. Diethylcarbamazine citrate is almost nontoxic and fairly effective. Give 2–3 mg/kg orally 3 times daily for 14–21 days. To prevent severe allergic symptoms, which may be provoked early in therapy as microfilariae are rapidly killed, start treatment with small doses and increase the dosage over 3–4 days. When the eyes are involved, particular caution is necessary, starting with a single daily dose of 0.25 mg/kg. Use antihistamines to control allergic symptoms.

One course of diethylcarbamazine will eradicate the infection in about 40% of patients and halt progression in the remainder. Two or 3 courses will cure almost all cases.

2. Sodium suramin is more effective than diethylcarbamazine in eradicating infection in a single course, but it has the disadvantage of potential renal toxicity (proteinuria, casts, red cells). Renal disease is a contraindication. Give 20 mg/kg as a 10% solution in distilled water IV every 4–7 days to a total of 10 doses. Start treatment with a test dose of 0.2 gm.

B. Surgical Measures: Surgical removal of nodules is not curative but removes many adult worms and is particularly justifiable when nodules are located close to the eyes. Nodulectomy may also be indicated for cosmetic reasons.

Prognosis

With chemotherapy, progression of all forms of the disease usually can be checked. The prognosis is unfavorable only for patients seen for the first time with already far-advanced ocular onchocerciasis.

Duke BOL: Onchocerciasis. Br Med J 1:301, 1968.

Woodruff AW & others: Papers and discussion on onchocerciasis. Trans R Soc Trop Med Hyg 60:695, 1966.

10. FILARIASIS

Essentials of Diagnosis

- Lymphangitis of the legs and genitals; obstructive lymphatic disease.
- Recurrent episodes lacking in periodicity.
- Characteristic microfilariae in blood.
- Leukocytosis with marked eosinophilia.
- Positive skin test to Dirofilaria antigen.
- Positive indirect hemagglutination and bentonite flocculation tests.

General Considerations

Filariasis is caused by infection with filarial

worms that produce microfilariae and parasitize the blood and lymphatic systems and involve muscles, serous cavities, and connective tissues. The 2 principal human pathogens are *Wuchereria bancrofti* and *Brugia malayi.* Both are transmitted by mosquitoes (*W bancrofti* by Culex and Aedes and *B malayi* by Anopheles and Mansonia). *W bancrofti* infection is widely prevalent in the tropics and subtropics throughout the world; *B malayi* is found mostly in India, Ceylon, and Southern Asia. Microfilariae are ingested by the mosquito vector and migrate to the thoracic muscles; larvae are deposited on the skin of humans close to the bite of the mosquito. The larvae migrate into the puncture wound and pass to the lymphatics, where they reside for approximately 1 year, reaching maturity in the interval. Adults reside in the lymphatics of the extremities and genitals, where they give rise to microfilariae which reach the circulation. Microfilariae of *W bancrofti* are in the peripheral blood at night (an exception is a nonnocturnal variety in the South Pacific). *B malayi* may show nocturnal periodicity but can be subperiodic (present at all times but more plentiful at night).

Man is the only definitive host for both filariae, except for a zoonotic strain of *B malayi* found infecting wild cats in northern Malaya. *B malayi* tends to occur in regions along coastlines dotted with multiple ponds bearing water plants of the genus Pistia, in which Mansonia mosquitoes breed.

Other species of filarial worms infect man but are of little consequence clinically. These include *Dipetalonema perstans* (African and South American tropics), *Mansonella ozzardi* (West Indies and Central and South America), and worms of the genus Dirofilaria (southern USA, especially Florida), including the common heartworm of dogs, *D immitis.*

Clinical Findings

A. Symptoms and Signs: Three clinical forms are apparent in children: the asymptomatic, the inflammatory, and the obstructive stages.

Asymptomatic infection is observed with both *W bancrofti* and *B malayi.* Children are exposed early in life and may exhibit microfilariasis in the blood without symptoms. By age 6, most children will be affected in endemic regions. Physical examination may reveal moderate lymphadenopathy, commonly of the inguinal nodes but not limited to this group. With death of the adult worms, the disease is "cured" and microfilariae disappear.

Inflammatory disease is probably related to hypersensitivity to antigens or products of the living and dead adult worms. Localized areas of lymphangitis involving the lower extremities and episodes of epididymitis, orchitis, and funiculitis are common. Systemic manifestations include fever, chills, vomiting, and malaise lasting for days or weeks. Abscesses occasionally occur in areas where adult worms have died. A chronic proliferative fibroblastic reaction eventually results in signs of obstructive lymphatic disease.

The obstructive stage develops in only a portion of those infected with filariae. Obstructive filariasis is a slow, chronic, progressive state resulting in edema of the affected parts. Elephantiasis results from multiple channel obstruction and can terminate in gross distortion of the extremities and genitalia. Recurrent inflammatory episodes may punctuate the progressive obstructive signs. Lymphatic rupture can result in the extrusion of lymph into serous cavities or organs (chyluria, chylous ascites, hydrocele).

B. Laboratory Findings: Eosinophilia in children may vary between 5–25% early in the disease. With progression and reduction of inflammatory episodes, the eosinophil count falls.

Microfilariae may be found in night blood specimens in the asymptomatic form as well as in the inflammatory form, but decrease as the obstructive phase progresses. Differentiation of *W bancrofti* and *B malayi* from nonpathogenic microfilariae requires an experienced observer. Adult worms can be identified in biopsy specimens, but biopsies should be performed judiciously to avoid damage to lymphatic channels.

Antibody determinations may be useful when microfilariae cannot be identified. The skin test employs Dirofilaria antigen and has a 10% false-positive response. Indirect hemagglutination and bentonite flocculation tests are under development.

Differential Diagnosis

During the inflammatory stage, diagnosis may be difficult, and many common childhood infections must be considered. In endemic areas or with a history of a stay in such areas, the presence of fever, lymphangitis, and lymphadenitis associated with eosinophilia should suggest filariasis. Various inflammatory lesions of the genitalia (gonorrhea, mumps orchitis, epididymitis) must be differentiated. Elephantiasis is strongly suggestive of filariasis but must be differentiated from hernia or hydrocele, Milroy's disease, venous thrombosis, or lesions resulting in anasarca or dependent edema (congestive heart failure, nephrosis, hepatic disease).

Prevention

Control of mosquitoes and human sources is necessary. Insecticide control of mosquitoes and attempts to reduce breeding areas are useful. Diethylcarbamazine therapy in humans results in a diminishing reservoir for mosquito transmission.

Treatment

A. General Measures: Rest and relocation in a cooler climate appear to aid in alleviation of inflammatory episodes. All secondary infections—particularly those affecting the lymphatics, such as streptococcal infections—should be diagnosed promptly and treated vigorously. Inflammatory genital lesions in the male are relieved by suspension of the affected part.

B. Surgical Measures: Plastic surgical correction of the involved genitalia may be accomplished with good results. Surgical treatment of limbs is unsatisfactory. Drainage of chyle, when it results in discomfort or reduced function, may be useful on a temporary basis.

C. Specific Treatment: Diethylcarbamazine citrate is the drug of choice. The dose is 2 mg/kg orally 3 times daily for 14–21 days. Allergic reactions are minimized by reducing each dose in relation to the occurrence and severity of prior reactions. The drug kills microfilariae but has little effect on the adult worms. Relapses can occur 3–12 months after a course of therapy, and retreatment over a period of 1–2 years is often necessary. Obstructive filariasis is not benefited by drug therapy.

Prognosis

In asymptomatic disease, the prognosis is excellent in young children. With progression, relocation can result in improvement provided the disease is in its early stages and is mild. Severe elephantiasis requires surgical correction, which may have a satisfactory result in the genital region but a poor result if extremities are involved.

Wijetunge HPA: Clinical manifestations of early bancroftian filariasis. J Trop Med Hyg 70:90, 1967.

Wilson T: Filariasis in Malaya: A general review. Trans R Soc Trop Med Hyg 55:107, 1961.

11. TROPICAL EOSINOPHILIA
(Tropical Pulmonary Eosinophilia)

Tropical eosinophilia is characterized by chronic or recurrent cough, exertional dyspnea, and wheezing, especially nocturnal. Generalized lymphadenitis and splenomegaly may occur. Fever is uncommon. Chest x-ray usually shows miliary mottling or other forms of interstitial infiltration. Marked leukocytosis, predominantly eosinophilic, is a diagnostic feature. Since mild to moderate eosinophilia is common in children where tropical eosinophilia is prevalent, an absolute eosinophil count of 4000/cu mm or more is generally considered an essential diagnostic criterion. Counts of 2000–4000/cu mm are equivocal, and lower counts speak against this diagnosis.

This disease is prevalent in the southwestern Pacific islands, southeastern and southern Asia, central and northwestern Africa, and some parts of South America. It may occur at any age but is uncommon in infants and very young children. It is believed to be due to infection with an unknown species of filaria. Microfilariae have been demonstrated in biopsies of lymph nodes, liver, and lung but not in the peripheral blood.

Treatment with the antifilarial drug diethylcarbamazine is usually effective. The recommended dosage is 10–15 mg/kg/day orally in 3 divided doses for 5 days. In case of recurrence or treatment failure, the course may be repeated for 10–20 days.

Ateshian B: Tropical eosinophilia: Radiographic lung field patterns and how to obtain them. Radiol Technol 46:84, 1974.

Charters AD & others: Tropical pulmonary eosinophilia in migrants in western Australia. Med J Aust 2:1195, 1972.

Mongotra ML & others: Tropical pulmonary eosinophilia in children. Indian Pediatr 10:559, 1973.

12. ANGIOSTRONGYLOSIS
(Eosinophilic Meningitis)

The rat lungworm *Angiostrongylus cantonensis* has an intermediate host in mollusks. Most important among them are the amphibious snails of the genus Pila, found in gardens and fresh waters on the Pacific islands and in southeastern Asia. Larvae in these snails, when ingested raw, infect man, and the developing parasites migrate through the liver and lungs to reach the CNS. After an incubation period of about 1–4 weeks, signs and symptoms of meningitis develop as well as eosinophilic pleocytosis of CSF. The parasite may occasionally be seen in CSF. The disease is usually self-limited but may be prolonged or fatal.

This infection has been reported from Taiwan, Hawaii, several other Pacific islands, Thailand, and Australia. It may occur at any age. Avoidance of raw mollusks in the diet is the best preventive measure. In addition to the meningitic form, an ocular form of disease also has been reported.

Alicata JE, Jindrak K: *Angiostrongylosis in the Pacific and Southeast Asia.* Thomas, 1970.

Punyagupta S & others: Eosinophilic meningitis in Thailand. Am J Trop Med Hyg 19:950, 1970.

CESTODE INFECTIONS

1. TAENIASIS & CYSTICERCOSIS

Essentials of Diagnosis

- Abdominal discomfort, pain, or diarrhea (taeniasis).
- Passage of segments (proglottids) or ova of tapeworm per rectum (taeniasis).
- Demonstration of cysticerci in tissue biopsy specimens or on x-ray (cysticercosis).

General Considerations

Taeniasis may be caused by the beef tapeworm (*Taenia saginata*) or pork tapeworm (*T solium*). The adult worms reside in the alimentary canal of man. The mature segments passed per rectum discharge ova in feces and soil which are then ingested by cattle and pigs. The hatched larvae develop into encysted forms mainly in the skeletal muscles (cysticercosis). When man consumes raw or undercooked meat, the larvae are liberated and develop into adults in the small intestine. The worm attaches itself to the mucosa by its scolex, with suckers and (in *T solium*) a double ring of eversible hooks.

Human cysticercosis is caused by the larvae of *T solium*. It occurs as a result of ingestion of eggs, which hatch in the intestines, or from internal autoinfection following reverse peristalsis and release of eggs from a broken segment of gravid *T solium* in the duodenal area. The swallowed or released eggs hatch, and the hexacanth larvae then penetrate the gastric or intestinal wall, enter the blood stream, and migrate into muscle and other tissues.

Both of these disorders are worldwide in distribution. They are more prevalent in areas where control over the quality of meat is inadequate.

Clinical Findings

A. Symptoms and Signs: In the majority of tapeworm infections there are no symptoms other than the passage of segments in feces—sometimes up to several dozen a day per worm—seen as white motile bodies about 1–2 cm long and 5 mm thick. Occasionally, the proglottid moves out of the rectum and crawls on the skin of the thigh—especially *T saginata,* whose segments are more muscular than the flaccid *T solium* segments.

Infants are not infected since they are not exposed. Toddlers and older children may harbor the infection for years. Abdominal pain, diarrhea, excessive appetite, failure to gain weight, abdominal distention, and anorexia may occur. Symptoms may be related to the number of worms present.

Most cases of cysticercosis go undiagnosed since there are few or no symptoms. The development of subcutaneous or muscle nodules is often the sole manifestation. After several years the cysticerci calcify and appear as opacities on x-ray. Cysticerci in the brain may remain silent or may cause symptoms and signs of epilepsy, brain tumor, hydrocephalus, and basal meningitis. In the eye they may cause uveitis, retinal detachment, and hemorrhage. The diagnosis is difficult to confirm except when nodules are available for biopsy or are visible in radiographs. The presence of *T solium* in the gut is of diagnostic significance.

B. Laboratory Findings: The diagnosis is confirmed by the demonstration of the proglottids or eggs. Eggs may be seen in fecal smears or may be detected on the perianal skin by the method used in the diagnosis of enterobiasis (see above). They are globular, 30–60 μm in diameter, with a double wall showing radial striations and an embryo with 6 hooklets (hexacanth).

If a proglottid is compressed between 2 glass slides, the main lateral branches of the uterus may be examined. *T saginata* has more than 15 and *T solium* fewer than 14 such branches to each side.

Eosinophilia is mild or absent in most cases.

Treatment

A. Taeniasis: Until recently, quinacrine was the best drug available though not completely satisfactory. Aspidium oleoresin (extract of male fern) is more effective but more toxic and not recommended for children. The introduction of warm hypertonic salt solutions into the duodenum has been successfully used but is too cumbersome for general use.

Niclosamide is the best available drug for all tapeworm infections. In the USA it is available only through the Parasitic Disease Drug Service, Center for Disease Control, Atlanta (Telephone: 404-633-3311). Toxicity is slight or absent in therapeutic doses. The drug is given orally in doses of 1 gm for children 2–8 years of age, 1.5 gm for children over 8, and 2 gm for adults—on an empty stomach on the morning following a light nonresidue supper. A saline cathartic is recommended after 2 hours only in *T solium* infection to prevent spillage of ova into the intestines, which may lead to cysticercosis.

An alternative drug (investigational in the USA for taeniasis) of high efficacy is paromomycin. The dosage is 45 mg/kg (total) to be given orally in 4 divided amounts at intervals of 4 hours. A saline cathartic is recommended in *T solium* infection (see above).

Quinacrine may be given in doses of 10–15 mg/kg orally up to a maximum of 800 mg, either as a single dose or in 2 divided doses 1 hour apart on an empty stomach in the morning as in niclosamide therapy. The purpose of dividing the dose is to prevent vomiting, but antiemetics may be given prior to administration, or sodium bicarbonate (200 mg) may be given with the drug. A saline cathartic is recommended in both types of taeniasis, since quinacrine only paralyzes the worm and does not kill it.

If segments are not passed per rectum for at least 3 months, that is sufficient evidence of complete expulsion of the worms.

B. Cysticercosis: There is no specific treatment for cysticercosis. Operative removal of cysticerci is of value when individual lesions cause symptoms.

Prognosis

The prognosis is good in taeniasis. In cerebral cysticercosis, the prognosis is less favorable: Symptoms may disappear after a variable interval, or heavy infections may result in death.

Dixon HBF, Hargreaves WH: Cysticercosis (*T solium*). Q J Med 13:107, 1944.

Nieto D: Cysticercosis of the nervous system: Diagnosis by means of the spinal fluid complement fixation test. Neurology 6:725, 1956.

Pawlowsky Z, Schultz MG: Taeniasis and cysticercosis (*Taenia solium*). Adv Parasitol 10:269, 1972.

Proctor EM: Identification of tapeworms. S Afr Med J 46:234, 1972.

Warren KS, Mahmoud AAF: Algorithms in the diagnosis and management of exotic diseases: Tapeworms. J Infect Dis 134:108, 1976.

WHO: Research needs in taeniasis-cysticercosis. (Memorandum.) Bull WHO 53:67, 1976.

2. HYMENOLEPIASIS

Hymenolepis nana commonly infects children; *H diminuta* does so rarely. *H diminuta* is a rat tapeworm with cysticercoid stages in fleas and insects. Children acquire the infection by eating insect-contaminated grains. *H nana* occurs in South and Southeast Asia, North Africa, southern Europe, South America, and the southern United States. It is primarily a human parasite, with another strain very commonly found in mice which is questionably infective for man. *H nana* may be passed to man by infected grain beetles and other insects, but it also has the unique ability to infect man directly by its eggs without passing through a developmental (cysticercoid) stage in an intermediate host. The eggs hatch in the intestinal lumen and the larvae penetrate the villi, where they form the larval stage, then return to the gut lumen, attach, and mature to become adult tapeworms. Fecal-oral contamination is necessary for infection of fresh human hosts.

Unlike other tapeworms, *H nana* is very small (2–5 cm), and numerous worms may be present in the intestine. Infection is usually asymptomatic, but diarrhea and abdominal pain may occur. The diagnosis is confirmed by detecting eggs in feces. They appear oval, rarely globular, 40–60 μm, and double-walled without radial striations; as with other tapeworms of man, the embryo has 6 hooklets.

Niclosamide has recently been used with success in the treatment of hymenolepiasis and is the drug of choice (for dosage see under Taeniasis). Alternatively, paromomycin may also be used (see under Taeniasis).

Quinacrine was until recently the recommended drug, but it is only moderately effective. (For dosage, see Taeniasis.) Hexylresorcinol may be tried if quinacrine fails (see Trichuriasis). Tetrachlorethylene may be of value in some cases (see Hookworm Disease).

Since none of the above drugs kills the eggs, a second course of therapy should be administered after an interval of 10 days to eliminate the newly developing worms.

Beaver PC, Sodeman WA: Treatment of *Hymenolepis nana* (dwarf tapeworm) infection with quinacrine hydrochloride (Atebrin). J Trop Med Hyg 55:97, 1952.

Wittner M, Tanowitz H: Paromomycin therapy of human cestodiasis with special reference to hymenolepiasis. Am J Trop Med Hyg 20:433, 1971.

3. DIPHYLLOBOTHRIASIS

Human infection with the broad fish tapeworm, *Diphyllobothrium latum,* occurs in the Scandinavian, Baltic, and Mediterranean regions, in Japan, and around the Great Lakes region of the USA and Canada. One or more adult worms lives inside the human intestine, attached to the mucosa by its scolex with twin sucking grooves. Adults and children are infected.

The ova develop in copepod crustaceans (Diaptomus), which are eaten by fish. The larvae develop further in the muscle and connective tissues of the fish. Pike, salmon, trout, and barbels may become infected. Man acquires the infection by consuming raw or undercooked fish. Smoking or ordinary kippering does not destroy the larvae.

In many cases the infection remains silent. No segments (proglottids) are passed per rectum. Abdominal pain, vomiting, diarrhea, and nutritional deficiency occur occasionally.

The diagnosis is made by the detection of ova in stools. They are oval, operculated, 45 × 70 μm, with a brownish operculated shell enclosing several granulated, tightly packed yolk cells.

In fewer than 1% of cases—but a higher percentage in Finland—progressive macrocytic, megaloblastic anemia occurs as a result of vitamin B_{12} deficiency. The megaloblastic anemia may be complicated by spinal cord lesions.

Quinacrine, hexylresorcinol, and tetrachlorethylene are moderately effective against this worm (see Hymenolepiasis). Niclosamide (see Taeniasis) has replaced these older drugs. Paromomycin also appears to be effective.

In the majority of instances of megaloblastic anemia, the expulsion of the worms results in a hematologic remission. In severe cases, cyanocobalamin (vitamin B_{12}) may be given parenterally in a single dose of 15–30 μg by deep subcutaneous or IM injection. Oral cyanocobalamin is of little value until after the expulsion of the worms.

Nagahana M & others: Treatment of *Taenia saginata* and *Diphyllobothrium latum* infections with bithionol. Am J Trop Med Hyg 15:351, 1966.

Rausch RL, Hilliard DK: Studies on the helminth fauna of Alaska. XLIX. The occurrence of *Diphyllobothrium latum* (Linnaeus 1758) in Alaska, with notes on other species. Can J Zool 48:1201, 1970.

Von Bonsdorff B & others: Vitamin B_{12} deficiency in carriers of the fish tapeworm, *Diphyllobothrium latum.* Acta Haematol (Basel) 24:15, 1960.

4. ECHINOCOCCOSIS

Essentials of Diagnosis

- Cystic tumor of liver or lung; rarely, of kidney, bone, brain, and other organs.
- Urticaria and pruritus secondary to rupture of cyst.
- Eosinophilia.
- Protoscoleces, brood capsules, or daughter cysts in lesion.
- Elevated titers on indirect hemagglutination (> 1:400) or bentonite flocculation (> 1:5) tests.
- Positive skin test (Casoni).

General Considerations

Echinococcus granulosus is a tapeworm that infects dogs and some cats and other carnivores. The adult worm lives in the intestines, and eggs are excreted in the feces. Man serves as an intermediate, never a final host. When eggs from dog feces are ingested by a child, the embryo hatches out and passes into intestinal lymphatics, reaching various parts of the body via the circulation. A cyst develops in the organ where the embryo settles. There is a predilection for the liver (60–70%) and the lungs (20–25%). A unilocular spherical cyst is the most common expression of the infection. It grows over a period of years and may reach 10 inches in diameter, although most are between 0.5 and 3 inches. A well-defined structure exists in the cyst. Infection with *E multilocularis* results in cysts which are multilocular or alveolar, without the heavy enclosing capsule which typifies the unilocular cyst of *E granulosus* and prevents rapid, uncontrolled growth as is seen in *E multilocularis.*

Clinical Findings

A. Symptoms and Signs: Clinical findings are dependent upon several phenomena: pressure by the enlarging cysts, erosion of blood vessels, and circulation of sensitizing parts of the cyst or worm. Cysts in the liver present as slowly growing tumors. Jaundice may be present if biliary obstruction occurs. Most cysts are in the right lobe, extending downward into the abdomen; one-fourth are on the upper surface and may go undetected for many years.

Hemorrhage may result from erosion. Omental torsion is also observed.

Pulmonary cysts rarely produce pressure symptoms but may erode into a bronchus, resulting in cough and atelectasis.

Rupture of a cyst and discharge of its contents may result in sudden episodes of coughing if in the lung. Asthma, urticaria, and pruritus may be observed. The sputum is blood-tinged and frothy and contains bits of the cyst and worm. Common signs in pulmonary cyst rupture are coughing, dyspnea, hemoptysis, chest pain, and increase in pulse and respiratory rates.

Cysts of the brain may produce focal neurologic signs and convulsions; of the kidney, hematuria and pain; of bone, pain.

B. Laboratory Findings: In suspected cases of echinococcosis with allergic manifestations, a search for protoscoleces, brood capsules, or daughter cysts should be made. Specimens for examination will depend on the site of the cyst but include sputum or bronchoscopic aspirates, urine, ascitic fluid or pleural fluid, and CSF.

Eosinophilia occurs irregularly and to a variable extent.

Serologic tests can assist both in the diagnosis of hydatid cyst and in evaluation of the success of cystectomy. It is best to use more than one type of immunodiagnostic test and to bear in mind that the diagnostic titer varies in different laboratories. The bentonite flocculation test is positive at 1:5, as is the comple-ment fixation test. The immunohemagglutination test is usually considered positive at 1:400. When secondary echinococcosis is present, the titers are usually much higher. In one series of 26 surgically proved cases with secondary daughter cysts, the geometric mean titers were 1:95 for the complement fixation test, 1:414 for the latex agglutination test and 1:39,810 for the immunohemagglutination test. All of these immunodiagnostic tests remain high for at least 1 year following surgery, even when successful. They drop significantly by 3–4 years postoperatively and are usually negative by the tenth year. If the parasite has not been completely removed at operation, the tests remain higher. Continued presence of the parasite should be suspected when titers remain at or above 1:40 for complement fixation, 1:160 for latex agglutination, or 1:25,600 for immunohemagglutination. The immunohemagglutination titer takes longer to drop under all circumstances. Note also that the intradermal (Casoni) test remains positive for many years longer than the serologic tests. Furthermore, while positive in 85% of cases, there is a high (18%) rate of false-positive tests.

C. X-Ray Findings: X-ray of the chest may reveal the cyst. Special studies of the CNS may reveal evidence of an intracranial mass and increased pressure. Calcified cysts in any organ may be noted; destruction of bony structure is visible in osseous lesions.

Differential Diagnosis

Hydatid cysts in any site may be mistaken for a variety of malignant and nonmalignant tumors or for abscesses, both bacterial and amebic. In the lung, a cyst may be confused with an advanced tubercular lesion. Syphilis may also be confused with echinococcosis. Allergic symptoms arising from cyst leakage may resemble those associated with many other diseases.

Complications

Sudden rupture of a cyst leading to anaphylaxis and sometimes death is the most important complication of echinococcosis. If the patient survives the rupture, he still faces the danger of multiple secondary cyst infections arising from seeding of daughter cysts. Segmental lung collapse, secondary infections of cysts, secondary effects of increased intracranial pressure, and severe renal damage due to kidney cysts are other potential complications.

Treatment

The only definitive treatment is surgical removal of the intact cysts, preferably preceded by inoculation into the cyst of hydrogen peroxide, Lugol's iodine, glycerin, or formalin. A recent advance in surgical technic is the freezing of the cyst wall and instillation of silver nitrate immediately prior to removal.

Often, however, the presence of a cyst is only recognized when it begins to leak or when it ruptures. Such an event calls for vigorous treatment of allergic symptoms or emergency management of anaphylactic shock. In cases where spillage of hydatid cyst fluid at surgery is recognized or inevitable and in the inoperable case, mebendazole should be tried. Numerous reports of cure or amelioration have been published. The dose is higher than used for other helminths, and the danger of rupture of cysts due to degeneration from the drug must be considered. The literature referenced should be consulted before such treatment is contemplated.

Prognosis

Patients may live for years with relatively large hydatid cysts before their condition is diagnosed. Liver and lung cysts often can be removed surgically without great difficulty, but for cysts in sites less accessible to surgery the prognosis is less favorable. The prognosis is always grave in secondary echinococcosis and with alveolar cysts. About 15% of patients with echinococcosis eventually die because of the disease or its complications.

Abrishami MA, Ziai M: Shock, urticaria and a right upper quadrant abdominal mass. Clin Pediatr (Phila) 14:602, 1975.

Bonakdarpour A: Echinococcus disease: A report of 112 cases from Iran and a review of all cases from the United States. Am J Roentgenol Radium Ther Nucl Med 99:660, 1967.

Ekrami Y: Surgical treatment of hydatid disease of the liver. Arch Surg 111:1350, 1976.

Heath DD, Chevis RAF: Mebendazole and hydatid cysts. Lancet 2:218, 1974.

Kammerer WS, Judge DM: Chemotherapy of hydatid disease (*Echinococcus granulosus*) in mice with mebendazole and bithionol. Am J Trop Med Hyg 25:714, 1976.

Kaya U & others: Intracranial hydatid cysts: Study of 17 cases. J Neurosurg 42:580, 1975.

Lewis JW Jr & others: A review of echinococcal disease. Ann Surg 181:390, 1975.

Nourmand Aziz: Hydatid cysts in children and youths. Am J Trop Med Hyg 25:845, 1976.

Romanoff H, Krausz M: Surgical aspects of pulmonary hydatid disease and report of a familial hydatidosis. Int Surg 60:361, 1975.

Saidi F, Nazarian I: Surgical treatment of hydatid cysts by freezing of cyst wall and instillation of 0.5 per cent silver nitrate solution. N Engl J Med 284:1346, 1971.

Todorov T & others: Antibody persistence after surgical treatment of echinococcosis. Bull WHO 53:407, 1976.

Williams JF & others: Current prevalence and distribution of hydatidosis with special reference to the Americas. Am J Trop Med Hyg 20:224, 1971.

TREMATODE INFECTIONS

1. PARAGONIMIASIS, CLONORCHIASIS, FASCIOLIASIS, & FASCIOLOPSIASIS

Paragonimiasis, caused by the lung fluke *Paragonimus westermani,* occurs in East and Southeast Asia, parts of Africa, and in South America. Man and carnivorous animals acquire the infection by consuming uncooked crabs and other crustacea, the intermediate hosts carrying encysted larvae.

Clonorchiasis and fascioliasis are caused by the Oriental liver fluke *Clonorchis sinensis* and the sheep liver fluke *Fasciola hepatica.* The former occurs in East and Southeast Asia and the latter is worldwide. Ingestion of raw fish containing encysted Clonorchis larvae or fresh aquatic plants with attached encysted Fasciola larvae results in infections.

Fasciolopsis buski, the giant intestinal fluke of man, causes fasciolopsiasis, found in East and Southeast Asia. The encysted larvae remain attached to water plants as in the case of Fasciola.

Clinical Findings

A. Paragonimiasis: The young lung flukes digested free of their cysts migrate from the intestines to the lungs, where they mature and form cystic lesions with fibrous walls, often 2 worms to a cyst. Fibrous nodules also appear around masses of eggs. The usual symptoms are cough with copious brownish sputum and frequent hemoptysis. In heavy infections the worms are also found in various abdominal viscera and even in the brain. In such instances, abdominal pain, dysentery, and convulsive and paralytic disease may occur. X-ray changes in the lungs and clubbing of the fingers are common. The diagnosis depends on the demonstration of ova in sputum or feces.

B. Clonorchiasis and Fascioliasis: The hatched worms of these liver flukes migrate from the intestine to mature in the liver bile ducts. Most infections remain asymptomatic. Fever, upper abdominal pain, hepatomegaly, jaundice, urticaria, and eosinophilia in varying combinations are the early features in heavy and continued infections, especially in older children. Cholangitis, cholecystitis, and cholelithiasis may occur in episodes. Cirrhosis of the liver is a late complication. The diagnosis is confirmed by the demonstration of ova in feces or duodenal aspirate.

C. Fasciolopsiasis: The flukes inhabit the duodenum and the jejunum. The usual symptoms are abdominal pain and diarrhea. Gradually, progressive malnutrition, ascites, and generalized edema appear. Severe and untreated infections may cause death. The diagnosis is confirmed by the presence of ova in feces.

Treatment

A. Paragonimiasis, Clonorchiasis, and Fascioliasis: Bithionol, 10 mg/kg orally in 3 divided doses on alternate days for 10–15 doses, is recommended for paragonimiasis. Emetine hydrochloride, 1 mg/kg/day IM for 5–7 days, or dehydroemetine (perhaps more effective and less toxic) at the same dosage, is usually recommended for fascioliasis. An alternative drug is bithionol (above dosage) or chloroquine, 10 mg/kg orally daily for 3 weeks. It may be advisable to give one course each of both drugs. Treatment of clonorchiasis is often difficult and temporary. Chloroquine, bithionol, or gentian violet—or all 3—may be effective.

B. Fasciolopsiasis: Intestinal fluke infection may

be treated with either oral hexylresorcinol or tetrachlorethylene. These drugs are discussed under trichuriasis and hookworm disease, respectively. Other useful drugs include dehydroemetine or emetine (see under Amebiasis), bithionol as for paragonimiasis, or chloroquine as for fascioliasis.

Ashton WLG & others: Human fascioliasis in Shropshire. Br Med J 3:500, 1970.

Ehrenworth L, Daniels RA: Clonorchiasis sinensis: Clinical manifestations and diagnosis. Ann Intern Med 49:419, 1958.

Hardman EW & others: Fascioliasis: A large outbreak. Br Med J 3:502, 1970.

Lammler G: Chemotherapy of trematode infections. Pages 153–251 in: *Advances in Chemotherapy.* Vol 3. Goldin A & others (editors). Academic Press, 1968.

Neghime A, Ossandon M: Ectopic and hepatic fascioliasis. Am J Trop Med Hyg 23:545, 1943.

Nwokolo C: Paragonimiasis in eastern Nigeria. J Trop Med Hyg 67:1, 1964.

Warren KS, Mahmoud AAF: Algorithms in the diagnosis and management of exotic diseases. XXI. Liver, intestinal, and lung flukes. J Infect Dis 135:692, 1977.

2. SCHISTOSOMIASIS
(Bilharziasis)

Essentials of Diagnosis

- A transient itchy papular rash following exposure to fresh water.
- Fever, urticaria, joint pain, cough, lymphadenitis, eosinophilia.
- Anorexia, loss of weight, diarrhea or dysentery.
- Hematuria [usually terminal], painful micturition.
- Demonstration of ova in stools, urine, or rectal biopsy specimen.

General Considerations

Schistosomiasis is caused by the blood flukes *Schistosoma haematobium, S japonicum,* or *S mansoni. S haematobium* is prevalent in tropical and subtropical Africa and some parts of western Asia. *S japonicum* occurs in East and Southeast Asia. *S mansoni* is common in tropical Africa and South America.

The infective swimming larvae (cercariae) are found in fresh water. When in contact with human skin, they penetrate, invade the blood vessels, migrate to the liver, and finally move up the mesenteric vessels to specific final preferred sites. Respectively, the preferential sites of *S haematobium, S japonicum,* and *S mansoni* are the vesical venous plexus, the draining veins of the small intestine, and those of the large bowel. They mature in the liver, mate, and migrate to these sites where the females lay eggs. The eggs escape into the perivascular tissues, cause inflammatory lesions, and exude into the lumens of the bladder and bowel. This is accompanied by extravasation of blood.

The eggs that escape in urine and feces hatch in fresh water and the ciliated larvae (miracidia) enter and develop in the appropriate fresh water intermediate snail host. The parasite multiplies in the snail, and after 3–4 weeks large numbers of cercariae issue forth and seek the skin of new final hosts—human for *S haematobium,* human or rodent for *S mansoni,* and human, cattle, dog, or many other final hosts for *S japonicum.*

Clinical Findings

In highly endemic areas, large proportions of the population may be infected, with many showing no symptoms, but discharging eggs. Symptoms follow heavy and continued exposure. The diagnosis is readily suspected in endemic areas. Otherwise, a history of residence in endemic areas is of great value in alerting the pediatrician.

A. Symptoms and Signs: Irritation of the skin may occur at sites of cercarial entry with a transient itchy papular rash. During the ensuing migration of the larvae, fever and urticaria may occur. The larvae may escape into the alveoli, causing cough and hemoptysis. Liver and spleen gradually enlarge and become tender. After lodgement of the flukes in their favorite venous plexuses, fever and toxemia occur and last for several days to weeks. In bladder infection, painful and frequent micturition and hematuria are common. Bladder stones and incontinence of urine may follow. Secondary pyelonephritis, ureterovesical reflux, and anatomic changes in the ureters demonstrable by intravenous urograms are common. In the intestinal types, abdominal pain, diarrhea (often bloody), and progressive abdominal enlargement due to increasing splenomegaly and ascites occur.

B. Laboratory Findings: The diagnosis should be confirmed by the demonstration of schistosome eggs in feces or urine. *S japonicum* eggs are seen only in feces. *S mansoni* eggs are frequently seen in feces and occasionally in urine. If there are no eggs in feces and urine, rectal biopsy specimen may reveal *S mansoni* eggs. *S haematobium* eggs are frequently seen in urine and occasionally in feces.

The eggs of *S mansoni* and *S haematobium* measure about 140×60 μm and those of *S japonicum* about 90×70 μm. *S haematobium* eggs have a terminal spine, whereas the eggs of *S mansoni* and *S japonicum* have a lateral hook or spine, though it is often hidden or hard to see clearly in the smaller eggs of *S japonicum.*

An intradermal test is available and is of value especially in *S japonicum* infection.

Marked eosinophilia is common.

Complications & Sequelae

The complications and sequelae of *S haematobium* infection are anemia, renal calculi, ascending bacterial infection of the urinary tract, strictures and fistulas, lymphedema of the genitalia, uremia, hypertension, and malignancy of the bladder. Schistosomal granulomas in the female genital tract or in the spinal cord (with paraplegia) have been described.

Anemia, cirrhosis of the liver, portal hypertension, and bleeding from esophageal varices may occur in alimentary forms of schistosomiasis. Pulmonary hypertension and cor pulmonale may occur late in S mansoni infections.

Severe nutritional deficiencies and death are not uncommon in unchecked and heavy infections.

Prevention

In endemic areas, prevention of infection by avoiding skin contact with contaminated fresh water (bathing, wading) is of paramount public health importance.

Treatment

A. General Measures: It is important to look for and treat intercurrent bacterial or parasitic infections and nutritional deficiencies. For fibrotic and calcified lesions in the older child, especially of the urinary tract, corrective surgery should be done to relieve symptoms or arrest the progression of renal damage. Splenectomy and portacaval shunt are palliative measures in advanced alimentary schistosomiasis.

B. Specific Measures:

1. Antimony compounds—Antimony potassium or sodium tartrate is recommended only for S japonicum infections. It is given intravenously as a freshly prepared 0.5% solution. Injections are given on alternate days, starting with 4 ml on the first day and increasing by 2 ml on alternate days up to 14 ml, and continued at this level (ie, 14 ml on alternate days) until 200–250 ml have been given to children under 40 kg and 300 ml to those over 40 kg. It must be given very slowly, avoiding leakage into perivascular tissue. The patient must rest in bed during the injection and for several hours afterward. When intravenous therapy is difficult, stibophen (see below) may be given intramuscularly as for S haematobium or S mansoni infections.

One of the following antimonials is recommended in the treatment of S haematobium and S mansoni infections:

Antimony sodium dimercaptosuccinate is given for S haematobium and S mansoni in total doses of 40–60 mg/kg for children under 20 kg and 30–50 mg/kg for older children in 5 or 6 IM injections, 1–2 injections per week. Persistent rash or fever and excessive vomiting are indications for a temporary suspension of therapy.

Stibophen is given IM as a 6.3% aqueous solution in doses of 1 ml/15 kg, not exceeding 5 ml per injection. A test dose of 0.5 or 1 ml is given first and the dose increased in 2–3 steps. A short course consists of 8 injections and a long course consists of 5 injections per week for 4 weeks. Recurrent vomiting, proteinuria, and joint pains call for cessation of therapy.

Antimony lithium thiomalate is given IM on alternate days to a total of 40–45 ml for children under 15 years. The first dose is 0.5 ml; thereafter, give 2 ml for children under 10 and 2.5–3 ml for those above.

2. Niridazole—This drug is less effective than the antimonials but far less toxic. The results are best with S haematobium, somewhat less good for S mansoni, and nil for S japonicum. The daily dose is 25 mg/kg (maximum, 1.5 gm) in 2 divided doses daily for 7 days. It is the drug of choice for nonantimonials against S haematobium and an alternate choice for S mansoni.

3. Hycanthone methanesulfonate—Give 3 mg/kg (base) as a single IM dose, or, in the form of enteric-coated tablets of the base drug only (not the mesylate), 2–3 mg/kg/day for 5 days. This drug may cause anorexia, nausea, and vomiting in about half of patients and abdominal colic in one-fourth. It is useful only for S mansoni and S haematobium infections. Prior hepatic disease is a contraindication to its use.

Prognosis

The prognosis is good in mild infections and in heavy symptomatic infections treated early. Otherwise, the prognosis is poor, especially with involvement of the lungs, liver, spleen, and urinary tract.

Berberian DA & others: A comparison of oral and parenteral activity of hycanthone and lucanthone in experimental infections with Schistosoma mansoni. Am J Trop Med Hyg 16:487, 1967.

Cheng TH: Schistosomiasis in mainland China. Am J Trop Med Hyg 20:26, 1971.

Da Cunha AS & others: Manifestações de intolerância ao hycanthone no tratamento da esquistossomose mansoni. Rev Inst Med Trop Sao Paulo 13:213, 1971.

Farid Z & others: Hepatotoxicity after treatment of schistosomiasis with hycanthone. Br Med J 2:88, 1972.

Fernandez A, Steigmann F, Villa F: Schistosomiasis: Mimicry of gastrointestinal diseases. Am J Gastroenterol 40:482, 1963.

Forsyth DM, MacDonald G: Urological complications of endemic schistosomiasis in school children. Part 1. Usagara School. Trans R Soc Trop Med Hyg 50:171, 1965.

Foster R & others: Comparative studies of the action of mirasan, lucanthone, hycanthone and niridazole against S mansoni in mice. Ann Trop Med Parasitol 65:45, 1971.

Hartman PE & others: Hycanthone: A frameshift mutagen. Science 172:1058, 1971.

Jordan P: Chemotherapy of schistosomiasis. Bull NY Acad Med 44:245, 1968.

Jordan P, Webbe G: Human Schistosomiasis. Heinemann, 1969.

Mostofi FK (editor): Bilharziasis. Springer-Verlag, 1967.

Warren KS, Newill VA: Schistosomiasis: A Bibliography of the World's Literature From 1852 to 1962. 2 vols. Western Reserve Univ Press, 1967.

•   •   •

General References

Adams ARD, Maegraith BG: *Clinical Tropical Diseases,* 5th ed. Blackwell, 1971.

Brown HW: *Basic Clinical Parasitology,* 3rd ed. Appleton-Century-Crofts, 1969.

Faust EC & others: *Craig and Faust's Clinical Parasitology,* 8th ed. Lea & Febiger, 1970.

Jawetz E, Melnick JL, Adelberg EA: *Review of Medical Microbiology,* 12th ed. Lange, 1976.

Katz M: Parasitic infections. J Pediatr 87:165, 1975.

Knight R & others: Progress report: Intestinal parasites. Gut 14:145, 1973.

Maegraith BG: *Exotic Diseases in Practice.* Heinemann, 1965.

Maegraith BG, Gilles HM (editors): *Management and Treatment of Tropical Diseases.* Blackwell, 1971.

Marcial-Rojas RA (editor): *Pathology of Protozoal and Helminthic Diseases With Clinical Correlation.* Williams & Wilkins, 1971.

Meyers FH, Jawetz E, Goldfien A: *Review of Medical Pharmacology,* 5th ed. Lange, 1976.

Trowell HC, Jelliffe DB: *Diseases of Children in the Subtropics and Tropics,* 2nd ed. Arnold, 1970.

Wilcocks C, Manson-Bahr PEC: *Manson's Tropical Diseases,* 17th ed. Williams & Wilkins, 1972.

28...
Infections: Mycotic

Vincent A. Fulginiti, MD

ACTINOMYCOSIS

Essentials of Diagnosis

- Chronic suppurative lesions of the skin, with sinus tract formation.
- "Sulfur granules"—actinomyces colonies 1–2 mm in diameter—found in pus from lesion.
- Gram-positive hyphae.
- Association with gram-negative bacteria.
- Isolation of organism from sulfur granule or pus.

General Considerations

Human actinomycosis is almost always caused by *Actinomyces israelii*. Although traditionally classified as a fungus, *A israelii* is actually a bacterium.* The symptoms and course of the diseases produced resemble those of the chronic mycoses, but successful therapy with antibacterial antibiotics is more in keeping with the true nature of these organisms.

The organism is a frequent oral and dental saprophyte, and infection is endogenous. Actinomycosis is characteristically a chronic, slowly progressive disease.

Clinical Findings

A. **Symptoms and Signs:** Three forms of the disease are recognized: cervicofacial, thoracic, and abdominal.

1. Cervicofacial actinomycosis (lumpy jaw)—Granulomas appear in the mandible or maxilla and are of dental or oral origin. These break down and suppurate, and may seal over but do not heal. Sinus tracts form and reform, and without treatment the disease has a chronic unremitting course.

2. Thoracic actinomycosis—This form is heralded by fever (often of septic nature), pleural pain, cough, and weight loss. Mucopurulent or sanguineous sputum or sinus tract drainage may be present. Dullness to percussion and signs of consolidation may be present, and sinus tracts may communicate with the skin.

3. Abdominal actinomycosis—Usually begins with inflammation of the appendix and weight loss. Fever,

*Discussed in this chapter by convention. See also Nocardiosis, p 837.

chills, and vomiting over a protracted course are associated with painful, palpable masses.

B. **Laboratory Findings:** Identification of typical sulfur granules and gram-positive hyphae in secretions should lead to culture of *A israelii*.

C. **X-Ray Findings:** With bony involvement, periostitis and osteomyelitis are visible on x-ray examination. Heavy hilar and basilar infiltration is characteristic of pulmonary actinomycosis.

Differential Diagnosis

Actinomycosis must be distinguished from fungal diseases causing similar manifestations (culture); pulmonary, intestinal, or lymphatic tuberculosis (PPD, isolation of mycobacteria, response to therapy); and lymphomas (biopsy, absence of sinuses, blood or bone marrow changes). Bacterial infection of the cervical lymph nodes, bones, chest, or abdomen can usually be differentiated on the basis of culture, acuteness, and response to therapy.

Complications

Extension of the infection from the primary site to contiguous structures (irrespective of anatomic limits) results in osteomyelitis, brain abscess, hepatic or renal involvement, abscesses, and sinus tracts.

Treatment

A. **Specific Treatment:** Penicillin is the drug of choice. Daily doses range up to 2 million units in infants and up to 20 million units in older children. Initial intravenous therapy followed by intramuscular and then by oral administration must usually be continued for as long as 1–1½ years. Broad spectrum antibiotics and sulfadiazine are useful adjuncts but should not be used alone.

B. **General Measures:** Surgical excision is frequently necessary, particularly with chronic, multiple sinus tracts. Preoperative therapy with penicillin is always indicated.

Prognosis

Penicillin therapy has greatly improved the prognosis. Unless the course has been prolonged and complications such as brain abscess or meningitis have appeared, recovery is the rule. Convalescence may be prolonged.

Coodley EL: Actinomycosis: Clinical diagnosis and management. Postgrad Med 46:73, Aug 1969.

Peabody JW, Seabury JH: Actinomycosis and nocardiosis. Am J Med 28:99, 1960.

Clin Pediatr (Phila) 11:178, 1972.

Slavin RG, Laird TS, Cherry JD: Allergic bronchopulmonary aspergillosis in a child. J Pediatr 76:416, 1970.

ASPERGILLOSIS

Opportunistic infection due to *Aspergillus fumigatus* and other species of this genus is rare in childhood. These organisms are found commonly in nature, particularly in decaying vegetation. A number of cases have occurred in children receiving corticosteroids or immunosuppressive drugs; other predisposing causes include chronic bronchopulmonary disease, tuberculosis, and morphologic abnormalities of the respiratory tract.

A chronic course is characteristic, and a history of long-standing symptoms may be elicited. Fever, productive cough, and increasing lassitude often precede cavitary pulmonary changes. Pulmonary infection may become disseminated to other viscera, often with a fatal outcome. Mucopurulent sputum or hemoptysis is frequently present. Chronic otomycosis is manifested by obstruction of the auditory canal with a plug composed of fungus, wax, and epithelial debris. In the absence of bacterial infection, the canal is dry. There are no laboratory aids to the diagnosis save for culture of the fungus or identification of hyphae in sodium hydroxide preparations from specimens of sputum, pus, or ear curettage.

In recent years, a variety of syndromes have been recognized in association with this organism, particularly allergic pulmonary disease, endophthalmitis following eye surgery, and disseminated disease.

Pulmonary symptoms resemble those of allergic asthma. Patients with true asthma may also have clinical exacerbation upon exposure to aspergillus. The diagnosis is suggested by positive immediate-type skin tests and by the presence and increase in titer of serum precipitins and other antibodies. Transient infiltrates may be seen on x-ray examination of the lungs and may be due to bronchial plugging with the organisms in association with bronchospasm. Therapy is symptomatic; a few patients seem to benefit from desensitization.

Amphotericin B (Fungizone) systemically has little place in the therapy of aspergillosis. Surgical resection of pulmonary fungal masses may be coupled with local instillation of amphotericin B. Disseminated disease and endophthalmitis may be treated with amphotericin B but with little hope of success; many of these organisms are resistant to the serum levels of this antibiotic usually achieved, and the fulminant nature of the disease process may preclude successful therapy.

Pennington JE: Successful treatment of aspergillus pneumonia in hematological neoplasia. N Engl J Med 295:426, 1976.

Phillips WL, Shenker IR: Pulmonary aspergillosis in childhood.

NORTH AMERICAN BLASTOMYCOSIS

Blastomyces dermatitidis, a budding yeast form in human infection, is present in soil, but its exact mode of transmission is not known. The disease is widely distributed in North and Central America, with a high prevalence in the Mississippi Valley. Childhood illness is uncommon.

There are 2 basic forms—pulmonary and cutaneous—and a disseminated form that may arise from either and is characterized by chronic suppurative bronchopulmonary disease with insidious and often prolonged (months) early symptoms of cough, fever, weight loss, increasing chest pain, and hoarseness. Purulent or bloody sputum may be present. With dissemination, cutaneous lesions, bone pain, chills, and sweats become apparent. CNS symptoms are heralded by severe headache, and focal neurologic signs, particularly paralysis, are common.

Cutaneous lesions are usually single, beginning as a nodular papule on an exposed surface and gradually ulcerating and failing to heal. Multiple sites may be present and are all associated with pulmonary disease. Spread is believed to be via the blood stream. The individual lesion has a raised border with a multiply abscessed crater. Purplish discoloration is frequent, and small abscesses can be found in the border.

Dissemination results in involvement of the brain, kidneys, bones, skin, and subcutaneous tissues. Symptoms referable to these tissues in a patient with chronic pulmonary infection should lead one to suspect blastomycosis.

A positive blastomycin skin test reaction indicates contact with the organism. A rise in complement fixation titer occurs in paired sera.

Iodides and diamidines have been employed with variable success. Amphotericin B (Fungizone) by intravenous infusion may be helpful (see Chapter 37). Surgical drainage and excisional therapy are of limited benefit but may be useful in selected cases and as an adjunct to antifungal therapy.

Mild forms of the pulmonary disease may exist, but the usual clinically apparent case, if untreated, usually disseminates, leading to death.

Busey J: North American blastomycosis. Ariz Med 34:392, 1977.

Parker JD & others: A decade of experience with blastomycosis and its treatment with amphotericin B. Am Rev Respir Dis 99:895, 1969.

Turner DJ, Wadlington WB: Blastomycosis in childhood: Treatment with amphotericin B and a review of the literature. J Pediatr 75:708, 1969.

CANDIDIASIS

Essentials of Diagnosis

- Plaque-like and ulcerative lesions of the oral mucosa.
- Vulvovaginitis, skin fold infections, paronychia; pulmonary, CNS, and disseminated disease.
- A compatible clinical picture, a susceptible host, and the repeated finding of oval, budding yeasts in clinical specimens should establish the diagnosis.

General Considerations

Candida albicans is the major human pathogen of the genus. It is a ubiquitous, dimorphic fungus which usually reproduces by budding. The yeast forms are vegetative; in most human tissue infections, the mycelial form is observed. Although many host defense factors have been described, no consistent relationship to infection or disease has been established. Delayed hypersensitivity to candida appears to be important in that clinically significant disease states are almost always associated with a lack of skin test reactivity.

C albicans exists as a normal inhabitant of the gastrointestinal flora, and its growth is held in check by the presence of other members of the flora. With the exceptions of thrush in neonates and vaginitis in pregnant women, it seldom produces disease in healthy individuals. Reduction in host defenses or a significant change in the indigenous flora results in overgrowth of candida and can lead to local and systemic disease. Thus, lymphopenic immunologic deficiencies, the use of corticosteroids or other immunosuppressive therapy, and the administration of antibiotics all may result in systemic candidiasis. Candidiasis is also commonly associated with diabetes mellitus. Topical candidiasis may occur in areas of the skin macerated or exposed to excessive moisture (eg, the diaper area).

Clinical Findings

A. Symptoms and Signs:

1. Oral candidiasis—White patches with superficial mucosal ulceration appear on the entire oral and pharyngeal mucosa and frequently result in loss of appetite, difficulty in swallowing, and even respiratory distress. Individual lesions are surrounded by intensely red areolas; occasionally, in severe forms, coalescence occurs. The illness may be seen in neonates or even 1–2 weeks later.

A new form of oropharyngeal candidiasis has been associated with the use of beclomethasone dipropionate inhalations in the treatment of asthma. Clinical signs may be seen in 5–10% of patients; as many as 4–8 times this number are colonized. This incidence is higher than that associated with oral corticosteroid use and may reflect the higher local concentrations or the increased potency of this agent.

2. Skin infection—Diaper dermatitis is common, with an intensely red, "scorched" appearance extending to the perianal and anterior abdominal areas. Sharp demarcation is sometimes evident. Scaling, weeping lesions, vesicles, pustules, and papules are occasionally present. Satellite lesions are frequent.

Vulvovaginitis may present with the above changes plus a thick, often yellowish exudate associated with itching (often intense).

3. Pulmonary infection—*C albicans* pneumonia (uncommon) tends to occur only in diseases associated with deficiency or abnormalities of lymphocyte function. On the other hand, candida is commonly isolated from sputum or on autopsy, and it is sometimes difficult to determine what etiologic role candida played in the pneumonia. This is especially true if antibiotics or corticosteroids have been administered. Symptoms include low-grade fever, chronic cough, and mucoid or mucosanguineous sputum. Rales, signs of pleuritis, and effusion may be present.

4. Other forms—Meningitis, endocarditis, pyelonephritis, and candidemia are seen. All of these forms are limited to patients who are rendered susceptible by therapy with antibiotics, corticosteroids or other immunosuppressive agents, or underlying disease.

A chronic progressive granulomatous skin lesion, occasionally associated with oral candidiasis, is characterized by horny excrescences.

Paronychia and onychia due to candida are observed in children as part of the clinical illness characterized by hypoadrenalism, hypoparathyroidism, pernicious anemia, and steatorrhea. Candidiasis usually precedes the other manifestations, but all combinations are seen.

Candidiasis has also been implicated in diarrheal illness associated with watery stools and abdominal cramping pain but no blood or mucus in the stools. This isolated form of the disease responds to minimal (3–4 days) oral therapy with nystatin.

B. Laboratory Findings: Direct examination of scrapings, pus, or sputum will reveal ovoid, budding yeast cells in large numbers. With tissue invasion, typical mycelial elements may be found.

The organism is readily cultured on the usual laboratory media or on Sabouraud's medium.

A skin test is available, but the ubiquitousness of the fungus and the large number of positive reactions precludes its clinical usefulness. Furthermore, lymphopenic states associated with a high incidence of candidiasis are frequently characterized by anergy to candida extract injected intradermally.

Serology is of little use in diagnosis.

Differential Diagnosis

Characteristic mucosal or skin lesions, isolation of the fungus, and response to therapy establish the diagnosis in most cases. To be differentiated are agranulocytic mucosal lesions, herpes simplex, herpangina, contact or allergic dermatitis, avitaminosis, bacterial infections, and toxic or drug eruptions of the skin.

Complications

Dissemination from oral and skin infection is the

most serious complication. The severity of candidal infection is directly related to the type of underlying disease and the amount of therapy with antibiotics, corticosteroids, or immunosuppressive agents.

Treatment

Mild candidiasis is usually a benign disease that is easily treated with a single course of topical gentian violet or nystatin (Mycostatin) (see Chapter 37). Sodium caprylate, various propionates, and potassium permanganate have also been used for skin lesions. The diaper area should be kept dry and open to the air if possible. Bland powder should be applied to prevent accumulation of moisture.

The visceral, systemic, and chronic forms of candidiasis are more difficult to treat because of the underlying disease process or because it is necessary to continue antibiotic, corticosteroid, or immunosuppressive therapy for other reasons. In these forms of candidiasis, amphotericin B (Fungizone) may have to be employed adjunctively (see Chapter 37). Whenever possible, modification or elimination of predisposing causes should be attempted.

The introduction of flucytosine (Ancobon) has improved the outlook for some patients with severe candidiasis. Used alone or in conjunction with amphotericin B, flucytosine has produced cures or improvement in patients with disseminated disease, urinary tract infections, and other forms of candidiasis. Unfortunately, it is a toxic drug; leukopenia, thrombocytopenia, nausea, diarrhea, and disturbance in liver function are among the more common adverse effects.

An experimental drug, miconazole, has recently been employed successfully in the treatment of severe candidiasis. Miconazole is a synthetic imidazole derivative with a broad spectrum of antifungal and antibacterial activity. Intravenous administration may be associated with phlebitis. It is anticipated that this drug will soon be available commercially.

Some investigators have been successful in treating the underlying immunodeficiency and secondarily benefiting the patient with candidiasis. Immunotherapy, usually directed at correcting disorders of cell-mediated immunity, has included bone marrow transplantation and administration of transfer factor.

Prognosis

Most superficial forms are self-limited and, with topical therapy, curable. In some cases, only suppression is achieved, and the disease recurs upon discontinuing antifungal therapy.

The prognosis is usually grave in systemic or visceral forms of the disease.

Bayer AS & others: Candida meningitis. Medicine 55:477, 1976.

Goldstein E, Hoeprich PD: Problems in the diagnosis and treatment of systemic candidiasis. J Infect Dis 125:190, 1972.

Harder EJ, Hermans PE: Treatment of fungal infections with flucytosine. Arch Intern Med 135:231, 1975.

Kane JG & others: Diarrhea caused by candida. Lancet 1:335, 1976.

Katz ME, Cassileth PA: Disseminated candidiasis in a patient with acute leukemia: Successful treatment with miconazole. JAMA 237:1124, 1977.

Mazumdar PK, Marks MI: *Candida albicans* infections in hospitalized children. Clin Pediatr (Phila) 14:123, 1975.

Milne LJR, Crompton GK: Beclomethasone dipropionate and oropharyngeal candidiasis. Br Med J 2:797, 1974.

Montes LF & others: Chronic mucocutaneous candidiasis. JAMA 221:156, 1972.

Roe DC, Haynes RE: *Candida albicans* meningitis successfully treated with amphotericin B. Am J Dis Child 124:926, 1972.

Sheft D, Shrago G: Esophageal moniliasis. JAMA 213:1859, 1970.

COCCIDIOIDOMYCOSIS

Essentials of Diagnosis

- Primary pulmonary form: Fever, pleuritis, productive cough, anorexia, weight loss, and (in 10%) generalized macular skin rash.
- Erythema nodosum and multiforme with arthralgia ("desert rheumatism").
- Extrapulmonary form: Traumatic site, indurated ulcer 1–3 weeks later, regional adenopathy.
- Disseminated lesions in skin, bones, viscera, and meninges.
- Sporangia (30–60 μm) in pus, sputum, CSF, etc.
- Gray, cottony growth on Sabouraud's medium.
- Delayed type skin test reaction (induration more than 5 mm) to coccidioidin.
- Precipitin (early, 1–4 weeks) and complement-fixing (late, 6–12 weeks) antibodies develop.

General Considerations

Coccidioidomycosis is caused by the dimorphic fungus *Coccidioides immitis.* The infective forms (arthrospores) are found in soil in the lower Sonoran life zone, and the disease is endemic in parts of California, Arizona, New Mexico, Texas, Mexico, and South America. Infection is acquired by inhalation or skin inoculation. Many rodents are naturally infected. The human disease is not contagious, but laboratory infections can occur from cultured coccidioides.

Almost two-thirds of infections are asymptomatic; of the remainder, less than 0.5% will disseminate.

Clinical Findings

A history of residence or travel in an endemic area is essential to the diagnosis. The incubation period of 7–28 days seems to be directly related to the intensity of exposure; brief and minimal exposure is associated with a longer interval. Children in agricultural communities are at risk.

A. Symptoms and Signs: The primary forms of

coccidioidomycosis are usually pulmonary and rarely dermal. Severity varies from a mild upper respiratory illness to a severe influenza-like syndrome. In the latter, fever is prominent and may be prolonged. Associated symptoms include pleural pain, myalgia, headache, severe lassitude and malaise, anorexia with weight loss; cough, which may be productive of clear to purulent sputum; and arthralgia ("desert rheumatism"). Milder forms of the disease are associated with milder symptoms of brief duration. Skin rashes may be prominent, with 10% of patients exhibiting a generalized erythematous macular eruption early in the illness. A few patients will develop tender, indurated nodules on the lower extremities (erythema nodosum), and a more generalized pleomorphic rash (erythema multiforme).

Apart from fever and skin eruptions, physical findings are usually few and limited to the lungs. Rales, signs of consolidation, and a pleural friction rub may be noted.

An indolent indurated ulcer at the site of skin trauma is observed in primary dermal coccidioidomycosis. Regional lymphadenopathy is usually present.

Chronic pulmonary coccidioidomycosis may be asymptomatic. Some patients complain of chest pain and cough, and a few produce sputum, which may be bloody. The pulmonary lesion is cavitary and may elicit signs of consolidation or, if it is subpleural, may rupture and cause empyema or pneumothorax.

Dissemination may be heralded by a biphasic course with recurrence and extension of symptoms following initial improvement. However, dissemination may occur rapidly in the primary illness. Symptoms are similar to the primary illness but more severe and persistent. Also, signs referable to the organs involved will appear (eg, meningitic signs in CNS involvement).

Dissemination in children may be of the limited variety. Following an initial pulmonary or asymptomatic infection, typical symptoms of osteomyelitis may occur. A single lesion, usually in the long bones but also sometimes in the skull, pelvis, and mandible, appears on x-ray as a sharply demarcated osteolytic opacity. Diagnosis may be confirmed by (1) high complement fixation titers, (2) little or no skin test reactivity, and (3) identification of the organism in curetted material from the osseous lesion. Rarely, dissemination may be limited to another site such as the meninges, the kidney, a lymph node, or the skin. Isolation of the organism from these sites establishes the diagnosis. The mandibular form is a special instance of coccidioidomycosis in that it produces a very indolent osteomyelitis requiring a surgical approach with or without the local instillation of amphotericin B. All other forms must be treated with systemic amphotericin B. In addition, the meningeal form requires instillation of amphotericin B into the subarachnoid space, usually by direct cisternal puncture and occasionally via a reservoir placed in communication with the ventricles. In contrast to the visceral dissemination forms of this disease, the limited dissemination can be cured or converted to a chronically present but relatively

asymptomatic process. For example, we have observed survival of 4 and 14 years, respectively, in 2 children with meningeal coccidioidomycosis. Both required initial courses of amphotericin B and repetitive intracisternal administration of this antibiotic. Most patients with the single bone lesion characteristic of limited dissemination respond to amphotericin B or surgical curettage of the lesion (or both). There is some experimental evidence that establishment of effective cell-mediated immunity by transfer factor administration can result in cure of the limited dissemination forms of this disease.

B. Laboratory Findings: Direct examination of pus, CSF, sputum, or other clinical specimens treated with sodium hydroxide may reveal the characteristic sporangia (30–60 μm). India ink may be useful for contrast, but staining is of no value. The fungus can be cultured on Sabouraud's agar, but the slants should be sealed and never opened to avoid laboratory infections. *C immitis* grows rapidly, and gray, cottony colonies appear in a few days. Occasionally, mouse inoculation will aid in diagnosis.

Precipitating antibodies appear in the first to third weeks of infection and disappear by 4–6 weeks. Complement-fixing antibodies develop much later, if at all. Mild and asymptomatic illness is associated with no complement-fixing antibodies; moderate to severe illness is associated with a complement-fixing antibody rise which disappears in 6–8 months; and disseminated illness is associated with a persistent and high titer of complement-fixing antibodies. The presence of complement-fixing antibody in CSF is diagnostic of meningitis.

A skin test with coccidioidin results in an area of induration more than 5 mm in diameter within 2–21 days after onset. In patients with allergic manifestations (erythema nodosum), extreme skin sensitivity is present and the coccidioidin should be diluted 10–100 times before testing. Reactivity may persist for years in convalescence but may decrease or disappear with dissemination.

The sedimentation rate is elevated during the acute phase. An intense eosinophilia has been described just prior to dissemination.

C. X-Ray Findings: Roentgenologic evidence of pneumonia, pleural effusion, granuloma, or cavitation may be present at various stages of the pulmonary disease. Osteomyelitis may be noted.

Differential Diagnosis

Coccidioidomycosis must be distinguished from acute viral and bacterial pneumonias and acute tuberculosis. The chronic pulmonary lesion must be distinguished from chronic tuberculosis and malignancy. The disseminated forms will resemble diseases of the organs involved (osteomyelitis, meningitis, etc).

Complications

These are primarily pulmonary, with pleural effusion, empyema, pneumothorax, or combinations occurring in association with a subpleural cavity.

Treatment

A. Specific Measures: There is no universally effective drug. Amphotericin B (Fungizone) may be of value in individual cases, particularly with dissemination. (See Chapter 37.) In the meningitic form, systemic amphotericin B alone is of little benefit. Intracisternal administration of amphotericin B, initially on a daily basis and subsequently at intervals of 1–6 weeks, may result in prolonged survival.

Miconazole, a synthetic imidazole, has been successful in the therapy of severe coccidioidomycosis. As yet an experimental agent, miconazole may offer effective therapy with minor side-effects, a major advance in antifungal therapy.

B. General Measures: Most children with pulmonary coccidioidomycosis require little therapy. They may feel ill for a day or 2 and limit their own activities. Rarely does one need to treat the cough or chest pain. Bed rest is required only for children with severe symptoms or excessive fatigue. It is surprising how active children with this disease can be despite severity of symptoms and chest findings.

C. Surgical Measures: Surgery may be indicated in cavitary lesions or with chronic draining sinuses. Amphotericin B should be administered prior to and for 4 weeks following excisional surgery.

Prognosis

Complete recovery is the rule for all but a very few patients. Those with disseminated disease are at greatest risk, and as many as 50% died prior to the availability of amphotericin B. Blacks and Filipinos appear to be at greater risk of dissemination (10 times the rate for whites) and, therefore, a fatal outcome. Meningitis and diffuse disseminated disease carry the worst prognosis. An increasing complement-fixing antibody titer and a decrease or reversion of a positive skin test are unfavorable prognostic signs.

Doto IL & others: Coccidioidin, histoplasmin, and tuberculin sensitivity among school children in Maricopa County, Arizona. Am J Epidemiol 95:464, 1972.

Richardson HB, Anderson JA, McKay BM: Acute pulmonary coccidioidomycosis in children. J Pediatr 70:376, 1967.

Seabury J: Coccidioidomycosis. In: *Disorders of the Respiratory Tract in Children,* 2nd ed. Vol 1. *Pulmonary Disorders.* Kendig EL Jr (editor). Saunders, 1972.

Sieber O, Larter W, Fulginiti V: Limited extrapulmonary coccidioidomycosis as a form of disseminated disease in children. In: *Coccidioidomycosis: Current Clinical & Diagnostic Status.* Ajello L (editor). Symposia Specialists, Florida, 1977.

Sieber O & others: *Coccidioides immitis* osteomyelitis of the mandible in an infant. J Oral Surg 35:721, 1977.

Stevens DA & others: Miconazole in coccidioidomycosis. 2. Therapeutic and pharmacologic studies in man. Am J Med 60:191, 1976.

Werner SB & others: An epidemic of coccidioidomycosis among archeology students in northern California. N Engl J Med 286:507, 1972.

Winn WA: Long term study of 300 patients with cavitary-abscess lesions of the lung of coccidioidal origin. Dis Chest 54:268, 1968.

CRYPTOCOCCOSIS

Cryptococcus neoformans is a spherical fungus found worldwide in soil and in the old excreta of pigeons. It is an opportunistic organism that is frequently associated with seriously altered host mechanisms, eg, leukemia. It is commonly found at autopsy. Humans are probably infected by inhalation.

Systemic cryptococcosis may result in widespread infection. Particular sites of localization include the CNS, eyes, skin, and bone. Skin lesions vary from papules to ulcerative abscesses. Bony lesions are indurated and painful and result in extensive local destruction, although periosteal proliferation is minimal or absent.

Several forms of the disease exist. Most commonly observed is the insidious cryptococcal meningitis. Recurrent or progressive headache, changes in personality and ambition, dizziness, and vomiting herald the onset of meningeal infection. The patient may have mild fever, slight nuchal rigidity, and alteration in lower extremity reflexes. Signs of progressive increase in intracranial pressure follow, with papilledema, cranial nerve paresis, and optic atrophy. The symptoms usually progress slowly over a period of several months, but chronic forms may last for years.

Sporadic cases of acute pulmonary cryptococcosis are seen, and asymptomatic granulomas are frequently detected at necropsy. Thus, it is likely that the lungs are the portal of entry for the fungus.

Clinical laboratory specimens are usually very mucoid owing to the capsule of the fungus. Direct visualization of the 5–20 μm fungi is enhanced by India ink contrast. Any specimen containing cellular debris should be digested with 10% sodium hydroxide. Culture from pus, sputum, bone marrow, or CSF is possible. When CSF is inoculated, care must be taken to use sufficient volume. As much as 2–20 ml should be inoculated into a single culture, as the fungus cell content may be quite low.

Chest x-rays may reveal solitary or multiple lesions; bone films may show areas of osteolysis.

Amphotericin B (Fungizone) (see Chapter 37) is of proved value, and its use (intravenously or intrathecally) may result in complete cure. Surgical excision may be of adjunctive value.

Flucytosine (Ancobon) offers additional therapy. Patients have received both amphotericin B and flucytosine. Flucytosine is toxic, with leukopenia, thrombocytopenia, nausea, diarrhea, and disturbance in liver function all having been reported.

Miconazole may be useful in cryptococcal disease. This synthetic imidazole is currently being investigated in various forms of the disease.

The disease process may be relatively acute or may progress slowly over a period of several years. In the chronic forms, remissions and exacerbations are frequent. The disseminated and meningeal forms are frequently fatal.

Gauder JP: Cryptococcal cellulitis. JAMA 237:672, 1977.

Harder EJ, Hermans PE: Treatment of fungal infections with flucytosine. Arch Intern Med 135:231, 1975.

McDonald R & others: Cryptococcal meningitis. Arch Dis Child 45:417, 1970.

Robert F, Durant JR, Gams RA: Demonstration of *Cryptococcus neoformans* in a stained bone marrow specimen. Arch Intern Med 137:688, 1977.

Sakowitz AJ, Sakowitz BH: Disseminated cryptococcosis. JAMA 236:2429, 1976.

HISTOPLASMOSIS

Essentials of Diagnosis

- History of residence in or travel to endemic areas.
- Pulmonary calcification.
- Hepatosplenomegaly, anemia, leukopenia.
- Positive skin test.
- Isolation of organism or identification in smears (2–4 μm oval budding yeasts with narrow neck).

General Considerations

Histoplasmosis is caused by the dimorphic fungus *Histoplasma capsulatum.* Its tissue form is a budding oval yeast, 2–4 μm in diameter. Benign histoplasmosis was first noted in tuberculin-negative individuals with pulmonary calcifications. Such individuals were histoplasmin reactive (positive). The endemic areas include central and eastern USA. The fungus is found in soil, especially when enriched by bat feces. It is believed that infection is acquired by inhalation, and over 65% of children acquire asymptomatic infections in the endemic areas.

Clinical Findings

A history of residence or travel to the endemic areas is essential. Heavy contact with potentially infected soil or excreta (bat feces) may provide an etiologic clue.

A. Symptoms and Signs: Three forms of infection are recognized: asymptomatic benign infection, pneumonia, and disseminated disease.

1. Asymptomatic infection—The diagnosis is made by observation of pulmonary calcifications in the absence of delayed hypersensitivity to other antigens and a positive histoplasmin skin test.

2. Histoplasmal pneumonia—This form of the disease is manifested by nonproductive cough, chest pain, hemoptysis, and dyspnea. Cyanosis and hoarseness may also be noted. Influenza-like symptoms may also occur, with fever, muscle and joint pains, and malaise. Night sweats and weight loss may simulate tuberculosis. Physical signs may be absent, or typical findings of pneumonia (rales, bronchial breathing, etc) may be observed. A chronic pulmonary disease may be seen in adults but almost never in children.

3. Disseminated histoplasmosis—The disseminated form of the disease has all of the pulmonary features plus signs and symptoms referable to the lymphatic system. Thus, hepatosplenomegaly, severe wasting, and generalized lymphadenopathy occur. Ulceration of the gastrointestinal and respiratory tracts occurs occasionally. Pallor may be a prominent finding.

B. Laboratory Findings: Anemia and leukopenia, often profound, occur in the disseminated form. Isolation of the fungus provides a specific diagnosis. This usually is unrewarding in the benign infection, although rarely the organism may be found in the urine. Examination of sputum, urine, biopsy material, bone marrow, or blood may yield the organism in the disseminated form. Morphologically, *H capsulatum* appears as 2–4 μm oval cells on a smear stained with Giemsa's or Wright's stain. A large vacuole and crescent-shaped eosinophilic masses of cytoplasm may be visible in the larger end of the ovoid. If budding is observed, the neck is seen to be narrow and may appear as a separate ovoid. Such cells are identified within monocytes or macrophages but often are found free. Upon culture (with agar at 20–30° C), the organism may be isolated and specifically identified. Mouse inoculation is an extremely sensitive method for isolation of histoplasma. Complement fixation and precipitin antibody tests are available. Both are positive in the first few weeks after infection and remain elevated only with dissemination.

C. X-Ray Findings: Pulmonary calcifications, solitary or multiple, may be noted in an asymptomatic child. In acute pulmonic disease, bilateral bronchial pneumonia is the rule. Miliary distribution occasionally occurs.

Differential Diagnosis

Pulmonary histoplasmosis with or without symptoms must be differentiated from tuberculosis. The use of skin tests and serologic and isolation technics permits differentiation. The disseminated form of the disease mimics miliary tuberculosis and leukemia. Differentiation is based upon isolation of the organism. Serology may be helpful if the disease is not fulminant.

Complications

Benign and mild symptomatic infections require no specific therapy, and recovery is the rule. With concomitant disease (lymphatic malignancies, tuberculosis) or with immunosuppressive therapy, dissemination may occur.

Treatment

Benign or mild forms require no treatment. Selective extirpative surgical therapy may be of benefit in localized pulmonary disease. Amphotericin B (Fungizone) appears to be effective. (See Chapter 37.)

Prognosis

In benign or mild forms, the prognosis is excellent for recovery and complete healing. Chronic infection may result from more marked pulmonary disease. Disseminated histoplasmosis has a variable course and severity. Fulminant histoplasmosis, histoplasmosis associated with concomitant tuberculosis or malignancy, or histoplasmosis occurring in a patient receiving immunosuppressive therapy has a very poor prognosis.

Crawford SE: Histoplasmosis in infants and children. GP 30:78, Jan 1964.

Fosson AI, Wheeler WE: Short term amphotericin B treatment of severe childhood histoplasmosis. J Pediatr 86:32, 1975.

Holland P, Holland NH: Histoplasmosis in early infancy. Am J Dis Child 112:412, 1966.

Shearer WT & others: Presumptive histoplasmosis presenting as cerebellar ataxia with spontaneous recovery. Pediatrics 57:150, 1976.

Tesh RB & others: Histoplasmosis in children. Pediatrics 33:894, 1964.

NOCARDIOSIS

Nocardiosis is infrequent in childhood. It is caused by *Nocardia asteroides,* an aerobic, gram-positive, partially acid-fast actinomycete.* Pulmonary infection is common and may lead to chronic pneumonia or dissemination to the meninges or brain. Typical gram-positive, short-branching rods or coccal forms are seen which are also acid-fast. Culture establishes the diagnosis.

The sulfonamides are the drugs of choice (see Chapter 37).

Bach MC & others: Pulmonary nocardiosis. JAMA 224:1378, 1973.

*A bacterium, not a fungus. Discussed in this chapter by convention since *N asteroides* (like *Actinomyces israelii*) was thought for many years to be a fungus.

Ballenger CN, Goldring D: Nocardiosis in childhood. J Pediatr 50:145, 1957.

Beamon BL & others: Nocardial infections in the United States, 1972–1974. J Infect Dis 134:286, 1976.

Murray JF & others: The changing spectrum of nocardiosis. Am Rev Respir Dis 83:315, 1961.

SPOROTRICHOSIS

Sporotrichosis is caused by *Sporotrichum schenckii.* Localized lymphatic sporotrichosis may follow a prick with a thorn or splinter which results in an ulcer or nodule followed by others along the route of lymphatic return from the injured part. Dissemination to the skin and mucosa can occur, but the viscera are usually spared. Diagnosis is best accomplished by culture of aspirates or drainage from local lesions or nodes.

Potassium iodide is said to be effective, although some cases may require amphotericin B (Fungizone) (see Chapter 37). Potassium iodide can be administered orally as the saturated solution. The dose is variable. Initially, give 3–5 drops 3 times daily after meals. Increase the dose to 40 drops 3 times daily by adding 1 drop per dose. Continue therapy for 2 weeks or until signs of disease activity have disappeared. Then reduce the dose by 1 drop per dose until 5 drops is reached, at which time therapy is discontinued. *Note:* If signs of iodism appear, the dosage must be reduced. Potassium iodide is indicated only in sporotrichosis and not in other fungal diseases.

Chandler JW & others: Childhood sporotrichosis. Am J Dis Child 115:368, 1968.

Hanrahan JB, Erickson ER: Sporotrichosis in western Pennsylvania. JAMA 197:814, 1966.

Orr ER, Riley HD: Sporotrichosis in children: Report of 10 cases. J Pediatr 78:951, 1971.

•   •   •

General References

Bennett JE: Chemotherapy of systemic mycoses. (First of 2 parts.) N Engl J Med 290:30, 1974.

Conant NF & others: *Manual of Clinical Mycology,* 3rd ed. Saunders, 1971.

Dalldorf G (editor): *Fungi and Fungous Diseases.* Thomas, 1962.

Dubos RJ, Hirsch JG: *Bacterial and Mycotic Infections of Man,* 4th ed. Lippincott, 1965.

Emmons CW & others: *Medical Mycology,* 2nd ed. Lea & Febiger, 1970.

Fetter BF & others: *Mycoses of the Central Nervous System.* Williams & Wilkins, 1967.

Halde C: Systemic mycoses. Chap 23 in: *Current Medical References,* 6th ed. Chatton MJ, Sanazaro PJ (editors). Lange, 1970.

Hildick-Smith G & others: *Fungus Diseases and Their Treatment.* Little, Brown, 1964.

Lewis GM & others: *An Introduction to Medical Mycology.* Year Book, 1958.

Salvin SB: Immunologic aspects of the mycoses. Prog Allergy 7:213, 1963.

Sweany HC (editor): *Histoplasmosis.* Thomas, 1960.

Wilson JW, Plunkett OA: *The Fungous Diseases of Man.* Univ of California Press, 1965.

29...
Emergencies & Accidents*

John D. Burrington, MD

INITIAL EMERGENCY EXAMINATION & MANAGEMENT

Initial Management

A. Emergency Measures:

1. Ensure adequate ventilation—

a. Clear the upper airway. Pull the tongue forward and insert an airway. Draw the chin forward with the patient supine by inserting the second and third fingers behind the angles of the mandibles. Check for gum or loose teeth. Suction mucus or blood. If indicated, insert an endotracheal tube or perform tracheostomy.

b. Administer oxygen if necessary.

c. Institute artificial respiration if necessary.

d. Close sucking wounds of thorax.

2. Cardiac resuscitation if necessary.

3. Stop hemorrhage with direct pressure. Examine for concealed hemorrhage into the thorax, abdomen, pelvis, or soft tissues.

4. Treat shock promptly. Begin lactated Ringer's injection at 10 ml/kg/hour through a plastic cannula carefully secured in a vein. Correct acidosis.

5. Avoid spinal cord damage. Maintain normal alignment of the vertebrae in both examination and transportation. Assume cervical spine injury in unconscious patient until x-rays are obtained.

B. Follow-Up Measures:

1. Splint and elevate fractures.

2. Dress open wounds.

3. Adjust intravenous fluids as indicated by color, pulse, and blood pressure.

4. Check urine sediment, volume, and specific gravity.

5. Obtain baseline hematocrit and specimen for blood bank.

Initial Rapid Survey Examination

A. History:

1. Present illness—Prodrome, onset, recent illness, progression of symptoms, environment, medicines, syringes, etc. In case of injury, elicit exact details.

2. Past history—Previous attacks, chronic illness, habits, medications, occupation (student, part-time employment, etc). Examine patient's personal effects

*Other medical emergencies are discussed in appropriate chapters elsewhere in this book. Poisoning, including snakebite, spider bite, scorpion bite, and insect stings, is discussed in Chapter 30. Drowning is discussed in Chapter 12.

(diabetic or epileptic identification card, prescription labels, etc).

B. Physical Examination:

1. General Observations—Note position of body and extremities, evidence of external or internal bleeding, skin color, rate and quality of pulse and respiration, temperature, blood pressure (both arms), state of consciousness, and unusual odors. Note neck vein distention; check pulsation in major arteries, paradoxic pulse.

2. Head, neck, and eyes—Injuries of skull and face, neck rigidity, breath aroma, appearance of pupils and reaction to light, ophthalmoscopic examination in coma, fluid or blood from ears or nose, mucous membranes of mouth, position of trachea, crepitation in the neck, rigidity of neck muscles.

3. Chest—Note pattern of breathing, retraction, paradoxic motion, bruising, sucking sounds. Test chest wall stability with gentle anteroposterior and lateral compression. Check trachea for mediastinal shift. Listen and percuss for breath sounds, dullness, mediastinal crunch, murmurs, or increased cardiac dullness.

4. Abdomen—External evidence of injury, distention, presence of rigidity or tenderness, bowel sounds. Percuss bladder and other palpable or percussable organs. Measure abdominal girth at navel.

5. Back—Examine for injuries. Maintain normal alignment of vertebrae.

6. Extremities—Note position, deformity, color, and pulses in extremities. Check active and passive motion. Compress wings of ilium; palpate symphysis pubica and examine perineum for hematoma, genital injury, or extravasated urine.

7. Neurologic examination—Deep and superficial reflexes, flaccidity or rigidity; response to pinprick or noxious stimuli. Elicit cranial nerve abnormalities when possible.

CARDIAC ARREST

Begin resuscitation when peripheral pulse not palpable or pulse < 60/minute. Irreversible CNS damage will occur within 4 minutes after circulatory failure. Whether the arrest is secondary to ventricular fibrillation or standstill (asystole) is of no immediate consequence. Initial resuscitative measures are identical in both circumstances.

Treatment

Initial treatment is directed at restoring circulation and oxygenation of tissues.

A. Heart Massage:

1. Begin closed chest cardiac massage immediately at 60–80/minute. The tendency is to pump too fast. (See Technic, below, and Fig 29–1.)

2. Open heart massage is indicated only in the operating room if closed chest massage is unsuccessful.

B. Pulmonary Ventilation: Must be initiated immediately. (See Technic, below, and Fig 29–2.)

1. Patients often aspirate vomitus or secretions before cardiac arrest. Always clear the throat and trachea before beginning positive pressure breathing.

2. Mouth-to-mouth breathing is the most efficient of the commonly available methods of administering immediate artificial respiration. The mask and bag method is most efficient (Fig 29–4).

3. Endotracheal intubation should be initiated as soon as equipment is available. Add oxygen until normal color returns.

C. Intravenous Fluids: Introduce an 18 gauge or larger plastic cannula into a vein. A central venous catheter can be introduced via the basilic vein at the elbow or via the external jugular. Begin lactated Ringer's injection and add plasma or blood as indicated. If arrest has occurred, give 0.9 M sodium bicarbonate according to the following formula:

$$\text{Weight (in kg)} \times 0.3 \times 10 = \text{ml of 0.9 M sodium bicarbonate}$$

This assumes a base deficit of 10 and should be repeated every 3–5 minutes during resuscitation. All other measures will fail if acidosis is not corrected.

D. Electrocardiogram: Determine by ECG whether the heart is in ventricular fibrillation or asystole.

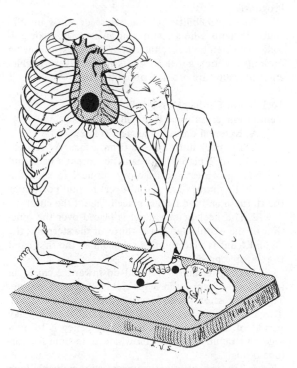

Figure 29–1. Technic of closed chest cardiac massage. (Heavy circle in heart drawing shows area of application of force. Circles on supine figure show points of application of electrodes for defibrillation.)

E. **Management of Fibrillation**: (See Technic, below, and Fig 29—1.) Use of a defibrillator is indicated.

F. **Management of Asystole**:

1. Correct acidosis with 0.9 M sodium bicarbonate as above.

2. Strike the chest sharply with the fist 2 or 3 times.

3. Ensure adequate ventilation.

4. Single electric shocks from a defibrillator may initiate contraction.

5. Calcium has an inotropic action and should be used if asystole continues. Give 1 ml of 10% calcium gluconate by direct intracardiac injection or through a central venous catheter.

6. For persistent asystole, epinephrine, 1—3 ml of 1:10,000 solution by direct intracardiac injection, may restore the heartbeat.

7. Once a regular heartbeat and palpable peripheral pulses have been established, determine arterial pH, P_{O_2}, P_{CO_2}, and base deficit. Repeat these determinations at least hourly until the patient's condition has stabilized since resuscitation may wash metabolic acids out of tissues and lead to profound acidosis.

8. Plan on endotracheal intubation and assisted or controlled ventilation for at least several hours after resuscitation from cardiac arrest.

9. Watch carefully for cardiac tamponade and pneumothorax if direct intracardiac medications have been given.

Prognosis

The reversibility of the arrest depends on the cause. Patients who arrest during an acute hypoxic episode can often be resuscitated. Cardiac arrest following prolonged shock and acidosis is not easily reversible, and the results are often disappointing.

Technics of Cardiac Massage, Pulmonary Ventilation, & External Defibrillation

A. **External Cardiac Massage**: (Fig 29—1.)

1. The back must be on a firm surface. A "resuscitation board," placed between the patient's back and the bed, provides a satisfactory surface. In small infants, both thumbs are placed over the mid portion of the sternum and the fingers placed behind the chest.

2. The heel of one hand is placed over the junction of the middle and lower thirds of the sternum; the second hand is placed on the dorsum of the first hand to reinforce pressure.

3. The sternum is pressed downward 2 cm in an infant or 3—5 cm in an older child, 60 times a minute. The compression phase is very fast (about 0.4 second). This is followed by a rapid release and then a delay period of about 0.6 seconds. The tendency is to massage too rapidly and not allow adequate time for cardiac filling.

4. The test of effective massage is a palpable femoral or carotid pulse.

5. If only one physician is available, he should interrupt cardiac massage every 30 seconds and inflate

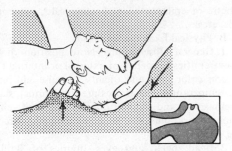

The operator takes his position at the patient's head.

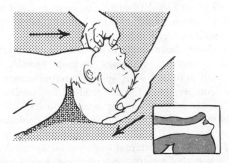

With the right thumb and index finger he displaces the mandible forward by pressing at its central portion, at the same time lifting the neck and tilting the head as far back as necessary to establish airway. Beware of cervical spine fracture.

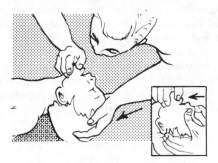

The victim's mouth is opened by downward and forward traction on the lower jaw or by pulling down the lower lip.

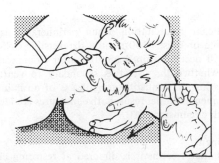

After taking a deep breath, the operator immediately seals his mouth around the mouth and nose of the victim and exhales until the chest of the victim rises.

Figure 29—2. Technic of mouth-to-mouth insufflation.

the lungs several times by the mouth-to-mouth technic.

B. Pulmonary Ventilation:

1. The mouth-to-mouth technic is the most efficient of the commonly available means of achieving immediate ventilation.

a. Position the patient flat on his back and extend his neck gently; he may have apnea from cervical spine injury.

b. Clear the oropharynx and pull the tongue forward.

c. If there is evidence of aspiration and suction is immediately available, aspirate both mainstem bronchi.

d. Occlude the nostrils.

e. Cup the patient's lips and exhale into the patient's mouth.

f. Continue a rate of 40 breaths per minute in newborns or 20 breaths per minute in older children.

2. Hand AMBU bags (Fig 29–4) are advantageous because the physician can more easily observe the patient's response and because 100% oxygen can be delivered. The manual resuscitator consists of a pliable bag, nonrebreathing valve, and face mask. Effective positive pressure ventilation can be achieved by applying the mask firmly over the nose and mouth and squeezing the bag, which recoils promptly to the full position when released. Oxygen can be administered if desired by attaching the oxygen tubing to the air intake valve at the end of the bag. The manual resuscitator should be available in ambulances, coronary care and intensive care units, and wherever there might be victims of heart attack, cardiac arrest, suffocation, drowning, etc.

3. Wherever oxygen and an AMBU (self-inflating) bag are available, there should be a laryngoscope and an assortment of endotracheal tubes.

4. For emergency endotracheal intubation, select a tube the size of the patient's small finger. For elective intubation, use a tube the size of his index finger.

5. The criteria of adequate ventilation are chest excursion and breath sounds, improvement in nail bed and skin color, and serial determinations showing normal arterial blood gases and pH.

C. External Defibrillation:

1. Place one electrode in the second intercostal space of the right sternal border and a second electrode in the 4th intercostal space of the left midaxillary line (Fig 29–1). Be sure that adequate electrode paste has

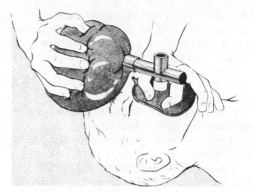

(1) Lift the victim's neck with one hand.
(2) Tilt head backward into maximum neck extension. Remove secretions and debris from mouth and throat and pull the tongue and mandible forward as required to clear the airway.
(3) Hold the mask snugly over the nose and mouth, holding the chin forward and the neck in extension as shown in diagram.
(4) Squeeze the bag, noting inflation of the lungs by the rise of the chest wall.
(5) Release the bag, which will expand spontaneously. The patient will exhale and the chest will fall.
(6) Repeat steps 4 and 5 approximately 12 times per minute.

Figure 29–4. Portable manual resuscitator.

been applied and that no personnel are touching the patient at the time of defibrillation.

2. Begin in the low ranges of 50 watt-seconds and increase in increments of 25 watt-seconds (values are for DC defibrillators).

3. If single shocks are ineffective, attempt paired shocks at intervals as short as the defibrillator will allow.

4. Be sure that no one is touching the patient during defibrillation.

5. Be sure that electrodes are discharged before setting them aside.

Aberdeen E: Artificial airways in children. Surg Clin North Am 54:1155, 1974.

Lefer AM: Role of corticosteroids in the treatment of circulatory response. Clin Pharmacol Ther 11:630, 1970.

Resnekov L: Electroconversion of cardiac dysrhythmias. Am Heart J 78:581, 1970.

Riker WL: Cardiac arrest in infants and children. Pediatr Clin North Am 16:661, 1969.

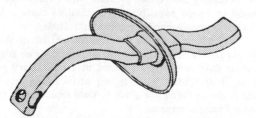

Figure 29–3. Airway for use in mouth-to-mouth insufflation. The larger airway is for adults. The guard is flexible and may be inverted from the position shown for use with infants and children.

SHOCK

Shock is a clinical syndrome characterized by prostration and hypotension resulting from a profound depression of vital cell functions associated with or secondary to poor tissue perfusion. If cellular function is not improved, shock becomes irreversible and death will ensue even though the initiating cause of the shock is corrected.

Clinical Findings

Early signs of shock are tachycardia, pallor, agitation, confusion, and thirst. As shock progresses, the patient will become less and less responsive and eventually comatose.

The skin is pale, mottled, and cold. The nail beds are cyanotic, and local and peripheral edema may occur. Poor capillary filling and decreased skin turgor can be demonstrated. Tachypnea indicates hypoxemia or acidosis.

Newborns in shock appear lethargic, pale, and slightly gray. Late shock may be manifested by a decrease in skin temperature, particularly of the extremities.

Immediate Treatment of Shock

(1) Position the patient flat. Elevation of the legs is helpful except in instances of respiratory distress, when it is contraindicated.

(2) Try to determine the cause of shock.

(3) Establish a patent upper airway and administer oxygen by mask or nasal catheter. If the clinical condition deteriorates, consider the use of an endotracheal tube and intermittent positive pressure breathing.

(4) Establish an intravenous site with a large bore catheter (No. 18 or larger).

(5) Initiate fluid therapy with lactated Ringer's injection or isotonic saline solution at a rate calculated to restore one-fourth of the patient's blood volume in 1 hour (about 15–20 ml/kg).

(6) Establish a central venous pressure monitor in all cases of shock that are not easily reversible.

(7) Monitor urine volume and specific gravity.

(8) Consider an arterial catheter as a useful guide to monitoring pressure and as a source of specimens for blood gases and arterial pH.

Treatment of Specific Types of Shock

A. Hypovolemic (Hemorrhagic) Shock: This is defined as a reduction in the size of the vascular compartment, with a falling blood pressure, poor capillary filling, and a low central venous pressure. Treatment consists of preventing further fluid loss and volume replacement of existing losses. Vasopressors should not be used until blood volume has been restored. The choice of fluid used as a volume expander depends on the cause of the hypovolemia. In most instances, lactated Ringer's injection is the preferred solution.

1. Blood loss—Whole blood is the replacement fluid of choice for shock due to hemorrhage. Type-specific blood is strongly recommended; however, unmatched type O Rh-negative blood has been used without causing serious transfusion reactions in emergency situations. The rate of blood replacement is judged by the rate of blood loss, the patient's response, and a rising central venous pressure. Hemorrhagic shock is usually accompanied by marked metabolic acidosis, which must be corrected with sodium bicarbonate solution.

Acute blood loss can be safely replaced with isotonic crystalloid solutions such as lactated Ringer's injection. Albumin infused into patients in shock rapidly "leaks" out of capillaries and becomes sequestered in the alveoli and interstitial spaces.

2. Burns—Even in the case of extensive burns and severe crush injuries, most experimental evidence favors use of crystalloid alone. Packed red cells should be added as soon as they are available to keep the hematocrit above 30% to maintain oxygen-carrying capacity.

Dextran should be used sparingly since it is probably the saline in which it is suspended that is most helpful in reversing shock. Dextran can interfere with platelet function and potentiate bleeding. It is also excreted in the urine and produces artificially high urine specific gravity.

3. Pressor agents—Only cardiotonic drugs that also improve tissue perfusion should be used. Isoproterenol, 1–2 mg in 500 ml of saline solution, and dopamine, 5 µg/kg/minute, are the alternative drugs of choice. Dopamine is usually preferred because it improves renal perfusion.

4. Dehydration—Isotonic salt solutions are indicated in all instances of dehydration, including hypertonic dehydration, when there is an absolute depletion of body salt and fluid even though there is a relative hypertonicity. Lactated Ringer's injection or 0.5 N saline solution with added sodium bicarbonate (30 mEq of $NaHCO_3$ per 500 ml bottle) should be started at a rate of 25–35 ml/kg/hour IV until skin turgor improves and electrolyte values can be obtained.

B. Cardiogenic Shock: This is defined as shock resulting from decreased cardiac output, eg, due to cardiac tamponade, trauma to the myocardium, myocarditis, abnormal rates and rhythm, and biochemical abnormalities.

1. Cardiac tamponade is usually secondary to fluid collection in the pericardial space, but it can also occur secondary to constrictive pericarditis. The only effective treatment is to relieve the tamponade by evacuating the pericardial space or surgically excising the pericardium. Temporary treatment can be achieved by increasing the venous pressure with a transfusion of blood or blood substitutes. Vasodilators cause a drop in venous pressure and are contraindicated.

2. Patients with cardiogenic or persistent shock should have a Swan-Ganz catheter passed via an arm or jugular cutdown. When wedged in a pulmonary arteriole, it accurately reflects left atrial filling pressure and is a more sensitive guide to fluid replacement than central venous pressure.

3. Myocarditis results from viral infections and toxins secondary to bacterial infections.

4. Abnormal heart rate and rhythm result in decreased cardiac output.

a. Marked sinus bradycardia can occur during

anesthesia, particularly when associated with surgery of the neck and thorax. Sinus bradycardia can be blocked with atropine, 0.01 mg/kg as a single IM dose. The minimum dose for newborns is 0.15 mg regardless of weight. The maximum dose for older children is 0.6 mg.

    b. Atrioventricular block may occur secondary to inflammatory disease, surgical trauma, or ischemic injury to the conduction system. Prednisolone, 1 mg/kg/day IV or IM in 4 equally divided doses, may be useful in such conditions. If slowing persists, the ventricular rate can often be increased with isoproterenol, 3–5 μg/kg/minute by IV drip. The infusion is then adjusted according to the pulse response.

    c. Ventricular arrhythmias may be secondary to hypoxia, acidosis, or myocarditis. Procainamide, 50 mg/kg/day IV, is useful in controlling premature ventricular contractions. (For discussion of defibrillation, see Cardiac Arrest, above.)

    5. Biochemical disturbances can result in decreased cardiac output. These include acidosis, hypoxia, and hyperkalemia. (See Chapter 35.)

    C. Bacteremic (Endotoxin, Septic) Shock: This type of shock occurs when overwhelming sepsis and circulating bacterial toxins result in peripheral vascular collapse. Clinical recognition depends on the toxic appearance of the patient, often in association with purpura, splinter hemorrhages, hepatosplenomegaly, and jaundice. While adequate treatment of bacterial shock depends on proper antibiotic therapy of the primary infection, correction of fluid and electrolyte abnormalities is essential to successful resuscitation. Other procedures are useful in supporting the patient with bacterial shock:

    1. Crystalloid and colloid should be administered to keep central venous pressure within the range of 10–14 mm Hg.

    2. When bacteremic shock is due to gram-negative organisms, corticosteroids should be used early. Give prednisolone, 2–4 mg/kg/day IV, or hydrocortisone, 10–40 mg/kg/day IV.

    3. Hypotension often persists in spite of a high central venous pressure. However, tissue perfusion is more important than arterial pressure per se. Isoproterenol, 1 mg in 500 ml of saline solution, or dopamine, 5 μg/kg/minute, by IV drip, will often give adequate peripheral perfusion even though arterial pressure is as much as 20 mm Hg below normal systolic pressure. Levarterenol (Levophed) is rarely used in shock since it elevates central arterial pressure partly by inducing profound vasoconstriction, with resulting decrease in tissue perfusion.

    4. Heparin is of value when bacterial infections are complicated by disseminated intravascular coagulation (DIC).

    D. Anaphylactic Shock: This is an extreme form of allergy or hypersensitivity to a foreign substance which results in circulatory and respiratory distress. The diagnosis is established by a history of exposure to an antigen and by clinical signs of respiratory distress and circulatory collapse. Urticaria and angioneurotic edema are often present. The pathophysiologic mechanisms involve the release of histamine, serotonin, and bradykinins and their effects on various body tissues. The net effect of these compounds is to cause arteriolar dilatation, venular constriction, increased capillary permeability, and bronchial constriction. Such physiologic changes cause marked hypovolemia and respiratory distress.

    1. If shock is precipitated by a drug given intramuscularly, apply a tourniquet proximal to the site of injection tight enough to restrict venous return but not interrupt arterial flow.

    2. Give epinephrine, 1:1000 aqueous solution, 0.1 ml/kg IM immediately. Follow with 0.1 ml/kg IV and repeat in 20 minutes if the response is not satisfactory. (If cardiac arrest occurs, treat as outlined above.)

    3. Give antihistamines, eg, diphenhydramine, 5 mg/kg/day in 4–6 divided doses by IV push over a 5–10 minute interval.

    4. Give prednisolone, 2 mg/kg/day IV in 4–6 divided doses.

    5. For treatment of respiratory distress or wheezing, give aminophylline, 12 mg/kg/day by IV drip in 4 divided doses every 6 hours.

    6. Secretions should be suctioned and may require repeated bronchoscopy. Laryngeal edema may necessitate intubation followed by tracheostomy.

    7. Hypovolemia should be treated vigorously with isotonic saline solution at rates of 25 ml/kg/hour until the patient voids or the central venous pressure monitor indicates a rise to normal values.

    E. Neurogenic Shock: This includes all forms of shock in which interruption of the normal neuronal control results in decreased cardiac output and vascular tone. There is usually a history of exposure to anesthetic agents, spinal cord injuries, or ingestion of barbiturates, narcotics, or tranquilizers. Examination reveals abnormal reflexes and muscle tone, tachycardia and tachypnea, and low blood pressure. The pathophysiologic mechanism is loss of vessel tone with subsequent expansion of the vascular compartment, resulting in relative hypovolemia. Many anesthetic agents have a direct effect on the myocardium which causes a decrease in cardiac output.

    1. Fluids–Neurogenic shock responds well to volume therapy. Give isotonic saline solution, 25 ml/kg/hour IV, until peripheral circulation and skin turgor improve.

    2. Vasopressors–Vascular tone can be improved by several drugs which have a primary effect on vessels and little or no effect on the myocardium. They should be administered only if fluid therapy is not successful. Give either of the following:

    a. Methoxamine, 0.25 mg/kg IM as a single dose, or 0.08 mg/kg IV given over a 10–15 minute interval.

    b. Phenylephrine, 0.1 mg/kg IM as a single dose.

    3. Isoproterenol, 1 mg in 500 ml of saline solution by IV drip, markedly improves perfusion but does not elevate blood pressure. Circulating fluid volume must be expanded before starting an isoproterenol drip.

F. Shock Due to Miscellaneous Causes:

1. Following pulmonary embolism—Shock secondary to pulmonary emboli is rare in pediatrics, but the possibility should be considered if there is a fracture or significant soft tissue injury followed by symptoms of chest pain, dyspnea, cyanosis, and signs of right heart failure. Treatment is supportive, with oxygen and analgesics. If hypotension occurs, isoproterenol is the drug of choice since it provides a bronchodilator effect. If right heart failure develops, a rapid-acting digitalis preparation such as digoxin should be given. The digitalizing dose of digoxin is 0.05 mg/kg IV or IM. The maintenance dose is about one-fifth the digitalizing dose.

2. Respiratory disease—Respiratory disease due to any cause can result in sufficient hypoxia to cause shock. Shock of this nature is reversible only to the extent that the lung disease is reversible, and treatment should be directed toward the primary pulmonary disorder. Oxygen and alkali therapy will only temporarily improve the patient's condition.

3. Metabolic shock—Shock may be secondary to a number of metabolic conditions, such as adrenocortical insufficiency and diabetic acidosis.

Prognosis

With prompt and effective emergency care for both the shock itself and the underlying condition, the immediate prognosis is excellent. If, however, resuscitation is delayed or if the pH has fallen below 7.0, initial resuscitation may be successful but long-term survival is unlikely.

Gabel RA: Cardiopulmonary resuscitation. Am Fam Physician 7:69, Feb 1973.

Goldberg AH: Cardiopulmonary arrest. N Engl J Med 290:381, 1974.

Herman CM: Advances and newer concepts of shock. Pages 1–51 in: *Surgery Annual.* Cooper P, Nyhus LM (editors). Appleton-Century-Crofts, 1972.

Sonnenschein H: Endotoxin shock. Clin Pediatr (Phila) 10:240, 1971.

Stiehm ER: Recognition and management of shock in pediatric patients. Curr Probl Pediatr 3:3, 1973.

TRAUMA

FIRST AID

General Principles

(1) Determine the extent of injury quickly but thoroughly.

(2) Treat immediately such life-endangering conditions as cardiac arrest, airway obstruction by blood or vomitus, arrhythmias or serious bleeding, and shock.

(3) Improvise dressings, splints, and transportation, and arrange for prompt definitive treatment.

Evaluation of the Patient

A. History: Take a sufficient history to ascertain the degree and type of damage and any serious underlying medical problems, eg, cardiac disease or diabetes mellitus.

B. Physical Examination: Examine the patient thoroughly after major trauma.

1. External wounds—Control bleeding promptly (see below).

2. Respiratory distress—Stridor and suprasternal or intercostal retraction indicate airway obstruction. Shortness of breath may be due to chest injury or shock. Respiratory depression may occur in head injury or in severe shock. Cyanosis is due to poor oxygenation from any cause. Check the position of the trachea; a shift indicates either collapse of one lung or tension pneumothorax in contralateral thorax.

3. Shock—Typical signs are faintness, agitation, pallor; cool, moist skin; thirst, air hunger; and a weak, usually rapid pulse.

4. Fractures and dislocations—Palpate carefully from head to foot. Move all joints cautiously, and exert gentle pressure on the spine, chest, and pelvis. Pain, swelling, ecchymosis, deformity, and limitation of motion are classical signs of fracture and dislocation. Few or none of these may be apparent immediately after injury.

5. Brain and spinal cord damage—Assess CNS injury by noting state of consciousness, position and motion of limbs, gross skin sensation, and ability to move extremities actively.

6. Internal injury—Overt localizing signs are often minimal. Hypovolemic shock in the absence of external bleeding or extensive soft tissue trauma suggests internal hemorrhage. Chest pain with respiratory distress and abdominal pain with signs of peritoneal irritation point to visceral injury.

Management of External Bleeding

A. Major Arterial Bleeding: Serious bleeding is usually due to the laceration of a major artery. Speed is essential.

1. Direct pressure on the wound will reduce or stop the flow.

2. Compression of the major artery proximal to the wound may make local pressure effective, permit grasping of a bleeder with a hemostat, or allow time for fashioning a pressure dressing.

3. Do not use a tourniquet unless direct pressure on the wound fails to control bleeding. *Caution:* Faulty use of a tourniquet on an extremity may cause irreparable vascular or neurologic damage. Tourniquets can be improvised from rubber tubing, rope, neckties, belts, handkerchiefs, stockings, strips of cloth, or other suitable materials. Keep the tourniquet exposed and release it briefly at least every 30 minutes. Record time of each release.

B. Venous and Minor Arterial Bleeding: These can be controlled by direct pressure on the wound with sterile gauze or a clean cloth and by elevation of the part.

Management of Respiratory Distress

A. When Due to Airway Obstruction:

1. Remove secretions and foreign material from the mouth and throat. Use suction if available.

2. Hold up the patient's chin or pull out his tongue when relaxation of the tongue and jaw obstruct the hypopharynx, as in comatose patients.

3. Tracheostomy may be necessary if a foreign body or edema obstructs the larynx.

B. When Due to Other Causes: Maintain a clear airway, treat the underlying cause, and administer oxygen if available.

C. In Respiratory Arrest: Clear the airway and institute artificial respiration by mouth-to-mouth insufflation. Intubate the trachea and control ventilation when possible.

Management of Shock

Anticipate and prevent shock by the measures outlined above.

(1) Control hemorrhage and such contributing causes as exposure and pain.

(2) Keep the patient comfortably warm in the recumbent, slightly head-down position. Avoid rapid position changes.

(3) Splint fractures and apply traction if necessary to relieve pain. Pneumatic splints are compact and light. When inflated to 35–40 mm Hg, they immobilize the fracture and control local edema. Check peripheral circulation frequently.

(4) Transport as gently and as quickly as possible to a hospital.

(5) If profound or progressive shock develops, give lactated Ringer's injection, blood, or plasma as soon as possible.

Control of Pain

Distinguish fear and excitement from real pain. Severe injuries frequently cause surprisingly little discomfort. Immobilization of injured parts often relieves distress. *Note:* Narcotics are contraindicated in coma, head injuries, and respiratory depression. Morphine sulfate, 0.1 mg/10 lb IV, or meperidine, 0.05 mg/lb IV, will relieve pain and anxiety. The intravenous route is quick and sure; peripheral vasoconstriction may delay absorption of a subcutaneous or intramuscular injection and will lead to overdosage if multiple injections are later absorbed at the same time. The intravenous dosage is about one-tenth of the intramuscular dosage. Inform other attendants that the patient has received morphine and record the time and dosage on a note or tag affixed to the patient's wrist or ankle.

Care of Open Wounds

(1) Remove gross foreign debris; apply a dry, sterile dressing or a clean cloth and secure it firmly in place. Note if bone is exposed.

(2) Do not place antiseptic solutions or antibacterial powders in the wound.

(3) Arrange for the earliest possible cleansing, debridement, and closure under aseptic conditions.

Transportation of Injured Patients

Improper methods of moving patients can increase injuries. Lift severely injured patients with care (see above), and improvise stretchers from blankets, boards, and doors when necessary. (See accompanying illustrations.) Transport the following types of cases in the recumbent position, on a stretcher, preferably in an ambulance: head and internal injuries; fractures of the spine, pelvis, and long bones of the lower extremities; shock; and major wounds in general. The physician administering first aid is morally and in some areas legally responsible for ensuring the safe transfer of the patient to a medical facility or to another physician.

EMERGENCY ROOM WORK-UP

Examine accident victims promptly and thoroughly. Record history and findings in accurate detail. Obtain the following information in cases of acute injury.

Identification

Obtain as much of this as possible from the family or from adults accompanying the child.

(1) Patient's name, address, phone number, age, sex, and race.

(2) Date and exact time brought to emergency room.

(3) Brought to emergency room by (give name and address).

(4) Referring physician (name and address).

(5) Next of kin (name and address).

(6) If injured at school, record the name, address, and phone number of the school and the name of the school's insurance carrier.

History of Injury

(1) Date and exact time of accident.

(2) Where and how it occurred.

(3) Accurate description of the mechanism of injury, including symptoms, subsequent course, and treatment given.

(4) Note and record exact medications and doses that have been administered.

(5) In major injuries, take a complete general history.

Physical Examination

(1) In minor injuries, describe accurately the local findings. Line drawings are frequently helpful in showing the location and configuration of wounds.

(2) Severe trauma commonly causes multiple injuries, and symptoms may not become manifest for many hours. Palpate such patients carefully and completely in order not to overlook occult fractures and visceral damage.

Laboratory Examination

(1) In major injuries determine the hematocrit,

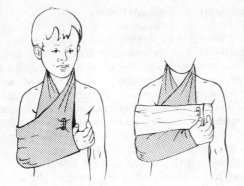

Figure 29—5. Method of application of sling and swathe.

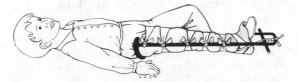

Figure 29—6. Keller-Blake half-ring splint for transportation of patient with fracture of thigh or leg. Spanish windlass on a Collins hitch.

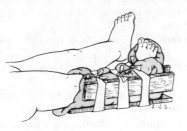

Figure 29—7. Reinforcement of pillow splint for transportation of patient with injury of ankle and foot.

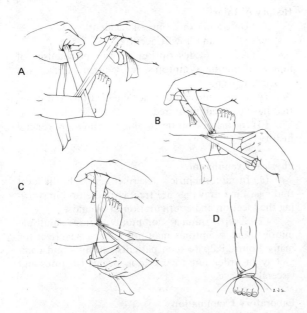

Figure 29—8. Method of tying Collins hitch.

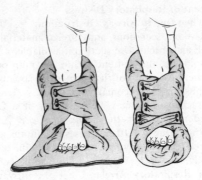

Figure 29—9. Method of application of pillow splints.

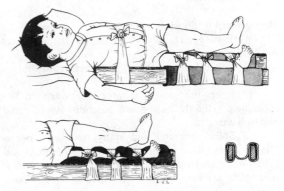

Figure 29—10. Padded board splints for transportation of patient with fracture of thigh and leg. Outer board extends to axilla.

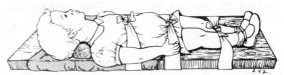

Figure 29—11. Board or door used for transportation of patient with injured spine.

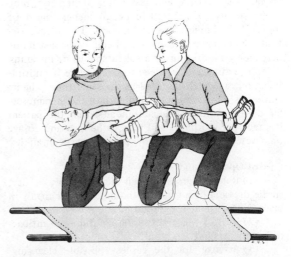

Figure 29—12. Method of lifting injured patient onto stretcher.

hemoglobin, white blood count, and differential count, and perform a urinalysis.

(2) Group and cross-match for blood transfusion as required.

(3) Obtain appropriate x-rays. All sites of suspected fracture should be x-rayed as soon as the patient's condition permits.

(4) Special laboratory tests as indicated.

Diagnostic Impression & Differential Diagnosis

Signature of examiner
Date and hour of examination

Disposition

(1) Discharge; date of return visit.
(2) Referral (name and address of physician).
(3) Hospital admission.

ABDOMINAL INJURIES

Nonpenetrating Abdominal Injuries

May be accompanied by varying degrees of shock, hemorrhage, or peritonitis. The nature and direction of injury should be ascertained. Serial examinations are imperative. Pass a nasogastric tube and aspirate the stomach contents. Test for blood. Leave on suction. Measure abdominal girth at the navel. After initial x-rays, consider peritoneal lavage if the patient is comatose. Insert an Angiocath or Rochester needle 2 cm below the navel and run in 10 ml/kg of normal saline. Siphon fluid by lowering the bottle to the floor.

A. Liver Rupture: Manifestations are due to hemorrhage, shock, and possible bile peritonitis. Liver rupture is characterized by a history of injury followed immediately or after a few hours by right upper quadrant pain, tenderness, and signs of hemorrhage. Shock and rapid exsanguination may occur. The white blood count is elevated.

B. Splenic Rupture: Manifestations are due to hemorrhage and shock. Splenic rupture is characterized by a history of injury followed immediately or after days (subcapsular hemorrhage) by left upper quadrant and shoulder pain, rebound tenderness, muscle rigidity, signs of bleeding (including shifting dullness), a mass in the left upper quadrant, and shock. Often there is no associated rib fracture. The white blood count is elevated. Spontaneous rupture may occur with malaria, leukemia, or infectious mononucleosis.

C. Intestinal Rupture: Manifestations are due to localized peritonitis or to gangrene of the bowel following a mesenteric tear with impairment of blood supply. Characterized by history of injury followed by symptoms due to peritonitis, anemia, or gangrene of bowel. Upright x-rays of the abdomen or chest show free air under the diaphragm, ileus, and free fluid in the abdomen.

D. Kidney Rupture: Manifestations are due to perirenal bleeding and urinary extravasation or intra-

renal bleeding. Characterized by a history of injury followed by flank pain, hematuria, local costovertebral angle tenderness, swelling, muscle spasm, a palpable mass, nonshifting flank dullness, shock, and ecchymosis. An intravenous urogram is valuable for confirmation and to determine the extent of injury.

E. Bladder Rupture: Manifestations are due to local injury with intra- or extraperitoneal extravasation of urine or blood. Rupture is caused by trauma to a full bladder or by a pelvic fracture. Characterized by history of injury to the lower abdomen, followed by persistent pain, suprapubic tenderness, muscle spasm, inability to urinate, or hematuria. Signs of free fluid in the peritoneal cavity may be present. A boggy suprapubic mass may be felt or percussed. X-rays of the pelvis should be taken to determine if fracture has occurred. A cystogram is the most dependable test for bladder injury: instill sterile radiopaque contrast fluid and take anteroposterior and oblique views. (The capacity of the bladder in a 1-year-old child is 75–100 ml; in an adult, 250–300 ml.)

F. Urethral Rupture: Manifestations depend upon the segment of urethra involved; extravasation of urine or blood may be around the bladder, in the anterior abdominal wall, periprostatic, or perineal. An abdominal or perineal injury is followed by pain, blood at the urethral meatus, difficulty in voiding, and signs of extravasation (see above). Urethrograms (5–20 ml radiopaque material instilled into urethra by catheter) should be taken to confirm and localize the site of rupture. A catheter may not pass the area of urethral injury. Never try to force a catheter.

Penetrating Abdominal Injuries

All penetrating abdominal injuries must be explored in the operating room. A minute entry wound may mask extensive internal damage. The patient should have all clothing removed and be carefully examined for entry and exit wounds and for evidence of associated injuries or bleeding contributing to shock. Symptoms, signs, and laboratory evidence of severe hemorrhage must be evaluated promptly so that lifesaving surgery may be done—in spite of shock, if necessary.

The status of the patient depends upon (1) the organs involved, as suggested by the type and direction of the injury and specific symptoms and signs; (2) the severity of hemorrhage, shock, and peritonitis; (3) the time elapsed since injury; and (4) treatment already administered.

Symptoms and signs of specific organ involvement are reviewed above. Manifestations of hemorrhage and shock are reviewed on p 841.

Freeark RJ: Penetrating wounds of the abdomen. N Engl J Med 291:185, 1974.

Reid IS: Renal trauma in children. Aust NZ J Surg 42:260, 1973.

Sinclair MC: Major surgery for abdominal and thoracic trauma in childhood and adolescence. J Pediatr Surg 9:155, 1974.

Talbert JL, Rodgers BM: Acute abdominal injuries. Pediatr Ann 5:35, 1976.

PERINEAL INJURIES

Perineal injuries most often result from falls on a bicycle seat, falls in a bath tub, or sexual assault.

Injuries to the labia often cause bruising, edema, and urinary retention. Have the child attempt to urinate while sitting in a tub of warm water. Catheterization is rarely necessary.

Vaginal injuries require thorough examination under sedation or anesthesia. If associated with fever, abdominal pain, lower abdominal tenderness, or free air in the abdomen, the abdomen must be explored. Otherwise, lacerations can be sutured loosely and the patient begun on sitz baths.

Urethral injuries are rare if the pelvis is not fractured or the symphysis pubica disrupted.

Testicular pain following trauma should suggest torsion of the testes or the appendix testis. Rupture of the tunica albuginea is rare. Persistence of pain for 1–2 hours after trauma is indication for exploration of the testes. In torsion of the testis, the testis is tense and tender and the cord may be thick and shortened. Torsion of the appendix testis may follow trauma or activities such as bicycle or horseback riding. The earliest sign is a tender, firm, palpable nodule. Later, the entire testis becomes larger because of effusion into the tunica vaginalis. The scrotum is often red on the involved side. Surgery reduces morbidity and shortens convalescence, but the disease is self-limited.

CHEST INJURIES

External evidence of injury may not be present.

Rib Fracture
Localized pleuritic pain (sharp pain with breathing), localized severe pain with pressure at the fracture site, crepitus with respiration, or pain with compression of sternum or lateral chest. Pleural friction rub may be present. Examine for fluid (hemothorax) and pneumothorax.

Flail Chest
If several adjacent ribs are broken in 2 or more places, this portion of the chest may move paradoxically with respiration. With inspiration, the segment is sucked in, limiting expansion of the lung on the involved side. Flail chest is characterized by pain, dyspnea, cyanosis, and paradoxic motion of the involved segment. Immediate immobilization is required. This may require endotracheal intubation and support with a positive pressure ventilator. There is often an associated pneumothorax or hemothorax.

Pneumothorax
Pneumothorax is classically characterized by dyspnea, cyanosis, chest lag, absence of fremitus, hyperresonance, and absence of breath and voice sounds on the involved side. Upright chest x-ray will confirm the diagnosis and show any associated blood or fluid in the pleural space. Pneumothorax is classified as spontaneous, traumatic, tension, or open.

A. Spontaneous Pneumothorax: Usually in older children; rupture of bleb with leakage of air into the pleural cavity; source of leak usually seals spontaneously. Characterized by a sudden onset of dyspnea, pleuritic pain, respiratory lag, hyperresonance, and absent breath and voice sounds on the involved side. Symptoms and signs do not progress. Often complicates an asthmatic attack or cystic fibrosis.

B. Tension Pneumothorax: Failure of the lung leak to seal may produce a one-way valve effect leading to an increasing amount of air in the pleural space with each breath. This causes mediastinal shift, rapidly progressive dyspnea and cyanosis, and physical findings as noted above. Marked intrathoracic pressure may prevent hyperresonance. Tension pneumothorax may result from lung trauma (penetrating wounds) or may occur with spontaneous pneumothorax. Air must be aspirated immediately through a needle or chest tube. Crepitus may develop over the neck or chest wall.

C. Open Pneumothorax: Characterized by the presence of an open wound, severe respiratory distress with cyanosis, audible sucking sounds, and ingress or egress of frothy, blood-tinged fluid with each breath. The opening must be closed *at once* with an airtight bandage and the patient placed on the injured side. Vaseline gauze covered with a bulky bandage will usually suffice.

Hemothorax
Signs of pleural fluid as evidenced by absent fremitus, loss of resonance, absent breath and voice sounds, and tracheal shift to the opposite side, together with general symptoms of hemorrhage following chest injury; may be associated with pneumothorax. Physical findings of coexisting pneumothorax may obscure those of hemothorax. Confirm by needle aspiration after upright chest x-ray.

Penetrating Wounds of Chest
May be closed or open.

A. Closed Wounds: A minute point of entry may be associated with extensive intrathoracic damage. Check for rib fracture, pneumothorax, hemothorax, subcutaneous (palpation) or mediastinal emphysema (crunching sound with each heartbeat), and cardiac contusion (ECG).

B. Open Wounds: Open wounds inevitably produce critical pneumothorax; see above.

Cardiac Injury
May consist of simple contusion, a penetrating wound, valve rupture, or cardiac tamponade. Contusion may be associated with arrhythmia or nonspecific ECG findings. Rupture occurs most commonly in the aortic valve and is manifested by a loud, "cooing" diastolic murmur; signs of acute left heart failure may be present.

Cardiac tamponade due to blood in the pericardial sac progresses to limitation of diastolic filling of the heart with resultant progressive narrowing of pulse pressure, increase in pulse rate, paradoxic pulse, engorged neck veins, and eventually critically low cardiac output. Pericardial paracentesis may be lifesaving.

Pulmonary Contusion

Chest trauma is often associated with hemorrhage into contused areas of lung. This appears as floccular or large densities on x-ray. The patient becomes progressively cyanotic and agitated. Blood may be present in the tracheal aspirate. Increased pulmonary shunting leads to a progressive rise in P_{CO_2} and a fall in P_{O_2}. Administration of oxygen by mask or nasal catheter may help, but the patient often requires endotracheal intubation and positive pressure ventilation. Oxygen concentration should be just adequate to maintain an arterial P_{O_2} of 60–80 mm Hg. Prolonged exposure to high concentrations of oxygen can lead to permanent lung damage. Treat with salt restriction, furosemide (Lasix), 1 mg/2.5 kg IV, and maintenance fluids. Pulmonary contusion is completely reversible.

Ruptured Bronchus

Persistent pneumothorax after placement of a chest tube, air in the mediastinum, and hemoptysis should suggest traumatic rupture of a bronchus. In children, this can occur without rib fracture. Bronchoscopy is indicated as soon as possible if this diagnosis is suspected.

Haller JA, Shermeta DW: Acute thoracic injuries in children. Pediatr Ann 5:71, 1976.
Sinclair MC: Major surgery for abdominal and thoracic trauma in childhood and adolescence. J Pediatr Surg 9:155, 1974.
Webb WR: Thoracic trauma. Surg Clin North Am 54:1179, 1974.

ARTERIAL OCCLUSION

A cold, pale, pulseless extremity following trauma suggests arterial occlusion. This may be from direct penetration or division, from local pressure, or from entrapment in a fracture site. Once the patient is stable and the fractured extremity has been placed in traction, persistent signs and symptoms demand immediate arteriography to demonstrate the site of occlusion. Corrective surgery within 4 hours can save the limb.

Arterial occlusion can occur in the newborn. Emboli from the occluding ductus arteriosus or umbilical arteries are the usual cause, although iatrogenic complications of umbilical artery catheterization may occur. The limb appears pale at first, and then cyanotic or mottled. Pulses are absent below the occlusion. The extremity may swell. If there are no specific contraindications to anticoagulation, immediate therapy consists of heparin, 100 units/kg body weight IV every 4 hours, to maintain a clotting time 3–4 times normal. If symptoms progress, embolectomy must be attempted and can be successful in the neonate.

FRACTURES

Clinical manifestations of fracture include pain, local tenderness, ecchymosis, deformity due to swelling and bone displacement, impaired function, abnormal motion, and crepitus at the site of fracture. In some instances, only pain is present. Simple inspection is often diagnostic. X-ray confirmation is mandatory. Evaluate sensory changes and voluntary motion of joints distal to the fracture for evidence of nerve damage. Check distal portion of extremity for evidence of impaired blood supply.

Splint fracture, elevate extremity, and apply ice to control swelling. Reduction and casting are never emergency procedures.

Spinal Injuries

Vertebral fractures and spinal cord injuries are suggested by the nature of the injury, back pain, and abnormal position or mobility of the neck, back, or extremities. All unconscious patients or those who complain of back or neck pain should be treated as potential spinal cord injury cases. Every effort should be made to maintain the normal alignment of the spine in both examination and transportation. Never transport such patients in a sitting or semireclining position; use a flat stretcher without a pillow. By asking the patient to move his toes, legs, and hands, one can roughly determine the presence of significant cord injury and its approximate location. Loss of sensation to pain will further identify the level of the cord injury.

LACERATIONS

All lacerations sufficiently deep to penetrate the skin must be thoroughly explored. When possible, place the extremity in about the same position it was in when injury occurred. This may reveal more extensive injury than previously suspected.

Organic iodine solutions such as povidone-iodine (Betadine, Isodine) are excellent cleansing solutions that will not cause tissue injury. Clean the skin thoroughly around the laceration. Then inject sufficient 0.5% procaine or lidocaine to achieve good anesthesia before cleansing the depths of the wound. All clots and debris must be removed.

Remove all dead fat, muscle, and fascia with sharp scissors or scalpel. Debride the edges of the wound if they are ragged, crushed, or heavily impregnated with grease or dirt. The edges should be straight, clean, and bleeding freely.

Interrupted sutures of fine silk or nylon give the best cosmetic results. They should be evenly placed and should approximate the edges accurately. Sutures should not be tighter than necessary to give skin edge approximation.

Give a tetanus toxoid booster as indicated.

Lacerations heal faster and with less scarring if the extremity is at rest. Use splints, slings, and bed rest as necessary.

See patient in 24 hours. Check the edges of the wound for erythema, drainage, or undue tenderness. Warn the parents what to look for.

The face is very vascular and rarely under tension. Remove half of the stitches on the third day and the rest on the 5th day. Support with Steri-Strips if in doubt. The hands, arms, and neck usually heal in 7 days. The feet, knees, pretibial areas, and shoulder require 10–14 days to heal.

EXTREMITY AMPUTATION

Stop major bleeding by pressure around the ends of the stump. Retrieve the extremity if feasible for possible reimplantation. First attention must always be to the patient; he may be neglected in the haste of retrieving the limb.

Treat blood loss and associated injuries.

FINGER INJURIES

Door Injuries
Car doors and metal cabinet doors may partially amputate a fingertip. The terminal phalanx is usually fractured and the nail bed is usually avulsed.

Cleanse the area thoroughly, realign all viable tissue, and approximate skin loosely with 3 or 4 sutures. Splint the digit and protect with sling.

These injuries often become infected and must be checked frequently. If infection develops, remove sutures near the site of infection and begin frequent soaks. Use antibiotics as indicated by cultures.

Finger Amputations
Amputated fingertips should not be sewed on if more than just skin is lost. A child's fingertip has an amazing capacity for regeneration, and no viable bone should be removed from a denuded finger. Simple debridement and dressing the open portion of the wound will give the best ultimate functional and cosmetic results.

If an entire finger is amputated, it may be possible to reattach it using microsurgical technics on the digital vessels and nerves.

Illingworth CM: Trapped fingers and amputated fingertips in children. J Pediatr Surg 9:853, 1974.

INTRAORAL INJURIES

Children who fall with lollipop sticks, pea shooters, rulers, etc in their mouths are likely to sustain intraoral lacerations or punctures.

Examination
A tongue blade and flashlight are usually the only equipment required. Hold the child supine with arms held tightly to the side of the head. It may be necessary to grasp the tip of the patient's tongue to pull it forward when the laceration is on the tongue.

Treatment
Most linear lacerations or punctures in the buccal mucosa, tonsillar pillar, or posterior pharynx require no therapy. They heal as well without sutures as they do with them. The specific indications for suturing under anesthesia are (1) through and through injury to the soft palate, (2) the presence of a flap of mucoperiosteum lifted off the hard palate, and (3) crepitus in the neck indicating deep puncture. Tongue lacerations are usually inflicted by the child's incisors. These too will heal without sutures in most cases. Lacerations through the edge of the tongue, producing a triangular flap, are best sutured with plain catgut.

EMERGENCIES DUE TO LOCAL INFECTIONS & INFLAMMATION

Paronychia
Paronychia is a staphylococcal infection around the base or side of a fingernail. There is usually a history of nailbiting. Drain under digital block using 0.5% lidocaine or procaine anesthesia. Soak the hand twice daily in warm water until healing occurs. Protect the hand with a sling.

Felon
This consists of an infection, usually staphylococcal, in the pulp space of a finger. It often follows sliver or thorn injury to the finger pad. It is very painful and can progress to ischemic necrosis of the terminal phalanx.

Treatment consists of drainage by lateral incision deep into the pulp space after adequate digital block anesthesia. Soak the digit frequently in warm water and protect the hand with a sling.

Testicular Pain
If the diagnosis of the cause of persistent testicu-

lar pain is in doubt, explore the testes as soon as possible because of the high incidence of torsion of the testes (see p 848).

Orchitis may be secondary to mumps. Check the history and draw acute phase serum for antibody titer determination. Treat with bed rest, fluids, and analgesics as necessary.

Epididymitis is uncommon in children who have no urinary tract infection or catheter. The epididymis can often be felt and is tense and tender. Treat urinary infection as indicated and check the prostate for prostatis.

Groin Abscesses

Adenopathy below the groin crease is usually secondary to sepsis in the foot or leg. Adenopathy above the groin crease is usually secondary to diaper rash or vulval lesions. Enlargement of nodes above the groin crease may be confused with incarcerated hernia or hydrocele of the cord.

If the diagnosis is not clear, exploration of the groin is indicated. If the swelling is clearly a lymph node enlargement, treat for 10 days with penicillin and drain only when fluctuant.

Urinary Retention

Urinary retention is rare in children. The most common cause is chronic constipation, resulting in a large fecal concretion that presses on the bladder neck. Prolapse of an ectopic ureterocele can cause retention, as can tumors such as rhabdomyosarcoma of the prostate or cystosarcoma phyllodes. Metastases of neuroblastoma to the meninges as leukemic infiltrate can cause urinary retention by spinal cord compression. There is usually associated paralysis of the anal sphincter.

Catheterization is rarely necessary except in cases of tumor or spinal cord compression.

BATTERED CHILD SYNDROME*
(CHILD ABUSE & NEGLECT)

Essentials of Diagnosis

- Unexplained or inadequately explained signs of trauma.
- Multiple fractures at different stages of healing.
- Failure to thrive that responds to nutritional therapy alone.

Injuries Frequently Associated With Abuse

(1) Burns when the pattern does not match the history given.

*This section is prepared by Barton D. Schmitt, MD.

(2) Fractures, especially chip fractures of long bones.

(3) Subdural hematomas secondary to shaking injuries.

(4) Whipping with a belt or electric cord.

(5) Hair pulling with scalp hematoma.

(6) Ear twisting, resulting in ecchymosis in ear.

(7) Ruptured tympanic membrane from ear boxing.

(8) Retinal hemorrhage.

(9) Multiple abrasions and bruises of differing ages.

(10) Cigarette burns, dunking burns.

(11) Slap marks on the cheek.

(12) Healing fractures of different ages.

General Considerations

Child abuse can be defined as a lack of reasonable care and protection of children by their parents, guardians, or relatives. The prevalence of physical abuse is approximately 500 cases per million population per year. Therefore, in a city of 100,000 people, about 50 new cases can be detected per year. When neglect cases are vigorously reported, their number will equal the above figures.

The abused child is often an infant. Young children are at greater risk because they are demanding, defenseless, and nonverbal. Estimates of the usual age for child abuse are that one-third occur under 1 year of age, one-third from ages 1–3, and one-third over age 3.

The laws on child abuse are clear. In every state of the USA, reporting of suspected cases of child abuse by the physician is mandatory, and penalities exist for failing to report. The laws also protect the physician from liability suits regarding release of confidential information. Despite these laws, physicians sometimes go to great lengths to avoid diagnosing child abuse. They often fear that detection and reporting of child abuse will require them to personally treat this complex psychosocial problem. The responsibility for proper treatment rests with the child protective agency in the community—not with the physician. The critical role of the physician is case-finding.

Classification

A. Physical Abuse: Approximately 10% of alleged accidents in children under age 6 are due to physical abuse. These injuries can occur in several ways.

1. Injury in anger—Misbehavior makes parents angry. Some parents hit the child before they can control themselves.

2. Harsh punishment—Some parents attempt to discipline children in painful ways. This type of corporal punishment is not acceptable to society when it results in an injury that requires medical attention or when it leaves bruises.

3. Deliberate assault or murder—This occurs rarely. Such parents are usually psychotic.

B. Nutritional Deprivation: Caloric deprivation is the most common cause of underweight in infancy. Over 50% of cases of failure to thrive are due to this cause. Many of these children also have developmental delays due to emotional deprivation. Older children who are emotionally deprived occasionally develop deprivation dwarfism (see Chapter 24).

C. Sexual Abuse: Sexual abuse can be defined as any sexual exploitation of a child under 18 years of age by a family-related adult. Sexual abuse includes incest, oral-genital contact, sodomy, molestation, digital manipulation, etc. Incest often remains undiagnosed unless the physician looks carefully at the reasons behind unexplained urinary tract infections or vaginitis or running away by a young girl. A stepfather or a mother's boyfriend living in the home is more likely than a natural father to be involved in this kind of problem. Incest requires reporting to child welfare and separation from the offending adult.

D. Emotional Abuse: Emotional abuse involves the continual scapegoating, terrorizing, and rejection of a specific child. Such treatment mutilates the developing personality. Proving this type of child abuse is nearly impossible. Perhaps it is fortunate that these children are eventually physically abused, abandoned, or imprisoned in their rooms. At this point, the child can be legally removed from his destructive environment.

E. Medical Care Neglect: When a child with a chronic disease has serious deterioration in his condition or frequent emergencies because the parents repeatedly ignore medical recommendations for home treatment, reporting and foster placement may be indicated.

F. Intentional Drugging or Poisoning: This rare type of child abuse can be defined as the deliberate drugging of children by adult caretakers. This includes drugging them with sedatives intended for use by adults or sharing narcotics or other dangerous drugs with them.

Etiology

Most parents who abuse their children were also abused as children. They are often lonely, immature, isolated, unloved, depressed, and angry people. The parent who batters his child has poor impulse control; the parent who starves his child may have relatively good impulse control but can deny the needs of his child. An overlap between caloric deprivation and physical abuse can occur.

Parents who abuse children come from all racial, religious, geographic, socioeconomic, and educational backgrounds. The abuser is a parent or step-parent in 90% of cases, a boyfriend in 5% of cases, an unrelated baby-sitter in 4% of cases, and a sibling in 1% of cases. Either parent can be responsible, although the father is more likely to be the offender when several children are harmed. In cases of failure to thrive, the mother is almost always responsible.

Clinical Findings

Child abuse should be considered in any of the following medical problems: skin bruises, soft tissue swellings, fractures, dislocations, tender extremities, burns, head injuries, subdural hematomas, unexplained seizures, unexplained comas, undernutrition problems, or "crib deaths." Lacerations are uncommon as an isolated finding.

A. Symptoms: The diagnosis of child abuse is usually confirmed by the presence of several of the following suggestive factors:

1. The injury is completely unexplained or only vaguely explained.

2. The accident as described is bizarre or implausible.

3. There is a discrepancy between the type of accident and the child's developmental age.

4. There is a discrepancy between the accident and the physical findings.

5. Accidents have been repeated.

6. The parents have delayed in seeking medical care.

7. The parents disappear during admission; they rarely visit; or they don't ask about discharge.

8. A history of anorexia, recurrent vomiting, or recurrent diarrhea is not confirmed in the hospital setting (especially in the case of infants who fail to thrive).

B. Signs:

1. Pathognomonic skin lesions include lash marks, cigarette burns, grab marks, cord loop marks, belt buckle marks, human bites, tie marks, strap marks, choke marks, or bruises of the frontal dental ridge due to forced feeding of a crying baby.

2. An injury that could not have been self-inflicted (eg, a dunking burn).

3. Multiple old and new signs of trauma.

4. Retinal hemorrhages mean severe shaking if they are present without a skull fracture or scalp bruise.

5. Obvious fear of a parent.

6. Failure to thrive.

7. Signs compatible with neglect (eg, long nails, rampant diaper rash, unwashed, bald occiput).

8. Signs of emotional deprivation (eg, blank face, marked withdrawal, no complaint on venipuncture).

C. X-Ray Findings: Radiographic evidence of multiple fractures at different stages of healing is diagnostic of physical abuse. If a single injury is present, abuse can be suspected when metaphyseal chip fractures or exuberant periosteal reactions are found. When the initial film is normal, a follow-up film 2 weeks later will often confirm the suspicion of a nondisplaced epiphyseal fracture by demonstrating metaphyseal fragmentation and callus formation. Any case in which a child is brought into the hospital dead on arrival is an indication for total body x-rays in addition to autopsy.

D. Diagnostic Trial of Caloric Rehabilitation: The diagnosis of failure to thrive secondary to nutritional deprivation is confirmed by rapid weight gain on unlimited feedings in the hospital. The same milk that was used at home is preferred. Accurate daily weights are essential. A rapid gain can be defined as greater than 45 gm/day for a sustained period or a gain that is strikingly greater than seen during a similar interval at home. The infant usually responds within 2 weeks. The same personnel should feed the child to the extent that this is possible.

E. Consultations: The child with developmental delay may need a baseline developmental quotient assessed by a developmental pediatrician or a psychologist.

F. Family Assessment: Certain psychosocial factors are usually present in abusive families. A psychiatrist, social worker, or specially trained pediatrician can gather this information. Even when the child's injury is explained and plausible, this assessment should be done if (1) the child is under 6 months of age, (2) the injury was major and required hospitalization, or (3) the child is an accident repeater. The inquiry should establish the following:

1. The parents' stability—How is the mother doing? (Depressed, overwhelmed, etc?) Does either parent have violent temper outbursts?

2. The mother-child relationship—Can the parent say anything positive about the child? Is there a bond of love with the child?

3. Discipline—What does the parent expect of the child? Are the expectations realistic? Does the child cause problems—eg, crying, eating, toilet training? What discipline is necessary?

4. Crisis—Was there a family crisis at the time of the injury—eg, moving, sick baby, absent husband, new pregnancy?

5. Rescue source—Does the parent have someone to talk to? Does the parent have someone to count on? (This is unlikely if there are marital problems and no extended family.)

G. Cases at High Risk for Fatal Outcome: The physician must make every effort to identify which physically abused children are in imminent danger of being killed. He may need to urge the Child Welfare Department to intervene more aggressively in these cases. Without question, all of these children should be initially placed under foster care. The following danger signals should be unfailingly heeded:

1. Life-threatening abuse (eg, multiple injuries, head injuries, or internal injuries).

2. Premeditated or sadistic injuries (eg, many burns).

3. Deliberate poisoning.

4. Any physical abuse of a child under 1 year of age.

5. A repeated episode of abuse after initial report and intervention.

6. An abused child with a sibling who has been killed by the parents.

7. Dangerous parent (eg, psychotic, suicidal, sociopathic).

8. A child who is extremely fearful of returning home.

Differential Diagnosis

Rare bone disorders may resemble nonaccidental trauma (eg, osteogenesis imperfecta, scurvy, syphilis), but a skilled radiologist can easily differentiate these entities. In children who fail to thrive, laboratory tests for rare malabsorptive disorders (eg, celiac disease) should be withheld until after an adequate trial of feeding.

Treatment

A. General Measures: The following 11 steps are recommended when a physician sees a child who may have been abused:

1. Hospitalize the child—The purpose of hospitalization is to protect the child until the safety of the home can be evaluated. The extent of the injuries is not relevant to this requirement. The reason given to the parents for hospitalization is that, "His injuries need to be watched." It is not helpful to mention to the parents the possibility of nonaccidental trauma until the child is safely hospitalized. If the parents refuse hospitalization, a court order can be obtained.

2. Treat the child's injuries—Once the child is in the hospital, the medical and surgical problems should be cared for in the usual manner. Orthopedic consultation is commonly needed. Ophthalmologists, neurologists, neurosurgeons, and plastic surgeons are occasionally consulted.

3. Obtain necessary laboratory tests—Every suspected case under 5 years of age should receive a skeletal survey. The x-ray findings may establish a definite diagnosis of nonaccidental trauma. Over age 5, x-rays should be obtained only if the history of injury or the physical findings point to bone trauma. If there are unexplained bruises or a history of "easy bruising," one should obtain a "bleeding disorder screen" (platelet count, bleeding time, partial thromboplastin time, prothrombin time, and thrombin time). If there are visible physical findings, photographs may be considered.

4. Maintain a helping approach to the parents—This is the hardest step. It is natural to feel angry with these parents, but expressing anger is very damaging to parent cooperation. Confrontation, accusation, and interrogation must be avoided. The primary physician must see or phone these parents daily. They become suspicious quite easily if communication is not optimal. If the child is brought in dead or with multiple life-threatening injuries, the parent must receive an emergency psychiatric evaluation because he may be psychotic or suicidal.

5. Report to Child Welfare by phone within 24 hours—Tell the parents the diagnosis and the need to report it before doing so. Tell them, "Your explanation for the injury is insufficient. I am obligated by law to report all suspicious injuries in children." The physician must also tell the parents of the subsequent visit by a child welfare worker. He can add that the police will not be involved, that the matter will be kept confidential, and that everyone's goal is to help them find better ways of dealing with their child.

6. Report to Child Welfare in writing within 48 hours—The official report should be written by a physician and should contain the following data:

a. The alleged cause of the present injury.

b. Physical findings and x-ray results.

c. Concluding statement about why this represents nonaccidental trauma.

7. **Request hospital social worker consultation within 48 hours**—This referral can be explained as "hospital policy." The social worker does the in-depth psychosocial interview to determine overall family problems, environmental problems, the safety of the home, the state of the marriage, how disturbed the parents are, and how likely they are to accept therapy. In severe or complex cases, the social worker may request a psychiatric evaluation. This helps to uncover the 10% of parents who are very dangerous because they are sociopathic or psychotic. Child Welfare Services carries out its own home evaluation concurrently.

8. **Attend child protection team dispositional conference**—The social worker, pediatric consultant, house staff, child welfare worker, police representative, psychiatrist, and any other community agencies involved with the family should meet within 1 week of admission. All evaluations should have been completed. All possible suspects (including baby-sitters, neighbors, siblings, boyfriends) should have been interviewed. At this meeting, an attempt is made to list all of the family's problems in the case being reviewed. A joint decision is then reached regarding the best immediate and long-range plans for each problem. Based on the assessed safety of the home, a decision must be made about whether to have the child observed with the parent's cooperation or to request the court to order temporary foster home placement or court-enforced supervision. In very serious cases, the team may decide to urge the court to terminate parental rights and make the child available for adoption.

9. **Discharge the patient when Child Welfare authorizes it**—The physician is obligated to keep the child in a protected environment until Child Welfare carries out the legal decisions of the child protection team. If the child is well and the temporary custody hearing is pending, Child Welfare can be asked to place the child temporarily in a receiving home.

10. **Follow-up of physical status by the pediatrician**—The battered child needs more frequent well child care than the average child. He should be seen once a week for a while. He needs follow-up to detect any recurrence of physical abuse. If he has sustained head injury, he needs follow-up for mental retardation, spasticity, and subdural hematomas. If he has experienced nutritional deprivation, he needs careful monitoring of weight gain.

11. **Follow-up and treatment of psychosocial problems by Child Welfare**—The pediatrician should not feel responsible for restoration of these multiproblem families to emotional health. Child Welfare is primarily responsible for provision of psychotherapy, for home visits, and for finding the patient who becomes "lost to follow-up." The pediatrician can contribute to the therapeutic process by giving the parent his telephone number to call "if things get rough." It is best if the parent has several helping people available as lifelines. After the parent calls, Child Welfare should be notified that the parent is upset and urgently needs help.

B. **Psychotherapy**: The parents in child abuse cases usually do not accept interpretive psychotherapy and respond better to therapists who can reach out. Home visits are often necessary. Professional therapists are not always required. Laymen have been trained as parents' aides or homemakers. Other battering parents have been helped by group therapy. Day care centers are very important in giving the mother a part of her day free from her child.

C. **Legal Aspects of Management**:

1. **Dependency hearing**—A dependency petition is a legal instrument that permits the child protective agency to request temporary custody of an abused child. If the petition is sustained by the court, the child becomes a ward of the state. The court can then insist that psychotherapy, marital counseling, or certain changes in the home be carried out. The parents cannot legally remove their child from the state during this period of time. This court-enforced supervision is usually reviewed after 6 months.

2. **Foster placement**—If the home is considered dangerous for the child, he should be placed in a foster home. However, the ultimate goal is to reunite the family. In 90% of cases in one large state where this problem has been extensively studied, the children are returned to their own homes after the court has observed improvement in the parents. Only 10% of cases require termination of parental rights or long-term foster placement.

3. **Police intervention**—Police are rarely needed in child abuse cases except to provide court holds at night or on weekends. Arrests, interrogations, or public incriminations by the police are detrimental to helping these parents. These cases should be managed by the juvenile court system and the Protective Services Division of Child Welfare or its equivalent.

Prevention

There are many types of behavior that suggest to the newborn nursery or maternity ward staff that a mother will have difficulty with her baby and possibly be abusive. Factors that might arouse concern include drug addiction, a history of serious mental illness, a lack of maternal attachment as indicated by poor cuddling or lack of eye contact with the baby, disparaging remarks about the baby, postpartum depression, and infrequent visiting if the mother is discharged earlier than the baby. Extremely adverse prognostic factors are serious abuse or death of a sibling or overt spanking of a newborn baby.

The minimal postdischarge follow-up on all such babies should include a visit 2 days after discharge by a public health nurse and a visit 2 weeks after discharge to a primary physician. Both of these professionals should be designated by name well in advance of discharge and the parents so informed. Medical visits during the first year should continue at intervals more frequent than those provided for routine well child care, and the public health nurse should visit as frequently as necessary. Special emphasis should be placed on discipline counseling, close follow-up on acute illnesses, frequent telephone calls, uninterrupted availability of crisis nurseries, and day care arrangements as the child becomes older. This type of nurturing, reaching-out approach can help some parents to become adequate who otherwise would continue to be physically and psychically abusive toward their children.

Prognosis

The highest priority in child abuse treatment is to prevent repeated injuries to the child. In cases of child abuse where the child is returned to his parents without any intervention, 5% are killed and 35% suffer permanent physical damage from repeated abuse. The untreated survivors also have emotional problems. Physically abused children often relate violently to the world when they grow up; emotionally deprived children often relate only shallowly to people. Early detection and intervention are mandatory in this syndrome.

Caffey J: On the theory and practice of shaking infants. Am J Dis Child 124:161, 1972.

Gillespie RW: The battered child syndrome: Thermal and caustic manifestations. J Trauma 5:523, 1965.

Helfer RE, Kempe CH (editors): *The Battered Child,* 2nd ed. Univ of Chicago Press, 1974.

Helfer RE, Kempe CH (editors): *Child Abuse and Neglect—The Family and the Community.* Ballinger, 1976.

Kempe CH, Helfer RE (editors): *Helping the Battered Child and His Family.* Lippincott, 1971.

Martin HP (editor): *The Abused Child.* Ballinger, 1976.

Rausen AR (editor): Symposium on child abuse. Pediatrics (Suppl) 51:771, 1973.

Schmitt BD, Kempe CH: The pediatrician's role in child abuse and neglect. Curr Probl Pediatr 5:3, March 1975.

EMERGENCIES DUE TO PHYSICAL AGENTS*

BURNS

A second degree burn of 10% or more of the body surface in a child under 1 year of age or of 15% of the body surface in an older child is a serious injury and requires hospitalization for proper treatment. Initial management is the most important factor in survival.

Classification & Characteristics of Burn Wounds

A. First Degree: Involves superficial epidermis

*Drowning is discussed in Chapter 12.

(partial thickness burn). The skin area is pink or red in appearance, blanches with pressure, and is painful to touch. Causes include sunburn, scalds, and distant flash fires.

B. Second Degree: Involves entire epidermis (partial thickness). The skin is red, blistered, or moist with exudate, and painful to pinprick or touch. Causes include scalds and flash fires.

C. Third Degree: Involves dermis or underlying fat, muscle, or bone (full thickness). The skin is white, dry or charred, and painless. Causes include scalds from live steam, open flame burns, or contact with chemicals or electric current.

Treatment of Minor Burns

First degree burns and second degree burns of less than 10% of the body surface that do not involve the hands, the feet, the perineum, or the face can be treated on an outpatient basis with plain petrolatum or antibiotic-impregnated gauze and clean dressings, which should be changed every 48 hours. All children with burns of the hands and most children with burns of the feet should be hospitalized so that proper splinting of the extremity and careful local wound care can be performed. Burns of the face need close observation for airway obstruction and careful local wound care to avoid infection and scarring.

When seen in the emergency room, a child with scalds of about 10% of his body surface area should have a baseline hematocrit determined. If he is to be treated as an outpatient, urine specific gravity should be determined at 24 hours and again at 48 hours to ensure adequate hydration. Dead skin and broken blisters should be cleansed and debrided. Sterile dressings of pigskin or bismuth tribromophenate (Xeroform) gauze should be changed daily for 2–3 days until healing is complete.

Treatment of Major Burns

Major burns are second or third degree burns involving more than 10% of the body surface.

A. Emergency Measures:

1. Cool the burned area immediately by running cool water over it.

2. Transport the child wrapped in a clean sheet to a hospital.

3. If analgesia is needed, give meperidine, 1 mg/kg subcut, or morphine, 0.05 mg/kg subcut, and make certain that a written record of the amount given stays with the patient when he is transported to the hospital. Avoid all opiates in children with flame burns because of possible lung damage.

4. Begin fluid replacement if hospitalization will be delayed for several hours after injury.

B. Definitive Measures:

1. Treatment of burned area—

a. Using sterile technic (with gown, gloves, cap, and mask), remove burned clothing and carefully examine the patient for other injuries. Determine his general condition.

b. In facial burns, verify the patency of the airway and evaluate the need for tracheostomy or endotracheal tube.

c. Clean the wound of all grease and ointments, using dilute povidone-iodine (Betadine, Isodine) solution or mild soap. Uncover blisters if topical antibiotics are to be used (see below).

d. Record areas of second and third degree burn as percentage of total body area, using the chart as adapted from Lund & Browder (Fig 29–13). (The "rule of nines" is useful in adult burns but does not apply to children.)

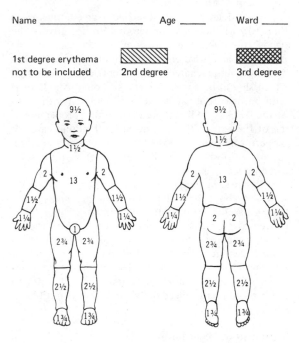

Infant Less Than One Year of Age

Name _____   Age _____   Ward _____

1st degree erythema not to be included   2nd degree   3rd degree

Variations from Adult Distribution in Infants and Children (in Percent).

	New-born	1 Year	5 Years	10 Years
Head	19	17	13	11
Both thighs	11	13	16	17
Both lower legs	10	10	11	12
Neck	2			
Anterior trunk	13			
Posterior trunk	13			
Both upper arms	8	These percentages remain constant at all ages.		
Both lower arms	6			
Both hands	5			
Both buttocks	5			
Both feet	7			
Genitals	1			
	100			

Figure 29–13. Lund and Browder modification of Berkow's scale for estimating extent of burns. (The table under the illustration is after Berkow.)

2. Fluid administration—

a. Place a large bore catheter in a vein. If a central catheter can be placed via the external jugular, subclavian, or cephalic vein, it can be used to obtain central venous pressure readings.

b. Record urine output and specific gravity. Catheterization is rarely necessary.

c. Type and cross-match blood. Do a complete blood count and determine serum electrolytes.

d. Calculate fluid requirements (see Chapter 35) and begin fluid replacement.

3. Prevention of infection—

a. Administer tetanus toxoid or hyperimmune serum if not immunized.

b. Culture burn wound and nose and throat secretions.

c. Begin penicillin G for 3 days to control streptococcal infections.

d. Apply topical anti-infective agents.

4. Topical burn therapy—A variety of topical agents are available for control of wound sepsis. Silver sulfadiazine (Silvadene) and 0.5% silver nitrate have proved safest, and both provide excellent bacteriostasis. However, *no topical agent is a substitute for frequent local cleansing and debridement.*

Silver nitrate must be used in 0.5% aqueous solution. Hyponatremia and hypochloremia can be a problem, but monitoring urinary sodium helps determine the adequacy of sodium chloride replacement; a urinary sodium concentration of 40 mg/liter or more indicates adequate NaCl replacement.

Silver nitrate dressings must be kept moist since the dressings are no longer bacteriostatic if allowed to dry. Dressings must be changed daily to allow cleansing and debridement of the burned tissue.

Silver sulfadiazine is prepared in a vanishing cream base and can be applied to any burned area. There is little pain, and allergic reactions are rare. The cream is best covered with bulky dressings in small children since they tend to rub it off on the bedsheets. All old caked Silvadene must be washed off prior to applying fresh Silvadene.

Fresh or frozen pig skin has been widely utilized in treating second degree burns and in preparing third degree burns for grafting. (The skin is available commercially from the Burn Treatment Skin Bank, Phoenix, AZ 85034.)

C. General Measures: Withhold food and oral fluids for 24–48 hours. A nasogastric tube is desirable to reduce gastric acid until ileus subsides. Frequent determinations of urine volume and specific gravity are helpful in controlling fluid replacement. Frequent hematocrit measurements are also helpful in judging the state of hydration.

Boswick JA (editor): Symposium on burns. Surg Clin North Am 50:1191, 1970.

Lee YC: Early heterografting of partial-thickness burns. J Trauma 12:818, 1972.

Polk HC Jr, Stone HH: *Contemporary Burn Management.* Little, Brown, 1971.

HEAT STROKE

Heat stroke is rare in children but may occur with prolonged exposure to high ambient temperatures that results in failure of the thermoregulatory mechanism. In temperate climates, newborn infants, especially the sick and premature, have suffered from heat stroke when placed in cots next to radiators that have suddenly been turned on. Strenuous sports such as football played with heavy padding may also produce heat stroke.

Symptoms and signs include headache, dizziness, nausea, visual disturbances, convulsions, and loss of consciousness. Rectal temperature may exceed 42° C (107.6° F); the pulse is rapid, irregular, and weak; and the skin is hot, flushed, dry, and incapable of sweating. Plasma and extracellular water volume and composition are normal.

Treatment

Place the child in a cool place and remove all clothing. Bring the rectal temperature down to 39° C (102.2° F) by fanning after sprinkling with water, by ice packs, or by immersion in cold water. Do not bring the temperature below 39° C. When that temperature is reached, discontinue antipyretic therapy.

Massage all 4 extremities to maintain peripheral circulation.

Avoid sedation. Give maintenance fluids, electrolytes, and calories intravenously.

Treat shock if present.

Avoid reexposure to similar conditions.

Eichler AC: Heat stroke. Am J Surg 118:855, 1969.
Sohar E: Heatstroke caused by dehydration and physical effort. Arch Intern Med 122:159, 1969.

HEAT EXHAUSTION

Heat exhaustion is due to excessive depletion of plasma and extracellular volume as a result of sweating profusely in a high ambient temperature. Chloride losses are more critical than water losses, which explains the high risk of this condition in patients with cystic fibrosis in hot weather.

Headache and muscle cramps are common, especially in the calves. Perspiration is profuse, and there is weakness, dizziness, and stupor. The skin is pale and cool, and the temperature is normal or low. The tongue is dry, the eyes may be sunken, and the subcutaneous tissues have an inelastic quality due to loss of extracellular water. Oliguria is present, and sometimes hypotension. The condition is liable to occur in children with unusual salt losses, eg, those with cystic fibrosis or salt-losing renal diseases. It may also occur in healthy active children who replace sweat losses with water and not salt. Therefore children undergoing strenuous physical exertion in hot weather should satisfy thirst with water containing one-fourth tsp of salt to the pint. Certain proprietary drinks are pleasantly flavored, eg, Gatorade.

Treatment

Extracellular fluid volume should be restored intravenously and maintenance fluid and electrolytes given according to the principles outlined in Chapter 37. In severe heat exhaustion, a volume of isotonic lactated Ringer's injection equal to 8% of the body weight should be given intravenously over 24 hours, with two-thirds administered in the first 6 hours. Maintenance water should be 600 ml/sq m/24 hours and maintenance sodium 6 mEq/kg/24 hours until hydration is normal.

Nadel ER & others: Mechanisms of thermal acclimation to exercise and heat. J Appl Physiol 37:515, 1974.
Schwartz E & others: Heat strain in hot and humid environment. Aerosp Med 43:852, 1972.

COLD INJURY
(Frostbite)

The severity of a frostbite injury depends on several factors: (1) The intensity of the cold exposure (a function of both temperature and wind velocity*) as well as increased rate of heat loss from the tissues due to contact with water or metal and restrictive or tight clothing proximal to the involved area. (2) Duration of exposure to cold is important in the progression of frostbite from superficial to deep involvement. (3) The rate of rewarming. Severe tissue damage will occur if the area is warmed too slowly or warmed and then refrozen. Thawing should not be attempted until facilities are available to properly rewarm the frostbitten tissue.

Clinical Findings & Classification

Cold injury is characterized by loss of sensation of affected parts and white, cold skin over affected areas in a child with a history of cold exposure.

A. First Degree (Frost Nip): Erythema of the skin and edema of the part but without blister formation. No significant tissue damage.

B. Second Degree: Blister and bulla formation.

C. Third Degree: Necrosis of the thick layers and subcutaneous tissues without loss of the part.

D. Fourth Degree: Complete necrosis with gangrene and loss of the affected part.

Complications

Complications include necrosis of the affected area and bacterial infection through broken skin. Late

---

*Eg, 15° F when there is no wind has a "cooling power" of 15°; with winds of 25 mph, the cooling power would be −22° F at the same thermometer reading.

sequelae involving frostbitten areas and lasting months to years have included persistent pain, hyperhidrosis, skin tenderness, cold sensitivity, and retarded epiphyseal growth.

Treatment

A. Frost Nip: Treat by local warming.

B. Superficial and Deep Frostbite:

1. Loosen any garments which restrict blood flow.

2. Remove any wet garments which are in contact with the skin.

3. Cover the involved area with dry bulky garments.

4. Elevate the affected area.

5. Protect the part from trauma. Do not rub frostbitten tissue, for this macerates the area and causes further damage.

6. Rewarming—Transport the patient to a warm environment and rewarm the frostbitten area by immersion in a large volume of water preheated to 37.8–40.6° C (100–105° F) for about 20 minutes.

a. Rewarming with an oven, fire, or other source of dry heat should not be attempted, since unequal exposure will result in tissue burns.

b. Analgesics may be required during the rewarming period.

c. Low molecular weight dextran given during the rewarming phase prevents red cell and platelet agglutination and promotes tissue perfusion. An adequate dose is 1 gm/kg given once as a 5–10% solution IV.

7. Place the patient at bed rest with the part elevated.

8. Maintain local hygiene by whirlpool baths twice a day for 20 minutes at body temperature.

9. Avoid all surgical procedures on cold-injured skin. Do not remove or puncture bullae or blisters.

10. Sympathectomy and paravertebral block are of little value.

11. Amputation of a necrotic limb should be postponed 2–3 months until optimal healing has occurred. If uncontrolled infection supervenes, early amputation may be required.

Prognosis

With proper therapy, full recovery is the rule. Complications of infections are unusual in frostbite cases.

Jarrett JR & others: Cold injury. Mo Med 67:169, March 1970.

Lapp N, Juergens JL: Frostbite. Mayo Clin Proc 40:932, 1965.

Vellar ID: Four cases of pedal cryopathy. Med J Aust 1:64, 1970.

ELECTRIC SHOCK & ELECTRIC BURNS

The danger of injury from electric shock depends upon the voltage and the frequency. Alternating current is more dangerous than direct current. At a frequency of 25–300 cycles, voltages below 230 volts can produce ventricular fibrillation. High voltages (which may be encountered in television circuits) produce respiratory failure. Faulty wiring of home appliances may lead to electric shock. In homes with young children, it is advisable to install occlusive safety outlets in the play area.

Electric Shock

Consciousness is rapidly lost. If the current continues, death from asphyxia due to ventricular fibrillation or respiratory arrest occurs within a few minutes.

Interrupt the power source or knock wire away from the skin with a dry piece of wood or other nonconducting material and institute external cardiac massage or mouth-to-mouth respiration, depending on whether asphyxia is cardiac or respiratory. Supply oxygen if available and institute appropriate treatment for shock.

Electric Burns

Momentary contact, particularly with a high-voltage outlet, will lead to localized, sharply demarcated, painless gray areas without associated inflammation of the skin. The examiner should search for a second area of grayness where the current has left the body. Sloughing occurs after a few weeks. With simple burns, the skin should be cleansed and a dry dressing applied. Deeper burns should be treated with silver sulfadiazine (Silvadene) (see p 856) under an occlusive dressing. Management is the same as for other types of burns. Infection occurs less often with electric burns, but reconstructive surgery for scarring after healing may be required.

Toddlers and young children may sustain electric burns of the mouth by biting an electric cord. They are rarely electrocuted because the circuit is completed locally in the mouth. There is a local slough of tissue on the seventh to tenth days that may lead to brisk bleeding. The defect should be allowed to heal by scarring and the corner of the mouth revised later.

Baxter CR: Present concepts in the management of major electrical injury. Surg Clin North Am 50:1401, 1970.

Lievens JB: Electrical accidents. Community Health (Bristol) 2:88, 1970.

Robinson DW & others: Electrical burns: A review and analysis of 33 cases. Surgery 57:385, 1965.

Thomson GH, Juckes AW, Farmer AW: Electrical burns to the mouth in children. Plast Reconstr Surg 35:466, 1965.

IRRADIATION REACTIONS

The effects of radiation may develop during or after the course of therapeutic x-ray or radium administration or after any exposure to ionizing radiation (eg, x-rays, neutrons, gamma rays, alpha or beta particles). The harmful effects of radiation are determined by the degree of exposure, which in turn depends upon not only the quantity of radiation delivered to the body but also the type of radiation, which tissues of the body are exposed, and the duration of exposure. Three hundred to 500 R (400–600 rads) of x-ray or gamma radiation applied to the entire body at one time would probably be fatal. (For purposes of comparison, a routine chest x-ray delivers about 0.3 R.) Tolerance to radiation is difficult to define, and there is no firm basis for evaluating radiation effects for all types and levels of irradiation.

Andrews GA & others: Clinical and biological consequences of nuclear explosions. Practitioner 207:331, 1971.

ACUTE (IMMEDIATE) RADIATION EFFECTS ON NORMAL TISSUES

Diagnosis

A. Injury to Skin and Mucous Membranes: Irradiation causes erythema, depilation, destruction of fingernails, or epidermolysis, depending upon the dose.

B. Injury to Deep Structures:

1. Hematopoietic tissues—Injury to the bone marrow may cause diminished production of blood elements. Lymphocytes are most sensitive, polymorphonuclear leukocytes next most sensitive, and erythrocytes least sensitive. Damage to the blood-forming organs may vary from transient depression of one or more blood elements to complete destruction.

2. Blood vessels—Smaller vessels (the capillaries and arterioles) are more readily damaged than larger blood vessels. If injury is mild, recovery occurs.

3. Gonads—In males, small single doses of radiation (200–300 R) cause temporary aspermatogenesis and larger doses (600–800 R) may cause sterility. In females, single doses of 200 R may cause temporary cessation of menses and 500–800 R may cause permanent infertility. Moderate to heavy radiation of the embryo in utero results in injury to the fetus or in embryonic death and abortion.

4. Lungs—High or repeated moderate doses of radiation may cause pneumonitis.

5. Salivary glands—The salivary glands may be depressed by radiation, but relatively large doses may be required.

6. Stomach—Gastric secretion may be temporarily (occasionally permanently) inhibited by moderately high doses of radiation.

7. Intestines—Inflammation and ulceration may follow moderately large doses of radiation.

8. CNS—The brain and spinal cord may be damaged by high doses of radiation because of impaired blood supply.

9. Resistant structures—The normal thyroid, pituitary, liver, pancreas, adrenals, and bladder are relatively resistant to radiation. Peripheral and autonomic nerves are highly resistant to radiation.

C. Systemic Reaction (Radiation Sickness): The basic mechanisms of radiation sickness are not known. Anorexia, nausea, vomiting, weakness, exhaustion, lassitude, and in some cases prostration may occur, singly or in combination. Radiation sickness associated with x-ray therapy is most likely to occur when the therapy is given in large dosage to large areas over the abdomen, less often when given over the thorax, and rarely when therapy is given over the extremities. With protracted therapy, this complication is rarely significant. The patient's emotional reaction to the illness or to the treatment plays an important role in aggravating or minimizing such effects.

Prevention

Persons handling radiation sources can minimize exposure to radiation by recognizing the importance of time, distance, and shielding. Areas housing x-ray and nuclear materials must be properly shielded. Untrained or poorly trained personnel should not be permitted to work with x-ray and nuclear radiation. Any unnecessary exposures, diagnostic or therapeutic, should be avoided. X-ray equipment should be periodically checked for reliability of output, and proper filters should be employed. When feasible, it is advisable to shield the gonads, especially of young persons. Fluoroscopic examination should be performed as rapidly as possible, using an optimal combination of beam characteristics and filtration; the tube-to-table distance should be at least 18 inches, and the beam size should be kept to a minimum required by the examination. Special protective clothing may be necessary to protect against contamination with radioisotopes. In the event of accidental contamination, removal of all clothing and vigorous bathing with soap and water should be followed by careful instrument (Geiger counter) check for localization of ionizing radiation.

Treatment

There is no specific treatment for the biologic effects of ionizing radiation. The success of treatment of local radiation effects will depend upon the extent, degree, and location of tissue injury. Treatment is supportive and symptomatic.

A systemic radiation reaction following radiation therapy (radiation sickness) is preferably prevented, but when it does occur it is treated symptomatically and supportively. The antinauseant drugs, eg, dimenhydrinate (Dramamine), 100 mg 1 hour before and 1 hour and 4 hours after radiation therapy, may be of value. Whole blood transfusions may be necessary if anemia is present. Transfusion of marrow cells has been employed recently. Disturbances of fluid or electrolyte balance require appropriate treatment. Antibiotics may be of use for secondary infection.

DELAYED (CHRONIC) EFFECTS OF EXCESSIVE DOSES OF IONIZING RADIATION

Diagnosis

A. Somatic Effects:

1. Skin scarring, atrophy, and telangiectases, obliterative endarteritis, pulmonary fibrosis, intestinal stenosis, and other late effects may occur.

2. Cataracts may occur following irradiation of the lens.

3. Leukemia may occur, perhaps only in susceptible individuals, many years following radiation.

4. The incidence of neoplastic disease is increased in persons exposed to large amounts of radiation, particularly in areas of heavy damage.

5. Microcephaly and other congenital abnormalities may occur in children exposed in utero, especially if the fetus was exposed during the first 4 months of pregnancy.

B. Genetic Effects: Alteration of the sex ratio at birth (fewer males than females) suggests genetic damage. The incidence of congenital abnormalities, stillbirths, and neonatal deaths when conception occurs after termination of radiation exposure is apparently not increased.

Treatment

See treatment of acute radiation reactions.

BITES

ANIMAL BITES

Animal bites are important as potential sources of pyogenic and anaerobic infections. In these cases, wounds should be treated by conventional surgical cleansing and debridement as necessary. A special problem, present largely in the minds of parents, is the possibility of rabies. Even though only 1–2 cases of rabies occur each year in the USA, about 30,000 individuals receive antirabies treatment each year. The decision to use rabies vaccine or hyperimmune serum is a difficult one. These products have been associated with numerous side reactions, and some cases of disability and death have resulted from their use. For further discussion, see Chapter 25.

Treatment

Wash and irrigate animal bite wounds with soap and water and then with povidone-iodine (Betadine, Isodine).

Dog bites are usually associated with severe crushing injuries because of the animal's powerful jaws. All devitalized tissue should be debrided and the edges of the wound excised to give clean, square edges. The wound can then be closed as any laceration of equivalent size.

Cat bites are usually on the hand, and the sharp, needle-like teeth are likely to penetrate the periosteum of the digit. These wounds should be cleansed carefully but left open. Warm soaks 2–3 times a day stimulate local circulation and prevent the puncture wound from sealing until healing is complete. Many domestic pets harbor *Pasteurella multocida* in their mouths. This anaerobe produces an infection resembling streptococcal cellulitis.

Ampicillin is an appropriate antibiotic for most bites by household pets.

If the patient has been immunized against tetanus, give a tetanus toxoid booster (0.5 ml subcut). If the child has not been immunized, give human tetanus immune globulin, 4 units/kg subcut.

Specific antirabies treatment should be given after careful individual consideration. See Chapter 25 for details.

Chambers GH & others: Treatment of dog-bite wounds. Minn Med 52:427, 1969.

Harris D: Dog bites: An unrecognized epidemic. Bull NY Acad Med 50:981, 1974.

Thomson HG & others: Small animal bites: The role of primary closure. J Trauma 13:20, 1973.

HUMAN BITES

Most human bites inflicted by children on playmates are superficial and require only local hygiene for prompt healing.

Deep bites extending below subcutaneous tissue levels should be treated vigorously since a wide variety of pathogenic organisms are present in the human mouth. Most are sensitive to penicillin G or ampicillin.

Swabbings should be collected for culture.

Treatment

A. Local Measures:

1. Cleanse the wound with soap and water and irrigate vigorously. For deep wounds, force large quantities of sterile water into the wound with a syringe.

2. Surgically debride the wound as indicated.

3. Do not suture skin over a bite wound.

B. Specific Measures for Deep Wounds: Give full doses of broad spectrum antibiotics. Combinations of penicillin, kanamycin, and colistin provide a wide coverage for most organisms. After the results of cultures have been received, specific antibiotic therapy can be instituted.

Paton BC: Bites: Human, dog, spider, and snake. Surg Clin North Am 43:537, 1963.

● ● ●

General References

Gans SL (editor): Symposium on surgical pediatrics. Pediatr Clin North Am 16:529, 1969.

Smith CA: *The Critically Ill Child.* Saunders, 1972.

Varga C & others: *Handbook of Pediatric Medical Emergencies,* 4th ed. Mosby, 1968.

30 . . .
Poisoning

Barry H. Rumack, MD

Poisonings, the fourth most common cause of death in children, result from the complex interaction of the agent, the child, and the family environment. The peak incidence is at age 2; and most of these episodes are not actual poisonings but ingestions that do not produce toxicity. Accidents occur most often in children under 5 years of age as a result of insecure storage of drugs, household chemicals, etc. Repeated poisonings may be a sign of a family problem requiring intervention on the child's behalf, although 25% of children will have a second episode of ingestion of a toxic substance within a year following the first one. Accidental poisonings are unusual after age 5. "Poisonings" in older children and adolescents usually represent manipulative or genuine suicide attempts. Toxicity may also result in this group following the use of drugs or chemicals for their mind-altering effects.

PHARMACOLOGIC PRINCIPLES
OF TOXICOLOGY

In the evaluation of the poisoned patient it is important to compare the anticipated pharmacologic or toxic effects with the clinical presentation of the patient. If the history, for example, is that the patient ingested phenobarbital 30 minutes ago but the clinical examination reveals dilated pupils, tachycardia, dry mouth, absent bowel sounds, and active hallucinations, then clearly the major toxicity is anticholinergic and therapy should be given accordingly.

Knowledge of the pharmacokinetics of the toxic agent will help the physician to plan a rational approach to definitive care after necessary life-supporting measures have been instituted.

LD_{50}, MLD

Many health professionals, when confronted with an episode of ingestion of a potentially poisonous agent, are eager to look up the LD_{50} or the MLD (minimum lethal dose) because they think this information will help them decide whether or not the child is going to be ill. Unfortunately, such information is seldom of value since it is usually impossible to tell how much the child has ingested, how much has been absorbed, the metabolic status of the patient, or where the patient's response to the agent will fall in the normal distribution curve. Furthermore, these values are often not valid in humans even if the history is accurate.

Half-Life (T½)

Knowledge of the T½ of an agent that has been taken in an overdose amount is often of value in planning therapy. For example, the therapeutic T½ of salicylates is approximately 2 hours, whereas the T½ in overdosages is 24–30 hours. Clearly, effective measures to enhance excretion of the salicylate will be useful in decreasing the duration of toxicity.

Volume of Distribution (V_D)

The volume of distribution (V_D) of a drug represents the percentage of the body mass in which a drug is distributed. It is obtained by dividing the amount of drug absorbed by the blood level. With aspirin, for example, this is roughly equivalent to the body water volume and can be expressed as 0.6 liters/kg body weight, 60% of body weight, or 42 liters in an adult. V_D is variously described by any of these terms. (See Table 30–1.) In general, drugs which are significantly protein-bound or are water-soluble are not distributed with a volume much above that of total body water. Ethchlorvynol, a lipophilic drug, on the other hand, distributes well beyond total body water. Since the calculation produces a volume above body weight (300 liters in an adult, 500% of body weight in children), this figure is frequently referred to as *apparent* volume of distribution, a designation shared by many lipophilic drugs.

When a drug is differentially concentrated in body lipids and has a high volume of distribution, only a small proportion of the ingested drug will be in the body water and thereby accessible to diuresis or dialysis. On the other hand, a drug which is water-soluble and has a low volume of distribution may cross the dialysis membrane well and also respond to diuresis.

Metabolism & Excretion

The route of detoxification of an agent—correlated with other information—will help in making therapeutic decisions. Methanol, for example, is metabolized to a toxic product. This metabolic step may be

Table 30—1. Some examples of pK_a and V_D.

Drug	pK_a	Diuresis	Dialysis	Approximate V_D
Amobarbital	7.9	No	No	200–300% body weight
Amphetamine	9.8	Acid	Yes	60% body weight
Aspirin	3.5	Alkaline	Yes	60% body weight
Chlorpromazine	9.3	No	No	40–50 liters/kg (2800–3500% body weight)
Codeine	8.2	No	No	5–10 liters/kg
Desipramine	10.2	No	No	30–40 liters/kg (2100–2800% body weight)
Ethchlorvynol	8.7	No	No	5–10 liters/kg (350–700% body weight)
Glutethimide	4.5	No	No	10–20 liters/kg (700–1400% body weight)
Isoniazid	3.5	Alkaline	Yes	61% body weight
Methadone	8.3	No	No	5–10 liters/kg (350–700% body weight)
Methicillin	2.8	Yes	Yes	60% body weight
Phenobarbital	7.4	Alkaline	Yes	75% body weight
Phenytoin	8.3	No	No	60–80% body weight
Tetracycline	7.7	No	No	200–300% body weight

blocked by the administration of ethanol. Long-acting barbiturates are partially metabolized in the liver but are primarily excreted in the urine, which means that forced diuresis will be an effective therapeutic measure. Secobarbital, a short-acting barbiturate, while also metabolized in the liver, is poorly excreted in the urine, and forced diuresis is therefore ineffective.

Blood Levels

Care of the poisoned patient should never be guided solely by the results of laboratory measurements. Treatment should be directed first against the clinical signs and symptoms, followed by more specific therapy based on laboratory determinations. The laboratory pathologist should be given whatever information he needs regarding the history and the class of the suspected toxic agent (sedative-hypnotic, opiate, amphetamine, etc), so that the specific agent can be identified as rapidly as possible. The laboratory should know its own normal levels of therapeutic ranges so that interpretation of results can be rational.

Handling of Specimens

A. Vomitus and Gastric Lavage Fluid: Collect and send to the laboratory initial material produced in separate containers plus an aliquot of the remainder. Include any material that appears to be pill fragments.

B. Blood: Ask the laboratory pathologist specifically what type of container and anticoagulant are desired before drawing the sample.

C. Urine: Collect an initial sample—if possible, 100 ml—for analysis and then begin a timed 6–12 hour collection, which may be useful in determining the rate of excretion of the agent.

GENERAL TREATMENT OF POISONING

The first contact in the case of possible poisoning by ingestion involving a child under age 5 will usually be over the telephone. Proper handling of the situation by phone can significantly reduce morbidity and prevent unwarranted or excessive treatment.

After initial telephone advice has been given, a decision is made about whether or not the child should be seen. If the child is brought to the office or hospital emergency room, life-sustaining measures are introduced, followed by definitive therapy.

Initial Telephone Contact

Evaluate the urgency of the situation and decide whether immediate emergency transportation to a health facility is indicated. Transportation of seriously poisoned patients should be by competent emergency rescue personnel who have suction, oxygen, and other equipment available to provide or continue emergency procedures. Determine whether the patient is in immediate danger, potential danger, or no danger.

Basic information that should be *written down* at the first telephone contact includes the patient's name, age, weight, address and telephone number, and the time elapsed since ingestion or other exposure.

Type of Ingestion

This information is usually given by the parent in the first few words of the call. (*Example:* "My little boy just swallowed the vitamin pills!") After a decision is made about whether the ingestion is a dangerous one and basic information has been obtained, the physician should develop more details about the suspected toxic agent. It may be difficult to obtain an accurate history. For example, an empty bottle of iron tablets may have rolled out of sight under the couch, and the mother may then assume that the empty vitamin bottle means that only the vitamin capsules have been swallowed. Obtain names of drugs or ingredients, manufacturers, prescription numbers, names and phone numbers of prescribing physician and pharmacy, etc. Find out whether the substance was shared among several children, whether it had been recently purchased, who had last used it, how full it was, and how much was spilled if any.

PREVENTING CHILDHOOD POISONINGS

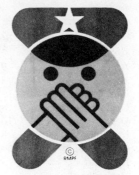

"OFFICER UGG"

Each year, thousands of children are accidentally poisoned by medicines, polishes, insecticides, drain cleaners, bleaches, household chemicals, and garage products. It is the responsibility of adults to make sure that children are not exposed to potentially toxic substances.

Here are some suggestions:

(1) Insist on safety closures and learn how to use them properly.
(2) Keep household cleaning supplies, medicines, garage products, and insecticides out of the reach and sight of your child. Lock them up whenever possible.
(3) Never store food and cleaning products together. Store medicine and chemicals in original containers and never in food or beverage containers.
(4) Avoid taking medicine in your child's presence. Children love to imitate. Always call medicine by its proper name. Never suggest that medicine is "candy"–especially aspirin and children's vitamins.
(5) Read the label on all products and heed warnings and cautions. Never use medicine from an unlabeled or unreadable container. Never pour medicine in a darkened area where the label cannot be clearly seen.
(6) If you are interrupted while using a product, take it with you. It only takes a few seconds for your child to get into it.
(7) Know what your child can do. For example, if you have a crawling infant, keep household products stored above floor level, not beneath the kitchen sink.
(8) Keep the phone number of your doctor, Poison Center, hospital, police department, and fire department or paramedic emergency rescue squad near the phone.

FIRST AID FOR POISONING

Always keep syrup of ipecac and Epsom salt (magnesium sulfate) in your home. The former is used to induce vomiting and the latter may be used as a laxative. These drugs are used sometimes when poisons are swallowed. Only use them as instructed by your Poison Center or doctor, and *follow their directions for use.*

INHALED POISONS
If gas, fumes, or smoke have been inhaled, immediately drag or carry the patient to fresh air. Then call the Poison Center or your doctor.

POISONS ON THE SKIN
If the poison has been spilled on the skin or clothing, remove the clothing and flood the involved parts with water. Then wash with soapy water and rinse thoroughly. Then call the Poison Center or your doctor.

SWALLOWED POISONS
If the poison has been swallowed and the patient is awake and can swallow, give the patient only water or milk to drink. Then call the Poison Center or your doctor. *CAUTION:* Antidote labels on products may be incorrect. Do not give salt, vinegar, or lemon juice. Call before doing anything else.

POISONS IN THE EYE
Flush the eye with lukewarm water poured from a pitcher held 3–4 inches from the eye for 15 minutes. Call the Poison Center or your doctor.

DOCTOR_____ POISON CENTER_____ AMBULANCE_____

POLICE_____ FIRE DEPARTMENT_____ HOSPITAL_____

(This page may be reproduced and used for purposes of education in poison prevention. Courtesy of Rocky Mountain Poison Center, Denver, Colorado.)

Bring the Poison to the Hospital

If the patient is to be seen in the emergency department, everything in the vicinity of the patient suspected to be a cause of toxicity should be brought with him.

Initial Therapy Over the Phone

Treatment at home should include external and internal decontamination if appropriate.

A. External:

1. Skin—If the patient has been exposed to an insecticide or has spilled a caustic agent on the skin, the area should be immediately flooded with water and washed well with soap and a soft washcloth or sponge.

2. Eye—Irrigation of the eye with plain water should begin *before* the patient arrives at the emergency room. Use plain tap water—do not try to neutralize acids or alkalies. Have the head held back over the sink and direct a gentle stream of water into the eye from the tap, or pour water into the eye from a drinking glass or pitcher. Irrigation should be continued for 15—20 minutes. Then transport the patient to the hospital for ophthalmologic examination.

B. Internal: Milk or water should be immediately administered to any patient who has ingested a strongly acid or alkaline agent. Do not induce vomiting in patients who are comatose or convulsing or who have lost the gag reflex. If the patient can be seen at the hospital in less than 20 minutes, then it is probably useful only to administer a few glasses of water and wait to administer syrup of ipecac in the emergency room. If vomiting occurs en route, the vomitus should be retained for further analysis. If emesis is induced on the way to the hospital, syrup of ipecac should be administered as described in the section on prevention of absorption (see p 867).

Poison Information

Data on ingredients of commercial products and medications can usually be obtained from the regional poison information center. Be sure that the source utilized is up to date. Many sources of information on poisonous ingredients are outdated simply because manufacturers change the ingredients in some of their products as often as every 3—6 months. *POISINDEX* is a quarterly publication that offers current data about toxic ingredients based on computer contact with over 7000 manufacturers. The manufacturer of the product can be called (collect) for information about toxic ingredients. It is important to have the actual container at hand when calling the manufacturer so that information about serial numbers, label colors, etc can be conveyed. In some cases, the experience of the company physician may be of value in management. *Caution:* Antidote information on labels of commercial products is frequently incorrect and may contain bad advice such as administration of an acidic agent like vinegar to a child who has ingested a caustic substance.

Follow-Up

In over 95% of cases of ingestion of potentially toxic substances by children, a trip to the hospital is not required. If it is decided that an ingestion is not toxic or that vomiting induced at home is the only treatment required, it is important to call the parent at 1 and 4 hours after an ingestion. If the child has actually ingested an additional unknown agent and is gradually becoming comatose, a change in management may be instituted, including transportation to the hospital. An additional call should be made 24 hours after the ingestion to begin the process of poison prevention.

Poison Prevention Over the Telephone

This may be instituted with a few simple questions about storage of hazardous substances in unsafe locations. The following is a partial list of potentially poisonous substances that must be stored safely if there are small children in the home: drain cleaning crystals or liquid, dishwasher soap and cleaning supplies, paints and paint thinners, medicines, garden spray and other insecticide materials, automobile products.

If it seems that there are problems that may lead to further episodes of hazardous exposure of small children to potential poisons, it will be useful to arrange an appointment with the parent to discuss the matter or to send a public health nurse to the home to examine storage practices and make suitable arrangements to improve the situation.

PREVENTION OF POISONING

A major goal of pediatricians is to reduce the number of accidental ingestions in the high-risk age group under 5 years. A systematic poison education effort should be part of the routine care of every patient. Awareness of potential hazards and raising of consciousness among parents have been made easier through the character known as "Officer Ugg" (see p 864). Parents of very young children are encouraged to search the house and identify all hazardous substances. As the child is gradually taught the meaning of the face, then parents and children can play "poison policeman" and together identify hazardous substances. Children are taught to imitate the face and cover their mouths whenever confronted with a potential poison, whether or not the sticker face is attached. Use of this symbol is available free of royalty obligations from the Rocky Mountain Poison Foundation, 1722 Prudential Plaza, Denver 80202.

The chart entitled "Preventing Childhood Poisonings," reproduced on p 864, may be copied from this book and given to parents along with a bottle of syrup of ipecac at the 6-month check-up.* Reinforcement should occur at the 1-year check-up to make certain

---

*No request for permission to reproduce the chart is necessary provided it is done without modification.

that adequate poison-proofing measures have been instituted and maintained.

INITIAL EMERGENCY ROOM CONTACT

If the decision has been made to see the child in the hospital, or if the patient has bypassed the initial phone call and is brought to the hospital emergency room—as in the case of many severe ingestions or adolescent overdoses—the following steps should be followed:

Make Certain the Patient Is Breathing

This is sometimes overlooked in the emergency room frenzy of getting intravenous lines started and searching for treatment protocols. The adequacy of tidal volume should be checked, normal being 10—15 ml/kg.

Treat Shock

Initial therapy of the hypotensive patient should consist of laying the patient flat and administering colloids, blood, or isotonic solutions. Because of potential interaction and toxicity, vasopressors should be reserved for poisoned patients in shock who do not respond to these standard measures.

Treat Burns

Burns may occur following exposure to strong acid or strong alkaline agents or petroleum distillates. Burned areas should be cleaned and debrided if extensive and fully decontaminated by flooding with sterile saline solution or water. Skin decontamination should be performed in a patient with cutaneous exposure. Emergency department personnel working on a critically ill patient who has been contaminated with (for example) an organophosphate insecticide should themselves be decontaminated if their skin or clothing has been exposed to the agent. So-called "barbiturate burns" require treatment as for any other kind of burn. These bullous lesions, usually on the fingers, may occur following exposure to a wide variety of sedating agents.

Take a Pertinent History

The history should be taken from family, friends, or the patient if old enough and sufficiently alert to give useful answers to questions. It may be crucial to determine all of the kinds of toxicants in the home: ill family members with toxic medications, chemicals associated with hobbies, occupations of family members, purity of the water supply, unusual eating or medication habits, or other clues to the possible cause of poisoning.

Coma, Hyperactivity, & Withdrawal

It is useful to determine the level of coma, degree of hyperactivity, or severity of withdrawal symptoms as a means of assessing the efficacy of treatment.

A. Determine the Level of Coma: Coma is graded on a scale of 0—4:

0   Asleep but can be aroused and can answer questions.
1   Comatose; withdraws from painful stimuli; reflexes intact.
2   Comatose; does *not* withdraw from painful stimuli; most reflexes intact; no respiratory or circulatory depression.
3   Comatose; most or all reflexes absent; no depression of respiration or circulation.
4   Comatose; reflexes absent; respiratory depression with cyanosis, circulatory failure, or shock.

B. Determine the Degree of Hyperactivity:

1+ Restlessness, irritability, insomnia, tremor, hyperreflexia, sweating, mydriasis, flushing.
2+ Confusion, hyperactivity, hypertension, tachypnea, tachycardia, extrasystoles, sweating, mydriasis, flushing, mild hyperpyrexia.
3+ Delirium, mania, self-injury, marked hypertension, tachycardia, arrhythmias, hyperpyrexia.
4+ Above plus convulsions, coma, circulatory collapse.

C. Determine the Severity of Narcotic Withdrawal Symptoms: Score the following findings on a scale of 0—2:

Diarrhea	Insomnia
Dilated pupils	Lacrimation
Gooseflesh	Muscle cramps
Hyperactive bowel	Restlessness
sounds	Tachycardia
Hypertension	Yawning

A score of 1—5 represents mild, 6—10 moderate, and 11—15 severe withdrawal symptoms.

Seizures, which are unusual in narcotic withdrawal, indicate severe withdrawal problems.

DEFINITIVE THERAPY OF POISONING

Antidotes

There are few specific antidotes. Many of these agents are discussed in the section on treatment of specific agents. A few poisons that may require immediate antidotal therapy are listed here:

Poison	Antidote
Carbon monoxide	Oxygen
Cyanide	Amyl nitrite (pediatric dosage), sodium thiosulfate
Nitrites and nitrates	Treat methemoglobinemia with methylene blue
Organophosphate or carbamate insecticides	Atropine
Anticholinergics	Physostigmine
Narcotics	Naloxone (Narcan)
Methanol, ethylene glycol	Ethanol

Prevention of Absorption

A. Emesis: Induced vomiting is *contraindicated* in a patient who is comatose or convulsing or who has lost the gag reflex; in a patient who has ingested strong acids or strong bases; or in one who has ingested a hydrocarbon. However, in the case of petroleum distillates, vomiting should be induced if more than 1 ml/kg has been ingested, if they contain heavy metals, or if the solvent is a CNS depressant.

1. Ipecac method—Adult dose, 30 ml; pediatric dose, 15 ml. Give orally and repeat once only in 20 minutes if necessary. The procedure is as follows:

a. Give ipecac orally.

b. Follow with large amounts of water or whatever fluid the child will drink (ipecac on an empty stomach is "like squeezing an empty balloon").

c. Keep the patient ambulatory.

d. After 15 minutes, stimulate the patient's throat, if necessary, to induce vomiting.

2. Other emetics—The only approved oral emetic agent is syrup of ipecac. Use of sodium chloride may lead to lethal hypernatremia. Apomorphine is contraindicated in pediatric practice. Other emetic agents are not as effective as syrup of ipecac and should be avoided.

B. Lavage: If the patient is becoming unconscious, is unconscious, is convulsing, or has lost the gag reflex, gastric lavage following endotracheal or nasotracheal intubation should be performed rather than induced vomiting. Lavage is less effective than emesis if a small (8–16F) tube is utilized but not if the recommended 28–36F Ewald tube is used. The tube should be inserted orally, and lavage should be with warm saline solution in a small child to avoid hyponatremia or hypothermia. Save the initial aspirate for laboratory determination and lavage until the returns have been clear for 1 liter.

Emesis and lavage recover an average of about 30% of the stomach contents. While this may be helpful in reducing the amount of toxin available for absorption, it means that approximately 70% of an ingested dose will remain. Additional measures such as charcoal and cathartics should be instituted to prevent further absorption.

C. Charcoal: Thirty grams of charcoal should be made into a slurry with water. The mixture will keep without affecting the activity of the charcoal. A few milliliters of cherry syrup may be added just prior to oral administration to increase palatability. The patient may regurgitate some of the charcoal, but 70% is usually retained. Charcoal acts as a marker of intestinal transit; once charcoal appears in the stool, it is unlikely that further absorption of drug will occur.

D. Catharsis: *Caution:* Do not give cathartics containing magnesium to patients in renal failure. Pneumonitis and "mineral oil pneumonia" may occur following aspiration of oil-based cathartics.

Give either magnesium sulfate (Epsom salt), 30 gm orally for an adolescent or 250 mg/kg orally for a child, or sodium sulfate (Glauber's salt) in a similar dosage. A convenient alternative is Fleet's Phospho-Soda, 15–30 ml diluted 1:4, with the entire amount administered to an adolescent and one-fourth the amount administered to a child.

Enhancement of Urinary Excretion

Urinary excretion of absorbed toxins can be hastened by forced acid or alkaline diuresis, or dialysis (hemodialysis or peritoneal dialysis).

A. Diuresis: Forced diuresis is often useful in serious poisonings if the drug is excreted in the urine in active form. The technic should not be used unless it is specifically indicated, as it may increase the likelihood of cerebral edema, a common cause of death in poisonings.

Excretion of any of the following can be hastened by forced diuresis:

Alcohol	Other renally cleared
Amphetamines (acid)	drugs
Bromides	Phenobarbital (alkaline
Isoniazid (big anion	diuresis)
gaps; alkalinization	Salicylates (alkaline di-
needs will be massive)	uresis)
Jequirity beans (alka-	Strychnine (acid diure-
line diuresis)	sis)

Hypertonic or pharmacologic diuretics should be given along with adequate fluids. The usual urine flow is 0.5–2 ml/kg/hour; with forced diuresis, urine flow should increase to 3–6 ml/kg/hour. Alkaline or acid diuresis should be chosen on the basis of the toxin's pK_a, so that ionized drug will be trapped in the tubular lumen and not reabsorbed. (See Table 30–1.) Thus, if the pK_a is less than 7.0, alkaline diuresis is appropriate; if it is over 8.0, use acid diuresis. Osmotic load is also important, and either type of diuretic should be given at intervals. Proximal reabsorption will occur if adequate osmotic load is not maintained in the tubule. The pK_a is usually supplied with general drug information.

1. Alkaline diuresis can usually be accomplished with bicarbonate. It is well to observe for potassium depletion, in which case administration of potassium citrate, which has both potassium and considerable alkalinizing ability, may be used. It is also available orally as K-Lyte "fizzies," which are a quite palatable form. Follow serum K^+ and observe for ECG evidence of K^+ deficiency.

2. Acid diuresis may be accomplished with ascorbic acid, arginine, or ammonium chloride, all of which may be given intravenously or orally.

a. Ascorbic acid may be given in doses of 0.5—1 gm orally or IV as needed to obtain acid urine (pH 4.5—5.5).

b. Ammonium chloride may be given in a total dose of 2—6 gm/day or 75 mg/kg/dose in 4 divided doses. It comes as solution for intravenous use or as tablets or syrup for oral administration.

c. Mannitol diuresis may accomplish an acid urine without any additional measures.

B. Dialysis: Hemodialysis (or peritoneal dialysis if hemodialysis is unavailable) is useful in the poisonings listed below. Dialysis should be considered part of supportive care if the patient satisfies any of the following criteria:

1. Clinical criteria—

a. Stage 3 or 4 coma or hyperactivity caused by a dialyzable drug which cannot be treated by conservative means.

b. Hypotension threatening renal or hepatic function which cannot be corrected by adjusting circulating volume.

c. Apnea in a patient who cannot be ventilated.

d. Marked hyperosmolality which is not due to easily corrected fluid problems.

e. Severe acid-base disturbance not responding to therapy.

f. Severe electrolyte disturbance not responding to therapy.

g. Marked hypothermia or hyperthermia.

2. Immediate dialysis indicated regardless of clinical condition—

a. Ethylene glycol.

b. Methanol.

c. Heavy metals in soluble compounds.

d. Heavy metals after chelating in patients in renal failure.

3. Dialysis indicated on basis of condition of patient—(In general, dialyze if patient is in coma deeper than level 3.)

Alcohols	Bromides	Paraldehyde
Ammonia	Calcium	Potassium
Amphetamines	Chloral hydrate	Quinidine
Anilines	Fluorides	Quinine
Antibiotics	Iodides	Salicylates
Barbiturates	Isoniazid	Strychnine
(long-acting)	Meprobamate	Thiocyanates
Boric acid		

(Other drugs may be dialyzable, but the information should be verified prior to institution of dialysis therapy.)

4. Dialysis not indicated except for support— Therapy consists of intensive care.

Antidepressants (tricyclics and MAO inhibitors also)	Barbiturates (short-acting)
	Chlordiazepoxide (Librium)
Antihistamines	Diazepam (Valium)

Digitalis and related drugs	Oxazepam (Serax)
Diphenoxylate with atropine (Lomotil)	Phenothiazines
	Phenytoin (Dilantin)
Heroin and other opiates	Synthetic anticholinergics
Methaqualone (Quaalude)	and belladonna compounds
Methyprylon (Noludar)	

Amphetamines respond better to acid diuresis, but dialysis should be considered if the response is not adequate.

While the long-acting barbiturates (cleared by the kidneys) are more readily dialyzable than the short-acting ones (cleared by the liver), dialysis may be helpful if the patient satisfies the criteria for supportive dialysis needs as outlined above.

Salicylates generally respond very well to intensive alkaline diuretic therapy, but, if complications such as renal failure or pulmonary edema develop, peritoneal dialysis with 5% albumin may be helpful.

Peritoneal dialysis and *exchange transfusion* may be more useful in small children than hemodialysis. Again, the main purpose of these procedures may not be removal of the poison but restoration of fluid or acid-base balance. The infant who has been poisoned and whose serum sodium is rising because of excess bicarbonate administration may be helped considerably by an exchange transfusion even if little poison is removed.

Except in the case of the "immediate" (see above, ¶ B 2 a–d) list, dialysis should *not* be performed as initial therapy but only when the criteria listed above are met.

Hemoperfusion

Perfusion of blood through charcoal- or resin-filled devices, while still experimental, is gradually becoming more widely available in many centers. These technics will probably allow removal of many substances previously considered nondialyzable because of strong lipid solubility or large molecular size.

MANAGEMENT OF SPECIFIC COMMON POISONS

Unless otherwise directed, syrup of ipecac should be given to all conscious patients poisoned by the substances listed in the following section. Gastric lavage is usually indicated for comatose patients after an endotracheal tube is inserted. Apomorphine should not be used because of the high incidence of complications.

ACETAMINOPHEN

Acetaminophen is an analgesic antipyretic contained in numerous preparations often accessible to children. In prescribed doses the drug is a safe and effective agent for relief of fever and pain. In overdosage, acetaminophen can cause severe hepatotoxicity. Toxicity in adults and adolescents is well recognized, but overdosage in children under age 5 rarely appears to cause significant toxic reactions.

Acetaminophen is normally metabolized in the liver. A small percentage of the drug goes through a pathway leading to a toxic metabolite. Normally, this nucleophilic reactant is removed harmlessly by conjugation with glutathione. In overdosage, the supply of glutathione becomes exhausted, and the metabolite may bind covalently to hepatic macromolecules to produce necrosis.

Treatment is based upon supplying a surrogate glutathione. Cysteamine has been used extensively in Britain with good success but is not available in the USA. Acetylcysteine (Mucomyst) may also be used and appears to be less toxic than cysteamine and just as effective. This drug, which is currently the subject of a nationwide study, is administered to patients whose acetaminophen levels plot in the toxic range on the nomogram (Fig 30−1).

The dose is 140 mg/kg orally diluted to a 5% solution in sweet fruit juice or carbonated soft drink. After this loading dose, 70 mg/kg should be administered orally every 4 hours for 3 days. SGOT, SGPT, serum bilirubin, and plasma prothrombin time should be followed closely, and, if the patient develops hepatic encephalopathy, supportive measures should be provided and acetylcysteine withdrawn.

Peterson RG, Rumack BH: Treating acute acetaminophen poisoning with acetylcysteine. JAMA 237:2406, 1977.

Prescott LF & others: Cysteamine, methionine, and penicillamine in the treatment of paracetamol poisoning. Lancet 2:109, 1976.

Rumack BH, Matthew H: Acetaminophen poisoning and toxicity. Pediatrics 55:871, 1975.

ALCOHOL, ETHYL
(Ethanol)

Alcoholic beverages, tinctures, cosmetics, and rubbing alcohol are common sources of poisoning in children. Concomitant exposure to other depressant drugs increases the seriousness of the intoxication. (Blood levels cited are for adults; comparable figures for children are not available. In most states, alcohol levels of 50−80 mg/100 ml are considered compatible with impaired faculties, and levels of 80−150 mg/100 ml are considered evidence of intoxication.)

50−150 mg/100 ml: Incoordination, slow reaction time, and blurred vision.

150−300 mg/100 ml: Visual impairment, staggering, and slurred speech. Marked hypoglycemia may be present.

300−500 mg/100 ml: Marked incoordination, stupor, hypoglycemia, and convulsions.

> 500 mg/100 ml: Coma and death except in individuals who have developed tolerance.

Complete absorption of alcohol by the stomach and small bowel requires 30 minutes to 6 hours depending upon the volume, the presence of food, the time spent in consuming the alcohol, etc. The rate of metabolic degradation is constant (about 10 ml of 50% alcohol per hour in an adult). Less than 10% is excreted in the urine. One ml/kg of absolute ethanol results in a peak blood level of about 100 mg/100 ml in 1 hour after ingestion.

Treatment

Supportive treatment, including aggressive management of hypoglycemia and acidosis, is usually the only measure required. Glucagon does not correct the hypoglycemia because hepatic glycogen stores are reduced. If the patient is conscious, vomiting should be induced with syrup of ipecac. Although forced diuresis increases the clearance rate of ethanol, it is not usually indicated as it increases the chance of cerebral edema. If a short-acting diuretic is used, ethacrynic acid (Edecrin) should probably not be used since it is thought to inhibit alcohol dehydrogenase. Monitoring of blood gases and oxygen administration are indicated in serious overdoses because death is usually caused by respiratory failure. In severe cases, cerebral edema should be treated with dexamethasone, 0.1 mg/kg IV every 4−6 hours. Peritoneal dialysis and hemodialysis are indicated in life-threatening intoxication.

Beard JD: Fluid and electrolyte abnormalities in alcoholism. Psychosomatics 11:502, 1970.

Hammond K, Rumack B, Rodgerson D: Blood ethanol. JAMA 226:63, 1973.

Seixas FA: Alcohol and its drug interactions. Ann Intern Med 83:86, 1975.

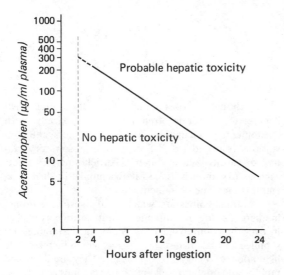

Figure 30−1. Semilogarithmic plot of plasma acetaminophen levels vs time. (Reprinted, with permission, from Rumack BH, Matthew H: Pediatrics 55:871, 1975.)

Sellers EM, Kalant H: Alcohol intoxication and withdrawal. N Engl J Med 294:757, 1976.
Seppälä M & others: Ethanol elimination in a mother and her premature twins. Lancet 1:1188, 1971.

AMPHETAMINES & RELATED DRUGS

Acute poisoning. Amphetamine poisoning is common because of the widespread availability of "diet pills" and the use of "speed" by adolescents. Symptoms include CNS stimulation, anxiety, hyperactivity, hyperpyrexia, hypertension, abdominal cramps, nausea and vomiting, and inability to void urine. A toxic psychosis indistinguishable from paranoid schizophrenia may occur.

Chronic toxicity. Amphetamines are common causes of dependency and perhaps addiction. Chronic users develop such a high tolerance that more than 1500 mg of intravenous methamphetamine can be used daily. Hyperactivity, disorganization, and euphoria are followed by exhaustion, depression, and coma lasting 2–3 days. Upon awakening, the patient is ravenously hungry. Heavy users, taking more than 100 mg a day, have restlessness, incoordination of thought, insomnia, nervousness, irritability, and visual hallucinations. Psychosis may be precipitated by the chronic administration of high doses of the drug. Depression, weakness, tremors, gastrointestinal complaints, and suicidal thoughts occur frequently.

Treatment
Because chlorpromazine (Thorazine) (0.5–1 mg/kg every 30 minutes as needed) brings about dramatic decreases in hyperactivity in intoxication, it is used in the management of intoxication. However, if ingestion of STP, MDA, or DMT is suspected, diazepam (Valium) should be used instead of chlorpromazine because of the risk of hypotension with the latter drug. When combinations of amphetamines and barbiturates (diet pills) are used, the action of the amphetamines begins first, followed by a rebound depression caused by the barbiturates. In these cases, particularly, treatment with additional barbiturates is contraindicated because of the risk of respiratory failure. Emesis or lavage, charcoal, and cathartics should be used followed by forced acid diuresis as described earlier in the chapter.

Chronic users may be withdrawn rapidly from amphetamines. On the other hand, if amphetamine-barbiturate or amphetamine-phenothiazine combination tablets have been used, the barbiturates or phenothiazines must be withdrawn gradually to prevent withdrawal seizures. Psychiatric treatment should be considered.

Cohen S: Amphetamine abuse. JAMA 231:414, 1975.
Griffith JD & others: Dextroamphetamine: Evaluation of psychotomimetic properties in man. Arch Gen Psychiatry 26:97, 1972.

ANESTHETICS, LOCAL

Intoxication caused by local anesthetics may be associated with CNS stimulation, anxiety, delirium, shock, convulsions, and death.

Local anesthetics used in obstetrics cross the placental barrier and are not efficiently metabolized by the fetal liver. Mepivacaine, lidocaine, and bupivacaine can cause fetal bradycardia, neonatal depression, and death. Prilocaine causes methemoglobinemia, which should be treated if levels in the blood exceed 40% or if the patient is symptomatic.

Accidental injection of mepivacaine (Carbocaine) into the unborn baby's head during caudal anesthesia has caused neonatal asphyxia, cyanosis, apnea, bradycardia, convulsions, and death.

Treatment
If ingested, induced vomiting should be followed by activated charcoal. Any contaminated mucous membranes should be carefully cleansed. Oxygen administration, with assisted ventilation if necessary, is indicated. Methemoglobinemia is treated with methylene blue, 1%, 0.2 ml/kg IV over 5–10 minutes; this should dramatically relieve the cyanosis. Exchange transfusion is indicated in a newborn with mepivacaine toxicity. Therapeutic levels of mepivacaine, lidocaine, and procaine are less than 5 μg/ml.

Meffin P, Long GJ, Thomas J: Clearance and metabolism of mepivacaine in the human neonate. Clin Pharmacol Ther 14:218, 1973.
Murphy PJ, Wright JD, Fitzgerald TB: Assessment of paracervical nerve block anesthesia during labor. Br Med J 1:526, 1970.
Rosefsky JB, Petersiel ME: Perinatal deaths associated with mepivacaine paracervical block anesthesia in labor. N Engl J Med 278:530, 1968.

ANTIHISTAMINES

Although antihistamines typically cause CNS depression, children often react paradoxically with excitement, hallucinations, delirium, tremors, and convulsions followed by CNS depression, respiratory failure, or cardiovascular collapse. Anticholinergic effects such as dry mouth, fixed dilated pupils, flushed face, and fever may be prominent.

Antihistamines are widely available in the home, in allergy, cold, and antiemetic preparations as well as in over-the-counter sedatives. Many antihistamines are supplied in sustained-release forms, which increases the likelihood of dangerous overdoses. They are absorbed rapidly and metabolized by the liver, lungs, and kidneys. A potentially fatal dose of most antihistamines is 25–50 mg/kg, or 20–30 tablets of the most commonly used antihistamines.

Treatment

Activated charcoal should be used to delay drug absorption. Emetics may be ineffective if the antihistamine is structurally related to phenothiazines. A saline cathartic is indicated for sustained-release preparations. Physostigmine, 0.5–2 mg IV, dramatically reverses the central and peripheral anticholinergic effects of antihistamines. Diazepam (Valium), 1–2 mg/kg IV, can be used to control seizures. Forced diuresis is not helpful. Exchange transfusion with 5% albumin should be considered in very severe intoxications, since most antihistamines are highly protein-bound and are concentrated in the serum.

Nigro SA: Toxic psychosis due to diphenhydramine hydrochloride. JAMA 203:301, 1968.

Rumack BH & others: Ornade and anticholinergic toxicity, hypertension, hallucinations and arrhythmia. Clin Toxicol 7:573, 1974.

Wallace AR, Allen E: Recovery after massive overdose of diphenhydramine and methaqualone. Lancet 2:1241, 1968.

ARSENIC

Acute poisoning. Abdominal pain, vomiting, watery and bloody diarrhea, cardiovascular collapse, paresthesias, neck pain, garlic odor on breath, difficulty in walking, and exfoliative dermatitis occur. Convulsions, coma, and anuria are later signs. Inhalation may cause pulmonary edema. Death is the result of cardiovascular collapse.

Chronic poisoning. Anorexia, generalized weakness, giddiness, colic, abdominal pain, polyneuritis, dermatitis, nail changes, alopecia, and anemia often develop.

Arsenic is commonly used in insecticides (fruit tree or tobacco sprays), rodenticides, weed killers, and wallpaper. It is well absorbed primarily through the gastrointestinal and respiratory tracts, but skin absorption may occur. Arsenic can be found in the urine, hair, and nails by laboratory testing.

Poisoning with arsenic trioxide, an insoluble precursor of most arsenicals, is associated with a 12% mortality rate. Highly toxic soluble derivatives of this compound, such as sodium arsenite, are frequently found in liquid preparations and can cause death in as many as 65% of victims. The alkyl methanearsonates found in "persistent" or "preemergence" type weed killers (eg, Ortho Crabgrass Killer) are relatively less soluble and do not cause deaths. Poisonings with a liquid arsenical preparation which does not contain alkyl methanearsonate compounds should be considered potentially lethal. Patients with any clinical signs other than minor gastrointestinal irritation should be treated until laboratory tests indicate it is no longer necessary.

Treatment

In acute poisoning, induce vomiting and put activated charcoal into the stomach. Then give dimercaprol (BAL), 2.5 mg/kg IM, immediately and follow with 2 mg/kg IM every 4 hours. After 4–8 injections, dimercaprol should be administered twice daily for 5–10 days. The dimercaprol-arsenic complex is dialyzable. Penicillamine (Cuprimine), 100 mg/kg orally to a maximum of 1 gm/day in 4 divided doses, should be used instead of BAL after the first day or even immediately if the patient is not acutely ill.

Dimercaprol is not effective in the treatment of arsine gas intoxication, which should be treated by exchange transfusion, followed by hemodialysis if there is renal damage. Vomiting should always be induced.

Chronic arsenic intoxication should be treated with penicillamine. Collect a 24-hour baseline urine specimen and then begin chelation. If the 24-hour urine arsenic is > 50 μg, continue chelation for 5 days. After 10 days, repeat the 5-day cycle once or twice depending on how soon urine arsenic falls below 50 μg/24 hours.

Done AK: . . . and old lace. Emergency Med 5:246, 1973.

Peterson RG, Rumack BH: Arsenic poisoning treated with D-penicillamine. J Pediatr 91:661, 1977.

BARBITURATES

A patient who has ingested barbiturates in toxic amounts can present with a variety of findings including confusion, poor coordination, coma, miotic or fixed dilated pupils, increased or (more commonly) decreased respiratory effort, etc. Respiratory acidosis is commonly associated with pulmonary atelectasis, and hypotension frequently occurs in severely poisoned patients. Ingestion of more than 6 mg/kg of long- or 3 mg/kg of short-acting barbiturates is usually toxic; however, chronic users of barbiturates can tolerate blood levels up to 25 mg/100 ml.

Treatment

If the patient is awake, activated charcoal and induced vomiting are indicated. Careful conservative management with emphasis on maintaining a clear airway, adequate ventilation, and control of hypotension is critical in these patients. Since phenobarbital is excreted unchanged by the kidney, forced alkaline diuresis is useful and often eliminates the need for dialysis. If the patient develops increasing respiratory acidosis after initial improvement during forced alkaline diuresis, pulmonary edema ("shock lung") is suggested and may require dialysis or hemoperfusion if the blood level is high. Forced alkaline diuresis or hemodialysis is not of significant help in the treatment of poisoning with short-acting barbiturates.

Analeptics are contraindicated.

Bloomer HA: A critical evaluation of diuresis in the treatment of barbiturate intoxication. J Lab Clin Med 67:898, 1966.

Gröschel D, Gerstein A, Rosenbaum J: Skin lesions as a diagnostic aid in barbiturate poisoning. N Engl J Med 283:409, 1970.

Hadden J & others: Acute barbiturate intoxication. JAMA 209: 893, 1969.

Matthew H: Barbiturates. Clin Toxicol 8:495, 1975.

BELLADONNA ALKALOIDS
(Atropine, Scopolamine, Stramonium, Asthmador, Jimsonweed, & Potato Leaves)

Patients with atropinism have been characterized as "red as a beet, dry as a bone, and mad as a hatter." Common complaints include dry mouth, thirst, decreased sweating with hot, dry, red skin, high fever, and tachycardia which may be preceded by bradycardia. The pupils are dilated and vision is blurred. Speech and swallowing may be impaired. Hallucinations, delirium, and coma are common. Leukocytosis may occur, confusing the diagnosis.

The onset of symptoms is quite rapid, but symptoms usually last only 3–4 hours unless large overdoses have been taken. Atropinism has been caused by normal doses of atropine or homatropine eyedrops, especially in children with Down's syndrome. Many common plants and over-the-counter sleeping medications contain belladonna alkaloids.

Treatment

Emesis or lavage should be followed by activated charcoal and cathartics. Physostigmine, 0.5–2 mg IV (can be repeated every 30 minutes as needed), dramatically reverses the central and peripheral signs of atropinism. Neostigmine is ineffective because it does not enter the CNS. High fever must be controlled. Catheterization may be needed if the patient cannot void.

Gowdy JM: Stramonium intoxication: Review of symptomatology in 212 cases. JAMA 221:585, 1972.

Mikolich JR, Paulson GW, Cross CJ: Acute anticholinergic syndrome due to Jimson seed ingestion. Ann Intern Med 83:321, 1975.

Rumack BH: Anticholinergic poisoning: Treatment with physostigmine. Pediatrics 52:449, 1973.

BORIC ACID

Boric acid is a worthless antiseptic which has been commonly used to treat diaper rash and burns. It is rapidly absorbed through broken skin and is potentially toxic to all organs, especially the CNS, kidneys, and pancreas. About half of the ingested dose will be excreted in the first 24 hours. The estimated lethal dose in children is 5–6 gm. The amount of boric acid present in baby powder is relatively safe, but other boric acid preparations should be discarded.

Anorexia, weight loss, and mild diarrhea are the most common initial findings. Later, the "boiled lobster" skin, a characteristic erythematous exfoliating rash which desquamates in 1–2 days, is seen. Fever, vomiting, dehydration, anuria, and convulsions are commonly associated with the rash. CNS signs (irritability, high-pitched cry, exaggerated startle reflex, and opisthotonos) are common in children.

Treatment

Unless contraindicated, induced vomiting followed by catharsis should be used to remove ingested boric acid. If boric acid is being absorbed through the skin or mucous membranes, it should be removed with water and its use discontinued. Ten percent glucose in water given intravenously will induce diuresis. Anticonvulsants may be needed. Peritoneal dialysis and hemodialysis are more effective than exchange transfusion in severe boric acid poisoning.

Baliah T, McLeish HP, Drummond KN: Acute boric acid poisoning. Can Med Assoc J 101:166, 1969.

Levin S: Diapers. S Afr Med J 44:256, 1970.

CARBON MONOXIDE

The degree of toxicity correlates well with the carboxyhemoglobin level. Symptoms are more severe if the patient has exercised, taken alcohol, or lives at a high altitude. Normal blood may contain up to 5% carboxyhemoglobin.

The most prominent early clinical effect is headache. Other symptoms occur in relation to levels as follows:

Saturation of Blood	Symptoms
0–10%	None.
10–20%	Tightness across forehead; slight headache; dilatation of cutaneous vessels.
20–30%	Headache; throbbing in temples.
30–40%	Severe headache; weakness and dizziness; dimness of vision; nausea and vomiting; collapse and syncope; increased pulse and respiratory rate.
40–50%	As above, plus increased tendency to collapse and syncope; increased pulse and respiratory rate.
50–60%	Increased pulse and respiratory rate; syncope; Cheyne-Stokes respiration; coma with intermittent convulsions.
60–70%	Coma with intermittent convulsions; depressed heart action and respiration; death possible.
70–80%	Weak pulse, depressed respiration; respiratory failure and death.

Proteinuria, glycosuria, elevated serum transaminase levels, or ECG changes (including S–T segment and T wave abnormalities, atrial fibrillation, and interventricular block) may be present in the acute phase. Myocardial infarction most commonly occurs about a week after an acute serious exposure. Permanent cardiac, liver, renal, or CNS damage occasionally occurs. Even in extremely severe poisoning, CNS damage may be completely reversible, although months may be required for total recovery.

Treatment

The half-time of carbon monoxide in room air is approximately 200 minutes; in 100% oxygen, it is 40 minutes. After the level has been reduced to near zero, therapy is aimed at the nonspecific sequelae of anoxia. The addition of CO_2 is more hazardous than beneficial. A hyperbaric chamber (if readily available) at 2–2.5 atmospheres of oxygen is the ideal treatment. Hypothermia appears to be a useful adjunct to therapy. Dexamethasone, 0.1 mg/kg IV or IM every 4–6 hours, should be started to combat cerebral edema.

The patient should be closely observed for at least a week following a severe acute poisoning because myocardial infarction, pulmonary edema, and myoglobinuria may occur during convalescence.

Anderson TB: Natural gas: Unnatural causes. Lancet 1:466, 1970.

Gore I: Treatment of carbon-monoxide poisoning. Lancet 1:468, 1970.

Smith JS, Brandon S: Morbidity from acute carbon monoxide poisoning at three-year follow-up. Br Med J 1:318, 1973.

Zikria BA & others: What is clinical smoke poisoning? Ann Surg 181:151, 1975.

CAUSTICS

1. ACIDS
(Hydrochloric, Nitric, & Sulfuric Acids; Sodium Bisulfate)

Strong acids are commonly found in metal and toilet bowl cleaners, batteries, etc. Sulfuric acid is the most toxic and hydrochloric acid is the least toxic of these 3 substances. However, even a few drops can be fatal if aspirated into the trachea.

Painful swallowing, mucous membrane burns, bloody emesis, abdominal pain, respiratory distress due to edema of the epiglottis, thirst, shock, and renal failure can occur. Coma and convulsions sometimes are seen terminally. Residual lesions include esophageal, gastric, and pyloric strictures as well as scars of the cornea, skin, and oropharynx.

Treatment

Emetics and lavage are contraindicated. Water or milk is the ideal substance to dilute the ingestant because a heat-producing chemical reaction does not occur. Alkalies should not be used. The use of gas-forming carbonates is contraindicated since they increase the likelihood of perforating an already weakened stomach wall. Burned areas of the skin, mucous membranes, or eyes should be washed with copious amounts of warm water. Olive oil should not be applied to denuded areas unless the surgeon concurs. Opiates for pain and antibiotics may be needed. Treatment of shock is often necessary. An endotracheal tube may be required to alleviate laryngeal edema. Esophagoscopy should be performed if the patient has significant burns or difficulty in swallowing. Acids are more likely to produce gastric burns than esophageal burns. Corticosteroids may be of use.

2. BASES
(Clorox, Purex, Sani-Clor, Drano, Liquid-Plumr, Clinitest Tablets)

Alkalies produce more severe injuries than acids do. Some substances, such as Clinitest Tablets or Drano, are quite toxic, while the chlorinated bleaches (3–6% solutions of sodium hypochlorite) are not as toxic as formerly thought. When sodium hypochlorite comes in contact with the acid pH of the stomach, hypochlorous acid, which is very irritating to the mucous membrane and skin, is formed. However, the rapid inactivation of this substance prevents systemic toxicity from developing. If a chlorinated bleach is mixed with a strong acid such as a toilet bowl cleaner, chloramine, which is extremely irritating to the eyes and respiratory tract, is produced.

Alkalies can cause burns of the skin, mucous membranes, and eyes. Respiratory distress may be due to edema of the epiglottis, pulmonary edema resulting from inhalation of fumes, or pneumonia. Mediastinitis or other intercurrent infections or shock can occur. Perforation of the esophagus or stomach is rare.

Treatment

The skin and mucous membranes should be cleansed with copious amounts of water. A local anesthetic can be instilled in the eye if necessary to alleviate blepharospasm. The eye should be irrigated for at least 20–30 minutes. Ingestions should be treated with water or milk as a diluent. Routine esophagoscopy is no longer indicated to rule out burns of the esophagus due to chlorinated bleaches unless an unusually large amount has been ingested or the patient is symptomatic. The absence of oral lesions does not rule out the possibility of laryngeal or esophageal burns following granular alkali ingestion. A 3-week course of corticosteroids in high doses (dexamethasone, 10 mg initially, then 1 mg every 4 hours) is indicated for the treatment of esophageal burns. Bougienage may be helpful in selected cases. Antibiotics may be needed if mediastinitis is likely, but they should not be used prophylactically.

Burrington JD: Clinitest burns of the esophagus. Ann Thorac Surg 20:400, 1974.

Haller JA Jr & others: Pathophysiology and management of acute corrosive burns of the esophagus. J Pediatr Surg 6:578, 1971.

Leape LL & others: Hazard to health: Liquid lye. N Engl J Med 284:578, 1971.

Rumack BH, Burrington JP: Antidotal therapy of caustic reactions. Clin Toxicol 11:27, 1977.

CONTRACEPTIVE PILLS

The only known toxic effects following acute ingestion of oral contraceptive agents are nausea, vomiting, and vaginal bleeding in girls.

COSMETICS & RELATED PRODUCTS

The relative toxicities of commonly ingested products in this group are listed in Table 30–2.

Permanent wave neutralizers may contain bromates, peroxides, or perborates. Bromates have been removed from most products because they can cause nausea, vomiting, abdominal pain, methemoglobinemia, shock, hemolysis, renal failure, and convulsions. Four gm of bromate salts are potentially lethal. Poisoning is treated by induced emesis or gastric lavage with 1% sodium thiosulfate followed by demulcents to relieve gastric irritation. Sodium thiosulfate, 1%, 100–500 ml, can be given IV, but methylene blue should not be used to treat methemoglobinemia in this situation because it increases the toxicity of bromates. Dialysis is indicated in severe bromate poisoning. Perborate can cause boric acid poisoning.

Fingernail polish removers used to contain toluene or aliphatic acetates, which produce CNS irritation and depression. They now usually have an acetone base, which does not require treatment.

Table 30–2. Relative toxicities of cosmetics and similar products.

High toxicity	Low toxicity
Permanent wave neutralizers	Perfume
	Hair removers
Fingernail polish remover	Deodorants
	Bath salts
Moderate toxicity	
Fingernail polish	**No toxicity**
Metallic hair dyes	Liquid make-up
Home permanent wave lotion	Vegetable hair dye
	Cleansing cream
Bath oil	Hair dressing (non-alcoholic)
Shaving lotion	
Hair tonic (alcoholic)	Hand lotion or cream
Cologne, toilet water	Lipstick

Cobalt, copper, cadmium, iron, lead, nickel, silver, bismuth, and tin are sometimes found in metallic hair dyes. In large amounts, they can cause skin sensitization, urticaria, dermatitis, eye damage, vertigo, hypertension, asthma, methemoglobinemia, tremors, convulsions, and coma. Treatment for ingestions is to administer demulcents and the appropriate antidote for the heavy metal involved.

Home permanent wave lotions, hair straighteners, and hair removers usually contain thioglycollic acid salts, which cause irritation and perhaps hypoglycemia.

Shaving lotion, hair tonic, hair straighteners, cologne, and toilet water contain denatured alcohol, which can cause CNS depression and hypoglycemia.

Deodorants usually consist of an antibacterial agent in a cream base. Antiperspirants are aluminum salts, which frequently cause skin sensitization. Zirconium oxide can cause granulomas in the axilla.

Chronic inhalation of hair sprays containing synthetic and natural resins has reportedly caused thesaurosis (hilar lymphadenopathy and diffuse pulmonary infiltration) as well as ocular irritation and keratitis.

Arena JM: *Poisoning: Toxicology, Symptoms, Treatments,* 3rd ed. Thomas, 1974.

CYANIDE

Cyanide poisoning may cause a bitter, burning taste with an odor of bitter almonds on the breath, salivation, nausea (usually without vomiting), anxiety, confusion, vertigo, giddiness, stiffness of the lower jaw, coma, convulsions, opisthotonos, paralysis, dilated pupils, cardiac irregularities, and transient respiratory stimulation followed by respiratory failure. A prolonged expiratory phase is characteristic.

Cyanide is commonly used in rodenticides, metal polishes (especially silver), electroplating, and photographic solutions as well as in fumigation products. Aqueous solutions are readily absorbed through the skin, mucous membranes, and lungs, but alkali salts are toxic only when ingested. Lethal doses vary greatly with the individual, but death has usually been associated with ingestion of 200–300 mg of the sodium or potassium salt, or blood cyanide levels of 0.26–3 mg/100 ml. Death usually occurs within minutes following inhalation but may be delayed several hours following ingestion.

Treatment

If the patient is apneic or has gasping respirations, artificial respiration must be started immediately. The patient should inhale amyl nitrite for 15–30 seconds of every minute while a sodium nitrite solution is being prepared for intravenous injection. Amyl nitrite alone is not adequate treatment because the maximum methemoglobin level obtainable in this way is about 5%.

Table 30—3. Pediatric dosages of sodium nitrite and sodium thiosulfate.

Hemoglobin	Initial Dose 3% Sodium Nitrite (ml/kg)	Initial Dose 25% Sodium Thiosulfate (ml/kg)
8 gm/100 ml	0.22 ml (6.6 mg)	1.1 ml
10 gm/100 ml	0.27 ml (8.7 mg)	1.35 ml
12 gm/100 ml*	0.33 ml (10 mg)	1.65 ml
14 gm/100 ml	0.39 ml (11.6 mg)	1.95 ml

*Normal child.

Cyanide kits (Lilly Stock No. M76) which contain instructions *(for use in adults)* should be carried in all emergency vehicles. Intravenous sodium nitrite is given first followed immediately by sodium thiosulfate. Doses for children are in Table 30—3. Oxygen increases the effects of nitrites and thiosulfates but is not adequate treatment by itself. It should be continued after the thiosulfate is given because methemoglobinemia decreases the ability of blood to carry oxygen. Exchange transfusion or infusion of whole blood is indicated if methemoglobin levels rise over 50%.

The patient should be observed for 24--48 hours since toxicity may reappear. If a relapse occurs, the patient should be retreated using one-half of the above doses of sodium nitrite and sodium thiosulfate.

Berlin CM Jr: The treatment of cyanide poisoning in children. Pediatrics 46:793, 1970.
Hillman B & others: The use of dicobalt edetate (Kelocyanor) in cyanide poisoning. Postgrad Med J 50:171, 1974.

DIGITALIS & OTHER CARDIAC GLYCOSIDES

Manifestations include nausea, vomiting, diarrhea, headache, delirium, confusion, and occasionally coma. Cardiac irregularities such as atrial fibrillation, paroxysmal atrial tachycardia, and atrial flutter often occur. Death usually is the result of ventricular fibrillation.

Toxic reactions occur with doses of digoxin greater than 0.07 mg/kg.

Transplacental intoxication by digitalis has been reported. An accurate radioimmunoassay for digitalis is now available.

Treatment

If vomiting has not occurred, induce emesis or provide lavage followed by charcoal cathartics. Potassium should not be given in acute overdosage unless there is laboratory evidence of hypokalemia. In acute overdosage, hyperkalemia is more common.

The patient must be monitored carefully for ECG changes. The correction of acidosis will better demonstrate the degree of potassium deficiency present. In some cases, phenytoin (Dilantin), beta-adrenergic blocking agents such as propranolol (Inderal), or pro-

cainamide (Pronestyl) are necessary to correct arrhythmias. A pacemaker may be needed.

It has recently been noted that digoxin has an enterohepatic circulation. The use of oral binding agents such as cholestyramine resin (Cuemid, Questran) has been suggested in massive digitalis overdoses.

Hobson JD, Zettner A: Digoxin serum half-life following suicidal digoxin poisoning. JAMA 223:147, 1973.
Rumack BH & others: Phenytoin (diphenylhydantoin) treatment of massive digoxin overdose. Br Heart J 36:405, 1974.
Smith TW & others: Reversal of advanced digoxin intoxication with Fab fragments of digoxin-specific antibodies. N Engl J Med 294:797, 1976.

DIPHENOXYLATE HYDROCHLORIDE
(Lomotil)

Lomotil is a combination of diphenoxylate hydrochloride, a synthetic narcotic, and atropine sulfate. Early signs of Lomotil intoxication are due to its anticholinergic effect and consist of fever, facial flush, tachypnea, and lethargy. However, the miotic effect of the narcotic predominates. Later, hypothermia, increasing CNS depression, and loss of the facial flush occur. Seizures are probably secondary to hypoxia. Small amounts of Lomotil are potentially lethal when ingested by children; it is contraindicated as a drug under age 2.

Treatment

After an adequate airway has been established with an endotracheal tube, gastric lavage may be useful because of the prolonged delay in gastric emptying time. Narcotics are not adsorbed by activated charcoal, but atropine is. Naloxone (Narcan), 0.01 mg/kg IV, should be given. A transient improvement in respiratory status may be followed by respiratory depression because the duration of action of diphenoxylate is considerably longer than that of the antagonists. The anticholinergic effects do not usually require treatment but can be reversed temporarily by the use of physostigmine, 0.5—2 mg IV.

Rumack BH, Temple AR: Lomotil poisoning. Pediatrics 53:495, 1974.

DISINFECTANTS & DEODORIZERS

1. NAPHTHALENE

Naphthalene is commonly found in mothballs as well as in disinfectants and deodorizers commonly used in bathrooms, toilets, and garbage cans.

Naphthalene's toxicity is often not fully appreciated. It is absorbed not only when ingested but also through the skin and lungs. Naphthalene is very soluble in oil and relatively insoluble in water. It is potentially hazardous to store baby clothes in naphthalene because baby oil is an excellent solvent which increases absorption of the drug through the skin.

Metabolic products of naphthalene cause a severe hemolytic anemia similar to that due to primaquine toxicity 3–7 days after ingestion. Other physical findings include nausea, vomiting, diarrhea, jaundice, oliguria, anuria, coma, and convulsions. The urine may contain hemoglobin, protein, and casts.

Treatment

Induced vomiting should be followed by a saline cathartic. Forced alkaline diuresis prevents blocking of the renal tubules by acid hematin crystals. Repeated small blood transfusions may be necessary to bring the hemoglobin level up to 60–80% of normal. Corticosteroids are said to be useful in minimizing naphthalene hemolysis. Anuria may persist for 1–2 weeks and still be completely reversible.

2. p-DICHLOROBENZENE & PHENOLIC ACIDS

Disinfectants and deodorizers containing p-dichlorobenzene or sodium bisulfate are much less toxic than those containing naphthalene. Disinfectants containing phenolic acids are highly toxic, especially if they contain a borate ion. Phenol precipitates proteins and causes respiratory alkalosis followed by metabolic acidosis. Some phenols cause methemoglobinemia.

Local gangrene occurs after prolonged contact with tissue. Phenol is readily adsorbed from the gastrointestinal tract, causing diffuse capillary damage and, in some cases, methemoglobinemia. Pentachlorophenol, which has been used in terminal rinsing of diapers, has caused infant fatalities.

The toxicity of alkalies, quaternary ammonium compounds, pine oil, and halogenated disinfectants varies with the concentration of active ingredients. Wick deodorizers are usually of moderate toxicity. Iodophor disinfectants are the safest. Spray deodorizers are not usually toxic because a child is not likely to swallow a very large dose.

Manifestations of acute ingestion include diaphoresis, thirst, nausea, vomiting, diarrhea, cyanosis, hyperactivity, coma, convulsions, hypotension, abdominal pain, and pulmonary edema. Acute liver or renal failure may develop later.

Treatment

Activated charcoal should be used prior to emesis or gastric lavage. Castor oil dissolves phenol and retards its absorption. Mineral oil and alcohol are contraindicated because they increase the gastric absorption of phenol. A saline cathartic should follow the castor oil. The metabolic acidosis must be carefully managed. Anticonvulsants or measures to treat shock may be needed.

Because phenols are absorbed through the skin, exposed areas should be irrigated copiously with water.

Arena JM: *Poisoning: Toxicology, Symptoms, Treatments,* 3rd ed. Thomas, 1974.

George JN, Miller DR, Weed RI: Heinz body hemolytic anemias. NY State J Med 70:2574, 1970.

GLUTETHIMIDE
(Doriden)

Patients may have nystagmus, mydriasis, dry mouth, ileus, and CNS depression manifested by absent deep tendon reflexes, coma, and either hypothermia or hyperpyrexia. Respiratory depression with normal respiratory rates, sudden apnea, and alternating levels of consciousness occur. The anticholinergic effects of glutethimide often predominate in children.

There is a narrow range between therapeutic and toxic blood levels. Doses exceeding 25–50 mg/kg are toxic in children. Blood levels greater than 3 mg/100 ml are generally associated with coma and serious illness. Glutethimide levels usually fall at a rate of 1.5–2 mg/100 ml/day. As in any other sedative poisoning, coma often is prolonged and varies in depths from moment to moment, but patients usually awake when blood levels decline to 1.5 mg/100 ml, although in some cases the patient awakens at levels higher than at the beginning of coma.

Treatment

Meticulous conservative management is the most successful approach and consists of adequate lavage and administration of activated charcoal and magnesium sulfate. Forced diuresis, peritoneal dialysis, and hemodialysis (including lipid dialysis) have not been helpful in reducing the duration of coma or the morbidity or mortality rate, although enhanced excretion of inert metabolites of the drug has been demonstrated. Fluids should be used cautiously because there is an increased likelihood of pulmonary or cerebral edema.

Chazan JA, Garella S: Glutethimide intoxication: A prospective study of 70 patients treated conservatively without hemodialysis. Arch Intern Med 128:215, 1971.

Comstock EG: Glutethimide intoxication. JAMA 215:1668, 1971.

Hansen AR & others: Glutethimide poisoning: A metabolite contributes to morbidity and mortality. N Engl J Med 292:250, 1975.

Vestal RE, Rumack BH: Glutethimide dependence: Phenobarbital treatment. (Correspondence.) Ann Intern Med 80:670, 1974.

Wright N, Roscoe P: Acute glutethimide poisoning: Conservative management of 31 patients. JAMA 214:1704, 1970.

HYDROCARBONS
(Petroleum Distillates, Kerosene, Benzene, Turpentine, Charcoal Lighter Fluid, Gasoline, Etc)

Ingestion causes irritation of mucous membranes, vomiting, blood-tinged diarrhea, respiratory distress, cyanosis, tachycardia, and fever. Although 10 ml are potentially fatal, patients have survived ingestion of several ounces of petroleum distillates. The more aromatic and the lower the viscosity rating of a hydrocarbon, the more toxic it is. Benzene, gasoline, kerosene, and red seal oil furniture polish are the most dangerous. A dose exceeding 1 ml/kg is likely to cause CNS depression. A history of coughing or choking, as well as vomiting, suggests aspiration with resulting hydrocarbon pneumonia, an acute hemorrhagic necrotizing disease which usually develops within 24 hours of the ingestion and resolves without sequelae in 3–5 days. However, several weeks may be required for resolution of a hydrocarbon pneumonia. Pneumonia may be caused by a few drops of petroleum distillate being aspirated into the lung or by absorption from the circulatory system. Pulmonary edema and hemorrhage, cardiac dilatation and arrhythmias, hepatosplenomegaly, proteinuria, and hematuria can occur following large overdoses. Hypoglycemia is occasionally present. A chest film may reveal pneumonia shortly after the ingestion. An abnormal urinalysis in a child with a previously normal urinary tract suggests a large overdose.

Treatment
Both emetics and lavage should be avoided if only a small amount has been ingested. It is impossible to do a "cautious gastric lavage" unless a cuffed endotracheal tube is inserted. Under these circumstances, gastric lavage may be done using saline or 3% sodium bicarbonate solution. Following lavage, magnesium or sodium sulfate should be left in the stomach. (Mineral oil should not be given because it is capable of causing a low-grade lipoid pneumonia.)

Emetics are probably preferable to gastric lavage if massive ingestion has occurred. Epinephrine should not be used since it may affect an already sensitized myocardium. Analeptic drugs are contraindicated. The usefulness of corticosteroids is debated, and antibiotics should be reserved for patients with infections. Oxygen and mist are helpful.

Bergeson PS & others: Pneumatoceles following hydrocarbon ingestion: Report of three cases and a review of the literature. Am J Dis Child 129:49, 1975.

Ng RC & others: Emergency treatment of petroleum distillate and turpentine ingestion. J Am Coll Emerg Phys 6:4, 1977.

INSECTICIDES

The petroleum distillates or other organic solvents used in these products are often as toxic as the pesticide. Unless otherwise indicated, induced vomiting or gastric lavage is warranted after insertion of an endotracheal tube.

DePalma AE, Kwalich DS, Zukerberg N: Pesticide poisoning in children. JAMA 211:1979, 1970.

Hayes WJ: *Clinical Handbook on Economic Poisons.* US Department of Health, Education, and Welfare, 1963.

1. CHLORINATED HYDROCARBONS
(Aldrin, Carbinol, Chlordane, DDT, Dieldrin, Endrin, Heptachlor, Lindane, Toxaphene, Etc)

Signs of intoxication include salivation, gastrointestinal irritability, abdominal pain, nausea, vomiting, diarrhea, CNS depression, and convulsions. Inhalation exposure causes irritation of the eyes, nose, and throat, blurred vision, cough, and pulmonary edema.

Chlorinated hydrocarbons are absorbed through the skin, respiratory tract, and gastrointestinal tract. These compounds or their metabolic products are chronically stored in fat. Decontamination of skin (tincture of green soap) and evacuation of the stomach contents are critical. All contaminated clothing should be removed. Castor oil, milk, and other substances containing fats or oils should not be left in the stomach as they increase absorption of the chlorinated hydrocarbons. Convulsions should be treated with diazepam (Valium), 0.1–0.3 mg/kg IV. Epinephrine should not be used as it may cause cardiac arrhythmias.

2. ORGANIC PHOSPHATE
(CHOLINESTERASE-INHIBITING) INSECTICIDES
(Chlorthion, Co-Ral, DFP, Diazinon, Malathion, Para-oxon, Parathion, Phosdrin, TEPP, Thio-TEPP, Etc)

Dizziness, headache, blurred vision, miosis, tearing, salivation, nausea, vomiting, diarrhea, hypoglycemia, cyanosis, sense of constriction of the chest, dyspnea, sweating, weakness, muscular twitching, convulsions, loss of reflexes and sphincter control, and coma can occur.

The clinical findings are the result of cholinesterase inhibition, which causes an accumulation of large amounts of acetylcholine. The onset of symptoms is within 12 hours of the exposure. Red cell cholinesterase levels should be measured as soon as possible. (Some normal individuals have a low serum cholinesterase level.) Normal values vary in different laboratories. A screening test apparatus for cholinesterase levels (Unopette #5820, Becton, Dickinson & Co, Rutherford, NJ 07070) should be available in every hospital emergency room. In general, a decrease of red cell cholinesterase to below 25% of normal indicates significant exposure to organophosphate insecticides and is an indication for treatment with pralidoxime.

Repeated low-grade exposure may result in sudden, acute toxic reactions. This syndrome usually occurs after repeated household spraying rather than agricultural exposure.

Although all organophosphates act by inhibiting cholinesterase activity, they vary greatly in their toxicity. Parathion, for example, is 100 times more toxic than malathion. The toxicity is influenced by the specific compound, the type of formulation (liquid or solid), the vehicle, and the route of absorption (lungs, skin, or gastrointestinal tract).

Treatment

Atropine plus a cholinesterase reactivator, pralidoxime (Protopam), is a chemical antidote for organophosphate insecticide poisoning. After establishing a clear airway and eliminating any cyanosis, large doses of atropine should be given and repeated every few minutes until signs of atropinism are present. An appropriate starting dose of atropine is 2–4 mg IV in an adult and 0.05 mg/kg in a child. The patient should receive enough atropine to stop secretions (approximately 10 times the normal dose). As much as 50 mg of atropine per 24 hours may be needed in an adult.

Because atropine antagonizes the parasympathetic effects of the organophosphates but does not alter the muscular weakness, pralidoxime should also be given immediately in more severe cases and repeated every 8–12 hours as needed (1 gm IV for older children and 250 mg IV for infants at a rate of no more than 500 mg/minute). Pralidoxime should be used in addition to—not in place of—atropine if red cell cholinesterase is less than 25% of normal. Pralidoxime is probably not useful later than 36 hours after the exposure. Morphine, theophylline, aminophylline, succinylcholine, and tranquilizers of the reserpine and phenothiazine types are contraindicated. Hyperglycemia is common.

Decontamination of the skin (including nails and hair) and clothing with soapy water is extremely important. Decontamination of the skin must be done carefully to avoid abrasions, which increase organophosphate absorption significantly.

Melby TH: Prevention and management of organophosphate poisoning. JAMA 216:2131, 1971.

Nelson DL, Crawford CR: Organophosphorus compounds: The past and the future. Clin Toxicol 5:223, 1972.

3. CARBAMATES
(Carbaryl, Sevin, Zectran, Etc)

Carbamate insecticides are reversible inhibitors of cholinesterase. The usual laboratory procedures used to determine red cell cholinesterase will not show a depression after carbamate exposure. The reversal is often so rapid that measurements of blood cholinesterases are near normal, whereas β-naphthol, a metabolite, is present in significant amounts. The signs and symptoms of intoxication are similar to those associated with organophosphate poisoning but are generally less severe. Atropine in large doses is sufficient treatment. Pralidoxime should not be used with carbaryl (Sevin) poisoning but is of value with other carbamates. In combined exposures to organophosphates, give atropine but reserve pralidoxime for cases in which the red cell cholinesterase is depressed below 25% of normal.

4. BOTANICAL INSECTICIDES
(Raid, Black Flag Bug Killer, Black Leaf CPR Insect Killer, Flit Aerosol House and Garden Insect Killer, French's Flea Powder, Etc)

Pyrethrins, allethrin, ryania, and rotenone do not commonly cause signs of toxicity. Antihistamines, short-acting barbiturates, and atropine are helpful when needed.

INSECT STINGS
(Bee, Wasp, & Hornet)

Insect stings are painful but not usually dangerous; however, these insects cause more deaths in the USA than snakes do. Deaths from insect stings are usually due to severe allergic reactions. Bee venom, for example, has hemolytic, neurotoxic, and histamine-like activities which can on rare occasions cause hemoglobinuria and severe anaphylactoid reactions. If possible, a tourniquet should be applied above the bite and the stinger removed, being careful not to squeeze the venom sac. Epinephrine, 0.01 ml/kg of 1:1000 solution, should be administered IV or subcut above the site of the sting. Three to 4 whiffs from an isoproterenol (Isuprel) aerosol inhaler may be given at 3–4 minute intervals as needed. Corticosteroids (hydrocortisone, 100 mg IV) or diphenhydramine (Benadryl), 1.5 mg/kg IV, are useful ancillary drugs but have no immediate effect. Ephedrine or antihistamines may be used for 2 or 3 days to prevent recurrence of symptoms.

A patient who has had a potentially life-threatening insect sting should be desensitized against the hymenoptera group since the honey bee, wasp, hornet, and yellow jacket have common antigens in their venom.

For the more usual stings, cold compresses, aspirin, and diphenhydramine (Benadryl), 1 mg/kg orally, are useful.

Russell F & others: Insect and scorpion bites and stings. JAMA 224:131, 1973.

IRON

Five stages of intoxication occur following iron intoxication: (1) Hemorrhagic gastroenteritis, which occurs 30–60 minutes after ingestion and may be associated with shock, acidosis, coagulation defects, and coma. This phase usually lasts 4–6 hours and is commonly followed by a 6–24 hour asymptomatic period. (2) Phase of improvement during which patient looks better. Lasts 2–12 hours. (3) Delayed shock may occur 12–48 hours after ingestion and is usually associated with a serum iron level greater than 500 mg/100 ml. Metabolic acidosis, fever, leukocytosis, and coma may also be present. (4) Liver damage with hepatic failure. (5) Residual pyloric stenosis, which usually develops at least 4 weeks after the ingestion.

Ferrous sulfate is approximately 20% elemental iron. The average lethal dose is about 200–250 mg of iron/kg, but deaths in small children have been caused by as little as 600 mg of iron. Although the correlation between serum iron and clinical symptoms is not good, it appears that serum iron levels greater than the total serum iron-binding capacity (300–500 μg/100 ml) are necessary to produce severe symptoms.

Once iron is absorbed from the gastrointestinal tract, it is not normally eliminated in feces but may be partially excreted in the urine, giving it a red color prior to chelation. A reddish discoloration of the urine suggests a serum iron level greater than 350 μg/100 ml. Abdominal x-ray will show radiopaque tablets remaining in the gastrointestinal tract, but finely dispersed iron will often not be identified.

Treatment

Shock must be treated in the usual manner. After inducing vomiting, leave sodium bicarbonate or Fleet's Phospho-Soda (15–30 ml diluted 1:2 with water) in the stomach to form the insoluble phosphate or carbonate. Deferoxamine (Desferal), a specific chelating agent for iron, is a useful adjunct in the treatment of severe iron poisoning, but it should not replace careful conservative management. When given parenterally, it forms a soluble complex which is excreted in the urine. It is contraindicated in patients with renal failure unless dialysis can be used.

Deferoxamine should not be delayed in serious cases of poisoning until serum iron levels are available. Intravenous administration is indicated if the patient is in shock, in which case it should be given at a rate not to exceed 15 mg/kg/hour for 8 hours. Rapid intravenous administration causes hypotension, facial flushing, urticaria, tachycardia, and shock. The dose may be repeated every 18 hours if clinically indicated. Deferoxamine, 1–2 gm IM every 3–12 hours, may be given if clinically indicated. Blood levels of deferoxamine given intramuscularly and intravenously are about equal in 15 minutes if the patient is not in shock. The drug should not be given orally.

Hemodialysis, peritoneal dialysis, or exchange transfusion can be used to increase the excretion of the dialyzable complex, if necessary. Urine output should be monitored and urine sediment examined for evidence of renal tubular damage. Initial laboratory studies should include blood typing and cross-match, total protein, serum iron, total iron-binding capacity, serum sodium, potassium, chloride, CO_2, pH, and liver function tests. Serum iron levels fall rapidly even if deferoxamine is not given.

After the acute episode, liver function studies and an upper gastrointestinal series are indicated to rule out residual damage.

James JA: Acute iron poisoning: Assessment of severity and prognosis. J Pediatr 77:117, 1970.

Propper RD, Shurin SB, Nathan DG: Reassessment of the use of desferrioxamine B in iron overload. N Engl J Med 294:1421, 1976.

Westlin WF: Deferoxamine as a chelating agent. Clin Toxicol 4:597, 1971.

LEAD

Clinical Findings

Lead poisoning causes weakness, irritability, weight loss, vomiting, personality changes, ataxia, constipation, headache, transient abdominal pain, opaque flakes in the gastrointestinal tract, and a "lead line" on the gums and in many bones at the metaphyseal area. Late manifestations consist of retarded development, convulsions, and coma associated with increased intracranial pressure. The latter is a medical emergency.

Plumbism usually occurs insidiously in children under 5 years of age. The most likely sources of lead include pica involving flaking leaded paint, artist's paints, fruit tree sprays, leaded gasoline, solder, brass alloys, home-glazed pottery, and fumes from burning batteries. Only paint containing < 1% lead is safe for interior use (furniture, toys, etc). Repetitive ingestions of small amounts of lead are far more serious than a single massive exposure.

Toxic reactions are likely to occur if more than 0.5 mg of lead per day is absorbed, but fatality usually does not occur unless more than 0.5 gm/day is absorbed. Only uncombined lead is removed by deleading agents. Children under 2 years of age have a poor prognosis, whereas children who develop peripheral neuritis without evidence of mental retardation or encephalitis usually recover completely.

Laboratory tests are necessary to establish a diagnosis of plumbism. Urinary coproporphyrins or, preferably, red cell δ-aminolevulinic acid dehydratase levels are satisfactory screening tests. Urine lead levels are the definitive test. The 24-hour urinary lead level exceeds

80 μg/day without treatment and should increase to >
1.5 mg/day on any one of the first 3 days on calcium
edathamil or penicillamine therapy (or both). Dehydration and acidosis may falsely lower urinary lead levels.
Glycosuria, proteinuria, hematuria, and aminoaciduria
occur frequently. Blood lead levels usually exceed 80
μg/100 ml in symptomatic patients. Blood lead levels
exceeding 40 μg/100 ml on 2 occasions warrant further
investigation. Abnormal blood and urinary lead levels
should be repeated in asymptomatic patients to rule
out laboratory error. Specimens must be meticulously
obtained in acid-washed containers. A normocytic,
slightly hypochromic anemia with basophilic stippling
of the red cells and reticulocytosis is usually present in
plumbism. Stippling of red blood cells is absent in
cases of sudden massive ingestion.

The CSF protein is moderately to markedly elevated, and the CSF white cell count is usually less than
100 cells/ml. CSF pressure is usually elevated. Lumbar
punctures must be performed very cautiously to prevent herniation of the brain stem in patients with encephalopathy.

Treatment

Induced vomiting followed by a saline cathartic is
indicated. Combination therapy with dimercaprol
(BAL), 4 mg/kg/dose every 4 hours IM, and calcium
disodium edathamil, 12.5 mg/kg/dose (maximum dose,
75 mg/kg/day) IV or IM starting with the second dose
of dimercaprol, should reduce the mortality rate of
acute lead encephalopathy to < 5%. Penicillamine
(Cuprimine), 100 mg/kg/day (maximum, 1 gm), should
be added as soon as the patient can take oral medication. This treatment is indicated for a symptomatic
patient or one with a blood lead level of 100 μg/100
ml. It should be started as soon as urine flow is initiated. If urine flow is delayed over 4 hours, simultaneous hemodialysis must be started. Unless the patient
is severely affected, 50 mg/kg/day of calcium disodium
edathamil (EDTA) is an adequate dose which is less
likely to damage the kidneys or cause hypercalcemia.
Elevated lead levels will usually return to normal in
3–5 days when the combination method is used; this is
rarely true when calcium disodium edathamil is used
alone. After a 2-day pause, another course of treatment can be given if desired, again including oral penicillamine. Dimercaprol can be used with complete
renal shutdown but not in patients with severe hepatic
insufficiency. Dimercaprol (but not calcium disodium
edathamil) increases the fecal excretion of lead. The
development of lacrimation, blepharospasm, paresthesias, nausea, tachycardia, and hypertension suggests a
toxic reaction to dimercaprol. Iron should not be given
to patients being treated for plumbism since it forms a
toxic substance with dimercaprol.

If the blood lead level is 80–100 μg/100 ml, calcium disodium edathamil and dimercaprol can be
given for 2 days and then replaced with penicillamine
orally for 5 days if there is no lead in the gut, or
calcium disodium edathamil can be given alone for 5
days or dimercaprol and calcium disodium edathamil

can be given concomitantly for 3 days.

A brief course of edathamil or a longer course of
penicillamine is indicated for lead levels of 60–80
μg/100 ml. Chelation therapy is not indicated for lead
levels below 60 μg/100 ml unless there is additional
evidence of toxicity.

Anticonvulsants may be needed. Mannitol or
corticosteroids are indicated in patients with encephalopathy. Fluid intake should be restricted. One expert
investigator feels that surgical decompression is contraindicated, but others disagree. Hypothermia and
corticosteroid therapy have not altered mortality rates
significantly. A high-calcium, high-phosphorus diet and
large doses of vitamin D remove lead from the blood
by depositing it in the bones.

Urinalysis should be done daily; serum calcium
and phosphorus and BUN every 2 days. Calcium gluconate given intravenously as a 10% solution is helpful in
controlling the colic which sometimes occurs.

A public health team should evaluate the source
of the lead. Necessary corrections should be completed
before the child is returned home.

Chisolm JJ Jr, Barrett MB, Mellits ED: Dose-effect and dose-
    response relationships for lead in children. J Pediatr
    87:1152, 1975.
Klein M & others: Earthenware containers as a source of fatal
    lead poisoning. N Engl J Med 283:669, 1970.
Lin-Fu JS: Undue absorption of lead among children. N Engl J
    Med 286:702, 1972.
Specter MJ; Guinee VF, Davidow B: The unsuitability of ran-
    dom urinary delta aminolevulinic acid samples as a screen-
    ing test for lead poisoning. J Pediatr 79:799, 1971.

MEPROBAMATE
(Miltown, Equanil)

Respiratory depression, coma, cardiac arrhythmias, and occasional convulsions associated with
hyperexcitability occur. Death is the result of cardiac
or respiratory failure.

Meprobamate is a general depressant, anticonvulsant, and muscle relaxant which causes habituation and
a withdrawal syndrome. In addition to being detoxified in the CNS and liver by an acetylation process,
meprobamate is excreted unchanged in the urine.
There are genetic variations in the rate of acetylation
which are of great significance in patients who have
taken massive overdoses of meprobamate. People who
are rapid acetylators tolerate higher serum levels without toxicity. Serum meprobamate levels of 10–20
mg/100 ml are usually associated with severe toxicity.
However, toxicity may occur at much lower levels in
patients who are slow acetylators.

Treatment

Gastric lavage is not very effective because meprobamate is highly insoluble in water. Delayed gastric
emptying is common, and the drug is absorbed slowly

from the gastrointestinal tract. Induced vomiting is indicated if the patient is awake and should be followed by charcoal and a saline cathartic. Patients who show an initial improvement may relapse and die as a result of delayed absorption from concretions of meprobamate in the stomach.

Treatment in mild intoxications is supportive. If the patient deteriorates rapidly or develops deep coma with seizures or cardiac arrhythmias, hemodialysis, peritoneal dialysis, or forced alkaline diuresis is indicated.

Schwartz HS: Acute meprobamate poisoning with gastrotomy and removal of a drug-containing mass. N Engl J Med 295:1177, 1976.

MERCURY

Mercury poisoning is manifested by a metallic taste, thirst, severe vomiting, bloody diarrhea, cough, pharyngeal and abdominal pain, dyspnea, pulmonary embolization, dermatitis, corneal ulcers, nephrosis, renal failure, hepatic damage, ulcerative colitis, and shock. Acrodynia occurs in children after chronic exposure to small amounts of mercury in diaper rash ointments and teething lotions.

Chronic inorganic mercury poisoning causes salivation, loosening of teeth, bad oral odor, gingivitis, mouth ulcerations, dermatitis, fatigue, loss of memory, irritability, apprehension, tremors, decreased visual acuity and night vision, and staggering and slurred speech ("mad hatter syndrome"). Both organic and inorganic mercury poisoning can cause similar physical signs, although organic mercury intoxication characteristically causes dysarthria, ataxia, and constricted visual fields.

Elevated mercury levels have recently been noted in tuna and swordfish, and human mercury poisoning has been attributed to eating large amounts of contaminated swordfish. Mercury is a possible constituent of antiseptics, cathartics, diuretics, fumigants, and fungicides. All forms of mercury are potentially poisonous, but organic mercurials are generally less toxic than inorganic mercurials because they are poorly absorbed. The small amount of metallic mercury from a thermometer is nontoxic because it is not well absorbed.

Treatment

Activated charcoal should be followed by induced vomiting and a saline cathartic. Dimercaprol (BAL) as for lead poisoning (see above) is often used. (Edathamil is contraindicated.) Penicillamine (Cuprimine), 100 mg/kg/day orally (maximum, 1 gm), is as effective as BAL. Demulcents and analgesics are indicated, as well as correction of fluid and electrolyte imbalances. Hemodialysis may be indicated for renal failure but not for removal of mercury.

Eyl TB: Alkylmercury contamination of foods. JAMA 215:287, 1971.

Javett SN, Kaplan B: Acrodynia treated with D-penicillamine. Am J Dis Child 115:71, 1968.

Kark RAP & others: Mercury poisoning and its treatment with N-acetyl-D,L-penicillamine. N Engl J Med 285:1, 1971.

Teitelbaum DT, Ott JE: Elemental mercury self-poisoning. Clin Toxicol 2:243, 1969.

MUSHROOMS

Many toxic species of mushrooms are difficult to separate from edible varieties. Symptoms vary with the species ingested, the time of year, the stage of maturity, the quantity eaten, the method of preparation, and the interval since ingestion. A mushroom that is toxic to one individual may not be toxic for another. Drinking alcohol and eating certain mushrooms may cause a reaction similar to that seen with disulfiram (Antabuse) and alcohol. Cooking destroys some toxins but not the deadly one produced by *Amanita phalloides,* which is responsible for 90% of deaths due to mushroom poisoning. Mushroom toxins are absorbed relatively slowly. Onset of symptoms within 2 hours of ingestion suggests muscarinic toxin, whereas a delay of symptoms for 6–48 hours after ingestion strongly suggests Amanita poisoning. Patients who have ingested *A phalloides* may relapse and die of hepatic or renal failure following initial improvement.

Mushroom poisoning may be manifested by muscarinic symptoms (salivation, vomiting, diarrhea, cramping abdominal pain, tenesmus, miosis, and dyspnea), coma, convulsions, hallucinations, hemolysis, and hepatic and renal failure.

Treatment

Induce vomiting and follow with activated charcoal and a saline cathartic. If the patient has muscarinic signs, give atropine, 0.05 mg/kg IM (0.02 mg/kg in toddlers) and repeat as needed (usually every 30 minutes) to keep the patient atropinized. Atropine, however, is only used when there are cholinergic effects and not for all mushrooms. Hypoglycemia is most likely to occur in patients with delayed onset of symptoms. It is important, if at all possible, to specifically identify the mushroom if the patient is symptomatic. Local botanical gardens, university departments of botany, and societies of mycologists may be able to help. Supportive care is usually all that is needed except in the case of *A phalloides,* where thioctic acid or hemodialysis may be indicated.

Beargie RA: Beware of mushroom poisoning. Consultant, pp 44–47, April 1967.

Litton W: The most poisonous mushrooms. Sci Am 232:90, March 1975.

Mitchell DH: Poisonous mushrooms. In: *POISINDEX: An Emergency Poison Management System.* Rumack BH (editor). Micromedex, Denver, Colorado, 1975.

Rumack BH, Salzman E: *Mushroom Poisoning, Diagnosis and Treatment.* CRC Press, 1978.

NARCOTICS & SYNTHETIC CONGENERS*
(Heroin, Methadone, Morphine, Codeine, Propoxyphene)

Physicians may be called upon to treat various narcotic problems, including drug addiction, withdrawal in a newborn infant, and accidental overdoses. Accidental ingestions of propoxyphene (Darvon) and diphenoxylate (in Lomotil) are frequent.

Unlike other narcotics, methadone is readily absorbed from the gastrointestinal tract. Drug abusers often use the intravenous route of administration. Most narcotics, including heroin, methadone, meperidine, morphine, and codeine, are excreted in the urine within 24 hours and can be readily detected.

The treatment of a narcotic addict—who usually is a demanding, manipulating, and irritating patient—is often quite difficult. If an addict seeks medical help, the physician must decide whether to treat the patient or refer him to another physician.

Narcotic addicts often have other medical problems, including cellulitis, abscesses, thrombophlebitis, tetanus, infective endocarditis, tuberculosis, hepatitis, malaria, foreign body emboli, thrombosis of pulmonary arterioles, diabetes mellitus, obstetric complications, and peptic ulcer.

Treatment of Overdosage

Children receiving an overdose of opiates can develop respiratory depression, stridor, coma, increased oropharyngeal secretions, sinus bradycardia, and urinary retention. Methadone is less likely to cause miosis than other narcotics. Pulmonary edema rarely occurs in children; deaths usually result from respiratory arrest and cerebral edema. Convulsions may occur with propoxyphene overdosage.

The treatment of choice is naloxone (Narcan), 0.01 mg/kg IV, which rapidly produces a marked improvement without causing respiratory depression. The dose can be safely repeated and increased as needed. Nalorphine (Nalline) is an older drug with a respiratory depressant effect of its own. It should no longer be used. An improvement in respiratory status may be followed by respiratory depression since the depressant action of narcotics may last 24–48 hours while the antagonist's duration of action is only 2–3 hours. Give intravenous fluids cautiously, since narcotics exert an antidiuretic effect and may precipitate cerebral or pulmonary edema.

Withdrawal in the Addict

The severity of withdrawal signs should be evalu-

*Diphenoxylate (Lomotil) poisoning is discussed above in alphabetic sequence.

ated as explained on p 866.

Diazepam (Valium), 10 mg every 6 hours orally, has been recommended for the treatment of mild narcotic withdrawal in ambulatory adolescents. Ambulatory or hospitalized patients with moderate or severe withdrawal signs can be given the same dose of diazepam intramuscularly. Diazepam is recommended because it is nonhepatotoxic, nonmutagenic, does not affect the fetus when given to pregnant women, and is a good anticonvulsant. Diazepam therapy can be discontinued when the withdrawal score falls below 2. Diphenoxylate (Lomotil) is used to treat severe diarrhea and abdominal cramps. Chloral hydrate is the drug of choice for insomnia.

Methadone maintenance is not usually recommended for adolescents, although it may be used for withdrawal purposes. One method of administration is to give methadone orally every 12 hours, starting with a 25 mg dose and decreasing the amount by 5 mg every 12 hours. When the dose of methadone is 10 mg, add 3 tablets of diphenoxylate with atropine (Lomotil) 3 times daily for 1 day followed by 2 tablets 3 times daily for 2 days. If signs of withdrawal recur, 10 mg of methadone orally or diazepam (orally or IM) are given.

The abrupt discontinuation of narcotics (cold turkey method) is not recommended and may cause severe physical withdrawal signs.

Withdrawal in the Newborn

A newborn infant in narcotic withdrawal is small for his gestational age and demonstrates yawning, sneezing, decreased Moro reflex, hunger but uncoordinated sucking action, jitteriness, tremor, constant movement, a shrill, protracted cry, increased tendon reflexes, convulsions, vomiting, fever, watery diarrhea, cyanosis, dehydration, vasomotor instability, and collapse. The onset of symptoms commonly begins in the first 48 hours but may be delayed as long as 8 days depending upon the timing of the mother's last fix and her predelivery medication. The diagnosis can be easily confirmed by identifying the narcotic in the urine of the mother and baby.

Several methods of treatment have been suggested for narcotic withdrawal in the newborn. Phenobarbital, 8 mg/kg/day IM or orally in 4 doses for 4 days and then reduced by one-third every 2 days as signs decrease, may be continued for as long as 3 weeks. Paregoric is given in gradually increasing doses until a clinical response is seen—2–4 drops/kg orally every 4–6 hours, increasing to as high as 20–40 drops/kg/day if necessary—and then lowered gradually as the signs diminish. Methadone is not recommended in neonates.

It is not clear whether prophylactic treatment with these drugs decreases the complication rate. The mortality rate of untreated narcotic withdrawal in the newborn may be as high as 45%.

Arena JM: Two current poisonings: Methadone and tricyclic drugs. Pediatrics 51:919, 1973.

Ingall D, Zuckerstatter M: Diagnosis and treatment of the passively addicted newborn. Hosp Pract 5:101, Aug 1970.

Litt I, Colli A, Cohen M: Diazepam in the management of heroin withdrawal in adolescents: Preliminary report. J Pediatr 78:692, 1971.

Lovejoy FH Jr, Mitchell AA, Goldman P: The management of propoxyphene poisoning. J Pediatr 85:98, 1974.

Martin WR: Naloxone. Ann Intern Med 85:765, 1976.

Reddy AM, Harper RG, Stern G: Observations on heroin and methadone withdrawal in newborn. Pediatrics 48:353, 1971.

NITRITES, NITRATES, ANILINE, & PENTACHLOROPHENOL

Nausea, vertigo, vomiting, cyanosis (methemoglobinemia), cramping abdominal pain, tachycardia, cardiovascular collapse, tachypnea, coma, shock, convulsions, and death are possible manifestations of nitrite or nitrate poisoning.

Nitrite and nitrate compounds found in the home include amyl nitrite, nitroglycerin, pentaerythritol tetranitrate (Peritrate), sodium nitrite, nitrobenzene, and pyridium. High concentrations of nitrites in water or spinach have been the most common cause of nitrite-induced methemoglobinemia. Symptoms do not usually occur until 40–50% of the hemoglobin has been converted to methemoglobin. A rapid test is to compare a drop of normal blood with the patient's blood on a dry filter paper. Brown discoloration of the patient's blood indicates a methemoglobin level of more than 15%.

Treatment

After administering activated charcoal, induce vomiting and follow by a saline cathartic. Decontaminate any affected skin with soap and water. Oxygen and artificial respiration may be needed. If the blood methemoglobin level exceeds 40% or if levels can not be obtained, give 0.2 ml/kg of 1% solution of methylene blue IV over 5–10 minutes. Avoid perivascular infiltration since it causes necrosis of the skin and subcutaneous tissues. A dramatic change in the degree of cyanosis should occur. Transfusion is occasionally necessary. Epinephrine and other vasoconstrictors are contraindicated. If reflex bradycardia occurs, atropine can be used to block it.

Bakshi SP, Fahey JL, Pierce LE: Sausage cyanosis: Acquired methamoglobinemic nitrite poisoning. N Engl J Med 277:1072, 1967.

McDermott JH: Health aspects of toxic materials in drinking water. Am J Public Health 61:2269, 1971.

PHENOTHIAZINES
(Chlorpromazine [Thorazine], Prochlorperazine [Compazine], Trifluoperazine [Stelazine], Etc)

Extrapyramidal crisis. Episodes characterized by torticollis, stiffening of the body, spasticity, poor speech, catatonia, and inability to communicate although conscious are typical manifestations. These episodes usually last a few seconds to a few minutes but have rarely caused death. Extrapyramidal crises may represent idiosyncratic reactions and are aggravated by dehydration. The signs and symptoms occur most often in children who have received prochlorperazine (Compazine). They are commonly mistaken for psychotic episodes.

Overdose. Lethargy and deep prolonged coma commonly occur. Promazine, chlorpromazine, and prochlorperazine are the drugs most likely to cause respiratory depression and precipitous drops in blood pressure. Occasionally, paradoxical hyperactivity and extrapyramidal signs as well as hyperglycemia and acetonemia are present. Seizures are uncommon.

Phenothiazines are rapidly absorbed from the gastrointestinal tract and bound to tissue. They are principally conjugated with glucuronic acid and excreted in the urine.

Treatment

Extrapyramidal signs are dramatically alleviated within minutes by the slow intravenous administration of 1–5 mg/kg of diphenhydramine (Benadryl). No other treatment is usually indicated. Dialysis is contraindicated.

Patients with overdoses should be treated conservatively. An attempt should be made to induce vomiting with apomorphine after administration of activated charcoal. Charcoal adsorbs chlorpromazine and probably other phenothiazines very well. Emetics are often unsuccessful in this situation because phenothiazines are potent antiemetics; gastric lavage, therefore, may be the only practical way to remove gastric contents. A large amount of intravenous fluid without vasopressor agents is the preferred method of treating tranquilizer-induced neurogenic hypotension. If a pressor agent is required, norepinephrine (levarterenol) should be used. Epinephrine should *not* be used because phenothiazines reverse epinephrine's effects.

Barry D, Meyskens FL Jr, Becker CE: Phenothiazine poisoning: A review of 48 cases. Calif Med 118:1, Jan 1973.

Davies DM: Treatment of drug-induced dyskinesias. Lancet 1:567, 1970.

Thomas J: Fatal case of agranulocytosis due to chlorpromazine. Lancet 1:44, 1970.

PLANTS

Many common ornamental, garden, and wild plants are potentially toxic. Small amounts of a plant may cause severe illness or death. These effects usually involve the cardiovascular, gastrointestinal, and central nervous systems and the skin. Table 30–4 lists the most toxic plants, symptoms and signs of poisoning, and treatment.

Hardin JW, Arena JM: *Human Poisoning From Native and Cultivated Plants,* 2nd ed. Duke Univ Press, 1974.

Kozma JJ: *Killer Plants: A Poisonous Plant Guide.* Milestone Publishing Co., 1969.

Table 30–4. Poisoning due to plants.*

	Symptoms and Signs	Treatment
Autumn crocus (colchicine)	Abdominal cramps, severe diarrhea, CNS depression, and circulatory collapse. Occasionally, oliguria and renal shutdown. Delirium or convulsions occur terminally.	Fluid and electrolyte monitoring. Abdominal cramps may be relieved with meperidine or atropine.
Caladium (arum family) Dieffenbachia, calla lily, dumbcane (oxalic acid)	Burning of mucous membranes and airway obstruction secondary to edema caused by calcium oxalate crystals.	Accessible areas should be thoroughly washed. Corticosteroids relieve airway obstruction. Apply cold packs to affected mucous membranes.
Castor bean plant (ricin—a toxalbumin)	Mucous membrane irritation, nausea, vomiting, bloody diarrhea, blurred vision, circulatory collapse, acute hemolytic anemia, convulsions, uremia.	Fluid and electrolyte monitoring. Saline cathartic. Forced alkaline diuresis will prevent complications due to hemagglutination and hemolysis.
Foxglove and cardiac glycosides	Nausea, diarrhea, visual disturbances, and cardiac irregularities (eg, heart block).	See treatment for digitalis drugs in text (p 875).
Jequirity bean (abrin—a toxalbumin)	Nausea, vomiting, abdominal and muscle cramps, hemolysis and hemagglutination, circulatory failure, respiratory failure, and renal and liver failure.	Symptomatic. Renal failure can be prevented by alkalinizing the urine. Gastric lavage or emetics are contraindicated because the toxin is necrotizing. Saline cathartics are indicated.
Jimsonweed: See Belladonna Alkaloids, p 872.		
Larkspur (ajacine, delphinium, delphinidine)	Nausea and vomiting, irritability, muscular paralysis, and CNS depression.	Symptomatic. Atropine may be helpful.
Monkshood (aconite)	Numbness of mucous membranes, visual disturbances, tingling, dizziness, tinnitus, hypotension, bradycardia, and convulsions.	Activated charcoal, oxygen. Atropine is probably helpful.
Oleander (dogbane family)† (oleandrin)	Nausea, bloody diarrhea, respiratory depression, tachycardia, and muscle paralysis.	Symptomatic. See treatment for poisoning with digitalis drugs in text (p 875).
Poison hemlock (coniine)	Mydriasis, trembling, dizziness, bradycardia, CNS depression, muscular paralysis, and convulsions. Death is due to respiratory paralysis.	Symptomatic. Oxygen and cardiac monitoring equipment are desirable. Assisted respiration is often necessary. Give anticonvulsants if needed.
Rhododendron (andromedotoxin)	Abdominal cramps, vomiting, severe diarrhea, muscular paralysis, CNS and circulatory depression. Hypertension with very large doses.	Atropine can prevent bradycardia. Epinephrine is contraindicated. Antihypertensives may be needed.
Yellow jessamine (active ingredient, gelsemine, is related to strychnine)	Restlessness, convulsions, muscular paralysis, and respiratory depression.	Symptomatic. Because of the relation to strychnine, forced acid diuresis and diazepam (Valium) for seizures would be worth trying.

*Many other plants cause minor irritation but are not likely to cause serious problems unless large amounts are ingested. See Hardin JW: Poisonous plants. In: *POISINDEX: An Emergency Poison Management System.* Rumack BH (editor). Micromedex, Denver, Colorado, 1975.

†Done AK: Ornamental and deadly. Emergency Med 5:255, April, 1973.

PSYCHOTROPIC DRUGS

Psychotropic drugs consist of 4 general classes: stimulants (amphetamines), depressants (narcotics, barbiturates, etc), antidepressants and tranquilizers, and hallucinogens (LSD, etc).

The following clinical findings are commonly seen in patients abusing drugs:

Stimulants. Agitation, euphoria, grandiose feelings, tachycardia, fever, abdominal cramps, visual and auditory hallucinations, mydriasis, coma, convulsions, and respiratory depression.

Depressants. Emotional lability, ataxia, diplopia, nystagmus, vertigo, poor accommodation, respiratory depression, coma, apnea, and convulsions. Dilatation of conjunctival blood vessels suggests marihuana ingestion. Narcotics cause miotic pupils and occasionally pulmonary edema.

Antidepressants and tranquilizers. Hypotension, lethargy, respiratory depression, coma, and extrapyramidal reactions.

Hallucinogens and psychoactive drugs. *Belladonna alkaloids* cause mydriasis, dry mouth, nausea, vomiting, urinary retention, confusion, disorientation, paranoid delusions, hallucinations, fever, hypotension, aggressive behavior, convulsions, and coma. *Psychoactive drugs* such as LSD cause mydriasis, unexplained bizarre behavior, hallucinations, and generalized undifferentiated psychotic behavior.

See also other entries discussed in alphabetic sequence in this chapter.

Management of the Patient Who Abuses Drugs

Only a small percentage of the persons using drugs come to the attention of physicians; those who do are usually suffering from adverse reactions such as panic states, drug psychoses, homicidal or suicidal thoughts, and respiratory depression which could not be satisfactorily managed by friends.

Even with cooperative patients, an accurate history is difficult to obtain. The user often does not really know either the dose or the specific drug or drugs he has been taking. "Street drugs" are almost always adulterated with one or more other compounds. Multiple drugs are often taken together, making it impossible to clinically define the type of drug. Friends may be a useful source of information. A drug history is most easily obtained in a quiet spot by a gentle, nonthreatening, honest examiner.

The general appearance, skin, lymphatics, cardiorespiratory status, gastrointestinal tract, and CNS should be stressed during the physical examination since they often provide clues suggesting drug abuse. A drug history should not be taken from an adolescent in the presence of his parents.

Although it is desirable to know the specific drug taken, it is often impossible to obtain this information. Hallucinogens are not life-threatening unless the patient is frankly homicidal or suicidal. A specific diagnosis is usually not necessary to manage the patient; instead, the presenting signs and symptoms are treated. Does the patient appear intoxicated? Does he seem to be in withdrawal? Is he having a "flashback" experience? Does he have some illness or injury (eg, head trauma) that is being masked by a drug? (Remember that an obvious "hippie" who is a known drug user may still be hallucinating because he has meningoencephalitis.)

The signs and symptoms in a given patient are a function of not only the drug and the dose but also the level of acquired tolerance, the "setting," the patient's physical condition and personality traits, the potentiating effects of other drugs, and many other factors.

The most common drug problem in most hospital emergency rooms is the "bad trip," which is usually a panic reaction. This is best managed by "talking the patient down" and minimizing auditory and visual stimuli. It is helpful to communicate a light mood and join with the patient in his trip while trying to focus on realities. If a negative response occurs, quickly change the subject. The physician should not attempt to use "street language" unless he is comfortable with it. A friend of the patient can often help by sitting with him. Trips may last 8 hours or more. The physician's job is not to end the trip but to help the patient over the bad sensations he is experiencing.

Drugs are often unnecessary and may complicate the clinical course of a patient with a panic reaction. Although phenothiazines have been commonly used to treat "bad trips," they should be avoided if the specific drug is not known since they may cause a precipitous drop in blood pressure if STP has been taken or paradoxical hyperactivity which makes management difficult. Diazepam (Valium), 20 mg orally every 30 minutes as necessary, is the drug of choice if a sedative effect is required. Physical restraints are rarely if ever indicated and usually increase the patient's panic reaction.

For treatment of life-threatening drug abuse, consult the section on the specific drug elsewhere in this chapter and the section on general management at the beginning of the chapter.

After the acute episode, the physician must decide whether psychiatric referral is indicated; in general, patients who have made suicidal gestures or attempts and adolescents who are not communicating with their families should be referred. On the other hand, adolescents who are "experimenting" with drugs often do not need psychiatric referral.

Consroe PF: Treatment of acute hallucinogenic drug toxicity: Specific pharmacological intervention. Am J Hosp Pharm 30:80, 1973.

Eastman JW, Cohen SN: Hypertensive crisis and sudden death associated with phencyclidine poisoning. JAMA 231:1270, 1975.

Gabel M: Treatment for ingestion of LSD. J Pediatr 81:634, 1972.

Hollister LE: Marihuana in man: Three years later. Science 172:21, 1971.

Marijuana. The Medical Letter 18:69, 1976.

Teitelbaum DT: Poisoning with psychoactive drugs. Pediatr Clin North Am 17:557, 1970.

Tjio J, Panke W, Kurland A: LSD and chromosomes: A controlled experiment. JAMA 210:849, 1969.

SCORPION BITES

Scorpion bites are common in arid areas of the southwestern USA. Scorpion venom is more toxic than most snake venoms, but only minute amounts are injected. Although neurologic manifestations of the bite may last a week, most clinical signs subside within 24–48 hours.

Bites by less toxic scorpion species cause local pain, redness, and swelling. Bites by more toxic species cause tingling or burning paresthesias at the site of the bite which tend to progress up the extremity, plus throat spasm, a feeling of a thickening of the tongue, restlessness, muscular fibrillation, abdominal cramps, convulsions, urinary incontinence, and respiratory failure.

A specific antiserum for scorpion bites is available from Laboratories "MYN," S.A., Av. Coyoacan 1707, Mexico 12, D.F. In addition, calcium gluconate, 10% solution, 5–20 ml IV, relieves muscular cramps. Hot compresses of sodium bicarbonate will soothe the bitten area. Sedation and corticosteroids may be indicated.

The prognosis for life is good except in infants and young children.

Bartholomew C: Acute scorpion pancreatitis in Trinidad. Br Med J 1:666, 1970.

Gueron M & others: Cardiovascular manifestations of severe scorpion sting: Clinicopathologic correlations. Chest 57:156, 1970.

Zlotkin E & others: Recent studies on the mode of action of scorpion neurotoxins: A review. Toxicon 7:217, 1969.

SNAKEBITE

Considering the lethal potential of venomous snakes, human morbidity and mortality are surprisingly low. The outcome depends on the size of the child, the site of the bite, the degree of envenomation, and the effectiveness of treatment.

Poisonous snakebites are most common and most severe in the early spring. Children in snake-infested areas should wear boots and long trousers, should not walk barefoot, and should be cautioned not to explore under ledges or in holes where a snake might be hiding.

Ninety-eight percent of poisonous snakebites in the USA are caused by pit vipers (rattlesnakes, water moccasins, and copperheads). A few are caused by elapids (coral snakes), and occasional bites occur from cobras and other nonindigenous exotic snakes kept as pets. Snake venom is a complex mixture of enzymes, peptides, and proteins which may have predominantly cytotoxic, neurotoxic, hemotoxic, or cardiotoxic effects but other effects as well. The snake seldom uses all its venom in a single bite. Up to 70% of bites by pit vipers do not result in venom injection.

Pit viper venom is predominantly cytotoxic and hemotoxic, causing a severe local reaction with pain, discoloration, and edema, as well as hemorrhagic effects. Peripheral and central neurologic abnormalities can also occur. Convulsions are common in children.

Swelling and pain occur soon after rattlesnake bite and are a certain indication that envenomation has occurred. During the first few hours, swelling and ecchymosis extend proximally from the bite. The bite is often obvious as a double puncture mark surrounded by ecchymosis. Hematemesis, melena, hemoptysis, and other manifestations of coagulopathy develop in severe cases. Respiratory difficulty and shock are the ultimate causes of death. Even in fatal rattlesnake bite, there is usually a period of 6–8 hours between the bite and death; there is, therefore, usually enough time to start effective treatment.

Coral snake envenomation causes little local pain, swelling, or necrosis, and systemic reactions are often delayed for 10 hours, although children may convulse within 1 hour after being bitten. The early signs of coral snake envenomation include bulbar paralysis, dysphagia, and dysphoria; these may appear in 5–10 hours and may be followed by total peripheral paralysis and death in 24 hours.

Snakebites are an important hazard in many parts of the world; in India there are thought to be over 30,000 deaths per year from cobra bites. The general principles outlined here apply to any bite, but specific therapy will naturally vary between species.

Treatment

The treatment of snakebite envenomation is controversial, but the following approach seems most useful.

A. Emergency (First Aid) Treatment: The most important first aid measure is reassurance. If possible, clean the wound with a germicidal preparation. Splint the affected extremity and minimize the patient's motion. Tourniquets are of questionable value, and ice packs are contraindicated.

Incision and suction are useful only if done soon after envenomation. Because most bites are into the deep subcutaneous layer or muscle, small skin incisions are not effective. In making an incision, consideration must be given to the danger of damaging underlying tendons, nerves, or vessels. Incision is not effective for coral snake bites.

B. Definitive Medical Management: Blood should be drawn for typing and cross-match, hematocrit, clotting time and platelet function, and serum electrolyte determinations. Close monitoring of the hematocrit and electrolytes is indicated. The massive destruction of red cells may be associated with hyperkalemia.

Establish 2 secure intravenous sites for the administration of antivenin, blood, and other medications.

Specific antivenin is indicated only when definite signs of severe envenomation are present. Polyvalent pit viper antivenin and coral snake antivenin (Wyeth Laboratories) are widely available from drugstores. Coral snake antivenin can also be obtained on an emergency basis from state epidemiologists, and is stockpiled (mainly in the southeastern USA) at over 75 locations, including the Center for Disease Control, Atlanta–telephone (404) 633-3311.

After horse serum sensitivity tests (see Chapter 5) are negative, antivenin should be given intravenously and can be given at any desired concentration or rate. Ten to 100 ml may be required. (Antivenin should not be given intramuscularly or subcutaneously because it is slow-acting, inefficient, and impossible to control if adverse reactions occur. Antivenin injected into the bite site has little effect.) If anaphylaxis occurs despite negative skin tests, it will occur at the onset of treatment. Epinephrine, 0.3 ml of 1:1000 solution, should be drawn up in a syringe before antivenin is administered. Horse serum sensitivity must be reevaluated if another course of antivenin is required over 36 hours after the first. The hemorrhagic tendency, pain, and shock are rapidly improved by adequate amounts of antivenin.

Codeine, 1–1.5 mg/kg/dose orally, or meperidine (Demerol), 0.6–1.5 mg/kg/dose orally or IM, is occasionally necessary to control pain during the first 24 hours. Cryotherapy is contraindicated since it commonly causes tissue damage severe enough to necessitate amputation. Early physiotherapy minimizes contractions. In rare cases, fasciotomy to relieve pressure within muscular compartments is required to save the function of a hand or foot. The evaluation of function as well as of pulses will better predict the need for fasciotomy. Corticosteroids (hydrocortisone, 1–2 gm IV every 4–6 hours) are useful in the treatment of serum sickness or anaphylactic shock and may be useful treatment by themselves, especially if the patient is already sensitive to antivenin. Ampicillin (200 mg/kg/day orally) is given to treat gram-negative infections which are often associated with snakebite.

A fluid tetanus toxoid booster is adequate if the patient was previously immunized against tetanus. If the patient has not completed his primary immunizations, 250 units of tetanus immune globulin (human) should be given IM. Tetanus antitoxin is not given if tetanus immune globulin is available.

Glass TG: Early debridement in pit viper bites. JAMA 235:2513, 1976.
Reid HA: The principles of snakebite treatment. Clin Toxicol 3:473, 1970.
Russell FE & others: Snake venom poisoning in the United States: Experience with 550 cases. JAMA 233:841, 1975.
Sadan N, Soroker B: Observations on the effects of the bite of a venomous snake on children and adults. J Pediatr 76:711, 1970.

SOAPS, HEXACHLOROPHENE, & DETERGENTS

1. SOAPS

Soap is made from salts of fatty acids. Some toilet soap bars contain both soap and detergent. Ingestion of soap bars may cause vomiting and diarrhea, but they have a low toxicity.

Dilute with milk or water. Induced emesis is unnecessary.

2. HEXACHLOROPHENE

Hexachlorophene is an antibacterial agent which is found in soaps, detergents, creams, etc. It is also dispensed as a 3% solution (pHisoHex). Cleansing of extensive areas of burned or abraded skin with pHisoHex and the application of pHisoHex wet dressings has resulted in a significant degree of absorption, CNS irritation, and convulsions. pHisoHex should be thoroughly cleaned off with water or saline to minimize its absorption.

pHisoHex placed in a cup or glass has also been confused with milk of magnesia and formula, resulting in ingestion, absorption of large amounts of the agent, and deaths. Nausea, vomiting, diarrhea, abdominal cramps, convulsions, dehydration, and shock have occurred following ingestion of pHisoHex.

Induce vomiting and carefully monitor fluid and electrolyte balance. Anticonvulsants, vasoconstrictors, and sedatives may be needed.

Hexachlorophene–Its use in the nursery. Pediatrics 51 (Suppl): 329, 1973.
Lockhart JD: How toxic is hexachlorophene? Pediatrics 50:229, 1972.

3. DETERGENTS

Detergents are nonsoap synthetic products used for cleaning purposes because of their surfactant properties. Commercial products include granules, powders, and liquids. Electric dishwasher detergent granules are very alkaline and can cause caustic burns. Low concentrations of bleaching and antibacterial agents as well as enzymes are found in many preparations. Although these pure compounds are moderately toxic, the concentration used is too small to significantly alter the product's toxicity although occasional primary or allergic irritative phenomena have been noted in housewives and in employees manufacturing these products.

There are 3 general types of detergents: cationic, anionic, and nonionic.

Cationic Detergents (Zephiran, Diaperene, Ceepryn, Phemerol)

Nausea, vomiting, collapse, coma, and convulsions may occur. The estimated fatal dose is approximately 1 gm of pure product/sq m of body area. Death is most likely in the first 4 hours, as cationic detergents are rapidly inactivated by tissues and ordinary soap.

Induce vomiting and follow with a saline cathartic. Ordinary soap is an effective antidote for unabsorbed cationic detergents. Anticonvulsants may be needed. Analeptics are likely to aggravate seizures and should not be used.

Anionic Detergents

Most common household detergents are anionic— Tide, Cheer, etc. Laundry compounds (All, etc) have water softener (sodium phosphate) added, which acts as a corrosive and may reduce ionized calcium. Anionic detergents irritate the skin by removing natural oils. Although ingestion causes diarrhea, intestinal distention, and vomiting, no fatalities have been reported. The LD_{50} in animals ranges from $1-5$ gm/kg.

The only treatment usually required is to discontinue use if skin irritation occurs. Induced vomiting is not indicated following ingestion of electric dishwasher detergent because of its strong alkalinity. Dilute with water or milk. Give 5 ml of 10% calcium gluconate IV if the patient has hypocalcemia.

Nonionic Detergents (Tritons X-45, X-100, X-102, X-144 & Brij Products)

These compounds include lauryl, stearyl, and oleyl alcohols and octyl phenol. They have a minimal irritating effect on the skin and are nontoxic when swallowed.

Deichmann WB, Gerarde HW: Hazards of alkaline laundry detergents. JAMA 220:1014, 1972.

Enzyme detergents. (Editorial.) Br Med J 1:518, 1970.

Jeven JE: Severe dermatitis and "biological" detergents. Br Med J 1:299, 1970.

Newhouse ML & others: An epidemiological study of workers producing enzyme washing powders. Lancet 1:689, 1970.

SPIDER BITES

At least 50 species of spiders have been implicated in human spider bites, but most toxic reactions in the USA are caused by the black widow spider (*Latrodectus mactans*) and the North American brown recluse (violin) spider (*Loxosceles reclusus*). Many spider venoms have common chemical and pharmacologic properties. Positive identification of the spider is helpful since many spider bites may mimic those of the brown recluse spider.

Black Widow Spider

The black widow spider, which is endemic to nearly all areas of the USA, causes most of the deaths due to spider bites. The initial bite may be hemorrhagic and associated with a sharp fleeting pain. Local and systemic muscular cramping, abdominal pain, nausea and vomiting, and shock can occur. Convulsions are more commonly seen in small children. Systemic signs of black widow spider bite are often confused with other causes of acute abdomen. Although paresthesias, nervousness, and transient muscle spasms may persist for months in survivors, recovery from the acute phase is generally complete within 3 days.

Antivenin is no longer in general use because of the self-limiting nature of the injury and the danger of serum sickness with its use. Give $5-20$ ml of 10% calcium gluconate IV to relieve muscle cramps. Hydrocortisone, $25-100$ mg IV, or diazepam may be useful. Morphine or barbiturates may occasionally be needed for control of pain or restlessness, but they increase the possibility of respiratory depression.

Local treatment of the bite is not helpful.

Brown Recluse Spider (Violin Spider)

The North American brown recluse spider is most commonly seen in the central and midwestern areas of the USA. Its bite characteristically produces a localized reaction with progressively severe pain within 8 hours. The initial bleb on an erythematous ischemic base is replaced by a black eschar within a week. This eschar separates in $2-5$ weeks, leaving a poorly healing ulcer which may result in keloid formation. Systemic signs include cyanosis, morbilliform rash, fever, chills, malaise, weakness, nausea and vomiting, joint pains, hemolytic reactions with hemoglobinuria, jaundice, and delirium. Fatalities are rare. Fatal disseminated intravascular coagulation due to the brown recluse spider has recently been reported.

Hydrocortisone sodium succinate (Solu-Cortef), 1 gm/24 hours IV, is indicated for systemic complications. Hydroxyzine (Atarax, Vistaril), 1 mg/kg/day IM, is reportedly useful because of its muscle relaxant, antihistaminic, and tranquilizing effects. The advisability of total excision of the lesion at the fascial level to minimize necrosis is debatable.

Arena JM: *Poisoning: Toxicology, Symptoms, Treatments,* 3rd ed. Thomas, 1974.

Bolton M: The brown spider bite. J Kans Med Soc 71:197, 1970.

Frazier CA: *Insect Allergy: Allergic and Toxic Reactions to Insects and Other Arthropods.* Warren Green, 1969.

Russell FE, Waldron WG: Spider bites, tick bites. Calif Med 106:247, 1967.

Vorse H: Disseminated intravascular coagulopathy following fatal brown spider bite. J Pediatr 80:1035, 1971.

STRYCHNINE

Strychnine poisoning is characterized by restlessness, apprehension, perceptual difficulties, and simultaneous contraction of all muscles, resulting in opisthitonos, respiratory depression, cyanosis, and a characteristic tetanic contraction of the face (risus sardonicus). The patient is conscious throughout the convulsion and is in great pain. Complete muscle relaxation frequently occurs between convulsions. The onset of symptoms is 10–20 minutes after exposure.

Strychnine can be found in household products such as rodenticides, tonics, and cathartics. It is also occasionally added to hallucinogenic drugs. Deaths have been reported after ingestion of as little as 15 mg.

Treatment

If the patient is seen before the onset of symptoms, vomiting should be induced after administration of activated charcoal, which is a very efficient adsorber of strychnine. Apomorphine should be used to induce vomiting since ipecac is also adsorbed by activated charcoal. Convulsions can be controlled with diazepam (Valium), 0.1–0.3 mg/kg to a maximum of 10 mg. External stimulation should be minimized. Forced acid diuresis is very helpful since strychnine is not significantly protein-bound and is present in large concentration in the serum. It is rapidly cleared in the urine. The hyperacute nature of strychnine intoxication makes hemodialysis impractical.

Maron BJ, Krupp JR, Tane B: Strychnine poisoning successfully treated with diazepam. J Pediatr 78:697, 1971.
Teitelbaum DT, Ott JE: Management of strychnine intoxication. Clin Toxicol 3:267, 1970.

THYROID PREPARATIONS
(Desiccated Thyroid,
Sodium Levothyroxine [Synthroid])

Ingestion of the equivalent of 50–150 gr of desiccated thyroid can cause signs of hyperthyroidism, including irritability, mydriasis, hyperpyrexia, tachycardia, and diarrhea. Maximal clinical effect occurs about 9 days after ingestion—several days after the PBI has fallen dramatically.

Induce vomiting. Chlorpromazine (Thorazine) is useful if the patient develops clinical signs of toxicity because of its adrenergic and anticholinergic activity.

Funderburk SJ, Spaulding JS: Sodium levothyroxine (Synthroid) intoxication in a child. Pediatrics 45:298, 1970.

TRICYCLIC ANTIDEPRESSANTS

These agents (amitriptyline [Elavil], imipramine [Tofranil], etc) are utilized in adolescents and adults as antidepressants. In children, imipramine especially is used in the management of enuresis. Unfortunately, these drugs have a very low toxic:therapeutic ratio,

and in a young child even a moderate overdose can have a disastrous effect similar to overdoses with atropine or belladonna alkaloids. The 5 features of tricyclic antidepressant overdosage which make it more of a problem than other drugs with anticholinergic properties are arrhythmias, coma, convulsions, hypertension (and, later, hypotension), and hallucinations. These may be life-threatening and require rapid intervention. Standard procedures such as emesis, lavage, and catharsis should be used. If the patient has symptoms–dry mouth, tachycardia, etc–an ECG should be taken. If there is any arrhythmia, the patient should be admitted and monitored until free of irregularity for 24 hours. Another indication for monitoring is tachycardia of more than 110/minute plus additional findings of anticholinergic toxicity. The onset of arrhythmias is rare beyond 24 hours after ingestion.

Treatment of the 5 major problems consists of intensive supportive measures followed by administration of physostigmine in the following doses:

Child under 12: 0.5 mg IV over 60 seconds. If there is no effect, the dose may be repeated at 5-minute intervals to a maximum of 2 mg. Repeat as necessary only for life-threatening situations.

Adult and adolescent: 2 mg IV over 60 seconds. If there is no effect, repeat in 10 minutes to a maximum dose of 4 mg. Repeat for life-threatening situations.

Physostigmine is a dangerous drug that must be given slowly to avoid iatrogenic convulsions. It is contraindicated in asthma, vascular gangrene, or urinary tract obstruction.

Propranolol or phenytoin may be used if physostigmine is ineffective for treatment of arrhythmias. Alkalinization with sodium bicarbonate, 0.5 mEq/kg IV, may dramatically reverse arrhythmias. Bicarbonate should be administered with physostigmine to all patients with significant arrhythmias to achieve a plasma pH of 7.5–7.6. Forced diuresis is contraindicated. A QRS interval greater than 100 msec specifically identifies patients with major tricyclic antidepressant overdosage.

Hypotension is a major problem since tricyclic antidepressants block the reuptake of catecholamines. This may produce a rebound hypotension following initial hypertension. Treatment with physostigmine is not effective. Infusion of sodium bicarbonate, 0.5 mEq/kg, to produce a plasma pH of 7.5 or 7.6, will help avert hypotension. Vasopressors are generally ineffective, and the mortality rate is 60% in patients with hypotension who prove unresponsive to initial fluids.

Biggs JT & others: Tricyclic antidepressant overdose: Incidence of symptoms. JAMA 238:135, 1977.
Burks JS & others: Tricyclic antidepressant poisoning: Reversal of coma, choreoathetosis, and myoclonus by physostigmine. JAMA 230:1405, 1974.

Rumack BH: Anticholinergic poisoning: Treatment with physostigmine. Pediatrics 52:449, 1973.

VITAMINS

Accidental ingestion of excessive amounts of vitamins rarely causes significant problems. Occasional cases
of hypervitaminosis A and D do occur, however, particularly in patients with poor hepatic or renal function.
The fluoride contained in many multivitamin preparations is not a realistic hazard since a 2- or 3-year-old
child could eat 100 tablets, containing 1 mg of sodium
fluoride per tablet, without producing serious symptoms. Iron poisoning has been reported with multiple
vitamin tablets containing iron.

Armstrong GD: Vitamin ingestions. National Clearinghouse Poison Control Center Bull 1–6, April–June, 1972.
Morrice G: Papilledema and hypervitaminosis A. JAMA
213:1344, 1970.
Seelig MS: Vitamin D and cardiovascular, renal, and brain damage in infancy and childhood. Ann NY Acad Sci 147:539,
1969.

WARFARIN

Warfarin is used as a pesticide. It causes hypoprothrombinemia and capillary injury. It is readily absorbed from the gastrointestinal tract but is absorbed
poorly through the skin. One to 2 mg/kg/day (or 0.5 kg
of rat bait at one ingestion) are required to cause
severe toxic effects in humans. Warfarin is more toxic
to dogs. A prothrombin time is helpful in establishing
the severity of the poisoning. Chloral hydrate poten-
tiates the hypoprothrombinemic effect of warfarin.

Treatment consists of induced vomiting followed
by a saline cathartic. If bleeding occurs or the prothrombin time is prolonged, give 10–50 mg of vitamin K IV.

Filmore SJ, McDevitt M: Effect of coumarin compounds on the
fetus. Ann Intern Med 73:731, 1970.
Monro P: Iatrogenic encephalopathy. Postgrad Med J 46:327,
1970.
Sellers EM: Potentiation of warfarin-induced hypoprothrombinemia by chloral hydrate. N Engl J Med 283:827, 1970.

•   •   •

General References

A Directory of Information Resources in the United States:
General Toxicology. Library of Congress, US Government
Printing Office, 1969.
AMA Drug Evaluations, 3rd ed. American Medical Association,
1977.
Arena JM: Poisoning: Toxicology, Symptoms, Treatments, 3rd
ed. Thomas, 1974.
Aviado DM: Krantz and Carr's Pharmacologic Principles of
Medical Practice, 8th ed. Williams & Wilkins, 1972.
Billups NF: American Drug Index. Lippincott, 1977.
Browning E: Toxicity and Metabolism of Industrial Solvents.
Elsevier, 1965.
Browning E: Toxicity of Industrial Metals, 2nd ed. Butterworth,
1969.
Childhood poisoning: Prevention and first-aid management.
Leading article. Br Med J 4:483, 1975.
Dreisbach RH: Handbook of Poisoning: Diagnosis & Treatment,
9th ed. Lange, 1977.
Gleason MN, Gosselin RE, Hodge HC: Clinical Toxicology of
Commercial Products, 4th ed. Williams & Wilkins, 1976.
Goodman LS, Gilman A: The Pharmacological Basis of Thera-
peutics, 5th ed. Macmillan, 1975.

Hamilton A, Hardy HL: Industrial Toxicology, 3rd ed. Publish-
ing Sciences Group, Inc., 1974.
Handbook of Nonprescription Drugs, 5th ed. The American
Pharmaceutical Association, 1977.
Hardin JW, Arena JM: Human Poisoning From Native and Culti-
vated Plants. Duke Univ Press, 1969.
Hayes WJ: Clinical Handbook on Economic Poisons. US Depart-
ment of Health, Education, & Welfare, 1963. [Available
through most state health departments.]
Kozma JJ: Killer Plants: A Poisonous Plant Guide. Milestone
Publishing Co., 1969. [Available from the author: Direc-
tor, Poison Control Center, Passavant Memorial Area Hos-
pital, Jacksonville, Ill.]
Matthew H, Lawson AA: Treatment of Common Acute Poison-
ings, 3rd ed. Livingstone, 1975.
Meyler L, Herxheimer A: Side Effects of Drugs. Vol 7. Excerpta
Medica, Amsterdam, 1972.
Rumack BH: POISINDEX: An Emergency Poison Management
System. Micromedex, Denver, Colorado. [Published quar-
terly.]
Samter M, Parker CW: Hypersensitivity to Drugs. Vol 1.
Pergamon Press, 1972.

31 . . .
Neoplastic Diseases

David G. Tubergen, MD, & Charlene P. Holt, MD

Cancer is the most common cause of death due to disease in children over the age of 1 year. Malignant diseases occur in about 10 per 100,000 children per year and account for about 4000 deaths annually. Leukemias and lymphomas constitute about 40% of pediatric malignant diseases, with the solid tumors, chiefly sarcomas, making up the remaining 60%. The signs and symptoms of pediatric malignancy may be subtle. Any mass—solid, cystic, or mixed—should be considered malignant until a definitive histologic diagnosis is established or until specific therapy directed at another cause has resulted in its disappearance within the expected period.

The causes of cancer in children remain elusive. Genetic disorders play an important role in some cases, eg, retinoblastoma and the tumors associated with neurofibromatosis. Chromosomal excess, as in trisomy 21, or chromosomal instability, as in Fanconi's hypoplastic anemia, is associated with an increased incidence of malignancy. Somatic growth disturbances, as seen in hemihypertrophy, may be associated with liver, kidney, or adrenal tumors.

A wide variety of immunologic deficiencies have been associated with an increased incidence of many types of cancer. This may reflect a decrease in the host's surveillance mechanism against transformed cells or may result in prolonged exposure to oncogenic agents as a consequence of failure to mount an adequate immune response. Our lack of information regarding the causes of cancer makes prevention virtually impossible and emphasizes the importance of early detection and specific diagnosis followed by aggressive treatment.

Once malignancy is suspected or diagnosed, there are several considerations that affect the ultimate outcome. The initial evaluation requires determination of the nature of the malignancy and the precise extent of disease. Since many pediatric tumors fit the broad description of "small cell neoplasm," the pathologic material should be examined by pediatric pathologists using special stains, histochemical technics, and electron microscopy when necessary. Determination of the extent of disease requires a knowledge of potential metastatic sites and selected utilization of many radiographic, isotopic scanning, and ultrasonic technics as well as biochemical and biopsy procedures. The surgeon must not only have sound judgment and expert technical skills; he must also include with his operative notes an accurate description of the extent of tumor involvement and the location and extent of local metastases or extensions. These observations are critical to further therapeutic planning.

Therapy is multidisciplinary and ideally involves a surgeon, a radiation therapist, and a pediatric oncologist before therapy is started. Certainly once the diagnosis has been made, a comprehensive treatment plan must incorporate all 3 major modalities. The significant progress that has been made in the management of several pediatric cancers as a result of aggressive multimodal therapy emphasizes the importance of this approach and the advantage of beginning treatment in a medical center where personnel and facilities are available to implement this concept. The primary physician serves several roles as a member of this team: as the diagnostician best situated to facilitate early detection; as the person administering therapy in the home community; as the physician most likely to observe early complications or toxic reactions; and as counselor to the patients and their families.

The current goal of cancer chemotherapy is to cure the patient. This implies an aggressive approach, as will be evident in the following pages. Chemotherapeutic agents fall into several general classes based on mode of action, and almost all programs utilize combinations of agents of differing actions in an attempt to increase tumor kill. This can only happen, of course, if each agent has some activity against the tumor in question. Ideally, the agents used together should have nonadditive toxicities. In other words, one attempts to use combinations with additive or synergistic antitumor effects and nonadditive toxic effects. In the treatment of solid tumors, the concept of adjunctive chemotherapy is important to achieve better results. In the case of many tumors, microscopic metastases are already present at the time of initial therapy, and local treatment alone will not be curative. Owing to the growth characteristics of small tumor implants and probably because of their relatively better blood supply, these microscopic tumors appear more susceptible to drugs than are clinically obvious metastases. In beginning chemotherapy, then, one should reason that metastasis has already occurred because the potential for cure is greater at this time than if one waits for clinical metastases to appear. In the management of some tumor types, the efficacy of drug therapy against microscopic residual disease lessens the need for extensive local tumor bed irradiation.

Table 31–9 lists the commonly used chemotherapeutic agents, the tumors for which they are used, and the most common toxicities.

LEUKEMIA

1. ACUTE LYMPHOBLASTIC LEUKEMIA

Essentials of Diagnosis

- Pallor, petechiae, purpura, fatigue, fever, bone pain.
- Hepatosplenomegaly, lymphadenopathy.
- Thrombocytopenia, normal or low hemoglobin.
- Diagnosis confirmed by bone marrow examination.

General Considerations

Acute lymphoblastic leukemia (ALL) comprises about 85% of leukemias in childhood. About 12% of cases are acute myeloblastic or monoblastic and 3% are chronic granulocytic leukemia. Acute stem cell leukemia and acute undifferentiated leukemia are terms used to denote leukemia cells with slightly different morphologic characteristics, but clinically these leukemias behave as acute lymphoblastic leukemia.

The peak incidence of onset of acute lymphoblastic leukemia is at 4 years of age, but the disease may occur at any time during childhood. Before the advent of chemotherapy, this disease was usually fatal within 3–4 months, with virtually no survivors 1 year after diagnosis. Current estimates are that over half of children receiving aggressive combination chemotherapy and early CNS irradiation may be expected to survive free of disease for 5 years or longer. Not all patients have the same likelihood of achieving long-term remission. Those with the best prognosis are 3–7 years of age with white counts at presentation of less than 10,000/cu mm. Patients who present with a white blood cell count over 50,000/cu mm or have CNS involvement initially have the poorest prognosis. The leukemic cells of approximately 15% of patients have surface characteristics of thymus-dependent lymphocytes. These patients tend to have higher white counts; many of them are adolescents; and mediastinal masses may be present on chest x-ray. This group of patients is less likely to achieve prolonged remission.

Clinical Findings

A. Symptoms and Signs: The variable presenting complaints of children with acute leukemia are referable to organ infiltration and marrow replacement with malignant cells that crowd out normal elements of the marrow. The absence of red cell precursors leads to anemia, which may make the child pale, listless, irritable, and chronically tired. The lack of mature granulocytes makes the child more susceptible to infection, and a history of repeated infections prior to a definitive diagnosis of leukemia is not unusual. The thrombocytopenia predisposes to bleeding episodes: epistaxis, petechiae, hematomas, or life-threatening hemorrhage. Organs may be infiltrated by disease and not function properly; may cause discomfort because of their large size; or may cause symptoms due to pressure on other structures.

Organ infiltration, especially of the kidney, may cause significant dysfunction. This may result in serious uric acid toxicity when therapy is initiated and must be assessed prior to treatment.

B. Laboratory Findings: The white count at presentation is below normal in one-third of patients, normal in another third, and elevated in the remainder. Thrombocytopenia is present in about 85% of patients, and varying degrees of anemia are reported in almost that many. The peripheral blood smear may or may not demonstrate the malignant cells. The diagnosis is established by bone marrow examination, which shows a homogeneous infiltration of blast cells replacing the normal elements. Special stains may be useful in classification of the various types of leukemia, and T and B lymphocyte markers should be sought on the lymphoblasts. Elevated serum lactic acid dehydrogenase and an elevated sedimentation rate are nonspecific findings. An elevated serum uric acid level requires careful monitoring and treatment (see below).

Diagnostic Work-Up

A. Complete History and Physical Examination: Important features of the history are a family history of cancer, drugs used, radiation exposure, immunizations, and infectious diseases.

B. Laboratory Studies:

1. Complete blood count, platelet count, reticulocyte count, prothrombin time, and bone marrow aspiration or biopsy (or both).

2. Lumbar puncture with study of a special Wright-stained smear of the sediment for blast cells; sugar and protein determinations.

3. BUN; serum creatinine, uric acid, bilirubin, GOT, alkaline phosphatase, proteins, sodium, potassium, lactic acid dehydrogenase, and immunoglobulins.

4. Urinalysis.

5. Cultures and smears of mouth, throat, blood, bone marrow, skin lesions, urine, CSF, and stool should be taken immediately if infection is suspected. Fungal and viral cultures and serologic tests should also be done when needed.

6. PPD intermediate strength skin test and endemic fungal skin tests.

C. X-Ray Studies: A chest x-ray should be obtained to look for mediastinal enlargement. Bone films of areas of pain will help rule out osteomyelitis, and some oncologists obtain an intravenous urogram before starting therapy to assess renal size and function.

D. Psychosocial Evaluation: An inventory of the patient's and family's strengths, coping abilities, and economic status is helpful in anticipating problems.

Differential Diagnosis

Early in the course of the disease, leukemia may produce signs and symptoms similar to those of rheumatic fever, rheumatoid arthritis, viral diseases such as infectious mononucleosis or hepatitis, or other neoplastic diseases such as neuroblastoma or histiocytosis X. The peripheral blood picture may be indistinguishable from that of aplastic anemia.

Specific Treatment

The goal of therapy is to eradicate the disease or, at a minimum, to produce a prolonged period free of disease. Therapy can be divided into (1) systemic therapy, consisting of induction and maintenance phases, and (2) treatment of the CNS.

A. Systemic Therapy: The theoretical objective of antileukemic therapy is elimination of lymphoblasts from the body. A child weighing 20–30 kg may present with a tumor weighing approximately 1 kg, which represents about 10^{12} cells. Current technics do not permit us to detect the disease when the number of cells is approximately 10^9 or fewer, thus making it impossible to determine whether the objective is being approached.

Induction therapy is designed to achieve a complete remission, ie, absence of detectable tumor tissue and normal bone marrow and peripheral blood counts. This generally requires 3–6 weeks of therapy and can be achieved in 85–95% of patients. The drugs most commonly used are vincristine, 1.5 mg/sq m IV once a week, and a corticosteroid given daily, usually prednisone, 40 mg/sq m orally in 3 divided doses, or, less commonly, dexamethasone, 6 mg/sq m orally in 3 divided doses. Asparaginase in doses of 6000 units/sq m IM given 3 days a week for 9 doses has been included in several large studies, but this drug is available only as an investigational agent. Once remission has been achieved, some programs call for 2–3 weeks of more intensive chemotherapy with other agents in an attempt to further reduce the tumor burden. This has been called the consolidation phase.

Maintenance therapy is designed to prevent reappearance of the disease. Current information indicates that therapy should be continued for at least 2½ years, but the optimal duration has not yet been established. The most common maintenance programs are with mercaptopurine, 50–75 mg/sq m orally daily, plus methotrexate, 15–20 mg/sq m orally once or twice weekly. Cyclophosphamide, 200 mg/sq m orally once weekly, has been added to the above. Some programs add periodic (1–3 months) "mini-inductions" with vincristine and 5–14 days of a corticosteroid to attempt to eliminate cells that develop resistance to the other agents.

An alternative maintenance program utilizes "pulse" type therapy with intensive treatment for 6 days out of each 3 weeks. Vincristine, 2 mg/sq m, and doxorubicin, 30 mg/sq m, are given IV on the first day, followed by dexamethasone, 18 mg/sq m orally in 3–4 divided doses, and mercaptopurine, 225 mg/sq m orally in 3–4 divided doses for the next 5 days. Doxorubicin is stopped after a cumulative dose of about 400 mg/sq m because of its cardiac toxicity, and the patient then receives methotrexate for 5 days in addition to the other drugs.

In any treatment program the dosages of drugs must be carefully adjusted to the patient's tolerance. The goals are to give the maximum tolerated amounts of drugs while preventing unacceptable toxicities or the hazards of severe marrow depression, particularly infections associated with profound neutropenia. This generally means maintaining the white count between 2000–3000/cu mm and the absolute neutrophil count above 1000/cu mm.

B. Central Nervous System Leukemia: In the absence of specific therapy directed at leukemic cells within the CNS, as many as 50% of children with acute lymphoblastic leukemia may develop clinical CNS involvement. The symptoms are most commonly headache, stiff neck, vomiting, and lethargy and may include cranial nerve palsies, hyperphagia and rapid weight gain, polydipsia, and polyuria. Physical examination may show papilledema; in younger children, a skull x-ray may reveal spread cranial sutures. The diagnosis is established by Wright-stained cytocentrifuge preparations of spinal fluid, which demonstrate the presence of lymphoblasts. Occasional patients will have definite symptoms of CNS leukemia without detectable lymphoblasts in the CSF; in others, unequivocal lymphoblasts will be present in the absence of any associated symptoms.

CNS leukemia appears to originate from leukemia cells that gain access to the CNS early in the course of the disease. Many of the antileukemic drugs do not penetrate the blood-brain barrier in adequate concentrations, and the cells can proliferate in the CNS while the disease is being controlled systemically.

Overt CNS leukemia can be prevented by "prophylactic" treatment. This can be accomplished by the use of cranial irradiation, 2400 rads, with cobalt or the linear accelerator, plus intrathecal methotrexate, 12 mg/sq m diluted to 3–5 ml in preservative-free saline or sterile water given 3–6 times concomitantly with the irradiation (maximum single dose of intrathecal methotrexate is 15 mg). The amount of spinal fluid withdrawn should equal the volume injected. Such treatment will reduce the incidence of overt CNS symptoms from as high as 50% to 5–10%. It does, of course, expose a significant number of children who would not develop CNS disease to irradiation, but at present there is no better alternative.

If overt CNS disease develops, the use of intrathecal methotrexate given twice weekly for 4–6 doses will usually relieve the symptoms and clear the spinal fluid of lymphoblasts. However, the disease tends to recur within a few months, and total eradication is rarely achieved. Cytarabine may also be used intrathecally, and a repeated course of irradiation may be

used to control the debilitating symptoms. Oral corticosteroids may also offer some temporary relief. If
CNS disease develops, a bone marrow examination is
needed because systemic relapse may also be present.

The best means of achieving long-term survival is
by prolongation of the first remission. If bone marrow
relapse occurs, second and third remissions are obtainable in 40–70% of children using vincristine and corticosteroids. Maintenance drugs may then consist of
combinations including cytarabine, cyclophosphamide,
daunorubicin, doxorubicin, asparaginase, or newer
experimental agents.

Immunotherapy using BCG or other means designed to stimulate the host's resistance to his malignancy are experimental methods which thus far have
not proved to be of significant benefit.

Supportive & Adjunctive Treatment

A. Massive Tumor Tissue: Uric acid nephropathy,
which can be fatal, can occur during initial therapy in
the presence of leukemic leukocytosis, massive hepatosplenomegaly, mediastinal mass, or compromised renal
function due to infiltrates. In some patients, hyperuricemia is present prior to therapy. Prevention of uric
acid nephropathy depends upon decreasing uric acid
production by the use of a xanthine oxidase inhibitor,
increasing uric acid solubility in urine by keeping the
urine pH above 6.5, and ensuring a large urine volume.
These measures are important for the first 3–7 days of
therapy.

Hyperphosphatemia and hypocalcemia may occur
with rapid tumor destruction. On occasion, it will be
symptomatic and require temporary calcium supplementation. Specific drugs and dosages are as follows:

1. Allopurinol, 100 mg/sq m orally 3 times a day.
This should be started 24 hours before beginning specific antileukemic therapy.

2. Provide 2–3 liters/sq m of fluids daily orally or
IV. Avoid potassium-containing parenteral solutions
during the stage of tumor catabolism.

3. Maintain a careful record of fluid intake and
urinary output.

4. Alkalinize the urine with sodium bicarbonate,
3–4 gm/sq m/day orally in 4–6 divided doses. Increase
the dose if needed to maintain a urine pH of 7.0 or
greater. If the patient cannot tolerate sodium bicarbonate, an alkaline urine can be obtained with acetazolamide.

5. Measure urine pH of each voiding at the bedside to ensure adequate alkalinization.

6. Perform a daily urinalysis and measure BUN
and serum uric acid, potassium, calcium, and phosphorus daily for 3 days or until normal levels are reported.

7. Regular diet for age with no added salt.

B. Hepatic Dysfunction: When there is evidence
of hepatic dysfunction as manifested by elevated enzymes or bilirubin or prolonged prothrombin time,
vincristine toxicity is more likely since vincristine is
excreted by the liver. Subsequent doses of vincristine
may need to be reduced if toxicity is moderate to
severe.

C. Infection: Cultures of blood and bone marrow
and smears and culture of the pharynx, nasopharynx
(if no bleeding), rectal swabs, and urine should be
taken on admission and repeated as necessary. Gram-
stained smears of infected lesions and body orifices
should be examined immediately. Full doses of appropriate bactericidal antibiotics should be used as soon as
infection is suspected. If paronychia or other skin
infections occur, 0.3 ml saline should be injected and
aspirated for smear and culture. Do not wait for
"pointing." Urinary tract infections may exist without
pyuria in the granulocytopenic child. Do not delay
antibiotic chemotherapy. Suspect *Escherichia coli,*
klebsiella-enterobacter, or staphylococcal infection if
the child has been receiving penicillin. Therapy should
be initiated with broad spectrum combinations such as
carbenicillin plus gentamicin or carbenicillin plus cephalothin. Tobramycin may also be useful. Therapy
should be given intravenously. Prolonged antibiotic
therapy should be avoided.

The organisms responsible for infections in leukemic children are almost always their own skin or enteric organisms. This has 2 important implications:
"Reverse" precautions are unlikely to reduce the incidence of infections beyond that obtained by good
hand washing (and tends to make good medical and
nursing care more difficult to provide), and prolonged
use of antibiotics may modify the gut flora and select
for increasingly resistant organisms.

In the severely neutropenic child with sepsis,
transfusions of granulocytes may be extremely useful.
Once started, they should be used for at least 4–6 days
or until the patient's own neutrophils appear in the
blood in adequate numbers.

Pneumocystis carinii pneumonia may be treated
with pentamidine given cautiously intravenously or
with trimethoprim-sulfamethoxazole (co-trimoxazole;
Bactrim, Septra) orally. Recent evidence indicates that
pneumocystis infection may be prevented in susceptible patients by daily low-dosage trimethoprim therapy. Fungal infections require prolonged treatment
with amphotericin B given intravenously.

The classical symptoms of infection may be
masked by immunosuppressive chemotherapy. Children may have life-threatening infections with rubeola
and varicella. Parents, teachers, and school nurses need
to be educated regarding notification of the physician
when the child shows symptoms of infection or has
been exposed to contagious diseases. Zoster immune
globulin (available only from authorized CDC representatives) or convalescent plasma given within 48 hours
of exposure may prevent or modify varicella. No live
virus vaccines should be given to leukemic children or
to children receiving immunosuppressive therapy.

D. Thrombocytopenia: The patient with thrombocytopenia is at risk of bleeding. Bleeding episodes
involving difficult to control epistaxis, gastrointestinal
bleeding, or signs and symptoms of CNS hemorrhage
(retinal hemorrhage is an important finding) should
receive platelet transfusions. Prophylactic platelet
transfusion is usually not indicated in thrombocytope-

nic patients who are not bleeding, although some clinicians give platelets prior to lumbar puncture. Patients with fever and infection tend to have more frequent serious bleeding episodes, and platelet transfusions may be indicated on a prophylactic basis.

E. Additional Precautions:

1. A "no salt added" diet is prescribed when the patient is on corticosteroids.

2. Avoid deep venipunctures or lumbar puncture, intramuscular injections, and instrumentation with catheters, laryngoscopes, etc in children with bleeding tendencies. Avoid tight clothing.

3. Avoid administration of barium sulfate during vincristine therapy, and give the child fruit, fruit juice, and plenty of liquids to help prevent constipation due to vincristine. Stool softeners may be indicated.

4. For nausea and vomiting, give antiemetics orally (or as suppositories) and fluids if needed.

5. Good nutrition and well-balanced meals are essential. Providing extra fluids on the day before and the day of cyclophosphamide therapy helps decrease bladder toxicity.

F. Psychologic Support of Patient and Family: The emotional impact of the diagnosis of leukemia is usually overwhelming and affects the entire family. A thorough discussion with the parents regarding diagnosis, prognosis, therapy, toxic reactions to drugs, and their own role in the care of the child is mandatory initially and throughout the course of the disease. Psychologic problems are common in the patient's siblings, and anticipatory guidance is needed.

What to tell the patient depends upon the maturity of the child and the judgment of physicians and family about the problems at hand. The authors recommend frank discussion of the disease with the adolescent patient. The discussion should be factual and honest, emphasizing the hopeful aspects and offering reassurance that progress is being made.

Psychologic guidance may be needed for siblings, parents, and patient, and appropriate professional consultation should be obtained.

Prognosis

Many centers are now reporting greater than 50% projected 5-year survival rates with various programs which have in common aggressive combination chemotherapy, radiation therapy with or without drugs to treat occult CNS disease, and the use of intensive supportive therapy as needed. It is likely that we will now begin to see significant numbers of long-term survivors. The word "cure" as applied to leukemia is difficult to define.

See references below.

2. ACUTE NONLYMPHOCYTIC LEUKEMIA

The acute nonlymphocytic leukemias include acute myeloblastic leukemia, acute monoblastic leuke-

mia, and leukemias whose morphologic features suggest both cell lines, the myelomonocytic leukemias.

The clinical features are similar to those of acute lymphoblastic leukemia, and the supportive care is basically the same. Therapy is more difficult, with different drugs, and produces remission rates of about 50–70% and a median duration of remission of about 12 months. Some centers are performing bone marrow transplants on these children when a suitable donor is available. A few instances of long-term survival have been reported.

See references below.

3. CHRONIC MYELOCYTIC LEUKEMIA

Chronic myelocytic leukemia (CML) of the adult form that demonstrates the Philadelphia (Ph) chromosome is treated with busulfan (Myleran), beginning with 5–8 mg/sq m/day orally and reducing the dosage to 2–4 mg/day when the white count reaches 15,000/cu mm. The white count should remain between 5000–10,000/cu mm, and the dosage is adjusted as necessary to achieve this response.

The juvenile non-Philadelphia chromosome (Ph-negative) form of chronic myelocytic leukemia is seen in younger children. Bleeding secondary to thrombocytopenia, organomegaly, and repeated infections makes this form of disease difficult to control clinically. Attempts at various forms of chemotherapy have not been successful. Transient relief of pressure symptoms has been accomplished by splenic irradiation with ^{60}Co. Splenectomy has resulted in longer survival times in a few patients.

Alavi JB & others: Clinical trial of granulocytic transfusions for infection in acute leukemia. N Engl J Med 296:706, 1977.

Aur R & others: Comparison of two methods of preventing central nervous system leukemia. Blood 42:349, 1973.

Bodey GP (editor): Infectious complications in hematological diseases. Clin Hematol 5:2, June 1976. [Entire issue.]

Furman L & others: Development of an effective treatment program for childhood acute lymphocytic leukemia: A preliminary report. Med Pediatr Oncol 2:157, 1976.

Mauer AM, Simone JV: The current status of the treatment of childhood acute lymphoblastic leukemia. Cancer Treatment Reviews 3:17, 1976.

O'Reagan S & others: Electrolyte and acid-base disturbances in the management of leukemia. Blood 49:345, 1977.

Simone JV: Management of childhood leukemia. Postgrad Med 55:225, May 1974.

Zippin C, Cuttler S, Lum D: Time trends in survival in acute lymphocytic leukemia. J Natl Cancer Inst 54:581, 1975.

LYMPHOMAS

1. HODGKIN'S DISEASE

Essentials of Diagnosis

- Lymphadenopathy.
- Hepatomegaly with or without splenomegaly.
- Fever, night sweats, fatigue, weight loss, generalized pruritus.

General Considerations

The clinical course of Hodgkin's disease has been favorably altered by advances in diagnostic technics that have improved our understanding of the disease and by the application of combined modality therapy. Optimal results depend on precise definition of the extent of disease and selection of therapy based on these results.

The histologic classification currently used is shown in Table 31–1. Nodular sclerosing Hodgkin's disease is the type most commonly seen in the second decade. Hodgkin's disease is less frequent in the first decade but has occurred in children as young as 3 years. The mixed cellularity type is more common in younger children. The response to therapy is nearly equal in these 2 types. Lymphocyte-depleted Hodgkin's disease is less common and is much less responsive to therapy.

Clinical and pathologic staging of the disease is carried out according to the Ann Arbor classification (Table 31–2). The subclassification of (A) absence or

Table 31–1. Histologic classification of Hodgkin's disease.

Designation	Distinctive Features	Relative Frequency
Lymphocyte predominance	Abundant stroma of mature lymphocytes, histiocytes, or both; no necrosis; Reed-Sternberg cells may be sparse.	10–15%
Nodular sclerosis	Nodules of lymphoid tissue partially or completely separated by bands of doubly refractile collagen of variable width; atypical Reed-Sternberg cells in clear spaces ("lacunae") in the lymphoid nodules.	20–50%
Mixed cellularity	Usually numerous Reed-Sternberg and atypical mononuclear cells with a pleomorphic admixture of plasma cells, eosinophils, lymphocytes, and fibroblasts; foci of necrosis commonly seen.	20–40%
Lymphocyte depletion	Reed-Sternberg and malignant mononuclear cells usually, though not always, numerous; marked paucity of lymphocytes; diffuse fibrosis and necrosis may be present.	5–15%

Table 31–2. Staging classification for Hodgkin's disease. (Ann Arbor classification.)

Stage I	Involvement of a single lymph note region (I) or a single extralymphatic organ or site (I$_E$).
Stage II	Involvement of 2 or more lymph node regions on the same side of the diaphragm (II) or localized involvement of an extralymphatic organ or site (II$_E$).
Stage III	Involvement of lymph node regions on both sides of the diaphragm (III) or localized involvement of an extralymphatic organ or site (III$_E$) or spleen (III$_{SE}$).
Stage IV	Diffuse or disseminated involvement of one or more extralymphatic organs with or without associated lymph node involvement. The organs involved should be identified by a symbol.
	A = Asymptomatic. B = Fever, sweats, weight loss > 10% of body weight.

(B) presence of systemic symptoms (fever, night sweats, or loss of over 10% of body weight) is also of prognostic value, and for a given stage treatment may be more aggressive in the presence of systemic symptoms.

Clinical Findings

A. Symptoms and Signs: The most common presentation in Hodgkin's disease is painless enlargement of lymph nodes. The most common site of involvement is in the cervical node areas. The involved nodes are firm or rubbery, often matted together and nontender to palpation. They may cause symptoms by compressing other structures such as a chronic cough due to tracheal compression from a large mediastinal mass. Extranodal disease may occur in any organ. Symptoms may be absent but may include anorexia, fatigue, weight loss, night sweats, and pain upon ingesting alcohol. Generalized pruritus may occur but is no longer a symptom that puts the patient into a B stage.

B. Laboratory Findings: Hematologic findings are often normal but may include anemia, elevated or depressed leukocytes and platelets, and sometimes modest eosinophilia. The sedimentation rate and the serum copper level may be elevated. With hepatic involvement, the serum levels of alkaline phosphatase, GOT, and GPT may be elevated. Many patients have tumors that take up gallium, and in these patients the gallium scan may help identify areas of involvement. Gallium scanning does not differentiate between Hodgkin's disease and inflammatory tissue, and its usefulness is limited in the subdiaphragmatic area.

Immunologic abnormalities may occur, primarily in the cell-mediated system, with anergy to the common delayed hypersensitivity antigens. Coombs-positive hemolytic anemia and abnormal immunoglobulin levels have also been described.

The diagnosis is established by histologic examination of an excised lymph node or other involved tissue. After the diagnosis is made, bone marrow biopsy and radiologic examinations, including lymphangiography, are done. This is then followed in almost all cases by pathologic staging, which involves laparotomy with multiple abdominal lymph node biopsies, liver biopsy, wedge bone marrow biopsy, and splenectomy and may include moving the ovaries laterally to remove them from the contemplated radiation field.

C. X-Ray Findings: Chest x-ray may show parenchymal or mediastinal nodal disease. Skeletal survey may show bone involvement. The intravenous urogram may show deviation of the ureter or bladder; a lateral view is often helpful to show anterior displacement. Lymphangiography may reveal "foamy" filling defects in an enlarged node, which implies tumor involving the node. Allergy to iodides and severe pulmonary disease are contraindications to lymphangiography.

Complications

Patients with Hodgkin's disease have an increased susceptibility to herpes zoster and fungal infections. Therapy may induce acute toxicities which include nausea, vomiting, anorexia, alopecia, bone marrow suppression, and radiation pneumonitis. The patient must be carefully monitored so that necessary adjustments can be made in treatment. Chronic toxic effects of therapy include retardation of bone growth and an increased incidence of second malignancies. The splenectomy which is done as part of pathologic staging is associated with a 10% incidence of sepsis, most commonly pneumococcal, which can occur days to years after the splenectomy. These septic episodes have a high mortality rate. All such splenectomized patients should be put on prophylactic antibiotics to prevent sepsis.

The psychologic effects of this disease and its treatment in the adolescent age group require good rapport between the patient, the family, the school, and the physician.

Treatment

Following establishment of the patient's stage of disease, therapy is planned by the chemotherapist and radiation therapist. Optimum results will be obtained by a radiation therapist skilled in the treatment of growing children by means of megavoltage irradiation. Combination chemotherapy is vastly superior to single agent therapy. Several combinations have been used effectively, including mechlorethamine, vincristine (Oncovin), procarbazine, and prednisone (MOPP); cyclophosphamide, vincristine (Oncovin), procarbazine, and prednisone (COPP); and lomustine (CCNU), vinblastine, procarbazine, and prednisone. New programs using doxorubicin and bleomycin also appear promising. The dosage, frequency of administration, and duration of therapy depend upon the patient's tolerance to therapy and the stage of disease.

In general, for stage IA or IIA disease, treatment may consist of extended field irradiation alone or may employ irradiation only of clinically involved areas plus chemotherapy. We favor the latter and would use 6-monthly courses of lomustine, vinblastine, procarbazine, and prednisone. In stages IB or IIB, extended field irradiation is followed by 6 months of chemotherapy. In stage IIIA disease, therapy is initiated with 3 cycles of chemotherapy and the patient then receives total nodal irradiation. Following hematologic recovery, chemotherapy is resumed for a total of 9 courses.

Stage IIIB or stage IV disease is treated with 12 courses of chemotherapy plus irradiation to areas of bulky disease. If lungs or liver is involved, these organs are also irradiated as tolerated.

The goal of therapy is to eradicate malignant tissue. Recurrences in nonirradiated areas may require further irradiation. The various chemotherapy programs are not cross-resistant, and second prolonged remissions often can be obtained.

Prognosis

The 5-year survival rate of pathologically staged and aggressively treated patients with stage IA and IIA disease is about 90%. Most of these will be without relapse, and a high proportion are curable. In more advanced stage IIIA disease, the 5-year survival rate is about 70%, and even in stage IV disease, survival of more than 2 years with no evidence of disease can be achieved in a majority of cases.

Bloomfield CD & others: Combined chemotherapy with cyclophosphamide, vinblastine, procarbazine, and prednisone (CVPP) for patients with advanced Hodgkin's disease. Cancer 38:42, 1976.

Chilcote RR & others: Septicemia and meningitis in children splenectomized for Hodgkin's disease. N Engl J Med 259:798, 1976.

Donaldson SS & others: Pediatric Hodgkin's disease II: Results of therapy. Cancer 37:2435, 1976.

Kaplan H: *Hodgkin's Disease.* Harvard Univ Press, 1972.

Lanzkowsky P & others: Staging laparotomy and splenectomy: Treatment and complications of Hodgkin's disease in children. Am J Hematol 1:393, 1976.

Smith KL, Rivera G: Comparison of the clinical course of Hodgkin's disease in children and adolescents. Med Pediatr Oncol 2:361, 1976.

2. NONHODGKIN'S LYMPHOMA

The non-Hodgkin's lymphomas form a relatively diverse group of malignancies of the lymphoid organs. Recent advances in our understanding of normal lymphocyte subpopulations have enabled Lukes and others to clarify the origin of these malignancies and to modify the classification developed by Gall and Rappaport. Lymphoma cells may carry the membrane markers of T (thymus-dependent) lymphocytes, the surface markers of immunoglobulin-producing B lymphocytes, or no distinctive markers (null cells). Table 31–3 presents the classification of non-Hodgkin's lymphomas used at Denver Children's Hospital.

The convoluted cell type of lymphoma is associated with T cell surface markers. Patients with this disease often have a mediastinal mass, and the disease tends to involve bone marrow early. This disease ap-

Table 31–3. Classification of non-Hodgkin's lymphoma in children.

Morphologic Classification	Immunologic Markers (Expected)	Rappaport's Classification
Convoluted cell type	T cell	Undifferentiated
Immunoblastic type	T or B cell	Histiocytic
Burkitt's type	B cell	Poorly differentiated, Burkitt's type
Lymphoblastic type	Null, T, or B cell	Lymphocytic, poorly differentiated
Multiphasic type		
Histiocytic	Monocyte (?)	Histiocytic
Unclassified	Null, T, or B cell	Unclassifiable

pears very closely related to, if not identical with, T cell leukemia and shares with that disease an excellent early response to therapy but a relatively short remission and a generally fatal outcome within 2 years.

Burkitt's lymphoma is a lymphoma involving the B lymphocyte line. It is responsible for over half the pediatric cancer deaths in Uganda and Central Africa, and in that area the Epstein-Barr virus appears to play an important role in tumor development. Its prevalence is much less in the USA, where it tends to present with primary abdominal involvement and an extremely aggressive pattern of spread to viscera, marrow, and bones.

Clinical Findings

A. Symptoms and Signs: The non-Hodgkin's lymphomas in general are more common in boys than in girls, and the single most common site of origin is in the lymphoid structures of the intestinal tract, usually in the ileocecal area. The most common presentation in these children is with symptoms of an acute surgical abdomen. Disease originating elsewhere generally presents as nontender lymph node involvement, which may produce symptoms due to compression. CNS involvement consists of symptoms due to cord compression or increased intracranial pressure.

B. Laboratory Findings: The evaluation is similar to that used in patients with Hodgkin's disease except that routine laparotomy and splenectomy are not done. The evaluation permits a clinical stage to be assigned as outlined in Table 31–4. Owing to the frequency of CNS involvement, lumbar puncture with careful cytologic examination of the fluid needs to be done on all patients.

Table 31–4. Clinical staging of non-Hodgkin's lymphoma

Stage I	One single site.
Stage II	Two or more sites on the same side of the diaphragm.
Stage III	Disseminated disease without involvement of bone marrow or CNS.
Stage IV	Any of the above with involvement of bone marrow or CNS.

Treatment

The lymphomas are sensitive to both chemotherapy and irradiation. Recent results suggest that longer survival can be achieved with combination chemotherapy and the use of megavoltage irradiation to areas of bulk disease. The use of CNS therapy prior to clinical CNS involvement—as has been shown to be effective in acute lymphoblastic leukemia—is recommended. The best results to date have been reported by Wollner and her associates. The current program for non-Hodgkin's lymphoma at Denver Children's Hospital and the University of Colorado Medical Center employs monthly courses of bleomycin, 5 mg/sq m on days 1 and 8 (given in every other course); vincristine, 1.5 mg/sq m on days 1 and 8; prednisone, 40 mg/sq m/day for 14 days; doxorubicin, 40 mg/sq m on day 1 only of each course (up to a cumulative dose of 300–400 mg); and mechlorethamine, 3 mg/sq m on days 1 and 8. Patients receive cranial irradiation and 3 doses of intrathecal methotrexate during the third course of therapy. Fifteen courses of therapy are given, with carmustine (BCNU), 100 mg/sq m, being substituted for doxorubicin when the cumulative maximum dose of the latter is reached. Other combinations have also been useful in producing remissions.

Prognosis

Wollner reports 2-year survival rates in excess of 70%. Most series do not report such high survival figures, but a small number of long-term survivors are seen in most series. Leukemic conversion is a frequent preterminal event.

Hutter JJ & others: Non-Hodgkin's lymphoma in children: A correlation of CNS disease with initial presentation. Cancer 36:2132, 1975.

Murphy SB, Frizzera G, Evans AE: A study of childhood non-Hodgkin's lymphoma. Cancer 36:2121, 1975.

Sullivan MP: Treatment of lymphoma. Cancer 35 (Suppl):991, 1975.

Wollner N & others: Non-Hodgkin's lymphoma in children: A comparative study of two modalities of therapy. Cancer 37:123, 1976.

NEUROBLASTOMA

Essentials of Diagnosis

- Asymptomatic abdominal mass, subcutaneous nodules, posterior mediastinal mass, and organomegaly.
- Fever, anemia, weakness, "black eyes," proptosis, opsoclonus, diarrhea, and hypertension.
- Bone pain, paraplegia, and ataxia.

General Considerations

Neuroblastoma is a tumor arising from cells in the sympathetic ganglia and adrenal medulla. It is the third most frequent pediatric neoplasm. Clinically, the survival rates are much better in children under 2 years of age, in children with extra-adrenal tumor, and in those with localized disease. These tumors may spontaneously regress in 5–10% of cases. In routine autopsies of infants under 3 months of age dying of other causes, neuroblastoma in situ in the adrenal is seen 40 times more frequently than expected, suggesting a high rate of spontaneous regression or differentiation.

Immunologic factors may be very significant in understanding the biology of neuroblastoma. Many tumors show infiltration with lymphocytes and plasma cells. The colony inhibition test (Hellström) has shown the lymphocytes of neuroblastoma patients, and in some cases of their mothers as well, to react against neuroblastoma cells in tissue culture.

Clinical staging of extent of disease is the basis of therapeutic planning. The system developed by Evans is shown in Table 31–5.

Clinical Findings

A. Symptoms and Signs: The child most commonly presents at about age 2 with a palpable abdominal mass, although the tumor may present at any time from neonatal life to adolescence. Symptoms depend upon the extent of disease at the time of diagnosis. Bone pain, weight loss, and fever may be the presenting complaints. Newborn infants may present with subcutaneous nodules and adrenal masses with marrow involvement. Early diagnosis depends on keeping the disease in mind so that obscure presentations will not be missed.

B. Laboratory Findings: Anemia and thrombocytopenia may be present secondary to marrow replacement by neuroblasts which may mimic leukemia.

The urinary excretion of catecholamines is elevated in the majority of patients. A 24-hour urine collection for vanilmandelic acid (VMA) should be done preoperatively. This test is useful in following the patient if levels are elevated initially. If the VMA levels increase during follow-up, recurrence may be suspected and reevaluation is advised. Urinary cystathionine is increased in 50% of children with neuroblastoma; it is independent of VMA excretion and may offer additional diagnostic help if VMA levels are normal.

Measurement of other urinary catecholamines is sometimes useful.

C. X-Ray Findings: Chest x-ray, skeletal survey, and intravenous urography aid in preoperative staging of the disease. Angiography may aid the surgeon in identifying the extent of the tumor and its blood supply; the tumor may be extremely vascular. Bone scanning may detect skeletal metastases before gross lesions on x-rays can be observed.

Treatment

Therapy involves the combined use of surgery, irradiation, and chemotherapy. Initial surgical efforts are directed at removal of as much of the primary tumor as possible. The massive size of some tumors precludes a vigorous surgical approach, and only a biopsy may be advisable. Following radiation and chemotherapy, a second surgical procedure may permit more definitive removal. Chemotherapy with drugs such as vincristine, cyclophosphamide, doxorubicin, and dacarbazine produces remissions in about 80% of patients. No definite increase in permanent tumor eradication can be ascribed to the drugs, however.

Infants under 1 year of age with stage IV-S disease have a generally good prognosis, with 80% or more 2-year disease-free survival. These infants may need little if any therapy of any kind to effect a cure.

Prognosis

Approximately two-thirds of children with neuroblastoma after age 2 years have widely disseminated disease at the time of diagnosis. Death due to the tumor occurs rapidly in over 90%, although chemotherapy may provide brief remissions. In children under age 2, the prognosis is significantly better.

Evans AE & others: Factors influencing the survival of children with nonmetastatic neuroblastoma. Cancer 38:661, 1976.

Gerson J, Koop E: Neuroblastoma. Semin Oncol 1:35, 1974.

Jaffe N: Neuroblastoma: Review of the literature and an examination of factors contributing to its enigmatic character. Cancer Treatment Rev 3:61, 1976.

Koop E, Schnaufer L: The management of abdominal neuroblastoma. Cancer 35 (Suppl):905, 1975.

Table 31–5. Clinical staging of neuroblastoma (Evans).

Stage I	Tumors confined to the organ or structure of origin.
Stage II	Tumors extending in continuity beyond the organ or structure of origin but not crossing the midline. Regional lymph nodes on the ipsilateral side may be involved.
Stage III	Tumor extending in continuity beyond the midline. Regional lymph nodes bilaterally may be involved.
Stage IV	Remote disease involving skeleton, parenchymatous organs, soft tissues, or distant lymph node groups. (See IV-S.)
Stage IV-S	Tumors which would be stage I or II except for the presence of remote disease confined to one or more of the following sites: liver, skin, and bone marrow (without radiographic evidence of bone metastases on complete skeletal survey).

WILMS'S TUMOR

Essentials of Diagnosis

- Asymptomatic abdominal mass or abdominal pain.
- Hematuria, genitourinary anomalies, aniridia.
- Hypertension, fever.

General Considerations

Wilms's tumor follows neuroblastoma in frequency

of occurrence of pediatric solid tumors. It is believed to be embryonal in origin, develops within the kidney parenchyma, and enlarges with distortion and invasion of the adjacent renal tissue. This tumor may be associated with congenital anomalies, and patients should be evaluated for Wilms's tumor if the following entities occur: hemihypertrophy, aniridia, ambiguous genitalia, hypospadias, undescended testes, duplications of the ureters or kidneys, horseshoe kidney, or Beckwith's syndrome.

Wilms's tumor more commonly presents as an abdominal mass—in contrast to renal tumors in adults, which usually present with hematuria. The incidence of bilateral Wilms's tumor is 2%. Metastases to liver and lungs are present in 25% of patients under 2 years of age at the time of diagnosis; in children over 2 years of age, 50% show spread of disease at diagnosis.

Several systems of tumor staging exist for Wilms's tumor. The system used at The Children's Hospital in Denver and at the University of Colorado Medical Center is shown in Table 31—6.

Clinical Findings

A. Symptoms and Signs: Children with Wilms's tumor may be asymptomatic, and a mass may be felt by the parent while dressing or washing the child or, less commonly, by a physician on a routine well baby examination. Occasionally, a tumor may be ruptured by a fall or trauma to the abdomen with symptoms of an acute surgical abdomen.

B. Laboratory Findings: Complete blood count, reticulocyte count, platelet count, and bone marrow examination are needed as baselines for staging and for following therapy. Wilms's tumor rarely metastasizes to bone marrow, whereas neuroblastoma does so frequently. Urinalysis and urine culture may reveal hematuria or infection. BUN and serum creatinine, uric acid,

---

Table 31—6. Staging of Wilms's tumor (Denver).

Stage I	Tumor confined to kidney.
	A. Tumor limited to kidney and less than 6 cm in size without renal capsule involvement.
	B. Tumor limited to kidney and greater than 6 cm in size with extension to renal capsule.
Stage II	Tumor confined to renal fossa.
	A. Local extension beyond renal capsule but no invasion of adjacent viscera or metastasis.
	B. Tumor in renal vessels.
	C. Positive lymph nodes at renal hilus.
Stage III	Tumor confined to abdomen.
	A. Invasion of adjacent viscera by direct extension only (ie, diaphragm, spleen, colon, stomach, pancreas, liver).
	B. Metastases confined to abdomen only. Tumor ruptured at time of surgery with peritoneal dissemination. Primary tumor not resectable.
	C. Involvement by tumor of vena cava; bilateral Wilms's tumor.
Stage IV	Disseminated tumor. Distant metastases outside abdomen (lungs, bone, bone marrow, etc).

---

bilirubin, alkaline phosphatase, lactic acid dehydrogenase, and GOT are other baseline studies of importance for following treatment. Erythropoietin levels are followed in some centers and may aid in detecting tumor activity.

C. X-Ray Findings: Posterior-anterior, lateral, and oblique views of the chest should be taken to search for pulmonary metastases. Intravenous urograms to define the tumor mass and an inferior venacavagram to rule out vascular invasion are suggested. A liver scan is helpful to rule out hepatic metastases.

Treatment

In 1956, a 47% cure rate with total excision of Wilms's tumor was reported. It is now proper to use a transabdominal approach to allow early ligation of the renal vessels, to avoid manipulation of the tumor, and to examine the abdominal viscera, nodes, and opposite kidney for staging. Silver clips should be placed at tumor margins.

Radiation therapy to the renal fossa postoperatively increased the survival rate in some series to 60%. Therapy with megavoltage equipment is begun following surgery. Dosages of 2000—3500 rads are given, depending on the age of the patient and the stage of the tumor. If the tumor is ruptured, the entire abdomen should be treated using lead shields to protect the remaining kidney. The entire vertebral body is treated to prevent scoliosis if the spine is included in the radiation field. Radiation hepatitis may occur in the treatment of right-sided Wilms's tumor, and the early chemotherapy doses may need to be adjusted downward.

In 1966, survival rates of 89% were reported when chemotherapy with dactinomycin was added to surgery and radiation therapy in 53 patients with operable tumors; 53% survival rates were reported in 15 children presenting with metastases. Chemotherapy with vincristine and dactinomycin in courses of 6—12 weeks has been effective, with tolerable toxicity. Radiation and chemotherapy are given concurrently; wound healing and adequate nutrition are important factors in following patients postoperatively. Chest films, complete blood counts, and renal function studies should be monitored during therapy. The duration of therapy depends on the patient's age and the extent of the disease.

The following treatment methods are those in use at The Children's Hospital Oncology Center and the University of Colorado Medical Center in Denver. Postoperative treatment (based on staging) with radiation and chemotherapy is begun as soon as possible after recovery from surgery or when the diagnosis is established—usually within 72 hours.

Stage IA: No chemotherapy or radiation therapy.

Stage IB: No radiation therapy. Chemotherapy: under 1 year of age, give vincristine, 1.5 mg/sq m/dose, and dactinomycin, 0.4 mg/sq m per dose IV once weekly for 6 weeks. In children over 1 year of age, the above 6-week course is followed by vincristine every other week for 3 doses and the entire cycle is then repeated for a total of 6 months of chemotherapy.

Stages II and IIIA: Radiation therapy is given to the tumor bed in stage II and to the entire abdomen in IIIA. Chemotherapy consisting of 13-week courses of vincristine and dactinomycin as described above is given for 1 year.

Stages IIIB and IV: Radiation therapy is given to the entire abdomen in stage IIIB. In stage IV, it is individualized because of the varied anatomic locations of metastases. Chemotherapy consists of the same basic 13-week course of vincristine and dactinomycin continued for a total of 2 years. In addition, during the first year, doxorubicin, 20 mg/sq m, is given IV on weeks 6 and 10 of each course.

Prognosis

The 2-year disease-free survival rate is about 80% in patients with tumor extending beyond the kidney by contiguity but without apparent hematogenous spread. It is about 90% in patients with tumor confined to the kidney, and in this group patients under 2 years of age do better than older patients. Even in patients with metastatic disease, an aggressive approach is rewarded with a significant number of cures.

D'Angio GJ & others: The treatment of Wilms' tumor: Results of the National Wilms' tumor study. Cancer 38:633, 1976.

Everson R, Fraumeni J: Declining mortality and improving survival from Wilms' tumor. Med Pediatr Oncol 1:3, 1975.

Wolff J: Advances in the treatment of Wilms' tumor. Cancer 35:901, 1975.

HEPATIC TUMORS

Essentials of Diagnosis

- Abdominal mass.
- Weight loss, malaise, fever.
- Nausea, vomiting, diarrhea, rarely jaundice.
- Liver function studies usually normal; mild to moderate anorexia, hyperlipemia, osteoporosis, elevated α-fetoprotein, masculinization.

General Considerations

Hepatic carcinoma is the most common malignancy in the newborn period, although hepatic malignancy in general is a rare tumor. A survey of the Surgical Section of the American Academy of Pediatrics revealed data on 375 children with liver tumors over a period of 10 years: 252 (67%) were malignant; of these, 129 (51%) were hepatoblastoma and 98 (39%) hepatocellular carcinoma. The leading benign tumors were hemangioma (38 cases), hamartoma (37 cases), and hemangioendothelioma (16 cases).

Hepatic tumors declined in incidence after a peak in the first year of life, although hepatocellular carcinoma showed a substantial increase in incidence during

Table 31–7. Staging of hepatic tumors (Denver).

Stage I	Unicentric lobar lesion < 6 cm resectable.
Stage II	Unicentric lobar lesion > 6 cm:
	A. Margin clear.
	B. Margin involved.
	C. Multicentric, one lobe.
Stage III	Multicentric, both lobes involved.
Stage IV	Metastatic disease:
	A. Direct extension to adjacent viscera.
	B. Distant spread.

adolescence. Children with tyrosinemia are particularly susceptible to these tumors.

Industrial exposure to vinyl chloride has recently been reported to cause angiosarcoma of the liver. Norethandrolone and other androgenic hormones used in the treatment of aplastic anemias have recently been associated with benign and malignant tumors.

Clinical Findings

A. Symptoms and Signs: A painless, firm right upper quadrant mass is the most common finding; anorexia, weight loss, fever, or (rarely) jaundice may be the initial complaint.

B. Laboratory Findings: The workup should include specific inquiries about chemical or drug exposure or hepatitis in addition to bone marrow examination, reticulocyte count, and renal and liver function studies, including serum bilirubin, protein electrophoresis, serum alkaline phosphatase, serum lactate dehydrogenase, and tests for hepatitis-associated antigen titer and α-fetoprotein.

C. X-Ray Findings: Radiologic examination includes posterior-anterior, lateral, and oblique chest films, an intravenous urogram, skeletal and liver scans, and angiography in some cases.

D. Surgical Staging: Personnel at The Children's Hospital Oncology Center in Denver have developed a clinical staging system based on stage, resectability, and extent of tumor (Table 31–7). Surgery must always be considered after the extent of disease has been assessed.

Treatment

In 1970, a review of primary childhood hepatic cancers revealed no 3-year survivors in a group of 20 children age 3 months to 17 years. A surgical adjuvant multidrug regimen was designed for these patients based on stage of disease. The initial results have been encouraging (see Holton reference, below):

Stage I:
Surgery.
Vincristine, 1.5 mg/sq m IV weekly for 6 weeks.
Cyclophosphamide, 200 mg/sq m IV weekly for 6 weeks.
Fluorouracil, 200 mg/sq m IV weekly for 6 weeks.
No maintenance.

Stages IIA, B, C:

Surgery.

Chemotherapy as for stage I for 6 weeks, then—

Maintenance chemotherapy with the same 3 drugs every 2 weeks for 1 year, and then discontinue.

Stages III and stages IVA, B, C:

Surgery if resectable, followed by—

Vincristine, 1.5 mg/sq m IV weekly for 6 weeks and then every 2 weeks.

Cyclophosphamide, 300 mg/sq m IV weekly for 6 weeks and then every 2 weeks.

Fluorouracil, 300 mg/sq m IV weekly for 6 weeks, then every 2 weeks.

Maintenance chemotherapy for 2 years.

Add doxorubicin (starting on week 6), 40 mg/sq m IV every 4 weeks, with the above, for a total dose of 550 mg/sq m because of cardiac toxicity.

Almersjö O & others: Accuracy of diagnostic tools in malignant hepatic lesions: A comparative study using serum tests, angiography, scintiscanning, and laparotomy. Am J Surg 127:663, 1974.

Block BJ: Angiosarcoma of the liver following vinyl chloride exposure. JAMA 229:53, 1974.

Clatworthy HW, Schiller M, Grosfeld JL: Primary liver tumors in infancy and childhood: 41 cases variously treated. Arch Surg 109:143, 1974.

Holton CP, Burrington JD, Hatch EI: A multiple chemotherapeutic approach to the management of hepatoblastoma. Cancer 35:1083, 1975.

Matsumoto Y & others: Response of alpha-fetoprotein to chemotherapy in patients with hepatomas. Cancer 34:1602, 1974.

SOFT TISSUE TUMORS

Tumors arising in tissues of mesodermal origin may be malignant or benign. Histologically, they are of connective, fatty, or muscle tissue origin. The most common clinical complaint is of a painless lump that may arise at any site. These lumps should not be "watched" for long periods of time; surgical consultation with excisional biopsy is warranted. These tumors are too often diagnosed by means of incisional biopsy, which may disseminate the tumor and make a potentially curable lesion a widespread disease.

The malignant soft tissue tumors are rhabdomyosarcoma, malignant mesenchymoma, and fibrosarcoma.

1. RHABDOMYOSARCOMA

Rhabdomyosarcoma is the most common type of sarcoma among the somatic soft tissues of children. It is most commonly found in the first 2 decades of life and is an embryonal tumor. The 4 histologic types (with definite overlapping) are embryonal, alveolar, botryoid, and pleomorphic. Common sites of occurrence are the head and neck, extremities, orbits, and pelvic regions. The histologic pattern is variable and may be related to the site, ie, if arising in a luminal structure such as the bladder or nasopharynx where there is poor support, the tumor may assume a gelatinous or botryoid ("grapelike") appearance, in contrast to the fleshy sarcomatous tumor within the body of a muscle bundle in an extremity, where a more alveolar pattern with cross-striations may be noted. This tumor is often misdiagnosed as neuroblastoma; special electron microscopic studies may be needed for clarification and show primitive Z bands in the myofibrils.

Chest x-ray, intravenous urograms, and bone marrow examination should be done. Rhabdomyoblasts may appear in the marrow as primitive "tadpole" cells. Creatine phosphokinase and lactic acid dehydrogenase may be elevated. Renal and liver function studies should be obtained as baselines.

Treatment must be coordinated with staging. Staging is done according to a scheme developed for a nationwide cooperative therapy trial (Table 31–8).

Cures are rare when single therapeutic modalities are used because of the tumor's microscopic local extensions and early infiltration of blood and lymphatic vessels. Surgical procedures should be designed to produce wide margins of normal tissue, but amputations or mutilating procedures need not be employed. Megavoltage therapy in the range of 4000–6000 rads is used locally for any residual disease or, in initially inoperable lesions, may precede surgical extirpation. Chemotherapeutic agents with demonstrated effectiveness include dactinomycin, cyclophosphamide, vincristine, doxorubicin, and dacarbazine.

Treatment

Group I: Surgery followed by vincristine, cyclophosphamide, and dactinomycin for 1 year.

Group II: Surgery, local irradiation, and vincristine, cyclophosphamide, and dactinomycin for 2 years.

Group III: Chemotherapy with vincristine, dactinomycin, and cyclophosphamide is given for 4–6 weeks. Once sufficient tumor shrinkage has occurred,

Table 31–8. Staging of rhabdomyosarcoma.

Group I	Localized disease, completely resected: (a) Confined to muscle or organ of origin. (b) Infiltration outside the muscle or organ of origin, but regional nodes not involved.
Group II	(a) Grossly resected tumor with microscopic residual disease. (b) Regional disease completely resected. (c) Regional disease grossly resected but with evidence of microscopic residual.
Group III	Incomplete resection or biopsy with gross residual disease.
Group IV	Distant metastases present at diagnosis.

the residual tumor and involved regional nodes are resected. Radiation therapy to the area of involvement is then administered, and chemotherapy is resumed and given for a total of 2 years.

Group IV: Chemotherapy employing vincristine, cyclophosphamide, dactinomycin, doxorubicin, and decarbazine; then, after 2–3 months, the possibility of surgery, with or without irradiation therapy of mass lesions, is considered.

Prognosis

Group I patients have a greater than 90% chance of long-term survival. With only microscopic residual disease and no regional spread, about 70% of children will survive for 3 years. With regional or distant metastases at the time of diagnosis, the long-term survival rate drops to about 30%.

Ghavimi F & others: Multidisciplinary treatment of embryonal rhabdomyosarcoma in children. Cancer 35:677, 1975.

Holton C & others: Extended combination therapy of childhood rhabdomyosarcoma. Cancer 32:1310, 1973.

Jereb B & others: Local control of embryonal rhabdomyosarcoma in children by radiation therapy when combined with concomitant chemotherapy. Int J Radiat Oncol Biol Phys 1:217, 1976.

Pratt C, Fleming I, Hustu O: Multimodal therapy of childhood rhabdomyosarcoma. Proc Am Assoc Cancer Res 103:29, 1971.

Suit H, Russell W, Martin R: Sarcoma of soft tissue: Clinical and histopathologic parameteres and response to treatment. Cancer 35:1478, 1975.

2. MALIGNANT MESENCHYMOMA

This tumor consists of 2 or more anaplastic mesenchymal elements. It is the second most frequent soft tissue cancer. It may be found in any superficial soft tissue as well as viscera.

Since the most common differentiated element is the rhabdomyosarcoma, treatment is as above.

Mayer C & others: Malignant mesenchymoma in infants. Am J Dis Child 128:847, 1974.

3. FIBROSARCOMA

Fibrosarcoma may be found as a nodule of varying size which invades locally and may metastasize to the lung. It may be present at birth but more commonly is noted in the first year of life. A variant called neurilemoma, arising in the nerve sheath, may be seen in Recklinghausen's disease.

Surgical excision is the treatment of choice. The prognosis is good, though local recurrence and distant spread may occur. Patients may then be treated as rhabdomyosarcoma patients with drugs and radiation.

BRAIN TUMORS

Brain tumors comprise about 20% of malignant disease in pediatrics. Two-thirds of these tumors arise in the infratentorial region. The most common histologic types are cerebellar astrocytoma, medulloblastoma, and brain stem glioma. Symptoms may be generalized as a result of increased intracranial pressure secondary to obstruction of normal CSF flow or may be localized to the involved area of brain. In young children, the sutures may spread in response to increased pressure, and rapid head enlargement may occur. Headaches and vomiting—especially soon after rising in the morning—and lethargy are the most common symptoms of increased pressure. Papilledema is found in older children with increased pressure but may be absent in infants when the sutures spread to provide decompression.

In addition to a careful neurologic examination, skull x-rays, brain scan, and CT scan are important noninvasive diagnostic tests. Cerebral angiography and pneumoencephalograms contribute to precise tumor localization.

Therapy depends upon the tumor type. Cerebellar astrocytomas can often be totally excised, and no other therapy is indicated. With incomplete removal of more aggressive lesions, radiotherapy may be added. The 10-year survival rate is about 65%. Chemotherapy is not of proved effectiveness in primary management but may play a role in tumor recurrence.

Medulloblastoma is radiosensitive. Following surgery to reduce the tumor burden, radiation therapy is given to the primary and to the entire neuraxis because of the predilection of the tumor to metastasize to other areas of the brain and spinal cord via the CSF. This therapy may produce 25% 10-year survival rates. Chemotherapy trials with vincristine, nitrosoureas, podophyllin derivatives, and procarbazine as single agents and in various combinations are under way in an attempt to improve survival.

Brain stem gliomas are usually not amenable to operation, and biopsy may not be feasible. Radiation therapy may produce survivals ranging from a few months in high-grade tumors to 3–5 years in low-grade ones. Chemotherapy with nitrosoureas and methotrexate, either intrathecally or in high doses by the intravenous route, has caused tumor regression, but the role of drugs is not established.

Crist WM & others: Chemotherapy of childhood medulloblastoma. Am J Dis Child 130:639, 1976.

Mealey J, Hall PV: Medulloblastoma in children. J Neurosurg 46:56, 1977.

Shapiro WR: Chemotherapy of primary malignant tumors in children. Cancer 35:965, 1975.

Walker MD: Malignant brain tumors: A synopsis. CA 25:3, 1975.

Table 31—9. Antineoplastic agents commercially available in common use.

Agent	Dosage and Route	Indications	Toxicity
Cyclophosphamide (Cytoxan)	75—100 mg/sq m/day orally or 300 mg/sq m/week IV.	Leukemia, Hodgkin's lymphoma, neuroblastoma, sarcomas, retinoblastoma, hepatoma, rhabdomyosarcoma, Ewing's sarcoma.	Nausea, vomiting, anorexia, alopecia, bone marrow depression, hemorrhagic cystitis.
Cytarabine (cytosine arabinoside, Cytosar)	100—300 mg/sq m/week IV or IM; 5—50 mg/sq m once or twice weekly intrathecally for CNS leukemia until CSF clears.	Acute myeloblastic and acute lymphocytic leukemia.	Nausea, vomiting, anorexia, bone marrow depression, hepatotoxicity.
Dactinomycin (Cosmegen)	0.4 mg/sq m/week IV in 6 doses in phases with varying rest periods.	Wilms's tumor, sarcomas, rhabdomyosarcoma.	Nausea, vomiting, anorexia, bone marrow depression, alopecia, chemical dermatitis if leakage at intravenous site, tanning of skin if used with radiation therapy.
Doxorubicin (Adriamycin)	40—75 mg/sq m IV every 21 days, not to exceed 550 mg/sq m total dose.	Acute lymphoblastic and myelocytic leukemia, lymphoma, Hodgkin's, Wilms's, neuroblastoma; ovarian or thyroid carcinoma, Ewing's, osteogenic, rhabdomyosarcoma, other soft tissue sarcomas.	Alopecia, stomatitis, esophagitis, nausea, vomiting, severe chemical cellulitis and necrosis if extravasated; bone marrow suppression, myocardial damage if dose exceeds 550 mg/sq m; monitor ECG.
Fluorouracil (Efudex)	300—360 mg/sq m IV. Dosage should be scheduled based upon the specific disease stage. Maximum dose: 800 mg/day.	Hepatoma, gastrointestinal carcinoma.	Nausea, vomiting, oral ulceration, bone marrow depression, gastroenteritis, alopecia, anorexia.
Lomustine (CCNU, CeeNu)	100—130 mg/sq m orally every 6 weeks.	Brain tumors, Hodgkin's disease.	Nausea and vomiting, alopecia, stomatitis, hepatic toxicity. Bone marrow suppression with 4—6 week delay in onset.
Mercaptopurine (Purinethol)	50—100 mg/sq m/day orally.	Acute myeloblastic and acute lymphocytic leukemia.	Nausea, vomiting, rare oral ulcerations, bone marrow depression.
Methotrexate	15—20 mg/sq m orally twice a week until relapse. Give 12 mg/sq m/week intrathecally for CNS leukemia until CSF clears.	Acute lymphocytic leukemia, CNS leukemia, lymphomas, choriocarcinoma, brain tumors, Hodgkin's disease.	Oral ulcers, gastrointestinal irritation, bone marrow depression, hepatotoxicity. Do not use in presence of impaired renal function.
Prednisone	40 mg/sq m/day orally in 3 divided doses for 4—6 weeks.	Acute myeloblastic and lymphocytic leukemia, lymphoma, Hodgkin's disease, bone pain from metastatic disease, CNS tumors.	Increased appetite, sodium retention, hypertension, provocation of latent diabetes or tuberculosis, osteoporosis.
Procarbazine (Matulane)	100—125 mg/sq m/day orally for 4—6 weeks depending on schedule.	Hodgkin's disease, lymphomas.	Nausea, vomiting, anorexia, bone marrow depression (3-week delay). Do not give with narcotics or sedatives; has "disulfiram effect." Monitor liver and renal function.
Vincristine (Oncovin)	1.5 mg/sq m/week IV for 4—6 weeks, then every 2 weeks. Maximum dose: 2 mg.	Acute lymphocytic and myeloblastic leukemia, lymphoma (Hodgkin's), rhabdomyosarcoma, Wilms's tumor, neuroblastoma, Ewing's sarcoma, retinoblastoma, hepatoma, sarcomas, osteosarcoma, brain tumors.	Alopecia, constipation, abdominal cramps, jaw pain, paresthesia, myalgia and muscle weakness, neurotoxicity, decrease in deep tendon reflexes, chemical dermatitis. Do not use in presence of severe liver impairment.

BONE TUMORS

A variety of benign and malignant tumors may originate in bone. Bones are also common sites of metastatic disease. The principal symptoms of bone tumors, whether primary or metastatic, are pain and swelling. A fracture may first call attention to an area of cortical destruction due to cancer. The diagnosis must be based on careful and complete clinical evaluation and examination of an adequate biopsy specimen. Two tumor types are sufficiently common to warrant specific discussion.

Ewing's sarcoma occurs most commonly in the long bones of the lower extremities and in the pelvis. Radiographically, it shows cortical bone destruction, often with periosteal elevation and an "onion skin" appearance beneath the periosteum. It must be differentiated from neuroblastoma, rhabdomyosarcoma, and non-Hodgkin's lymphoma. Metastasis occurs to other bones and to the lungs and may be present at diagnosis in one-third of patients. Ewing's sarcoma is treated with radiation doses of 6000–8000 rads over a 6- to 8-week period and with combination chemotherapy for 2 years employing vincristine, cyclophosphamide, and doxorubicin, with dactinomycin substituting for doxorubicin after a dose of 300–400 mg/sq m of the latter has been given. If metastatic lesions are present, these are also irradiated. In patients without overt metastasis, 75% or more should live 3 years with no evidence of recurrent disease.

Osteogenic sarcoma is the most common malignant bone tumor in the pediatric age group. It is most frequently seen during adolescence and usually occurs in long bones, with the distal femur, proximal tibia, and proximal humerus being the most common sites. The diagnosis is made by biopsy, and the therapeutic approach is jointly planned after a careful review of the x-ray and histologic findings and the bone scan results.

Therapy for this tumor is undergoing rapid change. The traditional and still most widely used surgical approach is amputation above the joint proximal to the involved bone or, in the case of femoral lesions, disarticulation of the hip. This is followed by intensive chemotherapy with vincristine, high doses of methotrexate with folinic acid rescue, and doxorubicin. Chemotherapy extends over a period of 2 years. In some centers, carefully selected patients are being treated either with 10,000 rads of electron beam therapy to the entire bone containing the primary or by en bloc resection of the tumor followed by prosthetic replacement in an attempt to avoid the problems of amputation. Current results indicate that aggressive chemotherapy and surgery with or without irradiation may permit a 2-year disease-free survival of 60%.

Jaffe N: The potential of combined modality approaches for the treatment of malignant bone tumors in children. Cancer Treatment Rev 2:33, 1975.

Nesbit ME: Ewing's sarcoma. CA 26:174, 1976.

Rosen G & others: Chemotherapy resection and prosthetic bone replacement in the treatment of osteogenic sarcoma. Cancer 37:1, 1976.

Sutow WW & others: Multidrug chemotherapy in the primary treatment of osteosarcoma. J Bone Joint Surg 58A:629, 1976.

● ● ●

General References

Evans AE: Pediatric tumors. Semin Oncol 1:1, March 1974. [Entire issue.]

Evans AE, D'Angio GJ, Koop CE (editors): Symposium on pediatric oncology. Pediatr Clin North Am 23:1, Feb 1976. [Entire issue.]

Franhauser R, Luginbuhl H, McGrath J: Tumors of the nervous system. Bull WHO 50:53, 1974.

Holland J, Frei E: *Cancer Medicine.* Lea & Febiger, 1973.

Jones PG, Campbell PE: *Tumours of Infancy and Childhood.* Lippincott, 1976.

Pochedly C (editor): Cancer in childhood I. Pediatr Ann 3:6, May 1974. [Entire issue.]

Pochedly C (editor): Cancer in childhood II. Pediatr Ann 3:4, June 1974 [Entire issue.]

Proceedings of the American Cancer Society's National Conference on Childhood Cancer. Cancer 35 (Suppl):863, 1975.

Sutow W, Vietti T, Fernbach D: *Clinical Pediatric Oncology.* Mosby, 1973.

32...
Allergic Disorders

David S. Pearlman, MD

Allergic disorders include a variety of local and systemic manifestations which commonly are ultimate expressions of the union between antigen and antibody. Although this union triggers the chain of events that culminates in the clinical allergic reaction, nonimmunologic factors are important in modifying this chain of events. In some instances, nonimmunologic factors can be completely responsible for clinical reactions indistinguishable from immunologically induced reactions (eg, urticaria caused by histamine-releasing drugs such as codeine and polymyxin B).

Allergic reactivity is normal. The reaction that results from the transfusion of mismatched blood is an allergic reaction; the repeated injection of antitoxin in the form of foreign serum often leads to the development of serum sickness; and contact with poison ivy frequently causes an allergic dermatitis. Some forms of allergic reactivity, however, occur only in certain members of the population. These disorders (which include allergic rhinitis, asthma, and atopic dermatitis) are called *atopic disorders,* signifying an unusual form of reactivity for which there is some unknown predisposition.

GENERAL PRINCIPLES OF DIAGNOSIS

By definition, allergic reactions stem from an antigen-antibody interaction; identification of these participants is of prime importance both in the diagnosis and in the therapy of allergic disorders. It is often difficult to identify the antigens (allergens) responsible for a particular clinical disorder, but the most helpful procedure by far is a thorough and detailed history. Tests for the presence of a specific antibody which will implicate specific allergens are helpful but are never a substitute for a thorough history.

Antibodies differ in their biologic activities. Since certain types of antibodies are involved in some disorders and others in different disorders, it is essential to select the appropriate immunologic test for the disorder being investigated. In atopic disorders, reaginic or skin-sensitizing antibody is important.* The usual immunologic test for this type of antibody is the scratch or intradermal skin test. In this test, the union of skin-sensitizing antibody with antigen is responsible for the liberation of histamine, which in turn induces local vasodilatation and edema with consequent wheal and erythema ("hive") formation. As with all immunologic tests, the presence of antibody does not itself signify its clinical importance since antibody can often be identified in the absence of any clinical symptoms. When correlated with the history, however, the results of skin tests for this type of antibody can be highly informative.

Skin-sensitizing antibody plays no significant role in contact dermatitis. In this type of disorder, cellular immunity (delayed hypersensitivity), which also characterizes the tuberculin reaction, is responsible. Unlike the wheal and erythema response, delayed hypersensitivity reactions are characterized by infiltration around the allergen of a variety of cells, including sensitized lymphoid cells, which cause tissue destruction by other mechanisms. In contact dermatitis, "patch testing" (placing the suspected allergen in direct contact with the skin for 24—48 hours under cover of a "patch") is used to detect the presence of specific sensitivity to the allergen.

The presence of a particular antibody does not always identify the cause of a given allergic disorder, ie, the presence of antibody is necessary but not in itself sufficient to produce allergic symptoms. The suspicion of the clinical importance of an allergen, however, may be confirmed by the use of a "provocative test," ie, challenging a given individual with the suspected allergen and observing the response. In a sense, "patch testing" in contact dermatitis is a provocative test since this is both the route of sensitization and the point of reaction. Inhalation of pollens and molds by patients with asthma or hay fever and the feeding of milk to patients with suspected milk allergy are other examples of provocative tests. However, since allergic sensitivity can be inordinately great, provocative testing is potentially dangerous and should not be used routinely. Provocative tests may prove a relationship between the provoking substance and a clinical reaction, but they do not necessarily establish that the reaction is allergic. For example, in children with lactase deficiency, milk may elicit gastrointestinal symptoms similar to those of milk allergy.

*The major portion of reaginic antibody activity appears to reside in the IgE fraction, and IgE levels are often elevated in atopic disorders.

GENERAL PRINCIPLES OF TREATMENT

Environmental Control of Exposure

Since the clinical allergic reaction stems from the union of antigen with antibody, avoidance of the offending antigen is the most effective means of therapy of all allergic disorders. In many instances, complete avoidance of identified allergens is impossible, but it is frequently feasible to reduce the incidence and severity of reactions by minimizing the contact. Many nonimmunologic factors can precipitate or aggravate atopic disorders (eg, irritating smoke, or cold air in asthma) and avoidance of such known or suspected irritants is also of prime importance in the therapy of allergic disorders.

Sample directions for environmental control of common allergens. The following refers mainly to the patient's bedroom, but the principles are applicable to the rest of the house as well.

(1) House dust is a common offender. The accumulation of dust may be minimized by the avoidance of dust catchers and dust producers such as wool (in rugs, blankets), flannel (in bedding, pajamas), upholstered furniture, toys stuffed with plant or animal products, chenille (bedspreads, drapes, and rugs), cotton quilts, stuffed cotton pads, and venetian blinds.

(2) Rooms should be dusted daily with a damp or oiled cloth. The room should be cleaned thoroughly at least once a week—never with the patient present.

(3) All forced air ducts, which frequently contain dust and molds and tend to stir up room dust, should be sealed off. An electric radiator may be substituted as a source of heat, if necessary. If pollenosis is a problem, windows should be kept closed during the pollen seasons. Air cleaners (central or room) and refrigerated air conditioners may be usefully employed. Automatic humidifiers with provision for humidity not to exceed 40% can be helpful in dry climates and winter time heating systems.

(4) Plant products (kapok, cotton) and animal products (feathers, horse and cow hairs) commonly used for pillows, stuffing of furniture, toys, bedding, and hair pads for rugs should be eliminated. Alternatively, all mattresses, box springs, and pillows in the bedroom should be completely enclosed in impermeable plastic or rubber casings. Inexpensive casings may be obtained from department stores; better quality encasings may be obtained from Allergy-Free Products for the Home, 1162 West Lynn, Springfield, Missouri 65802, or 224 Livingston Street, Brooklyn, NY 11201; or from Allergen-Proof Encasings, Inc, 1450 E 363rd Street, Eastlake, Ohio 44094. Especially if plastic casings are used, they should be checked periodically for tears or punctures. Furniture, bedding, and clothes stuffed solely with synthetic products (eg, Dacron pillows) or rubber are permissible; the latter, however, may harbor molds. Toys stuffed with old nylon stockings or synthetic foam, with plain nonfuzzy cotton or synthetic coverings, are very satisfactory.

(5) Cleaning equipment, wool, and fur coats should not be kept in or near the child's room or closet.

(6) Basements and attics, particularly if unfinished, are forbidden territory for an atopic child.

(7) Sensitization to animals develops so frequently in atopic individuals that close contact with animals of any sort should be avoided. If there is any reason to suspect already existing sensitivity, it is important to rid the environment completely of animals.

Hyposensitization

If avoidance of offensive allergens is not possible, specific hyposensitization is sometimes attempted. The value of hyposensitization is limited mainly to atopic disorders and to severe insect allergy. There are a variety of hyposensitization procedures, but the same general principle applies to all: Extremely small amounts of allergen are injected subcutaneously at frequent intervals and in increasing amounts until a "top dose" is reached; this is usually the highest tolerated dose of a given allergen extract, or that amount which induces a state of clinical hyporeactivity to the allergen as demonstrated after natural contact. When perennial therapy is adopted, the top tolerated dose is used as a maintenance dose, with carefully regulated lengthening of intervals (by not more than an additional week at a time) up to 6 weeks, as tolerated.

Most allergists agree that the majority of well selected patients with pollen asthma (or hay fever) are significantly improved after 1–2 years of therapy on a "perennial" injection regimen of aqueous antigens, and there is evidence to substantiate the beneficial effects of hyposensitization even in perennial asthma. The effectiveness of therapy is dose-related. Repository therapy using alum-precipitated extracts (Allpyral, Center-Al) are useful mainly in increasing the antigen dosage in individuals who are extremely sensitive to small amounts of aqueous antigen. Theoretically, fewer injections of alum-precipitated material are required to reach a maintenance dose of antigen, and maintenance injections need to be given less frequently. However, information on the efficacy of this form of therapy is not as complete as that relating to aqueous therapy. Mold hyposensitization therapy is believed to offer significant protection, but adequate documentation of this is lacking. The value of hyposensitization against house dusts is substantiated; it appears beneficial but is no substitute for good environmental control. The use of bacterial extracts is controversial; the rationale for their effectiveness consists mainly of testimonial evidence, and the good results reported have not been duplicated in well-controlled studies.

Drug Therapy (Table 32–1)

A variety of drugs are effective in the treatment of allergic disorders. However, inappropriate use of drugs may aggravate the reaction, and a thorough understanding of the pharmacologic actions of these drugs is essential. The principal groups include adrenergic agents, antihistamines, methyl xanthines, expec-

Table 32—1. Preparations and dosages of drugs commonly used in allergic disorders.

Agent	Dosage
Adrenergic agents	
Epinephrine aqueous, 1:1000	0.01 ml/kg subcut or IM up to 0.25 ml. (May repeat at 20-minute intervals—total of 3 doses.)
Terbutaline (Bricanyl)	0.01 ml/kg subcut or IM up to 0.25 ml. (May repeat at 20-minute intervals—total of 2 doses.)
Sus-Phrine 1:200	0.1—0.2 ml subcut every 8—12 hours. (Shake well before administering.)
Ephedrine sulfate	0.5—1 mg/kg/dose orally, 4—6 times a day.
Pseudoephedrine hydrochloride (Sudafed)	1 mg/kg/dose orally, 4—6 times a day.
Metaproterenol (Alupent, Metaprel)	10—20 mg every 6—8 hours.
Terbutaline (Brethine, Bricanyl)	2.5 mg every 8 hours. (Not recommended for persons under age 12 by the manufacturer.)
Adrenergic aerosols	
Isoproterenol sulfate (Medihaler-Iso)	1—2 inhalations from pressurized aerosol. May use as often as once every 3—4 hours but not on a regular basis. *Avoid excessive use.*
Isoproterenol hydrochloride (Isuprel Mistometer, Norisodrine)	
Isoproterenol hydrochloride plus phenylephrine (Duo-Medihaler)	
Isoetharine methanesulfonate (Bronkometer)	
Metaproterenol (Alupent, Metaprel) (not recommended for persons under age 12 by the manufacturer)	
Isoetharine, 1% (Bronkosol-II)	0.25—0.5 ml diluted with 1 ml water and administered by hand or compressor-driven nebulizer.
Isoproterenol hydrochloride solution, 1:200, for nebulization	4—5 drops diluted with 1 ml water and administered by hand or compressor-driven nebulizer.
Drugs with antihistaminic activity	
Diphenhydramine hydrochloride (Benadryl)	1 mg/kg/dose orally, 4 times a day.
Injectable	25—50 mg IV (slowly) or IM (ampules, 50 mg/ml; vials, 10 mg/ml).
Chlorpheniramine maleate (Chlor-Trimeton)	0.1 mg/kg/dose orally, 4 times a day.
(Teldrin, Chlor-Trimeton Repetabs)	0.1—0.2 mg/kg/dose orally, twice a day.
Injectable	4—8 mg IV (slowly) or IM (10 mg/ml in 1 ml vials; 100 mg/ml in 2 ml vials).
Brompheniramine maleate (Dimetane)	0.1 mg/kg/dose orally, 4 times a day.
Tripelennamine hydrochloride (Pyribenzamine)	0.5—1 mg/kg/dose orally, 4 times a day.
Hydroxyzine (Atarax, Vistaril)	0.2—0.5 mg/kg/dose orally, 3 times a day.
Cyproheptadine (Periactin)	0.05 mg/kg/dose orally, 3—4 times a day.
Combination drugs for allergic rhinitis and conjunctivitis	
Phenylephrine and chlorpheniramine (Novahistine)	Elixir: ½—1 tsp every 4 hours. Forte capsules: 1 capsule every 8 hours (older children).
Pseudoephedrine and triprolidine (Actifed)	Syrup: ½—2 tsp 3 times a day depending on age. Tablets: ½—1 tablet 3 times a day depending on age.
Pseudoephedrine and carbinoxamine (Rondec)	Drops: ¼—1 dropperful, 4 times a day (infants). Syrup: ½—1 tsp, 4 times a day (older children). Tablets: ½—1 tablet 4 times a day (older children).
Phenylpropanolamine, pyrilamine, and pheniramine (Triaminic)	Drops: 5—10 drops 3 times a day (infants). Syrup: ½—2 tsp, 4 times a day depending on age. Juvulets: 1—2 tablets, 4 times a day (older children).
Sedatives	
Chloral hydrate	15 mg/kg orally or rectally every 6—8 hours (maximum, 1 gm/dose).
Expectorants	
Potassium iodide, saturated solution (1 gm KI/ml)	25 mg/kg/day orally in 3—4 doses.
Guaifenesin (glyceryl guaiacolate, Robitussin)	1 tsp every 4—6 hours.
Xanthines	
Aminophylline, theophylline (Choledyl, Elixophylline, Quibron, Slo-phyllin, Theodur, Theospan)	IV: 4—6 mg*/kg every 4—6 hours (infuse over 10- to 20-minute period). Oral: 4—6 mg*/kg every 6 hours. Longer acting preparations (eg, Choledyl Caps or Slo-phyllin Gyrocaps) can be used every 8—12 hours. Rectal: Enema, Fleet's or Somophylline, 4—6 mg*/kg every 6 hours.

*Refers to theophylline dose.

Table 32—1 (cont'd). Preparations and dosages of drugs commonly used in allergic disorders.

Agent	Dosage
Adrenal glucocorticoids	
Most rapid therapeutic effect follows intravenous or oral administration, but there may be no perceptible effect for hours. In acute situations, high doses of corticosteroids (eg, 100–200 mg hydrocortisone or 40–80 mg Solu-Medrol every 4–6 hours) are generally employed the first day and the dose tapered as rapidly as possible to maintenance levels or withdrawn completely.	
Approximate equivalents of activity: 100 mg hydrocortisone = 4 mg dexamethasone = 25 mg prednisolone = 20 mg methylprednisolone.	
Intravenous preparations	
Hydrocortisone sodium succinate (Solu-Cortef)	100 mg vials.
Dexamethasone-21-phosphate (Decadron)	Each ml contains 4 mg dexamethasone-21-phosphate (in 1 ml and 5 ml vials).
Methylprednisolone (Solu-Medrol)	40 mg/ml in 1 ml vials.
Prednisolone-21-phosphate (Hydeltrasol)	20 mg/ml in 2 and 5 ml vials.
Dermatologic preparations	
Fluocinolone acetonide (Synalar)	0.025% cream or ointment and 0.01% cream.
Flurandrenolone (Cordran)	0.05% and 0.025%.
Cort-Dome cream	0.125% up to 2% hydrocortisone in acid mantle base.
Topical inhalational preparations (for steroid-dependent asthma)	
Beclomethasone dipropionate (Vanceril)	Not to exceed 3 inhalations (150 μg 4 times a day). (Generally not recommended under 6 years of age.)
Cromolyn sodium (Aarane, Intal)	20 mg capsules—1 capsule by inhalation 4 times a day or just prior to exercise or contact with other asthma precipitating agents (preventive only). (Not recommended by manufacturer for children under 5 years.)

torants, oxygen, and adrenal corticosteroids. The selection of drugs obviously depends upon the pathologic processes involved.

A. Adrenergic Agents: As a group, adrenergic agents exhibit many different pharmacologic effects. Their usefulness in allergic disorders depends mainly on their ability to constrict blood vessels and relax other smooth muscle. The manifestations of many allergic reactions are due, at least in part, to chemical mediators such as histamine and acetylcholine which produce varying degrees of vasodilatation, edema, and smooth muscle spasm. Adrenergic agents are the principal pharmacologic antagonists of these chemical mediators and at times may even reverse their effects completely. However, the pharmacologic properties of adrenergic drugs as a group are not shared uniformly by all members of the group, and these drugs cannot be used interchangeably to produce a given effect. In rhinitis, for example, phenylephrine, an effective vasoconstrictor but a poor smooth muscle dilator, would be especially useful. Isoproterenol, on the other hand, although devoid of vasoconstrictor action, is the most effective bronchodilator of the group and is useful in asthma. In asthma and in anaphylaxis—in which vasodilatation, edema, and asthma may all be a problem—epinephrine, which is a potent antagonist of all of these effects, is the drug of choice.

Adrenergic drugs are not always effective in a given disorder and are not without undesirable effects. Epinephrine resistance may occur in severe asthma, for example, and its use in such cases may actually aggravate the disorder by increasing the patient's anxiety and contributing to venous congestion and mucus plug-

ging. The injection of epinephrine in the face of severe hypoxemia and acidosis may produce cardiac arrhythmia or arrest. Adrenergic aerosols, although frequently effective in acute asthma, may also severely aggravate asthma if used excessively. Aerosols containing adrenergic drugs should be used cautiously and only as adjuncts to other appropriate pharmacologic management of asthmatic patients.

B. Antihistamines: The antihistamines act through competition with histamine for receptor sites, thereby preventing histamine from exerting its activity. Antihistamines are particularly useful in urticaria, anaphylaxis, and allergic rhinitis; for reasons not well understood, they may not be effective in certain other syndromes such as asthma and atopic dermatitis, in which vascular reactions are certainly involved. Although antihistamines may be very useful in severe allergic disorders, they are not the drug of first choice in medical emergencies due to allergic reactions but may be administered after epinephrine has been given. Antihistamines have antipruritic properties, however, and are useful in atopic dermatitis and in contact dermatitis, in which histamine may play a major role. The sedation which occurs as a side-effect, although undesirable in many instances, may be an advantage in others.

The transition between the antihistamines and the anticholinergic group of drugs is a subtle one, and many agents classified as one have both actions. For example, antihistamines in general have a mild atropine-like drying effect; and many tranquilizers, particularly the phenothiazines and hydroxyzine (Atarax), are especially good antihistamines. Because of their antihistaminic actions, these tranquilizers have been found useful in some conditions in which antihistamines are helpful (eg, urticaria).

C. **Methyl Xanthines:** Theophylline and its ethylenediamine derivative, aminophylline, are effective bronchodilators which appear to act at a different point but in the same pathway through which epinephrine exerts its smooth muscle dilating effect. The improper use of these agents has been associated with severe toxic reactions, in some cases resulting in death. Overdosage frequently occurs following the use of rectal suppositories and as a result of failure to appreciate the variability of rate and extent of absorption with different routes of administration. Toxic reactions include headache, palpitations, dizziness, stomach ache, nausea and vomiting, excessive thirst, and hypotension. *Nausea and stomach ache may be related to the alcohol or other vehicle used for the drug but can also represent a CNS-mediated toxic effect of the drug.* The diuretic action of theophylline or aminophylline should always be kept in mind when calculating fluid needs, particularly since dehydration may be part of the clinical problem in an asthmatic attack. When used properly, theophylline and aminophylline are valuable drugs with a bronchodilating effect equal to that of any of the adrenergic agents. There is great individual variation in the metabolism of methyl xanthines, and dosage must be highly individualized. Optimal therapeutic blood levels of theophylline are considered to be between $10-20$ $\mu g/ml$ serum or plasma, with levels over 20 $\mu g/ml$ more likely to be associated with drug toxicity. Average dosages likely to achieve levels in this range are 25 ± 5 mg/kg/day until about age 8, then 20 ± 5 mg/kg/day until about age 16; thereafter, average daily dosage is closer to 12 ± 3 mg. The daily dosage can be divided into $3-4$ doses (every $6-8$ hours).

Rectal administration of theophylline in fluid form usually results in prompt and efficient absorption of the drug that may be almost as efficient as intravenous administration. Absorption from rectal suppositories tends to be slow and erratic. Effective drug levels can be achieved by the oral route, and the oral route is the route of choice for chronic administration of methyl xanthines.

D. **Expectorants:** Expectorants such as iodides and guaifenesin (glyceryl guaiacolate) are used mainly in bronchial asthma to liquefy thick, tenacious mucus, but it is not clear whether the therapeutic effectiveness of these agents is in fact due to their expectorant action. Iodides seem more effective than guaifenesin and are relatively nontoxic, but—especially with prolonged use—goiter, salivary gland inflammation, gastric irritation, skin eruptions, and acne may occur. Acne is rarely provoked before adolescence. *Note:* It is important to keep in mind that adequate hydration is essential to effective expectoration. In general, expectorant preparations containing narcotics should not be used in asthma.

E. **Corticosteroids:** Adrenal glucocorticoids have been used in the treatment of all of the allergic disorders. Their effectiveness is apparently due to their "anti-inflammatory" actions. They are most useful in disorders of delayed hypersensitivity (such as contact dermatitis) and in asthma. The untoward side-effects of prolonged corticosteroid administration (eg, growth suppression, myopathy, Cushing's syndrome, hypertension, peptic ulcer [controversial], diabetes, and electrolyte imbalance) limit their use mainly to those conditions that are refractory to other measures or are life-threatening. Even then, however, their slow onset of action (even when given intravenously) precludes first-choice administration of these drugs in acute allergic emergencies. Most allergic syndromes are amenable to other forms of therapy, and the systemic use of the corticosteroids usually is unnecessary. When chronic use is necessary, alternate-day corticosteroid therapy with a short-acting preparation (eg, prednisone) in the early morning every other day should be attempted. Alternatively, for asthma, beclomethasone by inhalation can be considered. There are virtually no advantages to the use of corticotropin over the glucocorticoids themselves when glucocorticoid action is deemed necessary in treating allergic disorders.

The main indications for the use of systemic corticosteroids are severe, acute life-threatening asthma and control of chronic severe disorders such as asthma and atopic dermatitis which are refractory to other appropriate therapy. In some instances, administration of a short course of corticosteroids for self-limiting allergic disorders (eg, serum sickness) may be warranted.

Topical corticosteroids are extremely effective anti-inflammatory agents in the control of allergic dermatitis—mainly contact dermatitis and atopic dermatitis. Topical application is the preferred route of administration in such disorders. Of particular promise in the treatment of chronic asthma are adrenergic aerosols such as beclomethasone dipropionate (Vanceril). Other similar agents such as flunisolide, betamethasone valerate, and triamcinolone acetonide are being tested or are available outside the USA for use in asthma or allergic rhinitis.

F. **Sedatives:** Sedatives have been grossly misused in asthma and have been responsible for the deaths of some asthmatics. Although the psyche undoubtedly exerts a significant influence on asthma and other allergic disorders, the anxiety associated with extreme asthma is more often a reflection of the severity of the respiratory distress than the main cause of it. Sedatives which suppress the respiratory center (as the barbiturates do) should not be used in the therapy of severe asthma. If sedatives are necessary, chloral hydrate may be used (Table 32–1).

G. **Oxygen:** Oxygen is extremely important in the treatment of severe asthma. Hypoxemia usually occurs early in the course of moderately severe or severe asthma, much in advance of any detectable cyanosis. Oxygen is potentially very drying and should be humidified when administered. Excessively high concentrations of oxygen should be avoided since they can lead to atelectasis or lessening of respiratory drive.

H. Antibiotics: There are no special indications for the use of antibiotics in allergic disorders. Antibiotics should of course be used when evidence of bacterial infection exists. However, their excessive use in children with allergic disorders should be avoided to reduce the risk of sensitization to these drugs.

Erythromycin seems to be one of the least sensitizing antibiotics and offers good coverage against many respiratory pathogens.

I. Cromolyn Sodium (Aarane, Intal): This drug is an adjunct in the management of severe asthma. Its mode of action is to block release of pharmacologic mediators such as histamine resulting from antigen-antibody interaction, and it is useful in the prevention of chronic severe asthma. However, it does not reverse tissue changes induced by these mediators and is therefore of no value in the treatment of acute asthmatic paroxysms. It is useful in blocking exercise-induced asthma. It currently is undergoing trials for use in preventing food-induced allergic reactions, allergic rhinitis, and conjunctivitis, with promising results.

Avner SE: β-Adrenergic bronchodilators. Pediatr Clin North Am 22:129, 1975.

Falliers CJ: Cromolyn sodium (disodium cromoglycate) prophylaxis. Pediatr Clin North Am 22:141, 1975.

Johnstone DE: The case for hyposensitization: Its rationale and justification. Pediatr Clin North Am 22:239, 1975.

Leifer KN, Wittig HJ: The beta-2 sympathomimetic aerosols in the treatment of asthma. Ann Allergy 35:69, 1975.

Morris H: Corticosteroids in asthma. Pages 105–130 in: *Annual Review of Allergy, 1972.* Frazier CA (editor). Medical Examination Publishing Co., 1973.

Norman PS: Specific therapy in allergy. Med Clin North Am 58:111, 1974.

Pearlman DS: Allergic disorders. Chap 19, pages 333–369, in *Immunologic Disorders in Infants and Children.* Stiehm ER, Fulginiti VA (editors). Saunders, 1973.

Pearlman DS: Antihistamines: Pharmacology and clinical use. Drugs 12:258, 1976.

Pearlman DS: Rationale for therapy of allergic disorders. Pediatr Clin North Am 22:101, 1975.

MEDICAL EMERGENCIES DUE TO ALLERGIC REACTIONS

Skin testing, hyposensitization with allergen extracts, drugs, vaccines, toxoids, sera, blood transfusions, and insect bites and stings are the most common causes of severe allergic reactions. Anaphylactic shock, angioedema, and bronchial obstruction, alone or in combination, are the principal life-threatening manifestations of severe allergic reactions. Lightheadedness, paresthesias, sweating, flushing, palpitations, and urticaria may precede or accompany severe reactions.

Prevention

Prevention consists mainly of avoiding allergens known or believed to be responsible for allergic reactions. A history suggestive of a reaction to a given drug is an indication for the selection of an alternative and unrelated drug for therapeutic use. Skin tests should be performed *cautiously* before foreign serum is administered.

Treatment

A. Emergency Measures: Immediate treatment is essential for successful management of these reactions.

1. Epinephrine, 1:1000, 0.2–0.4 ml, should be injected IM without delay. This may be repeated at intervals of 15–20 minutes as necessary. If the reaction is due to the recent injection of a drug, serum, or other substance, a tourniquet should be applied proximal to the injection. If the offending substance has been injected intradermally or subcutaneously, absorption of the material may be delayed further by injecting epinephrine, 0.1 ml subcut, near the site of injection. Subsequent therapy depends partly upon the response.

2. Antihistamines (Table 32–1) should be given intramuscularly or intravenously. When intravenous infusions are used, they should be given over a period of 5–10 minutes since untoward reactions, particularly hypotension, have been induced by too rapid administration.

3. Theophylline is useful when bronchospasm occurs. Further treatment of bronchial obstruction is discussed under Asthma.

4. Tracheostomy may be lifesaving in cases of profound laryngeal edema.

5. Fluids—Since anaphylactic shock is in part produced by hypovolemia secondary to massive exudation of intravascular fluid, maintenance of a proper volume by intravenous fluids (isotonic saline, 5% dextrose in water, or 5% dextrose in saline) is particularly important.

B. Follow-Up Measures:

1. Adrenal corticosteroids have little place in the treatment of acute reactions but may be employed with persistent severe reactions. The onset of action of these drugs is slow (hours, even by intravenous administration). If used, they should be given only after epinephrine and antihistamines have been administered.

2. Mild sedation may also be indicated.

C. Hyposensitization for Insect Bites: Individuals who have experienced serious reactions following an insect sting should be hyposensitized. A polyvalent vaccine consisting of bee, wasp, yellow jacket, and hornet antigens is commercially available and is recommended over species-specific antigen. The efficacy of whole body extract vaccines, which contain little undenatured venom, has recently been questioned. Unfortunately, venom is not commercially available for treatment. Hypersensitivity to insect allergens is often so great that testing and therapy are best left to physicians experienced in dealing with insect allergy. Treatment kits for anaphylactic reactions should be available for immediate use in individuals with insect hypersensitivity and should be kept in the home or taken along by a responsible person when the sensitive person travels in an area likely to be infested with the offensive insects. The single most important item in such a kit is epinephrine.

Barr SE: Insect sting allergy. Cutis 17:1069, 1976.

Kelly JF, Patterson R: Anaphylaxis: Course, mechanisms, and treatment. JAMA 227:1431, 1974.

Reisman RE, Arbesman CE: Stinging insect allergy: Current concepts and problems. Pediatr Clin North Am 22:185, 1975.

ATOPIC DISORDERS*

Certain individuals are predisposed to allergic rhinitis, asthma, or atopic dermatitis. The incidence tends to be familial, but little is known about the constitutional factors responsible. Sensitization is usually to substances considered to be innocuous for other people. Animal danders, feathers, kapok (used as stuffing in mattresses and toys), and house dusts are the most common perennial allergens. Emanations of house dust mites (high in mattress flock) and of cockroaches (abundant in poor housing situations) may be important factors contributing to the allergenicity of house dust. Many varieties of trees, grass and weed pollens, and molds cause atopic disorders in a more or less seasonal incidence. Foods and a number of other substances may contribute to perennial or seasonal problems. Atopic individuals commonly become sensitized to one or more of these sensitizing substances, and "environmental control" (see above) is therefore recommended for any child with an atopic syndrome. Particular emphasis is placed on the bedroom.

Diagnosis

The diagnosis of atopic disease is based primarily on the clinical findings. Laboratory procedures (including skin testing) can be very helpful but should be interpreted in the light of the history and physical findings. To arrive at a diagnosis of any or all atopic diseases, a detailed history and complete physical examination are essential. More than one atopic disease (precipitated in many instances by the same allergens) may be present, and a history of familial atopic disorders or of other past or present atopic symptoms is especially useful. The following is a guideline for the overall history and physical examination. Indicated laboratory procedures will be included under individual atopic diseases.

A. **History:**

1. Chief complaint of patient.

2. Specific allergen sensitivity, or any atopic disease in other family members, past or present (asthma, allergic rhinitis, atopic dermatitis).

3. Details of development of first episode (eg, infection), change in environment (family move,

*Atopic dermatitis is discussed in Chapter 8.

acquisition of pets or toys, different household furnishings), season of year, ingestion of "new" food, special occasions, emotional and social upheavals.

4. Circumstances of subsequent and most recent episodes (as above).

5. Associated atopic or other allergic diseases (past or present), especially allergic rhinitis, bronchial asthma, "allergic cough," atopic dermatitis, food intolerance, "allergic rashes," angioedema.

6. History of pneumonia, bronchiolitis, "croup," recurrent ear infections, sinusitis, removal of tonsils and adenoids.

7. Food-related symptoms, eg, vomiting, colic, diarrhea, abnormal stools, abdominal pain, skin rashes, headache.

8. Presence of "continuity symptoms," eg, itchy or stuffy nose, night cough, breathlessness, cough or wheezing (with exercise, laughter, crying, "frustration"), fatigue, irritability.

9. Wheezing, cough, rashes, or nose, ear, or eye symptoms following contact with the following:

a. Animals, especially house pets and household furnishings or clothing of animal origin (feather pillows, hair rug pads, mohair [goat], felt [rabbit and cow hair], wool).

b. Seasonal agents—In winter, predominantly house dust and respiratory infections; in spring, trees; in late spring to early summer, grasses; in late summer to early fall, weeds.

c. Seasonal sources of pollen, eg, flowers, grass mowing, harvesting, play or work in weed patches.

d. Mold, eg, outside seasonal molds (wet, warm periods), moldy foods, mildew, old storage areas (attics, damp basements).

e. Cosmetics, eg, bubble bath, hair spray, facial cosmetics, shampoos, soaps, enzyme detergents.

10. Emotional and social factors and habits—Family structure, general attitudes and behavior; family, school, and social adjustments; temper tantrums, enuresis.

B. **Physical Examination:** A complete physical examination is essential. The following signs deserve special emphasis:

1. General appearance for state of nourishment and physical development, including weight and height; degree of activity; signs of fatigue; sneezing; cough and its character; dyspnea.

2. Attitudes, responses, and relationships of patient to parents, physician, nurses, etc; general level of intelligence.

3. Vital signs—Blood pressure, temperature, pulse rate, and character of respirations.

4. Skin—Rashes, pallor, cyanosis, temperature changes, sweating, degree of dryness.

5. Eyes—"Allergic pleats" (lower lid edema, eye-shadowing), conjunctival injection, blebs, itching, cataracts (in severe, long-standing atopic dermatitis), blepharitis (from chronic rubbing), tearing.

6. Nose—Itching ("allergic salute," "bunny nose," nasal crease), excoriation of nares, hyperemia, mucosal edema, polypoid changes, purplish pallor,

excessive serous or mucoid discharge.

7. Ears—With allergic rhinitis, retraction of drums; with recurrent serous otitis media, hearing loss, changes in drum (immobility, distortion, retraction, fullness, opacity, narrow and "chalky" malleus), evidence of fluid in middle ear; discharge in canal uncommon.

8. Mouth—For palatal malformations, character of speech, "canker sores," changes in tongue (geographism, grooving).

9. Throat—Presence and appearance of tonsils and pharyngeal lymphoid tissue, appearance of mucosal epithelium (anterior pillars, soft palate, pharyngeal wall), nasopharyngeal secretions.

10. Chest—Configuration ("barrel chest," "pigeon breast," prominent Harrison's grooves—all may be present in long-standing asthma), evidence of hyperinflation, pattern of breathing, development and use of accessory muscles for respiration (eg, hypertrophy of pectorals, trapezii, sternocleidomastoids), retractions.

11. Lungs—Relationship to inspiratory-expiratory cycle of gross or auscultatory wheezes (including after exercise and forced expiration), rhonchi and their pitch, rales, degree and equality of air exchange; degree of resonance and level and movement of diaphragm.

12. Heart—Tachycardia, size, accentuation of pulmonic second sound (for evidence of pulmonary hypertension in asthma).

13. External genitalia—Vulvitis (girls in pollen season), meatal ulcer (boys with contact dermatitis).

14. Signs of associated infections—Pyoderma, purulent nasal or ear discharge, purulent bronchial secretions, significant adenopathy.

C. Supplementary Diagnostic Procedures:

1. Skin tests—In all atopic disorders, skin testing for the presence of reaginic antibody is a potentially useful procedure in identifying allergens. As a general rule, atopic individuals have reaginic antibody to many antigens, and the finding of multiple positive skin tests tends to confirm a suspicion of atopy. Scratch testing should be done first since it is less likely than intradermal testing to cause severe reactions in very sensitive individuals. Intradermal testing is about 100 times more sensitive than scratch testing. The tests are read at the peak of the urticarial reaction, which is usually within 15—20 minutes. If scratch tests are negative, intradermal tests (on an extremity) may be used. Skin testing is a potentially dangerous procedure in highly sensitive individuals, and epinephrine and a tourniquet should always be at hand.

A positive skin test reaction consists of an erythema, wheal, and flare (triple response) to "scratch" or intracutaneously injected allergens. In interpreting the skin tests and assessing their clinical significance, the following should be kept in mind: (1) Diluent control should always be used for comparison. (2) Infants may react predominantly with flaring; older children, with wheal and flare reactions. (3) Mild reactions (1—2+) are less likely to be clinically significant than more strongly positive (pseudopodic wheal) reactions. Also,

a positive reaction elicited by scratch or puncture testing is more likely to be clinically significant than a positive test which can be elicited only by intradermal testing. (4) When a skin test does correlate with clinical sensitivity, the size of the reaction cannot be taken as an index of the severity of the clinical syndrome. (5) False-positive and false-negative reactions to foods are especially common, particularly in older children. (6) A definitely positive skin test means only that reaginic antibody is present in the skin. It may reflect a past, present, or potential clinical hypersensitivity manifest as one or more of the atopic diseases; on the other hand, the patient may never develop an atopic disease due to the specific allergen. (7) In a child with allergic rhinitis and allergic asthma, a positive skin test may be clinically relevant to one but not necessarily to all the allergic disorders present. (8) Up to 10% of nonatopic individuals may have positive skin reactions to a few allergens, especially house dust.

2. The Prausnitz-Küstner reaction—Passive transfer of antibody by injecting serum from a sensitized individual into the skin of a nonsensitized individual, followed by local challenge of the transfer site with the suspected allergen, is occasionally employed when skin testing is not feasible. This has been largely supplanted by the RAST test (see below).

3. Conjunctival tests are infrequently used and appear to offer little advantage in testing.

4. Provocative testing may be employed but is not recommended as a routine procedure for any potentially severe disorder such as asthma. Provocative tests are most valuable in determining clinical sensitivity to foods. Elimination and subsequent challenge with the following may be especially revealing: (1) Foods eaten more or less daily (unless there is a history of vomiting or angioedema involving the mouth and throat immediately following ingestion), eg, cow's milk, legumes, cereal grains, potatoes, chocolate, eggs. (2) Foods eaten less often, eg, nuts, peanuts, fish or seafood, sunflower seeds, and melons—if vomiting and angioedema have not occurred. In most cases, the parent or patient is already aware of the relationship between allergen and reaction if severe asthma or angioedema has immediately followed ingestion.

Procedure for provocative testing. After environmental factors are stabilized, withhold all suspected foods for at least 3 weeks; then challenge with a single food. Repeated offerings for a few days may be necessary to establish a hypersensitivity reaction.

Direct provocative inhalant testing is potentially hazardous and is best performed in a hospital setting. Exposure to the "natural" casual contacts of the patient with the inhalant allergens is very helpful in definitive diagnosis and usually bears permissible risk.

5. Eosinophilia—Increased numbers of eosinophils in the blood or bodily secretions (nasal, gastrointestinal) are frequently present in a variety of allergic conditions, especially in atopic disorders, and the presence of eosinophilia may strengthen a suspicion of allergic diathesis. Nasal eosinophilia is practically diagnostic of allergic rhinitis, but eosinophilia itself is by no means pathognomonic of other clinical allergies. Conversely, the absence of eosinophilia does not rule out allergy, particularly since a variety of factors (eg, concurrent infection) may suppress eosinophilia. The degree of eosinophilia correlates inversely with the degree of control of allergic and nonallergic asthma. Nasal eosinophilia in infants up to 3 months of age is considered normal.

6. Other tests—Numerous other tests (leukocyte histamine release in vitro, in vitro basophil degranulation test, the radioallergosorbent test, the induction of blast transformation of peripheral blood lymphocytes by antigen in vitro, the skin window test) have been employed in attempts to identify allergens which may be responsible for particular allergic reactions. In some cases (eg, the induction of blast transformation in lymphocytes), the validity of the test for implicating allergens is questionable; others are more promising and may aid in the identification of problem allergens. Of some promise is the radioallergosorbent test (RAST), which measures the amount of specific reaginic antibodies in serum, eg, the antiragweed antibodies of the IgE class; and the radioimmunosorbent test (RIST), which measures the concentration of IgE immunoglobulin in the blood. The RAST correlates well with skin testing, although it is somewhat less sensitive. Its main advantages include the ability to test individuals difficult to test by skin testing (eg, in extensive dermatitis) and safety, and the test should be especially useful in testing for severe drug hypersensitivity when the appropriate problematic antigens can be identified. The number of antigens available for testing is limited, however, and, considering the expense involved and delay in obtaining results, it is a less preferable technic than skin testing. Elevated IgE levels as measured by RIST or PRIST (paper RIST) suggest an atopic disorder, but the correlation is so imperfect that this is not a generally useful screening procedure. Greatly elevated IgE levels in infancy (> 2 SD above the mean) are highly predictive of an atopic diathesis, and elevated levels of IgE in "bronchiolitis" strongly suggest the diagnosis of a reactive airway disorder (asthma).

7. Controversial technics for diagnosis and treatment—Intracutaneous end point titration, sublingual and serial intracutaneous provocative titration tests, cytotoxic tests, and sublingual desensitization all have been claimed by some to be of value in diagnosing and treating allergic disorders. Their merit is yet to be validated scientifically, and they remain technics of unproved value at the present time.

8. Prophylaxis of atopic disorders—There is evidence that avoidance of cow products, eggs, wheat, and chicken during the first 9 months of life significantly lessens the likelihood of development of allergic rhinitis and asthma. Recently, evidence has been presented also that a diet excluding cow products, fish, and eggs for the first 6 months of life coupled with general environmental precautions minimizing house dust and animal dander contact is associated with a diminished likelihood of developing atopic dermatitis,

at least in the first year. It seems prudent, therefore, to institute dietary and environmental restrictions mentioned above in the first few months of life in children with a strong family history of atopy.

Aas K: Diagnosis of immediate type respiratory allergy. Pediatr Clin North Am 22:33, 1975.

Baer H: In vitro methods in allergy. Med Clin North Am 58:85, 1974.

Golbert T: A review of controversial diagnostic and therapeutic techniques employed in allergy. J Allergy Clin Immunol 56:170, 1975.

Halpern SR & others: Development of childhood allergy in infants fed breast, soy, or cow milk. J Allergy Clin Immunol 51:139, 1973.

Hannaway PJ, Hyde JS: Scratch and intradermal skin testing: A comparative study in 250 atopic children. Ann Allergy 28:413, 1970.

Johnstone DE, Dutton AM: Dietary prophylaxis of allergic disease in children. N Engl J Med 274:715, 1976.

Lecks HI, Kravis LP: The allergist and the eosinophil. Pediatr Clin North Am 16:125, 1969.

Matthew DJ & others: Prevention of eczema. Lancet 1:321, 1977.

Minor TE & others: Viruses as precipitants of asthmatic attacks in children. JAMA 227:292, 1974.

Norman PS: Antigens that cause atopic disease. Chap 44 in: *Immunological Diseases,* 2nd ed. Samter M (editor). Little, Brown, 1971.

BRONCHIAL ASTHMA
("Reactive Airway Disorder")

Essentials of Diagnosis

- Paroxysmal or chronically exacerbating dyspnea characterized by bilateral wheezing, prolongation of expiration, "air trapping," and hyperinflation of the lungs.

- Restoration of abnormal pulmonary function to (or significantly toward) normal by injection of epinephrine, inhalation of adrenergic aerosols, or other therapeutic measures.

- Eosinophilia of sputum and blood (common).

- Positive immediate skin test reactions to provoking allergens (common but not necessary).

- Attacks of dyspnea and wheezing caused by specific antigens, infectious agents, irritants, emotional upsets, or exercise.

General Considerations

Bronchial asthma is a largely reversible obstructive process predominantly of the lower pulmonary tract caused by mucosal edema, increased and unusually viscid secretions, and constriction of the bronchial tree. Especially in protracted asthmatic episodes, the obstructive pathologic changes may cause not only hypoxemia but retention of CO_2 and respiratory acidosis.

The incidence of asthma has been reported to be less than 10% of the total population but to constitute 26–63% of all atopic diseases. Before adolescence, boys are affected twice as frequently as girls. Onset is common in early childhood (but asthma frequently begins in adulthood). In the majority of cases in childhood, the onset is by the seventh year.

In many patients, offensive allergens cannot be identified by history or suggested by skin testing, and IgE-mediated allergy, at least, does not appear to be related to the pathogenesis of the disorder in such individuals. Even when allergens contribute to or are major precipitants of asthma, "allergy" rarely is the sole significant factor involved. The most common allergens causing asthma in children are inhalants: house dust and its usual ingredients of old kapok, cotton linters, indoor molds, insects, epidermals (especially feathers and the hair and danders of cats, dogs, horses, cattle, rabbits, and sheep), airborne pollens (trees, grasses, weeds), and out-of-doors seasonal molds. Foods occasionally provoke asthma, especially in infants, but this is less common in later childhood. The most common food allergens are egg white, cow's milk, fish, and foods of seed origin, eg, nuts, legumes, chocolate, and wheat and other cereal grains. It is probable that foods act as allergens in fewer than 10% of cases. The same allergens that cause asthma frequently cause allergic rhinitis in the same patient; many children with initial hay fever develop asthma, but there are divergent opinions regarding the number who do so (eg, 7% versus 60% in 2 different series).

The central feature of asthma is an extraordinary hyperreactivity of the tracheobronchial tree to various chemical mediators (eg, acetylcholine, histamine, prostaglandins) and, in turn, various insulting agents or events which cause their activation or liberation. In addition to allergic reactions, numerous factors trigger or aggravate asthma, principally upper and lower respiratory tract infections. The specific role of bacterial organisms and their products in the precipitation of asthma is a disputed question. Other triggering factors are rapid changes in temperature or barometric pressure, the common air pollutants in cities, cooking odors, smoke, paint fumes, exercise, and emotional upheavals. Psychologic factors appear to be important in some cases but are seldom the sole cause. Aspirin idiosyncrasy can be a cause of asthma in childhood as well as in adult life.

Clinical Findings

A. History: Onset may be as early as the first few weeks of life. In infancy in particular, the first attack usually is associated with an upper respiratory tract infection or "bronchiolitis." As age increases, there is a progressively greater tendency for initial and subsequent episodes to be associated with inhalants, pollens, and molds.

A history of atopic dermatitis or allergic rhinitis is often obtainable. A family history of atopic diseases (especially allergic rhinitis and bronchial asthma) is often present and is helpful in arousing suspicion of the diagnosis. Asthma can (and all too frequently does) occur in the absence of overt wheezing, and complaints may range from frequent "chest congestion" to recurrent cough. A careful physical examination, including chest auscultation on a forced expiratory maneuver rather than on simple tidal volume, or pulmonary function tests, can be revealing, especially when the patient is experiencing clinical discomfort.

B. Progressive Symptoms and Signs: (During an acute severe attack or if an attack is prolonged.)

1. Flushed, moist skin; pallid cyanosis; dry mucous membranes.

2. Restlessness, apprehension, fatigue, drowsiness, coma.

3. Distressing cough, dyspnea, increasing prolongation of expirations, high-pitched rhonchi and wheezes throughout the chest (diminishing in intensity as the obstruction becomes more severe), secretions (variable but decreasing in amount with ensuing dehydration), hyperinflation of the chest, poor air exchange, or areas of imperceptible air exchange.

4. Increasing tachycardia; initially, there may be mild hypertension; ultimately, hypotension; rarely, signs of cardiac failure.

5. Initially good and prompt response to epinephrine or other adrenergic drugs or methyl xanthines. If the attack is quite prolonged, the response to the above drugs may be poor.

C. Special Clinical Findings:

1. Episodes of asthma in association with infections are frequently insidious in onset and prolonged; those due to specific identifiable allergens tend to be acute in onset and brief if the causative agent is removed.

2. Bronchial asthma in infants (under 2 years of age) deserves special comment. The first attack usually follows by a few days the onset of a respiratory infection; some degree of wheezing may persist for prolonged periods and becomes worse with subsequent "colds."

3. In infants, the predominant symptoms may be dyspnea, excessive secretions, noisy and rattly breathing, cough, and, in many cases, some intercostal and suprasternal retractions—rather than the typical pronounced expiratory wheezes that occur in older children. Initial and repeated diagnoses of these episodes are apt to be "croup," "bronchiolitis," and "pneumonia." Evidence of infection (viral) is often present.

4. Cough frequently is a presenting symptom, with or without wheezing. Asthma can exist *without overt wheezing,* and "subclinical" wheezing may be detected only by careful physical examination including auscultation on a forced vital capacity maneuver, examination during an episode of "chest congestion," or pulmonary function testing.

5. A syndrome of paroxysmal cough, presumably tracheal in origin ("irritable trachea," "allergic cough"), occurs and may be difficult to differentiate from true asthma, particularly since bronchodilator drugs are sometimes effective in this condition. In this condition, wheezing generally does not occur and signs of

lower respiratory tract obstruction are lacking. The condition frequently is provoked by a (viral?) respiratory infection, and allergic factors may or may not play a role.

D. Laboratory Findings: Eosinophil accumulations (eg, clumps of eosinophils in a nasal or sputum smear) and peripheral blood eosinophilia are commonly found but are often absent in infection or if corticosteroids are being given.

Hematocrit can be elevated with dehydration, as in prolonged attacks, or in severe chronic disease. In severe asthma, the first sign is hypoxemia without CO_2 retention. Respiratory acidosis and increased CO_2 tension may ensue. (Moderately severe hypoxemia may occur with low CO_2 tension due to a combination of hyperventilation and ventilation-perfusion disturbances.)

E. X-Ray Findings: Bilateral hyperinflation, bronchial thickening and peribronchial infiltration, and areas of densities (patchy atelectasis or associated bronchopneumonia) may be present. (Patchy atelectasis is common and often misread as pneumonitis.) The pulmonary arteries may also appear prominent.

F. Pulmonary Function Studies: (See Chapter 12.) Increased airway resistance with a decrease in flow rates, decreased vital capacity (VC), and increased functional residual capacity (FRC) and residual volume (RV). The first 3 may be normal in asymptomatic intervals, but frequently there is residual hyperinfiltration chronically.

G. Skin Testing: Positive skin reactions (immediate wheal and flare reactions) to injected allergens are frequently present (supportive evidence only).

H. Provocative Tests:

1. Food—Positive clinical reactions usually occur within hours after ingestion. Foods causing low-grade hypersensitivity reactions may not induce a reaction for a few days and are difficult to document.

2. Inhalants—A positive clinical reaction usually occurs immediately after inhalation but may not occur until a few hours after challenge. Asthma may occasionally be provoked by skin testing with the appropriate allergens.

Differential Diagnosis*

Bronchial asthma may be confused with middle and lower respiratory tract infections (eg, laryngotracheobronchitis, acute bronchiolitis, bronchopneumonia, and pertussis), especially in the very young.

Nasal "wheezes" may be transmitted to the chest (especially in infants) from upper airway edema, increased secretions, or other obstructing factors such as allergic rhinitis, upper respiratory tract infections, adenoidal hypertrophy, foreign body, choanal stenosis, and nasal polyps (incidence high in cystic fibrosis).

Congenital laryngeal stridor is usually associated with other anomalies.

In tracheal or bronchial foreign body, dyspnea or wheezing is usually of sudden onset; on auscultation,

*See also Other Allergic Pulmonary Disorders, p 927.

the wheezes are usually but not always unilateral. Characteristic x-ray findings are not always present.

The differentiation between bronchial asthma and cystic fibrosis is made on the basis of high sweat sodium and chloride, a history (often present) in cystic fibrosis of serious pulmonary infections since birth, a personal and family history of associated intestinal disturbances with profuse, bulky stools, and pancreatic enzyme deficiency. There is evidence, however, for a significant reactive airway (asthmatic) component with or without allergic precipitant in many children with cystic fibrosis, and it is clear that cystic fibrosis and asthma can coexist.

Tracheal or bronchial compression by extramural forces may resemble asthma and may be due to foreign body in the esophagus, aortic ring, anomalous vessels, or inflammatory or neoplastic lymphadenopathy.

Chronic recurrent bronchial asthma may lead to invalidism, both organic and psychologic, barrel chest, and distensive emphysema; atelectasis and massive pulmonary collapse; mediastinal emphysema and pneumothorax; and death due to respiratory insufficiency or improper medication (oversedation, misuse of adrenergic aerosols, theophylline, tranquilizers, narcotics). Sudden death may occur as a result of unknown causes other than respiratory insufficiency. Although asthma often is defined as a "reversible" obstructive airway disorder, chronic moderately severe to severe asthma may, in time, have a significant irreversible element.

Treatment of Mild & Moderate Asthma

As is true of all atopic diseases, bronchial asthma can be controlled but not cured.

A. Specific Measures: Insofar as possible, the patient should avoid contact with proved or suspected irritants and allergens in the environment. (See Environmental Control of Exposure, above). Hyposensitization therapy is generally believed to be justified for patients whose allergens cannot be avoided, eg, pollens, seasonal molds, and house dust.

B. General Measures: General management should be directed in a comprehensive fashion to include the measures listed below. Depending upon the frequency and severity of asthma in a given child, some or all of these measures may be used, mainly with the onset of an asthmatic attack or as a constant regimen—especially during the times of year when asthma is most severe.

1. Education—The patient must be educated to live optimally with his chronic problem. Complete understanding of all recommendations made is essential.

2. Liquefaction and expectoration of mucus—Maintain adequate hydration by encouraging oral fluid intake, or give intravenous fluids if necessary. Expectorants may be used as necessary. Adrenergic aerosols may be used twice daily followed by postural drainage or every 2–6 hours, depending upon the severity of asthma and the tolerance of the patient.

3. Bronchodilatation—The main bronchodilating

drug recommended is theophylline or aminophylline. Bronchodilating adrenergic drugs (oral, aerosol) can be added cautiously if theophylline alone is not adequate.

4. Correction of metabolic acidosis, if present, by providing an adequate energy source to diminish ketosis (eg, 5% dextrose IV), food if tolerated, and bicarbonate (see below).

5. Corticosteroids—In severe acute asthma or in chronic asthma unresponsive to other measures, adrenal glucocorticoids may be indicated (see below). If chronic use of corticosteroids is necessary for adequate control of asthma, alternate-day prednisone or other short-acting equivalent given before 8:00 a.m. on alternate days should be attempted. Beclomethasone dipropionate (Vanceril) by topical aerosol can be considered as an alternative, given in a dosage of up to 600 μg/day. Before resorting to chronic steroid therapy, cromolyn sodium, 20 mg by inhalation 4 times daily, should be given a therapeutic trial for at least 1 month.

6. Antibiotics—If there is evidence of bacterial infection, appropriate antibiotics should be given. However, leukocytosis up to 15,000/cu mm is common in severe asthma without any evidence of bacterial infection. Patchy atelectasis can be confused with pneumonitis on x-ray.

7. In children with chronic or recurrent asthma, breathing and fitness exercises under the guidance of a properly trained physical therapist may assist the patient in aborting some attacks of asthma and improving muscular functions of the thoracic cage.

8. Exercise should be encouraged rather than restricted. Exercise-induced bronchospasm can be ameliorated, if necessary, by theophylline given 1–2 hours before exercise, with or without cromolyn sodium or adrenergic aerosol (metaproterenol is recommended) just prior to exercise.

9. Children with frequent overt asthma attacks (eg, 1 or 2 per week) and evidence of more or less constant pulmonary obstruction should be on constant pharmacologic therapy. A daily regimen stimulating coughing and encouraging expectoration (eg, postural drainage at least twice a day) may be useful. Cromolyn sodium (Aarane, Intal), 20 mg 4 times daily by inhalation, may be considered for chronic symptomatic asthma, alone or in addition to constant theophylline therapy.

Treatment of Severe Asthma (Status Asthmaticus, Intractable Asthma)

This is a medical emergency!

A. Emergency Care: Epinephrine (1:1000 aqueous solution, 0.1–0.3 ml subcut) is the drug of first choice. It may be repeated at 20-minute intervals for a total of 3 doses. If the response to epinephrine is good but relatively short-lived, a longer acting epinephrine preparation (eg, Sus-Phrine) may then be employed. If a response to epinephrine is not apparent by the second or third injection, discontinue the drug since excessive use of epinephrine, particularly in the face of "epinephrine resistance," may actually aggravate asthma. The lack of therapeutic response to 2 or 3 injec-

tions of epinephrine is sometimes used as the criterion for "status asthmaticus." Relative or apparent complete lack of responsiveness to epinephrine ("epinephrine fastness") may be due to hypoxemia and acidosis, bronchial obstruction with thick mucus plugs, pneumothorax, or simply severe asthma. Epinephrine sensitivity may improve after initiation of other therapy.

B. Hospital Care: If signs are relatively early, an overnight stay may suffice.

1. Give 5% dextrose solution with 0.2% saline intravenously at the first sign of resistance to epinephrine or with poor fluid intake, vomiting, or dehydration. (Use 1½ times maintenance fluid requirements.) Particularly if steroids are used, remember to add potassium (10–20 mEq/liter of IV fluid).

2. Give moisturized oxygen (by mask or nasal prongs—not by tent) at a flow rate of approximately 4 liters/minute. All patients with acute severe asthma will be hypoxemic, largely as a result of the ventilation/perfusion imbalance which is an integral part of "asthma."

3. Give aminophylline, 4–6 mg/kg, in intravenous tubing over a 10–20 minute period (if not used in previous 4 hours) and repeat every 4–6 hours, or give as a constant infusion beginning with a loading dose of 4–6 mg/kg over 15 minutes and then 0.6–1 mg/kg/hour.*

4. Take an arterial or venous blood sample for pH and an arterial sample for P_{CO_2} and P_{O_2} determinations. Early in the course of an asthmatic paroxysm, the patient usually hyperventilates and blows off CO_2, with a resultant low Pa_{CO_2}. As the severity of the episode increases, the patient may become fatigued and may be unable to perform the necessary work, contributing to an increasing Pa_{CO_2}. (A "normal" as well as increased Pa_{CO_2} in acute severe asthma, in other words, is an indication of respiratory failure.) Continued close monitoring of blood gases and pH is essential to proper management of severe asthma. (Determination of gases or pH on capillary blood generally is unreliable.)

5. Correction of acidosis (pH 7.3 or below) with sodium bicarbonate should be attempted. With the increased work of breathing and hypoxemia, there may be metabolic acidosis due to lactic acid production. This may be compensated by a respiratory alkalosis due to hyperventilation. The appropriate bicarbonate

---

*In patients receiving chronic theophylline therapy, use *at least* the usual total daily maintenance dose infused over a 24-hour period. Theophylline blood levels of 10–20 μg/ml serum are considered "therapeutic." Average total daily dosages of theophylline to achieve therapeutic levels (divided into 4–6 doses daily) are listed below, but there is much individual variation in requirements:

Age	Average Total Daily Dose ± SD
Infancy to 8 years	25 ± 5 mg/kg
8–16 years	20 ± 5 mg/kg
Over 16 years	12 ± 3 mg/kg

dose may be calculated by means of the following formula:

$$\text{mEq bicarbonate needed} = \text{Negative base excess} \times$$
$$0.3 \times \text{Body weight in kg}$$

The bicarbonate can be given rapidly by the intravenous route.* Arterial or venous pH should be redetermined 5–10 minutes later, and further correction of acidosis, using bicarbonate, should be considered at that time if necessary. In respiratory failure, in the absence of a pH determination, 2 mEq/kg body weight may be infused initially.

6. Give isoproterenol, 1:200 by inhalation (or other adrenergic aerosols) every 2–4 hours followed by postural drainage *as tolerated*. (The proper use of aerosolized adrenergic agents early in the course of acute severe asthma may obviate the need for injected epinephrine.)

7. Corticosteroids–If the patient is already receiving corticosteroids, do not withdraw but increase the dose temporarily. Corticosteroids may be withheld in attacks of mild to moderate severity responding satisfactorily to the other treatment measures. However, they should be used at once when the asthmatic attack is of sufficient severity to be life-threatening or when the patient has been on prolonged daily corticosteroid therapy (at least 2 weeks) in the past year. If it is decided that corticosteroids are to be used, one of the following should be given intravenously in the following initial doses every 4 hours around the clock: (1) Hydrocortisone sodium succinate (Solu-Cortef), 100 mg. (2) Prednisolone sodium phosphate (Hydeltrasol), 20 mg. (3) Dexamethasone sodium phosphate (Decadron), 4 mg. (4) Solu-Medrol, 20 mg. (Add at least usual daily potassium requirements to intravenous fluids.)

With amelioration of symptoms, the dose should be decreased as rapidly as possible. (If the patient has not been on prolonged corticosteroid therapy within the past year, the corticosteroids can be discontinued abruptly rather than tapered. It is frequently feasible to use high doses of corticosteroids for 48 hours or less.)

8. Give antibiotics as indicated.

9. Chloral hydrate, 15 mg/kg rectally, may be given for restlessness or apprehension.

10. In respiratory failure unresponsive to the above therapy, intravenous isoproterenol therapy or assisted ventilation by a mechanical respirator may be required. Failure to respond to the above measures can be defined as 2 arterial P_{CO_2} determinations above 45 mg Hg over a 15- to 30-minute period. This is the indication for insertion of an indwelling arterial catheter if that has not been done. If the steady state arterial P_{CO_2} remains above 45 mm Hg in the blood drawn from the indwelling line, this is an indication for the initiation of a continuous isoproterenol infusion. *Such*

an infusion should be undertaken only in an intensive care unit where continuous cardiac and blood pressure monitoring facilities are available. An additional intravenous line should be started for the isoproterenol so that it is not infused into the only existing line. The infusion should be started at a rate of 0.1 μg/kg/ minute and increased by this amount every 10–15 minutes until there is clinical improvement or until the heart rate approaches 200 beats/minute. The development of significant arrhythmias is an indication for decreasing the rate of isoproterenol infusion. If a favorable response occurs, it is necessary to very slowly wean the patient from the isoproterenol, decreasing the rate of infusion over a period of 30–36 hours. Rebound bronchospasm may occur if the rate is decreased too rapidly.

If the arterial P_{CO_2} remains high or continues to increase despite the continuous isoproterenol infusion, endotracheal intubation should be performed and assisted ventilation initiated. A volume respirator capable of producing high inspiratory pressures should be used. Since these patients have prolonged expiratory times as a result of the marked airway resistance, it is necessary to set an adequate expiratory time on the ventilator to avoid further air trapping within the lung. The need for assisted ventilation for status asthmaticus in children has been reduced since the introduction of the continuous isoproterenol infusion. *Intubation and assisted ventilation should be performed only by medical personnel trained in such technics.*

C. Precautions in Therapy: Note the following "don'ts":

1. Don't use narcotics or barbiturates. (They depress the respiratory center. Tranquilizers may do the same in the presence of severe hypoxemia.)

2. Don't use epinephrine excessively. (The patient has probably already had too much; it tends to thicken secretions, depletes glycogen stores, and increases apprehension.)

3. Don't use adrenergic aerosols excessively. (They may aggravate asthma. Discontinue if responsiveness to aerosol therapy is not apparent.)

D. Follow-Up Therapy:

1. **Fluids**–When the patient is improved and is able to take fluids and oral medications, continue humidification and give oral fluids in the form of fruit juices with added sugar, eg, grape, apple, pineapple, carbonated drinks (but not fluids containing caffeine and chocolate). Give no milk or iced drinks.

2. **Drugs**–The following medications are of value at this stage:

a. Adrenergic aerosol every 3–6 hours, followed by postural drainage for 20 minutes.

b. Theophylline orally every 6 hours (dosage according to weight).

c. Saturated solution of potassium iodide, 25 mg/kg/day, may be tried.

d. If corticosteroids have been started, withdraw after 48 hours or taper gradually and discontinue as soon as possible.

---

*Sodium bicarbonate for injection may be obtained in ampules or multidose vials which contain approximately 1 mEq/ml.

Prognosis

There is no evidence that bronchial asthma can be cured, and the old adage still holds: "Once an asthmatic, always an asthmatic." However, the prognosis for symptom-free control in childhood asthma is fairly good. The majority of asthmatic children have less symptomatic asthma in their teens, and some appear to lose any asthmatic symptomatology for life. Unfortunately, however, only a minority (probably less than 30%) fall into this category, and—more often than not—it is the pediatrician rather than the disorder that the child outgrows. Many have persistent significant though often unrecognized chronic pulmonary obstruction and others later redevelop symptomatic obstruction.

Recent reports indicate that in the past 25 years the morbidity and mortality rates in asthma may have increased, but it is not clear whether this increase is due to the diagnosis of more cases of "infectious" or "intrinsic" asthma, increased air pollution, the use of isoproterenol aerosols, or corticosteroid therapy. Mortality statistics indicate that a high percentage of deaths have been due to indiscriminate use of sedatives, narcotics, and aminophylline, but many also are from undertreatment. In the pediatric age group, the highest mortality rates have been reported in infants with onset of asthma under 2 years of age.

"Continuity" symptoms of night cough, breathlessness, and provocation of wheezing with exercise or stress are usually indicative of more serious disease than occasional, spontaneous, and brief attacks due to recognizable allergens (eg, epidermals, kapok, pollens) with symptom-free periods in between. Infection-related asthma beginning in early childhood, uncomplicated by allergic factors, tends to have a better prognosis than asthma in which allergy plays an important role.

Bierman CW, Pierson WE: The pharmacologic management of status asthmaticus in children. Pediatrics 54:245, 1974.

Cotton EK, Parry WH: Treatment of status asthmaticus and respiratory failure. Pediatr Clin North Am 22:163, 1975.

Downes GJ & others: Intravenous isoproterenol infusion in children with severe hypercapnia due to status asthmaticus. Effects on ventilation, circulation, and clinical score. Crit Care Med 1:63, 1973.

Falliers CJ: Aspirin and subtypes of asthma: Risk factor analysis. J Allergy Clin Immunol 52:141, 1973.

Lecks HI: Explosive asthma in the infant and young child under two years. Clin Pediatr (Phila) 15:135, 1976.

McIntosh K: Bronchiolitis and asthma: Possible common pathogenetic pathways. J Allergy Clin Immunol 57:595, 1976.

Mellis CM, Phelan PD: Asthma death in children: A continuing problem. Thorax 32:29, 1977.

Reed CE: Epidemiology and natural history. Pages 291–300 in: *New Directions in Asthma.* American College of Chest Physicians, 1975.

Williams HE, McNicol KN: The spectrum of asthma in children. Pediatr Clin North Am 22:43, 1975.

ALLERGIC RHINITIS

Essentials of Diagnosis

- Chronic or recurrent nasal obstruction; itching and sneezing (frequently paroxysmal) with seromucoid discharge. There may be accompanying conjunctival injection and itching, with or without tearing. Bilateral "vacuum" headaches often present.
- Mucosal hyperemia to purplish pallor and edema of nasal mucous membranes; polypoid changes of turbinates may occur.
- Eosinophilia of nasal secretions when symptomatic. (May be absent with infections, or possibly with corticosteroid therapy.)
- Positive immediate skin test reactions to provoking allergens (supportive evidence only).

General Considerations

Allergic rhinitis is the most common atopic disease, perhaps because the nose is anatomically and physiologically vulnerable to inhalant allergens. The pathologic changes are chiefly hyperemia, edema, goblet cell and connective cell proliferation, cellular infiltration (especially with eosinophils and lymphocytes), and exudation of serous and mucoid secretions, all of which lead to variable degrees of nasal obstruction, rhinorrhea, and pruritus. Inhalant allergens are principally responsible for causation of symptoms, but food allergens on occasion may provoke rhinitis.

Classification

Allergic rhinitis may be classified as perennial or seasonal (hay fever), but these 2 entities frequently occur concomitantly. Children with allergic rhinitis seem to be more susceptible to upper respiratory infections, which in turn intensify the symptoms of existing allergic rhinitis.

A. Perennial Allergic Rhinitis: Perennial allergic rhinitis occurs to some degree all year long but is usually more severe in winter. Characteristically, it "blows up" when forced air heating systems are turned on in the fall, causing increased exposure to house dusts. Nasal stuffiness, frequent sniffing, or constant rhinorrhea with evidence of mild to moderate itching (frequent nose rubbing) are often the dominant symptoms, although more severe symptoms, including paroxysmal sneezing, may occur. Sneezing is often most pronounced in the morning shortly after waking. Symptoms may be related to periods of shedding of hair of house pets (early fall and early spring), redecoration procedures, and changes in home furnishings. Greater exposure to house dust during the winter months is due to increased indoor activities, the use of winter blankets and wool or hairy clothing, dry air and heating systems which raise, disperse, and circulate dust, and indoor housing of pets.

This disease frequently begins before the second year of life. It often accompanies bronchial asthma and may be provoked by the same allergens. Dental abnormalities and disturbances in dental arch growth and malocclusion have been attributed to longstanding perennial allergic rhinitis.

B. Seasonal Allergic Rhinitis (Hay Fever): Hay fever occurs seasonally as a result of exposure to specific wind-borne pollens. The major important pollen groups in the temperate zones are trees (late winter, early spring), grasses (spring to early summer), and weeds (late summer to early fall). Seasons may vary significantly in different parts of the country. Mold spores may also be a significant cause of seasonal allergic rhinitis, principally in the summer and fall.

The age at onset is generally later than for perennial allergic rhinitis. Hay fever is rare before age 1; in most cases it begins after 3 years of age. Worsening or extension of pollen sensitivities over a period of several years after onset can be expected.

Clinical Findings

A. Symptoms and Signs: Nasal obstruction is manifested by mouth breathing, snoring, difficulty in nursing or eating, nasal speech, and inability to clear the nose with blowing. Nasal seromucoid secretions are increased, with anterior drainage, sniffling, "nasal stuffiness," postnasal drip, and loose cough. Nasal itching leads to nose rubbing ("allergic salute," "bunny nose"), nose-picking, epistaxis, and sneezing. Eye manifestations consist of itching, unilateral or bilateral tearing, conjunctival injection, lid edema, "allergic pleats," and eye shadows. There may be headache or a feeling of fullness. Palatal and pharyngeal itching may occur as well as pharyngeal soreness or irritation and hoarseness. Lassitude or frank fatigue often occurs during problematic seasons.

The symptoms and signs of perennial allergic rhinitis and hay fever differ little except for seasonal incidence and, in hay fever, severe intense itching, coryza, and sneezing. Examination shows decreased or absent patency of nasal airways, increased seromucoid discharge anteriorly and posteriorly (usually more serous in seasonal rhinitis), and excoriation of the nares. The mucous membranes range from reddened with little edema to pale blue, swollen, and boggy, with dimpling in the turbinates or pedunculated polyps. Increased pharyngeal lymphoid tissue from chronic pharyngeal drainage or enlarged tonsillar and adenoid tissue may be present. Bleeding points or ulceration may be seen on the anterior nasal septum. A horizontal crease may be seen extending across the lower third of the nose due to frequent upward rubbing of the nose. Malocclusion (overbite), presumably due to excess pressure of digit sucking to relieve palatal itching, may be seen in long-standing cases.

The florid conjunctival injection, coryza, intense itching of the eyes and nose, and violent sneezing experienced by older children and adults are not so commonly seen in young children. Paroxysmal sneezing, however, is a frequent symptom even in young children.

B. Laboratory Findings: Eosinophilia can be demonstrated on smears of nasal secretions or blood (usually higher in seasonal than perennial rhinitis.) The technic of examination of nasal secretions is as follows:

1. Obtain nasal secretions by having the patient blow onto a piece of wax paper or by nasal swab; spread on a microscope slide and allow to dry.

2. Cover the slide with Hansel's stain for 1−2 minutes.

3. Add enough distilled water to take up staining solution and allow to stand 1 minute.

4. Wash with distilled water.

5. Flood with 95% ethanol and drain off immediately; allow to dry.

6. Examine under the oil immersion objective. (Look for consistently greater than 5% eosinophils, or accumulation [clumps] of eosinophils.)

C. Skin Testing: Positive immediate reactions to scratch or intradermal tests with offending allergens.

D. Provocative Tests: Positive on ingestion or inhalation of offending allergens.

E. X-Ray of Paranasal Sinuses: Sinusitis may accompany allergic rhinitis and is frequently demonstrable on x-ray (mucosal thickening, fluid levels, or complete opacification of sinuses). Vigorous treatment is indicated until there is complete resolution of x-ray as well as clinical findings.

Differential Diagnosis

These disorders must be differentiated from the common cold, other infectious diseases (eg, purulent rhinitis and sinusitis, congenital syphilis), adenoidal hypertrophy, foreign bodies (usually unilateral), nasal polyposis with cystic fibrosis or aspirin idiosyncrasy, choanal stenosis or atresia, nasopharyngeal neoplasms, palatal malformations (eg, congenitally high arch, cleft palate), and "vasomotor rhinitis."

Treatment

A. Specific Measures: Avoid exposure to proved allergens insofar as is reasonably possible. (See Environmental Control of Exposure, above.)

1. Perennial allergic rhinitis—Hyposensitization should be considered when symptoms are severe and other symptomatic measures have failed; when the disease is definitely associated with recurrent serous otitis media and hearing loss; or when it is accompanied by significant seasonal allergic rhinitis. The main allergen for which hyposensitization might be of benefit in perennial allergic rhinitis is house dust.

2. Hay fever—Hyposensitization may be beneficial in seasonal rhinitis due to specific allergens identified by clinical history and skin tests. It should be reserved for cases which have become progressively worse and cannot be controlled by antihistamines or adrenergic drugs (or both), or those which are accompanied by asthma. There is controversial evidence that hyposensitization for hay fever may prevent the onset of asthma; some allergists therefore favor hyposensitization therapy in all children with hay fever in whom an inciting allergen can be identified.

B. General Measures:

1. Give antihistamines with or without vasoconstricting adrenergic drugs by mouth. (Table 32–1.)

2. Treat associated infections.

3. Avoid all nasal topical drugs except for minimal use of decongestants (eg, phenylephrine) for severe episodes. Corticosteroids (topical or systemic) should be used only for short periods in polypoid states or severe nasal obstruction not controllable by other means.

4. Surgical removal of nasal polyps is indicated if other measures fail.

Prognosis

A. Perennial Allergic Rhinitis: Unless specific allergens can be identified and eliminated from the environment or diet (unusual cases), this atopic disease tends to be very protracted. As the child grows older—presumably because of increasing caliber of the nasal airway and if polypoid growths do not appear—nasal obstruction may become less troublesome.

B. Seasonal Allergic Rhinitis: Hay fever patients tend to repeat their seasonal symptoms if exposure to offending allergens is high. On moving to a region devoid of specific allergens, they may be free of seasonal allergic rhinitis for 1–3 years but frequently acquire new pollen hypersensitivities from airborne pollens in the areas to which they move. (*Example:* On moving to the Rocky Mountain region from mideastern USA, patients usually become less symptomatic to ragweed because of low exposure but acquire hypersensitivity to tumbleweeds and sages.)

About 70% of patients seem to improve significantly on hyposensitization therapy over a 2–4 year period. About 25% of boys seem to improve spontaneously during adolescence; girls often get worse during these years (and may also develop seasonal rhinitis for the first time during adolescence). Continued hyposensitization with prolongation of intervals between infections (if possible) or resumption of a previous injection program may be necessary in some patients.

Miller DL, Friday GA: Allergic diseases of the nose and middle ear in children. Pediatr Ann 5:483, 1976.

Norman PS, Lichtenstein LM: Allergic rhinitis: Clinical course and treatment. Chap 48, pages 840–858, in: *Immunological Diseases,* 2nd ed. Samter M (editor). Little, Brown, 1971.

Tennenbaum JI: Allergic rhinitis. Chap 6, pages 161–195, in: *Allergic Diseases, Diagnosis and Management.* Patterson R (editor). Lippincott, 1972.

RECURRENT SEROUS OTITIS MEDIA ASSOCIATED WITH ALLERGY
("Glue Ear")

Essentials of Diagnosis

- Recurrent or protracted nonpurulent otitis media characterized by episodes of mild to moderate hearing loss with or without earaches.
- Presence of viscid secretions within the middle ear; decreased mobility of tympanic membranes.
- Nasal eosinophilia (common).
- Positive immediate skin test reaction to offending allergens (supportive only).
- Occurrence of symptoms with inhalation or ingestion of provoking allergens.

General Considerations

Recurrent serous otitis media is probably a misnomer since the secretions within the middle ear are more mucoid than serous. In some cases, this entity is thought to be an extension of the pathologic changes of allergic rhinitis (edema and increased secretory activity of the mucosa) involving the eustachian tubes and the epithelial lining of the middle ear. The result is episodic obstruction of the eustachian tubes, metaplastic mucosal changes, accumulation of viscid secretions within the middle ear, decreased mobility with or without fullness or retraction of the tympani, hearing loss, often earache and ear plugging, and, sometimes, rupture of the tympani. Hearing loss and frequent "colds" are common complaints.

This entity is most common in small children and is seldom seen after 8 years of age. Some cases previously believed to be due to inadequately treated acute or subacute otitis media of infectious origin or primary hypertrophy of adenoid tissues are now thought to be part of an allergic diathesis. The atopic young child seems to be particularly prone to the development of serous otitis media. The middle ear probably is not a "shock organ" for allergy per se for there is little evidence that allergy-associated serous otitis media exists in the absence of allergic rhinitis. Etiologic allergens are those responsible for the rhinitis. Intercurrent ear infections are common in this disorder and tend to complicate the underlying problem. Although allergic factors appear to be important in many cases of serous otitis media, most cases do not appear to be associated with "allergy."

Clinical Findings

A. Symptoms and Signs: In addition to the existence of allergic rhinitis, the incidence of recurrent episodes of infectious otitis media is high. Recurrent episodes of ear plugging and earaches since infancy are frequently reported; there may be complaints of "popping" sounds in the ears. Rupture of the drum and discharge of mucoid secretions in the ear canal are uncommon.

Hearing impairment is recurrent and variable (usually mild to moderate); audiographic changes are usually variable and for the most part reversible. Difficulties in social and school adjustment due to hearing loss are often encountered.

Vertigo seems to be rare.

The tympani may be scarred, distorted, full, very retracted, opaque, and amber to bluish in color, and movement of the tympanic membrane is limited. Chalky appearance and narrowing of the malleus are prominent signs. Tympanic bleb formation is sometimes present. A fluid level or "bubbles" behind the tympani may be observed. Occasionally, the ears may appear normal.

B. Laboratory Findings: Eosinophilia of nasal secretions (see Allergic Rhinitis, above) is often present. Smears of middle ear secretions are usually negative for eosinophils and other cells.

C. Audiometry: A bilateral hearing loss of up to 10–40 dB in all frequencies (usually reversible with treatment) may be present.

D. Skin Testing: Positive immediate skin reactions to provoking allergens supports the presumption of an allergic cause.

Differential Diagnosis

This entity must be differentiated from viral otitis media, inadequately treated bacterial otitis media, anomalies of the eustachian tube and nasopharynx, hypertrophy of adenoidal tissue due to nonallergic causes, growths in the nasopharynx (eg, nasal polyps, carcinoma), or otosclerosis in late childhood.

Complications & Sequelae

Complications include permanent hearing loss, recurrent chronic infectious otitis media and its sequelae, and learning and social adjustment problems.

Treatment

The treatment of recurrent serous otitis media in which an allergic cause is suspected is as outlined for allergic rhinitis (see above), with the following additional considerations: (1) ENT consultation as required, eg, when the question of intubation and drainage of the middle ear arises. (2) Special schools may be necessary in cases of hearing loss. (3) Elimination of identified causative allergens and daily use of antihistamines coupled with decongestants. (4) Prompt treatment of bacterial infections of ears and nose. (5) Hyposensitization with proved inhalant allergens must be considered if elimination of allergens and drug therapy are of little benefit. (6) Provision of adequate and controlled humidification (40%). (7) A milk-free diet trial should be considered.

Adenoidectomy gives poor results. Myringotomy or intubation gives temporary improvement.

Prognosis

The problem of recurrent serous otitis media appears to diminish with age. With appropriate treatment, the long-term prognosis appears excellent.

The benefit of hyposensitization against inhalant allergens has not been proved for serous otitis media but presumably should help control the underlying rhinitis, and therefore the otitis. There is no substantial evidence for the value of hyposensitization with microbial antigens.

Goodhill V: Chronic middle ear effusion. Pages 92–114 in: *Modern Trends in Diseases of the Ear, Nose and Throat.* Ellis M (editor). Butterworth, 1972.

Miller DL, Friday GA: Allergic diseases of the nose and middle ear in children. Pediatr Ann 5:483, 1976.

Murray AB & others: A survey of hearing loss in Vancouver school children. Part 2. The association between secretory otitis media and enlarged adenoids, infections, and nasal allergy. Can Med Assoc J 98:995, 1968.

Rapp DJ, Fahey IF: Allergy and chronic secretory otitis media. Pediatr Clin North Am 22:259, 1975.

FOOD ALLERGY

Allergic reactions can be provoked by food antigens in virtually any tissue of the body containing blood vessels, smooth muscle, or mucous and secretory epithelium. A wide variety of signs and symptoms are encountered many of which may appear extremely vague. Significant serious reactions include anaphylaxis, acute angioedema of the upper airway, and severe bronchial asthma provoked especially by eggs, shellfish, trout, cow's milk (see Chapter 16), walnuts, peanuts, pork, melons, and certain seeds (sesame, sunflower). Such reactions usually occur within 1–2 hours. Other symptom complexes of lesser consequence can also occur in response to a variety of common foods. These are more likely to appear after several hours.

Classification

"Syndromes" which may be induced by hypersensitivity to foods include the following:

A. Angioedema: (Often accompanied by urticaria.) In mild cases, periorbital and lip edema, a few hives, mild arthralgia, malaise; in severe cases, tongue, pharyngeal, and laryngotracheal edema and joint swelling. Death may occur from asphyxia. (See Medical Emergencies Due to Allergic Reactions.)

B. Anaphylaxis: Immediate reaction with lightheadedness to syncope, flushing to pallor, paresthesias, generalized itching (especially palms and soles), palpitations, and tachycardia; symptoms and signs of pulmonary edema, bronchial asthma, and vascular collapse. (See Medical Emergencies Due to Allergic Reactions.)

C. Gastrointestinal Intolerance: In mild cases, nausea, diarrhea, flatulence, bloating, and abdominal discomfort; in severe cases, forceful vomiting, severe colic, bloody and mucoid diarrhea, and dehydration. Prolonged episodes of gastrointestinal intolerance can result in malnutrition and growth retardation.

D. Perennial Allergic Rhinitis, Bronchial Asthma, Atopic Dermatitis, Urticaria: See elsewhere in this chapter.

E. Tension-Fatigue Syndrome: A combination of fatigue, lassitude, irritability, sleeplessness, disturbed behavior, disinterest, pallor, "shadowy" eyes with "allergic pleats," "run-down feeling," and sometimes generalized headache with vague abdominal complaints has been reported. This syndrome may be associated with other atopic or allergic disorders. It may be related to inhalant allergens but frequently seems to be provoked by foods commonly and abundantly eaten, eg, cow's milk, cereal grains, chocolate, eggs, pork. The diagnosis of this syndrome is frequently difficult and is one of exclusion of many other mild and chronic disease states, particularly in a patient who has no other evidence of allergic disease. Whether these food-associated symptoms are mediated by an allergic mechanism is not clear. Claims that salicylates, dyes, and other food ingredients may add to hyperactivity in children with minimal brain dysfunction are controversial, and in the occasional child who does appear to be benefited by restricted diets (eg, the "Feingold diet") there is no evidence of an allergic reaction to the foodstuffs involved.

F. Migraine: In addition to other causes, certain foods may precipitate a migrainous episode. A true hypersensitivity reaction is questioned. Certain foods such as chocolate, cheeses, liver, and some wines and beers in which significant amounts of vasoactive amines have been found have been demonstrated to precipitate migraine.

Clinical Findings

A. History; Symptoms and Signs: See above, the section on history in the discussion of atopic disorders; and individual disorders.

B. Laboratory Findings:

1. Eosinophilia of stool mucus may be present in cases of gastrointestinal intolerance but may be a normal finding in the first 3 months of life; blood eosinophilia may occur.

2. Skin testing for food hypersensitivity often is unrevealing; however, large positive reactions can give an important lead to responsible allergens, especially those provoking a reaction of rapid onset, eg, angioedema, anaphylaxis, and severe gastrointestinal symptoms. Use scratch tests only.

3. Provocative food tests are important in the less serious entities. Elimination, challenge, and rechallenge must be relied upon for definitive diagnosis. In immediate or very serious reactions such as angioedema, anaphylaxis, and bronchial asthma, the causative food is usually known by the patient or parents or can be identified by the physician with the aid of a history. Food challenges and food skin testing would be hazardous in these situations. In the less serious and more obscure symptom entities, the likely food is a common one (eg, milk, cereal, chocolate); the suspected food should be withdrawn for a minimum of 3 weeks before challenge.

Differential Diagnosis of Important Symptoms

A. Gastrointestinal Intolerance: Differentiate from cystic fibrosis, pyloric stenosis, celiac disease, acute or chronic intestinal infections, gastrointestinal malformations, carbohydrate enzyme deficiencies (eg, lactase), and irritable bowel syndrome.

B. Angioedema of the Upper Airway: Differentiate from acute epiglottitis and foreign body in upper airway.

C. Tension-Fatigue Syndrome: Because the symptomatology is often vague, the differential diagnosis is often not specific. Connective tissue disorders (early phase), low-grade chronic infections, nutritional and metabolic disorders, leukemia (early), chronic poisonings, and hypochondriasis must be considered.

Treatment

Treatment consists of eliminating the offending food, but with specific advice for ensuring the nutritional adequacy of the diet. If milk or a comparable milk substitute is withdrawn from the diet for over 1 month in infants or over 2 months in older children, the daily maintenance requirement of calcium should be administered (see Chapter 4). *Note:* To be condemned—especially in the growing child—is the unnecessary and unjustified restriction of many foods over an indefinite period merely because they *might* be involved or happened to give a positive skin test reaction.

Treat specific signs or symptoms as indicated.

Prognosis

The prognosis is good if the offending food can be identified. In some of the vague chronic syndromes this may not be possible, in which case the patient will remain symptomatic. In the severe syndromes, the responsible food is usually known and can be avoided.

Frier S: Pediatric gastrointestinal allergy. Pages 107–126 in: *Clinical Immunology—Allergy—in Pediatric Medicine.* Brostoff J (editor). Blackwell, 1973.

Goldstein GB, Heiner DC: Clinical and immunologic perspectives in food hypersensitivity: A review. J Allergy 46:270, 1970.

Johnstone DE: Office management of food allergy in children. Ann Allergy 30:173, 1972.

May CD: Food allergy. Chap 17, pages 435–458, in: *Infant Nutrition,* 2nd ed. Fomon SJ (editor). Saunders, 1974.

CONTACT DERMATITIS

Essentials of Diagnosis

- Erythematous, papular eruption which may progress to include vesiculation, bulla formation, and denudation.
- Mild to intense pruritus.
- Eruption confined more or less to areas of direct skin contact with allergen.

General Considerations

Contact dermatitis is a delayed hypersensitivity reaction of the skin. The allergen is believed to conjugate locally with skin tissue elements. Sensitization after initial contact requires at least a few days and frequently takes much longer, but an already sensitized individual may react to contact with the allergen in as little as 24 hours. Fur, leather and fabric dyes, formalin, dye intermediates, soaps, enzymes in detergents, rubber compounds and impurities, insecticides and fungicides, cosmetics, topical antibiotics and other drugs, vegetable oleoresins and mineral oils, weeds, flowers, foods, wool, silk, rayon, and plastics are among the most common offenders in contact dermatitis. Although most contact is local, dermatitis can be induced systemically in an already sensitized individual by ingestion of the antigen.

Clinical Findings

A. History: A history of contact with possible allergens appropriate to the distribution of the lesions, in conjunction with the appearance of the lesions, may be sufficient for the diagnosis or may serve only as a starting point for further investigation. Itching is the rule, is frequently intense, and may precede the onset of observable lesions.

B. Physical Examination: The appearance and distribution of the lesions are the main criteria for diagnosis. The eruption may be confined to areas of contact with the offending allergen, and the inflammation sharply demarcated from normal skin. With more severe and chronic eruptions, however, dissemination may occur as a result of scratching and repeated contact with the allergen. If the eruption is mild, only erythema with some papulation may be present; more intense reactions include vesiculation with denudation of skin and frank weeping. Exfoliative dermatitis and secondary infection can also occur. There may be evidence of excoriation reflecting the pruritic nature of these lesions. With chronic dermatitis, skin thickening may be present.

C. Patch Testing: Patch testing with suspected allergens can be used to identify the contactants involved. In general, patch testing should not be performed when the dermatitis is active since this procedure may exacerbate the dermatitis. Patch testing kits of common contact allergens can be obtained from a variety of firms dealing with allergenic materials. The patch testing procedure is briefly as follows:

1. Material is applied to a gauze patch and secured to a nonhairy portion of the skin with adhesive tape (or an adhesive substitute in tape-sensitive persons).

2. The patch is removed after 48 hours—or sooner if itching, pain, or burning develops. The patch should be kept dry and remain securely fastened to the skin during the contact period.

3. The test is read 24—48 hours after removal of the patch. A positive test is one in which there is definite evidence of dermatitis which persists 24 hours or more. (A hand lens is helpful in interpreting mild or questionable reactions.) A control patch test should be employed. Be certain that the testing material is not itself a primary irritant. Solutions and oils can be soaked into the gauze; ointments and creams are merely smeared on the gauze.

Differential Diagnosis

Seborrheic dermatitis, atopic dermatitis, scabies, papular urticaria, nummular eczema, dermatophytoses, and candidiasis may at times be confused with contact dermatitis.

Prevention

Sensitizing substances should be avoided to the extent possible. Inflamed skin is more susceptible to sensitization than normal skin, and one must regard virtually any substance applied to the skin as potentially sensitizing; a test application of a "new" topical agent to a very limited area is advised before more extensive use.

Hyposensitization is not generally successful and presents a number of problems. Moreover, the striking beneficial effects of a brief course of local or systemic corticosteroid treatment virtually nullify justification for hyposensitization at the present time.

Treatment

A. Early Treatment:

1. Terminate exposure to the contactant.

2. Burow's solution (Domeboro powder or tablet, 1 package or tablet to 1—2 pints of water), or potassium permanganate, 1:6000 (0.3 gm tablet plus 2 quarts of water), soaks may be used in the early stage of treatment, especially if oozing is present, to diminish itching.

B. Mild Dermatitis: Zinc oxide paste or calamine lotion may be used.

C. Severe Dermatitis: Creams containing corticosteroids—particularly the fluorinated corticosteroids—are helpful. These should be applied liberally and frequently so as to keep the inflamed areas covered at all times. In unusual circumstances, when the dermatitis is extremely severe and extensive, systemic corticosteroids should be considered. A short course of systemic corticosteroids followed by topical corticosteroid administration is frequently helpful in controlling acute severe contact dermatitis (eg, poison ivy dermatitis). In severe cases, a course of 3—4 weeks may be necessary. Pastes, ointments, and creams should not be applied to weeping skin.

D. General Measures:

1. Avoid all secondary irritants to the skin, eg, wool, detergents.

2. Treat infection, if present. Early, potassium permanganate solution may be employed instead of Burow's solution. Topical treatment may be sufficient, but with extensive lesions systemic antibiotic therapy must be used. Topical antibiotics should not be used because they have potential for sensitization.

3. Give antihistamines orally for pruritus. Colloidal soaks, such as starch baths, may be employed with extensive dermatitis.

DeWeck AL: Contact eczematous dermatitis. Pages 669–680 in: *Dermatology in General Medicine.* Fitzpatrick TB & others (editors). McGraw-Hill, 1971.

Fisher AA: *Contact Dermatitis,* 2nd ed. Lea & Febiger, 1973.

Hjorth N, Fregert S: Contact dermatitis. Pages 305–385 in: *Textbook of Dermatology.* Rook A & others (editors). Blackwell, 1972.

SERUM SICKNESS

Essentials of Diagnosis

- Fever, malaise.
- Skin rash (usually urticarial).
- Local or generalized lymphadenopathy, polyarthralgia, or polyarthritis is frequent.
- History of recent administration of foreign serum or drug.

General Considerations

Antibiotics—particularly penicillin—have largely replaced foreign serum as the principal cause of serum sickness. In addition to antibiotics and foreign sera, vaccines, toxoids, and virtually any injectable foreign substance may cause this disorder. It may occur after the first encounter with a substance, usually requiring 7–10 days for sufficient sensitization to occur. Reexposure to the antigen in an already sensitized individual may result in symptoms as early as 1–4 days later. In unusually sensitive individuals, exposure to antigen may result in anaphylactic shock. Administration of antigen or, in atopic individuals, natural exposure (eg, to horse allergens) may sensitize an individual to the antigen without inducing clinically apparent symptoms.

Clinical Findings

A. Symptoms and Signs: This disorder usually begins with a low-grade fever and malaise which are followed to a variable extent by skin rash, lymphadenopathy, polyarthritis, and neurologic symptoms. Skin rashes occur in over 90% of cases. Most commonly, the skin rash is urticarial with an accompanying severe pruritus (which may precede the urticaria), but other erythematous eruptions may occur. Development of a localized erythematous or frankly urticarial reaction may first occur at the injection site. Lymphadenopathy may be localized to an area which drains the injection site or it may be generalized. Neurologic lesions, when they occur, are most commonly those of peripheral neuritis, but there may be CNS involvement as well. Gastrointestinal symptoms sometimes occur.

B. Laboratory Findings: Leukopenia may occur early, followed later by leukocytosis. Eosinophilia is not common but does occur. Proteinuria and microscopic hematuria may be seen.

Prevention

The patient should always be questioned about a history of previous reactions before the administration of drugs, sera, or other injectable foreign substances. (In atopic individuals, a history of respiratory allergy induced by contact with an animal from which the serum to be administered has been derived is strongly suggestive that the patient may react adversely.)

Since foreign sera are highly sensitizing, skin tests with the serum should be performed if a history of previous contact or suspected allergy is obtained. Caution is required, since anaphylactic reactions after skin tests have been known to occur. Scratch testing should be done first, followed by intradermal testing with a 1:20 dilution of the scratch test material. Unfortunately, the reliability of the skin test in predicting clinical sensitivity is much less than desired; both false-positive and false-negative reactions occur. Conjunctival tests are also unreliable.

Treatment

Treatment consists mainly of the discontinuance of the drug or other offending agent, the use of antihistamines with or without adrenergic drugs, and, in more severe and prolonged cases, administration of adrenal corticosteroids. When angioneurotic edema, bronchial constriction, and vascular collapse occur, epinephrine and theophylline may be lifesaving. (See Medical Emergencies Due to Allergic Reactions, above.) Joint pain, pruritus, and high fever may be amenable to treatment with aspirin. Sedation may also be in order.

Prognosis

In most cases serum sickness subsides in less than a week, but on occasion it may be more prolonged. The symptoms usually abate with the clearance of offending antigen from the circulation; persistence, therefore, suggests continued exposure.

Arbesman CE, Reisman RE: Serum sickness and human anaphylaxis. Chap 20 in: *Immunological Diseases,* 2nd ed. Samter M (editor). Little, Brown, 1971.

DRUG ALLERGY

Drugs are so widely used that drug reactions of one type or another are commonplace. *Toxic drug reactions* are due to the inherent pharmacologic properties of the drug and are most frequently encountered after drug overdosage. Some individuals exhibit inordinate sensitivity to the recognized pharmacologic effects of a drug, however, and may therefore develop toxicity after administration of amounts that are usually nontoxic. *Drug idiosyncrasy* is an unusual response to the pharmacologic action of the drug (eg, hyperactivity rather than sedation following the administration of phenobarbital). This paradoxic reaction to barbiturates is not uncommon in patients with atopy. *Allergic reactions to drugs,* on the other hand, are independent of the drug's pharmacologic action and, as is true of all allergic reactions, are the result of antigen-antibody interaction. The allergen may not be the drug administered but a metabolic derivative of it produced in the body. Although the immunologic reaction is highly specific, cross-reactions with chemically related drugs are not infrequent. Allergy to one sulfonamide, for example, is often associated with allergy to many other sulfonamides, and there is potential cross-reactivity among the various kinds of penicillins.

The manifestations of drug allergy are extremely varied, and virtually all allergic syndromes can be produced by drugs. The most common manifestations are skin eruptions (see Chapter 8) and fever.

In recent years, various syndromes related to reactivity to aspirin have been recognized, predominantly in adults but also in children. The reactions appear to be nonallergic, based rather on some peculiar biochemical idiosyncrasy. Production of nasal polyposis, severe aspirin-induced bronchospasm, and rhinitis with sinusitis have been well publicized, but a more subtle bronchospastic influence also has been documented in many children with asthma. Urticaria or angioedema also occurs in association with rhinitis and nasal polyposis, generally without bronchospasm in the urticarial forms.

Although any drug is a potential sensitizer, some, particularly penicillin and the sulfonamides, are more often associated with allergic reactions than others. The likelihood of sensitization is increased by repeated exposure. It is also probable that parenteral administration is more sensitizing than oral administration. Topical administration of drugs, especially over inflamed skin, is particularly sensitizing.

Exposure to sunlight may activate skin reactions to photosensitizing drugs such as sulfonamides, tetracycline antibiotics, and topically applied coal tar products.

In questioning a patient about drug reactions, it should be remembered that certain drugs such as benzathine penicillin G remain in the body for a long time. Reactions to a single depot injection of penicillin have been known to last for months.

With the exception of patch testing in contact dermatitis, skin testing has usually been a disappointing procedure in identifying or predicting drug allergy. The reasons are many, and in some cases at least the allergic reaction is due to a metabolically altered form of the drug. In the case of penicillin, some of the offensive metabolic derivatives have been identified. When these substances are used in skin testing, prediction of allergic reactions on the basis of a skin test reaction is more successful. However, these reagents are not readily available, and until the exact allergens in other drugs are identified and preparations containing the appropriate allergens become widely available, skin (and RAST) testing for drug allergy cannot be considered a reliable procedure. The basis for "hypersensitivity" reactions to urographic or other radiocontrast material is unknown, and skin testing to predict reactivity to these agents is unreliable.

The history of previous reactions to drugs remains the best means of diagnosing drug sensitivity. This is often difficult, however, and in any instance in which a reaction to a drug is questionable an alternative drug should be used (if possible) and the patient advised to avoid the drug even though a definite drug allergy has not been established.

Treatment

Regardless of the manifestation, the treatment of drug allergy includes discontinuance of the offending drug at the first sign of an adverse reaction and making certain that further contact with the drug is avoided. Small amounts of drugs to which a patient may be sensitive may be found in vaccines, foods, and other substances. Individuals with extreme hypersensitivity to a given drug should be warned, therefore, of other hidden sources of contact with the drug. Although desensitization has been used successfully, it is not recommended, and the physician is better advised to substitute a chemically unrelated drug for the offending drug.

Symptomatic treatment is usually effective. Patients suspected of being reactive to a radiocontrast dye should be pretreated with steroids and antihistamines if the use of the dye is considered necessary.

Prognosis

The prognosis is good, especially with early identification.

DeSwarte RD: Drug allergy. Chap 16, pages 393–493, in: *Allergic Diseases, Diagnosis and Management*. Patterson R (editor). Lippincott, 1972.

Kasik JE, Thompson JS: Allergic reactions to antibiotics. Med Clin North Am 54:59, 1970.

Nelson H: Allergic reaction to drugs. (Part 1.) Special problems in drug allergy. (Part 2.) Adv Asthma Allergy 3:18, 1976; 4:22, 1977.

Samter M, Parker CW: *Hypersensitivity to Drugs*. Pergamon Press, 1972.

Schatz M & others: The administration of radiographic contrast media to patients with a history of a previous reaction. J Allergy Clin Immunol 55:358, 1975.

Settipane GA, Pudupakkam RK: Aspirin intolerance. 3. Subtypes, familial occurrence, and cross-reactivity with tartrazine. J Allergy Clin Immunol 56:215, 1975.

URTICARIA

Essentials of Diagnosis

- Multiple (occasionally single) macular lesions, consisting of localized edema (wheal) with surrounding erythema.
- Pruritus, frequently intense.

General Considerations

Urticaria is a vascular reaction of the upper dermis consisting mainly of vasodilatation and perivascular transudation, resulting in the classical "hive" or wheal and flare. Lesions are characteristically pruritic. Ordinarily, this vascular reaction is due to the liberation of histamine, but other mediators may be involved.

Urticarial reactions are usually transient (hours) but have been known to persist for months or more. They may be the sole allergic manifestation or may represent only a part of the clinical picture, as in serum sickness. Emotional tension may be a precipitating factor. *Angioedema* is essentially an urticarial reaction of the lower parts of the dermis, resulting in the production of a more diffuse edema.

Hereditary angioneurotic edema is a rare syndrome characterized by periodic bouts of angioedema frequently involving one or more extremities but other anatomic areas as well. It is inherited as an autosomal dominant trait and appears to be related to a deficiency of C1 esterase and kinin inhibitor. There is no good evidence that an allergic mechanism is involved. Characteristically, pruritus is absent in this disorder.

Cholinergic urticaria, which is uncommon, seems to occur in some individuals during and following exercise, increased environmental heat, and emotional stress. Characteristically, the lesions appear as extremely small wheals accompanied by a large bright-red flare. Abdominal cramps, diarrhea, increased sweating, and headache may also occur.

Clinical Findings

A. History: The history is of prime importance in ascertaining the possible cause. The most common causes of urticaria include the following:

1. Drugs, hyposensitization extracts, vaccines, toxoids, and hormone preparations.

2. Infections—Bacterial (especially staphylococci, group A beta-hemolytic streptococci), parasitic, fungal, and viral, including viral hepatitis.

3. Foods (especially eggs, milk, wheat, chocolate, pork, shellfish, fresh water fish, berries, cheese, and nuts) and food dyes and other food additives.

4. Inhalants, pollens, molds.

5. Insect bites—Papular urticaria is a term given to a syndrome characterized by multiple papules resembling insect bites, found especially on the extremities. It is thought to be due to hypersensitivity to the bites of fleas, mites, mosquitoes, lice, or bedbugs.

6. Psychologic factors.

7. Physical factors (cold, heat), histamine liberators, and dermographia should be considered.

B. Symptoms and Signs: Urticarial lesions characteristically appear as erythematous areas with a pale center and usually occur in large numbers. Pruritus is the rule and is frequently intense; it may precede the appearance of the lesions. Pruritus is not as characteristic of angioneurotic edema (giant hives), however, which occurs most often as a solitary lesion or in conjunction with multiple urticaria. When urticaria involves the laryngeal area, it may be a threat to life.

Dermographia may be symptomatic and occurs in approximately 10% of allergic patients.

In addition to the history, diagnostic procedures may include drug elimination, dietary elimination of suspected foods and their challenge, and a thorough search for infection elsewhere in the body. Skin testing more often than not is of little value in urticaria.

Differential Diagnosis

Urticaria is a prominent feature of mastocytosis (urticaria pigmentosa) and may occur in systemic diseases such as lupus erythematosus, various liver diseases, lymphoma, and leukemia.

Treatment

Treatment consists mainly of the detection and elimination of the appropriate allergens, when possible, and psychotherapy if indicated. Aspirin should be avoided altogether, as it may secondarily aggravate the urticaria. Antihistamines are usually the most useful therapeutic agents in urticarial disorders, but adrenergic agents with vasoconstrictor properties can be a useful adjunct. Epinephrine is especially effective when rapid relief is needed. Hydroxyzine (Atarax, Vistaril) has been reported to be effective in some instances in which antihistamines are not, eg, chronic urticaria and dermatographia. Cyproheptadine (Periactin) is most effective in some patients with cold urticaria. Mild sedation may also be indicated.

Adrenal corticosteroids are sometimes used in the more chronic form of urticaria but are reserved for more refractory cases. They generally are not required in the management of acute urticaria or angioneurotic edema.

Topical medications generally are not effective.

Prognosis

Except for life-threatening laryngeal edema, the prognosis is good. Identification of the offending agent is most important.

Epstein JH: Photoallergy. Arch Dermatol 106:741, 1972.

Fink JN: Urticaria and physical allergy. Chap 13, pages 341–354, in: *Allergic Diseases, Diagnosis and Management.* Patterson R (editor). Lippincott, 1972.

Mathews KP: A current view of urticaria. Med Clin North Am 58:185, 1974.

Sheffer A: Urticaria and angioedema. Pediatr Clin North Am 22:193, 1975.

Thompson JS: Urticaria and angioedema. Ann Intern Med 69:361, 1968.

Warin RP, Champion RH (editors): *Urticaria.* Saunders, 1974.

OTHER ALLERGIC PULMONARY DISORDERS

Various pulmonary disorders either known or thought to stem from an allergic reaction to inhaled or ingested antigens have been described. In some cases, evidence implicating an allergic mechanism in the pathogenesis of the disease is substantial; in others, the role of allergic mechanisms is mainly conjectural.

A syndrome thought to be related to *cow's milk hypersensitivity* has been described which consists of recurrent pulmonary infiltrates, wheezing, chronic cough, chronic or frequent otitis media and rhinorrhea, and iron deficiency anemia related to excessive gastrointestinal blood loss. Gastrointestinal symptoms (diarrhea, vomiting) and poor weight gain are also features of this disorder which is seen in children chiefly in the first 2 years of life. Some of these children have evidence of pulmonary hemosiderosis, and blood eosinophilia is sometimes seen. Multiple precipitins to cow's milk can be demonstrated, but the significance of this finding is controversial. Dietary elimination of cow's milk antigens is followed by improvement of the disorder, although symptoms also have been reported to subside spontaneously.

Extrinsic allergic alveolitis (hypersensitivity pneumonitis) is an inflammatory reaction involving principally the alveoli and characterized clinically by malaise, fever, chills, cough, and dyspnea. Tissue damage stems from a hypersensitivity reaction to any of a variety of inhaled organic dusts or of fungi which may or may not also be infective. The disease is seen predominantly in adults as a result of occupational exposure to large concentrations of certain antigens (eg, proteinaceous material from bird droppings in bird fancier's lung; thermophilic actinomycetes from hay in farmer's lung or from contaminated air conditioners), but it can occur at any age. Pulmonary allergic aspergillosis, with or without tissue invasion by the organism, is seen with some frequency in Great Britain but is rare in the USA. These diseases occur principally in adults but have been reported in children also. The onset may be insidious or acute. Symptoms—particularly in the acute onset form—typically occur 4—8 hours after exposure to the offending antigen. In asthmatic individuals, wheezing also may be a part of the picture, with involvement of reagin-mediated mechanisms as well. Rales may be heard, but physical findings referable to the lungs may be minimal. Chest x-ray reveals a variable pattern, with mottled densities or infiltrates early in the disease and a picture of interstitial fibrosis in more chronic cases. Pulmonary function studies reveal a restrictive defect with diminished diffusing capacity (Pa_{O_2} may be decreased, but Pa_{CO_2} is usually normal). Treatment consists mainly of avoiding the offensive inhalants. Glucocorticoids may be extremely helpful in minimizing the hypersensitivity reaction early in the disease. Accompanying fungal infection must also be treated (eg, amphotericin in aspergillosis). If recognized early, lesions are largely reversible and the prognosis is excellent. With chronic severe disease, pulmonary fibrosis may result, leading to severe respiratory insufficiency and death.

An association between *tissue and blood eosinophilia* and *pulmonary infiltrates* has been observed in various disorders (eg, asthma, pulmonary allergic aspergillosis, connective tissue diseases) and is thought to reflect an allergic pathogenesis in these disorders. Pulmonary infiltrates with eosinophilia (PIE) sometimes occur as an apparently distinct clinical entity characterized by mild (mainly cough) to absent clinical symptoms and fleeting pulmonary infiltrates which, on x-ray, appear to migrate from one area of the lungs to another over a few days (often called Löffler's syndrome). A number of drugs (especially sulfonamides and nitrofurantoin), parasites (eg, ascaris), and other antigens have been implicated at times in the production of this syndrome, but frequently no cause can be found. The disorder is generally self-limited, lasting less than a month; but more severe forms may be seen (eg, in many cases of so-called tropical eosinophilia associated with filariasis), and the tissue reaction may proceed to pulmonary fibrosis. Corticosteroids may be extremely beneficial, particularly early in the reaction, and should be used when the severity of the disorder warrants.

Heiner DC: Pulmonary hemosiderosis. Chap 30, pages 336—351, in: *Diseases of the Respiratory Tract in Children,* 2nd ed. Vol 1. *Pulmonary Disorders.* Kendig EL Jr (editor). Saunders, 1972.

Lake WW, Salvaggio JE, Beuchner HA: Infiltrative "hypersensitivity" lung disease. Chap 13, pages 252—294, in: *Annual Review of Allergy 1973.* Frazier CA (editor). Medical Examination Publishing Co., 1974.

Rosenow EC III: The spectrum of drug-induced pulmonary disease. Ann Intern Med 77:977, 1972.

Slavin RG: Allergic bronchopulmonary aspergillosis. Pages 543—546 in: *Allergic Diseases, Diagnosis and Management.* Patterson R (editor). Lippincott, 1972.

TRANSFUSION REACTIONS

Essentials of Diagnosis

- Fever and chills during or after transfusion.
- Urticarial reaction with or without lymphadenopathy, joint pains, fever, hypotension, asthma.

General Considerations

The incidence of transfusion reactions is high—estimates ranging up to 20%. A common form is a febrile reaction which may be related to contamination with bacterial or other pyrogenic products or which may accompany hemolytic reactions or reactions in which transfused leukocytes are destroyed by anti-leukocyte antibodies present in the recipient. Urticarial reactions have been reported to occur in 1—3% of transfusions and are said to be more common in atopic individuals. Citrate toxicity, manifested largely as tetany and vascular collapse progressing at times to death, is an unusual complication of transfusion therapy. The transmission of serum hepatitis is also a potential problem, but careful screening of donors has helped to reduce the incidence of transmission.

Transfusion of mismatched blood may have any of the following adverse effects: symptoms and signs of intravascular or extravascular hemolysis; ischemia or bleeding; or a reaction involving antibodies formed to

IgA, especially in IgA-deficient recipients. Allergic reactions to mismatched transfused blood may result from passive sensitization of the recipient through blood from a donor who is sensitive to foods, drugs, inhalants, or other allergens, or from the infusion of allergen present in donor's plasma to which the recipient is sensitive. Hemolytic reactions are among the most severe transfusion reactions and are associated with a high mortality rate.

Clinical Findings

A. Symptoms and Signs: Chills and fever are particularly common and may be associated with septicemia, hemolytic reactions, or reactions due to the presence of leuko-agglutinins, especially if the patient has received multiple transfusions. Symptoms of hemolytic reactions may also include headache, nausea and vomiting, apprehension and anxiety, facial flushing, a feeling of warmth along the vein into which blood is being transfused, and abdominal or chest pains. Hypotension, oliguria, and frank renal failure with anuria may result.

Urticarial reactions with accompanying pruritus frequently occur without other symptoms but may also occur in conjunction with anaphylactic and hemolytic reactions. Anaphylactic reactions, which may include bronchial obstruction, hypotension, or laryngeal edema, are seen rarely. With allergic reactions, eosinophilia is sometimes noted.

B. Laboratory Findings: With hemolytic reactions, free hemoglobin is usually present in detectable amounts in the serum almost immediately and may also be found in the urine; serum bilirubin levels may become elevated within hours, as may methemoglobin levels also. The white blood count may be high or low. A Coombs test (direct and indirect) performed on posttransfusion recipient's blood should reveal the presence of antibody reactive with cells of the recipient or donor. In addition, red cell agglutinates can sometimes be seen in a sample of the recipient's blood. Agglutinins to other formed blood elements or antibody to donor immunoglobulins may be found.

Prevention

Antihistamines (Table 32–1) given 1 hour before the blood transfusion may be used prophylactically to decrease the incidence and severity of allergic reactions. This procedure has reportedly been very effective, but it would seem to make more sense to administer antihistamines only to those patients who develop allergic symptoms rather than to use the drugs routinely. Used prophylactically, *antihistamines do not completely eliminate the possibility of a severe transfusion reaction.* Problems consequent to the administration of hemolyzed blood can largely be avoided with proper inspection of the blood and equipment prior to transfusion.

Treatment

Treatment consists chiefly of immediate discontinuation of the transfusion and maintenance of adequate blood volume and pressure by means of intravenous fluids and pressor amines. Other ancillary measures depend upon the degree and nature of the reaction.

Urticaria with pruritus unaccompanied by other signs or symptoms does not necessarily contraindicate continuing the transfusion, as is the case with mild febrile reactions.

The treatment of urticarial reactions, angioedema, laryngeal edema, asthma, serum sickness, and anaphylactic shock has been described elsewhere.

Epinephrine, 1:1000, 0.2–0.4 ml IM, remains the most important single drug early in the treatment of severe acute allergic reactions. Antihistamines may also be given intravenously. Corticosteroids have also been recommended for the treatment of allergic and hemolytic transfusion reactions, but their efficacy in acute reactions is questionable.

For citrate toxicity, treatment consists of discontinuation of the transfusion and *slow* administration of calcium chloride (5%) or calcium gluconate (10%), 5–20 ml IV.

With hemolytic reactions, recipient and donor blood should be retyped and cross-matched and recipient blood cross-matched against other possible donors. If the hemolytic reaction is severe—and in the absence of cardiac failure, severe dehydration, intracranial bleeding, or renal failure—mannitol, 0.3 gm/kg of 20% solution IV over 10–15 minutes, should be given in addition to intravenous fluids in order to ensure adequate urine flow. This procedure may be repeated once in 2 hours if adequate urine flow is not attained in this time.

Plasma expanders may be necessary to treat hypotension due to hypovolemia.

Corticosteroids—eg, hydrocortisone sodium succinate (Solu-Cortef), 4 mg/kg—should be added to intravenous fluids and infused over a 4- to 6-hour period.

Prognosis

The prognosis depends on the nature and degree of the reaction. Hemolytic reactions must be kept in mind since they are associated with a high fatality rate.

Baker RJ, Nyhus LM: Diagnosis and treatment of immediate transfusion reaction. Surg Gynec Obst 130:665, 1970.

Hossaini AA, Boyan CP: Transfusion reactions. Internat Anesth Clin 10:227, 1972.

Masouredis SP: Hazards of transfusion therapy. Pages 1314–1319 in: *Hematology.* Williams WJ & others (editors). McGraw-Hill, 1972.

Rudowski WJ: Complications associated with blood transfusion. Progr Surg 9:78, 1971.

● ● ●

General References

Aas K: *The Biochemical and Immunological Basis of Bronchial Asthma.* Thomas, 1972.

Feingold BF (editor): *Introduction to Clinical Allergy.* Thomas, 1973.

Patterson R (editor): *Allergic Diseases, Diagnosis and Management.* Lippincott, 1972.

Samter M (editor): *Immunological Diseases,* 2nd ed. Little, Brown, 1971.

Samter M, Durham OC: *Regional Allergy of the United States, Canada, Mexico, and Cuba.* Thomas, 1955.

Sheldon JM, Lovell RG, Matthews KP: *A Manual of Clinical Allergy,* 2nd ed. Saunders, 1967.

Sherman WB: *Hypersensitivity: Mechanisms and Management.* Saunders, 1968.

Speer F, Dockhorn RJ (editors): *Allergy and Immunology in Childhood.* Thomas, 1973.

Van Der Wert PJ: *Mold Fungi and Bronchial Asthma.* Thomas, 1958.

Weiss EB, Segal MS (editors): *Bronchial Asthma, Mechanisms and Therapeutics.* Little, Brown, 1976.

33...
Genetic & Chromosomal Disorders, Including Inborn Errors of Metabolism

Arthur Robinson, MD, Stephen I. Goodman, MD, & Donough O'Brien, MD, FRCP

I. GENETIC & CHROMOSOMAL DISORDERS

Recent developments in the science of genetics have greatly increased our understanding of the basic processes of heredity. Genetics is an essential discipline for an understanding of human biology; it helps to unify the physician's concept of disease and has increasing relevance to his clinical experience.

THE CELL

The central structure of any living cell is its complement of genes (located on the chromosomes) within the cell nucleus and consisting of a molecule whose 3-dimensional structure is that of a double helix. This molecule, deoxyribonucleic acid (DNA), is the chief constituent of the gene, which has a dual function: (1) to replicate itself (the central act of biologic reproduction); and (2) to be responsible, through the enzymes, for specific aspects of the cell's metabolism.

The information residing within a specific gene is necessary to permit synthesis of the polypeptide, a linear array of amino acids, which forms a segment of a protein. The enzymes, which are proteins, are necessary as catalysts for chemical reactions in the cell. This is in accord with the Beadle-Tatum "one gene, one enzyme" hypothesis.

A series of consecutive triplet pyrimidine and purine base pairs in the linear DNA chain code for, and are colinear with, the series of consecutive amino acids in the polypeptide chain. Many of the details of how this information is transcribed and translated have been worked out; and protein synthesis has even been observed in vitro in a cell-free system.

The majority of the genes are probably not "structural," ie, not responsible for the production of specific proteins, but are regulatory. These latter genes permit the cell to respond sensitively to its environment and to differentiate into the various kinds of cells within the organism. This has been shown in bacteria and is probably true in man, although this has yet to be proved.

CELL DIVISION

The cell cycle can be roughly divided into 4 periods (Fig 33–1): (1) S, the period of DNA replication; (2) M, the period of cell division; and (3) G1 and (4) G2, the periods separating S and M in which protein synthesis may occur.

Cell division is of 2 types: meiosis, a form of cell division limited to those cells (germ cells or gametes) which participate in sexual reproduction; and mitosis, a form of asexual division occurring in somatic cells.

Meiosis occurs during gametogenesis (Fig 33–2). During the first meiotic division, homologous chromosomes are arranged in pairs (synapsis) along the equatorial plate, permitting genetic recombination, a process essential to human variability and evolution. The 2 homologues then separate and move to opposite poles (disjunction). Unlike the situation which exists in mitosis, described below, division occurs between (not through) the centromeres. As a result, the daughter cells have one member of each chromosome pair (haploid). Following the first meiotic (reduction) division, a second division, mitotic in character, occurs. Hence

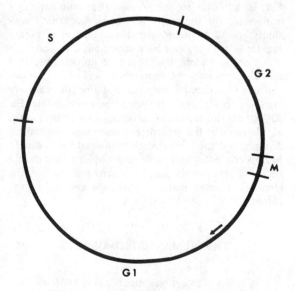

Figure 33–1. Diagram of the life cycle of a mammalian cell.

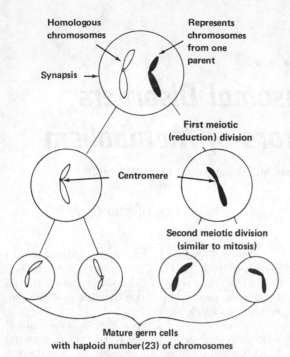

Figure 33–2. Diagrammatic representation of meiosis, demonstrating the conversion from the diploid somatic cell to the haploid gamete.

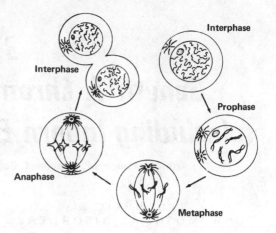

Figure 33–3. Diagram demonstrating the various stages of the mitotic cycle.

the mature germ cells, both sperm and ova, have the haploid number of 23 chromosomes. After fertilization, the fertilized egg (zygote) has the full diploid chromosome complement of somatic cells, 46.

It is worth stressing that, during the first meiotic division, chance alone determines which member of a chromosome pair, the maternally or paternally derived one, will migrate to a given pole. This permits 2^{23} different combinations of chromosomes in the gametes and, in addition to the process of recombination, is responsible for the major part of human genetic variability. No 2 humans, with the exception of monozygotic twins, have ever been genetically identical.

During *mitosis,* the DNA coils up tightly so that the chromosomes become short and thick, which explains why they are only visible during this relatively brief segment of the cell cycle. During metaphase (Fig 33–3), the shortened chromosomes arrange themselves on the spindle; the centromere undergoes longitudinal division; and the separated chromosomal halves disjoin to opposite poles before the cell divides into 2 daughter cells. This permits the 2 daughter cells to have the identical genetic material that was present in the parent cell.

THE HUMAN CHROMOSOMES

A new era in cytogenetics began in 1956 with the discovery, by Tjio and Levan, that the human chromo-

somal number was 46. Since then, this field has advanced with explosive rapidity. Its importance to medicine may be judged by the fact that grossly abnormal karyotypes occur in about 1% of human live births.

Since the chromosomes can only be delineated during mitosis, it is important to examine human material containing many cells in a dividing state. The only tissue in the body where this condition exists to any degree is the bone marrow. Because bone marrow is not readily available for routine biopsy, it becomes necessary to utilize tissue culture technics to stimulate rapid in vitro growth, so that many cells in mitosis may be examined. The period of culture varies with the tissues sampled. The lymphocytes of the blood, being most readily available, are most commonly cultured, requiring 3 days of growth in the presence of phytohemagglutinin (PHA), a mitogenic agent.

Chromosomes prepared from cultures consist of 2 arms separated by a light-staining centromere by which they are normally attached to the spindle. Because the DNA has already replicated (in the S period), each arm consists of 2 identical chromatids. Chromosomes may be designated, according to the position of the centromere, as metacentric, submetacentric, and acrocentric (nearly terminal centromere). The 10 acrocentrics are satellited.

The human somatic cell has 22 pairs of autosomes and 2 sex chromosomes. The female, being the homogametic sex, has 2 X chromosomes; the heterogametic male has one X and one Y (Figs 33–4 and 33–5).

The system for numbering and ordering the chromosomes adopted in 1960 by an international study group meeting in Denver is now used throughout the world. Although there is some difficulty in clearly distinguishing individual pairs within a given grouping, especially in suboptimal preparations, the "Denver system" has greatly simplified communication among cytogenetic laboratories in all countries. The finding, with the help of autoradiography, that chromosome replication in the S period occurs in a definite order

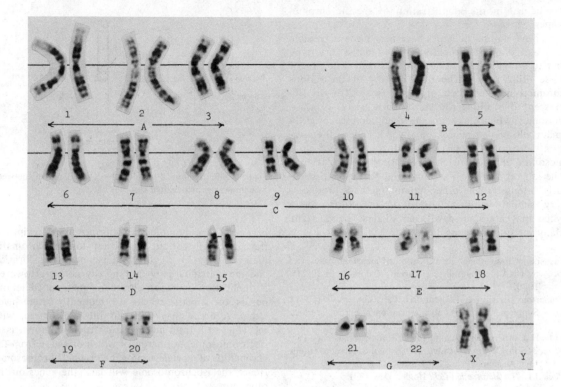

Figure 33—4. Female human chromosomes (Giemsa banding).

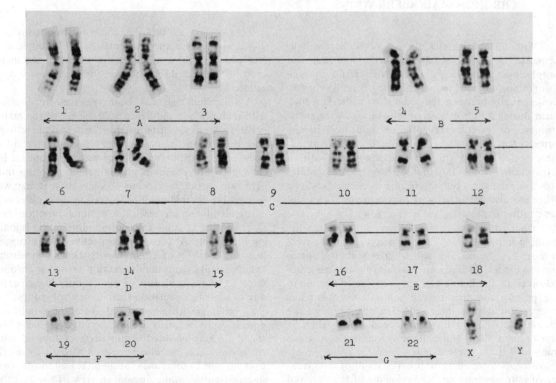

Figure 33—5. Male human chromosomes (Giemsa banding).

has helped in the identification of specific chromosomes.

New staining technics have now made it possible to identify all of the chromosomes in the karyotype and to arrange them in homologous pairs. The first of these utilizes the differential affinity of the various chromosomes and parts of chromosomes for the fluorescent dye, quinacrine mustard. Segments of chromosomes which take up the dye fluoresce brightly under ultraviolet microscopy whereas the other segments do not. This gives the individual pairs of chromosomes unique and characteristic banding patterns. The long arm of the Y chromosome fluoresces particularly intensely. The other staining methods produce a very similar banding pattern on the chromosomes when they are stained with an alkaline Giemsa stain. Many variants are being described.

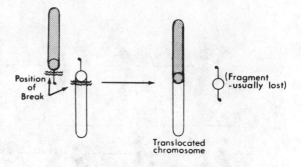

Figure 33–6. Reciprocal translocation (Robertsonian) between 2 nonhomologous satellited chromosomes.

Caspersson T & others: Identification of human chromosomes by DNA-binding fluorescent agents. Chromosoma 30:215, 1970.
Hamerton JL, Klinger HP (editors): Paris Conference (1971), Supplement (1975): Standardization in human genetics. Birth Defects 11(9):1, 1975. [Entire issue.]
Lubs H & others: New staining methods for chromosomes. Page 345 in: *Methods in Cell Biology.* Vol 6. Prescott D (editor). Academic Press, 1973.
Puck TT: *The Mammalian Cell.* Holden-Day, 1971.

between 2 nonhomologous chromosomes (reciprocal translocation) without significant loss of chromatin material (Fig 33–6), this is a balanced translocation and the individual is phenotypically normal. However, if duplication or loss of chromatin material (deletion) occurs, the somatic effects are frequently severe—even lethal. A break may occur at the centromere, with rehealing to form a metacentric structure known as an isochromosome, both arms of which originate from the chromatids of a single arm of the original chromosome. Hence the isochromosome will lack the genes on the other arm.

CHROMOSOMAL ABERRATIONS

With current technics, the cytogeneticist is able to recognize 2 classes of abnormality: numerical and morphologic. *Numerical abnormalities* are due to nondisjunction, ie, the failure of the chromosomes to divide equally between the 2 daughter cells. This may occur during either meiosis or mitosis, ie, during gametogenesis or as a postzygotic phenomenon. In the former eventuality, 2 types of gametes will be formed: those which lack a chromosome and those with an extra chromosome. If either of these gametes unites with a normal germ cell, the resulting conceptus will be either monosomic or trisomic for the involved chromosome rather than having the normal pair.

When the nondisjunction is postzygotic, the resulting individual may be a mosaic, ie, he may have 2 or more cell populations which differ in their chromosomal number. Mosaicism may also be due to chromosome lag, the failure of a chromosome to migrate to one pole of the dividing cell and its subsequent loss from one of the daughter cells. The phenotype of the mosaic individual will then depend upon when in development the nondisjunction occurred and which anlage had the aneuploid cells.

Morphologic aberration is the result of the breakage of chromosomes and the rejoining of the damaged ends in new ways. When such a rearrangement occurs

CAUSE OF CHROMOSOMAL ABERRATIONS

As many as 0.5% of human live births and 25–50% of spontaneous abortions are aneuploid, a fact which marks nondisjunction as one of the major causes of human disease whose origin requires investigation.

Nondisjunction has been observed to increase with maternal age and hence with the age of the maternal ova. An explanation of this "maternal age effect" may be that the ovary contains a full complement of oocytes at birth, at which time meiotic prophase has already begun. These oocytes remain in prophase until ovulation, which may occur 40 years later. It may well be that the completion of oogenesis in these older cells is attended by an increased risk of nondisjunction.

Another possible cause of nondisjunction is ionizing irradiation. At least 3 retrospective studies suggest that the mothers of children with Down's syndrome (which results from nondisjunction involving chromosome 21) have a history of significantly higher exposure to ionizing irradiation than do control groups.

Patients with a variety of aneuploid conditions, especially those with Down's syndrome, have been found to have elevated serum titers of thyroid autoantibodies. This has also been true of their close relatives, in whom there may be an increased incidence of so-called autoimmune disease. In view of the fact that several epidemiologic studies have revealed that aneuploidy tends to occur in clusters in both time and space in a manner suggestive of viral epidemics, some have suggested that nondisjunction may occur more frequently as a result of a specific viral insult in those genetically predisposed to autoimmune disease.

Recent studies on the occurrence of nondisjunction of the X chromosome have thus far provided presumptive evidence that nonrandom environmental causes of nondisjunction exist.

Viral infections, both in vivo and in vitro, have been shown to cause chromosomal breaks with or without abnormal rehealing. In 3 diseases—congenital aplastic anemia (Fanconi), Bloom's dwarfism, and ataxia-telangiectasia—an increased incidence of chromosomal breakage has been found. Whether viral infections are involved in the etiology of these breaks is unknown. All 3 of these diseases are associated with an increased risk of malignancy.

Finally, a variety of chemical agents, especially drugs, have been implicated as causes of chromosomal breakage. In many cases, the data are conflicting and a final conclusion has not yet been reached. If these drugs do, in fact, break chromosomes, their influence on the production of congenital malformations is also not yet known.

Alberman E & others: Parental exposure to x-irradiation and Down's syndrome. Ann Hum Genet 36:195, 1972.

Atkin NB: Chromosomes in human malignant tumors. In: *Chromosomes and Cancer*. German J (editor). Wiley, 1974.

Carr DH, Gedeon M: Population cytogenetics of human abortions. In: *Population Cytogenetics*. Hook EB, Porter IH (editors). Academic Press, 1977.

Cohen MM, Hirschhorn K, Frosch WA: Cytogenetic effects of tranquilizing drugs in vivo and in vitro. JAMA 207:2425, 1969.

German J: Bloom's syndrome. 2. The prototype of genetic disorders predisposing to chromosomal instability and cancer. In: *Chromosomes and Cancer*. German J (editor). Wiley, 1974.

Goad W & others: Incidence of aneuploidy in a human population. Am J Hum Genet 28:62, 1976.

CHROMOSOMAL DISEASES

Numerical abnormalities may involve either the sex chromosomes or the autosomes, predominantly the former. Gross autosomal imbalances produce severe phenotypic disturbances and, particularly when they involve loss of chromosomal material, are usually incompatible with life.

DERMATOGLYPHICS

In persons with a variety of congenital malformations, and especially in those with chromosomal dis-

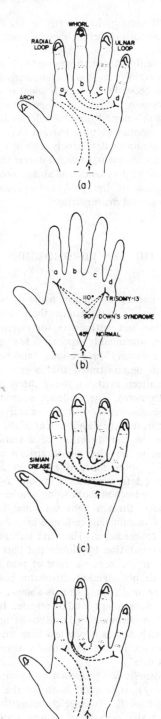

Figure 33—7. Abnormal palm prints. Schematic representation of *(a)* normal hand; *(b)* atd angle in normal person and in patients with Down's and trisomy 13 syndrome; *(c)* dermatoglyphic pattern in a patient with Down's syndrome; *(d)* dermatoglyphic pattern in a patient with trisomy 18 syndrome. (Reproduced from Porter IH: *Heredity and Disease*. McGraw-Hill, 1968. Copyright © 1968. Used with permission of McGraw-Hill Book Company.)

ease, the dermatoglyphic patterns, ie, the fingerprints, palm prints, and foot prints, deviate from the normal (Fig 33–7).

Since the fine dermal ridges on the hands and feet begin to develop in their characteristic patterns between the second and fourth months of embryogenesis, deviations from normal embryonic development during this period may be reflected in abnormalities of the dermatoglyphic pattern. As a result, the presence of abnormal dermatoglyphics in a patient suggests some developmental trauma during the second to fourth months of pregnancy and should prompt a careful examination of the patient for associated, less obvious, congenital malformations.

THE SEX CHROMOSOMES

Unlike Drosophila, in which the fly with the XO pattern is the male, in the human the Y chromosome is necessary (but not sufficient) for maleness. The Y chromosome presumably contains few genes other than those necessary to produce "maleness." It has recently been demonstrated that a gene for the so-called H-Y antigen exists on the Y chromosome (close to the centromere). The evidence suggests that this gene may be concerned with the primary determination of sex through the development of the undifferentiated gonad in the direction of a testicle. The X chromosome, on the other hand, carries many X-linked ("sex-linked") genes, most of which are not involved with either sex determination or sex development.

The X chromosome has some unique characteristics that have thrown light on some fundamental properties of mammalian cells and have been of great importance to medicine. The first indication of this was the demonstration by Moore and Barr of a sexual dimorphism in the somatic cells of man which consisted of a deeply staining chromatin body in some cells of the normal female and its absence in the male (Fig 33–8). Subsequent studies revealed that humans may have 0–4 chromatin (Barr) bodies and that the number of such bodies is one less than the number of X chromosomes in the individual's karyotype (the "nuclear sex rule").

A hypothesis was proposed by Lyon and Russell (independently) to account both for the above phenomenon and for the "dosage compensation" effect—the fact that the amount of protein produced by a given X-linked gene such as the one for antihemophilic globulin is independent of the number of X chromosomes the individual has (eg, the female with 2 X chromosomes does not produce twice as much antihemophilic globulin as the male with only one). They suggested that only one X chromosome in any cell is fully active and that all others are genetically inactive during the major part of the cell's life cycle. Moreover, the hypothesis suggests that, early in embryogenesis (about the tenth to twelfth day in man), a random

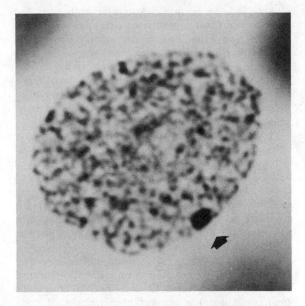

Figure 33–8. Nucleus of cell obtained from the buccal mucosa, demonstrating the densely staining chromatin body. Arrow points to chromatin body.

choice is made by each somatic cell about which X will remain active. Thereafter, the same X will remain active for all future progeny of a given cell. The normal female would then constitute a mosaic of clones with respect to the identity of the active X chromosome.

Much evidence has been accumulated to support the basic validity of the Lyon-Russell hypothesis. At present, it is thought that the Barr body represents the genetically inactive (or, more probably, the partially genetically inactive) X chromosome. Autoradiography has demonstrated that the various chromosome pairs have specific patterns of replication. The X chromosomes are remarkable for the degree of asynchrony they show in their patterns of replication, one of them being the last chromosome to replicate its DNA during the S period of the cell cycle. Whenever X polysomy (an increased number of X chromosomes) exists, all but one of the X chromosomes replicates late; and when one of the two X chromosomes has a morphologic abnormality, it too (with rare exceptions) is late in replicating. The Barr body, then, is thought to represent the genetically inactive, late-replicating X chromosome. When one of the X chromosomes is morphologically abnormal and hence late-replicating, the corresponding chromatin body may be abnormal in size.

The Lyon-Russell hypothesis provides an explanation for the observation that abnormalities of X chromosomal constitution are more likely to be compatible with life and to be associated with less severe phenotypic defects than those of autosomes.

A second type of sexual dimorphism which has the same significance as the Barr body is the "drumstick" on the nucleus of polymorphonuclear leukocytes (Fig 33–9). The presence of at least 6 of these in

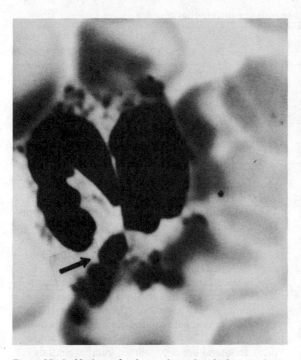

Figure 33—9. Nucleus of polymorphonuclear leukocyte. Arrow points to "drumstick."

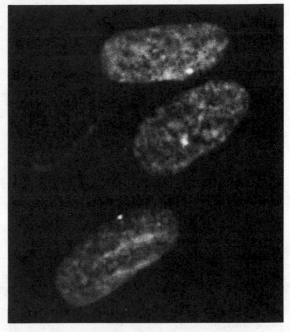

Figure 33—10. Fluorescent Y bodies in nuclei cells obtained from the umbilical cords of newborn males.

500 polymorphonuclear leukocytes reflects chromatin positivity in the blood. A discrepancy between the "drumstick" condition and the sex chromatin status as determined by buccal smear reflects mosaicism.

The Barr test has become an effective means of screening patients for sex chromosomal abnormalities. The test may be performed rapidly by means of a buccal smear. Normal males have less than 3% positive cells in their buccal smears, whereas normal females have 25–50% positive cells. Intermediate counts suggest mosaicism. Recently, the amniotic membrane stripped from the placenta has been utilized to great advantage in screening populations of newborns for abnormalities of the X chromosomes.

The affinity of the long arm of the Y chromosome for fluorescent dyes is also being used in screening newborns for abnormalities of the Y chromosome by looking for the "Y body" in interphase cells (Fig 33–10).

Bergsma D (editor): New chromosomal and malformation syndromes. Birth Defects 11(5), 1975. [Entire issue.]

Greensher A & others: Screening of newborn infants for abnormalities of the Y chromosome. J Pediatr 79:305, 1971.

Lyon FL: Mechanisms and evolutionary origins of variable X-chromosomal activity in mammals. Proc R Soc Lond [Biol] 187:243, 1974.

Smith OW: *Recognisable Patterns of Human Malformation*, 2nd ed. Saunders, 1976.

Wachtel S & others: Expression of H-Y antigen in human males with two Y chromosomes. N Engl J Med 293:1070, 1975.

DISEASES OF THE SEX CHROMOSOMES
(See Table 33–1.)

About 0.25% of all live infants born at term and about 1% of the inmates of institutions for the retarded have sex chromosomal anomalies. Examination of the chromatin status can identify most of them.

Indications for Examining the Sex Chromatin

An incidence of sex chromosomal anomalies of 0.35% has been found in a survey of 40,000 newborns born in 2 Denver hospitals. Since most of the abnormal cases would not have been diagnosed by physical examination alone, it may eventually be desirable for obstetric services to establish the chromatin status of all newborns at birth by routine examination of the amniotic membranes.

Sex chromatin examination is especially indicated in the following cases:

(1) All individuals, including newborns, with any abnormalities of the external genitalia, including micro-orchidism.

(2) All those with mental retardation.

(3) All sterile individuals.

(4) All females with primary amenorrhea.

(5) All female newborns with somatic abnormalities suggestive of Turner's syndrome, eg, lymphedema of the dorsa of the feet, cubitus valgus, coarctation of the aorta, webbing of the neck.

Table 33–1. Other diseases involving sex differentiation.

Lesion and Disease	Chromosome Number	Symptoms
XX male. Sex chromatin positive.	46	Like Klinefelter's or partial feminization, as in true hermaphrodite. Usually does not have a eunuchoid build.
45,X/46,XY male pseudohermaphrodite, "mixed gonadal dysgenesis." Sex chromatin negative.	45/46	A variable degree of Turner's phenotype with infantile female secondary sex characteristics and a variable amount of masculinization of the genitals. Tendency to develop gonadoblastomas.
"Pure" gonadal dysgenesis, 46,XY male pseudohermaphroditism. Sex chromatin negative.	46	Tall female with underdeveloped secondary sex characteristics, streak gonads, primary amenorrhea, and sterility. Tendency to develop gonadal tumors.
Testicular feminizing syndrome, male pseudohermaphroditism, 46,XY. Sex chromatin negative.	46	Tall, well feminized, sterile female with testes. Probably an "end organ" insensitivity to androgens. May be suspected in sterile adult females with primary amenorrhea and in girls with bilateral inguinal hernias. Inherited most probably as an X-linked recessive disease. Tendency to develop gonadal tumors.
True hermaphrodite, 46,XX; 46,XY or 46,XX/46,XY (the latter possibly due to an ovum being fertilized by 2 sperm).	46	Varying degrees of abnormal phenotypic sexual indeterminacy. May have ovum on one side, testis on the other (lateral hermaphrodite) or ovotestis on one (unilateral) or both sides (bilateral hermaphrodite). In lateral hermaphrodites, internal genitals usually conform to gonad on that side. External genitals may vary widely.

(6) Older girls with hypoplastic nipples, short stature, facies suggestive of Turner's syndrome, and inguinal or femoral hernia.

(7) Females with inguinal hernias.

Eller E & others: Prognosis of newborns with X-chromosomal abnormalities. Pediatrics 47:681, 1971.

Harris JS, Robinson A: X chromosome abnormalities and the obstetrician: The value of routine nuclear sexing of newborn infants. Am J Obstet Gynecol 109:574, 1971.

Tennes K & others: The early childhood development of 17 boys with sex chromosome anomalies: A prospective study. Pediatrics 59:574, 1977.

TURNER'S SYNDROME
(Gonadal Dysgenesis)

Essentials of Diagnosis

- Short stature, primary amenorrhea, and sexual infantilism in adults.
- "Streaked" gonads and partial or complete X-chromosomal monosomy (Fig 33–11) are found at all ages.

General Considerations

Turner's syndrome has an incidence of about 1:3000 live births, but the "45,X anomaly" is 40 times as common in spontaneous abortions. The occurrence

of some of the somatic stigmas of the disease varies greatly from case to case. Most cases are chromatin-negative.

Clinical Findings

The family history is noncontributory except that an increased incidence of twinning has been reported in families with gonadal dysgenesis. Birth weight tends to be low (especially for those with webbed neck and coarctation of the aorta). Newborns often display lymphedema, especially of the lower parts of the legs and the distal arms. This may last for several years.

A. Symptoms and Signs: The characteristic findings are sexual infantilism and primary amenorrhea in a postpubertal female, shortness of stature, low birth weight, congenital lymphedema, cubitus valgus, a small "turned down" mouth, low hair line, retrognathia or micrognathia, webbing of the neck, and short neck. Other abnormalities may include coarctation of the aorta, pigmented nevi, deep-set nail beds, and hypoplastic nails. The IQ is usually normal, although many of these patients have perceptual difficulties and space blindness or have trouble with numbers (dyscalculia). Congenital malformations of the urinary tract are common, especially horseshoe kidneys and double ureter and pelvis. In addition, there may be "shield chest" combined with widely spaced nipples, abnormalities of the spine (epiphysitis), retardation of bone age, and osteoporosis. The growth rate throughout childhood is slow, and the ultimate height is usually 52–59 inches. Occasional patients have been reported who menstru-

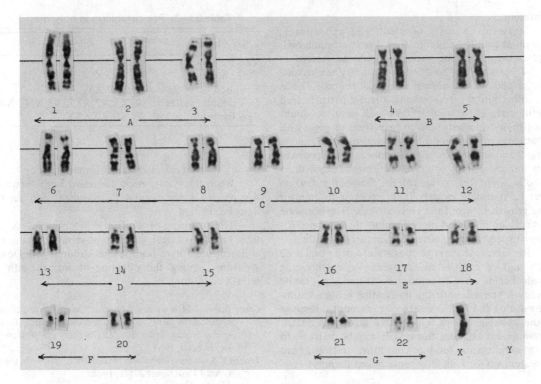

Figure 33–11. 45,X karyotype of girl with Turner's syndrome.

ate and have normal height; these are probably chromosomal mosaics. Two reportedly 45,X females have borne normal children.

B. Laboratory Findings: Sex chromatin is usually negative. 45,X/46,XX mosaicism is not uncommon; in these cases there may be some chromatin-positive cells but a lower percentage (< 20%) than one would normally expect to find. Occasionally the buccal smear is chromatin-positive but the bodies look particularly large; this suggests that the patient has an X-isochromosome of the long arm of the 46,X,i(X$_q$)* sex chromosomal constitution. If, on the other hand, the chromatin bodies look small, the patient may have an X-deletion X or X-isochromosome of the small arm 46,X,i(X$_p$)* constitution.

In the typical case the karyotype reveals a 45,X condition. Mosaicism (45,X/46,XX or 45,X/46,XX/47,XXX)* is not rare. In these cases the phenotype may be modified so that many of the characteristic clinical findings are absent. Even mosaics, however, are likely to have "streak" gonads and primary amenorrhea.

Patients with 46,X,i(X$_q$) usually have typical Turner's phenotypes. In addition, they have an increased incidence of Hashimoto's thyroiditis. When a deletion of part or all of the long arm of one X chromosome occurs, many of the characteristic signs

*Terminology adopted by Paris Conference on the Human Chromosomes (1971).

and symptoms, including shortness of stature, are absent, but amenorrhea and the sterility which results from dysgenetic gonads persists.

Urinary FSH excretion is elevated by the 13th to 14th year. Prior to this, FSH may be higher than normal for the age.

The gonads appear as long, slender white "streaks" in the broad ligaments. They are composed of wavy connective tissue without any germinal epithelium.

C. X-Ray Findings: X-ray studies often reveal rarefaction of the bones, especially in the hands, feet, and spine, where epiphysitis may also be present. Bone age is only slightly retarded. Intravenous urography will often reveal urinary tract anomalies.

Differential Diagnosis

Turner's syndrome must be ruled out in all cases of females with shortness of stature, amenorrhea, webbing of the neck, or coarctation of the aorta. The diagnosis depends on the buccal smear and the chromosomal analysis. Patients with pseudohypoparathyroidism may have many of the stigmas of gonadal dysgenesis.

Complications & Sequelae

These relate primarily to the dangers of coarctation of the aorta when that is present. Rarely, the dysgenetic gonads may become neoplastic (gonadoblastoma). Sexual infantilism and the perceptual motor difficulties to which these patients are prone may have concomitant psychologic hazards.

Treatment

Treatment consists of identifying and treating perceptual problems before they become established. Replacement hormone therapy should be started at 12–14 years of age to develop secondary sex characteristics and permit normal menstrual periods. This is psychologically most important. Teenage patients need careful counseling so that they will have no doubt about their femininity and to help them to cope with the stigmas of their condition. The need for hormone therapy should be carefully explained. Some pediatricians initiate therapy at about 10 years of age with an anabolic agent (eg, oxandrolone, 0.1 mg/kg/day) in order to stimulate growth. It is important to monitor bone growth to avoid too rapid advance. The hormone is usually given for a 4-month period, then stopped for 4 months, and then restarted for another 4 months.

Replacement therapy consists of a daily oral dose (1.25 mg) of conjugated estrogens. Vaginal bleeding usually begins after 3–6 months. At that time, cyclic therapy is started, with the medication being administered during the first 3 weeks of each month. Because of the possible risk of endometrial carcinoma related to unopposed estrogen therapy, it may be desirable to use a combination oral contraceptive (estrogen and progesterone) for long-term replacement therapy.

Prognosis

The prognosis for life is good, limited only by complications such as coarctation of the aorta. Sterility is permanent.

De la Chapelle A: Cytogenetical and clinical observations in female gonadal dysgenesis. Acta Endocrinol 40 (Suppl 65), 1962.
Nakashima I, Robinson A: Fertility in a 45,X female. Pediatrics 47:770, 1971.
Zergollern L: Cytogenetic variations of Turner's syndrome. Clin Genet 10:374, 1976.

POLYSOMY X SYNDROME (XXX & XXXX)

The incidence of this syndrome in newborns is about 0.12% (significantly higher among retardates). These patients are phenotypic females with 2 or more sex chromatin bodies. In an as yet undetermined proportion of cases, there is underdevelopment of secondary sex characteristics, primary or secondary amenorrhea, and mild mental retardation. Occasional patients have epicanthus, transverse palmar lines, and curved little fingers.

All phenotypic females with mild mental retardation, epicanthic folds, transverse palmar lines, or primary or secondary amenorrhea should have buccal smears.

Treatment is supportive. Cyclic hormone therapy is indicated for older girls with underdeveloped second-

Table 33–2. Sex chromatin in polysomy X.

Sex Chromatin	Karyotype
Two bodies	47,XXX
Three bodies	48,XXXX
Four bodies	49,XXXXX
Few double bodies	46,XX/47,XXX; 45,X/47,XXX
Few triple bodies	45,X/48,XXXX

ary sex characteristics and amenorrhea.

When the syndrome is diagnosed in the newborn, the prognosis for mental development and fertility must be guarded.

The offspring of women with polysomy X have thus far had normal sex chromosomal constitutions, although there have been several children with Down's syndrome among the offspring of women with the tetra-X condition.

Court Brown WM & others: Abnormalities of the sex chromosome complement in man. Medical Research Council Special Report Series 305. Her Majesty's Stationery Office, London, 1964.
Tennes K & others: A developmental study of girls with trisomy X. Am J Hum Genet 27:71, 1975.

KLINEFELTER'S SYNDROME

Essentials of Diagnosis

- Micro-orchidism due to prepubertal testicular atrophy, azoospermia, and sterility in the adult (about 4 patients with this syndrome are said to have been fertile).
- Elevated urinary gonadotropins in puberty. 47,XXY chromosomal constitution (Fig 33–12).
- Chromosomal variants are occasionally seen.

General Considerations

The incidence in the newborn population is roughly 1:500, but it is about 1% in groups of male retardates and 3% in males seen at infertility clinics. The maternal age at birth is often advanced. The diagnosis is rarely made before puberty except as a result of screening tests for sex chromatin. Unlike gonadal dysgenesis, this lesion is rarely found in spontaneous abortions.

Clinical Findings

A. Symptoms and Signs: The characteristic findings do not usually appear until after puberty. Therefore, it is improper to stigmatize a child with a 47,XXY karyotype with a diagnosis of Klinefelter's syndrome. The most that can be said is that such a child is at an unmeasurable increased risk of developing the syndrome during adolescence. Micro-orchidism

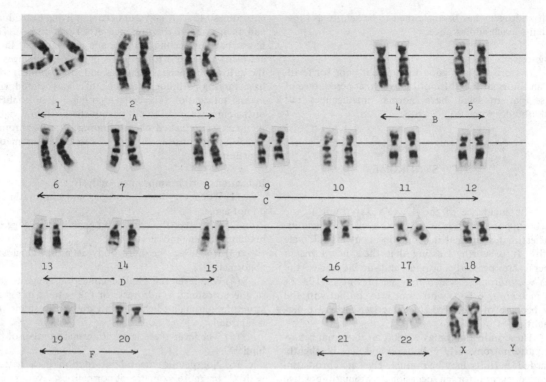

Figure 33—12. 47,XXY karyotype of man with Klinefelter's syndrome.

associated with otherwise normal external genitalia, azoospermia, and sterility is almost invariable in diagnosed cases. Gynecomastia, subnormal IQ, diminished facial hair, lack of libido and potency, and a tall, eunuchoid build are frequent. In chromosomal variants with 3 and 4 X chromosomes, mental retardation is severe and radioulnar synostosis may be present as well as anomalies of the external genitalia and cryptorchidism. In the XXXXY cases, these findings are especially prominent, as well as microcephaly, hypertelorism, epicanthus, prognathism, and incurved fifth fingers.

The adult XXYY patient tends to be taller and more retarded than the average XXY patient.

In general, the physical and mental abnormalities in Klinefelter's syndrome increase with the number of sex chromosomes.

B. Laboratory Findings: Sex chromatin is positive. Twenty to 40% of the cells of the buccal mucous membrane usually have one Barr body, although 2 and 3 Barr bodies may be found in individuals having one of the rare variants of Klinefelter's syndrome with more than 2 X chromosomes.

The majority of cases have a 47,XXY constitution. However, rare variants may have 48,XXXY, 49,XXXXY, 49,XXXYY, and 48,XXYY. A variety of mosaics containing combinations of the above and including 46,XY/47,XXY mosaicism have been reported. Some of these latter have been fertile and not mentally defective.

Urinary excretion of gonadotropins is high in adults, the levels being comparable to those found in postmenopausal women.

Histology of the testis in the adult is characterized by hyalinization and atrophy of the majority of seminiferous tubules, with large clumps of abnormal Leydig cells in between. A marked deficiency of germ cells (spermatogonia) has been found also in prepubertal patients (even in a 10-month-old child).

Differential Diagnosis

Chromatin-positive Klinefelter's syndrome must be differentiated from 2 chromatin-negative varieties: postpubertal testicular atrophy and germ cell aplasia. In both cases the diagnosis can be made by buccal smear for sex chromatin and testicular biopsy.

Adolescent obesity with delayed puberty and Prader-Willi syndrome may be confused with Klinefelter's syndrome. In both cases, the sex chromatin determination, absence of a eunuchoid build, and absence of true testicular atrophy should rule out Klinefelter's syndrome.

Complications & Sequelae

These patients may be more prone to a variety of conditions, including antisocial personality (especially sex crimes), schizophrenia, male breast cancer, asthma, and thyroid disease.

Treatment

Treatment consists of supportive care for the psychologic stresses of the disease and, occasionally, plastic surgery for gynecomastia. Recently, therapy with androgens has been claimed to be helpful as these patients reach adolescence.

Prognosis

The prognosis is good for life but poor for fertility and normal IQ. It is not known what percentage of these patients will have normal intelligence, but undoubtedly some do.

XYY SYNDROME

The incidence of the 47,XYY karyotype in the newborn population is as yet unknown, although current estimates are that it occurs in about 1:1000 male births. It is worth stressing that these newborns in general are perfectly normal and do *not* have the "XYY syndrome," which may be present in 10% of tall men (over 6 feet) who come into conflict with the law because of their grossly defective, aggressive personalities.

These individuals may exhibit an abnormal behavior pattern from early childhood and may be slightly retarded. Fertility may be normal. They are chromatin-negative except for an occasional chromatin-positive individual with a 48,XXYY karyotype. Hence, these patients are not identified by examination of the sex chromatin. However, they can be identified by a buccal smear stained for the fluorescent "Y body."

There is no treatment. Many males with an XYY are normal. Long-term problems may relate to IQ and environmental stress. Occasionally, therapy with estrogens such as Depo-Provera has been reported to be helpful.

Caldwell P & others: The XXY (Klinefelter's) syndrome in children: Detection and treatment. J Pediatr 80:258, 1972.
Court Brown WM: Males with an XYY chromosome complement. J Med Genet 5:341, 1968.
Hook EB: Behavioral implications of the human XYY genotype. Science 179:139, 1973.
Marinello MJ & others: A study of the XYY syndrome in tall men and juvenile delinquents. JAMA 208:321, 1969.
Witkin HA & others: Criminality in XYY and XXY men. Science 193:547, 1976.

AUTOSOMAL DISEASES
(See Table 33–3.)

Man is even more susceptible to autosomal disorders than to abnormalities of the sex chromosomes. Uniform autosomal monosomy is not compatible with life and has been observed only in spontaneously aborted fetuses. Similarly, only trisomy of the small autosomes (13, 18, and 21) occurs in living individuals and then only in the presence of serious disease. The newer banding technics have made us aware that there are many patients with minor morphologic changes of the autosomes (partial trisomies and monosomies) who have varying pathologic features, often associated with mental retardation. The belief that many abnormalities of the chromosomes do not permit the birth of a viable infant is strengthened by the finding of gross chromosomal aberrations in 30–50% of cases of spontaneous abortion.

Indications for Chromosomal Analysis

(1) Whenever the phenotypic and chromatin sex do not agree.

(2) Whenever the chromatin examination suggests sex chromosome mosaicism.

(3) Whenever the Barr body is morphologically abnormal.

(4) Whenever the clinical condition suggests one of the autosomal syndromes, or the patient has gross structural anomalies involving a variety of systems and is retarded.

(5) Whenever there is an abnormal number of "Y bodies."

(6) Nonspecific mental retardation in a patient with 2 or more somatic abnormalities, even minor ones.

Bergsma D (editor): New chromosomal and malformation syndromes. Birth Defects 11(5), 1975. [Entire issue.]
Lewandowski R Jr, Yunis JJ: New chromosomal syndromes. Am J Dis Child 129:515, 1975.
Polani PE: Autosomal imbalance and its syndromes, excluding Down's. Br Med Bull 25:81, 1969.
Stenchever MA & others: Testicular feminization syndrome: Chromosomal, histologic, and genetic studies in a large kindred. Obstet Gynecol 33:649, 1969.

DOWN'S SYNDROME

Essentials of Diagnosis

- Slow development, characteristic facies, short stature, abnormal dermatoglyphics.
- Trisomy 21 or chromosomal translocation.

General Considerations

The term Down's syndrome is preferred to mongolism since the latter term is descriptively inaccurate and is offensive to some. The most constant characteristic of the disease is mental retardation. IQs may vary between 20 and 80, with the great majority being between 45 and 55. The incidence of Down's syndrome has been dropping with the lowering of the average maternal age. Whereas about 10% of pregnant women were over 35 years of age 2 decades ago, currently only about 3.5% are. In the author's series,

Table 33—3. Other diseases of the autosomes.

Lesion and Disease	Symptoms
Deletion of long arm of chromosome 22—the Ph[1] chromosome. The deleted segment is translocated onto the terminal portion of the long arm of a "C-group" chromosome, usually No. 9.	Chronic granulocytic leukemia. The chromosomal abnormality is present in the bone marrow in 95% of cases. Less often, it is also present in cells cultured from the peripheral blood.
Bloom's dwarfism: multiple chromosome breaks, quadriradial figures, occasionally "pulverization" of chromosomes.	Dwarfism, chronic erythematous rash, tendency to malignancy, especially leukemia. Inherited as a single gene autosomal recessive. Increased chromosomal breaks may be seen in close relatives.
Congenital aplastic (Fanconi's) anemia: increased number of chromosomal breaks; chromosomes probably more susceptible to breakage by virus (especially SV40).	Skeletal (especially upper extremities) and hematopoietic abnormalities, increased hemoglobin F. Anemia often does not appear until 6—10 years of age. Hyperpigmentation, sexual and mental retardation, and microcephaly may also be present. Autosomal recessive inheritance.
Trisomy 8 mosaicism (46/47+8).	Mild to moderate mental retardation, strabismus, large ears, upturned nose, thick everted lower lip, high-arched palate, micrognathia, vertebral anomalies, genitourinary anomalies, thick bulging skin with deep furrows (especially on hands and feet), restricted movement of some small and large joints. Absence of patellas is very characteristic.
46,XY(XX),18q— Partial deletion of long arm of No. 18.	Mental retardation, microcephaly, midfacial dysmorphia, prominent antihelix, atretic ear canals, "carp-shaped" mouth, cryptorchidism, long, tapering fingers. IgA often absent.
46,XY(XX),13q— Partial deletion of long arm of No. 13.	Mental retardation, failure to thrive, microcephaly, hypertelorism, ptosis, microphthalmia and colobomas, hypoplastic or absent thumbs, occasional retinoblastoma, congenital heart disease, genitourinary abnormalities.
46,XY(XX),4p— Partial deletion of short arm of No. 4.	Severe mental retardation, microcephaly, epicanthi, coloboma, beaked nose, cleft palate, micrognathia, inguinal hernia, hypospadias, growth deficiency of prenatal onset.
46,XY(XX),18p— Partial deletion of short arm of No. 18.	Variable mental retardation, micrognathia, flat nasal bridge, low-set and large ears, short hands.
Partial trisomy 22 (22q+).	Coloboma (cat's eye), anal atresia, severe mental retardation, hypertelorism, antimongoloid slant, abnormal ears, genitourinary anomalies, congenital heart disease.

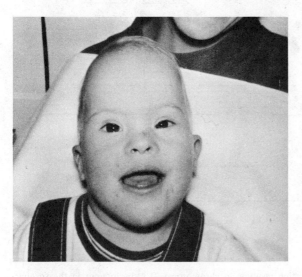

Figure 33—13. Facies of a child with Down's syndrome.

Down's syndrome currently occurs in about one in 900 newborns, whereas the less recent literature states its incidence to be about one in 600 newborns. The patient's mother's age at the time of conception and the nature of the chromosomal malformation are important in genetic counseling.

Clinical Findings

A. **Symptoms and Signs:** The principal findings are a small, brachycephalic head, flat nasal bridge, ruddy cheeks, dry lips, large protruding "scrotal" tongue, small ears, oblique palpebral fissures which narrow laterally, epicanthic folds, occasional Brushfield spots, and a short fleshy neck. Irregular development of teeth is common; in about one-third of cases, the upper lateral permanent incisors are missing or defective. About one-third have congenital heart disease, most often an endocardial cushion defect or other septal defect. Patients tend to have short, stubby, spade-like hands with transverse palmar ("simian") lines and abnormal dermatoglyphics (see below).

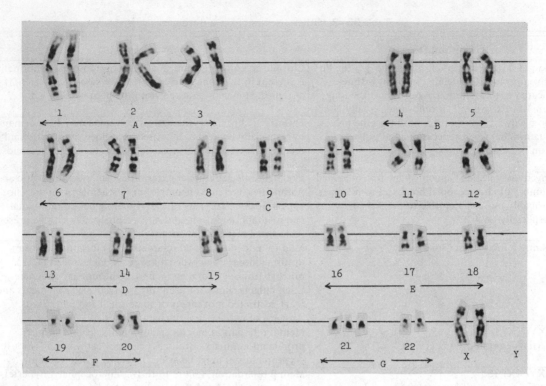

Figure 33—14. Karyotype of Down's syndrome: 47,XX,+21.

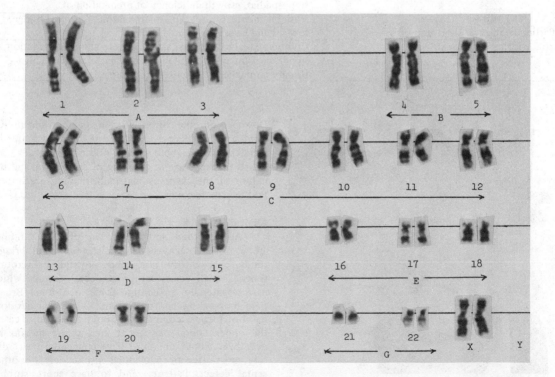

Figure 33—15. Karyotype demonstrating an unbalanced translocation resulting in chromosome 21 being present in the trisomic state. 46,XX,-14,+t(14;21)(p11;q11).

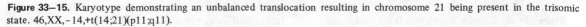

Generalized hypotonia is often present, as well as umbilical hernia. There is often a cleft between the big toe and second toe. Sexual development is retarded. The affected newborn is prone to have a third fontanel, prolonged physiologic jaundice, polycythemia, and a transient leukemoid reaction. "Cutis marmorata" is often present.

Patients with Down's syndrome display an increased sensitivity to the mydriatic effects of atropine instilled into the conjunctiva.

Dermatoglyphic patterns are characteristic. In general, the dermal ridges are poorly formed, and the frequencies of arches, radial and ulnar loops on the fingers, the distal location of the axial triradius on the palm, and the hallucal pattern on the sole of the foot differ from normals. Ford-Walker has combined frequency data on dermatoglyphic patterns on the fingers, palms, and soles into a "dermal index" which delineates 3 ranges—"mongol," "normal," and "overlap." A single flexion crease on the fifth finger is often found.

B. Laboratory Findings: The chromosomal abnormalities are pathognomonic. The great majority of cases (95%) have 47 chromosomes with trisomy of 21 (Fig 33–14). However, about 4% of sporadic cases have 46 chromosomes, including an abnormal translocated chromosome formed as a result of centric fusion between 2 acrocentric chromosomes,* one of which is chromosome 21 (Fig 33–15). On the other hand, about one-third of the familial cases have a translocation. Ten percent of patients whose mothers are younger will have these "interchange" lesions, whereas this is true in only 3% of those with older mothers.

Mosaicism of the 46/47 type can also occur in persons with Down's syndrome. This may result in milder symptoms, especially in higher than expected IQ. Apparently normal mothers of affected children have occasionally been mosaics.

Although increased levels of leukocyte alkaline phosphatase have been reported, there has been a marked overlap in the distribution of patients and controls. This and increased levels of other enzymes (galactose-1-phosphate uridyl transferase and glucose-6-phosphate dehydrogenase) are probably nonspecific effects of a variation in the metabolism of leukocytes which occurs in association with Down's syndrome. However, the gene for superoxide dismutase has been localized to chromosome 21 and does show the expected dosage effect in trisomy 21 patients.

Total serum proteins are usually in the low normal range. Serum albumin is low but gamma globulin is often elevated.

Decreased urinary excretion of xanthurenic and indoleacetic acids after a tryptophan load is indicative of some abnormality of tryptophan metabolism.

C. X-Ray Findings: X-rays of the pelvic bones of affected infants reveal flattening of the inner edges of the ileum and widening of the iliac wings. The "iliac index" is one-half the sum of both acetabular and iliac

*Fusion between 2 centromere regions—a Robertsonian translocation.

angles. This index is low (below 65) in about 80–90% of infants under 9 months of age with Down's syndrome (over 80 in the controls).

Skull x-rays often reveal brachycephaly, with flattening of the occiput. The sinuses may be absent or poorly developed. X-rays of the hand show shortening of the metacarpal bones and phalanges. The second phalanx of the little finger, in particular, is often abnormally small.

Differential Diagnosis

Most of the individual signs and symptoms of Down's syndrome also occur in the normal population, and the diagnosis is based on the presence of a *combination* of symptoms. Other autosomal trisomies, and occasionally girls with the triple X syndrome, may have many similar findings. The dermatoglyphics, sex chromatin status, and chromosomal analysis will differentiate the latter from Down's syndrome.

Complications

Leukemia (not the transient leukemoid reaction of the newborn) is 20 times more common than normal in individuals with Down's syndrome. These patients are very susceptible to intercurrent infections and are subject to the complications of congenital heart disease when they have it.

Prevention

In general, Down's syndrome is not familial and the risk of having an affected child in a sibship varies with maternal age (1:2000 for mothers under 25; 1:50 for mothers 35–39 years of age; 1:20 over 40 years of age). These figures are fairly accurate for families with trisomy 21 but much too low when one of the parents is a balanced translocation carrier.

In counseling parents who have produced one child with Down's syndrome about the risk of having a second affected child, the prognostic accuracy can be improved by studying the karyotypes of the affected child and the parents. Several different situations may be present:

A. Child Has Trisomy 21, Parents Have Normal Karyotypes: The risk is only slightly greater than for parents in the general population (1–2%).

B. Trisomic Child, One Parent Mosaic: The risk will depend upon the degree of gonadal mosaicism of the affected parent. A rough estimate will be half of the proportion of abnormal cells in fibroblast cultures of the cells obtained from the parent.

C. Child Has 14/21 (D/G) Translocation, Parents Have Normal Karyotypes: The risks are unknown but should be considered slightly increased.

D. Child has 14/21 Translocation, One Parent a Balanced Translocation Carrier:

1. When the mother is the carrier, about 15% of the children will be affected, one-third will be carriers, and the remainder completely normal.

2. When the father is the carrier, there is a 3–5% chance of having another affected child and half of the apparently unaffected children may be carriers.

E. Child Has a 21/22 (G/G) Translocation:

1. Both parents have normal karyotypes—The prognosis is roughly the same as under (A), although there is some evidence that advancing paternal age may increase this risk slightly.

2. One parent carries the translocation—If it is an isochromosome of 21 (21/21), the risk is 100%. If it is a 21/22 translocation, the risk is as in (D).

Treatment

No form of medical treatment has been shown to have much merit. Therapy is directed toward specific problems, eg, cardiac surgery or digitalis for heart problems, antibiotics for infections, checking thyroid function, special education and occupational training, etc. These children should be helped to make the most of their limited abilities. Infant stimulation programs are helpful and early institutionalization is not recommended. Support of the parents is important.

Chemke J, Robinson A: The third fontanelle. J Pediatr 75:617, 1969.

Mikkelsen M, Stene J: Genetic counselling in Down's syndrome. Hum Hered 20:457, 1970.

Penrose LS: The causes of Down's syndrome. Adv Teratol 1:9, 1966.

Penrose LS, Smith GF: *Down's Anomaly*. Little, Brown, 1966.

Smith DW, Wilson AA: *The Child With Down's Syndrome*. Saunders, 1973.

TRISOMY 18 SYNDROME
(E₁ Trisomy)

Essentials of Diagnosis

- Mental retardation, failure to thrive, hypertonicity.
- Abnormal dermatoglyphics.
- Trisomy of chromosome 18 or, occasionally, an unbalanced translocation involving chromosome 18.

General Considerations

This disease has an incidence of about 1:4500 live births, and there is an approximately 1:3 sex ratio (male:female). The mean maternal age is advanced. Affected individuals usually die in early infancy, although occasional patients survive into childhood.

Clinical Findings

A. Symptoms and Signs: Trisomy 18 is characterized by failure to thrive, low birth weight, mental retardation, hypertonicity, prominent occiput, low-set, malformed ears, micrognathia, abnormal flexion of the fingers (index over third), equinovarus or "rocker bottom" feet, short sternum and narrow pelvis, congenital heart disease (often ventricular septal defect or patent ductus arteriosus), and inguinal or umbilical hernias. There is an increased occurrence of single umbilical arteries.

Dermatoglyphics show simple arches on fingers, a single flexion crease on the fifth finger, and transverse palmar lines.

B. Laboratory Findings: In place of uniform trisomy 18, chromosomal analysis occasionally reveals mosaicism for trisomy 18 or an unbalanced translocation involving a third number 18 and a chromosome of the 13–15 group. Rarely, double trisomies have been found in which trisomy X or trisomy 21 is present in addition to trisomy 18.

C. X-Ray Findings: X-ray often reveals gross retardation of osseous maturation, eventration of the diaphragm, and kidney abnormalities.

Differential Diagnosis

Trisomy 18 is differentiated from trisomy 13, in which failure to thrive, congenital heart disease, and retardation are also present. In the latter condition, the shape of the head; eye, ear, and palatal anomalies; dermatoglyphics; and the occurrence of apneic spells are all different. Other causes of failure to thrive must be considered.

Complications

Complications are related to associated lesions. Death is often due to heart failure or pneumonia.

Treatment

There is no treatment other than general supportive care.

Prognosis

Death usually occurs in infancy, although occasional patients have lived into early childhood.

Taylor AI: Autosomal trisomy syndromes: A detailed study of 27 cases of Edwards' syndrome and 27 cases of Patau's syndrome. J Med Genet 5:227, 1968.

TRISOMY 13
(D Trisomy)

The incidence of this disorder is about 1:5000 live births, and 60% of the patients are female. The mean maternal age is high. Death usually occurs by the second year of life, usually as a result of heart failure or infection.

The symptoms and signs consist of failure to thrive, mental retardation, arhinencephaly, sloping forehead, eye deformities (anophthalmia, colobomas), low-set ears, cleft lip and palate, capillary hemangiomas, deafness, apneic spells, seizures, polydactyly or syndactyly, and congenital heart disease (usually ventricular septal defect). Other abnormal findings may include hyperconvex, narrow fingernails, flexed and overlapping fingers, "rocker bottom" feet, retroflexible thumbs, urinary tract anomalies, umbilical hernia, and cryptorchidism or bicornuate uterus.

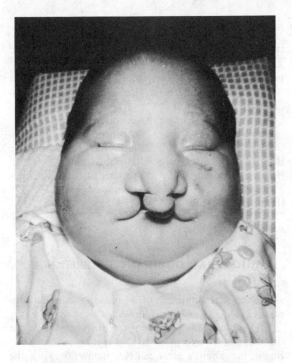

Figure 33–16. Facies of an infant with trisomy 13.

Although most patients have trisomy 13 (D trisomy), occasional patients are mosaic, and there are rare cases of an unbalanced (D/D) translocation with one of the parents carrying a similar translocation in the balanced state. Multiple projections and abnormal lobulation of the neutrophils are often present. Grossly elevated fetal hemoglobin and the presence of embryonic Gower's hemoglobin often occur.

Trisomy 18 patients are more hypertonic than these infants, and the head shape is different. The diagnosis of trisomy 13 should be considered in all cases of failure to thrive associated with retardation and palatal anomalies.

Other forms of the first arch syndrome are differentiated by the absence of a sloping forehead and the usual absence of other generalized malformations.

Treatment is supportive. Since on occasion it is necessary to decide immediately after birth how extensive and definitive therapy should be for a severely malformed infant, an immediate confirmation of this diagnosis (as well as one of trisomy 18) can be arrived at by direct examination of mitotic figures obtained from bone marrow. Prevention in the form of genetic counseling is indicated when one of the parents carries a balanced translocation, in which case the risks for future affected children are high (as in the analogous situation in Down's syndrome).

Taylor AI: Autosomal trisomy syndromes: A detailed study of 27 cases of Edwards' syndrome and 27 cases of Patau's syndrome. J Med Genet 5:227, 1968.

CRI DU CHAT ("CAT CRY") SYNDROME

The incidence of this syndrome is not known. It occurs more commonly among females. Life expectancy is not seriously curtailed. The dimensions of the deleted chromosomal fragment are variable, which explains the variations observed in the phenotype.

Symptoms and signs consist of severe mental retardation, low birth weight, failure to thrive, microcephaly, hypertelorism, obliquity of palpebral fissures, epicanthic folds, low-set ears, a broad, flattened nasal bridge, "moon-like" facies, and micrognathia. The cry has a unique mewling quality like that of a kitten. It has a sharp timbre and plaintive tonality when emitted on expiration. It is due to small, flaccid, and somewhat rudimentary laryngeal structures and becomes less typical as the child gets older.

These patients often have repeated respiratory infections and persistent feeding problems. Breathing may be difficult. Hypospadias, cryptorchidism, and curved little fingers have been reported.

Chromosomal analysis shows deletion of part of the short arm of chromosome No. 5. This is occasionally replaced by a "ring" chromosome No. 5 or by a translocation.

Dermatoglyphics are often abnormal, with distal axial triradii. Transverse palmar lines may be present.

Because of the lack of specificity of many of the symptoms associated with abnormalities of the autosomes, all children with severe mental retardation, microcephaly, and failure to thrive enter into the differential diagnosis.

Newborn infants with various kinds of weak cry and laryngeal stridor may be differentiated by the fact that the "cat cry" is an expiratory sound and that an affected baby has the associated malformations.

Few cases have been familial. However, when one parent carries a balanced translocation involving chromosome No. 5 with deletion of the short arm, the risks are increased as in Down's syndrome.

Supportive care is all that can be given.

"NEW" CHROMOSOMAL SYNDROMES

A variety of new syndromes have recently been described, primarily because of the greater diagnostic accuracy resulting from the chromosomal banding technics. By and large, many of these comprise a group of patients with more subtle chromosomal defects in whom one of the parents often has a balanced translocation. This makes possible the prevention of future children with the same phenotype through prenatal diagnosis (see Table 33–3).

Carr DH: Chromosomal errors and development. Am J Obstet Gynecol 104:327, 1969.
Lewandowski RC Jr, Yunis JJ: New chromosomal syndromes. Am J Dis Child 129:515, 1975.

THE GENE

The genes, which occur in pairs in somatic cells, occur at similar sites on the homologous chromosomes. The members of a pair, although they encode for the same function, are not always the same but may constitute alternate forms (alleles). When the homologues are the same, the individual is said to be "homozygous" for the gene; if they are different, he is "heterozygous." Since the male has only one X chromosome, he is said to be "hemizygous" for X-linked genes.

GENE EXPRESSION

Most of what is currently known about a gene stems from how it expresses itself—its phenotype.

The phenotypic expression of a gene is the result of an interaction between the gene and its environment. The latter, in addition to the surrounding nucleoplasm and cytoplasm, includes the rest of the genome* which may have a modifying effect on the expression of a particular gene. It is this interaction that results in the variable severity of genetic diseases (expressivity) and occasionally completely prevents the expression of a defective gene (penetrance). The primary gene product, a protein, is least affected by environmental conditions. Hence, one of the criteria for determining that a gene product is primary is complete penetrance and little variation in expressivity. This would be true, for example, of hemoglobin S, a protein which is the direct result of a single mutation in the gene which produces the beta polypeptide chain of hemoglobin. An important point in clinical genetics is that the defective gene which is not expressed at all (nonpenetrant) can still be passed on to offspring, where it may be expressed.

SINGLE GENE DEFECTS

Diseases which are due to defects in a single gene are said to be "autosomal" or "X-linked" depending on whether the defective gene is located on an autosome or X chromosome. If the disease is present when the defective gene is present either in the heterozygous or in the homozygous state, it is a dominantly inherited disease. If, however, it is present only when the gene involved is in the homozygous state, it is a recessively inherited disease.

*Genetic complement.

Table 33—4. Some dominantly inherited diseases (autosomal).

Achondroplasia	Intestinal polyposis
Isolated cleft palate (when due to a genetic defect)	Marfan's syndrome
	Muscular dystrophy (facio-scapulohumeral type)
Ehlers-Danlos syndrome	
Epidermolysis dystrophica hereditaria	Neurofibromatosis
	Osteogenesis imperfecta
Gardner's syndrome	Porphyria, hepatic form
Hereditary spherocytosis	Retinoblastoma
Hidrotic ectodermal dysplasia	Treacher Collins' syndrome
	Tuberous sclerosis
Huntington's chorea	

AUTOSOMAL DOMINANT INHERITANCE

Some characteristics of dominantly inherited diseases (Table 33—4) are as follows:

(1) One of the parents of the propositus will have the disease. An exception to this is a mutation occurring in the parent's germ cell (see below) or when the disease in the parent was either not penetrant or of a greatly diminished expressivity.

(2) There is a 50% risk of involvement in each sibling of an affected individual.

(3) The disease is usually not so serious as a recessively inherited disease.

(4) Either sex may be affected.

(5) The pedigree tends to be "vertical," ie, there are affected individuals in several generations.

AUTOSOMAL RECESSIVE INHERITANCE

Some characteristics of recessively inherited diseases (Table 33—5) are as follows:

(1) The disease tends to be rare and more severe than many dominantly inherited conditions.

(2) Affected individuals tend to be in the same generation.

(3) Normal parents are carriers.

(4) The rarer the trait, the greater the incidence of consanguinity in the parents.

(5) There is a 25% risk of involvement of the sibs of an affected individual.

(6) Either sex may be affected.

(7) The pedigree is usually "horizontal," ie, affected individuals are in the same generation.

X-LINKED (SEX-LINKED) DISEASE

When a gene is located on the X chromosome, it is said to be X-linked (sex-linked). A disease due to a

Table 33–5. Some recessively inherited diseases (autosomal).

Albinism
Chondroectodermal dysplasia
Congenital afibrinogenemia
Cystic fibrosis of the pancreas
Endemic goitrous cretinism
Epidermolysis bullosa dystrophica (severe recessive form)
Familial amaurotic idiocy
Familial nonhemolytic jaundice with kernicterus
Galactosemia
Gaucher's disease
Glycogen storage disease
Hurler's syndrome
Ichthyosis congenita
Maple syrup urine disease
Microcephaly
Morquio's syndrome
Niemann-Pick disease
Phenylketonuria
Sickle cell anemia
Thalassemia
Virilizing adrenal hyperplasia
Wilson's disease
Xeroderma pigmentosa

Table 33–7. X-linked recessively inherited diseases.

Aldrich's syndrome
Color blindness
Glucose-6-phosphate dehydrogenase deficiency
Hemophilia A
Hemophilia B
Hereditary anhidrotic ectodermal dysplasia
Lesch-Nyhan syndrome
Lowe's oculocerebrorenal syndrome
Microcephaly (some types)
Pseudohypertrophic muscular dystrophy (Duchenne)
Agammaglobulinemia
"Kinky hair" syndrome (Menkes)

single gene defect, which is inherited in an X-linked fashion, may be inherited either as an X-linked dominant or X-linked recessive.

X-linked dominant traits are rare (Table 33–6). They have the following characteristics:

(1) The hemizygous male will exhibit the full disease. None of his sons will be involved. All of his daughters will be involved, but will show a milder form of the disease. There will be a 50% risk of involvement in each of his daughter's children.

(2) The homozygous female will have severe disease, and all of her children will be involved.

(3) The heterozygous female will have a milder form of disease, and there will be a 50% chance in all of her children, regardless of sex, of their being involved.

The X-linked recessive form of disease (Table 33–7) will have the following characteristics:

(1) Affected individuals are nearly always males.

(2) The mother is usually a carrier. She transmits the disease to half of her sons, ie, there is a 50% chance that each of her sons will be involved.

(3) One-half of a carrier mother's daughters will be carriers. All of an affected father's daughters will be carriers.

Table 33–6. X-linked dominant inheritance.

Hereditary hematuria: some types
Vitamin D-resistant rickets: some types
Xg(a) blood group

(4) The uninvolved sons do not transmit the disease.

(5) There is no father-son transmission.

MUTATION

The word mutation means a sudden change in genotype. In the case of a gene, this is a point mutation to distinguish it from more gross changes in chromosomal structure. A mutation occurring in a germ cell will result in a child who differs at the given genetic locus from his parents. This mutant gene, however, will be passed on to the descendants of the individual having the mutation in the same manner as any other gene. It is obvious that mutations can only be recognized when the trait exhibits itself in the heterozygous condition—in other words, is dominantly inherited.

The causes of mutation are not completely known, although some factors, particularly high-energy radiation, which increase the rate of mutation are recognized.

SPORADIC OCCURRENCE OF DISEASE

It is especially important to investigate sporadic cases of disease occurring in a family when it is known that the disease is usually due to a single gene defect. The following causes should be considered:

(1) Mutation occurring in one of the parents. If this is true, then the disease should be dominantly inherited in the offspring of the affected individual; and, since the mutant event was a point mutation occurring in one germ cell, the parents of the affected individual are not at an increased risk that further affected children will result from conceptions involving other, nonmutated germ cells.

(2) The disease is a rare recessive. Both parents are healthy carriers, and any future children that the

parents have will run the usual 25% risk of being involved.

(3) The disease is a phenocopy, ie, a predominantly environmentally determined disease which mimics a genetic disease. An example of this would be the microcephaly occurring as part of the rubella syndrome versus genetically determined microcephaly.

(4) The disease is dominantly inherited but has low penetrance, and has for this reason skipped the previous generation. It is possible that if one were to examine the parents by very sensitive technics, some abnormal manifestation might be found to show that they were, in fact, involved.

(5) One must always consider the possibility in sporadic cases of genetic diseases that there may be illegitimacy and that one of the supposed parents is not really the parent.

SEX-LIMITED DISEASE

A sex-limited disease is one which is actually autosomally inherited but which, because of factors in the environment such as the presence of certain sex hormones, is expressed only in one sex. An example of this is baldness, which is inherited as an autosomal dominant but occurs predominantly in the male.

POLYGENIC DISEASE
(Multifactorial Inheritance)

In addition to those traits which are due to the inheritance of a single gene, there are many traits and genetically determined diseases which are multifactorial in origin. Many of these traits occurring in the general population do not sharply divide the population up into those who have and those who do not have the trait but exhibit a continuous variability representing a varying interaction between a genotype of a certain composition and an environment. The inheritance of certain characteristics such as blood pressure, intelligence, and height is multifactorial.

A number of relatively common defects and diseases that are clearly familial cannot be made to fit *all* the expectations for single gene (autosomal) inheritance. These discontinuous manifestations (Table 33-8) have been recognized during the last 4 decades to be examples of the multifactorial inheritance of a continuously distributed variable (liability or susceptibility). When the combination of genetic susceptibility and toxic environmental factors exceeds a developmental threshold, the defect or disease becomes manifest.

Cleft of the secondary palate is an example of such a threshold having been exceeded. In order for

Table 33–8. Some common polygenically determined diseases.

Cleft lip and palate
Anencephaly/meningomyelocele
Pyloric stenosis
Congenital dislocated hips
Diabetes
Asthma

the palate to close, the palatal shelves must move from a vertical position alongside the tongue to a horizontal one above the tongue so that their medial edges may fuse. A variety of factors are involved in the timing of these embryologic events. Any delay will prevent meeting of the edges at the critical time (the threshold), and a cleft palate will result.

Some of the characteristics of this type of inheritance may be listed as follows:

(1) Increased risk of recurrence in relatives of the index case.

(2) Recurrence risks for all first-degree relatives (those with 50% of their genes in common) are the same. However, risks for second-degree relatives (grandchildren, nieces and nephews, aunts and uncles) and still more distant relatives drop off greatly in a nonlinear fashion.

(3) Increased risk of recurrence after 2 affected children. This is in marked contrast to single gene inheritance.

(4) Increased recurrence risk with increased severity of the defect. The risk of recurrence in future siblings of a child with cleft lip or palate is greater if the index case has bilateral cleft lip and palate (5.6%) than if he has a unilateral cleft lip (2.6%).

(5) Sex of index case (proband) may affect the recurrence risk. In defects that occur more frequently in one sex than the other, when the index case is of the less frequently affected sex, it must be assumed that susceptibility is greater and thus the risk for recurrence is greater. Pyloric stenosis occurs more commonly in males. If a female has it, the risk for recurrence increases significantly.

Unfortunately for the practical application of genetics to medicine, the more common diseases tend to be etiologically heterogeneous and due to many genetic and environmental factors. As a result, genetic counseling about these conditions is not as simple as it is when discussing the aforementioned diseases in which simple types of inheritance occur.

EMPIRIC RISK FIGURES

Where the pattern of inheritance is obscure, as in diseases in which a number of genes interacting with the environment seem to be responsible, it becomes difficult to provide accurate risk rates. In this case so-

Table 33–9. Empiric risks for some congenital diseases.

Mental deficiency of unknown cause: Incidence 3:100
  Risks among siblings
    Both parents normal, 15% defective
    One parent defective, 35% defective
    Both parents defective, 85% defective

Anencephaly and spina bifida: Incidence 1:100
  Male:female = 1:3. Incidence increases with maternal age and parity, and also in firstborn of very young mothers.
  Risk of repeat = about 3%. Risk of abnormal child or abortion = 25%.

Hydrocephalus: Incidence 1:2000 newborns
  Occasional X-linked recessive
  Often associated with meningocele or spina bifida
  May be nongenetic (toxoplasmosis, aminopterin, x-ray)
  Chance of repeat of some CNS anomaly = 3%
  Chance of repeat of hydrocephalus = 1%

CNS malformations in general: Incidence 29:10,000
  Siblings 6 times more likely to have CNS malformation
  Stillborn and abortion rates increased

	Cleft lip ± cleft palate (%)	Cleft palate (%)
Incidence	0.1	0.04
Negative family history	4	2
Normal parents; relatives involved	4	4
2 affected children	9	7
1 affected parent; no affected children	4	6
1 affected parent; 1 affected child	17	15

Congenital heart disease: Incidence 2:1000
  Neither parent involved, 1.4–1.8% risk of repeat*
  One parent involved, 5% risk of repeat*

Diabetes: Incidence 5:100
  One parent involved, 15% risk of repeat*
  Both parents involved, 25–75% risk of repeat*

Pyloric stenosis
  Male index patients:
    Brothers   3.2% ⎫ 10 times greater than normal risk
    Sons   6.8% ⎭
    Sisters   3.0% ⎫ 20 times greater than normal risk
    Daughters   1.2% ⎭
  Female index patients:
    Brothers   13.2% ⎫ 35 times greater than normal risk
    Sons   20.5% ⎭
    Sisters   2.5% ⎫ 70 times greater than normal risk
    Daughters 11.1% ⎭

Clubfoot: Incidence 1:1000 (male: female = 2:1)
  Sibling risk = 3–8%

Congenital dislocated hip: Incidence 1:1000
  Siblings of index case, 40 times greater than normal risk
  Aunts, uncles, nephews, nieces (of index case), 4 times greater than normal risk

---

*Many exceptions.

called empiric risk figures must be used. These are obtained by perusing the literature and finding pooled data on a large number of families with the disease. It is important to remember that these figures represent averages which may have little meaning in a specific case. However, they are the best available. It is also well to remember, in counseling, that where the pattern of inheritance is not clear a risk of a repeat is generally about one in 20, a figure much lower than the risks which must be quoted when single gene defects are involved (Table 33–9).

II. INBORN ERRORS OF METABOLISM

In his Croonian Lecture to the Royal College of Physicians of London in 1908, Sir Archibald Garrod described 4 diseases—alkaptonuria, cystinuria, albinism, and pentosuria—at the same time coining the term inborn errors of metabolism. Since then, there has been a prodigious increase in our understanding of the molecular mechanisms of genetic misinformation. Technical developments in fields such as gas chromatography and mass spectroscopy have also extended diagnostic possibilities to other areas of intermediary metabolism than amino acids and lipids.

Most of these conditions are rare autosomal recessive traits. However, inexpensive screening procedures and the potential for confirmatory identification and treatment as well as wider acceptance of termination of pregnancy following antenatal diagnosis have made them an important group of pediatric diseases. Some of the better known and more common syndromes are described below or in Tables 33–11 and 33–12. Others are described elsewhere in this book—eg, the hyperbilirubinemias in Chapter 18, glucose-6-phosphate dehydrogenase deficiency and the hemoglobinopathies in Chapter 14, the immune globulin disorders in Chapter 15, and the lipid storage diseases in Chapter 21.

DISORDERS OF CARBOHYDRATE METABOLISM*

GALACTOSEMIA

The term galactosemia now denotes 2 conditions of galactose intolerance, one due to galactose-1-phos-

---

*A good general reference is Cornblath M, Schwartz R: *Disorders of Carbohydrate Metabolism in Infancy,* 2nd ed. Saunders, 1976.

phate uridyl transferase deficiency and the other due to galactokinase deficiency.

1. GALACTOSE-1-PHOSPHATE URIDYL TRANSFERASE DEFICIENCIES

Although many enzyme variants with differing activities are now known such as the Indiana, Hammarsen, Negro, Kelly, Rennes, unstable, and much more common Duarte variants, classical galactosemia occurs only when there is virtual absence of galactose-1-phosphate uridyl transferase activity. The resulting accumulations of galactose-1-phosphate in the liver, brain, and proximal convoluted tubules of the kidney cause hepatic parenchymal failure, mental retardation, and the renal Fanconi syndrome. The accumulation in the lens of galactitol, a reduction product of galactose, produces cataracts.

The disorder is inherited as an autosomal recessive trait with an incidence of approximately one in 40,000 live births; the carrier frequency is thus 1:200. Although no simple and inexpensive carrier detection method is available, carriers can be detected through assay of erythrocyte galactose-1-phosphate uridyl transferase activity. In utero diagnosis of the deficiency in an affected fetus can be made on the basis of the activity of this enzyme in cultured amniotic cells.

Clinical Findings

A. Symptoms and Signs: In the severe form of the disease the onset is with vomiting and diarrhea in the newborn period after a milk feeding. The infant becomes jaundiced and develops hepatomegaly. Without treatment, death frequently occurs in a few days. Cataracts usually develop within 2 months in untreated cases, and hepatic cirrhosis is progressive.

Not all cases are severe, as shown by the occasional identification of a patient with galactosemia in mental institution surveys. Mental retardation occurs unless treatment is given and seems to be irreversible. Clinical and laboratory evidence of the disease abates gradually with effective treatment.

B. Laboratory Findings: Laboratory findings in infancy include galactosuria, hypergalactosemia, proteinuria, and aminoaciduria. The simplest way to make the diagnosis is by the Beutler fluorescent screening test. Elevated serum galactose levels, especially after a galactose load, help to confirm the diagnosis but are technically hard to perform. Moreover, galactose loading may lead to severe hypoglycemia and is not advised. Specific confirmation of defective red cell galactose-1-phosphate uridyl transferase activity must always be carried out. Normal levels are ≥ 300 international milliunits (ImU)/gm hemoglobin; in galactosemia, they are < 8 ImU/gm hemoglobin.

Neonatal screening for galactosemia is in fairly wide use, but there is some doubt whether the classical case is picked up more quickly by this means or by clinical suspicion. Probably both approaches are justified.

Treatment

A galactose-free diet should be instituted as soon as the diagnosis is made. In the USA, regimens based on hydrolysates such as Nutramigen with added Dextri-Maltose have proved satisfactory. For the detailed implementation of such a regimen, the reader should consult the references given below.

The efficacy of the diet should be monitored by measuring red cell galactose-1-phosphate concentration, which should not exceed 2 mg/100 ml packed red cell lysate. However, results must be corroborated with dietary history as in certain conditions galactose-1-phosphate can be produced endogenously from UDP-galactase. Avoidance of galactose should be lifelong in severe cases, although there is some increased tolerance with age. Mothers of identified cases are advised to take a galactose-free diet during subsequent pregnancies.

Prognosis

With prompt institution of a galactose-free diet, the prognosis for life is excellent. Long-term follow-up still suggests, however, that the majority of severely affected individuals suffer some intellectual impairment.

Chacho CM & others: Unstable galactose-1-phosphate uridyl transferase: A new variant of galactosemia. J Pediatr 78:454, 1971.

Hsia DYY (editor): *Galactosemia.* Thomas, 1969.

Komrower GM & others: Long term follow-up of galactosemia. Arch Dis Child 45:367, 1970.

Segal S: Disorders of galactose metabolism. Chap 8, pages 160–181, in: *The Metabolic Basis of Inherited Disease,* 4th ed. Stanbury JB, Wyngaarden JB, Fredrickson DS (editors). McGraw-Hill, 1978.

Tedesco TA & others: The genetic defect in galactosemia. N Engl J Med 292:737, 1975.

2. GALACTOKINASE DEFICIENCY

Increasing numbers of patients with galactosemia and galactosuria due to galactokinase deficiency are being described. Such individuals show no renal, hepatic, or CNS disease but do develop cataracts, often within the first few months of life, and the condition should thus be suspected in any child with cataracts. Confirmation is made by identifying the presence of galactosuria and by demonstrating galactokinase deficiency in erythrocytes or cultured skin fibroblasts. The cataracts may regress upon institution of a galactose-free diet. The disorder is transmitted as an autosomal recessive trait and may be as common as galactosemia due to galactose-1-phosphate uridyl transferase deficiency. Heterozygotes have mild galactose intolerance and an increased incidence of cataracts.

Beutler E & others: Galactokinase deficiency as a cause of cataracts. N Engl J Med 288:1203, 1973.

Gitzelman R: Additional findings in galactokinase deficiency. J Pediatr 87:1007, 1975.

Olambiwounu NO & others: Galactokinase deficiency in twins: Clinical and biochemical studies. Pediatrics 53:314, 1974.

HEREDITARY FRUCTOSE INTOLERANCE

In this autosomal recessive disorder, there is deficient cleavage of fructose-1-phosphate into glyceraldehyde and dihydroxyacetone phosphate by fructose-1-phosphate aldolase. Affected individuals are symptom-free except after the ingestion of fructose, when hypoglycemia appears as well as failure to thrive, vomiting, jaundice, hepatomegaly, proteinuria, generalized aminoaciduria, and tyrosyluria. While the untreated condition can progress to death in liver failure, treatment is simple and consists of removal of fructose-containing foods from the diet. In fact, as less severely affected individuals grow up, they may recognize the association of nausea and vomiting with fructose-containing foods and selectively avoid them.

The diagnosis is supported by the demonstration of fructosuria following an oral fructose load. Hypoglycemia and hypophosphatemia following fructose loading (24 gm/sq m) is diagnostic, and the same is true of demonstration of greatly reduced activity of hepatic fructose-1-phosphate aldolase on biopsy.

Treatment consists of eliminating cane sugar from the diet. If the disorder is recognized early enough, the prospects for normal intellectual and somatic development are good. Fructose-1,6-diphosphatase deficiency is another form of fructose intolerance, which usually presents as neonatal hypoglycemia.

Levin B & others: Fructosaemia. Am J Med 45:826, 1968.

Melancon SB & others: Metabolic and biochemical studies in fructose 1,6-diphosphatase deficiency. J Pediatr 82:650, 1973.

Rennert OM, Greer M: Hereditary fructosemia. Neurology 20:421, 1970.

GLYCOGEN STORAGE DISEASES

Glycogen is a branched chain polysaccharide which is stored in liver and muscle. The usual end-to-end linkage in the molecule, which may contain about 10,000 glucosyl residues, is between carbon atoms 1 and 4. The branching links, however, are formed by a1,6-glucosidic bonds. About half of the bulk of the molecule is made up of free-end chains which are 7–10 glucosyl units long.

In the synthesis of glycogen, glucose is phosphorylated first in the 6 and then in the 1 position. Uridine diphosphoglucose is then formed by the enzyme UDPG pyrophosphorylase. In the next step, activated by glycogen synthetase, a glucosyl unit is added to the growing chain in a 1:4 bond. At the same time, the branching enzyme amylo-1,4:1,6-transglucosidase dislodges appropriate terminal chain segments and reattaches them in the 1,6 position. In the breakdown of glycogen, a small amount of glucose is liberated by the action of the debranching enzyme amylo-1,6-glucosidase; however, the bulk of the molecule is broken down to glucose-1-phosphate by phosphorylase. The activity of the latter enzyme is subject to a complex control mechanism initiated by glucagon and epinephrine and dependent on cyclic AMP.

About 10 different disorders of glycogen synthesis and breakdown have been described and the specific enzymic defects identified. In the hepatic form, the diagnosis is suggested by growth failure and hepatomegaly with a tendency to fasting hypoglycemia. Other types predominantly affect muscle glycogen. These include acid maltase deficiency with cardiomegaly and macroglossia and muscle phosphorylase and phosphofructokinase deficiency, where the most striking features are easy fatigability and muscle weakness and stiffness.

Precise diagnosis is dependent on liver or muscle biopsy and appropriate biochemical tests. Treatment is for the most part symptomatic. In the more severe hepatic forms, some good results have been reported following continuous nighttime high-carbohydrate feeding.

Angelini C, Engel AG, Titus JL: Adult acid maltase deficiency: Abnormalities in fibroblasts cultured from patients. N Engl J Med 287:498, 1972.

Fernandes J & others: Hepatic phosphorylase deficiency. Arch Dis Child 49:186, 1974.

Greene HL & others: Continuous nocturnal intragastric feeding: A new management for type I glycogen-storage disease. N Engl J Med 294:423, 1976.

Moses SW, Gutman A: Inborn errors of glycogen metabolism. In: *Advances in Pediatrics.* Vol 19. Schulman I (editor). Year Book, 1972.

THE HYPOGLYCEMIAS

Impaired ability to sustain normal serum glucose levels is a common metabolic problem in infancy and childhood. Precise definitions are difficult, so that diagnosis and treatment are designed to detect and treat either hyperinsulinism or disorders of glycolysis, gluconeogenesis, and absorption.

Table 33–10 sets out many of the recognized forms of infantile hypoglycemia and summarizes the differential diagnosis. The special importance of this group of disorders is worth repeated emphasis, namely, that failure to diagnose and treat correctly can lead to significant permanent cerebral damage.

Table 33—10. Guide to the diagnosis of hypoglycemic states.

Causes and Types	Diagnosis	References
Newborn period		
Infants of diabetic mothers, prematurity, placental insufficiency, intracranial injury, sepsis, erythroblastosis fetalis, neonatal cold injury, cessation of intravenous glucose	Clinical history and serum glucose determination. Increased K_g (see p 1047) following intravenous glucose may predict severe cases.	See General References. Also Pediatrics 58:10, 1976.
Cardiomegaly and neonatal hypoglycemia		Acta Paediatr Scand 60:295, 1970.
Metabolic disorders in older infants and children (disorders of glycolysis) Glycogen storage diseases (see p 953)	Ideally, specific enzyme assay on liver biopsy.	N Engl J Med 294:423, 1976.
Glucagon deficiency		
Glucagon-resistant and hypoalaninemic ketotic hypoglycemia	Hypoglycemia with ketonuria. Hypoglycemia induced by ketosis. Small for gestational age infants. Some respond to diazoxide.	Arch Dis Child 46:295, 1971; J Clin Invest 50:730, 1971.
Hypopituitarism with or without hyperinsulinism	Clinical history and supportive laboratory evidence. HGH levels unresponsive to arginine.	
Hypoadrenocorticism	Clinical history and supportive laboratory evidence.	
Primary liver disease	Poor response to glucagon and epinephrine.	
Malnutrition	Rarely < 20 mg/100 ml, but serious if associated with hypothermia, coma, and bacterial or parasitic infection.	Lancet 1:171, 1970.
Catechol insufficiency (Zetterström type)	Defective catechol response to hypoglycemia.	Pediatrics 59:215, 1961.
Other disorders of hexose metabolism Galactosemia (see p 951)	Screen for red cell UDPgal transferase deficiency.	
Fructose intolerance (see p 953)	Hypoglycemia after fructose load. Test for specific aldolase deficiency.	
Fructose-1,6-diphosphatase deficiency	Acidosis and hypoglycemia on fasting; glycerol and fructose provoke hypoglycemia.	Lancet 2:13, 1970; J Pediatr 82:650, 1973.
Induced by lactose and other monosaccharides	Flat oral glucose tolerance test. Hypoglycemic response to lactose.	J Pediatr 77:595, 1970.
Induced by glycerol	Poor response to glycogen. 1 gm/kg of glycerol produces sustained hypoglycemia.	Diabetes 22:292, 1973.
Phosphoenolpyruvate carboxykinase deficiency	Severe infantile hypoglycemia. Fatty changes in liver and kidney.	Pediatr Res 8:910, 1974.
Disorders of glyconeogenesis Idiopathic spontaneous hypoglycemia	Increased insulin sensitivity as shown by insulin/glucose tolerance test (see p 1048).	
Hyperinsulinism	Often but not always an excessive insulin response to a glucagon, tolbutamide, or epinephrine tolerance test. Prompt and exaggerated hypoglycemic response to glucose loading.	
Islet cell hyperplasia, nesidioblastosis	Increased K_t on intravenous glucose tolerance test.	N Engl J Med 296:1323, 1977.
Islet cell adenoma or adenocarcinoma	Irregular hyperinsulinemia after a glucose load. May have paradoxic response to diazoxide. May only be diagnosed at exploratory laparotomy.	Arch Pathol 89:208, 1970.
Some extrapancreatic tumors		N Engl J Med 278:177, 1968.
Beckwith's syndrome	Associated with macroglossia, microcephaly, hepatomegaly, somatic gigantism, omphalocele.	N Engl J Med 275:236, 1966.
Prediabetes	Delayed hypoglycemia following oral glucose tolerance test; later, glucose intolerance.	N Engl J Med 274:815, 1965.
Leucine sensitivity	Positive leucine sensitivity test.	N Engl J Med 267:1057, 1962.
Maple syrup urine disease	Presence of typical smell, neurologic symptoms, acidosis, branched chain ketoaciduria.	Acta Paediatr Scand 61:81, 1972.
Miscellaneous disorders Hypothyroidism	Clinical history; serum glucose levels.	
Primary neurologic disorders	Clinical history; serum glucose levels.	
Reye's syndrome	Clinical picture of encephalopathy, hepatomegaly, and acidosis.	Am J Dis Child 125:809, 1973.

Table 33–10 (cont'd). Guide to the diagnosis of hypoglycemic states.

Causes and Types	Diagnosis	References
Miscellaneous disorders (cont'd)		
Chronic diarrhea	Especially with enteric infection.	Lancet 2:1311, 1970.
Familial glucocorticoid deficiency	Body pigmentation, normal growth.	Arch Dis Child 50:291, 1975.
L-Asparaginase	In therapy for leukemia.	N Engl J Med 282:732, 1970.
Methylmalonic aciduria	Specific organic aciduria.	N Engl J Med 295:1136, 1976.
Toxic		
Salicylates	Positive ferric chloride test; elevated blood salicylates.	Am J Dis Child 108:171, 1964.
EDTA		Lancet 2:637, 1961.
Sulfonylureas	History of diabetes in the mother.	Arch Dis Child 45:696, 1970.
Manganese	Has been used in treatment of diabetes.	Nature 194:188, 1962.
Biotin deficiency	Vomiting, glossitis, and scaly dermatitis.	Life Sci 8:299, 1969.

Clinical Findings

A. Symptoms and Signs: Symptoms of hypoglycemia are quite variable. In the newborn, especially, there may be none, or the infant may show difficulty in feeding, apathy, hypothermia, pallor, cyanosis, a weak cry, and, later, episodes of tremors, eye rolling, or actual convulsions. The fontanel is sometimes distended, and there may be cardiomegaly in severe cases. In older children, the usual symptoms are those of faintness, headache, sweating, and feeling hungry. Patients may look pale and complain of muscle pains and paresthesia; they may become irritable and drowsy and ultimately develop convulsions. Clinical response to restoration of normal serum glucose levels is usually rapid at all ages unless neurologic involvement is marked.

B. Laboratory Findings:* Hypoglycemia is usually defined as a serum glucose level of ≤ 20 mg/100 ml in the premature and ≤ 30 mg/100 ml in newborn or older infants. The possibility of this diagnosis always warrants complete laboratory evaluation, which can usually be done as an elective procedure. Where toxic or other specific cause is indicated, the diagnosis is that of the supposed underlying condition. In other cases, the following procedure is suggested:

1. After 3 days of a high-carbohydrate diet, the child is admitted to the hospital and, after an overnight fast, is given a standard glucose test lasting 4 hours. This is followed immediately after the last sample by a glucagon tolerance test. An abrupt fall in blood sugar between 30 minutes and 60 minutes is indicative of hyperinsulinism, including leucine sensitivity: late hypoglycemia at 3–4 hours suggests the delayed hyperinsulinemia of prediabetes. A flat curve may suggest malabsorption. A normal glucagon tolerance test indicates adequate hepatic glycogen and serves also as a screening test for normal glycolytic mechanisms.

2. On the second day, an insulin/glucose tolerance test should be given to evaluate the homeostatic responses to induced hypoglycemia. This test is safer than the insulin sensitivity test since it is less likely to induce severe hypoglycemia. Even so, it should only be

*See Chapter 38 for details of the tests discussed in this section.

done with an intravenous drip of 0.5 N saline set up so that 50% dextrose can be administered promptly if required. A positive test indicates failure of normal glycolysis or gluconeogenesis. The previous glucagon tolerance test will differentiate between the 2 processes.

3. Special tests—

a. Tests for galactosemia, glycogen storage disease, fructose intolerance, fructose-1,6-diphosphatase deficiency, and glycerol sensitivity should be performed as indicated by the clinical history.

b. Leucine loading test for leucine sensitivity when the history suggests that hypoglycemia follows protein loading. Hyperinsulinism with reactive hypoglycemia during an oral GTT may be seen.

c. Start a ketogenic diet (Colle E, Ulstrom J: J Pediatr 64:632, 1964) if the patient is small for gestational age at birth and the history suggests a relationship between hypoglycemia and ketosis. Oral administration of medium chain triglycerides may also produce symptoms.

Complications

Uncontrolled hypoglycemic episodes may lead to progressive cerebral damage, with epilepsy and developmental retardation. In cases where a pancreatectomy has been performed, diabetes is an occasional complication.

Treatment

Treatment is directed at counteracting the imbalance in glucose homeostasis; it is not necessarily specific to the nature of the imbalance. The following program can be used as a guide.

A. Toxic Causes: Discontinue drug, provide high carbohydrate intake.

B. Newborn: Treat initially with 5 or 10% dextrose infusion. This sometimes does not prevent hypoglycemia and may occasionally provoke hypoglycemia if suddenly discontinued. Prednisone, 5 mg/day orally, glucagon, 15 μg/kg every 4 hours IM, or epinephrine, 1:200 (Sus-Phrine), 0.005 ml/kg IM, may sometimes be required for a few days in addition to a glucose infusion. Fructose can be used instead of glucose in equimolar amounts. It is less likely to cause reactive hypoglycemia if temporarily discontinued.

C. Idiopathic Hypoglycemia of Infancy: Treat acute episodes with glucagon, 15 μg/kg IM, repeated, if necessary, in 30 minutes. At the same time, give 10% dextrose in 0.5 N saline at a rate of 100 ml/kg/24 hours.

For long-term therapy, a high-protein intake with frequent small high-carbohydrate feedings may be successful. If this fails, prednisone, 1–2 mg/kg/day orally in 2 or 3 divided doses, may be helpful. Finally, diazoxide (Hyperstat), 6–12 mg/kg/day orally in 2 doses, may be given. If all these measures fail, subtotal pancreatectomy should be considered.

D. Leucine Sensitivity: Restrict protein intake to < 1.5 gm/kg/day (provided growth is adequate) and give frequent high-carbohydrate feedings. Diazoxide or prednisone may also be helpful.

E. Ketotic Hypoglycemia: Test urine routinely, using nitroprusside (Acetest) papers for acetone, and treat incipient ketosis with frequent high-carbohydrate feedings and snacks. In infection, administer glucose intravenously and, as in other cases, have glucagon available in the home should severe hypoglycemia develop.

F. Hyperinsulinism: The delayed inappropriate hyperinsulinism of early diabetes should be treated by carbohydrate restriction in the diet. Pancreatic or extrapancreatic insulin-secreting tumors should be removed. In the case of simple hyperplasia, 85% of the pancreas should be removed.

G. Failure of Glycogenolysis: In glycogen storage disease, give frequent carbohydrate feedings. Surgical shunting procedures may help (see Glycogen Storage Diseases, above).

H. Galactosemia, Fructose-1,6-diphosphatase Deficiency, Fructose Intolerance: Avoid appropriate monosaccharide in diet.

I. Deficient Pressor Amine Response: Apply measures as under C (above), but also try ephedrine, 0.5–1 mg/kg orally 3 times a day.

Prognosis

Treatment may be complex but is usually successful. Symptoms of hypoglycemia may persist into adult life.

Cornblath M, Schwartz R: Page 82 in: *Disorders of Carbohydrate Metabolism in Infancy.* Saunders, 1967.
Greenberg RE, Christiansen RD: The critically ill child: Hypoglycemia. Pediatrics 46:915, 1970.
Hypoglycaemia in infancy and childhood. Br Med J 3:130, 1971.
Mereu TR & others: Diazoxide in the treatment of infantile hypoglycemia. N Engl J Med 275:1455, 1966.
Pagliara A: Hypoglycemia in infancy and childhood. (2 parts.) J Pediatr 82:365, 559, 1973.

DISORDERS OF AMINO ACID METABOLISM

The development of column chromatographic technics for the detection and quantitation of amino acids in biologic fluids has enormously expanded the possibilities of laboratory diagnosis and treatment of one rare but important group of inborn errors of metabolism, ie, those involving the amino acids. Most of these disorders are summarized briefly in Tables 33–11 and 33–12. A few of special interest or importance are described in the following paragraphs.

PHENYLKETONURIA & THE HYPERPHENYLALANINEMIAS

Essentials of Diagnosis

- Serum phenylalanine levels persistently in excess of 20 mg/100 ml after the first few days of life with low serum tyrosine levels.
- Phenylalanine levels can only be lowered by a special low-phenylalanine formula.
- Tolerance to phenylalanine is very poor, and serum levels rise rapidly with any increase in intake. Tolerance is unchanged with increasing age.
- Untreated cases excrete phenylpyruvic and o-hydroxyphenylacetic acid in the urine and show a positive ferric chloride test.

General Considerations

Probably the most studied and best known disorder of amino acid metabolism, phenylketonuria was first recognized in 1934 by Følling in 10 severely retarded children who excreted phenylpyruvic acid in the urine. The disorder is due to diminished activity of phenylalanine hydroxylase, a complex enzyme system which converts phenylalanine to tyrosine and is transmitted as an autosomal recessive trait with a frequency of approximately one in 10,000 live births. The biochemical block leads to hyperphenylalaninemia and to the formation and excretion of such alternative phenylalanine metabolites as phenylacetylglutamine and phenylpyruvic, phenyllactic, phenylacetic, and o-hydroxyphenylacetic acids. The clinical picture includes severe mental retardation, a "mousy" odor of the urine, light complexion and eczema, hyperactivity, and seizures. While decreased pigmentation is thought to be due to inhibition of melanin synthesis by hyperphenylalaninemia, the biochemical basis of the CNS dysfunction remains unclear. Postulated mechanisms have included inhibition of cerebroside, sulfatide, dopamine, and serotonin synthesis by phenylalanine and inhibition of brain pyruvate kinase by phenylpyruvic acid.

Early favorable results on phenylketonuric children treated from early infancy with a diet low in phenylalanine led to the development of programs which were designed to detect hyperphenylalaninemia early in life, the notion being that phenylalanine restriction would then prevent the severe neurologic consequences. In general terms, this expectation has been fulfilled.

Present data suggest that diagnosis should be established and diet therapy begun before 3 months of age—hence the necessity for newborn screening, which is usually performed in the first few days of life. Because about 10% of newborns with classical phenylketonuria will not be hyperphenylalaninemic during the first 3–4 days of life, optimal case-finding requires either that screening be done somewhat later (eg, 2 weeks) or that a second test (eg, between 2 and 6 weeks) be added to the usual screening procedure.

A. The Enzyme Defect: The 3 cosubstrates of phenylalanine hydroxylase are L-phenylalanine, atmospheric oxygen, and tetrahydrobiopterin; the products of the reaction are L-tyrosine, water, and the quininoid form of dihydrobiopterin. The latter is then reconverted to tetrahydrobiopterin by dihydropteridine reductase. In classical phenylketonuria, the mutant enzyme is phenylalanine hydroxylase, and little or no residual activity is demonstrable; in the less severe hyperphenylalaninemias, significant residual activity (10–20%) is present. Two rare variants are due in one case to dihydropteridine reductase deficiency and in the other to a combined hydroxylation deficiency of phenylalanine and tryptophan.

B. Genetic Considerations: All of the hyperphenylalaninemias and phenylketonurias are inherited as autosomal recessives; some are true homozygous traits, while others probably represent heterozygosity for 2 different mutant alleles at the same locus.

Since phenylalanine hydroxylase activity is not normally present in fibroblasts in cultured amniotic cells, its absence cannot be used as an index of fetal disease; phenylketonuria thus cannot be diagnosed in utero. However, dihydropteridine reductase activity is normally present in these cells, and the diagnosis of hyperphenylalaninemia due to the absence of such activity probably can be made antenatally.

There is no absolutely reliable test for the carrier state. It appears that the easiest approach is through analysis of fasting serum phenylalanine and tyrosine concentrations followed, in unclear situations, by phenylalanine loading.

Clinical Findings

In infants, one of the earliest manifestations of phenylketonuria is vomiting. Another is a "mouse-like" odor of the urine and sweat, which contains excessive amounts of phenylacetic, phenyllactic, and phenylpyruvic acids. By 1 year of age, the untreated phenylketonuric infant is often quite obese. The excessive accumulation of phenylalanine also impairs melanin production: thus, the untreated phenylketonuric individual is often lighter complexioned than his unaffected relatives. For example, Negroes, Orientals, and Spanish individuals have been noted to have brown hair; eczema is also common. Neurologic impairment is usual but not universal. Most are mentally retarded and hypertonic and have hyperactive reflexes. Seizures and tremors may be noted. Some have autistic or psychotic manifestations. Because this is an inherited disorder, a family history of phenylketonuria or of some of the above manifestations may also be helpful.

Differential Diagnosis

The diagnosis of phenylketonuria in a severely retarded older child with typical biochemical and physical characteristics is straightforward, but in the newborn period, especially when there is no family history, the condition must be differentiated from other forms of hyperphenylalaninemia. The causes of hyperphenylalaninemia in the newborn period are summarized below.

A. Classical Phenylketonuria: Persistent elevation of serum phenylalanine > 20 mg/100 ml, with normal or low serum tyrosine, and urine excretion of phenylpyruvic and *o*-hydroxyphenylacetic acids. Poor tolerance to oral phenylalanine throughout life. Serum tyrosine does not rise after a phenylalanine load. Phenylalanine restriction lowers serum phenylalanine and is indicated.

B. Mild Phenylketonuria: The criteria for classical phenylketonuria are met except that tolerance for phenylalanine is higher. Diet therapy is necessary to prevent mental retardation. The disorder probably represents allelic variation at the phenylalanine hydroxylase locus.

C. Transient Phenylketonuria: The criteria for classical phenylketonuria are met except that phenylalanine intolerance disappears at some time during the first years of life. Diet therapy is necessary during the period of phenylalanine intolerance. This probably also represents allelic variation at the phenylalanine hydroxylase locus.

D. Dihydropteridine Reductase Deficiency: The criteria for classical phenylketonuria are met, but seizures and psychomotor retardation progress even on diet therapy. The use of levodopa and 5-hydroxytryptophan may be warranted. The defect and its carrier state are definable in cultured fibroblasts.

E. Hyperphenylalaninemia: Serum phenylalanine is consistently below 15 mg/100 ml on a normal protein intake, serum tyrosine rises after a phenylalanine load, and phenylketones are not excreted. Dietary treatment is not required.

F. Tyrosinemia of the Newborn: Hyperphenylalaninemia is accompanied by an even greater hypertyrosinemia. This is most common in premature infants, is due to immaturity of phenylalanine hydroxylase and *p*-hydroxyphenylpyruvic acid oxidase, and is probably benign (see section on tyrosinemia).

G. Maternal Phenylketonuria: The heterozygous (for PKU) offspring of phenylketonuric mothers have transient hyperphenylalaninemia after birth; virtually all are retarded and microcephalic. Diet therapy is not indicated, although the phenotype suggests a need for

Table 33–11. Selected inborn errors of amino acid metabolism.*

Disorder	Enzyme Defect	Biochemical Features	Clinical Features and Treatment
Sulfur amino acids			
Cystathioninuria	Cystathioninase	Cystathioninuria	Variable: from normal phenotype to mental retardation and congenital anomalies, probably coincidental. Vitamin B_6 in large amounts decreases cystathionine excretion.
Homocystinuria[1]	Cystathionine synthase	Hypermethioninemia, homocystinuria	Marfan-like appearance, ectopia lentis, thromboembolic phenomena, mental retardation, schizophrenia. Homocystinuria sometimes responsive to large amounts of pyridoxine.
	Defective synthesis of methyl-B_{12}	Homocystinuria, low or normal serum methionine, methylmalonic aciduria	Variable: from mild mental retardation and schizophrenia to severe acidosis and failure to thrive. Homocystinuria can be lessened by betaine, the methylmalonic aciduria by vitamin B_{12} in large doses.
	Methylene tetrahydrofolate reductase[2]	Homocystinuria, low or normal serum methionine	Schizophrenia, mental retardation, seizures.
Cystinuria	Renal and gut transport of cystine and dibasic amino acids	Dibasic aminoaciduria and normal serum amino acids	Cystine renal calculi. Treat with high water intake, alkalies, and penicillamine.
Cystinosis[3]	Cystine sequestration in lysosomes, cause unknown	Generalized aminoaciduria, phosphaturia; cystine crystals in cornea, bone marrow, and kidney	Variable: classical form with diabetes insipidus and renal Fanconi syndrome, progressive glomerular failure with death in uremia. Treat kidney failure with renal transplant.
Branched-chain amino acids			
Maple syrup urine disease	See text.		
Isovaleric acidemia	Isovaleryl-CoA dehydrogenase	Isovaleric acid and isovalerylglycine in urine	Odor of sweaty feet. Course varies from severe neonatal acidosis to recurrent vomiting and metabolic acidemia. Treat with a low-protein diet.
β-Methylcrotonylglycinuria	β-Methylcrotonyl-CoA carboxylase	β-Methylcrotonylglycine and β-hydroxyisovaleric acid in urine	Retardation, urine odor of cat urine, vomiting, metabolic acidemia. Some patients respond to biotin in large amounts.
α-Methyl-β-hydroxybutyric aciduria[4]	α-Methylacetoacetyl-CoA ketothiolase(?)	α-Methyl-β-hydroxybutyric, α-methylacetoacetic acids, and tiglylglycine in urine. Occasionally hyperglycinemia and hyperglycinuria.	Episodic vomiting and metabolic acidemia in childhood. Treat with low-protein diet.
Propionic acidemia	Propionyl-CoA carboxylase	Propionic, β-hydroxypropionic, and methylcitric acids in urine. Hyperglycinemia and hyperglycinuria.	Recurrent vomiting and severe metabolic acidosis. One of the ketotic hyperglycinemia syndromes. Some patients respond to biotin in large amounts.
Methylmalonic aciduria	See text.		
Imino acids			
Hyperprolinemia Type I	Proline oxidase	Hyperprolinemia; proline, hydroxyproline, and glycine in urine	Variable. Association with familial nephritis and mental retardation may be fortuitous.
Type II[5]	Δ^1-Pyrroline-5-carboxylic acid dehydrogenase	Same as above but with Δ^1-pyrroline-5-COOH and Δ^1-pyrroline-3-OH-5-COOH in urine. Positive urine test with o-aminobenzaldehyde.	Variable association with seizures and mental retardation.
Hydroxyprolinemia	Hydroxyproline oxidase	Hydroxyprolinemia, hydroxyprolinuria	Variable association with mental retardation.
Iminoglycinuria	Renal (and gut) transport of imino acids and glycine	Proline, hydroxyproline, and glycine in urine with normal serum amino acids	None.

Table 33–11 (cont'd). Selected inborn errors of amino acid metabolism.*

Disorder	Enzyme Defect	Biochemical Features	Clinical Features and Treatment
Histidine			
Histidinemia	Histidase	Histidinemia, histidinuria, imidazolpyruvic aciduria	Mild mental retardation frequent, slurred speech. Biochemical control possible by low-histidine diet but clinical effects uncertain.
Formiminoglutamic aciduria	Glutamate formiminotransferase	N-Formiminoglutamic aciduria	Variable. Mental retardation and hematologic changes compatible with folate deficiency are not constant.
Lysine and tryptophan			
Hyperlysinemia Periodic	(?)L-Lysine dehydrogenase	Hyperlysinemia and hyperammonemia with protein intake	Protein intolerance with episodic vomiting, seizures, and coma. Treat with low-protein diet.
Persistent	Lysine:a-ketoglutarate reductase	Hyperlysinemia and hyperlysinuria	Inconstant association, possibly fortuitous, with mental retardation.
Saccharopinuria	Saccharopine dehydrogenase	Hyperlysinemia and hyperlysinuria, saccharopinuria	Mental retardation, short stature.
Tryptophanuria	Tryptophan pyrrolase	Tryptophanuria (variable)	Mental retardation, photosensitive rash, cerebellar ataxia. Treat with nicotinic acid(?).
Hydroxykynureninuria	Kynureninase	3-Hydroxykynurenine in urine	Mild mental retardation, photosensitive rash.
a-Ketoadipic aciduria[6]	a-Ketoadipate dehydrogenase	a-Aminoadipic acidemia and aciduria, a-ketoadipic aciduria	
Glutaric aciduria[7]	Glutaryl-CoA dehydrogenase	Glutaric and β-hydroxyglutaric acids in urine	Mental retardation, dystonia, athetosis, intermittent metabolic acidosis. Treat with low-protein diet(?).
Hartnup disease	Renal (and gut) transport of neutral amino acids	Neutral aminoaciduria with normal serum amino acids, indoluria, and indicanuria	Variable mental retardation, pellagra-like skin rash, ataxia. Treat with nicotinic acid.
Phenylalanine			
Phenylketonurias	See text.		
Hyperphenylalaninemias	See text.		

*If no references are given, the reader should consult the following general references: (1) Nyhan WL (editor): *Heritable Disorders of Amino Acid Metabolism: Patterns of Clinical Expression and Genetic Variation.* Wiley, 1974. (2) Scriver CR, Rosenberg LE: *Amino Acid Metabolism and Its Disorders.* Saunders, 1973.

[1] N Engl J Med 291:537, 1974.
[2] Biochem Biophys Res Commun 46:905, 1972.
[3] Department of Health, Education, and Welfare. Pages 225–232 in: Publication No. (DHEW) 72-249, 1972.
[4] Clin Chim Acta 57:269, 1974.
[5] Science 185:1053, 1974.
[6] Clin Chim Acta 58:257, 1975.
[7] Biochem Med 12:12, 1975.

phenylalanine restriction in women with phenylketonuria during pregnancy.

H. Miscellaneous Hyperphenylalaninemics:

1. Phenylalanine transaminase deficiency.

2. Combined phenylalanine and tryptophan hydroxylase deficiency.

3. Phenylketonuria with cystathioninuria.

Treatment

Treatment is aimed at limiting the intake of the essential amino acid phenylalanine to allow normal growth and development without producing neurologic impairment, an approach made possible by the availability of a low-phenylalanine milk substitute (Lofenalac). Since excessive restriction of phenylalanine may produce bone changes, anemia, and retardation of growth and development, it is essential to monitor the treatment closely through serial serum phenylalanine determinations as well as by ascertaining general health, growth, development, and nutritional intake. Such coordination of care is frequently best done at clinics where specialists in each of these areas are in attendance. Although dietary treatment is most effective when initiated during the first few months of life, it is sometimes beneficial in reversing maladaptive behavior such as hyperactivity and excessive lethargy when started later in life.

There is considerable difference of opinion about when phenylalanine restriction should be discontinued, some authorities contending that dietotherapy can be safely terminated at 4–5 years of age while others advocate continuous dietary restriction throughout childhood and adolescence. As noted above, adult phenylketonuric females merit special attention during pregnancy.

Prognosis

Children treated promptly after birth and properly managed in terms of phenylalanine and tyrosine homeostasis develop well physically and have a good but less than normal expectation for intellectual development.

Acosta PB & others: *Dietary Management of Inherited Metabolic Diseases.* Department of Pediatrics, Emory University School of Medicine, 1976.

Bartholomé K & others: A new variant of phenylketonuria. Pediatrics 59:757, 1977.

Bickel H, Hudson FP, Wolff LI: *Phenylketonuria and Some Other Inborn Errors of Amino Acid Metabolism.* Thieme Verlag, Stuttgart, 1971.

Committee on Nutrition, American Academy of Pediatrics: Special diets for infants with inborn errors of metabolism. Pediatrics 57:783, 1976.

Frankenburg WK: Maternal phenylketonuric implications for growth and development. J Pediatr 73:560, 1968.

Smith I, Clayton BE, Wolff OH: New variant of phenylketonuria with progressive neurological illness unresponsive to phenylalanine restriction. Lancet 1:1108, 1975.

TYROSINEMIA

The normal metabolism of tyrosine is by transamination to *p*-hydroxyphenylpyruvic acid (*p*HPPA) followed by oxidation to homogentisic acid by *p*-hydroxyphenylpyruvic acid oxidase; homogentisic acid is then oxidized to fumaric and acetoacetic acids. The tyrosinemias are disorders in which defects in this pathway result in high serum concentrations of tyrosine (tyrosinemia) and urinary excretion of various tyrosine metabolites like *p*-hydroxyphenylpyruvic and *p*-hydroxyphenyllactic acids (tyrosyluria). The most important forms of tyrosinemia are summarized below.

A. Tyrosinemia of the Newborn: Tyrosinemia of the newborn (serum tyrosine 6 mg/100 ml) is due to immaturity of *p*-hydroxyphenylpyruvic acid oxidase and is thus especially common in premature infants; it is accentuated by vitamin C deficiency and high protein intake. Recovery of enzyme activity is usually quite sudden and may occur at any time between a few days and 3 months of age.

Tyrosinemia in this condition may be reduced by lowering protein intake to 2 gm/kg/day or by ascorbic acid (50–100 mg/day), and this may be important for 2 reasons: (1) to differentiate the condition from the causes of tyrosinemia described below, and (2) because the relation of prolonged tyrosinemia (> 6 weeks) to CNS damage is unclear.

B. Hereditary Tyrosinemia: Hereditary tyrosinemia is an inherited syndrome of progressive hepatic parenchymal damage, renal tubular dystrophy with generalized aminoaciduria and hypophosphatemic rickets, hypermethioninemia, mild tyrosinemia, and tyrosyluria. The course may be rapidly fatal in infancy or somewhat more chronic. It has become apparent that this clinical picture is nonspecific and may occur with a number of disorders, including those caused by deficiencies in fructose-1-phosphate aldolase (hereditary fructose intolerance), galactose-1-phosphate uridyl transferase (galactosemia), fructose-1,6-diphosphatase, and fumaryl aceto-acetase.

C. Hypertyrosinemia (Oregon Type): This disorder is probably due to inherited deficiency of hepatic cytosol tyrosine aminotransferase and is characterized by profound tyrosinemia (35–50 mg/100 ml), a syndrome of palmar and plantar keratoses and corneal dystrophy (Richner-Hanhart syndrome) whose severity fluctuates with the elevation of serum tyrosine, and mental retardation.

Treatment

At present there is only tentative evidence that transient *p*HPPA deficiency in the newborn leads to any neurologic impairment. However, there have been animal studies that show an effect of tyrosinosis on myelination. It seems reasonable, therefore, to use a low-protein formula until enzyme activity is restored and to ensure an adequate vitamin C supplement.

In the groups with liver damage, control with a low-phenylalanine and low-tyrosine diet (50 mg of each per kg/24 hours) now seems mandatory.

Conference on hereditary tyrosinemia. Can Med Assoc J 97:1045, 1967.

Mamunes P & others: Intellectual deficits after tyrosinemia in term neonates. Pediatr Res 8:344, 1974.

Rizzardini M, Abeliuk P: Tyrosinemia and tyrosinuria in low birth weight infants. Am J Dis Child 121:182, 1971.

MAPLE SYRUP URINE DISEASE
(Branched Chain Ketoaciduria)

Maple syrup urine disease is due to generalized deficiency of the enzymes that catalyze oxidative decarboxylation of the keto acid derivatives of the branched chain amino acids leucine, isoleucine, and valine. The keto acids of leucine and isoleucine contribute to the characteristic odor, while only the keto acid of leucine has been implicated in CNS dysfunction. Many variants of this disorder have been described, including mild, intermittent, and thiamine-dependent forms.

In the classical form, patients are normal at birth but soon develop the characteristic odor, lethargy, feeding difficulties, coma, and seizures. If the diagnosis is not made and diet therapy begun, most will die in the first month of life. Peritoneal dialysis may be necessary in initial therapy. Oral bicarbonate is also useful in the amelioration of acidotic episodes in the older treated child.

Diet therapy in this condition is directed toward restriction of intake of branched chain amino acids, all of which are essential, to amounts necessary for normal growth and development. If such treatment is begun prior to about 10 days of age, normal growth and development can be achieved. Problems include (1) maintenance of dietary restriction throughout life—unlike phenylketonuria, in which a normal diet can be instituted after myelination is complete; (2) necessity for and cost of biochemical monitoring; and (3) hyperleucinemia and CNS symptoms accompanying catabolic episodes during infections.

This rare disorder is transmitted as an autosomal recessive trait. It can be diagnosed during fetal life on the basis of absent branched chain keto acid decarboxylase activity in cultured amniotic cells. There is no accurate and cheap test for mass carrier detection.

Acosta PB & others: *Dietary Management of Inherited Metabolic Diseases.* Department of Pediatrics, Emory University School of Medicine, 1976.

Dancis J, Hutzler J, Rokhones T: Intermittent branched chain ketonuria. N Engl J Med 267:84, 1967.

Management of maple syrup urine disease in Canada. Can Med Assoc J 115:1005, 1976.

Scrivner CR & others: Thiamine responsive maple syrup urine disease. Lancet 1:310, 1971.

DISORDERS OF THE UREA CYCLE

The urea cycle is a series of 5 enzymes which convert ammonia to one of the amino groups in urea. Inherited deficiency of one of the first enzymes in the sequence (carbamyl phosphate synthetase and ornithine transcarbamylase) usually presents in infancy with a syndrome of episodic vomiting, hyperammonemia, and neurologic signs (coma, seizures, etc) which can lead to early death. A more benign course, characterized only by mental retardation, is more usual in deficiencies of argininosuccinic acid synthetase (citrullinemia), argininosuccinic acid lyase (argininosuccinic aciduria), and arginase (argininemia).

Diagnosis is based on the presence of hyperammonemia and specific aminoacidemia or aminoaciduria (in citrullinemia, argininosuccinic aciduria, and argininemia) and specific enzyme assay. Treatment, which is variably effective, is through use of a low-protein diet (about 1 gm/kg/day).

With the exception of ornithine transcarbamylase deficiency, which is inherited in X-linked fashion, all of these disorders are inherited as autosomal recessive traits. Citrullinemia, argininosuccinic aciduria, and argininemia can probably be diagnosed in utero; carbamyl phosphate synthetase deficiency and ornithine transcarbamylase deficiency cannot.

Batshaw M, Bruslow S, Mackenzie W: Treatment of carbamyl phosphate synthetase deficiency with keto analogues of essential amino acids. N Engl J Med 292:1085, 1975.

Carton D & others: Argininosuccinic aciduria. Acta Paediatr Scand 58:528, 1969.

Corbeel LM & others: Periodic attacks of lethargy in a baby with ammonia intoxication. Arch Dis Child 44:681, 1969.

Dancis J & others: Familial hyperlysinemia. J Clin Invest 48:1447, 1969.

Hommes FA & others: Carbamylphosphate synthetase deficiency. Arch Dis Child 44:688, 1969.

Morrow G & others: Citrullinuria with defective urea production. Pediatrics 40:465, 1967.

O'Brien D, Goodman SI: The critically ill child: Acute metabolic disease. Pediatrics 46:620, 1970.

CONGENITAL METHYLMALONIC ACIDURIA

Four essential amino acids (L-threonine, L-valine, L-isoleucine, and L-methionine) are metabolized through D-methylmalonyl-CoA. Under normal conditions, this compound is converted to L-methylmalonyl-CoA by methylmalonyl-CoA racemase and then to succinyl-CoA by methylmalonyl-CoA isomerase, an enzyme which requires deoxyadenosyl-B_{12} as coenzyme. Congenital methylmalonic aciduria can be caused by deficiencies of methylmalonyl-CoA racemase, methylmalonyl-CoA isomerase, or enzymes that function in the synthesis of deoxyadenosyl-B_{12}.

There are at least 2 different diseases in the latter category: (1) one that affects only the synthesis of deoxyadenosyl-B_{12} and (2) one that affects the synthesis of both deoxyadenosyl-B_{12} and methyl-B_{12}. The latter is the coenzyme for N^5-methyltetrahydrofolate methyltransferase, an enzyme necessary for the conversion of homocysteine to methionine.

Clinical symptoms in methylmalonic aciduria depend on the location and severity of the enzyme block. Those with severe blocks present with acute, life-threatening metabolic acidemia early in infancy or with metabolic acidemia, vomiting, and failure to thrive during the first few months of life. Children with less severe blocks may show only moderate mental retardation. Laboratory findings include hyperglycinemia and hyperglycinuria, a positive methylmalonic aciduria screening test, the presence of methylmalonic acid in the urine on organic acid chromatography, and, in the case of an appropriate block in B_{12} metabolism, hypomethioninemic homocystinuria.

Patients with enzyme blocks in B_{12} metabolism usually respond to massive (1 mg/day) doses of vitamin B_{12}, while nonresponders require protein restriction and correction of their rather constant metabolic acidemia.

All types of methylmalonic aciduria described to date are transmitted as autosomal recessive traits. The disorder can be diagnosed in utero by demonstrating defective conversion of propionate to CO_2 in cultured amniotic fluid cells.

Giorgio AJ, Luhby AL: A rapid screening test for the detection of congenital methylmalonic aciduria in infancy. Am J Clin Pathol 52:374, 1969.

Kang ES, Snodgrass PJ, Gerald PS: Methylmalonyl coenzyme A racemase defect: Another cause of methylmalonic aciduria. Pediatr Res 6:875, 1972.

Kaye CI & others: In vitro "responsive" methylmalonic acidemia: A new variant. J Pediatr 85:65, 1974.

Mahoney MJ, Rosenberg LE: Inherited defects of B_{12} metabolism. Am J Med 48:584, 1970.

Morrow G & others: Congenital methylmalonic acidemia: Enzymatic evidence for two forms of the disease. Proc Natl Acad Sci USA 63:191, 1969.

DISORDERS OF PURINE & PYRIMIDINE METABOLISM

Hereditary Orotic Aciduria

Orotate phosphoribosyltransferase and orotidylate decarboxylase are sequential and (physically complexed) enzymes in the biosynthesis of uridine monophosphate, and absence of one or both activities leads to an autosomal recessive condition characterized by failure to thrive, hypochromic anemia with megaloblastic changes in the marrow, and increased urine excretion of orotic acid. The enzyme defect may be demonstrated in tissue biopsy, erythrocytes, and cultured skin fibroblasts.

Two types have been described: one in which both enzyme activities are deficient (type I) and one in which only decarboxylase activity is deficient (type II). Although the former situation was once thought due to mutation of a regulator gene, both types are in fact due to decarboxylase mutations. The type I mutation does not allow proper aggregation of phosphoribosyltransferase and decarboxylase subunits, so that both activities appear to be deficient, whereas the type II mutation affects only its active site and not aggregation.

Treatment with uridine results in hematologic remission and improvement in growth.

Brown GK, O'Sullivan WJ: The subunit structure of the orotate phosphoribosyltransferase-orotidylate decarboxylase complex from human erythrocytes. Biochemistry. [In press.]

Kelley WN, Smith LH Jr: Hereditary orotic aciduria. Chap 46, pages 1045–1071, in: *The Metabolic Basis of Inherited Disease*, 4th ed. Stanbury JB, Wyngaarden JB, Fredrickson DS (editors). McGraw-Hill, 1978.

Adenosine Deaminase Deficiency

Adenosine deaminase (ADA) is the enzyme responsible for the conversion of adenosine to inosine in the purine salvage system. The autosomal recessive disorder due to its deficiency chiefly affects the immune system, causing the most common form of combined immunodeficiency disease, a syndrome characterized by the onset of severe infections early in life, lymphopenia, and deficiency of both B- and T cell-mediated immunity. Without treatment, patients die at age 2 years or after.

The combined immunodeficiency disease caused by this enzymopathy may be distinguished from ADA-positive forms by (1) enzyme assay on lymphocytes, erythrocytes, or cultured fibroblasts; (2) the presence of various radiologic abnormalities of pelvis, spine, and ribs; and (3) the presence in the thymus of Hassall's corpuscles and differentiated thymic epithelium.

Unlike the ADA-positive forms of combined immunodeficiency disease, which respond only to bone marrow or fetal liver transfusions, enzyme replacement by repeated transfusions of normal irradiated erythrocytes rapidly restores and maintains immunocompetence in the ADA-negative patient.

Meuwissen HJ & others: Combined immunodeficiency disease associated with adenosine deaminase deficiency. J Pediatr 86:169, 1975.

Polmar SH & others: Enzyme replacement therapy for adenosine deaminase deficiency and severe combined immunodeficiency. N Engl J Med 295:1337, 1976.

Purine Nucleoside Phosphorylase Deficiency

Purine nucleoside phosphorylase (PNP) is the enzyme responsible for the respective conversions of inosine, guanosine, and xanthosine to hypoxanthine, guanine, and xanthine in the purine salvage system, and the autosomal recessive disease caused by its deficiency is, like ADA deficiency (see above), primarily one of the immune system. In this situation, however, only T cell-mediated immunity is severely deficient, and the clinical condition is characterized by recurrent infections, hypochromic anemia with megaloblastic changes in the bone marrow, lymphopenia, hypouricemia, and hypouricosuria. Erythrocytes and cultured fibroblasts are completely deficient in PNP activity.

Cohen A & others: Abnormal purine metabolism and purine overproduction in a patient deficient in purine nucleoside phosphorylase. N Engl J Med 295:1449, 1976.

Giblett ER & others: Nucleoside-phosphorylase deficiency in a child with severely defective T-cell immunity and normal B-cell immunity. Lancet 1:1010, 1975.

Hypoxanthine-Guanine Phosphoribosyltransferase Deficiency (Lesch-Nyhan Syndrome)

Hypoxanthine-guanine phosphoribosyltransferase (HGPRT) is the enzyme that converts the purine bases hypoxanthine and guanine to IMP and GMP, respectively, and the X-linked recessive disorder due to its complete deficiency is characterized by CNS dysfunction and purine overproduction with hyperuricemia and hyperuricosuria. Depending on the residual activity of the mutant enzyme, male hemizygotes may be severely retarded and show choreoathetosis, spasticity, and compulsive, mutilating lip and finger biting, or may present with only gouty arthritis and urate ureterolithiasis. The enzyme deficiency can be demonstrated in erythrocytes, fibroblasts, and cultured amniotic cells; this disorder can thus be diagnosed with certainty in utero.

Although the cause of the CNS dysfunction in Lesch-Nyhan syndrome remains obscure, the absent or less severe CNS manifestations of PNP deficiency (where HGPRT is functionally inactive because of lack of substrate) suggest that the problem is related to the accumulation of substrate or metabolites behind the block.

Allopurinol and probenecid may be given to reduce hyperuricemia, but they do not affect neurologic status.

Cohen A & others: Abnormal purine metabolism and purine overproduction in a patient deficient in purine nucleoside phosphorylase. N Engl J Med 295:1449, 1976.

Kelley WN, Wyngaarden JB: The Lesch-Nyhan syndrome. Chap 44, pages 1011–1036, in: *The Metabolic Basis of Inherited Disease,* 4th ed. Stanbury JB, Wyngaarden JB, Fredrickson DS (editors). McGraw-Hill, 1978.

DISORDERS OF MUCOPOLYSACCHARIDE & LIPID METABOLISM

The lysosome is the cellular organelle responsible for the degradation of complex macromolecules. When one of its specific hydrolases is genetically altered so as to become inactive, the substrate of the enzyme accumulates in the lysosomes of tissues degrading it, thus causing the characteristic clinical picture. Depending on the nature of the stored material, disorders of this type fall into 2 main groups: mucopolysaccharidoses and lipidoses.

Table 33–12. Disorders of lysosomal hydrolases. (See also Table 21–6.)*

Disorder	Enzyme Defect	Mucopolysaccharides In Urine	Clinical Features
Hurler's syndrome	α-Iduronidase	Heparatin sulfate and dermatan sulfate	Autosomal recessive. Mental retardation, hepatosplenomegaly, umbilical hernia, coarse facies, corneal clouding, skeletal changes with gibbus.
Scheie's syndrome	α-Iduronidase (allele to Hurler mutant but probably more residual activity to natural substrate)	Dermatan sulfate and lesser amounts of heparatin sulfate	Autosomal recessive. Corneal clouding, stiff joints, normal intellect.
Hunter's syndrome	Sulfoiduronate sulfatase	Heparatin sulfate and dermatan sulfate	X-linked recessive. Variable mental retardation, coarse facies, hepatosplenomegaly. Corneal clouding and gibbus not present.
Sanfilippo syndrome Type A	Sulfamidase	Heparatin sulfate	Autosomal recessive. Severe mental retardation with comparatively mild skeletal changes, visceromegaly, and facial coarseness. Types A and B *cannot* be differentiated clinically.
Type B	α-N-Acetylglucosaminidase	Heparatin sulfate	
Morquio's syndrome	N-Acetylhexosamine-6-sulfatase	Keratosulfate	Autosomal recessive. Severe skeletal changes, platyspondylisis, corneal clouding.
Maroteaux-Lamy syndrome Type A	N-Acetylgalactosamine-4-sulfatase	Dermatan sulfate	Autosomal recessive. Coarse facies, growth retardation, severe skeletal deformities with gibbus, corneal clouding, hepatosplenomegaly, normal intellect. Types A and B *cannot* be differentiated clinically.
Type B	Unknown	Dermatan sulfate	
β-Glucuronidase deficiency[1]	β-Glucuronidase	Chondroitin sulfates A and C	Autosomal recessive. Varies from mental retardation, skeletal changes with gibbus, corneal clouding, and hepatosplenomegaly to much milder course.
Mannosidosis[2]	α-Mannosidase	None	Autosomal recessive. Varies from severe mental retardation, coarse facies, short stature and skeletal changes, and hepatosplenomegaly to mild facial coarseness, retardation, and loose joints. Hearing loss common.
Fucosidosis[3]	α-Fucosidase	None	Autosomal recessive. Variable: coarse facies, skeletal changes, hepatosplenomegaly, occasional angiokeratoma corporis diffusum.
I-cell disease[4]	Multiple cytosomal hydrolases	None	Similar to Hurler's disease.

*For further details, refer to McKusick VA: *Heritable Disorders of Connective Tissue,* 4th ed. Mosby, 1972. See also specific references:
[1] J Pediatr 86:388, 1975.
[2] Acta Paediatr Scand 62:555, 1973.
[3] J Pediatr 84:727, 1974.
[4] Pediatrics 54:797, 1974.

MUCOPOLYSACCHARIDOSES

Mucopolysaccharidoses are characterized by mucopolysacchariduria and by the storage of products of partial mucopolysaccharide digestion in lysosomes throughout the body. Features of these conditions are given in Table 33−12, which also includes some closely related diseases not associated with mucopolysacchariduria.

Diagnosis of these conditions, usually suspected on clinical grounds, can be confirmed by any of a number of tests which screen for mucopolysacchariduria. The specific mucopolysaccharides excreted

Table 33−13. Clinical features of lipidoses.

Disorder	Enzyme Defect	Clinical Features
Niemann-Pick disease	Sphingomyelinase	Autosomal recessive. Acute neuronopathic form most common and especially frequent in Eastern European Jews. Accumulation of sphingomyelin in lysosomes of cells of reticuloendothelial system and CNS. Onset at 3−6 months of age with hepatosplenomegaly, mental retardation, and cherry-red spot on retina. Death by 1−4 years.
Metachromatic leukodystrophy	Arylsulfatase A	Autosomal recessive; late infantile form most common. Accumulation of sulfatide in white matter. Onset at age 1−4 years with disturbances of gait (ataxia), motor incoordination, and dementia. Death usually in first decade.
Krabbe's disease (globoid cell leukodystrophy)	Galactocerebroside, β-galactosidase	Autosomal recessive. Globoid cells in white matter and myelin deficiency. Onset at 3−6 months of age with seizures, irritability, and retardation. Death by 1−2 years.
Gaucher's disease	Glucocerebroside, β-glucosidase	Autosomal recessive. Acute neuronopathic form: Accumulation of glucocerebroside in lysosomes of cells of reticuloendothelial system and CNS. Onset at age 6 months with hepatosplenomegaly, mental retardation, cherry-red spot on retina, and Gaucher's cells on biopsy. Death by 1−2 years. Chronic form: Especially frequent in Eastern European Jews. Accumulation of glucocerebroside in lysosomes of reticuloendothelial system. Hepatosplenomegaly and flask-shaped osteolytic bone lesions. Often compatible with normal life expectancy.
GM$_1$ gangliosidosis	β-Galactosidase	Autosomal recessive. Accumulation of GM$_1$ ganglioside in lysosomes of reticuloendothelial system and CNS. Infantile form: Patient abnormal at birth with dysostosis multiplex, hepatosplenomegaly, mental retardation, and cherry-red spot on retina. Death by 2 years. Juvenile form: Normal development to 1 year of age, then ataxia, weakness, dementia, and occasional inferior beaking of the vertebral bodies of L1 and L2. Death by 4−5 years.
GM$_2$ gangliosidosis, Tay-Sachs disease,* Sandhoff's disease	β-N-Acetylhexosiminidase	Automosomal recessive. Tay-Sachs disease 100 times more common in Eastern European Jews than in other groups; Sandhoff's disease is pan-ethnic. The A isoenzyme is deficient in Tay-Sachs disease; the A and B isoenzymes are deficient in Sandhoff's disease. Phenotypes identical, with accumulation of GM$_2$ ganglioside in lysosomes of CNS. Onset at 3−6 months of age with hypotonia, hyperacusia, retardation, and cherry-red spot on retina. Death by 2−3 years.
Fabry's disease	α-Galactosidase	X-linked recessive. Accumulation of digalactoglucoceramide in lysosomes of endothelial cells, corneal epithelium, glomeruli, and peripheral Schwann cells. Angiokeratoma corporis diffusum, corneal opacities, glomerular failure, and periodic crises of pain in extremities. Death from complications of vascular disease in fifth decade. Clark JTR & others: N Engl J Med 284:233, 1971.
Wolman's disease	Acid lipase	Autosomal recessive. Accumulation of cholesterol esters and triglycerides in lysosomes of reticuloendothelial system. Onset in first weeks of life with gastrointestinal symptoms and hepatosplenomegaly. Death by 3−6 months. Enlargement and calcification of the adrenals is constant. Young EP: Arch Dis Child 45:664, 1970.
Refsum's disease	. . .	Autosomal recessive. A rare disorder characterized by peripheral neuritis with motor and sensory involvement, retinitis pigmentosa, ataxia, deafness, visual field restriction, cerebellar ataxia, and ichthyotic skin lesions. There is a defect in the oxidation of exogenous phytanic acid (3,7,11,15-tetramethylhexadecanoic acid), which accumulates in the blood and tissues. Dietary restriction of phytanic acid is helpful.

*Carrier detection and ante-natal diagnosis are available for all of the above conditions and have been especially publicized in relation to Tay-Sachs disease. Physicians requiring diagnostic assistance should call Dr. David Wenger (303) 394-7249.

can then be determined by chromatographic (thin layer or ion exchange) technics. Especially when parents are considering having additional children, enzyme diagnosis is mandatory and can be made on tissue biopsy (eg, liver), cultured skin fibroblasts, or peripheral leukocytes. Most of these disorders can be diagnosed in utero through appropriate enzyme assays on cultured amniotic cells.

McKusick VA: *Heritable Disorders of Connective Tissue,* 4th ed. Mosby, 1972.

LIPIDOSES

Lipidoses are characterized by lysosomal accumulation of lipids. Features of these conditions are given in Table 33–13, which may duplicate somewhat the material in Table 21–16.

When suspected, diagnosis may be confirmed by approximate enzyme assays in biopsy specimens, cultured skin fibroblasts, and peripheral leukocytes. Most can be diagnosed in utero by appropriate enzyme assays on cultured amniotic cells.

Hers HG, Van Hoff F (editors): *Lysosomes and Storage Diseases.* Academic Press, 1973.
Malone MJ: The cerebral lipidoses. Pediatr Clin North Am 23:303, 1976.
O'Brien JS: Ganglioside storage diseases. In: *Advances in Human Genetics.* Vol 3. Harris H, Hirschhorn K (editors). Plenum Press, 1972.
Stanbury JB, Wyngaarden JB, Fredrickson DS (editors): *The Metabolic Basis of Inherited Disease,* 4th ed. McGraw-Hill, 1978.
Stokke OG, Eldjarn L: Biochemical and dietary aspects of Refsum's syndrome. In: *Peripheral Neuropathy.* Dych PJ, Thomas PK (editors). Saunders, 1975.

DISORDERS OF THE PLASMA LIPOPROTEINS

The intravascular transport of lipids is mediated via 2 protein-binding systems: one for free fatty acids and one involving lipoproteins. Free or unesterified fatty acids are the main currency of energy in the body during the postabsorptive state. They circulate as an albumin-fatty acid complex and are derived in part from enteric absorption of fatty acids with less than 12 carbons, but mainly from the triglyceride stores from which they are released by a series of complex homeostatic mechanisms. Primary disorders of this system are very rare and are not further discussed in this section.

Other lipids—primarily glycerides but also phospholipids, cholesterol, and the fat-soluble vitamins—are transported in the plasma in lipoprotein complexes. There are 4 main subdivisions of these lipoproteins characterized by their basic apoprotein, electrophoretic mobility, density, molecular size, and composition as shown in Table 33–14.

Exogenous glycerides are derived from the intestine. Ingested triglyceride is broken down by pancreatic lipase to micelles of monoglyceride and fatty acid. The short chain fatty acids move directly across the mucosal cell to the portal vein. The longer chain fatty acids and monoglycerides also enter the mucosal cell, where hydrolysis is completed and where triglycerides are resynthesized. The latter pass into the blood stream via the thoracic duct and are carried as chylomicrons to adipose tissue, liver, heart, and other organs, where they are immediately hydrolyzed as they enter the cells. In fasting plasma, the glyceride content is derived primarily from the liver.

Transport of cholesterol within the body is quantitatively much less than free fatty acids or glycerol. Exogenous cholesterol moves to the liver in the chylo-

Table 33–14. Percentage composition of plasma lipoproteins.*

	Protein	Cholesterol	Phospholipid	Glyceride	Electro-phoresis	
Chylomicrons (exogenous glyceride)	1	4	5	90		chylo
Low density or beta lipoproteins	25	40	25	10		β
Very low density or prebeta lipoproteins (endogenous glyceride)	5	20	20	55		pre β
High density or alpha lipoproteins	50	20	25	5		a

*For normal values, see Chapter 38.

microns. From then on, transport of endogenous and exogenous cholesterol is on the alpha or beta lipoproteins. The phospholipids—mainly phosphatidyl choline and sphingomyelin—are also carried on the alpha and beta lipoproteins. Their biologic role is unclear but they are believed to stabilize the lipoprotein:plasma water interface.

The protein components of the alpha and beta lipoproteins are called A and B proteins. They are important in relation to conditions where there is an inborn deficiency of these proteins.

THE LIPOPROTEIN DEFICIENCY SYNDROMES

Familial Alpha Lipoprotein Deficiency (Tangier Disease)

This rare inherited condition was first identified in a kindred from Tangier Island in Chesapeake Bay. The most characteristic clinical features are the large lobulated tonsils with their red, orange, or yellowish banding. Hepatosplenomegaly and lymphadenopathy are .common. Neurologic complications, including loss of pain and temperature sensation and peripheral neuropathy, are reported.

Plasma cholesterol levels are abnormally low, and alpha and prebeta lipoprotein bands are about 8% of normal on electrophoresis; levels in the parents are about 50% of normal. Serum triglycerides are normal or modestly elevated. The diagnosis can be confirmed by finding typical foam cells in the bone marrow or rectal mucosa. The appearance of the tonsils, together with hypo-alphaproteinemia, is unique except for LCAT deficiency (see below).

Tonsillectomy may be required because of their size. Treatment is not otherwise indicated, although, in time, CNS complications may constitute a significant handicap.

Koler RS & others: Familial α-lipoprotein deficiency (Tangier disease) with neurological abnormalities. Lancet 1:1341, 1967.

Lecithin: Cholesterol Acyltransferase (LCAT) Deficiency

LCAT deficiency is a rare inborn error of metabolism characterized by hypertriglyceridemia and hypercholesterolemia with lipid deposits in the corneas, proteinuria, and normochromic anemias. There is an almost complete absence of the normal alpha and prebeta lipoprotein bands on electrophoresis.

Serum phospholipids (especially lecithin) are increased to a greater extent than cholesterol. Only 3–4% of cholesterol is esterified; this is due to the absence of the enzyme transferring the acyl group from lecithin to cholesterol to form lysolecithin.

Norum VR & others: Familial plasma lecithin:cholesterol acyl transferase deficiency. Acta Med Scand 188:323, 1970.

Abetalipoproteinemia

This rare autosomal recessive condition is manifested in early infancy with failure to thrive and steatorrhea. Later in life, neurologic deficits include weakness, nystagmus, and posterior column, pyramidal tract, and cerebellar signs. Retinitis pigmentosa is also described.

Cholesterol and phospholipid levels are all extremely low, and chylomicrons are not formed after fat ingestion. Fasting glyceride levels are also abnormally low. Lipoprotein electrophoresis shows no chylomicron band and no beta or prebeta bands. Characteristically, the red blood cells demonstrate acanthocytosis.

Low cholesterol levels with steatorrhea are also found in celiac disease but without acanthocytosis, neurologic findings, or the typical lipoprotein pattern. In cystic fibrosis, there are respiratory symptoms and an elevated sweat chloride. In IgA deficiency, the immunoglobulin change can be measured.

The patient should be given a low-fat diet, but medium chain triglycerides are helpful as an additional source of calories. Supplements of water-soluble vitamin A (5000 IU/day) and vitamin D (500 IU/day) should be given.

Neurologic complications shorten life expectancy. A variant with normal TG levels is described.

Gotto AM & others: On the protein defect in abetalipoproteinemia. N Engl J Med 284:813, 1971.
Herbert PN, Gotto AM, Fredrickson DS: Familial lipoprotein deficiency (abetalipoproteinemia, hypobetalipoproteinemia, and Tangier disease). Chap 28, pages 544–588, in: *The Metabolic Basis of Inherited Disease,* 4th ed. Stanbury JB, Wyngaarden JB, Fredrickson DS (editors). McGraw-Hill, 1978.

Hypobetalipoproteinemia

A small number of patients have been reported with reduction of serum beta lipoprotein concentrations to 10–50% of normal with decreased serum levels of cholesterol, phospholipids, and glycerides. Acanthocytosis and neurologic symptoms may be seen. The condition must be differentiated from hypobetalipoproteinemias secondary to the celiac syndrome or the thalassemia trait.

A syndrome has also been described with low α- and β-lipoprotein, raised cholesterol and triglycerides, retardation, and hepatomegaly.

Van Buchem FS & others: Congenital β-lipoprotein deficiency. Am J Med 40:794, 1966.

THE FAMILIAL HYPERLIPOPROTEINEMIAS

There have been many classifications of these disorders based on clinical, biochemical, and inheritance characteristics. No one approach is completely satisfactory. The one used here, based on lipoprotein electrophoresis patterns, is that of Fredrickson and is perhaps the best known. The problems of classification are well illustrated by the newly described condition of "familial combined hyperlipidemia" in which affected individuals may show types II, IV, or V lipoprotein phenotypes with relatives demonstrating any combination of elevated serum beta (LDL) or prebeta (VLDL) lipoproteins.

The primary lipoproteinemias are a group of heritable disorders of serum lipoprotein components; the secondary hyperlipoproteinemias are a reflection of a number of disorders such as nephrosis, hypothyroidism, and obstructive liver disease.

Dietschy JM, Wilson JD: Regulation of cholesterol metabolism. (3 parts.) N Engl J Med 282:1128, 1179, 1241, 1970.

Motulsky AG: The genetic hyperlipidemias. N Engl J Med 294:823, 1976.

Type I. Familial Hyperchylomicronemia (Lipoprotein Lipase Deficiency)

The onset is usually early in life, with bouts of abdominal pain. Later, moderate hepatosplenomegaly is noted and the retinal vessels are seen to be especially pale. Small cutaneous xanthomas are common.

The serum is characteristically lactescent, and on standing the chylomicrons rise to the top as a creamy layer on the plasma. Serum protein electrophoresis shows a great increase in the chylomicron band and a decrease in the alpha and beta bands. Postheparin lipoprotein lipase activity is reduced from the normal range of 240–600 nEq/ml of free fatty acids to 20–40 nEq/ml. The test is carried out following administration of 0.1 mg/kg of heparin IV by taking 15-minute samples from 0–90 minutes for lipoprotein lipase activity determination. Activity is maximal at 15 minutes.

Hyperglycemia and glycosuria have been reported but are not common (as in type IV; see below).

Hyperchylomicronemia usually decreases on a low-fat diet (< 0.2 gm/kg/day). The alpha and beta lipoprotein bands will increase somewhat, and the prebeta band which carries endogenous triglyceride will increase further. Caloric intake can be supplemented on a low-triglyceride diet (< 0.5 gm/kg/day) by giving medium chain triglycerides, either as a milk formula (Portagen) or as a special diet using MCT oil.

Episodes of abdominal pain, which may be accompanied by pancreatitis, can be controlled on this regimen, and so can the hepatosplenomegaly. There is no increased risk of atherosclerosis. The diagnosis is consistent with a normal life.

Ford S & others: Familial hyperchylomicronemia. Am J Med 50:536, 1971.

Schotz MC & others: A rapid assay for lipoprotein lipase. J Lipid Res 11:68, 1970.

Type IIA. Familial Hyperbetalipoproteinemia; Essential Familial Hypercholesterolemia

Familial hyperbetalipoproteinemia is the commonest lipoprotein disorder of childhood and is inherited as an autosomal dominant. The basic defect may be a lack of the normal LDL receptor on the cell membrane resulting in a failure of the feedback inhibition of cholesterol synthesis. Evidence of hypercholesterolemia in at least one parent is essential to the diagnosis. The most striking clinical manifestations in homozygotes are the xanthomatous deposits in tendons (particularly the Achilles tendon), over extensor surfaces of knees, hands, and elbows, and in pressure or trauma areas such as the buttocks. Xanthomas of the eyelids (xanthelasma) and corneal arcus are also common. Coronary atherosclerosis may be an early and life-threatening complication. Heterozygotes usually have no abnormal physical findings prior to the onset of early atherosclerosis.

mg/100 ml have been seen at 3 months of age. As with the appearance of xanthomas, the age at which hypercholesterolemia develops varies considerably, the more fulminating cases being seen in association with inheritance of the gene from both parents. Total cholesterol levels in childhood vary with age and methodology, but any level > 240 mg/100 ml should be considered abnormal. Homozygotes usually have levels in excess of 600 mg/100 ml, and levels are elevated in the parents. Serum phospholipid is moderately elevated but not to the same extent as cholesterol, and in some cases there may be a modest elevation of endogenous prebeta glycerides. Lipoprotein electrophoresis shows a characteristic intense increase in the beta band, with lipoprotein cholesterol exceeding 210 mg/100 ml. Hypercarotenemia is also seen because of the increased beta lipoprotein.

Hyperbetalipoproteinemia is reported in hypothyroidism, in obstructive liver disease, and in nephrosis. Florid xanthomatosis is, however, very rare in children with these conditions, and the differential diagnosis in the light of other evidence of thyroid, liver, or renal disease is easy to make.

A history of coronary infarction before age 50 in either parent is the best screening test for this disease. Neonatal cholesterol values do not seem to be helpful.

Treatment possibilities are as follows:

A. Dietary Management: With the overall proviso that the diet should be palatable and contain adequate protein and calories, it is justifiable to limit the fat intake to 20% of calories, depending primarily on vegetable or polyunsaturated fats. Increasing dietary polyunsaturates is more important than reducing dietary cholesterol. Obesity, if present, should be controlled.

B. Drug Therapy:

1. Cholestyramine (Cuemid, Questran) is a resin which bonds bile acids, prevents their reabsorption, and, in turn, enhances the hepatic conversion of cholesterol to more bile acids. The dose is 0.3 gm/kg/day orally, but the drug is unpleasant to take and may cause steatorrhea. In some cases, the effect is to remove feedback inhibition of endogenous cholesterol synthesis, and levels rise.

2. D-Thyroxine (Choloxin) in a dose of 0.15 mg/kg/day orally sometimes lowers cholesterol levels, but this drug is contraindicated in the presence of cardiac disease.

3. Clofibrate (Atromid-S) inhibits the synthesis of mevalonic acid from acetate in the cholesterol synthesis pathway. The initial dose is 1 gm/sq m/24 hours orally in 3 or 4 divided doses; it may be justified to increase this to the limit of tolerance. Complications include leukopenia, mild hepatic damage, polyphagia, weakness, and muscle cramps. The drug is variably effective in type IIA disease in children.

4. Nicotinic acid, 0.15 mg/kg/day orally, may lower cholesterol levels. The mechanism is not understood but may relate to liver damage. Liver function tests should be followed closely.

5. There is some early evidence that a portacaval shunt will substantially lower serum cholesterol levels. The mechanism is not at present understood.

Ahrens AH: Homozygous hypercholesterolemia and the portacaval shunt. Lancet 2:449, 1974.

Brown MS & others: Familial hypercholesterolemia: A genetic defect in the low density lipoprotein receptor. N Engl J Med 294:1386, 1976.

Chase HP & others: Screening for hyperlipidemia in childhood. JAMA 230:1535, 1974.

Fredrickson DS, Goldstein JL, Brown MS: The familial hyperlipoproteinemias. Chap 30, pages 604–655, in: *The Metabolic Basis of Inherited Disease,* 4th ed. Stanbury JB, Wyngaarden JB, Fredrickson DS (editors). McGraw-Hill, 1978.

Yeshurun D & others: Drug treatment of hyperlipidemia. Am J Med 60:379, 1976.

Type IIB. Familial Combined Hyperlipoproteinemia

Some hypercholesterolemic patients have elevations of endogenous triglyceride (VLDL) as well as LDL. Many of these have come to be regarded as a separate autosomal dominant clinical entity. Relatives may show elevations of cholesterol, triglyceride, or both. In childhood the diagnosis may be confusing because the hypertriglyceridemia is expressed before the hypercholesterolemia. The group may also include other phenotypes, resulting in elevation of serum cholesterol and triglyceride levels. Some type IIA patients will have environmentaly elevated triglycerides (as found with inadequate exercise or obesity). Some type IV patients will have secondary hypercholesterolemia as prebetalipoprotein is normally converted in part to betalipoprotein, which then results in elevated cholesterol levels. It is wise to look at the height of elevation of the 2 lipids and the life style of the patient in attempting to separate contaminating phenotypes from true "familial combined hyperlipoproteinemia." Parent phenotypes may also be helpful. Subjects with combined hyperlipoproteinemia usually manifest characteristics of the type IV disorder—impaired glucose tolerance, obesity, and hyperuricemia—and not characteristics of the type IIA disorder such as skin xanthomas. Patients should be treated as for the type IV disorder. After types IIA and IV, this disorder is third in frequency in children.

Glueck CJ & others: Familial combined hyperlipoproteinemia. Metabolism 22:1403, 1973.

Type III. Hyperbetalipoproteinemia

Type III hyperbetalipoproteinemia is an autosomal recessive condition which has not been described in childhood; in late adolescence, it would be distinguished by the small papular xanthomas on palm creases and fingertips, the tubero-eruptive lesions at the elbows, and, in the laboratory, by the opalescent serum with increased cholesterol and glyceride. Lipoprotein electrophoresis shows an intense conjoined broad beta and prebeta band. Estrogen treatment may be of value.

Chait A & others: Type III hyperlipoproteinemia. Lancet 1:1176, 1977.

Type IV. Familial Hyperprebetalipoproteinemia

This is a common form of hyperlipoproteinemia in adults and is also seen in childhood. It is characterized by turbid plasma and an increase in endogenous glyceride with a marked increase in the prebeta band on serum lipoprotein electrophoresis and a decrease in the alpha and beta bands. There are no chylomicrons on a low-fat diet. Hyperuricemia is common, and in most cases the lipemia is carbohydrate-induced. The condition may be secondary to uncontrolled diabetes, type I glycogen storage disease, idiopathic hypercalcemia, hypoparathyroidism, nephrosis, and obesity. If a patient does not fast for 12 hours before testing, a false diagnosis may be made.

Treatment consists of providing 40% of calories as fat, primarily polyunsaturated, and restricting carbohydrate sufficiently to reduce endogenous hyperlipemia. Nicotinic acid and clofibrate (Atromid-S) may also be helpful (see under type IIA, above).

Type V. Familial Hyperprebetalipoproteinemia With Hyperchylomicronemia

This condition is usually not seen until adult life, but it has been reported in childhood. Clinically, patients tend to be obese and to have a family history of diabetes. There are widespread xanthomas with lipemia retinalis, hepatosplenomegaly, and foam cells in the bone marrow. On lipoprotein electrophoresis, there is an increase in both endogenous and exogenous glyceride (chylomicrons), and cholesterol levels may also be elevated. Lipoprotein lipase activity is normal. Cases of type IV hyperlipoproteinemia and familial combined hyperlipidemia may occur in the kindred.

Treatment consists of reducing weight by caloric and fat restriction. Clofibrate (Atromid-S) and nicotinic acid may also be helpful.

Kwiterovich PO & others: Type V hyperlipoproteinemia in childhood. Pediatrics 59:513, 1977.

• • •

GENETIC COUNSELING

The most direct application of the advances in our understanding of basic genetic mechanisms is in the provision of genetic advice or genetic counseling. The advice usually stems from an inquiry about whether a given disease is likely to recur in the family, and its primary purpose is thus to help people make responsible decisions about reproduction. Other questions may relate to the desirability of cousin marriage, the risk of having children when the parents are at advanced ages, the effects of hallucinatory drugs, or the possible hazards of ionizing radiation.

Genetic counseling is expensive but is an effective way of diminishing society's burden of chronic disease, which is far more expensive.

The prime requisite for giving advice is the possession of all available facts about the patient and the disease. In order to give genetic advice, the physician must ask himself the following questions:

(1) What is the disease in the propositus? This requires the most accurate diagnosis available.

(2) Is the disease hereditary or is it a phenocopy, eg, Is the cleft palate due to abortifacients? Is the mental deficiency due to a birth injury? Is the pseudohermaphroditism due to the use of oral progestins?

FAMILY HISTORY

History taking is a fundamental tool in every physician's armamentarium. In genetic counseling, however, there are points in the family history which should be stressed in order to pinpoint the genetic factors involved:

(1) **Parental age:** Mention has already been made of the maternal age effect, ie, the increasing risk of nondisjunction and the increasing risk of other congenital malformations with increasing parental age. Elevated paternal age has recently been associated with an increased incidence of dominant mutations.

(2) **Siblings:** Their age, sex, and state of health is important. The larger the number of unaffected sibs, the less likely the condition is to be due to a single segregating gene.

(3) **Consanguinity:** The chance of both parents carrying the same rare recessive gene is greater if they are related. The likelihood of the patient's disease being recessively inherited is thus increased in the presence of consanguinity. Consanguinity rates in the general population have been decreasing throughout the world, being about 0.05% in the USA. Among the parents of children with albinism, however, there is a consanguinity rate of about 20%. This fact should be borne in mind when one is asked, "Should I marry my cousin?"

(4) **Radiation history:** The deleterious effect of x-irradiation on the embryo has been well documented. In addition, there occur genetic effects of irradiation such as point mutations, chromosomal breaks with abnormal healing, and increased incidence of nondisjunction. These effects are likely to occur prior to conception during gametogenesis. For this reason a history of radiation exposure to the gonads of either parent prior to conception is important. Because of the nature of gametogenesis in the female, inquiries should be made concerning exposure of the mother to x-ray at a time when she herself was an embryo.

(5) **History of exposure to drugs and virus infections early in pregnancy:** A positive history of exposure to a known teratogen may help in determining whether genetic or environmental factors were etiologically important in the child's disease.

(6) **History of previous pregnancies in the family:** Many abortions in the family may suggest the carrier state of a translocation chromosome, which should then be looked for in the patient. Similarly, diabetes or "prediabetes" should be ruled out.

(7) **Construction of a pedigree:** The diagrammatic representation of the family history helps one decide whether a disease is familial and, if so, whether it follows one of the single gene patterns of inheritance, ie, the vertical patterns of dominant inheritance, the horizontal pattern of recessive inheritance, or the oblique pattern of X-linked recessive inheritance. The larger the pedigree, the more typical the pattern (Fig 33–17). A pedigree also helps identify other family members who may be at risk and be unaware of it.

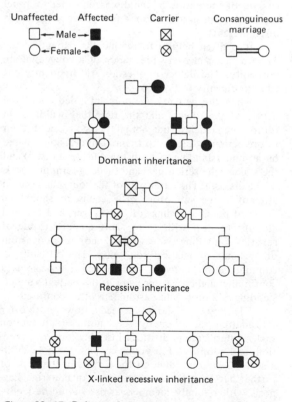

Figure 33–17. Pedigrees demonstrating various types of single gene inheritance.

PHYSICAL EXAMINATION

In addition to the physical examination that is performed on the affected patient for diagnostic purposes, it is frequently desirable to examine the parents and the unaffected siblings of the patient in order to pick up cases where expressivity is diminished. This is important in determining whether a gene mutation has occurred in a parental germ cell, a fact which changes risk figures greatly. Sometimes a laboratory test on the parents, such as a blood phosphorus level when the patient has vitamin D-resistant rickets, will bring to light an expression of a previously unrecognized defective gene in a seemingly normal parent.

Finally, the literature on a specific disease should be carefully reviewed in order to determine the usual type of transmission and, if this is not clear, to estimate the empiric risks. This is particularly helpful if the patient's pedigree data are not too complete.

NATURE OF ADVICE

Counseling should be given with both parties present. Knowledge of the cultural, religious, and educational background of the family is helpful. Advantage should be taken of the opportunity for a thorough discussion of the nature of the disease in order to dispel the store of misinformation, anxiety, and guilt that is often present.

It is often helpful to remind the patient of the 3–5% chance in every pregnancy of a congenital abnormality. The defect in question will frequently not add significantly to this risk.

When the patients are fully informed about the nature of the disease and the risks they will incur in future pregnancies, the actual decision about their future action is left up to them. This decision is based on an understanding of both the odds (a statistic) and the stakes (the seriousness and the long-term prognosis of the disease). The latter part of the counseling should attempt to be supportive. The counselor should be aware of possible feelings of guilt, anger, and fear and attempt to deal with them. This supportive side of genetic counseling is essentially no different from other kinds of medical counseling. The difficulty in communication between patient and physician is a continuing challenge, especially as the patient's understanding of a probability estimate is often confused.

The physician should be ready, however, to offer information on alternatives to normal reproduction such as sterilization, artificial insemination, contraception, and adoption. For young couples it may be desirable to delay reproduction for 5 years in the hope of further developments in treatment or intrauterine diagnosis. Other family members at risk should be identified and, if possible, counseled. The counselor in general attempts to be nondirective in counseling, even though this is often misunderstood and resented by the patient, who is accustomed to being told what to do by the physician. An earnest attempt is made by the counselor to help the patient arrive at what the patient determines is an appropriate decision.

The above type of preconceptional counseling, which is generally retrospective, in the sense that the question usually relates to the risk of a couple having a second affected child, may often lead into *prospective* counseling, ie, in the identification of other individuals in the kindred who may be at risk of a genetic disease but are unaware of their risk because they have not yet borne affected children. It is an important responsibility of the counselor and the primary care physician to communicate with these individuals after the necessary permission is obtained from the patient.

Another type of prospective counseling is genetic screening—either (1) of the general population of newborns (as for phenylketonuria or hypothyroidism) in order to diagnose and treat disease early enough to prevent serious and irreversible symptomatology; or (2) of a defined population (as for Tay-Sachs disease), in order to identify those at risk of having an affected child before tragedy occurs. Essential features of these procedures are that people be fully informed prior to being tested; that rights to privacy be carefully guarded; and that those who are at risk have adequate counseling. Occasionally, those *not* at risk also need counseling, since many are made needlessly anxious by virtue of having been screened. The psychologic implications of being "branded" as a carrier must be considered in counseling carriers. It has been helpful to remind these individuals that we all carry several potentially harmful genes.

Genetic counseling may be postconceptional as well as preconceptional. In the former case, the question to be answered is, "Should pregnancy be interrupted?" In most cases the investigative procedure is similar to what has been discussed above, and the patient is told the probability of the unborn child being affected, which may be from 1% to 50%. On the basis of this figure, one must decide whether there is a valid genetic indication for interrupting pregnancy.

INTRAUTERINE DIAGNOSIS

Intrauterine diagnosis constitutes the greatest single advance in medical genetics of the last decade. It usually converts the probability of fetal disease to a certainty, giving the pregnant woman much more secure information on which to act.

Several methods of intrauterine diagnosis are currently being used or are becoming available as follows:

(1) X-ray: Only for significant risk of gross skeletal lesions.

(2) Ultrasound: For diagnosis of anencephaly, hydrocephaly, polycystic kidneys, twins, fetal death.

(3) Fetoscopy: Permits direct visualization of the

Table 33–15. Some biochemical disorders which can be diagnosed antenatally.

Argininosuccinic aciduria	Juvenile GM_1 gangliosidosis
Branched chain ketoaciduria	Ketotic hyperglycinemia
Cystathionine synthase deficiency	Krabbe's syndrome
Cystinosis	Lesch-Nyhan syndrome and variants
Fabry's disease	Mannosidosis
Fucosidosis	Metachromatic leukodystrophy
Galactokinase deficiency	
Galactosemia	Methylmalonic aciduria
Gaucher's disease (infantile)	Niemann-Pick disease
Generalized gangliosidosis	Orotic aciduria
Hunter's and Hurler's syndromes	Pompe's disease
	Refsum's disease
Hypervalinemia	Sandhoff's disease
I-cell disease	Sanfilippo's syndrome
Isovaleric acidemia	Tay-Sachs disease

fetus by insertion of appropriate endoscopic tube into the uterus. This procedure, still in an experimental stage, will identify gross structural malformations and will make possible the sampling of fetal blood for the intrauterine diagnosis of hemoglobinopathies.

(4) Aminography: A radiopaque substance is introduced into the uterus and attaches to fetal skin. An x-ray may then outline the fetus and demonstrate structural abnormalities such as meningomyelocele. The efficacy of this procedure has been questioned.

(5) Amniocentesis: This is currently the most widely used form of antenatal diagnosis.

The procedure of amniocentesis has made possible intrauterine diagnosis for some diseases—in particular, the cytogenetic diseases and those biochemical diseases that can be diagnosed by assaying for a specific enzyme on cultured fetal cells obtained from amniotic fluid (Table 33–15). The procedure consists of the suprapubic insertion of a needle into the uterine cavity at about 15 weeks of pregnancy and the aspiration of 15–20 ml of sterile amniotic fluid. Thus far, the complications have been few. For this reason, it seems reasonable to perform the procedure when the risk of diagnosable fetal disease exceeds 1%.

The indications for amniocentesis are as follows:

(1) Either parent is a carrier of a balanced translocation. The risk of an affected child is about 3–15% depending upon which parent is the carrier.

(2) A previous child with trisomy 21. The risk of a repeat may be as high as 2%, especially for mothers under 30.

(3) Parents are carriers of an autosomal recessively inherited disease that can be diagnosed in utero (Table 33–14).

(4) Mother is a carrier of an X-linked recessively inherited disease which cannot be diagnosed in utero (eg, muscular dystrophy, hemophilia A). However, the risk of being affected is 50% if the fetus is a male and close to zero if a female.

(5) Maternal age over 35 years (in some clinics, the indication is maternal age over 40 years).

(6) A pregnant woman who is at increased risk of having a child with a neural tube defect (anencephaly, meningomyelocele). The level in the amniotic fluid of alpha-fetoprotein, the predominant protein in fetal serum, is significantly higher than normal in 90% of affected fetuses. When anencephaly is suspected, ultrasound examination of the uterine contents may often reveal an absent or disturbed fetal head.

(7) A single gene dominant condition for which there is currently no marker diagnosable in utero but where the gene is closely linked (on the chromosome) to another gene (such as the gene for a blood group) for which there is a diagnosable marker in utero. Myotonic dystrophy, the nail-patella syndrome, and a dominant form of congenital cataract so far are the only disorders in which a close linkage useful for antenatal diagnosis has been established.

An important preliminary to the actual procedure of amniocentesis is genetic counseling. During this session, a pedigree is obtained and examined for other conditions which might be of importance. This session is utilized to describe in detail the procedure, potential complications, and what can and what cannot be learned from it. The patient must be made aware that there is no guarantee of a normal child.

Ultrasonography is usually employed prior to the procedure in order to rule out a missed abortion or twinning and to locate the placenta, which one hopes not to puncture, although this is not always possible.

The extracted amniotic fluid contains fetal cells which are cultured in vitro so that karyotyping and enzyme assays can be performed. The noncellular part of the fluid is assayed for α-fetoprotein. The procedure usually takes 2½–3 weeks to complete.

CONCLUSION

Who should give genetic counseling? The primary care physician who knows the family, its attitudes, and its social and financial stresses may be the best person to provide counseling. Ideally, genetic counseling—an important form of preventive medicine—should be part of primary care. The primary care physician may not have the training in medical genetics, the facilities for sophisticated laboratory tests, the acquaintance with rare syndromes, or the considerable amount of time necessary to do the complete job but nevertheless should be in a position to reinforce the counseling that is provided by the genetics clinic, which should be a satellite clinic of the main clinic at the university medical center staffed by a medical geneticist, genetic associate, and public health nurse.

It is clear that the general public is largely unaware of the existence of genetic counseling and its benefits. A greater public education effort is required to make these services available to those who need them.

Bergsma D (editor): Human gene mapping 3. Birth Defects 12(7), 1976. [Entire issue.]

Childs B: Approaches to genetic counseling. Ann NY Acad Sci 240:132, 1975.

Fraser FC: Genetic counseling. Am J Hum Genet 26:636, 1974.

Riccardi VM, Robinson A: Preventive medicine through genetic counseling: A regional program. Prev Med 4 (2):126, 1975.

GLOSSARY OF
GENETIC TERMS

Alleles: Genes that occupy homologous loci on homologous chromosomes. An individual can never have more than 2 allelic genes at a given locus.

Aneuploid: This refers to the chromosomal number of a cell population which is not an integral multiple of the haploid number.

Autosomes: All of the chromosomes other than the 2 sex chromosomes.

Chromatids: The 2 halves resulting from the longitudinal division of a chromosome through the centromere, each consisting of a double helix of DNA. Pictures of metaphase chromosomes will usually show sister chromatids on each side of the centromere and joined together at the centromere.

Consanguinity: The blood relationship of 2 individuals. It usually refers to a married couple.

Crossing-over: The physical process of exchange between chromatids in synapsis, which permits the process of recombination. This has the result that genes lying in one chromosome are not always passed on together to the descendants.

Diploid: The double set of chromosomes in the somatic cells of the organism. The diploid number in man is 46.

Gametes: The mature germ cells which have the haploid set of chromosomes.

Genotype: The genetic constitution of an organism.

Haploid: One-half of the diploid complement of chromosomes, in which only one chromosome of each homologous pair is present. The haploid number in man is 23.

Isochromosome: A morphologically abnormal chromosome which results from an abnormal "horizontal" division of the centromere, instead of its normally vertical division, during mitosis. The result is that the chromosome is metacentric, with the centromere in the center. The 2 arms of the chromosome arise from 2 homologous chromatids. Such a chromosome would possess a double set of genes from the arm of the parent chromosome which supplied the chromatids, and would be lacking the genes normally provided by the other arm of the parent chromosome.

Karyotype: The chromosomal constitution of an individual, as typified by the systematized array of the chromosomes of a single cell prepared by photography.

Meiosis: A form of cell division in which the haploid gametes are produced from diploid cells.

Monosomy: Having only one chromosome of a particular homologous pair, instead of 2.

Mosaic: An individual whose tissues are of two or more genetically different kinds, usually of different chromosomal constitution.

Phenocopy: A nongenetic condition which mimics that produced by a certain genotype.

Phenotype: The manifest constitution of an individual as determined by careful examination. This is the result of an interaction between his genetic makeup and the environment.

Proband or propositus: The index case, or starting case, from which a genetic investigation is undertaken.

Satellite: These are small deeply staining bodies situated at the end of the short arm of an acrocentric chromosome and separated from it by a short distance.

Trisomy: The presence of any single chromosome in 3 homologous forms, rather than the usual 2.

●   ●   ●

General References

Bergsma D (editor): Contemporary genetic counseling. Birth Defects 9:1, April 1973.

Carr DH: Chromosomal abnormalities in clinical medicine. Chap 1 in: *Progress in Medical Genetics.* Vol 6. Steinberg AG, Bearn AG (editors). Grune & Stratton, 1969.

Holt SB: *The Genetics of Dermal Ridges.* Thomas, 1968.

McKusick VA: *Mendelian Inheritance in Man,* 4th ed. Johns Hopkins Univ Press, 1975.

Milunsky A (editor): *The Prevention of Genetic Disease and Mental Retardation.* Saunders, 1975.

Nyhan WL (editor): *Amino Acid Metabolism and Genetic Variation.* McGraw-Hill, 1967.

O'Brien D, Goodman SI: The critically ill child: Life-threatening metabolic disease in infancy. Pediatrics 45:620, 1970.

Penrose LS, Smith GF: *Down's Anomaly.* Little, Brown, 1966.

Reisman LE, Matheny AP Jr: *Genetics and Counseling in Medical Practice.* Mosby, 1969.

Scriver CR, Rosenberg LE: *Amino Acid Metabolism and Its Disorders.* Saunders, 1973.

Smith DW: *Recognizable Patterns of Human Development,* 2nd ed. Saunders, 1976.

Stanbury JB, Wyngaarden JB, Fredrickson DS (editors): *The Metabolic Basis of Inherited Disease,* 4th ed. McGraw-Hill, 1978.

Symposium on treatment of amino acid disorders. Am J Dis Child 113:1, 1967.

Thompson J, Thompson M: *Genetics in Medicine.* Saunders, 1966.

34...
Diagnostic & Therapeutic Procedures

Ronald W. Gotlin, MD, & Henry K. Silver, MD

The care of children optimally does not end with diagnosis and treatment but includes an understanding of the specific procedures referable to this age group.

This chapter records those methods which have proved to be useful and effective. No claim is made of originality, and all possible pediatric procedures have not been included.

We recognize what may appear to be a lack of sufficient emphasis regarding the comfort and feelings of our pediatric patient and his parents. Were it not for limited space, we would continually reiterate the importance of patience and understanding when conducting procedures in children.

PREPARATION OF THE PATIENT & ORIENTATION OF THE PROCEDURE TEAM

With any diagnostic or treatment procedure, proper positioning and restraint are of greatest importance.

In the majority of cases, failure to complete a procedure is directly related to undue haste in preparing the patient. Young patients often have levels of apprehension and fear that do not lend themselves to "classic" adult physician-patient understanding; competence needs to be developed to balance reassurance and determination to carry out a procedure. This should be done by individualizing the approach for each patient.

Patience and adequate preparation are also necessary when dealing with understandably anxious parents. A few words of explanation to concerned family members will be most reassuring. In general, procedures go more smoothly when parents are not in the procedure room. However, in the event that a parent wants to be present, forcible ejection from the scene may be associated with harmful effects both to the patient and to the procedure team and it is usually advisable to allow the parent to remain under these circumstances. If parents are allowed to remain in the room, they should not be asked to become part of the procedure team or to play an active part in restraining the patient.

Most procedures should have consent from parents. As full an explanation as possible, even to children as young as 3 years, should be given to the patient.

RESTRAINT & POSITIONING

The physician should acquaint himself with various methods of properly restraining and positioning a patient. It is usually very difficult and sometimes dangerous to attempt any procedure on an unrestrained young patient. Before actually starting a procedure, the physician should be certain that all necessary items of equipment are available and arranged for immediate use.

The commonly employed method of restraint and immobilization is shown in the accompanying illustration (Fig 34–1). Following immobilization of any extremity, the fingers or toes should be examined for adequate circulation by noting the temperature, color, and capillary pressure in the nail bed.

When total body restraint is necessary, the physician must be certain before and during the procedure that cardiorespiratory function has not been impaired. To assist in doing this, a stethoscope may be taped to the anterior chest of the patient to permit frequent evaluation.

Local subcutaneous infiltration with procaine or lidocaine (Xylocaine) before performing a lumbar puncture, bone marrow aspiration, or thoracic, pericardial, or peritoneal aspiration is frequently necessary and advisable. Whenever drugs are employed, a history of previous reactions to the drugs should be ascertained and equipment (suction apparatus, oral airway or endotracheal intubation device, laryngoscope, tourniquet, and epinephrine, 1:1000 solution) should be readily available to manage the rare but dangerous untoward reaction that may occur.

Following any procedure, the physician should personally observe the child long enough to be certain that he has not developed any untoward reaction.

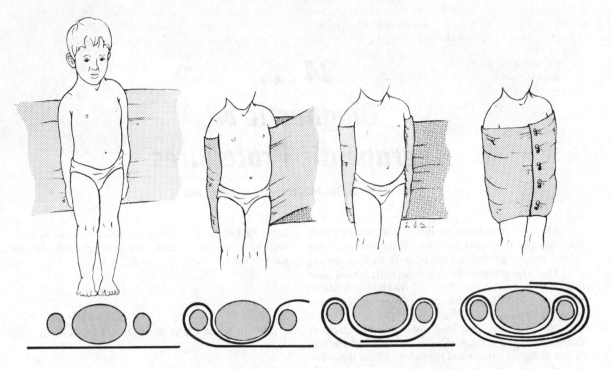

Figure 34—1. Body restraint. This method can also be employed to leave an extremity available for venipuncture.

DIAGNOSTIC PROCEDURES

COLLECTION & PROCESSING OF BLOOD SAMPLES

1. VENIPUNCTURE

The antecubital, femoral, and external or internal jugular veins are used most frequently for venipuncture and withdrawal of blood, but the sagittal sinus may be used if necessary. Venipuncture of the femoral and internal jugular veins may be associated with serious complications (see below), particularly in the neonate, and should be avoided if possible. The sagittal sinus has been employed in some countries. In some instances, blood may be withdrawn from other veins in the extremities.

Large, accessible veins are best for purposes of injection. *Caution:* Do not inject materials into internal jugular, sagittal sinus, or other deep veins.

The skin should be cleansed thoroughly and a disinfectant (eg, an iodinated organic compound or isopropyl alcohol) applied. Clean off iodine with alcohol and allow skin to dry before doing vein puncture for blood culture. Iodinated solutions should not be used when blood is to be tested for various iodinated compounds, and alcohol should be avoided when blood is

drawn for alcohol levels. When blood is obtained for culture and for various tests, it should be put into media-containing tubes or bottles before being placed in vacutainer tubes since the latter may not be sterile.

Antecubital Vein Puncture

If available, the antecubital vein should be used for venipuncture in larger infants and children; frequently it may be entered readily in small infants.

A soft elastic tourniquet is applied proximal (cephalad) to the vein and the venous pattern observed. Dilatation of a vein may be facilitated by local

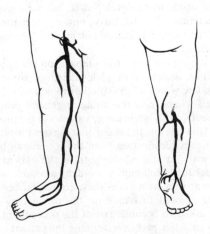

Figure 34—2. Veins of leg and foot.

warming in a wash basin or sink (preferred) or with warm moist towels. The wearing of red-tinted goggles by the operator may make the venous pattern more readily visible.

A short, sharp-beveled, 20 or 22 gauge needle (disposable syringes and needles are recommended) applied firmly to an appropriate-sized syringe is used.

The skin is entered with the needle at an approximately 10–30 degree angle with the bevel up. If gentle suction is applied to the syringe barrel, blood will be aspirated as the vessel is entered. Blood should be withdrawn gently and rapidly to avoid clotting and hemolysis. In a struggling patient, the use of a needle and catheter (eg, scalp vein assembly) attached to the syringe will lessen leverage between the vein and needle. When the required quantity of blood has been obtained, the tourniquet is released and the needle withdrawn quickly. After the needle is removed, a dry sterile cotton ball is applied with pressure over the puncture site and held for approximately 3 minutes or until any evidence of bleeding has subsided. To avoid excessive hemolysis, the needle should be removed from the syringe and the stopper taken out of vacuum tubes prior to expelling the blood from the syringe into the specimen tube.

Femoral Vein Puncture (Fig 34–3)

This is a hazardous precedure, particularly in the newborn, and should be employed only in emergencies.

Place the child on a flat, firm table. Abduct the leg so as to expose the inguinal region. Locate the femoral artery by its pulsation. The vein lies immediately medial to it. Be certain of the position of the femoral pulse at the time of puncture. Prepare the skin carefully with an antiseptic solution and carry out the procedure using strict sterile precautions. Insert a short-beveled needle, 20 or 21 gauge, into the vein (perpendicularly to the skin) about 3 cm below the inguinal ligament; use the artery as a guide. If blood does not enter the syringe immediately, withdraw the needle slowly, gently drawing on the barrel of the syringe; the needle sometimes passes through both walls of the vein, and blood is obtained only when the needle is being withdrawn. Use a large enough syringe to produce adquate suction to assist in withdrawing the blood.

After removing the needle, exert firm, steady pressure over the vein for 3–5 minutes. If the artery has been entered, check the limb periodically for several hours.

Dangers: Following femoral vein puncture, osteomyelitis of the femur and abscess of the hip may occur. Arteriospasm which has resulted in serious vascular compromise of the extremity, particularly in the debilitated and dehydrated infant, has been reported secondary to arterial puncture or venipuncture. When arteriospasm occurs, it may sometimes be relieved by application of heat or by the subcutaneous administration of 2% procaine hydrochloride proximal to the site of puncture.

External Jugular Vein Puncture (Fig 34–4)

Wrap the child firmly so that arms and legs are adequately restrained. The wraps should not extend higher than the shoulder girdle. Place the child on a flat, firm table so that both shoulders are touching the table; the head is rotated fully to one side and extended partly over the end of the table so as to stretch the vein. Adequate immobilization is essential.

Use a very sharp No. 20 or 22 gauge needle or a No. 21 scalp vein needle with attached catheter (see above) for withdrawing blood. The child should be crying and the vein distended when entered. First thrust the needle just under the skin; then enter the vein. Pull constantly on the barrel of the syringe and be certain that air is not drawn into the vein during aspiration.

After removing the needle, exert firm pressure over the vein for 3–5 minutes while the child is in a sitting position.

Figure 34–3. Femoral vein puncture.

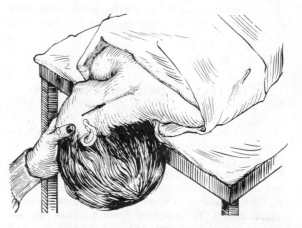

Figure 34–4. External jugular vein puncture.

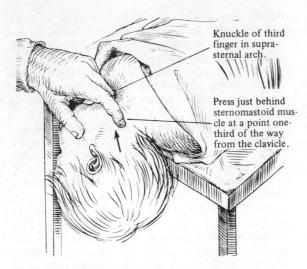

Knuckle of third finger in suprasternal arch.

Press just behind sternomastoid muscle at a point one-third of the way from the clavicle.

Figure 34—5. Direction of needle for internal jugular vein puncture.

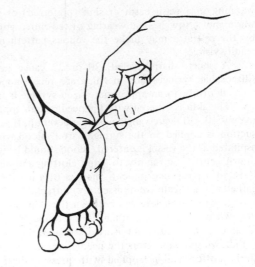

Figure 34—6. Heel puncture.

Internal Jugular Vein Puncture (Fig 34—5)

Prepare the child as for an external jugular vein puncture. Insert the needle beneath the sternocleidomastoid muscle at a point marking the junction of its lower and middle thirds. Aim at the suprasternal notch and advance the needle until the vein is entered. Avoid the trachea and the upper pleural space. Do not use this method in the presence of a hemorrhagic diathesis.

If no blood is obtained on inserting the needle, withdraw slowly and continue to pull gently on the barrel of the syringe. Not infrequently the needle passes through both walls of the vein and blood is obtained only when the needle is being withdrawn.

After completing the procedure, remove the needle and exert firm pressure over the area for 3—5 minutes with the child in a sitting position so as to reduce pressure in the vein.

Dangers: When properly performed, complications are rare. However, careless deep probing of the internal carotid vessel may result in injury to the trachea, vagus nerve, and pleura; the pleural cavity may be entered, and respiratory complications have been reported.

2. COLLECTION OF CAPILLARY BLOOD

The majority of determinations may be made on blood obtained from a finger and heel stick. An expertly performed heel stick (Fig 34—6) is much less traumatic for a small infant than is a femoral puncture and has the additional advantage that it may be repeated frequently and does not have the same risk of complications. The ear lobe is not a satisfactory site since puncture here may be associated with excessive bleeding which may be relatively difficult to control.

To ensure the formation of discrete drops of blood without hemolysis or clotting, the skin should first be wiped with ether. A free flow of blood without squeezing or "milking" is required. The small vein posterior to the medial malleolus is likely to bleed freely and should be used whenever possible. When blood is to be obtained from the heel, make a careful and deliberate puncture with a No. 11 Bard-Parker blade or a Hagedorn needle rather than a rapid stick as employed on the fingertip.

Collection of capillary blood may be difficult, and proficiency may be gained only after prolonged practice. In our laboratory the blood is collected in small glass tubes under a layer of mineral oil.

The flow of blood can be arrested by applying pressure with a sterile cotton ball. The site of puncture should be examined several times during the next 1—2 hours for evidence of oozing or ecchymoses.

3. ARTERIOPUNCTURE

Arteriopuncture is routinely employed in studying blood gas concentration and hemoglobin saturation and in measuring arterial blood pressure. The brachial, radial, and temporal arteries are entered most readily; the umbilical artery may be employed in the newborn period.

Procedure

A. Branches of the Superficial Temporal Artery: A No. 23—25 gauge scalp vein infusion set is employed for catheterization (Fig 34—7). The infant is restrained as described on p 973. The neonate receiving oxygen should remain in the incubator during arteriopuncture and efforts should be made to maintain a constant oxygen concentration.

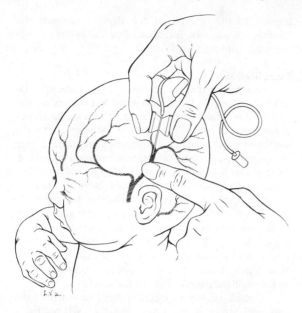

Figure 34–7. Scalp arteries suitable for blood sampling in infants. Note that the artery is palpated during cannulation. This helps immobilize the artery.

A 1 ml gas-tight syringe (eg, Hamilton Co.) is attached to the end of the scalp vein catheter and the system is filled with heparinized saline (1–2 units/ml). Either the frontal or parietal branch of the temporal artery is palpated, and the scalp hair shaved over the course of the artery. The area is cleaned with 1% iodine, and the iodine solution is removed with alcohol. With the palpating finger partially immobilizing the artery, the needle is inserted into the artery with the bevel up. After the pulsatile flow of bright-red oxygenated blood has cleared the system of solution, the syringe is connected and the sample is collected. The needle is withdrawn, and pressure is maintained over the artery for 5 minutes. If more than one sample is to be obtained, the line is cleared with heparinized saline and a 3-way stopcock is employed to close the line between samplings. The needle is taped in place, and the infant is secured appropriately. If a hematoma occurs during any part of the procedure, the needle is removed and pressure is applied over the artery until the bleeding has stopped.

B. Radial and Brachial Arteries: Either of these vessels may be entered in an older child. The radial artery is preferable since it is relatively immobile in its position at the wrist and since it does not course with an accompanying vein. If the brachial artery is selected, it is entered either in the antecubital fossa or just proximal to the antecubital fossa along the anteromedial aspect of the arm. These vessels may be cannulated as described above under temporal artery cannulation, or a tuberculin syringe with a 25 gauge needle containing 1 drop of heparin may be employed to obtain single or repeated samples.

Dangers: Firm pressure should be applied for at least 10–15 minutes after withdrawal of the blood specimen to avoid hematoma formation. Temporary or persistent arteriospasm with serious vascular compromise may occur, leading to sloughing of the skin. Distal obstruction of an artery due to the inadvertent injection of clots into the vessel during arteriopuncture has been reported. Arteriospasm may be relieved by the application of heat or by the subcutaneous administration of 2% procaine proximal to the site of puncture.

Schlueter MA & others: Blood sampling from scalp veins in infants. Pediatrics 51:120, 1973.

UMBILICAL VESSEL CATHETERIZATION

The use of an indwelling catheter in an umbilical artery or vein has become a common procedure in hospital nurseries. Catheterization of the artery generally provides a more useful source of diagnostic information and is safer than catheterization of the more frequently used umbilical vein.

Indications*
A. Diagnostic Procedures:
1. To obtain blood samples for analysis (particularly blood gas and pH analysis).
2. To measure intravascular pressures (arterial and venous).
3. Cardiac catheterization and angiocardiography.
B. Therapeutic Procedures:
1. Exchange transfusion.
2. Administration of fluids, blood, antibiotics, electrolytes, alkali (sodium bicarbonate), etc. The use of a Millipore filter in the infusion apparatus (eg, Abbott, Travenol) is recommended to reduce the chances of introduction of infection.

Procedure
The catheter should be made of flexible, nontoxic radiopaque material that will not kink when advanced through a vessel and will not collapse during blood withdrawal. Nonwettable material and a single, smooth-surfaced end hole reduce clot formation. A #3.5 (Aloe Medical Corporation) catheter is used for infants weighing less than 1500 gm and a #5 for larger infants. Dead space of the catheter system should be determined prior to catheterization.

The infant is loosely restrained, warmed (preferably under an overhead radiant heater), and the procedure carried out under sterile conditions.

*Because of the risks of serious complications, the use of peripheral veins is preferable to catheterization of umbilical vessels for routine blood withdrawal or infusion of therapeutic agents. However, when umbilical vessels are already catheterized for other reasons, use of the catheter obviates further peripheral vein puncture or capillary puncture during the exchange transfusion procedure.

In normal infants, arterial constriction may prevent catheterization after the first 15–30 minutes of life. (In the presence of hypoxia and acidosis, arterial constriction is usually diminished).

A standard cut-down tray is opened, and the wide end of the umbilical artery catheter is cut off so that the blunt needle adapter fits snugly into the catheter. Discarding the wide end and utilizing the needle adapter reduces the catheter capacity. A sterile syringe is filled with flushing fluid (eg, heparinized saline) and attached to a 3-way stopcock and, in turn, to the umbilical catheter. The entire system is filled with flushing fluid.

An assistant may elevate the umbilical cord by the cord clamp while the operator prepares the cord and adjacent skin with 1% iodine solution, which should then be removed with alcohol to prevent an iodine burn of the skin. All areas of the skin should be inspected for the presence of iodine solution. The area is then draped. A purse-string suture (taking care not to puncture the umbilical vessels) or a loop of umbilical tape is placed at the base of the umbilical cord and tied loosely in order to control bleeding if necessary. The cord is then cut 1–1.5 cm above the skin with scissors or a scalpel blade.

The 2 thick-walled, round arteries and the single, thin-walled vein are identified. The rim of the cut vessel is grasped with a pointed forceps or mosquito clamp. The lumen of the vessel is then dilated with the tips of the forceps. Initially, the lumen may allow only one tip to enter. Both tips may then be inserted and allowed to spread, further dilating the vessel. The fluid-filled catheter is inserted into the lumen of the artery or vein and advanced. Any obstruction to advancement usually can be overcome by steady, gentle pressure. Forceful probing may lead to increased arteriospasm in the artery or perforation of the vein or artery. If the obstruction in one of the arteries cannot be overcome, the catheter should be removed and an attempt made to catheterize the other umbilical artery. If a similar obstruction occurs, the catheter should be removed and filled (0.1–0.2 ml) with 1–2% lidocaine (Xylocaine) in epinephrine. The catheter should be reinserted up to the obstruction and the lidocaine injected. This usually relaxes the arteriospasm after 1–2 minutes and allows the catheter to advance.

Frequent aspiration will demonstrate blood return. In arterial catheterization, the tip may be left at the bifurcation of the aorta (approximately at the level of the third lumbar vertebra on x-ray), but fewer minor complications (blanching and cyanosis) occur when it is advanced so that the tip is above the level of the diaphragm (at the 12th thoracic vertebra—confirmed roentgenographically). Since thrombosis occurs in almost all cases, low arterial catheter placement will reduce the risk of emboli entering vessels proximal to the lower extremities.

The catheter is tied in place by means of a purse-string suture at the base of the cord, securing the ends of the suture to the catheter, and the catheter taped to the infant's abdomen. An antibiotic ointment is applied to the stump and the stump examined frequently for signs of infection. Routine systemic antibiotics are not indicated.

Complications

The principal complications of this procedure are infection ("prophylactic" systemic antibiotics do not reduce the incidence of infection), hemorrhage, vasospasm (placement of the arterial catheter above the diaphram is not associated with this complication once placement is complete), and thrombosis and embolism. Thrombosis is common in arterial catheterization, but vascular occlusion is unusual and is minimized by catheter placement above the diaphragm; thrombosis is also common (3–33%) in venous catheterization. Embolization occurs when air or clots are introduced, usually as a result of careless technic. Vascular perforation is a rare complication of portal vein catheterization. Vascular and tissue damage may occur secondary to the rapid infusion of hypertonic solutions.

Complications are exceedingly rare when the umbilical artery is employed and the catheter tip is placed in the abdominal aorta above the aortic bifurcation and below the renal arteries (L1–L2).

Anagnostakis D & others: Risk of infection associated with umbilical vein catheterization: A prospective study in 75 newborn infants. J Pediatr 86:759, 1975.
Krishnamoorthy KS & others: Paraplegia associated with umbilical artery catheterization in the newborn. Pediatrics 58:443, 1976.
Pollock AA: Scalp-vein needle and infection. N Engl J Med 293:560, 1975.

URINE COLLECTION

Midstream Catch

The "midstream catch," is a useful screening method for urine collection with minimal bacterial contamination. In both infants and toilet-trained children, the genital area is thoroughly cleansed with hexachlorophene detergent. The toilet-trained child obtains a portion of the midstream urine in a sterile container; the infant is observed after a feeding and before voiding. A portion of the urine passed spontaneously is obtained. Alternatively, the infant may be held upside down and the spinal reflex of Perez elicited by stroking the back along the paravertebral muscles. Spontaneous voiding usually occurs within 5 minutes. The stream is directed into a sterile container. All "positive" urine cultures must be confirmed by either sterile catheterization or suprapubic aspiration (see below).

Attached Receptacle Method

A. Equipment: Pediatric Urine Collector (a Sterilon product), a plastic bag with a round opening surrounded by an adhesive surface to adhere to the skin, may be used. After application the diaper may be reapplied.

Urine may also be collected with a bird cup (for girls) or test tube (for boys) fitted in a specimen band.

B. Procedure: Remove diaper. Fit test tube or cup into band. Place child on his back and adjust band and container. Pin band tightly around child with safety pins. Prop up in bed in semi-Fowler position. Restrain arms and legs with diapers if necessary. Remove restraints and band as soon as specimen is obtained.

If a specimen is to be used for culture, the genitalia should first be cleansed thoroughly with soap and water and a mild disinfectant. Whenever possible a midstream specimen (see above) should be obtained. Catheterization is seldom necessary and should be avoided if possible.

For collection of a 24-hour specimen, the chamber of a plastic infusion set may be used. Cut the chamber and cover the rim with adhesive tape to prevent injury. Insert the penis into the tube and tape the tube against the pubic area. Prop the child in bed in the semi-Fowler position. This apparatus may be kept in place for several days without undue discomfort or irritation of the skin.

Clean Catch Method

The male prepuce and glans of the penis or the opening of the female urethra and external vaginal vestibule are cleansed by gentle scrubbing with hexachlorophene (pHisoHex). (In the event that the male is uncircumcised, the foreskin should first be retracted.) Benzalkonium chloride (Zephiran) sponges (1:750) are then employed for several more cleansings. If the patient is old enough, he is instructed to void into the sterile container; as soon as urine is passed, the container is sealed and sent immediately for laboratory analysis.

Metabolic Bed (Fig 34–8)

The metabolic bed is a crib in which the mattress has been replaced by a taut synthetic cloth mesh. The infant or young child is maintained without a diaper in

the crib, and any urine that is passed flows through the mesh and onto a sloping surface beneath the crib. Children can usually tolerate the mesh for periods up to 24–48 hours without difficulty. This and similar devices have largely replaced the test tube and bird cup methods of urine collection in many hospitals.

Catheterization of the Urinary Bladder

Catheterization is seldom necessary. When it is used, sterile technic, including the use of sterile gloves and towels and adequate antiseptic preparation with hexachlorophene (pHisoHex) and benzalkonium chloride (Zephiran), should be employed.

If catheterization is necessary, catheters measuring 3–6 mm in diameter are usually satisfactory for most patients. A No. 5 feeding tube may be used for all age groups beyond the newborn period. Catheters made of inert Silastic or Teflon coated materials are preferred. They may be either straight or indwelling. The latter are double lumen tubes with an inflatable balloon near the distal opening. When inflated, removal is prevented until the bulb is deflated. This type of catheter is employed when continuous urine collection is necessary. If a retention catheter is employed, it should be changed at least every 2 days or replaced by a suprapubic cystocatheter. Acetic acid (0.25%) may be employed for bladder irrigation when a heavy urinary sediment is present. The urethral orifice and surrounding area should be cleaned at regular intervals and an appropriate antibiotic ointment (eg, polymyxin B-bacitracin-neomycin [Neosporin]) applied.

The patient is placed supine on a bed or table and immobilized and restrained when necessary. The skin is cleansed and the catheter is inserted into the external urethra. In the male, the penis is held initially at a right angle to the body, and in the female the labia majora and minora are widely separated. The female urethra is somewhat **C**-shaped and is more easily traversed than the relatively acute-angled male urethra. Trauma to the urethra or bladder can be minimized by using a catheter of the proper size and by gentle technic.

Suprapubic Percutaneous Bladder Aspiration

This method is particularly useful when a sterile urine sample is necessary (eg, suspected urinary tract infection). It is indicated in selected cases but does not lend itself to routine use.

The bladder *must* be full before the procedure is attempted. Cooperative patients should be urged to drink liberal quantities of fluid without voiding. In others, the bladder should be enlarged to palpation and percussion above the pubis before an attempt is made to aspirate urine. Local anesthesia may be used but is generally not necessary.

A. Procedure:

1. Prepare the skin carefully with an antiseptic solution, using strict sterile precautions. Remove hair if necessary.

2. Firmly introduce a sterile No. 21, long (4½ inch), spinal needle with obturator in place 1 or 2 cm above the pubis in the midline, with the needle perpen-

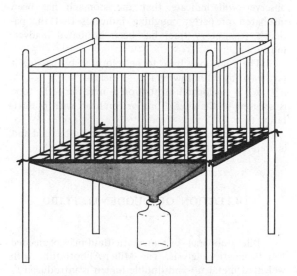

Figure 34–8. Metabolic bed (crib).

dicular to the skin. In an infant, a 2 inch No. 21 gauge needle is sufficient, and the obturator is not essential. After the skin and anterior wall have been penetrated, the tip of the needle will be lying against the bladder.

3. With a quick, firm motion, enter the bladder for a distance of 3—4 cm.

4. Remove the obturator and aspirate the urine with a sterile syringe.

5. After urine has been obtained, withdraw the needle with a single, swift motion.

6. Cover the area with a small sterile gauze dressing, and observe the patient carefully after the procedure.

B. Dangers: When the procedure is performed as outlined above, complications are uncommon. Trantients. Failure to obtain urine usually indicates either that the bladder was not full or that the needle did not bladder was either not full or that the needle did not enter the bladder but passed to one side. The procedure may be repeated.

COLLECTION OF NASOPHARYNGEAL FLUID

Nasopharyngeal secretions are frequently collected for culture in upper respiratory infections. In the newborn period, removal of fluid from the pharynx is frequently necessary after birth; passage of a nasopharyngeal tube and DeLee suction apparatus is helpful in excluding choanal atresia.

Fluid is easily obtained with the use of an ordinary polyvinyl feeding tube to which a syringe has been attached for suction. The tube is introduced into either nostril or into the oral cavity and directed downward as necessary, applying gentle suction with the syringe.

GASTRIC ASPIRATION

Aspiration of the gastric contents of all newborn infants should be performed at the time of the initial examination; simultaneously, the possibility of choanal atresia may also be excluded and esophageal patency assured. A positive culture of the gastric fluid or a finding of polymorphonuclear cells on stained smear may provide evidence of newborn sepsis. Intestinal distention may be temporarily relieved by this procedure.

Infants and children unable to cooperate are restrained in the supine position. A cooperative older child is best intubated in the sitting position, with neck and chin held forward without flexion or extension of the neck. When restraint is necessary, the patient is placed on his left side after insertion of the nasogastric tube, allowing the stomach to assume a dependent position. When the danger of pulmonary aspiration is present (ie, toxic ingestions), the patient should be placed with his head in a dependent position while

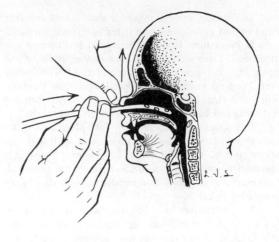

Figure 34—9. Inserting the nasogastric tube.

gastric aspiration is being carried out. In ingestions, use one orogastric tube (Ewald). If there is danger of aspiration, the patient should be intubated with an inflated cuffed orotracheal or endotracheal tube in place.

The desired tube length is determined by measuring the distance from the patient's nose to the xiphoid process and adding 4 inches. This point is marked on the tube and another mark is made approximately 6 inches distal to that point for reference. The tube is lubricated and introduced into one nasal passage and directed posteriorly while the tip of the nose is held up (Fig 34—9). The tube is then advanced for a distance of 2—3 inches as the patient swallows water. If the tube coils, it is best to remove it entirely and start over. To minimize coiling, the tube may be made stiff by prior cooling in ice. After passage of the tube, aspiration with a syringe is attempted. If gastric fluid is not obtained, air or sterile water is introduced while an assistant auscultates over the area of the stomach. A characteristic "gurgling" noise heard by the second observer will indicate that the stomach has been intubated properly; coughing indicates that the patient's respiratory tract has been intubated inadvertently.

The tube may have to be relocated by passing it farther or by withdrawing it 1—2 inches.

When prolonged intubation is necessary, the tube is secured to the cheekbone or forehead with nonirritating tape.

As an alternative, the oral route may be used and is preferable in the newborn.

COLLECTION OF DUODENAL FLUID

Bile, duodenal, or pancreatic fluid may be needed for diagnostic analysis. The Miller-Abbott tube with weighted metal tip and double lumen is introduced as described above for gastric aspiration, and the gastric contents are aspirated with the patient placed on his right side. The tube is advanced approximately 6 inches and the patient asked to remain in that position for 30–60 minutes. In this position, the normal stomach will pass the tube beyond the gastric pylorus and into the duodenum. The appearance of bile and change in pH of the aspirated duodenal fluid or roentgenographic visualization of the metal tip verifies proper positioning of the tube.

OBTAINING SPINAL FLUID

The 4 procedures for the collection of CSF are lumbar, subdural, cisternal, and ventricular punctures. Lumbar puncture is most frequently used for obtaining CSF for diagnostic purposes. It may be performed in either the lateral recumbent or sitting position.

Lumbar Puncture in Newborn & Small Infants
The sitting position is preferable in an infant and may be achieved by sitting the patient backward in a modified "infaseat" or "potty" chair. A small pillow or blanket between the abdomen and the back of the chair will increase the flexion of the back. When restraints are required, changes in cardiorespiratory activity should be monitored. When the lateral recumbent position is elected, the surface on which the child is placed should be firm and flat. The infant is best restrained by holding his legs between the fourth and fifth fingers and his arms between the second and third fingers. The head is supported with the thumbs, and the holder may readily evaluate the child for evidence of respiratory distress.

Lumbar Puncture in Children & Older Infants
Restrain the patient in the lateral recumbent position on a firm flat table (Fig 34–10). Prepare the skin surrounding this area as for a surgical procedure with iodine and alcohol or other suitable antiseptic. Iodine should be thoroughly removed to avoid the possibility of iodine arachnoiditis.

Drape the area with sterile towels or a special drape. Infiltrate the skin and subcutaneous tissues with 1% procaine (not necessary in infants and young children).

Pertinent landmarks are the spinous processes and iliac crests. The line joining the tops of the iliac crests passes through the fourth spinous process. The space above (third) and 2 spaces below (fourth and fifth) are the sites of choice for puncture.

The operator sits with the puncture site at eye level and the light adjusted to shine over his operating hand. The needle and obturator are inserted into the chosen vertebral space in the exact midline and perpendicular to the plane of the body. The needle is directed toward the umbilicus with the bevel facing the operator. In older children, a distinct "give" is usually felt when the dura is pierced; if in doubt, remove the stylet

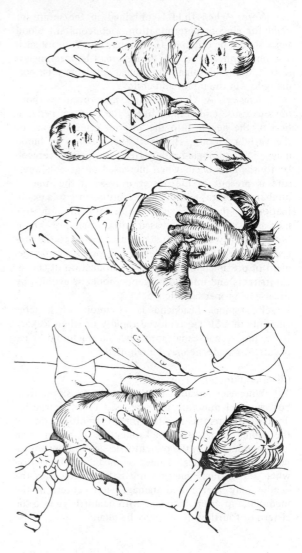

Figure 34–10. *Above:* Restraining the infant for lumbar puncture. *Below:* Lumbar puncture with assistance of nurse. (Drapes omitted to show positioning.)

and examine the needle hub for the appearance of fluid. Gentle suction with a small syringe may be required in the small infant or in the case of purulent meningitis.

When fluid is obtained, the 3-way stopcock and manometer are attached and the stopcock opened. Pressure measurements are made before collection (opening pressure) and at the completion of collection (closing pressure). In addition, the presence of pressure changes with compression of the neck veins (Queckenstedt's test) is indicative of patency between the intracranial system and cerebrospinal canal.

After the closing pressure is obtained, the needle is removed with a quick deliberate movement and pressure applied for several minutes with a sterile sponge over the puncture site. Pressure measurements are usually meaningless in the struggling, crying patient.

Note: When fluid is obtained in the infant or child for glucose determination, a concomitant blood sugar should be obtained for comparison. Without such a comparison, a low CSF glucose may be meaningless since blood and spinal fluid sugar levels may be normally low in the infant and child.

Dangers: A "bloody tap" may occur without obvious cause and is most likely the result of penetration of the needle into the anterior venous plexus of the vertebral body. However, the presence of blood may be a pathologic finding. Herniation of the cerebellar tonsils may occur when increased intracranial pressure is present in the posterior fossa at the time of lumbar puncture; preoperative ophthalmoscopic examination of the retina may be helpful in indicating increased pressure. Increased intracranial pressure is not necessarily an absolute contraindication to the procedure if provision is made for neurosurgical management of possible complications. Introduction of chemical irritants and infectious agents should be avoided by the use of proper technic.

Postspinal headache is common when large amounts of CSF are removed rapidly or when leakage from the spinal canal into the subarachnoid space occurs. An analgesic may be required.

Cisternal Puncture

Whenever possible, the lumbar route is preferred, but cisternal puncture may be used to advantage for drainage and treatment when there is an obstruction of the spinal canal. Cisternal puncture is easier than lumbar puncture in the patient with marked opisthotonos, and there is less danger of medullary impaction when the intracranial pressure is high. However, the needle may pierce and damage vital centers in the medulla, and arterial damage with hemorrhage into the cistern or fourth ventricle may be fatal.

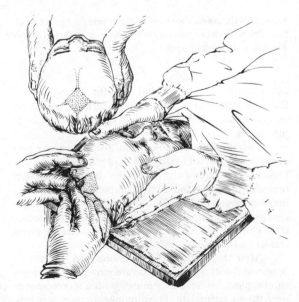

Figure 34—11. Subdural puncture.

Subdural Puncture (Fig 34—11)

Following CNS infection or trauma, bilateral subdural taps are frequently performed to determine the presence of, and remove, a subdural collection of fluid.

The anterior two-thirds of the scalp are shaved and sterile precautions are observed. The patient is restrained as shown.

Insert a short 19 or 20 gauge lumbar puncture needle with a very short bevel for a distance of 0.2—0.5 cm at the extreme lateral corner of the fontanel or farther out through the suture line, depending on the size of the fontanel. The needle is advanced in a Z pattern to minimize later leakage of CSF. A hemostat clamped on the needle will prevent the operator from going too deep. Piercing the tough dura is easily recognized. Normally, not more than a few drops (up to 1 ml) of clear fluid are obtained. If a subdural hematoma is present, the fluid will be grossly xanthochromic or bloody and more abundant. For children over age 2, a trephine opening usually is necessary.

Repeat the procedure on the other side. Do not remove more than 15—20 ml of fluid at any one time.

Remove the needle, exert firm pressure for a few minutes, and apply a sterile collodion dressing.

Note: Hemorrhage may occur if the needle causes a laceration of a tiny vein communicating with the sagittal sinus. This may result in subsequent taps yielding xanthochromic fluid from the blood introduced during the preceding procedures. Fistulous drainage is prevented by covering the orifice with a sterile collodion dressing.

BONE MARROW ASPIRATION

Bone marrow puncture is indicated in the diagnosis of blood dyscrasias, neuroblastoma, lipidosis, reticuloendotheliosis, and lupus erythematosus and to obtain culture material. The procedure should be performed with extreme caution when a defect of the clotting mechanism is suspected.

Sites for Punctures

The sites of choice for different age groups are listed in Table 34—1.

A. Iliac Crest: The site of choice for children is

Table 34—1. Sites for bone marrow puncture.

Site	Age to Which Adaptable
Anterior iliac crest	Any age
Posterior iliac crest	Any age
Femur	Birth to 2 years
Spinous vertebral process	2 years and older
Sternum	6 years and older
Tibia	Birth to 2 years

*Reproduced, with permission, from Hughes WT: *Pediatric Procedures.* Saunders, 1964.

the posterior iliac crest. Restrain the child on his abdomen with a rolled sheet placed under his hips. Locate the iliac crest and enter at a spot approximately 1–2 cm posterior to the midaxillary line and approximately 1 cm below the crest.

B. Sternal Marrow: Seldom used in children.

C. Tibia: Between the tibial tubercle and the medial condyle over the anteromedial aspect. Recommended by some for infants.

D. Lumbar Spinous Process: In the midline.

Procedure

The patient should be adequately restrained. Sedation is often necessary for children. Prepare the skin surrounding the area as for a surgical procedure. Scrub and wear sterile gloves. Infiltrate with 1% procaine solution through the skin and subcutaneous tissues to the periosteum.

Insert a short-beveled needle with stylet in place perpendicular to the skin, through the skin and tissues, down to the periosteum. (Use a 21 gauge lumbar puncture needle for infants, an 18 or 19 gauge special marrow needle with a short bevel for older children.) Push the needle through the cortex, using a screwing motion with firm, steady, and well controlled pressure. Some "give" is usually felt as the needle enters the marrow; the needle will then be firmly in place.

Immediately fit a dry syringe (20–50 ml) onto the needle and apply strong suction for a few seconds. A small amount of marrow will come up into the syringe; this should be smeared on glass coverslips or slides for subsequent staining and counting.

Remove the needle after withdrawing marrow, exert local pressure for 3–5 minutes or until all evidence of bleeding has ceased, and apply a dry dressing.

COLLECTION OF FLUID FROM BODY CAVITIES

Thoracentesis

Used for removing pleural fluid for diagnosis or treatment, to inject antibiotics in cases of empyema, or to induce or relieve pneumothorax.

A. Site: Locate the fluid or air by physical examination and by x-ray if necessary. If entering the base, locate the bottom of the uninvolved lung as a guide so that the puncture will not be below the pleural cavity.

B. Equipment: Use an 18 to 19 gauge needle with a very short bevel and a sharp point. The needle and a 10 or 20 ml syringe are attached to a 3-way stopcock (10 ml syringe is easier). If much fluid is to be removed, it can be pumped through a rubber tube attached to the sidearm of the stopcock, thereby avoiding leakage of air into the pleural space.

C. Procedure: When possible, the patient should be in a flexed position and leaning forward against a chair back or bed stand. If too ill to sit, he can lie on his uninvolved side on a firm, flat surface with a small pillow under his chest to widen the upper interspaces.

Use strict sterile precautions; scrub and wear sterile gloves. Prepare the skin surgically and use suitable drapes, preferably a large drape with a hole in the center. Infiltrate into the skin and down to the pleura with 1% procaine. A 3-way stopcock is attached to the aspiration needle, a section of rubber tubing is applied to the sidearm, and a 10 ml syringe is applied to the hub.

Insert the needle through an interspace, passing just above the edge of the rib. The intercostal vessels lie immediately below each rib. With gentle aspiration of the syringe, the needle is advanced a few millimeters at a time until the pleural space is reached. It is usually not difficult to know when the pleura is pierced: suction on the needle at any stage will show whether or not fluid has been reached. In cases of long-standing infection, the pleura may be thick and the fluid may be loculated, necessitating more than one puncture site. To prevent accidental penetration of the lung after the needle is in place, apply a surgical hemostat to the needle adjacent to the skin. Pleural fluid is apt to coagulate unless it is frankly purulent, and an anticoagulant should be added after removal to facilitate examination. If a large amount of fluid is present, it should be removed slowly at intervals, 100–500 ml each time, depending on the size of the patient.

D. Dangers: Complications of this procedure include introduction of a new infection, pneumothorax or hemothorax from tearing of the lung, hemoptysis, syncope (pleuropulmonary reflex or air embolus), and pulmonary edema (from too rapid removal of large amounts of fluid). Careful sterile technic will decrease the risk of introducing infection. Hemodynamic imbalance is unlikely when only small quantities are removed slowly. Air embolism will not occur if the stopcock is closed so that air cannot enter. Insertion of the needle into a blood vessel, heart, liver, and spleen can be prevented by proper selection and positioning of the puncture site. Pneumothorax should not occur if care is taken to avoid advancing the needle beyond the point where fluid should be present.

If the patient starts to cough, the needle should be removed.

Pericardiocentesis (Fig 34–12)

Pericardiocentesis is indicated for the diagnosis and treatment of purulent pericarditis or to relieve cardiac embarrassment due to collection of large amounts of blood or other fluid. The procedure is contraindicated if pericardial or myocardial adhesions are suspected.

A. Site: The puncture site is determined by physical or x-ray examination. The common site of aspiration is the fourth left interspace, 1–2 cm inside of the left outer border of percussion dullness or x-ray shadow. Other sites of entrance are just outside the apical pulsation; from below, in the chondroxiphoid angle; and occasionally from the back if a very large collection has collapsed the lung against the posterior chest wall.

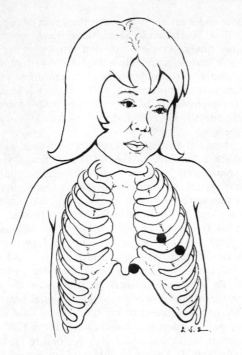

Figure 34-12. Sites of needle insertion for pericardiocentesis.

B. Procedure: The patient sits forward at a 60 degree angle supported by bed or pillows. Using sterile technic, infiltrate the skin and subcutaneous tissues with 1% procaine. Connect a 50 ml syringe, 3-way stopcock, and 18 gauge needle. Insert the needle slowly at the lower border of the interspace just above the edge of the rib, directing it posteriorly and toward the spine. Aspirate, and then turn the stopcock to discharge fluid via the rubber tubing. When fluid is being aspirated with ease, attach a surgical clamp to the needle next to the skin to prevent the needle from slipping farther.

Continuous monitoring of the pulse and blood pressure is necessary during the removal of small increments of fluid. The needle is removed in one quick movement and pressure applied to the puncture site to ensure that air does not enter the pericardial or pleural space.

C. Dangers: Cardiac arrhythmias and penetration of the heart or coronary vessels have been reported to have resulted from pericardiocentesis.

Peritoneal Paracentesis

This procedure can be used as a therapeutic measure to remove excessive fluid in cases of nephrotic syndrome or hepatic cirrhosis or diagnostically for evidence of blood or intestinal contents. In cases of known or suspected trauma, a puncture in each of the 4 quadrants of the abdomen may be made ("4 quadrant tap") in search of blood or intestinal contents. Infrequently, peritoneal paracentesis may be used as a diagnostic measure to obtain bacteriologic specimens in peritonitis, but this involves the danger of punctur-

ing the distended bowel, which frequently is adherent to the abdominal wall. Electrolyte solutions, albumin, blood, and antibiotics may be administered by the peritoneal route. Peritoneal dialysis may be of value for renal insufficiency and in the treatment of certain poisonings.

A. Procedure: Use an 18 or 19 gauge needle with a short bevel and a sharp point. The skin is cleansed and surgical safeguards employed to avoid peritoneal infection. A local anesthetic is injected and a small incision is made in the skin with a surgical knife. Enter at a level about halfway between the symphysis and the umbilicus in the lower quadrant or in the midline. The needle should enter obliquely to avoid leakage afterward. Ascitic fluid will flow out readily. Pus may require aspiration.

B. Dangers: Perforation of the intestine has resulted when the intestines are distended or adhesions are present. Perforation of the bladder has resulted when the bladder is not empty. The removal of excessive amounts or excessively rapid removal of fluid may result in circulatory embarrassment. Peritonitis from the introduction of infectious agents has been observed; "prophylactic" antibiotics are no substitute for proper surgical technic and are usually not indicated.

THERAPEUTIC PROCEDURES

ADMINISTRATION OF FLUIDS

The administration of fluids may be necessary in a number of clinical situations. The available routes of administration are as follows: (1) Alimentary: Oral, gastric (gavage or gastrostomy), rectal. (2) Intravascular: Intravenous, intra-arterial. (3) Hypodermoclysis. (4) Intraosseous. (5) Intraperitoneal. (6) Intramuscular.

1. ALIMENTARY ROUTE

Oral

When available, the alimentary tract is the route of choice for the administration of all nutrients and fluids with the exception of blood. When the oral-gastric avenue is not competent, intubation of the stomach and duodenum is safe and easily accomplished.

Rectal

The rectal route may be used for diagnosis (culture or roentgenologic examination with barium), for cleansing (fecal impaction), or for therapy (administration of fluids, electrolytes, or drugs).

Because the vascular drainage of the rectum does

not enter the portal system, the liver is bypassed and administered fluids and drugs that are absorbed can enter the systemic circulation directly without hepatic conjugation or detoxification. The portal bypass may be avoided by administering fluids into the colon by high enema or colonic flush.

A. Procedure: The older patient is placed in either the left lateral recumbent or the knee-chest position. The small infant may be placed on his back with his legs flexed and elevated. A rectal examination should be performed initially to rule out the presence of a foreign body. A rectal catheter of appropriate size is lubricated and introduced beyond the anal sphincter. Fluid (preferably warmed) is administered by the gravity method, holding or taping the buttocks together if necessary to prevent the loss of fluid.

B. Dangers: Rectal perforation, particularly in the small infant, is not rare but can be avoided with the use of a soft rubber catheter.

2. INTRAVENOUS ROUTE

Intravenous Therapy by the Gravity Method

For most infants and children a standard gravity apparatus or special equipment (Vacoset, to deliver fluids slowly, and Pedatrol, which permits controlled administration of fluid) should be used for giving large amounts of fluid slowly over a long period. Fluids are

best administered through a 21 or 23 gauge needle. In the neonate, a precision controlled infusion set (eg, Howard pump) is ideal.

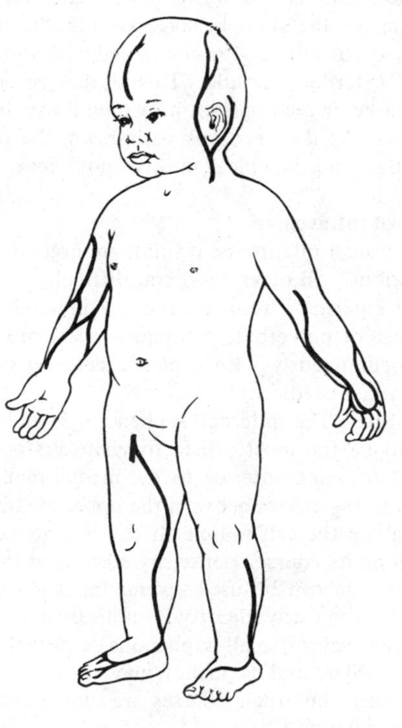

A. Site: (Figs 34–13, 34–14, 34–15, 34–16) For small infants, a scalp vein or one on the wrist, hand, foot, or arm will usually be most convenient. The superficial veins of the scalp do not have valves, and fluids may therefore be infused in either direction. Any accessible vein may be used in an older child. If a

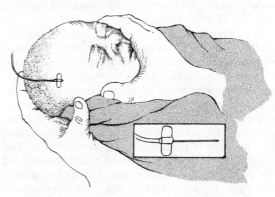

Figure 34–14. Intravenous fluids into scalp vein.

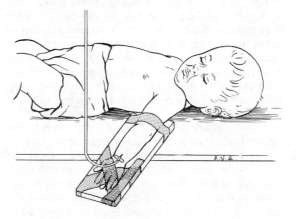

Figure 34–15. Intravenous fluids into wrist vein.

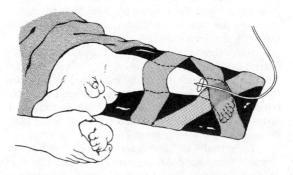

Figure 34–16. Intravenous fluids into ankle vein.

Figure 34–13. Superficial veins used most frequently for intravenous infusion.

vein cannot be entered, blood may be given intra-peritoneally in an emergency.

B. Equipment: A gravity apparatus is used with a closed drip bulb in the tubing not far below the container so that it will hang perpendicularly. The bulb should be one-fourth to one-third full and the connected tubing free of air. Flow is regulated by a screw clamp on the tubing.

C. Procedure: Use a Pediatric Scalp Vein Infusion Set (Cutter or Abbott) with a 21 gauge needle and rubber finger grip connected to plastic tubing or a short 21–24 gauge needle.

A syringe is attached to the catheter and the system is filled with saline. The skin over the area is prepared with an antiseptic and the tourniquet applied snugly but not tightly enough to impede arterial pressure. Warming in water or gentle percussion over the vein will enhance distention of the vein. (Holding a fiberoptic light under a hand or foot is useful in locating veins in infants.) The vein is stabilized by stretching the skin over it proximal to the puncture site. The needle is introduced bevel up and parallel to the long axis of the vein at a point just beneath the skin. A characteristic "give" is perceptible, and blood usually flows back into the catheter and syringe. In the infant, venous pressure may be low and blood return not appreciated until negative pressure is applied with the syringe. The tourniquet is released and the winged tabs of the scalp vein set are held stable with the free hand. Very gentle pressure is applied to the syringe barrel to ensure patency of the system. If the syringe does not function easily, pressure should not be increased but merely maintained. Initial resistance is not uncommon and has been attributed to "spasm" of the vessel. After a few seconds, the vein may open and saline will flow easily from the syringe.

The winged tabs are secured by taping; the syringe is removed and the scalp needle catheter is connected to an air-free gravity type infusion apparatus with a drip bulb. Final restraints are applied when necessary and the flow rate adjusted. Tape the needle firmly in place. Sandbags will be useful in securing the head, and sandbags or a padded board are employed to immobilize the hand and arm.

Superficial veins of the scalp of infants under the age of 2 years are easily visualized and can be distinguished from the superficial arteries of the scalp by palpation. When these veins are used, special care in cleansing the skin is mandatory since they communicate with the dural sinuses.

An ordinary rubber band will usually suffice as a tourniquet.

D. Rate: The rate can be calculated by counting the number of drops per minute delivered from the bottle. If a Pedatrol microdrop bulb is employed, drops/minute = ml/hour. When the adult set is used, drops/minute × 4 = ml/hour.

E. Precautions: *The rate of flow should be checked frequently.* An accurate record must be kept of the amount of fluid added. For small infants (particularly those who were prematurely born), never per-

mit more than one-third of the daily fluid requirements to be in the container at any one time. It is advisable to remove the needle and change location each 48–72 hours to avoid phlebitis. If possible, avoid hypertonic solutions.

For the patient receiving fluids in an extremity, use foam rubber to maintain the limb in a position of comfort. Inspect the limb at regular intervals for evidence of undue pressure and circulatory embarrassment.

Intravenous Therapy by the Pump Method

In some infants, veins may be too small for the administration of fluids by the gravity method despite maximum elevation of reservoir bottle; in these cases, the solution can be pumped in slowly by syringe and a 3-way stopcock. With a needle and syringe on the terminal stopcock, one operator enters the vein and maintains the needle in the proper position. A second person "pumps" the solution in with a syringe on the second stopcock inserted farther up the tubing. If only one person is available, he can pump from the terminal stopcock. Twenty to 30 ml/kg body weight (except blood and plasma) may be administered slowly over the course of several minutes.

Percutaneous Catheterization

Catheterization of either a vein or an artery may be performed percutaneously by inserting a large bore, thin-walled needle into a relatively large vein and then threading a catheter through the needle and into the vein.

The needle is withdrawn and the catheter secured by taping to the skin. Leakage around the puncture site may occur but may be eliminated with the use of a Buffalo (Sterilon) needle. This device reverses the needle-catheter relationship, providing a needle within a catheter. As the needle is withdrawn, the puncture site is not reduced and leakage does not occur.

Cut-Down Intravenous

For small infants—or if fluids are urgently needed by a seriously ill older child and difficulty is encountered in entering a vein—expose a vein surgically and tie a piece of polyethylene tubing in place or enter the vein subcutaneously with a plastic catheter equipped with an inner needle stylet.

A. Site: The internal saphenous vein has been found to be the most satisfactory site. Its position is constant, running anterior to the medial malleolus of the tibia to the groove between the upper medial end of the tibia and the calf muscle. It can be entered at any point along its course. Hence, by starting at the ankle, the same vein can be used several times if necessary. The novice can easily identify it on his own leg first.

Other veins (small saphenous, external jugular, median basilar, and cephalic) may also be used for "cut-downs," but their courses are more variable and difficult to define.

B. Equipment:

1. Sterile solution, container, tubing, drip bulb,

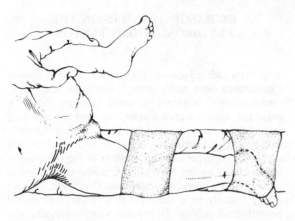

Figure 34—17. Position and taping of leg for cut-down incision.

and clamp are prepared as for continuous venoclysis.

2. Thin polyethylene tubing with the end cut on the slant is easiest to use and least irritating. A 19 gauge tubing is preferred, but tubing as small as 22 gauge may be used.

C. Procedure:

1. Preparation—Apply a tourniquet, cleanse the skin, and drape the leg as for a surgical procedure, using sterile precautions. The foot can be securely taped to a sandbag or board splint (Fig 34—17). Make a large wheal with 1 or 2% procaine solution in the skin over the vein.

2. Incision—With a scalpel, make an incision about 1 cm long just through the skin. The incision should be at a right angle to the direction of the vein. Using small, curved, sharp-pointed scissors or fine forceps, spread the incision widely.

3. Identifying the vein—The vein is usually seen lying on the fascia. Some dissection of subcutaneous fat may be necessary. Insert a curved clamp to the periosteum and bring the vein to the surface (Fig 34—18). Be certain it is a vein, not a nerve or tendon, by observing for the passage of blood. Using a small hook (eg, strabismus hook), dissect the vein free for a

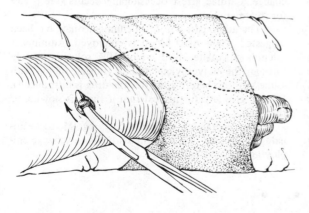

Figure 34—18. Isolation of vein for cut-down intravenous. (Drapes not shown.)

length of 1.5—2.5 cm. In small infants the vein is small and fragile, and great care must be taken in handling it.

4. Placing ties—Using No. 00 black silk, tie the vein off at the extreme distal (lower) end of the exposed portion. Leave the ends of the suture long so that they may be used later for traction. At the proximal end of the vein, loop a piece of suture loosely around the vein.

5. Nicking the vein—Using a fine-pointed scissors, sterile razor blade, or sharp-pointed scalpel blade, make a small incision through the wall of the vein a few millimeters above the lower ligature. Make certain that the lumen has been entered by lifting the vein on the handle of the hook or other instrument used so as to flatten it and draw it taut. Release tourniquet after tubing is in the vein.

6. Fixing the cannula—Insert the polyethylene tubing for a distance of at least 2 cm. Blood will usually drip from it; if not, note whether a small amount of the solution can be injected easily with a syringe and rubber adapter without producing a wheal or filling the incision site. Tie the upper proximal suture firmly around the vein and tubing to hold it in place. Connect the tubing from the reservoir of fluid to the polyethylene tubing in the vein with care to avoid pulling and tearing the vein.

7. Closing the wound—Close the wound with fine silk sutures which are removed in 3—4 days. The tubing must be firmly strapped in place. When using a needle or cannula, a pad of gauze under the hub will keep it in alignment with the vein. Cover the wound with gauze and roller bandage. Avoid restraint, which interferes with adequate circulation or causes pressure lesions.

The needle is withdrawn and the catheter secured by taping to the skin.

Filston HC, Johnson DG: Percutaneous venous cannulation in neonates and infants: A method for catheter insertion without "cutdown." Pediatrics 48:896, 1971.

3. HYPODERMOCLYSIS

For Small Infants

A. Site: For small infants, hypodermoclysis may be given by syringe, using the subcutaneous tissues of the anterior and posterior axillary folds, the medial aspect of the mid-thigh, the upper back in the area of the inferior aspect of the scapula, or the lower abdominal wall. In most instances, the intravenous route is preferred since hypodermoclysis may be associated with erratic absorption or a shift in body fluids.

B. Equipment: A 20 or 50 ml syringe and a 20 gauge needle. Use only isotonic solutions.

C. Procedure: After aspirating to make certain that a blood vessel has not been entered, inject slowly; if the center of the injected area becomes pale, change the position of the needle point. Gentle massage will help to diffuse the fluid into the tissues. (Hyaluronidase may be used to facilitate spread and absorption.) In infants, up to 50 ml can be injected in each site at one time. Rigid aseptic precautions are necessary. The infant must be restrained to prevent bending or breaking the needle.

D. Dose: Thirty to 40 ml/kg body weight at one time. Larger amounts can be given over a longer period by a gravity apparatus with a Y-tube and 2 needles.

For Older Children

For older children, fluids by hypodermoclysis are best given slowly in the outer aspect of the mid-thigh by a gravity apparatus, using a Y-tube and 2 needles.

4. INTRAOSSEOUS THERAPY

Intraosseous (into the bone marrow) administration of fluids is a form of intravenous therapy. The effluent vessels of bone marrow provide a rapid and relatively complete drainage into the systemic circulation. However, the obvious consequences of infection preclude its general use.

5. INTRAPERITONEAL THERAPY

Isotonic fluids and blood may be administered by the intraperitoneal route, but the intravenous route is generally preferred.

6. INTRAMUSCULAR THERAPY

Intramuscular injections may be given into the upper outer quadrant of the gluteal area. With the child prone on a flat surface, locate the head of the greater trochanter of the femur and the posterior superior iliac spine. Direct the needle perpendicular to the table or bed in this space cephalad to the head of the trochanter.

Other satisfactory sites include (1) the anterolateral aspect of the thigh (use a 1 inch needle), with the needle directed downward at an oblique angle toward the bone; or (2) the ventral gluteal muscles, to the center of an area outlined by locating the anterior iliac tubercle, placing the index finger on the tubercle, and extending the middle fingertip along the crest of the ileum as far as possible, forming a triangle. The needle is directed slightly toward the iliac crest.

EXCHANGE TRANSFUSION FOR ERYTHROBLASTOSIS FETALIS

After an adequate preparation of the infant (respirations and temperature stabilized and maintained, gastric contents removed, proper restraint), drape the umbilical area. Cut off the cord about ½ inch or less from the skin. Control any bleeding. Identify the vein (the 2 arteries are white and cordlike; the single vein is larger and thin-walled). If the vein cannot be visualized in the cord stump, make a small transverse incision above the umbilicus. Cannulate the vein gently (usually to a distance of 6–8 cm) with naked polyethylene tubing. Determine venous pressure and maintain below 10 cm of water with the child at rest.

Selection & Amount of Blood

Employ sterile packaged equipment specifically prepared for this procedure (eg, Pharmaseal Laboratories).

Use freshly collected heparinized blood (preferred) or blood preserved with anticoagulant acid-citrate-dextrose (ACD). Blood should be less than 5 days old and should be warmed before use. Give twice the blood volume (BV = 85–100 ml/kg) for a complete 2-volume exchange. In Rh- sensitized infants, use type O Rh-negative blood. If the infant is ABO sensitized, use type O, Rh-specific blood to which Witebsky anti-A and anti-B substance is added.

Remove blood in 10–20 ml amounts and save the first aliquot for laboratory studies. Replace with an equivalent amount of blood. When the infant is severely affected, a full exchange should not be attempted immediately after birth. Instead, small doses of sedimented erythrocytes should be given, alternating with slow withdrawal of the infant's blood until the venous pressure is less than 10 cm of water. Determine the pulse rate every 20–30 ml exchanged and the venous pressure every 100 ml exchanged; if venous pressure is elevated, gradually establish a deficit (10–100 ml). If hemorrhagic manifestations, respiratory distress, yawning, pallor, or cyanosis develop, discontinue the exchange. Cardiac arrest occasionally occurs (see p 839 for treatment).

The administration of calcium gluconate has been suggested when ACD blood is employed. Administer calcium gluconate, 1–2 ml of 10% solution, slowly through the polyethylene tubing (rinsing tubing with saline solution before and after the drug is introduced). Do not give any further calcium if there is slowing of the pulse.

Give protamine sulfate, 0.5–1 mg IM, to terminate the heparin effect at the end of an exchange employing heparinized blood.

• • •

General References

Barnett HL: *Pediatrics,* 15th ed. Appleton-Century-Crofts, 1972.

DeSanctis AG, Varga C: *Handbook of Pediatric Medical Emergencies,* 4th ed. Mosby, 1968.

Gellis SS, Kagan BM: *Current Pediatric Therapy 6.* Saunders, 1973.

Hughes WT Jr: *Pediatric Procedures.* Saunders, 1964.

Klein JO, Gellis SS: Diagnostic needle aspiration in pediatric practice. Pediatr Clin North Am 18:219, 1971.

Vaughan VC III, McKay RJ, Nelson WE (editors): *Nelson Textbook of Pediatrics,* 10th ed. Saunders, 1975.

Shirkey HC (editor): *Pediatric Therapy,* 5th ed. Mosby, 1975.

Silver HK, Kempe CH, Bruyn HB: *Handbook of Pediatrics,* 12th ed. Lange, 1977.

35...
Fluid & Electrolyte Therapy

Donough O'Brien, MD, FRCP

I. PHYSIOLOGY OF THE FLUID SPACES IN CHILDHOOD

ELECTROLYTES

An electrolyte is any low molecular weight substance which, when dissolved in water, renders the solution capable of conducting an electric current. Conductivity is made possible because electrolytes in solution exist as ions and, therefore, have positive or negative charges. Positively charged ions are called cations (eg, Na^+, K^+, Ca^{++}), and negatively charged ions are called anions (eg, Cl^-, HCO_3^-). In any solution, the number of positive and negative charges is equal. Certain ions have more than one positive or negative charge, the number of charges per ion being the valence of the ion.

Molecular weight can be calculated as the sum of the weights of the individual atoms in a molecule. When expressed in grams, the value is known as a gram mol, and a solution containing 1 gram mol/liter is said to be 1 molar. If an ion has a valence of 2, then 1 mol of that ion can combine with 2 mols of any univalent reactant. Or, in other words, a 1 molar solution of a univalent ion also contains 1 equivalent (Eq) per liter. It is sometimes also referred to as a 1 normal solution. If the ion is divalent, then a 1 molar solution will contain 2 equivalents and be twice normal (2 N). Electrolytes are customarily expressed as milliequivalents per liter (mEq/liter) of solution, 1 mEq being equal to 0.001 Eq.

The following formulas may be used to interconvert grams (gm), milligrams (mg), moles (mol), and millimoles (mmol) to mEq.

$$\text{mEq/liter} = \frac{\text{gm/liter} \times 1000}{\text{Molecular wt}} \times \text{Valency}$$

$$\text{mEq/liter} = \frac{(\text{mg/dl} \times 10) \text{ or mg/liter}}{\text{Molecular wt}} \times \text{Valency}$$

$$\text{mEq/liter} = \text{mol/liter} \times 1000 \times \text{Valency}$$

$$\text{mEq/liter} = \text{mmol/liter} \times \text{Valency}$$

BODY FLUIDS, MEMBRANES, & OSMOLALITY

Of the total water in the body (TBW), roughly two-thirds are intracellular (ICW) after early infancy and the remainder is extracellular (ECW). Between the ECW and ICW lie all the cell membranes of the body, which may be considered as one large, aggregate membrane. This so-called cell membrane possesses 2 qualities of importance to clinicians: (1) It is water-permeable, and (2) it concentrates Na^+ into the ECW and K^+ into the ICW by virtue of a membrane-associated Na^+-K^+ "pump."

Water molecules cross the cell membrane constantly and equally in both directions; hence, the volumes of the ECW and ICW do not change. Particles dissolved in the water interfere with the movement of water molecules and thus lower the number which find "pores" in the membrane and cross to the opposite side. The number of dissolved particles per number of water molecules must therefore be equal on both sides of the cell membrane, or a net transfer of water or particles (or both) would result. If the membrane is impermeable to certain solute particles, addition of such particles to one side will lower the number of water molecules leaving that side and the number of water molecules entering from the opposite side will then be greater. A net transfer of water will occur until the ratio of particles to water molecules has again been equalized on both sides. The number of dissolved particles per number of water molecules is seldom computed as such, but a closely related value, osmolality, is employed. Osmolality is customarily expressed as mOsm/liter* of water.

The forces generated by separating solutions of differing osmolalities by a semipermeable membrane may be substantial and will cause the transfer of water or particles or both. Much evidence exists that osmolality is the same throughout the TBW. Osmolality is often referred to as tonicity, and solutions which contain approximately 285 mOsm/kg are referred to as isosmolal, isotonic, or occasionally as normal. ("Normal" in this sense does not imply equivalents/liter.)

---

*mOsm/liter = mmol/liter $\times$ number of particles formed when 1 molecule dissolves, eg, 1 for glucose, 2 for NaCl, 3 for $MgCl_2$.

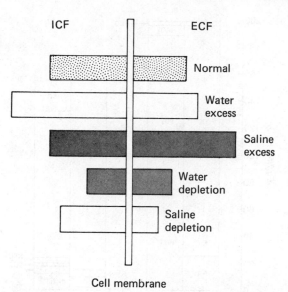

Figure 35–1. Changes in water distribution between ICF and ECF.

Table 35–1. Blood and plasma volume formulas.*

Boys

Blood volume in ml/kg = 75.7 − 0.114 × wt in kg

Blood volume in ml/sq m = 697 × surface area (in sq m) + 1312

Girls

Blood volume in ml/kg = 82.4 − 0.374 × wt in kg

Blood volume in ml/sq m = 360 × surface area (in sq m) + 1575

Plasma volume = blood volume × $\left(1 - \dfrac{0.95 \times Hct}{100}\right)$

Whole body hematocrit = True venous hematocrit × 0.95

*From Cropp JA: J Pediatr 78:220, 1971.

Solutions containing less than or more than 285 mOsm/kg are spoken of as hypo- or hyperosmolal or hypo- or hypertonic, respectively. Osmolality can be changed by selectively adding or taking away water, or by selectively adding or taking away solute particles. It is generally true that isosmolality (ie, 285 mOsm/kg) of the body fluids is optimal.

Some of the consequences of the cell membrane's ability to concentrate Na^+ into the extracellular fluid (ECF) and K^+ into the intracellular fluid (ICF) are shown in Fig 35–1.

EXTRACELLULAR FLUID

1. COMPONENTS

The components of the ECF are (1) plasma, (2) interstitial fluid, (3) connective tissue, cartilage, and bone fluids, and (4) transcellular fluids.

Plasma

After early infancy, the plasma constitutes about one-sixth of the ECF volume, about one-twelfth of the TBW, and about one-twentieth of the weight of the patient (Table 35–1). It is separated from the interstitial fluid by the endothelial membranes lining the blood vessels. Endothelium allows the immediate passage of water and very rapid passage of ions but confines most of the albumin and globulin molecules to the intravascular compartment proper. This is presumably due to the large size of the protein molecules. The plasma proteins consist mostly of albumin of approximately 60,000 mol wt and globulins ranging in mol wt from 180,000–1,000,000. The albumin molecules, though smaller, are much more numerous and contribute roughly three-fourths of the osmotic pressure attributable to the plasma proteins. This is frequently called colloid osmotic pressure. Compared to the osmotic pressure due to the more numerous low molecular weight electrolyte molecules of the plasma (eg, Na^+, K^+, Cl^-, HCO_3^-), the colloid osmotic pressure is negligible and constitutes only about 1 mOsm out of 285. Nevertheless, this difference plays a critical role in the maintenance of plasma volume.

Plasma is delivered to capillary beds under hydrostatic pressure. This pressure forces fluid out of the intravascular compartment into the interstitial fluid, concentrating the plasma proteins and raising the colloid osmotic pressure in the capillaries. As hydrostatic pressure falls and colloid osmotic pressure rises with further passage down the capillaries, a point is reached where the fluid, initially exuded, is reabsorbed back into the capillaries.

Interstitial Fluid (ISF)

The ISF may be regarded as an ultrafiltrate of plasma. Thus, the concentrations of Na^+, K^+, HCO_3^-, and Cl^- in ISF closely resemble those of plasma, and for all practical purposes plasma electrolyte analyses reflect interstitial fluid composition.

The ISF is the perfusate of the cells. Its composition is regulated chiefly by renal and pulmonary action on plasma. It represents a fluid "space" or "compartment" of considerable volume and therefore acts as a buffer against changes occurring in the much smaller plasma compartment. Excessive volume of ISF is manifested as edema. When ISF volume is diminished, the clinical signs include poor skin turgor, sunken eyes, depressed fontanels, and small tongue size. The ISF is thus an integral component of soft tissue structure.

Connective Tissue, Cartilage, & Bone Water

No particular symptoms are known to derive specifically from alterations in these fluids.

Transcellular Fluids

Transcellular fluids are body fluids which have been directly elaborated by cells. The fluids involved are spinal and ventricular fluid, bile, the humors of the eye, synovial fluid, and gastrointestinal fluids. Ordinarily, these fluids comprise less than 2% of TBW. The volume of gastrointestinal fluids, however, can expand enormously, creating a fluid pool of considerable size and importance.

2. CONTROL OF THE ECF

A wide variety of mechanisms play a role in the control of the composition and volume of the ECF. The most important ones are discussed below.

Thirst

Thirst is the perception of the need to drink, and control mechanisms operate with astonishing precision. ECF volume deficits evoke thirst, and the organism will use water to control volume at the expense of osmolality. Many fluid balance problems arise when thirst cannot be perceived, communicated, or satisfied.

Aldosterone

This potent, adrenocortical hormone acts to enhance the tubular resorption of Na^+. Aldosterone secretion plays an important role in the control of ECF volume, as this depends mainly on the amount of Na^+ that it contains.

Antidiuretic Hormone (Vasopressin, ADH)

ADH acts to enhance renal resorption of water and thus allows formation of a concentrated urine of small volume. ADH is secreted from the posterior pituitary after synthesis in the anterior hypothalamus. ADH secretion, causing antidiuresis, is promoted by an increase in osmolality, a decrease in plasma (or ECF) volume, emotional stress (pain, fear, rage), exercise, and a number of drugs, including morphine, ether, barbiturates, nicotine, histamine, acetylcholine, and epinephrine. ADH secretion is inhibited, causing diuresis, by dilution of body fluids, distention of the left atrial wall, and alcohol.

INTRACELLULAR WATER

The bulk of the body water is intracellular, and for technical reasons quantitative assays are difficult, although it is sometimes of value to assay striated muscle biopsies for sodium, potassium, and magnesium content to give an approximation of their concentration in intracellular water.

It is clearly inappropriate to conceive of intracellular water as a simple homogeneous solution. As

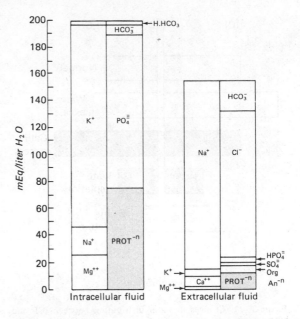

Figure 35—2. Electrolyte composition of intracellular and extracellular water.

yet, however, there is no useful information about regional differences in the volume and composition of intracellular water as between cytoplasm and organelles.

DISTRIBUTION OF BODY WATER WITH AGE

An understanding of fluid and electrolyte problems requires an understanding of certain differences in ionic composition between extracellular and intracellular water (Fig 35—2), bearing in mind that the proportions of TBW in the various compartments vary with age (Table 35—2).

Table 35—2. Distribution of body water with age (in percentage of total body weight).

Age	Total (TBW)	Extra-cellular (ECW)	Intra-cellular (ICW)
0–11 days	77.8 (69–84)	42 (34–53)	34.5 (28–40)
11 days–6 months	72.4 (63–83)	34.6 (28–57)	38.8 (20–47)
6 months–2 years	59.8 (52–72)	26.6 (20–30)	34.8 (28–38)
2–7 years	63.4 (55–73)	25 (21–30)	40.4 (31–53)
7–16 years	58.2 (50–64)	20.5 (18–26)	46.7

ACID-BASE PHYSIOLOGY

Definitions

An acid is a substance which, when in solution, dissociates into hydrogen ions (H^+) and anions (A^-). Acids are, therefore, hydrogen ion donors, and a strong acid dissociates more completely than a weak acid. Acidity is thus directly proportionate to the concentration of hydrogen ions in solution. In contrast, a base dissolved in water yields anions that react with hydrogen ions to remove them from solution. A base is consequently a hydrogen ion acceptor, and the strength of a base is proportionate to its affinity for H^+.

Acidity and alkalinity are not independent of one another; the product of $[H^+] \times [OH^-]$ is constant. Thus, a rise in $[H^+]$ (or acidity) is accompanied by an equivalent fall in $[OH^-]$ (or alkalinity) and vice versa.

The acidity of body fluids has come to be described not in terms of $[H^+]$ but by another term, pH, which is equal to $-\log [H^+]$. This relationship may be rewritten as follows:

$$pH = \log \frac{1}{[H^+]}$$

Hence, it can be seen that as acidity or $[H^+]$ rises, pH falls, and vice versa.

The pH of arterial blood is normally 7.40 ± 0.02.

When the pH of blood is 7.40, the $[H^+]$ is only 0.04 μEq/liter. At that pH, the buffer acids and buffer bases are present in milliequivalents per liter, making buffer acid and buffer base molecules many times more numerous than hydrogen ions.

Normal Control

Normal fine control of pH is achieved by 3 mechanisms. The first is the normal buffering capacity of the body fluid (except gastric fluid). A buffer is a mixture of a weak acid and its conjugate base. In the equilibrium $H_2CO_3 \rightleftharpoons HCO_3^- + H^+$, carbonic acid ($H_2CO_3$) is a weak acid and bicarbonate ion (HCO_3^-) is the conjugate base. In a buffer, or buffered solution, the weak acid is called a buffer acid and the weak base is called a buffer base. Buffers tend to ameliorate the effect of adding hydrion to a solution.

The second mechanism is the respiratory control of carbonic acid as the most important buffer acid.

The third homeostatic mechanism is the kidneys' ability to conserve bicarbonate, the principal buffer base, and to excrete H^+ into the urine against a gradient and in exchange for Na^+ as well as NH_4. The action of the last 2 mechanisms is slower than buffering.

Relationships Between pH, P_{CO_2}, Serum $[HCO_3^-]$, & Other Buffers

Acid-base relationships are governed by the following equation:

$$pH = pK + \log \frac{[\text{Buffer base}]}{[\text{Buffer acid}]}$$

Because 53% of all blood buffering is in the bicarbonate system and because it is this system which is predominantly altered in acid-base disorders, this equation can be conveniently rewritten as follows:

$$pH = 6.1 + \log \frac{[HCO_3^-]s}{0.03 \, P_{CO_2}}$$

A complete evaluation of acid-base status thus requires a knowledge of 2 of its 3 variables: pH, serum bicarbonate, and P_{CO_2}.

Some understanding is still required of the interchangeability between bicarbonate and nonbicarbonate buffers in the blood. The latter are primarily erythrocyte hemoglobin and, to a lesser extent, anionic groups on plasma proteins, and phosphates.

Consider the second equation:

$$H_2CO_3 + Hb^- = HCO_3^- + HProt$$

An increase in H_2CO_3 or P_{CO_2} will shift the reaction to the right. This will reduce $[Hb^-]$ and increase the $[HCO_3^-]$. The sum of $[Hb^-] + [HCO_3^-]$ or "total buffer base" is not changed, however. The same is also true in reverse, ie, total buffer base is independent of P_{CO_2}. Normal values for total buffer base are about 46–50 mEq/liter: it has, however, become popular instead to use the term "base excess" for deviations from normal values. The interrelationship of all these buffer systems, however, cannot be expressed in one simple equation, and a nomogram (Fig 35–3) is therefore used. Again, this requires knowing 2 of the 3 variables (pH, P_{CO_2}, and $[HCO_3^-]s$) as well as knowing hemoglobin concentration.

In "metabolic" acidosis or alkalosis, where the changes are due to loss or excess of buffer base, therapy can be based on changes in serum bicarbonate concentration $[HCO_3^-]s$. The Siggaard-Andersen nomogram (Fig 35–4) is useful in determining the metabolic component in mixed respiratory and metabolic situations such as may be seen in salicylate intoxication. Other nomograms also help to separate the respiratory and metabolic components.

Total body buffering capacity is only about 20% in the blood, about 30% in extracellular water, and 50% in intracellular water. However, therapy can be successfully based on an estimate of total body water and of the base excess in plasma.

LABORATORY MEASUREMENT OF ACID-BASE DISTURBANCES

pH

Whole blood or plasma pH is measured using a micro glass electrode and an extended scale pH meter.

P_{CO_2}

In most clinical laboratories, P_{CO_2} is calculated

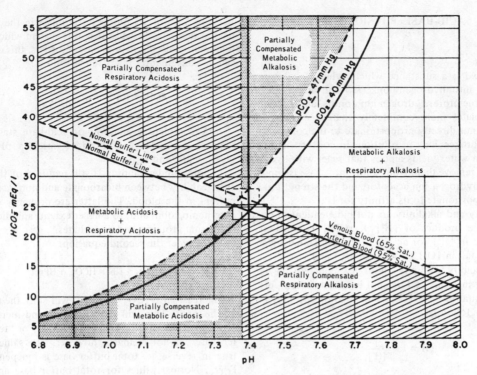

Figure 35—3. The relation of blood pH to plasma bicarbonate in acidosis and alkalosis. (Reproduced, with permission, from Pickering DE, Fisher DA: *Fluid and Electrolyte Therapy*. Medical Research Foundation of Oregon, 1959.)

from the pH and $[HCO_3^-]_S$. It can also be measured directly with a special electrode.

$[HCO_3^-]_S$

This is determined volumetrically by measuring the total CO_2 evolved from a plasma sample after the addition of lactic acid. Total plasma CO_2 is about 5% higher than $[HCO_3^-]$ because it includes dissolved CO_2.

With automated equipment, $[HCO_3^-]$ is measured as the effect of evolved CO_2 on the color change in a weak phosphate buffer containing phenol red.

II. GENERAL PRINCIPLES OF FLUID & ELECTROLYTE MANAGEMENT

All plans for the repair of fluid and electrolyte distortions are based on calculations first of maintenance requirements and then of volume and qualitative changes (correctional requirements).

MAINTENANCE REQUIREMENTS

Maintenance requirements are the fluids and electrolytes which must be given to maintain homeostasis for the next balance period (usually 24 hours). Predictions must be made for (1) sensible and insensible losses, (2) urinary output, (3) gastrointestinal (or other) losses, and (4) sufficient calories to prevent undue expenditure of the patient's own energy stores.

SENSIBLE & INSENSIBLE LOSSES

Table 35—3 lists approximate sensible and insensible losses. Both sweating and pulmonary losses must be considered.

Sweating

When planning ordinary sensible and insensible losses, no Na^+ is allocated, only free water, since most sweat Na^+ is normally reabsorbed within the duct.

When sweating becomes profuse, the duct's capacity to reabsorb Na^+ is saturated, and sweat is then produced which contains significant amounts of Na^+. Patients with cystic fibrosis have a limited capacity to reabsorb Na^+ in their excretory ducts and may require additional Na^+ to sustain body $[Na^+]$ in the presence of continued heavy sweating.

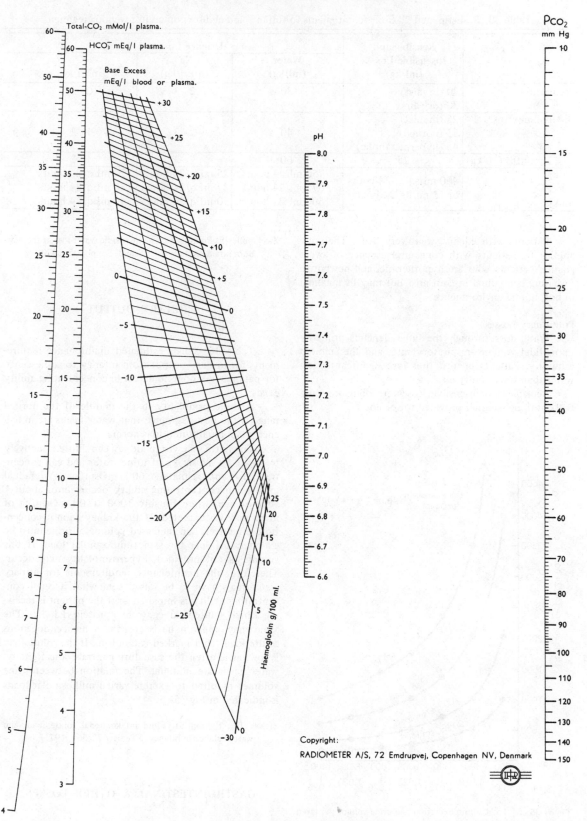

Figure 35–4. Siggaard-Andersen alignment nomogram.
(Reproduced by permission of the copyright holder, Radiometer A/S, Copenhagen.)

Table 35–3. Estimated 24-hour requirements for infants and children on an intravenous regimen.

	Sensible and Insensible Losses (ml/kg)	Urinary Losses		
		Water (ml/kg)	Na⁺ (mEq/kg)	K⁺ (mEq/kg)
Prematures	20 (in mist) 30 (dry air)	30	2–3	0–2
Birth–2 months	25 (in mist) 35 (normal) 45 (hypermetabolic)	40	2–3	1–2
2–12 months (10 kg)	25	60	2–3	1–2
15 kg 30 kg 45 kg	400 ml/sq m/24 hours or 13 ml/kg/24 hours	750 ml/24 hours 1075 ml/24 hours 1500 ml/24 hours	25 mEq/24 hours 37 mEq/24 hours 50 mEq/24 hours	20 mEq/24 hours 30 mEq/24 hours 40 mEq/24 hours

Patients with edema sweat very little. The same applies to patients with congenital absence of sweat glands, patients who are hypothermic, and newborns. Sweating is minimal in cool mist but may be maximal in hot, humid environments.

Pulmonary Losses

Water loss through the lungs depends primarily upon tidal volume, respiratory rate, and the ambient humidity. Patients in mist thus lose significantly less water than those in dry air.

Sensible and insensible losses are obligatory and will continue whether provided for or not.

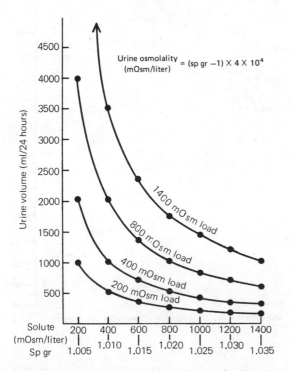

Figure 35–5. Total solute excretion and urine volume per given sp gr. (Redrawn and reproduced, with permission, from Bland JH: *Clinical Recognition and Management of Disturbances of Body Fluids.* Saunders, 1956.)

Zweymuller E, Preining O: The insensible water loss of the newborn infant. Acta Pediatr Scand, Suppl 205, 1970.

URINARY OUTPUT

Table 35–3 lists estimated maintenance requirements for urinary output from infancy to adolescence for patients in whom no defect in concentrating ability exists.

A urine osmolality in the middle of the normal range is the best assurance that water needs are in balance when renal function is normal.

The normal newborn kidney can dilute effectively to about 50 mOsm/kg of urine water and can concentrate to approximately 600 mOsm/kg. A gradual increase in concentrating ability occurs until about 1 year of age, when roughly 1000–1200 mOsm/kg of urine may be excreted. If the kidney cannot concentrate effectively, an increased volume of urine must be excreted to clear the same milliosmolar load. If this volume is not provided, hyperosmolality may occur. Therefore, the maintenance requirements for urinary water may have to be raised somewhat if renal concentrating ability is impaired or if the patient is receiving a high solute load, eg, from a protein-rich diet. The same may apply if he is creating a high endogenous solute load from marked catabolism. If the solute load is low, as is often the case during intravenous therapy, water needs are minimal. The relation between urine volumes required to excrete varied milliosmolar loads is indicated in Fig 35–5.

Ziegler EE, Fomon SJ: Fluid intake, renal solute load, and water balance in infancy. J Pediatr 78:561, 1971.

GASTROINTESTINAL & OTHER LOSSES

The most satisfactory guide for estimating anticipated gastrointestinal losses is the previous day's

Table 35—4. The approximate concentration of electrolytes (mEq/liter) in fluids obtained from the gastrointestinal tract.*

Fluid Type	Sodium	Potassium	Chloride	Total HCO$_3^-$
Stomach	20–120	5–25	90–160	0–5
Duodenal drainage	20–140	3–30	30–120	10–50
Biliary tract	120–160	3–12	70–130	30–50
Small intestine				
Initial drainage	100–140	4–40	60–100	30–100
Established	4–20	4–10	10–100	40–120
Pancreatic	110–160	4–15	30–80	70–130
Diarrheal stool	10–25	10–30	30–120	10–50

*Because of the wide range of normal values, specific analyses are suggested in long-term cases.

volume and trend. This requires that nasogastric fluid, biliary fistula fluid, etc be analyzed for electrolyte composition. However, adjustments always have to be made to adapt to the clinical situation.

For example, patients with ileus or pyloric obstruction may initially be estimated to lose gastric fluid at the rate of 20 ml/kg/24 hours until bowel activity returns. This fluid contains approximately 100 mEq/liter of NaCl and 10 mEq/liter of KCl.

Patients with gastroenteritis may lose large quantities of fluid and electrolytes in diarrheal stools. Nevertheless, the estimate of gastrointestinal losses may be zero, for as soon as patients are sustained intravenously and given nothing by mouth, stooling usually ceases altogether.

Biliary fistulas, intra-abdominal drains, thoracic drains, and even CNS drains occasionally produce obligatory fluid loss that must be taken into account in calculating maintenance requirements.

CALORIES

If maintenance requirements are given as 5% glucose solutions, no additional source of calories need be added provided that such a regimen is not continued for longer than 2–3 days and the patient's caloric needs are not markedly increased, as in salicylate intoxication or the respiratory distress syndrome of prematurity. In these instances, 10% glucose in water may be substituted. Maintenance fluids given as 5% glucose solutions contain few calories, but they provide enough to prevent the patient from being hungry; they exert a substantial protein-sparing effect; and they prevent ketosis. Ordinarily, all intravenous fluids should contain at least 5% glucose. If water restriction is in force, however, insufficient protein-sparing calories will be administered if only 5% glucose is given. Fifteen to 20% glucose may then be used—if need be, with ethyl alcohol. Such solutions rapidly inflame veins and shorten the life of an intravenous site. If oral intake is allowed, cookies and candy may provide excellent therapy.

A special section of this chapter is devoted to the problem of prolonged intravenous alimentation.

Table 35—5 illustrates how 24-hour maintenance requirements are calculated for a 10 kg, 1-year-old child in normal fluid and electrolyte balance. (Data from Table 35—3.)

REPAIR OF EXISTING DEFICITS OR SURPLUSES

Calculations must be designed to correct both volume and qualitative distortions. In theory, adjustments should apply to all the body water compartments; however, knowledge of changes in the intracellular water in disease is limited because of the technical difficulties of measurement. From a practical viewpoint, therefore, correctional changes are applied as extracellular water, and there is experimental evidence that sodium may temporarily substitute for potassium as the main intracellular cation. Clinical response certainly justifies this approach. In making calculations, independent appraisals are made for (1) ECF volume changes and (2) qualitative changes in osmolality, acid-base balance, and electrolyte potassium balance.

Table 35—5. Twenty-four-hour maintenance requirements in a 1-year-old, 10 kg child.

	Fluid		Na$^+$		K$^+$		Cl$^-$	
	ml/kg	ml	mEq/kg	mEq	mEq/kg	mEq	mEq/kg	mEq
Estimated insensible losses	25	250	...	...	...	...	...	...
Estimated urinary losses	60	600	3	30	2	20	5	50
Totals	...	850	...	30	...	20	.	50

I. Changes in the Volume of Body Fluids

EXTRACELLULAR FLUID DEPLETION

Clinical Features

Depletion of ECF, usually due to gastroenteritis, is one of the most common clinical problems in pediatrics. The symptoms and signs vary with the severity of fluid depletion. Skin turgor begins to be lost after 3–5% of the body weight is lost as isotonic ECF. The patient is thirsty, and urinary output is reduced. With a 10% loss of body weight, skin turgor becomes strikingly depressed, the eyes become sunken and soft, the fontanel, if present, is sunken, and the sutures in the skull may become prominent. Pulse rate is increased and pulse volume diminished. Orthostatic hypotension may occur in older children. Fever, oliguria, a dry mouth, diminished tearing, and lethargy are present. The skin, however, is pink, and the capillary refill time is prompt. The hematocrit is elevated. When over 10% of the body weight is lost as ECF, the above signs become more prominent, but the hallmark of this end stage of acute ECF depletion is progressive cardiovascular collapse. Tachycardia increases, pulse volume decreases further, and the skin becomes cool and pale. A peculiar mottling of the skin occurs and is an ominous sign. Osmolality and $[Na^+]_s$ may remain normal up to the time of death.

Treatment

The treatment of ECF depletion is prompt restoration of a normal ECF volume. In severe cases, maintenance of the intravascular volume with plasma, isosmolal albumin solution, dextran, or any other suitable plasma expander takes first priority. Isotonic saline or lactated Ringer's injection may also be given as an interim measure to sustain peripheral circulation.

Once an adequate plasma volume is assured, the objectives of treatment are (1) to ensure a continuing adequate intake of calories, water, and electrolytes for maintenance or to compensate for other special losses; (2) to restore the remaining ECF deficit; and (3) to correct qualitative distortions of ECF homeostasis, such as acidosis and K^+ depletion (see below). The volume deficits may amount to 5–10% of the body weight. Where this is so, an extracellular water-like fluid should be given intravenously rapidly enough to halve the volume deficit in under 2 hours or until skin turgor, sunken eyes, and lethargy are substantially improved. In less severe cases, fluid restoration should be planned in such a way that the volume deficit is half-corrected during the first 8 hours and fully corrected by 24–48 hours.

In severe malnutrition, especially in infants, skin turgor may be markedly depressed in the absence of fluid depletion. Caution should be exercised lest such patients receive needless overexpansion of their ECF compartments.

In shigella dysentery, neurotoxins may cause dramatic lethargy, with eye rolling and stupor in the absence of correspondingly severe signs of ECF depletion. The sodium needs are obviously not determined solely by the state of consciousness.

In patients with cardiac failure, ECF replacement should be achieved more cautiously. In an emergency, fluids may be given intraperitoneally or subcutaneously.

EXTRACELLULAR FLUID EXCESS

The accumulation of excess extracellular water, whether due to retention of water or salt and water or to a proportion shift between ECF and ICF, constitutes edema. The various forms are described below.

Systemic Edema

By the time edema has become manifest, significant ECF excess is already present. Rapid weight gain with no change in $[Na^+]$ indicates accumulation of ECF and may be the only sign available until edema appears. Edema fluid is an ultrafiltrate of plasma, and its presence implies sodium excess.

Edema fluid is mobile and is distributed to the most dependent portions of the body. Children may have periorbital edema upon arising in the morning which disappears in a short time as the edema fluid is redistributed. Paroxysmal nocturnal dyspnea may occur when edema fluid within the legs is added to the circulation upon lying down, giving rise to acute episodes of pulmonary edema. Pulmonary edema is generally the most serious complication of systemic edema.

Edema of Hypoproteinemia

Significant hypoproteinemia (albumin concentration less than about 2 gm/100 ml) is usually accompanied by edema. This comes about in 2 ways. First, inadequate albumin concentrations cause the colloid osmotic pressure of plasma to fall below that necessary to reabsorb fluid filtered from capillaries under hydrostatic pressure. Second, the resulting decrease in plasma volume activates the renin-angiotensin-aldosterone system and increases the renal tubular reabsorption of sodium.

The "Third Space" Phenomenon

A special situation exists when edema fluid is sequestered in a particular location and can no longer readily exchange with the plasma. Such an accumulation of fluid is called a "third space." Examples include ascites, lymphedema, dermal sequestration in burns, and bowel edema in enterocolitis.

In all these instances, the third space must be allowed to form and sufficient isotonic saline or other ECF substitute made available. However, any third space may rapidly return its borrowed sodium to the circulation, as is frequently seen 3–4 days after a severe burn. The resulting volume distortion may be sufficient to cause pulmonary edema.

ICF to ECF Shifts

Occasionally in renal failure, a shift occurs in the distribution of water between extracellular and intracellular fluid, and children will become edematous without any change in total body water.

Treatment

The treatment of ECF excess depends upon whether the edema fluid is generalized or localized (third space) and whether or not serious hypoproteinemia exists (causing "obligate" edema).

Treatment involves the restriction of both dietary and parenteral Na$^+$ and water. A good example is the control of anuric or oliguric renal failure, where dialysis may also be used to control ECF volume. If rapid correction of edema is desired, these diuretics (alone or in combination) may be employed: furosemide (Lasix), 1–2 mg/kg/day; hydrochlorothiazide (Hydro-Diuril), 2 mg/kg/day; and spironolactone (Aldactone), 2 mg/kg/day.

Neither sodium restriction nor diuretic therapy should be used in a patient in otherwise satisfactory fluid balance in order to alleviate a third space. In treating a third space, provide for it when it forms, beware of it when it resolves, and treat its cause whenever possible.

The treatment of edema due to hypoproteinemia usually consists of treatment of the primary disease. Administration of parenteral albumin is rational, but rapid administration is to be avoided lest the plasma volume be overexpanded by a sudden influx of interstitial fluid. Combinations of intravenous protein administration, diuretics (particularly furosemide), and sodium restriction are usually effective but seldom provide more than transient benefit unless protein can ultimately be retained in the plasma.

II. Changes in the Composition of Body Fluids

DISORDERS OF OSMOLALITY

1. HYPONATREMIA

Hyponatremia Due to Water Overload

Patients with normal renal function can ordinarily excrete a sudden water load with relative ease. However, many patients with impaired renal function and virtually all patients with acute renal failure or total obstructive uropathy are unable to tolerate water loading. Such patients are prone to develop hyponatremia with great rapidity and often make this fact known with an unexpected seizure. Treatment consists of water restriction, relief of urinary tract obstruction, and hypertonic saline only to control convulsions.

Hyponatremia With Normal ECW Volume

If a patient receives vasopressin (ADH) either iatrogenically or from inappropriate endogenous secretion, the urine output falls and the urine concentration increases. Thirst is unaffected, and the patient, if allowed access to water, will drink. As water is retained, the serum osmolality and serum sodium concentrations begin to fall. After 1–3 days, sufficient ECF volume expansion has occurred to inhibit aldosterone secretion, and a saline diuresis occurs which normalizes the ECF volume but leaves the osmolality and serum sodium concentration low. Administration of isotonic or hypertonic saline may result in transient rises of $[Na^+]_S$ but is quickly followed by brisk saline diuresis. Restriction of water can prevent this and will rectify the situation once it has developed.

The most common cause of this disorder is inappropriate secretion of vasopressin in the face of a normal ECF volume. Vasopressin is secreted in a variety of intracranial diseases, including tumors, head injuries, hydrocephalus, and meningitis. It also occurs with a variety of intrathoracic disorders varying from pneumonia to cystic fibrosis. Drugs such as barbiturates, ether, morphine, and histamine may have this effect, and strong emotional stress, rage, fear, and pain, as well as surgery, occasionally initiate this inappropriate chain of events.

Hyponatremia is seldom associated with significant signs or symptoms until Na$^+$ concentrations fall below 120 mEq/liter. If hyponatremia develops gradually, anorexia, apathy, and mild nausea and vomiting may be the only symptoms. If it develops rapidly, headache, mental confusion, muscular twitching, eventual delirium, and, finally, convulsions occur. The signs and symptoms are related almost as much to the rate at which the hyponatremia developed as to the severity achieved. Extremely low Na$^+$ concentrations (90–110 mEq/liter) invariably cause CNS dysfunction but are not incompatible with either survival or recovery. CNS dysfunction due to rapid onset hypo-osmolality is sometimes called water intoxication.

Treatment consists of water restriction. Administration of isotonic or hypertonic saline solution results in overexpansion of the ECF. Hypertonic saline should be reserved for severe water intoxication with frank CNS disturbance. An occasional patient is helped by administration of ethanol, 7% solution, 20 ml/kg/24 hours, to inhibit ADH secretion.

Hyponatremia With Diminished ECW Volume

Depletion of the ECF in gastroenteritis, vomiting, adrenal insufficiency, renal salt-losing states, diabetic ketoacidosis, etc calls into play a number of mechanisms which act to protect plasma volume. Aldosterone conserves Na$^+$, thirst prompts the patient to drink, renin and catecholamines help to maintain blood pressure, and decreased glomerular filtration rate enhances both Na^+ and water resorption. In addition to the above, vasopressin is secreted, and as a result the organism will conserve water alone to maintain an adequate plasma volume at a lower than normal osmolality, if necessary. In the presence of a lowered ECF volume, renal clearance of free water (C_{H_2O}) is strikingly impaired. Thus, even though the organism is hypo-osmolal, excess water is now conserved. Rigid restriction of water will cause severe oliguria and will tend to normalize the osmolality, but it is poor treatment for the patient. If water alone is made available to the patient, he will drink water when sodium is needed.

The signs and symptoms are those typical of ECF depletion, ie, thirst, tenting skin, dehydrated appearance, dry mucous membranes, tachycardia, and oliguria.

Therapy is directed toward restoring a normal ECF volume by the administration of normal ECF-like fluids. This is usually associated with a water diuresis from the ICF compartment and rapid resolution of the hyponatremic state. If the hyponatremia is severe, correction of ECF depletion by saline may be combined with free water restriction.

Hyponatremia With Expanded ECW Volume

This type of hyponatremia is by far the most serious and most difficult to treat. The presence of hyponatremia in combination with edema implies that the osmoregulatory mechanisms have been reset at a lower level. It occurs with severe heart failure, liver disease, renal failure, or occasionally CNS disease. If the underlying circulatory disturbance can be corrected, hyponatremia with edema usually resolves spontaneously. These patients may have gross edema and therefore a high total body Na^+ content.

The signs and symptoms are overshadowed by those of the underlying disease. Edema is obvious, and both the $[Na^+]$ and osmolality are low.

Vigorous water restriction should be instituted despite complaints of thirst.

The Dysequilibrium Syndrome

Any sudden reduction in serum osmolality—as, for example, in acute intravenous water overloading, in too rapid dialysis, or with overly prompt reduction of glucose levels in diabetic acidosis—will produce an osmotic gradient between the intracalvarial and other extracellular fluid spaces. Water will move into the brain quicker than sodium moves out, leading to acute nausea, vomiting, headaches, and convulsions.

Artifactual Hyponatremia

Plasma ordinarily contains about 93% water and 7% solids. The serum sodium concentration may be affected by the amount of solid present. Marked hyperproteinemia or hyperlipidemia may thus cause falsely low serum sodium concentrations. Osmolality, as determined by freezing point depression, is not significantly affected by this phenomenon. In children this is most common in diabetes and nephrotic syndrome.

2. HYPERNATREMIA

Hypernatremia always implies a deficit of water with respect to solute throughout the entire body. Therefore, it always indicates hyperosmolality. It may arise primarily from too little water or too much solute but is usually due to a combination of both. Hypernatremia is said to exist whenever the $[Na^+]_S$ exceeds 148 mEq/liter. Values over 160 mEq/liter are serious, yet patients have survived $[Na^+]_S$ in excess of 190 mEq/liter. Serious hypernatremia frequently causes intracerebral bleeding, brain damage, and subsequent mental retardation, convulsions, and death.

Hypernatremia Due to Primary Inability to Maintain Normal Body Water Content

A. Inadequate Water Intake: Patients who are denied access to water (or are unable to retain water, as in diabetes insipidus) are at risk of developing hypernatremia. Renal water conservation becomes extreme, but sensible and insensible water losses through the skin and lungs are unavoidable and, if continued, may cause hypernatremia. Unconscious or mentally retarded patients are unable to communicate thirst and may develop water deficiency hypernatremia in spite of normal osmoregulatory capability.

B. Defective Osmoregulation: Tumors in or near the anterior hypothalamus, the third ventricle, or the cerebral aqueduct and certain other lesions associated with noncommunicating hydrocephalus may destroy the perception of thirst.

Patients with hypothalamic or hypophyseal diabetes insipidus, although generally thirst-perceptive, are at risk of developing hypernatremia if denied access to water or overloaded with solute.

Also at risk are patients with nephrogenic (vasopressin-resistant) diabetes insipidus and those with chronic hypercalciuria or chronic hypokalemia, both of which cause a vasopressin-resistant clinical picture similar to diabetes insipidus. In recovery from acute tubular necrosis, a water-losing state may exist.

C. Extrarenal Water Loss: Large sensible and insensible water losses occurring through the skin and lungs may predispose to hypernatremia. Patients with burns over large areas, prolonged high fevers, heat exhaustion (occasionally), hyperpnea due to diabetic ketoacidosis or salicylism, and patients with tracheostomies are all at risk.

Hypernatremia Due to Primary Salt Overloading

Salt overloading most commonly occurs when salt is accidentally used instead of sugar in making up the formula. In severe cases, the symptoms, signs, and treatment are the same as in hypertonic dehydration.

If the mistake is detected early in an otherwise healthy infant, serum sodium levels may be restored by giving hydrochlorothiazide, 2 mg/kg/24 hours for 1 or 2 days. Peritoneal dialysis has also been used.

Hypernatremia Due to Water Loss in the Presence of Solute Gain

A. Hypernatremia Due to Infantile Diarrhea: This type of hypernatremia begins by lowering the ECF volume. The usual mechanisms of sodium and water conservation (thirst, vasopressin secretion, and aldosterone secretion) are called into play. If the patient is fed a high sodium load, hypernatremia may develop.

B. Hypernatremia Due to Large Solute Loads: The solute load required to produce hypernatremia need not be particularly rich in NaCl. Tube feeding of protein-rich foods to an unconscious patient or an infant creates a heavy solute load for renal excretion and results in an osmotic diuresis with the loss of much more water than salt. Hypernatremia may quickly follow if additional water is not provided. Chronic glycosuria in uncontrolled diabetes mellitus occasionally leads to hypernatremia in this fashion, as does overzealous therapy with mannitol or the absorption of the breakdown products of a gastrointestinal hemorrhage.

The signs and symptoms are referable to CNS dysfunction. Irritability, twitching, mental confusion, stupor, irregular respirations, frank convulsions, and eventually coma may occur. Thirst is severe, but the patient may be unable to swallow solid foods owing to the dryness of his mucosa. Weight loss may amount to 20–25% of body weight. There may be moderate fever due to lack of substrate with which to sweat.

Skin turgor may be normal, but the skin often feels "doughy" and inelastic. Subcutaneous fat may feel stiff or unusually firm. Pulse and blood pressure are usually normal. The hemoglobin tends to rise, MCV decreases, and the hematocrit changes little. BUN may be greatly elevated (> 100 mg/100 ml). Red cells, hyaline and granular casts, and protein appear in the urine.

Treatment consists of restoring deficits in ECW with isotonic solutions followed by slow, careful reduction of the $[Na^+]_S$ at a rate that should not exceed 15 mEq/24 hours. This is best accomplished by administering solutions which contain sodium concentrations about 60 mEq less than the patient's $[Na^+]_S$, with the rate of administration being governed by frequent laboratory determinations of $[Na^+]_S$. The $[Na^+]_S$ should never be lowered rapidly because doing so may precipitate convulsions. The administration of hypertonic saline solution may be helpful if convulsions do occur.

Patients with hypernatremia frequently have metabolic acidosis. Rapid alkalinization with sodium bicarbonate should not be attempted unless the acidemia is severe, since alkalinization enhances CNS irritability. Hypocalcemia commonly accompanies hypernatremia, although the reason for it is not clear. Therapy with calcium is, however, seldom necessary.

Lastly, not all patients with hyperosmolality have hypernatremia. The presence of large quantities of glucose may osmotically draw water into the plasma from the cells. The presence in the blood of 100 mg/100 ml of glucose is approximately equivalent to 3 mEq/liter added to the $[Na^+]_S$. A patient with a blood glucose concentration of 800 mg/100 ml and a $[Na^+]_S$ of 140 mEq/liter thus has about the same osmolality as a patient with a $[Na^+]_S$ of 156 mEq/liter. These changes are a complication of intravenous alimentation. Urea also contributes to osmolality, and uremia is frequently associated with a hyperosmolal state. However, because urea readily crosses cell membranes, shrinkage of the ICF volume does not occur.

Finberg L: Hypernatremia (hypertonic) dehydration in infants. N Engl J Med 289:196, 1973.

POTASSIUM DISORDERS

Physiology

The total body potassium (TBK^+) of a 20 kg child is normally about 900 mEq. Roughly 20 mEq of this is in extracellular fluid; the remainder is intracellular. The $[TBK^+]$ has been measured by whole cadaver analysis and by counting the naturally occurring $^{40}K^+$ in whole body counters in "background-free" rooms. Ninety to 95% of the total body K^+ is more or less freely exchangeable, and this quantity, the "exchangeable K^+," may be assessed by following the 24- to 48-hour dilutional distribution of an injection of $^{40}K^+$ or $^{42}K^+$. Tissue $[K^+]$ may be investigated in muscle biopsy specimens, but such studies require rather broad inferences in their interpretation. $[K^+]_S$ is the only simple potassium determination available in most laboratories and is usually the only direct assessment of $[K^+]$ available to the physician. Red blood cell $[K^+]$ does not reflect total body or intracellular $[K^+]$.

The preponderance of K^+ lies within cells—about 60% of it specifically within skeletal muscle cells. Expressed as $[K^+]$/kg body weight, $[TBK^+]$ correlates well with total body water, lean body mass, and fatfree dry solid. The correlation of $[TBK^+]$ with weight falls off in obese patients and in those with malnutrition due to starvation or wasting illness. Postpubertal females tend to have less $[K^+]$/kg of body weight than postpubertal males, owing chiefly to differences in total body fat content. Neonates contain roughly 35–40 mEq/kg, a value which increases gradually to 50–55 mEq/kg in adult males and changes little throughout life in females.

Maintenance of normal $[K^+]_S$ is primarily dependent upon the Na^+-K^+ pump at the cell membrane. The normal skeletal muscle $[K^+]$ approximates 150–160 mEq/liter cell water. For comparison, in extracellular fluid the $[K^+]$ is normally only 4.5–5 mEq/liter.

The second most important regulator of $[K^+]$ is the kidney. The normal kidney is able to excrete a large load of K^+ but is poorly equipped to conserve K^+ on short notice. A massive crush injury which damages the integrity of large numbers of cell membranes and causes renal shutdown due to myoglobinuria and shock is, as might be expected, one of the quickest ways to dangerously elevate the $[K^+]_S$.

The distribution of K^+ between ICF and ECF is dependent upon ECF pH. Alkalemia promotes entry of K^+ into cells and lowers $[K^+]_S$. Acidemia, on the other hand, promotes exit of K^+ from cells and may raise $[K^+]_S$ if renal K^+ excretion lags behind. Nevertheless, the presence of symptoms or ECG changes (see below) which are referable to a potassium disturbance should always be taken seriously regardless of whether or not acid-base abnormalities are, in part, responsible.

When glycogen deposition occurs, K^+ enters cells and the serum level tends to fall. This is one of the factors explaining the low $[K^+]_S$ seen in diabetics following institution of insulin therapy. The Na^+-K^+ pump requires energy in the form of ATP. Uncoupling of oxidative phosphorylation, therefore, evokes rises in $[K^+]_S$.

$[K^+]_S$ may be raised artifactually in a number of ways. Hemolysis of red cells occurring between the time of sampling and centrifuging is well known and requires that blood drawn for $[K^+]_S$ determination be handled gently. Elevations of $[K^+]_S$ in patients with acute intravenous hemolysis are more difficult to evaluate. Storing of blood samples on ice (without freezing) is followed by rises in $[K^+]_S$. Blood with a grossly elevated leukocyte count (as in leukemia) may show artifactual elevations in $[K^+]_S$ due to damage of the leukocytes during clotting. Platelets are also rich in K^+, and thrombocythemic blood samples may show hyperkalemia if clotting is allowed to occur. The simple alternative is to do $[K^+]$ determinations on fresh plasma rather than serum.

Renal Aspects of [K⁺] Control

Under normal circumstances, the K^+ filtered by the glomerular membrane is mostly reabsorbed in the proximal tubule. Most of the potassium excreted is the product of distal tubular secretion. The quantity secreted by the distal tubular cells appears to result from an exchange with Na^+ from the distal tubular urine.

The amount of K^+ secreted also appears to depend on there being an adequate amount of Cl^- (or other directly reabsorbable anion) in the glomerular filtrate.

This may be more clearly understood by considering 2 glomerular filtrates: one contains 130, 105, and 25 mEq/liter of Na^+, Cl^-, and HCO_3^-, respectively. The other contains only 85 mEq/liter of Cl^- plus 20 mEq/liter of nonreabsorbable anion (A^-). In the first filtrate, 105 mEq of Na^+ are resorbed by active transport and at the same time 105 mEq Cl^- are resorbed passively to maintain electroneutrality. The 25 mEq/liter of $NaHCO_3$ are also absorbed (see p 493). All the Na^+ has now been resorbed. In the second filtrate only 85 mEq of NaCl may be resorbed, leaving 25 mEq of $NaHCO_3$ and 20 mEq of NaA. A 25 mEq/liter H^+ exchange for Na^+ occurs as before, but further H^+ secretion will now meet with an increasing H^+ gradient so that K^+ rather than H^+ will be exchanged for Na^+ across the inner tubule membrane. Tubular

potassium loss is thus proportionate to the tubular content of nonreabsorbable anion. It is for this reason that potassium losses should be replaced as potassium chloride and not with some salt such as potassium gluconate.

If dietary K^+ intake is totally curtailed, K^+ excretion will continue, decreasing only gradually for 2–3 weeks, by which time a significant negative K^+ balance will exist. The finding of a lowered urinary $[K^+]$ strongly implies that a K^+ depleted state exists and virtually excludes a renal K^+ wasting condition as the cause.

A number of factors enhance the renal secretion of K^+. Hypochloremia (eg, due to vomiting, prolonged nasogastric suction, $AgNO_3^+$ treatment of burns, chloriduria or diuretic therapy) has been mentioned. Adrenal corticosteroids, by causing renal retention of Na^+, increase the quantity of Na^+ reaching the distal tubules and invoke wastage of K^+. If dietary Na^+ intake is minimized, corticosteroid-induced K^+ loss ceases. Diuretics of many types—in particular, thiazides, mercurials, and acetazolamide—effectively enhance the secretion of K^+.

Potassium Depletion

When 10–20% of the TBK^+ of the patient has been lost, symptoms of apathy and muscular weakness ensue. Paresthesias and tetany are occasionally seen. If the depletion worsens, the muscular weakness extends to a flaccid paralysis, eventually interfering with respiration. Extracellular replacement of K^+ may suffice to bring about dramatic but temporary relief from the muscular disability of K^+ depletion, but only as long as the K^+-containing infusion is running.

During serious K^+ depletion, typical ECG changes occur. These include T wave depression, the appearance of a U wave, and eventually ST segment depression. The Q–T interval may appear prolonged if a Q–U interval is mistakenly measured instead. A number of arrhythmias occur (Fig 35–6).

In the kidney, concentrating ability is impaired and a clinical picture similar to that of diabetes insipidus is produced which gives rise, occasionally, to hypernatremia. Tubular degeneration is seen on renal biopsy. Of the effects of hypokalemia, this is the slowest to resolve after proper therapy, and 2–3 weeks may be required for restoration of normal renal function. K^+ depletion also predisposes to digitalis intoxication, and a $[K^+]_S$ determination is always indicated when digitalis toxicity exists.

The treatment of K^+ depletion is to restore a $[K^+]_S$ sufficient to dispel any signs of muscular weakness or ECG abnormalities and to return the $[TBK^+]$ to normal. Such replacement may require several days.

Chronic K^+ depletion frequently complicates hypochloremic metabolic alkalosis. Until the Cl^- deficiency is corrected, administered K^+ continues to be wasted. The administration of KCl, therefore, corrects both the metabolic alkalosis and the K^+ depletion at the same time. The administration of K^+ with virtually any other anion (see above) effectively corrects neither. A variety of K^+-containing foods and juices provide excellent oral

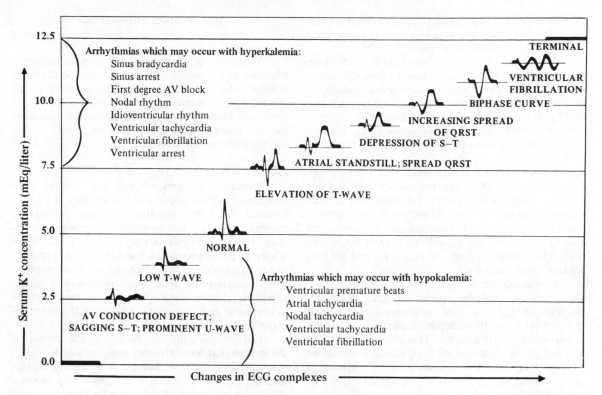

Figure 35—6. Rough correlation between $[K^+]_S$ and the ECG. In hyperkalemia, the cardiotoxicity at a given $[K^+]_S$ becomes more marked by a decrease of $[Na^+]_S$. Thus, with severe hyponatremia, far-advanced cardiotoxicity may be seen with a $[K^+]_S$ of 7.5 mg/liter. (Reproduced, with permission, from Krupp MA, Chatton MJ [editors] : *Current Medical Diagnosis & Treatment 1974.* Lange, 1974.)

medication for this purpose (Table 35—6).

Changes in pH effect changes in the distribution of K^+ between intracellular and extracellular fluid. Acidemia causes K^+ to leave cells and enter the ECW, raising the $[K^+]_S$. Alkalemia causes the reverse. A normal $[K^+]_S$ in the presence of acidemia, therefore, suggests that K^+ depletion exists and that rapid correction of pH may be followed by a brisk fall in $[K^+]_S$. This is commonly seen during correction of diabetic ketoacidosis and acidosis which attends diarrhea. The deposition of glycogen also sequesters substantial amounts of K^+ in such instances.

Up to 5 mEq/kg/24 hours of additional KCl may be given to infants and small children as a correctional measure (in addition to maintenance K^+); 1—2 mEq/kg/24 hours may be given to older children. As K^+ depletion is corrected, the amount and especially the rate of administration should be lowered lest hyperkalemia occur. Actually, intravenous K^+ therapy in excess of that required for maintenance is not necessary to relieve symptoms of K^+ depletion; therefore, K^+ depletion should be treated without haste.

All intravenous K^+ should be evenly infused throughout the 24-hour balance period. If concentrations of K^+ greater than 40 mEq/liter are present in any bottle of intravenous solution, there should be a maximum rate and laboratory control. Concentrated K^+ solution must never be given by intravenous "push."

Hyperkalemia

The symptoms and signs of hyperkalemia are few. They include muscle weakness and, occasionally, tetany or paresthesias with ascending central paralysis. The major toxic symptoms and signs are cardiac in origin. ECG changes include tenting and then elevation of T waves, spreading of the QRS complex, atrial arrest, and, finally, a sine wave followed by ventricular fibrillation and death. These changes, with their attendant arrhythmias, are shown in Fig 35—6.

The extent of treatment required depends upon

Table 35—6. Juices high in potassium.

	Approximate Content*	
	mEq	mg
Apple juice	2.5	100
Apricot juice	2.4	94
Pineapple juice	3.5	140
Grape juice	3	120
Grapefruit juice	4	150
Orange juice	5	190
Prune juice	6.5	260
Tomato juice	6	230

*½ cup quantities (120 ml)

the severity of the hyperkalemia, the ECG findings, the electrolyte profile of the serum, and the predicted behavior of the underlying disorder.

Ordinarily, $[K^+]_S$ values less than 6.5 mEq/liter require little more than curtailment of all K^+ intake. However, such levels might cause serious concern if, for example, QRS complex widening were noted, if the $[Na^+]_S$ were low, if alkalemia existed, if a previous value indicated a sharp rate of rise of $[K^+]_S$, if acute renal failure had occurred, or if digitalis toxicity were evident.

Serious hyperkalemia (levels greater than 8 mEq/liter) or serious ECG changes (widened QRS complexes, heart block, ventricular arrhythmias, etc) warrant vigorous measures. These are aimed at accomplishing 4 objectives: (1) counteracting the depolarization of cardiac muscle, (2) shifting K^+ from serum into cells, (3) ridding the body of excess K^+, and (4) preventing tissue catabolism.

Depolarization of cardiac muscle may be effectively counteracted for several minutes by administration of Ca^{++}. A slow intravenous infusion of 0.2–0.5 ml/kg of 10% calcium gluconate is given over a period of 2–10 minutes. The infusion should be stopped at the first sign of bradycardia. It should be stressed that while Ca^{++} infusion may be lifesaving, it has no effect on $[K^+]_S$ and its cardiac effects are of brief duration.

K^+ may be shifted into cells by administration of sodium in high amounts, by raising the pH with HCO_3^-, and by promoting the deposition of intracellular glycogen with glucose. $NaHCO_3$ is usually marketed in hypertonic form in ampules which contain 44.6 mEq/50 ml. One to 3 ml/kg (at ampule strength) is given over a 5- to 20-minute time span by intravenous infusion. Ten to 20% glucose solutions may also be infused over 30–60 minutes at a dose of 1 gm/kg body weight. The effects of these measures may persist for several hours.

K^+ may be removed from the body by oral or rectal administration of ion exchange resins in their Na^+ or Ca^{++} cycles. For example, 0.2 gm/kg of sodium polystyrene sulfonate (Kayexalate) is mixed with 3–4 ml of water or syrup per gram of resin and given orally or by intragastric tube; or 1 gm/kg of resin is mixed into a loose slurry with water and administered as a well mixed retention enema into the sigmoid or descending colon, where it is held for 4–8 hours and then flushed out with isotonic saline solution. In an emergency $[K^+]_S$ may be rapidly lowered by the administration of insulin, 0.25 unit/kg subcutaneously, or 0.1 unit/kg intravenously. Each unit of insulin should be covered by 3 gm of glucose given orally or intravenously.

Peritoneal dialysis—or, preferably, hemodialysis—may be used to rid the body of K^+ but only at some increased risk and a significant cost in time.

The administration of maximal calories is of great value in minimizing tissue catabolism.

Lastly, whenever hyperkalemia occurs, stop the administration of all oral and parenteral K^+.

MAGNESIUM DISORDERS

Magnesium is the fourth most abundant cation in the body and is second only to potassium in the intracellular water and soft tissues. Approximately 1/2 of the total body magnesium is contained in bone; the remainder exists primarily in the intracellular water of the soft tissues, where it acts as a cofactor in a wide spectrum of enzymic reactions.

Clinical Findings

Clinically, hypomagnesemia can present with muscular weakness and wasting, irritability, a positive Chvostek sign with a negative Trousseau sign, vertigo, tremors, and, in the newborn especially, convulsions. Hypomagnesemia (serum levels < 1 mEq/liter) is seen in the newborn as a familial condition or with hypoparathyroidism; in older infants and children, with malabsorption syndromes, protein-calorie malnutrition, chronic renal disease, and renal tubular dystrophies; and in diabetic acidosis and hyperparathyroidism.

Hypermagnesemia may be seen in the newborn if the mother has been given magnesium sulfate and in older children in renal failure. It is usually asymptomatic, but levels of over 6 mEq/liter may produce drowsiness and levels of over 10 mEq/liter may cause respiratory failure and heart block.

Treatment

Hypomagnesemia can be treated by administering 2 mEq/kg (0.5 ml $MgSO_4$, 50% w/v aqueous solution USP) twice daily IM. Oral therapy can be sustained initially by 3 mEq/kg/daily. Magnesium gluconate, 42 gm/liter w/v, will give 1 mEq/5 ml.

Hypermagnesemia only requires treatment in renal failure, where, at levels > 7 mEq/liter, it would justify dialysis.

Niklasson E: Familial early hypoparathyroidism associated with hypomagnesemia. Acta Pediatr Scand 59:715, 1970.

O'Brien D: Treatment of magnesium deficiency in childhood. In: Gellis SS, Kagan BM: *Current Pediatric Therapy 7.* Saunders, 1976.

Stromme JH: Familial hypomagnesemia. Acta Pediatr Scand 58:433, 1969.

ACID-BASE DISORDERS

1. CHRONIC RESPIRATORY ACIDOSIS

Chronic respiratory acidosis involves a gradual impairment of the rate of CO_2 removal by the lungs, with a consequent trend to low blood pH. It can arise with normal lungs as a result of CNS damage or when skeletal or chest wall deformities prevent normal lung volume changes during the respiratory cycle. More typically, chronic respiratory acidosis results from primary pulmonary disease.

Disease entities in which chronic respiratory acidosis is seen include bulbar poliomyelitis, advanced muscular dystrophy, polymyositis, osteogenesis imperfecta, rickets, chronic severe asthma, and cystic fibrosis.

Clinically, the patient is dyspneic, shows peripheral cyanosis with clubbing of the fingernails, and may be uncooperative, disagreeable, depressed, and occasionally confused. Laboratory data typically show pH values only slightly below normal (7.27–7.35). The P_{CO_2} is, by definition, abnormally high, and base excess values are significantly elevated above normal (+3 to +15 mEq/liter). The elevated base excess values derive from augmented renal conservation of HCO_3^-, a so-called "compensatory mechanism" which acts to prevent dangerous depressions in pH.

Treatment

Treatment consists of correcting the ventilatory problem to the fullest possible degree, making sure that adequate oxygenation is achieved, and occasionally providing sufficient quantities of $NaHCO_3$ to effect near-complete compensation, ie, to normalize the pH in the presence of an abnormally high P_{CO_2}. Na^+ administration should be carefully controlled in the presence of cardiovascular complications.

2. ACUTE RESPIRATORY ACIDOSIS

Acute respiratory acidosis involves an abruptly developing retention of CO_2 and consequent H_2CO_3 elevation, as a result of which blood pH may fall abruptly. Acute respiratory acidosis can result from a variety of causes: perfusion failure (due to cardiac arrest, ventricular fibrillation), respiratory failure (due to CNS damage, poliomyelitis), upper airway obstruction (due to croup, epiglottitis, aspiration of foreign body), lower airway obstruction (due to asthma, aspiration of vomitus), and ventilation/perfusion disturbances (due to hyaline membrane disease).

Clinically, the patient is acutely air hungry; chest wall retraction may be evident; accessory muscles of respiration may be in use; and the patient is commonly dusky or frankly cyanotic.

Laboratory data include an elevated P_{CO_2}; a lowered arterial blood pH, occasionally to levels below 7.0; and a variable depression in base excess which usually ranges from −5 to −15 mEq/liter. The acidemia results directly from acute hypercapnia.

A greater hypobasemia is observed in premature and newborn infants with acute respiratory acidosis. This is chiefly because prematures have larger ISF volumes (on a percentage basis) than older children and adults.

Treatment

The management of acute respiratory acidosis depends upon the underlying cause. In cases due to acute upper airway obstruction, relief of the obstruction may be the only measure required. If it is impossible to correct the lesion, adequate ventilation should be provided by mouth-to-mouth resuscitation, mechanical ventilation, etc. If artificial ventilation is not feasible, therapy with buffer base may be started. The buffer base of choice is $NaHCO_3$, and whenever possible it is given until the blood pH has been restored to normal. This is frequently impossible when the P_{CO_2} has risen above about 70 mm Hg owing to the intolerably large Na^+ loads required. Most authorities feel that the hazards of rapid correction are significant and recommend several hours of $NaHCO_3$ infusion to alleviate acute acidemia of respiratory origin. $NaHCO_3$ should not be administered as it comes from ampules but diluted to near isosmolality (150 mEq/liter).

3. RESPIRATORY ALKALOSIS

Respiratory alkalosis is characterized by hyperventilation which lowers the P_{CO_2} below normal and thereby tends to raise the pH of blood above normal. The hyperventilation is nearly always the result of abnormal CNS stimulation and thus is usually seen in one of 3 clinical settings: hysterical hyperventilation, salicylate or salicylamide poisoning, or irritative CNS disorders such as meningitis and encephalitis.

Clinically, the patient may experience paresthesias about the fingers, toes, and lips. He may complain of dizziness, faintness, palpitations, heart pain, and even a band-like feeling about the chest. Hypocalcemic tetany is occasionally observed, and susceptible patients may have convulsions. Hyperventilation is usually apparent, and in salicylate intoxication this may mimic the Kussmaul respirations seen in diabetic ketoacidosis.

Laboratory data are helpful. The P_{CO_2} is depressed, occasionally to levels as low as 10 or 15 mm Hg. Arterial pH values above 7.65 are sometimes reported. Acutely, the base excess tends to be normal or slightly low. With greater chronicity (several days), base excess values as low as −15 mEq/liter may be observed. Whether such depressions in base excess derive from a compensatory process is not known, although hypocapnia stimulates red cells to produce abnormally large quantities of lactic acid.

Treatment

The management of respiratory alkalosis depends upon the disorder. If hysterical hyperventilation is the cause, simple rebreathing into a paper bag followed by administration of tranquilizers or psychotherapy (or both) usually suffices. If the disorder is caused by salicylate intoxication, management consists of suitable fluid and electrolyte administration to enhance excretion of the drug. If the patient is younger than about 5 years of age, metabolic acidosis with significant acidemia may soon supervene. Accordingly, zealous treatment of respiratory alkalosis due to salicylate intoxication is seldom practiced. Prolonged irritative CNS lesions may require administration of 2–4% CO_2. Apparatus designed to increase dead space or to allow partial rebreathing may be helpful. Careful laboratory monitoring of acid-base values is essential. The most effective therapy is usually directed at the underlying lesion.

4. METABOLIC ACIDOSIS

Metabolic acidosis is that primary pathophysiologic process which tends to lower the pH of blood by causing abnormal production or retention of strong nonvolatile acid or by enhancing the loss of buffer base.

A wide variety of illnesses are associated with metabolic acidosis. Abnormal acid production is seen, eg, in diabetic or starvational ketoacidosis, lactic acidosis due to tissue hypoxia or metabolic poisoning, and ingestion of a large number of acidic or acidogenic products such as NH_4Cl, ethylene glycol, etc. Diminished acid excretion is seen in renal failure, primary renal tubular dystrophies of several kinds, and in renal hypoperfusion due to dehydration, shock, and other causes. Abnormal base loss causes metabolic acidosis in occasional diarrheal states (especially cholera) in which the stools are strongly alkaline. Biliary fistulas and certain HCO_3^- wasting nephropathies also produce metabolic acidosis by this route.

Regardless of the route, the clinical and laboratory pictures are similar. There is significant hypobasemia. Base excess values as low as -23 mEq/liter are occasionally encountered. There is usually a brisk compensatory hyperventilation, but compensation is seldom, if ever, complete. Arterial blood pH values lower than 7.0 are sometimes found.

Treatment

Management consists of the administration of $NaHCO_3$ and appropriate treatment of the underlying disorder. There is no advantage to using lactate, phosphate, citrate, or tromethamine instead of $NaHCO_3$. Once the pH approaches 7.25 or 7.30, then the rate of correction may be tapered. The compensatory hyperventilation which usually attends serious metabolic acidosis ordinarily requires 1–2 days to abate once hypobasemia has been resolved. If full correction of hypobasemia is undertaken in the first few hours of treatment, a transient (though seldom severe) respiratory alkalosis may occur. As usual, acid-base therapy is directed toward achieving a blood pH of 7.40 and then keeping the pH at that level.

In most cases, the objective is to correct the base excess in extracellular fluid within 24 hours. The dose of $NaHCO_3$ is calculated according to the following formula:

Dose of $NaHCO_3$ (mEq) = 0.3 × body weight (kg) × base excess. This formula usually provides a dose of bicarbonate that fully corrects the negative base excess if given on 2 successive days.

When calculating the total daily requirement, equivalent amounts of sodium and chloride must be deducted from maintenance or replacement solutions.

5. METABOLIC ALKALOSIS

Metabolic alkalosis is caused by losses of excessive quantities of strong, nonvolatile acid or excessive gains of buffer base. The most frequent cause of metabolic alkalosis is loss of gastric fluid (HCl) via nasogastric tube or vomiting. Vomiting due to pyloric obstruction (eg, pyloric stenosis) is especially prone to cause metabolic alkalosis since the acidic emesis fluid is not contaminated with pancreatic (alkaline) fluid.

Any condition which selectively depletes the patient of Cl^- is prone to cause a metabolic alkalosis in which hypokalemia, hypochloremia, hyperkaluria, and paradoxical aciduria are prominent features. Besides vomiting and nasogastric suction, diuretics, silver nitrate treatment of burns, and certain chronic diarrheas ("chloridorrheas") are well known causes.

Likewise, any condition which selectively conserves Na^+ without selectively conserving Cl^- results in the same syndrome, the only difference being a normal $[Cl^-]_S$. Examples include Calcagno's syndrome, adrenal 11β-hydroxylase deficiency, and certain juxtamedullary tumors of the kidney.

The laboratory picture is classical and consists of elevated blood pH, elevated base excess, and normal to very slightly elevated P_{CO_2}. Respiratory compensation appears to be limited, however, by oxygen need. A common denominator underlies most cases of metabolic alkalosis, viz, a widened gap between $[Na^+]_S$ and $[Cl^-]_S$ (see p 1000).

Treatment

The mainstay of management is the administration of Cl^-. A common misconception exists that K^+ is essential to treat the alkalosis. This is now known not to be so. Cl^-, as NaCl, KCl, or NH_4Cl, will correct the alkalosis. K^+ plus Cl^- is required to repair the K^+ depletion. Potassium gluconate, acetate, citrate, and bicarbonate have all been shown to be ineffective in treating either the K^+ depletion or the metabolic alkalosis.

PLANNING & ADMINISTRATION OF INTRAVENOUS FLUIDS

WRITING INTRAVENOUS FLUID ORDERS

Once maintenance and correctional requirements have been calculated and combined into 24-hour totals, intravenous fluid orders may be written. Some rounding-off of numbers is permissible in older children, but small infants should receive intravenous fluids almost exactly as calculated. Unless emergency considerations dictate otherwise, the 24-hour totals are evenly administered over a 24-hour balance period. The necessity for regular review of fluid orders in the light of clinical changes and ongoing laboratory data cannot be overestimated.

The sequence number and composition of each bottle should be stated in the orders and on the bottles themselves.

It is preferable that intravenous infusions for small children be constituted in a number of small bottles rather than a single large one. If 24-hour totals are mixed in a single bottle and then delivered to the patient by way of a smaller increment chamber (eg, Pedatrol or Metriset), then a hemostat should be placed between the large reservoir bottle and the increment chamber. As a general rule, quantities exceeding 150 ml should not be connected to children under 2 years of age, nor should quantities greater than 250 ml be connected to children under 5, nor quantities greater than 500 ml to children under 10.

All orders for intravenous fluids should contain specific instructions regarding the rate of infusion for each bottle. It is convenient to use a microdrop apparatus which delivers 60 drops/ml. When this is done, microdrops/minute equals ml/hour, and the rate of infusion may be readily calculated. A number of calibrated intravenous pumps are in use. Bottles containing K^+ should contain instructions regarding the maximum rate of infusion lest a nurse fall behind schedule and try to catch up.

All orders for intravenous fluid therapy should be accompanied by orders to record careful daily weights and intake and output.

All output, whether gastric fluid or urine, should be saved and measured at the end of each therapy period. All empty or partly emptied intravenous fluid bottles should also be saved for the duration of each period.

ROUTES OF PARENTERAL FLUID ADMINISTRATION

A variety of routes other than the intravenous one are available for administration of parenteral fluids. These include hypodermoclysis, proctoclysis, and the intraperitoneal and intramedullary (bone marrow) routes. These are poor substitutes for intravenous infusion. Scalp vein needles have been perfected to such a degree that the above routes are seldom if ever indicated. If a vein cannot be found and it is important to use intravenous fluids, a venous cutdown should be performed.

HAZARDS IN THE ADMINISTRATION OF INTRAVENOUS FLUIDS

Infection is usually preventable with proper hygiene and rotation of sites. If an intravenous or cutdown site becomes infected, the site should be changed and appropriate therapy begun.

Sloughing can occur due to extravasation of hypertonic fluids, inadvertent administration into an artery, or pressure necrosis. Adequate padding is essential, especially beneath the heel when veins in the dorsum of the foot are used.

Rapid injection of certain substances may be fatal. K^+-induced ventricular fibrillation is a well known hazard. Rapid Ca^{++} infusion may cause cardiac arrest which is preceded by bradycardia. Ca^{++} infusions should never be given without monitoring the pulse. NH_4Cl or any NH_4^+-containing salt should never be given to patients with liver disease and should never be injected rapidly. A slow, even infusion over 24 hours, at a rate well below 0.1 mEq/kg/minute, does not exceed the normal hepatic clearance of NH_4^+. Sudden death may occur if given otherwise. Tromethamine (THAM-E) causes respiratory arrest if rapidly infused and offers no advantages over $NaHCO_3$.

KEEPING AN INTRAVENOUS INFUSION RUNNING

A variety of means may be employed to prolong the usable life of an intravenous site. Adequate immobilization of the site is extremely important, and so is nontraumatic insertion of the needle. This may sometimes be facilitated by warming the extremity around the vein and by the infiltration of small amounts of 1% lidocaine (Xylocaine).

Metal needles last longer than plastic catheters. Whichever is used, constant vigilance must be maintained for signs of phlebitis or infection. Silastic (silicone rubber) tubing has been useful in large and small veins.

Hypertonic solutions should be avoided.

The addition of 100 units of heparin and 1 mg of prednisolone to each liter of intravenous solution lengthens the life of a vein without causing significant systemic effects.

SOLUTIONS COMMERCIALLY AVAILABLE FOR PEDIATRIC INTRAVENOUS USE

Carrier Solutions

Dextrose, 2.5%, 250 ml
Dextrose, 5%, 250, 500, and 1000 ml
Dextrose, 10%, 500 ml
Dextrose, 20%, 500 ml
Dextrose, 50%, 50 and 500 ml
Water, 20, 250, and 500 ml

Straight Solutions

Lactated Ringer's injection, 500 ml (contains sodium, 130 mEq/liter, potassium, 4 mEq/liter, calcium, 3 mEq/liter, chloride, 109 mEq/liter, and lactate, 28 mEq/liter)
Dextrose, 2.5%, and sodium chloride, 0.45%, 250 and 500 ml
Dextrose, 5%, and sodium chloride, 0.45%, 250 and 500 ml
Dextrose, 5%, and sodium chloride, 0.9%, 250 and 500 ml
Dextrose, 10%, and sodium chloride, 0.9%, 500 ml
Sodium lactate, 1/6 M, 500 ml
Dextrose, 5%, and ethanol, 5% or 10%

Concentrated Electrolytes

(For Use in Carrier Solutions)
Sodium bicarbonate, 44.6 mEq in 50 ml
Ammonium chloride, 3 mEq/ml in 30 ml
Potassium chloride, 2 mEq/ml in 10 or 20 ml
Sodium chloride, 3 mEq/ml in 30 ml
Potassium phosphate, 3 mEq/ml in 10 ml

Special Solutions

Volume Expander: Dextran, 10% in 0.9% sodium chloride solution
Osmotic Diuretic: Mannitol, 15%, 150 and 500 ml
Amino Acids: Freamine II contains 39 gm of protein equivalent in 500 ml. L-Amino acid concentrations (in gm/100 ml) are isoleucine, 0.59; leucine, 0.77; lysine acetate, 0.87; methionine, 0.45; phenylalanine, 0.48; threonine, 0.34; tryptophan, 0.13; valine, 0.56; alanine, 0.60; arginine, 0.31; histidine, 0.24; proline, 0.95; serine, 0.50; glycine, 1.7; and cysteine hydrochloride, < 0.02.
The electrolyte content is sodium, 10 mEq/liter, and phosphate, 20 mEq/liter (31 mg/100 ml).
For Peritoneal Dialysis: In mEq/liter: Na^+, 141; Ca^{++}, 3.5; Mg^{++}, 1.5; Cl^-, 101; lactate, 45. (Eg, Impersol.) Dextrose 1.5% or 4.25%.

SPECIAL CLINICAL SITUATIONS

BURNS
(See also Chapter 29.)

Burns are the third commonest cause of accidental death in childhood (after automobile accidents and drownings). Many thousands of burned children who do not die have to endure prolonged and painful hospitalization, with complications and after-effects that may go on for many years. These tragedies are the worse because so many are preventable.

The management of severe burns, ie, burns involving more than 15% of body surface, is primarily a surgical responsibility and ideally carried out in a special burn center. Details of care are given in Chapter 29, and this section is concerned only with the fluid and electrolyte problems.

Fluid and electrolyte abnormalities in burned patients can present a major challenge for a number of reasons. Capillary leakage into the burned areas in the first 48 hours may substantially diminish blood volume. Myoglobinuria from electrical burns and hemoglobinuria from initial hemolysis may also contribute to poor renal perfusion and oliguria or anuria. Acute tubular necrosis or renal cortical necrosis can also occur if there is hypotension.

The immediate need is to expand plasma volume, and this was for many years treated with colloid infusions by the modified Brooke formula, which allowed (0.5 ml colloid + 1.5 ml ECF-like fluid) × % area burned (up to 50%) × body weight in kg as ml of correction fluid for the first 24 hours. The modern tendency is to use colloid-free solutions initially. These tend to increase initial edema but also permit easier resorption of the third space.

Table 35–7. Percentage of body surface area in infants and children. (After Berkow.)

	Newborn	1 year	5 years	10 years
Head	19	17	13	11
Both thighs	11	13	16	17
Both lower legs	10	10	11	12
Neck	2			
Anterior trunk	13			
Posterior trunk	13			
Both upper arms	8	These percentages remain constant at all ages.		
Both lower arms	6			
Both hands	5			
Both buttocks	5			
Both feet	7			
Genitals	1			
	100			

The fluid and electrolyte plan should include maintenance needs, including the need for a urine flow of at least 1 ml/kg/hour, and recognition of the loss of plasma volume. It is usually necessary to catheterize the patient, to install a central venous pressure line, and to have a separate catheter access for fluids into a large vein. A convenient routine is to give isotonic lactated Ringer's injection or equivalent solution, 3 ml per % area burned per kg of body weight per 24 hours, plus at least 1500 ml/sq m/24 hours of additional fluid containing calories and maintenance sodium and potassium. Serum protein concentration should still be maintained at $\geqslant 3.5$ gm/100 ml. The appropriateness of the plan is checked by repeatedly monitoring serum electrolytes and proteins, body weight, urine flow, and osmolality.

If the plasma hematocrit rises above 50%, if central venous pressure falls, or if urine flow drops below 0.5 ml/kg/hour, then the rate of infusion of isotonic lactated Ringer's injection should be increased to as much as 300 ml/sq m/hour. If this fails, plasma volume must be sustained by colloid, initially giving 1 gm/kg of albumin.

Half of the first 24-hour allocation should be given in the first 8 hours. Subsequent therapy must be planned on the basis of clinical and laboratory progress.

ANURIA & OLIGURIA

The principles of conserving extracellular water homeostasis in renal failure are the same irrespective of etiology or duration. Careful attention to detail may sustain life for several weeks without the necessity of peritoneal or hemodialysis. Treatment of the primary condition, when possible, is implicit.

The first rule is to keep meticulous input and output records that are clear to both physicians and nursing staff. Reconciliation of these records must be made at regular intervals, never exceeding 24 hours. In difficult problems, calculations should be made on an 8-hour basis. Apart from reports of clinical changes, it is necessary to chart urine volume, patient's weight, and, if possible, plasma pH and levels of Na^+, K^+, Cl^-, and HCO_3^-. It may also be helpful to know the ionic composition of any urine, gastric fluid, etc.

The most difficult problem is to provide calories and to manipulate electrolyte distortions within a limited water intake. A suitable water allowance is 400 ml/sq m/24 hours; to this may be added the volume of passed urine in the previous calculation period plus the volume of any other extraneous losses. Water should be given as 20% dextrose. Electrolyte losses are replaced. Correction problems are dealt with as indicated elsewhere in this chapter. Hyperosmolality or hypernatremia is a considerable problem as it restricts alkali administration unless extracellular water is present in increased amounts. This is of no concern in

the short term but may require dialysis if sustained. Hypo-osmolality requires treatment, but at the same time it affords an opportunity to counteract acidosis with parenteral bicarbonate administration. Hyperkalemia is usually satisfactorily managed by potassium restriction. Resins by enema will remove 1 mEq/gm. If necessary, dialysis may be used, and insulin, 0.1 unit/kg IV, may be given in an emergency. Low potassium levels are particularly likely to occur in the period immediately following recovery from acute tubular necrosis. Treatment consists of administering potassium in amounts necessary to restore extracellular levels to the normal range. Acidosis is treated with bicarbonate in the usual manner; it is more important to contain acidosis than normal extracellular water volume unless cardiac failure is present.

The indications for abandoning medical treatment for dialysis are a deteriorating clinical state and intractable acidosis or hyperkalemia.

Finally, it is essential not to neglect caloric intake. Where anuria is complete and due to acute tubular damage which promises to be relatively short-lived (ie, less than 2 weeks), it is advisable to depend entirely on the intravenous route for the first week. Thereafter, if good electrolyte control has been achieved or if some urine flow exists, hard candy and renal cookies can be allowed with some oral water intake—also products such as Cal-Power.

SALICYLATE POISONING

Publicity regarding accidental poisoning and the use of childproof containers has made salicylate poisoning a less common event than it used to be. Serious intoxication still occurs and must be regarded as an emergency.

Salicylates uncouple oxidative phosphorylation, leading to increased heat production, excessive sweating, and, in turn, to dehydration. They also interfere with glucose metabolism and may cause hypo- or hyperglycemia. Respiratory center stimulation is also an early effect.

Clinical & Laboratory Findings

Patients are usually hyperventilating, sweating, dehydrated, febrile, and may have vomiting and diarrhea. In severe cases, disorientation, convulsions, and coma are often present.

The severity of intoxication can in some measure be judged by the serum salicylate levels (Fig 35–7). High levels are always dangerous irrespective of clinical signs, and low levels may be misleading as regards severity. It should be remembered that the normal fluorimetric assay also measures salicyl conjugates such as salicylamide whose toxic effects are less severe. Other laboratory values usually indicate metabolic acidosis despite the hyperventilation, low serum K^+ values, and often abnormal serum glucose levels.

Treatment

Treatment is directed at removing residual gastric salicylate and facilitating urinary excretion by giving alkali and restoring normal extracellular water volumes and intracellular potassium, hydrion, and glucose levels. Comatose patients should be catheterized.

A. Mild Intoxication: Mild poisoning in a child or toddler may only be manifested by hyperventilation. Syrup of ipecac or gastric lavage should be used to remove residual salicylates, and plentiful fluids should be given orally.

B. Moderate Intoxication: When levels are moderate or high (Fig 35–7) but there is no dehydration, gastrointestinal symptoms, or CNS signs, the child should be admitted to hospital and given 1.5 times the normal maintenance quantity of fluids containing increased potassium, up to 40 mEq/liter for 24 hours. Serum electrolytes, glucose, and salicylates should be monitored in tandem with the clinical state.

C. Severe Intoxication: This occurs when there is hyperpyrexia, severe metabolic acidosis, hypertonic dehydration, disturbances of glucose metabolism, and CNS complications.

Shock may have to be treated, and assisted ventilation will occasionally be needed if there is respiratory depression. Cool sponging or a cooling blanket will control temperature elevation. Fluid and electrolyte therapy should follow the principles already set forth. The calculated intravenous solution should aim to replace 50% of the ECW loss in the first 24 hours and give 1.5 times the normal maintenance amounts of water and sodium. The total amount of water should be at least 3000 ml/sq m/24 hours and should contain at least 35 mEq/liter of $NaHCO_3$. Once urine flow is established, the potassium content should be maintained at 40 mEq/liter. One-half of the total volume should be given over the first 8 hours and the remaining 24 hour allocation over the next 16 hours. Intravenous fluids on succeeding days will be dictated by the results of monitoring serum electrolytes, acid-base status, glucose and salicylate levels, and urine sodium, potassium, pH, and osmolality.

Hemodialysis or hemoperfusion over charcoal may be valuable in extreme cases.

Hill JB: Salicylate intoxication. N Engl J Med 288:1113, 1973.
Segar WE: Salicylate intoxication. In: *The Critically Ill Child*, 2nd ed. Smith CA (editor). Saunders, 1977.

PREOPERATIVE & POSTOPERATIVE FLUID & ELECTROLYTE MANAGEMENT

Surgery in a child should, if possible, be deferred until fluid and electrolyte balance has been achieved and his general nutritional status is optimal.

Special problems can be corrected according to instructions given elsewhere in this chapter. The following points should be considered.

(1) Complete volume replacements in plasma and ECF prior to surgery. Correct all electrolyte distortions.

(2) Arrange a planned review of fluid, electrolyte, and caloric balance for the operative and postoperative period.

(3) Except for minor procedures, use an intravenous infusion for at least 24 hours postoperatively.

(4) Maintenance fluid and electrolytes should be given evenly over the period of the operation. Whole blood is replaced in proportion to operative losses.

(5) The carrier vehicle for water and electrolytes should be 10% dextrose to provide minimum calories until normal alimentation is restored. Prolonged parenteral feeding is discussed at the end of this chapter.

PYLORIC STENOSIS

The main problem in pyloric stenosis is that repeated vomiting of gastric contents without diarrhea leads to extracellular water depletion complicated by excessive potassium and chloride losses and metabolic alkalosis.

Consider the example of a typical case in a 3-week-old male infant weighing 3 kg and with the following serum values: Na^+, 140 mEq/liter; K^+, 3.5 mEq/liter; Cl^-, 85 mEq/liter; HCO_3^-, 44 mEq/liter; pH, 7.60; base excess, +19 mEq/liter; and P_{CO_2}, 45 mm Hg.

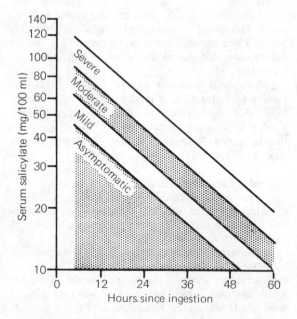

Figure 35–7. Nomogram relating serum salicylate concentration and expected severity of intoxication at varying intervals following ingestion of a single dose of salicylate. (Redrawn and reproduced, with permission, from Done AK: Salicylate intoxication. Pediatrics 26:800, 1960.)

An infusion of isotonic NaCl is begun at once. Thirty minutes later, when 100 ml have been infused, his skin turgor is much improved and his listlessness diminished.

Basic maintenance and correctional requirements are now calculated (Tables 35—8 and 35—9).

The above case represents an example of moderate (10%) ECW depletion with hypokalemic, hypochloremic metabolic alkalosis due to vomiting from pyloric stenosis. After allowing for the initial 100 ml of saline, the rest of the 24 hour requirement was dispensed and given in equal measure over the remainder of the period. Practically, it amounted to 400 ml of 0.8 N saline with 15 mEq of KCl added. On the following day, clinical dehydration had disappeared and all laboratory values were normal except the pH, which was 7.5; the base excess, which was +4 mEq/liter; and the [K$^+$], which was still slightly low at 4 mEq/liter. Basic maintenance requirements plus a KCl correctional allowance of 2 mEq/kg were given for an additional day, following which all values were normal and surgery was performed.

INTESTINAL OBSTRUCTIONS

In intestinal obstruction the bowel is distended with gas and accumulates substantial volumes of fluid. With continued vomiting there is a variable loss of sodium, potassium, chloride, and hydrogen, leading to reduced extracellular volume with changes in pH and ionic composition. These should be corrected according to the principles established elsewhere in the chapter, but the following guidelines should be observed.

(1) Maintain careful records of laboratory data, weight, etc and renew fluid and electrolyte balance at regular intervals.

(2) Delay surgery until these disturbances are corrected unless it is an emergency.

(3) Maintain continuous nasogastric suction, recording volume and, if necessary, ionic composition and pH of aspirated fluid. This will relieve distention. Give all fluids and calories intravenously until bowel sounds have returned postoperatively and the patient is free of distention and vomiting.

(4) Start alimentation as small frequent feedings, giving not more than one-fourth of the daily requirements by this route in the first 24 hours. Start with water or 0.225% saline in 10% dextrose, and then give fruit juices or milk before starting any solids.

ACUTE INFANTILE GASTROENTERITIS

This is perhaps the most common fluid and electrolyte problem in pediatric practice. The principles of management are illustrated by the following case.

A 1-year-old child is brought to the hospital with a history of profuse watery diarrhea of 2 days' duration. He has vomited virtually all oral intake. On physical examination, his rectal temperature is 39.4° C (103° F), pulse 160 but easily palpated, respiratory rate 56 and deep, weight 8 kg, and blood pressure 84/54. The fontanel is depressed, his eyes are sunken and frequently roll aimlessly, his oral mucosa is dry but not parched, his tongue is small, and his skin turgor is diminished but his skin is pink. Laboratory data are as follows: hematocrit, 45%; [Na$^+$]$_S$, 138 mEq/liter; [K$^+$]$_S$, 4 mEq/liter; [Cl$^-$]$_S$, 106 mEq/liter; pH, 7.15; base excess, −20 mEq/liter; and P$_{CO_2}$, 24 mm Hg.

Fluid and electrolyte diagnoses are as follows:

(1) ECF depletion (severe), equal to approximately 10% of body weight.

(2) Metabolic acidosis (severe), with acidemia, hypobasemia, and compensatory hypocapnia.

(3) K$^+$ depletion. (Note the low-normal [K$^+$]$_S$ in the presence of a low pH.)

Fluid and electrolyte requirements are estimated as shown in Tables 35—10 and 35—11.

PARENTERAL ALIMENTATION

Over the last decade, intravenous alimentation has been used with increasing frequency for the nutritional support of low birth weight infants, for patients with chronic diarrhea and other inflammatory bowel disease, after surgery of the bowel, and as a means of restricting nitrogen but not calories in renal failure. In addition, the development of the cuffed Silastic small bore (0.1 mm) Broviac subclavian catheter has made it possible to continue parenteral alimentation for months or even years after massive bowel resections.

COMPOSITION OF BASIC SOLUTION

The most commonly used solutions are based on free amino acids and glucose, with minerals and vitamins added. In general, they do not contain iodine, biotin, zinc, or copper, and these nutrients may have to be added. Essential fatty acids must also be given (see discussion of Intralipid, below). The solution given here is one that can be easily dispensed in any well equipped hospital pharmacy. Ideally, it should be prepared in 24-hour batches since prescription changes may be required. Where the procedure is carried out at home, however, as with the Broviac catheter, weekly dispensing is satisfactory if the solutions are refrigerated. A laminar air flow table should be used to ensure sterility. However, if such a unit is not available, solu-

Table 35—8. Basic maintenance requirements for the first 24 hours in the example (pyloric stenosis) cited above. (Data in part from Table 35—3.)

	ml/kg	ml	Na⁺/kg	Na⁺	K⁺/kg	K⁺	Cl⁻/kg	Cl⁻
Estimated insensible losses	25	75	...	...	...	...	...	...
Estimated urine output	40	120	3	9	3	9	6	18
Estimated continuing gastro-intestinal losses*	(20)	(60)	(2)	(6)	(0.2)	(0.6)	(2.2)	(6.6)
Maintenance totals		195		9		9		18

*Given only if vomiting continues. It usually does not continue once feedings are started unless there is a continuing gastritis.

Table 35—9. Correctional requirements in the example (pyloric stenosis) cited above.

	Volume 5% Dextrose	Na⁺	K⁺	Cl⁻	HCO₃⁻
Volume loss 10% ECW*	300	51	...	51	...
Acid-base	Will be self-correcting with NaCl				
K⁺ (2 mEq/kg)	...	...	6	6	...
Correctional total	300	51	6	57	...
Total 24 hour requirements	495	60	15	75	...

*100 ml were given initially and are included in this figure.

Table 35—10. Basic maintenance requirements for the first 24 hours in the example (acute infantile gastroenteritis) cited below.

	Fluid		Na⁺		K⁺		Cl⁻	
	ml/kg	ml	mEq/kg	mEq	mEq/kg	mEq	mEq/kg	mEq
Estimated insensible losses	25	200	...	...	...	...	...	...
Estimated urinary output	60	480	3	24	2	16	5	40
Estimated gastro-intestinal losses	...	...	...	...	...	...	...	...
Totals	...	680	...	24	...	16	...	40

Table 35—11. Correctional requirements in the example (acute infantile gastroenteritis) cited below.

	Fluid	Na⁺	K⁺	Cl⁻	HCO₃⁻
ECW-like fluid (10% body weight)	800	72*	...	72	...
Potassium (2 mEq/kg/24 hours)	...	...	16	16	...
Acid-base (0.3 × body weight × base excess)	...	48*	...	...	48
24-hour totals (maintenance plus correction)	1480	144	32	128	48

*Note that part of the 120 mEq of Na⁺ needed to make 800 ml of ECW-like fluid is given as NaCl and part as NaHCO₃.

In actual practice, the above fluids should probably be given rapidly at first and the rate then tapered as clinical improvement is noted.

Table 35—12. Composition of basic solution.

Component	Ordered Concentration	Provided as:	Volume (ml) per liter
Amino acids	2%	Freamine II	235
Glucose	20%	50% dextrose	400
Sodium	35 mEq/1liter	NaCl, 4 mEq/ml	2.5
		Sodium acetate, 3 mEq/ml	7.5
Potassium	24.6 mEq/liter	KC1, 2 mEq/ml	5
		Potassium phosphate: 4.4 mEq K and 3 mmol P/ml (Abbott)	3.3
Calcium	7.5 mEq/liter	Ca gluconate, 0.45 mEq/ml	16.7
Magnesium	2.5 mEq/liter	50% Mg SO_4	0.62
Multivitamin infusion (MVI)	1 ml/liter	MVI concentrate	1
Folic acid	200 µg/liter	Folvite diluted to 500 µg/ml	0.4
Vitamin B_{12}	50 µg/liter	Sytobex, 100 µg/ml	0.5
Sterile water			qs ad 1000

tions may be assembled using syringes with Millipore filter attachments. Table 35—12 gives a standard solution which, when given in a volume of 130 ml/kg/24 hours, provides 2.5 gm/kg/24 hours of protein equivalent and about 110 kcal/kg/24 hours.

It is usual practice to start at lower glucose concentrations, and in small infants it may also be necessary to use lower initial amino acid concentrations. Phosphate content should also be reduced in the newborn.

The regimen given in Table 35—13 is standard.

Once a glucose concentration of 200 gm/liter at a flow rate of 100 ml/kg/day has been achieved, further increases in flow rate will be done ad libitum depending upon clinical indications to a maximum of 105 ml/kg/day. Flow rate increments should be 10 ml/kg/day. Similarly, the glucose concentration may be increased by 10 gm/liter increments to a maximum of 250 gm/liter.

MANAGEMENT

Insertion of the catheter is a surgical procedure done under sterile conditions. A Silastic catheter, 0.025 inch inner diameter and 0.047 inch outer diameter, is inserted into the external jugular vein and advanced until it reaches the junction of the superior

Table 35—13. Glucose administration flow rates.

Glucose	Flow Rate
100 gm/liter	60 ml/kg/day × 1 day
100 gm/liter	80 ml/kg/day × 2 days
100 gm/liter	100 ml/kg/day × 2 days
125 gm/liter	100 ml/kg/day × 2—3 days
150 gm/liter	100 ml/kg/day × 2—3 days
175 gm/liter	100 ml/kg/day × 2—3 days
200 gm/liter	100 ml/kg/day × 2—3 days

vena cava and the right atrium. This position should be confirmed by fluoroscopy. The other end of the catheter is then drawn back through a subcutaneous tunnel to emerge through the skin in the right parietal area. The skin opening should be inspected daily.

The following is an outline of management principles.

A. Infusion Apparatus:

1. Give nothing but the alimentation fluid through the catheter.

2. Do not add anything to the alimentation bottle.

3. Do not draw or infuse blood through the alimentation catheter.

4. Change the alimentation bottle and infusion set at least once every 24 hours.

5. Change the intravenous tubing, including the Buratrol and infusion pump tubing, once every 24 hours.

6. Change the dressing around the catheter, using sterile technic with gloves, at least every 2 days. Use povidone-iodine ointment around the catheter.

7. Procedure when the catheter is to be removed: (a) Draw a blood culture through the catheter prior to removal; (b) prepare the skin around the catheter with povidone-iodine, pull out the catheter, cut off the tip with sterile scissors, and send the tip in a culture tube for culture; and (c) draw a peripheral blood culture if infection is suspected on clinical grounds.

B. Clinical Course:

1. Strict intake and output records must be kept.

2. Each urine should be tested for specific gravity, sugar, acetone, and protein.

3. Dextrostix determinations should be done initially at every shift for 4 days. When changes in flow rate or of glucose concentration occur, Dextrostix testing should also be done at each shift. Thereafter, Dextrostix determinations should be performed daily.

4. Blood glucose concentrations should be measured daily for the first 4 days and 12 hours after any change in flow rate or carbohydrate concentration of the infusate. Blood glucose should also be assayed if

Table 35—14. Monitoring summary.

Variables	Suggested Frequency	
	Week 1	Week 2 On
Growth variables		
Weight	Daily	Daily
Length	Weekly	Weekly
Occipitofrontal circumference	Weekly	Weekly
Metabolic variables		
Blood measurements		
Dextrostix and blood glucose	See text.	See text.
Plasma electrolytes	Daily for 5 days	Every 3 days
Blood acid-base status	Daily for 5 days	Every 3 days
Blood urea nitrogen	Daily for 5 days	Every 3 days
Ca^{++}, P, Mg^{++}	Days 1, 3, 6	Weekly
Total protein	Days 1, 3, 6	Weekly
Liver function tests (SGOT, SGPT, LDH)	Days 1, 3, 6	Weekly
Alkaline phosphatase	Days 1, 3, 6	Weekly
Ammonia	Clinical indications	Clinical indications
Urine measurements		
Volume	Daily	Daily
Glucose	Void	Twice a day
Specific gravity or osmolarity	Void	Twice a day
General measurements		
Infusate volume	Daily	Daily
Oral intake (if any)	Daily	Daily
Prevention and detection of infection		
Clinical observations (general status, temperature, etc)	Daily shift	Daily
Complete blood count with differential	Twice a week and on clinical indications	Clinical indications
Culture	Clinical indications	Clinical indications

the Destrostix is > 200 mg/100 ml or if ≥ 1% glycosuria occurs. In such situations, the flow rate of the infusate should be temporarily reduced by half and fluid requirements compensated by peripheral infusion. This avoids osmotic diuresis and dehydration. Suspicion of sepsis should also be entertained.

5. Electrolytes, BUN, and serum pH should be obtained each day for the first 5 days and then every third day thereafter. These same parameters should be obtained within 12 hours after any alteration in flow rate.

6. Serum or plasma calcium, phosphorus, magnesium, total protein, SGOT, SGPT, LDH, and alkaline phosphatase determinations should be obtained at the time of initiating the infusion, on the third and sixth days of the infusion, and then once a week. The one exception is that 2 days after any change in flow rate, these values should again be measured.

7. Because of the difficulty of obtaining adequate samples, blood ammonia levels should be obtained only on clinical indication. However, the physician should be alert to the possibility of ammonia intoxication in any infant with lethargy, pallor, temperature instability, poor growth, elevated liver enzymes, acidosis, azotemia, or a blood urea nitrogen < 6 mg/100 ml.

8. A complete blood count should be obtained twice weekly.

9. Administrations of packed cells or whole blood

should be done on clinical indication and to maintain a hematocrit greater than 30%. The routine or empiric administration of blood or plasma is not indicated.

10. Because the infusate, as designed, does not include essential fatty acids or trace metals, a careful detection protocol must be instituted and prescription changes made if indicated.

11. Parenteral nutrition should be discontinued, if possible, with the patient on good oral intake and should be tapered gradually over 1—2 days. Careful observation for rebound hypoglycemia after abrupt termination of total parenteral nutrition is mandatory.

12. A thorough laboratory flow sheet must be maintained at the patient's bedside.

C. Monitoring Summary: See Table 35—14.

COMPLICATIONS

The complications of total parenteral nutrition can be divided into those related to the catheter itself and the metabolic problems associated with this method of management.

Catheter-Related Complications

Catheters may be initially malpositioned if fluoroscopic verification is not used, and they may become dislodged if not carefully protected. Clots may develop around the tip of the catheter, especially if there is any pump malfunction, and this in turn may lead to pulmonary embolization or superior vena caval thrombosis. Infection is a frequent complication usually due to some lapse in technic, eg, failure to change the tubing or to give proper attention to dressings.

If there is clinical evidence of infection of the catheter, it should be removed, the tip cultured, and a new one inserted. The organisms most often involved are from the normal body flora, ie, *Staphylococcus aureus, Streptococcus viridans,* proteus, klebsiella, and *Escherichia coli.* Saprophytes such as candida and aspergillus and weakly pathogenic organisms such as serratia may also be involved.

Metabolic Complications

A. Glucose: Many patients are already malnourished with consequent glucose intolerance, so that it is wise to increase glucose concentrations gradually.

Hypoglycemia is also a complication which is most liable to occur if the rate of glucose administration is suddenly slowed. Therapy should always be discontinued slowly.

B. Nitrogen: Hyperammonemia may result from inadequate arginine intake. Azotemia may occur if the amino acid load is excessive. Changes may also be seen in the serum aminogram, with elevated levels of methionine and, less importantly, of threonine, valine, and glycine. Such changes do not seem to be harmful. The need for taurine in alimentation of small infants seems now to be established, even though this amino acid is still not generally included in the formulation.

C. Anemia: The constant infusion of a hypertonic solution may cause mild hemolytic anemia. This should be monitored by weekly blood counts. The presence of anisocytosis and serum haptoglobin saturation with hemoglobin are sensitive indications of hemolysis. Transfusions with packed cells may be required occasionally.

D. Psychologic Problems: Older children who have been encouraged to eat in order to maintain their nutritional status may become depressed at becoming dependent on intravenous nutrition. Psychiatric help to allow them to ventilate their feelings is often effective. Parents should be encouraged to hold infants receiving intravenous nutrition so that normal emotional attachments can develop.

E. Other Complications: Acidosis from the use of amino acid hydrochlorides, copper and zinc depletion, and biotin and essential fatty acid deficiencies all need to be watched for.

INTRAVENOUS FAT

Intralipid is a preparation of soybean oil emulsified with egg yolk phosphatide which had been used extensively in Europe over the last decade. The preparation now in use in the USA contains 10% fat of which 50% is linoleic acid. Intravenous fat is a useful source of calories when only a peripheral vein is available which may be damaged by the high osmolality of isocaloric glucose solutions. Present evidence, however, is that fat is somewhat less effective in protein sparing than glucose.

Intravenous fat is commonly given in the treatment or prophylaxis of essential fatty acid deficiency, which is a definite hazard of intravenous alimentation based on glucose and amino acid infusions only. It usually presents as areas of dry scaly skin and desquamation on the dorsum of the foot, in the axillas, or on the anterior chest wall. When serum fatty acids are measured there is a fall in the ratio of linoleic acid ($18:2\ \omega6$) to oleic acid ($18:1\ \omega9$) with an absolute fall in linoleic and arachidonic acid ($20:4\ \omega6$) levels. 11-Eicosatreinoic acid ($20:3\ \omega9$), an abnormal metabolite of oleic acid, may appear (see Chapter 38 for normal values).

Intralipid cannot be mixed with other infusates because of the risk of breaking the emulsion. For this reason, it is usually given "piggy back" into a side arm of the infusion set just before the venous insertion. The rate of administration should not exceed 3 gm/kg/24 hours of fat or 30 ml/kg/24 hours of emulsion. The actual requirement of intralipid during long-term parenteral alimentation is not known; ideally, it should account for 5–10% of the daily caloric intake. Giving about 15% of calories once a week in Intralipid is more economical and appears to be satisfactory. The effectiveness of the cutaneous application of linoleic acid, 2–3 mg/kg/24 hours, deserves to be further explored.

Intralipid should not be given to infants with respiratory problems because it may diminish pulmonary perfusion or to those with serum bilirubins > 5 mg/100 ml because of the risk of bilirubin displacement from albumin.

Heird WC, Winters RW: Total parenteral nutrition: The state of the art. J Pediatr 86:2, 1975.

• • •

General References

Gamble JL: Early history of fluid replacement therapy. Pediatrics 11:554, 1953.

Winters RW: *The Body Fluids in Pediatrics.* Little, Brown, 1973.

36 . . .
Drug Therapy

Henry K. Silver, MD
With Revisions & Additions By
Robert G. Peterson, MD, PhD, & Barry H. Rumack, MD

INTRODUCTION

Precautions

Older children should never be given a dose greater than the adult dose. Adult dosages are given below to show limitation of dosage in older children when calculated on a weight basis. All drugs should be used with caution in children, and dosage should be individualized. In general, the smaller the child, the greater the metabolic rate; this may increase the dose needed. Dosage may also have to be adjusted for body temperature (metabolic rate is increased about 10% for each degree centigrade); for obesity (adipose tissue is relatively inert metabolically); for edema (depending on whether the drug is distributed primarily in extra-cellular fluid); for the type of illness (kidney and liver disease may impair metabolism of certain substances); and for individual tolerance (idiosyncrasy). The dosage recommendations on the following pages should be regarded only as estimates; careful clinical observations and the use of pertinent laboratory aids are necessary. Established drugs should be used in preference to newer and less familiar drugs.

Drugs should be used in early infancy only for significant disorders. In both full-term and premature infants, detoxifying enzymes may be deficient or absent; renal function relatively inefficient; and the blood-brain barrier and protein binding altered.

Dosages have not been determined as accurately for newborn infants as for older children.

At any age, oliguria requires a reduction of dosage of drugs excreted via the urine.

Whenever possible, reference should also be made to the printed literature supplied by the manufacturer or other recent authoritative sources, particularly for drugs that are used infrequently.

Determination of Drug Dosage*

Dosage rules based on proportions of the adult dose are not entirely satisfactory but have been widely used in the past and may serve as a rough guide. Dosage based on surface area is probably the most accurate method of estimating the dose for a child.

*To convert dose in gm/kg to dose in gr/lb, multiply gm dosage by 7.

Table 36–1. Determination of drug dosage from surface area.*

Weight		Approximate Age	Surface Area (sq m)	% of Adult Dose
kg	lb			
3	6.6	Newborn	0.2	12
6	13.2	3 months	0.3	18
10	22	1 year	0.45	28
20	44	5.5 years	0.8	48
30	66	9 years	1	60
40	88	12 years	1.3	78
50	110	14 years	1.5	90
65	143	Adult	1.7	102
70	154	Adult	1.76	103

*If adult dose is 1 mg/kg, dose for 3-month-old infant would be 2 mg/kg.

See also section on Special Considerations in Pediatric Drug Dosage, below.

A. Surface Area: (See Table 36–1 and Figs 36–1 and 36–2.)

$$\text{Child dose} = \frac{\text{Surface area of child in sq m} \times \text{Adult dose}}{1.75}$$

or

Surface area in sq m × 60 = Percentage of adult dose.

Formula for calculating approximate surface area in children:

$$\text{Surface area (sq m)} = \frac{4W + 7}{W + 90}$$

where W is weight in kg.

A variety of formulas have been proposed for converting adult dosages to pediatric dosages. Those presented below have been widely used but are not, in general, as accurate as formulas based on surface area or volume of distribution.

B. Clark's Rule: Based on weight, for children over 2 years.

$$\text{Child dose} = \frac{\text{Weight in lb} \times \text{Adult dose}}{150}$$

C. Bastedo's Rule: Based on age.

$$\text{Child dose} = \frac{(\text{Age in years} \times \text{Adult dose}) + 3}{30}$$

D. Cowling's Rule:

$$\text{Child dose} = \frac{\text{Age at next birthday} \times \text{Adult dose}}{24}$$

E. Young's Rule: Based on age.

$$\text{Child dose} = \frac{\text{Age in years} \times \text{Adult dose}}{\text{Age in years} + 12}$$

F. Dose in mg/kg if Adult Dose is 1 mg/kg (After Leach & Wood):

Age:	Adult	1
	12 years	1.25
	1−7 years	1.5
	2 weeks−1 year	2

Administration of Drugs

A. Route of Administration:

1. Oral—Tablets may be crushed between spoons and given with chocolate, honey, jam, or maple or corn syrup. Many regularly prescribed drugs are commercially available in special pediatric preparations. The parent should be warned that the attractively flavored drug must be kept out of reach of children in the home.

a. Avoid administering drugs with important foods.

b. The powdered drug should be mixed in the vehicle and held between 2 layers, not floated on the top.

c. Attempt to administer the entire dose in 1 spoonful.

2. Parenteral—Parenteral administration of certain drugs may sometimes be necessary, especially in the hospital. Its use as a matter of convenience should be evaluated in the light of the psychic trauma which may result.

3. Rectal—Rectal administration is often very useful, especially for home use. (Rectal dosages are approximately twice the amount given orally.) The physician must make certain, however, that rectal absorption is adequate before depending upon this route for a specific drug. Drugs may be given rectally in corn starch (not more than 60 ml); they are best given through a tube, but an enema bulb may be used. Some drugs are prepared in suppository form.

B. Flavoring Agents for Drugs: Drugs for children should not be so flavorful that they are sought out as "candy." Syrups are more useful as flavoring agents than alcoholic elixirs, which have a burning taste.

Refusal of Medications

The administration of a drug to a child requires tact and skill. The parent or nurse should proceed as if protest is not anticipated. Persuasion before it is necessary sets the stage for struggle. The child must understand that the drug will be given despite protest, but great care should be exercised in a struggling child to avoid aspiration.

SPECIAL CONSIDERATIONS IN PEDIATRIC DRUG DOSAGE

When treating children by means of drugs, the pediatrician must not only be aware of the correct dosage and indications but must also take into account optimal frequency of administration as well as rates of absorption, metabolism, and elimination, which may vary widely at different ages and under different conditions. The following approach to rational drug administration in the pediatric age group takes into account various states of renal function, liver metabolism, and body size which affect drug dosage in children.

Therapeutic Range

Determination of plasma levels of drugs can be extremely useful in monitoring therapy. For some drugs (eg, digoxin, theophylline, phenobarbital), the plasma level is well correlated with the drug's physiologic effect and is easier to determine than the physiologic effect itself. For other classes of drugs (eg, antibiotics, anticoagulants, insulin), it is more important to measure the physiologic effect: serum bactericidal level, prothrombin time, blood glucose, etc.

The therapeutic range is defined as the range of plasma levels for any given drug at which the majority of a treated population will receive the drug's intended therapeutic benefit without experiencing serious toxic side-effects. Table 36−2 lists the therapeutic ranges for some drugs commonly used in pediatric practice. Drug toxicity can be expected when plasma levels exceed the therapeutic range.

To obtain a therapeutic level for a particular drug, one must take into account the distribution of the drug throughout the body, whereas maintenance of a therapeutic level requires consideration of elimination processes.

Volume of Distribution

Following the intravenous administration of a drug, plasma levels will fall rapidly as the drug is distributed from the vascular compartment to the extracellular, cellular, CNS, and other "compartments" of the body. Its final concentration in the plasma will be dependent upon the dilution of the drug in the various body spaces. Mathematically, this is expressed as

$$\text{Plasma level} = \frac{\text{Dose}}{\text{Volume of distribution}}$$

Since different drugs have differing solubilities in the body fluids or bind to tissues to varying degrees,

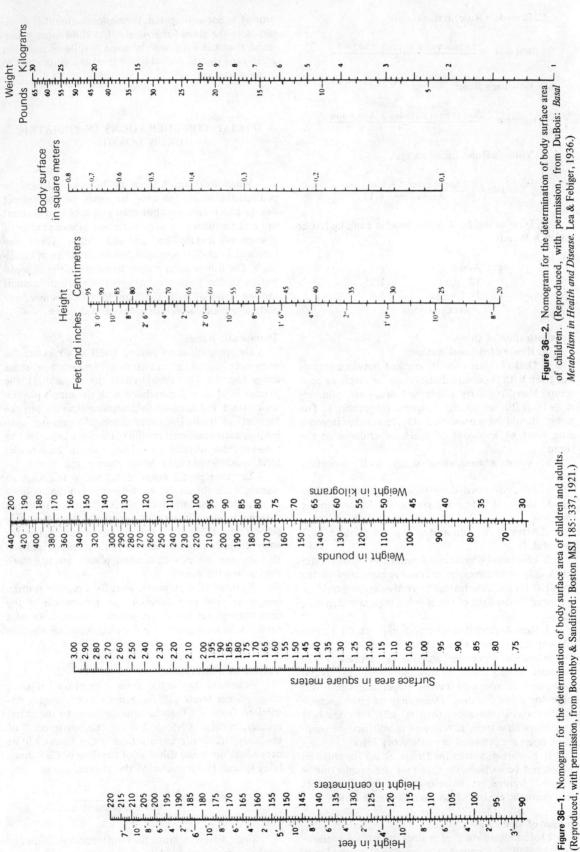

Figure 36–2. Nomogram for the determination of body surface area of children. (Reproduced, with permission, from DuBois: *Basal Metabolism in Health and Disease.* Lea & Febiger, 1936.)

Figure 36–1. Nomogram for the determination of body surface area of children and adults. (Reproduced, with permission, from Boothby & Sandiford: Boston MSJ 185: 337, 1921.)

Table 36–2. Therapeutic blood levels.*

Acetaminophen (Tylenol)	10–20 µg/ml†
Amobarbital (Amytal, Tuinal)	< 5 µg/ml
Aprobarbital (Alurate)	< 5 µg/ml
Bromide	< 500 µg/ml
	< 6 mEq/l
Bupivacaine (Marcaine)	< 100 ng/ml
Butalbital (Fiorinal)	⩽ 5 µg/ml
Carbamazepine (Tegretol)	3–6 µg/ml
Chloramphenicol	15–30 µg/ml
Digoxin (Lanoxin)	0.9–2.4 ng/ml
Ethanol	1000 µg/ml
	("under the influence")
Ethchlorvynol (Placidyl)	10 or 20 µg/ml
Ethosuximide (Zarontin)	40–80 µg/ml
Glutethimide (Doriden)	< 4 µg/ml
Hexobarbital	< 5 µg/ml
Lidocaine (Xylocaine)	< 100 ng/ml (newborn)
	1.5–2.5 µg/ml (adult)
Meprobamate (Equanil, Miltown)	5–20 µg/ml
Methsuximide (Celontin) as the metabolite N-des methsuximide	10–40 µg/ml
Methyprylon (Noludar)	< 5 µg/ml
Pentobarbital (Nembutal)	< 5 µg/ml
Phenobarbital	15–30 µg/ml
Phensuximide (Milontin)	10–20 µg/ml
Phenytoin (diphenylhydantoin, Dilantin)	< 10–20 µg/ml
Primidone (Mysoline)	< 10 µg/ml
Procainamide (Pronestyl)	4–6 µg/ml
Quinidine	3–5 µg/ml
Salicylate	< 350 µg/ml
Secobarbital (Seconal, Tuinal)	5 µg/ml
Sulfisoxazole (Gantrisin)	100 µg/ml
Theophylline	7–20 µg/ml

*Therapeutic level or range for drugs which can be routinely analyzed.
†Conversions: 1 µg/ml = 1 mg/liter. 1 µg/ml = 0.1 mg/100 ml.

the volume of distribution (V_D) will vary from drug to drug. Table 36–3 gives the V_D values for a number of commonly used drugs. With the therapeutic level (from Table 36–2) and the volume of distribution (from Table 36–3), one can calculate the appropriate dose for a number of drugs as follows:

$$\text{Dose (mg/kg)} = \text{Plasma level (mg/liter)} \times V_D \text{ (liters/kg)}$$

Although the V_D is determined from data gathered after intravenous use, it is also a valuable constant for use with oral or intramuscular preparations. Provided the drug's absorption is complete, there is little difference between a slow intravenous infusion and an intramuscular injection. In an instance where an immediate effect is desired but intramuscular absorption is poor (eg, digoxin, phenytoin, diazepam), the slow intravenous route is preferred.

Renal Elimination

Maintenance of a therapeutic level requires that drugs be administered in amounts equivalent to their elimination. Charged or polar drugs (eg, penicillins, aminoglycosides) are directly excreted by the kidneys, and there is little danger of drug accumulation unless the drug is given more frequently than every half-life. Thus, the recommendation for dosage interval for this type of drug is approximately every 1–2 half-lives. When drugs are eliminated by renal processes alone, a steady state will be reached after approximately 5 half-lives, and the plasma level will depend upon the dose and volume of distribution of the drug as outlined above.

Recommendations for dose and frequency of administration of a large number of pediatric medications are given in Drug Dosages for Children (below).

Hepatic Elimination

Nonpolar drugs are first metabolized in the liver to make them polar and are then excreted by the kidneys. A steady state plasma level will be achieved only when the dose given is equivalent to the amount of drug metabolized in the interval between doses.

In deciding on dosages of drugs metabolized in the liver, care must be exercised to make certain that an amount of drug given at a particular frequency does not overwhelm the liver's capacity to metabolize it during the prescribed interval. Fig 36–3 demonstrates the effect of increasing dosage for a drug such as phenytoin upon the plasma level of the drug. As can be observed, one can determine a safe maximum dose (indicated by arrow) above which drug accumulation rapidly occurs. This dose corresponds to the maximum capacity of the liver for metabolism of this drug.

Drug toxicity can occur rapidly with drugs requiring hepatic elimination. When plasma levels in the upper portion of the therapeutic range are required, frequent plasma determinations should be utilized to avoid drug accumulation.

An example is as follows: A 20 kg child receiving phenytoin has a plasma level of 18 µg/ml 4 hours following a daily oral dose. Just prior to the next dose (given at 24-hour intervals), a plasma level is 10 µg/ml. One can estimate the amount metabolized by this child and, therefore, the appropriate maintenance dose by means of the following equation:

Table 36–3. Approximate volumes of distribution.

| Drug | V_D (liters/kg) | |
	Newborn	Children
Acetaminophen	. . .	0.35
Amobarbital	. . .	1.29
Caffeine	0.90	0.90
Digoxin	7.5	15.0
		(7.5 for adolescent)
Furosemide	0.20	0.25
Phenobarbital	0.75	0.75
Phenytoin	0.75	0.75
Salicylates	. . .	0.60
Theophylline*	0.69	0.46

*Dose calculated for theophylline should be multiplied by 1.25 if aminophylline is to be used (salt effect on molecular weight).

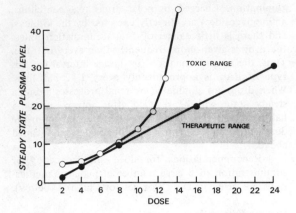

Figure 36–3. Plot (○ – ○) represents plasma level as a function of increasing dosage of any drug eliminated by hepatic metabolism. Arrow indicates dose at which rapid accumulation of drug occurs. This quantity of administered drug equals capacity of liver metabolism. Dosages above this level cause further rapid increase in plasma level. Plot (● – ●) shows data observed with drugs eliminated directly by the kidney without metabolism; observe the difference.

Fall in plasma level = 8 mg/liter
V_D = 20 kg × 0.75 liter/kg = 15 liters
Dose = 15 liters × 8 mg/liter = 120 mg

120 mg was eliminated in 20 hours, or 144 mg would be eliminated in 24 hours. The appropriate dose of phenytoin for this child is 144 mg or 7.2 mg/kg given every 24 hours.

Table 36–4. Principal routes of drug elimination.

Renal	Liver
Aminoglycosides	Acetaminophen*
Digoxin	Alcohol
Furosemide	Caffeine
Penicillins	Digitoxin (75%)
Phenobarbital (25%)	Phenobarbital (75%)
	Phenytoin
	Salicylates
	Theophylline*

*Liver metabolism is rapid, and kinetics appear to be similar to those of drugs excreted by primary renal elimination.

Table 36–4 outlines examples of drugs which are eliminated by the 2 routes discussed above.

SUMMARY

The therapeutic ranges for a number of drugs are presented in Table 36–2. The measurement of plasma levels during therapy will facilitate the regulation of dosage to produce therapeutic effects without toxicity. Drugs whose elimination is dependent chiefly upon hepatic metabolism require special surveillance. Drug Dosages for Children (below) lists a number of drugs used in pediatric patients along with the appropriate dose and frequency for each.

DRUG DOSAGES FOR CHILDREN

Acetaminophen (Tempra, Tylenol): 10 mg/kg/dose in 6 doses orally. Under 1 year, 60 mg/dose; 1–3 years, 60–120 mg/dose; 3–6 years, 120 mg/dose; 6–12 years, 240 mg/dose. (Adult = 0.3–0.6 gm 6 times daily.)

Acetazolamide (Diamox): 5–30 mg/kg/day orally every 6–8 hours. (Adult = 5 mg/kg/day.) For hydrocephalus: 20–55 mg/kg/day orally in 2 or 3 divided doses. (For anticonvulsant use, see p 560.)

Acetylsalicylic acid: See Aspirin.

ACTH: See p 695. Aqueous: 1.6 units/kg/day in 3 or 4 doses IV, IM, or subcut. Gel: 0.8 units/kg/day IM.

Actinomycin D: See Dactinomycin.

Adanon: See Methadone.

Adrenalin: See Epinephrine.

Adroyd: See Oxymetholone.

Aerosporin: See Polymyxin B, p 1041.

Albumin, salt-poor: 0.5–1 gm/kg as 25 gm/100 ml solution (up to 100 ml) IV. (Adult = 50 gm/day IV.)

Aldactone: See Spironolactone.

Aldomet: See Methyldopa.

Aluminum hydroxide gel: 15–30 ml orally with meals.

Amantadine (Symmetrel): See p 1043.

Amethopterin: See Methotrexate.

Amidon: See Methadone.

Aminophylline: (1) Orally, 2–6 mg/kg/dose. (Adult = 0.25 gm.) (2) IV, 2–6 mg/kg; 9 mg/kg/day in isotonic saline as maintenance. (3) Rectally, 6 mg/kg/dose. (Adult = 0.5 gm.) Do not repeat in less than 6 hours. *Caution* in younger children.

Aminosalicylic acid (PAS): See p 1039.

Ammonium chloride: 75 mg/kg/day orally in 4 doses. Single expectorant dose, 0.06–0.3 gm orally/dose. (Adult = 0.3 gm.) For urine acidification, 60–75 mg/kg/day orally. (Adult = 4 gm/day.)

Amobarbital sodium (Amytal): 3–12 mg/kg IV (slowly) or IM. (Adult = 0.125–0.5 gm.) Use freshly prepared 10% solution and give slowly. Try smaller dose first. Orally, 6 mg/kg/day, every 8 hours.

Amphetamine sulfate (Benzedrine): 0.5 mg/kg/day in 3 doses orally (not over 15 mg/day). (Adult = 5–15 mg.) (For anticonvulsant use, see p 560.)

Amphotericin B (Fungizone): 0.25 mg/kg/day IV slowly. Increase to 1–1.5 mg/kg/day diluted 1 mg in 10 ml. (Adult = 50–100 mg IV daily.) *Caution:* Toxic. (See also p 1039.)

Ampicillin: See p 1037.

Amytal: See Amobarbital sodium.

Anadrol: See Oxymetholone.

Ancobon: See Flucytosine, p 1040.

Anhydrohydroxyprogesterone: See Ethisterone.

Ansolysen: See Pentolinum.

Antepar (piperazine): See pp 814 and 815.

Apomorphine: Not indicated in pediatric practice.

Apresoline: See Hydralazine.

AquaMephyton: See Phytonadione.

Aralen: See Chloroquine.

Aramine: See Metaraminol.

Arfonad: See Trimethaphan.

Aristocort: See Triamcinolone, p 696.

Ascorbic acid (vitamin C): See pp 89, 92, and 109.

Asparaginase: 5000–10,000 IU/sq m IV daily to weekly.

Aspirin: Analgesic, 65 mg/year of age/dose. (Adult = 0.3–0.65 gm.) For rheumatic fever, 65–130 mg/kg/day to maintain a blood level of 20–30 mg/100 ml. (Adult = 6–8 gm.) As antipyretic: up to 30–65 mg/kg/day. Obtain blood levels for higher doses.

AT 10: See Dihydrotachysterol.

Atabrine: See Quinacrine.

Atarax: See Hydroxyzine.

Atropine sulfate: 0.005–0.02 mg/kg/dose subcut or orally. Maximum total dose: 0.4 mg. (Adult = 0.3–1 mg.) *Caution.*

Azathioprine (Imuran): 3–5 mg/kg/day orally.

Azulfidine: See Salicylazosulfapyridine.

Bactrim: See Trimethoprim-sulfamethoxazole, p 1042.

BAL: See Dimercaprol, p 880.

Banthine: See Methantheline.

Belladonna tincture: 0.1 ml/kg/day orally in 3 divided doses. (Adult = 0.6 ml 3 times daily.) Do not give over 0.6 ml/dose or 3.5 ml/day.

Benadryl: See Diphenhydramine.

Benemid: See Probenecid.

Bentyl: See Dicyclomine.

Benzedrine: See Amphetamine sulfate.

Betamethasone: See p 696.

Bethanechol chloride (Urecholine Chloride): (1) Orally, 0.6 mg/kg/day in 3 divided doses. (Adult = 10–30 mg 3–4 times daily.) (2) Subcut, 0.15–0.2 mg/kg/day. (Adult = 2.5–5 mg.)

Bicillin (benzathine penicillin G): See p 1038.

Bisacodyl (Dulcolax): 0.3 mg/kg orally or rectally.

Blood: Packed erythrocytes, 15 ml/kg IV (not over 300 ml). Whole, 15–22 ml/kg IV as single transfusion. (Adult = 500 ml.)

Bonine: See Meclizine.

Brewers' yeast (dried yeast tablets): 5–30 gm 3 times daily.

Brompheniramine (Dimetane): Children under 6 years: 0.1 mg/kg/day. Children over 6 years: 4 mg 3–4 times daily. (Adult = 4–8 mg 3–4 times daily.)

Busulfan (Myleran): 0.06 mg/kg/day orally. (Adult = 2 mg 1–3 times daily.)

Cafergot P-B: See p 565.

Calciferol (ergocalciferol, vitamin D_2): 25–200 thousand units/day.

Calcium chloride (27% calcium): Newborn: 0.3 gm/kg/day orally as a 2–5% solution. Infants: 1–2 gm/day as dilute solution. Children, 2–4 gm/day. (Adult = 2–4 gm 3 times daily.) *Caution:* See p 84.

Calcium EDTA: See EDTA (edathamil).

Calcium gluconate (9% calcium): (1) Orally: Infants, 3–6 gm/day. Children, 6–10 gm/day in divided doses as a 5–10% solution. (Adult = 8 gm 3 times daily.) (2) IV, 0.1–0.2 gm/kg/dose (not over 2 gm) as a 10% solution. Inject slowly and stop if bradycardia occurs. (Adult = 5–10 ml.) *Caution.*

Calcium lactate (13% calcium): 0.5 gm/kg/day in divided doses orally in dilute solution. (Adult = 4–8 gm 3 times daily.)

Calcium mandelate: 2–8 gm daily orally, depending on age. (Adult = 3 gm 4 times daily.)

Carbamazepine (Tegretol): See p 560.

Carbarsone: 10 mg/kg/day in divided doses.

Carbenicillin: See p 1037.

Castor oil: Infants, 1–5 ml/dose orally. Children, 5–15 ml/dose orally. (Adult = 15–60 ml orally.)

Cefazolin (Kefzol): See p 1036.

Celestone: See Betamethasone, p 696.

Celontin: See Methsuximide.

Cephalothin (Keflin): See p 1036.

Charcoal, activated: 10 gm mixed in water.

Chloral hydrate: Hypnotic: 12.5–50 mg/kg as single dose orally or rectally (not over 1 gm). (Adult = 0.5–2 gm.) Sedative: 4–20 mg/kg as single dose rectally or orally (not over 1 gm). (Adult = 0.25–1 gm.) May be repeated in 1 hour to obtain desired effect, and then may be repeated every 6–8 hours.

Chlorambucil (Leukeran): 0.1–0.2 mg/kg/day. (Adult = 0.2 mg/kg.)

Chloramphenicol (Chloromycetin): See p 1039.

Chlordiazepoxide (Librium): Over 6 years, 0.5 mg/kg/day orally in 3–4 doses.

Chloromycetin: See Chloramphenicol, p 1039.

Chloroquine (Aralen): 10 mg/kg/day orally.

Chlorothiazide (Diuril): 7–40 mg/kg/day in 2 divided doses orally. (Adult = 0.5–1 gm once or twice daily.)

Chlorpheniramine (Chlor-Trimeton, Teldrin): Infants, 1 mg 3–4 times daily. Children, 0.35 mg/kg/day in 4 doses orally or subcut. (Adult = 2–4 mg 3–4 times daily; long-acting, 8–12 mg 2–3 times daily.)

Chlorpromazine (Thorazine): (1) Orally, 0.5 mg/kg every 4–6 hours. (2) IM, up to 5 years: 0.5 mg/kg every 6–8 hours as necessary (not over 40 mg/day). 5–12 years: not over 75 mg/day. (3) Rectally, 2 mg/kg. (Adult = 10–50 mg.)

Chlorpropamide (Diabinese): Initially: 8 mg/kg/day in 3 divided doses. (Adult = 250 mg/day.) *Caution.*

Chlor-Trimeton: See Chlorpheniramine.

Cholestyramine (Cuemid, Questran): Children under 6 years: dose not yet established. Children over 6 years: 240 mg/kg/day orally in 3 divided doses. (Adult = 4 gm 3–4 times daily.)

Citrovorum factor: 1–6 mg/day orally. (Adult = 3–10 mg.)

Codeine phosphate: (1) Orally, 0.8–1.5 mg/kg as a single sedative or analgesic dose; 3 mg/kg/day. (Adult = 8–60 mg.) (2) Subcut, 0.8 mg/kg. (Adult = 30 mg.) (3) For cough, 0.2 mg/kg/dose.

Colace: See Dioctyl sodium sulfosuccinate.

Colistimethate: See Colistin, p 1039.

Colistin (Coly-Mycin): See p 1039.

Coly-Mycin: See Colistin, p 1039.

Compazine: See Prochlorperazine.

Corticosteroids: See p 696.

Corticotropin: See ACTH and p 698.

Cortisone: See p 696.

Cosmegen: See Dactinomycin.

Cotazym (pancreatic replacement): 0.3–0.6 mg with each feeding. (Adult = 3 capsules with meals.)

Cuemid: See Cholestyramine.

Cuprimine: See Penicillamine.

Curare: See Tubocurarine.

Cyclizine (Marezine): 3 mg/kg/day in 3 divided doses orally.

Cyclophosphamide (Cytoxan): 2–8 mg/kg/day orally or IV for 7 or more days or 20–50 mg/kg/dose once a week. (See also p 904.)

Cyproheptadine (Periactin): 0.25 mg/kg/day orally in 3 or 4 doses. (Adult = 12–16 mg/day.)

Cytarabine (cytosine arabinoside, Cytosar): 2 mg/kg/day by direct injection. 0.5–1 mg/kg/day by infusion. (See also p 904.)

Cytomel: See Triiodothyronine.

Cytosar: See Cytarabine.

Cytosine arabinoside: See Cytarabine.

Cytoxan: See Cyclophosphamide.

Dactinomycin (actinomycin D; Cosmegen): 0.015 mg/kg/day IV for 5 days. (Same as adult dose.) (See also p 904.)

Daraprim: See Pyrimethamine.

Darvon: See Propoxyphene.

Decadron: See Dexamethasone, p 696.

Decapryn succinate: See Doxylamine succinate.

Deferoxamine mesylate (Desferal): 20 mg/kg IM (preferred) or IV infusion slowly as initial dose.

Delalutin: See Hydroxyprogesterone caproate.

Delatestryl: See Testosterone enanthate.

Delestrogen: See Estradiol valerate.

Deltra: See Prednisone, p 696.

Demerol: See Meperidine.

Dendrid: See Idoxuridine.

Depo-Provera: See Medroxyprogesterone acetate.

Desferal: See Deferoxamine.

Desoxycorticosterone: See p 696.

Dexamethasone: See p 696.

Dexedrine: See Dextroamphetamine.

Dextroamphetamine (Dexedrine): 2–15 mg/day in 3 divided doses orally. (Adult = 5–15 mg/day.) (See also p 560.)

Dextromethorphan (Romilar): 1 mg/kg/day orally.

Dextropropoxyphene: See Propoxyphene.

Diamox: See Acetazolamide.

Dianabol: See Methandrostenolone.

Diazepam (Valium): 0.12–0.8 mg/kg/day orally in 4 divided doses. IV (slowly), 0.04–2 mg/kg as single dose. (Adult = 2–10 mg 2–4 times daily.) (See also p 561.)

Dicodid: See Hydrocodone.

Dicyclomine (Bentyl): Infants: 5 mg as syrup 3 or 4 times daily. Children: 10 mg 3 or 4 times daily. (Adult = 10–20 mg 3 or 4 times daily.)

Diethylcarbamazine (Hetrazan): (1) 15 mg/kg/day in a single dose for 4 days for ascariasis. (2) 6 mg/kg/day in 3 divided doses for filariasis.

Diethylstilbestrol: See Stilbestrol.

Digitalis preparations: See p 334.

Dihydrotachysterol (AT 10): 1–4 ml (1.25 mg/ml) orally daily initially; 0.5–1 ml 3–5 times weekly as maintenance. (Adult = 4–10 ml initially and then 1–2 ml.)

Diiodohydroxyquin (Diodoquin): 40 mg/kg/day orally in 2–3 doses. (Adult = 0.2 gm/15 lb/day.)

Dilantin: See Phenytoin.

Dimenhydrinate (Dramamine): 1–1.5 mg/kg/dose orally. (Adult = 50–100 mg.)

Dimercaprol (BAL): See p 880.

Dimetane: See Brompheniramine.

Dimocillin: See p 1038.

Dioctyl sodium sulfosuccinate (Colace, Doxinate): 3–5 mg/kg/day in 3 divided doses orally. (Adult = 60–480 mg daily.)

Diodoquin: See Diiodohydroxyquin.

Diodrast: See Iodopyracet.

Diphenhydramine (Benadryl): 4–6 mg/kg/day orally in 3–4 divided doses; 2 mg/kg IV over 5 minutes as an antidote for phenothiazine toxicity. (Adult = 100–200 mg/day orally.)

Diphenoxylate (in Lomotil): Older children: 2.5 mg 2 or 3 times daily and decrease dose as relieved. (Adult = 5 mg 3–4 times daily and reduce.)

Diuril: See Chlorothiazide.

Doxinate: See Dioctyl sodium sulfosuccinate.

Doxylamine succinate (Decapryn): 2 mg/kg/day orally.

Dramamine: See Dimenhydrinate.

Dulcolax: See Bisacodyl.

Durabolin: See Nandrolone.

Edathamil: See EDTA.

Edetate: See EDTA.

Edrophonium chloride (Tensilon): Test dose for infant: 0.2 mg/kg IV. Give only one-fifth of dose slowly initially; if tolerated, give remainder. (Adult = 5–10 mg IV.) Have atropine available as antidote.

EDTA (edathamil, edetate): 12.5 mg/kg IM (in solution containing procaine, 0.5–1.5%).

Ephedrine sulfate: 0.5–1 mg/kg/dose orally. May repeat every 4–6 hours. (Adult = 25 mg.) 0.2 mg/kg every 6 hours IM; 50 mg/1000 ml IV, adjusting drip rate to patient's response.

Epinephrine solution, 1:1000 (aqueous): 0.01–0.025 ml/kg (maximum dose: 0.5 ml) subcut. (Adult = 0.5–1 ml.)

Epinephrine solution, 1:200 (aqueous) (Sus-Phrine): 0.05–0.1 ml subcut, one dose only. Use smallest effective dose.

Equanil: See Meprobamate.

Ergotamine-caffeine: See Cafergot P-B, p 565.

Erythrocin: See Erythromycin, p 1040.

Erythromycin: See p 1040.

Esidrix: See Hydrochlorothiazide.

Estinyl: See Ethinyl estradiol.

Estradiol valerate (Delestrogen, Lastrogen): 10 mg/month IM for teenage girl. (Adult = 10–20 mg IM every 2–3 weeks.)

Ethambutol (Myambutol): See p 1040.

Ethinyl estradiol (Estinyl): 0.02–0.05 mg/dose orally 1–3 times daily for teenage girl. (Adult = 0.05 mg 1–3 times daily.)

Ethisterone (anhydrohydroxyprogesterone, Lutocylol, Pranone, Progestoral): 5–25 mg/day orally. (Same as adult dose.)

Ethosuximide (Zarontin): Under 6 years, 250 mg/day orally as starting dose. Over 6 years, 250 mg twice daily as starting dose. (See also p 561.)

Ethotoin (Peganone): 25–75 mg/kg/day orally in divided doses. (Adult = 0.5 gm orally 4–6 times daily.) (See also p 561.)

Ferrous salts: Medicinal iron. 4.5–6 mg/kg of elemental iron in 3 divided doses. (See also pp 92 and 380.)

Flaxedil: See Gallamine.

Flucytosine (Ancobon): See p 1040.

Fluorescein: 2 ml of 5% solution IV. (Adult = 3—4 ml of 20% solution.)

9α-Fluorocortisol (Florinef): See p 696.

Fluorouracil: Adults: 15 mg/kg daily for 4 days, not to exceed 1 gm/day. If no toxicity occurs, give 7.5 mg/kg on 6th, 8th, 10th, and 12th days of treatment. Discontinue at end of 12th day even if no toxicity is apparent. May repeat in 6 weeks after last injection of previous course if no toxicity is reported.

Fluoxymesterone (Halotestin, Ultandren): Up to 0.15 mg/kg/day orally in 2 divided doses in prepuberal children and up to 0.1 mg/kg/day in puberal children. (Adult = 2—10 mg/day.)

Fluprednisolone: See p 696.

Folic acid: 0.2—1 mg/day orally. (Adult = 10—15 mg/day.)

Fulvicin: See Griseofulvin, p 1040.

Fungizone: See Amphotericin B.

Furadantin: See Nitrofurantoin, p 1041.

Furazolidone (Furoxone): 5 mg/kg/day in 4 divided doses.

Furosemide (Lasix): Children: 1 mg/kg IV, IM, or orally. (Adults = Diuretic: 40—80 mg in a.m. Hypertension: 40 mg twice daily.)

Furoxone: See Furazolidone.

Gallamine (Flaxedil): 1 mg/lb IV.

Gammacorten: See Dexamethasone, p 696.

Gamma globulin: See pp 115 and 475.

Gantrisin: See p 1042.

Garamycin: See Gentamicin, p 1035.

Gemonil: See Metharbital, p 560.

Gentamicin (Garamycin): See p 1035.

Geocillin: See Carbenicillin, p 1037.

Geopen: See Carbenicillin, p 1037.

Glucagon: (1) Newborn, 0.025—0.1 mg/kg as single dose IV. Try smaller dose first. May repeat in 30 minutes. (2) Older child, 0.25—1 mg subcut, IM, or IV as single dose. Maximum dose is 1 mg.

Gold sodium thiosulfate: 1 mg/kg/week.

Gonadotropin, chorionic: 500—1000 units 2—3 times/ week for 5—8 weeks IM.

Griseofulvin (Fulvicin): See p 1040.

Guanethidine (Ismelin): 0.2 mg/kg/day orally as single dose. Increase dose at weekly intervals by same amount. (Adult = 10 mg daily. Larger doses possible for hospitalized adults.) *Caution.*

Haldol: See Haloperidol.

Haloperidol (Haldol): Children: contraindicated in children under 12 years of age; safety is not yet established. (Adults: no more than 15 mg/day. Initial: 1—2 mg 2 or 3 times daily. Maintenance: 1—2 mg 3—4 times daily.)

Halotestin: See Fluoxymesterone.

Heparin: (1) IV, 0.5 mg/kg/dose. This may be repeated every hour. One mg/kg every 4 hours is recommended for intravascular clotting. Control with clotting time. (Adult = 50 mg.) (2) Subcut, 4 mg/kg. Will prolong clotting time for 20—24 hours.

Herplex: See Idoxuridine.

Hetrazan: See Diethylcarbamazine.

Hexylresorcinol (Caprokol): 0.1 gm/year of age orally. Do not give over 1 gm. (Adult = 1 gm.)

Histadyl: See Methapyrilene.

Histamine: Provocative test: 0.02 mg/sq m IV. *Caution:* Phentolamine should be available.

HN2: See Mechlorethamine.

Hyaluronidase (Wydase): 500 viscosity units or 150 turbidity-reducing units in 1 ml sterile water or saline at site of fluid administration.

Hycodan: See Hydrocodone.

Hydralazine (Apresoline): (1) Orally, 0.15 mg/kg/dose 4 times daily. Increase to tolerance. (2) IV or IM alone: 1.5—3.5 mg/kg/day in 4—6 divided doses. (Adult, initial parenteral dose = 20—40 mg; single oral dose = 100 mg.)

Hydrochlorothiazide (Esidrix, HydroDiuril): One-tenth of chlorothiazide dose. (Adult = 25—200 mg/ day.)

Hydrocodone (Dicodid, Hycodan): 0.6 mg/kg/day orally in 3—4 doses. (Adult = 5—10 mg.)

Hydrocortisone: See p 696.

HydroDiuril: See Hydrochlorothiazide.

Hydroxyprogesterone caproate (Delalutin): 125 mg IM for teenage girl.

Hydroxyzine (Atarax): 1—2 mg/kg/day orally in 3 divided doses. Preoperatively, 1 mg/kg/day IM. (Adult = 25—50 mg 3 times daily.)

Hyoscine: See Scopolamine.

Idoxuridine (Dendrid, Herplex, Stoxil): 50 mg/kg/day by continuous IV drip over 4 days for newborn. (Adult maximum = 600 mg/kg total dose.)

Ilosone: See Erythromycin, p 1040.

Ilotycin: See Erythromycin, p 1040.

Imferon: See Iron-dextran complex, p 381.

Imipramine (Tofranil): Children: not generally recommended for children under 6 years. Initial dose of 25 mg/day; may increase according to response and tolerance. Generally not more than 75 mg/day for adolescents. (Adults = 75 mg initially, increased up to 150 mg daily.) *Caution.*

Imuran: See Azathioprine.

Inderal: See Propranolol.

Insulin: See p 708.

Iodine solution, strong (Lugol's solution): 1–10 drops daily for 10–21 days.

Iodochlorhydroxyquin (Vioform): 0.25 gm orally 3 times daily for 14 days.

Iodopyracet (Diodrast): 35% for IV urography and retrograde aortography. 70% for IV angiocardiography. 7% in saline with hyaluronidase for subcut injection.

Ipecac syrup: 15–20 ml/dose orally. (Adult = 20 ml.) Give water. Ambulate. Repeat in 20 minutes if necessary. Recover dose (lavage) if not vomited. (Adult = 15 ml.) *Caution:* Never use fluidextract of ipecac as emetic.

Iron: See pp 92 and 380. See also Ferrous salts, above.

Iron-dextran complex (Imferon): See p 381.

Ismelin: See Guanethidine.

Isoniazid: 15–20 mg/kg/day (up to 30 mg if necessary) divided into 3–4 doses. Maximum, 300 mg/day. (See also p 1040.)

Isonorin: See Isoproterenol.

Isoproterenol hydrochloride (Many trade names): 2–10 mg/dose sublingually 3 times daily for older children (not oftener than every 3–4 hours). Oral inhalation, 5–15 breaths of 1:200 solution (not more than 0.5 ml). (Adult = 15 mg sublingually 4 times daily.)

Isoproterenol sulfate: 1:200 or 1:400, 1–2 inhalations.

Isuprel: See Isoproterenol hydrochloride.

Kanamycin (Kantrex): See p 1035.

Kantrex: See Kanamycin, p 1035.

Kaopectate: 3–6 years, 1–2 tbsp; 6–12 years, 2–4 tbsp.

Kayexalate: See Sodium polystyrene sulfonate.

Keflin: See Cephalothin, p 1036.

Kefzol: See Cefazolin, p 1036.

Kenacort: See Triamcinolone, p 696.

Konakion: See Phytonadione.

Lasix: See Furosemide.

Lastrogen: See Estradiol valerate.

Latrodectus antivenin: 2.5 ml IM, repeated in 1 hour if symptoms have not markedly improved.

Leucovorin calcium: See Citrovorum factor.

Leukeran: See Chlorambucil.

Levarterenol: See Norepinephrine.

Levophed: See Norepinephrine.

Levothyroxine sodium: 0.1 mg levothyroxine sodium = 65 mg thyroid USP = 25–30 μg triiodothyronine. (See also pp 678 and 681.)

Lidocaine (Xylocaine): 1 mg/kg IV slowly for arrhythmia. Repeat as needed. (For anticonvulsant use, see p 561.) (Adult = 50–100 mg IV *slowly.*)

Lincocin: See Clindamycin, p 1039.

Lincomycin (Lincocin): See Clindamycin, p 1039.

Liothyronine: See Triiodothyronine.

Liquid petrolatum, liquid paraffin: See Mineral oil.

Liver injection, crude: 2 ml/day IM. (Same as adult dose.)

Lomotil: See Diphenoxylate.

Lugol's solution: See Iodine solution, strong.

Lypressin (lysine-8 vasopressin; Syntopressin): 30–55 units/day as a nasal spray.

Magnesium hydroxide: See Milk of magnesia.

Magnesium sulfate: As anticonvulsant or for hypertension: 0.1–0.4 ml/kg of 50% solution IM every 4–6 hours if renal function is adequate; or 10 ml (100 mg)/kg IV slowly as 1% solution. *Caution:* Check blood pressure carefully and have calcium gluconate available. As cathartic: 250 mg/kg/dose orally.

Mandelamine: See Methenamine mandelate.

Mannitol (Osmitrol): Test dose for oliguria, 0.2 gm/kg IV. Edema, 1–2.5 gm/kg IV over 2–6 hours. Cerebral edema, 1–2.5 gm/kg over a period of 30 minutes to 6 hours.

Marboran: See Methisazone, p 1043.

Marezine: See Cyclizine.

Matulane: See Procarbazine hydrochloride.

Mebaral: See Mephobarbital, p 560.

Mebendazole: 100–200 mg/day as single oral dose.

Mechlorethamine (HN2, Mustargen, nitrogen mustard): Inject slowly, diluted, 0.1 mg/kg/day for 4 days IV. (Same as adult dose.)

Mecholyl: See Methacholine.

Meclizine (Bonine): 2 mg/kg every 6–12 hours orally. (Adult = 25–50 mg.)

Medrol: See Methylprednisolone, p 696.

Medroxyprogesterone acetate (Depo-Provera): Children under 4 years, 100–150 mg per injection every 2 weeks. Children over 4 years, 150–200 mg per injection every 2 weeks.

Mellaril: See Thioridazine.

Menadiol sodium diphosphate (vitamin K analogue; Synkayvite): 1 mg IM. Not for infants. (Adult = 3–6 mg.)

Menadione sodium bisulfite (Hykinone): 1 mg IM. (Adult = 0.5–2 mg IM.)

Mepacrine: See Quinacrine.

Meperidine (Demerol): 0.6–1.5 mg/kg IM or orally as single analgesic dose; up to 6 mg/kg/day. (Adult = 50–100 mg.)

Mephentermine (Wyamine): 0.4 mg/kg orally, IM, or slowly IV as single dose. (Adult = 15–20 mg IM.)

Mephenytoin (Mesantoin): 3–10 mg/kg/day orally. Start smaller dose and gradually increase. (Adult = 0.1–0.3 gm 3 times daily.) (See also p 561.)

Mephobarbital: See p 560.

Meprobamate (Equanil, Miltown): Over 3 years: 7–30 mg/kg/day in 2–3 doses orally. (Adult = 400–800 mg 3 times daily.)

Mercaptopurine (6-MP, Purinethol): 2.5–4 mg/kg/day orally in 3 divided doses. (Same as adult dose.) *Caution.* (See also p 904.)

Mesantoin: See Mephenytoin.

Mestinon: See Pyridostigmine.

Metaraminol (Aramine): 0.04–0.2 mg/kg subcut or IM; 0.3–2 mg/kg in 500 ml solution as IV infusion. (Titrate by effect or by blood pressure readings.) (Adult = 2–10 mg IM, 0.5–5 mg IV.)

Methacholine (Mecholyl): For arrhythmia in young child, 0.1–0.4 mg/kg subcut or IM. May be increased by 25% every 30 minutes. Oral starting dose: about 18 times greater.

Methacycline: See p 1042.

Methadone (Adanon, Amidon): 0.7 mg/kg/day orally in 4–6 doses for analgesia.

Methandrostenolone (Dianabol): 0.04 mg/kg/day orally. (Adult = 2.5–5 mg daily.)

Methantheline (Banthine): 4–8 mg/kg/day orally or IM in 4 divided doses. (Adult = 50–100 mg 3 times daily.)

Methapyrilene (Histadyl, Thenylene): 0.2–0.3 mg/kg up to 5 times daily. (Adult = 50 mg/dose.)

Metharbital (Gemonil): See p 560.

Methdilazine (Tacaryl): 0.3 mg/kg/day orally in 2 doses.

Methenamine mandelate (Mandelamine): 60 mg/kg/day orally in 4 divided doses. Maintain acid urine. (Adult = 1–1.5 gm 4 times daily.) (See also p 1041.)

Methicillin: See p 1038.

Methimazole (Tapazole): 0.4 mg/kg/day in 3 divided doses. Maintenance, half of initial dose. (See also p 680.) (Adult = 15–60 mg.)

Methionine: 250 mg/kg/day orally in 3–4 divided doses. (Adult dose to acidify urine: 12–15 gm/day orally.)

Methisazone (Marboran): See p 1043.

Methocarbamol (Robaxin): 40–65 mg/kg/day orally in 4–6 divided doses. (Adult = 1.5–2 gm 3–4 times daily.)

Methotrexate (amethopterin): (1) Orally or IM, 0.12 mg/day. (Adult = 5–10 mg/day.) (2) Intrathecally, 0.25–0.5 mg/kg/week. (3) IV, 3–5 mg/kg as single dose every other week. *Caution:* Toxic. (See also p 904.)

Methoxamine (Vasoxyl): 0.25 mg/kg IM as single dose. (Adult = 15 mg IM.)

Methsuximide (Celontin): 20 mg/kg/day orally in divided doses. (Adult = 300 mg 1–3 times daily.) (See also p 560.)

Methylatropine nitrate: 1:10,000 alcoholic solution. Initial dose: 0.05 mg; increase to 0.3 mg as necessary subcut. (Adult = 1–3 mg.)

Methylcellulose: 0.5 gm at bedtime.

Methyldopa (Aldomet): 2–4 mg/kg IV initially. Double dose in 4 hours if no effect. Dilute in 50–100 ml fluid and infuse over 30–60 minutes. Children: 10 mg/kg/day orally in divided doses every 6 hours, increasing at 2-day or greater intervals to 65 mg/kg/day. For crises, 20–40 mg/kg/day in divided doses every 6 hours, continuing with oral doses when controlled. *Caution.* (Adult = 250 mg 3 times daily initially; adjust at 2- to 7-day intervals.)

Methylene blue: 0.1–0.2 ml/kg/dose of 1% solution slowly IV. (Adult = 100–150 mg.)

Methylphenidate (Ritalin): 0.25–0.75 mg/kg/dose orally. (Adult = 10 mg 3 times daily.) *Caution.*

Methylphenylethylhydantoin: See Mephenytoin.

Methylprednisolone: See p 696.

Methyltestosterone (Metandren, Oreton): 0.08–0.15 mg/kg/day sublingually. (Adult = 5–10 mg.)

Methysergide (Sansert): Children: dosage has not been established. (Adult = 4–8 mg/day.) Do not continue for more than 6 months; interrupt for 3–4 weeks and begin again. Precede drug-free interval with dosage reduction.

Meticorten: See Prednisone, p 696.

Metrazol: See Pentylenetetrazol.

Milk of magnesia: 0.5–1 ml/kg/dose orally. (Adult = 30–60 ml.)

Milontin: See Phensuximide.

Miltown: See Meprobamate.

Mineral oil: 0.5 ml/kg/dose orally. (Adult = 15–30 ml.)

Mintezol: See Thiabendazole, p 1042.

Morphine sulfate: 0.12–0.2 mg/kg every 4 hours as necessary subcut (no more than 10 mg/dose). (Adult = 10–15 mg.) Infants, start with half the dose. IV, 0.2 mg/kg/dose. May repeat.

6-MP: See Mercaptopurine.

Mustargen: See Mechlorethamine.

Myambutol: See Ethambutol, p 1040.

Mycifradin: See Neomycin, p 1035.

Mycostatin: See Nystatin, p 1041.

Myleran: See Busulfan.

Mysoline: See Primidone.

Nalidixic acid (NegGram): See p 1041.

Nalline: See Nalorphine.

Nalorphine (Nalline): 0.1–0.2 mg/kg/dose IV or IM. Repeat in 15 minutes if necessary. Use IV for shocky infant. Naloxone is drug of choice.

Naloxone (Narcan): 0.01 mg/kg/dose. Larger dosage usually required for propoxyphene poisoning. Short duration. Repeat every 15–30 minutes as needed.

Nandrolone (Durabolin): Infants: 12.5 mg every 2–4 weeks IM. Children: 25 mg every 2–4 weeks IM.

Narcan: See Naloxone.

NegGram: See Nalidixic acid, p 1041.

Nembutal: See Pentobarbital.

Neobiotic: See Neomycin, p 1035.

Neo-Cultol: 4 ml at bedtime.

Neolin: See Benzathine penicillin G, p 1038.

Neomycin (Mycifradin, Neobiotic): See p 1035.

Neostigmine (Prostigmin): (1) Orally, 0.25 mg/kg/dose. (Adult = 15 mg.) (2) IM, 0.025–0.045 mg/kg/dose. (Adult = 0.25–1 mg.) For myasthenia test, 0.04 mg/kg/dose IM. *Caution:* Atropine should be available.

Neo-Synephrine: See Phenylephrine.

Niacinamide (nicotinamide): See Niacin (p 89) and p 108.

Nicotinamide (niacinamide): See Niacin (p 89) and p 108.

Nilevar: See Norethandrolone.

Nitrofurantoin (Furadantin): See p 1041.

Nitrogen mustard: See Mechlorethamine.

Noctec: See Chloral hydrate.

Norepinephrine (levarterenol, Levophed): Start at 0.05 µg/kg/minute and titrate rate by blood pressure. (See also p 690.)

Norethandrolone (Nilevar): 0.4–0.8 mg/kg/day orally. (Adult = 30–50 mg daily.)

Norisodrine: See Isoproterenol hydrochloride and sulfate.

Nystatin (Mycostatin): See p 1041.

Omnipen: See p 1037.

Oncovin: See Vincristine, p 904.

Opium tincture, camphorated: See Paregoric.

Oreton: See Methyltestosterone.

Osmitrol: See Mannitol.

Ouabain (strophanthin): 0.01 mg/kg IV. Give half the dose initially. Check ECG frequently.

Oxacillin: See p 1038.

Oxandrolone: 0.05–0.1 mg/kg/day orally.

Oxymetholone: 1–3 mg/kg/day orally. (2.5 mg for children weighing less than 20 kg and 3.75 mg for those over 20 kg.)

Pancreatin (pancreatic enzymes): 0.3–0.6 gm with each feeding. Increase as necessary. (Adult = 2.5 gm.)

Papaverine: 1–6 mg/kg/day orally, IV, or IM in 4 divided doses. (Adult = 0.1 gm.)

Paradione: See Paramethadione, p 561.

Paraldehyde: (1) Orally, 0.1–0.15 ml/kg/dose. (Adult = 4–16 ml.) (2) Rectally, 0.3–0.6 ml/kg/dose in 1 or 2 parts of vegetable oil. (Adult = 16–32 ml.) (3) IM, 0.1 ml/kg as single anticonvulsant dose (not over 10 ml). (Adult = 4–10 ml.) (4) IV, 0.02 ml/kg *very slowly.* (Adult = 1–2 ml.) *Caution:* IM administration may cause fat necrosis; IV administration may cause respiratory distress or pulmonary edema. Do not use plastic equipment.

Paramethadione (Paradione): See p 561.

Paramethasone: See p 696.

Parathyroid injection: 50–300 units subcut or IM, and then 20–40 units every 12 hours. (Adult = 20–100 units daily.)

Paregoric: 0.06 ml/month of age up to 12 months. 5-year-old, 2 ml. May repeat every 3–4 hours if no drowsiness or respiratory depression. (Adult = 4 ml.) *Caution.*

PAS: See Aminosalicylic acid, p 1039.

Pediamycin: See Erythromycin, p 1040.

Peganone: See Ethotoin.

Penbritin: See p 1037.

Penicillamine (Cuprimine): Infants over 6 months: 250 mg/kg/day. Older children: 1 gm/day in 4 doses orally.

Penicillins: See p 1037.

Pentetrazol: See Pentylenetetrazol.

Pentobarbital (Nembutal): 1–1.5 mg/kg orally. Up to 3–5 mg/kg as single sedative dose. (Adult = 100 mg.)

Pentolinium (Ansolysen): (1) Orally, 1 mg/kg/day. (Adult = 20–200 mg 3 times daily.) (2) IM or subcut, 0.035–0.15 mg/kg dose. (Adult = 2.5–10 mg.) Start smaller dose and increase gradually.

Pentothal: See Thiopental.

Pentylenetetrazol (Metrazol, Pentetrazol): 20 mg/kg/ dose diluted IV slowly. *Caution.*

Periactin: See Cyproheptadine.

Permapen: See p 1038.

Pethidine hydrochloride: See Meperidine.

Phenacemide (Phenurone): 20–30 mg/kg/day orally. 5–10 years, 0.25 gm 3 times daily orally initially. (Adult = 0.5 gm 2–4 times daily.) (See also p 561.)

Phenergan: See Promethazine.

Phenobarbital: As sedative, 0.5–2 mg/kg as single dose orally every 4–6 hours. Anticonvulsant: 3–5 mg/kg/dose IM (IV only with extreme caution). **Epilepsy:** Starting doses: under 3 years, 16 mg 3 times daily; 3–6 years, 32 mg twice daily; over 6 years, 32 mg 3 times daily. (Adult = 30 mg.) **Hypnotic:** 3–6 mg/kg/dose orally. (Adult = 100–200 mg.)

Phenobarbital sodium: (1) Subcut or IM, 4–10 mg/kg as anticonvulsant. (2) Orally, 1–5 mg/kg as single sedative dose. (Adult = 15–100 mg.) (3) IM or rectally, 1 mg/kg as single sedative dose. (Adult = 30 mg.) (4) Rectally, 3–5 mg/kg as anticonvulsant. Acts more rapidly than phenobarbital. (Adult = 0.3 gm.)

Phenoxymethyl penicillin: See p 1038.

Phensuximide (Milontin): 20–40 mg/kg/day orally in divided doses. (Adult = 0.5–1 gm 2–3 times daily.) (See also p 561.)

Phentolamine (Regitine): (1) Test dose: 0.1 mg/kg IV. *Caution.* (2) Therapeutic, 5 mg/kg/day orally in 4 divided doses.

Phenurone: See Phenacemide.

Phenylephrine (Neo-Synephrine): 0.1 mg/kg IM or subcut; 1 mg/kg/day orally in 6 divided doses; 3–10 mg orally for nasal vasoconstriction. (Adult = 10–25 mg.)

Phenylpropanolamine (Propadrine): 2–4 ml of syrup every 4 hours.

Phenytoin (Many trade names): 2–8 mg/kg/day orally in 1 to 2 divided doses. IV, 1–5 mg/kg/day slowly; not to exceed 5 mg/minute in infants. (Adult = 0.3–0.5 gm/day.) (See also p 560.)

Physostigmine: 1–2 drops of 0.25 or 0.5% solution or ointment several times daily.

Phytonadione (vitamin K$_1$, AquaMephyton, Konakion, Mephyton): Prophylactic dose, 0.5–5 mg IM; therapeutic dose, 5–10 mg IM, IV, or orally. (Mephyton for oral use; others for parenteral use.)

Pilocarpine: 0.5, 1, and 2% as eyedrops; 0.1 mg/kg as single IM or subcut dose.

Piperazine (Antepar): See pp 814 and 815.

Piperoxan (Benodaine) hydrochloride: Test dose, 0.25 mg/kg IV slowly. (Same as adult dose.)

Pitressin and Pitressin Tannate: See Vasopressin injection and Vasopressin tannate injection.

Pituitary, posterior, powder: Small pinch (approximately 40–50 mg) nasally 4 times daily as necessary. (Adult = 30–60 mg 2–3 times daily.)

Plasma: 10–15 ml/kg IV.

Polycillin: See p 1037.

Polymyxin B (Aerosporin): See p 1041.

Posterior pituitary: See Pituitary, posterior.

Potassium chloride: See pp 607 and 1002.

Potassium iodide (saturated solution): 0.1–0.3 ml orally in cold milk or fruit juice. (Adult = 0.3 ml.)

Povan: See Pyrvinium pamoate.

Pralidoxime (Protopam): 25–50 mg/kg as 5% solution IV.

Pranone: See Ethisterone.

Prednisolone: See p 696.

Prednisone: See pp 696 and 904.

Primidone (Mysoline): 12–24 mg/kg/day. Under 8 years, start with 125 mg twice daily; over age 8, 250 mg twice daily. Increase slowly as necessary. (Adult = 250 mg as initial dose.)

Priscoline: See Tolazoline.

Pro-Banthine: See Propantheline.

Probenecid (Benemid): Initial dose, 25 mg/kg, then 10 mg/kg every 6 hours orally. (Adult = 1–2 gm initially, then 0.5 gm every 6 hours.)

Procainamide (Pronestyl): (1) Orally, 8–15 mg/kg every 4–6 hours. (2) IM, 6 mg/kg every 4–6 hours. (3) IV, for emergency use only: 2 mg/kg slowly over a 4- to 20-minute period. Monitor by continuous ECG and blood pressure recording every minute.

Procarbazine (Matulane): 8 mg/kg orally as initial dose. *Caution.*

Prochlorperazine (Compazine): 0.25–0.375 mg/kg/day orally or rectally in 2–3 doses. (Adult = 25 mg rectally twice daily or 5 mg orally 3–4 times daily.) IM, 0.25 mg/kg/day. *Caution:* Avoid overdosage; irritating to tissue.

Progesterone: See Ethisterone.

Progestoral: See Ethisterone.

Promethazine (Phenergan): As antihistaminic, 0.5 mg/kg orally at bedtime; 0.1 mg/kg orally 3 times daily. For nausea and vomiting, 0.25–0.5 mg/kg rectally or IM. For sedation, 0.5–1 mg/kg IM.

Pronestyl: See Procainamide.

Propadrine: See Phenylpropanolamine.

Propantheline (Pro-Banthine): 1–2 mg/kg/day orally in 4 divided doses after meals. (Adult = 15–30 mg 3–4 times daily.)

Propoxyphene (Darvon): 3 mg/kg/day orally. (Adult = 32–65 mg 3–4 times daily.)

Propranolol (Inderal): 0.01–0.15 mg/kg/dose as slow push IV. Oral dose is 0.5 to 1 mg/kg/day every 6 to 8 hours. Tetralogy spells may require dosage to 0.25 mg/kg IV.

Propylthiouracil: 6–7 mg/kg/day in 3 divided doses at intervals of 8 hours. Maintenance: one-third to one-half initial dose. (See also p 679.)

Prostaphlin: See p 1038.

Prostigmin: See Neostigmine.

Protamine sulfate: 2.5–5 mg/kg, then 1–2.5 mg/kg IV. Newborn: 1–2.5 mg/kg IM or IV. (Adult = 50 mg every 4–6 hours IV.)

Protopam: See Pralidoxime.

Pseudoephedrine hydrochloride (Sudafed): 4 mg/kg/day in 4 doses.

Purinethol: See Mercaptopurine.

Pyrantel pamoate (Combantrin): See p 815.

Pyribenzamine: See Tripelennamine.

Pyridostigmine (Mestinon): 7 mg/kg/day orally in 6 doses. Increase as necessary. (Average adult dose = 600 mg/day.)

Pyrimethamine (Daraprim): 12.5 mg weekly (in syrup).

Pyronil: See Pyrrobutamine.

Pyrrobutamine (Pyronil): 0.6 mg/kg/day. (Adult = 15 mg 3–4 times daily.)

Pyrvinium pamoate (Povan): 5 mg/kg/day. (Same as adult dose.)

Questran: See Cholestyramine.

Quinacrine (mepacrine, Atabrine): Giardiasis, 8 mg/kg/day for 5 days in 3 doses orally. (Maximum, 300 mg/day.) Tapeworm, 15 mg/kg in 2 doses orally. (Maximum, 800 mg.)

Quinidine: Test dose: 2 mg/kg orally. If tolerated, give 3–6 mg/kg every 2–3 hours. (Adult = 200 mg.) Therapeutic dose: 30 mg/kg/day orally in 4–5 divided doses.

Quinine sulfate: 1 year: 0.13 gm orally 3 times daily. 5–10 years: 0.3–0.6 gm 3 times daily. (Adult = 0.6 gm 3 times daily for 5–7 days.)

Regitine: See Phentolamine.

Reserpine (Serpasil, etc): (1) Orally, 0.005–0.03 mg/kg/day in 4 doses. (2) IM, 0.02–0.07 mg/kg every 12–24 hours. Initially, try smaller dose (except in life-threatening situations) and double in 4–6 hours if response is inadequate. May give with hydralazine (Apresoline). (Adult = 0.1–0.5 mg orally daily.)

Ritalin: See Methylphenidate.

Robaxin: See Methocarbamol.

Romilar: See Dextromethorphan.

Rondomycin (methacycline): See p 1042.

Salamid: See Salicylamide.

Salicylamide (Salamid, Salrin): 65 mg/kg/day in divided doses or 65 mg/year of age/dose orally 3 or 4 times daily. (Adult = 0.3–0.6 gm orally 3–4 times daily.)

Salicylazosulfapyridine (Azulfidine): 50–100 mg/kg/day orally at 4- to 6-hour intervals. (Adult = 1 gm 4–6 times daily.)

Salrin: See Salicylamide.

Sansert: See Methysergide.

Scopolamine: 0.006 mg/kg as single dose orally or subcut.

Secobarbital sodium (Seconal): (1) Orally, 2–6 mg/kg as a single sedative or light hypnotic dose. (Adult = 100 mg.) (2) Rectally, 6 mg/kg as a minimal hypnotic dose. (Adult = 200 mg.)

Seconal: See Secobarbital sodium.

Septra: See Trimethoprim-sulfamethoxazole, p 1042.

Serpasil: See Reserpine.

Sodium bicarbonate: See pp 68 and 1005.

Sodium nitrite: 10 mg/kg for every 12 gm/100 ml hemoglobin. May repeat one-half dose in 30 minutes. (See also p 875.)

Sodium phosphate: 150–200 mg/kg/dose orally. (Adult = 4–8 gm.)

Sodium polystyrene sulfonate (Kayexalate): Children: 1 mEq potassium/gm resin. Calculate dose on basis of desired exchange. Instill rectally in 10% glucose. May be administered every 6 hours. (Adult = 15 gm orally 1–4 times daily in small amount of water or syrup; 3–4 ml/gm resin.)

Sodium salicylate: As a single analgesic or antipyretic dose, 65 mg/year of age orally. (Adult = 0.3–0.6 gm.) For rheumatic fever, 90–130 mg/kg/day orally to maintain a blood level of 20–30 mg/100 ml. (Adult = 0.3–4 gm.)

Sodium sulfate: 150–200 mg/kg/dose orally. Give as 50% solution. (Adult = 8–12 gm.)

Sodium thiosulfate: See p 875.

Spectinomycin: See p 1035.

Spironolactone (Aldactone): (1) Diagnostic test: 0.5–1.5 gm/sq m/day in divided doses orally. (2) Edema and ascites: 1.7–3.3 mg/kg/day orally in divided doses. Start with smaller dose. *Caution.* (Adult = 25 mg 3–6 times daily orally.)

Stanozolol (Winstrol): 0.1 mg/kg/day orally.

Staphcillin: See p 1038.

Stilbestrol: 0.1–1 mg/day orally. (Adult = 0.5–1 mg.)

Stoxil: See Idoxuridine.

Streptomycin: See p 1035.

Strophanthin: See Ouabain.

Sudafed: See Pseudoephedrine hydrochloride.

Sulfisoxazole (Gantrisin): See p 1042.

Sulfonamides: See p 1042.

Sus-Phrine: See Epinephrine solution, 1:200.

Symmetrel: See Amantadine, p 1043.

Synkayvite: See Menadiol sodium diphosphate.

Synthroid Sodium: See Levothyroxine sodium.

Tapazole: See Methimazole, p 680.

Tegretol: See Carbamazepine, p 560.

Tempra: See Acetaminophen.

Tensilon: See Edrophonium chloride.

Testosterone: (1) Testosterone enanthate (Delatestryl): 200 mg IM every 4 weeks for teenage male. (2) Testosterone cyclopentylpropionate: 50–200 mg IM every 2–4 weeks for teenage male. (3) Testosterone propionate in oil: 10–50 mg 2–6 times a week IM for adult or teenage male. (4) Testosterone microcrystals in aqueous suspension: 100 mg IM every 2–3 weeks. (5) Testosterone pellets: 300 mg approximately every 3 months.

    Tetracyclines: See p 1042.

Tetraethylammonium chloride (Etamon): Test dose, 250 mg/sq m IV. *Caution:* Phentolamine should be available. (Adult = 10–15 mg/kg IV or IM.)

Theophylline: 10 mg/kg/day orally in 2–3 divided doses.

Thiabendazole (Mintezol): See p 1042.

Thiamine: See p 89.

Thiopental (Pentothal): 10–20 mg/kg rectally *slowly* for basal anesthesia.

Thioridazine (Mellaril): Children 2–12 years: 0.5–3 mg/kg/day (maximum). Older children: 20–40 mg/day. Not for children under 2 years. (Adult = 20–200 mg/day. Psychosis: 200–800 mg/day.)

Thorazine: See Chlorpromazine.

Thyroid: See p 678.

L-Thyroxine sodium: See Levothyroxine sodium.

Tigan: See Trimethobenzamide.

Tofranil: See Imipramine.

Tolazoline (Priscoline): *Potent vasodilator!* Up to 5 years, 2–10 mg; over 5 years, 5–15 mg orally or IM. Increase by 2–10 mg every 4 hours as necessary until flush or "goose-pimples" appear. (Adult = 12.5 mg 3 times daily.)

Toluidine blue: Initial dose: 2.5–7.5 mg/kg/day IV. Subsequent dose: 2–5 mg/kg/day IV. (Adult = 6–8 mg/kg.)

Triamcinolone: See p 696.

Tribromoethanol (Avertin): 65–100 mg/kg rectally. (Adult = 60 mg/kg.) Not over 8 gm should be given.

Trichlormethiazide: 0.03–0.1 mg/kg/day orally. (Adult = 2–8 mg daily.)

Tridione: See Trimethadione, p 561.

Triethylenemelamine (TEM): Initial dose: 5 mg/day orally. Subsequent dose: 1 mg/day or 0.04 mg/kg orally. (Adult = 5 mg, then 2.5 mg.) *Caution.*

Triiodothyronine (liothyronine, Cytomel): 25–30 μg are equivalent to 65 mg thyroid USP or 0.1 mg levothyroxine sodium.

Trimethadione (Tridione): See p 561.

Trimethaphan (Arfonad): Adult = 1–15 mg/minute IV.

Trimethobenzamide (Tigan): 15 mg/kg/day in divided doses. Children weighing less than 15 kg, one-half suppository (100 mg) 3 times daily. Children over 15 kg, 100 mg 3 times daily orally or 100–200 mg 3 times daily rectally.

Trimethoprim-sulfamethoxazole (Bactrim, Septra): See p 1042.

Tripelennamine (Pyribenzamine): 3–5 mg/kg/day orally in 3–6 divided doses. Maximum, 300 mg/day. (Adult = 50 mg 3–4 times daily.)

Trobicin: See Spectinomycin, p 1035.

Tubocurarine (curare): 0.2–0.4 mg/kg/day IM or subcut. *Caution.* (Adult = 6–9 mg.)

Tylenol: See Acetaminophen.

Unipen: See p 1038.

Urea: (1) 0.8 gm/kg/day in 3 divided doses orally. (Adult = 8 gm.) (2) 0.5–1 gm/kg IV over a period of 30–60 minutes. (Adult = 1–1.5 gm/kg.)

Urecholine Chloride: See Bethanechol chloride.

Valium: See Diazepam.

Vancocin: See Vancomycin, p 1043.

Vancomycin (Vancocin): See p 1043.

Vasopressin (Pitressin) injection: 0.125–0.5 ml (20 units/ml) IM. Short duration. (Adult = 0.25–0.5 ml.)

Vasopressin (Pitressin) tannate injection: 0.2–1 ml (5 units/ml in oil) every 2–4 days as necessary IM. Start with smaller dose and increase. Effective 1–3 days. (Adult = 0.3–1 ml.)

Vasoxyl: See Methoxamine.

Velban: See Vinblastine.

Versenate (edathamil): See EDTA.

Vinblastine (Velban): 0.1–0.2 mg/kg/week as single dose IV. (Adult = 0.1–0.15 mg/kg IV weekly.)

Vincristine (Oncovin): See p 904.

Vioform: See Iodochlorhydroxyquin.

Viokase (pancreatic replacement): 0.3–0.6 gm with each feeding. (Same as adult dose.)

Vitamins: See pp 89, 91, and 92.

Vitamin A: See pp 89, 92, and 103.

Vitamin C: See pp 89, 92, and 109.

Vitamin D: See pp 89 and 104.

Vitamin D$_2$ (calciferol): 25–200 thousand units/day.

Vitamin K$_1$: See Phytonadione.

Wyamine: See Mephentermine.

Wydase: See Hyaluronidase.

Xylocaine: See Lidocaine.

Zarontin: See Ethosuximide.

● ● ●

General References

Gellis SS, Kagan BM: *Current Pediatric Therapy 6.* Saunders, 1973.

Goodman LS, Gilman A: *The Pharmacological Basis of Therapeutics,* 5th ed. Macmillan, 1975.

Physicians' Desk Reference to Pharmaceutical Specialties and Biologicals, 31st ed, 1977. Medical Economics Co., 1977.

Shirkey HC (editor): *Pediatric Therapy,* 5th ed. Mosby, 1975.

Silver HK, Kempe CH, Bruyn HB: *Handbook of Pediatrics,* 12th ed. Lange, 1977.

Word B (editor): *A Paediatric Vade-Mecum,* 8th ed. Lloyd-Luke, 1974.

Ziai M, Janeway A, Cooke RE: *Pediatrics.* Little, Brown, 1969.

37 . . .
Anti-infective Chemotherapeutic Agents & Antibiotic Drugs

Anne S. Yeager, MD, & C. Henry Kempe, MD

Success in the use of antibiotics depends upon (1) identification of the pathogens to be eliminated; (2) selection of the therapeutic agent or agents most active against the pathogen (Table 37–1), which frequently requires the use of sensitivity tests; (3) selection of the appropriate route of administration in order to achieve maximum contact of the drug with the pathogen; and (4) administration of a sufficient amount of drug to reach and destroy the pathogen.

Resistance may develop (1) if strains in the bacterial population which are genetically resistant to the agent being used become dominant by selection; (2) if "spontaneous" mutation to a state of resistance should occur; or (3) by transmission from other organisms by means of episomes.

Newer Antibiotics

Methicillin, oxacillin, nafcillin, cloxacillin, and dicloxacillin are resistant to staphylococcal penicillinase and are used in the treatment of infections due to penicillin-resistant staphylococci. When used in proper dosage, drugs in this group are effective against penicillin-sensitive strains of staphylococci but are unnecessarily expensive; penicillin remains the drug of choice for penicillin-sensitive staphylococci.

Cefazolin, a cephalosporin for parenteral administration, has the same spectrum as cephalothin, but higher blood levels are achieved and last longer in comparison with cephalothin when both are given in the same dosage. The currently recommended dosage, however, is less than the dosage of cephalothin usually used in serious infections. Cephalexin is an improved oral cephalosporin which has the same spectrum as other members of this class of drugs and achieves better blood levels than previously available oral cephalosporins. It should not be relied upon for initiation of therapy in serious infections but is of use in urinary tract infections if the organism is sensitive.

Clindamycin, in addition to being effective against gram-positive cocci, appears to give as adequate coverage of anaerobic organisms as chloramphenicol. Pseudomembranous colitis has been associated with clindamycin administration. This serious complication appears to be much more common in adults than in children and is also more common after oral than after parenteral administration. Although useful, clindamycin should be prescribed under circumstances in which the patient can be carefully observed. Oral administration to outpatients with mild infections should be discouraged until more is known about the incidence of adverse side-effects in children.

Rifampin is an effective drug against *Mycobacterium tuberculosis* and also is useful in the treatment of carriers of *Neisseria meningitidis* who are in household contact with young children and infants to whom they pose a potential threat. In the therapy of tuberculosis, rifampin should be used in conjunction with other drugs and, in children, is generally indicated only if isoniazid resistance is suspected.

New Aminoglycosides; Problems in Prescribing

Tobramycin and gentamicin are aminoglycosides useful in the therapy of pseudomonas and other gram-negative infections. These 2 drugs are very similar in dosage rate, route of excretion, and toxicity. They have a narrow therapeutic-toxic ratio. Amikacin is also effective against pseudomonas as well as most other gram-negative organisms. The ability to achieve higher blood levels with amikacin may widen the therapeutic-toxic ratio and make the drug easier to use. Whether amikacin will be more clinically efficacious than the other aminoglycosides remains to be shown. At present, amikacin should probably be reserved for patients who have been shown to have infections due to organisms which are resistant to kanamycin, gentamicin, and tobramycin or who are housed in nurseries, intensive care units, or other areas which are encountering nosocomial infection with drug-resistant strains.

Blood levels of aminoglycosides show more scatter at a standard dose than is desirable, and any dose recommendations should be regarded as "best guesses." The dosages listed in the text are either absolute doses per day or per mg/kg/day. A more rational method would be to calculate the dosage on the basis of surface area, and this will be done as experience with these drugs accumulates.

Dosages in Newborns & Prematures

In premature and full-term newborn infants, caution is necessary to prevent overdosage in order to avoid causing serious and permanent damage. However, undertreatment is a definite risk if doses are not adjusted as the infant's renal function matures.

"Newborn" antibiotic dosages usually are recom-

Table 37—1. Choice of anti-infective agents.

Organism (and Gram Reaction)	Drug(s) of First Choice	Drug(s) of Second Choice
Actinomyces (+)	Penicillin	Tetracyclines, sulfonamides
Bacillus anthracis (+)	Penicillin	Tetracyclines, erythromycin
Bacteroides (−)*	Chloramphenicol, clindamycin	Penicillin, tetracyclines
Bordetella pertussis (−)	Erythromycin	Ampicillin
Brucella (−)	Tetracyclines + streptomycin	Kanamycin
Candida albicans	Nystatin, amphotericin B	Flucytosine
Chlamydiae (agents of lymphogranuloma venereum, psittacosis, and trachoma)	Tetracyclines	Chloramphenicol, sulfonamides
Clostridia (+)	Antitoxin + penicillin	Erythromycin, kanamycin
Corynebacterium diphtheriae (+)	Antitoxin + penicillin	Erythromycin, lincomycin
Enterobacter (−)*	Kanamycin, gentamicin, amikacin, chloramphenicol	Polymyxin, colistin, tetracycline + streptomycin
Erysipelothrix (+)	Penicillin	Tetracyclines, erythromycin
Escherichia coli (−)*	Gentamicin, ampicillin, kanamycin, cephalexin, cephalothin	Tetracyclines, polymyxin, colistin, sulfonamides
Francisella tularensis (−)	Streptomycin + tetracycline	
Haemophilus influenzae (−)*	Chloramphenicol, ampicillin	Streptomycin, sulfadiazine
Klebsiella pneumoniae (−)*	Kanamycin, gentamicin, cephalothin, cephalexin, cefazolin	Polymyxin, colistin, tetracycline + streptomycin
Leptospira icterohaemorrhagiae	Tetracyclines	Penicillin
Listeria monocytogenes (+)	Ampicillin, tetracyclines	Penicillin
Mycobacterium leprae (+)	Sulfones	Solasulfone, sulfonamides, diphenylthiourea, sulfoxone, rifampin
M tuberculosis (+)*	Isoniazid + rifampin or Isoniazid + (PAS + streptomycin) or ethambutol† In meningitis: Isoniazid + rifampin ± streptomycin	Ethionamide, pyrazinamide, cycloserine, viomycin
Mycoplasma pneumoniae	Tetracyclines, erythromycin	
Neisseria gonorrhoeae (−)	Penicillin + probenecid	Ampicillin + probenecid, spectinomycin, tetracyclines
N meningitidis (−)	Penicillin	Ampicillin, chloramphenicol
Nocardia (+)*	Sulfonamides + cycloserine	Sulfonamides + agent chosen by sensitivity tests
Proteus mirabilis (−)*	Ampicillin, penicillin	Cephalothin, kanamycin, gentamicin
Proteus vulgaris, P morganii, *P rettgeri* (−)*	Kanamycin, gentamicin, amikacin	Chloramphenicol
Pseudomonas aeruginosa (−)*	Tobramycin, amikacin, carbenicillin	Polymyxin B, colistin, kanamycin, gentamicin, tetracyclines
Rickettsiae (−)	Chloramphenicol (+ corticosteroids for Rocky Mountain spotted fever)	Tetracyclines
Salmonella other than *S typhi* (−)*	Ampicillin, gentamicin	Chloramphenicol, cephalothin, tetracyclines, kanamycin
S typhi (−)*	Chloramphenicol, amoxicillin	Trimethoprim-sulfamethoxazole
Serratia (−)*	Amikacin or gentamicin + carbenicillin	Chloramphenicol
Shigella (−)*	Ampicillin, cephalothin	Tetracyclines
Spirillum minus (−)	Penicillin	Tetracyclines
Staphylococcus (+)* if sensitive	Penicillin	Erythromycin, cephalothin, cephalexin
Staphylococcus (+) if resistant to penicillin*	Methicillin, nafcillin, oxacillin, dicloxacillin, cloxacillin	Cephalothin, cefazolin, clindamycin, erythromycin, kanamycin
Streptococcus (+) (group A, B, and nonenterococcal group D)	Penicillin	Erythromycin, cephalothin, ampicillin, clindamycin
S faecalis (+)* (group D enterococci)	Penicillin + streptomycin, ampicillin	Cephalothin
S (Diplococcus) pneumoniae	Penicillin	Cephalothin, erythromycin, clindamycin
Treponema pallidum	Penicillin	Cephalothin, erythromycin
Yersinia pestis (−)	Streptomycin + tetracycline	

*Sensitivity tests usually indicated.

†Ethambutol should be used with caution in children too young to complain of or be tested for changes in visual acuity.

Table 37—2. Use of antibiotics in patients with renal failure.*

Drug	Principal Mode of Excretion or Detoxification	Approximate Half-Life in Serum		Proposed Dosage Regimen† in Renal Failure‡	
		Normal	Renal Failure	Usual Initial Dose	Give Half the Initial Dose at Interval Of
Penicillin G	Tubular secretion	0.5 hours	10 hours	70,000 units/kg	8–12 hours
Ampicillin	Tubular secretion	0.5 hours	10 hours	50 mg/kg	8–12 hours
Methicillin	Tubular secretion	0.5 hours	10 hours	50 mg/kg	6–8 hours
Cephalothin	Tubular secretion	0.8 hours	15 hours	35 mg/kg	12 hours
Streptomycin	Glomerular filtration	2.5 hours	3–4 days	10 mg/kg	3–4 days
Kanamycin§	Glomerular filtration	3 hours	3–4 days	7.5–10 mg/kg	3–4 days
Gentamicin§	Glomerular filtration	2.5 hours	3–4 days	1.5–2 mg/kg	3–4 days
Vancomycin	Glomerular filtration	6 hours	8–9 days	10 mg/kg	8–10 days
Polymyxin B§	Glomerular filtration	5 hours	2–3 days	1.5 mg/kg	3–4 days
Colistimethate	Glomerular filtration	3 hours	2–3 days	2.5 mg/kg	3–4 days
Chloramphenicol	Liver and glomerular filtration	3 hours	4 hours	30 mg/kg	8 hours
Erythromycin	Liver and glomerular filtration	1.5 hours	5 hours	20 mg/kg (IV)	8 hours
Clindamycin	Glomerular filtration and liver (?)	4 hours	8 hours	5 mg/kg (orally)	8 hours

*This table should be used only as a guide. Serum killing power or μg/ml should be measured when possible, as well as minimal inhibitory concentration (MIC) of drug for specific organism.

†IV or IM unless otherwise specified.

‡Considered here to be marked by creatinine clearance of 10 ml/minute or less.

§See Kunin C: Antibiotic usage in patients with renal impairment. Hosp Pract 1:141, Jan 1972.

mendations for the first 7 days of life in a full-term infant and not for the first 6 weeks of life referred to as the perinatal period. Failure to recognize that there is a marked increase in excretion of drugs such as penicillin G, methicillin, ampicillin, gentamicin, and kanamycin by the second week of life and to increase drug dosages at this time will result in unsatisfactory blood levels as well as clinical failure. The need for higher drug dosages in infants 8 or more days old is especially important if therapy of gram-negative infections, including meningitis, is to be successful. Whatever the age of the child, about 30 times as much ampicillin is required in blood or CSF to kill a sensitive *Escherichia coli* strain as is required to kill a sensitive *Haemophilus influenzae* strain. Some strains of group B streptococci are 50 times more resistant to penicillin G than group A strains. Marginal penicillin levels in the CSF will result if the infant's increasing ability to excrete penicillin is not taken into account.

An increasing ability to excrete cephalothin is also seen throughout the first week of life and is similar in extent to that which occurs with ampicillin. Indications for the use of cephalothin in the neonatal period are rare, however, because the drug does not penetrate into CSF and therefore does not protect bacteremic patients from meningitis.

The small, sick, premature infant who is neither "just born" nor old enough in chronologic age to be considered "term" remains in no-man's-land, and drug dosages should probably be intermediate between those used for prematures who are less than 3 days of age and those used for term babies who are more than 7 days of age.

Precautions in Oliguric Children (Table 37—2)

Regular drug dosages are too high for children with reduced renal function. Dosage and time schedules must be adjusted to renal output in the case of the more toxic agents (amikacin, gentamicin, kanamycin, tobramycin, colistin, and polymyxin).

PEDIATRIC ANTIMICROBIAL THERAPEUTIC AGENTS

The aminoglycosides and cephalosporins are grouped together in sections 1 and 2, respectively. The penicillin derivatives are listed under penicillin in section 3 according to whether they are sensitive or resistant to penicillinase. All other drugs are individually listed in alphabetical order in section 4.

1. AMINOGLYCOSIDES

Amikacin (Amikin)

Use: Active against most gram-negative organisms, including most strains of pseudomonas and serratia.

Dosage (IM or IV):

Newborn: 15 mg/kg/day in divided doses every 12 hours. (IV dose not well established.)

Child: 22.5 mg/kg/day in divided doses every 8 hours.

Adolescent: 22.5 mg/kg/day in divided doses every 8 hours.

Gentamicin (Garamycin)

Use: Gram-negatives including pseudomonas, proteus, and serratia. Some activity against coagulase-positive staphylococci. Relatively inactive against pneumococci, streptococci, and anaerobic organisms.

Dosage:

IM:

Newborn, premature under 3 days old: 6 mg/kg/day in divided doses every 8–12 hours.

Newborn, premature over 3 days old and full-term: 7.5 mg/kg/day in divided doses every 8 hours.

Child: 7.5 mg/kg/day in divided doses every 6–8 hours.

Adolescent: 5 mg/kg/day in divided doses every 6–8 hours.

IV: The dose should be given over a 1-hour period because of possible curare-like effects if administered too rapidly. The dosage is the same as for IM administration.

Intraventricular: 4 mg/day (gives CSF levels of 3–50 µg/ml or more 24 hours after injection).

Intrathecal: 2.5–4 mg/day.

Toxicity: Irreversible vestibular damage has occurred, most often in uremic patients, and is related to excessive plasma levels. Transient proteinuria, elevated BUN, oliguria, azotemia, macular skin eruption, and elevated SGOT.

Comment: Dosage schedule for uremic patients should be modified. Should be used with caution in patients receiving other ototoxic drugs. Overall toxicity is probably the same as or less than kanamycin. *Caution:* Parenteral therapy should be reserved for serious pseudomonas infections, hospital-acquired infections, and life-threatening infections of unknown but suspected gram-negative origin. If cultures later are positive for an organism sensitive to penicillin, methicillin, cephalothin, ampicillin, or kanamycin, therapy should be changed to one of these drugs. Every effort should be made to use this drug as little as possible in order to discourage the development of drug resistance. Serum levels should be measured in any patient requiring long-term therapy as blood levels are variable despite standard dose in mg/kg. Blood levels of 6–8 µg/ml are usually necessary to control serious infections. Levels of > 10–12 µg/ml may be toxic to the eighth nerve. In young children, peak serum levels of less than 5 µg/ml are common on currently recommended doses. After measurement of serum levels, dose increases may be necessary in serious gram-negative infections. Oral therapy is recommended only for nursery outbreaks of diarrhea due to enteropathogenic *E coli.*

Kanamycin (Kantrex)

Use: Bactericidal for coliforms, proteus, some pseudomonas, staphylococci, mycobacteria. Of use in special circumstances in some vibrio, salmonella, and shigella infections.

Dosage:

Oral: Not absorbed. Used for sterilization of bowel. 50–100 mg/kg/day in divided doses every 6 hours.

IM or IV:

Newborn, premature: Up to 3 days old, 7.5 mg/kg every 12 hours; over 3 days old, 10 mg/kg every 12 hours.

Newborn, full-term: Up to 7 days old, 10 mg/kg every 12 hours; over 7 days old, 10 mg/kg every 8 hours.

Child: 30 mg/kg/day in divided doses every 8 hours.

Adolescent: 1 gm/day in divided doses every 12 hours (for serious infection, give 2 gm/day for a short time).

Intrathecal: 5–8 mg/day (up to 20 mg/day has been used).

Toxicity: Limit use to 10 days. Irreversible deafness occurs after prolonged administration of high doses. (Cumulative ototoxicity with other ototoxic drugs occurs.) Nephrotoxicity is transient unless prior renal impairment was present.

Comment: Modify dosage and use with caution in oliguric patients. Measurement of blood levels is desirable.

Neomycin (Mycifradin, Neobiotic)

Use: Parenteral uses superseded by penicillinase-resistant penicillins.

Comment: Because neomycin therapy can result in the development of disaccharide deficiency, it is no longer recommended for therapy of enteropathogenic *E coli* (EPC). For the individual case, oral polymyxin, colistin, or kanamycin is suggested. The sensitivities of prevalent EPC strains differ in different parts of the country. Gentamicin is recommended only for nursery outbreaks of enteropathogenic *E coli.*

Spectinomycin (Trobicin)

Use: *Neisseria gonorrhoeae.*

Dosage (IM):

Adolescent: 2 gm as a single dose.

Comment: This drug is in the same class of drugs as streptomycin and kanamycin. Toxicity reported after a single dose includes urticaria, dizziness, nausea, chills, fever, and insomnia.

Streptomycin Sulfate

Use: *Mycobacterium tuberculosis, Haemophilus in-*

fluenzae, some gram-negatives. Synergistic with penicillin against enterococci. Resistance develops quickly.

Dosage:

IM:

  Newborn: 10–20 mg/kg/day. Use with caution.

  Child: 20 mg/kg every 12–24 hours.

  Adolescent: 1 gm every 12–24 hours.

Toxicity: Damage to vestibular apparatus. Fatal CNS and respiratory depression. Bone marrow depression, renal toxicity, hypersensitivity, superinfection.

Comment: Should never be used as the only drug. Dihydrostreptomycin is toxic to the eighth nerve and should not be used.

Tobramycin

Use: Most *Escherichia coli,* enterobacter, klebsiella, proteus, and pseudomonas strains.

Dosage (IM or IV):

  Child: 7.5 mg/kg/day in divided doses every 8 hours (not well established).

  Adolescent: 4 mg/kg/day in divided doses every 8 hours.

Toxicity: Renal and eighth nerve (similar to gentamicin).

Comment: Excretion and dosage are similar to those of gentamicin. Some pseudomonas strains are more sensitive to tobramycin than to gentamicin; hence, tobramycin may be more clinically effective than gentamicin at the same concentration in μg/ml. With this possible exception, these 2 drugs are very similar. Gram-negative strains which are resistant to gentamicin but sensitive to tobramycin occur but are relatively rare. More commonly, gentamicin-resistant strains are also resistant to tobramycin.

2. CEPHALOSPORINS

Use

Equivalent to penicillin against gram-positive organisms except enterococcus, which is relatively insensitive. Highly resistant to staphylococcal penicillinase. Effective against some *Escherichia coli,* indole-negative proteus, most klebsiellae, and many strains of *Haemophilus influenzae.* Ineffective against pseudomonas and most strains of serratia and enterobacter. When used for gram-negative infections, sensitivities should be determined in each case.

Comment

There are no significant differences among cephalosporins with regard to sensitivity of the different species of bacteria. Cephalosporins do not penetrate CSF well and should not be used for therapy of meningitis. Cephalosporins have been used as penicillin substitutes in penicillin-sensitive persons but should be

used with caution. Anaphylaxis has been reported but is rare clinically, although the incidence of "sensitivity" to cephalothin as demonstrated by in vitro tests in penicillin-sensitive persons is high. The reason for this discrepancy is not known at present. In comparison with cephaloridine, these 3 members of this class of drugs are relatively nontoxic to the kidneys. Owing to its greater renal toxicity and lack of significant therapeutic advantage, cephaloridine is no longer recommended. Blood levels obtained with the oral cephalosporins are adequate for gram-positive organisms but in general should not be relied on for therapy of systemic gram-negative infections or for initial therapy in seriously ill persons. Urine levels are adequate for the therapy of gram-negative infections with sensitive organisms. Cefazolin has a longer serum half-life than cephalothin, and higher blood levels are achieved when it is used at the same dosage on a mg/kg basis. Synergistic action may occur when cephalosporins are used in conjunction with the aminoglycosides for some gram-negative strains.

Cefazolin (Ancef, Kefzol)

IM or IV:

  Newborn: Do not use.

  Child: 25–100 mg/kg/day in divided doses every 6–8 hours.

  Adolescent: 2–6 gm/day (up to 12 gm in serious infections).

Toxicity: Renal toxicity has been proved in experimental animals in doses of 300 mg/kg or more.

Cephalexin (Keflex)

Oral:

  Child: 50–100 mg/kg/day in divided doses every 6–8 hours.

  Adolescent: 1–2 gm/day in divided doses every 6–8 hours.

IM or IV: Not available.

Toxicity: Nausea, vomiting, diarrhea, elevated SGOT, rash, pruritus.

Cephalothin (Keflin)

Oral: Not absorbed.

IM or IV:

  Newborn: 60–150 mg/kg/day in divided doses every 4–6 hours.

  Child: 100–300 mg/kg/day in divided doses every 4–6 hours.

  Adolescent: Up to 12 gm/day (up to 24 gm in serious infections).

Toxicity: Pain on injection, drug fever, sterile abscesses, positive direct Coombs test, idiopathic thrombocytopenic purpura, brown-black Clinitest response (normal glucose oxidase).

3. THE PENICILLINS

All penicillins are cross-allergenic. The mechanism of action of the tetracyclines and chloramphenicol is antagonistic to that of the penicillins.

In serious infections, all penicillins should be given in divided doses at least every 4 hours.

Until skin testing materials are commercially available, the following method may be used to desensitize the patient when penicillin must be used in the presence of possible penicillin sensitivity: (1) scratch test, 100 units/ml; (2) scratch test, 10,000 units/ml; (3) intradermal injection, 0.1 ml of solution of 1000 units/ml; (4) if no reaction occurs, proceed with continuous intravenous therapy.

Penicillinase Sensitive

Ampicillin, amoxicillin, hetacillin, carbenicillin, penicillin G, procaine penicillin G, benzathine penicillin G, phenoxymethyl penicillin.

A. Ampicillin, Amoxicillin, Hetacillin:

Use: Gram-positive cocci, except for penicillinase-producing staphylococci, *Neisseria meningitidis, N gonorrhoeae,* and listeria. Most *Haemophilus influenzae* are sensitive, but resistant strains appear to be increasing. Fifty to 80% of strains of *Escherichia coli,* some salmonellae, shigellae, and 90% of *Proteus mirabilis* are sensitive. *Enterobacter aerogenes* and klebsiellae are usually resistant.

Toxicity: Generally of low toxicity. Diarrhea, skin rash (especially in mononucleosis), drug fever, and superinfection occur.

Comment: Hetacillin is hydrolyzed in the body to ampicillin, which appears to be the active agent. Amoxicillin is slightly less active than ampicillin against shigellae and *H influenzae* and slightly more active against enterococci and *Salmonella typhi.* Amoxicillin achieves about twice the blood level as is attained at the same dose of ampicillin. Less diarrhea may occur with amoxicillin than with ampicillin.

A loading dose of 50–100 mg/kg of ampicillin is desirable in serious infections. Five hundred milligrams of ampicillin contain about 1.7 mEq Na^+. Ampicillin levels in the CSF drop after the third day in meningitis as the pleocytosis decreases; the drug should be given parenterally for the entire course. Higher blood levels are achieved on oral administration if the drug is given in the fasting state. Peak blood levels following oral administration are in the range of 1 μg/ml, which is sufficient for sensitive gram-positive organisms but inadequate for systemic infections with gram-negative organisms. Higher levels are achieved in urine. In intravenous solutions, ampicillin is not stable; it should be reconstituted immediately prior to use. Hetacillin is more stable after reconstitution than ampicillin.

Dosage:

Ampicillin (Alpen, Omnipen, Penbritin, Polycillin, Totacillin)
Oral (infant, child, adolescent): 50–150 mg/kg/day in divided doses every 6 hours.
IM or IV:
Newborn: 100–300 mg/kg/day in divided doses every 4–6 hours. By 7–10 days of age, excretion of ampicillin is such that per kg doses should be increased to those used in the young infant.
Child, adolescent: 150–400 mg/kg/day in divided doses every 4 hours.
Amoxicillin (Amoxil, Larocin, Polymox)
Oral:
Child: 25–100 mg/kg/day in divided doses every 8 hours.
Adolescent: 750–1500 mg/day in divided doses every 8 hours.
Hetacillin (Versapen-K)
Oral:
Child: 25–40 mg/kg/day in divided doses every 6–8 hours.
IM or IV:
Child, adolescent: 25–40 mg/kg/day.

B. Carbenicillin (Geocillin, Geopen):

Use: Covers principally pseudomonas, indole-positive proteus, and some strains of serratia.
Dosage:
Oral (carbenicillin indanyl sodium):
Child: 50–100 mg/kg/day.
Adolescent: 4 gm/day.
IM: Do not use.
IV (carbenicillin disodium):
Newborn: 400 mg/kg/day (not well established).
Child: 500–600 mg/kg/day in divided doses every 2–4 hours.
Adolescent: Up to 30 gm/day.
Toxicity: Bleeding diathesis secondary to platelet dysfunction. SGOT rises have been reported and may be due to anicteric hepatitis as well as muscle necrosis after intramuscular injection.
Comment: High doses are required. The oral form is useful only in urinary tract infections. Of value in pseudomonas infections in patients with compromised renal function (toxicity low). Probably synergistic with gentamicin. Because of the rapid development of resistance and the difficulty of treating systemic infections, intravenous carbenicillin should be used only in combination with an aminoglycoside. Contains 4.7 mEq Na^+ per gram.

C. Penicillin G, Potassium or Sodium Salt:

Use: Gram-positive and gram-negative cocci, gram-positive bacilli. In high doses, some gram-negative bacilli.
Dosage:
Oral (child, adolescent): 100–400 thousand units/dose in 5 doses one-half hour before meals.

IM (child, adolescent): 20—50 thousand units/ kg/day in divided doses every 4—6 hours.

IV:

Newborn under 7 days old: 200,000 units/kg in divided doses every 4—6 hours. Run in over at least 20 minutes (see comment).

Newborn over 7 days old: 400,000 units/kg in divided doses every 4 hours. Run in over 20 minutes (see comment).

Child: 20—400 thousand units/kg/day in divided doses every 4—6 hours.

Adolescent: 5—20 million units.

Toxicity: Hypersensitivity (anaphylaxis, urticaria, rash, drug fever). Change in bowel flora, candidiasis, diarrhea, hemolytic anemia, hematuria, interstitial nephritis. Neurotoxic in very large doses.

Comment: Some group B streptococci require 0.5 U/ml of penicillin G for inhibition. This compares to the $\leqslant$ 0.009 U/ml required to inhibit group A streptococci. These higher penicillin G doses are unlikely to cause seizures in the newborn if the dose is administered over a 20 minute period. Not all group B streptococcal infections will respond to these increased newborn doses. High concentration in the urine makes this agent useful in treatment of some urinary tract infections with gram-negative rods. One million units of potassium penicillin G contain 1.7 mEq K^+. Avoid pushing large doses of potassium salt, as in initiating therapy for meningitis; use sodium salt instead. 1.7 units = 1 μg penicillin G. Because of exceedingly rapid excretion, administration of a dose every 2 hours or a constant infusion may be desirable in the treatment of some infections.

D. Procaine Penicillin:

Dosage (IM):

Newborn: 50,000 units/kg/day. Avoid if possible since it causes sterile abscesses, does not achieve therapeutic levels in the CSF, and also contains 120 mg procaine/300,000 units penicillin G, which may be toxic.

Child, adolescent: 100—600 thousand units every 12—24 hours.

E. Benzathine Penicillin:

1. Benzathine penicillin G (Bicillin L-A, Neolin, Permapen)—

Dosage: 1.2 million units IM every 25—27 days.

Comment: The preferred drug for rheumatic fever prophylaxis. Increasing the dose gives a more sustained rather than a higher blood level. (Penicillin cannot be detected in CSF after administration of this form.) In acute illness, the procaine penicillin in Bicillin C-R may be desirable.

2. Benzathine penicillin, 600,000 units, and penicillin G procaine, 600,000 units (Bicillin C-R); benzathine penicillin, 900,000 units, and penicillin G procaine, 300,000 units (Bicillin C-R 900/300)—

Dosage: 1.2 million units IM.

Comment: Used for treatment of acute streptococcal infections. Do not use for rheumatic fever prophylaxis.

F. Phenoxymethyl Penicillin (Compocillin V, Pen-Vee, V-Cillin):

Dosage (oral):

Newborn: 50—170 mg/kg in divided doses every 6 hours.

Child: 1—6 gm in divided doses every 6 hours.

Adolescent (serious infections): More than 6 gm/day in divided doses every 4—6 hours.

Comment: 125 mg = 200,000 units.

Penicillinase Resistant

Cloxacillin (Tegopen), dicloxacillin (Dynapen, Veracillin), methicillin (Dimocillin, Staphcillin), nafcillin (Unipen), oxacillin (Prostaphlin).

Use: Penicillinase- and nonpenicillinase-producing staphylococci. These penicillins probably are somewhat less effective than penicillin G for pneumococci and streptococci. Enterococci are insensitive.

Dosage:

Oral:

Cloxacillin: 50—100 mg/kg/day in divided doses every 6 hours.

Dicloxacillin: 25—100 mg/kg/day in divided doses every 6 hours.

Methicillin: Do not use.

Nafcillin: Do not use.

Oxacillin: 50—100 mg/kg/day in divided doses every 6 hours.

IM or IV:

Newborn, premature: Methicillin, 100 mg/kg/ day in divided doses every 6—8 hours for the first 7 days.

Newborn, full-term: Methicillin, 200—250 mg/kg/ day in divided doses every 6 hours for the first 7 days.

Child: Methicillin or nafcillin, 250—300 mg/kg/ day in divided doses every 4 hours.

Adolescent: Methicillin or nafcillin, 4—12 gm/ day.

Toxicity: Hypersensitivity; kidney damage, hematuria (thought to be hypersensitivity phenomena) in all age groups with methicillin and in infants with oxacillin. Hematuria not reported to date in patients treated with nafcillin alone. Reversible bone marrow depression occurs.

Comment: Deterioration of methicillin in dextrose in water or normal saline solution is rapid and lessened by adding 3 mEq/liter $NaHCO_3$. If therapy is initiated with a drug in this class because of suspected penicillin resistance, therapy should be changed to penicillin G when sensitivity to this agent is shown. One gram of methicillin contains 2.5 mEq Na^+. Nafcillin causes a false-positive sulfosalicylic acid reaction for urinary protein.

4. ANTIMICROBIAL AGENTS
(In Alphabetical Order)

Aminosalicylic Acid (PAS; PAS-C)
Use: Tuberculosis.
Dosage (oral):
Child: PAS: 250–300 mg/kg/day in divided doses every 6 hours; for salts of PAS, increase dose by 25%. PAS-C: 150 mg/kg/day in divided doses every 6 hours.
Adolescent: PAS: 12 gm/day; PAS-C: 8 gm/day.
Toxicity: Gastrointestinal symptoms, hypersensitivity (skin, fever, genital), renal irritation, goitrogenic, hematologic, hepatic.
Comment: Avoid or reduce dosage by half when renal function is impaired. Stop drug at first sign of skin rash. PAS-C usually causes less gastric irritation than PAS.

Amphotericin B (Fungizone)
Use: Active against a variety of fungi (candida, cryptococcus, blastomyces, sporotrichum, coccidioides, histoplasma).
Dosage (infant, child, adolescent):
IV: 0.5–1.5 mg/kg/day or every other day, given over 4–6 hours. Begin as 0.25 mg/kg/day.
Intrathecal, intraventricular, or cisternal: 0.5–1 mg in 10 ml spinal fluid every other day. Begin with 0.1 mg and increase.
Toxicity: Chills, fever, malaise. Significant renal, hepatic, and bone marrow damage. Thrombophlebitis, calcifications.
Comment: Indicated only in severe systemic fungal infections. Administration of corticosteroids before the daily dose is given may ameliorate side-effects. Blood levels are variable (Am J Med 45:405, 1968).

Chloramphenicol (Chloromycetin)
Use: Bacteriostatic for a wide range of gram-positive and gram-negative organisms, rickettsiae, and chlamydiae. Active against most species of bacteroides and anaerobic streptococci.
Dosage:
Oral (crystalline):
Child: 50–100 mg/kg/day in divided doses every 6 hours. The palmitate form is poorly absorbed.
Adolescent: 50 mg/kg/day in divided doses every 6 hours.
IM: Intramuscular injection should not be used since absorption is poor.
IV (succinate):
Newborn, premature: 25 mg/kg/day as a single dose once every 24 hours. This drug should be avoided in premature infants. If used, serum levels should be followed to avoid toxicity initially and to avoid inadequate dosage as renal and liver functions mature. Peak

blood levels of 15–20 µg/100 ml may be sufficient for infections other than meningitis. Blood levels of 30 µg/ml may be necessary to attain adequate spinal fluid levels in gram-negative meningitis.
Newborn, full-term: 25–50 mg/kg/day in divided doses every 12 hours.
Child: 50–100 mg/kg/day in divided doses every 6–8 hours.
Adolescent: 50–100 mg/kg/day.
Toxicity: In newborns up to 4 months of age, vasomotor collapse (gray syndrome). Irreversible aplastic anemia (one in 60,000 cases) and reversible suppression of granulocyte production. Gastrointestinal symptoms, stomatitis, candidal infections. Allergy, hepatitis, optic neuritis, and neurologic abnormalities occur rarely.
Comment: Should not be used when an equally effective drug is available. Mechanism of action is antagonistic to that of penicillin. Diffuses better than most penicillins (eyes, CSF). Uses include treatment of cases of haemophilus meningitis due to ampicillin-resistant strains, meningococcal meningitis in penicillin-sensitive persons, bacteroides infections, typhoid fever, and peritonitis.

Clindamycin (Cleocin)
Use: Common anaerobic organisms, including various species of bacteroides and anaerobic streptococci. Most aerobic gram-positive cocci are sensitive, but clindamycin is relatively ineffective against *Streptococcus faecalis, Neisseria gonorrhoeae, N meningitidis,* and *H influenzae.*
Dosage:
Oral:
Child: 8–20 mg/kg/day in divided doses every 6–8 hours.
Adolescent: 0.6–1.8 gm/day in divided doses every 6 hours.
IV: (Do not use in infants less than 1 month old.)
Child: 25–40 mg/kg/day in divided doses every 6–8 hours.
Adolescent: 1.8 gm/day in divided doses every 6–8 hours.
Toxicity: Gastrointestinal disturbances, pseudomembranous colitis, rash (10%), thrombophlebitis, sterile abscess.
Comment: This drug is structurally similar to lincomycin, with somewhat better and more rapid absorption after oral dosage and greater activity in vitro against staphylococci and pneumococci. It is no more effective against group A streptococci than erythromycin. If diarrhea develops, the drug should be terminated or the patient should be examined by sigmoidoscopy to rule out pseudomembranous colitis. Pseudomembranous colitis appears to be an uncommon complication of therapy in children.

Colistin (Coly-Mycin M, Coly-Mycin S)
Use: *Pseudomonas aeruginosa;* some *Escherichia*

coli, enterobacter, and klebsiella. Proteus and gram-positive organisms are resistant.

Dosage:

Oral: Colistin sulfate: Not absorbed. 15 mg/kg/day in divided doses every 8 hours.

IM: Sodium colistimethate:

Newborn less than 1 week old: 1.5–5 mg/kg/day in divided doses every 12 hours.

Child: 5–10 mg/kg/day in divided doses every 6–12 hours given deep into a muscle.

Adolescent: 2.5–5 mg/kg/day in divided doses every 6–12 hours.

Toxicity: Proteinuria, cylindruria, hematuria, increased BUN (reversible). Paresthesias, ataxia, drowsiness, confusion. Fever, rash, pain at injection site.

Comment: May be used orally for enteropathogenic *E coli* infections. Use with care if renal function is abnormal. Gains access to CSF only when used in doses greater than 10 mg/kg/day, so that other drugs should be used for CSF infection. Do not use intrathecally because the preparation contains dibucaine.

Erythromycin (Erythrocin, Ilotycin, Ilosone, Pediamycin)

Use: Gram-positive cocci, clostridia, *Haemophilus influenzae, Bordetella pertussis, Corynebacterium diphtheriae*, rickettsiae, brucella, some bacteroides. Resistance of some group A streptococci and some pneumococci has been reported, although this is rare at present. May be of use in chronic bronchitis, cystic fibrosis, and some urinary tract infections because of action against L forms. Probably as effective as tetracycline for symptomatic relief of mycoplasmal infections, although the organisms continue to be shed.

Dosage:

Oral:

Newborn: 20–40 mg/kg/day in divided doses every 12 hours.

Child: 30–50 mg/kg/day in divided doses every 6 hours.

IM or IV:

Newborn: 10 mg/kg/day in divided doses every 12 hours.

Child: 10–20 mg/kg/day in divided doses every 6 hours (over a 20- to 60-minute period if given IV).

Adolescent: 1–2 gm/day. Higher doses could be used in severe infections.

Toxicity: Painful injection, gastrointestinal symptoms, candidiasis, drug fever. Estolate (Ilosone) is associated with intrahepatic cholestatic jaundice when treatment is for more than 10 days.

Comment: Do not use concomitantly with lincomycin or clindamycin.

Ethambutol (Myambutol)

Use: Tuberculosis.

Dosage (oral; adolescent): 15 mg/kg/day; retreatment, 25 mg/kg/day for 60 days, then 15 mg/kg/day.

Toxicity: Retrobulbar neuritis (3%). Patients should be routinely followed with monthly examination of visual acuity and color discrimination. Anaphylactoid reactions. Peripheral neuritis. Hyperuricemia.

Comment: Experience in the pediatric age range is limited.

Flucytosine (Ancobon)

Use: Antifungal agent active against some strains of candida, *Cryptococcus neoformans, Torulopsis glabrata.*

Dosage (oral; infant, child, adolescent): Give orally, 150 mg/kg/day in divided doses every 6 hours.

Comment: 90% of drug is excreted in urine. Drug resistance has been reported during therapy. Sensitivity studies are indicated. Currently it is suggested that patients on therapy be followed with creatinine or BUN, SGOT, alkaline phosphatase, hemoglobins, and white counts.

Griseofulvin (Fulvicin, Grifulvin, Grisactin)

Use: Tinea species, microsporum, trichophyton. Ineffective against candida, cryptococcus, blastomyces, histoplasma, and coccidioides.

Dosage (oral):

Griseofulvin (regular size):

Child: 20 mg/kg/day in divided doses every 6–12 hours.

Adolescent: 1 gm/day in divided doses every 6–12 hours.

Grisactin (microcrystalline):

Child: 10 mg/kg/day in divided doses every 6–12 hours.

Adolescent: 0.5 gm/day in divided doses every 6–12 hours.

Toxicity: Leukopenia and other blood dyscrasias, headache, incoordination and confusion, gastrointestinal disturbances, rash (allergic and photosensitivity), renal damage, lupus-like syndrome.

Comment: Do not use in patients with hepatocellular failure or porphyria.

Isoniazid (INH, Niadox, Nydrazid)

Use: Tuberculosis.

Dosage:

Oral:

Newborn: Dosage is not well established, but there is some evidence that INH may compete with bilirubin for albumin-binding sites in newborns. BCG vaccination is often a better alternative for the child of a tuberculous mother than INH prophylaxis.

Child: 10–20 mg/kg/day in divided doses every 6–24 hours. Give no more than 500 mg/day.

Adolescent: 300–500 mg/day.

IM:

Child: 10–20 mg/kg/day in divided doses every 12 hours.

Adolescent: 5 mg/kg/day in divided doses every 12 hours up to 300 mg/day.

Toxicity: Hepatitis; neurotoxic as a result of pyridoxine deficiency. Gastrointestinal symptoms, seizures, hypersensitivity.

Comment: Avoid use with preexisting liver disease. Although it is generally stated that addition of pyridoxine is unnecessary in children, exceptions to this rule occur. Routine supplementation with pyridoxine is recommended.

Lincomycin (Lincocin): See Clindamycin.

Methenamine Mandelate (Mandelamine)

Use: Genitourinary infections. Not effective against proteus.

Dosage (oral):

Child: 100 mg/kg immediately and then 50 mg/kg/day given in divided doses every 6–8 hours.

Adolescent: 4 gm/day in divided doses every 6–8 hours.

Comment: Urine should be kept acid.

Metronidazole (Flagyl)

Use: Trichomoniasis, giardiasis, amebiasis.

Dosage (oral; adolescent): 250 mg every 8 hours.

Toxicity: Nausea, anorexia, and other gastrointestinal intolerance; glossitis and stomatitis; leukopenia; dizziness, vertigo, ataxia; urticaria, pruritus. See p 804 for a comment on other adverse effects.

Comment: Has been used in the therapy of giardiasis and in the treatment of amebic dysentery in children in doses up to 40 mg/kg/day.

Nalidixic Acid (NegGram)

Use: Useful in gram-negative urinary tract infections with *Escherichia coli,* enterobacter, klebsiella, and proteus. Pseudomonas is generally resistant.

Dosage (oral):

Child: 40–50 mg/kg in divided doses 4 times daily; may be reduced to 20–25 mg/kg/day for maintenance.

Adolescent: 4 gm/day in divided doses every 6 hours; may be reduced to 2 gm/day for maintenance therapy.

Toxicity: Gastrointestinal symptoms, hypersensitivity (pruritus, rash, urticaria, eosinophilia), seizures, pseudotumor cerebri, pneumonitis.

Comment: Toxicity is low, and the drug may be used for months. Resistance may develop. Use cautiously in patients with liver disease or those with impaired renal function. Do not use in children under 1 month of age or for infections other than those of the urinary tract.

Nitrofurantoin (Furadantin)

Use: Many gram-negative organisms are susceptible to concentrations achieved in urine.

Dosage (oral):

Newborn: 1.5 mg/kg/day.

Child: 5–7 mg/kg/day. Reduce dosage to 2.5–5 mg/kg/day after 10–14 days.

Adolescent: 400 mg every day in divided doses every 6 hours.

Toxicity: Primaquine-sensitive hemolytic anemia, peripheral neuropathy, rash, chills, fever, myalgia-like syndrome, cholestatic jaundice.

Comment: Used only for urinary tract infections.

Nystatin (Mycostatin)

Use: *Candida albicans* and other yeasts.

Dosage:

Oral (not absorbed):

Newborn: 200–400 thousand units/day.

Child: Under 2 years old, 400-800 thousand units/day. Over 2 years old, 1–2 million units/day in divided doses every 6–8 hours.

Eye and skin: 100,000 units/gm.

Toxicity: None.

Polymyxin B (Aerosporin)

Use: Pseudomonas, some other gram-negative bacteria as determined by sensitivities on the specific organisms.

Dosage:

Oral: Not absorbed. 10–20 mg/kg/day in divided doses every 4–6 hours.

IM or IV:

Newborn: 3.5–4 mg/kg/day in divided doses every 6 hours.

Child: 3.5–5 mg/kg/day in divided doses every 6–8 hours (dosage not to exceed 200 mg/day).

Adolescent: 2.5 mg/kg/day in divided doses every 6 hours.

Intrathecal or intraventricular: 2–5 mg every other day.

Toxicity: Pain at injection site; neurotoxicity (paresthesias, ataxia, drowsiness); nephrotoxicity (cylindruria, hematuria, proteinuria, increased BUN); fever, rash.

Rifampin (Rifadin, Rimactane)

Use: Neisseria, mycobacterium, gram-positive cocci.

Dosage: Not available in solution; even capsules are unstable.

For treatment of tuberculosis (oral):

Child: Place contents of 300 mg capsule in 1 tbsp applesauce or pudding. Each teaspoon equals 100 mg. Administer 20 mg/kg/day; mix freshly each time.

Adolescent: 600 mg/day.

For treatment of carriers of *N meningitidis* (oral):

Child: 20 mg/kg/day divided every 12 hours for 2 days.

Adult: 1200 mg/day divided every 12 hours for 2 days.

Toxicity: Hepatotoxic in animals. SGOT should be followed when used with isoniazid.

Comment: The most striking contribution of rifampin has been in the care of patients infected with resistant strains of *Mycobacterium tuberculosis.* The main indications for its use in children are (1) contact with an adult with a drug-resistant strain, (2) isoniazid intolerance, (3) isoniazid resistance, and (4) meningitis due to *M tuberculosis.* Although the results have been remarkably good, when used alone the development of resistance is rapid; therefore, the drug should always be used in combination with one or 2 drugs to which the organisms are sensitive. In addition, rifampin is effective in eliminating the carrier state due to *Neisseria meningitidis,* but the development of rifampin resistance is relatively common.

Sulfonamides: Sulfadiazine, Sulfisoxazole (Gantrisin), Sulfamethoxazole (Gantanol), Trisulfapyrimidines USP

Use: Bacteriostatic against gram-positive and gram-negative organisms. Approximately 80% of shigellae are resistant. Nocardia.

Dosage (for sulfadiazine, triple sulfas, and sulfisoxazole):
   Oral:
      Newborn: Avoid usage.
      Child: 120–150 mg/kg/day in divided doses every 6 hours.
      Adolescent: 2–4 gm/day in divided doses every 6 hours.
   IV:
      Newborn: Do not use.
      Child: 120 mg/kg/day in divided doses every 6–12 hours; alkaline urine.

Dosage (oral, for sulfamethoxazole):
   Child: 50 mg/kg/day in divided doses every 12 hours.
   Adolescent: 1–3 gm/day in divided doses every 8–12 hours.

Toxicity: Crystalluria (mechanical urinary obstruction): *Keep fluid intake high.* Hypersensitivity (fever, rash, hepatitis, lupus-like state, vasculitis). Neutropenia, agranulocytosis, aplastic anemia, thrombocytopenia. Hemolytic anemia in individuals deficient in glucose-6-phosphate dehydrogenase. (G6PD deficiency is seen in association with sickle cell anemia.)

Comment: Sulfadiazine is preferred for CNS infections as diffusion into CSF is better. Sulfamethoxazole is intermediate-acting and has a slightly greater propensity for causing urinary sediment abnormalities. Long-acting preparations (Kynex, Madribon, Sulfameter) are occasionally associated with serious reactions.

   Useful in urinary tract infections and rheumatic fever prophylaxis. (Should not be used for group A streptococcal infections.)

Tetracyclines (Many trade names.)

Use: Gram-positive and gram-negative bacteria, rickettsiae, chlamydiae, *Mycoplasma pneumoniae,* brucella, bacteroides. Many gram-negative bacteria are resistant.

Dosage (for tetracycline, chlortetracycline, oxytetracycline):
   Oral:
      Child: 20–40 mg/kg/day in divided doses every 6 hours. Do not give with milk.
      Adolescent: 1–2 gm/day in divided doses every 6 hours.
   IM:
      Child: 15–25 mg/kg/day in divided doses every 12 hours; achieves poor levels; painful.
      Adolescent: 250–300 mg/day in divided doses every 8–24 hours.
   IV: Do not use.

Dosage (oral, for demecycline [demethylchlortetracycline, Declomycin] and methacycline [Rondomycin]):
   Newborn: Do not use.
   Child: 12 mg/kg/day in divided doses every 6 hours.
   Adolescent: 600 mg/day in divided doses every 6–12 hours.

Toxicity: In children under 7 years of age, tetracyclines cause damage to teeth and bones. Deposition in teeth and bones of premature and newborn infants can result in enamel dysplasia and growth retardation. Outdated tetracyclines can produce Fanconi's syndrome. Pseudotumor cerebri, bulging fontanels. Nausea, vomiting, diarrhea, stomatitis, glossitis, proctitis, candidiasis, and overgrowth of staphylococci in bowel. Disturbed hepatic and renal function. Drug fever, rash, photosensitivity.

Comment: Cross-resistance among the tetracyclines is complete. Minocycline, however, offers an advantage at this time over other tetracyclines in the therapy of carriers of *N meningitidis,* but it has been reported to cause vestibular dysfunction with high frequency.

Thiabendazole (Mintezol)

Use: Ascaris, trichuris, enterobius, ancylostoma, *Necator americanus,* cutaneous larva migrans, strongyloides.

Dosage: Give orally 25 mg/kg twice a day up to a total daily dose of 3 gm/day: for 4 days for trichuris; for 2 days for ascaris, ancylostoma, *N americanus,* strongyloides, and cutaneous larva migrans; and for 1 day for enterobius and repeat for 1 day 7 days later.

Toxicity: Anorexia, nausea, vomiting, dizziness, angioneurotic edema, pruritus.

Trimethoprim-Sulfamethoxazole (Co-trimoxazole; Bactrim, Septra)

Use: A combination agent with a wide range of activity against gram-positive and gram-negative organisms. In general, more active than the sulfonamides alone.

Dosage:
   Oral:
      Newborn: Not recommended.

Infant, child: Trimethoprim, 8–10 mg/kg/day, and sulfamethoxazole, 40–50 mg/kg/day, given in divided doses every 12 hours. Combination tablets contain 80 mg trimethoprim and 400 mg sulfamethoxazole. (For serious gram-negative infections and for therapy of *Pneumocystis carinii* infections, give trimethoprim, 20 mg/kg/day, and sulfamethoxazole, 100 mg/kg/day, in divided doses every 6–8 hours.)

Adolescent: 160 mg trimethoprim plus 800 mg sulfamethoxazole every 12 hours.

Parenteral: Not available.

Toxicity: Kernicterus in neonates, gastrointestinal irritation, bone marrow depression, allergic reactions. Should not be used in patients with renal or liver disease or blood dyscrasias, patients with a history of hypersensitivity to sulfonamides, or those with G6PD deficiency. Use in pregnancy is not recommended since large doses are teratogenic in animals.

Comment: Most promising therapeutic areas are in chronic or recurrent urinary tract infections with sensitive organisms. Possibly beneficial in certain salmonella infections and in *Pneumocystis carinii* infections.

Vancomycin (Vancocin)

Use: Staphylococci, other gram-positive cocci, clostridia, corynebacteria. Main use is in treatment of staphylococcal enterocolitis and methicillin-resistant staphylococcal infection.

Dosage:

Oral: Not absorbed. 2–4 gm/day in divided doses every 6 hours.

IV:

Child: 40 mg/kg/day in divided doses every 6 hours.

Adolescent: 2–3 gm/day in divided doses every 6 hours.

Toxicity: Painful when given intramuscularly; do not use. Troublesome symptoms during intravenous administration include rash, chills, thrombophlebitis, and fever. Concomitant administration of corticosteroids may be necessary. Nephrotoxicity and irreversible ototoxicity have occurred. Does not interfere with the action of any known antibiotic.

Comment: Before the advent of the penicillinase-resistant antibiotics, vancomycin was used successfully in the treatment of subacute bacterial endocarditis, osteomyelitis, and serious soft tissue infections. High oral doses are exceedingly effective in staphylococcal enterocolitis.

ANTIVIRAL CHEMOTHERAPY

Few therapeutic agents are available for viral infections. The following drugs have limited usefulness.

Amantadine (Symmetrel)

Use: Limited to prophylactic administration during identified A_2 influenza virus epidemics. Of no therapeutic value. Does not appear to interfere with immunity induced by vaccination.

Dosage (oral):

Child, 1–9 years: 2–4 mg/lb/day (do not exceed 150 mg/day) in 2 or 3 doses.

Child, 9–12 years: 200 mg/day in 2 doses (total dose).

Adolescent: 200 mg/day in 1 or 2 doses.

Toxicity: CNS irritability (nervousness, insomnia, dizziness, lightheadedness, drunken feelings, slurred speech, ataxia, inability to concentrate). Occasional depression and feelings of detachment; blurred vision (heightened with higher dosage, 300–400 mg/day, in elderly); less commonly, dry mouth, gastrointestinal upset, skin rash. Rarely, tremors, anorexia, pollakiuria, nocturia.

Idoxuridine (Dendrid, Herplex, Stoxil) & Adenine Arabinoside (Vira-A, Vidarabine)

Use: At present, limited to acute superficial herpes simplex or vaccinia virus keratitis. Should be administered under an ophthalmologist's supervision. Some prefer concomitant local corticosteroid administration.

Dosage (for idoxuridine): Solution (0.1%) should be used initially; place 1 drop in each infected eye every hour while awake and every 2 hours at night; with definite improvement, decrease to every 2 hours around the clock and continue treatment for 3–5 days after healing appears to be complete. Ointment (0.5%): Instill 5 times a day (every 4 hours), with last dose at midnight.

Dosage (for vidarabine): Ointment (3%) is administered 5 times a day (every 3 hours).

Toxicity: Too frequent administration leads to small punctate defects in the cornea.

Methisazone (Marboran)

Use: In smallpox prophylaxis if given in first 9 days after exposure; in therapy of complications of vaccination, especially eczema vaccinatum.

Dosage (oral):

Child, adolescent: Give a loading dose of 250 mg/kg/day orally followed by 50 mg/kg every 6 hours for 3 full days. An antiemetic should be given with the drug.

Toxicity: Vomiting, immediate gastric irritation, and late (5–6 hours) CNS stimulation. Short courses of therapy are not associated with other effects, but patients should be observed for hematologic and hepatic toxicity.

•   •   •

General References

American Thoracic Society, American Lung Association, Center for Disease Control: Preventive therapy of tuberculous infection. Morbid Mortal Wkly Rep 24:71, 1975.

Baldwin DS: Renal failure and interstitial nephritis due to penicillin and methicillin. N Engl J Med 279:1245, 1968.

Bauer DJ & others: Prophylaxis of smallpox with methisazone. Am J Epidemiol 90:130, 1969.

Bennett WM & others: Guide to drug usage in adult patients with impaired renal function. JAMA 223:991, 1973.

Brown CH & others: The hemostatic defect produced by carbenicillin. N Engl J Med 291:265, 1974.

Committee on Drugs, American Academy of Pediatrics: Infants of tuberculous mothers: Further thoughts. Pediatrics 42:393, 1968.

Council on Drugs, American Medical Association: Evaluation of a broad-spectrum anthelmintic—thiabendazole. JAMA 205:172, 1968.

Cutler RE: Correlation of serum creatinine concentration and kanamycin half-life. JAMA 209:539, 1969.

Darrell JH: Carbenicillin resistance in *Pseudomonas aeruginosa* from clinical material. Br Med J 3:141, 1969.

Drutz DJ: Treatment of disseminated mycotic infections. Am J Med 45:405, 1968.

Emerson BB & others: *Hemophilus influenzae* type B susceptibility to 17 antibiotics. J Pediatr 86:617, 1975.

Grossman ER: Tetracyclines and permanent teeth: The relation between dose and tooth color. Pediatrics 47:567, 1971.

Howard JB, McCracken GH: Reappraisal of kanamycin usage in neonates. J Pediatr 86:949, 1975.

Jawetz E, Melnick JL, Adelberg EA: *Review of Medical Microbiology,* 13th ed. Lange, 1978.

Kagan BM: *Antimicrobial Therapy,* 3rd ed. Saunders, 1974.

Kaiser AB: Seroepidemiology and chemoprophylaxis of disease due to sulfonamide-resistant *Neisseria meningitidis* in a civilian population. J Infect Dis 130:217, 1974.

Kaye D & others: The unpredictability of serum concentrations of gentamicin: Pharmacokinetics of gentamicin in patients with normal and abnormal renal function. J Infect Dis 130:150, 1974.

Klastersky J & others: Comparative clinical study of tobramycin and gentamicin. Antimicrob Agents Chemother 5:133, Feb 1974.

Kunin CM: Antibiotic usage in patients with renal impairment. Hosp Pract 1:141, Jan 1972.

Markowitz SM: Nafcillin-induced agranulocytosis. JAMA 232:1150, 1975.

McCracken GH: Pharmacological basis for antimicrobial therapy in newborn infants. Am J Dis Child 128:407, 1974.

Milner RDG & others: Clinical pharmacology of gentamicin in the newborn. Arch Dis Child 47:927, 1972.

Pickering LK & others: Comparative evaluation of cefazolin and cephalothin in children. J Pediatr 85:842, 1974.

Reynolds AV & others: Newer aminoglycosides—amikacin and tobramycin: An in vitro comparison with kanamycin and gentamicin. Br Med J 3:778, 1974.

Salmon JH: Ventriculitis complicating meningitis. Am J Dis Child 124:35, 1972.

Sanjad SA & others: Nephropathy: An underestimated complication of methicillin therapy. J Pediatr 84:873, 1974.

Southern P: Meningococcal meningitis. N Engl J Med 280:1163, 1969.

Tedesco FJ & others: Clindamycin-associated colitis: A prospective study. Ann Intern Med 81:429, 1974.

Vall-Spinosa A: Rifampin in the treatment of drug resistant *Mycobacterium tuberculosis* infections. N Engl J Med 283:616, 1970.

Vogelstein B, Kowarski A, Lietman PS: The pharmacokinetics of amikacin in children. J Pediatr 91:333, 1977.

38 . . .
Interpretation of Biochemical Values*

Donough O'Brien, MD, FRCP, & Keith B. Hammond, MS, FIMLT

SAMPLE COLLECTION

Blood

Laboratory personnel should be responsible for all sample collections, although this is not as important in older children, in whom venipunctures are simple. Fingersticks are satisfactory in older infants, but heelsticks should always be used in newborns and young infants.

Materials and supplies taken to the bedside are as follows:

Iodophor solution (150 ppm) and sterile gauze swabs.

Disposable lancets (eg, Becton-Dickinson Long Point "Microlance").

Rimless blood-collecting tubes, 9 × 35 mm, capped with a rubber cap.

Microhematocrit tubes, heparinized, 1.15 mm internal diameter.

Screw-cap vials containing 3 mg of potassium oxalate and 3 mg of sodium fluoride.

The skin should be cleansed with iodophor solution and dried with a sterile gauze swab.

In order to prevent hemolysis of the sample and contamination with tissue fluid, it is essential to obtain a free flow of blood. This may require gentle "milking" but never squeezing. The small vein running posteriorly to the internal malleolus is likely to yield a free flow and should be used whenever it can be located. A careful and deliberate puncture should be made. The blood should be allowed to drip into the collecting tube. It is permissible to touch the top of the tube against the drop, but the skin surface should never be in contact with the tube since hemolysis will occur. Directly after collection, a dry gauze swab is placed on the puncture site and pressure applied for a short time. When blood flow has ceased, a dressing is placed over the puncture site.

The tube of blood is covered with a piece of parafilm and the specimen is labeled appropriately.

*Normal values of most of the substances discussed in this chapter are given in Table 38–2 (alphabetically arranged). Normal values for peripheral blood (Table 38–3) are included in this chapter for convenience of reference.

On return to the laboratory, the sample is allowed to stand for approximately 30 minutes from the time of collection and then is centrifuged for about 5 minutes. If desired, the plasma or serum may then be transferred to one or more polyethylene microcentrifuge tubes (450 μl capacity) for ease of handling. These tubes have the added advantage that their narrow bore minimizes concentration of such small samples by evaporation.

Approximately 0.2 ml of whole blood should be allowed for each test described below even though much less is required in many cases. For example, 0.1 ml of plasma or serum will suffice for a combined sodium, potassium, chloride, and CO_2 determination. Samples for pH or hematocrit are collected into heparinized capillary tubes and samples for glucose and xylose into screw-capped vials containing fluoride-oxalate.

Stools

Random stool samples should be sent directly to the laboratory. Twenty-four-hour or longer collections should be placed in a clean, preweighed, 1 gallon paint can and stored in the freezer.

Urine

Random urine samples should be sent immediately to the laboratory. Timed collections should be directly stored in a freezer or at 4° C after acidification with concentrated hydrochloric acid to pH 2.0 or less.

Cerebrospinal Fluid

Samples of CSF should always be sent immediately to the laboratory. At least 2 tubes are required: one for protein and glucose and one for cell count, differential count, culture, stained smear for bacteria, and animal inoculation. A third tube is needed if a serologic test for syphilis is required.

Serum Separators

A recent advance in the design of blood collection tubes for pediatrics is the Becton-Dickinson Microtainer serum separator, which is gaining popularity in many pediatric laboratories. This tube is made of polypropylene and is 45 × 6 mm (inner dimensions). Rulings on the side of the tube indicate approximate blood volumes of 200 and 600 μl (0.2–0.6 ml). At the bottom of the tube there are approximately 100 μl of an inert silicone material which, after centrifugation, separates serum from cells. The cap of the tube is penetrated by a glass capillary filling device. Blood specimens are collected by heelstick or fingerstick directly into the capillary collector, which drains easily into the tube; the cap containing the capillary is then discarded and a plug-style cap substituted which eliminates a portion of the clot adhering to the cap. For the silicone material to form a clear barrier between cells and serum, a relative centrifugal force of at least 6000 g for 90 seconds is required.

The advantages of this type of collection device are the enhanced yield of serum compared with conventional technics and elimination of the need to transfer the sample into a second or third container. Values for potassium and enzyme concentrations have been shown to remain constant for up to 24 hours while allowing the serum to remain in contact with the silicone barrier.

Hicks JM, Rowland GL, Buffone GJ: Evaluation of a new blood-collecting device ("Microtainer") that is suited for pediatric use. Clin Chem 22:2034, 1976.

INSTRUMENTATION FOR THE PEDIATRIC CLINICAL LABORATORY

Until relatively recently, the amount of sample required for many automated analytical systems in use in clinical laboratories was greatly in excess of that available from most pediatric patients. In the past few years, a variety of new instruments have been introduced which require only a few microliters of sample. The incentive for manufacturers to produce instruments of this kind has been due primarily to the high cost of reagents currently in use for many assays and the consequent desire of pathologists and clinical chemists to reduce reagent volumes. Some of the currently available instruments that have special application for pediatric clinical laboratories because of their small sample requirements are discussed below.

Sodium & Potassium

Although apparently satisfactory ion-sensitive electrodes have been developed which form the basis for some analytical systems for the determination of electrolytes in blood and urine, the instrument of choice for the measurement of serum sodium and potassium is still the flame photometer. A variety of flame photometers are commercially available and are capable of performing simultaneous sodium and potassium determinations on as little as 10 μl of serum with a high degree of accuracy and precision.

Chloride & CO₂

The standard method for the microdetermination of CO_2 in plasma has for many years utilized the

Natelson Microgasometer. Although it is accurate, this technic is time-consuming and requires that technologists work with large quantities of mercury. An innovation is the Chloride/CO_2 Analyzer (Beckman Instrument Corp.), which can measure both chloride and CO_2 content in approximately 45 seconds using 10 μl of serum. CO_2 is liberated from the sample with an acid reagent, the gas then diffusing across a membrane into the buffer solution. The resulting rate of change in hydrogen ion concentration is monitored by means of a pH electrode and converted to actual CO_2 concentration on a digital display. The chloride concentration is measured simultaneously, using conventional coulometric titration. The instrument is now used in many pediatric clinical chemistry laboratories in the USA.

Osmolality

Freezing point determinations have been used for the determination of osmolality in body fluids for many years. The recent introduction of an instrument that can measure osmolality by vapor pressure determination on as little as 5 μl of sample (Wescor Vapor Pressure Osmometer) has facilitated the performance of these assays on pediatric patients. Clinicians should be aware that volatile compounds occasionally encountered in plasma (eg, ethanol) which result in elevated osmolality as measured by freezing point depression have no such effect in this newer technic.

Enzymes

Most clinical laboratories now utilize spectrophotometric rate measurements of enzyme activity in preference to the older and less specific end-point technics. A variety of instruments now exist that enable these assays to be performed on small quantities of serum, making them appropriate for pediatric use. Perhaps the most versatile of these are the centrifugal analyzers. These analytical systems make use of centrifugal force to mix sample and reagents and are capable of recording changes in absorbance in the rapidly rotating cuvettes, making possible the simultaneous assay of several samples in a very short space of time. A minicomputer is then used to convert the data into a report. While these systems obviously lend themselves readily to enzyme rate measurements, they are also used for a wide variety of other commonly performed assays including glucose, urea nitrogen, creatinine, bilirubin, total protein, albumin, and phosphorus. They have also recently been used for measuring immunoglobulins and anticonvulsant drug levels on very small samples of serum.

Werner M (editor): *Microtechniques for the Clinical Laboratory: Concepts and Applications.* Wiley, 1976.

SOURCES OF ERROR

Awareness of the possibility of error is important to the interpretation of laboratory data. All good laboratories have a reasonably accurate idea of the intrinsic error of their methods. One source of error of increasing concern to laboratory scientists is that due to drug interference. An understanding of the way in which certain pharmacologic agents alter the actual or measured levels of many constituents in biologic fluids is extremely valuable.

Caraway WT: Accuracy in clinical chemistry. Clin Chem 17:63, 1971.

Young DS, Pestaner LC, Gibberman V: Effects of drugs on clinical laboratory tests. Clin Chem 21:1D, 1975.

TESTS OF CARBOHYDRATE METABOLISM

Glucose in Serum, Plasma, & Cerebrospinal Fluid

A. Specimen and Test Requirements: 0.2 ml serum, CSF, or plasma. The patient should be fasted. Cells should be separated within 20 minutes. Plasma from heparinized blood must be precipitated at once.

B. Normal Values: Newborn, 30–80 mg/dl; older children, 60–105 mg/dl.

C. Interpretation: The most reliable methods are enzymatic. These methods are now adaptable to all forms of automated equipment, and the retention of reducing methods has no justification. Particularly attractive to the pediatric laboratory is the measurement of glucose by the rate of oxygen consumption in the presence of glucose oxidase. This procedure avoids many of the interferences to which catalase, the second enzyme of most glucose oxidase methods, is prone.

Kadish AH: Determination of urine glucose by measurement of rate of oxygen consumption. Diabetes 18:467, 1969.

Oral Glucose Tolerance Test

A. Specimen and Test Requirements: Give 1.75 gm/kg of glucose as corn syrup or as a 20% solution with flavoring after 3 days of high-carbohydrate intake followed by an overnight fast. Children under 2 years of age should be given 2 gm/kg of glucose. Commercial products are available.

Take blood samples fasting and then at 30, 60, 90, 120, and 150 minutes for serum glucose determination. In cases of suspected carbohydrate-reactive hypoglycemia, post-fasting samples should be taken at 2, 3, 4, and 5 hours.

Collect urine prior to the test and after 1 and 2 hours to test for glycosuria. The criteria for the range of normal response are that the 30-minute level should be < 180 mg/dl and that fasting levels should be restored at 90–120 minutes.

Because the relatively large doses of glucose used in this test may lead to nausea and vomiting, corn

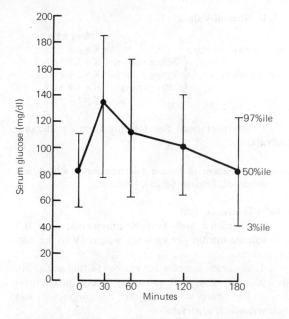

Figure 38–1. Serum glucose percentile levels after 1.75 gm/kg glucose orally.

syrup may be preferable. This could lead to error in the presence of a maltase deficiency. The glucose should be dissolved in ice cold water or soda water in a volume of 150 ml/sq m and flavoring added to make it palatable. Commercially prepared glucose solutions are available under various trade names.

B. Normal Values: The normal limits of glucose tolerance in children are shown in Fig 38–1.

C. Interpretation: Diminished glucose tolerance (elevated blood sugar values) is usually indicative of diabetes mellitus, but it may also be seen in states associated with excess anterior pituitary or adrenocortical hormones and with liver disease. An abrupt fall in serum glucose after the initial rise is sometimes seen with hyperinsulinism. Criteria for abnormality vary (see p 705), but 3 levels over the 97th percentile or a sum of the fasting, 30, 60, and 120 minute levels > 625 would be considered positive.

Intravenous Glucose Tolerance Test

A. Specimen and Test Requirements: The patient should be fasted for 6 hours if under 6 months of age; otherwise, for about 12 hours.

Inject rapidly into a vein 0.66 ml 50% glucose solution per kg body weight. Collect blood every 4–5 minutes for 30–45 minutes for serum glucose measurement. From the calculation of glucose assimilation a constant (K) is determined as follows:

$$K = \frac{\log_{10} C_1 - \log_{10} C_2}{t_1 - t_2} \times 230.3$$

where C_1 and C_2 are serum glucose levels in mg/dl at times t_1 and t_2 in minutes, respectively.

B. Normal Values:

		Mean ± SD
6 months to 10 years		K = 2.8 ± 0.6
10–15 years	before puberty	K = 2.7 ± 0.8
	during puberty	K = 2.1 ± 0.7
	after puberty	K = 1.9 ± 0.4
Adult		K = 1.7 ± 0.3

C. Interpretation: See interpretation for the oral test (above).

Loeb H: Variations in glucose tolerance during infancy and childhood. J Pediatr 68:237, 1966.

Insulin Tolerance Test

A. Specimen and Test Requirements: Give 0.1 unit soluble insulin per kg body weight IV to the fasting patient.

Take serum samples for glucose fasting and at 20, 40, 60, 90, and 120 minutes. Safety precautions should be observed as in the insulin/glucose test (below), which is preferable.

B. Interpretation: Failure of the serum glucose to rise significantly after 20 minutes indicates pituitary or adrenal insufficiency.

Insulin/Glucose Tolerance Test

A. Specimen and Test Requirements: This test was developed as a somewhat safer means of detecting insulin sensitivity than the insulin tolerance test.

Administer 0.05 unit soluble insulin per kg body weight IV after an overnight fast. At 30 minutes, give 0.8 gm glucose per kg body weight orally in flavored aqueous solution. Collect samples for serum glucose fasting and after 30, 60, 90, 120, and 180 minutes. Glucagon and sterile 50% glucose should be on hand in case of a hypoglycemic reaction.

B. Interpretation: Failure of the serum glucose to rise after 30 minutes is indicative of insulin sensitivity.

Engel FL: The insulin glucose tolerance test. J Clin Invest 29:151, 1950.

Glucagon Tolerance Test

A. Specimen and Test Requirements: This overall test of glycogenolysis is used in the diagnosis of glycogen storage disease and other liver diseases.

Administer 20 µg glucagon per kg of body weight IV to the fasting patient. Take samples for serum glucose determination fasting and at 10, 20, and 40 minutes.

B. Interpretation: Normal persons show a blood glucose rise of 50–100 mg/dl with a peak at 40 minutes and a return to normal by 2 hours.

Marks V: Glucagon test for insulinoma. J Clin Pathol 21:346, 1968.

Prednisone Glucose Tolerance Test

A. Specimen and Test Requirements: Perform a standard glucose tolerance test after giving 6 mg/sq m

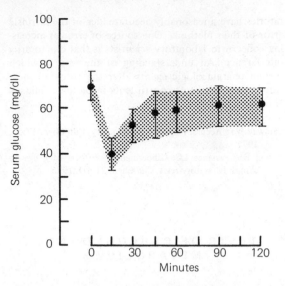

Figure 38–2. Serum glucose levels in children after 20 mg/kg of tolbutamide intravenously.

of prednisone orally 8½ and 2 hours before the first fasting sample.

B. Normal Values: As for Oral Glucose Tolerance Test.

C. Interpretation: This test is used in the detection of glucose intolerance in prediabetics among close relatives of known diabetics with a view to considering treatment with the sulfonylureas.

Rull JA & others: Levels of plasma insulin during cortisone glucose tolerance tests in "nondiabetic" relatives of diabetic patients. Diabetes 19:1, 1970.

Oral Tolbutamide Tolerance Test

A. Specimen and Test Requirements: Blood samples for glucose determinations are taken 20 minutes after an oral dose of 20 mg/kg tolbutamide with 1.2 gm/sq m of sodium bicarbonate to facilitate absorption. The tolbutamide may be given intravenously, but there is an increased risk of hypoglycemia.

B. Normal Values: Serum glucose levels should fall to between 20 and 40% of fasting in 20 minutes.

C. Interpretation: A fall of less than 15% at 20 minutes indicates insulin insufficiency. A fall greater than 50% by 20 minutes and to less than 70% of fasting at 90–120 minutes indicates hyperinsulinism. (See Fig 38–2.)

Cunningham GC: Tolbutamide tolerance test in hypoglycemic children. Am J Dis Child 107:714, 1966.

TESTS FOR FLUID & ELECTROLYTE & ACID-BASE DISORDERS

Bicarbonate or Total CO_2 in Plasma

A. Specimen: 0.03 ml heparinized plasma taken under oil.

B. Normal Values: 18–33 mmol/liter.

C. Interpretation: (See Chapter 35.) Low values indicate metabolic acidosis or respiratory alkalosis. Elevated values indicate metabolic alkalosis or respiratory acidosis. It is usually advisable to have a simultaneous blood pH reading.

Various authors: Acta Anaesthesiol Scand (Suppl) 37:10, 24, 27, 1970.

Blood & Plasma Volume

A. Specimen and Test Requirements: Evans blue dye or radioiodinated serum albumin (RISA) is injected intravenously, and samples of heparinized whole blood are drawn after allowing time for equilibration in the plasma volume. Technical details should be left to the laboratory.

B. Normal Values: See Table 38–2.

C. Method: The Evans blue dye and RISA methods are both simple dilution technics.

D. Interpretation: There is a definite role for the determination of blood volume in clinical work—particularly in judging the risk of transfusions in anemic patients and in assessing blood volume in diabetic acidosis, renal failure, severe burns, etc.

Cropp GJA: Changes in blood and plasma volumes during growth. J Pediatr 78:220, 1971.

Body Water: Total, Extracellular, & Intracellular

A. Specimen and Test Requirements: For total body water, deuterium oxide (D_2O) is injected intravenously and allowed to equilibrate for 3 hours. Plasma water is distilled off under vacuum and the D_2O concentration measured by its specific infrared absorbance. For extracellular water, a potassium bromide dilution technic is used. Bromide is measured polarographically.

B. Normal Values: See Table 38–2.

C. Interpretation: A measurement of total body water or extracellular water is occasionally of great value in renal failure and in other situations where an accurate appraisal of a severe fluid and electrolyte disturbance is important for therapy.

Cheek DB & others: Body water, height and weight during growth of normal children. Am J Dis Child 112:312, 1966.

Serum Calcium

A. Specimen: 0.1 ml serum, preferably fasting.

B. Normal Values: 4.4–5.3 mEq/liter.

C. Method: Atomic absorption spectrophotometry.

D. Interpretation: Elevated values (between 6–9 mEq/liter) may be seen in idiopathic hypercalcemia, vitamin D intoxication, hyperparathyroidism, sarcoidosis, *Pneumocystis carinii* pneumonia, and in the blue diaper syndrome. Low levels are seen in hypoparathyroidism, in pseudohypoparathyroidism, secondary to hypophosphatemia in chronic renal failure, in all forms of rickets, in postacidotic hypocalcemia, in hypoalbuminemia, in infantile tetany, and as a result of corticosteroid therapy.

Rodgerson DO: Measurement of serum calcium. Clin Chem 14:1207, 1968.

Serum Chloride

A. Specimen: 0.1 ml serum or plasma.

B. Normal Values: 97–104 mEq/liter.

C. Interpretation: The measurement of serum chloride, particularly in association with CO_2 content, offers in children a good index of acidosis, alkalosis, and the overall osmolality of the extracellular water provided excessive lipidemia is not present. Low values are found in pyloric stenosis and other instances of persistent vomiting; in overhydration, including states of inappropriate vasopressin secretion; and in rarer states where the intracellular tonicity has changed with a resultant migration of sodium and chloride into the cell. Somewhat high values normally occur in the thirsted infant at around the fourth day of life. High chloride values are also found in hyperchloremic renal acidosis, in hypertonic dehydration, and in some cases of diabetes insipidus. Salt retention may also occur in cerebral lesions, although it is more often associated with low serum chloride levels. Neurogenic hypochloremia may have a renal component. In some cases, end organ insensitivity to DOCA has been noted without other evidence of renal dysfunction.

Serum Magnesium

A. Specimen: 0.1 ml serum.

B. Normal Values: 1.2–1.6 mEq/liter.

C. Method: Atomic absorption spectrophotometry.

D. Interpretation: Abnormally low levels may be found in gastroenteritis, the malabsorption syndromes, protein and calorie malnutrition, and in the renal tubular dystrophies or chronic renal disease. Low levels are occasionally seen in the newborn who is "twitchy" with or without hypocalcemia and also in diabetic acidosis and hyperparathyroidism. The associated clinical findings are muscular weakness and wasting, instability, tetany, vertigo, ataxia, tremors, and ultimately convulsions.

Elevated serum magnesium levels are most commonly encountered in chronic renal failure.

Disorders of magnesium metabolism in infancy. Br Med J 4:373, 1973.

Osmotic Pressure

A. Specimen: 0.2 ml serum or urine.

B. **Normal Values:** 270–285 mOsm/liter serum.

C. **Interpretation:** Osmolality can be measured in terms of freezing point depression. It is primarily a measure of the serum tonicity and parallels serum sodium. Measurement of urine osmolality is a useful guide to water balance. Measurement of osmotic pressure by vapor pressure determination is a recent improvement in technic that is discussed on p 1046.

pH of Whole Blood

A. **Specimen:** 0.03 ml heparinized whole blood.

B. **Normal Values:** 7.38–7.42 at 37° C.

C. **Interpretation:** Measures acidemia or alkalemia (in conjunction with serum bicarbonate levels).

Suutarinen T: Acid-base balance in the normal child. Acta Anesthesiol Scand (Suppl) 37:28, 1970.

Serum Phosphorus, Inorganic

A. **Specimen:** 0.1 ml serum, preferably fasting.

B. **Normal Values:** 4.4–5.6 mg/dl.

C. **Interpretation:** Elevated plasma phosphorus levels are found in chronic renal disease, hypoparathyroidism, pseudohypoparathyroidism, and tetany of the newborn, where the elevation is caused by excessive phosphorus retention. The tetany found in infants of diabetic mothers is often normophosphatemic.

Low plasma phosphorus is encountered in rickets associated with malabsorption syndromes, in renal tubular dystrophies, postacidotic hypocalcemia, primary hyperparathyroidism, and in patients taking corticosteroids.

Kratiab AK, Forfar JO: Calcium, phosphorus and glucose levels in mother and newborn infant. Biol Neonate 15:26, 1970.

Serum Potassium

A. **Specimen:** 0.1 ml plasma or serum.

B. **Normal Values:** 4.1–5.6 mEq/liter.

C. **Interpretation:** High serum potassium levels occur in renal failure, respiratory distress syndrome, adynamia episodica hereditaria, and adrenal insufficiency. Low potassium is associated with congenital or acquired alkalosis and may result from persistent vomiting or diarrhea and from potassium-losing renal conditions.

Serum Sodium

A. **Specimen:** 0.1 ml plasma or serum.

B. **Normal Values:** 136–143 mEq/liter.

C. **Interpretation:** Serum sodium levels are obtained as a guide to serum osmolality. They are conspicuously low in adrenal insufficiency. The difference between the serum sodium level and the sum of the bicarbonate and chloride levels is an index of the degree of organic aciduria.

TESTS OF ENDOCRINE FUNCTION

ANTERIOR PITUITARY FUNCTION

The anterior pituitary gland is responsible for the elaboration of 7 tropic hormones: (1) follicle-stimulating hormone (FSH); (2) luteinizing or interstitial cell-stimulating hormone (LH, ICSH); (3) adrenocorticotropic hormone (ACTH, corticotropin); (4) thyrotropin (TSH); (5) somatotropin or human growth hormone (HGH); (6) luteotropic hormone or prolactin (LTH); and (7) melanocyte-stimulating hormone (MSH). Pituitary gonadotropic activity (an estimation of both FSH and LH) may be helpful in the evaluation of hypopituitarism, premature sexual development, and suspected cases of Turner's and Klinefelter's syndromes.

ACTH levels may be measured directly or indirectly. The metyrapone (Metopirone) stimulation and dexamethasone suppression tests described briefly below may be used to assess ACTH function and reserve.

Thyrotropic hormone (TSH) is now easily measured using radioimmunoassay and is available in many hospital and commercial laboratories at relatively low cost. Human-specific thyroid stimulator (formerly called LATS) bioassay is available in some university and commercial laboratories. (Normal values: TSH, 1–10 μU/ml; human-specific thyroid stimulator, none detectable in normal serum.)

Assays of growth hormone are readily available. The mean plasma levels of HGH in fasting children and young adults were 1.5–5 ng/ml and 1.9 ± 0.2 ng/ml, respectively. Levels during sleep, insulin hypoglycemia, or L-arginine infusion normally rise to 77 ng/ml.

Mace JW & others: Sleep related human growth hormone release. J Clin Endocrinol 34:339, 1972.

ADRENAL FUNCTION

The basic measure of adrenal glucocorticoid activity is the 24-hour urinary excretion of 17-hydroxycorticosteroids. Low levels are an absolute indication of hypoadrenalism, but normal values are obtained with low adrenal and pituitary reserve. Metyrapone (Metopirone) inhibits cortisol production and thereby cortisol feedback control of the pituitary. This leads to an increase in endogenous ACTH production and, secondarily, to increased levels of urinary hydroxycorticosteroids. The metyrapone test is therefore an estimate of hypothalamic-pituitary competence. If pituitary function is found to be normal, the corticotropin stimulation test can be used to measure adrenal reserve.

In cases of hyperadrenocorticism (Cushing's

syndrome) and in the adrenogenital syndrome, the urinary corticosteroids are elevated and cannot usually be suppressed by small doses of dexamethasone (eg, 1.3 mg/sq m/24 hours for 3 days). Failure to suppress urinary corticosteroids with 3.75 mg/sq m/24 hours for 3 days is an indication of an autonomous adrenal adenoma, carcinoma, or pituitary neoplasm.

In cases of adrenogenital syndrome, 24-hour urine levels of 17-ketosteroids and pregnanetriol are substantially elevated.

Brief details of the corticotropin stimulation, metyrapone, and dexamethasone suppression tests are given below. In all cases, at least 2 preliminary 24-hour urine samples should be collected for baseline 17-hydroxycorticosteroid assays. No special precautions need be taken other than to refrigerate samples pending the assays.

Plasma cortisol levels determined by competitive protein binding are now available in many hospital and commercial laboratories. Isolated values are not diagnostic of adrenal function but may be used with stimulation and suppression tests described below. Because there is considerable diurnal variation in plasma values of cortisol, samples are taken between 8:00 and 9:00 a.m., at which time 15–20 μg/dl is normal.

ACTH Stimulation Test

A. Specimen and Test Requirements: After 2 baseline 24-hour control collections, give 250 μg synthetic ACTH (Cortrosyn, Synacthen) in 250 ml isotonic saline over a period of 8–12 hours, beginning at 8:00 a.m., or 20 mg/sq m corticotropin gel IM every 9–12 hours for 4 days. Collect 24-hour urine samples for 4 days following intravenous corticotropin or during intramuscular treatment, and measure 17-hydroxycorticosteroids.

A screening ACTH test may be performed by using 250 μg synthetic ACTH as IV bolus. Plasma cortisol values are determined prior to and 30 and 60 minutes after the injection.

B. Normal Values and Interpretation: Normally, ACTH stimulation produces a 3- to 5-fold increase over baseline levels in both plasma and urine. An abnormal response indicates hypoadrenocorticism. A normal response excludes primary hypoadrenocorticism.

Melly JC: Assessment of adrenocortical function. N Engl J Med 285:735, 1971.
Speckart PF, Nicoloff JT, Bethune JE: Screening for adrenocortical insufficiency with cosyntropin (synthetic ACTH). Arch Intern Med 128:761, 1971.

Metyrapone (Metopirone) Test

A. Specimen and Test Requirements: After 2 baseline 24-hour control collections or two 8:00 a.m. control plasma 11-deoxycortisol determinations, give metyrapone, 300 mg/sq m orally (never < 250 mg or > 750 mg) every 4 hours for 6 doses. Then collect two 24-hour urine samples on the first and second days following the last dose of the drug for 17-hydroxycorticosteroid assay.

B. Normal Values and Interpretation: The normal rise should be 2.5- to 3-fold, indicating normal pituitary and adrenal response. An abnormal test in the presence of a normal ACTH stimulation test indicates hypopituitarism.

Spark RF: Simplified assessment of pituitary-adrenal reserve: Measurement of serum 11-deoxycortisol and cortisol after metyrapone. Ann Intern Med 75:717, 1971.

Dexamethasone Suppression Test

A. Specimen and Test Requirements: After 2 consecutive 24-hour urine collections have been made, give 1.25 mg/sq m/24 hours of dexamethasone orally in 4 divided doses for 3 days.

B. Normal Values: See Table 38–2 (17-hydroxycorticosteroids, 17-ketosteroids, and pregnanetriol).

C. Interpretation: If suppression of urinary hydroxycorticosteroids to a level of < 1.5 mg/24 hours or to < 50% of control values does not occur, increase the dose to 3.75 mg/sq m/24 hours and repeat the test. This is used to differentiate adrenal hyperplasia and adrenogenital syndrome (suppressible) from adrenal carcinoma, adenoma, or pituitary neoplasm (nonsuppressible).

Kendall JW, Sloop PR: Dexamethasone: Suppressible adrenocortical tumor. N Engl J Med 279:532, 1968.

URINARY FREE CORTISOL

This is the most helpful test in the diagnosis of hyperadrenocortisolism. It is not useful in the diagnosis of hypoadrenocortisolism. A 24-hour urine collection is necessary.

Staleche H: Normal values of free urinary cortisol in infants and children. Horm Metab Res 5:64, 1973.

THYROID FUNCTION

Thyroid function can be appraised by the measurement in serum of thyroxine (T_4), the triiodothyronine resin uptake test ($T_3 R$), and thyroid-stimulating hormone (TSH).

T_4 in Serum

A. Specimen: 0.2 ml serum.

B. Normal Values: 3.2–6.4 μg/dl (as T_4 I).

C. Interpretation: Radioimmunoassays have now replaced most other methods and have the advantage of requiring smaller sample volumes. T_4 levels are elevated in hyperthyroidism and are low in hypothyroidism. Patients receiving certain drugs (eg, salicylates, phenytoin) have falsely low levels, while estrogens (pregnancy, oral contraceptives, newborns) produce elevated values. (See Table 38–2 for normal T_4 values in newborns.)

T_3 Resin Uptake in Serum

A. Specimen: 0.2 ml serum or plasma.

B. Normal Values: 45–60% resin uptake (values vary with laboratory).

C. Interpretation: The basis of the T_3 resin uptake test is as follows. Plasma thyroid-binding globulin is normally partly saturated with T_4 and, to a very small extent, with T_3. The affinity for T_4, however, is greater than for T_3, so that if excess T_3 is added it does not displace the T_4. In the in vitro test, the added T_3 is labeled with ^{131}I and, after a period of equilibration, the residual unbound T_3 is adsorbed onto one of a variety of resins and the proportion of the original activity is measured.

In hypothyroidism, thyroid-binding globulin is relatively unsaturated and most of the labeled T_3 becomes attached to the protein, giving a low resin uptake value. The converse is true in hyperthyroidism. Drugs which compete with T_4 and T_3 plasma protein binding sites, eg, salicylates and phenytoin, will create a falsely elevated T_3 resin uptake value. Low values are obtained in the newborn period due to the effect of maternal estrogens during pregnancy.

HUMAN SPECIFIC THYROID STIMULATOR

Human specific thyroid stimulator (previously called long-acting thyroid stimulating hormone) bioassay is available in some university and commercial laboratories. (Normal values: None detectable in normal serum.)

SCREENING & DIAGNOSTIC PROCEDURES FOR INBORN ERRORS OF METABOLISM

Amino Acids in Urine & Plasma

A. Specimens: 0.5 ml of a random urine acidified to pH 2.0; 0.1 ml serum.

B. Normal Values: See Table 38–1.

C. Interpretation: Disturbances of amino acid metabolism fall into 2 broad categories. In the first group, the changes in serum or urine amino acid levels are secondary to some other condition. Wilson's disease, galactosemia, chronic renal disease, rickets, scurvy, protein malnutrition, the renal tubular dystrophies, and heavy metal poisoning belong in this group. The increase in total urinary amino acid excretion may be striking, but the pattern of amino acids

seen on paper chromatography usually reflects a generalized aminoaciduria and has little diagnostic value; measurement of total urinary amino acid nitrogen (expressed as $\mu mol/kg/24$ hours) may be helpful.

In a second group, aminoaciduria or aminoacidemia reflects more precisely some inherited defect affecting the metabolism or transcellular movement of one or more amino acids. Improving technology for the precise measurement of amino acids and the increased use of screening technics in newborns and other special risk groups (institutionalized children, epileptics, psychotic children, etc) are now bringing to light new syndromes.

Scriver CR & others: Simple screening of plasma for aminoacidopathies. Lancet 1:230, 1964.

Chromatography of Sugars in Biologic Fluids

A. Specimens: 0.5 ml of a random urine acidified to pH 2.0; 0.1 ml serum.

B. Normal Values: Small amounts of hexoses and pentoses may be excreted by the normal person. For example, normal urine may contain up to 5 mg glucose/dl or 3 mg xylose/dl. Most tests for reducing sugars are insensitive to concentrations below 100 mg/dl, so that most pathologic meliturias require chromatography for their detection.

C. Interpretation:

1. Glycosuria—Diabetes, certain cerebral lesions, corticosteroid "diabetes," nephrosis, and primary and secondary renal tubular dystrophies.

2. Lactosuria—In milk-fed infants, up to 30 mg/dl; gastroenteritis, steatorrhea, and hepatitis.

3. **Lactosuria, galactosuria, and fructosuria**—Acute hepatitis, gastroenteritis, and rickets. It has been reported also in pyloric stenosis.

4. Fructosuria—Up to 20 mg/dl may normally be present in infants. Abnormal amounts may also be detected in diabetes, hepatitis, Wilson's disease, and mercury poisoning. Infantile fructosuria may also arise as a syndrome associated with vomiting, sweating, hypoglycemia, and variable aminoaciduria, proteinuria, and hypophosphatemia.

5. Galactosuria—Up to 15 mg/dl may normally be present in small infants. Increased amounts may occur in children with galactosemia after galactose loads, although loading is not advised as a diagnostic test. Galactosuria may be present also in hepatitis.

6. Sucrosuria—Up to 15 mg/dl may be present in the urine of infants on alimentary loading. Sucrosuria is present also in pancreatic disease and has been described in a syndrome associated with hiatal hernia and mental retardation.

Wright SW & others: Studies on carbohydrates in body fluids. Am J Dis Child 93:173, 1957.

Screening Test for Galactosemia

A reliable screening test for galactosemia has been devised using 25 μl of heparinized blood. The test depends on the fluorescence formed when uridyl trans-

Table 38—1. Normal values of amino acids and other ninhydrin-positive substances in plasma* and urine.†

	Newborn Plasma (Wk. 1)	Premature Plasma (Wk. 6)	Premature Urine (Wk. 6)	Full Term Plasma (Wk. 6)	Full Term Urine (Wk. 6)	Years 2–12 Plasma	Years 2–12 Urine	Adult Plasma	Adult Urine	% Tubular Reabsorption Infancy	% Tubular Reabsorption Childhood	% Tubular Reabsorption Adult
Phosphoethanol-amine	tr	...	...	...	...	...	.08–.28	...	...	...	...	...
Taurine	.01–.20	.05–.08	.03–.08	.02–.11	.01–.18	.06–.11	.76–1.9	.05–.08	0.4–1.3	96–98	93–95	72–95
Hydroxyproline		tr–.08	1.1–2.1	tr	0.7–2.6	...	0	0–tr	0	‡	...	...
Aspartic acid	tr–.02	.01–.02	tr–.04	.008–.02	tr–.32	.004–.02	tr–.07	.004–.01	.03–.09	§	92–99	85–98
Threonine	.04–.05	.15–.33	0.9–1.9	.17–.23	.67–1.4	.04–.10	.04–.17	.09–.14	.09–.14	71–91	92–99.5	97–99
Serine	.04–.30	.10–.16	0.8–1.3	.16–.20	1.1–2.3	.08–.11	.09–.34	.08–.11	.09–.31	54–86	92–99	97–99
Asparagine Glutamine	0.3–2.1	.40–.44	0.5–1.5	.36–.57	1.1–2.0	.06–.47	.04–.75	.4–.5	.17–.48	90–96	98–99.9	99+
Proline	.02–.43	.10–.31	0.6–1.7	.40–.48	0.7–5.4	.07–.15	tr–.04	.15–.25	0	53–94	99.5–100	99+
Glutamate	tr–.26	.08–.14	.02–.13	.06–.21	.04–.62	.02–.25	.01–.13	.05–.20	.008–.16	95–99	98.5–99.8	99+
Citrulline	...	.04–.07	.02–.17	tr–.04	tr–.04	...	tr–.03	tr–.03	0–tr	92–98	...	99+
Glycine	.05–.44	.12–.21	2.5–4.2	.18–.24	3.7–8.4	.12–.22	.33–1.5	.15–.24	.40–.90	15–63	93–99	94–99
Alanine	.04–.44	.20–.39	0.5–0.7	.46–.52	1.2–2.1	.14–.30	.04–.35	.35–.37	.09–.27	87–92	99–99.9	99+
α-Amino adipic	...	0	0.1–.23	0	.17–.23	...	...	0	0–.02	‡	...	‡
α-Amino butyric	tr–.07	0–tr	tr	tr–.02	0	...	tr–.06	.01–.03	.01–.04	‡	...	99
Valine	.03–.32	.12–.22	tr–0.2	.32–.35	.10–.16	.13–.28	tr–.08	.05–.08	tr–.05	98–99+	99.6–99.9	99+
Homocitrulline	...	tr	.13–.37	0	.12–.24	...	...	0	.02–.04	‡	‡	‡
1/2 Cystine	.02–.07	tr–.07	.04–.25	0	.14–.34	...	...	0	.02–.08	60–90	...	99+
Cystathionine	...	.005–.01	.09–.12	0–tr	.11–.17	...	...	0	.01–.02	35–65	...	‡
Methionine	tr–.08	.02–.04	.08–.14	.03–.05	.12–.14	.01–.02	.01–.04	.01–.04	.02–.04	85–97	98.3–99.7	98–99+
Isoleucine	.01–.09	.04–.08	.03–.07	.08–.12	.10–.16	.03–.08	.01–.07	.05–.08	.01–.04	96–99+	99.2–99.9	99+
Leucine	.01–.18	.1–.5	.04–.08	.14–.22	.15–.18	.06–.18	.02–.11	.10–.14	.02–.05	97–99+	99.6–99.9	99+
Tyrosine	.05–.30	.1–.4	.17–.60	.11–.21	.22–.38	.03–.07	.03–.12	.04–.07	.06–.10	93–99	98.2–99.3	98–99+
Phenylalanine	.02–.12	.05–.07	.08–.13	.06–.12	.11–.14	.03–.06	.01–.11	.04–.07	.04–.07	94–99	98.8–99.7	99+
β-Alanine	...	0	0	0	0	.02–.05	tr	0	0	...	...	...
BAIB	...	0	.09–.16	0	.17–.42	...	0–.19	0	.01–.09	...	...	...
Methylglycine	...	...	...	...	...	< .01	< .05	...	...	...	...	...
Hydroxylysine	...	0	.13–.27	0	.05–.11	...	...	0	0–.02	‡	...	...
GABA	tr–0.1	0	0–tr	0	0–tr	...	...	0	tr	...	...	‡
Ornithine	.01–.22	.08–.11	0–.08	.07–.10	.05–.08	.03–.09	.01–.03	.58–.90	tr	96–99+	99.5–99.8	99+
Lysine	.05–.35	.08–.15	0.2–0.6	.21–.34	0.7–1.4	.07–.15	.04–.21	.16–.18	.02–.20	81–96	98.5–99.8	99+
1-Methylhistidine	...	0	0	0	0–.03	...	...	0	.58–.90	...	...	...
Histidine	tr–.13	.05–.13	.34–.83	.05–.08	0.8–1.8	.02–.08	.11–1.0	.06–.07	.15–.53	30–80	90.3–98.4	92–98
3-Methylhistidine	...	0	0	0	0–.07	...	...	0	.08–.28	...	...	...
Arginine	tr–.12	tr–.07	0	.04–.10	tr–0.1	.02–.09	.01–.04	.03–.06	.02–.20	99+	99–99.9	99+

*Measured in μmol/ml (fasting).
†Measured in μmol/min/1.73 sq m.

‡0–trace in plasma but significant amounts in urine.
§Detectable in plasma but not in urine except in traces.

ferase converts galactose-1-phosphate to UDP galactose.

Beutler E, Baluda MC: Screening test for galactosemia. J Lab Clin Med 68:137, 1966.

Diagnostic Test for Galactosemia

A. Specimen: 1 ml heparinized blood cooled in ice water.

B. Normal Values: Galactose-1-phosphate uridyl transferase, 308–475 ImU/gm hemoglobin.

C. Interpretation: Homozygotes for galactosemia are < 8 ImU/gm hemoglobin. In Duarte variants and heterozygotes, the levels are 142–225 ImU/gm.

Tedesco TA, Mellman WJ: The UDPglu consumption assay for gal-1-P uridyl transferase. Page 66 in: *Galactosemia*. Hsia DYY (editor). Thomas, 1969.

Hypothyroidism (See Chapter 24.)

A variety of approaches are acceptable. Perhaps the best approach for an individual hospital is to measure cord blood TSH levels, using a T_4 filter paper disk from the phenylketonuria test to confirm. For mass screening, blood on filter paper disks should be screened for T_4 and confirmed by TSH. This will select 1:500 infants, but only 15% or less of these will have hypothyroidism on final testing.

Mucopolysaccharides

A. Specimens: 5 ml of urine for screening test; a 24-hour urine sample for chromatographic test.

B. Normal Values: See Table 38–2.

C. Interpretation: In the last few years, a group of diseases have come to be identified which are now recognized to be associated with specific defects of lysosomal enzymes. Previously, they had been grouped together under the name of Hurler's syndrome, although they represented cases with a wide range of skeletal deformities, corneal clouding, hepatosplenomegaly, and intellectual impairment. As might be expected in an essentially connective tissue disorder, vascular and joint tissues may also be involved.

A satisfactory screening test for excess mucopolysaccharides in urine is available which depends on a precipitate formed in the presence of a buffered acid-albumin reagent. More specific assay uses a saline gradient and column chromatography of urine. Specific enzyme assays will probably be increasingly used.

Ferric Chloride Test for Phenylketonuria

A. Specimen: 5 ml urine.

B. Method: Add 10% ferric chloride solution, drop by drop, to 5 ml of urine in a test tube. Initially, a precipitate of ferric phosphate may form which may require filtering. A purple color is produced by both acetoacetic acid and salicylates, but the former color is heat-labile. A green color develops in the presence of phenylpyruvic acid. Other compounds reacting with ferric chloride are listed below.

C. Compounds Reacting in Ferric Chloride Test:

1. Metabolites—

Phenylpyruvic acid: green

p-Hydroxyphenylpyruvic acid: green fading rapidly

a-Ketobutyric acid (oasthouse syndrome): purple going to brownish red

3-Hydroxyanthranilic acid: brown

Urocanic acid (histidinemia): green

Homogentisic acid: very dark brown

Xanthurenic acid (pyridoxine disorders): dark green going to brown

Branched chain ketoacids (maple syrup urine): gray-green

Pyruvic acid: yellow-brown

Melanin: black

Acetoacetic acid: red-brown, red

Imidazole pyruvic acid (histidinemia): blue-green

1-Methylhistidine: slow green

2. Drugs—

Salicylates: purple

Phenothiazines: purple

Aminosalicylic acid: red-brown

Histidinuria Screening Test

A. Specimen: 1 ml random urine.

B. Interpretation: Excess histidine in urine will inhibit the formation of blue color given by biscyclohexane in the presence of copper. The screening test must be confirmed by a quantitative measurement of serum histidine.

Gerber MG: A simple screening test for histidinuria. Pediatrics 213:40, 1969.

Levy HL & others: A simple indirect method of detecting the enzyme defect in histidinemia. J Pediatr 75:1056, 1969.

Methylmalonic Aciduria Screening Test

The following simple screening test for the presence of methylmalonic acid in urine is based on the formation of a green diazo derivative:

Fifty μl of urine are added to 0.75 ml of 0.1% *p*-nitroaniline in 0.16 N hydrochloric acid. Aqueous sodium nitrite, 0.5%, 0.25 ml, and 1 M sodium acetate buffer, pH 4.3, 1 ml, are added, and the mixture is incubated for 1 minute in a boiling water bath. A green color appears at concentrations greater than 100 mg/dl of methylmalonic acid. This is sufficiently sensitive to detect cases of methylmalonate isomerase deficiency. Confirmation requires gas chromatography.

Giorgio AJ, Luhby AL: Rapid screening test for methyl malonic aciduria. J Clin Pathol 52:374, 1969.

Nitroprusside Cyanide Screening Test for Cystine & Homocystine in Urine

Acidify 5 ml of urine with 0.5 ml of 1 N hydrochloric acid, add 2 ml of fresh 5% sodium cyanide solution, and let stand at room temperature for 30 minutes. Then add 1 ml of fresh 5.5% sodium nitroprusside solution. A definite purple color indicates the presence of excess amounts of cystine, homocystine, or β-mercaptolactate cysteine disulfide. Faintly positive reactions may occur in older normal children, and more definite ones in small premature infants in the first trimester of life.

Orotic Aciduria Screening Test

A. Specimen: 0.5 ml random urine.

B. Method: Orotic acid is converted by bromine water and ascorbic acid to barbituric acid. The latter forms a yellow compound with Ehrlich's reagent. Histidinuria may produce a false-positive test.

C. Interpretation: The test is valid for the detection of hereditary orotic aciduria and also as confirmation of hyperammonemia due to ornithine transcarbamylase deficiency.

Rogers LE, Porter FG: Hereditary orotic aciduria. II. A urinary screening test. Pediatrics 42:423, 1968.

TESTS OF LIVER FUNCTION

Alkaline Phosphatase

A. Specimen: 0.05 ml serum.

B. Normal Values: See Table 38—2.

C. Interpretation: Alkaline phosphatase is a lysosomal enzyme whose activity is found to be increased in 2 groups of diseases: those affecting liver function, and those in which there is involvement of osteoblastic activity in the bones. In hepatic disease, increased plasma alkaline phosphatase is generally accepted as an indication of biliary obstruction. In the second group, serum phosphatase activity is increased in primary hyperparathyroidism, in secondary hyperparathyroidism owing to chronic renal disease, in the various forms of rickets, and in osteitis deformans juvenilia—whether these be due to vitamin D deficiency, malabsorption, or renal tubular dystrophies. Levels may also be increased in Recklinghausen's disease with bone involvement and in a variety of malignant infiltrations of bone. Low values are found in hyperthyroidism and in the rare condition known as idiopathic hypophosphatasia, where it is associated with rickets and the excretion of excess phosphoethanolamine in the urine.

Derren JJ & others: Alkaline phosphatase. N Engl J Med 270:1277, 1969.

Acid Phosphatase
A. Specimen: 0.1 ml serum.
B. Normal Values: 8.6–13 IU/liter.
C. Interpretation: Serum acid phosphatase levels are elevated to about twice normal in Gaucher's disease. Elevations are also found in acute and chronic thrombocytopenic purpuras. Acid phosphatase activity is greatly reduced in a syndrome associated with early severe progressive neurologic disease.

Blood Ammonia
A. Specimen: 1 ml plasma collected in a heparinized tube in ice cold water.
B. Normal Values: 45–80 μg/dl.
C. Interpretation: Ammonia is produced by bacterial action in the bowel and absorbed into the portal circulation. It is also produced endogenously by the deamination of amino acids. Ammonia levels are of some value in gauging the severity or prognosis of liver failure, especially in Reye's syndrome, but are essential in the diagnosis of inborn errors in the Krebs-Henseleit urea cycle.

Conn HD: Sources and significance of blood ammonia. Yale J Biol Med 41:33, 1968.

Bilirubin in Serum
A. Specimen: 0.05 ml serum.
B. Normal Values: See Table 38–2.
C. Interpretation: Bilirubin is produced by the destruction of hemoglobin and is then converted in the liver to its diglucuronide for excretion in the bile. The unconjugated form is elevated in hemolytic diseases, in acute hepatitis, and in hereditary glucuronyl transferase deficiency. The conjugated form is elevated in acute and chronic hepatitis as well as in obstructive liver disease.

Robinson SH: The origins of bilirubin. N Engl J Med 279:143, 1968.

Copper in Biologic Fluids
A. Specimens: 0.1 ml serum; 24-hour urine acidified to pH 2.0.
B. Normal Values: See Table 38–2.

C. Interpretation: Approximately 98% of circulating serum copper is bound to a blue alpha$_2$ globulin, ceruloplasmin. The remaining 2% exists in 2 forms: most is loosely bound to albumin, whereas the remainder exists as free ionic copper.

In Wilson's disease, urinary copper is increased and there is a decrease in serum copper and ceruloplasmin levels. In cirrhosis of the liver, urine copper is also elevated, but serum copper and ceruloplasmin (alpha$_2$ copper-binding protein) are increased. Serum copper oxidase assay is simple and specific since it relates closely to serum copper and ceruloplasmin levels, whose estimation is complex.

Wilson's disease should always be excluded as a cause of chronic liver disease in children. There is some recent evidence that, in a small number of cases of Wilson's disease, copper oxidase levels may be normal. Liver copper is the best index of Wilson's disease.

Slovis T & others: The varied manifestations of Wilson's disease. J Pediatr 78:578, 1971.

Bromsulphalein Excretion Test
A. Specimen and Test Requirements: The patient should be fasting. Give 5 mg/kg Bromsulphalein in sterile 5% solution IV over a period of 1 minute. Draw a blood sample at 45 minutes. The test requires 0.1 ml serum. The method assumes a plasma volume of 50 ml/kg.
B. Normal Values: < 10% retention in children.
C. Interpretation: This is essentially a test of both the glutathione conjugating ability of the liver and the excretion of conjugates; outside of this specific role, it is a generally less useful test of liver function than enzyme assays and serum electrophoresis, especially in children. Bromsulphalein conjugates of glutamic acid and cysteine are also found in the bile.

Lindquist B, Paulson L: BSP elimination in infants and children. Acta Paediatr Scand 48:223, 1959.

Serum Cholesterol
A. Specimen: 0.1 ml serum.
B. Normal Values: See Table 38–2.
C. Interpretation: Plasma cholesterol in the normal child varies within wide limits, and for this reason its estimation has a rather limited application. The level is elevated in diabetes, nephrosis, hypothyroidism, and biliary obstruction, as well as in idiopathic hypercholesterolemia and hyperlipidemia; it is depressed in hyperthyroidism, hepatitis, and sometimes in severe anemia or infection. In none of these instances does the measurement of serum cholesterol rank as more than a subsidiary test; in nephrosis, for example, serum protein electrophoresis provides a substantially more sensitive index of diagnosis and progress.

Rafstedt S: Serum lipids and lipoproteins in infancy and childhood. Acta Paediatr Scand 44(Suppl 102):1, 1955.

Gamma Glutamyl Transpeptidase (GGTP)

A. **Specimen:** 0.1 ml serum.

B. **Normal Values:** See Table 38–2.

C. **Interpretation:** This enzyme is present in kidney, pancreas, liver, and prostate, with the kidney showing the highest activity. Testis, epididymis, spleen, lung, bowel, placenta, and thyroid also contain significant amounts of enzyme.

The measurement of serum GGTP is a sensitive test for liver disease, particularly in biliary obstruction. However, elevations of this enzyme are not confined to a single category of liver disease and may be found in the majority of liver disorders. The test is particularly useful in screening for liver disease, and in the non-jaundiced patient it is superior to alkaline phosphatase, leucine aminopeptidase, 5'-nucleotidase, and transaminases. Liver disease is unlikely to be present if the plasma level is completely normal. However, because of the lack of specificity for hepatic tissue, the converse may not be true.

Rosalki SB: Gamma glutamyl transpeptidase. Vol 17, p 53, in: *Advances in Clinical Chemistry.* Bodansky O, Latner AL (editors). Academic Press, 1975.

Lactate Dehydrogenase, Serum & Cerebrospinal Fluid

A. **Specimen:** 0.1 ml serum or CSF.

B. **Normal Values:** See Table 38–2.

C. **Interpretation:** Lactate dehydrogenase (LDH) is one of the increasing number of enzymes that can be separated into different protein fractions possessing the same substrate specificity. Each of the 5 common isozymes of LDH has been shown to be a tetramer comprised of combinations of 2 polypeptide chains, A and B. The enzyme shows an organ specificity, so that the predominant isozyme (60%) in heart muscle, type 1, appears in increased concentration in the serum following cardiac infarction, traveling in the neighborhood of albumin upon electrophoresis. On the other hand, the greatest serum LDH activity in hepatitis is in the slowest moving band, type 5. In myopathies, types 3, 4, and 5 are increased.

Levels of total serum LDH activity 2–5 times normal have been reported in progressive forms of chronic hepatitis and hepatic cirrhosis. Abnormally high values have been detected in certain blood diseases, including sickle cell anemia, the hemolytic crisis in favism, acute acquired hemolytic anemia, and, particularly, in untreated pernicious anemia, in which levels more than 10 times normal are found. The serum LDH level is normal in anemias due to blood loss or iron deficiency.

LDH activity may be increased in the CSF following birth injury, results varying from 22–600 IU/liter in infants suspected of intracranial pathology.

Serum Leucine Aminopeptidase

A. **Specimen:** 0.1 ml serum.

B. **Normal Values:** 15–50 IU/liter.

C. **Interpretation:** Increases in the level of serum leucine aminopeptidase are associated (with the exception of pregnancy) almost exclusively with diseases of the liver, biliary tract, or pancreas. The determination has a special place in pediatric clinical chemistry in the differentiation of neonatal hepatitis and biliary atresia. In this respect, it ranks with rose bengal sodium I 131 as a diagnostic test. In neonatal hepatitis, values generally less than 120 IU/liter are recorded, but in atresia 90% are above this level.

Rutenburg AM & others: Serum leucine amino peptidases. Am J Dis Child 103:47, 1962.

Transaminase in Serum & Cerebrospinal Fluid

A. **Specimen:** 0.1 ml serum or CSF.

B. **Normal Values:** See Table 38–2.

C. **Interpretation:** The transaminases, as widely distributed intracellular enzymes, are raised in the serum in various kinds of tissue destruction, after major surgery, and in myopathies, but primarily in hepatitis and other forms of active liver disease. (The SGOT level in CSF following intracranial damage is 2.5–10.5 IU/liter.) High values are found in the newborn period; thereafter, values are remarkably uniform.

TESTS OF PANCREATIC & ENTERIC FUNCTION

Serum Amylase

A. **Specimen:** 0.1 ml serum or heparinized plasma.

B. **Normal Values:** 6–33 Close-Street units/dl.

C. **Interpretation:** Elevated levels of serum and urine amylase have been used as an index of pancreatitis following trauma or as a complication of mumps or infectious mononucleosis. In the above conditions, the serum amylase levels may initially exceed 250 Close-Street units. Levels may be increased in chronic pancreatic obstruction, in bowel obstruction, and in peritonitis, but levels in serum do not exceed 120 units.

Absorption Tests for Lactase, Amylase, Maltase, & Sucrase Activity

A. **Specimens and Test Requirements:** 0.1 ml serum at start of test and at 30 minutes for glucose assay. The oral loading dose of maltose and starch should be the same as that of glucose (see p 1047). The dose for lactose and sucrose should be twice that amount. All carbohydrate is administered as a flavored 10% aqueous solution.

B. **Interpretation:** In normal children, there is a rise of over 50 mg/dl within 30 minutes. A rise of less than 20 mg/dl is suggestive of enzymatic defect.

Fat Absorption

A. **Specimen and Test Requirements:** The patient

is placed on a normal diet containing 35% of calories as fat. On the third day, a 24-hour stool collection is made.

B. **Normal Values:** See Table 38–2.

C. **Interpretation:** About 40% of triglyceride is completely hydrolyzed in the small bowel: a further 40% is hydrolyzed to mono- and diglyceride, and about 20% is unhydrolyzed. Hydrolysis reflects the action of pancreatic lipase on emulsified triglyceride formed in the presence of bile salts, on fatty acids, and on mono- and diglycerides. Long chain fatty acids (> C-16) are absorbed in the free state or as mono-glycerides into the mucosal cell, where they are resynthesized into triglyceride before passing into the lymph. Short chain fatty acids (< C-16, and especially < C-10) may be absorbed into mucosal cells in any form as mono-, di-, or triglyceride or in the free state. Within the cell, they may be resynthesized into triglyceride or become attached to albumin. In both ways they pass into the portal blood.

In children, excess stool fat is most commonly found in either cystic fibrosis of the pancreas or in the gluten-sensitive celiac syndrome. Other causes include obstructive liver disease which interferes with bile salt availability, chronic enteric infections, blind loop syndrome, small bowel resections, pancreatic achylias (including hereditary pancreatitis and absence of lipase), acrodermatitis enteropathica, abetalipoproteinemia, and hypoparathyroidism.

Anderson CM: Intestinal malabsorption in childhood. Arch Dis Child 41:571, 1966.

Free Fatty Acids in Plasma

A. **Specimen:** 0.1 ml heparinized plasma frozen immediately after collection.

B. **Normal Values:** See Table 38–2.

C. **Interpretation:** The "free" fatty acids (FFA) of plasma represent metabolically active lipid in the process of being transported, albumin-bound, from the fat depots to the tissues. It is now clear that FFA form a readily available source of energy that can be metabolized by many tissues, notably cardiac and skeletal muscle. The respiratory quotient of newborn infants indicates that during the third to fifth days of life energy is derived from sources which are 80–90% fat. Although cord blood FFA levels are significantly lower than those of the mother at the time of delivery, the highest values achieved under normal conditions are found during the first day after birth. There ensues a gradual fall over the following year to levels slightly above normal adult levels. Infants born of diabetic mothers have cord blood levels which do not differ significantly from those of infants born of normal mothers.

The turnover rate of plasma FFA has been reported as 28% per minute, equivalent to about 250 μEq/liter/minute. During exercise, the turnover rate increases and the absolute level falls.

Elevated levels are found in hyperthyroidism, which is associated with an accelerated mobilization of fat. Fasting also results in an increased plasma FFA level, particularly in children up to age 10. A 19-hour period of fasting caused values higher than those following a 14-hour fast. While the same was true of adults, the levels found were considerably lower. The trauma experienced by an individual with burns is associated with raised FFA in plasma; the more pronounced the trauma, the greater and more prolonged the elevation. Four patients with nondetectable glucose-6-phosphatase levels had raised fasting FFA levels, presumably as a result of the hypoglycemic tendency typical of this glycogen storage disease. In the study of lipid levels of well controlled juvenile diabetics aged 2–13 years, no difference was found in the FFA levels when compared with normal children of the same age group. Twelve children age 13 months to 4 years suffering from kwashiorkor and a group with marasmus exhibited elevated levels of FFA.

Total Fatty Acids in Plasma & Red Cells

A. **Specimen:** 2.0 ml of whole blood (EDTA).

B. **Normal Values:** See Table 38–2. These values were determined for 20 children and young adults 6–19 years of age in Dr H.P. Chase's laboratory.

C. **Interpretation:** The lipids present in plasma and red cell membranes (triglycerides, phospholipids, and cholesterol esters) can be extracted and saponified to free the constituent fatty acids. After methylation, these fatty acids can be separated and quantitated by gas-liquid chromatography.

Patients with essential fatty acid deficiencies usually show increased levels of 16:0, 16:1, 18:0, and 18:1. Levels of 18:2 (linoleic) and 20:4 (arachidonic) are usually decreased.

Lipase in Serum or Duodenal Secretion

A. **Specimen:** 0.1 ml serum or duodenal secretion.

B. **Normal Values:** 10–136 IU/liter (serum).

C. **Interpretation:** Traditionally, the assay of lipase in duodenal juice has been considered a diagnostic test for cystic fibrosis of the pancreas. However, it is apparent that pancreatic digestive secretions may be considerably diminished during and after any serious illness, whether enteric or not. There is also a rare condition of primary lipase deficiency.

Serum lipase levels are elevated in acute pancreatitis, a relatively common concomitant of mumps and glandular fever. In this condition, serum lipase levels tend to rise more slowly and, once elevated, to be more sustained than serum amylase levels. The difficulties and discomforts to the child of obtaining samples of duodenal juice, together with the effectiveness of the sweat chloride test, mean that this and similar enzyme tests are seldom now required in the diagnosis of fibrocystic disease.

Sweat Electrolytes

A. **Specimen:** At least 50 mg (0.05 ml) of sweat collected by pilocarpine iontophoresis.

B. **Normal Values:** See Table 38–2 under Chloride and Sodium.

C. Interpretation: A positive sweat test is an important parameter in the diagnosis of cystic fibrosis. Unfortunately the test is performed poorly in many clinical laboratories, particularly those where sweat analysis is infrequently requested. A properly performed sweat test should involve pilocarpine iontophoresis and a measurement of the volume of sweat collected. At low rates of sweating, the electrolyte concentration varies proportionately to the volume of sweat. A collection of less than 50 mg of sweat should be considered inadequate and the test repeated. The laboratory report should include the volume or weight of sweat obtained.

The sodium and chloride concentrations in sweat are consistently and markedly elevated in almost all cases of cystic fibrosis. However, because of the late development of the sweat glands, it is sometimes difficult to obtain sufficient amounts of sweat in the newborn period, and testing may need to be delayed until after 6 weeks of age.

Elevated sweat electrolytes may be found in a number of conditions in addition to cystic fibrosis, ie, untreated adrenal insufficiency, nephrogenic diabetes insipidus, and certain forms of ectodermal dysplasia.

Xylose Absorption

A. Specimen and Test Requirements: The test is performed as follows: The fasting child is given 10 ml/kg of a 5% solution of D-xylose and, subsequently, fasted and thirsted for 5 hours. Urine is collected over this period, and, after the total volume is recorded, an aliquot is preserved in the deep freeze. Blood samples are taken into fluoride-oxalate tubes before the test starts, at 30 minutes, and at 120 minutes.

B. Normal Values: See Table 38–2.

C. Interpretation: Xylose absorption is a technically simple, reliable, and informative gauge of upper small bowel absorption. This pentose is not digested in the bowel, but it is not clear whether it is absorbed in the small bowel solely by diffusion or by an active process involving phosphorylation or other specific enzymes. About 60% of absorbed xylose is metabolized via fructose-6-phosphate and through the Krebs cycle; the remainder is excreted within 5 hours in the urine. The test is primarily one of upper small bowel absorption.

Xylose absorption is normal in colitis, liver disease, and in primary pancreatic deficiencies. In children, it is abnormal in fibrocystic disease of the pancreas, indicating that the malabsorption in this state is not solely a reflection of deficient pancreatic enzymes.

Bunta H: Xylose test and its normal values in children. Kinderärztl Prax 38:507, 1970.

BIOCHEMICAL TESTS FOR UNDERNUTRITION

The following tests are useful in the detection of undernutrition and in other situations which are outlined below. (See also Table 4–9 for levels indicating deficiencies.)

Ascorbic Acid

A. Specimens: 1 ml fresh plasma; 4-hour fresh urine collections.

B. Normal Values: See Table 38–2.

C. Interpretation: Ascorbic acid determinations may be useful when scurvy occurs with rickets and the typical radiologic picture is consequently obscured.

Estimates of ascorbic acid in fasting serum provide a rather crude assessment of the scorbutic state. Levels below 0.15 mg/dl are suggestive. A more satisfactory procedure is to perform a tolerance test by giving 20 mg/kg of ascorbic acid (IV or IM) as a 4% solution in sterile pyrogen-free saline. A 4-hour sample should show levels in excess of 1.5 mg/dl after the intravenous load and in excess of 0.6 mg/dl after the intramuscular load.

In scurvy, the urine level of ascorbic acid following an oral loading dose is < 1% in 24 hours.

Serum Proteins

A. Specimen: 0.1 ml plasma.

B. Normal Values: See Table 38–2.

C. Interpretation: Changes in serum protein levels occur in many childhood diseases. Albumin is depressed where there is proteinuria and in the exudative enteropathies. Alpha proteins are elevated in acute and chronic infections, and the alpha$_2$ globulins characteristically merge with the beta band in the acute stage of idiopathic nephrosis. Gamma globulins are increased in infection, in some immunodystrophies, and especially in disseminated lupus erythematosus and related diseases. The gamma globulins are diminished in the agammaglobulinemias.

Vitamin A & Carotene in Serum

A. Specimen: 0.1 ml serum.

B. Normal Values: See Table 38–2.

C. Interpretation: Vitamin A is fat-soluble, so that estimations of its level in plasma can be a measure of fat absorption. Low fasting levels are found in undernourished children and in those with malabsorption syndromes. Increased levels are noted in vitamin A intoxication and in some cases of idiopathic hypercalcemia of infancy. The absorption of vitamin A palmitate is a gauge of lipase function and chylomicron absorption, whereas vitamin A alcohol absorption is an index of chylomicron absorption only. Tolerance tests are a more sensitive index of malabsorption than fasting levels. They may also be used to demonstrate the augmented absorption often seen in idiopathic hypercalcemia, when values for vitamin A may rise from fasting values of 72–200 µg/dl to 4-hour levels of 360–1070 µg/dl.

β-Carotene occurs widely in leafy vegetables and in certain other fruits and roots. It is rather less well absorbed than vitamin A and more dependent on the presence of bile. Synthesis of vitamin A from β-carotene is thought to occur in the mucosa. Hypocarotenemia is found in malabsorption syndromes, and abnormally high levels may occur from a high intake of yellow vegetables and, occasionally, in diabetes and hypothyroidism.

Vitamin E in Serum

A. **Specimen:** 0.1 ml serum.

B. **Normal Values:** See Table 38–2.

C. **Interpretation:** The small premature infant fed evaporated milk unsupplemented by vitamin E may, by the second month of life, have a serum tocopherol level below that which is known to produce in vitro hemolysis of red blood cells. It has also been shown that children with cystic fibrosis of the pancreas may have hypovitaminosis E, often in association with ceroid deposits in the intestinal musculature.

Other Useful Laboratory Parameters
Indicative of Malnutrition

Hemoglobin, < 10 gm/dl

Hematocrit, < 30%

Serum iron, < 30 µg/dl at 2 years to < 60 µg/dl at 12 years

Transferrin saturation, < 20%

Red cell folacin, < 140 ng/ml

Serum folacin, < 3 ng/ml

Urinary thiamine, < 120 (1–3 years), < 85 (4–6 years), < 60 (7–12 years) µg/gm creatinine

Urinary riboflavin, < 150 (1–3 years), < 100 (4–6 years), < 80 (7–15 years) µg/gm creatinine

Urinary iodine, < 25 µg/gm creatinine

Serum urea, < 8 mg/dl

Serum amylase, < 6 IU/dl

Chase JP & others: Nutritional status of migrant farm children. Am J Dis Child 122:316, 1971.

TESTS OF RENAL FUNCTION

Urine Ammonia

A. **Specimen and Test Requirements:** Timed specimens should be acidified with concentrated hydrochloric acid to pH 3.0 as collected, and refrigerated. The assay is a simple colorimetric one using Nessler's reagent.

B. **Normal Values:** See Table 38–2.

C. **Interpretation:** The estimation of urine ammonia is one gauge of the renal tubular capacity to excrete hydrogen ion. Thus, in states of acidosis unaccompanied by renal impairment (eg, starvation and diabetic acidosis), there may be as much as a 5-fold increase in urine ammonia. Normal excretion is about 12 µEq/minute/sq m, but this varies with diet. The ammonium ion is derived from glutamine in the tubule cell, and in chronic renal disease the limitation of this mechanism is one of the causes of acidosis. As with all tests of renal function, the expanded capacity of remaining normal renal tissue conceals overall diminished performance until this is extensive.

Peonides A: The renal excretion of hydrogen ions in infants and children. Arch Dis Child 40:33, 1965.

Creatine & Creatinine in Plasma & Urine

A. **Specimen:** 0.1 ml serum; timed urine acidified to pH 2.0 and refrigerated.

B. **Normal Values:** See Table 38–2.

C. **Interpretation:** Serum creatinine is used as an index of glomerular failure, as is the creatinine clearance (urine concentration × urine volume per minute ÷ plasma concentration). The latter value, which is generally less reliable than the inulin clearance, can also be used as a reference for calculating tubular reabsorption, eg, of amino acids or phosphorus. In muscular dystrophy, an increased urinary creatine coefficient and a decreased urinary creatinine coefficient may be diagnostically helpful. Creatinine excretion is not a reliable reference term in which to express the urinary content of other solutes.

Applegarth DA & others: Creatinine excretion in children. Clin Chem Acta 22:131, 1968.

Glomerular Filtration Rate

(See also discussion in Chapter 18.)

A. **Specimen:** 0.1 ml fasting serum.

B. **Normal Values:** 45–95 ml/minute/sq m.

Phosphorus, Tubular Reabsorption

A. **Specimen:** 0.1 ml serum; 1 ml urine.

B. **Normal Values and Interpretation:** The ratio of phosphorus and creatinine clearances can be used to calculate tubular reabsorption of phosphorus (TRP):

$$\% \, TRP = 100 \left[1 - \frac{(Urine \, P \times Plasma \, creatinine)}{(Plasma \, P \times Urine \, creatinine)} \right]$$

In normal subjects, the range is 78–97% reabsorption. This is greatly diminished in the phosphate-losing forms of vitamin D–resistant rickets.

Nordin BEL, Fraser R: Assessment of urinary phosphate excretion. Lancet 1:947, 1960.

Blood Urea Nitrogen

A. **Specimen:** 0.1 ml heparinized whole blood.

B. **Normal Values:** See Table 38–2.

C. **Interpretation:** Urea is excreted by the glomeruli and reabsorbed by the tubules. Raised levels in the plasma offer only a rather crude index of renal failure since glomerular destruction must amount to about 80% before urea is retained. The same comment may be made about the urea clearance test. It is important to remember, however, that the blood urea may be raised up to 50 mg/dl or even more in small infants receiving a high dietary nitrogen load. In these circumstances, diminished urea clearance does not indicate renal disease.

Uric Acid in Plasma

A. Specimen: 0.2 ml plasma.

B. Normal Values: See Table 38–2.

C. Interpretation: Elevated in rheumatoid arthritis, in renal failure, in leukemia during treatment, and in the hyperuricemia/mental retardation syndromes. Gout in childhood is very rare.

TESTS FOR MUSCLE DISEASE*

Serum Aldolase

A. Specimen: 0.2 ml serum.

B. Normal Values: See Table 38–2.

C. Interpretation: Fructose diphosphate aldolase cleaves fructose-1:6-diphosphate to dihydroxyacetone phosphate and glyceraldehyde-3-phosphate. A second aldolase, predominantly in the liver, forms dihydroxyacetone phosphate and glyceraldehyde from fructose-1-phosphate.

Serum aldolase determinations are useful in differentiating primary diseases of muscle (eg, pseudohypertrophic muscular dystrophy) from disorders in which the lesion is neurogenic (eg, amyotonia). The activity of this enzyme is also increased in infective hepatitis, myocardial infarction, acute pancreatitis, and severe hemolytic anemia. Levels in portal cirrhosis and obstructive jaundice are within normal limits. Fructose-1-phosphate aldolase is absent in hereditary fructose intolerance and lowered in Tay-Sachs disease.

Niebroz-Dobosz I & others: Blood enzymes in Duchenne's progressive muscular dystrophy and their correlation with the clinical and histological pictures. Acta Med Pol 11:387, 1970.

Serum Creatine Kinase

A. Specimen: 0.1 ml serum.

B. Normal Values: See Table 38–2.

C. Interpretation: At present the most reliable laboratory confirmation of muscular dystrophy is provided by the serum creatine phosphokinase (CPK) level. This test has a further use in that it gives a moderately reliable indication of whether a young woman with affected male siblings is a carrier of the severe X-linked form. The test is not helpful in identi-

*See also Lactate Dehydrogenase, p 1056.

fying persons heterozygous for the mild X-linked and autosomal recessive forms.

A refinement of this assay is provided by starch-gel electrophoresis of CPK isozymes: Muscular dystrophy patients show only the major and not the minor component. CPK activity is strikingly elevated in serum in hypothyroidism; it is diminished, but less obviously, in hyperthyroidism.

Cao A & others: Serum creatine phosphokinase isoenzymes in congenital hypoparathyroidism. J Pediatr 78:134, 1971.

Katz RM, Liebman W: Creatine phosphokinase activity in central nervous systemic disorders and infections. Am J Dis Child 120:543, 1970.

Wilkinson JH: Serum enzymes. CRC Crit Rev Clin Lab Sci 1:599, 1970.

TESTS FOR SALICYLISM & OTHER INTOXICATIONS

Toxicologic analyses should be carried out in a specialized laboratory. There are, however, a number of procedures in the diagnosis of common childhood ingestions which should be available in all clinical chemistry laboratories.

Serum Salicylate

A. Specimen: 0.1 ml serum.

B. Normal Values: Therapeutic levels should be less than 30 mg/dl.

C. Interpretation: The estimation of plasma salicylates is no longer required to control therapy in rheumatic fever. It is, however, of great importance in the management and diagnosis of salicylism. The prognosis appears to be related to the initial salicylate load. In judging both appropriate treatment and prognosis, a single salicylate level must be related to time since ingestion. Done has suggested a formula—$\log S_0 = \log S + 0.015T$—for calculation of the theoretical extrapolated zero-time salicylate level, S_0. This is based on measurements of salicylate half-life in serum and is derived from the serum salicylate level (S) and the time (T) in hours since ingestion. Figures for S_0 of 50 or less indicate no intoxication; 50–80, mild; 80–100, moderate; 100–160, severe; and greater than 160, usually fatal. Because of delayed absorption, levels in the first 6 hours after ingestion may not be maximal.

The conventional treatment of salicylism involves only the restoration of normal acid-base balance. In some instances, the additional use of acetazolamide may be justified. In severe toxicity, a slow exchange transfusion or peritoneal dialysis is an effective means of rapidly lowering tissue salicylate levels. Ready-made commercial solutions for dialysis are available (Peridal, Impesol). However, it has been shown that for peritoneal dialysis to be really effective the dialysate must contain albumin. A solution should therefore be made to contain 140 mEq Na$^+$/liter, 4 mEq K$^+$/liter, 4 mEq Ca^{++}/liter, 1.5 mEq Mg^{++}/liter, 103 mEq Cl$^-$/liter, 45 mEq lactate/liter, and 15 gm glucose/liter in 5% salt-free human albumin.

From a laboratory viewpoint, particular care should be taken in the choice of method for serum salicylate determination. Until recently, the methods based on the reaction of ferric nitrate with salicylate have been adequate. However, with the increasing availability of salicyl conjugates such as salicylamide, which are not estimated by ferric nitrate methods, these procedures should now be abandoned in favor of a method such as the fluorometric procedure which involves a hydrolysis step.

Done AK: Salicylate intoxication. Pediatrics 26:800, 1960.

Barbiturates

A. Specimen: 1 ml heparinized whole blood.

B. Normal Values: Therapeutic values of pentobarbital and secobarbital are 0.2–0.3 mg/dl; of phenobarbital (continuous treatment), 1–3 mg/dl. Lethal levels are in the region of 10 times the therapeutic values.

Glutethimide

A. Specimen: 1 ml heparinized whole blood.

B. Interpretation: Therapeutic levels are in the region of 0.5 mg/dl. Levels greater than 2 mg/dl are usually toxic, and levels above 6 mg/dl lethal.

Huttenlocher PR: Accidental glutethimide intoxication in children. N Engl J Med 269:38, 1968.

Urine Screening Tests*

A. Salicylate: Add 1–2 drops of 5% ferric chloride to 0.5 ml of urine. A violet color results if salicylates or phenothiazines are present. The color caused by salicylates is eliminated by the addition of 50% sulfuric acid, whereas that due to phenothiazines will persist.

B. Phenothiazines: Mix 0.5 ml of FPN reagent with 0.5 ml of urine. The development of a pink to violet color within 1 minute indicates the presence of phenothiazines. (FPN reagent is prepared by mixing 5 parts 5% ferric chloride, 45 parts 20% perchloric acid, and 50 parts 50% nitric acid.)

C. Imipramines: Mix 0.5 ml of Forrest reagent with 0.5 ml urine. Imipramine and desipramine cause a green color. (Forrest reagent is prepared by mixing 25 parts 0.2% potassium dichromate, 25 parts 30% sulfuric acid, 25 parts 20% perchloric acid, and 25 parts 50% nitric acid.)

D. Halogenated Hydrocarbons: Heat 1 ml of urine with 1 ml of 20% sodium hydroxide and 1 ml of pyridine at 100°C for 1 minute. A red color in the pyridine

layer is indicative of the presence of halogenated hydrocarbons. A negative control is essential.

E. *p*-Aminophenol: To 2 ml of urine add 2–3 drops of diluted hydrochloric acid, cool in ice, and add 2–3 drops each of 1% sodium hydroxide and alkaline *a*-naphthol. A red color results if phenacetin or N-acetyl-*p*-aminophenol metabolites are present.

THERAPEUTIC LEVELS OF ANTICONVULSANTS, ANTIBIOTICS, & OTHER DRUGS

Serum Theophylline

A. Specimen: 0.1 ml serum.

B. Safe Therapeutic Values: 10–20 μg/ml.

C. Interpretation: Theophylline plays an important role in the management of bronchial asthma. Optimal therapeutic serum concentrations of theophylline range from 10–20 μg/ml. Values greater than 20 μg/ml are often associated with signs of toxicity. Seizures, which are often intractable and potentially lethal, usually occur with serum concentrations higher then 40 μg/ml, though toxic symptoms are not universal even at this level.

Piafsky KM, Ogilvie RI: Dosage of theophylline in bronchial asthma. N Engl J Med 292:1218, 1975.

Weinberger MM, Bronsky EA: Evaluation of bronchodilator therapy in asthmatic children. J Pediatr 84:421, 1974.

Zwiech CW & others: Theophylline-induced seizures in adults. Ann Intern Med 82:784, 1975.

Blood Chloramphenicol

A. Specimen: 0.5 ml heparinized whole blood.

B. Safe Therapeutic Values: 12–22 μg/ml.

C. Interpretation: In the newborn, treatment with chloramphenicol is accompanied by the risk of shock and death ("gray baby syndrome") unless the blood levels of unconjugated drug are carefully monitored. Dosage should be controlled so that blood levels are not allowed to exceed 25 μg/ml. After the neonatal period, it is important to monitor blood levels to guard against bone marrow suppression.

Blood for chloramphenicol determination can be drawn at any time since there is relatively little variation in the blood level after the first 24 hours of therapy.

Serum or Plasma Sulfonamide

A. Specimen: 0.1 ml serum or plasma.

B. Safe Therapeutic Values: 1–10 mg/dl.

C. Interpretation: Blood sulfonamide levels are required only rarely in the control of therapy. Occasionally, however, this determination may be of value in differential diagnosis in a cyanotic infant with sulfhemoglobinemia or methemoglobinemia resulting from

---

Note: All of these tests are screening procedures and are subject to a variety of interferences. It is essential that the results of positive tests should be confirmed by more specific analysis.

sulfonamide intoxication. During therapy, blood should be drawn immediately before an oral or intravenous dose in order to make certain that a therapeutic level is being maintained.

Serum Phenytoin

A. **Specimen:** 2 ml serum or heparinized plasma.

B. **Safe Therapeutic Values:** 1.3—1.7 mg/dl.

C. **Interpretation:** Most patients whose seizures respond to the use of phenytoin show a correlation between seizure control and plasma level. Levels below 1 mg/dl usually provide poor seizure control. Manifestations of toxicity occur with blood levels greater than 2 mg/dl but can occur at lower blood levels, particularly in situations in which there is alteration of the degree of protein binding of the drug, eg, uremia. Serious impairment of consciousness occurs at blood levels greater than 3 mg/dl.

Letten J & others: Diphenylhydantoin metabolism in uremia. N Engl J Med 285:648, 1971.

Serum or Plasma Phenobarbital

A. **Specimen:** 1 ml serum or heparinized plasma.

B. **Safe Therapeutic Values:** 1.5—3 mg/dl.

C. **Interpretation:** In children with febrile convulsions, the required therapeutic level is over 1.5 mg/dl. A similar blood level is required for the control of grand mal seizures. Toxic symptoms are rare in persons who have been on the drug for some time since tolerance to the sedative effect of the drug develops rapidly. When these toxic symptoms are seen, the serum concentration is higher than 3 mg/dl. Hypersensitivity reactions requiring withdrawal of therapy occur rarely and are not related to the blood level.

Lennox-Buchthal MA: Febrile convulsions: A reappraisal. Electroenceph Clin Neurophysiol 32(Suppl):1—138, 1973.

Table 38—2. Normal and therapeutic values.

Acid-Base Measurements   (Whole Blood)
pH: 7.38—7.42 as of 14 minutes of age.
Pa_{O_2}: 65—76 mm Hg.
Pa_{CO_2}: 36—38 mm Hg.
Base excess: −2 to +2 mEq/liter, except in newborns (range, −4 to −0).

Acid Maltase   (Liver)
> 0.7 μmol/minute/gm wet tissue.

Acid Phosphatase   (Serum, Plasma)
Newborn: 7.4—19.4 IU/liter.
2—13 years: 6.4—15.2 IU/liter.
Adults: Males, 0.5—11 IU/liter; females, 0.2—9.5 IU/liter.

Albumin: See Proteins in Serum, below.

Aldolase
Newborns: 17.5—47.8 IU/liter at 37° C.
Children: 8.8—23.9 IU/liter at 37° C.
Adults: 4.4—12 IU/liters at 37° C.

Alkaline Phosphatase
Values in IU/liter at 37° C. Using p-nitrophenyl phosphate buffered with AMP (kinetic).

Age	Female	Male
Newborn (1—3 days)	95—368	95—368
2—24 months	115—460	115—460
2—5 years	115—391	115—391
6—7 years	115—460	115—460
8—9 years	115—345	115—345
10—11 years	115—437	115—336
12—13 years	92—336	127—403
14—15 years	78—212	79—446
16—18 years	35—124	58—331
Adults	39—118	41—137

Alkaline Phosphatase, Heat-Labile   (Serum, Plasma)
Up to 35% of total units heat-labile. Bone phosphatase is heat-labile.

Amino Acids: (Plasma, Urine)
See Table 38—1.

δ-Aminolevulinic Acid: See Porphyrins in Urine, below.

δ-Aminolevulinic Acid Dehydratase   (Whole Blood)
μg blood lead < 30 μg/dl: 10—54 units/ml red cells.

Amino Nitrogen   (Urine)
Older children: 129 μmol/kg/24 hours (range, 66—204 μmol/kg/24 hours).
Full-term newborns: About 3 times as high.
Values are higher in breast-fed than in cow's milk-fed babies.
Premature infants: Values are, on the average, 6 times as high.

Aminophylline   (Serum, Plasma)
10—20 μg/ml; great patient variability seen within the therapeutic range.

Ammonia   (Plasma, Urine)
Blood: 90—150 μg/dl in newborn; higher in premature and jaundiced infants; 0—60 μg/dl thereafter when drawn with proper precautions.
Urine: 2—11.5 months, 4.2—19.9 μEq/minute/sq m; 13 months to 16 years, 5.9—16.5 μEq/minute/sq m.

Amylase   (Serum, Plasma)
6—33 Close-Street units/dl.

Amylo-1,6-Glucosidase   (Liver)
Debrancher: > 1 μmol/minute/gm wet tissue.

a_1 Antitrypsin   (Serum, Plasma)
210—500 mg/dl.

Arsenic   (Urine)
< 50 μg/24 hours when collected into an acid-washed container.

Table 38—2 (cont'd). Normal and therapeutic values.

Ascorbic Acid (Plasma, Urine)
Plasma: 0.5–1 mg/dl.
Urine: > 5% of an oral 20 mg/kg loading dose/24 hours;
< 1% in scurvy.

Barbiturates (Serum, Plasma)
Phenobarbital: 1.5–3 mg/dl.

Bicarbonate or Total CO₂ (Serum, Plasma)
Total: 18–23 mmol/liter plasma.

Bilirubin (Serum, Plasma)
Peak bilirubin levels during newborn period.

Birth Weight	< 2001 g	2001–2500 g	> 2500 g
Number of Babies	379	1428	18,400

Total Bilirubin (mg/dl)	(Percent of Babies Exceeding This Level)		
> 20.0	8.2	2.6	0.8
> 18.0	13.5	4.6	1.5
> 16.0	20.3	7.6	2.6
> 14.0	33.0	12.0	4.4
> 11.0	53.8	23.0	9.3
> 8.0	77.0	45.4	26.1

After 1 month:
Conjugated: 0–0.3 mg/dl
Unconjugated: 0.1–0.7 mg/dl

Blood Volume
Prematures, 98 ml/kg; at 1 year, 86 (69–112) ml/kg; older children, 70 (51–86) ml/kg.

Bromsulphalein Test (Serum, Plasma)
Newborn infants in respiratory distress: Up to 30% retention.
Normal newborn infants: Up to 15%.
Thereafter: < 10% retention.

Calcium (Serum, Plasma)
4.4–5.3 mEq/liter.

Calcium (Urine)
4–8 mEq/24 hours during childhood (4–12 years).

Carbon Dioxide, Total (Serum, Plasma)
18–23 mmol/liter.

Carboxyhemoglobin
< 5% of total hemoglobin.

Carotene (Serum, Plasma)
At birth: About 70 μg/dl, rising to about 340 μg/dl at age 1.
At age 3½: About 150 μg/dl.
Thereafter: 100–150 μg/dl.

Ceruloplasmin (Serum, Plasma)
0.25–0.49 absorbance units in 1 cm path cells = 21–43 mg/dl.

Chloramphenicol (Whole Blood)
Therapeutic levels are 12–22 μg/ml. Levels in excess of 25 μg/ml may be dangerous in the newborn.

Chloride
Serum, plasma: 97–104 mEq/liter.
Breast milk: 11 (2.5–30) mEq/liter.
Cow's milk: 37 (20–80) mEq/liter.
Muscle: 20–26 mEq/kg wet fat-free tissue.
Spinal fluid: 120–128 mEq/liter.
Sweat: 96% of children, up to 30 mEq/liter; in the remainder, up to 50 mEq/liter. (Adults: Up to 70 mEq/liter.)

Cholesterol (Serum, Plasma)
Premature cord blood: 67 (47–98) mg/dl.
Full-term cord blood: 67 (45–98) mg/dl.
Full-term newborn: 85 (45–167) mg/dl.
3 days–1 year: 130 (69–174) mg/dl.
2–14 years: 188 (138–242) mg/dl.

Cholinesterase (Serum or Red Cells)
2.5–5 μmol/minute/ml serum (pseudocholinesterase).
2.3–4 μmol/minute/ml red cells.

Chymotrypsin
245–275 μg/ml intestinal juice.

Copper (Serum, Plasma)
Up to 6 months: < 70 μg/dl.
6 months–5 years: 27–153 μg/dl.
5–17 years: 94–234 μg/dl.
Adults: 70–118 μg/dl.

Copper (Urine)
Up to 30 μg/24 hours.

Copper (Liver)
< 20 μg/gm wet tissue.

Copper Oxidase (Serum, Plasma)
Same as Ceruloplasmin, above.

Cortisol (Serum, Plasma)
7:00–9:00 a.m.: 15–20 μg/dl.
2:00 p.m.: 10.5 ± 4.3 μg/dl.

Creatine (Serum, Plasma)
0.2–0.8 mg/dl.

Creatine (Urine)
18–58 mg/liter.

Creatine Kinase (Serum, Plasma)
Adult males: 30–210 IU/liter at 37° C.
Adult females: 20–128 IU/liter at 37° C.
Newborns (1–3 days): 40–474 IU/liter at 37° C.

Creatinine (Serum, Plasma)
Values in mg/dl.

Age	Female	Male
1 year	0.2–0.5	0.2–0.6
2–3 years	0.3–0.6	0.2–0.7
4–7 years	0.2–0.7	0.2–0.8
8–10 years	0.3–0.8	0.3–0.9
11–12 years	0.3–0.9	0.3–1.0
13–17 years	0.3–1.1	0.3–1.2
18–20 years	0.3–1.1	0.5–1.3

Table 38—2 (cont'd). Normal and therapeutic values.

Creatinine Clearance
(ml/minute/1.73 sq m) = 0.43 × Ht in cm ÷ plasma creatinine in ml/dl.

Digoxin (Serum, Plasma)
Children: 1.5—2.5 mg/ml.
Adults: 1—1.5 mg/ml.

2,3-Diphosphoglycerate (Whole Blood)
4.5—6 mmol/liter; normals vary with the method employed and with the altitude at which the patient resides.

Epinephrine (Urine)
0.2 (0.02—0.7) μg/kg/24 hours.

Erythrocyte Protoporphyrin, Free (Red Cells)
< μg FEP/gm hemoglobin

Erythrocyte Sedimentation (Citrated Whole Blood)
Rate, Micro
Up to 2 years: 1—5 mm/hour.
2 years to adulthood: 1—8 mm/hour.

Fats (Fecal)
< 5 gm/24 hours.

Fatty Acids, "Free" (Plasma)
Newborn: 905 ± 470 μEq/liter.
4 months—10 years: 699 ± 199 μEq/liter (14-hour fast); 966 ± 235 μEq/liter (19-hour fast).
Adults: 448 ± 140 μEq/liter (14-hour fast); 560 ± 157 μEq/liter (19-hour fast).

Fatty Acids, Total Esterified (Fasting)

	mg/dl (± 2 SD)	Percent of Total (± 2 SD)
Plasma		
16:0	42.6 ± 13	24.5 ± 4
16:1	4.1 ± 3	2.3 ± 1
18:0	19.9 ± 9	11.5 ± 5
18:1	36.5 ± 15	20.7 ± 4
18:2	51.5 ± 27	29.3 ± 10
20:3	4.0	2.3
20:4	16.2 ± 11	9.4 ± 6
Erythrocytes		
16:0	36.9 ± 12	23.4 ± 5
16:1	3.4	1.9
18:0	30.4 ± 17	19.8 ± 7
18:1	29.2 ± 18	18.0 ± 5
18:2	24.3 ± 24	14.1 ± 8
20:3	4.2 ± 3	2.6 ± 2
20:4	30.2 ± 16	19.4 ± 7

Ferritin (Serum)
7—140 μg/ml from 6 months to 15 years.

Fibrinogen (Plasma)
200—500 mg/dl.

Folic Acid
Serum: > 6 ng/ml.
Red cells: > 160 ng/ml.

Follicle-Stimulating Hormone (Urine)
(Pituitary Gonadotropins)
6—50 mouse uterine units/24 hours.

Galactose (Serum, Plasma)
Up to 20 mg/dl.

Galactose (Urine)
Up to 15 mg/dl on a milk diet.

Galactose-1-Phosphate (Heparinized Red Cells)
< 1 mg galactose-1-phosphate/dl packed erythrocyte lysate; slightly higher in cord blood.
Congenital galactosemic on a milk-free diet: < 2 mg/dl.
Congenital galactosemic taking milk: 9—20 mg/dl.

Galactose-1-Phosphate (Heparinized Red Cells)
Uridyl Transferase
Normal: 308—475 ImU/gm hemoglobin.
Heterozygous for Duarte variant: 225—308 ImU/gm hemoglobin.
Homozygous for Duarte variant: 142—225 ImU/gm hemoglobin.
Heterozygous for congenital galactosemia: 142—225 ImU/gm hemoglobin.
Homozygous for congenital galactosemia: < 8 ImU/gm hemoglobin.

Gamma Glutamyl Transpeptidase (Serum, Plasma)
Adult males: 9—69 IU/liter at 37° C.
Adult females: 3—33 IU/liter at 37° C.
Newborns (1—3 days): 13—198 IU/liter at 37° C.

Gastrin (Serum)
Normal: Under 100 pg/ml.
Indeterminate: 100—150 pg/ml.
Elevated: Over 150 pg/ml.

Glomerular Filtration Rate
Older children and adults: 130 (75—165) ml/minute/1.73 sq m. (These levels are reached by about 6 months.)
Newborns: About 50% of the above values.

Glucose (Serum)
Newborn: 20—80 mg/dl.

Glucose (Fluoride Plasma or Serum)
60—105 mg/dl (fasting).

Glucose-6-Phosphatase (Liver)
> 5 μmol/minute/gm wet tissue.

Glucose-6-Phosphate Dehydrogenase (Red Cells)
150—215 units/dl.

Glucose Tolerance Test: See under Insulin.

Growth Hormone (Serum)
After infancy, 0—5 ng/ml (fasting specimen). In response to

Table 38–2 (cont'd). Normal and therapeutic values.

natural and artificial provocation (eg, sleep, arginine, insulin hypoglycemia), > 8 ng/ml. In the newborn period, fasting GH levels are high (15–40 ng/ml) and responses to provocation variable.

Haptoglobin (Serum)
50–150 mg hemoglobin bound/dl.

Hematocrit
Birth: 44–64%.
14–90 days: 35–49%.
6 months–1 year: 30–40%.
4–10 years: 31–43%.

Hemoglobin (Plasma)
No more than 3 mg/dl.
A_2 hemoglobin: 2–3.5% of total hemoglobin.
A_1 C hemoglobin: 5–8% of total hemoglobin.

Hemoglobin, Fetal (Whole Blood)
Birth: 50–85% of total hemoglobin.
1 year: < 15% of total.
Up to 2 years: Up to 5% of total.
Thereafter: < 2% of total.

Homovanillic Acid (Urine)
Children: 3–16 µg/mg urine creatinine.
Adults: 2–4 µg/mg urine creatinine.

Human-Specific Thyroid Stimulator (Serum)
None detectable.

17-Hydroxycorticosteroids (Serum)
After 2 weeks: 10–15 µg/dl.

17-Hydroxycorticosteroids (Urine)
0–2 years: 2–4 mg/24 hours.
2–6 years: 3–6 mg/24 hours.
6–10 years: 6–8 mg/24 hours.
10–14 years: 8–10 mg/24 hours.

5-Hydroxyindoleacetic Acid (Urine)
0.35 (0.11–0.61) µmol/kg/7 hours. (Based on 15 well nourished, apparently healthy mentally defective children on a tryptophan load.)

Hydroxyproline, Total (Urine)
5–14 years: 38–126 mg/24 hours.

Immunoglobulins (Serum)
See Table 15–3.

Immunoglobulins (CSF)
Children: Up to 9% of total protein.
Adults: Up to 14% of total protein.

Insulin (Serum)
Normals based on 13 normal children given a 1.75 gm/kg oral glucose dose after 2 weeks on a high-carbohydrate diet.

Time	Glucose (mg/dl)	Insulin (µU/ml)	Phosphorus (mg/dl)
Fasting	56–96	5–40	3.2–4.9
30 min	91–185	36–110	2–4.4
60 min	66–164	22–124	1.8–3.6
90 min	68–148	17–105	1.6–3.6
2 hours	66–122	6–84	1.8–4.2
3 hours	47–99	2–46	2–4.6
4 hours	61–93	3–32	2.7–4.3
5 hours	63–86	5–37	2.9–4.4

Inulin Clearance
< 1 month: 50 (29–88) ml/minute/1.73 sq m.
1–6 months: 78 (40–112) ml/minute/1.73 sq m.
6–12 months: 106 (62–121) ml/minute/1.73 sq m.
> 1 year: 130 (78–164) ml/minute/1.73 sq m.

[131]I-Labeled Triolein Absorption Test
> 8% of ingested dose in total blood volume 4–6 hours after ingestion.

Iron (Serum, Plasma)
87–279 µg/dl by atomic absorption.
110–270 µg/dl at birth, falling in first 4–6 months, then rising to 59–175 µg/dl by 3 years by Fischer-Price.

Iron-Binding Capacity (Serum, Plasma)
250–400 µg/dl.

17-Ketogenic Steroids (Urine)
0–1 year: < 1 mg/day.
1–10 years: 1 mg/year of age/day.

Ketones (Serum)
Trace amounts of acetone may be found in normal serum. Levels are usually above 50 mg/dl in diabetic ketoacidosis.

17-Ketosteroids (Urine)
(Values in mg/24 hours.)
0–14 days: 0.5–2.5.
2 weeks–2 years: 0–0.5.
2–6 years: 0–2.
6–8 years: 0–2.5.
8–10 years: 0.7–4.

	Boys	Girls
10–12 years:	0.7–6	0.7–5
12–14 years:	1.3–10	1.3–8.5
14–16 years:	2.5–13	2.5–11

Lactate (Whole Blood)
1–1.8 mmol/liter after an overnight fast when drawn with special precautions.

Lactate Dehydrogenase (Serum, Plasma)
Adult males: 70–178 IU/liter at 37° C.
Adult females: 42–166 IU/liter at 37° C.
Newborns (1–3 days): 40–348 IU/liter at 37° C.
All children: 17–59 IU/liter at 37° C. (CSF)

Table 38–2 (cont'd). Normal and therapeutic values.

Lactate Dehydrogenase Isoenzymes
LDH$_1$ (heart): 24–34%.
LDH$_2$ (heart, red cells): 35–45%.
LDH$_3$ (muscle): 15–25%.
LDH$_4$ (liver [trace] , muscle): 4–10%.
LDH$_5$ (liver, muscle): 1–9%.

LATS   (Serum)
None detectable.

Lead   (Whole Blood)
< 50 μg/dl whole blood.

Leucine Aminopeptidase   (Serum, Plasma)
Newborn: 29–59 IU/liter.
1 month–adult: 15–50 IU/liter.

Lipase
Serum: 20–136 IU/liter based on 4-hour incubation.
Duodenal juice: 8000–35,000 IU/liter.

Lipoproteins   (EDTA Plasma)
Newborn:
    Alpha: 134 ± 9 (71–176) mg/dl.
    Beta: 103 ± 7.2 (51–158) mg/dl.
    Omega: 77 ± 4.9 (48–106) mg/dl.
    Total lipid: 314 ± 14 (170–440) mg/dl.
3–10 days:
    Alpha: 194 ± 12 (116–266) mg/dl.
    Beta: 277 ± 4.5 (215–320) mg/dl.
    Omega: 138 ± 7.4 (84–190) mg/dl.
    Total lipid: 608 ± 30 (430–760) mg/dl.
10 days–1 year:
    Alpha: 169 (67–281) mg/dl.
    Beta: 290 (122–450) mg/dl.
    Omega: 124 (51–247) mg/dl.
    Total lipid: 606 (240–800) mg/dl.
2–14 years:
    Alpha: 251· ± 9.7 (147–327) mg/dl.
    Beta: 412 ± 16 (225–541) mg/dl.
    Omega: 176 ± 90 (98–268) mg/dl.
    Total lipid: 838 ± 32 (490–1090) mg/dl.

Long-Acting Thyroid Stimulator   (Serum)
None detectable.

Magnesium   (Serum, Plasma, Red Cells)
Newborns: 1.5–2.3 mEq/liter.
Adults: 1.4–2 mEq/liter.
Red cells: 3.92–5.28 mEq/liter.

Mercury   (Urine)
< 50 μg/24 hours when collected in an acid-washed container.

Metanephrine   (Urine)
Children: 0.02–0.16 μg/mg urine creatinine.

Methemoglobin   (Whole [Oxalate-Fluoride] Blood)
0–0.3 gm/dl.

Milliosmols   (Serum, Plasma)
270–285 mOsm/liter plasma water.

Milliosmols   (Urine)
50–600 mOsm/liter in infancy.
50–1400 mOsm/liter in older children.

Mucopolysaccharides   (Urine)
Acid mucopolysaccharide screen should be negative. A positive screen after dialysis of the urine should be followed up with a thin-layer chromatogram for evaluation of the acid mucopolysaccharide excretion pattern.

Nonesterified Fatty Acids
See Fatty Acids, Free (above).

Norepinephrine   (Urine)
0.8 (0.4–1.6) μg/kg/24 hours.

Normetanephrine   (Urine)
Children: 0.05–0.6 μg/mg urine creatinine.

Osmotic Pressure   (Plasma)
270–285 mOsm/liter plasma water.

Osmotic Pressure   (Urine)
Infants: 50–600 mOsm/liter urine water.
Older children: 50–1400 mOsm/liter urine water.

Oxalates   (Urine)
0–50 mg/24 hours.

Oxygen Capacity of Blood
1.34 ml/gm hemoglobin.

Oxygen Saturation of Venous Blood
Newborn: 30–80%.
Thereafter: 65–85%.

Packed Cell Volume
Birth: 44–64%.
14–90 days: 35–49%.
6 months–1 year: 30–40%.
4–10 years: 31–43%.

PaCO$_2$ (Whole Blood)
40 mm Hg (at sea level).
36–38 mm Hg (Denver).

PaO$_2$ (Whole Blood)
65–70 mm Hg.

pH   (Whole Blood)
7.38–7.42 at 37° C.

Phenobarbital   (Serum, Plasma)
1.5–3 mg/dl.

Phenylalanine   (Serum, Plasma)
0.7–3.5 mg/dl.

Phenytoin   (Serum, Plasma)
1–2 mg/dl.

Phosphatase
See Acid Phosphatase and Alkaline Phosphatase, above.

Table 38—2 (cont'd). Normal and therapeutic values.

Phospholipid (Serum)
Cord blood: 48—160 mg/dl.
2—13 years: 166—247 mg/dl.
3—20 years: 193—338 mg/dl.

Phosphorus, Inorganic (Serum, Plasma)
Premature:
Birth: 5.6—8 mg/dl.
6—10 days: 6.1—11.7 mg/dl.
20—25 days: 6.6—9.4 mg/dl.
Full-term:
Birth: 5—7.8 mg/dl.
3 days: 5.8—9 mg/dl.
6—12 days: 4.9—8.9 mg/dl.
Children:
1 year: 3.8—6.2 mg/dl.
10 years: 3.6—5.6 mg/dl.
Adults:
3.1—5.1 mg/dl.

Phosphorus, Tubular Reabsorption:
78—97%.

Porphyrins (Urine)
δ-Aminolevulinic acid:
0—7 mg/24 hours.
Porphobilinogen:
0—2 mg/24 hours.
Coproporphyrin:
0—160 μg/24 hours.

Uroporphyrin:
0—26 μg/24 hours.

Porphyrins, Total (Plasma)
Adults: < 0.7 μg/dl. (Values for children are not available.)

Porphyrins (Red Cells)
Protoporphyrin (all ages): 15—100 μg/dl.
Coproporphyrin (all ages): 0.5—2 μg/dl.

Potassium
Plasma: 4.1—5.6 mEq/liter.
Cow's milk: 20—45 mEq/liter.
Breast milk: 17—17 mEq/liter.
Muscle: 160—180 mEq/kg fat-free tissue.
Red cells: 87.2—97.6 mEq/liter.

Pregnanetriol (Urine)
2 weeks—2 years: 0.02 (0—0.2) mg/24 hours.
2—16 years: 0.6 (0.3—1.1) mg/24 hours.

Procainamide (Pronestyl) (Serum, Plasma)
4—6 μg/dl.

Proline (Plasma, Serum)
37—74 μg/ml by colorimetric assay.

Proteins (Serum)
See accompanying chart.

Proteins in Serum*
(gm/dl)

	First Week		4 Months	12 Months		4 Years
	Premature	Full-Term	Premature	Premature	Full-Term	and Over
Total						
	5.29	5.97	5.76	6.47	6.41	6.79
	(4.32—7.63)	(4.65—7.41)	(4.74—6.17)	(5.8—7.12)	(6.08—6.72)	(6.15—8.1)
	SD 0.72	SD 0.8	SD 0.8	SD 0.47	SD 0.4	SD 0.43
Albumin						
	3.38	4.17	3.90	3.76	4.48	4.58
	(2.81—3.91)	(3.32—5.13)	(2.78—4.92)	(3.22—4.48)	(4.07—5.03)	(3.72—5.5)
	SD 0.35	SD 0.65	SD 0.53	SD 0.37	SD 0.28	SD 0.4
Alpha₁						
	0.21	0.17	0.23	0.35	0.22	0.22
	(0.13—0.47)	(0.12—0.32)	(0.05—0.45)	(0.19—0.46)	(0.15—0.35)	(0.12—0.3)
	SD 0.08	SD 0.04	SD 0.08	SD 0.09	SD 0.06	SD 0.06
Alpha₂						
	0.39	0.38	0.57	0.77	0.54	0.57
	(0.25—0.65)	(0.25—0.47)	(0.37—0.83)	(0.5—1.11)	(0.41—0.66)	(0.35—0.95)
	SD 0.12	SD 0.04	SD 0.13	SD 0.18	SD 0.13	SD 0.11
Beta						
	0.46	0.38	0.63	0.86	0.62	0.62
	(0.31—1.16)	(0.17—0.61)	(0.41—1.13)	(0.64—1.08)	(0.52—0.83)	(0.47—0.92)
	SD 0.07	SD 0.11	SD 0.14	SD 0.1	SD 0.12	SD 0.06
Gamma						
	0.85	0.87	0.43	0.72	0.55	0.81
	(0.48—1.56)	(0.4—1.41)	(0.12—0.67)	(0.33—1.2)	(0.45—9.66)	(0.53—1.2)
	SD 0.28	SD 0.26	SD 0.16	SD 0.22	SD 0.1	SD 0.24

*Values are for paper electrophoresis. Using cellulose acetate, mean albumin levels increase by 0.3 gm/dl and gamma globulin decreases by 0.2 gm/dl.

Table 38–2 (cont'd). Normal and therapeutic values.

Proteins (Spinal Fluid)
Total:
  Newborn: 40–120 mg/dl.
  1 month: 20–70 mg/dl.
  Thereafter: 15–40 mg/dl.
Gamma globulin:
  Children: Up to 9% of total.
  Adults: Up to 14% of total.

Pseudocholinesterase (Serum)
2.3–5 µmol/minute/ml serum.

Pyrophosphate (Serum)
40–80 µg/dl.

Pyrophosphate (Urine)
0.0042 × inorganic phosphorus/24 hours.

Pyruvate (Blood)
50.5–60.1 µmol/liter. (Resting adult males; arterial samples.)
56–112 µmol/liter. (Adult venous samples.)

Pyruvate Kinase (Red Cells)
7.3–14.7 units/gm hemoglobin.

Quinidine (Serum, Plasma)
2–4 mg/liter.

Serotonin (Serum, Plasma)
Children: 127–187 ng/ml.
Adults: 119–171 ng/ml.

Sodium
Serum: 136–143 mEq/liter.
Sweat: < 30 mEq/liter for 96% of all children; up to 60 mEq/liter for the remainder. (Adults: Up to 70 mEq/liter.)
Cow's milk: 22–26 mEq/liter.
Breast milk: 4.7–8.3 mEq/liter.
Muscle: 33–43 mEq/kg wet fat-free tissue.
Urine: 6–10 mEq/sq m, or 0.3–3.5 mEq/24 hours (infants); 5.6–17 mEq/24 hours (children and adults).

T₃ Uptake (Serum, Plasma)
45–60% resin uptake. (Note: Normal values may vary with method used. Decreased in hypothyroidism.)

T₄ Iodine (Serum, Plasma)
3.2–6.4 µg/dl by column chromatography.
7.3–12.3 in 10 full-term newborns 2–4 days old.
3.1–7 µg/dl by competitive protein binding assay.
6.1–19.1 µg/dl in 40 full-term newborns 2–4 days old.

T₄, "Free"
1–2.3 ng/dl.

Testosterone (Serum)
1–34 ng/dl in girls age 4–10.
20–80 ng/dl in boys age 4–10.

Theophylline (Serum, Plasma)
10–20 µg/ml, great patient variability seen within the therapeutic range.

Thyroid-Stimulating Hormone (Serum)
1–10 µIU/ml.

Transaminases (Serum)
[IU/liter at 37° C.]

	Adult Males	Adult Females	Newborns (1–3 days)
GOT	8–46	7–34	16–74
GPT	7–46	4–35	1–25

Triglycerides (Serum, Plasma)
Adult fasting: 74–172 mg/dl.

Trypsin
Duodenal juice: 160–180 µg activated trypsin/ml. Dilution of 1:12.5 or more digests gelatin.
Feces: Under age 1, dilution of feces of 1:100 or more digests gelatin.

TSH
1–10 µU/ml.

Tyrosine (Serum, Plasma)
Normal newborn: 0.2–4.8 mg/dl.
Adults: 0.6–1.6 mg/dl.

Urea Clearance
Premature: 3.5–17.3 ml/minute/1.73 sq m.
Newborn: 8.7–33 ml/minute/1.73 sq m.
2–12 months: 40–95 ml/minute/1.73 sq m.
2 years and over: > 52 ml/minute/1.73 sq m.

Urea Nitrogen (Serum, Plasma)
1–2 years: 5–15 mg/dl.
Therafter: 10–20 mg/dl.

Uric Acid (Serum, Plasma)
2–5.5 mg/dl.

Urobilinogen (Urine)
< 3 mg/24 hours.

Vanilmandelic Acid (VMA) (Urine)
Children: 31–135 µg/kg/24 hours, or 2–12 µg/mg urine creatinine.
Adults: 1–4 mg/24 hours, or 1.5–3 µg/mg urine creatinine.

Vitamin A (Serum, Plasma)
Rises from 40 µg/dl at birth to 70 µg/dl at age 1, then falls slowly to 40 µg/dl by age 2.

Vitamin B₁₂ (Serum, Plasma)
330–1025 pg/ml.

Vitamin C
Plasma: 0.5–1 mg/dl.
Urine: > 5% of an oral 20 mg/kg loading dose in 24 hours; < 1% in scurvy.

Vitamin E (Alpha-Tocopherol) (Serum, Plasma)
Should exceed 0.5 mg/dl.

Table 38—2 (cont'd). Normal and therapeutic values.

Xylose Absorption Test (Urine) (Mean 5-hour excretion expressed as percentage of ingested load.) Under 6 months: 11—30%. 6—12 months: 20—32%. 1—3 years: 20—42%. 3—10 years: 25—45%.	**Xylose Absorption Test (Cont'd)** Over 10 years: 25—50%. Or: % excretion K (0.2 × age in months) + 12. **Zinc** (Serum) 77—137 μg/dl by atomic absorption.

• • •

General References

Behrendt H: *Diagnostic Tests in Infants and Children,* 2nd ed. Lea & Febiger, 1962.

O'Brien D, Ibbott FA, Rodgerson DO: *Laboratory Manual of Pediatric Micro-biochemical Techniques,* 4th ed. Hoeber, 1968.

Table 38–3. Normal peripheral blood values at various ages.*

	1st day	2nd day	6th day	2 weeks	1 month	2 months	3 months	6 months	1 year	2 years	5 years	8–12 years	Adults	
													Males	Females
Red blood cells (millions/µl)	5.9 (4.1–7.5)	6 (4.0–7.3)	5.4 (3.9–6.8)	5 (4.5–5.5)	4.7 (4.2–5.2)	4.1 (3.6–4.6)	4 (3.5–4.5)	4.5 (4–5)	4.6 (4.1–5.1)	4.7 (4.2–5.2)	4.7 (4.2–5.2)	5 (4.5–5.4)	5.4 (4.6–6.2)	4.8 (4.2–5.4)
Hemoglobin (gm/dl)	19 (14–24)	19 (15–23)	18 (13–23)	16.5 (15–20)	14 (11–17)	12 (11–14)	11 (10–13)	11.5 (10.5–14.5)	12 (11–15)	13 (12–15)	13.5 (12.5–15)	14 (13–15.5)	16 (13–18)	14 (11–16)
White blood cells (per µl)	17,000 (8–38)		13,500 (6–17)	12,000 (5–16)	11,500 (5–15)	11,000 (5–15)	10,500 (5–15)	10,500 (5–15)	10,000 (5–15)	9,500 (5–14)	8,000 (5–13)	8,000 (5–12)	7,000 (5–10)	
PMNs† (%)	57	55	50	34	34	33	33	36	39	42	55	60	57–68	
Eosinophils (total) (per µl)	20–1000				150–1150		70–550	70–550					100–400	
Lymphocytes† (%)	20	20	37	55	56	56	57	55	53	49	36	31	25–33	
Monocytes† (%)	10	15	9	8	7	7	7	6	6	7	7	7	3–7	
Immature white cells (%)	10	5	0–1	0	0	0	0	0	0	0	0	0	0	
Platelets† (per µl)	350,000		325,000	300,000			260,000			260,000		260,000	260,000	
Nucleated red cells/ 100 white cells‡	0–10		0–0.3	0	0	0	0	0	0	0	0	0	0	
Reticulocytes (%)	3 (2–8)	3 (2–10)	1 (0.5–5)	0.4 (0–2)	0.2 (0–0.5)	0.5 (0.2–2)	2 (0.5–4)	0.8 (0.2–1.5)	1 (0.4–1.8)	1 (0.4–1.8)	1 (0.4–1.8)	1 (0.4–1.8)	1 (0.5–2)	
Mean diameter of red cells (µm)	8.6				8.1		5–7		7.4		7.4			7.5
MCV§ (fl)	85–125		89–101	94–102	90		80	78	78	80	80	82	82–92	
MCHC§ (%)	36		35	34				33		32	34	34	34	
MCH§ (pg)	35–40		36	31	30		27	26	25	26	27	28	27–31	
Hematocrit (%)	54±10		51	50	40		35	35	36	37	38	40	40–54	37–47

*Modified and reproduced, with permission, from Silver HK, Kempe CH, Bruyn HB: *Handbook of Pediatrics*, 12th ed. Lange, 1977.

†Usual or average values; considerable individual variation may occur.

‡Total nucleated red cells: first day, <1000/µl.

§MCV = mean corpuscular volume. MCHC = mean corpuscular hemoglobin concentration. MCH = mean corpuscular hemoglobin.

Index

METRIC SYSTEM PREFIXES
(Small Measurement)

In keeping with the decision of several scientific societies to employ a uniform system of metric nomenclature, the following prefixes have been used in this text:

k	kilo	10^3
c	centi	10^{-2}
m	milli	10^{-3}
μ	micro	10^{-6}
n	nano (formerly millimicro, mμ)	10^{-9}
p	pico (formerly micromicro, $\mu\mu$)	10^{-12}
f	femto	10^{-15}